TOPICAL TABLE OF CONTENTS

CLINICAL DISORDERS

MARCUS

Cardiac Imaging

A COMPANION TO BRAUNWALD's

HEART DISEASE

MARCUS Cardiac Imaging

SECOND EDITION

A COMPANION TO BRAUNWALD's HEART DISEASE

VOLUME 2

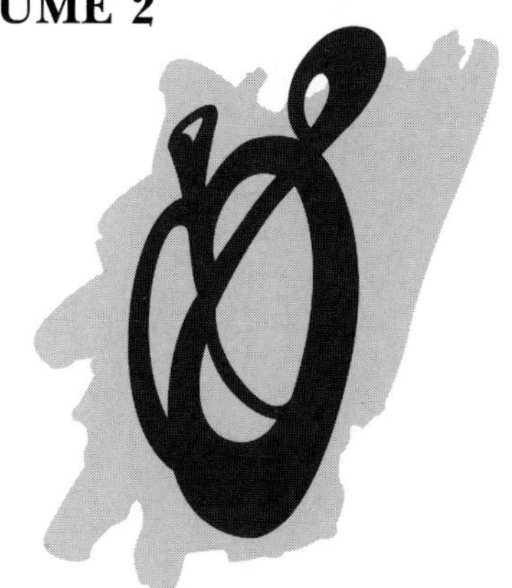

EDITOR IN CHIEF

DAVID J. SKORTON, M.D.
Professor of Medicine and Electrical and Computer Engineering
Co-Director, The University of Iowa Hospitals and Clinics Adolescent and Adult Congenital Heart Disease Clinic
Vice President for Research
The University of Iowa
Consulting Physician, Department of Veterans Affairs Medical Center
Iowa City, Iowa

ASSOCIATE EDITORS

HEINRICH R. SCHELBERT, M.D.
Professor of Pharmacology and Radiological Sciences
Vice Chair
Department of Molecular and Medical Pharmacology
UCLA School of Medicine
Principal Investigator, Laboratory of Structural Biology and Molecular Medicine
Medical Director, Nuclear Medicine Clinic
UCLA Medical Center
University of California at Los Angeles
Los Angeles, California

GERALD L. WOLF, Ph.D., M.D.
Professor of Radiology
Harvard Medical School
Director, Center for Imaging and Pharmaceutical Research
Massachusetts General Hospital
Boston, Massachusetts

BRUCE H. BRUNDAGE, M.D.
Professor of Medicine and Radiologic Sciences
UCLA School of Medicine
Chief, Division of Cardiology, Harbor-UCLA Medical Center
Scientific Director, Saint John's Cardiovascular Research Center
Torrance, California

CONSULTING EDITOR

EUGENE BRAUNWALD, M.D.
Hersey Professor of the Theory and Practice of Medicine
Harvard Medical School
Chairman, Department of Medicine
Brigham and Women's Hospital
Boston, Massachusetts

W.B. SAUNDERS COMPANY
A Division of Harcourt Brace & Company
PHILADELPHIA LONDON TORONTO
MONTREAL SYDNEY TOKYO

W.B. SAUNDERS COMPANY
A Division of Harcourt Brace & Company

The Curtis Center
Independence Square West
Philadelphia, Pennsylvania 19106

Library of Congress Cataloging-in-Publication Data

Marcus cardiac imaging: a companion to Braunwald's heart disease / David J. Skorton . . . [et al.]. — 2nd ed.

p. cm.

Rev. ed. of: Cardiac imaging / edited by Melvin L. Marcus . . . [et al.]. 1991.

Companion to: Heart disease / edited by Eugene Braunwald. 4th ed. ©1992.
Includes bibliographical references and index.

ISBN 0–7216–4687–5 (set)

1. Heart—Imaging. 2. Heart—Diseases—Diagnosis. I. Marcus, Melvin. II. Braunwald, Eugene. III. Heart Disease. [DNLM: 1. Diagnostic Imaging. 2. Heart Diseases—diagnosis. 3. Skorton, David J. WG 141 M322 1996]

RC683.5.I42C37 1996 616.1′20754—dc20

DNLM/DLC 95–19482

ISBN
Volume 1 0–7216–7127–6
Volume 2 0–7216–7128–4
Two-Volume Set 0–7216–4687–5

Marcus Cardiac Imaging:
A Companion to Braunwald's Heart Disease, Second Edition

Printed in the United States of America.

Last digit is the print number: 9 8 7 6 5 4 3 2 1

Dedications

In memory of my parents,
Pauline and Sam Skorton.

D.J.S.

To my wife, Barbara, my daughter, Kristina, and my son, Mark,
for their continued patience, support, and encouragement.

H.R.S.

To David, Darin, Alvera, Cindy, and Delia,
who supported my heart, especially in difficult times.

G.L.W.

To my wife, Rita,
for her constant, unselfish support and love,
without which none of this would have been possible.

B.H.B.

Contributors

NICOLE AEBISCHER, MD
Chef de clinique, Department of Cardiology, Centre Hôpitalier Universitaire Vaudois (CHUV), Lausanne, Switzerland
Echocardiographic Assessment of Ventricular Systolic Function

BENICO BARZILAI, M.D.
Associate Professor of Medicine, Washington University School of Medicine; Associate Physician, Barnes Hospital, St. Louis, Missouri
Ultrasonic Characterization of Cardiovascular Tissue

MALCOLM R. BELL, M.B.B.S.
Associate Professor of Medicine, and Consultant in Cardiovascular Diseases and Internal Medicine, Mayo Clinic and Foundation, Rochester, Minnesota
Measurement of Myocardial Perfusion Using Electron-Beam (Ultrafast) Computed Tomography

GEORGE A. BELLER, M.D.
Ruth C. Heede Professor of Cardiology and Professor of Internal Medicine, University of Virginia School of Medicine; Chief, Cardiovascular Division, Department of Internal Medicine, University of Virginia Health Sciences Center, Charlottesville, Virginia
Myocardial Imaging for the Assessment of Myocardial Viability

KEVIN S. BERBAUM, PH.D.
Adjunct Professor, Department of Radiology, University of Iowa, Iowa City, Iowa
Perceptual Aspects of Cardiac Imaging

DANIEL G. BLANCHARD, M.D.
Assistant Professor of Medicine, University of California, San Diego, School of Medicine; Director, Noninvasive Cardiac Laboratories, UCSD Medical Center, San Diego, California
Cardiac and Extracardiac Masses: Echocardiographic Evaluation

PAUL A. BOTTOMLEY, PH.D.
Russell H. Morgan Professor of Radiology, The Johns Hopkins University School of Medicine, Baltimore, Maryland
Cardiac Magnetic Resonance Spectroscopy: Principles and Applications

GARY M. BROCKINGTON, M.D.
Assistant Professor of Medicine, Tufts University School of Medicine, Boston; Director of Cardiac Pacing, Faulkner Hospital, Jamaica Plain, Massachusetts
Echocardiography in Pericardial Diseases

BRUCE H. BRUNDAGE, M.D.
Professor of Medicine and Radiological Sciences, UCLA School of Medicine; Chief, Division of Cardiology, Harbor-UCLA Medical Center; Scientific Director, Saint John's Cardiovascular Research Center, Torrance, California
Goals of Cardiac Imaging; Valvular Heart Disease; Myocarditis and Cardiomyopathy; Pericardial Disease; Diseases of the Great Vessels

RICHARD C. BRUNKEN, M.D.
Staff Physician, Department of Nuclear Medicine, The Cleveland Clinic Foundation, Cleveland, Ohio
Evaluation of Myocardial Substrate Metabolism in Ischemic Heart Disease

DENIS B. BUXTON, PH.D.
Associate Professor of Molecular and Medical Pharmacology, UCLA School of Medicine, Los Angeles, California
Principles of Myocardial Metabolism

EDWARD G. CAPE, PH.D.
Assistant Professor, University of Pittsburgh, Schools of Medicine and Engineering; Director, Cardiac Dynamics Laboratory, Division of Cardiology, Children's Hospital of Pittsburgh, Pittsburgh, Pennsylvania
Principles and Instrumentation for Doppler

MELVIN D. CHEITLIN, M.D.
Professor of Medicine, University of California, San Francisco; Chief of Cardiology Service, San Francisco General Hospital, San Francisco, California
The Chest Radiograph in the Adult Patient

MICHAEL P. CHWIALKOWSKI, Ph.D.
Professor, Department of Electrical Engineering, University of Texas, Arlington, Arlington, Texas
Quantitative Magnetic Resonance Imaging of the Heart

C. DAVID COOKE, M.S.E.E.
Assistant Professor of Radiology, Emory University School of Medicine, Atlanta, Georgia
Radionuclide Imaging: Principles and Instrumentation

JOHN MICHAEL CRILEY, M.D.
Professor of Medicine and Radiological Sciences, UCLA School of Medicine; Faculty, Division of Cardiology, Harbor-UCLA Medical Center, Torrance, California
Principles of Valvar Function

BIBIANA CUJEC, M.D.
Associate Professor of Medicine, University of Saskatchewan; Director, Echocardiography Laboratory Staff Cardiologist, Royal University Hospital, Saskatoon, Saskatchewan, Canada
Echocardiography in Pericardial Diseases

S. JAMES CULLOM, Ph.D.
Assistant Professor of Radiology, Emory University School of Medicine; Department of Mechanical Engineering, Georgia Institute of Technology; Associate Director, Nuclear Medicine Physics, Emory University Hospital, Atlanta, Georgia
Radionuclide Imaging: Principles and Instrumentation

JOHANNES CZERNIN, M.D.
Assistant Professor of Pharmacology and Medicine, Department of Molecular and Medical Pharmacology, UCLA School of Medicine, Los Angeles, California
Metabolic Imaging With Single-Photon Emitting Tracers

SETH T. DAHLBERG, M.D.
Assistant Professor, Departments of Nuclear Medicine and Medicine, University of Massachusetts Medical Center, Worcester, Massachusetts
Single-Photon Emitting Tracers for Imaging Myocardial Perfusion and Cell Membrane Integrity

ANTHONY N. DeMARIA, M.D.
Professor of Medicine, University of California at San Diego School of Medicine; Chief, Division of Cardiology, University of California at San Diego, San Diego, California
Cardiac and Extracardiac Masses: Echocardiographic Evaluation

LINDA L. DEMER, M.D., Ph.D.
Associate Professor of Medicine and Cardiology, UCLA School of Medicine; Chief, Division of Cardiology, UCLA Medical Center, Los Angeles, California
Evaluation of Myocardial Blood Flow in Cardiac Disease

ALBERT de ROOS, M.D.
Department of Diagnostic Radiology, University Hospital Leiden, Leiden, The Netherlands
Congenital Heart Disease Assessed With Magnetic Resonance Techniques

ROBERT R. EDELMAN, M.D.
Professor of Radiology, Harvard Medical School; Director of Magnetic Resonance, Beth Israel Hospital, Boston, Massachusetts
Magnetic Resonance Imaging Assessment of Ischemic Heart Disease

STEVEN R. FLEAGLE, B.S.E.E.
Technical Director, Cardiovascular Image Processing Laboratory, College of Medicine, The University of Iowa, Iowa City, Iowa
Quantitative Methods in Cardiac Imaging: An Introduction to Digital Image Processing

EDWARD D. FOLLAND, M.D.
Professor of Medicine, University of Massachusetts Medical School; Chief, Cardiology, and Director, Cardiac Catheterization Laboratory, Medical Center of Central Massachusetts, Worcester, Massachusetts
Echocardiographic Assessment of Ventricular Systolic Function

THOMAS L. FORCE, M.D.
Assistant Professor of Medicine, Harvard Medical School; Staff Cardiologist, Massachusetts General Hospital, Boston, Massachusetts
Echocardiographic Assessment of Ventricular Systolic Function

ELYSE FOSTER, M.D.
Associate Professor of Clinical Medicine and Anesthesia, and Associate Director, Adult Echocardiography Laboratory, University of California, San Francisco, California
Transesophageal Echocardiography

MICHAEL W. FRANK, M.D.
Instructor, Department of Surgery, Northwestern University Medical School, Chicago, Illinois
Principles of Myocardial Perfusion

E. A. FRANKEN, JR., M.D.
Professor of Radiology, University of Iowa, Iowa City, Iowa
Perceptual Aspects of Cardiac Imaging

JAMES R. GALT, PH.D.
Assistant Professor of Radiology, Emory University School of Medicine, Atlanta; Assistant Chief, Nuclear Medicine Service, Veterans Affairs Medical Center (Atlanta), Decatur, Georgia
Radionuclide Imaging: Principles and Instrumentation

ERNEST V. GARCIA, PH.D.
Professor of Radiology, Emory University School of Medicine; Director, Emory Center for Positron Emission Tomography (P.E.T.), Emory University Hospital, Atlanta, Georgia
Radionuclide Imaging: Principles and Instrumentation

EDWARD A. GEISER, M.D.
Professor of Medicine, Director, Echocardiography, and Associate Director, General Clinical Research Center, University of Florida, College of Medicine, Gainesville, Florida
Echocardiography: Physics and Instrumentation

EDWARD M. GELTMAN, M.D.
Professor of Medicine, Washington University; Director, Heart Failure–Transplant Program; Medical Director, Cardiac Diagnostic Laboratory, Barnes Hospital, St. Louis, Missouri
Assessment of Myocardial Perfusion and Metabolism in the Cardiomyopathies

RAYMOND J. GIBBONS, M.D.
Professor of Medicine, Mayo Medical School; Consultant, Cardiovascular Diseases, Mayo Clinic, Rochester, Minnesota
Equilibrium Radionuclide Angiography

STANTON A. GLANTZ, PH.D.
Professor of Medicine, University of California, San Francisco, San Francisco, California
Principles of Ventricular Function

ANTOINETTE S. GOMES, M.D.
Associate Professor of Radiology and Medicine, UCLA Medical Center, Los Angeles, California
Pulmonary Angiography

LEENA M. HAMBERG, PH.D.
Instructor in Radiology, Harvard Medical School; Medical Physicist, Massachusetts General Hospital, Boston, Massachusetts
Principles of Nuclear Magnetic Resonance Relaxation

SCOTT M. HANDLEY, PH.D.
Research Scientist, Washington University, St. Louis, Missouri
Ultrasonic Characterization of Cardiovascular Tissue

CHARLES B. HIGGINS, M.D.
Professor and Vice-Chairman, Radiology, School of Medicine, University of California, San Francisco, San Francisco, California
Contrast Agents for Cardiac Magnetic Resonance Imaging

JOHN W. HIRSHFELD, JR., M.D.
Professor of Medicine, University of Pennsylvania; Director, Cardiac Catheterization Laboratory, University of Pennsylvania Medical Center, Philadelphia, Pennsylvania
Radiographic Contrast Agents

MARK R. HOLLAND, PH.D.
Research Scientist, Washington University, St. Louis, Missouri
Ultrasonic Characterization of Cardiovascular Tissue

W. GREGORY HUNDLEY, M.D.
Cardiology Fellow, The University of Texas Southwestern Medical Center at Dallas, Parkland Hospital, Dallas, Texas
Quantitative Magnetic Resonance Imaging of the Heart

GEORGE J. HUNTER, M.D.
Assistant Professor of Radiology, Harvard Medical School; Assistant Radiologist, Massachusetts General Hospital, Boston, Massachusetts
Cardiomyopathies, Cardiac Masses, and Pericardial Disease: Value of Magnetic Resonance in Diagnosis and Management

TAREK S. HUSAYNI, M.D.
Director of Noninvasive Imaging, The Heart Institute for Children, Christ Hospital and Medical Center, Oak Lawn, Illinois
Ultrafast Computed Tomography Evaluation of Congenital Cardiovascular Disease in Children and Adults

GARY D. HUTCHINS, PH.D.
Associate Professor of Radiology, Indiana University School of Medicine, Indianapolis, Indiana
Imaging the Cardiac Autonomic Nervous System

JEFFREY M. ISNER, M.D.
Professor of Medicine and Pathology, Tufts University School of Medicine; Chief, Cardiovascular Research, St. Elizabeth's Medical Center, Boston, Massachusetts
Intravascular Ultrasound

LYNNE L. JOHNSON, M.D.
Professor of Medicine, Brown University School of Medicine; Director of Nuclear Cardiology, Rhode Island Hospital, Providence, Rhode Island
Imaging Acute Myocardial Necrosis (Monoclonal Antibodies and Technetium-99m Pyrophosphate)

MARYL R. JOHNSON, M.D.
Associate Professor of Medicine, Rush Medical College; Associate Medical Director, Rush Heart Failure and Cardiac Transplant Program, Rush-Presbyterian-St. Luke's Medical Center, Chicago, Illinois
Principles and Practice of Coronary Angiography

ALAN S. KATZ, M.D.
Assistant Professor of Medicine, Brown University School of Medicine; Director, Echocardiography Laboratory, The Miriam Hospital, Providence, Rhode Island
Echocardiographic Assessment of Ventricular Systolic Function

SANJIV KAUL, M.D.
Professor of Medicine, University of Virginia; Director, Cardiac Imaging Center, University of Virginia Medical Center, Charlottesville, Virginia
Myocardial Perfusion and Other Applications of Contrast Echocardiography

RICHARD E. KERBER, M.D.
Professor of Medicine, Department of Internal Medicine, University of Iowa Hospital and Clinics, Iowa City, Iowa
Echocardiography in Coronary Artery Disease; Myocardial Ischemia and Infarction

ALLAN L. KLEIN, M.D.
Associate Professor of Medicine, Health Science Center, Ohio State University, Columbus; Staff Cardiologist, Director of Cardiovascular Imaging Research, and Associate Director, Echocardiography Laboratory, The Cleveland Clinic Foundation, Cleveland, Ohio
Doppler-Echocardiographic Evaluation of Diastolic Function

FRANCIS J. KLOCKE, M.D.
Professor of Medicine and Director, Feinberg Cardiovascular Research Institute, Northwestern University School of Medicine, Chicago, Illinois
Principles of Myocardial Perfusion

ARTHUR J. LABOVITZ, M.D.
Professor of Medicine and Director of Echocardiography, St. Louis University School of Medicine, St. Louis, Missouri
Cardiomyopathies

JEFFREY A. LEPPO, M.D.
Professor of Medicine and Nuclear Medicine, and Clinical Director, Nuclear Medicine, University of Massachusetts Medical Center, Worcester, Massachusetts
Single-Photon Emitting Tracers for Imaging Myocardial Perfusion and Cell Membrane Integrity

NADJA M. LESKO, M.D.
Director of Radiology, Northern Hospital of Surrey County, Mt. Airy, North Carolina
Imaging of the Valves and Great Vessels

KERRY M. LINK, M.D.
Department of Radiology, Bowman Gray School of Medicine, Winston-Salem, North Carolina
Imaging of the Valves and Great Vessels

JAMSHID MADDAHI, M.D.
Professor of Molecular and Medical Pharmacology (Nuclear Medicine) and Radiological Sciences, University of California at Los Angeles School of Medicine, Los Angeles, California
Myocardial Perfusion Imaging for the Detection and Evaluation of Coronary Artery Disease

G. B. JOHN MANCINI, M.D.
Eric W. Hamber Professor, University of British Columbia; Head, Department of Medicine, Vancouver Hospital and Health Sciences Centre, Vancouver, British Columbia, Canada
Digital Angiography

WARREN J. MANNING, M.D.
Assistant Professor of Medicine and Radiology, Harvard Medical School; Associate Director, Non-Invasive Cardiac Imaging, and Co-Director, Cardiac MR Center, Beth Israel Hospital, Boston, Massachusetts
Magnetic Resonance Imaging Assessment of Ischemic Heart Disease

CYNTHIA H. McCOLLOUGH, Ph.D.
Assistant Professor of Radiologic Physics, Mayo Medical School; Consultant in Diagnostic Radiology, Mayo Clinic, Rochester, Minnesota
Ultrafast Computed Tomography: Principles and Instrumentation

PASCAL MERLET, M.D.
Head of Clinical Section, Service Hôpitalier Frédéric Joliot, Département de Recherche Médicale, Commissariat à l'Energie Atomique, Orsay, France
Positron Emission Tomography: Evaluation of Cardiac Receptors and Neuronal Function

JAMES G. MILLER, Ph.D.
Professor of Physics, Research Professor of Medicine, and Director, Laboratory for Ultrasonics, Washington University, St. Louis, Missouri
Ultrasonic Characterization of Cardiovascular Tissue

TODD D. MILLER, M.D.
Associate Professor of Medicine, Mayo Medical School; Consultant, Cardiovascular Diseases, Mayo Clinic, Rochester, Minnesota
Equilibrium Radionuclide Angiography

R. JOE NOBLE, M.D.
Clinical Professor of Medicine, Indiana University School of Medicine; Consultant in Cardiology, St. Vincent Hospital and Health Care Facility, Indianapolis, Indiana
A Clinician's Perspective: The Place of Imaging in Cardiac Diagnosis

LYLE J. OLSON, M.D.
Assistant Professor of Medicine, Mayo Medical School; Consultant, Division of Cardiovascular Diseases and Internal Medicine, Mayo Clinic and Mayo Foundation, Rochester, Minnesota
Valvular Heart Disease

NATESA G. PANDIAN, M.D.
Associate Professor of Medicine and Radiology, Tufts University School of Medicine; Director of Cardiovascular Imaging and Hemodynamic Laboratory, New England Medical Center, Boston, Massachusetts
Echocardiography in Pericardial Diseases

ELÉONORE PAQUET, M.D.
Associate Professor of Medicine, University of Montreal, Montreal Heart Institute, Montreal, Canada
Cardiomyopathies, Cardiac Masses, and Pericardial Disease: Value of Magnetic Resonance in Diagnosis and Management

ALFRED F. PARISI, M.D.
Professor of Medicine, Brown University School of Medicine; Chief of Cardiology, The Miriam Hospital, Providence, Rhode Island
Echocardiographic Assessment of Ventricular Systolic Function

ALAN S. PEARLMAN, M.D.
Professor of Medicine, University of Washington School of Medicine; Director, Echocardiography Laboratory, University of Washington Medical Center, President, American Society of Echocardiography, Seattle, Washington
Assessment of Systolic Function With Doppler Echocardiography

JULIO E. PÉREZ, M.D.
Professor of Medicine, Cardiovascular Division, Washington University School of Medicine; Director of Echocardiography and Physician, Barnes Hospital, St. Louis, Missouri
Ultrasonic Characterization of Cardiovascular Tissue

RONALD M. PESHOCK, M.D.
Professor, Radiology and Internal Medicine, University of Texas Southwestern Medical Center at Dallas, Southwestern Medical School, Dallas, Texas
Quantitative Magnetic Resonance Imaging of the Heart

STEVEN PORT, M.D.
Clinical Professor of Medicine, University of Wisconsin Medical School, Madison, Wisconsin
First-Pass Radionuclide Angiography

SIDNEY A. REBERGEN, M.D.
Department of Diagnostic Radiology, University Hospital Leiden, Leiden, The Netherlands
Congenital Heart Disease Assessed With Magnetic Resonance Techniques

STUART RICH, M.D.
Professor of Medicine, and Chief, Section of Cardiology, University of Illinois at Chicago Medical Center, Chicago, Illinois
Evaluation of Coronary Artery Disease by Electron-Beam Computed Tomography

RICHARD A. ROBB, PH.D.
Professor of Biophysics and of Computer Science, and Director, Biomedical Imaging Resource, Mayo Foundation and Clinic, Rochester, Minnesota
Ultrafast Computed Tomography: Principles and Instrumentation

JOHN A. RUMBERGER, PH.D., M.D.
Associate Professor of Medicine, and Consultant in Cardiovascular Diseases and Internal Medicine, Mayo Clinic and Foundation, Rochester, Minnesota
Measurement of Myocardial Perfusion Using Electron-Beam (Ultrafast) Computed Tomography

THOMAS RYAN, M.D.
Associate Professor of Medicine, and Director of Echocardiography, Duke University School of Medicine, Durham, North Carolina
Stress Echocardiography

MAYTHEM SAEED, D.V.M., PH.D.
Associate Professor of Radiology, University of California, San Francisco, School of Medicine, San Francisco, California
Contrast Agents for Cardiac Magnetic Resonance Imaging

COLLEEN SANDERS, M.D.
Associate Professor of Radiology, University of Alabama at Birmingham, Birmingham, Alabama
Role of Aortography in the Age of Imaging

DANY E. SAYAD, M.D.
Cardiology Fellow, University of Texas Southwestern Medical Center at Dallas, Parkland Memorial Hospital, Dallas, Texas
Quantitative Magnetic Resonance Imaging of the Heart

HEINRICH R. SCHELBERT, M.D., PH.D.
Professor of Pharmacology and Radiological Sciences, and Vice Chair, Department of Molecular and Medical Pharmacology, UCLA School of Medicine; Principal Investigator, Laboratory of Structural Biology and Molecular Medicine; Medical Director, Nuclear Medicine Clinic, UCLA Medical Center, University of California at Los Angeles, Los Angeles, California
Goals of Cardiac Imaging; Coronary Artery Disease; Metabolic Imaging With Single-Photon Emitting Tracers; Principles of Positron Emission Tomography; Evaluation of Myocardial Blood Flow in Cardiac Disease; Evaluation of Myocardial Substrate Metabolism in Ischemic Heart Disease; Appendix I: Radiation Dosimetry

NELSON B. SCHILLER, M.D.
Professor of Medicine, Radiology, Anesthesiology, and Director, Adult Echocardiography Laboratory, University of California, San Francisco, San Francisco, California
Transesophageal Echocardiography

HEIKO SCHÖDER, M.D., PH.D.
Postdoctoral Scholar, Department of Pharmacology, Division of Nuclear Medicine, UCLA School of Medicine, Los Angeles, California
Appendix I: Radiation Dosimetry

STEVEN L. SCHWARTZ, M.D.
Associate Professor of Medicine, Tufts University School of Medicine; Associate Director, Cardiovascular Imaging and Hemodynamic Laboratory, New England Medical Center, Boston, Massachusetts
Echocardiography in Pericardial Diseases

SATISH SHARMA, M.D.
Associate Professor of Medicine, Brown University School of Medicine; Chief of Cardiology, Veterans Administration Medical Center, Providence, Rhode Island
Echocardiographic Assessment of Ventricular Systolic Function

FLORENCE H. SHEEHAN, M.D.
Research Professor, Department of Medicine, Division of Cardiology, University of Washington, Seattle, Washington
Principles and Practice of Contrast Ventriculography; Applications of Contrast Ventriculography

DAVID J. SKORTON, M.D.
Professor of Medicine and Electrical and Computer Engineering, and Co-Director, The University of Iowa Hospitals and Clinics Adolescent and Adult Congenital Heart Disease Clinic, and Vice President for Research, The University of Iowa; Consulting Physician, Department of Veterans Affairs Medical Center, Iowa City, Iowa
Goals of Cardiac Imaging; Quantitative Methods in Cardiac Imaging: An Introduction to Digital Image Processing; Congenital Heart Disease; Cardiovascular Trauma; Ultrasonic Characterization of Cardiovascular Tissue

A. REBECCA SNIDER, M.D.
Pediatric Cardiologist, Baltimore, Maryland
Two-Dimensional and Doppler Echocardiography in the Evaluation of Congenital Heart Disease

HEINZ SOCHOR, M.D.
Professor of Cardiology, University of Vienna Medical School, Vienna, Austria
Metabolic Imaging With Single-Photon Emitting Tracers

STEVEN SOLOMON, PH.D.
Cardiovascular Research Institute, University of California, San Francisco, School of Medicine, San Francisco, California
Principles of Ventricular Function

KIRK T. SPENCER, M.D.
Assistant Professor of Medicine, University of Chicago, Chicago, Illinois
Echocardiography in Coronary Artery Disease: Myocardial Ischemia and Infarction

WILLIAM STANFORD, M.D.
Professor, Department of Radiology, College of Medicine, University of Iowa; Director, Cardiovascular Radiology, University of Iowa Hospitals and Clinics, Iowa City, Iowa
Evaluation of Cardiovascular Structure and Function With Electron-Beam Computed Tomography; The Great Vessels: Imaging by Electron-Beam Computed Tomography; Cardiac Masses and Pericardial Disease: Imaging by Electron-Beam Computed Tomography

WILLIAM J. STEWART, M.D.
Associate Professor of Medicine, Ohio State University; Director, Echocardiography Laboratory, and Co-Director, Cardiac Valve Management Center, Cleveland Clinic Foundation, Cleveland, Ohio
Intraoperative Echocardiography

JOHN R. STRATTON, M.D.
Professor of Medicine, Division of Cardiology, University of Washington; Staff Cardiologist, Seattle VA Medical Center, Seattle, Washington
Thrombosis Imaging With Indium-111–Labeled Platelets

ANDRÉ SYROTA, M.D., PH.D.
Professor of Biophysics and Nuclear Medicine, Université Paris Sud; Head of Service Hôpitalier Frédéric Joliot, Département de Recherche Médicale, Commissariat à l'Energie Atomique, Orsay, France
Positron Emission Tomography: Evaluation of Cardiac Receptors and Neuronal Function

DAVID M. SZCZESNIAK, M.D.
Resident, Mayo Clinic, Rochester, Minnesota
Imaging of the Valves and Great Vessels

DIETER SZOLAR, M.D.
Research Fellow, University of California, San Francisco, School of Medicine, San Francisco, California
Contrast Agents for Cardiac Magnetic Resonance Imaging

A. JAMIL TAJIK, M.D.
Chair, Division of Cardiovascular Diseases and Internal Medicine, Mayo Clinic and Foundation; Thomas J. Watson, Jr., Professor in Honor of Dr. Robert L. Frye, Mayo Medical School, Rochester, Minnesota
Valvular Heart Disease

JAMES D. THOMAS, M.D.
Professor of Medicine and Biomedical Engineering, The Ohio State University, Columbus; Director of Cardiovascular Imaging, Department of Cardiology, Cleveland Clinic Foundation, Cleveland, Ohio
Doppler-Echocardiographic Evaluation of Diastolic Function

BRAD H. THOMPSON, M.D.
Assistant Professor, Department of Radiology, University of Iowa College of Medicine, Iowa City, Iowa
The Great Vessels: Imaging by Electron-Beam Computed Tomography; Cardiac Masses and Pericardial Disease: Imaging by Electron-Beam Computed Tomography

BYRON F. VANDENBERG, M.D.
Associate Professor of Medicine, Department of Internal Medicine, The University of Iowa College of Medicine, Iowa City, Iowa
Ultrasonic Characterization of Cardiovascular Tissue

ERNST E. VAN DER WALL, M.D.
Department of Cardiology, University Hospital Leiden, Leiden, The Netherlands
Congenital Heart Disease Assessed With Magnetic Resonance Techniques

JOHN R. VOTAW, PH.D.
Assistant Professor of Radiology, Emory University, Atlanta, Georgia
Radionuclide Imaging: Principles and Instrumentation

ROBERT G. WEISS, M.D.
Associate Professor of Medicine and Radiology, Cardiology Division, The Johns Hopkins University School of Medicine; Attending Physician, The Johns Hopkins Hospital, Baltimore, Maryland
Cardiac Magnetic Resonance Spectroscopy: Principles and Applications

ROBERT M. WEISS, M.D.
Assistant Professor, Department of Internal Medicine, University of Iowa College of Medicine; Staff Cardiologist, University of Iowa Hospitals and Clinics and Department of Veterans Affairs Medical Center, Iowa City, Iowa
Evaluation of Cardiovascular Structure and Function With Electron-Beam Computed Tomography

ROBERT W. WEISSKOFF, PH.D.
Assistant Professor, Radiology, Harvard Medical School, Boston; Director of NMR Physics Research, Massachusetts General Hospital NMR Center, Charlestown, Massachusetts
Principles and Instrumentation for Cardiac Magnetic Resonance Imaging

MICHAEL F. WENDLAND, PH.D.
Associate Professor, University of California, San Francisco, School of Medicine, San Francisco, California
Contrast Agents for Cardiac Magnetic Resonance Imaging

JAMES S. WHITING, PH.D.
Adjunct Associate Professor, Department of Radiological Sciences, University of California, Los Angeles; Director, Department of Medical Physics and Imaging, Cedars-Sinai Medical Center, Los Angeles, California
Principles and Instrumentation for Radiography

DUWAYNE L. WILLETT, M.D.
Instructor of Internal Medicine, Division of Cardiology, The University of Texas Southwestern Medical Center at Dallas; Attending Physician, Cardiology, Zale Lipsky University Hospital and Parkland Hospital, Dallas, Texas
Quantitative Magnetic Resonance Imaging of the Heart

GERALD L. WOLF, PH.D., M.D.
Professor of Radiology, Harvard Medical School; Director, Center for Imaging and Pharmaceutical Research, Massachusetts General Hospital, Boston, Massachusetts
Goals of Cardiac Imaging; Principles of Nuclear Magnetic Resonance Relaxation

CHRISTOPHER J. WOLFKIEL, PH.D.
Research Assistant Professor of Medicine, and Director, Ultrafast CT Laboratory, University of Illinois at Chicago Medical Center, Chicago, Illinois
Evaluation of Coronary Artery Disease by Electron-Beam Computed Tomography

AJIT P. YOGANATHAN, PH.D.
Professor of Chemical, Mechanical and Bioengineering, Georgia Institute of Technology, Atlanta, Georgia
Principles and Instrumentation for Doppler

ELIAS A. ZERHOUNI, M.D.
Professor of Radiology and Biomedical Engineering, The Johns Hopkins University School of Medicine; Director, Thoracic Imaging and MRI, The Johns Hopkins Hospital, Baltimore, Maryland
Integrated Cardiac Magnetic Resonance Examination

DOUGLAS P. ZIPES, M.D.
Professor of Cardiology, Indiana University School of Medicine, Indianapolis, Indiana
Imaging the Cardiac Autonomic Nervous System

Foreword

The dramatic reductions in cardiovascular mortality and morbidity during the past three decades represent one of the major triumphs of twentieth-century medicine. Striking advances in three major areas are responsible—diagnosis, therapy, and prevention. The first of these, cardiac diagnosis, has improved almost entirely as a consequence of the spectacular developments in cardiac imaging. In the five years since the publication of the first edition of this book, the technologies available for cardiac imaging have progressed exponentially, and the contributions made by cardiac imaging to every aspect of cardiac care have expanded with unexpected rapidity.

As we approach the end of the century, it is clear that the public expectations of the medical profession are increasing. Patients, their families, and those who pay for medical care require first and foremost an accurate clinical assessment—not merely a diagnosis. In the case of patients with cardiac disease, both anatomic and functional evaluations are required, and clinicians now have a broad array of cardiac imaging techniques available to them for accomplishing these tasks. While this book presents the cardiologist, cardiovascular radiologist, and cardiovascular surgeon with the information required to use and interpret the entire gamut of contemporary imaging techniques, it goes much further by providing the understanding required to employ these complex and sometimes costly techniques intelligently. In an era of cost-conscious medicine, it is essential to select the appropriate technique without paying for unnecessary or redundant information. An entire new section of this edition, "Integrated Clinical Approach to Diagnosis Using Imaging Methods," guides clinicians to the specific technique required for addressing specific clinical issues.

This second edition is much more than a revision and an updating of an exemplary text. A new editor, Dr. Bruce H. Brundage, has joined the editorial group, and his influence on the second edition is clearly felt. Approximately one half of the chapters are new to this edition or were written by new authors, and both volumes are replete with spectacular new illustrations, which constitute the cornerstone of any work on imaging. The editors and authors of this book are not only technical experts but also experienced and thoughtful clinicians, and this combined expertise is interwoven throughout the text.

A number of excellent review articles, manuals, and texts are now available to aid physicians in the clinical applications of cardiac imaging. Rarely are such works also helpful in selecting the appropriate imaging technique for solving specific problems. In my estimation, none accomplishes these twin tasks with greater clarity, precision, and judgment than does the second edition of *Marcus Cardiac Imaging.* I am proud of its continued companionship to the new (fifth) edition of *Heart Disease: A Textbook of Cardiovascular Medicine.*

Eugene Braunwald, M.D.
Boston, Massachusetts

Preface

Imaging techniques continue to be immensely important in the management of patients with known or suspected cardiovascular disease. The widespread use of imaging technology in clinical diagnosis and the rapid development of new knowledge and methods in the research laboratory and at the bedside have dictated the need for an updated edition of this book. Virtually all modalities of cardiac imaging have experienced growth and development since the first edition of *Cardiac Imaging*. Echocardiographers have further embraced transesophageal echocardiography as an important method of assessing cardiac structure and function in the clinic, emergency room, and operating suite. The revised chapter on transesophageal echocardiography by Schiller and Foster is a lucid and comprehensive "textbook within a textbook" that will be useful to new and experienced echocardiographers alike. Intravascular ultrasound techniques are acquiring an increasingly important role and are discussed in a new chapter by Isner. All the other chapters in the echocardiography section have been updated and revised. Chapters on fast computed tomography have also been updated. In this section, the chapter by Rumberger and Bell is an extremely useful review of applicable principles of perfusion imaging. Radionuclide methods have focused to a greater extent on the assessment of myocardial viability, and this important area is discussed in a new chapter by Beller. Further experience with newer, technetium-based single-photon emitting radionuclides has necessitated extensive updating in Part 7. A new chapter by Dahlberg and Leppo discusses single-photon emitting tracers for assessing perfusion and cell membrane integrity. Also, imaging of myocardial neuronal activity with single-photon emitting tracers has further developed; the new chapter by Hutchins and Zipes provides a detailed account of this topic. Positron emission tomography (PET) continues to mature; the chapters on PET have been revised carefully. They emphasize new accomplishments and their clinical applications as well as the potential role of absolute myocardial blood flow measurements. The entire magnetic resonance imaging (MRI) section of the second edition has been extensively rewritten, including basic principles of relaxation, imaging, spectroscopy, contrast agents, and quantitation. A new chapter by Zerhouni summarizes the enormous amount of information that can be obtained in a 1-hour integrated cardiac MRI examination. The expanded MR glossary will be valuable for all students of this technology.

Although one thrust of the book continues to be sophisticated, *high-tech* imaging methods, we have attempted to further emphasize general issues that span different techniques and simpler methods. A new chapter by Cheitlin on the chest roentgenogram emphasizes the usefulness of this simple yet effective imaging method. An entirely new section, *The Integrated Clinical Approach to Diagnosis Using Imaging Methods,* is intended to help guide the busy clinician through the often bewildering maze of seemingly redundant diagnostic imaging choices. Finally, a new appendix has been added, detailing useful information on radiation dosimetry. In all, the book has undergone a major revision: Of the 73 chapters in this edition, 21 are by new authors, 14 are new chapters, and 1 appendix is new.

The features of the book that were popular in the first edition have been retained. The introductory section (Part 1) again features clear descriptions of the aspects of cardiovascular physiology relevant to imaging studies of cardiac function, perfusion, and metabolism as well as discussion of digital image processing and perceptual considerations in imaging. Each imaging modality is described comprehensively, from physics and instrumentation through clinical applications. Abundant use is made of figures, with full-color illustrations appearing in each volume. Finally, the reference lists have been updated to supply the reader with the latest information for further learning.

Dr. Eugene Braunwald continues to be an important force in the conceptualization and implementation of this project. We again gratefully acknowledge his inspiration and support during the preparation of this second edition of our text.

We also thankfully acknowledge Carolyn Frisbie, Catherine Dowty, Leah Voigt, Eileen Rosenfeld, and Diane Dalton for their efforts in organizational aspects of the project as well as manuscript preparation. We again were fortunate to work with Richard Zorab and his colleagues Nellie McGrew, Leslie E. Hoeltzel, Gina Scala, Mike Carcel, and others at W.B. Saunders Company; these consummate professionals guided us through the project with good humor and patience.

The second edition of the text is named *Marcus Cardiac Imaging* in acknowledgment and honor of the late Dr. Melvin L. Marcus, founding editor of the book. Mel Marcus' dedication to excellence in the principles and practice of cardiac imaging was an inspiration in the preparation of this second edition.

The text continues to target cardiologists, cardiology fellows, radiologists, nuclear medicine physicians, radiology trainees, cardiac surgeons, internists, and others who employ cardiac imaging methods with the ultimate goal of improvement in patient care.

David J. Skorton, M.D.
Bruce H. Brundage, M.D.
Heinrich R. Schelbert, M.D.
Gerald L. Wolf, Ph.D., M.D.

Contents

Volume 1

Color Plates 22 to 35 follow page 892.

PART

MAGNETIC RESONANCE IMAGING 5

CHAPTER

42 Principles of Nuclear Magnetic Resonance Relaxation

Leena M. Hamberg, Ph.D.
Gerald L. Wolf, Ph.D., M.D.

BASIC NUCLEAR MAGNETIC RESONANCE PHYSICS

In 1946, Bloch and Purcell, with their respective co-workers, independently demonstrated the phenomenon of nuclear magnetic resonance, or NMR.[1, 2] This discovery was quickly applied in physics and chemistry to study the structure of liquids and solids, but its application to anatomy and physiology awaited the development of a method of recording and converting NMR signals from a human subject into a readable image. In the early 1970s, Damadian, followed shortly by Lauterbur, developed such an imaging methodology based on the NMR characteristics of the hydrogen atom nucleus.[3, 4] The method usually depends on the presence of hydrogen, and so it is sometimes called proton imaging, but this technique has become known to the medical community at large as magnetic resonance imaging, or MRI.

Nuclear magnetic resonance is a quantum mechanical phenomenon, and, as such, it may be explained by using the language of quantum physics. However, for protons, which have a spin quantum number (I) of 1/2, the approach provided by classic mechanics is both valid and more readily understood. In this chapter, we use these two approaches interchangeably to translate the complex language of physics into intuitive scenes that help visualize the basic NMR events. A selection of basic texts covering a range of NMR topics, both simple and complex, is included in the bibliography for further reference.[5–11]

The proton in the nucleus of a hydrogen atom possesses angular momentum; it is said to have a "spin." Spin is quantized and characterized by a spin quantum number (I), which determines the number of orientations $(2 \times I + 1)$ that a nuclear magnetic moment can possess in a magnetic field. Therefore, for a proton, there exist two $(2 \times 1/2 + 1 = 2)$ different spin states that can be occupied. The permitted energy levels, in turn, are characterized by a magnetic quantum number whose values are determined by I according to the rule: $m_I = -I, -I + 1, \ldots, I - 1, I$. The possible values of m_I for a proton are 1/2 and $-1/2$. The nucleus of the hydrogen atom has a positive charge that is not located in the very center of the nucleus. Thus, when a proton rotates around its axis, the center of a positive charge revolves around a circular path and creates a magnetic field analogous to the field created by a current of electrons in a circular wire. This magnetic field is called nuclear magnetic moment (μ). The magnetic field is a vector quantity (here shown in **boldface** symbols) that has a magnitude and a direction. The direction of the nuclear magnetic moment lies along the rotation axis of the proton (Fig. 42–1*A*), and its magnitude is given by

$$\mu = \gamma hI/2\pi \quad (1)$$

where γ is the gyromagnetic ratio, h is Planck's constant, and I is the spin quantum number.

When a spinning proton is placed within an external magnetic field, $\mathbf{B_0}$, it attempts to line up with $\mathbf{B_0}$. Because of the laws of quantum mechanics, it can align either parallel or antiparallel with $\mathbf{B_0}$ (see Fig. 42–1*B*). These two alignments correspond to two possible nuclear energy states that the proton may take in an external magnetic field, the low-energy state (E_1) and the high-energy state (E_2), respectively (see Fig. 42–1*C*). The external magnetic field causes a torque on the proton, which makes it precess around the direction of the external field, with the motion of precession describing the surface of a cone. The rate of this precession is called the Larmor frequency, and it is proportional to the strength of the external field:

$$f_0 = \gamma B_0/2\pi \quad (2)$$

where f_0 is the Larmor frequency and γ is the gyromagnetic ratio. It is possible to induce transitions between the two energy states, E_1 and E_2, by introducing into the spin system characteristic electromagnetic radiation, the energy of which equals the energy difference between the two states:

$$\Delta E = E_2 - E_1 = hf_0 = \gamma hB_0/2\pi \quad (3)$$

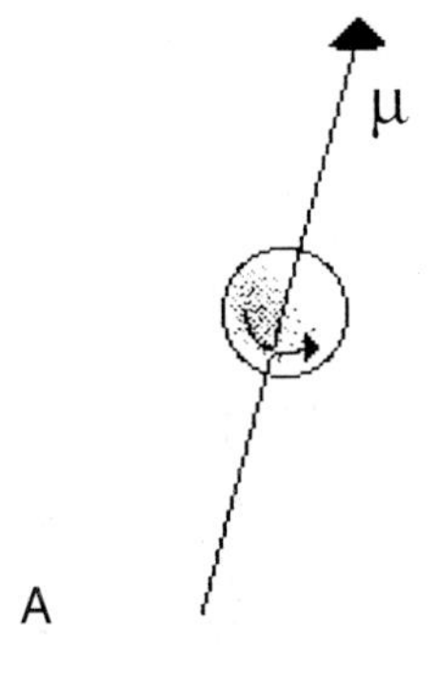

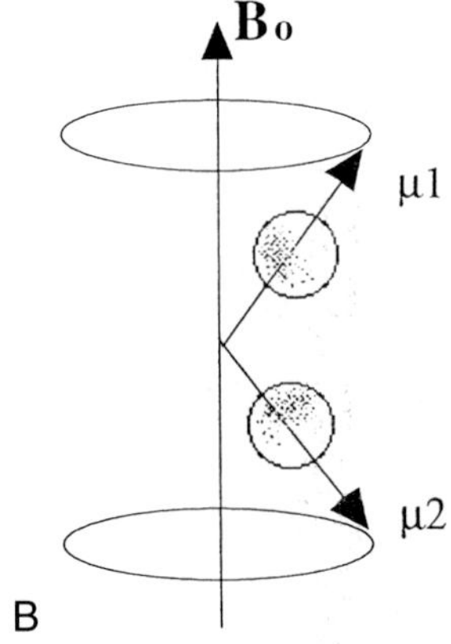

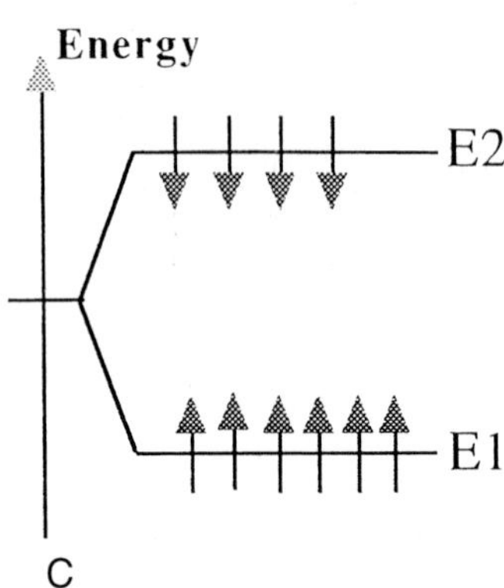

FIGURE 42–1. *A*, When placed in an external magnetic field ($\mathbf{B_0}$), a proton, or spin, starts to precess around it. The magnetic moment of the proton is described by a vector, μ, that has aligned parallel to $\mathbf{B_0}$. *B*, A proton (I = 1/2) may align either parallel or antiparallel to the $\mathbf{B_0}$; it has two different spin states corresponding to two different values of magnetic quantum number m_I. *C*, These two alignments are equivalent to two possible energy levels.

where γ is the gyromagnetic ratio, f_0 is the frequency, and h is Planck's constant. This phenomenon is called resonance. In a 1.5-Tesla magnetic field, the energy of electromagnetic radiation that is needed to induce transitions between the lower (E_1) and higher (E_2) proton energy levels is 0.264×10^{-6} eV.

Bulk Magnetization

In imaging, we deal with net magnetization rather than individual nuclear moments. In thermal equilibrium without an external field, the spins are in random motion and occupy the same energy level. When a spin system is under the influence of an external magnetic field, its protons distribute between the two permissible energy levels, E_1 and E_2, with a bias toward the lower one, because everything in nature moves toward the lowest possible energy state. The difference in the number of protons in the two energy levels is governed by Boltzmann statistics, and the ratio of the numbers of protons in the lower energy level to the number in the higher level is as follows:

$$N_{low}/N_{high} = \exp(hf_0/kT) = \exp(\gamma h B_0/2\pi) \approx 1 + hf_0/kT \quad (4)$$

where k is Boltzmann's constant and T is temperature in degrees Kelvin. If the total number of spins ($N_{total} = N_{low} + N_{high}$) is known, the difference in the number of spins between the low- and high-energy levels may be calculated as follows:

$$N_{effective} = N_{low} - N_{high} = N_{total}\, hf_0/2kT \quad (5)$$

These effective protons build up NMR signal, as measured in MRI. The greater the number of effective protons, the stronger the signal. The reason for the poor sensitivity of NMR imaging can now be understood, because the fractional excess of population in the lower energy level is extremely small. As can be seen in equations 4 and 5, the effective number of protons is proportional to the field strength; thus a higher magnetic field strength leads to a stronger NMR signal. If we assume that the total number of

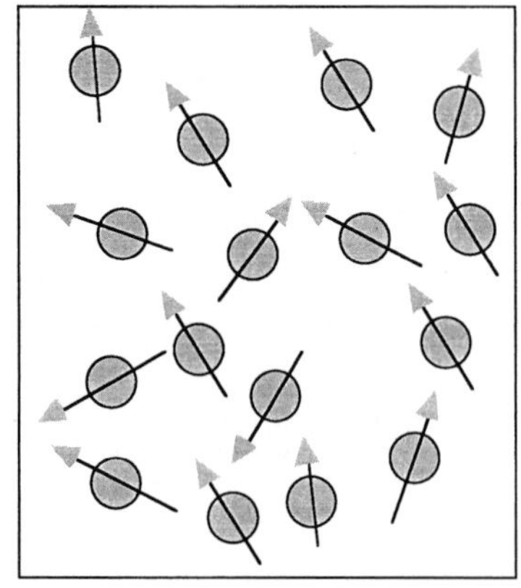

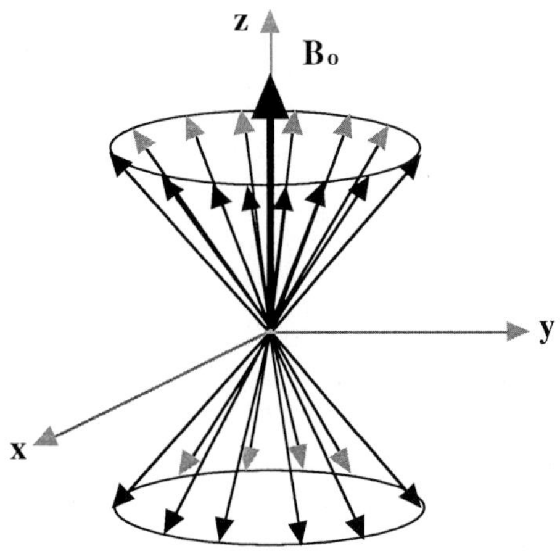

FIGURE 42–2. Net magnetization is a vector sum of all individual magnetic moment vectors, $\mathbf{M} = \Sigma\mu_i$. *A*, Without an external field the sum is zero, $\mathbf{M} = 0$, and there is no net magnetization. *B*, When the spin system is put into an external field (e.g., into a magnetic resonance scanner) the individual μ-vectors experience alignment with the field and the vector sum will be pointing to the preferred direction of the spins, that is, parallel to $\mathbf{B_0}$. Often, the coordinate system is defined so that $\mathbf{B_0}$ is parallel to the *z* axis, which is the case in this figure and throughout the text.

spins in a sample is 1 million, the effective number of spins that will produce the measured NMR signal is 1.7 at 0.5 Tesla and 5.2 at 1.5 Tesla (k = 1.380658 × 10^{-23} J/K; T = 293° K; h = 6.625 × 10^{-27} erg/Hz; f_0 = 21.3 MHz at 0.5 Tesla; f_0 = 63.9 MHz at 1.5 Tesla). Thus, the signal measured at 1.5 Tesla will be stronger than that measured at the lower 0.5-Tesla field, because the number of effective spins is three times greater in the former case.

The magnetic behavior of protons during imaging may be better explained by studying the behavior of the net magnetization, rather than individual magnetic moments. Net magnetization is defined as a vector sum of these individual nuclear magnetic moments:

$$\mathbf{M} = \Sigma \mu_i$$

It acts in a manner identical to that of the individual magnetic moments. In thermal equilibrium at room temperature, without an external field, the individual moments point in random directions, and their vector sum, **M**, is zero (Fig. 42–2*A*). When positioned in an external field, $\mathbf{B_0}$, the tiny nuclear magnetic fields align with $\mathbf{B_0}$ (parallel or antiparallel) and start to precess around $\mathbf{B_0}$. As explained earlier, more protons align with the external field than are opposed to it, and the net magnetization, **M,** also aligns with the external field (see Fig. 42–2*B*). As a vector, the net magnetization, **M,** may be divided into transverse (xy) and longitudinal (z) components. When individual nuclei precess and are out of phase, the individual magnetic moment vectors are distributed randomly over a surface of a double cone, with a slight excess of vectors pointing in the $\mathbf{B_0}$ direction. Because there is no net direction in the transverse (xy) plane and no phase coherence, the sum of individual **Mxy** vectors is zero. The result of this is that there is no magnetic field component in the xy plane, **Mxy** = 0. The net magnetization has only an **Mz** component, which points in the longitudinal or z direction; this phenomenon is referred to as equilibrium magnetization, $\mathbf{M_0}$.

Measurement of Nuclear Magnetic Resonance Signal and Free Induction Decay

Unfortunately, the longitudinal component of net magnetization, **Mz,** cannot be measured directly. Nuclear magnetic resonance receivers can only detect the transverse component of precessing magnetization, **Mxy,** that induces an electromotive force in the receiver coil. For this reason, at equilibrium, no signal is received from the patient in the scanner. To detect an NMR signal, the net magnetization, $\mathbf{M_0}$, must be tipped away from its equilibrium state along the *z* axis by irradiating the tissue with a burst of electromagnetic energy, which is done by using a temporary oscillating magnetic field, $\mathbf{B_1}$, that lies perpendicular to the $\mathbf{B_0}$ field. The frequency of oscillation of the $\mathbf{B_1}$ field must match the Larmor frequency of the sample to induce transitions between the two energy states and thereby change the direction of **M.** The burst of $\mathbf{B_1}$ energy is typically short in duration. Its frequency is in the radiofrequency part of the electromagnetic spectrum, and so it is also called an *RF,* or *radiofrequency, pulse.* The $\mathbf{B_1}$ field changes the direction of the net magnetization vector. At the end of the RF pulse, the angle between the *z* axis and the vector **M** is called the *tip angle* (α). Tip angle is dependent on both the duration (t_p) and the amplitude or strength (B_1) of the RF pulse and may be calculated as $\alpha = \gamma B_1 t_p$. An RF pulse is called a 90-degree pulse when the tip angle is 90 degrees; the magnetization vector **M** is then turned from the *z* axis exactly into the xy plane. In summary, therefore, at the end of the 90-degree pulse, $M_{xy} = M_0$ and $M_z = 0$. This equation is explained in Figure 42–3.

When a spin system is excited in such a way that the magnetization is placed in the xy direction, the signal is observed to disappear rapidly, a process called *free induction decay,* which reflects the behavior of transverse magnetization, which rapidly loses its coherence under these conditions. The free induction decay rate is mostly caused by local inhomogeneities of the magnetic field, leading to a loss of phase coherence, and it can be characterized by a relaxation time constant known as T2* (vide infra).

After the RF pulse is turned off, the spin system is left in an excited energy state that will discharge by emitting electromagnetic radiation with a frequency f_0. During the discharge, the net magnetization vector returns back to the equilibrium state (i.e., where $M_Z = M_O$). This return to equilibrium after RF pulse is called relaxation. The rate of return is determined by the spin system's relaxation properties.

Behavior of Net Magnetization During Relaxation

The two basic types of relaxation phenomena are spin-lattice, or longitudinal, relaxation and spin-spin, or transverse, relaxation. Both of these relaxation mechanisms are characterized by their own relaxation time constants, T1 for spin-lattice and T2 for spin-spin relaxation. The inverse values of T1 and T2, that is, 1/T1 and 1/T2, are called relaxation rates and are denoted by R1 and R2, respectively.

Let us study the behavior of net magnetization during each of these relaxation processes by using a spin system that is isolated from a biophysical environment. Later, we shall expand the notion to biologic tissues and the basic processes that make relaxation in different tissues distinctive.

To artificially simplify the motion of the magnetization vector, we are going to use the concept of a *rotating reference frame* (x′y′z′ frame), which is a coordinate system that rotates with the same frequency as the Larmor frequency of protons, f_0, which is also the same frequency as that of the $\mathbf{B_1}$ field. The *z* and *z′* axes

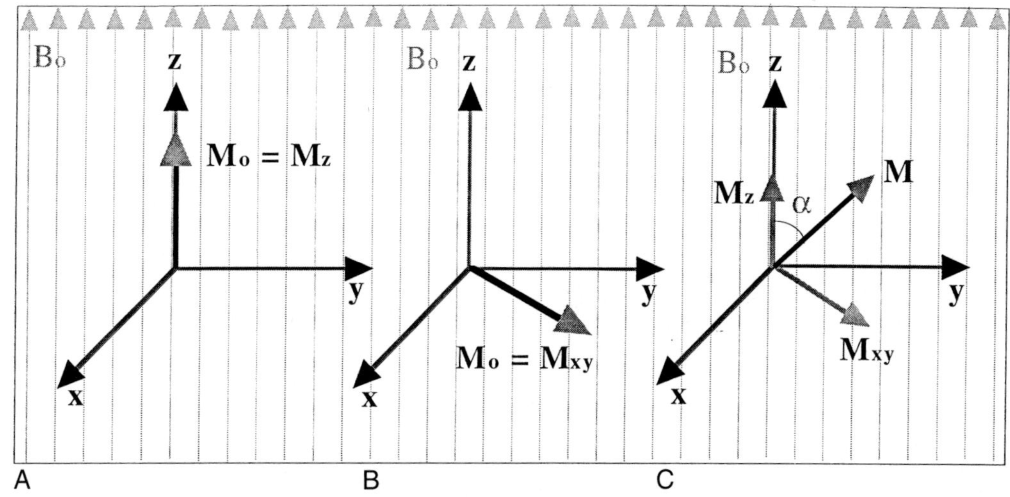

FIGURE 42–3. *A,* In equilibrium the net magnetization vector, $\mathbf{M_0}$, is parallel to $\mathbf{B_0}$. Because $\mathbf{B_0}$ is parallel to *z* axis and $\mathbf{M_0} = \mathbf{M_z}$. To observe an NMR signal, a transverse component of magnetization is needed, which is done with a burst of electromagnetic energy in radiofrequency range, called RF pulse. *B,* When the RF pulse is a 90-degree pulse, the magnetization is tipped to the xy plane and $\mathbf{M_{xy}} = \mathbf{M_0}$. *C,* If the pulse is an α-pulse (α < 90 degrees), the resultant magnetization **M** has z and xy components, both of which are smaller than $\mathbf{M_0}$.

are similar in both frames, whereas the x' and y' axes rotate with the frequency f_0. At equilibrium, when only $\mathbf{B_0}$ is present, the net magnetization vector, **M,** in the rotating reference frame is stationary and remains along the z' axis. When applied, the B_1 field acts like a stationary magnetic field that is perpendicular to the field $\mathbf{B_0}$ in the rotating reference frame. In the *laboratory reference frame* (xyz frame), a normal Cartesian coordinate system, the net magnetization vector travels toward the xy plane along a spiral path when disturbed from its equilibrium state by an RF pulse. In our artificial coordinate system (x′y′z′ frame), rotating synchronously with the $\mathbf{B_1}$ field, the movement of the net magnetization vector from the z' axis into the x′y′ plane may generally be described as a simple tilt from the z' axis into the x′y′ plane (Fig. 42–4).

T1, Spin-Lattice, or Longitudinal Relaxation

After the RF pulse, perturbation processes take place whereby the spin system relaxes and returns to thermal equilibrium by releasing excess energy into the surroundings, also known as the lattice. Induction of an NMR transition and transfer of spin energy to the lattice require that the nucleus experience a magnetic field fluctuating at the Larmor frequency. As the lattice is in thermal agitation, the magnetic dipoles it contains produce a fluctuating field with a wide frequency spectrum. Only a small fraction of this spectrum, however, corresponds to the Larmor frequency and thus contributes to relaxation processes. In fact, there are three principal types of magnetic interaction that result in these fluctuating fields. These are dipole-dipole interaction, the chemical shift anisotropic mechanism, and spin-rotation interaction. The most important of these, the dipole-dipole interaction, is attributable to the motion of neighboring magnetic dipoles creating a fluctuating magnetic field that the nucleus experiences. The two other types of interaction are less important, with the chemical shift anisotropic mechanism arising as a result of chemical shielding of the nucleus (described later) and, therefore, of the magnetic field acting on it, depend on the orientation of the molecule with respect to the B_0 field. This shielding arises from the electrons around the nucleus precessing in the B_0 field, thereby creating a weak secondary magnetic field that fluctuates as the molecule tumbles. Finally, the third mechanism, spin-rotation interaction, arises when a molecule rotates and generates a magnetic field, which couples with nuclear spin. A relaxation mechanism results when this coupling is interrupted, for instance, in the case of molecular collisions.

Longitudinal relaxation is described by the behavior of the z′ component of net magnetization, $M_{z'}$. Immediately after the 90-degree RF pulse, the net magnetization lies in the x′y′ plane with $M_{z'} = 0$ and $M_{x'y'} = M_0$. During the relaxation process, the $M_{z'}$ component steadily grows toward its equilibrium value M_O. The growth curve describing the continuous change in $M_{z'}$ is exponential in nature (Fig. 42–5A). The elapsed time in which $M_{z'}$ grows to 63 percent of its equilibrium value is defined as the T1 relaxation time, or longitudinal relaxation time, of the spin system. Any individual T1 relaxation time constant is field dependent and increases with the magnetic field.

T1ρ and Spin-Lattice Relaxation in Rotating Frame

T1ρ relaxation is similar to spin-lattice relaxation but is now measured in our rotating frame of reference along the direction of the so-called spin-lock field, B_L.[12–15] The method used to observe T1ρ is called a *spin-lock technique*, or forced transitory precession. After tipping the net magnetization, M, into the x′y′ plane with a 90-degree RF pulse, M is forced to stay along the y' axis, using the special spin-lock RF field, B_L. While the spin-lock field is on, relaxation of net magnetization M also takes place along the y' axis and is characterized by relaxation time constant T1ρ. T1ρ is analogous to T1 but is governed by the strength of the locking field, B_L, which is much weaker than B_0. T1ρ is the high-field analog of low-field T1 longitudinal relaxation time. This technique enables low-

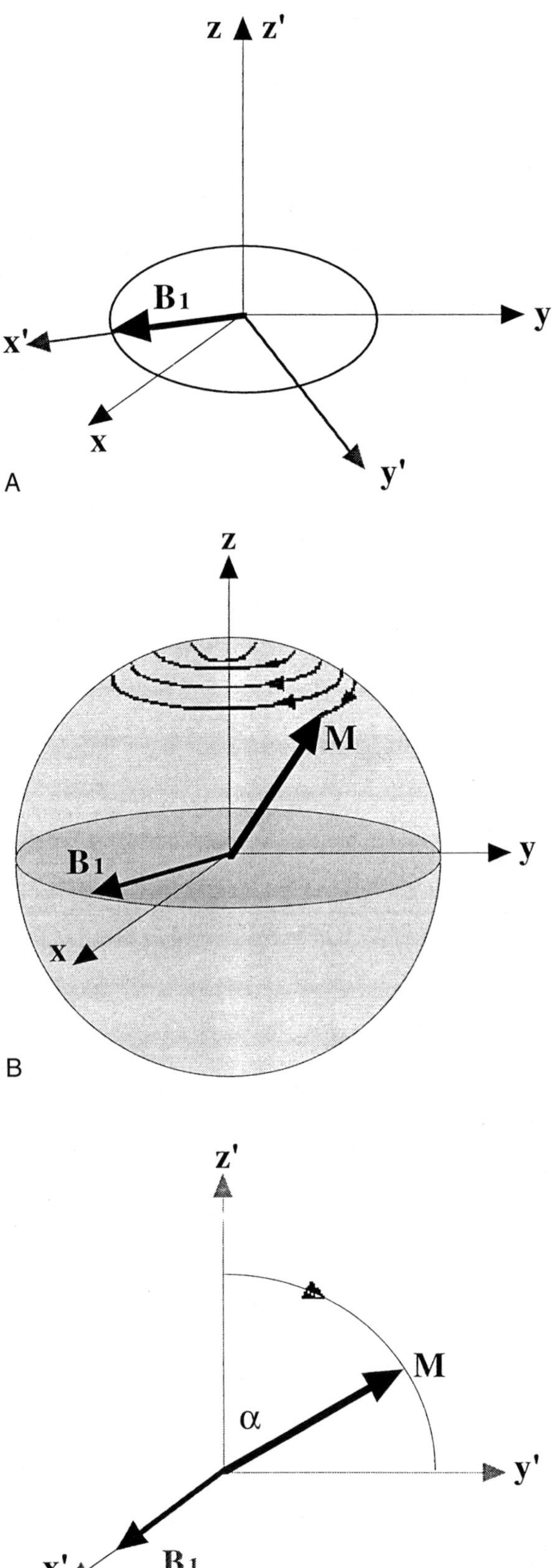

FIGURE 42–4. A, The definition of the rotating reference frame (x′y′z′ frame), as compared to that of the laboratory reference frame (xyz frame). Axes z and z' are common to both frames. Axes x' and y' rotate in the xy plane with the Larmor frequency of protons, f_0. *B,* The path of net magnetization vector during $\mathbf{B_1}$ field irradiation in the laboratory reference frame is a spiral on the surface of the ball with radius M. *C,* In rotating reference frame, the path of **M** is a simple tilt into the x′y′ plane in the case of a 90-degree pulse.

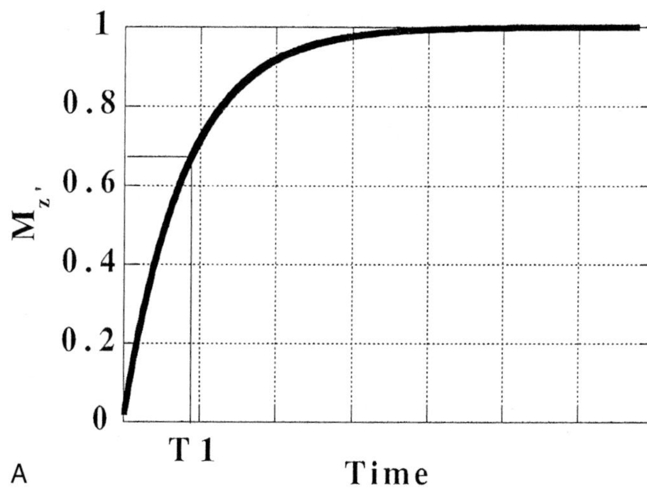

A

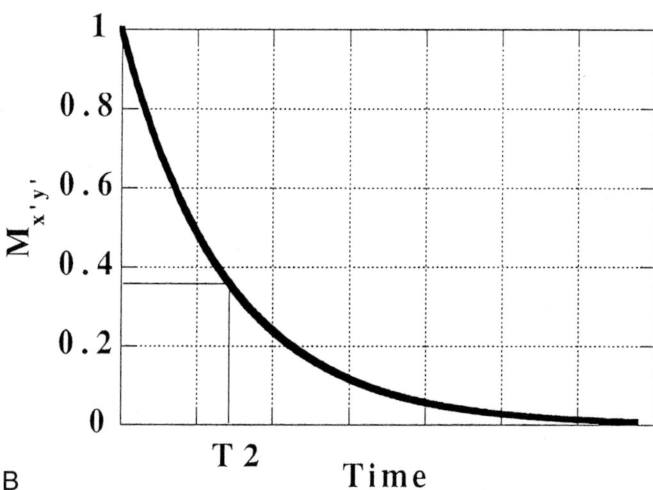

B

FIGURE 42–5. The behavior of the $M_{z'}$ and $M_{x'y'}$ components of a magnetization vector during relaxation of the spin system. *A,* The longitudinal, or T1, relaxation is defined with the behavior of the z′ component. The time it takes for an $M_{z'}$ component to reach 63 percent of its equilibrium value after a 90-degree pulse is T1, or longitudinal relaxation time. *B,* The transverse or T2 relaxation is defined with the behavior of x′y′ component. The point at which $M_{x'y'}$ has decreased to 37 percent of its original value defines the relaxation time, T2, for transverse relaxation.

field T1 values to be measured by the use of a high-field magnet, with all the advantages of the high-field magnet's signal-to-noise ratios. As we shall see, some biologic processes are better characterized at a low magnetic field, so this pulse sequence is potentially valuable.

T2, Spin-Spin, or Transverse Relaxation

During transverse, or spin-spin, relaxation, spins reciprocally exchange energy with no energy loss to the lattice. Under usual circumstances, spin-spin relaxation always occurs faster than spin-lattice relaxation (T2 < T1). Thus, additional mechanisms must exist for this type of relaxation. One of the most important additional mechanisms is chemical exchange. When an atom in some chemical location is replaced with another similar atom, the nuclear spin differs from the original one in terms of its phase of precession, and the resulting loss of phase coherence reduces transverse signal.

The behavior of the magnetization vector in the x′y′ plane after a 90-degree RF pulse is such as to progressively decrease its value from the maximum, $M_{x'y'} = M_O$, to zero (Fig. 42–5*B*). When the value of $M_{x'y'}$ has lost 63 percent of its original value M_O, the elapsed time is called T2, or the transverse relaxation time. During transverse relaxation, spins exchange energy between each other. The decrease of the x′y′ component is due to the gradual loss of phase coherence of precessional motion of individual protons, a phenomenon referred to as dephasing. Of course, T1 relaxation also eliminates transverse signal and is included in T2.

T2* Relaxation

T2 relaxation is the inherent transverse relaxation for the spin system in a perfectly homogeneous magnetic field B_0, where all spins in the system precess at the same frequency and only one Larmor frequency exists. However, in real life, a perfectly homogeneous magnetic field does not exist. MRI scanners inevitably contain field inhomogeneities of varying degrees, which results in individual proton vectors precessing at slightly different frequencies. These vectors are faster or slower, depending on whether they are in a locally stronger or weaker magnetic field, respectively. The net effect is that initial phase coherence is lost, and $M_{x'y'}$ decreases toward zero more rapidly; on measurement, the observed signal is weaker. The time constant that describes the decrease of $M_{x'y'}$, in the presence of field inhomogeneities, is called T2°. T2° may be defined as the transverse relaxation time that results from both inherent T2 effects and the effects of magnetic field inhomogeneities.

BIOLOGIC TISSUE RELAXATION

General Perturbation Processes

Thus far we have studied the basic processes of NMR physics by using either a single proton or a collection of isolated protons. In a biologic environment, protons experience slightly different magnetic fields that are caused by different physical and chemical surroundings.[16–19] A nucleus has an electron cloud around it that partially shields it from the applied field (B_0). As a consequence, a nuclear proton actually experiences a magnetic field smaller than B_0. Not only the electron cloud but also the presence of other nuclei (spin ≠ 0) within the same molecule or molecular subgroup influences the local field, B_{local}. The change in local magnetic field from B_0 to $B_0 + \Delta B$ shifts the resonance frequency of the proton from f_0 to $f_0 + \Delta f$; this change in frequency is called the chemical shift. In tissues, the chemical and physical environment changes from location to location, and protons at different sites precess at different local frequencies. Thus, they may relax differently. The relaxation of excited molecules is initiated by magnetic field fluctuations; thus potentially, relaxation may be induced by any process that is capable of causing local field fluctuations.

The local magnetic fields experienced by protons are not stable—they fluctuate over time. These fluctuations are generated by the translational and rotational movement of molecules, ions, and other protons within the same nucleus as well as by the movement of orbital electrons. To cause relaxation, fluctuations of local magnetic fields must match the local Larmor or resonance frequency. Generally, if molecules are free to move, field fluctuations are rapid. On the other hand, constrained molecular motion generally causes slow fluctuations. When molecules move very fast in an isotropic fashion (i.e., uniformly in all directions), the average field fluctuations are zero; this phenomenon is called motional narrowing. When the field fluctuations get slower and approach the Larmor frequency, they more effectively influence the protons and increase relaxation events. This influence is optimal when the field fluctuations exactly match the proton Larmor frequency. Factors such as temperature, viscosity, and binding affect the rate of molecular movement and, thus, the rate of field fluctuations and, ultimately, relaxation.

Water and Its Compartments

Because most of the hydrogen in soft tissues within the body is bound in water, the relaxation mechanisms of tissue are governed to a great extent by the relaxation processes of tissue water. The relaxation characteristics of tissue water are different from those of pure water. The differences arise largely from constraint on the movement of water molecules in tissue, which in turn is a response to the interactions of these molecules with other tissue constituents, such as macromolecules. Hydration shell formation results from the binding of water molecules to the surface of a macromolecule. Tissue water is often divided into three categories: free water, structured or intermediate water, and bound water (Fig. 42–6). Free water represents bulk water; that is, water molecules that are surrounded by other water molecules and are free to move. Bound water represents water molecules that are motionally restricted by virtue of their macromolecular binding. Structured or intermediate water is composed of motionally restricted water molecules that do not have complete motional freedom because of the influence of neighboring macromolecules but are not actually bound to them.

Brownian effects cause water molecules to be in constant, rapid motion. The parameter used to describe the extent of this motion is called the correlation time t_c; t_c is the time in which a molecule is fixed in one location before it collides with another molecule and changes its direction of movement. For a water molecule, this correlation time lies between 10^{-12} and 10^{-8} second and depends on the degree of binding experienced by the water molecule. Shorter times (picoseconds) reflect total freedom, whereas longer times imply some degree of binding. During an NMR measurement, a single water molecule may experience many different environments; the observed relaxation time constants can be considered the weighted averages of underlying individual relaxation time constants. If water molecules move within their environment solely by diffusion, then the distance (r) that a water molecule can travel in 700 msec (a typical T1 relaxation time in tissue) is about 68 μm, given by $r = \sqrt{6Dt}$, where D is the self-diffusion coefficient ($D = 1.1 \times 10^{-5}$ cm² per second in tissue) and t is the diffusion time (700 msec). As most cells have a radius of about 10 to 30 μm, water can experience the environments of several cells during this time. The diffusion radius for T2 relaxation is smaller, because the transverse relaxation times are shorter. For an average T2 of myocardium (~50 msec), this exploratory radius extends to only about 18 μm.[18]

Proton Exchange with Macromolecules

A small fraction of water, called bound water, is temporarily immobilized on the surface of macromolecules; in this microscopic environment, relaxation is markedly enhanced.[16, 20–24] Both T1 and T2 are very short for the macromolecular bound protons, and, in fact, the T2 process is so short that no imaging device can observe a signal from these protons. Thus, MRI is sensitive only to mobile protons. Binding at the macromolecular surface is a transient phenomenon, lasting only between 10^{-8} and 10^{-6} second. As described earlier, diffusion is a rapid event on the molecular scale. In combination, transient binding and rapid diffusion result in many water molecules experiencing assisted relaxation at the macromolecular surface.[23–25]

Recently, imaging techniques have been developed to use the *magnetization transfer* rate that occurs between bulk water and bound water as a contrast mechanism in NMR images.[15, 23, 25–28] Molecules in the free water pool move very rapidly and uniformly in all directions. This kind of movement results in the narrowing of the frequency spectrum, that is, so-called motional narrowing. A narrow frequency spectrum may be considered to occur simultaneously with uniform rates of precession, slow dephasing, and long transverse relaxation times, which describe the underlying physical phenomena in which, in the free water pool, rapid molecular movement results in a uniform rate of precession and slow dephasing. The width of the spectrum and the time constant of the free-induction decay (the duration of the measured free induction decay) are related via a mathematical operation called Fourier transformation. A narrow spectrum corresponds to a very long period of free induction decay, and vice versa.

By contrast, the tumbling of macromolecules is neither rapid nor isotropic, and their frequency spectrum is spread over a much larger range of frequencies. Indeed, it is possible to irradiate the protons bound to macromolecules separately from free protons by using a pulse of radiofrequency that is either above or below the resonant frequency range of free water protons (the frequency normally used for MRI) (Fig. 42–7A). After this offset irradiation,

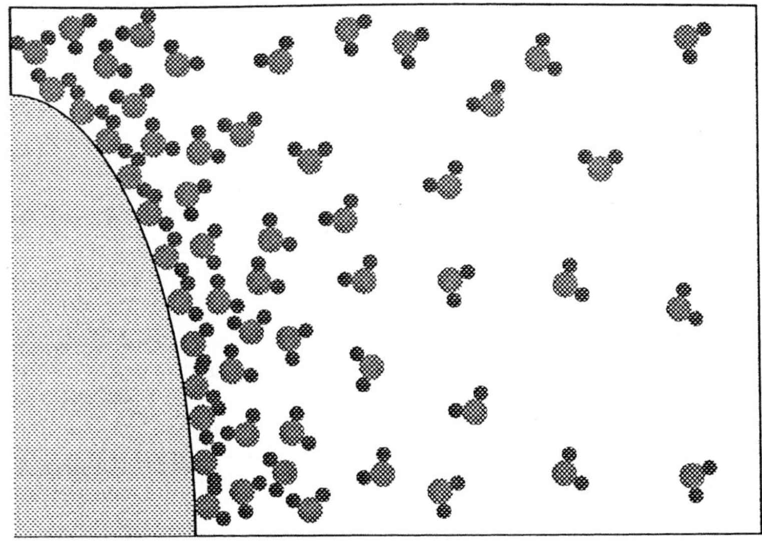

FIGURE 42–6. Tissue water is often divided into three compartments: free water, structured water, and bound water. The movement of water molecules in these different compartments is free, or partially restricted by the vicinity of a large macromolecule, or restricted because of the binding to the macromolecular surface. When the distance from the surface increases the speed of motion, the rotational frequency increases.

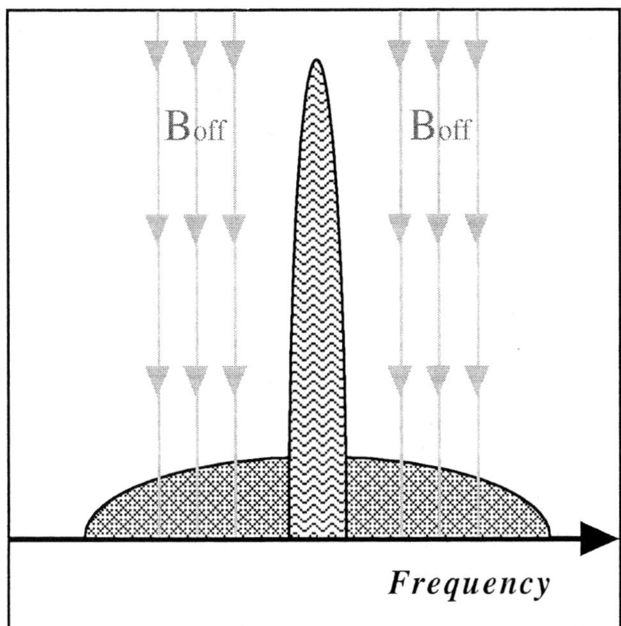

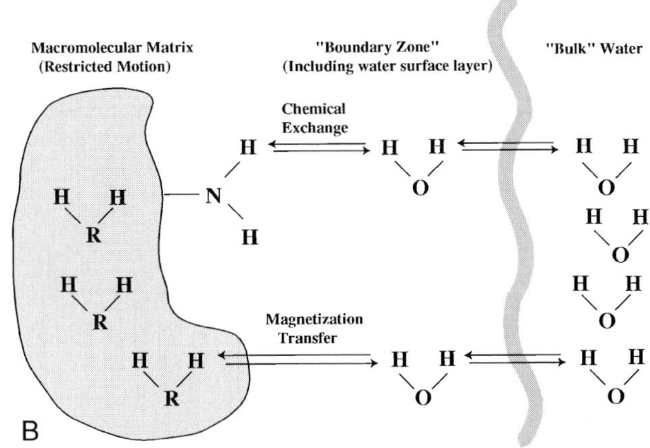

FIGURE 42–7. *A,* The resonance frequency range for macromolecular bound water pool is broader than the frequency range for free water pool that resonates with frequency f_0. This range makes it possible to irradiate the bound water pool separately from the free water pool, when an RF field is used, B_{off}, that has a radiofrequency that is either smaller or higher than f_0. *B,* Schematic diagram of water proton magnetization transfer in biologic tissues. Also depicted are the possible roles played by chemical exchange and by diffusion of water to and from the surface layer. (From Eng, J., Ceckler, T.L., Balaban, R.S.: Quantitative 1H magnetization transfer imaging in vivo. Magn. Reson. Med. 17:305, 1991; with permission.)

macromolecular protons become "saturated" (i.e., unable to generate an NMR signal). The exchange process between the free and the bound proton pools transfers saturated protons from the macromolecular zone to the free zone, and vice versa (see Fig. 42–7*B*). As a result, the measured NMR signal, which is mainly determined by mobile protons, decreases. This phenomenon is based on the proton exchange between the two pools and offers a unique way of studying the exchange processes. Thus, the tissues that transfer magnetization readily (i.e., white matter, renal cortex) lose more signal than adjacent tissues that do not exchange magnetization as rapidly (i.e., gray matter, cerebrospinal fluid, fat, muscle, and renal medulla). As a corollary, contrast agents that affect predominantly bulk water in the extracellular space remain independently effective, whereas water with a high magnetization transfer effect competes with the contrast effect. Each process is capable of producing selective tissue contrast.

Fat

Although protons are abundant in adipose tissue, they behave very differently from protons in water. Most of the protons are in a — CH_2 — form, and the electron cloud surrounding them causes their resonant frequency to be chemically shifted from the water peak by about 3.5 ppm. Proton exchange and cross-relaxation between fat and water are limited, because lipid molecules are hydrophobic. Both at the cellular level and within heterogeneous tissue, fat and water protons are separated, and the proton observed relaxation becomes biphasic. Storage fats in adipose tissue are nonpolar triglyceride molecules of intermediate size that rotate slowly in an isotropic fashion within their relatively homogeneous environment, which slows down the dephasing process so that T2 is almost equal to T1, itself fairly short. These factors show up as strong signals on both T1- and T2-weighted images, and where imaging is done with multiple 180-degree refocusing pulses, the fat signal is better sustained than the water signal.[29, 30] In brain, lipids are found predominantly in bilayer membranes. These membrane sheets prevent the lipid molecules from rotating in an isotropic fashion, resulting in such a short T2 that membrane lipids become invisible in MRI. In some tissues the fat fraction may change the relaxation behavior of tissue water because of the interaction between water and fat compartments; this has been proposed to be the case in white matter, where myelin or cerebrosides directly interact with water protons.[31, 32] Thus, T1 in white matter is shorter than would be expected purely because of its water content. There have been no reports of cardiovascular structures' exhibiting this phenomenon.

To address the chemical shift in water and fat frequencies, special pulse sequences can be designed to suppress the fat signal in the image, a technique called *fat suppression.* An example is the *short* (τ) *inversion recovery* sequence, whereby the time parameters are chosen to ensure that the signal from fat has reached its null point while that from other tissues still has magnitude and is visible.[33] Other methods of fat suppression use phase- or frequency-sensitivity methods to reduce the signal from fat to a low value, effectively removing it from an image.[34–36] Fat-suppression techniques are especially useful in cardiac imaging, where the presence of subpericardial fat can otherwise lead to the presence of significant artifacts.

Blood

In comparison with other tissues, blood has a relatively simple composition, with a water content higher and a protein content lower than those in other tissues. Because there are fewer macromolecules, the magnetization transfer effect is lower and extracellular contrast agents, such as gadolinium-diethylenetriamine-pentaacetic acid (GdDTPA), may be more effective. It should be emphasized at this stage that a prominent part of the tissue-contrast behavior of blood in magnetic resonance images arises from its motion, rather than from its relaxation properties. Normally, blood is in constant motion. Its movement within arteries and veins relative to voxel size and location during the period of pulsation required for imaging allows blood in the images to be visualized as white or black, an important feature in cardiac imaging. The long T1 of blood, caused by the slow recovery of protons, may result in saturation and thereby may limit blood signal relative to stationary tissue in circumstances in which magnetic resonance angiography is desired. On the other hand, both magnetization transfer pulse sequences and contrast agents can be used to exploit the differences between blood and adjacent stationary tissues.

Normal Versus Diseased Tissue

In normal tissues, the water content is tightly regulated within narrow boundaries, but in abnormal tissues, important changes in tissue-water content may, in fact, produce useful image contrast,

TABLE 42–1. MAGNETIC FEATURES OF HEMOGLOBIN AND ITS DEGRADATION PRODUCTS

Type of Hemoglobin or Degradation Product	Magnetic Feature
Oxyhemoglobin	No unpaired electrons Not paramagnetic
Deoxyhemoglobin	Four unpaired electrons Paramagnetic Shortens T2 when within red blood cell
Methemoglobin	Five unpaired electrons Strongly paramagnetic Shortens T1 because of PEDD* effects Shortens T2 when within red blood cell
Hemosiderin	Large, compact, crystalline iron core in protein shell Superparamagnetic Causes marked field inhomogeneity Shortens T2 much more than T1

*PEDD = proton-electron-dipole-dipole.

Note: In addition to the magnetic effects caused by the iron in heme listed above, the protein component of hemoglobin and its derivatives also mildly shortens T1 and T2.

From Roubidoux, M.A.: MR imaging of hemorrhage and iron deposition in the kidney. Radiographics 14:1033, 1994.

which is the case in edematous tissue. Generally, an increase in tissue-water content produces slower relaxation, because edema increases the bulk water content within host tissue, causing an increase in T1 and an even greater increase in T2. Edema does not contain many macromolecules, and magnetization transfer effect is therefore of little significance in edematous tissue. In intracellular edema, the relaxation effects are somewhat less significant than those in interstitial edema because of continued restriction in the movement of water molecules within the cell. In tissue in which macromolecules are reduced in number or broken down into smaller constituents, T1 and T2 relaxation rates are increased. An example of this situation is tissue necrosis with edema in myocardial infarction. By contrast, T1 and T2 rates decrease when macromolecules become cross-linked. This condition is seen with coagulation and chemical denaturing of tissue but is relatively uncommon in vivo.

In hemorrhage the NMR signal behavior changes dramatically as circumstances evolve.[37–39] The properties of a simple collection of stagnant blood are quite similar to the properties of normal blood. However, when the red blood cells become sediment, a layer of serum is formed with longer T1 and T2, and the red cell–rich fraction has shorter T1 and T2. As oxygen is extracted from the red cell hemoglobin and deoxyhemoglobin is thus formed, the interior of the cells becomes more paramagnetic. This sequence of events results in alterations in the local magnetic fields, called magnetic susceptibility variations, which cause the spins to dephase, reducing T2*. The change in T1 is not so prominent, and this so-called acute phase lasts about 18 to 24 hours (Table 42–1).

In the subacute phase, which lasts a few days, the red cell membranes lyse, and chemical processes change the hemoglobin to even more paramagnetically effective methemoglobin, resulting in shorter T1 and T2. At the same time, the susceptibility effect in this subacute phase is reduced as the compartmentation between cells and serum is destroyed. In the chronic stage, hemoglobin products are converted into hemosiderin and ferritin, which may be ingested locally by macrophages. Both processes produce high

Factors Affecting Image Contrast

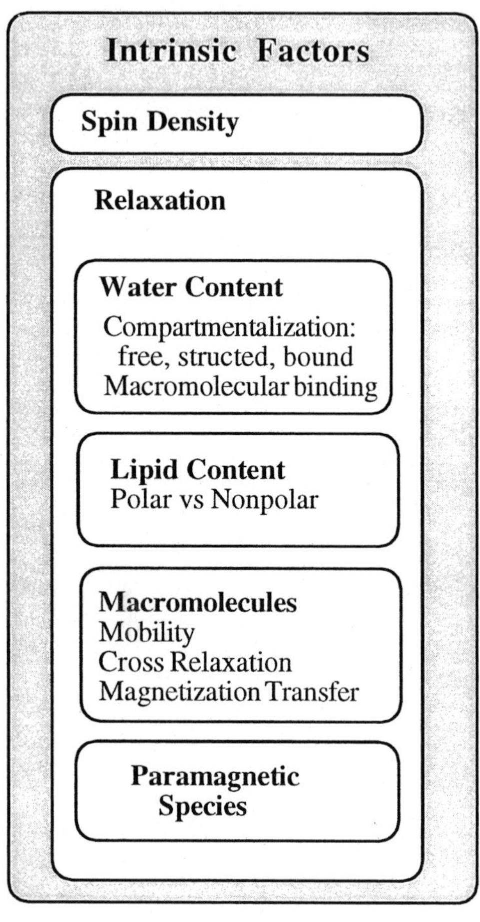

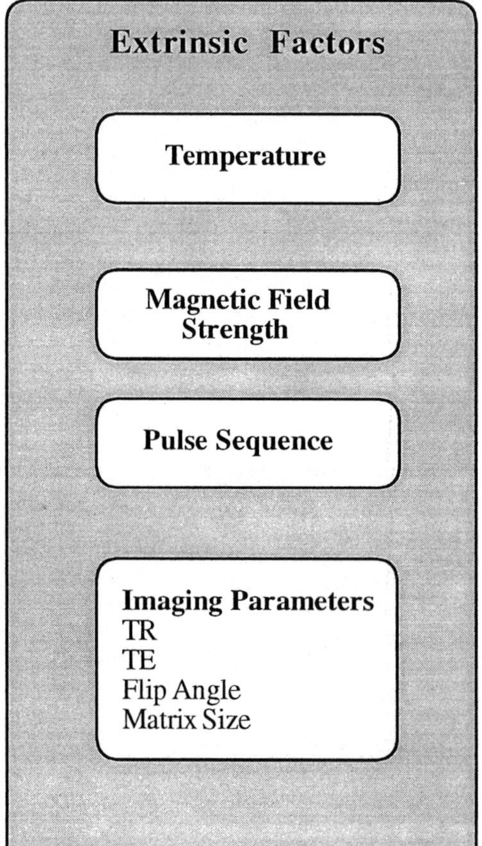

FIGURE 42–8. Magnetic resonance image contrast is defined by intrinsic tissue factors and by extrinsic factors. The intrinsic factors are tissue constants and may not be changed. On the contrary, many of the extrinsic factors may be changed during the imaging session, and they may be used to regulate the image contrast. Whether the tissue appears bright or dark in the image is a complicated function of all these different factors.

magnetic susceptibilities, which cause strong local dephasing in transverse-phase coherence, destroying the measured signals over a considerable distance. This final relaxation mechanism behaves like metal artifacts or superparamagnetic magnetic resonance contrast agents. (For a detailed discussion, see Chapter 44.)

Paramagnetic ions (those ions having an unpaired electron in their outer orbit) possess an electronic magnetic moment that is hundreds of times stronger than a nuclear moment. Even small amounts of paramagnetic ions influence the relaxation times substantially by causing strong fluctuations in local fields, thereby speeding up the relaxation process. This situation may exist in iron overload diseases, such as hemochromatosis or some forms of thalassemia, in which increased iron deposits are present in tissue, including myocardial tissue.

Other pathologies may lead to alteration of a normal tissue's relaxation properties. For instance, an inflammatory exudate (protein-rich) in the pericardial space, which may or may not be infected, decreases both the T1 and T2 relaxation times of a pericardial effusion, whereas a transudate (protein-poor) tends to increase T1 and T2 times toward the values observed with pure water. Other lesions with high water content tend to increase T1 and T2 times; for example, T2 values may rise above 80 msec in myocardium that is undergoing rejection after transplantation.

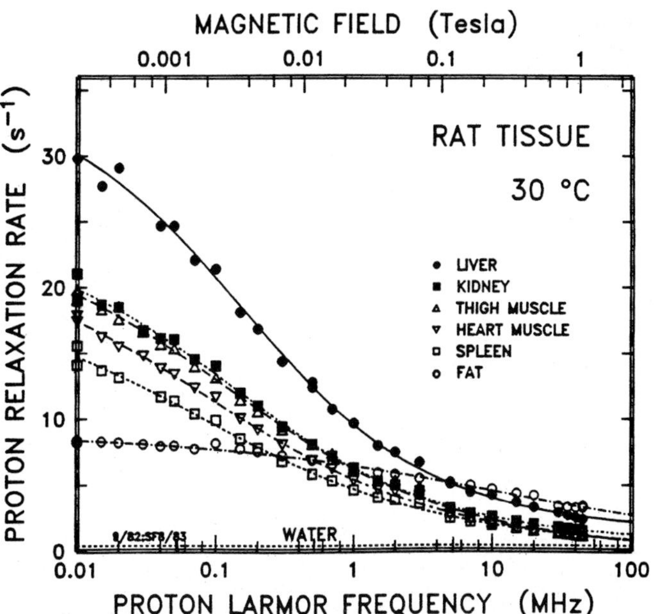

FIGURE 42–9. Change of proton relaxation rate with frequency; the dispersion of relaxation rate (1/T1) versus the Larmor frequency of the proton in fresh rat tissue studied at 30° C. Imaging frequencies range from 5 to 85 MHz, with magnetic field strengths of 0.12 to 2.0 Tesla. The relaxation of fat slows minimally as field increases, but macromolecular–water proton interaction causes other soft tissue to have a stronger field-dependent relaxation. (Courtesy of S. Koenig and R.D. Brown, III.)

IMAGING AND RELAXATION

In imaging, NMR signal intensity is determined by intrinsic tissue factors, spin density, and relaxation time constants of tissues, as well as by extrinsic factors, such as field strength and pulse sequence (Fig. 42–8). Intrinsic factors are tissue constants that may not be changed during the imaging session, whereas pulse sequence parameters may be used to emphasize one or more intrinsic tissue properties in the image. Spin density does not vary prominently from tissue to tissue but may lead to some contrast differences in magnetic resonance images. However, relaxation times T1 and T2 (Table 42–2) are more characteristic of different biologic compositions. T1 is magnetic field dependent (Fig. 42–9),[18, 40–42] which must be considered in determining the appropriate imaging sequence for a particular instrument.

Knowledge of tissue relaxation properties may be used to achieve the desired contrast between tissues under consideration.[43] Whether or not a given pixel appears bright or dark in the image depends on the pulse sequence used. The nature of the final images, T1-weighted, T2-weighted, or T2*-weighted, is determined by the dominant form of relaxation. The term "weighted" is used to emphasize the fact that NMR signal intensity is a complicated function of many parameters that cannot be totally separated; we can merely emphasize one or another. Signal intensity in each voxel is dependent on tissue homogeneity, and the signal intensity measured usually reflects an average behavior of many tissue components.

Simply put, the T2 weighting in an image is determined mainly by the selection of the echo time, TE, of the pulse sequence. TE is the time from the RF pulse, used to excite the spin system, to the moment when signal is measured. TE determines how long tissues may relax through T2 processes before the signal is captured. For a tissue with long T2, transverse relaxation is a slow process, and the transverse component of net magnetization, $M_{x'y'}$, will survive longer than in tissue with short T2. If TE is very short (not usually possible with routine imaging sequences), the measured signal is not influenced by T2 relaxation. When TE increases, T2 relaxation has enough time to modify measured signal intensities. This modification allows signal intensity differences between tissues of different T2 relaxation times to increase and thus to modify image contrast. Whatever the pulse sequence, echo time may always be seen as the period of opportunity for T2 relaxation processes to occur.

TABLE 42–2. PROTON RELAXATION PROPERTIES OF CARDIAC STRUCTURES*

	T1 (msec)	T2 (msec)
Myocardium	870	57
Adipose tissue	260	84
Blood	830	160
Valves and fibrous pericardium	200	22

*Approximate mean value at 60 MHz and 3° C.

T1 weighting is determined mostly by the selection of the repetition time, TR, of the pulse sequence. TR is the time from the beginning of the pulse sequence to the time when it is repeated. Within this time, the longitudinal component recovers from the minimum value gained after the RF pulse, toward the equilibrium value. When T1 relaxation time is short, as compared with TR, the $M_{z'}$ component of magnetization recovers quickly back to the equilibrium value, and the length of the $M_{z'}$ vector is the same as it was before the first excitation. However, if T1 relaxation is long, compared with TR, the $M_{z'}$ component does not recover its equilibrium value, and when excitation is repeated, the starting length of the $M_{z'}$ vector is smaller than its maximum value at equilibrium. By changing TR, it is possible to increase contrast in the image between short and long T1 tissues.

Imaging choices are never straightforward in real life; on the basis of selected imaging parameters, an image may be T1-weighted for some tissues but T2-weighted for others, depending on relaxation properties and the pulse sequence parameters selected. This occurs, for instance, in tissues having a very long T1, that is, fluids that generally show T1 contrast even in T2-weighted pulse sequences. Tissues with immobile protons and very short T2, such as bone, mainly evidence T2 properties, even in T1-weighted images. In cardiac imaging, extra difficulties exist that arise primarily from cardiac, blood, and respiratory motion. In selecting imaging parameters for electrocardiogram-gated, T1- or T2-weighted cardiac imaging, the effective TR (TR_{eff}), the one that actually determines image contrast, depends on the length of the cardiac cycle and may differ from the selected TR. An extra complication arises from the fact that the heart rate may change during imaging, and thus effective TR varies during an imaging sequence.

CONCLUSION

Relaxation phenomena result from transient radiofrequency perturbations of biologic tissue within a magnetic field. The relaxation characteristics of varying tissues serve as the basis for their contrast differentiation. For this reason, a proper understanding of the primary relaxation mechanisms, T1, T2, and T2*, is key to the accurate acquisition and interpretation of magnetic resonance images.

References

1. Purcell, E.M., Torrey, H.C., and Pound, R.V.: Resonance absorption by nuclear magnetic moments in a solid. Physiol. Rev. 69:37, 1946.
2. Bloch, F., Hansen, W.W., and Packard, M.E.: Nuclear induction. Physiol. Rev. 69:127, 1946.
3. Damadian, R.: Apparatus and method for detecting cancer in tissue. US Patent No. 3789832, filed March 17, 1972.
4. Lauterbur, P.C.: Image formation by induced local interactions: Examples employing nuclear magnetic resonance. Nature 242:190, 1973.
5. Farrar, T.C., and Becker, E.D.: Pulse and Fourier Transform NMR. Orlando, FL, Academic Press, 1971.
6. Mansfield, P., and Morris, P.G.: NMR imaging in biomedicine. New York, Academic Press, 1982.
7. Foster, M.A., and Hutchinson, J.M.: Practical NMR Imaging. Oxford, England, IRL Press, 1987.
8. House, W.V.: Theoretical basis for NMR imaging. *In* Partain, C.L., Price, R.R., Patton, J.A., et al. (eds.): Magnetic Resonance Imaging. Philadelphia, W.B. Saunders, 1988.
9. Partain, C.L., Price, R.R., Patton, J.A., et al.: The physical basis for NMR imaging. *In* Partain, C.L., Price, R.R., Patton, J.A., et al. (eds.): Magnetic Resonance Imaging. Philadelphia, W.B. Saunders, 1988.
10. Oldendorf, W., and Oldendorf, W.J.: MRI Primer. New York, Raven Press, 1991.
11. Talagala, S.L., and Wolf, G.L.: Principles of nuclear magnetic resonance. *In* Marcus, M.L., Schelbert, H.R., Skorton, D.J. et al. (eds.): Cardiac Imaging: A Companion to Braunwald's Heart Disease. Philadelphia, W.B. Saunders, 1991.
12. Lamminen, A.E., Tanttu, J.I., Sepponen, R.E., et al.: T1ρ dispersion imaging of diseased muscle tissue. Br. J. Radiol. 66:783, 1993.
13. Santyr, G.E., Fairbanks, E.J., Kelcz, F. et al.: Off-resonance spin locking for MR imaging. Magn. Reson. Med. 32:43, 1994.
14. Sepponen, R.E., Pohjonen, J.A., and Sipponen, J.T.: A method for T1ρ imaging. J. Comput. Assist. Tomogr. 9:1007, 1985.
15. Sepponen, R.: Rotating frame and magnetization transfer. *In* Stark, D.D., and Bradley, W.G.J. (eds.): Magnetic Resonance Imaging. St. Louis, Mosby–Year Book, 1992.
16. Koenig, S.H., Bryant, R.G., Hallenga, K., et al.: Magnetic cross relaxation among protons in protein solution. Biochemistry 17:4348, 1978.
17. Fullerton, G.D., and Cameron, I.L.: Relaxation of biological tissues. *In* Wehrli, F.W., Shaw, D., and Kneeland, J.B. (eds.): Biomedical Magnetic Resonance Imaging: Principles, Methodology and Applications. New York, VCH Publishers, 1988.
18. Wolf, G.L.: Biologic basis of proton relaxation. *In* Marcus, M.L., Schelbert, H.R., Skorton, D.J., et al. (eds.): Cardiac Imaging: A Companion to Braunwald's Heart Disease. Philadelphia, W.B. Saunders, 1991.
19. Fullerton, G.D.: Physiologic basis of magnetic relaxation. *In* Stark, D.D., and Bradley, W.G.J. (eds.): Magnetic Resonance Imaging. St. Louis, Mosby–Year Book, 1992.
20. Yang, H., and Schleich, T.: T1 discrimination contributions to proton magnetization transfer in heterogeneous biological systems. Magn. Reson. Med. 32:16, 1994.
21. Kuwata, K., Brooks, D., Yang, H., et al.: Relaxation-matrix formalism for rotating-frame spin-lattice proton NMR relaxation and magnetization transfer in the presence of an off-resonance irradiation field. J. Magn. Reson., Series B 104:11, 1994.
22. Gore, J.C., Brown, M.S., and Armitage, I.M.: An analysis of magnetic cross-relaxation between water and methylene protons in a model system. Magn. Reson. Med. 9:333, 1989.
23. Brooks, D., Kuwata, K., and Schleich, T.: Determination of proton magnetization transfer rate constants in heterogeneous biological systems. Magn. Reson. Med. 31:331, 1994.
24. Wolf, S.D., and Balaban, R.S.: Magnetization transfer contrast (MTC) and tissue water proton relaxation in vivo. Magn. Reson. Med. 10:135, 1989.
25. Eng, J., Ceckler, T.L., and Balaban, R.S.: Quantitative ^{1}H magnetization transfer imaging in vivo. Magn. Reson. Med. 17:304, 1991.
26. Grossman, R.I., Gomori, J.M., Ramer, K.N., et al.: Magnetization transfer: Theory and clinical applications in neuroradiology. Radiographics 14:279, 1994.
27. Hajnal, J.V., Baudouin, C.J., Oatridge, A., et al.: Design and implementation of magnetization transfer pulse sequences for clinical use. J. Comput. Assist. Tomogr. 16:7, 1992.
28. Haraldseth, O., Jones, R.A., Schjøtt, J., et al.: Early detection of regional myocardial ischemia in ex vivo piglet hearts: MR imaging with magnetization transfer. J. Magn. Reson. Imaging 4:603, 1994.
29. Constable, R.T., Anderson, A.W., Zhang, J., et al.: Factors influencing contrast in fast spin-echo imaging. Magn. Reson. Imaging 10:497, 1992.
30. Henkelman, R.M., Hardy, P.A., Bishop, J.E., et al.: Why fat is bright in RARE and fast spin-echo imaging. J. Magn. Reson. Imaging 2:533, 1992.
31. Koenig, S.H., Brown, III, R.D., Spiller, M.: Relaxometry of brain: Why white matter appears bright in MRI. Magn. Reson. Med. 14:482, 1990.
32. Kucharcyk, W., Macdonald, P.M., Stanisz, G.J., et al.: Relaxivity and magnetization transfer of white matter lipids at MR imaging: Importance of cerebrosides and pH. Radiology 182:521, 1994.
33. Bydder, G.M., Pennock, J.M., and Phil, M.: The short TI inversion recovery sequence: An approach to MR imaging of the abdomen. Magn. Reson. Imaging 3:251, 1985.
34. Szumowski, J., and Simon, J.: Proton chemical shift imaging. *In* Stark, D.D., and Bradley, W.G. (eds.): Magnetic Resonance Imaging. St. Louis, Mosby–Year Book, 1992.
35. Mao, J., Yan, H., Brey, W.W., et al.: Fat tissue and fat suppression. Magn. Reson. Imaging 11:385, 1993.
36. Simon, J.H., and Rubinstein, D.: Contrast-enhanced fat-suppression neuroimaging. Neuroimaging Clin. North Am. 4:153, 1994.
37. Thulborn, K.R., Sorensen, A.G., Kowall, N.W., et al.: The role of ferritin and hemosiderin in the MR appearance of cerebral hemorrhage: A histopathologic biochemical study in rats. Am. J. Neuroradiol. 11:291, 1990.
38. Janick, P.A., Hackney, D.B., Grossman, R.I., et al.: In vitro modeling of the magnetic resonance appearance of cerebral hemorrhage. Magn. Reson. Q. 7:57, 1991.
39. Bradley, W.G., Jr.: MR appearance of hemorrhage in the brain. Radiology 189:15, 1993.
40. Fischer, H.W., Rinck, P.A., and van Haverbeke, Y.: Nuclear relaxation of human brain gray and white matter: Analysis of field dependence and implications for MRI. Magn. Reson. Med. 16:317, 1990.
41. Bryant, R.G., Mendelson, D.A., and Lester, C.C.: The magnetic field dependence of proton spin relaxation in tissues. Magn. Reson. Med. 21:117, 1991.
42. Koenig, S.H., Brown, III, R.D., and Ugolini, R.: A unified view of relaxation in protein solutions and tissue, including hydration and magnetization transfer. Magn. Reson. Med. 29:77, 1992.
43. Wehrli, F.W., MacFall, J.R., and Prost, J.H.: Impact of the choice of operating parameters on MR imaging. *In* Partain, C.L., Price, R.R., Patton, J.A., et al. (eds.): Magnetic Resonance Imaging. Philadelphia, W.B. Saunders, 1988.

CHAPTER

43 Principles and Instrumentation for Cardiac Magnetic Resonance Imaging

Robert W. Weisskoff, Ph.D.

The previous chapter described the underlying physics, chemistry, and biology of the nuclear magnetic resonance phenomenon: the Larmor relation, relaxation times, and T1- and T2-weighted imaging. This chapter describes in greater detail how MR images are actually created, discusses the equipment that is used to create these images, and introduces some of the special techniques that are used for cardiac magnetic resonance imaging (MRI).

The first part of this chapter is devoted to explaining the theory of magnetic resonance (MR) image formation. Then follows a broad description of the general apparatus that is used to produce these images. The chapter closes with a discussion of instrumentation and techniques that have been developed specifically for cardiac MRI.

PRINCIPLES OF MAGNETIC RESONANCE IMAGING

Image formation in MRI is fundamentally quite different from other medical imaging modalities. One of the easiest ways of appreciating this difference is to think about the wavelength of medium used to create the images. For example, a microscope that uses visible light can resolve detail to something on the order of magnitude (i.e., within a factor of 10) of the wavelength of the light, or about 1/2 μm. The acoustic wavelength for 15 MHz ultrasound is 0.1 mm in tissue, which is on the same order of magnitude as its limiting resolution. In MRI, the radio waves that are used for imaging are many orders of magnitude larger. For example, at 1.5 Tesla (T), the Larmor frequency of protons is 64 MHz, corresponding to a wavelength of 5000 mm. Despite this huge wavelength (comparable to the size of the whole body), we easily make MR images with 1-mm resolution.

The key to MRI is not the wavelength of the radio waves; rather, it is the fact the resonance phenomenon is so precise that we can use it to image the protons based on differences in their resonance frequencies. As will be described later, by spatially varying this resonant frequency, we can identify the different protons and thus produce high-resolution MR images.

Spatial Encoding

This section discusses the most common method of MR image creation. Although it is not the original way that MR images were formed,[1] the overwhelming majority of MRI now uses this so-called "spin-warp"[2] method of image generation. In this method, encoding is performed independently (and somewhat differently) in the three orthogonal directions. As will be described at length later, after using the resonant property of MR to excite selectively one slab of protons, the magnetic field uniformity is purposely distorted to make the protons resonate at different frequencies in the two perpendicular directions. Frequency analysis (the Fourier transform) is then used to decode the proton densities.

Slice Selection

The first step in localization is the selective excitation of a *slice* of protons within the body. Recall from the previous chapter that protons tend to line up along the magnetic field, reaching equilibrium in a time of order T1. To image the protons, one must bring them out of this equilibrium by using a radiofrequency (RF) pulse. By transmitting radio waves precisely at the Larmor frequency equal to γB_0, where γ is the gyromagnetic ratio (42.58 MHz/Tesla for protons) and B_0 is the main magnetic field strength, the protons can be tipped into the transverse plane and can precess at their natural frequency. Excite the protons at the wrong frequency (i.e., transmit at a frequency different from the Larmor frequency) and nothing happens: the protons stay aligned with the magnet.

The trick to slice selection is to destroy the uniformity of the main magnetic field, so that protons have a Larmor frequency that varies with position. This is typically done by superimposing a linearly varying magnetic field on top of the uniform static field produced by the main magnet. This magnetic field *gradient* makes the Larmor frequency vary with positions. Figure 43–1, for example, shows the magnetic field and Larmor frequency as a function of position with and without this applied gradient.

Now, with this gradient applied, we transmit an RF wave composed of a limited spread of frequencies around the Larmor frequency of the magnet, γB_0. (Adding these frequencies together produces an RF pulse that has a shaped envelope.) Because the RF pulse contains only a limited number of frequencies, it can only excite those protons with those frequencies; hence, it excites a slice of protons. The thickness of this slice depends only on two things: the strength of the applied gradient and the spread of frequencies included in the RF pulse:

$$\Delta z = \frac{\Delta f}{\gamma G}$$

where Δz is the thickness of the slice (m), G is the strength of the gradient (T/m), and Δf is the spread of frequencies in the pulse (Hz). This relationship is illustrated in Figure 43–1.

This slice can be offset from the middle of the magnet by changing the center frequency of the RF pulse without changing its width. Again, because only the spins that are on resonance with the pulse will be excited, we see that the offset of the center of the slice, z_0, depends on offset from γB_0 of the transmitted frequency, f_0:

$$z_0 = \frac{f_0}{\gamma G}$$

Slice selection is depicted graphically in the usual short-hand notation used for describing MRI in Figure 43–2. This *pulse sequence* shows the temporal order of events that occur in the generation of an image. These diagrams show time running left to right. The slice selection process described above involves the RF channel and the slice-selection gradient. Essentially, what is graphed for the RF is the shape of the excitatory pulse happening in the presence of the gradient of magnetic field in the slice-selection direction. We call this gradient "G_s," although it is also commonly called G_z.

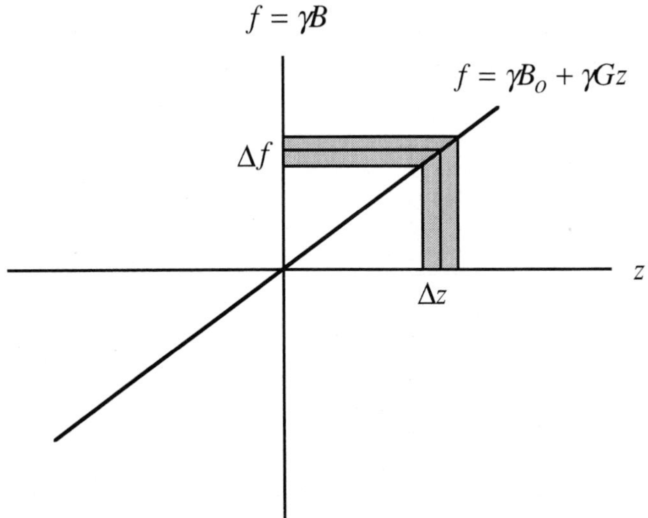

FIGURE 43–1. Principle of slice selection. When a spatially varying magnetic field is applied, the Larmor frequency of the protons becomes spatially dependent. This graph shows the Larmor frequency as a function of position in the presence of an added magnetic field gradient, G (mT/m), applied in the slice-selection direction. To excite a slab of protons of width Δz (m), the excitation pulse must have frequency width $\Delta f = \gamma G \Delta z$.

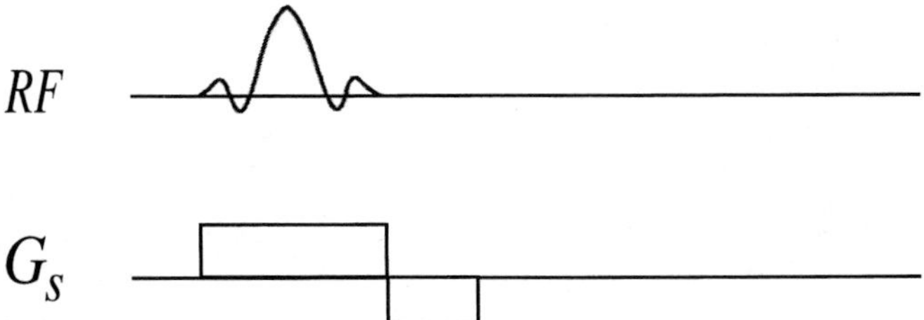

FIGURE 43–2. Pulse sequence diagram of slice selection. Pulse sequence diagrams are the shorthand descriptions of MRI techniques. For slice selection, we show the envelope of the RF waveform (a sinc-shape, that provides relatively uniform slice profile), playing out in the presence of a slice-selection gradient. The negative-going trapezoid after slice selection refocuses the spins, which are left dephased by slice selection.

Frequency Encoding

Once a desired slice of protons has been excited, the spins within that slice now must be spatially encoded to produce a tomographic image. We saw in slice selection that the resonant property of NMR was used to excite selectively only those protons within a physical slab on the patient. For the rest of the encoding we shall rely on the frequency-specific precession of the excited protons in order to image them.

Because it is somewhat more involved than simply making a "shadow" of the protons, two different ways of thinking about this imaging process are presented. In the first, we shall describe the encoding as a frequency-based projection analogous to x-ray computed tomography. In the second, the concept of "K-space" is introduced, in which the encoding is thought of as encoding the spatial frequencies (i.e., periodicity) of the object.

Projection Point of View

Frequency encoding relies on letting the protons precess at different frequencies, depending on their location in the magnet. Just as in slice selection, we use a magnetic field gradient (i.e., a magnetic field, which is applied in addition to the main field produced by the scanner, that varies linearly across the patient) to achieve this frequency dependence. However, this magnetic field varies at a right angle to the slice-selection direction. Figure 43–3 illustrates this idea.

Recall from the previous chapter that after excitation, the magnetization vector has been rotated into the transverse plane and now precesses at the Larmor frequency around the z axis. Imagine that we had a frequency detector that could let us listen to the protons precessing at one specific frequency. What would we hear when we listened in the presence of the frequency-encoding gradient illustrated in Figure 43–3?

If we listened right near the γB_0, we would hear a signal proportional to the number of protons that are spinning right near the middle of the magnet, shaded black in Figure 43–3*A*. Because the frequency-encoding gradient makes a field $B = B_0 + Gx$, where G is the strength of the frequency-encoding gradient (mT/m) and x is the position along the frequency-encoding axis ($x = 0$ is the middle of the scanner), we see that those protons that precess at a frequency near γB_0 must come from $x = 0$. The more protons there are near the middle of this slice, the bigger the signal right at γB_0.

On the other hand, if we listened at a frequency above γB_0, we would get a signal proportional to the number of protons at a position to the right of center, shaded black in Figure 43–3*B*. Thus, the amplitude of the signal at a frequency *f* Hz away from central magnet frequency (γB_0) is proportional to the number of spins at location x_f, where

$$x_f = \frac{f}{\gamma G}$$

To put real numbers in these equations, a typical transaxial

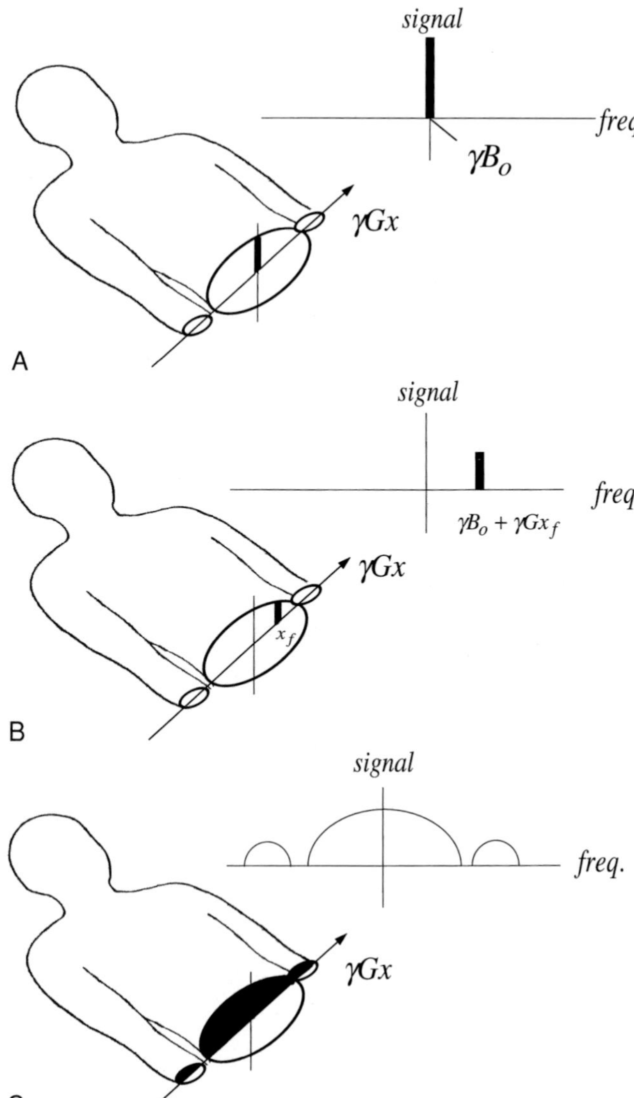

FIGURE 43–3. Frequency encoding. In the presence of a magnetic-field gradient, the different protons precess at different frequencies, depending on their position. The number of protons at different positions along the field gradients changes the intensity of the signal at each frequency. *A,* The protons at $x = 0$ precess at the Larmor frequency of the magnet, because $\gamma Gx = 0$. *B,* Because there are fewer protons at $x = x_f$, the signal at γGx_f is smaller than that in *A. C,* The composite signal from all the spins forms a projection of the object.

cardiac image might be taken with G = 7 mT/m. In the presence of this gradient, protons shifted 0.1 m (10 cm) to the right of center would precess at a frequency equal to (42.58 MHz/T) × (0.007 T/m) × (0.1 m), which equals 30 KHz.

The result of listening to *all* the frequencies is shown in Figure 43–3*C*. Because the signal at each frequency is proportional to the number of protons at that frequency, we see that a plot of the spectrum (i.e., a graph of amplitude versus frequency) is precisely a projection of the body along the *frequency-encoded direction.*

How do we listen to multiple frequencies simultaneously? Although humans can do this innately (listening to music, for example), the computer relies on a tool called the *Fourier transform,* or *FT.* The FT converts a time-varying signal into the frequencies that make it up. Thus, the time-varying signal that is produced by all the protons of a slice of the body precessing in the presence of the frequency-encoding gradient are decoded into its component frequencies by using the FT. The result of FT acting on this time data is a projection.

Figure 43–4 shows the pulse sequence, including frequency encoding. Two new channels are shown: G_r, depicting the presence of the frequency-encoding gradient, and data acquisition (DAQ), which defines when the scanner is listening to the protons' signals. This gradient is often called G_f (for "frequency-encode") or, as we have done here, G_r (for "read" gradients, because it "reads out" the spatially encoded information), or sometimes simply G_x.

K-Space Point of View

Although the frequency spectrum description of frequency encoding is the easiest to understand, there is an alternative way of thinking of the action of this gradient. This other description, although a little more abstract, is more useful when we add the third direction of spatial encoding.

The previous section described the NMR signal in the presence of the frequency-encoding gradient in terms of its frequency content: the spectrum *is* the projection. In this section, the actual time-domain signal will be described in greater detail.

Recall from the previous section that the protons are represented by a magnetization vector, and it is only the sum of these vectors that is ultimately detected. When adding vectors together, both the magnitude and the direction of the vectors matter. The *phase* of the vector is used interchangeably with the term "direction" when one is describing the transverse component of the magnetization vector. The whole idea of frequency encoding is to make the phase of protons different in different parts of the scanner at different times.

Most of the following discussion uses the simple model shown in Figure 43–5. Imagine eight groups of protons, equally spaced, and follow their transverse magnetization, shown as arrows on a clock face. The only signal that one can detect in MRI is the vector sum of all these arrows, which is made by placing the arrows sequentially tip to tail.

After excitation, all the spins are lined up, producing the maximal signal possible (point A in Fig. 43–5*A*). When the frequency-encoding gradient is turned on, the spins start to precess at different frequencies. As a result, the vector sum starts to decrease immediately and irreversibly (point B in Fig. 43–5*A*). Eventually, all the spins are out of phase, and the signal diminishes to zero (point C in Fig. 43–5*A*). Imagine, instead, that the initial spins were arranged as shown in Figure 43–5*B*, so that every other spin was absent. Although there would be a big initial peak at the

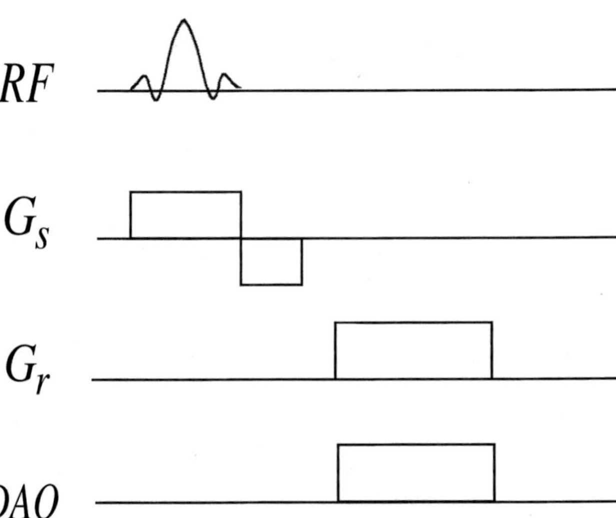

FIGURE 43–4. Pulse sequence diagram including frequency encoding. Continuation of Figure 43–2, now including frequency encoding. After selectively exciting the slab of protons (RF + G_s), a gradient in an orthogonal direction (G_r) produces a frequency-based projection of the object, which is the Fourier transform of the signal acquired during data acquisition (DAQ).

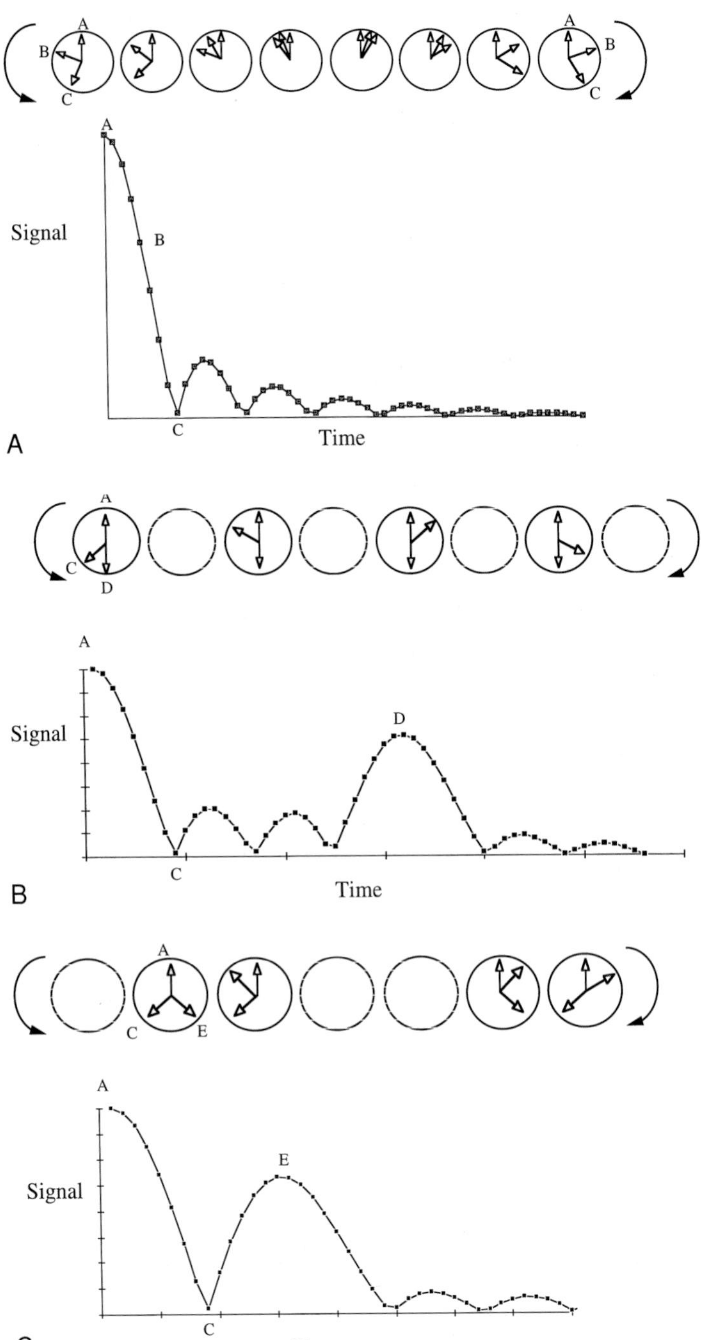

FIGURE 43–5. Frequency encoding and K-space. This figure demonstrates how frequency encoding can be thought of as encoding periodicity, or spatial frequency. *A*, Eight groups of spins in the presence of a frequency-encoding gradient. The gradient is such that the leftmost spins precess counterclockwise most rapidly, and the rightmost spins precess clockwise most rapidly. The signal is greatest when all the spins are lined up (A). As they begin to precess, they lose coherence, and their vector sum diminishes (B). Finally, at time C the net sum is zero. *B*, When every other spin is absent, the signal still goes to zero at point C. However, there is a second maximum, at point D, when the remaining spins come back into phase again. In *C*, which is less "wavy" than *B*, the spins come back into focus sooner.

beginning of frequency encoding, we also see that there would be a second peak at a later time as well. In this case, the spins all line up at 6 o'clock, although they have reached this point by very different paths. For example, the leftmost spins have gone nearly four full times around, whereas the spins nearest the middle have just gone around one-half turn. Why did we not get this peak in Figure 43–5*A*? Because although each of the spins present in Figure 43–5*B* is at 6 o'clock, each of the missing spins would have been at 12 o'clock, so that the net sum of all these spins would be zero. Thus, in Figure 43–5*B* this second peak occurs precisely because the would-be canceling spins are absent. In the third case, shown in Figure 43–5*C*, with an intermediate *spatial periodicity*, the second peak occurs somewhat earlier than that of Figure 43–5*B*. It appears that the frequency-encoding gradient produces signals in time that are related to the spatial gridding of the object. The more rapidly the spin density varies across the object, the later in time the second peak occurs. Thus, the gradient encodes the *spatial frequency* (i.e., periodicity) of the object.

This way of looking at frequency encoding is the exact parallel to the one described in the previous section, and both are correct. In the previous section, we found that the frequency-encoding gradient produced a spectrum of frequencies that represents the projection of the object. In this section, we found that the gradient also produces a signal that represents a projection of the spatial frequencies of the object. The FT mathematically explains the parallelism. Just as the FT of the signal provides its spectrum, the FT of an object provides its spatial frequencies. The description of an object in terms of its spatial frequencies is directly analogous to the description of a time-varying signal in terms of its component frequencies and accurately describes the MRI encoding process. This description, called the *K-space* formalism (e.g., Twieg[3]), helps explain MR image formation. For example, we see in Figure 43–5 that the *center of K-space* (the early time points) contains the information about the most slowly varying part of the object. The *edge of K-space* (the end time points) contains the information about the spatially most quickly varying parts of the object, in the sense that the object in Figure 43–5*B* varies more quickly than that in Figure 43–5*C*, which in turn varies more quickly than that in Figure 43–5*A*. The *resolution* (i.e., how well we can resolve spatial variation in the object) is thus equal to the distance out in K-space that we encoded. That is, the longer the gradient is on, or the greater its amplitude, the farther out in K-space we encode, and the greater the resolutions of the encoded MR image. Notice that this resolution does not depend on the static magnetic field and, thus, on the wavelength of the MRI radio waves. It is the parametrically encoded frequencies that give us resolution. As alluded to earlier, this parametrization is what sets MRI apart from other imaging modalities.

Phase Encoding

To finish the third direction of encoding, we cannot reuse the trick of frequency encoding. Adding another gradient in the orthogonal direction at the same time does not produce two dimensions of encoding: it simply frequency-encodes along the direction of the vector sum of the encoding gradients. However, there is a way we can use the phase of MR signal to encode the third direction. The K-space formalism above lets us think about this phase encoding quite simply.

We saw earlier that the effect of the applied gradient was to "move out" to a new position in K-space. In the frequency-encoding gradient, we continuously move across K-space because we have a gradient continuously applied. However, continuity is not required. For example, consider the situation shown in Figure 43–6. This figure shows signal from the same configuration of spins as that in Figure 43–5*B*. Instead of continuously applying the gradient, imagine that we stop the gradient at several points, as shown in Figure 43–6*A*. The protons will have evolved the same amount as in the continuously applied gradient case and, because there are no other fields present during the "off" periods in Figure 43–6*A*, the phase of the protons does not evolve during the off states. In fact, instead of encoding all the spatial frequencies during one excitation, we could even encode them across different excitations, as shown in Figure 43–6*B*. The key is to make sure that we end up acquiring the data on subsequent excitations at the correct spot in K-space. In Figure 43–6*B* we do this by changing the duration of gradient, but because all that matters is the phase of the protons' evolution, we could do this equally well by changing the amplitude, as shown in Figure 43–6*C*. In fact, the method sketched in Figure 43–6*C* is exactly how we perform the third dimension of spatial encoding: before the frequency encoding in the perpendicular direction, we phase-encode the signals to move each subsequent acquisition to a different part of K-space in the orthogonal direction.

A simplified 4 × 4 image acquisition is shown in Figure 43–7, adding in the new channel, called G_p, which is also called G_y in some references. Phase and frequency encoding are entirely parallel. The only difference is that phase evolves continuously in the frequency-encoding direction and in jerks along the phase-encoding direction. However, in both directions the information obtained at any given time is simply the spatial-frequency content of the object at that time, which is provided by the area under the gradient up to that time in each direction. A two-dimensional FT then takes this two-dimensional K-space information and produces the MR tomogram.

A "real" pulse sequence is shown in Figure 43–8*A*. There are two slight differences from what was shown previously. First, as a notational convenience, the phase-encoding gradient is shown as a multilevel block to represent its changes from excitation to excitation. The second is the addition of a *pre-encoding* pulse in the frequency-encoding channel before the actual frequency encoding. Most sequences use this offset so that the center of K-space is actually in the middle of the acquisition period, rather than at its edge. This shift is technically important, because it makes the images less sensitive to a variety of machine and body imperfections but does not change the concepts discussed earlier. The sequence shown in Figure 43–8 is a *gradient echo* sequence, which simply encodes the free-induction decay of the spins. By adding a 180-degree pulse before the readout, we would produce a *spin echo* sequence. The spin echo is coincident with the center of K-space for the spatial encoding. As described in the previous chapter, these sequences have different kinds of contrast, which are used for different applications in cardiac MRI.

Multislice Imaging

We saw earlier that multiple excitations are required to produce an MR image. As we saw in the previous chapter, the time between these excitations, *TR*, is a critical determinant of T1 contrast. Choosing TR ≤ T1 produces T1 weighting; TR >> T1 eliminates T1 weighting. In the heart, T1 ~ 800 msec, so to produce a 256 × 256 image requires at least 4 minutes, most of which is dead time between excitations. One useful way of spending this dead time is with the excitation of other slices. Because slice selection excites only those spins within one plane, the other spins are still available for imaging. The frequency and phase encoding do nothing to spins that are not excited (i.e., still longitudinal), so that the interleaved imaging of multiple slices is straightforward in MRI. This process is shown schematically in Figure 43–9. As we saw earlier, by changing the center frequency of the excitation pulse, different locations within the body are excited. In this way, the time to acquire many slices is the same as the time to acquire a single plane in the body.

Instrumentation for MRI

An MR scanner consists of many subsystems, orchestrated together precisely to produce diagnostic images. The primary systems are (1) a large magnet for polarizing the protons, (2) radiofrequency systems to excite and detect the protons, (3) gradient systems to provide the temporally and spatially varying magnetic fields for encoding, (4) a control computer for coordinating the various subsystems, and (5) an interface computer for setting up, displaying, and filming the results.

Magnets

A wide variety of magnets are used for MRI, with widely varying field strength, cost, and siting requirements. These magnets range from relatively low-field (0.064 to 0.2 T) permanent or electromagnets, which are relatively compact, to research behemoths at very high fields (4.0 T). However, the bulk of clinical work is currently performed between 0.5 and 1.5 T, primarily in superconducting magnet solenoids.

The sole purpose of the magnet is to produce a magnetic field large enough to align enough of the protons so that clinically useful images can be produced in a reasonable time. Despite this simple purpose, it remains the most costly single element of a commercial scanner and is ultimately the source of many of MRI's inconveniences.

Superconductors

It was realized early in the commercialization of MRI that the combination of high magnetic fields and large volume access needed for human imaging could be efficiently generated with superconducting technology. This is the case primarily because the power and cooling requirements for conventional electromagnets scale at least as the square of the magnetic field, and the stable generation of fields above 0.5 T, using either electromagnets or conventional magnets across a 1-m bore (large enough for a human), seemed unattainable. Superconducting wire, on the other hand, had been successfully used to produce small-bore (i.e., test tube–sized) analytical instruments for years. Superconductors, once energized, require no additional power to keep the current flowing in them, as long as their temperature is kept low enough. This temperature, however, is very low (about the temperature of deep outer space), and thus the magnets require, with only very recent

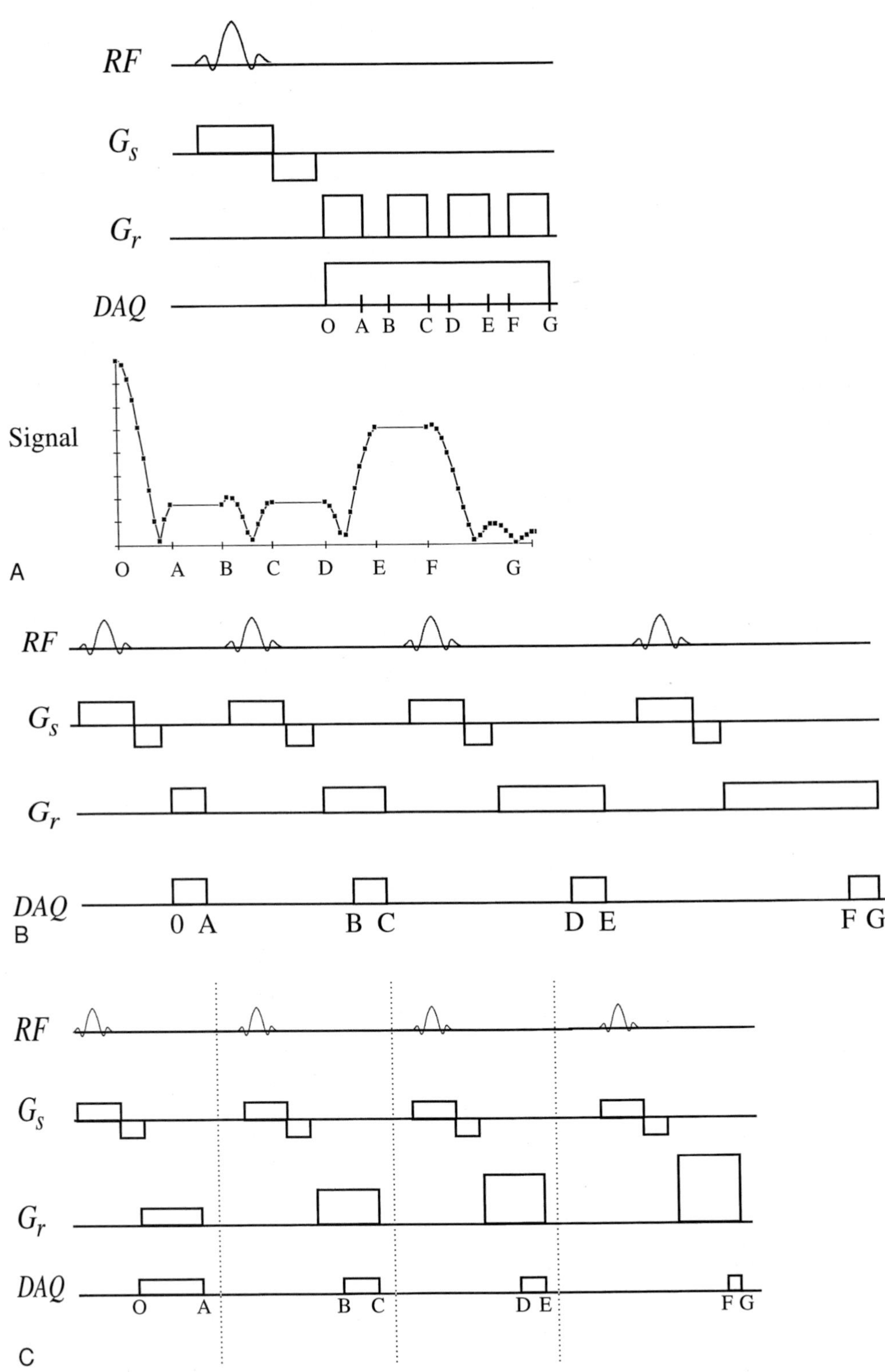

FIGURE 43–6. Discontinuous frequency encoding. This figure demonstrates that frequency encoding does not have to be continuous to have its desired effect. *A*, The pulse sequence and signal from the same configuration as in *B* but with multiple interruptions of the frequency-encoding gradient at time points A, C, and E is shown. The signal, and thus its trek across K-space, simply stop evolving when the gradients are turned off. *B*, A second kind of discontinuity, this time across excitations, is shown. Because the data acquisition (DAQ) is "on" during the same gradient histories as those in *A*, the signal is the same. Finally, in *C* the amplitude of the gradient is changed, rather than its duration. Because the net phase accumulated depends on the product of amplitude and time, the same signal as in *B* is produced.

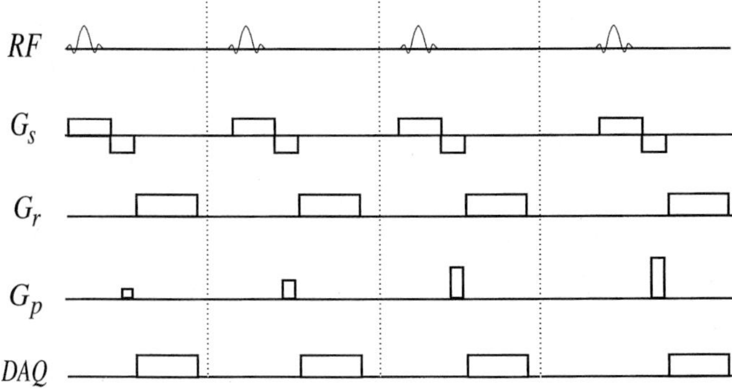

FIGURE 43–7. Image acquisition 4 × 4. This figure shows the sequence of pulses required to obtain a 4 × 4 image, covering the two dimensions of K-space, required to make a two-dimensional image. The frequency encoding (G_r) is the same for all four excitations, but the amplitudes in the phase-encoding direction (G_p) are progressively stepped to trace out a two-dimensional square in K-space.

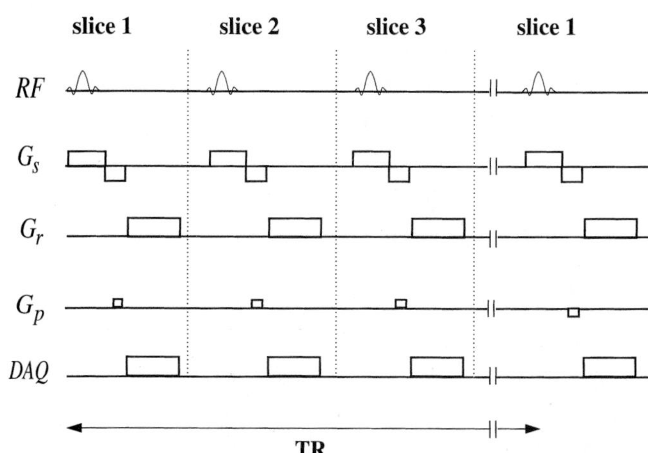

FIGURE 43–9. Multislice diagram. Many slices can often be imaged in the same length of time required to image one slice. Because the RF pulses are slice selective, they only minimally affect protons in other planes. As a result, adjacent slices can be imaged in the time between excitations (TR).

exceptions, cryogens to keep them cold, primarily helium or helium and nitrogen that have been liquefied.

Although this technology may seem exotic, the actual cost of cryogens and special superconducting materials is many times below the cost of power that would be required to run an electromagnet of the same field strength. In addition, as magnet construction and cooling technology become more and more advanced, cryogen consumption has become less and less a major cost in the operation of an MRI system.

The "standard" cylindrical-bore magnet is illustrated in Figure 43–10. The superconducting coils are arranged around the bore to make the most homogeneous field possible in the middle of the bore. The necessary uniformity of the field depends on how the scanner is used. Ultimately, poor uniformity produces poor images. For example, frequency encoding assumes that the static magnetic field is perfectly uniform, because it assumes that the only frequency differences between protons comes from the applied gradients. An error in magnetic field of ΔB produces a positional error of $\Delta B/G$, where G is the applied frequency-encoding gradient. Thus, in the presence of a gradient 7 mT/m, a nonuniformity of 7 μT translates into a 1-mm positional error. The degree of nonuniformity of the magnetic field is usually referred to colloquially as the *shim* of the magnet. For imaging purposes at 1.5 T, a shim of 5 ppm (i.e., 7.5 μT) would produce images with less than 1 mm of absolute positional error with the gradient described earlier. Spectroscopic applications (the use of nonwater protons and other MR-visible nuclei) or fat suppression can require much better homogeneity.

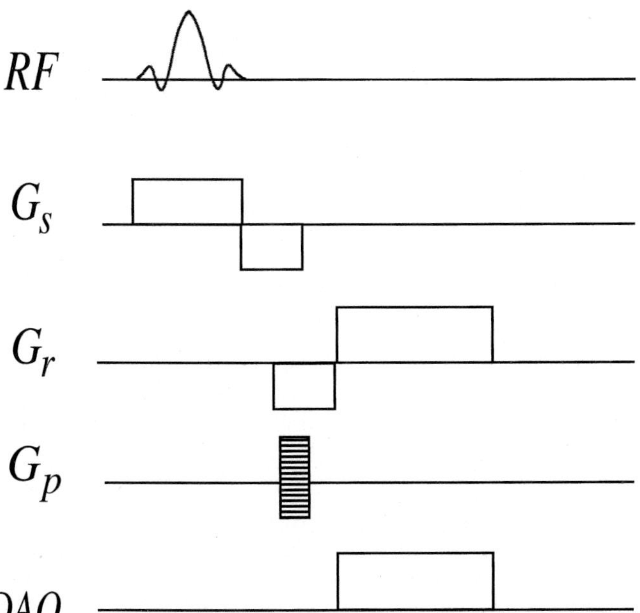

FIGURE 43–8. Full pulse sequence. Figure shows the pulse diagram for a gradient echo sequence. Pre-encoding lobes have been added for symmetric acquisitions.

Magnet Safety

The safety of MRI is always a topic of concern, especially because of the relative lack of known biologic effects of MRI. Although the specific concerns of safety are beyond the scope of this chapter (the interested reader should see reference 4), the largest source of hazard comes not from the imaging process but from the static field itself. The basic physics of magnetic fields makes it impossible to generate a completely contained magnetic field that has practical access for a patient. As a result, the field itself spills out from the scanner and into the scan room and beyond. Although this field itself does not present a known hazard to normal tissue, it can provide a potent hazard both for patients with implanted devices (i.e., pacemakers and neurostimulators are affected by even a weak magnetic field) and for the unwary scan room invader. The strong magnetic-field gradients attract ferromagnetic materials, and this attraction progresses, in the space of a few centimeters, from a small tug to an irresistible force. These fields are dangerous for patients with foreign objects either purposely placed (e.g., magnetic prostheses, heart valves) or accidentally acquired (shrapnel, metalworking shavings), as well as via the potentially lethal introduction of large metal objects (e.g., ladders, mops, screwdrivers) into the scan room by unwary staff. These dangers exist for scanners of all field strengths, and lower field strength magnets are not necessarily safer magnets, especially when safety precautions are lax around them. The field strength of a "low"-field scanner is still 1000 times the strength of the earth's field and, thus, is beyond the usual range of experience for most visitors.

Radiofrequency and Gradient Systems

After the magnet system, the next most specialized systems for MRI are the RF and gradient systems for exciting, detecting, and encoding the MR signals. Although these systems are specially engineered for MRI, they bear many similarities to technology used in other applications. For example, the RF systems are similar to those used for AM and amateur radio, and the gradient systems (at least the amplifiers) are similar to those used for high-power hi-fi systems.

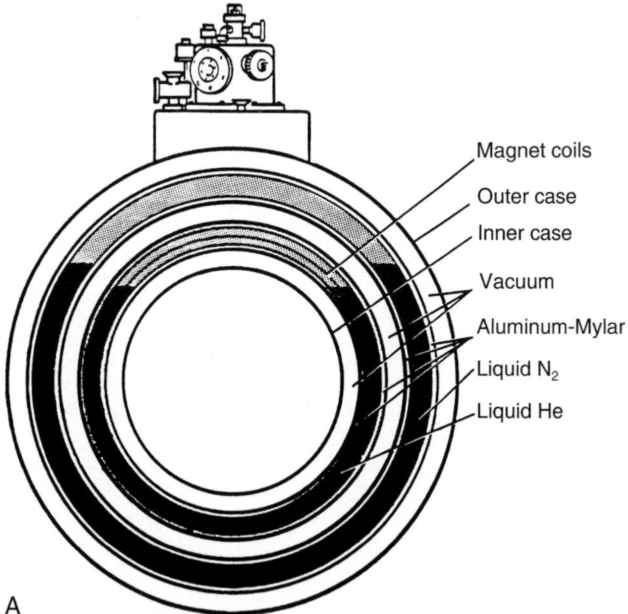

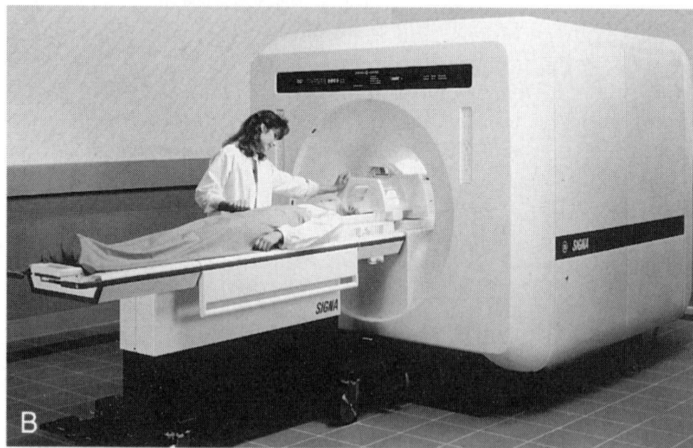

FIGURE 43–10. MRI magnet. *A* shows the cross-section of a typical superconducting solenoidal magnet. A liquid helium reservoir is used to cool the superconducting magnet coils that surround the patient bore. Although a liquid nitrogen reservoir is shown in this example, this portion is often replaced by a larger helium reservoir and an external compressor for additional refrigeration. *B* shows a typical MRI scanner; the cylindrical magnet is enclosed in the large box on the right. (Illustration courtesy of General Electric Medical Systems.)

Radiofrequency

The RF system needs both to transmit energy into the body and to detect the precessing protons after they have been excited. The site of both transmission and reception is a coil (or pair of coils) inside the magnet, surrounding the body. Like the protons themselves, this *RF coil* is tuned to resonate at the Larmor frequency of the magnet. The coil is sometimes called an "antenna," but this nomenclature is somewhat confusing. MRI takes place on distance scales that are short compared to the RF wavelength of the radio waves used, so that the normal antenna theory is inappropriate for MRI. Often, the same RF coil is used both to transmit the RF and to receive it after transmission. (An exception is "surface coils," described later.) However, the power differences are quite dramatic in these two modes. For example, at 1.5 T the body coil requires up to 20 kW of peak RF power on transmission. Most of this power, however, is lost in the patient's body. The power received from the nutating protons can be less than 1 mW, roughly five orders of magnitude smaller. As a result, several of the parts of the RF system play the important role of isolating the transmission side from the reception side, so that none of the many kilowatts going into the coil show up across the sensitive amplifier, whose function it is to make detectable the relatively feeble MR signal.

A simplified version of the RF chain is sketched in Figure 43–11. Going from left to right on that figure, the *modulator* takes the precision RF frequency source (near the Larmor frequency) and performs the waveform shaping required to produce, for example, slice-selection pulses. This low-power wave is then augmented through the *RF amplifier.* (This amplifier is usually enabled only during the actual excitation epochs to minimize the amount of spurious saturation caused by the transmitter.) The amplified wave is then fed through an *RF enclosure (or screen room),* designed to minimize leakage of extraneous noise both into and out of the RF coils and into a transmit-receive switch *(T/R switch),* whose function is to protect the sensitive output circuitry during high-power transmission. This switch is coupled to the *RF coil.* On reception, the T/R switch couples the RF coil (which is now listening) to the *preamplifier,* which takes the very low level signal and amplifies it sufficiently so as to take it out of the RF enclosure and into a *demodulator,* which takes the phase- and frequency-encoded MR signal back down to near audiofrequencies, where it is detected with the use of a set of analog-to-digital converters. Although the ultimate output of the system is digital, because a computer is ultimately responsible for the FT required for image generation and display, and the actual proton signal itself is an analog signal, other parts of the system can be either digital or analog. As a general rule, the fewer analog components the system has, the more drift- and instability-resistant it is, although there are plenty of exceptions to this rule.

Gradients

As we saw earlier, the crux of imaging is the encoding gradients. The actual devices used to create the magnetic field gradients are complex patterns of wire, whose ultimate aim is the generation of a magnetic field whose components vary in a very predictable way, approximating a pure magnetic-field gradient in the desired direction.

The *gradient coils* themselves, like the magnet, are large inductors. Unlike the case with the magnet, however, the resistance of the wires of the gradient coils is relatively unimportant. That is because, unlike the main magnet, the primary functions of the gradients is to change their field over time, as diagrammed in the pulse sequence. To see the relevance of the inductance and resistance of these coils, consider implementing the sequence described in Figure 43–8. For a typical scanner, the frequency-encoding period is about 10 msec. To get the 7 mT/m described in the example provided earlier usually requires about 70 A. For a coil resistance of 1/2 ohm, this represents about 1.2 kW of power. However, to switch 70 A through the coil involves putting voltage across the inductor: $V = L\ di/dt$, where L is the inductance of the coil. For a typical 1-mH coil, switching in 0.5 msec requires about 140 V. At peak, this switching requires a linear amplifier capable of producing 10 kW. Even with the use of switching-amplifier technology, the large voltage swing during ramping far exceeds the voltages required during the flat encoding period. As a result, minimizing the resistance of these coils beyond a certain point seems too costly to be effective.

These coils are driven by audio amplifiers, called *gradient amplifiers,* which most resemble very high-end stereo amplifiers. (This is not surprising, given that the gradient coil in the magnet bears some resemblance to a high-fidelity speaker.) The amplifiers or the coils, or the combination, can be referred to as the "gradients," depending on the context.

Gradient system performance usually directly affects the flexibility of an MRI system, in terms of minimum echo time, maximum number of slices per time, and so forth. The two most often quoted specifications are the maximum *gradient strength* (i.e., the maximum mT/m the system can generate, which translates, for a fixed encoding period, to maximum resolution or minimum TE) and minimum *rise time* to that strength. Cardiac, ventricular, and great vessel imaging are particularly demanding MRI tasks, primar-

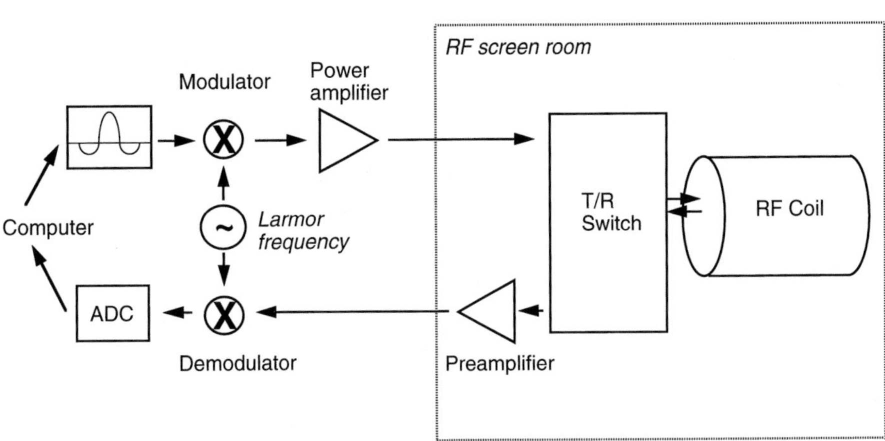

FIGURE 43–11. RF chain. Schematized block diagram of RF signal paths. Clockwise from the top right: the RF pulse shape (for slice selection) is generated by a pulse sequencer at audio frequencies, is modulated up to the (RF) Larmor frequency of the magnet, and is then amplified to create enough power to excite the spins in the body. This amplified signal is brought into the (RF-shielded) scan room and passed through a transmit-receive switch (T/R switch) that, under computer control, sends the RF power to the RF coil. The (much smaller) detected NMR signal is sent back to the T/R switch and, when excitation is completed, is provided to the input of the sensitive preamplifier. The T/R switch thus protects the preamplifier from the high-power transmitted pulses. This signal is ultimately demodulated back near audiofrequency, converted to digital data with the use of an analog-to-digital converter (ADC), and is sent back to the computer for analysis.

ily because of the difficulty in imaging moving systems. Gradient systems come in two types: shielded and unshielded, which refer the presence or absence of a second set of gradient coils, located radially outside the first, whose job it is to prevent a changing magnetic field from reaching the magnet itself.

Computer and Workstations

Because the generation of the MR images, like x-ray computed axial tomography scanning, is primarily a form of computed tomography, it comes as no surprise that computers form a crucial piece of the imaging technology. In addition to central imaging processing (the FT that converts the phase- and frequency-encoded K-space data into an MR image), computers orchestrate the control of scanner components, interact with the technologist running the instrument, and control the display and archiving of the resulting medical images. However, despite this central role, the computer hardware in MRI systems is, unlike the components described earlier, relatively unspecialized, which is because the general flexibility of computers allows the creation of specialized software that can be used on a variety of hardware systems. However, the creation of the software required for commercial scanners is a huge task and consumes a large fraction of the manufacturers' ongoing costs in their MRI systems.

The most recent crop of MRI scanners is moving more and more from the previous generation of minicomputers to workstation-like platforms, such as those used in hospitals and in industry for general high-performance computing. The relative increase in the performance-to-price ratios of these workstations is allowing for increasingly powerful image-processing tools to become easily implementable on MRI scanners. These implementations will be particularly relevant for cardiac MRI, for which sophisticated ray-tracing programs and automatic segmentation are likely to be critical to the more widely spread use of cardiac MRI, as such technology seems to be required for unsupervised extraction of clinically useful parameters (e.g., ejection fraction, myocardial mass, coronary artery angiograms) from cardiac MRI data.

SPECIAL INSTRUMENTATION FOR CARDIAC MAGNETIC RESONANCE IMAGING

In addition to the technology described for conventional MR imaging, cardiac MRI has special demands that require modifications in either hardware or software (pulse sequences) to image the heart and the great arteries. These technologies have been designed to deal with the two aspects of the heart that are, of course, critical to its function: beats and its ejectate flows. These motions take place on a time scale (60 to 100 times per minute) that is very fast relative to the time required to make an MR image (1 to 8 minutes). As a result, strategies for imaging the moving organ and moving blood have been developed. These strategies have two general approaches: hardware tricks for making the heart appear frozen, and software tricks to minimize the effects of motion that cannot be eliminated.

Cardiac Gating

The principal technique that has allowed NMR imaging of the heart is "cardiac gating," or the synchronization of the MR acquisitions to the cardiac cycle. The idea is the same as stroboscopic photography: by repetitively catching the same portion of the cardiac cycle, the phase-encoding process appropriately catches the heart, as if it were frozen. Figure 43–12 illustrates the timing of this process. As is shown in Figure 43–12*A*, each successive phase-encoded line is acquired at the same portion of the cardiac cycle. Multislice imaging is possible, although each slice is, of necessity, at a different phase of the cardiac cycle. Typically, 8 to 12 phases can be achieved in a single RR interval. Typical images with and without cardiac gating are shown in Figure 43–12*B* and *C*, respectively. As might be expected, the absence of cardiac triggering smears the heart unrecognizably.

Depending on the patient's rhythm, cardiac imaging can take either about the same time or somewhat longer than nongated imaging. For example, for a patient with a heart rate of 72 beats per minute, a 256 × 256 image, gated every heartbeat, will require about 4 minutes.

Arrhythmia and Gating

In practice, cardiac images seldom have the same, consistent image quality as scans of the brain. The three primary reasons for this inconsistency are a poorer signal-to-noise ratio, cardiac arrhythmia, and respiratory artifact. The signal-to-noise problems (especially compared with joint and central nervous system imaging) are dictated by the physics of MRI. The location of the heart centrally in the body, especially so in the larger patients that often make up the cardiac patient population, renders ineffective many of the tricks of clinical MRI, although some improvements are possible with the use of surface coils (see later text). Respiratory problems, too, can be handled in a variety of ways that have met with variable success in cardiac MRI, primarily because of the long acquisition times required. (See section on respiratory gating and respiratory-ordered phase encoding.) However, the problems attributable to arrhythmia, and even to normal beat-to-beat variations in cardiac cycle, are easy to understand.

The difficulty with RR variations is primarily a problem of variable T1 relaxation. Recall from the previous chapter that T1, or longitudinal relaxation time, is the period required for the protons, once put in a magnetic field, to reach 63 percent of their equilibrium magnetization. This is the same amount of time that it takes the spins, once excited to encode one line of K-space, to return to equilibrium. At 1.5 T, the T1 of the heart is roughly 800 msec, or comparable to the RR interval. As a result, when gating every RR interval, variations in the RR interval translate directly into variations in the magnetization available for each line of K-space. This variation is shown graphically in Figure 43–13. In this figure, we show how percent variability in the cardiac cycle translates into amplitude variations in the magnetization for imaging every, every other, and every third RR interval. Recall from the description of

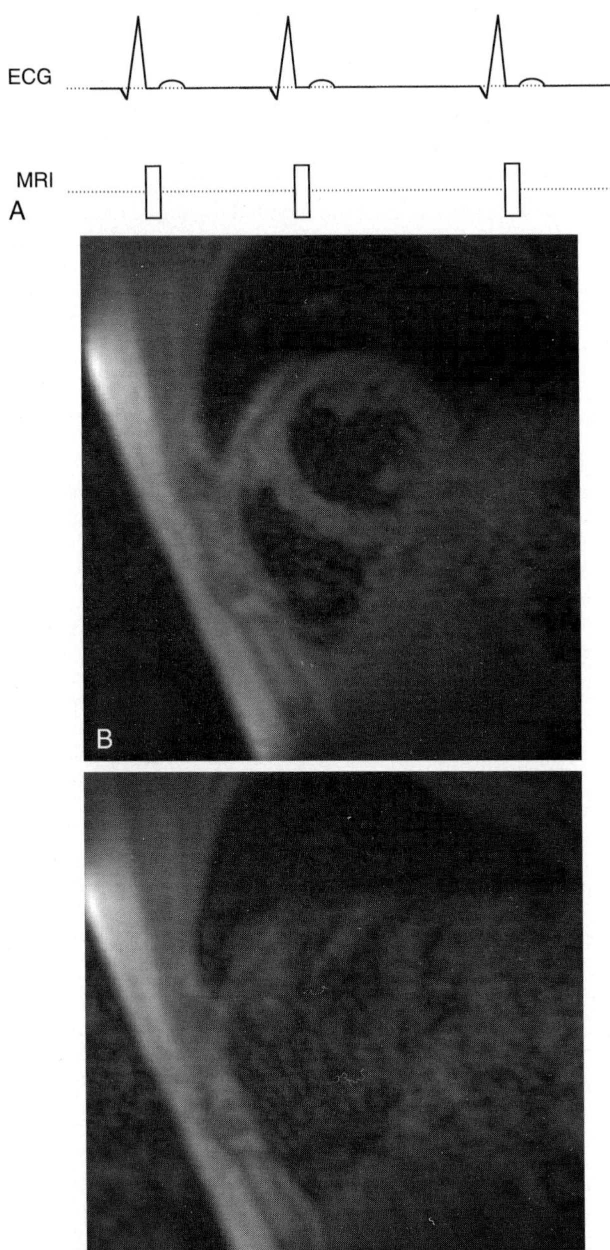

FIGURE 43–12. Cardiac gating. Cardiac images may be created by taking a normal imaging sequence (e.g., that in Fig. 43–9), triggering the beginning of each phase-encoded line to the same phase of the ECG signal. *A*, Schematic timing diagram, in which each box represents one phase-encoded acquisition (e.g., see Fig. 43–8) for a given slice. Multiple slices can be acquired, but each will be at a different phase of the cardiac cycle. *B*, Example of a gated, spin echo acquisition. *C*, Ungated acquisition in the same patient.

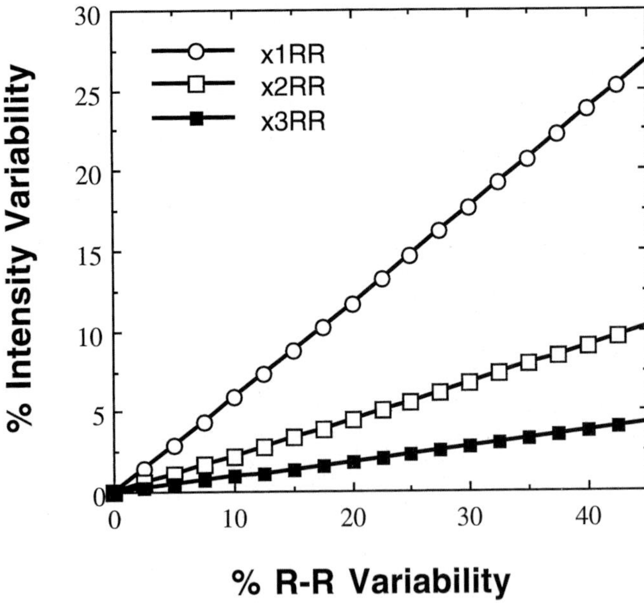

FIGURE 43–13. Cardiac cycle variability and MR image artifact. Cardiac cycle variability causes TR to fluctuate during image acquisition. Because T1 ~ RR interval, this variability leads to fluctuations in the heart magnetization and thus produces image artifacts. Imaging across several heartbeats reduces this T1 effect, although it also eliminates T1 contrast.

the imaging techniques above that each line of K-space is supposed to represent a separate encoding of the same object. When the intensity of the line of K-space changes with every excitation, the resulting image reconstruction is corrupted. The extent of this corruption depends on the degree of variability. It is easy to see that imaging every third interval all but eliminates this problem, and with cooperative patients it produces excellent results (see Fig. 43–14*A*). However, this multiplies the duration of the scan to unwieldy 12- to 18-minute lengths. In practice, rather than going to multiple RR gating, a more commonly used technique is to acquire multiple averages at a single RR interval. Because each acquisition is likely to have a different rate of arrhythmia, the variable timing of the cardiac cycle tends to average out, reducing the amount of image artifact. However, the duration of imaging is still quite long in these studies, averaging 10 to 12 minutes for a 192 × 256 image set, and can produce some blurring, as compared with the cross-RR study (see Fig. 43–14*B*).

Cine Acquisition

Whereas gating allows for single-phase imaging of multiple slices of the heart, imaging multiple phases of the same slice requires use of a different technique. Simply gating with short times (~50 msec) between acquisitions after each trigger to attempt multiphase, single-slice imaging exacerbates the timing problem described earlier, because the intensity of variations depends on T1/TR: the shorter the TR, the worse the problem.

Instead of multiple gating, a different technique was developed, called cine imaging (e.g., see reference 5). The idea is not to gate the acquisitions but rather to record the ECG signal and then phase-encode with sufficient density through the cardiac cycle to create, at the end of acquisition, a sampling of K-space sufficiently dense to reconstruct an image at each phase of the cardiac cycle. Because all the data are taken with a fixed TR, the magnetization reaches a steady state, and amplitude variations are eliminated. However, because the cardiac cycle varies throughout the acquisition, extra imaging time is required to obtain dense enough sampling of K-space. An example of cine images is shown in Figure 43–15.

The image contrast of cine acquisitions is different from that of

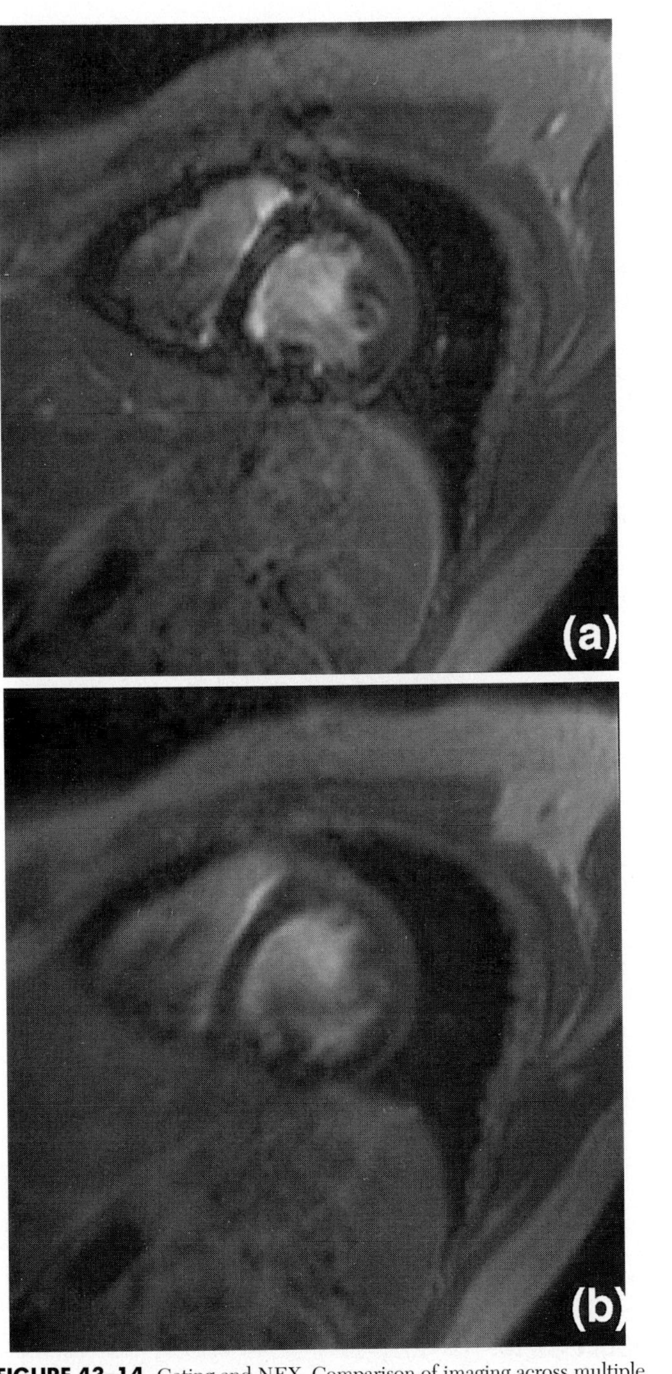

FIGURE 43–14. Gating and NEX. Comparison of imaging across multiple R waves. In the presence of RR variability, both strategies produce acceptable images of the heart. *A*, Each line of K-space is acquired every third heartbeat. *B*, Three averages, imaging every R wave. In this example, the cooperative patient was able to gate his breathing to the scanner in *A*, breathing every third heartbeat. As a result, *A* is also sharper due to the absence of respiratory blurring. These are spin echo images, using flow compensation (see Fig. 43–16), which makes the ventricular chamber bright.

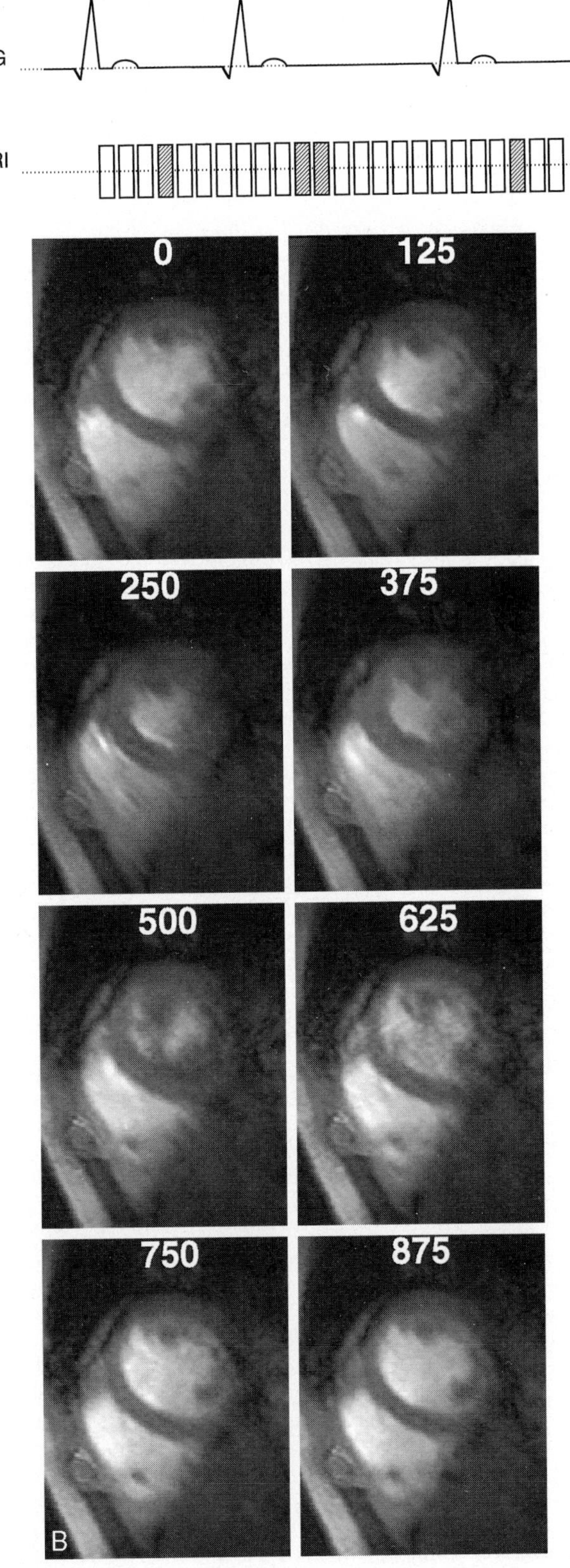

FIGURE 43–15. Cine cardiac imaging. *A*, Timing schematic for cine imaging. The imager scans continuously, acquiring the same line of K-space across the cardiac cycle before advancing to the next phase-encoding line. After acquisition, the data are binned with respect to the R wave, and with the use of interpolation when necessary, complete images can be reconstructed for each cardiac phase. For example, the shaded acquisitions may be used in the formation of a mid-diastolic image. *B*, Eight images from a typical cine acquisition. The images are labeled by their delay after R wave in milliseconds. Ventricular signal is typically bright on these images. Total acquisition time = 7 minutes.

the gated acquisitions, as can be seen from the comparison of Figures 43–13 and 43–15. The primary reason for these differences is the effect of flowing spins on image contrast. The short-TR gradient echo images are very T1-weighted: the flow of blood refreshes the apparent magnetization in these voxels, and thus blood appears bright. In the absence of flow, blood has a T1 that is somewhat longer than that of the myocardium. It is this flow-weighting that allows for the differentiation between the false and the true lumen in aortic dissections (e.g., see reference 6). The flow weighting has been used to advantage for cine imaging of the disordered flow that occurs both distal and proximal to valve stenoses (e.g., see reference 7). Cine-imaging techniques have been applied to imaging both the heart and the great vessels. However, in cases in which flowing blood is the important property, another methodologic trick has been used: flow compensation.

Flow Compensation

Because MR imaging depends sensitively on the phase of the protons to create an image, phenomena that affect the phase of the protons affect the quality of the images. The most common perturber of this phase is simple motion of spins in the presence of the imaging gradients. *Gradient moment nulling* has proved a useful technique for reducing the phase changes of these moving spins.

Refer back to Figure 43–8, and imagine a proton moving at velocity v in the left ventricle in the direction of the frequency-encoding gradient, G. In the time Δt between the pre-encode gradient and the read gradient, the protons will have moved some distance, $v\Delta t$. This displacement translates into a phase difference of $\gamma G(v\Delta t)\ \Delta t$. Notice that this velocity-induced phase increases as the velocity increases, and as the time Δt increases. If the velocity were the same on every excitation, the phase difference would have minimal impact and just show as a translation of the proton to a position $x \rightarrow x + v\Delta t$. Because phase encoding occurs earlier, there is no shift in this direction. As a result, flow along vessels oblique to the frequency-phase-encoding plane will have their spins displaced out of the vessel. However, either changes in velocity over time, or variations of velocity within the imaging voxel, will translate these phase differences directly into image artifact.

When the velocity changes over time, which it always does in the disordered flow near a stenosis or strong curvature, such as in the ascending aorta, the phase errors translate into smearing in the phase-encoding direction. The smearing goes in this direction because the *phase* of each proton is different from excitation to excitation and thus interferes with the phase-encoding process, which attempts to establish a specific phase evolution.

When the velocity, and thus the phase, varies within a voxel, because of swirling flow in ventricles or parabolic flow in the vessels, then the MR signal is disturbed even before it can be used for phase encoding. The relationship of this *intravoxel dephasing* to signal loss can be complex (e.g., see reference 8), but it is generally true that more phase variation tends to lead to more image artifact.

A way of reducing both velocity-induced phase shifts is with gradient moment nulling,[9] essentially rearranging the imaging gradients so that they have the same imaging effect but minimizing the velocity-induced phase shifts. The simplest version is illustrated in Figure 43–16, with its use in the heart illustrated for equal echo times. The 1-2-1 shape of the frequency-encoding gradient ensures that for constant velocity no net phase shift occurs at the center of K-space. This strategy can be generalized, 1-3-3-1 for acceleration nulling, 1-4-6-4-1 for jerk nulling, and so forth, but increasingly higher-order moment nulling tends to be a losing proposition. Because echo time is increased by the extra gradient lobes required for nulling, the assumption that the velocity, acceleration, jerk, and so forth are constant over the increasingly long echo time becomes a poorer and poorer assumption. Ordered flow tends to be well compensated by simple first-moment nulling; disordered flow tends to be disordered on time scales fast enough that higher-moment nulling is not particularly effective. As echo times become shorter and shorter (a product of improved gradient amplifier and coil technologies), the tradeoff between very short echo time, using a flow-*un*compensated sequence, and the somewhat longer echo time for a flow-compensated sequence becomes more and more complex.

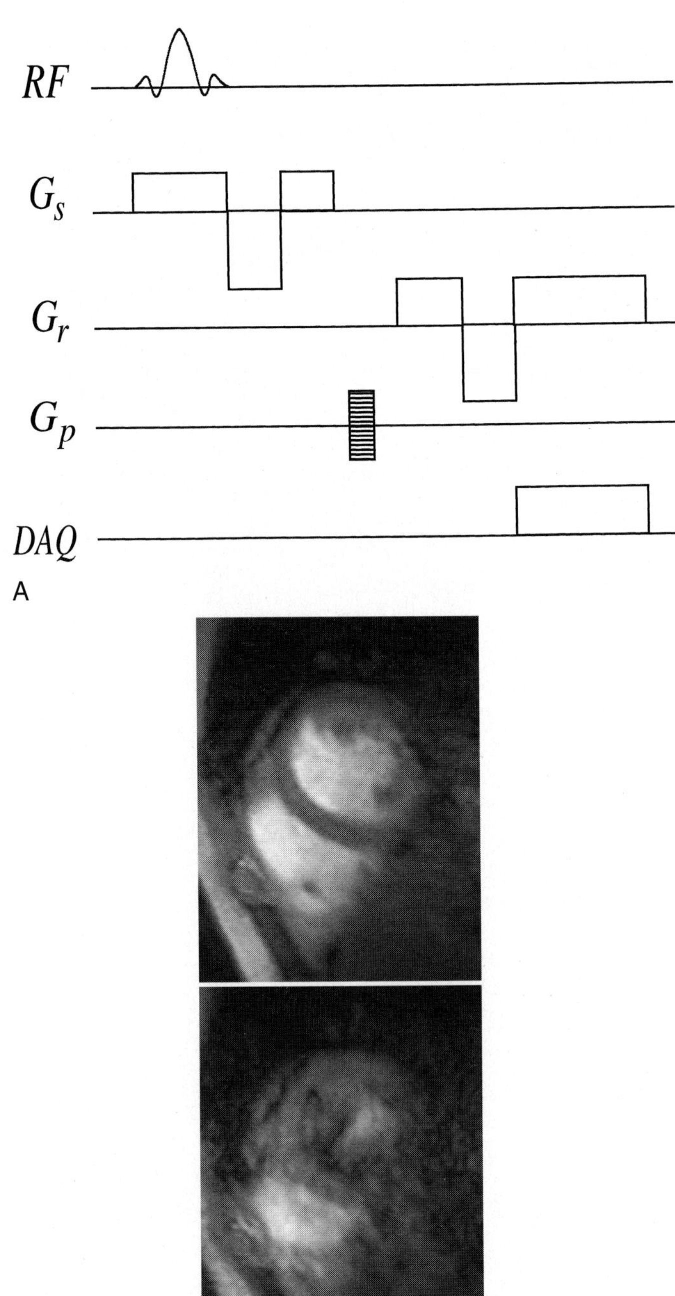

FIGURE 43–16. Flow compensation. Velocity-induced phase shifts can be minimized with the use of flow compensation. In *A*, the frequency and slice-selection gradients have been first-order nulled, so that spins moving at constant velocity produce no net additional phase shift. In *B*, one frame of a cine data set is shown with *(top)* and without *(bottom)* flow compensation. The contents of this (normal) ventricular chamber are much more uniform when flow compensation is used.

Respiratory Gating and Respiratory-Ordered Phase Encoding

Using ECG triggering and flow-compensation helps freeze cardiac-related motion but provides no assistance in reducing respiratory artifacts. As with cardiac gating, there are two general strategies to reduce chest motion: respiratory triggering and respiratory ordering, somewhat analogous to cardiac gating and cine imaging.

In respiratory triggering, a bellows placed across the patient's chest generates a respiratory cycle signal akin to an ECG signal. The scanner can then be triggered to image only during the coincidence of inspiration and R-wave. While this successfully eliminates breathing motion, it also increases the duration of the scan because of the relatively low frequency of respiration. A second strategy that requires no bellows is the use of multiple breath-hold intervals, scanning over a 5- to 20-second interval during breath-holds. This technique is compatible with both cardiac gating and cine imaging.

The alternative strategy is to order the phase encodings based on position in the respiratory cycle. This idea, sometimes called respiratory-ordered phase encoding, or ROPE, uses the sinusoidal property of the breathing to choose a "better" ordering. By grouping consecutive lines of K-space at the same portion of the respiratory cycle (rather than consecutively) so that K-space "appears" to have been acquired during one long breathing cycle, the phase smearing from random phase shifts can be reduced.

As with cardiac cycle variations, however, changes in the respiratory cycle affect the quality compensation provided by respiratory ordering. As a result, the alternative strategy of averaging multiple cycles, and having the patient breathe normally (but shallowly), has also found a degree of acceptance.

Surface Coils

Among the determinants of image quality is the raw signal-to-noise ratio available in the scan. In higher field MRI (0.5 T and above), the predominant source of noise is the body itself, so that careful design of RF coils optimized to anatomical structures has proved very profitable for image quality. It is no longer unusual to have separate coils for the brain, carotids, cervical spine, lumbar spine, knee, shoulder, hips, and so forth for clinical installations. The goal of these coils is to put the detector as near as possible to the anatomy of interest and to detect as little of the noise outside this area of interest as possible. Despite these advantages, there is no standard cardiac surface coil available, although a variety of local coils have been used in practice. Even though the heart has a relatively small volume (compared, for example, with the liver), its central location in the body and variable location across the patient population make a standardized coil difficult to construct. However, even suboptimal coils (e.g., a lumbar spine coil placed across the chest to image the heart,[10] also used in the cardiac images in this chapter) perform better than the standard body coil in many applications.

Echo Planar Imaging

One way of entirely eliminating cardiac motion is to image at a faster rate than that at which the heart itself is beating. Echo planar imaging (EPI), first described by Mansfield,[11] but only recently commercially available in the United States and Europe, attempts to do just this (e.g., see reference 12). By using rapidly oscillating frequency-encoding gradients, EPI collects all the lines of K-space after a single acquisition. Thus, unlike cardiac gating, which acquires each line of K-space at the same point after R-wave, or cine acquisition, which uses the ECG signal to allocate the acquired data to the appropriate point in the cardiac cycle, EPI acquires images quickly enough to produce whole images within any segment of the cardiac cycle.

In EPI, each frequency-encoded line takes 400 to 800 μsec, as opposed to 10 msec in conventional imaging, to squeeze in enough data to acquire a single image quickly enough. This rapid acquisition typically requires modification of many parts of the MR scanner. The gradient coil and gradient amplifiers are modified to produce the higher current and voltage required for these rapid acquisitions. The data acquisition and computer subsystems are also modified to extract and process these data quickly enough to provide useful data.

Because complete images are made from single excitations, EPI also should provide advantages in imaging the arrhythmic heart. It has been used to provide end-diastolic and end-systolic images in

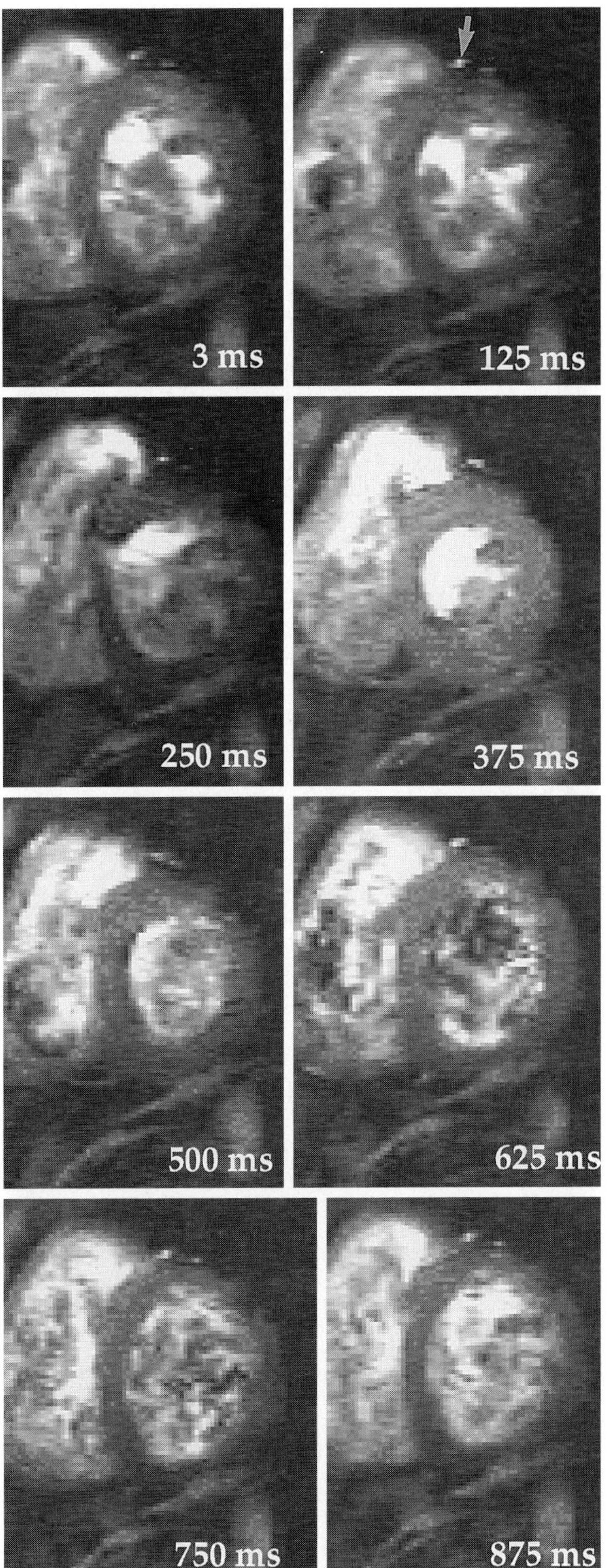

FIGURE 43–17. EPI imaging. Echo planar images during a single heartbeat. A 50-msec image was acquired every 125 msec. While the "nominal" resolution (field-of-view/matrix size) is actually worse than that of the cine images shown in Figure 43–15, certain small features are much easier to discern on these single-shot images. For example, the LAD *(arrow)* is easily visualized in this study, while beat-to-beat variability makes it much harder to visualize in the cine study. (Courtesy of Brigitte Poncelet, Ph.D., MGH-NMR Center, Charlestown, MA.)

a single breath-hold[10] that are amenable to automatic calculation of ejection fraction. Its increased availability in the clinical environment should provide continued development of cardiac MR techniques for assessing perfusion and function, as well.

Figure 43–17 shows an example of an EPI cardiac data set, displaying eight images progressively further advanced from R-wave. Unlike the cine images shown in Figure 43–15, these images were acquired within a *single* heartbeat.

SUMMARY

MRI is a powerful, although relatively complex, imaging modality that is unique among diagnostic techniques in its manner of image creation. By using the resonant behavior of the nuclei, and making this resonant frequency depend on position, the protons in the body can be imaged tomographically. Imaging the beating heart poses specific challenges to this complex process, for which novel technologies have been, and are continuing to be, developed to solve these problems. As will be described in the rest of the chapters in this section, the resulting technologies provide new windows on the anatomy and function of the heart and great vessels.

References

1. Lauterbur, P.C.: Image formation by induced local interactions: Examples employing nuclear magnetic resonance. Nature 242:190, 1973.
2. Edelstein, W.A., Hutchison, J.M.S., Johnson, G., et al.: Spin warp NMR imaging and applications to human whole-body imaging. Phys. Med. Biol. 25:751, 1980.
3. Twieg, D.B.: The k-trajectory formulation of the NMR imaging process with applications in analysis and synthesis of imaging methods. Med. Phys. 10:610, 1983.
4. Shellock, F., and Kanal, E.: Policies, guidelines, and recommendations for MR imaging safety and patient management. J. Magn. Reson. Imaging 1:97, 1991.
5. Sechtem, U., Pflugfelder, P., White, R., et al.: Cine MR imaging: Potential for the evaluation of cardiovascular function. AJR 148:239, 1987.
6. Dinsmore, R.E., Wedeen, V.J., Miller, S.W., et al.: MRI of dissection of the aorta: Recognition of the intimal tear and differential flow velocities. AJR 146:1286, 1986.
7. Drucker, E., Wedeen, V., Bradley, D., et al.: MR imaging flow velocity mapping of aortic regurgitation. Chicago, 73rd Annual Meeting of the Radiologic Society of North America, 1987, p. 236.
8. Wedeen, V., Weisskoff, R., and Poncelet, B.: MRI signal void due to in-plane motion is all-or-none. Magn. Reson. Med. 32:116, 1994.
9. Moran, P.: A flow velocity zeugmatographic interlace for NMR imaging in humans. Magn. Reson. Imaging 1:197, 1982.
10. Hunter, G., Hamberg, L., Weisskoff, R., et al.: Measurement of stroke volume and cardiac output within a single breath hold with echo-planary MR imaging. J. Magn. Reson. Imaging 4:51, 1994.
11. Mansfield, P.: Multi-planar image formation using NMR spin echos. J. Phys. C10:L55, 1977.
12. Cohen, M.S., and Weisskoff, R.M.: Ultra-fast imaging. Magn. Reson. Imaging 9:1, 1991.

CHAPTER

44 Contrast Agents for Cardiac Magnetic Resonance Imaging

Maythem Saeed, D.V.M., Ph.D.
Michael F. Wendland, Ph.D.
Dieter Szolar, M.D.
Charles B. Higgins, M.D.

Some of the earliest studies exploring the possible application of magnetic resonance imaging (MRI) in cardiovascular disease demonstrated unique capabilities for the evaluation of ischemic heart disease. In the early 1970s, Lauterbur and colleagues[1,2] found in excised canine hearts that magnetic resonance relaxation times are altered in infarcted regions. Several years later, in excised[3–5] and in situ beating hearts,[6–8] studies indicated that the changes in relaxation times are frequently sufficient to provide differential contrast between normal and infarcted myocardium on T2-weighted spin-echo images. Subsequently, several experimental[9–16] and clinical studies[17–19] have suggested that administration of magnetic resonance contrast agents can improve the contrast between normal and infarcted myocardium and reduce the time for detection. Early application of contrast-enhanced MRI involved primarily spin-echo techniques, which have been successfully used for detecting, characterizing, and sizing myocardial infarctions.

Despite this early interest in investigating the potential role of MRI in ischemic heart disease, at the present time MRI is infrequently used clinically for the evaluation of ischemic heart disease. The reason that MRI is so sparingly applied is that noninvasive imaging in ischemic heart disease is usually used to identify the presence of ischemic myocardium before infarction has occurred or the persistence of ischemia after infarction. This is customarily done with either rest-stress myocardial scintigraphy to identify perfusion defects or, increasingly, rest-stress two-dimensional echocardiography to identify regions of ischemia. Investigators have used coronary vasodilators, such as dipyridamole, dobutamine, and adenosine, coupled with cine MRI to induce regional dysfunction in potentially ischemic myocardium.[20–22] These coronary vasodilators cause regional imbalance in myocardial oxygen consumption and flow in regions supplied by a stenosed coronary artery. For the identification of hemodynamically significant stenosis, the results of stress cine MRI seem comparable to those of stress scintigraphy.[20, 21]

The development of fast MRI techniques, snapshot FLASH[23] and echo planar imaging[24] allows rapid measurement of magnetic resonance relaxation rate parameters and, when used in conjunction with a bolus-administered magnetic resonance contrast agent, allows the assessment of relative myocardial perfusion. For myocardial perfusion MRI to attain maximum clinical acceptance and utility, it will have to provide quantitative perfusion information. The assessment of myocardial perfusion represents an important advance in the diagnosis and treatment of ischemic heart disease. Other important goals for contrast-enhanced MRI are (1) to delineate ischemic but viable myocardium in the territory of stenosed or total coronary artery occlusion; (2) to discriminate between normal, stunned (viable but ischemic), and infarcted (dead) myocardial cells; (3) to document the success of reperfusion at the tissue level; and (4) to quantify the size of infarction at early stages.

MAGNETIC RESONANCE CONTRAST AGENTS

Magnetic Properties of Magnetic Resonance Contrast Agents

A diverse group of compounds have been employed experimentally to manipulate contrast of myocardium on magnetic resonance images. Most or all of these compounds can be grouped as either paramagnetic or superparamagnetic agents. The paramagnetic species contain at least one unpaired electron; the most commonly used in magnetic resonance contrast agents are paramagnetic metal atoms, gadolinium (III), dysprosium (III), manganese (II), and iron (III). The unpaired electron spin has a permanent magnetic dipole moment, which will align with and precess about an axis either parallel or antiparallel to the flux lines of an applied field. A slight excess of these spins (approximately 0.4 percent per tesla field strength) will be aligned with the field, and the net excess magnetization will add to the local magnetic field strength. Without an applied field, the electron magnetic moments are directionally randomized, and the bulk material has no net magnetization.

Superparamagnetic materials are very small bits of a ferromagnetic crystal. Each bit is a single crystal that is sufficiently small (<15 nm in diameter) that only a single magnetic domain is present.[25] Within each domain, the magnetic moments of all unpaired electrons are aligned together, and the sum of the electron magnetic moments can be considered as a single permanent magnetic dipole. In many ways a collection of such particles behaves analogously to a collection of paramagnetic atoms, which explains the origin of the term superparamagnetism. In both cases, the magnetic moments align with respect to an applied magnetic field, increasing the field strength or decreasing the temperature increases this alignment, and removing the applied field results in directional randomization of magnetic moments and no residual bulk magnetization.[25]

The local alterations in an applied magnetic field caused by the presence of these materials is referred to as the magnetic susceptibility. All matter exerts some alteration in the distribution of flux density when placed in a magnetic field. The vast majority of substances are diamagnetic and cause a local reduction in magnetic field strength. Materials that cause a local increase in field strength are either paramagnetic or ferromagnetic and contain unpaired electron spins. These features are described below in equation 1, where H is the applied magnetic field, B is the magnetic field within an object placed in the field H, and M is the induced magnetization within the object.

$$B = H + 4\pi M \qquad (1)$$

All three of these terms are vector fields. Dividing both sides of equation (1) by H:

$$B/H = 1 + 4\pi\, M/H \qquad (2)$$

yields the magnetic permeability (B/H) and the volume magnetic susceptibility (M/H). Thus, the magnetic susceptibility of a substance is the ratio of field strengths of the induced local field to the applied field and may be negative (for diamagnetic compounds) or positive (for paramagnetic or superparamagnetic compounds). The magnitude of the susceptibility is a function of the squared magnetic moment (μ_{eff}^2) of the atom and, for superparamagnetic agents, the strength of the external field. The magnetic lines of force that emanate from a magnetic dipole form closed loops (Fig. 44–1) so that centrally the field lines are directed along the magnetic moment vector, but at greater radial distance they loop back and point in the opposite direction. If an external magnetic field H is applied, the summation of the fields leads to a relatively larger magnetic field at the paramagnetic center and weaker fields in between. The introduction of material with a large magnetic susceptibility into tissue causes a change in magnetization (B) within the tissue and can produce large magnetic field gradients, both microscopic and macroscopic in extent, when the material is heterogeneously distributed.

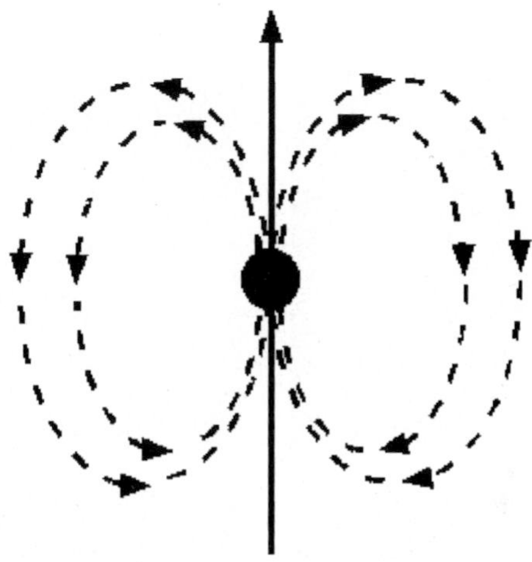

FIGURE 44–1. Depiction of the magnetic field lines in a single plane that emanate from a magnetic dipole. Magnetic lines of force *(dashed lines)* form closed loops that are centrally directed along the dipole moment *(arrow)* but that turn and point in the oposite direction at a greater distance from center. The toroidal topology of the field lines is obtained by rotating the figure about the magnetic moment vector. The magnetic field associated with each unpaired electron spin or ferromagnetic crystal is present regardless of the presence of an external magnetic field; the effect of the applied field is to order the orientations of the individual moments, which are otherwise randomly oriented.

Effect on Magnetic Resonance Imaging Signal Intensity

Paramagnetic and superparamagnetic contrast materials alter the signal of magnetic resonance images by two mechanisms: (1) facilitating the relaxation of nuclear spins of protons (T1 and T2), and (2) reducing the homogeneity of the applied magnetic field. These two mechanisms are active for all magnetic resonance contrast media, but usually one has the dominant effect. When the former mechanism is dominant, the agent is considered a relaxivity agent, whereas when the latter mechanism is more important, the compound is considered to be a susceptibility agent.[26]

Relaxivity agents exert an influence on contrast primarily by dipolar enhancement of relaxation rates (1/T1, 1/T2). The general theory for this interaction was described in early papers by Solomon, Bloembergen, and Morgan[27–30] and subsequently has been extensively studied in a variety of biologic settings. Excellent reviews are also available that describe this theory in detail, and the interested reader can refer to these.[31–34] The elements that are most relevant here are as follows: (1) Efficient relaxation enhancement requires very close contact between water protons and the metal atom (approximately 5 to 10 $\times$ 10^{-4} μm); thus, in tissues where water is compartmentalized, that agent only enhances relaxation of water molecules that can diffuse into the distribution volume of the agent. (2) The efficiency of relaxation enhancement is maximized when fluctuation in the local magnetic field experienced by the water proton is roughly equal to its precessional frequency (approximately 42.6 MHz/tesla). (3) Fluctuations in the experienced magnetic field are provided by molecular motion as well as dynamic changes in the induced field associated with the contrast agent.

Susceptibility agents alter signal intensity by reducing the homogeneity of the local magnetic field.[35–39] Water molecules within a magnetic field gradient exhibit a gradient of precessional frequencies, and the phase memory of the population of water molecules is reduced (shorter T2*). Consequently, signal intensity on spin echo, gradient echo, and echo planar MRI sequences would be reduced in regions where contrast agent is delivered. If the field gradient is constant over time and if water molecules were stationary, a refocusing radio-frequency pulse would completely restore the signal and no signal decrease would be observed on a spin-echo MRI sequence. However, water molecules are not stationary; random translation of water molecules (diffusion) during TE of a spin-echo MRI sequence prevents complete refocusing of the magnetic resonance signal and signal loss on spin-echo sequences.[35, 40, 41]

Although magnetic resonance contrast agents are usually characterized as being either relaxivity or susceptibility agents, neither type of agent is free from the other effect. All efficient T1 agents have a high magnetic susceptibility and can potentially be used to exert susceptibility contrast under appropriate imaging conditions. For example, gadolinium-based chelates can be used either as a relaxivity agent on T1-sensitive imaging sequences or as a susceptibility agent on T2*-sensitive sequences.[42–45] This novel feature of magnetic resonance contrast media has been used for the detection of regions of ischemia, where the ischemic region appears as a dark zone on T1-sensitive images and as a bright zone on T2*-sensitive images (Figs. 44–2 and 44–3). Likewise, agents considered as susceptibility agents cause some T1 enhancement, although the enhancement may be quite small. Dysprosium (Dy)-based chelates are used exclusively to provide susceptibility-dependent contrast but also cause weak T1 enhancement (relaxivity = 0.89 s^{-1} mM^{-1}) Superparamagnetic agents are very potent susceptibility agents in the heart[46–50] but also cause potent T1 enhancement and have been used successfully as relaxivity agents to delineate ischemic myocardium.[49]

Distribution of Magnetic Resonance Contrast Media in Myocardium

Paramagnetic metal atom is usually chelated to an organic molecule. The metal-ligand complex must be soluble in aqueous solution. The paramagnetic metal ion is responsible for altering magnetic resonance signal intensity, while the chelate serves to increase solubility of the metal, reduce its toxicity, direct its delivery to the region of interest, and facilitate its subsequent elimination. Paramagnetic agents may be prepared with a 1:1 stoichiometry (one metal atom per molecule of contrast agent) as in the clinically available agents gadolinium-diethylenetetramine-pentaacetic acid (Gd-DTPA [Magnavist, Schering AG]), gadolinium-hexapropyl-tetraazacyclododecane-triacetic acid (Gd-HP-DO3A [ProHance, Bracco SPA]), or Gd-DTPA-bismethylamide (Gd-DTPA-BMA [Omniscan, Nycomed]). Such compounds are generally quite small, having molecular weights less than 1000, and are able to freely diffuse from the blood into the myocardial interstitium. The pharmacokinetic properties of this class of magnetic resonance contrast

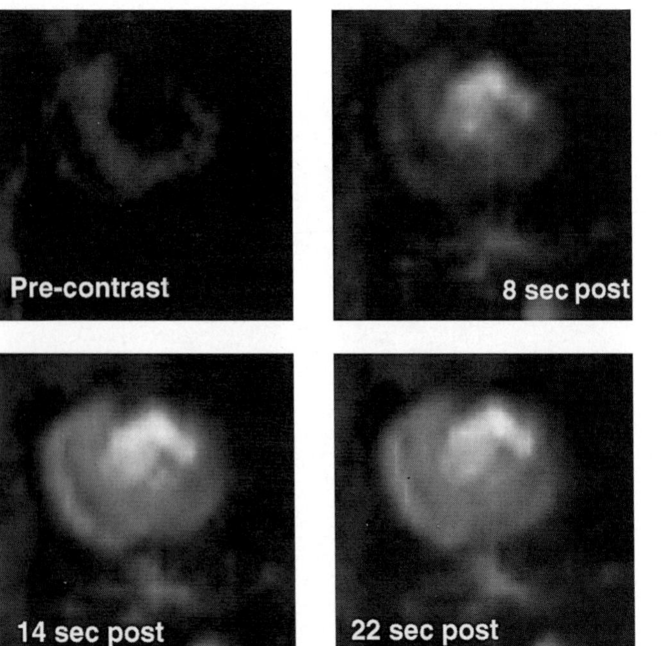

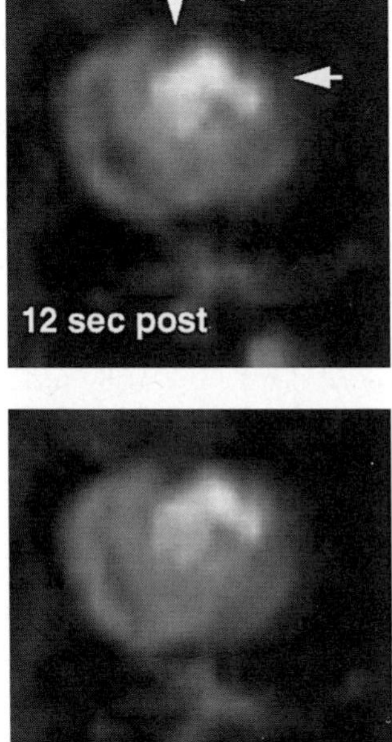

FIGURE 44–2. Selected inversion recovery echo planar magnetic resonance images (TR/TE/TI = 2000/10/700 msec) were acquired prior to *(top left)* and at 8, 12, 14, 22, and 30 seconds after the administration of 0.05 mmol/kg Gd-DTPA-BMA through the heart of a rat subjected to 2-hour coronary artery occlusion. Note that the infarcted region is shown as a region of low signal intensity—a "cold spot" *(arrows* in 12-second image).

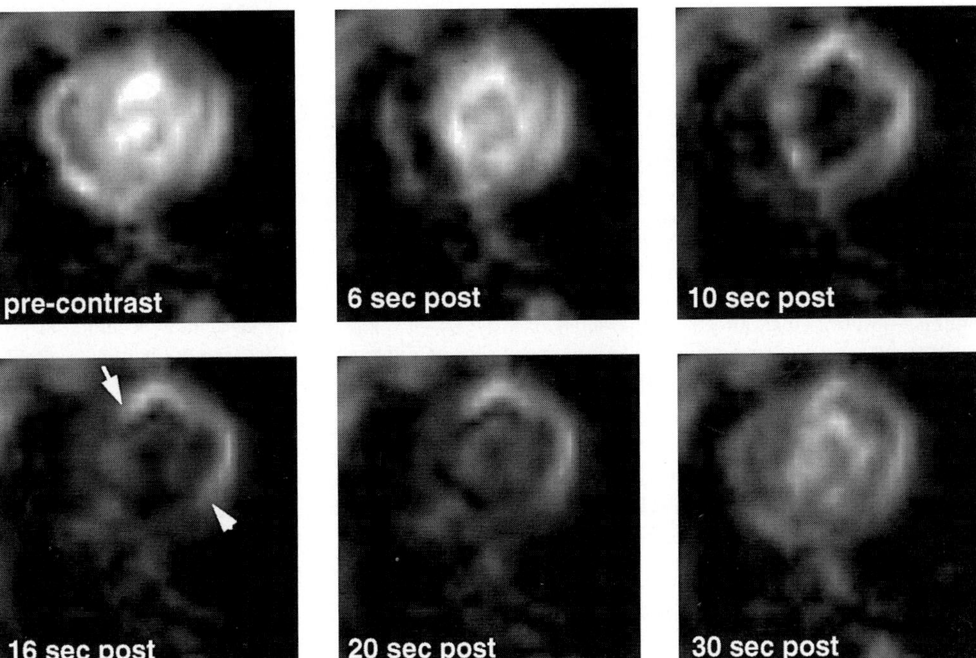

FIGURE 44–3. Selected gradient-recalled echo planar magnetic resonance images (TR/TE = 2000/10 msec) obtained from the same animal as shown in Figure 44–2. These images were acquired prior to *(top left)* and at 6, 10, 16, 20, and 30 seconds after the administration of 0.2 mmol/kg Gd-DTPA-BMA. Note that the ischemic region is shown as a hyperintense region—a hot spot (*arrows* in 16-second image).

media are similar to low-molecular-weight computed tomography agents. Most magnetic resonance agents have nonspecific biodistribution, which is determined by relative perfusion and capillary integrity.

Alternatively, many metal chelate complexes can be added to single macromolecules, such as albumin,[51, 52] polylysine,[53–55] dextran,[56] or synthetic cascade polymers.[57, 58] These agents have molecular weights between 15,000 and 100,000 and are retained in the blood pool much longer than are the smaller agents. Thus, the low-molecular-weight compounds are often referred to as extravascular or extracellular agents, since they do not enter the intracellular space, whereas the macromolecular compounds are classified as intravascular or blood pool agents. Macromolecular contrast media provide more efficient relaxation enhancement than low-molecular-weight agents in aqueous solution but their smaller distribution volume in the heart greatly limits signal enhancement on T1-weighted sequences.

Superparamagnetic agents are composed of an insoluble particulate suspension of crystalline iron oxide coated with an organic polymer, such as dextran or protein. Preparations of superparamagnetic particulates contain a large range of particle size, although different preparation techniques can yield particles of very small median size. These preparations have diverse properties, depending primarily on the size and composition of the iron oxide core and the nature of the polymer coat.[33, 59] Larger particles, such as AMI 25, are rapidly taken up by the reticuloendothelial system, whereas smaller particulates remain in the circulation much longer. Typically, these agents are much larger than paramagnetic compounds and are generally confined to the intravascular space while in the heart.

Since the presence of contrast agent in the heart is only evident indirectly from its effect on tissue water, the influence of dynamic water movement in tissue should also be considered along with the molecular distribution of the contrast agent. In normal myocardium, the distribution of water is almost homogeneous and is relatively freely movable across the capillary wall and cellular membrane. The extraction fraction of water is close to unity and is slightly sensitive to flow changes.[60] Low-molecular-weight agents are excluded from the intracellular compartment but are free to equilibrate throughout the interstitium. The volume of distribution of low-molecular contrast medium has been found to be approximately 30 percent of the myocardial volume.[61] However, when water exchange between any of these compartments is slow relative to the relaxation rate in the compartment with the longest T1, multiexponential longitudinal relaxation may result. Although these agents provide significant advantage over unenhanced magnetic resonance images, these agents distribute rapidly to the extravascular space and undergo early renal excretion. Macromolecular agents selectively enhance myocardium in proportion to their fractional blood volume.[62, 63] Gadolinium-DTPA-albumin and DTPA-polylysine have been used for characterization of myocardial injuries in rats.[52, 54, 64] This class of agents, however, has not yet been clinically tested.

Edema and an increase of interstitial proteins have been reported in infarcted myocardium, owing to an increase in capillary permeability, the loss of cellular integrity, and compression of the lymph system.[65, 66] Edema associated with myocardial infarction prolongs tissue relaxation times, resulting in higher signal intensity in infarcted regions than in normal myocardium on unenhanced T2-weighted spin-echo images.[15, 16] While edema develops rapidly after reperfusion of irreversibly injured myocardium, it is a much slower process in occlusive injury; coronary artery occlusion of 6 to 12 hours' duration is required for visualization of infarction on unenhanced images.[8, 67] On contrast-enhanced images of infarcted myocardium, marked hyperintensity of the injured zone indicates (1) delivery of the agent and (2) an enlarged distribution volume of the contrast agent in the hyperintense zone. The volume of distribution of magnetic resonance contrast agents is enlarged following cell death.[68, 69] In this case, contrast agents diffuse even into the intracellular space and cause much greater signal enhancement than that of normal myocardium. Preliminary investigations also demonstrated that estimation of volume of distribution with the use of contrast-enhanced MRI may provide a tool for evaluating the spatial extent and severity of local damage in cases of myocardial injuries.[70]

Cardiovascular Response

On conventional MRI, cardiotoxicity and osmotoxicity are minor complications of magnetic resonance contrast agents because of peripheral injection, small volume, and slow infusion. Acute and chronic toxicity of magnetic resonance contrast agents is related in part to their stability and clearance. Toxic effects from a metal complex can arise from (1) free metal ion or free ligand released by dissociation and (2) the intact metal complex. The toxicity of metal ions has been extensively reviewed.[71] Moreover, clinical usage of magnetic resonance contrast media has proved to be remarkably safe.[72–77]

In the current application of fast MRI, bolus administration of magnetic resonance contrast media is required. Accordingly, the potential hemodynamic effects of bolus must be considered. Several experimental studies in rats have demonstrated that ionic magnetic resonance contrast agents produce transient depression of cardiac performance, heart rate, and blood pressure when administered rapidly as a bolus.[78–82] This transient depression is partially attributed to the ability of the agents to reduce the ionic calcium in the blood.[82] Nonionic agents were found to produce minimal cardiovascular effects at the same dose levels.[78, 81] The severity of cardiovascular response following administration of ionic contrast agents depends on the dose, volume, osmolality, and site and duration of injection.

APPLICATIONS OF MAGNETIC RESONANCE CONTRAST AGENTS IN CARDIAC IMAGING

During the course of the last several years, multiple contrast-enhancing strategies for characterization of myocardial injuries have been examined. These strategies have included the following: (1) a single contrast agent for either T1, T2, or T2* enhancement, (2) a single magnetic resonance contrast agent followed by both T1- and T2*-sensitive sequences to monitor changes in myocardial signal intensity caused by both mechanisms, and (3) combination of two or more magnetic resonance contrast agents, given together.

Acute Coronary Occlusion

It has been shown that the major ultrastructural changes in ischemic (viable) myocardium following acute occlusion of a coronary artery consist of mild edema of the sarcoplasm and mitochondrial swelling, but no interstitial edema. Discrimination of jeopardized myocardium in the territory of the occluded vessel depends on the lengthened T2 relaxation rates that accompany interstitial edema. Consequently, there is no differential contrast between normal and ischemic myocardium on unenhanced magnetic resonance images early after occlusion.[62, 83–86]

The use of magnetic resonance contrast media partially ameliorates this difficulty by providing enhanced signal intensities in normally perfused regions.[42] Unfortunately, the combination of collateral flow and diffusion of the contrast media into the jeopardy zone limits the duration of differential contrast to less than 15 minutes after administration of gadolinium-based media.[83, 84] Thus, fast imaging sequences utilized early after contrast media injection are most effective in visualizing jeopardized myocardium immediately after coronary artery occlusion.

Recent reports have demonstrated that magnetic resonance perfusion imaging, in conjunction with multiple low doses of magnetic resonance contrast agents, provides effective definition of the territory of acutely occluded arteries.[44, 45, 87, 88] Contrast-enhanced echo planar and gradient-echo imaging have been used to detect regional ischemia in experimental models[44, 45, 63, 87–90] and in humans.[91–95] In a rat model of ischemia examined with inversion recovery and gradient-recalled echo planar imaging,[44, 45] there was no change in signal intensity in the territory of the occluded vessel after the administration of gadolinium-based magnetic resonance contrast agents, and the ischemic region was identified as a zone of either low "cold-spot" or high "hot-spot" signal (see Figs. 44–2 and 44–3), respectively. Similar results were obtained in dogs subjected to regional ischemia by acute occlusion of the left anterior descending coronary artery with the use of inversion recovery and driven equilibrium gradient-recalled sequences.[88] Figure 44–4 shows a region of ischemia in a dog subjected to acute occlusion of the left descending coronary artery on contrast-enhanced inversion recovery fast gradient–recalled echo images.

Although this technique provides definition of the ischemic region within a single section, it does not provide good coverage of the entire ischemic area. Coverage has recently been accomplished at the expense of temporal resolution of fast gradient–recalled echo imaging by acquiring images at multiple sections during the passage of the bolus (Fig. 44–5). Complete coverage of the heart may be compatible with the possibility of measuring perfusion with the use of echo planar imaging technique; this method would provide quantification of the size and extent of the ischemic region and perfusion deficit, information that is not available with the use of conventional MRI.[83–85, 88, 96]

Occlusive Myocardial Infarctions

Myocardial infarction is a complex and dynamic process. The progression of myocardial cell death may reach completion in a

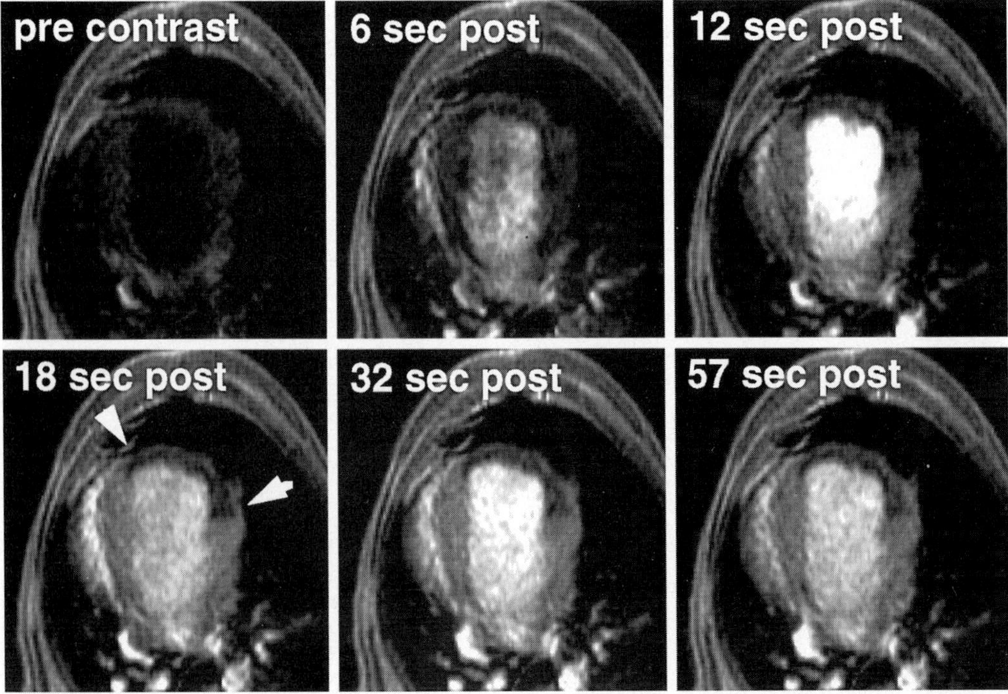

FIGURE 44–4. Inversion recovery-prepared fast gradient-recalled images (TI/TR/TE = 700/7.0/2.9 msec, and a flip angle = 7 degree) during the transit of 0.05 mmol/kg Gd-DTPA-BMA through the heart of a dog subjected to 10-minute left anterior descending coronary artery occlusion. Note that the ischemic region *(arrows)* is shown as a region of low signal intensity.

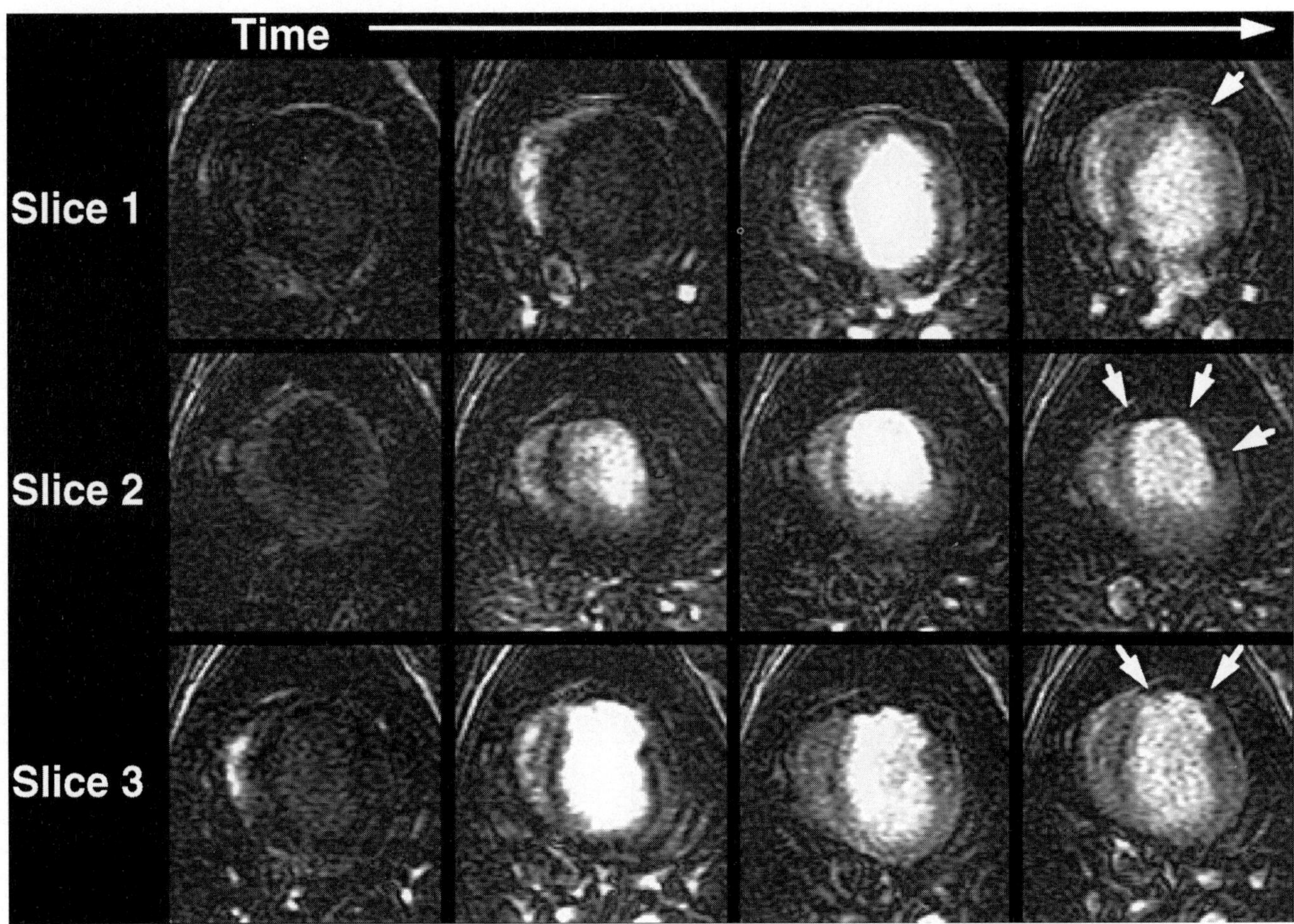

FIGURE 44–5. Multislice inversion recovery (IR)–prepared gradient-recalled echo images (TR/TE/TI = 6.9/2.3/600 msec) during the transit of 0.025 mmol/kg Gd-BOPTA/dimeg through the heart of a dog subjected to 10-minute left anterior descending coronary artery occlusion. Note that the ischemic region *(arrows)* is shown at all three slices as a region of low signal intensity. The middle slice shows the largest ischemic region.

matter of hours, but the process of repair requires 4 to 6 weeks. The formation of edema in the infarcted region requires several hours to days to develop in humans.[83–85, 88, 97] Previous clinical and experimental studies have shown that acute, subacute, or chronic myocardial infarction can be detected as a bright region on unenhanced T2-weighted spin-echo images.[17, 18, 97, 98] The increase in signal intensity in the infarcted region was attributed to the combination of interstitial edema and reduced motion in the infarcted zone. Thompson and co-workers[99] followed the healing process in patients with myocardial infarction over the course of 3 months, using MRI. They found that the signal intensity of the infarcted region evolved with the age of the infarction.

The administration of magnetic resonance contrast agents can improve the contrast between normal and acutely infarcted myocardium, reduce imaging time, and allow earlier definition of the injured region.[17, 19, 42, 83–85, 96, 98, 100–108] In a rat model, contrast-enhanced images of acute and subacute infarctions showed a bright peri-infarction zone.[54] Enhancement of the peri-infarcted region following the administration of gadolinium chelates has been noted as early as 3 to 5 hours (Fig. 44–6) in acute (1 day)[69] and subacute (10-day-old) myocardial infarctions.[13, 54, 103] The cause of this peri-infarction enhancement is unknown but could represent local hyperemia or edema, or both. Unlike animal models of occlusive infarction, acute and subacute myocardial infarctions in patients (Fig. 44–7) exhibit greater increases in signal intensity of the entire infarcted region versus normal myocardium on post–contrast-enhanced T1-weighted images.[17, 98] Interspecies differences in the anatomy of the coronary bed, chronicity of coronary disease, or age of the infarction may be responsible for the difference in the pattern of enhancement of occlusive infarctions.

Magnetic susceptibility agents have also proved to be useful for demarcation of occlusive infarctions in experimental models.[14, 87, 109] On T2-weighted spin-echo images, Dy-DTPA-BMA (0.3 to 1.0 mmol/kg) induced a marked decrease in signal intensity of normal myocardium, with a small decrease in signal of the infarcted region. The infarcted region can be visualized as a region of high signal intensity—a "hot spot".[14, 87]

The dual mechanisms of action (T1 and T2* contrast) of Gd-DTPA-BMA and Gd-BOPTA/dimeglumine were investigated with the use of conventional and fast imaging sequences.[43–45] Contrast-enhanced inversion recovery echo planar images provided clear delineation of the infarcted region as an area of low signal intensity (cold spot) after the injection of a low dose (0.05 mmol/kg) of gadolinium-chelate (see Fig. 44–2). At a higher dose (0.2 mmol/kg), the infarcted region was recognized as an area of high signal—a "hot spot" (see Fig. 44–3).[44, 45]

Reperfused Myocardial Infarctions

Discrimination between occlusive and reperfused myocardial infarctions has been a topic of considerable interest, with implications for the noninvasive imaging of patients undergoing reperfusion procedures. The appearances of occlusive and reperfused infarctions on contrast-enhanced images are different.[13, 103, 105] Reperfused infarction is intensely and homogeneously enhanced following administration of T1 contrast media[11–13, 102, 103, 105, 107] (Fig. 44–8).

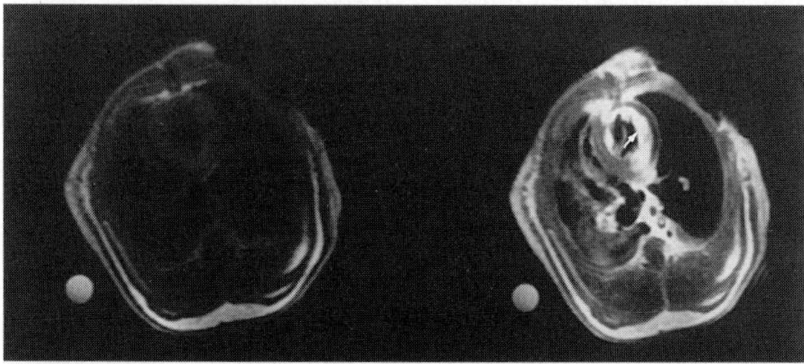

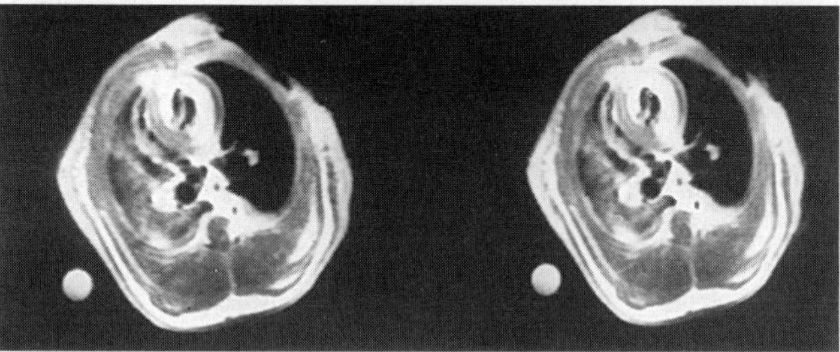

FIGURE 44–6. Electrocardiogram-gated T1-weighted spin-echo magnetic resonance images (TR/TE = 300/20 msec) obtained from a rat subjected to 3½ hours of coronary occlusion. Magnetic resonance images were acquired before *(top left)* and 3 minutes *(top right)*, 30 minutes *(bottom left)*, and 60 minutes *(bottom right)* after the administration of 0.2 mmol/kg Gd-DTPA-BMA. The infarcted region appears as a dark region (cold spot). A doughnut pattern of enhancement (peri-infarction region) is shown at the periphery of the infarcted region. A crescent area of high signal intensity adjacent to the endocardial layer of the infarcted wall represents slowly flowing blood in the cavity of the left ventricle *(arrow)*.

On the other hand, occlusive infarction demonstrates a markedly heterogeneous enhancement (see Fig. 44–6).

Recently, echo planar imaging has been employed to discriminate between occlusive and reperfused myocardial infarctions during bolus transit of Gd-BOPTA/dimeglumine. In rats subjected to occlusive infarction, inversion recovery echo planar images exhibited no change in signal intensity of the infarcted region, whereas normally perfused myocardium showed rapid signal enhancement during the first passage of the contrast agent. Reperfused infarcted myocardium was affected very differently. The reperfused region showed delayed signal enhancement and a subsequent gradual increase in signal intensity. By 2 minutes after injection, the signal of reperfused infarcted myocardium had increased to a greater degree than that of normal myocardium at the peak of the bolus effect.[104]

The findings of van Rossum and associates[107] in patients with myocardial infarction were in agreement with the experimental animal data. Unlike reperfused infarctions, occlusive infarctions have relatively lower signal intensity than does normal myocardium on Gd-DTPA-enhanced images. The difference is due to decreased delivery of Gd-DTPA to the territory of occluded artery. At early images (8 to 10 minutes), the researchers were able to discriminate occlusive infarctions from reperfused ones. On the other hand, de Roos and colleagues were unable to confirm these findings.[19] They found that in patients Gd-DTPA produced greater and more heterogeneous enhancement in occlusive infarcted regions compared with normal myocardium.[19, 101] Similar enhancement is observed on contrast-enhanced images in patients with subacute infarctions,[17, 18, 98] as demonstrated in Figure 44–7.

Size of Jeopardized or Infarcted Myocardium

Accurate sizing of jeopardized or infarcted areas can potentially provide valuable information for guiding therapeutic interventions aimed at limiting infarction size. Since MRI is a noninvasive tool, time-dependent responses to therapeutic intervention can be evaluated in individual subjects. In addition, certain physiologic and anatomical parameters, such as perfusion and infarction size, can be evaluated together in a single session with the use of contrast-enhanced MRI.

The size of reperfused infarction on gadolinium-enhanced magnetic resonance images was close to that obtained from histochemical morphometry in rats.[110] In occlusive infarction, Yu and associates[108] found a close correlation between unenhanced and dysprosium-enhanced T2-weighted images and the area in jeopardy measured by thallium-201 autoradiography, but not in infarction measured by histochemical staining. In dogs subjected to coronary occlusion, the infarction size measured on indium-111–enhanced images correlated well with that measured on gadolinium-enhanced images.[10] At the present time, it has not been demonstrated that both jeopardy and infarction can be quantified in a single preparation with the use of magnetic resonance techniques alone.

Recent animal studies from the authors' laboratory have suggested that contrast-enhanced MRI is also a suitable technique for assessing conditions that accentuate ischemic injury in hypertrophied hearts. T1-weighted imaging with the aid of magnetic resonance contrast agents accurately depicted the higher incidence of myocardial injury among animals with left ventricular hypertrophy as compared with normal after 25 minutes of coronary occlusion, followed by 1-hour reperfusion.[111] Furthermore, contrast-enhanced MRI proved to be useful in evaluating the effect of a calcium blocker in preserving myocardium at risk and reducing myocardial injury size in hypertrophied hearts.[112]

De Roos and co-workers[113] used Gd-DTPA–enhanced imaging to estimate infarction size in 21 patients who were or were not given thrombolytic therapy. It was found that the contrast provided by the agent allowed quantification of the infarction size, which was significantly ($P < .001$) smaller in patients with reperfusion versus those without reperfusion. Other studies have shown that infarction size measured on unenhanced and gadolinium-enhanced magnetic resonance images correlates well with thallium-201 single-photon emission computed tomography.[114]

MAGNETIC RESONANCE CONTRAST AGENTS FOR DETECTION OF MYOCARDIAL VIABILITY

The ability to noninvasively discriminate viable myocardium from nonviable myocardium following thrombolytic therapy has assumed considerable clinical significance. Stress thallium-201 scintigraphy has been proposed as a method of assessing myocardial viability. Diminished uptake of thallium-201 with stress and absent redistribution at 4 hours has been called scar, whereas a reduction in thallium-201 uptake followed by redistribution is considered a marker of myocardial viability.[115] Positron emission tomography also has the potential to differentiate between viable and nonviable myocardium in regions subjected to ischemia.[116] It may also be possible to determine myocardial cell viability with the use of magnetic resonance contrast media to probe membrane damage.[68, 70, 110]

Several years ago Thulborn and colleagues demonstrated that sonicating a suspension of red blood cells caused an increase in the T2 relaxation time.[35] The diminished relaxation rate was caused by converting a heterogeneous susceptibility distribution to a homogeneous one by removing cellular boundaries. This idea has recently been applied to the heart as one potential method for detecting the presence of nonviable myocardial cells in reperfused infarcted myocardium. The hypothesis, shown schematically in Figure 44–9, was that myocardial signal loss induced by Dy-DTPA-BMA is related to the cell viability; that is, cellular exclusion of Dy-DTPA-BMA is compromised as cell viability is lost. In normal myocardium, cell membranes act as a barrier and limit the distribution of the contrast agent to the extracellular space and thereby cause signal reduction (see Fig. 44–9*A*). Equilibrium distribution of the T2* contrast agent between extracellular and intracellular compartments results in a net loss of its effect (see Fig. 44–9*B*). This effect is evident on both spin-echo T2-weighted (Fig. 44–10)

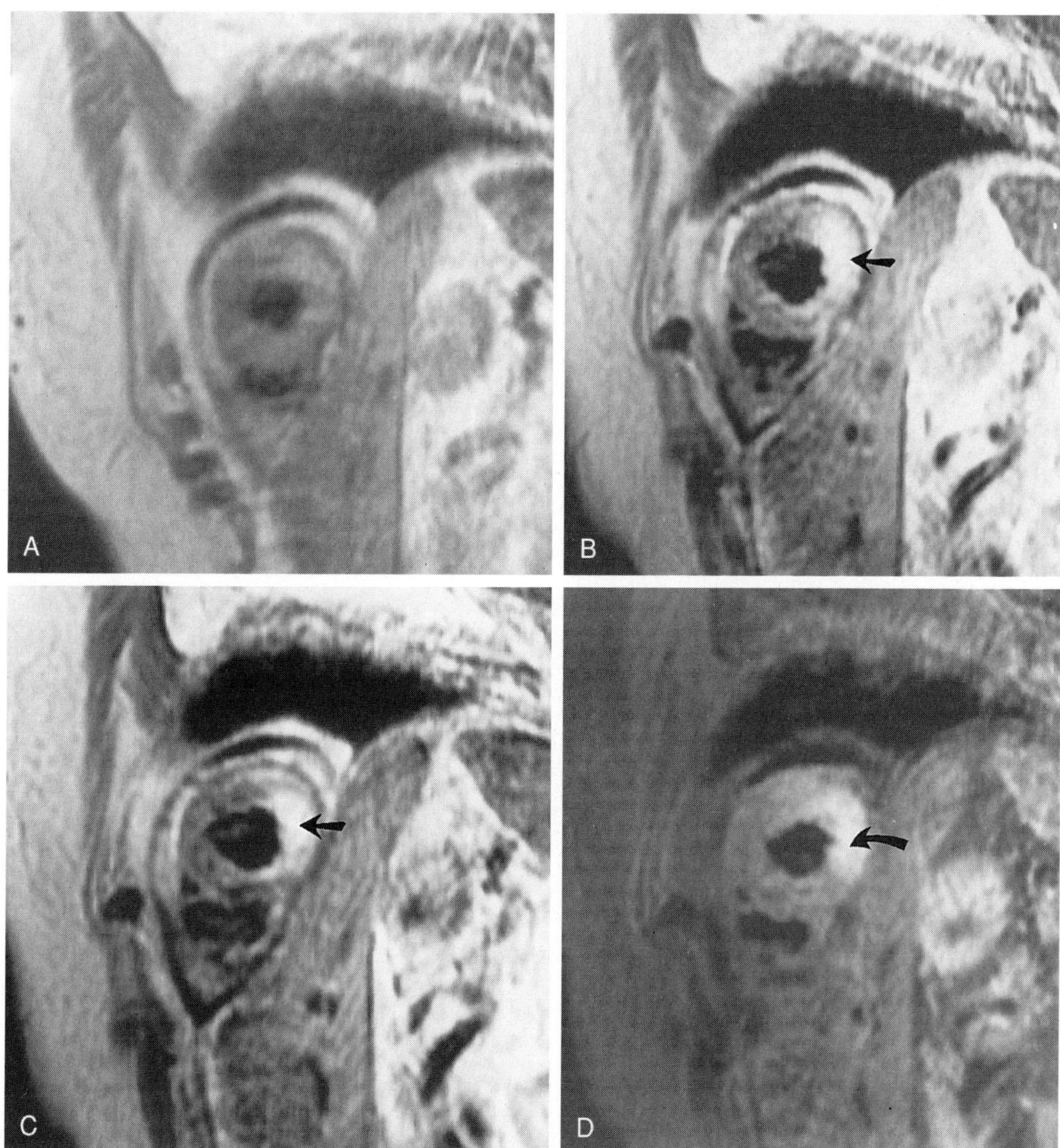

FIGURE 44–7. Short-axis T1-weighted spin-echo (TR/TE = 800/20 msec) magnetic resonance images acquired before *(A)* and 30 minutes *(B)* and 45 minutes *(C)* after the administration of 0.2 mmol/kg gadodiamide injection in a patient with subacute myocardial infarction. There was no clear evidence of infarction on the baseline image *(A)*. Administration of gadodiamide provides persistent demarcation of infarcted myocardium. The infarction appeared as a bright region for at least 45 minutes *(C)* after injection *(arrows)*. Excellent demarcation of infarction *(curved arrow)* is also seen on contrast-enhanced T1-weighted images with fat saturation *(D)*.

and gradient-echo T2*-weighted images (Fig. 44–11).[68, 110] In both studies, Gd-DTPA-BMA was used to document the restoration of flow in the reperfused region and the delivery of contrast agent, whereas Dy-DTPA-BMA was employed to probe myocardial viability.[68, 110] Since cell membrane damage is considered a lethal injury, alterations in the potency of susceptibility-dependent signal loss can be related to cell viability. Whether dysprosium exclusion predicts functional recovery, especially in stunned myocardium, will need to be addressed in future experiments.

MAGNETIC RESONANCE CONTRAST AGENTS FOR MYOCARDIAL PERFUSION

The most widely available clinical methods for the assessment of regional myocardial perfusion deficits are radionuclide scintigraphy and positron emission tomography. Contrast-enhanced magnetic resonance perfusion studies have recently been developed to allow noninvasive assessment of myocardial perfusion. Fast gradient–recalled echo and echo planar imaging are the techniques currently used for myocardial perfusion. Fast gradient–recalled echo imaging has the potential to acquire tomographic images at 1- to 3-second intervals, whereas echo planar imaging needs 30 to 50 msec. With small modifications in magnetic resonance pulse sequence, these techniques can be either T1- or T2-sensitive. It follows that appropriate magnetic resonance contrast agents for these studies are T1-enhancing agents and magnetic susceptibility agents, respectively.

Quantification of perfusion from first-pass profiles of bolus-administered contrast agent requires that, first, T1 or T2* values before and after contrast are monoexponential, and, second, change in 1/T1 or 1/T2* is a linear function of contrast agent concentration. When both assumptions hold true and both blood and tissue data are available, it is possible to convert bolus profiles to tissue residue and arterial input functions. It may be possible to convert such

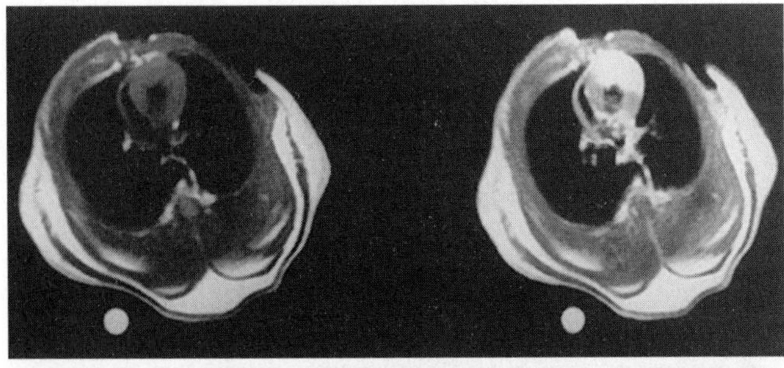

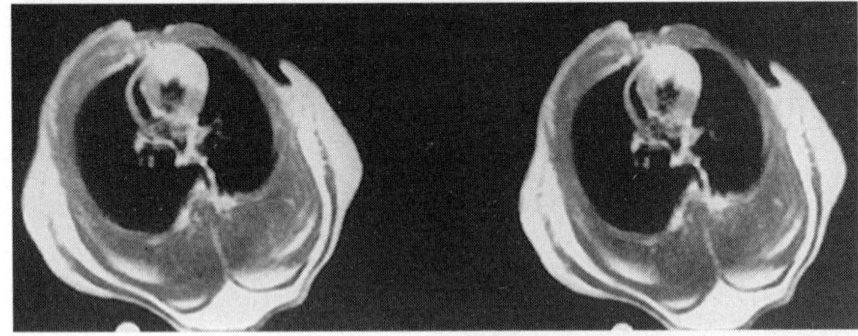

FIGURE 44–8. Electrocardiogram-gated T1-weighted spin-echo magnetic resonance images (TR/TE = 300/20 msec) obtained from a rat subjected to 2-hour coronary occlusion followed by 1½ hours of reperfusion. Magnetic resonance images were acquired before *(top left)* and 3 minutes *(top right)*, 30 minutes *(bottom left)*, and 60 minutes *(bottom right)* after the administration of 0.2 mmol/kg Gd-DTPA-BMA. Over the course of 60 minutes, the reperfused ischemically injured region (anterolateral left ventricular wall) was depicted as a region of high signal intensity (hot spot).

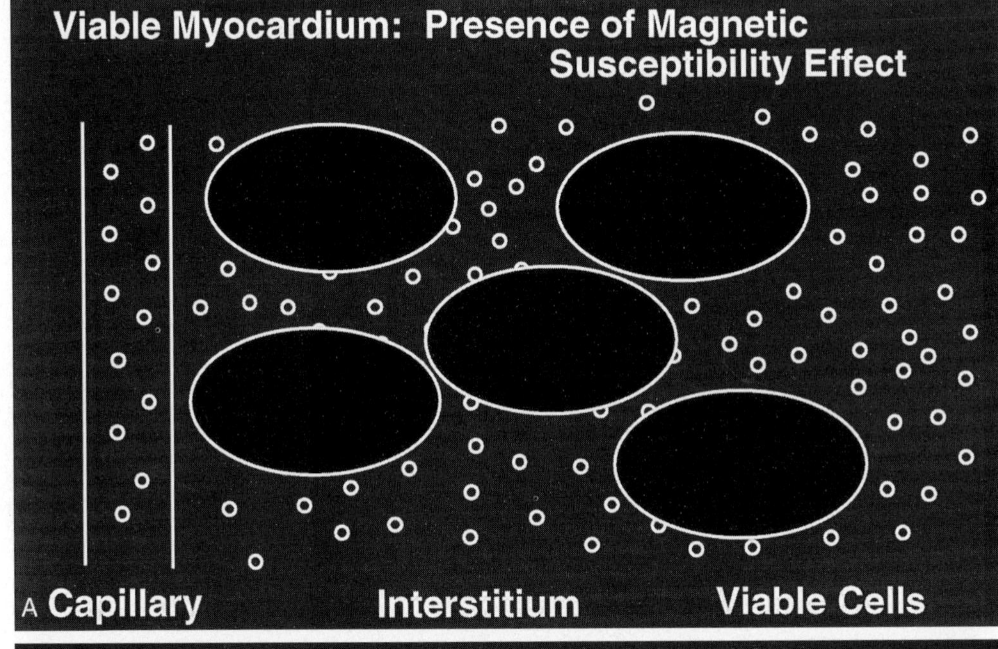

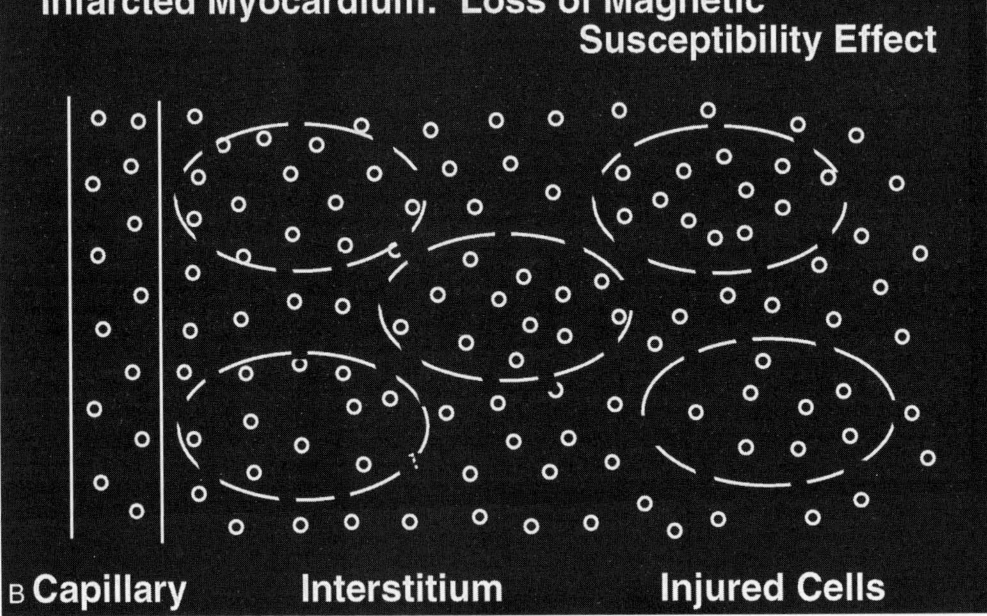

FIGURE 44–9. A schematic of the concept of the mechanism of action of Dy-DTPA-BMA in viable and infarcted myocardium. Dysprosium is excluded from viable cells *(A)* and is heterogeneously distributed and causes signal loss in the normal myocardium. In infarcted myocardium *(B)*, cell membrane integrity is damaged, and dysprosium diffuses into the cellular space and is homogeneously distributed throughout the damaged region. Water molecules in this region experience no field gradient, and the decrease in signal is much less than that in myocardium composed of viable cells.

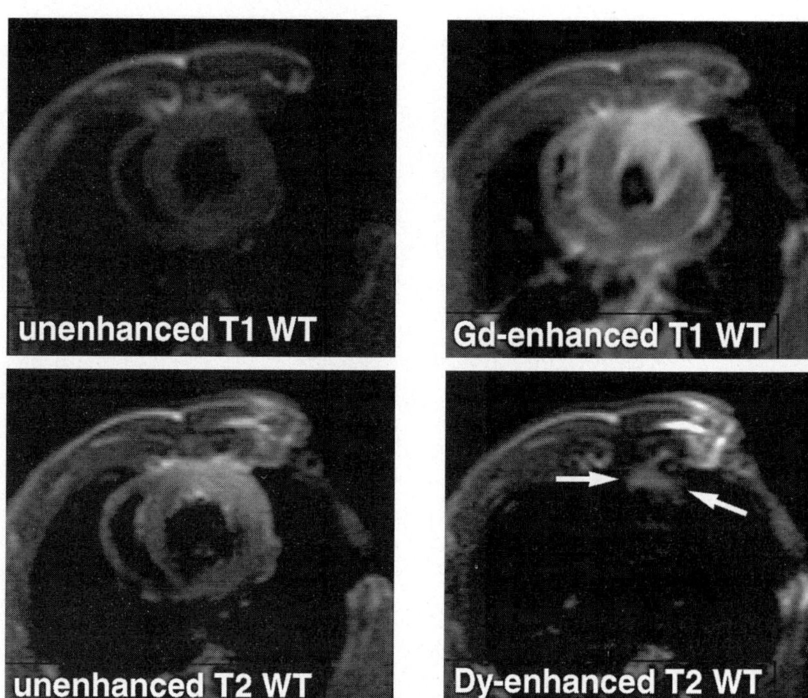

FIGURE 44–10. Magnetic resonance images acquired before and after the administration of Gd-DTPA-BMA and Dy-DTPA-BMA in a rat subjected to 2 hours of coronary occlusion followed by 2½ hours of reperfusion. *Top Left,* Unenhanced T1-weighted spin-echo image (TR/TE = 300/20 msec). *Top Right,* Gd-DTPA-BMA–enhanced T1-weighted image. On an unenhanced T2-weighted spin-echo image (TR/TE = 1500/60 msec), the infarcted region is shown as a bright region *(bottom left)* because of the presence of interstitial edema. *Bottom Right,* A Dy-DTPA-BMA–enhanced T2-weighted image. Reperfused infarcted myocardium is substantially enhanced compared with normal myocardium following Gd-DTPA-BMA. Dy-DTPA-BMA caused great reduction in signal intensity of normal myocardium, while that of reperfused infarction was moderately reduced, providing a depiction of the infarction as a visible area of relative hyperintensity *(arrows).*

profiles into blood flow parameters, as is currently done in CT, PET, and SPECT. However, it should be noted that substantial controversy exists concerning the validity of those two assumptions.[63, 89, 90, 117–121] Third, magnetic resonance contrast agents do not perturb the physiologic parameters being measured.

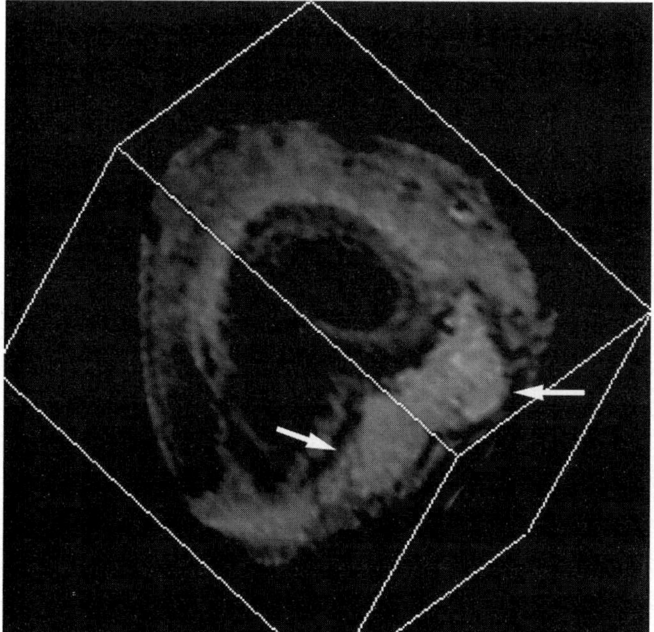

FIGURE 44–11. Three-dimensional gradient-recalled echo image (TR/TE = 600/15 msec) of a heart subjected to ischemia (1 hour) followed by reperfusion (1 hour). This constructed image was obtained from excised heart following administration of Dy-DTPA-BMA (1.0 mmol/kg). Note that the reperfused infarcted myocardium *(white arrows)* is clearly visualized as a hyperintense region compared with normal myocardium, as a result of greater signal loss in normal myocardium. This finding is consistent with the hypothesis that the failure of necrotic myocardial cells to exclude dysprosium chelate is responsible for the diminished potency of dysprosium to cause loss of magnetic resonance signal in reperfused infarcted but viable cells.

Experimental Models

Atkinson and colleagues[122] used inversion recovery–prepared fast gradient–recalled imaging to monitor the first pass of Gd-DTPA through Langendorff perfused isolated rat hearts subjected to regional ischemia. Contrast-enhanced images provided differential contrast between normal and ischemic myocardium. The first pass of gadolinium- and dysprosium-chelates through the heart has been monitored in dogs[88, 90, 123, 124] and rats.[43, 45, 87] In the authors' laboratory, dogs were studied with the use of a combination of inversion recovery–prepared and driven equilibrium–prepared fast gradient–recalled sequences, while in rats inversion recovery and echo planar images were used. On inversion recovery echo planar images (see Fig. 44–2) and gradient-echo images (see Figs. 44–4 and 44–5), administration of a low dose of gadolinium-chelates caused substantial enhancement in normal myocardium, whereas signal intensity of the ischemic region was unchanged. On gradient-recalled echo planar images (see Fig. 44–3) and driven equilibrium–prepared fast gradient–recalled sequences, administration of a high dose of gadolinium- or dysprosium-chelates caused substantial decrease in signal in normally perfused myocardium, while signal intensity of the ischemic region was less affected, and the ischemic region was visualized as an area of relatively high signal—a hot spot.[43, 45, 87] The quality of the images was higher on gadolinium-enhanced images than on dysprosium-enhanced images, and the ischemic region was clearly visualized on gadolinium-enhanced images.

Echo planar imaging appears to offer higher sensitivity to T2* weighting compared with spin-echo or fast gradient–recalled sequences. Kantor and co-workers[123] observed a reduction in myocardial signal intensity following the administration of Dy-DTPA or a high dose of Gd-DTPA on T2*-sensitive echo planar images. They also found that after dipyridamole infusion the magnitude of signal reduction was more profound and occurred earlier than in the baseline state. Coronary vasodilators have been routinely used in nuclear medicine to enhance the contrast between normal and hypoperfused myocardium. Using dipyridamole magnetic resonance perfusion imaging, investigators have demonstrated the feasibility of detecting hypoperfused myocardium under conditions of mild, moderate, and severe coronary stenosis.[89, 90] Wilke and associates[89] demonstrated in a canine heart a positive correlation between the alteration of myocardial signal intensity induced by Gd-DTPA

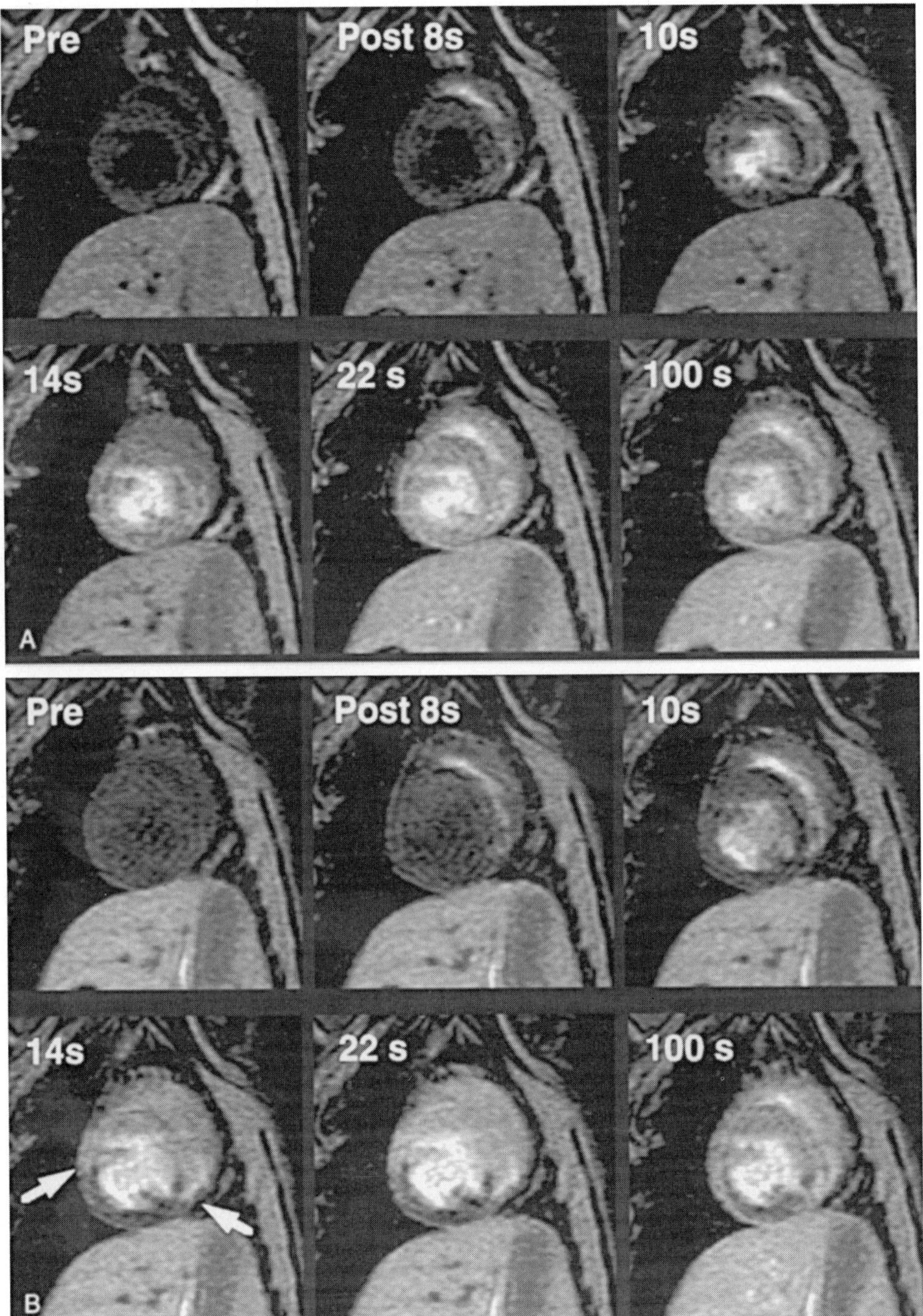

FIGURE 44–12. A, Inversion recovery (IR)–prepared GRE images (TR/TE/TI = 6.9/2.3/600 msec) during the transit of 0.05 mmol/kg Gd-BOPTA/dimeg through the heart of a dog subjected to nonocclusive left circumflex coronary artery stenosis in the basal state. Note that there is uniform enhancement of both normally perfused region and the area in jeopardy in the basal state. The territory of stenotic artery could not be defined during the transit of Gd-BOPTA/dimeg. *B*, IR-prepared gradient-recalled echo images (TR/TE/TI = 6.9/2.3/600 msec) during the transit of 0.05 mmol/kg of Gd-BOPTA/dimeg through the heart of the same dog following the infusion of dipyridamole, 0.1 mg/kg/min for 5 minutes. Note that the area in jeopardy (posterior wall of the left ventricle) is shown as a region of lower signal intensity *(arrow)* compared with normal myocardium (anterior wall). The territory of stenotic artery could clearly be defined during the transit of Gd-BOPTA/dimeg.

and absolute myocardial blood flow assessed by radiolabeled microspheres. In another study by the same group,[90] it was shown that myocardial blood flow and volume can be measured with the use of fast gradient–recalled sequence with macromolecular magnetic resonance contrast agent. Furthermore, Gd-DTPA-polylysine produced heterogeneous transmural enhancement on fast gradient–recalled images. This heterogeneous distribution of the agent may be attributed to variability in myocardial perfusion across the wall or capillary size and ordering.

In recent studies in the authors' laboratory, the use of dipyridamole has provided definition of hypoperfused regions during the first pass of gadolinium-based chelates. In the presence of critical stenosis (abolition of reactive hyperemic response), the hypoperfused region was not evident in the basal state (Fig. 44–12A).

When the flow was challenged by dipyridamole infusion, the hypoperfused region became visible during the first pass of Gd-BOPTA/dimeglumine (see Fig. 44–12*B*). This finding is in agreement with the well-established concept that hemodynamically significant stenosis is present when coronary reserve cannot be induced by vasodilatory stimulus.[125] In preliminary studies, Yeon and associates[126] and Taeymans and colleagues[127] used elegant techniques to evaluate the spatial relationship between signal enhancement defects due to impaired perfusion and spatial modulation of magnetization for assessment of function. They found that myocardial regions of perfusion deficit detected from the first pass of magnetic resonance contrast agent corresponded to regions with a contractile abnormality. Accordingly, fast MRI coupled with myocardial tagging techniques may allow noninvasive evaluation of myocardial perfusion, torsion, and regional wall stress and strain.

Human Studies

Pharmacologically induced coronary vasodilation with thallium-201 imaging, radionuclide angiography, or two-dimensional echocardiography is routinely used for detection of coronary artery stenosis and impairment of contractile function in myocardial segments distal to stenosis in patients. As with other techniques, investigators have demonstrated the utility of contrast-enhanced magnetic resonance perfusion images in healthy subjects[91, 128] and patients with coronary artery disease.[92–95, 120, 129–134] Perfusion MRI has been performed with or without coronary vasodilators. Preliminary data in patients with coronary artery disease have indicated that bolus administration of Gd-DTPA produces differential contrast between normal and ischemic myocardium on fast gradient–recalled imaging or echo planar imaging.[91, 92, 94, 120, 129, 130] Wilke and co-workers[120] found a delay in the enhancement of the area in jeopardy, whereas Manning and associates[92] found reduction in the peak enhancement and diminution in up-slope of the intensity-time curve in the area in jeopardy. Eichenberger and colleagues[93] and Schaefer and co-workers[94] also demonstrated the difference between normally perfused and hypoperfused myocardium in patients with coronary disease following the infusion of dipyridamole.

Lombardi and associates[131] studied eight patients with acute myocardial infarction, using contrast-enhanced fast gradient–recalled imaging and echocardiography. They found a close correlation between regional myocardial perfusion and contractility abnormalities after dobutamine infusion. Another group[95] used perfusion MRI in patients with healed myocardial infarction. This study has generated findings similar to those observed in different animal models of infarctions,[44, 45, 88] with myocardial regions perfused by occluded vessels displaying weak signal enhancement compared with normally perfused myocardium.

Hartnell and co-workers[134] studied 18 patients with ischemic coronary artery disease, using magnetic resonance perfusion imaging and magnetic resonance cineangiography before and during dipyridamole infusion. The results were compared with findings from perfusion scintigraphy and coronary angiography. The degree of accuracy of the combination magnetic resonance technique for detecting myocardial ischemia was similar to that of scintigraphy. Furthermore, the sensitivity of the combination of magnetic resonance technique for angiographically detecting significant coronary artery stenosis was 92 percent, and the specificity was 100 percent. For scintigraphy, the sensitivity was also 92 percent and the specificity was 100 percent. They concluded that a combination of stress magnetic resonance perfusion imaging and magnetic resonance ventriculography is feasible and that this technique can detect myocardial ischemia with an accuracy similar to that of scintigraphy. The authors have recently combined functional and perfusion MRI of patients with ischemic heart disease during the same magnetic resonance study (Fig. 44–13; see Fig. 44–12). In a group of patients with perfusion deficits previously demonstrated by thallium scintigraphy, breath-hold cine MRI has been used to display the extent of the deficit in wall thickening, while inversion recovery–prepared fast gradient echo imaging during the first pass of gadolinium-based magnetic resonance contrast agent demonstrated the perfusion deficit. Concordance has been shown between thallium deficit and functional and perfusion deficits as defined by MRI (Fig. 44–14).

Recently Edelman and Li[129] were the first to demonstrate the feasibility of using inversion recovery echo planar MRI in normal hearts of humans. Grist and colleagues[132] reported their initial experience in 10 patients with known coronary artery disease on rest-stress single-photon emission computed tomography with ^{201}Tl or ^{99m}Tc-sestamibi. They found that fixed and reversible perfusion defects can be identified following the infusion of dipyridamole contrast-enhanced multislice echo planar MRI. The results correlated with areas of abnormal perfusion detected on single-photon emission computed tomography perfusion study. Furthermore, Eichenberger and colleagues[93] used contrast-enhanced fast gradient echo imaging for the assessment of ischemic heart disease in 10 patients. They concluded that magnetic resonance perfusion imaging and magnetic resonance ventriculography are feasible and that this technique can detect myocardial ischemia.

Limitations

Magnetic resonance perfusion imaging measurement differs from the original indicator-dilution method in that magnetic reso-

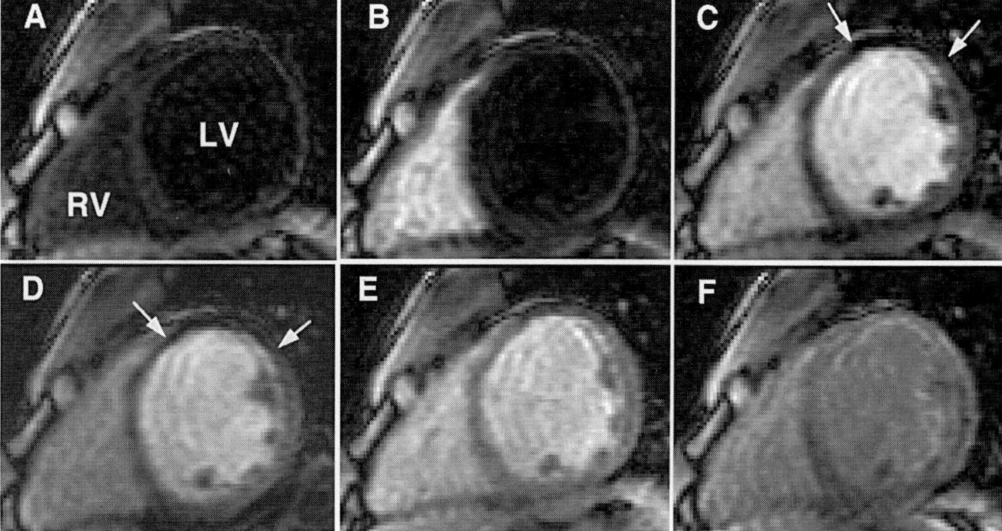

FIGURE 44–13. Perfusion scans in a patient with a fixed thallium defect in the anteroseptal region of the left ventricle. Contrast-enhanced fast gradient-recalled sequence shows a perfusion defect *(arrows)* in the anteroseptal and anterior regions.

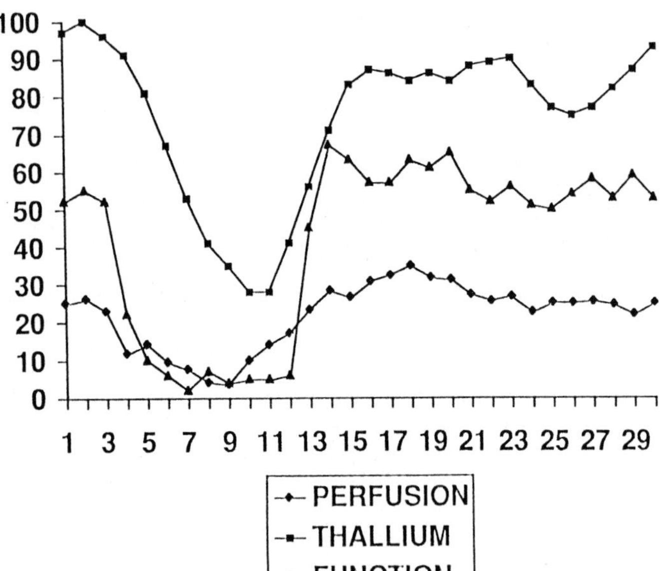

FIGURE 44–14. Comparison of thallium perfusion with magnetic resonance perfusion as shown on contrast-enhanced magnetic resonance perfusion images, and regional wall thickening as shown by cine MRI in a patient with a fixed thallium defect of the inferior segment of the left ventricle. The values were obtained from 30 segments (*x* axis) of the horizontal view of the left ventricle. Data are presented as a percentage of normal myocardium (*y* axis).

nance techniques do not directly measure quantities of contrast agents. Rather, one can infer the quantity of contrast agent from its effects on relaxation rate. The relaxation rate is not proportional to the concentration of the contrast agent in a compartmentalized environment.[135–138] The original formulation of indicator-dilution method was based on the ability to measure directly the indicator content at the entry and exit from the myocardium. On contrast-enhanced magnetic resonance images, the relaxation times (T1 and T2) of nearby water hydrogen in the capillaries can be lowered in the presence of contrast agent. The T1 value in other compartments (intracellular or interstitial) may then be lowered as a result of exchange of water between different compartments or because contrast agent can leak into these compartments.

Quantification of blood flow (perfusion) and volume is complicated by the fact that an ideal bolus of magnetic resonance contrast agent is difficult to achieve and the measured time dependence of signal intensity changes is a complex paradigm of organ transit function superimposed on arterial input function.[63, 91, 92] Previous studies have indicated that when magnetic resonance contrast agent is distributed throughout the extravascular space, enhanced T1 relaxation is not monoexponential.[135, 137] Any attempt to calculate myocardial flow from magnetic resonance contrast transit time or image pixel intensity must take into account the interdependence of transit time and blood volume. It is necessary to determine the contrast concentration in the aorta, the amount of the contrast agent retained in myocardium during the first pass, the complete transit time of the contrast agent through the capillary bed, changes in intravascular volume and interstitium, and the width of the contrast input function. The precise form of $\Delta R1$ function depends, however, not only on the integrity of local perfusion but also on the dilution and dispersion of the contrast medium bolus itself within the bloodstream.[139] If an arterial input function added to signal intensity changes over time, deconvolution analysis can then be used to find tissue clearance, the mean transit time through the capillary network, and ultimately the regional blood flow.[140] Further validations are necessary before definitive quantification of myocardial blood flow (ml/min/gm) can be obtained with the use of magnetic resonance perfusion imaging in patients. Although it is too early to predict whether magnetic resonance images of the first pass of contrast agents can be used to quantify myocardial perfusion, these methods currently provide high-quality images that clearly demonstrate the presence of a perfusion deficit and its extent.[141]

References

1. Lauterbur, P.C.: Image formation by induced local interactions: Examples employing nuclear magnetic resonance. Nature 242:19, 1973.
2. Lauterbur, P.C., Mendonca-Dias, M.H., and Rudin, A.M.: Augmentation of tissue water proton spin-lattice relaxation rate by in vivo addition of paramagnetic ions. *In* Dutton, P.L., Leigh, L.S., and Scarpa, A. (eds.): Frontiers of Biological Energetics. New York, Academic Press, 1978, pp. 752–768.
3. Higgins, C.B., Herfkens, R., Lipton, M.J., et al.: Nuclear magnetic resonance imaging of acute myocardial infarctions in dogs: Alterations in magnetic relaxation times. Am. J. Cardiol. 52:184, 1983.
4. Ratner, A.V., Okada, R.D., Newell, J.B., et al.: The relationship between proton NMR relaxation parameters and myocardial perfusion with acute coronary occlusion and reperfusion. Circulation 71:823, 1985.
5. Williams, E.S., Kaplan, J.I., Thatche,R.F., et al.: Prolongation of proton spin lattice relaxation times in regionally ischemic tissue from dog hearts. J. Nucl. Med. 21:449, 1980.
6. Pflugfelder, P.W., Wisenberg, G., Prato, F.S., et al.: Early detection of canine myocardial infarction by MRI in vivo. Circulation 70:587, 1985.
7. Wesbey, G., Higgins, C.B., Lanzer, P., et al.: Imaging and characterization of acute myocardial infarction *in vivo* by gated nuclear magnetic resonance. Circulation 69:125, 1984.
8. McNamara, M.T., Higgins, C.B., Schechtmann, N., et al.: Detection and characterization of acute myocardial infarction in man with the use of gated magnetic resonance imaging. Circulation 71:717, 1985.
9. Johnston, D.L., Thompson, R.S., Liu, P., et al.: Magnetic resonance imaging during acute myocardial infarction. Am. J. Cardiol. 57:1059, 1986.
10. Nishimura, T., Yamada, U., and Hayashi, M.: Determination of infarct size of acute myocardial infarction in dogs by magnetic resonance imaging and gadolinium-DTPA: Comparison with indium-111 antimyosin imaging. Am. J. Physiol. Imaging 4:83, 1989.
11. McNamara, M., Tscholakoff, D., Revel, D., et al.: Differentiation of reversible and irreversible myocardial injury by MR imaging with and without gadolinium-DTPA. Radiology 158:765, 1986.
12. Schaefer, S., Malloy, C.R., Katz, J., et al.: Gadolinium-DTPA–enhanced nuclear magnetic resonance imaging of reperfused myocardium: Identification of the myocardial bed at risk. Am. J. Cardiol. 12:1064, 1985.
13. Saeed, M., Wendland, M.F., Takehara, Y., et al.: Reperfusion and irreversible myocardial injury: Identification with a nonionic MR imaging contrast medium. Radiology 182:675, 1992.
14. Saeed, M., Wendland, M.F., Yu, K.K., et al.: Delineation of acute myocardial infarction with dysprosium DTPA-BMA: Influence of dose of magnetic susceptibility contrast medium. J. Am. Coll. Cardiol. 20:1634, 1992.
15. Tscholakoff, D., Higgins, C.B., Sechtem,U., et al.: MRI of reperfused myocardial infarct in dogs. AJR 146:925, 1986.
16. Tscholakoff, D., Higgins, C.B., Sechtem, U., et al.: Occlusive and reperfused myocardial infarcts: Effect of Gd-DTPA on ECG-gated MR imaging. Radiology 160:515, 1986.
17. Eichstadt, W.H., Felix, F., and Dougherty, R.C.: Magnetic resonance imaging at different stages of myocardial infarction using contrast agent gadolinium DTPA. Clin. Cardiol. 9:527, 1986.
18. Nishimura, T., Kobayashi, H., Ohara, Y., et al.: Serial assessment of myocardial infarction by using gated MR imaging and Gd-DTPA. AJR 153:715, 1989.
19. de Roos, A., van Rossum, A.C., van der Wall, E., et al.: Reperfused and nonreperfused myocardial infarction: Diagnostic potential of Gd-DTPA–enhanced MR imaging. Radiology 172:717, 1989.
20. Baer, F.M., Smolarz, K., Theissen, P., et al.: Identification of hemodynamically significant coronary artery stenosis by dipyridamole magnetic resonance imaging and ^{99m}Tc methoxyisohetlisonitrile-SPECT. Int. J. Cardiovasc. Imaging 9:133, 1993.
21. Pennell, D.J., Underwood, S.R., and Longmore, D.B.: Detection of coronary

artery disease using MR imaging with dipyridamole infusion. J. Comput. Assist. Tomogr. 14:167, 1990.
22. van Rugge, F.P., van der Wall, E.E., de Roos, A., et al.: Dobutamine stress magnetic resonance imaging for detection of coronary artery disease. J. Am. Coll. Cardiol. 22:431, 1993.
23. Haase, A.: Snapshot FLASH MRI: Applications to T1, T2, and chemical-shift imaging. Magn. Reson. Med. 13:77, 1990.
24. Mansfield, P.: Multiplanar image formation using NMR spin echoes. J. Phys. C. Solid State Phys. 10:L55, 1977.
25. Bean, C.P., and Livingston, J.D.: Superparamagnetism. J. Appl. Physics 30(Suppl.):120s, 1959.
26. Rosen, B.R., Belliveau, J.W., Vevea, J.M., et al.: Perfusion imaging with NMR contrast agents. Magn. Reson. Med. 14:249, 1990.
27. Solomon, I.: Relaxation processes in a system of two spins. Phys. Rev. 99:559, 1955.
28. Solomon, I., Bloembergen, N.: Nuclear magnetic interactions in the HF molecule. J. Chem. Phys. 25:261, 1956.
29. Bloembergen, N.: Proton relaxation times in paramagnetic solutions. J. Chem. Phys. 27:572, 1956.
30. Bloembergen, N., and Morgan L.O.: Proton relaxation times in paramagnetic solutions: Effects of electron spin relaxation. J. Chem. Phys. 34:842, 1961.
31. Burton, D.R., Forsen, S., Karlstrom, G., et al.: Proton relaxation enhancement (PRE) in biochemistry: A critical survey. Prog. NMR Spectroscopy 13:1, 1961.
32. Kowalewski, J., Nordenskiöld, L., Benetis, N., et al.: Theory of nuclear relaxation in paramagnetic systems in solution. Prog. NMR Spectroscopy 17:141, 1985.
33. Koenig, S.H., and Brown, R.D.: Field-cycling relaxometry of protein solutions and tissue: Implications for MRI. Prog. NMR Spectroscopy 22:487, 1985.
34. Lauffer, R.B.: Paramagnetic metal complexes as water proton relaxation agents for NMR Imaging: Theory and design. Chem. Rev. 87:901, 1987.
35. Thulborn, K., Waterton, J., Mathews, P., et al.: Oxygenation dependence of the transverse relaxation time of water protons in whole blood at high field. Biochim. Biophys. Acta 714:265, 1982.
36. Villringer, A., Rosen, B.R., Belliveau, J.W., et al.: Dynamic imaging with lanthanide chelates in normal brain: Contrast due to magnetic susceptibility effects. Magn. Reson. Med. 6:164, 1988.
37. Kennan, R.P., Zhong, J., and Gore, J.C.: Intravascular susceptibility contrast mechanisms in tissues. Magn. Reson. Med. 31:9, 1994.
38. Rosen, B.R., Belliveau, J.W., Aronen, H.J., et al.: Susceptibility contrast imaging of cerebral blood volume: Human experience. Magn. Reson. Med. 22:293, 1991.
39. Wismer, G.L., Buxton, R.B., Rosen, B.R., et al.: Susceptibility-induced MR line broadening: Applications to brain iron mapping. J. Comput. Assist. Tomogr. 12:259, 1988.
40. Albert, M.S., Huang, W., Lee, J.H., et al.: Susceptibility changes following bolus injections. Magn. Reson. Med. 29:700, 1993.
41. Chu, S.C., Xu, Y., Balschi, J.A., et al.: Bulk magnetic susceptibility shifts in NMR studies of compartmentalized samples: Use of paramagnetic reagents. Magn. Reson. Med. 13:239, 1990.
42. Saeed, M., Wendland, M.F., Yu, K.K., et al.: Dual effects of gadodiamide injection in depiction of the region of myocardial ischemia. J. Magn. Reson. Imaging 3:21, 1993.
43. Saeed, M., Wendland, M.F., Masui T., et al.: Dual mechanisms for change in myocardial signal intensity by means of a single MR contrast medium: Dependence on concentration and pulse sequence. Radiology 186:175, 1993.
44. Wendland, M.F., Saeed, M., Masui, T., et al.: Echo-planar MR imaging of normal and ischemic myocardium with gadodiamide injection. Radiology 186:535, 1993.
45. Yu, K.K., Saeed, M., Wendland, M.F., et al.: Real-time dynamics of an extravascular magnetic resonance contrast medium in acutely infarcted myocardium using inversion recovery and gradient-recalled echo-planar imaging. Invest. Radiol. 27:927, 1993.
46. Saini, S., Stark, D.D., Hahn, P.F., et al.: Ferrite particles: A superparamagnetic MR contrast agent for the reticuloendothelial system. Radiology 162:211, 1987.
47. Rozenman, Y., Zou, X., and Kantor, H.L.: Signal loss induced by superparamagnetic iron oxide particles in NMR spin-echo images: The role of diffusion. Magn. Reson. Med. 14:31, 1990.
48. Rozenman, Y., Zou, X.M., and Kantor, H.L.: Magnetic resonance imaging with superparamagnetic iron oxide particles for the detection of myocardial reperfusion. Magn. Reson. Imaging 9:933, 1991.
49. Canet, E., Revel, D., Forrat, R., et al.: Superparamagnetic iron oxide particles and positive enhancement for myocardial perfusion studies assessed by subsecond T1-weighted MRI. Magn. Reson. Imaging 11:1139, 1993.
50. Revel, D., Dandis, G., Pichard, J.B, et al.: MRI of acute myocardial infarction: Comparison of Gd-DPTA and superparamagnetic iron oxide particles (AMI-25). Radiology 177(Suppl.):219, 1990.
51. Schmiedl, U., Sievers, R.E., Brasch, R.C., et al.: Acute myocardial ischemia and reperfusion: MR imaging with albumin-Gd-DTPA. Radiology 170:351, 1989.
52. Schmiedl, U., Brasch, R.C., Ogan, M.D., et al.: Albumin labeled with Gd-DTPA: An intravascular contrast-enhancing agent for magnetic resonance blood pool and perfusion imaging. Acta Radiol. Suppl. 374:99, 1990.
53. Sieving, P.F., Watson, A.D., and Rocklage, S.M.: Preparation and characterization of paramagnetic polychelates and their protein conjugates. Bioconjugate Chem. 1:65, 1990.
54. Saeed, M., Wendland, M.F., Masui, T., et al.: Myocardial infarction: Assessment with an intravascular MR contrast medium. (Work in progress.) Radiology 180:153, 1991.
55. Vexler, V.S., Clement, O., Schmitt-Willich, H., et al.: Effect of varying the molecular weight of the MR contrast agent GdDTPA-polylysine on blood pharmacokinetics and enhancement patterns. J. Magn. Reson. Imaging 4:381, 1994.
56. Wang, S.C., Wikstrom, M.G., White, D.L., et al.: Evaluation of Gd-DTPA–labeled dextran as an intravascular MR contrast agent: Imaging characteristics in normal rat tissues. Radiology 175:483, 1990.
57. Wiener, E.C., Brechbiel, M.W., Brothers, H., et al.: Dendrimer-based metal chelates: A new class of magnetic resonance imaging contrast agents. Magn. Reson. Med. 31:1, 1994.
58. Adam, G., Neuerburg, J., Spüntrup, E., et al.: Gd-DTPA-cascade-polymer: Potential blood pool contrast agent for MR imaging. J. Magn. Reson. Imaging 4:462, 1994.
59. Fahlvik, AK, Klaveness, J, and Stark, DD.: Iron oxides as MR imaging contrast agents. J. Magn. Reson. Imaging 3:187, 1993.
60. Bol, A., Melin, J.A., Vanoverschelde, J.L., et al.: Direct comparison of [13-N] ammonia and [15-O] water estimates of perfusion with quantification of regional myocardial blood flow by microspheres. Circulation 87:512, 1993.
61. Judd, R.M., Resar, J.R., and Yin, F.C.P.: Rapid measurements of diastolic intramyocardial vascular volume. Am. J. Physiol. 265:H1038, 1993.
62. Brasch, R.C.: New directions in the development of MR imaging contrast media. Radiology 183:1, 1992.
63. Wilke, N., Kroll, K., Merkle, H., et al.: Regional myocardial blood volume estimated with MR first-pass imaging and polylysine-GdDTPA in the dog. J. Magn. Reson. Imaging 4(P):52, 1994.
64. Wolfe, C.L., Moseley, M.E., Wikstrom, M.G., et al.: Assessment of myocardial salvage after ischemia and reperfusion using magnetic resonance imaging and spectroscopy. Circulation 80:969, 1989.
65. Willerson, J., Watson, J., Hutton, I., et al.: Reduced myocardial reflow and increased coronary vascular resistance following prolonged myocardial ischemia in the dog. Circulation 36:771, 1975.
66. Dauber, I.M., VanBenthuysen, K.M., McMurtry, I.F., et al.: Functional coronary microvascular injury evident as increased permeability due to brief ischemia and reperfusion. Circ. Res. 66:986, 1975.
67. Fisher, M.R., McNamara, M.T., and Higgins, C.B.: Acute myocardial infarction: MR evaluation in 29 patients. AJR 148:247, 1987.
68. Geschwind, J.F., Wendland, M.F., Saeed, M., et al.: Identification of myocardial cell death in reperfused myocardial injury using a dual mechanisms of contrast enhanced magnetic resonance imaging. Acad Radiol. 1:319, 1994.
69. Pereira, R.S., Prato, F.S., Tong, C.Y., et al.: The relationship between myocardial viability and the distribution volume of Gd-DTPA in canine model of reperfusion and infarction injury. Proc. Soc. Magn. Reson. Med. 1492, 1994.
70. Wendland, M.F., Saeed, M., Lauerma, K., et al.: Alteration in T1 in normal and reperfused infarcted myocardium following GdBOPTA or GdDTPA on inversion recovery EPI. Proc. Soc. Magn. Reson. Med. 788, 1993.
71. Luckey, T.D., and Venugopal, B.: Metal Toxicity in Mammals. Vol. 1. New York, Plenum Press, 1977.
72. Sze, G., Brant-Zawadzki, M., Haughton, V.M., et al.: Multicenter study of gadodiamide injection as a contrast agent in MR imaging of the brain and spine. Radiology 181:693, 1991.
73. Sherwin, P.F., Hugo, F.P., Robison, R.O., et al.: Safety, tolerance, and pharmacokinetics of high doses of gadodiamide injection, a nonionic magnetic resonance imaging contrast agent. Acad. Radiol. 1:S2, 1994.
74. Runge, V.M., Bradley, W.G., Brant-Zawadzki, M.N., et al.: Clinical safety and efficacy of gadoteridol: A study in 411 patients with suspected intracranial and spinal disease. Radiology 181:701, 1991.
75. Runge, V.M., Dean, B., Lee, C., et al.: Phase III clinical evaluation of Gd-HP-DO3A in head and spine disease. J. Magn. Reson. Imaging 1:47, 1991.
76. Niendorf, H.P., Dinger, J.C., Haustein, J., et al.: Tolerance data of Gd-DTPA: A review. Eur. J. Radiol. 13:15, 1991.
77. Niendorf, H.P., Haustein, J., Cornelius, I., et al.: Safety of gadolinium-DTPA: Extended clinical experience. Magn. Reson. Med. 22:222, 1991.
78. Muhler, A., Saeed, M., Brasch, R.C., et al.: Hemodynamic effects of bolus injection of gadodiamide injection and gadopentetate dimeglumine as contrast media at MR imaging in rats. Radiology 183:523, 1992.
79. Muhler, A., Clement, O., Saeed, M., et al.: Gadolinium-ethoxybenzyl-DTPA, a new liver-directed magnetic resonance contrast agent: Absence of acute hepatotoxic, cardiovascular, or immunogenic effects. Invest. Radiol. 28:26, 1993.
80. Saeed, M., Li, H.T., Wendland, M.F., et al.: Comparison of cardiovascular response to ionic and nonionic magnetic resonance susceptibility contrast agents. Invest. Radiol. 29:319, 1994.
81. Li, H.T., Saeed, M., Wendland, M.F., et al.: Cardiovascular responses after ionic and nonionic magnetic resonance contrast media in rats with acute myocardial infarction. Invest. Radiol. 28:11, 1993.
82. Muhler, A., Saeed, M., Brasch, R.C., et al.: Amelioration of cardiodepressive effects of gadopentetate dimeglumine with addition of ionic calcium. Radiology 184:159, 1992.
83. Higgins, C.B., Saeed, M., and Wendland, M.F.: Contrast enhancement for the myocardium. Magn. Reson. Med. 22:347, 1991.
84. Higgins, C.B., Saeed, M., Wendland, M.F., et al.: Contrast media for cardiothoracic MR imaging. J. Magn. Reson. Imaging 3:265, 1993.
85. de Roos, A., and van Voorthuisen, A.E.: Magnetic resonance imaging of the heart: Perfusion, function, and structure. Curr. Opin. Radiol. 3:525, 1991.
86. Brasch, R.C.: Work in Progress: Methods in contrast enhancement for NMR imaging and potential applications. Radiology 147:781, 1983.
87. Wendland, MF, Saeed, M, Masui, T, et al.: First pass of an MR susceptibility contrast agent through normal and ischemic heart: Gradient-recalled echo-planar imaging. J. Magn. Reson. Imaging 3:755, 1993.
88. Saeed, M., Wendland, M.F., Lauerma, K., et al.: Detection of myocardial ischemia using first pass contrast-enhanced inversion recovery and driven equilibrium fast GRE imaging. J. Magn. Reson. Imaging 5:515, 1995.

89. Wilke, N., Simm, C., Zhang, J., et al.: Contrast-enhanced first pass myocardial perfusion imaging: Correlation between myocardial blood flow in dogs at rest and during hyperemia. Magn. Reson. Med. 29:485, 1993.
90. Wilke, N., Zhang, Y., Merkle, H., et al.: MR first pass imaging in the assessment of myocardial perfusion using a blood pool contrast agent. Proc. Soc. Magn. Reson. Med. 537, 1993.
91. van Rugge, F.P., Boreel, J.J., van der Wall, E.E., et al.: Cardiac first-pass and myocardial perfusion in normal subjects assessed by sub-second Gd-DTPA enhanced MR imaging. J. Comput. Assist. Tomogr. 15:959, 1991.
92. Manning, W.J., Atkinson, D.J., Grossman, W., et al.: First-pass nuclear magnetic resonance imaging studies using gadolinium-DTPA in patients with coronary artery disease. J. Am. Coll. Cardiol. 18:959, 1991.
93. Eichenberger, A.C., Schuiki, E., Köchli, D.V., et al.: Ischemic heart disease: Assessment with gadolinium-enhanced ultrafast MR imaging and dipyridamole stress. J. Magn. Reson. Imaging 4:425, 1994.
94. Schaefer, S., van Tyen, R., and Saloner, D.: Evaluation of myocardial perfusion abnormalities with gadolinium-enhanced snapshot MR imaging in humans: Work in progress. Radiology 185:795, 1992.
95. van Rugge, F.P., van der Wall, E.E., van Dijkman, P.R., et al.: Usefulness of ultrafast magnetic resonance imaging in healed myocardial infarction. Am. J. Cardiol. 70:1233, 1992.
96. Pettigrew, R.I.: Dynamic cardiac MR imaging: Techniques and applications. Radiol. Clin. North Am. 27:1183, 1989.
97. Been, M., Smith, M.A., and Ridgway, P.: Serial changes in the T1 magnetic relaxation parameter after myocardial infarction in man. Br. Heart J. 59:1, 1988.
98. Dulce, M.C., Duerinckx, A.J., Hartiala, J., et al.: MR imaging of the myocardium using nonionic contrast medium: Signal-intensity changes in patients with subacute myocardial infarction. AJR 160:963, 1993.
99. Thompson, R.C., Liu, P., Brady, T.J., et al.: Serial magnetic resonance imaging in patients following acute myocardial infarction. (See comments.) Magn. Reson. Imaging 9:155, 1991.
100. Pattynama, P.M.T., de Roos, A., van der Wall, E.E., et al.: Evaluation of cardiac function with magnetic resonance imaging. Am. Heart J. 128:595, 1994.
101. de Roos, A., Doornbos, J., van der Wall, EE., et al.: MR imaging of acute myocardial infarction: Value of Gd-DTPA. AJR 150:531, 1988.
102. Saeed, M., Wendland, M.F., Takehara, Y., et al.: Reversible and irreversible injury in the reperfused myocardium: Differentiation with contrast material-enhanced MR imaging. Radiology 175:633, 1990.
103. Saeed, M., Wagner, S., Wendland, M.F., et al.: Occlusive and reperfused myocardial infarcts: Differentiation with Mn-DPDP–enhanced MR imaging. Radiology 172:59, 1989.
104. Saeed, M., Wendland, M.F., Yu, K.K., et al.: Identification of myocardial reperfusion with echo planar magnetic resonance imaging: Discrimination between occlusive and reperfused infarctions. Circulation 90:1492, 1994.
105. van der Wall, E.E., de Roos, A., van Voorthuisen, A.E., et al.: Magnetic resonance imaging: A new approach for evaluating coronary artery disease? Am. Heart J. 121:1203, 1991.
106. van der Wall, E.E., van Dijkman, P.R., de Roos, A., et al.: Diagnostic significance of gadolinium-DTPA (diethylenetriamine penta-acetic acid) enhanced magnetic resonance imaging in thrombolytic treatment for acute myocardial infarction: Its potential in assessing reperfusion. Br. Heart J. 63:12, 1990.
107. van Rossum, A.C., Visser, F.C., van Eenige, M.J., et al.: Value of gadolinium-diethylene-triamine pentaacetic acid dynamics in magnetic resonance imaging of acute myocardial infarction with occluded and reperfused coronary arteries after thrombolysis. Am. J. Cardiol. 65:845, 1990.
108. Yu, K.K., Saeed, M., Wendland, M.F., et al.: Comparison of T1-enhancing and magnetic susceptibility magnetic resonance contrast agents for demarcation of the jeopardy area in experimental myocardial infarction. Invest. Radiol. 28:1015, 1993.
109. Saeed, M., Wendland, M.F., Tomei, E., et al.: Demarcation of myocardial ischemia: Magnetic susceptibility effect of contrast medium in MR imaging. Radiology 173:763, 1989.
110. Saeed, M., Wendland, M.F., Masui, T., et al.: Myocardial infarctions on T1- and susceptibility-enhanced MRI: Evidence for loss of compartmentalization of contrast media. Magn. Reson. Med. 31:31, 1994.
111. Lauerma, K, Saeed, M, Wendland, MF, et al.: The use of contrast-enhanced magnetic resonance imaging to define ischemic injury after reperfusion: Comparison in normal and hypertrophied hearts. Invest. Radiol. 29:527, 1994.
112. Lauerma, K., Saeed, M., Wendland, M.F., et al.: Evaluation of hypertrophic myocardium using gadoteridol enhanced MR imaging. Proc. Soc. Magn. Reson. Med. 544, 1993.
113. de Roos, A., Matheijssen, N.A.A., Doornbos, J., et al.: Myocardial infarct size after reperfusion therapy: Assessment by gadolinium-DTPA–enhanced MR imaging. Radiology 176:517, 1990.
114. Krauss, X.H., Van der Wall, E.E., Doornbos, J., et al.: Value of magnetic resonance imaging in patients with a recent myocardial infarction: Comparison with planar thallium-201 scintigraphy. Cardiovasc. Intervent. Radiol. 12:119, 1989.
115. Bodenheimer, M.M., Banka, V.S., Fooshee, C., et al.: Relationship between regional myocardial perfusion and the presence, severity and reversibility of asynergy in patients with coronary heart disease. Circulation 58:789, 1978.
116. Brunken, R., Schwaiger, M., Grover-McKay, M., et al.: Positron emission tomography detects tissue metabolic activity in myocardial segments with persistent thallium perfusion defects. J. Am. Coll. Cardiol. 557, 1987.
117. Tong, C.Y., Prato, F.S., Wisenberg, G., et al.: Techniques for the measurement of the local myocardial extraction efficiency for inert diffusible contrast agents such as gadopentate dimeglumine. Magn. Reson. Med. 30:332, 1993.
118. Diesbourg, L.D., Prato, F.S., Wisenberg, G., et al.: Quantification of myocardial blood flow and extracellular volumes using a bolus injection of Gd-DTPA: Kinetic modeling in canine ischemic disease. Magn. Reson. Med. 23:239, 1992.
119. Schwarzbauer, C., Syha, J., and Haase, A.: Quantification of regional blood volumes by rapid T1 mapping. Magn. Reson. Med. 29:709, 1993.
120. Wilke, N., Maching, T., Engels, G., et al.: Dynamic perfusion studies by ultrafast MR imaging: Initial clinical results from cardiology. Electromedica 58:102, 1990.
121. Shames, D.M., Kuwatsuru, R., Vexler, V., et al.: Measurement of capillary permeability to macromolecules by dynamic magnetic resonance imaging: A quantitative noninvasive technique. Magn. Reson. Med. 29:616, 1993.
122. Atkinson, D.J., Burstein, D., and Edelman, R.R.: First-pass cardiac perfusion: Evaluation with ultrafast MR imaging. Radiology 174:757, 1990.
123. Kantor, H.L., Rzedzian, R.R., Buxton, R., et al.: Contrast-induced myocardial signal reduction: Effect of lanthanide chelates on ultra high speed MR imaging. Magn. Reson. Imaging 12:51, 1994.
124. Schaefer, S., Lange, R.A., Gutekunst, D.P., et al.: Contrast-enhanced magnetic resonance imaging of hypoperfused myocardium. Invest. Radiol. 26:551, 1991.
125. Gould, K.L.: Noninvasive assessment of coronary stenosis by myocardial perfusion imaging during pharmacologic coronary vasodilatation: I. Physiologic basis and experimental validation. Am. J. Cardiol. 41:267, 1978.
126. Yeon, S.B., Reichek, N., Tallant, B.A., et al.: Imaging function and perfusion defects in myocardial infarction using magnetic resonance tagging and iron oxide contrast. Proc. Soc. Magn. Reson. Med. 371, 1991.
127. Taeymans, Y., Carlier, P.G., Gilles, R., et al.: MRI of acute myocardial infarction in dogs using dynamic contrast enhanced ultra-fast GE and tagging sequences. Proc. Soc. Magn. Reson. Med. 539, 1993.
128. Sakuma, H., O'Sullivan, M., Lucas, J., et al.: Effect of magnetic susceptibility contrast medium on myocardial signal intensity with fast gradient-recalled echo and spin-echo MR imaging: Initial experience in humans. Radiology 190:161, 1994.
129. Edelman, R.R., and Li, W.: Contrast-enhanced echo-planar MR imaging of myocardial perfusion: Preliminary study in humans. Radiology 190:771, 1994.
130. van Rossum, A.C., Keijer, T., Hofman, M., et al.: First-pass MRI of myocardial perfusion at rest and after pharmacologically induced vasodilation in patients with coronary artery disease. Proc. Soc. Magn. Reson. Med. 543, 1993.
131. Lombardi, M., Kvaerness, J., Soma, J., et al.: Snapshot gradient echo imaging at 0.5 T: A clinical study of perfusion deficits in acute myocardial infarctions. Proc. Soc. Magn. Reson. Med. 107, 1994.
132. Grist, T.M., Korosec, F.R., Fischer, D.J., et al.: Echo planar imaging in patients with myocardial perfusion abnormalities. Proc. Soc. Magn. Reson. Med. 106, 1994.
133. Klein, M.A., Collier, B.P., Hellman, R.S., et al.: Detection of chronic coronary artery disease: Value of pharmacologically stressed, dynamically enhanced turbo FLASH low angle shot MR images. AJR 161:257, 1993.
134. Hartnell, G., Cerel, A., Kamalesh, M., et al.: Detection of myocardial ischemia: Value of combined myocardial perfusion and cineangiographic MR imaging. AJR 163:1061, 1994.
135. Burstein, D., Taratuta, E., and Manning, W.J.: Factors in myocardial "perfusion" imaging with ultrafast MRI and Gd-DTPA administration. Magn. Reson. Med. 20:299, 1991.
136. Wendland, M.F., Saeed, M., Yu, K.K., et al.: Inversion recovery EPI of bolus transit in rat myocardium using intravascular and extravascular gadolinium-based MR contrast media: Dose effects on peak signal enhancement. Magn. Reson. Med. 32:319, 1994.
137. Mauss, Y., Grucker, D., Fornasiero, D., et al.: NMR compartmentalization of free water in the perfused rat heart. Magn. Reson. Med. 2:187, 1985.
138. Donahue, K.M., Burstein, D., Manning, W.J., et al.: Studies of Gd-DTPA relaxivity and proton exchange rates in tissue. Magn. Reson. Med. 32:66, 1994.
139. van Bruggen, N., Roberts, T.P.L., and Cremer, J.E.: The application of magnetic resonance imaging to the study of experimental cerebral ischemia. Cerebrovasc. Brain Metab. Rev. 6:180, 1994.
140. Rosen, B.R., Belliveau, J.W., Buchbinder, B.R., et al.: Contrast agents and cerebral hemodynamics. Magn. Reson. Med. 19:285, 1991.
141. Saeed, M., Szolar, D.H., Wendland, M.F., et al.: Detection of myocardial perfusion deficit and sizing of hypoperfused myocardium using first-pass contrast-enhanced inversion recovery and driven equilibrium fast GRE imaging. Proc. Soc. Magn. Reson. Med. 1408, 1995.

CHAPTER

45 Integrated Cardiac Magnetic Resonance Examination

Elias A. Zerhouni, M.D.

A comprehensive understanding of the heart in health and disease requires detailed knowledge of multiple functional parameters, such as integrity of the cardiac anatomy, adequacy of vascular supply during both rest and stress conditions, local and global mechanical function, and, ideally, underlying metabolism. These parameters are now obtained through a multiplicity of separate methods, including echocardiography, radionuclide imaging, coronary angiography, and magnetic resonance imaging (MRI).

To date, the primary clinical use of MRI has been in the evaluation of structural abnormalities of the heart, such as cardiac masses and congenital anomalies, and the long-term effects of myocardial infarction. Since its inception, however, MRI has been considered to have great potential to produce a more comprehensive evaluation of the cardiovascular system. The intrinsic multiplanar capabilities of MRI allow easy evaluation of anatomically complex structures. The intrinsic sensitivity of MRI to motion effects can be used advantageously to study flow patterns in vascular structures, including the coronary arteries. The high inherent tissue contrast obtainable with MRI allows sensitive detection of both endogenous and exogenous contrast agents in the intact human. In addition to the standard depiction of myocardial contraction, novel methods that use either tissue tagging or multidirectional phase encoding permit unique calculation of three-dimensional deformation within myocardial tissue during its entire contractile cycle.

Despite its enormous theoretical advantages, MRI has not yet achieved wide clinical acceptance because current scanners cannot perform a comprehensive cardiac study within reasonable examination times. Recent research and development of high-performance hardware and pulse sequences, however, now permit the formulation of more effective study protocols. Faster imaging sequences that require high-performance gradients have now been implemented successfully, and most manufacturers have improved the performance of imaging gradients to the point where routine, clinically effective, high-speed acquisitions can be obtained. This development has been greatly enhanced by the use of innovative pulse sequences, such as gated single breath-hold segmented K-space techniques and echo planar imaging (EPI). Although these advances have significantly improved the prospects for successful implementation of an integrated and time-efficient cardiac magnetic resonance examination, current scanners are still hampered by inadequate software design and slow computer systems that are being redesigned to allow nearly real-time interactive scanning. Now emerging is a consensus that dedicated high-speed scanners optimized for cardiovascular applications will be essential to the clinical success of cardiac MRI.

Pending successful development of these redesigned specific-use scanners, today it is nonetheless possible to perform comprehensive cardiac magnetic resonance examinations. Based on the author's experience, it is possible to formulate magnetic resonance examination strategies that answer most of the relevant questions in clinical cardiac imaging in a single examination. Although these protocols are likely to evolve over the near future, in line with technological developments, they foretell of the potential of using an integrated approach to clinical cardiac MRI. With the use of standardized imaging protocols that limit the examination to a minimum set of sequences and images while preserving the essential parameters needed for clinical assessment, it is possible to study anatomy, mechanical function, and tissue perfusion in about 1 hour.

The success of an integrated protocol depends, in great part, on the utilization of pulse sequences that are flexible enough to allow cine imaging in multiple arbitrary orientations from a single prescription. In addition, these sequences should permit detailed quantitative motion studies with the use of either myocardial tagging or multidirectional phase encoding. The same cine sequence modified in real time at the switch of user-defined control variables can also be employed for the assessment of perfusion with the use of exogenous contrast agents and coronary imaging. This sequence should allow single breath-hold acquisitions and should be compatible with multicoil array imaging for maximum signal-to-noise ratio. The author implemented this approach by developing a "master" cardiac imaging sequence based primarily on the segmented K-space approach initially proposed by Atkinson and Edelman. An optimization algorithm for arbitrary imaging angles was added to the sequence, and a user interface allows the operator to activate, without having to reload the sequence software, a series of imaging parameters, such as the number of phase-encode steps and their groupings and the addition of a tagging pattern in the x, y, or z directions. For a perfusion study, a single command can be activated, allowing acquisition of perfusion images following preparation by a train of RF pulses to reach steady state. This master sequence includes spectral fat saturation pulses to enable coronary imaging as well as slab saturation to eliminate signal from inflowing blood, when necessary. The development of such integrated "master" cardiac sequences is a key to the successful implementation of a comprehensive clinical cardiac examination. The author's current examination strategy comprises three separate steps: (1) the examination of mechanical function at rest and during pharmacologic stress, (2) the performance of an exogenous contrast-enhanced series with the use of clinically approved agents, and (3) a study of the proximal coronary vessels that focuses on the coronary territories suspected of being abnormal as determined by steps 1 and 2. All studies are performed with a specially developed cardiac multicoil array for maximum signal-to-noise ratio. On-line electrocardiogram and blood-pressure monitoring as well as pulse oximetry are always used. An indwelling intravenous catheter with saline perfusion via a calibrated magnetic resonance–compatible infusion pump is placed prior to the examination.

IMAGING OF GLOBAL AND LOCAL MECHANICAL FUNCTION

Electrocardiogram-gated segmented K-space cine acquisitions during suspended respiration provide views of the heart during systole and diastole at temporal resolution of 30 to 60 msec. Complete three-dimensional coverage of the myocardium in long and short axes can be accomplished with 12 to 18 breath-holds of a duration of 16 to 24 heartbeats with a standard gradient system and 3 to 6 breath-holds with multishot EPI capability. All the cine acquisitions are tagged with a DANTE-SPAMM scheme in a set of six parallel short-axis images and a set of six radially distributed long-axis images with a matrix of 256 by 110 and five phase groupings with TR of 6.5 msec and TE 2.3 msec, flip angle of 15 to 20 degrees (Fig. 45–1). Slab saturation is applied parallel to the image plane to decrease the signal from ventricular blood. Because tag persistence is dependent on the T1 relaxation time of myocardium, these image series are always obtained prior to injection of any contrast medium that shortens the T1 of myocardium.

With segmented multishot EPI, the acquisition of images is fast enough to allow both rest and post-dobutamine stress imaging with stages of 5 minutes each. At the present time, for validation and research purposes, the author selects patients who have already undergone dobutamine echo stress testing and does not exceed the dose of dobutamine at which wall motion abnormalities were observed with echocardiography. Other researchers have shown the feasibility of such studies with standard scanners. The author believes, however, that because of the requirement for on-line monitoring of wall motion to detect ischemia, such studies require high-speed acquisition capabilities.

These cine tagged images are viewed on-line for qualitative evaluation of myocardial contraction while the patient is being examined. The cine images are then analyzed off-line. After semi-automated segmentation of epicardial and endocardial contours and linear tags (Fig. 45–2), a three-dimensional finite element analysis of the *true* material deformation of the myocardium can be performed and spatially coregistered with the image data to provide a context-sensitive anatomical and functional data set (Fig. 45–3). All the usual parameters of global function, such as global and regional ejection fraction, ventricular mass, and wall stress, can then be easily extracted. Three-dimensional reconstruction at each point in time permits dynamic display of all strain parameters independent of global cardiac motion in a variety of formats (Fig. 45–4). Although myocardial tagging or three-dimensional phase encoding are the only existing methods that permit true noninvasive quantification of both global and local functional parameters, the issue of whether such a detailed analysis of mechanical function is of greater clinical value than simpler semiquantitative planar methods is still being investigated. Nonetheless, with improved scanners and image analysis methods, it is likely that the ability to more accurately quantify local function may find use in the development of more objective and operator-independent methods of measuring function during rest and graded levels of stress (Fig. 45–5). The development of such an inherently *quantitative stress test* could provide a more sensitive and objective method of detecting local ischemia than two-dimensional stress echocardiography, which suffers from the lack of spatial coregistration of myocardial regions at rest and during stress because of the change in the global shape of the heart during inotropic stress. The ability to quantitatively measure strain of the same *material* points rather than *image* points with MRI at rest and during stress is an unprecedented capability. The author has preliminarily shown that ischemic wall dysfunction can be demonstrated with MRI at levels of pharmacologic stress lower than those used with echocardiography. In addition, recovery of function in the regions surrounding infarcts can also be seen in the three-dimensional magnetic resonance

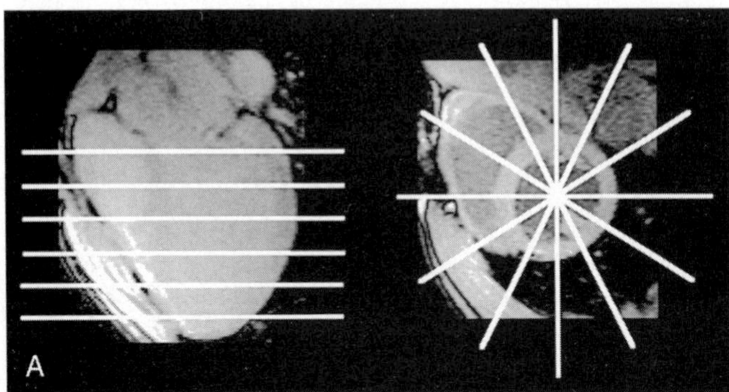

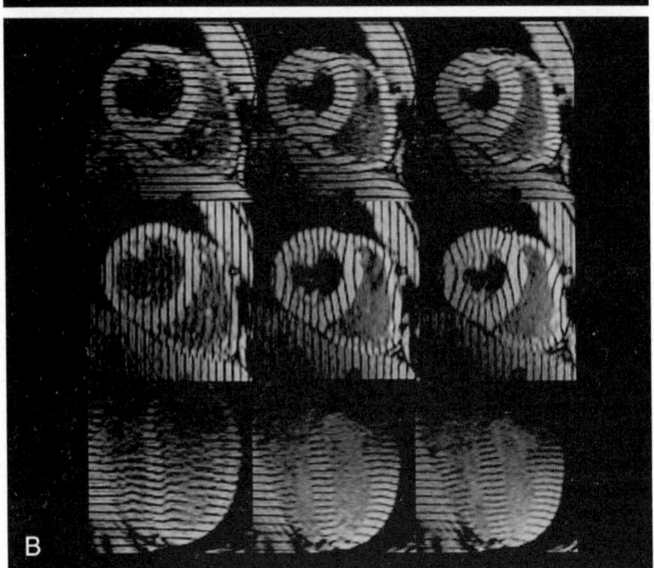

FIGURE 45–1. Acquisition protocol. *A*, Prescription planes for image acquisition. A series of parallel short-axis images followed by a series of radially distributed long-axis images are acquired to provide full anatomical coverage of the heart. *B*, Example of cine images with myocardial tagging. The top two rows show short-axis images, the bottom row a set of long-axis images.

strain data obtained during low-dose dobutamine stress, thus identifying stunned but viable myocardium (Fig. 45–6). Combined with concurrent measures of local perfusion at a spatial resolution greater than that achieved with radionuclide methods, such studies constitute a potentially powerful and cost-effective approach to the characterization of ischemia.

FIGURES 45–2 to 45–6. See Color Plates 22 and 23.

IMAGING OF TISSUE PERFUSION

At the present time, researchers obtain the most reliable results in clinical scanning with gadolinium-based contrast agents, using the T1-shortening effect of the agent with T1-sensitive pulse sequences. All the clinically approved magnetic resonance contrast media distribute freely within the vascular and extravascular extracellular spaces with a T1-shortening effect proportional to the concentration of gadolinium. Accurate in vivo quantitation of the local concentration of the agent via magnetic resonance images is, however, unlikely to be achieved because of exchange rate considerations between vascular and interstitial space and the complex influence of imaging parameters on signal intensity. Nonetheless, it appears that a semiquantitative approach may provide sufficient information for the sensitive detection of functionally ischemic regions prior to infarction and for the assessment of reperfusion after infarction.

The author's protocol for imaging of myocardial perfusion uses an image sequence that maximizes T1 contrast while preserving dynamic range and linearity of response to the concentration of gadolinium in both the ventricular cavity and the myocardium. To achieve these goals, the magnetization is first driven to saturation by a series of preparatory nonselective RF pulses followed by a segmented K-space spoiled gradient echo imaging sequence with a flip angle of 45 degrees and a matrix of 256 by 96 phase-encoded steps acquired in the same short-axis planes as those used for the functional images described earlier. By optimizing the RF saturation pulses, one can obtain two to three separate slices, depending on heart rate, in three successive heartbeats using 32 phase-encoded steps per heartbeat per image plane on a standard gradient system. Using multishot EPI, we can acquire six image planes in 2 to 4 heartbeats. Images are acquired as rapidly as possible following intravenous injection of the contrast medium. For the detection of suspected ischemia, contrast injection is performed immediately after the last stage of cine imaging during pharmacologic stress.

In patients with coronary flow restriction, transiently delayed opacification in the endocardial layer of the hypoperfused region is observed. The author's preliminary observations indicate that these zones of delayed enhancement correlate highly with the presence of flow-restricting lesions and that the amount of delay may predict the severity of the lesion. Encouragingly, these transient phenomena in the endocardium appear to last for periods of up to 30 to 60 seconds and thus are largely within the temporal resolution of current perfusion sequences (Fig. 45–7).

In patients with recent infarction, contrast agents provide insight into the status of tissue integrity in the ischemic region as well as an index of the effectiveness of reperfusion measures (Fig. 45–8). Central hypoenhancing zones that persist for several minutes in the infarct region have been shown to correlate with the "no-reflow" phenomenon in experimental canine models (Fig. 45–9). Late hyperenhancing regions, on the other hand, have been shown to correlate with the triphenyltetrazolium-chloride (TTC)–negative infarcted, nonviable myocardium both in humans with reperfused infarcts and in a canine model of infarction-reperfusion.

IMAGING OF THE CORONARY VESSELS

An important aspect of the cardiac magnetic resonance study is the ability to accurately coregister functional data in three dimensions. For instance, the perfusion images can be superimposed on the mechanical function images and transformed into a single function-perfusion map, since the same imaging planes are obtained for both. This capability is likely to enhance the interpretation and improve the accuracy of diagnosis. In addition, the finding of matched abnormal regions on tagged cine studies and perfusion studies in the same patient increases the likelihood of finding significant coronary flow restriction; such an improvement may ultimately lead to better patient selection for invasive coronary angiography. During the MRI examination one can tailor the mag-

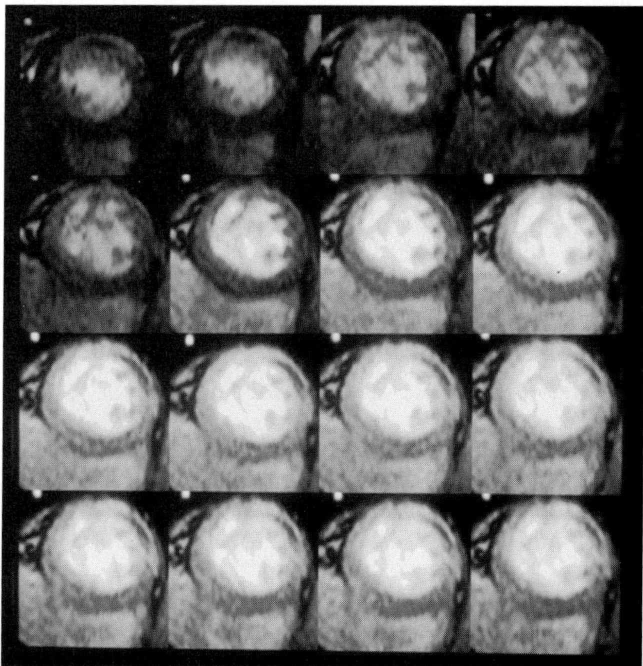

FIGURE 45–7. Endocardial ischemia. Contrast-enhanced study in a patient with proven circumflex coronary lesion and clinical history consistent with small infarct in the circumflex territory. Segmented driven equilibrium spoiled gradient-recalled acquisition at a temporal resolution of 3 heartbeats (1-cm-thick, 256 × 96 matrix, 28-cm field of view) shows the transit of an intravenously administered bolus of gadolinium DTPA. Note the presence of a crescentic-shaped subendocardial region of decreased signal intensity at 1 to 3 o'clock. The size of the abnormal signal region is seen to decrease over time.

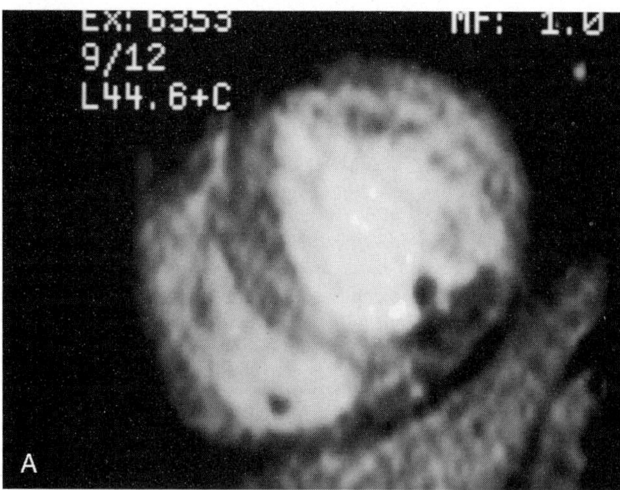

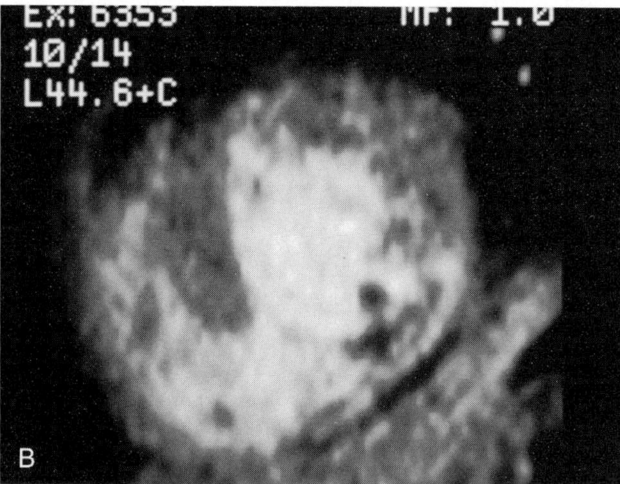

FIGURE 45–8. Reperfused infarction in a patient 48 hours after right coronary occlusion confirmed by angiography and treated with thrombolytic therapy and PTCA. Gadolinium-enhanced spoiled gradient-recalled images of a short-axis view of the heart using the same technique as that illustrated in Figure 45–7 and obtained at 1 minute *(A)* and 10 minutes *(B)* following bolus intravenous administration show a zone of persistent low-signal intensity at the center of the infarct region (4 to 5 o'clock). This central hypointensity area relates to the "no-reflow" region. Ten minutes after contrast administration, a zone of relative hyperintensity is seen from 3 to 8 o'clock, corresponding to infarcted but reperfused myocardium.

netic resonance coronary angiogram to the coronary vessel most likely to be responsible for the detected abnormality. This "guided" approach to coronary imaging with MRI is, the author believes, warranted because of the still-unreliable nature of magnetic resonance coronary angiography. In the author's experience, it has been difficult to obtain a satisfactory and complete depiction of all coronary vessels in one setting. The image resolution is still suboptimal for reliable "stand-alone" diagnosis of coronary lesions. The combination of functional and anatomical information in specific territories, however, is effective because the functional significance of any lesion can be assessed. Using surface coils, one can visualize the proximal 5 to 8 cm of the right coronary artery in more than 90 percent of patients, whereas success rates are more variable for the left main, left anterior descending, and circumflex arteries. Furthermore, lower success rates are experienced in female patients, owing to the smaller diameter of coronary arteries in women.

The method preferred by the author is scanning during diastole using fat-suppression with suspended respiration; the scan plane is oriented tangentially to the myocardial surface and a thick slice of 10 to 20 mm, 256 by 192 matrix, a flip angle of 15 to 20 degrees, and a field of view of 24 to 28 cm, with 16 phase-encode groupings is obtained (Fig. 45–10). This method allows direct visualization of the coronary vessel without the need for vessel segmentation from thin contiguous slices. This "tangential" scanning approach permits visualization of longer coronary segments in the region of suspected abnormality. Additional infusion of contrast material is sometimes required to better visualize more distal segments of the targeted vessel. At the present time, magnetic resonance coronary angiography remains the most challenging portion of the integrated cardiac MRI examination, and further progress is required for its widespread clinical applicability.

FIGURE 45–9. Reperfused infarction. A series of contrast-enhanced images over 15 minutes in a canine model of reperfusion shows a zone of subendocardial hypointensity from 30 seconds to 3 minutes corresponding to the "no-reflow" zone and a delayed surrounding zone *(arrow)* that enhances progressively from 2 to 15 minutes to become relatively hyperintense. This zone of delayed contrast enhancement corresponds to the reperfused but necrotic myocardium.

IMAGE ANALYSIS

The adequacy of image-analysis protocols for cardiac MRI remains a challenge. Off-line analysis still requires both time and operator interventions that limit the rapid availability of the information. Because of the complex and extensive amount of information generated during cardiac MRI, more efficient forms of data display and visualization that use state-of-the-art graphics computers are actively being developed. A promising approach, uniquely suited to MRI data, is the interactive display of both dynamic anatomical data and functional data derived from measurements of strain, perfusion, and coronary flow.

FUTURE POTENTIAL DEVELOPMENTS

Cardiac MRI is a very active field of investigation, and several new approaches are being proposed for studying myocardial function. It is clear that a period of increased experimentation will lead to rapid changes in the approach to the single-step comprehensive cardiac magnetic resonance examination. The exploitation of novel contrast mechanisms such as blood oxygen–dependent contrast (BOLD) may lead to more direct measurements of oxygenation at the tissue level. Perfusion measurements by spin tagging techniques also appear promising and may find a place in the examina-

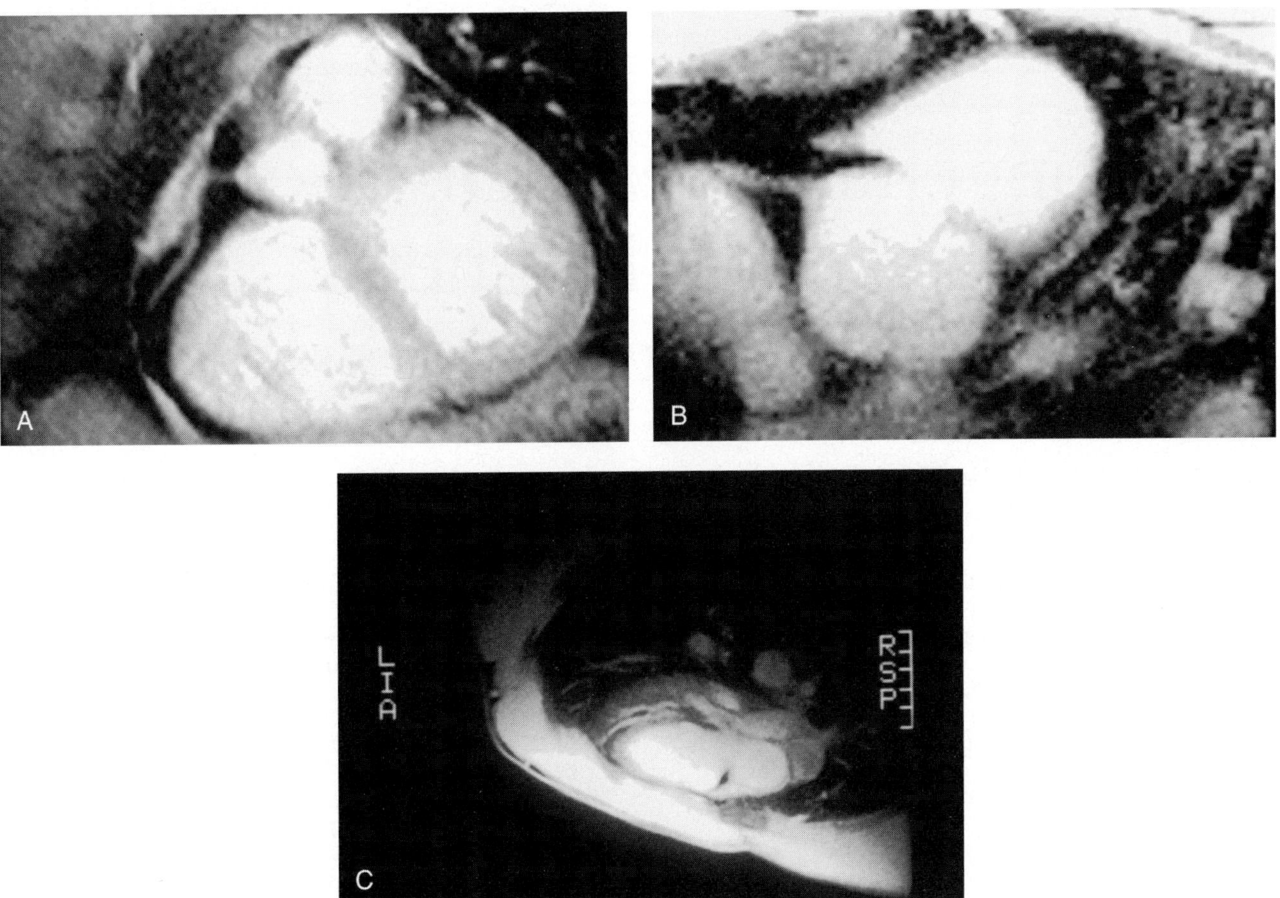

FIGURE 45–10. Coronary magnetic resonance angiography. Examples of right coronary magnetic resonance angiograms (*A* and *B*) and left anterior descending magnetic resonance angiograms (*C*) obtained with a surface coil and a single breath-hold technique.

tion protocol of the future. New contrast agents that use T2 contrast mechanisms or purely intravascular agents may play a prominent role. Cardiac spectroscopy, which is still a daunting technical challenge, may provide MRI with a metabolic dimension of great clinical value. The operator-independent nature of magnetic resonance examinations and its ability to accurately quantify multiple parameters of flow, perfusion, function, and anatomy at spatial and temporal resolutions unmatched by any other existing method are very likely to make MRI a cost-effective, high-diagnostic-value alternative in cardiac imaging.

CHAPTER

46 Congenital Heart Disease Assessed With Magnetic Resonance Techniques

Albert de Roos, M.D.
Sidney A. Rebergen, M.D.
Ernst E. van der Wall, M.D.

The number of patients with repaired congenital heart disease is steadily increasing, magnifying the strong clinical need for improved diagnostic methods to follow these patients over time. Long-term management is increasingly concerned with the growing numbers of postoperative patients, who continue to require medical surveillance over many years. It is estimated that there are between 500,000 and 600,000 adults with congenital heart disease in the United States, and each year another 10,000 children who have undergone surgical repair reach adulthood.[1]

The largest diagnostic category among patients who undergo repair is isolated ventricular septal defect, followed by tetralogy of Fallot. Imaging techniques are required to evaluate a wide spectrum of postoperative residua and sequelae after initial repair. The residua after reparative surgery for congenital heart disease include cardiac, vascular, or noncardiovascular abnormalities that are intentionally left behind at the time of reparative surgery. The sequelae encompass alterations or disorders that are intentionally incurred at the time of reparative surgery and are considered to be necessary and acceptable consequences of the operation.[2] Magnetic resonance (MR) imaging and spectroscopy provide a wide array of techniques for the evaluation of residua and sequelae after surgery for congenital heart disease that are unsurpassed by other noninvasive modalities.[3–5] The value of MR imaging is becoming firmly established in the follow-up of patients with a variety of congenital heart and great vessel abnormalities.[6] This acceptance is partly due to the complexity of the postoperative anatomy and function of, particularly, the right ventricle as well as to the limitations of the alternative imaging modalities that can be used in this category of patients. In these patients, echocardiography may be hampered by the presence of sternal wires and scar tissue, rib and chest malformations, and interposed lung tissue. Magnetic resonance imaging has unlimited access to the chest and is therefore well suited for the assessment of the heart and great vessels in any desired imaging plane with intrinsically three-dimensional capabilities. A stack of MR sections is commonly acquired to encompass the entire heart in contiguous imaging planes with a section thickness of 1 cm or less, allowing complete evaluation of the anatomy and function of both the ventricles and the atria without the need for geometric assumptions.

The value of this approach in presurgical planning of complex cardiovascular malformations has been compared with that of echocardiography and cardiac catheterization in a prospective study of a series of patients with heterotaxia syndrome.[5] In that study, MR imaging provided excellent anatomical and functional information that was in some patients not available with echocardiography or catheterization. However, cardiac catheterization is still required when determination of pulmonary vascular resistance is necessary for decision-making or when an interventional procedure is indicated.[5] Furthermore, until now MR imaging techniques have required data acquisition over many cardiac cycles with the use of electrocardiographic triggering and provided no real-time information, as with echocardiography. Recently, new MR imaging strategies have become available for high-speed image acquisition within one heartbeat. These imaging techniques provide real-time visualization of cardiac function and flow dynamics, alleviating the problems inherent to motion and cardiac arrhythmias. In this chapter the role of MR techniques in the evaluation of anatomy, function, flow, and metabolism is presented and its application in patients with some specific forms of congenital heart disease is discussed.

TECHNICAL OPTIONS OF MAGNETIC RESONANCE IMAGING AND SPECTROSCOPY

The array of MR techniques for the assessment of various aspects of congenital heart disease is steadily increasing. The fundamental aspects of MR imaging and spectroscopy have been summarized in previous chapters. In this chapter, the various options of MR imaging and spectroscopy that are relevant to the evaluation of congenital heart disease are addressed. Recently, there have been a number of developments in MR technology that will lead to increased clinical utility of MR techniques in cardiology. Magnetic resonance imaging provides high-resolution images without the use of ionizing radiation or contrast agents, while the technique is intrinsically sensitive to flow and motion.

Spin-Echo Magnetic Resonance Imaging

Multislice spin-echo MR imaging with triggering of the image acquisition by the electrocardiogram is the most commonly applied strategy to define the morphology of the heart and great vessels. Images are routinely obtained in the transverse plane, with additional imaging planes tailored to the cardiovascular structures under investigation (Fig. 46–1). The spin-echo images are acquired with relatively short repetition times (TR, dependent on the heart rate when electrocardiographic triggering is used) and short echo times (TE, 20 to 30 msec) with 2 to 4 averages to optimize the signal-to-noise ratio. This imaging sequence is especially well suited for defining anatomical detail but allows no assessment of dynamic cardiac events.[7] When a stack of spin-echo sections is acquired, each section corresponds to a different cardiac phase, without functional information of dynamic processes throughout the cardiac cycle.

Gradient-Echo Magnetic Resonance Imaging

In contrast with spin-echo techniques, gradient-echo MR imaging provides dynamic information on flow and cardiac function.[8]

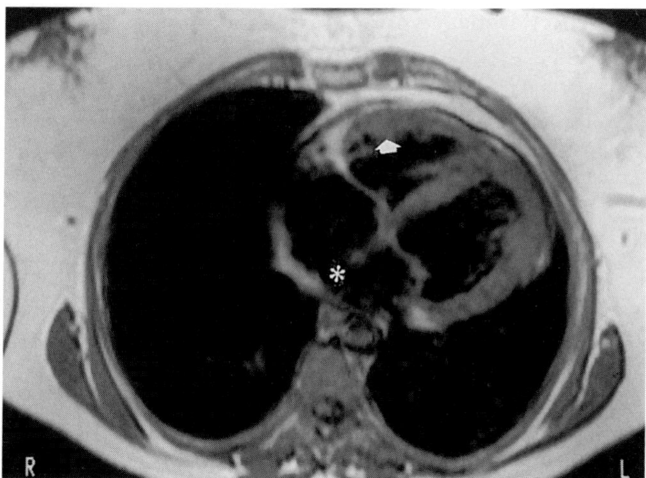

FIGURE 46–1. A transverse spin-echo image through the heart in a patient with an atrial septal defect *(asterisk)*. Note the signal void in the cardiac chambers, providing a natural contrast between the blood pool and cardiac structures. The free wall of the right ventricle *(arrow)* is markedly thickened owing to pulmonary hypertension.

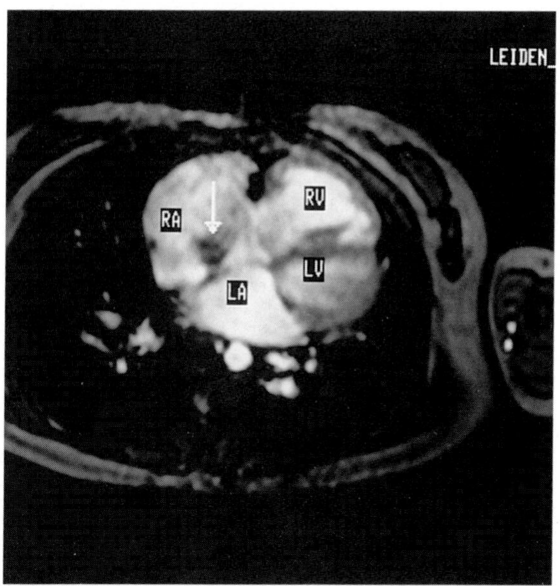

FIGURE 46–2. A transverse gradient-echo image through the heart in a patient with an atrial septal defect of the ostium secundum type, located in the region of the fossa ovalis. Note the high signal intensity of the blood pool in the cardiac chambers. A turbulent jet effect is emanating as a signal void from the central portion of the atrial septum, indicating a left-to-right shunt *(arrow)*. As a result of the left-to-right shunt, there is enlargement of the right atrium (RA) and right ventricle (RV). LA = left atrium; LV = left ventricle.

Gradient-echo images display flowing blood as bright signal intensity, whereas spin-echo images show flowing blood generally as dark signal or a signal void.[9] On gradient-echo cine displays disturbances of normal flow are evidenced as low-signal turbulent jet effects (Figs. 46–2 and 46–3). Gradient-echo images are acquired with high temporal resolution throughout the cardiac cycle by using short TR, short TE, and small flip angles.[7] However, the image acquisition is not real-time but requires, for example, 128 heart-

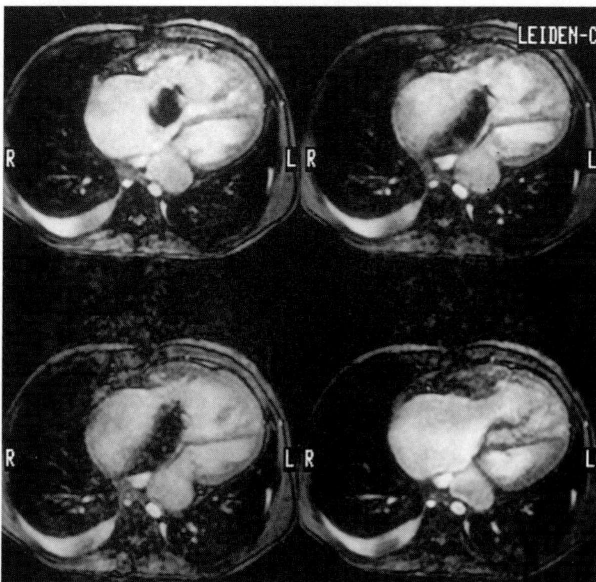

FIGURE 46–3. A series of four gradient-echo images throughout the cardiac cycle in a patient after Senning repair demonstrates a signal void originating at the level of the tricuspid valve and extending into the pulmonary-venous atrium, consistent with severe tricuspid valve insufficiency. Note the enlargement of the right ventricle and atrium. Pleural fluid is visible on the right side.

beats for images with 128 phase-encoding steps. The images can be displayed in a cine mode to reveal the dynamics of flow and other motion effects in a pseudo–real-time format. Artifacts inherent to gradient-echo techniques pose a problem when one images structures such as metallic implants or anatomical structures adjacent to the lung parenchyma because of susceptibility effects.

High-Speed Magnetic Resonance Imaging

Recently, ultrafast MR imaging sequences and real-time echo-planar techniques have been introduced into clinical practice.[10, 11] Fast imaging methods reduce image degradation from physiologic motion effects such as respiration and cardiac rotation during contraction, allowing improved evaluation of cardiovascular function. Ultrafast MR imaging allows image acquisition during a breath-hold within a one heartbeat interval. These rapid gradient-echo sequences operate with very short TR values, resulting in suboptimal image contrast. A prepulse is commonly applied to suppress the vascular signal and to provide T1-weighted contrast in the final image. To restore T1 and T2 image contrast, preparatory pulses are incorporated in the imaging sequence in the time interval before data collection starts. For example, this technique is applied to assess first-pass myocardial perfusion with the aid of various intravascular contrast agents used as perfusion markers.[12]

Echo-planar imaging (EPI) provides snapshot or multishot imaging with very short acquisition times of 20 to 100 msec per image, allowing real-time imaging of cardiac function and flow with acquisition rates of up to 50 images per second (Fig. 46–4).[11] In EPI, multiple segments of the image data are acquired from a single spin-echo or gradient-echo. The acquisition of an entire image after a single radiofrequency excitation is performed, for example, for a 128 phase-encoded image with 128 oscillations of the readout gradient. The readout gradient oscillates rapidly from positive to negative amplitude to form a train of gradient echoes that form around the envelope of the spin-echo induced by a single excitation. Each echo is differently phase-encoded by phase-encoded "blips" on the phase axis. EPI technology poses special demands on the gradient system and radiofrequency receiver of the MR scanner. With further technical development, EPI may become clinically applicable for multislice imaging of the entire heart within a single heartbeat. EPI images of the heart can be acquired without the need for electrocardiographic triggering in a free-run mode and displayed in a cine format to demonstrate dynamic processes such as valve function, flow, and perfusion.[13, 14]

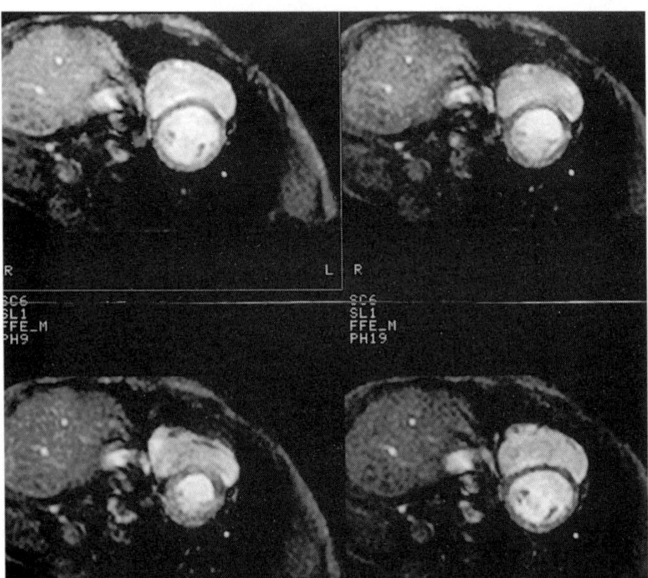

FIGURE 46–4. Multishot echo-planar short-axis images through the heart obtained with a 1.5 Tesla Philips NT15 MR scanner. Ten imaging sections with 21 cardiac phases per section were obtained to encompass the entire heart. Each imaging section with 21 phases and 36-msec temporal resolution was obtained during a 12-second breath-hold. Ten imaging sections with 21 phases for each level result in a total of 210 images, which are acquired during a 2-minute acquisition period.

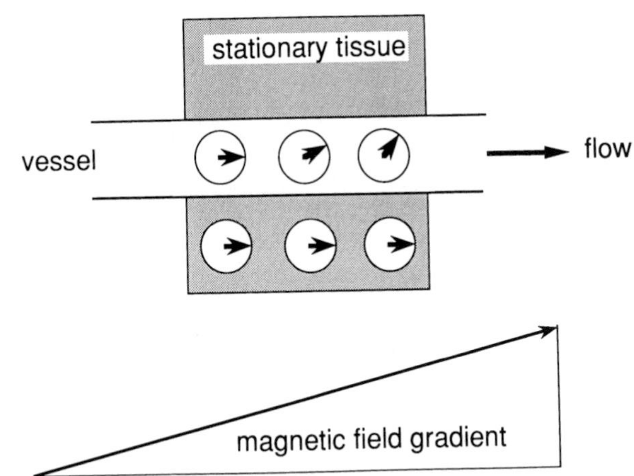

FIGURE 46–5. The principle of MR velocity mapping. Intravascular magnetic spins that move along magnetic field gradient accumulate a phase-shift that is proportional to flow velocity. In contrast, spins in stationary tissue do not acquire a phase change. (From Rebergen, S. A., Van der Wall, E. E., Doornbos, J., et al.: Magnetic resonance measurement of velocity and flow: Technique, validation, and cardiovascular applications. Am. Heart J. 126:1439, 1993, with permission.)

Fast spin-echo or turbo spin-echo MR imaging (TSE) allows the acquisition of high-quality T2-weighted MR images with substantial reduction in imaging time, compared with conventional T2-weighted MR sequences.[15] T2-weighted MR imaging is valuable in obtaining better characterization of the composition of tissue components. However, conventional T2-weighted approaches suffer from several artifacts due to motion during relatively long acquisition times. This problem may be overcome with the use of TSE acquisition. Reduced imaging time with electrocardiographically triggered TSE imaging is achievable because of the acquisition of multiple phase-encoding steps for each excitation in combination with the multislice mode. TSE imaging obviates the use of time-consuming conventional T2-weighted sequences, while maintaining high-quality T2 information for improved tissue characterization and improved definition of cardiac and mediastinal abnormalities.

Magnetic Resonance Angiography and Flow Mapping

Magnetic resonance angiography is based on a number of gradient-echo MR techniques that allow the visualization of flowing blood noninvasively. These techniques are categorized as time-of-flight (TOF) or phase-contrast (PC) methods, depending on the principle for visualization of flowing blood.[16] In the TOF method, the difference between the signal obtained from flowing blood and that from stationary tissue is due to the continuous wash-in of unsaturated blood and washout of saturated blood within an imaging section. This phenomenon, referred to as "flow-related enhancement," results in an image with bright vessels on a relatively dark background.[17] In the PC method, the difference in signal intensity between flowing blood and stationary tissue is based on velocity-induced phase shifts of moving spins in the presence of a magnetic field gradient (Fig. 46–5).[18, 19] In contrast with most MR imaging techniques, the images are not reconstructed from the amplitude, but from the phase of the MR signal. This approach allows the extraction of quantitative flow information, because the phase shift of flowing blood is proportional to its velocity. MR velocity mapping provides accurate measurement of flow velocity as well as flow volume in small or medium-sized vascular structures.

MR velocity mapping has been validated as an accurate technique both in vitro and in vivo.[20] This PC-based method is gaining widespread acceptance as a valuable technique for measuring flow in the aorta, pulmonary arteries, superior caval vein, pulmonary veins, and coronary circulation; flow across cardiac valves; and flow in other vascular structures throughout the body (Fig. 46–6).[21–23] Magnetic resonance velocity mapping correlates well with oximetry and with MR measurements based on ventricular volumetry for calculation of shunt size in patients with congenital heart defects, including atrial and ventricular septal defects, persistent ductus arteriosus, truncus arteriosus, and coronary–to–pulmonary artery fistulas.

Phosphorus-31 Magnetic Resonance Spectroscopy

Phosphorus-31 (^{31}P) MR spectroscopy is a noninvasive tool for the investigation of high-energy phosphate metabolism of the heart.[24, 25] Image-guided, localized ^{31}P spectra are obtained from the myocardium of the right and left ventricles with the use of a surface coil that is placed on the chest close to the myocardial region of interest. The ^{31}P spectrum contains information on the absolute concentration and ratios of multiple high-energy phosphate compounds that are critical to the energetics of the heart muscle (Fig. 46–7). The ^{31}P heart spectra disclose peaks of metabolites such as inorganic phosphate (Pi), phosphomonoesters (PME), phosphodiesters (PDE), and phosphocreatine (PCr), and peaks from adenosine triphosphate (ATP). The PME region in the spectra often includes 2,3-diphosphoglycerate contained in the blood pool of the heart muscle and cardiac chambers, overlapping the Pi peak. Furthermore, it may be technically problematic to distinguish myocardial and chest wall muscle contribution to the signal. However, when the Pi peak is resolved in the spectrum, the intracellular pH of the myocardium can be estimated from the distance between the peaks of Pi and PCr. Alterations in energy metabolism are fundamental to various disease processes that affect the heart. Under pathologic circumstances such as ischemia, the excess of PCr is consumed to replenish ATP by means of the creatine kinase reaction. Therefore, the PCr-to-ATP ratio and the PCr-to-Pi ratio are commonly used as markers for the metabolic status of the heart.

A few preliminary studies have explored the potential of ^{31}P MR spectroscopy in patients with congenital heart disease.[26–28] In an 8-month-old infant with congenital biventricular hypertrophy, reduced PCr-to-Pi and PCr-to-ATP ratios have been reported, compared with a single age-matched control subject.[28] This metabolic abnormality was found in both the myocardium and skeletal muscle. The reduced PCr-to-Pi ratio suggests that the mitochondria approach the maximal rate of aerobic energy production and that cardiac metabolism could be on the brink of being unable to aerobically meet energy demands. The PCr-to-Pi ratio of the myocardium was significantly raised after intravenous glucose or oral carbohydrate loading, indicating the potential of ^{31}P MR spectroscopy to evaluate optimization of therapy.

Phosphorus-31 MR spectroscopy has been applied to the evaluation of the metabolism of the right ventricle in a series of patients after a switch operation for transposition of the great arteries.[27] The PCr-to-ATP ratio of right ventricular myocardium appeared to be reduced in patients after repair for transposition, compared with that of left ventricular myocardium in normal subjects. Eventually, ^{31}P MR spectroscopy may help monitor right ventricular metabolism to detect right ventricular failure in patients after surgical correction of transposition of the great arteries. A reduction in the PCr-to-ATP ratio of the myocardium has also been reported in a small group of patients with cyanotic heart disease.[26] Eventually, these spectroscopic markers of myocardial metabolism may be used to plan the optimal timing for surgery in patients with congenital heart disease.

SEGMENTAL ANALYSIS OF MAGNETIC RESONANCE CARDIOVASCULAR ANATOMY

Magnetic resonance imaging is a comprehensive imaging technique for the assessment of congenital heart and great vessel pathology that uses the various MR techniques that are currently available.[29] The value of MR imaging in the evaluation of morphology of the heart and great vessels has been widely recognized.[30–32] An accurate diagnosis of anatomical anomalies can be achieved in more than 90 percent of patients with congenital heart disease.[33]

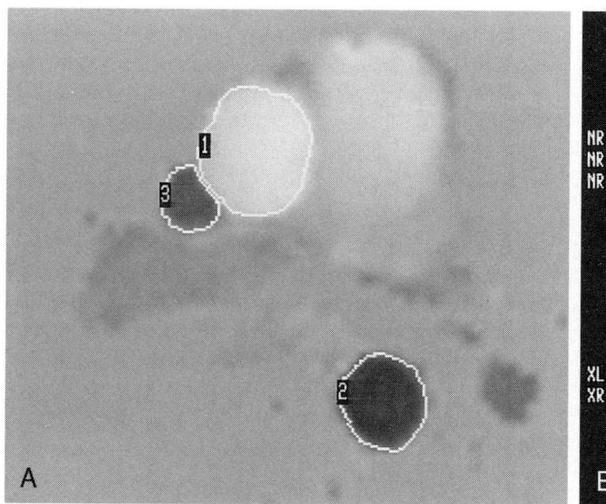

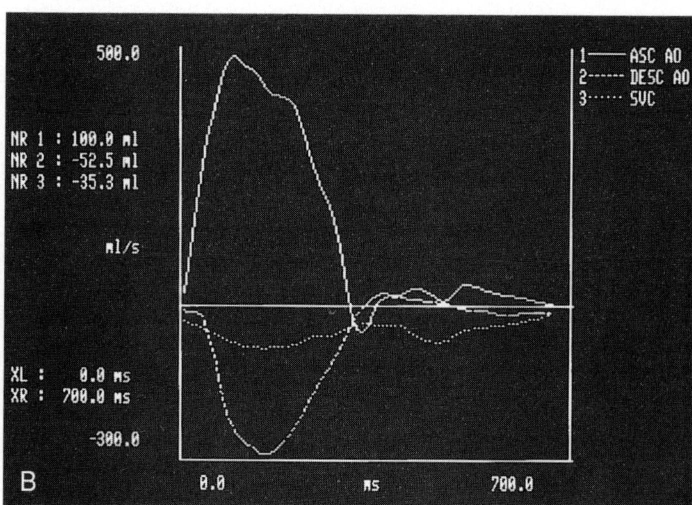

FIGURE 46–6. *A*, An MR velocity map at the level of the pulmonary artery perpendicular to the ascending aorta. Bright coloration indicates flow in the cranial direction, whereas dark coloration indicates flow in the caudal direction. Flow velocity and volume are derived from velocity maps by contouring the vessel of interest (tracing 1 = ascending aorta; tracing 2 = descending aorta; tracing 3 = superior vena cava). *B*, The corresponding velocity curves throughout the cardiac cycle are displayed. Volume flow (milliliters per second) is plotted against time after the R wave of the electrocardiogram. Instantaneous flow volumes measured from each velocity map are summed to give the stroke flow of each vessel. ASC AO = ascending aorta, DESC AO = descending aorta, SVC = superior vena cava. (*B* from Rebergen, S. A., Van der Wall, E. E., Doornbos, J., et al.: Magnetic resonance measurement of velocity and flow: Technique, validation, and cardiovascular applications. Am. Heart J. 126:1439, 1993, with permission.)

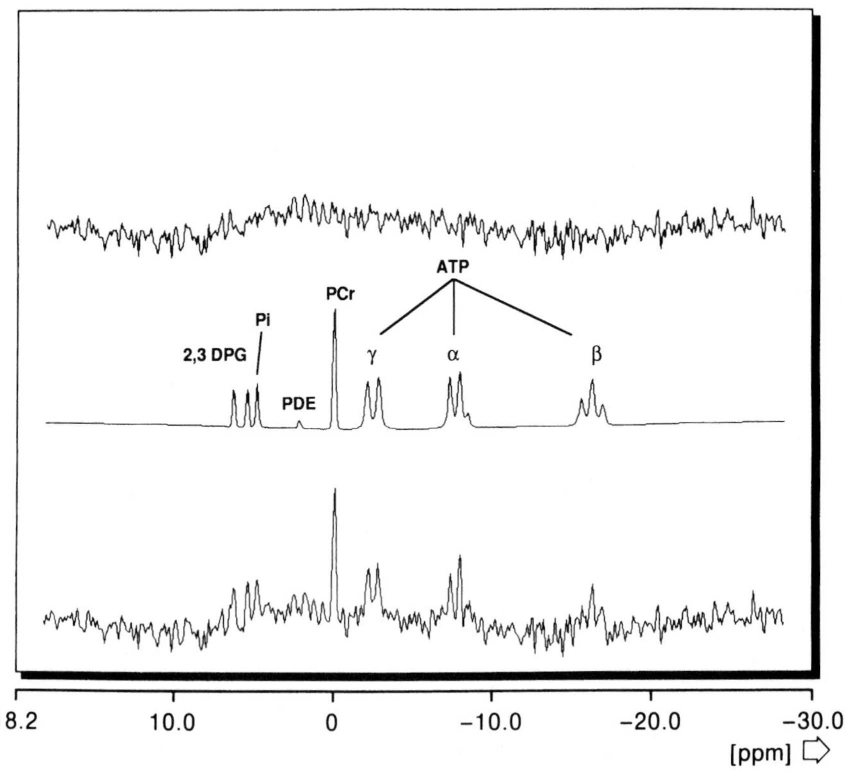

FIGURE 46–7. A phosphorus-31 MR spectrum from left ventricular myocardium in a patient with hypertrophic cardiomyopathy. The acquired spectrum *(bottom)*, simulated spectrum *(middle)*, and difference between the acquired and the simulated spectra *(top)* are shown. Note the resolution of Pi peak, allowing assessment of intracellular myocardial pH and PCr-to-Pi ratio as a measure of the energy reserve of the myocardium. 2,3 DPG = 2,3-diphosphoglycerate; Pi = inorganic phosphate; PDE = phosphodiesters; PCr = phosphocreatine; ATP = three peaks of adenosine triphosphate. (From De Roos, A., et al.: Cardiac metabolism in patients with dilated and hypertrophic cardiomyopathy: Assessment with proton-decoupled P-31 MR spectroscopy. Magn. Reson. Imaging 2:711, 1992. Copyright 1992, with kind permission from Elsevier Science, Ltd.)

Magnetic resonance imaging appears to be effective in both simple and complex cardiovascular malformations.

Analysis of the salient anatomical details in patients with complex cardiovascular malformations is accomplished to best advantage with the aid of a step-by-step analysis of the segmental anatomy.[34–36] The transverse multislice spin-echo series encompassing the heart and great vessels from the aortic arch to the level of the upper abdomen usually reveals all essential anatomical landmarks.[37]

The segment-by-segment approach includes the assessment of atrial situs, ventricular morphology, atrioventricular connections, the position and morphology of the great vessels, ventriculoarterial connections, and finally the evaluation of associated defects and postsurgical residua and sequelae.[38] Congenital cardiac malformations are categorized by the connections between these cardiac segments and by the assessment of additional defects.

After initial morphologic evaluation, the gradient-echo cine series is commonly obtained to assess cardiovascular flow and function tailored to the clinical situation and the malformation under investigation. The combined use of spin-echo and cine MR imaging in patients with complex cardiovascular malformations provides the most relevant information for presurgical planning.[5]

The value of the segmental approach is well illustrated below in a patient who was diagnosed as having abdominal situs inversus with levocardia, a common atrium, a single ventricle, double-inlet atrioventricular connection, transposition of the great arteries with dilation of the ascending aorta and infundibular pulmonary stenosis, left-sided inferior caval vein entering into the morphologic right atrium, and bilateral modified Blalock shunts with a malfunctioning shunt on the left side (Figs. 46–8, 46–9; see Figs. 46–11 and 46–12).

Situs Determination

The normal situation is atrial situs solitus, in which the morphologic right atrium is located on the right-side and the morphologic left atrium on the left-side of the patient. In atrial situs inversus, the mirror image of the normal situation is present. Generally, atrial situs is in accordance with abdominal or visceral situs. In situs solitus, the short main bronchus, the liver, and the inferior vena cava are right-sided structures, whereas the long main bronchus, the stomach, the spleen, and the abdominal aorta are located on the left side of the patient. The morphology of the main bronchi is usually well visualized on coronal spin-echo MR images and is a reliable indicator of atrial situs. Under normal conditions, the right pulmonary artery is located ventral to a relatively short right main bronchus, whereas the left pulmonary artery crosses over the left main bronchus. Situs ambiguus is diagnosed when symmetry of the main bronchi and pulmonary arteries is present. Situs ambiguus may occur as left-sided (or polysplenia syndrome) or right-sided (or asplenia syndrome) isomerism. Situs ambiguus is usually associated with complex cardiovascular malformations. In asplenia syndrome, bilateral short main bronchi, a large symmetric liver, absence of the spleen, and location of the inferior vena cava and abdominal aorta on the same side of the spine are encountered in conjunction with complex cardiac abnormalities. In polysplenia syndrome, the presence of bilateral long main bronchi, multiple spleens, and interruption of the hepatic segment of the inferior vena cava with azygos or hemiazygos vein continuation are characteristic.

The chest radiograph in the patient in Figure 46–8 reveals abdominal situs inversus as well as a short left-sided main bronchus and long right-sided main bronchus, confirming the presence of atrial situs inversus. In the patient with situs inversus in Figure 46–9, the morphologic right atrium with systemic venous drainage is located on the left side, whereas the morphologic left atrium with pulmonary venous drainage is located on the right side. The pulmonary veins can be defined with great accuracy by MR imaging techniques.[39]

The configuration of the atrial appendages may also be used on MR images to distinguish the morphology of the atria. The morphologic right atrium is characterized by an appendage with a triangular configuration and wide base of implantation into the atrial chamber. The morphologic left atrium has a tubular appendage with a narrow ostium to the main chamber. In most patients, the atrium connected to the inferior vena cava is the morphologic right atrium.

Ventricular Morphology

The anatomical location of a ventricular compartment or the wall thickness, by itself cannot be used as a marker for the morphology, because the ventricular position may be reversed in com-

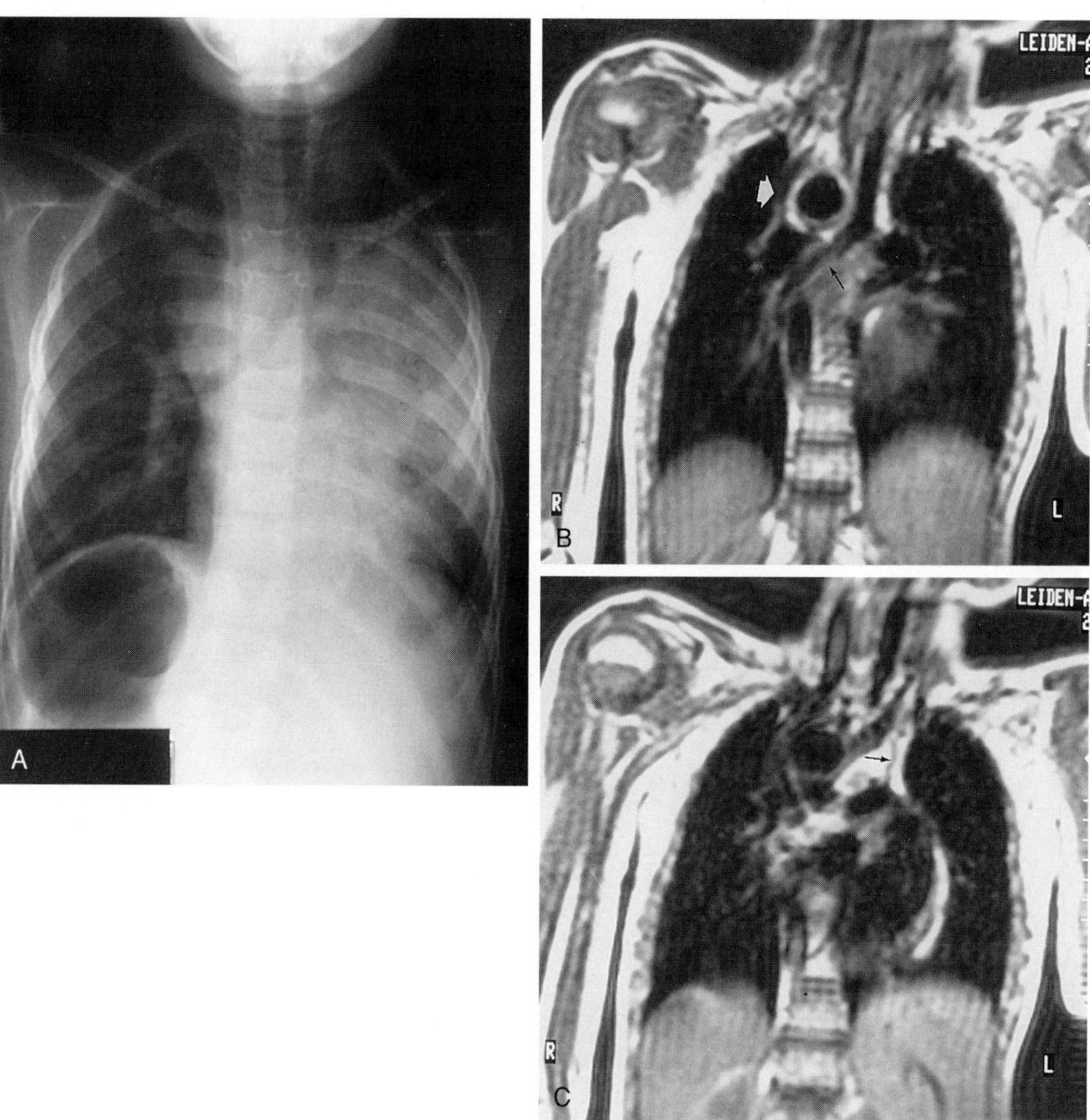

FIGURE 46–8. A chest radiograph *(A)* in a patient with complex cardiac malformation demonstrating situs inversus with levocardia and a right-sided aortic arch. Note the long right-sided bronchus and the short left-sided bronchus, indicating atrial situs inversus. The stomach is located on the right side of the patient, indicating abdominal situs inversus. The large vascular shadow on the right side of the trachea indicates a right-sided aortic arch. The cardiac apex is located on the left side of the patient, consistent with situs inversus with levocardia. Incidentally, note the extensive consolidations and air bronchograms in the parenchyma of the left lung. Coronal spin-echo MR images are shown for comparison in *B* and *C*. Note the long right-sided bronchus *(small arrow)*, the right-sided aortic arch, and a patent right-sided Blalock shunt *(large arrow)* in *B*. Note a tread-like, malfunctioning Blalock shunt *(small arrow)* on the left side, surrounded by bright mediastinal fat in *C*. The liver is located on the left side of the patient, consistent with abdominal situs inversus.

plex cardiac malformations and the wall thickness varies, depending on the loading conditions of the ventricle, which may be affected by many variables.[40]

The morphologic right and left ventricles can be distinguished on MR images in most patients by observing the different anatomical characteristics of both ventricles. Transverse spin-echo MR images at a midventricular level usually reveal the presence of the moderator band as a landmark for a morphologic right ventricle. The trabecular pattern of the right ventricle is coarse, while the interior of the left ventricle is smooth. Furthermore, the septal attachment of the atrioventricular valve of a morphologic right ventricle is closer to the cardiac apex than that for a morphologic left ventricle. Moreover, at the level of the ventricular outflow, the presence of a muscular infundibulum is a reliable anatomical marker for characterizing a morphologic right ventricle, even when the other landmarks are difficult to identify, as in a primitive ventricle (Fig. 46–10).[41] MR imaging is well suited for analyzing complex ventricular abnormalities.[42, 43]

In the patient with single ventricle, one ventricular compartment receives blood through both atrioventricular valves (Fig. 46–11). In these cases, assignment of ventricular morphology is based largely on the identification of the presence or absence of an infundibulum. When morphology cannot reliably be identified, the single ventricle is diagnosed as indeterminate type. After evaluation of atrial situs and ventricular morphology, the atrioventricular connections are defined.

Ventriculoarterial Connections

The aorta and pulmonary artery are defined by their usual branching pattern. The position and branching pattern of the aorta

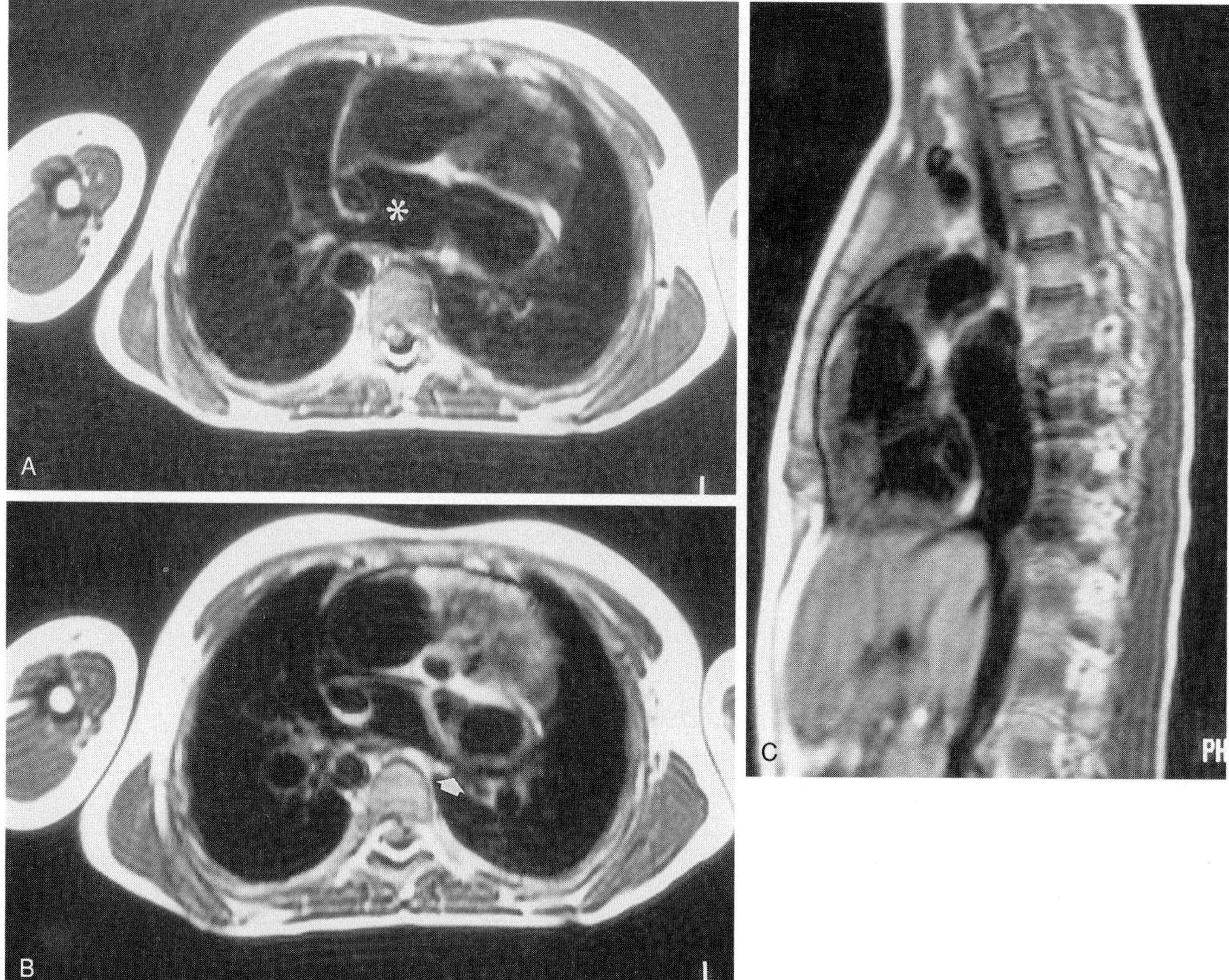

FIGURE 46–9. Transverse (*A* and *B*) and sagittal (*C*) spin-echo MR images through the heart in the same patient as in Figure 46–8, demonstrating pulmonary venous drainage and systemic venous drainage. In this patient with atrial situs inversus, the morphologic left atrium (*asterisk*) is located on the right side of the patient, whereas the morphologic right atrium is located on the left side of the patient. Two pulmonary veins enter the morphologic left atrium from the right-sided lung, whereas a single channel drains the left-sided lung (*arrow* in *B*). The inferior vena cava enters the dorsally located morphologic right atrium, as shown in *C*. The atrium connected to the inferior vena cava is generally the morphologic right atrium. Note also the large ascending aorta and the absence of pulmonary outflow consistent with pulmonary atresia. A large atrial septal defect is visualized in *A*, consistent with the diagnosis of a common atrium.

and pulmonary artery are well visualized on transverse spin-echo MR images at the base of the heart. Magnetic resonance imaging is useful in demonstrating concomitant large vessel abnormalities in patients with complex cardiovascular malformations.

Transposition of the great arteries is clearly depicted with the use of various imaging planes (Fig. 46–12). Congenitally corrected transposition is a congenital cardiac malformation defined by both discordant atrioventricular and ventriculoarterial connections. The morphologically right atrium communicates with the morphologically left ventricle through the mitral valve orifice, while the pulmonary artery originates from this ventricle. The morphologically left atrium communicates with the morphologically right ventricle through the tricuspid valve. The ascending aorta rises from the infundibulum of the right ventricle and is located to the left and anterior to the main pulmonary artery in situs solitus. The clinical utility of the segmental analysis of MR images in congenitally corrected transposition has been demonstrated.[37] Furthermore, MR imaging is well suited for diagnosing vascular rings and other aortic arch anomalies or pulmonary artery malformations.[44, 45]

Moreover, the utility of MR imaging for evaluating coarctation of the aorta has been established.[46, 47] Gradient-echo MR imaging and MR velocity mapping may also provide insight into the functional significance of coarctation of the aorta. Gradient-echo MR imaging may reveal abnormal flow patterns caused by the aortic coarctation as a signal void originating from the site of narrowing.[47] Magnetic resonance velocity mapping can be applied to the calculation of the pressure gradient across the coarctation with the aid of the modified Bernoulli equation. Because the pressure gradient is an indirect measurement of the severity of coarctation, MR velocity mapping of collateral blood flow below the coarctation provides a more direct assessment of the hemodynamic significance of the lesion, which may be critical in planning the operative approach.[48, 49]

ASSOCIATED DEFECTS AND POSTSURGICAL FINDINGS. The final step is to identify and characterize any associated defects or to define postoperative residua and sequelae (see Fig. 46–8*B* and *C*). Magnetic resonance imaging is very accurate in detecting atrial and ventricular septal defects.[31, 50, 51] The evaluation

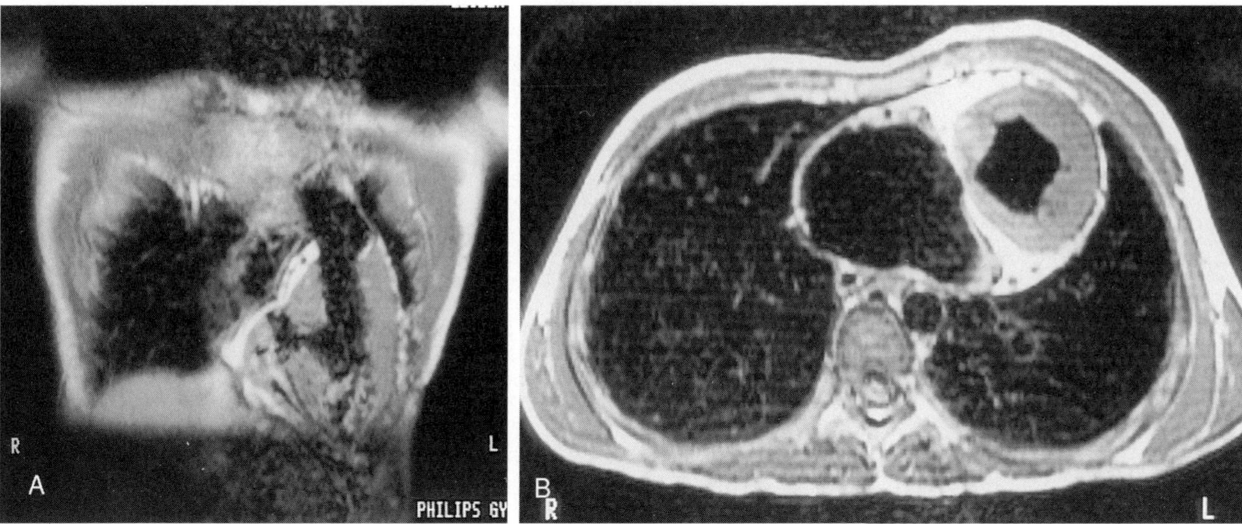

FIGURE 46–10. Coronal *(A)* and transverse *(B)* spin-echo MR images in a patient different from the one in Figures 46–8 and 46–9 demonstrate the presence of muscular infundibulum, which is characteristic for a morphologic right ventricle. In this patient with a single ventricle, assignment of ventricular morphology was based solely on the presence of a muscular infundibulum.

of ventricular septal defects can be improved with the use of gradient-echo MR imaging that demonstrates turbulent flow across the defect.[52]

MAGNETIC RESONANCE EVALUATION OF VENTRICULAR FUNCTION

Systolic Ventricular Function

The evaluation of global ventricular function depends on accurate measurement of ventricular volumes. Until now, transthoracic echocardiography has been the most widely applied technique for this purpose. However, the absence of appropriate acoustic windows and the requirement of geometric assumptions for volume measurements may limit its value. These geometric assumptions are of special concern when one measures right ventricular volumes.

Gradient-echo MR imaging is a three-dimensional technique that encompasses both the left and the right ventricles in multiple transverse or short-axis images.[53] The high temporal resolution is adequate to isolate end-diastolic and end-systolic time points (Fig. 46–13). Thus, ventricular volumetrics can be derived without the need for geometric assumptions.[54] This MR approach has been validated with cast studies and in patient studies, indicating its accuracy and ease of performance.[55] The degree of reproducibility of ventricular volumetrics is important when one follows patients

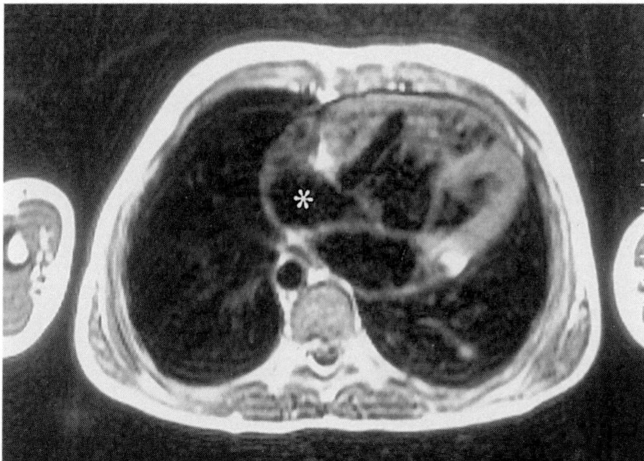

FIGURE 46–11. A transverse spin-echo MR image (same patient as in Figures 46–8 and 46–9) through the heart demonstrating a single ventricle that receives blood through both atrioventricular valves. Asterisk = morphologic left atrium.

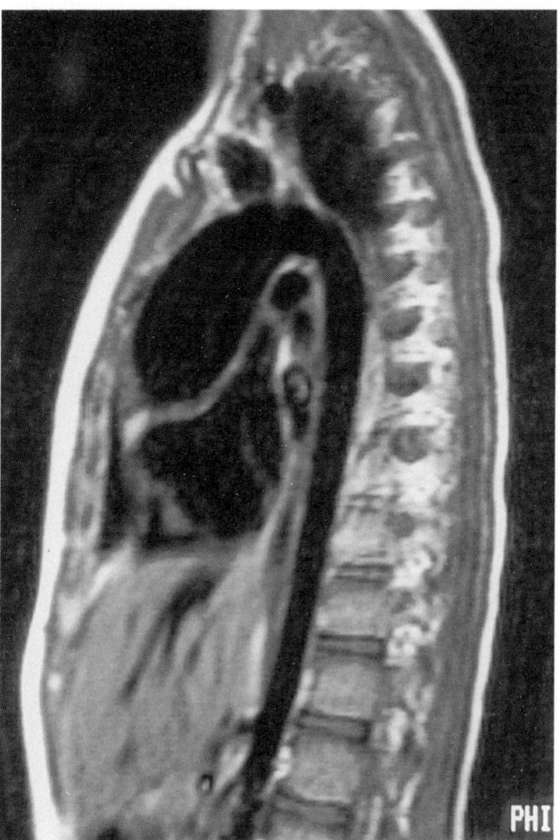

FIGURE 46–12. A sagittal spin-echo MR image through the chest (same patient as in Figures 46–8, 46–9, and 46–11) discloses the widened ascending aorta located directly behind the sternum. The aortic position indicates transposition of the great arteries.

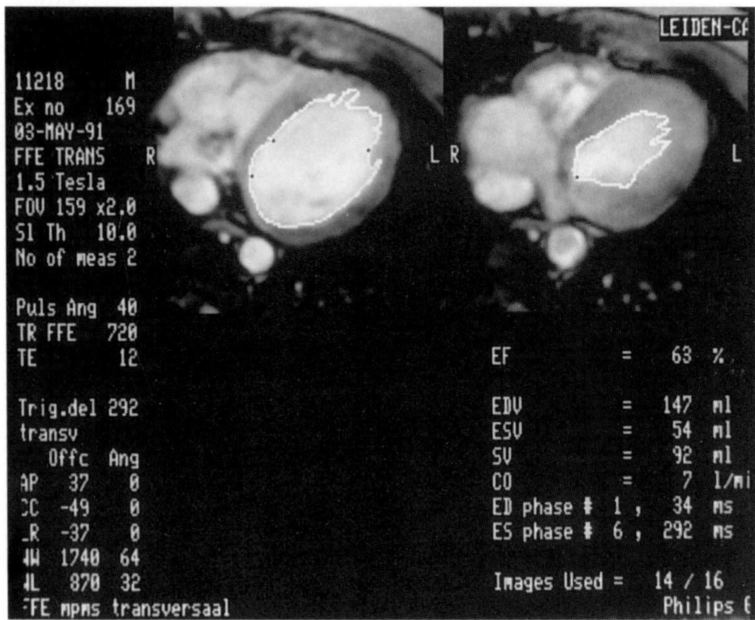

FIGURE 46–13. Transverse gradient-echo MR images demonstrate the end-diastolic (EDV, largest volume) and end-systolic (ESV, smallest volume) time points of the left ventricle from a series of images encompassing the entire cardiac cycle, with high temporal resolution. As indicated in the right lower panel, functional parameters can be calculated from these images. EF = ejection fraction; SV = stroke volume, CO = cardiac output.

over time. This issue has been addressed for MR imaging of the right and left ventricles with the use of variance component analysis.[56] Ventricular volume measurements with MR imaging appear to be more reproducible than those with other imaging modalities. MR imaging now appears to be emerging as the most accurate imaging modality for measuring ventricular volumes and myocardial mass.[57] However, especially with regard to the volume determination of the right ventricle, there is still room for improvement.[58, 59]

Wall Stress

The evaluation of systolic ventricular function can be further improved by combining volumes derived from MR imaging with blood pressure recordings.[60] This combination allows the quantification of wall stress, which is regarded as one of the primary determinants of cardiac function and oxygen demand at the myocardial level. Wall stress is defined as the force acting on the cross-sectional surface of the myocardial wall divided by its surface area. Mathematical models to determine wall stress take into account left ventricular cavity dimensions, wall dimensions, and cavitary blood pressure. Measurement of the wall stress according to the method of Arts and associates[61] appears to be more reproducible with MR imaging than the approach according to Sandler and Dodge.[62] The model of Arts and co-workers appears to be more realistic because it incorporates anisotropy of myocardial tissue as well as torsion of the left ventricle as an index of fiber stress. This model is based on changes in the dimensions of the entire ventricle, which can be measured accurately with MR imaging.[56]

Pressure-Volume Relations

Combining measurement of ventricular volumes derived from MR imaging with blood pressure recordings also allows evaluation of systolic function with the use of pressure-volume relations. Experimental studies have shown that MR-based analysis of the ventricular pressure-volume relationship is feasible for determining myocardial contractility.[63, 64] Global ventricular function is the result of the interaction between preload, afterload, and myocardial contractility. Preload is determined by the end-diastolic volume, whereas afterload is the load that the muscle fibers within the ventricular wall have to sustain during contraction. Contractility or inotropic state is the quantity that reflects the intrinsic contractile level of the myocardium. The end-systolic pressure-volume relationship in the pressure-volume diagram provides a direct measure of myocardial contractility (Fig. 46–14). This analysis is based on the observation that in the pressure-volume diagram, the left upper corners of the pressure-volume loops (end-systolic pressure-volume points) obtained at various loads at constant myocardial contractility reach the same, almost straight line, called the end-systolic pressure-volume relation. This line shifts to the left when there is an increase in inotropic state and to the right when a decrease in contractility occurs (see Fig. 46–14).[65] Measurement of the end-systolic pressure-volume relation is considered the most sophisticated index of myocardial contractility, owing to its relative independence from preload and afterload. In contrast, most other parameters, such as ejection fraction, strongly depend on loading conditions. For the assessment of this marker of contractility, accu-

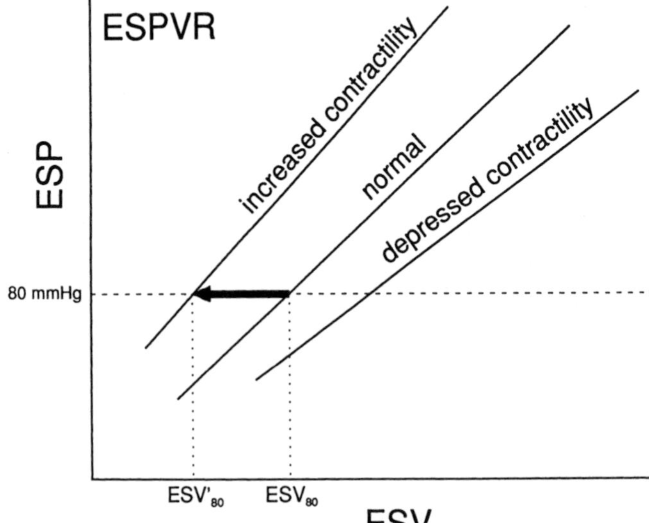

FIGURE 46–14. The end-systolic pressure-volume relation (ESPVR) of the left ventricle is shifted to the left or to the right by increases and decreases in myocardial contractility, respectively. The magnitude of this shift is quantified by recording the change in the volume intercept, ESV_{80}, at a fixed, arbitrary pressure of 80 mm Hg. An increase in contractility is indicated by a decrease in ESV 80. ESV = end-systolic volume; ESP = end-systolic pressure. (From Ross, J.: Cardiac function and myocardial contractility: A perspective. J. Am. Coll. Cardiol. 1:52, 1983. Reprinted with permission from the American College of Cardiology.)

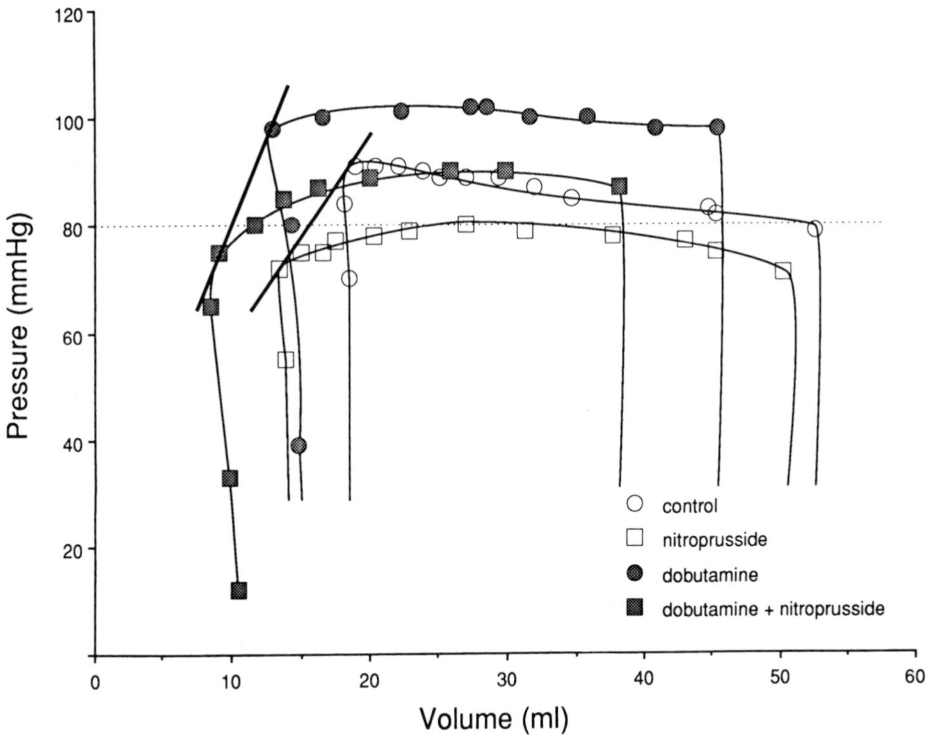

FIGURE 46–15. Pressure-volume loops under four different conditions in a pig model based on MRI volume data. Magnetic resonance volume samples were obtained every 26 to 28 msec and were then combined with invasive left ventricular pressure readings. By connecting the upper left corners (end-systolic pressure volume points) of the control loop and nitroprusside loop, the control end-systolic pressure-volume relation (ESPVR) at normal inotropic state was constructed *(solid line)*. The dobutamine ESPVR *(solid line)*, reflecting increased inotropic state, was determined from the dobutamine loop and the dobutamine-plus-nitroprusside loop. Note the leftward shift of the ESPVR during dobutamine infusion, as reflected in a decrease of the volume intercept at a pressure of 80 mm Hg. (From Pattynama, P. M. T.: Functional magnetic resonance imaging of the heart. Thesis, Leiden University, 1994, with permission.)

rate volume measurements of the ventricle are a prerequisite, which are provided by MR imaging. Magnetic resonance imaging appears to be as sensitive in detecting changes in myocardial contractility as the hitherto-used invasive conductance catheter method, which is regarded as the "gold standard."[64] With further development, MR imaging may be used for noninvasive analysis of pressure-volume relations of both the left and right ventricles (Fig. 46–15).

The clinical utility and accuracy of gradient-echo MR imaging of right and left ventricular volumes have been shown in normal children and in children with various types of congenital heart disease with abnormal loading conditions of the right ventricle.[66] The patient group included six patients with secundum type atrial septum defect, three patients with valvular pulmonary stenosis, seven patients who had undergone Senning operation for transposition of the great arteries, and eight patients with total correction of tetralogy of Fallot. Magnetic resonance imaging was successfully completed in all but two of the patients without the need for sedation. In addition, MR velocity maps were obtained at the level of the tricuspid valve, pulmonary artery, and aorta. The dimensional accuracy of the tomographic method can be validated against flow volume measurements (Figs. 46–16 and 46–17).[66]

Magnetic resonance imaging appears to be well suited to the evaluation of biventricular systolic function in children with complex cardiac morphology and abnormal loading conditions.

Diastolic Ventricular Function

Magnetic resonance imaging techniques may also allow evaluation of diastolic ventricular function.[67] Diastolic dysfunction may be defined as the inability of the left ventricle to fill at normal end-diastolic pressure. The filling of the left or right ventricle normally has a triphasic character, as defined by MR measurement of transmitral or transtricuspid flow.[68] An initial, rapid filling phase is followed by a second phase of diastasis with very slow diastolic filling and finally by a third phase of filling during atrial contraction. At very high heart rates, the first phase of rapid diastolic filling and the third phase of atrial contraction may merge. After closure of the aortic valve and before opening of the mitral valve, the left ventricle is relaxing during an interval called the isovolumic relax-

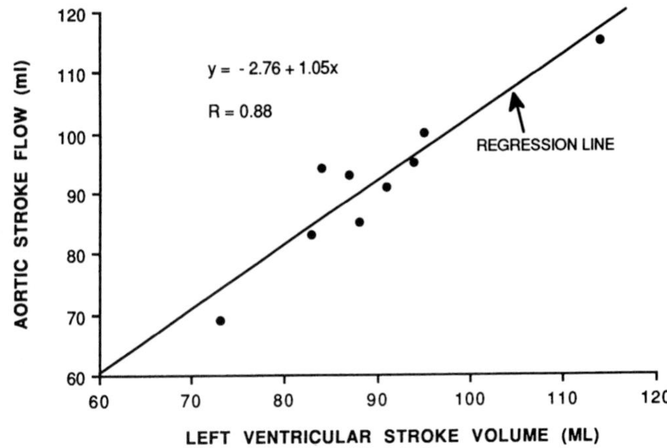

FIGURE 46–16. Comparison of aortic stroke volume measured with MR velocity mapping and left ventricular stroke volume measured with tomographic gradient-echo MRI. The good correlation between these basically different MR approaches provides internal validation of the reliability of the MR techniques.

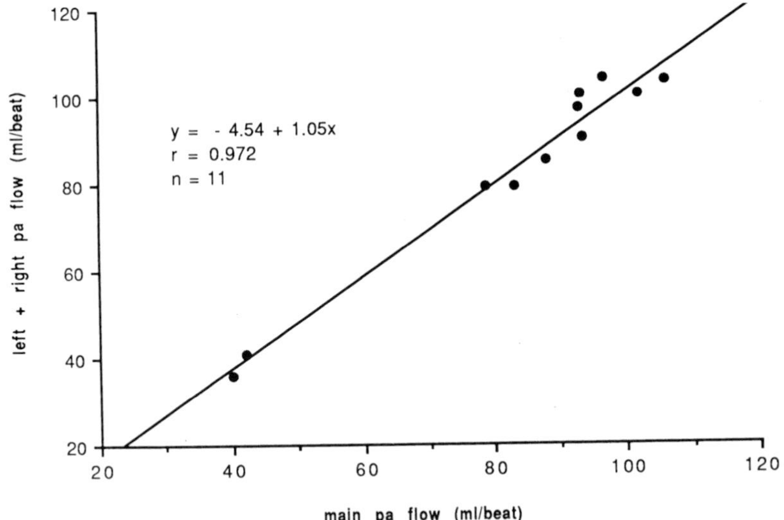

FIGURE 46–17. Total flow in the right and left pulmonary artery is compared to main pulmonary artery flow as measured with MR velocity mapping. The good correlation indicates that MR velocity mapping is reliable for the measurement of flow to both lungs separately. (From Rebergen, S. A., Ottenkamp, J., Doornbos, J., et al.: Postoperative pulmonary flow dynamics after Fontan surgery: Assessment with nuclear magnetic resonance velocity mapping. J. Am. Coll. Cardiol. 21:121, 1993. Reprinted with permission from the American College of Cardiology.)

ation time. The following rapid filling phase may be characterized by parameters such as peak filling rate, time-to-peak filling rate, acceleration and deceleration slope of the early filling peak, and the duration of the rapid filling period, whereas the atrial contraction may be quantified by the atrial filling velocity.

The isovolumic relaxation phase and the early filling phase are effected mainly by an active, energy-consuming process of relaxation, during which myofilament cross-bridges are detached. Other factors that contribute to the duration of the isovolumic relaxation phase and early filling are the pressure difference between the left atrium and the left ventricle, the inotropic state of the left ventricle, and the duration and synchronicity of the contraction. In contrast, the filling during atrial contraction is influenced mainly by atrial function and the passive physical properties of the left ventricle. Increased myocardial stiffness due to fibrosis or to pericardial thickening impairs the filling process during the last part of diastole.

Gradient-echo MR imaging offers the opportunity to evaluate regional wall motion dynamics over the cardiac cycle as a marker of regional diastolic function. Global diastolic function of both ventricles can be derived from time-volume curves obtained with gradient-echo MR imaging.[69]

Intracardiac Flow

Magnetic resonance velocity mapping techniques have been used to measure transmitral and transtricuspid flow as markers for diastolic ventricular function.[70] Measurements of flow velocities across the mitral valve by Doppler echocardiography to evaluate left ventricular diastolic filling are routinely performed. Doppler echocardiographic measurements of tricuspid flow for evaluation of right ventricular diastolic function may be more difficult. However, diastolic filling abnormalities of the right ventricle are of special significance in patients with postoperative congenital heart disease, in whom residual lesions of the right heart frequently occur. Magnetic resonance velocity mapping of tricuspid flow provides direct, accurate measurements of tricuspid flow velocities as well as volume flow (Fig. 46–18).[71] The tricuspid flow volume measured with MR velocity mapping agrees closely with tomographically measured right ventricular stroke volumes, providing internal validation of the accuracy and reproducibility of these measurements. Furthermore, the E:A ratio derived from MR peak flow velocities has proved to be similar to that determined with Doppler echocardiography.[71]

Thus, a variety of MR-derived measurements provide an opportunity to assess diastolic function of both the right and the left ventricles in patients with congenital heart disease.

MAGNETIC RESONANCE EVALUATION OF SPECIFIC CONGENITAL HEART DISEASES

Atrial Septal Defects

Atrial septal defect is the most common type of congenital heart disease in adults. The ostium secundum type is the most common form, located in the region of the fossa ovalis. Sinus venosus–type defects are often associated with anomalous return of the right upper pulmonary vein into the superior vena cava or right atrium. The ostium-primum atrial septal defect is part of the spectrum of atrioventricular septal defects. A definite diagnosis is often established with two-dimensional echocardiography with direct visualization of the septal defect and signs of right ventricular overload. Spin-echo MR techniques have been applied to the assessment of atrial septal defects (see Fig. 46–1).[51, 72] Magnetic resonance imaging is especially valuable in identifying partial anomalous pulmonary venous return in patients with sinus venosus–type atrial septal defect. This technique has a 95 percent accuracy for the detection of partial anomalous pulmonary venous return, which is better than that of echocardiography and angiography.[39] Blind analysis of MR images of the heart revealed a sensitivity and specificity of more than 90 percent for diagnosing atrial septal defects.[73] On spin-echo MR images, a secundum defect may be diagnosed unequivocally when a sharp and thickened edge is identified, but it may sometimes be difficult to differentiate between a true defect and a thin fossa ovalis.[30] Analysis of adjacent imaging sections and the use of additional imaging planes may help make the correct diagnosis. As a result of the left-to-right shunt, usually the right atrium, right ventricle, and pulmonary arteries are enlarged. Concomitant enlargement of the right side of the heart and pulmonary vasculature is easily identified in patients with an atrial septal defect.

Gradient-echo MR imaging may disclose a flow disturbance at the level of an atrial left-to-right shunt (see Fig. 46–2). Besides identification of a septal defect, knowledge of the amount of shunt flow is important for planning surgical options. Gradient-echo MR images also provide volumetrics of both ventricles, and the pulmonary-to-systemic flow ratio can be derived from the respective stroke volumes. Magnetic resonance velocity mapping of pulmonary and aortic flow is another accurate MR technique for the direct quantification of left-to-right shunts (Fig. 46–19).[74] The anatomical and functional assessment of atrial septal defects with these various MR techniques obviates the need for more invasive procedures and may provide a definite diagnosis when echocardiographic findings are equivocal.

In a series of 12 patients with suspected or proven atrial-level shunts, the combined use of gradient-echo MR imaging to measure biventricular stroke volumes and MR velocity mapping of as-

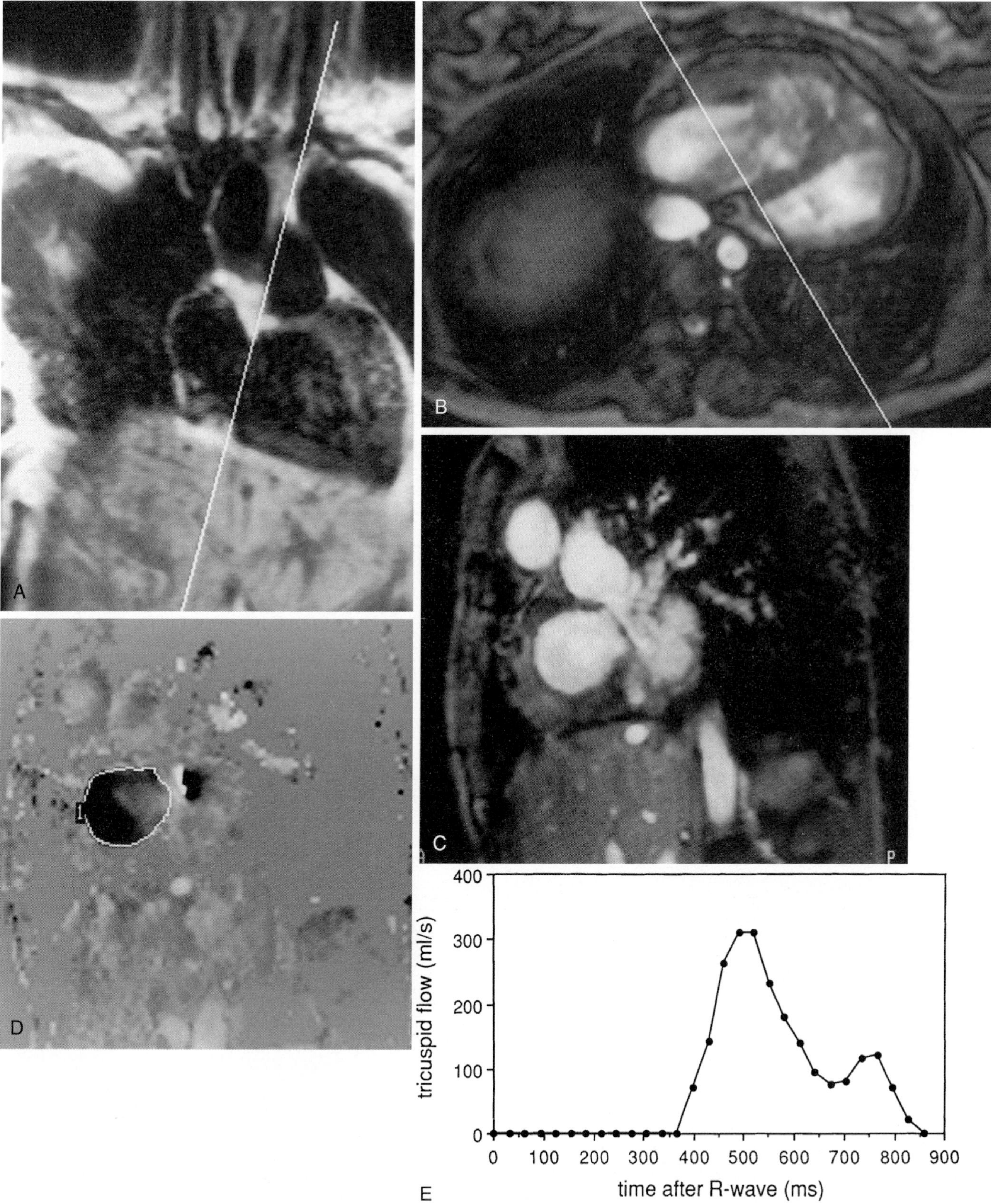

FIGURE 46–18. *A* to *E*, Illustration of the tricuspid flow mapping procedure. Coronal spin-echo MR image *(A)* through the right side of the heart indicates the plane of the tricuspid valve *(solid line)*. A transverse gradient-echo MR image *(B)* through the heart indicates the position of the tricuspid valve in the axial orientation *(solid line)*. By double-oblique angulation using the planes defined in *A* and *B*, a gradient-echo MR image *(C)* is acquired through the tricuspid valve perpendicular to the right ventricular inflow. The corresponding MR velocity maps *(D)* reveals an asymmetric flow pattern through the tricuspid orifice, as demonstrated by the differences in dark coloration. Tracing 1 = tricuspid valve orifice. From the velocity maps, a flow-versus-time curve *(E)* is constructed, revealing a large E wave and a small A wave. (From Rebergen, S. A., Helbing, W. A., Van der Wall, E. E., et al.: MR velocity mapping of tricuspid flow in healthy children and patients who have undergone Mustard or Senning repair. Radiology 194:505, 1995, with permission.)

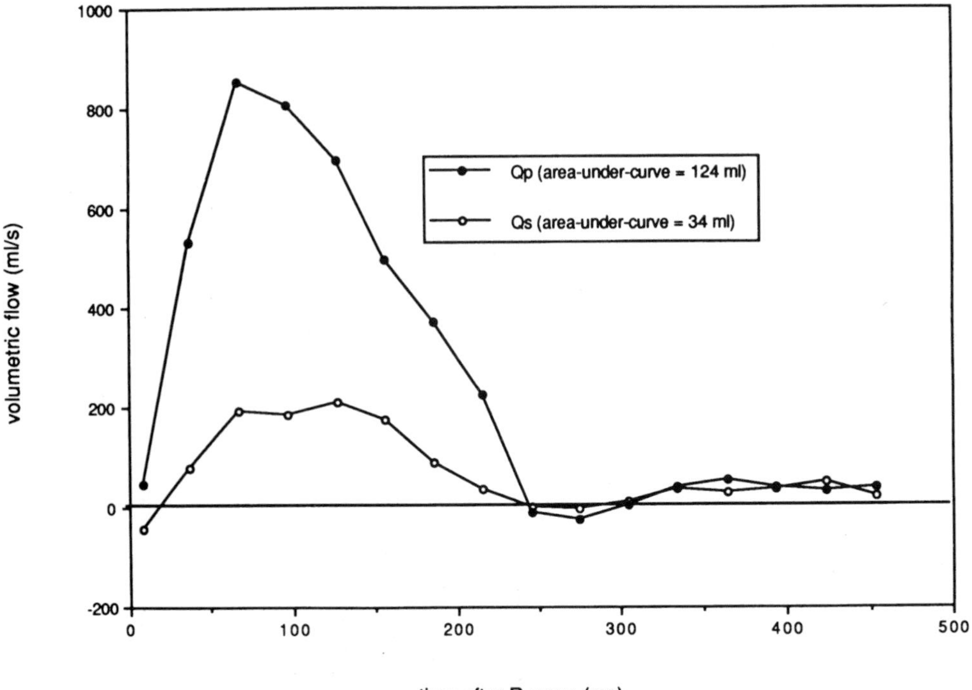

FIGURE 46–19. Aortic (Qs) and pulmonary (Qp) flow volume curves in a 23-year-old female patient with an atrial septal defect disclose a left-to-right shunt of approximately 1:4.

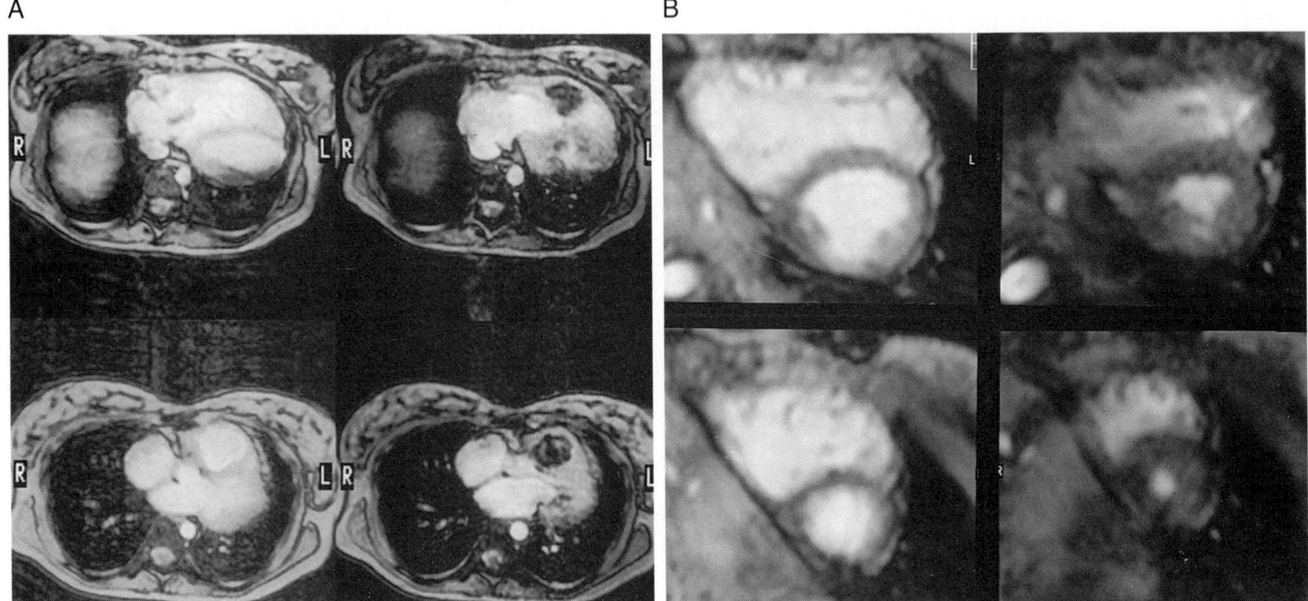

FIGURE 46–20. A series of four transverse gradient-echo MR images *(A)* selected from a set of images covering the entire cardiac cycle during systole *(left upper* and *left lower panels)* and diastole *(right upper* and *right lower panels)* in a patient with residual pulmonary insufficiency after surgery for tetralogy of Fallot. Note a signal void in the pulmonary outflow tract extending into the right ventricle during diastole, indicating the presence of severe regurgitant flow. *B*, Four gradient-echo MR images obtained in the short-axis orientation disclose marked enlargement of the right ventricle due to volume overload on the basis of pulmonary insufficiency. Biventricular function can be measured accurately with the use of gradient-echo images encompassing the ventricular compartments.

cending aortic and pulmonary artery flow revealed excellent correspondance between flow ratios and stroke volume ratios. In several patients with a suspected lesion, the diagnosis could be rejected on the basis of MR measurements of flow and stroke volumes.[75]

Although MR imaging techniques provide a complete evaluation of patients with atrial septal defects, it is unlikely that MR imaging will replace echocardiography for this indication. However, when echocardiographic findings are not conclusive, MR imaging is a good alternative method for confirming or rejecting the diagnosis of an atrial septal defect with a significant left-to-right shunt. When shunt flow is very limited, it may be difficult to detect a difference between aortic and pulmonary artery flows on the basis of MR flow measurements, because the method has an inaccuracy of approximately 6 percent. Another potential pitfall is the absence of a turbulent jet effect across the defect on gradient-echo MR images, limiting the value of this technique for the diagnosis of an atrial septal defect.

Shunt reversal may result when pulmonary hypertension develops over time with development of Eisenmenger physiology. Gradient-echo MR imaging may disclose shunt reversal by visualizing flow across the defect. Development of right ventricular hypertrophy occurs when pulmonary hypertension is present. Magnetic resonance imaging is particularly useful for evaluating the morphology and function of the right ventricle. Combining various MR techniques allows a complete evaluation of the anatomical characteristics of atrial septal defects as well as the functional consequences.

Postoperative Tetralogy of Fallot

In patients with tetralogy of Fallot, anterior displacement of the infundibular septum results in a ventricular septal defect and the development of infundibular pulmonary stenosis. Right ventricular hypertrophy is caused by right ventricular hypertension resulting from both the ventricular septal defect and pulmonary stenosis. The fourth component of the tetralogy is the aorta overriding onto the right ventricle. Surgical repair is aimed at relief of the right ventricular outflow obstruction and closure of the ventricular septal defect.

Despite improved surgical methods, pulmonary stenosis and pulmonary regurgitation are common postoperative sequelae after repair of tetralogy of Fallot (Fig. 46–20). Spin-echo and gradient-echo MR imaging are effective for the postsurgical evaluation of the anatomical and functional residua.

Pulmonary regurgitation is commonly found, especially when a transannular patch has been used for relief of outflow obstruction of the right ventricle. Controversy exists with regard to the significance of residual pulmonary regurgitation. On the one hand, it has been considered as a relative benign lesion that can be well tolerated over long periods of time.[76] On the other hand, researchers emphasize that pulmonary regurgitation-induced right ventricular volume overload may predispose to the development of ventricular arrhythmia, a risk factor for sudden death.[77]

The evaluation of the clinical significance of pulmonary regurgitation after Fallot repair has been hampered since there was no noninvasive modality that could accurately quantitate pulmonary volume flow. Magnetic resonance velocity mapping has been shown to be an accurate method for noninvasive, volumetric quantification of pulmonary regurgitation after surgical correction of tetralogy of Fallot.[78] In addition, multislice gradient-echo MR imaging is an accurate method for performing measurements of right ventricular volumes, without the limitations inherent to the complex geometry of the right ventricle (see Fig. 46–20*B*).[79, 80] The consequences of pulmonary regurgitation on right ventricular function in patients who have undergone Fallot repair can be comprehensively evaluated with combined use of MR velocity mapping and gradient-echo MR imaging (Figs. 46–21 to 46–23). Furthermore, the measurement of left and right ventricular stroke volumes based on the tomographic method can be used as an internal reference to validate the direct measurement of pulmonary flow (see Fig. 46–23).

This approach was explored in a study of 18 patients late after Fallot surgery, in which forward and regurgitant volume flows were measured directly in the main pulmonary artery with MR velocity mapping.[78] Pulmonary regurgitation volumes closely agreed with the difference between the corresponding right and left ventricular stroke volumes as measured tomographically by gradient-echo MR imaging (see Fig. 46–23). In that study,[78] MR velocity mapping results were compared with the estimated severity of pulmonary regurgitation as judged from Doppler echocardiography (Fig. 46–24). Both techniques agreed in patients in whom Doppler echocardiography revealed mild pulmonary regurgitation. However, from these initial results, it appears that when Doppler echocardiography shows moderate or severe regurgitation or when Doppler results are equivocal, reliable assessment of the severity of pulmonary regurgitation is problematic and may be measured more reliably with MR velocity mapping.

Thus, MR velocity mapping appears to be ideally suited for monitoring pulmonary regurgitation and right ventricular function, and this technique may aid in the planning of surgical intervention for residual pulmonary regurgitation following repair of tetralogy of Fallot.[78]

MAGNETIC RESONANCE EVALUATION OF PULMONARY FLOW DYNAMICS

Various operations have been devised to increase pulmonary blood flow in patients with congenital heart defects characterized by cyanosis and decreased pulmonary blood flow. Spin-echo MR imaging is a valuable technique for visualizing the anatomy of the pulmonary circulation and for evaluating surgical procedures aimed at the improvement of pulmonary blood flow.[81] Magnetic resonance imaging appears to be superior to echocardiography for determining the presence or absence of the confluence of the pulmonary arteries in patients with pulmonary atresia.[82, 83] Also, MR imaging has an advantage over angiocardiography in situations in which contrast medium cannot be delivered in an amount adequate for visualizing the pulmonary arteries in this category of patients. The size and patency of systemic–to–pulmonary artery shunts can be assessed with great detail by spin-echo MR imaging (see Fig. 46–8).[82]

Shunts and Conduits

Accurate diagnosis of obstruction in extracardiac conduits is well performed with the use of MR imaging techniques.[84] A variety of conduits exists for improvement of the pulmonary flow in patients with cyanotic heart disease. In Rastelli's operation a conduit establishes or improves the blood flow from the right ventricle to the pulmonary arteries. When a stenosis in the conduit is defined with spin-echo MR imaging, MR velocity mapping can be employed to calculate the pressure gradient across the obstructed conduit using the modified Bernouilli equation, in which the pressure gradient equals four times the peak velocity squared.[84, 85]

Fontan Operations

The Fontan procedure and its modifications are designed to direct total systemic venous return to the lungs.[86, 87] One modification consists of a direct atriopulmonary connection between the right atrium and the pulmonary artery. Another variation consists of an atrioventricular connection between the right atrium and the right ventricle, incorporating the pumping capability of the right ventricle into the pulmonary circulation (Fig. 46–25). The incorporation of the right ventricle in the Fontan circulation has been advocated on the basis of the concept that the right ventricle may grow over time, leading to improved pulmonary blood flow.[88, 89] Magnetic resonance velocity mapping has been used to elucidate

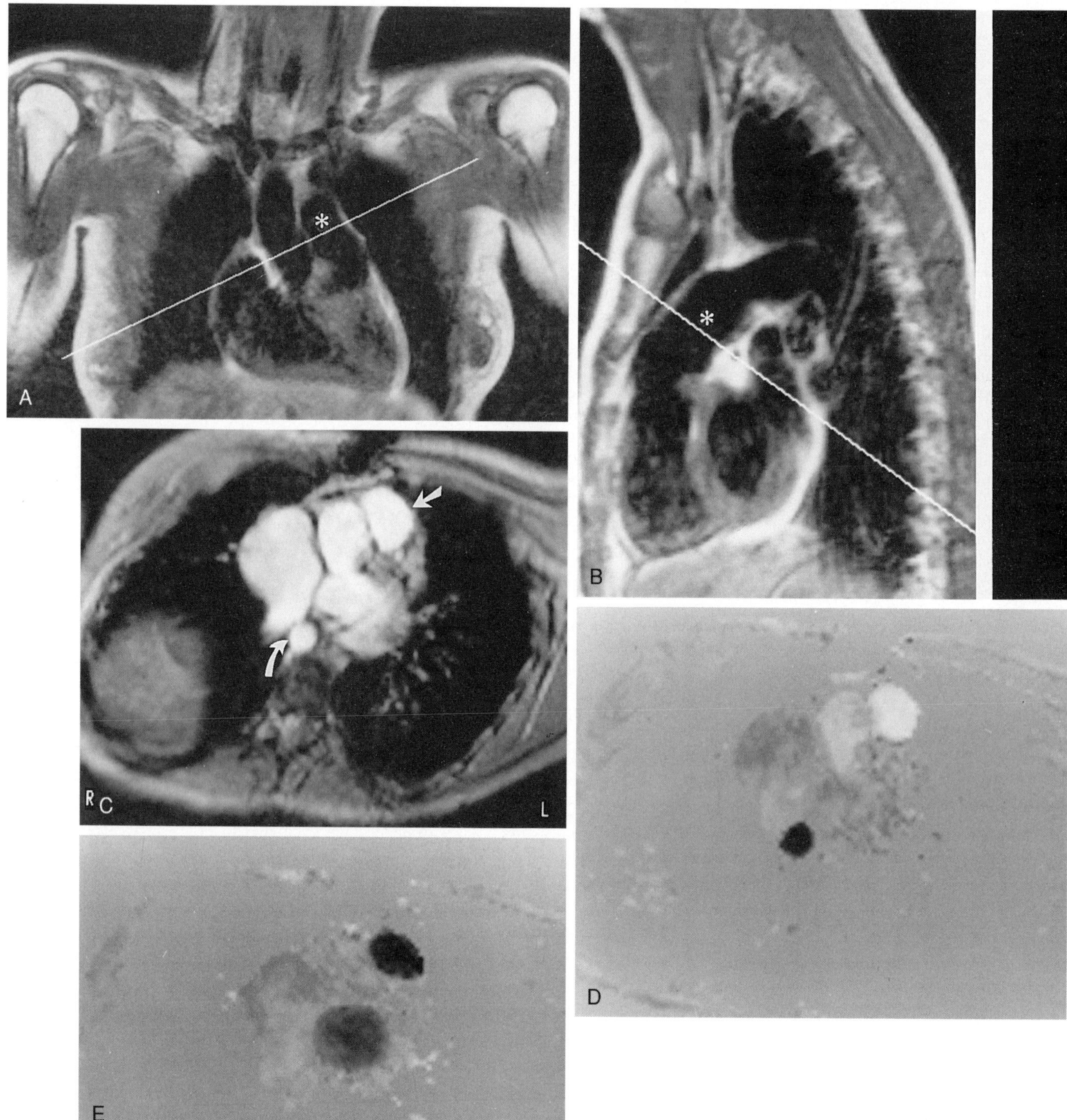

FIGURE 46–21. A coronal spin-echo MR image *(A)* discloses the orientation of the main pulmonary artery *(asterisk)*. The solid line perpendicular to the main pulmonary artery indicates the plane for MR velocity mapping. A sagittal spin-echo MR image *(B)* demonstrates the main pulmonary artery *(asterisk)* and the right ventricle. Again, the solid line indicates the plane for MR velocity mapping perpendicular to the pulmonary artery. By combining the angulation determined in *A* and *B*, a double-oblique gradient-echo MR image *(C)* is obtained perpendicular to the pulmonary artery. The pulmonary artery *(straight arrow)* and the right-sided descending aorta *(curved arrow)* are indicated. At the level selected in *C*, a series of MR velocity maps is acquired with high temporal resolution to measure flow in the pulmonary artery throughout the cardiac cycle. The MR velocity map in systole *(D)* reveals high-signal-intensity flow in the pulmonary artery toward the head. Low-signal-intensity flow in the descending aorta indicates flow in the opposite direction. An MR velocity map in diastole *(E)* reveals low-signal-intensity flow in the pulmonary artery in the caudal direction, indicating the presence of pulmonary regurgitation. (From Rebergen, S. A., Chin, J. G. J., Ottenkamp, J., et al.: Pulmonary regurgitation in the late postoperative follow-up of tetralogy of Fallot: Volumetric quantitation by nuclear magnetic resonance velocity mapping. Circulation 88[Part 1]:2257, 1993, with permission.)

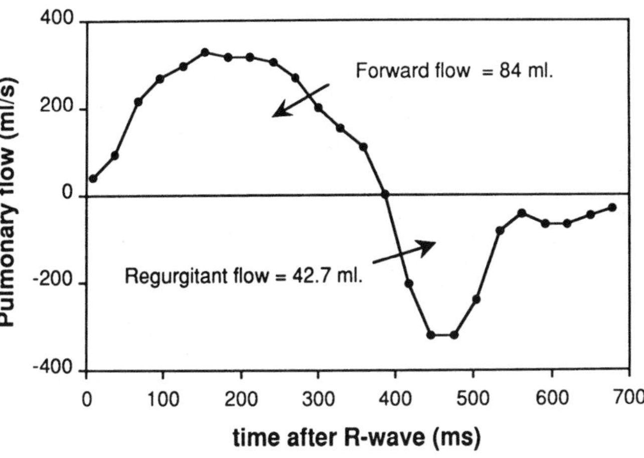

FIGURE 46–22. Volumetric pulmonary flow plotted against the time after the R wave of the electrocardiogram. The diastolic regurgitant flow volume approximates 50 percent of the systolic forward flow volume. (From Rebergen, S. A., Chin, J. G. J., Ottenkamp, J., et al.: Pulmonary regurgitation in the late postoperative follow-up of tetralogy of Fallot: Volumetric quantitation by nuclear magnetic resonance velocity mapping. Circulation 88[Part 1]:2257, 1993, with permission.)

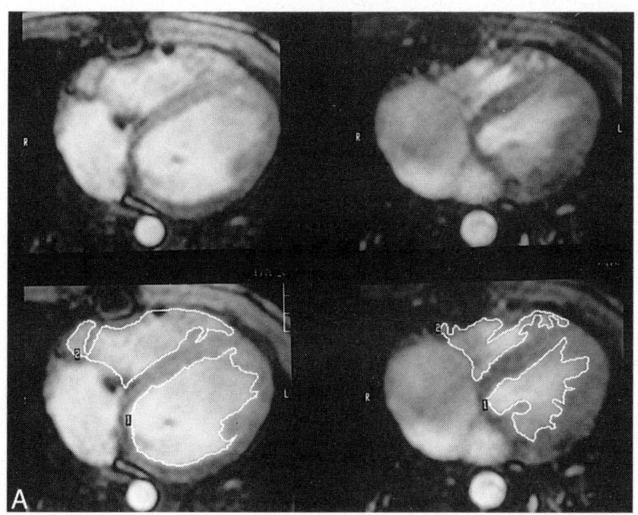

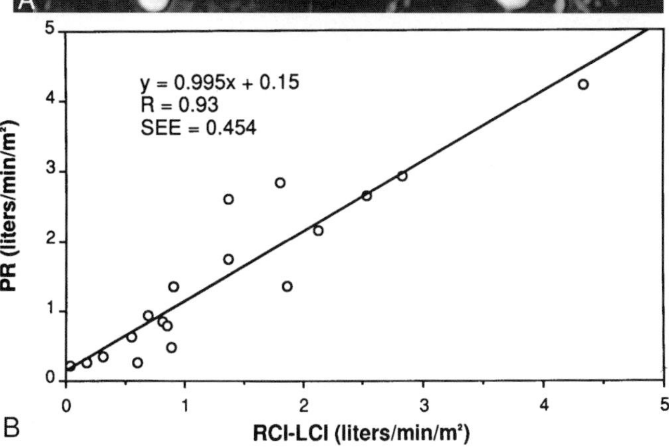

FIGURE 46–23. *A*, Axial gradient-echo MR images at end-diastole *(left upper panel)* and end-systole *(right upper panel)*. The lower panels show the same images with tracings of the left and right ventricular endocardial contours superimposed. Ventricular cavity areas obtained from a contiguous set of gradient-echo MR images are summed to yield ventricular volumes. *B*, Regression analysis of pulmonary regurgitation measured with MR velocity mapping (as illustrated in Figures 46–21 and 46–22) and the difference between left-sided (LCI) and right-sided cardiac index (RCI) measured with the tomographic approach (as illustrated in Figure 46–23*A*) reveal close agreement between these two intrinsically different techniques, providing internal validation of the reliability of the technique. (From Rebergen, S. A., Chin, J. G. J., Ottenkamp, J., et al.: Pulmonary regurgitation in the late postoperative follow-up of tetralogy of Fallot: Volumetric quantitation by nuclear magnetic resonance velocity mapping. Circulation 88[Part 1]:2257, 1993, with permission.)

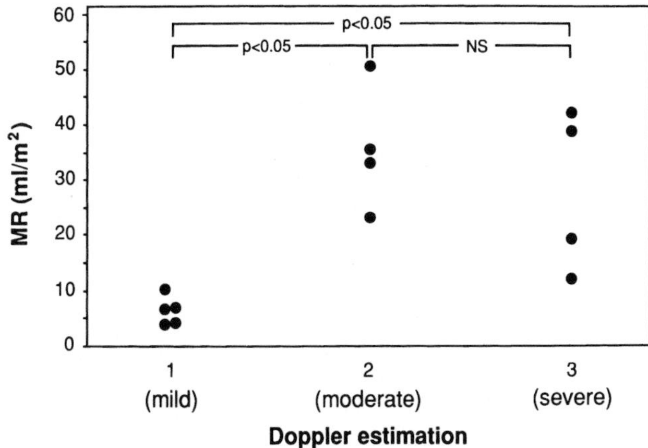

FIGURE 46–24. MR velocity mapping measurements of pulmonary regurgitation (PR) in each category and group of PR severity (1 = mild PR; 2 = moderate PR; 3 = severe PR) as differentiated semiquantitatively by Doppler echocardiography. The MR volumes measured in group 1 were significantly smaller than those in group 2 or group 3. However, the MR results measured in group 2 and group 3 were not significantly different from each other. (From Rebergen S. A., Chin, J. G. J., Ottenkamp, J., et al.: Pulmonary regurgitation in the late postoperative follow-up of tetralogy of Fallot. Volumetric quantitation by nuclear magnetic resonance velocity mapping. Circulation 88[Part 1]:2257, 1993, with permission.)

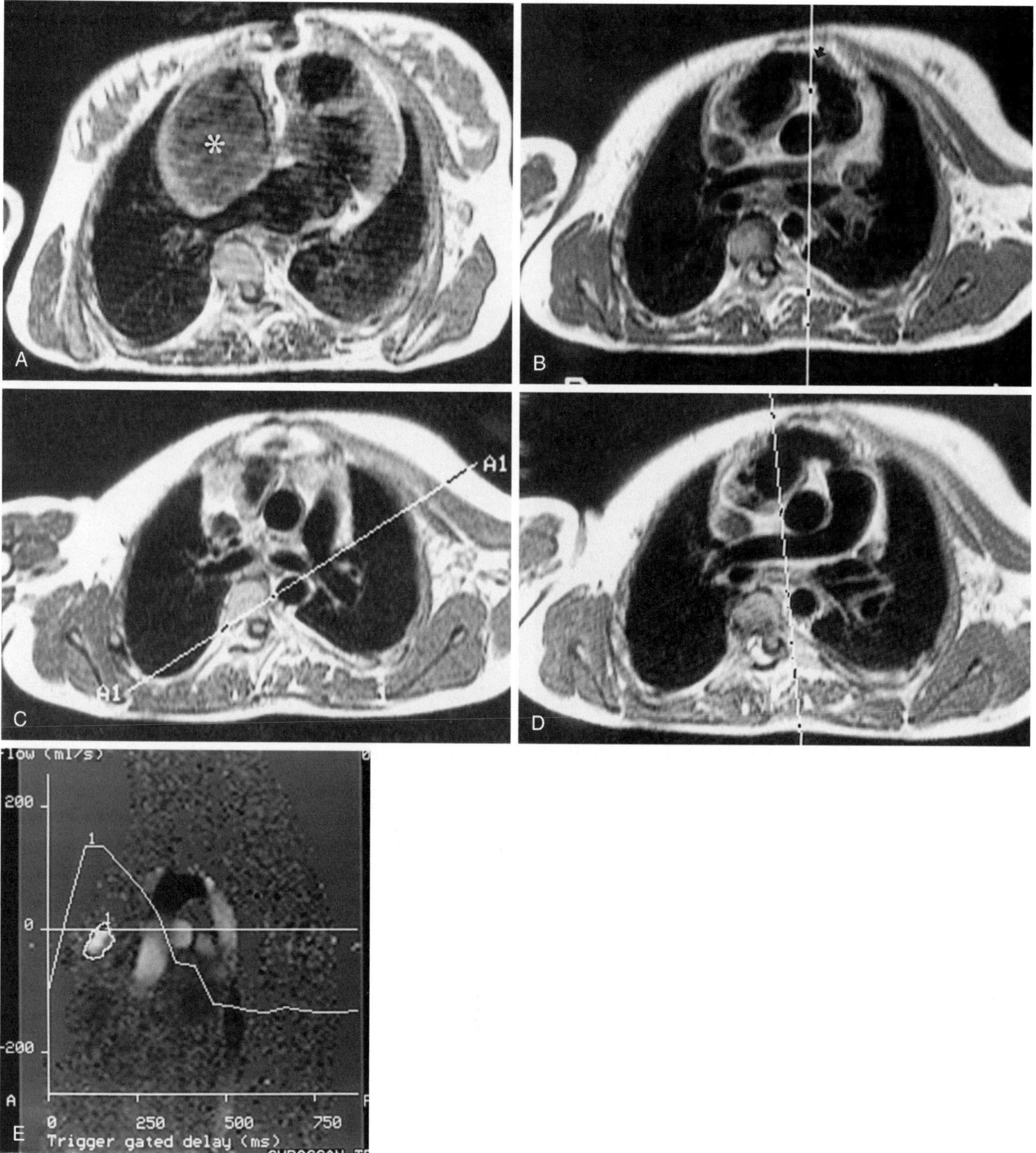

FIGURE 46–25. *A to E*, Evaluation of a Fontan operation in a patient with tricuspid atresia. Fatty replacement of the tricuspid valve plane is consistent with the diagnosis of tricuspid atresia *(A)*. Note enlargement of the right atrium *(asterisk* in *A)* with relative high signal intensity in the cavity due to flow-related enhancement. The widely patent connection of the right atrium and right ventricular outflow tract is shown in *B (arrow)*. The solid line indicates the plane for MR velocity mapping perpendicular to the atrioventricular connection. The solid line in *C* indicates the plane for MR velocity mapping perpendicular to the left pulmonary artery, whereas planning of a similar plane for the right pulmonary artery is shown in *D*. The resulting MR velocity map for the atrioventricular connection is shown in *E*. Note antegrade diastolic flow (area under the curve below zero line; 70 mL per cardiac cycle) in the conduit and systolic backflow (area under the curve above zero line; 20 cc per cardiac cycle) *(E)*. Therefore, effective forward flow through the conduit is 50 mL per cardiac cycle. The systolic forward flow as induced by right ventricular contraction through the main pulmonary artery is also 50 mL per cardiac cycle. The measured stroke flows for the right and left pulmonary arteries were 22 mL and 28 mL per cardiac cycle, respectively, equal to main pulmonary artery flow, demonstrating the accuracy and value of this method for evaluating the Fontan circulation.

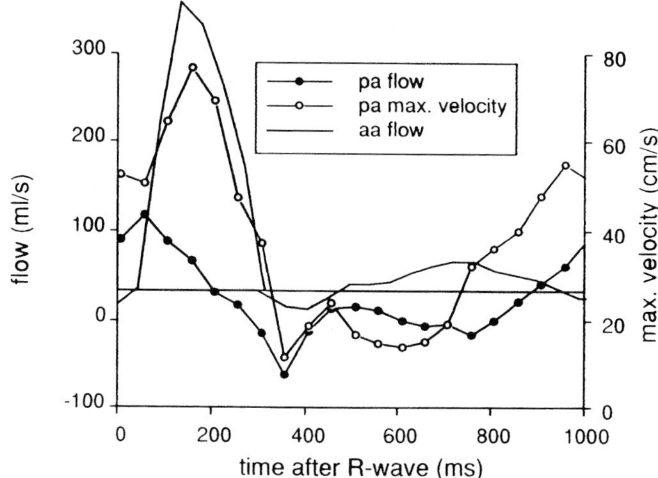

FIGURE 46–26. Magnetic resonance flow curves of the pulmonary artery in a patient with an atrioventricular Fontan connection. A presystolic peak of pulmonary volume flow is depicted, followed by a decrease in flow during ventricular systole. The timing of ventricular contraction is indicated by the aortic flow curve. Doppler velocity measurements and MR velocity mapping disclosed peak velocities at midsystole shortly after the R wave of the electrocardiogram, reflecting right ventricular contraction. The MR-based volume curves suggest that pulmonary flow is not significantly enhanced by right ventricular contraction, contrasting with the findings based on velocity measurements alone. (From Rebergen, S. A., Ottenkamp, J., Doornbos, J., et al.: Postoperative pulmonary flow dynamics after Fontan surgery: Assessment with nuclear magnetic resonance velocity mapping. J. Am. Coll. Cardiol. 21:121, 1993. Reprinted with permission from the American College of Cardiology.)

pulmonary flow patterns in patients who have undergone Fontan surgery with atriopulmonary as well as atrioventricular modifications of the operation.[90] In that study,[90] in all patients with an atriopulmonary Fontan connection, forward flow in the pulmonary artery was biphasic, reflecting the expected normal venous flow. Monophasic systolic pulmonary flow curves were detected in only half of the patients with atrioventricular Fontan connections, indicating right ventricular–dependent pulmonary blood flow. In the remaining half of the patients with an atrioventricular connection, the pumping capabilities of the right ventricle were not contributing to the Fontan circulation. In addition, it was shown that measurement of flow velocity alone may give a false impression of forward pulmonary flow and thus of the possible contribution of the right ventricle to the Fontan circulation (Fig. 46–26). Magnetic resonance velocity mapping uniquely provides reliable measurements of velocity as well as volume of pulmonary flow in patients with various modifications of Fontan procedures, being a tool for evaluating the success of Fontan surgery. The flow distribution to both lungs separately can also be measured with MR velocity mapping (see Fig. 46–17).[91] In normal volunteers, blood flow volume to the left lung appears to be significantly lower than flow to the right lung. Pulmonary flow after Fontan surgery appears to be preferentially oriented to the left lung, as demonstrated by MR velocity mapping.[90]

Pulmonary Hypertension

Assessment of pulmonary flow with the aid of MR velocity mapping may also provide insight into the presence and severity of arterial pulmonary hypertension.[92] Decreased pulmonary blood flow as well as lower peak systolic pulmonary flow velocities may be observed when pulmonary hypertension is present.[93] Furthermore, the signal intensity in the right pulmonary artery on spin-echo MR images appears to have a direct linear relationship with pulmonary vascular resistance in patients with congenital cardiovascular shunt lesions.[94]

MAGNETIC RESONANCE EVALUATION AFTER SENNING OR MUSTARD REPAIR

Ventricular Function

Mustard or Senning operations redirect the pulmonary venous return to the anatomical right ventricle in patients with transposition of the great arteries and subject the right ventricle to the loading conditions of a systemic ventricle (Fig. 46–27). The right ventricle is not ideally suited for systemic performance, and right ventricular failure may become evident in these patients. Magnetic resonance imaging may be of value in demonstrating baffle obstruction and in monitoring right ventricular systolic function in this category of patients (see Fig. 46–3). The ability of MR imaging to measure right ventricular diastolic function further qualifies this technique as a valuable tool for postsurgical evaluation of patients with congenital heart disease.[71] Because diastolic filling abnormalities may precede systolic dysfunction, the assessment of diastolic function may provide early information on the development of right ventricular dysfunction after Mustard and Senning operations.

Tricuspid Flow Patterns

Abnormal tricuspid flow patterns as demonstrated by Doppler echocardiography in patients who have undergone Mustard or Senning repair have been attributed to reduced compliance and

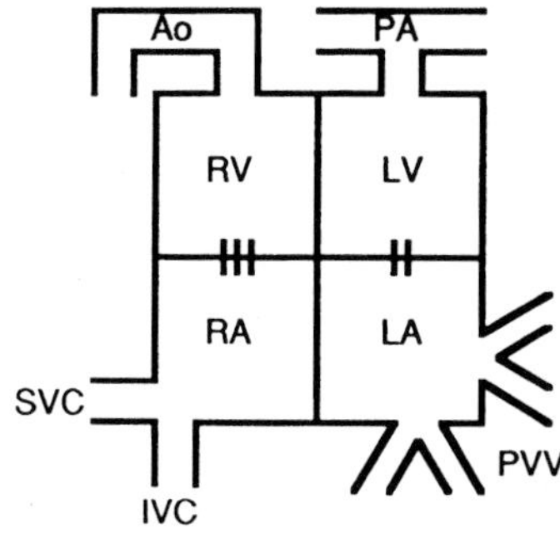

FIGURE 46–27. A diagram of transposition of the great arteries. The preoperative situation *(left)* illustrates the ventriculoarterial discordance. The situation after Mustard or Senning repair *(right)* shows the baffle (B) that directs the systemic venous return from the inferior and superior vena cava (IVC, SVC) to the mitral valve, left ventricle (LV), and pulmonary artery (PA). Oxygenated blood from the pulmonary veins (PVV) enters the neopulmonary venous atrium (PVA), reconstructed from the former left and right atriam (LA, RA), and is subsequently directed to the tricuspid valve, right ventricle (RV), and aorta (Ao). (From Rebergen, S. A., Helbing, W. A., Van der Wall, E. E., et al.: MR velocity mapping of tricuspid flow in healthy children and patients who have undergone Mustard or Senning repair. Radiology 194:505, 1995, with permission.)

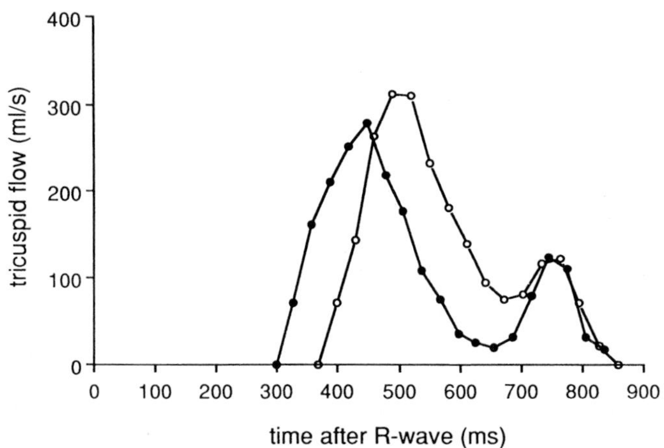

FIGURE 46–28. Tricuspid volume flow plotted against time after the R wave of the electrocardiogram in a normal child *(solid circles)* and in a patient after Senning repair *(open circles)* with similar ages and heart rates. Note the delayed onset of tricuspid flow and the slightly reduced relative contribution of atrial contraction to total forward flow in the patient. (From Rebergen, S. A., Helbing, W. A., Van der Wall, E. E., et al.: MR velocity mapping of tricuspid flow in healthy children and patients who have undergone Mustard or Senning repair. Radiology 194:505, 1995, with permission.)

impaired relaxation of the hypertrophied right ventricle. Rebergen and colleagues[71] have explored the use of MR velocity mapping of tricuspid flow in patients after Mustard or Senning repair. Abnormal tricuspid flow profiles can be demonstrated with MR velocity mapping in these patients (Fig. 46–28). Impaired myocardial relaxation generally results in a lower E peak velocity, a greater contribution of atrial contraction to ventricular filling, and therefore a smaller E:A ratio. In patients who have undergone Mustard or Senning repair, the time to peak E filling rate and normalized peak E filling rate were higher and peak A filling rate was lower, compared to a group of normal children with similar age, body surface area, and heart rate.

Diastolic Function

The contribution of atrial contraction to the diastolic filling was also reduced, an observation that is compatible with previous echocardiographic findings. A reduced compliance imposes a higher intraventricular pressure at the onset of atrial contraction, which may therefore be less effective. The prolonged time to peak filling rate agrees with the longer isovolumic relaxation time that has been reported in patients who have undergone Mustard or Senning repair. Magnetic resonance imaging allows comprehensive assessment of anatomy and both systolic and diastolic ventricular function after Mustard or Senning repair. Magnetic resonance imaging is developing into a complete tool for the evaluation of the postsurgical sequelae and residua in patients with congenital heart disease.

Acknowledgments

Parts of this chapter are based largely on the thesis by S. A. Rebergen. Furthermore, my colleagues J. Ottenkamp, J. Rohmer, J. G. J. Chin, P. M. T. Pattynama, P. Dendale, W. A. Helbing, A. Niezen, J. H. C. Reiber, A. V. G. Bruschke, and A. E. van Voorthuisen are acknowledged for helpful discussions and support.

References

1. Allen, H. D., Gersony, W. M., and Taubert, K. A.: Insurability of the adolescent and young adult with heart disease: Report from the Fifth Conference on Insurability, October 3–4, 1991. Circulation 86:703, 1992.
2. Perloff, J. K.: Congenital heart disease in adults: A new cardiovascular subspecialty. Circulation 84:1881, 1991.
3. Link, K. M., and Lesko, N. M.: Magnetic resonance imaging in the evaluation of congenital heart disease. Magn. Reson. Q. 7:173, 1991.
4. De Roos, A., and Van der Wall, E. E.: Magnetic resonance imaging and spectroscopy of the heart. Curr. Opin. Cardiol. 6:946, 1991.
5. Geva, T., Vick, W., Wendt, R. E., et al.: Role of spin echo and cine magnetic resonance imaging in presurgical planning of heterotaxy syndrome. Circulation 90:348, 1994.
6. Kersting-Sommerhoff, B. A., Seelos, K. C., Hardy, C., et al.: Evaluation of surgical procedures for cyanotic congenital heart disease by using MR imaging. AJR 155:259, 1990.
7. Doornbos, J., and De Roos, A.: Imaging strategy in cardiac magnetic resonance imaging. *In* Van der Wall, E. E., and De Roos, A. (eds.): Magnetic Resonance Imaging in Coronary Artery Disease. Dordrecht, Kluwer, 1991.
8. Chung, K. J., Simpson, I. A., Newman, R., et al.: Cine magnetic resonance imaging for evaluation of congenital heart disease: Role in pediatric cardiology compared with echocardiography and angiography. J. Pediatr. 113:1028, 1988.
9. Chung, K. J., Simpson, I. A., Glass, R. F., et al.: Cine magnetic resonance imaging after surgical repair in patients with transposition of the great arteries. Circulation 77:104, 1988.
10. Van Rugge, F. P., Van der Wall, E. E., Van Dijkman, P. R. M., et al.: Usefulness of ultrafast magnetic resonance imaging in healed myocardial infarction. Am. J. Cardiol. 70:1233, 1992.
11. Davis, C. P., McKinnon, G. C., Debatin, J. F., et al.: Normal heart: Evaluation with echo-planar MR imaging. Radiology 191:691, 1994.
12. Manning, W. J., Atkinson, D. J., Grossman, W., et al.: First-pass nuclear magnetic resonance imaging studies using gadolinium-DTPA in patients with coronary artery disease. J. Am. Coll. Cardiol. 18:959, 1991.
13. Guifoyle, D. N., Gibbs, P., Ordidge, R. J., et al.: Real-time flow measurements using echo-planar imaging. Magn. Reson. Med. 18:1, 1991.
14. Wendland, M. F., Saeed, M., Masui, T., et al.: Echo-planar MR imaging of normal and ischemic myocardium with gadodiamide injection. Radiology 186:535, 1993.
15. Seelos, K. C., Von Smekal, A., Vahlensieck, M., et al.: Cardiac abnormalities: Assessment with T2-weighted turbo spin-echo MR imaging with electrocardiogram gating at 0.5 T. Radiology 189:517, 1993.
16. Edelman, R. R.: Basic principles of magnetic resonance angiography. Cardiovasc. Intervent Radiol. 15:3, 1992.
17. Bradley, W. G.: Flow phenomena in MR imaging. AJR 150:983, 1988.
18. Mohiaddin, R. H., and Longmore, D. B.: Functional aspects of cardiovascular nuclear magnetic resonance imaging: Techniques and application. Circulation 88:264, 1993.
19. Rebergen, S. A., Van der Wall, E. E., Doornbos, J., et al.: Magnetic resonance measurement of velocity and flow: Technique, validation, and clinical applications. Am. Heart J. 126:1439, 1993.
20. Firmin, D. N., Nayler, G. L., Klipstein, R. H., et al.: In vivo validation of MR velocity imaging. J. Comput. Assist. Tomogr. 11:751, 1987.
21. Mohiaddin, R. H., Wann, S. L., Underwood, R., et al.: Vena caval flow: Assessment with cine MR velocity mapping. Radiology 177:537, 1990.
22. Mohiaddin, R. H., Amanuma, M., Kilner, P. J., et al.: MR phase-shift velocity mapping of mitral and pulmonary venous flow. J. Comput. Assist. Tomogr. 15:237, 1991.
23. Mohiaddin, R. H., Paz, R., Theodoropoulos, S., et al.: Magnetic resonance characterization of pulmonary arterial blood flow after single lung transplantation. J. Thorac. Cardiovasc. Surg. 101:1016, 1991.
24. Bottomley, P. A.: MR spectroscopy of the human heart: The status and the challenges. Radiology 191:593, 1994.
25. De Roos, A., Doornbos, J., Luyten, P. R., et al.: Cardiac metabolism in patients with dilated and hypertrophic cardiomyopathy: Assessment with proton-decoupled P-31 MR spectroscopy. J. Magn. Reson. Imaging, 2:711, 1992.
26. Keevil, S. F., Lewis, M. C., Garbutt, J. N., et al.: In vivo phosphorus-31 NMR spectroscopy of the myocardium in children with congenital heart abnormalities. *In* Book of Abstracts. Berkeley, CA, Society of Magnetic Resonance in Medicine, 1993, p. 1095.
27. Schröter, G., Stern, H., Habersbrunner, E., et al.: Energy and phospholipid metabolism in patients after atrial repair for transposition of the great arteries and cardiomyopathy. *In* Vienna, European Congress of Radiology, 1993, p. 903.
28. Whitman, J. R., Chance, B., Bode, H., et al.: Diagnosis and therapeutic evaluation of a pediatric case of cardiomyopathy using phosphorus-31 nuclear magnetic resonance spectroscopy. J. Am. Coll. Cardiol. 5:745, 1985.
29. Fellows, K. E., Weinberg, P. M., Baffa, J. M., et al.: Evaluation of congenital heart disease with MR imaging: Current and coming attractions. AJR 159:925, 1992.
30. Kersting-Sommerhoff, B. A., Diethelm, L., Teitel, D. F., et al.: Magnetic resonance imaging of congenital heart disease: Sensitivity and specificity using receiver operating characteristic curve analysis. Am. Heart J. 118:155, 1989.
31. Baker, E. J., Ayton, V., Smith, M. A., et al.: Magnetic resonance imaging of coarctation of the aorta in infants: Use of a high field strength. Br. Heart J. 62:97, 1989.
32. Bank, E. R., Aisen, A. M., Rocchini, A. P., et al.: Coarctation of the aorta in children undergoing angioplasty: Pretreatment and posttreatment MR imaging. Radiology 162:235, 1987.
33. Didier, D., Higgins, C. B., Fisher, M. R., et al.: Congenital heart disease: Gated MR imaging in 72 patients. Radiology 158:227, 1986.
34. Shinebourne, E. A., Macartney, F. J., and Anderson, R. H.: Sequential chamber localization: Logical approach to diagnosis in congenital heart disease. Br. Heart J. 41:327, 1976.
35. Tynan, M. J., Becker, A. E., Macartney, F. J., et al.: Nomenclature and classification of congenital heart disease. Br. Heart J. 41:544, 1979.
36. Van Praagh, R.: The importance of segmental situs in the diagnosis of congenital heart disease. Semin. Roentgenol. 20:254, 1985.
37. Guit, G. L., Bluemm, R., Rohmer, J., et al.: Levotransposition of the aorta: Identification of segmental cardiac anatomy using MR imaging. Radiology 161:673, 1986.

38. Higgins, C. B.: MRI of congenital heart disease. *In* Higgins, C. B. (ed.): Essentials of Cardiac Radiology and Imaging. Philadelphia, J. B. Lippincott, 1992.
39. Masui, T., Seelos, K. C., Kersting-Sommerhoff, B. A., et al.: Abnormalities of the pulmonary veins: Evaluation with MR imaging and comparison with cardiac angiography and echocardiography. Radiology 181:645, 1991.
40. Huggon, I. C., Baker, E. J., Maisey, M. N., et al.: Magnetic resonance imaging of hearts with atrioventricular valve atresia or double inlet ventricle. Br. Heart J. 68:313, 1992.
41. Kersting-Sommerhoff, B. A., Diethelm, L., Stanger, P., et al.: Evaluation of complex congenital ventricular anomalies with magnetic resonance imaging. Am. Heart J. 120:133, 1990.
42. Parsons, J. M., Baker, E. J., Anderson, R. H., et al.: Double-outlet right ventricle: Morphologic demonstration using nuclear magnetic resonance imaging. J. Am. Coll. Cardiol. 18:168, 1991.
43. Rebergen, S. A., Guit, G. L., and de Roos, A.: Double outlet left ventricle: Assessment with magnetic resonance imaging. Br. Heart J. 66:381, 1991.
44. Kersting-Sommerhoff, B. A., Sechtem, U. P., Fisher, M. R., et al.: MR imaging of congenital anomalies of the aortic arch. AJR 149:9, 1987.
45. Lowe, G. M., Donaldson, J. S., and Backer, C. L.: Vascular rings: Ten-year review of imaging. Radiographics 11:637, 1991.
46. Von Schulthess, G. K., Higashino, S. M., Higgins, S. S., et al.: Coarctation of the aorta: MR imaging. Radiology 158:469, 1986.
47. Simpson, I. A., Chung, K. J., Glass, R. F., et al.: Cine magnetic resonance imaging for evaluation of anatomy and flow relations in infants and children with coarctation of the aorta. Circulation 78:142, 1988.
48. Mohiaddin, R. H., Kilner, P. J., Rees, S., et al.: Magnetic resonance volume flow and jet velocity mapping in aortic coarctation. J. Am. Coll. Cardiol. 22:1515, 1993.
49. Steffens, J. C., Bourne, M. W., Sakuma, H., et al.: Quantification of collateral blood flow in coarctation of the aorta by velocity encoded cine magnetic resonance imaging. Circulation 90:937, 1994.
50. Didier, D., and Higgins, C. B.: Identification and localization of ventricular septal defect by gated magnetic resonance imaging. Am. J. Cardiol. 57:1363, 1986.
51. Lowell, D. G., Turner, D. A., Smith, S. M., et al.: The detection of atrial and ventricular septal defects with electrocardiographically synchronized magnetic resonance imaging. Circulation 73:89, 1986.
52. Sechtem, U., Pflugfelder, P., Cassidy, M. C., et al.: Ventricular septal defect: Visualization of shunt flow and determination of shunt size by cine MR imaging. AJR 149:689, 1987.
53. Higgins, C. B., Sechtem, U. P., and Pflugfelder, P.: Cine MR: Evaluation of cardiac ventricular function and valvular function. Int. J. Card. Imaging 3:21, 1988.
54. Kondo, C., Caputo, G. R., Semelka, R., et al.: Right and left ventricular stroke volume measurements with velocity-encoded cine MR imaging: In vitro and in vivo validation. AJR 157:9, 1991.
55. Cranney, C. B., Lotan, C. S., and Pohost, G. M.: Nuclear magnetic resonance imaging for assessment and follow-up of patients with valve disease. Circulation 84(Suppl. I):216, 1991.
56. Pattynama, P. M. T., Lamb, H. J. L., Van der Velde, E. A., et al.: Left ventricular measurements with cine and spin-echo MR imaging: A study of reproducibility with variance component analysis. Radiology 187:261, 1993.
57. Caputo, G. R., Suzuki, J. -I., Kondi, C., et al.: Determination of left ventricular volume and mass with use of biphasic spin-echo MR imaging: Comparison with cine MR. Radiology 177:773, 1990.
58. Doherty, N. E., Fujita, N., Caputo, G. R., et al.: Measurement of right ventricular mass in normal and dilated cardiomyopathic ventricles using cine magnetic resonance imaging. Am. J. Cardiol. 69:1223, 1992.
59. Pattynama, P. M. T., Lamb, H. J., Van der Geest, R., et al.: Reproducibility of measurements of right ventricular volumes and myocardial mass with MR imaging. Magn. Reson. Imaging 13:93, 1995.
60. Auffermann, W., Wagner, S., Holt, W. W., et al.: Noninvasive determination of left ventricular output and wall stress in volume overload and in myocardial disease by cine magnetic resonance imaging. Am. Heart J. 121:1750, 1991.
61. Arts, T., Veenstra, P. C., and Reneman, R. S.: Epicardial deformation and left ventricular wall mechanics during ejection in the dog. Am. J. Physiol. 243:H379, 1982.
62. Sandler, H., and Dodge, H. T.: Left ventricular tension and stress in man. Circ. Res. 13:91, 1963.
63. Pattynama, P. M. T.: Functional Magnetic Resonance Imaging of the Heart. Thesis, Leiden University, 1994.
64. Pattynama, P. M. T., De Roos, A., Van der Velde, E. T., et al.: Magnetic resonance imaging analysis of ventricular pressure-volume relations: Validation with the conductance method at rest and during dobutamine stress. Magn. Reson. Med. 1995 (in press).
65. Ross, J.: Cardiac function and myocardial contractility: A perspective. J. Am. Coll. Cardiol. 1:52, 1983.
66. Helbing, W. A., Rebergen, S. A., Maliepaard, C., et al.: Quantification of right ventricular function with magnetic resonance imaging in children with normal hearts and with congenital heart disease. Am. Heart J. 1995 (in press).
67. Fujita, N., Hartiala, J., O'Sullivan, M., et al.: Assessment of left ventricular diastolic function in dilated cardiomyopathy with cine magnetic resonance imaging: Effect of an angiotensin-converting enzyme inhibitor, benazepril. Am. Heart J. 125:171, 1993.
68. Mostbeck, G. H., Hartiala, J. J., Foster, E., et al.: Right ventricular diastolic filling: Evaluation with velocity-encoded cine MRI. J. Comput. Assist. Tomogr. 17:245, 1993.
69. Suzuki, J. -I., Chang, J. -M., Caputo, G. R., et al.: Evaluation of right ventricular early diastolic filling by cine nuclear magnetic resonance imaging in patients with hypertrophic cardiomyopathy. J. Am. Coll. Cardiol. 18:120, 1991.
70. Hartiala, J. J., Mostbeck, G. H., Foster, E., et al.: Velocity-encoded cine MRI in the evaluation of left ventricular diastolic function: Measurement of mitral valve and pulmonary vein flow velocities and flow volume across the mitral valve. Am. Heart J. 125:1054, 1993.
71. Rebergen, S. A., Helbing, W. A., Van der Wall, E. E., et al.: MR velocity mapping of tricuspid flow in healthy children and patients who have undergone Mustard or Senning repair. Radiology 194:505, 1995.
72. Dinsmore, R. E., Wismer, G. L., Guyer, D., et al.: Magnetic resonance imaging of the interatrial septum and atrial septal defects. AJR 145:697, 1985.
73. Diethelm, L., Déry, R., Lipton, M. J., et al.: Atrial-level shunts: Sensitivity and specificity of MR in diagnosis. Radiology 162:181, 1987.
74. Brenner, L. D., Caputo, G. R., Mostbeck, G. H., et al.: Quantification of left-to-right atrial shunts with velocity-encoded cine nuclear magnetic resonance imaging. J. Am. Coll. Cardiol. 20:1246, 1992.
75. Rebergen, S. A., Ottenkamp, J., Chin, J. G. J., et al.: Value of magnetic resonance velocity mapping for follow-up of grown-up postoperative congenital heart disease: XVth Congress of the European Society of Cardiology, Nice. Eur. Heart J. 14:1003, 1993.
76. Jones, E. L., Conti, C. R., Neill, C. A., et al.: Long-term evaluation of tetralogy patients with pulmonic valvular insufficiency resulting from outflow-patch correction across the pulmonic annulus. Circulation 47/48(Suppl. III):11, 1973.
77. Marie, P. Y., Marcon, F., Brunotte, F., et al.: Right ventricular overload and induced sustained ventricular tachycardia in operatively "repaired" tetralogy of Fallot. Am. J. Cardiol. 69:785, 1992.
78. Rebergen, S. A., Chin, J. G. J., Ottenkamp, J., et al.: Pulmonary regurgitation in the late postoperative follow-up of tetralogy of Fallot: Volumetric quantitation by nuclear magnetic resonance velocity mapping. Circulation 88(Part 1):2257, 1993.
79. Markiewicz, W., Sechtem, U., and Higgins, C. B.: Evaluation of the right ventricle by magnetic resonance imaging. Am. Heart J. 113:8, 1987.
80. Møgelvang, J., Stubgaard, M., Thomsen, C., et al.: Evaluation of right ventricular volumes measured by magnetic resonance imaging. Eur. Heart J. 9:529, 1988.
81. Formanek, A. G., Witcofski, R. L., D'Souza, V. J., et al.: MR imaging of the central pulmonary arterial tree in conotruncal malformation. AJR 147:1127, 1986.
82. Kersting-Sommerhoff, B. A., Sechtem, U., and Higgins, C. B.: Evaluation of pulmonary blood supply by nuclear magnetic resonance imaging in patients with pulmonary atresia. J. Am. Coll. Cardiol. 11:166, 1988.
83. Rees, R. S. O., Somerville, J., Underwood, S. R., et al.: Magnetic resonance imaging of the pulmonary arteries and their systemic connections in pulmonary atresia: Comparison with angiographic and surgical findings. Br. Heart J. 58:621, 1987.
84. Martinez, J. E., Mohiaddin, R. H., Kilner, P. J., et al.: Obstruction in extracardiac ventriculopulmonary conduits: Value of nuclear magnetic resonance imaging with velocity mapping and Doppler echocardiography. J. Am. Coll. Cardiol. 20:338, 1992.
85. Eichenberger, A. C., Jenni, R., and Von Schulthess, G. K.: Aortic valve pressure gradients in patients with aortic valve stenosis: Quantification with velocity-encoded cine MR imaging. AJR 160:971, 1993.
86. Fontan, F., and Baudet, E.: Surgical repair of tricuspid atresia. Thorax 26:240, 1971.
87. DeLeon, S. Y., Ilbawi, M. N., Idriss, F. S., et al.: Fontan type operation for complex lesions. J. Thorac. Cardiovasc. Surg. 92:1029, 1986.
88. Ottenkamp, J., Rohmer, J., Quaegebeur, J., et al.: Nine years' experience of physiological correction of tricuspid atresia: Long-term results and current surgical approach. Thorax 37:718, 1982.
89. Bull, C., De Leval, M. R., Stark, J., et al.: Use of a subpulmonary ventricular chamber in the Fontan circulation. J. Thorac. Cardiovasc. Surg. 85:21, 1983.
90. Rebergen, S. A., Ottenkamp, J., Doornbos, J., et al.: Postoperative pulmonary flow dynamics after Fontan surgery: Assessment with nuclear magnetic resonance velocity mapping. J. Am. Coll. Cardiol. 21:123, 1993.
91. Caputo, G. R., Kondo, C., Masui, T., et al.: Right and left lung perfusion: In vitro and in vivo validation with oblique-angle velocity-encoded cine MR imaging. Radiology 180:693, 1991.
92. Bogren, H. G., Klipstein, R. H., Mohiaddin, R. H., et al.: Pulmonary artery distensibility and blood flow patterns: A magnetic resonance study of normal subjects and of patients with pulmonary arterial hypertension. Am. Heart J. 118:990, 1989.
93. Kondo, C., Caputo, G. R., Masui, T., et al.: Pulmonary hypertension: Pulmonary flow quantification and flow profile analysis with velocity-encoded cine MR imaging. Radiology 183:751, 1992.
94. Didier, D., and Higgins, C. B.: Estimation of pulmonary vascular resistance by MRI in patients with congenital cardiovascular shunt lesions. AJR 146:919, 1986.

CHAPTER

47 Imaging of the Valves and Great Vessels

Kerry M. Link, M.D.
David M. Szczesniak, M.D.
Nadja M. Lesko, M.D.

Evaluation of the thoracic aorta is the leading indication for cardiovascular magnetic resonance imaging (MRI). The reasons for this are the excellent contrast and spatial resolution, large field of view (FOV), and multiplanar imaging capacity of MRI coupled with both static and functional imaging techniques. MRI combines the attributes of angiography, echocardiography, and computed tomography (CT) to make it the imaging modality of choice for most congenital anomalies and acquired diseases of the thoracic aorta.

BACKGROUND

Interpretation of congenital anomalies, normal variants, and acquired diseases requires a basic knowledge of the embryology, anatomy, and physiology of the thoracic aorta. The formation of the aorta is intimately related to the development of the heart, which begins about 20 days after fertilization and is complete in approximately 5 weeks. The thoracic aorta is composed of portions of the truncus arteriosus, aortic sac, and dorsal aortas and begins to develop when angiogenic cells appear on either side of the neural plate. These cells rapidly coalesce to form a pair of longitudinal vessels, the dorsal aortas, which parallel the course of the neural plate. The dorsal aortas join the inferior aspect of the developing endocardial or heart tubes. After the right and left endocardial tubes fuse, the inferior aspect of the newly developed single midline structure rotates 180 degrees posteriorly and cranially, bringing with it the dorsal aortas and forming the first pair of aortic arches. By 23 days, this process is complete. The most cranial aspect of the endocardial tube is the aorta sac. Superiorly, the sac joins the dorsal aortic arches. Inferiorly, the aorta sac joins the bulbus cordis, which in turn is connected to the ventricle (eventual left ventricle). The ventricle connects with the right and left atrium through the atrioventricular channel. Each atrium is joined to its respective sinus venosus.[1–3]

Next, the bulboventricular component of the endocardial tube undergoes exponential growth relative to the aortic sac superiorly and the atria inferiorly. This exponential growth results in a bowing or "looping" of the bulbus cordis and ventricle. The bend usually occurs to the right, resulting in a *d*- (dextro-) bulboventricular loop. The loop then undergoes a clockwise rotation (as viewed from the feet), which moves the bulbus cordis anterior to the ventricle. As a result, the aorta, specifically the aortic valve, will arise from the center of the heart base and to the right of the pulmonic valve, and it is therefore termed a *d*- (dextro-) aorta (Fig. 47–1). The

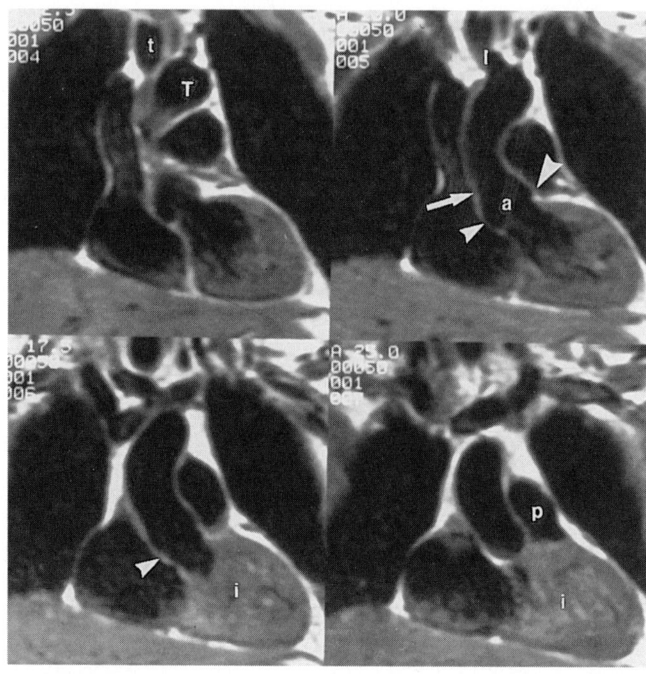

FIGURE 47–1. Sequential, 1-cm thick, electrocardiographically gated coronal images demonstrating the position of the *d*-aorta (a). It arises from the center of the cardiac base, posterior, inferior, and to the right of the pulmonic valve (p). *Arrow* = sinotubular junction; *small arrowhead* = right sinus of Valsalva; *large arrowhead* = left main coronary artery arising from left sinus of Valsalva; i = interventricular septum; I = innominate artery; T = transverse portion of aortic arch: t = trachea.

reverse of this situation occurs if the bulboventricular loop forms to the left and undergoes counterclockwise rotation. In this situation, the aortic valve is to the left of the pulmonic valve and is known as an *l*-aorta. The terms *d*- and *l*-aorta refer specifically to the position of the aortic valve in relation to the pulmonic valve and have nothing to do with the type of aortic arch.[1–3]

The bulbus cordis undergoes its own differentiation at about the same time and forms, from cranial to caudal, the truncus arteriosus, the conus cordis, and the right ventricle. The truncus arteriosus, aorta sac, and dorsal aortas will eventually form the semilunar valves, aortic root, ascending aorta, aortic arch, and descending thoracic aorta. The conus cordis and truncus arteriosus undergo a process of septation to form, respectively, the infundibulum and aortic annulus and the aortic and pulmonary channels. This is a complex process in which spiral ridges form within the cavities of these structures. As a result of this spiraling, the infundibulum and pulmonary artery arise anterior to the aorta, only to have the main pulmonary artery wrap around the aorta. The semilunar valves are formed when the proximal portions of the ridges, which form the septum between the aortic and pulmonary channels, and their free walls undergo a process of excavation. The leaflets are "scooped out" of the vessel wall and septum. The sinuses of Valsalva mark the area of excavation that formed the leaflets. The sinotubular junction (the point at which the top of the sinus joins the tubular portion or proximal aspect of the ascending aorta) marks the cranial end of the leaflets during systole[3] (see Fig. 47–1).

The transverse portion of the arch and the branch vessels are formed during another complex process, the development of the aortic arches. After the endocardial tube undergoes its 180-degree posterior and superior migration, the paired dorsal aortas form an aortic arch on both sides of the aorta sac, establishing the first of six pairs of dorsal (or embryonic) aortic arches. It is from the aortic sac that the aortic arches will develop and regress to finally form a single unilateral arch and the branch vessels. By the 25th day of development, the first aortic arches disappear except for remnant portions that form the maxillary arteries. The second arches develop and quickly disappear except for portions forming the stapedial arteries. The third arches are well developed at this time, and the fourth and six pairs are just beginning to form. By the 32nd day, the septation process of the conotruncal portion of the heart tube is complete. The septation extends into the aortic sac to form the distal portion of the ascending aorta, the innominate artery, and the transverse portion of the arch up to the left common carotid artery. The proximal portions of the sixth right and left arches form the right and left pulmonary arteries, respectively. The distal portions of the sixth arches form the right and left ductus arteriosus. The right ductus almost always disappears. At the same time, the dorsal aortas fuse to form a single descending aorta. The seventh intersegmental arteries arise from the dorsal arches just before their fusion to form the single descending aorta.[1–3] Edwards' hypothetical double aortic arch model is based on the development of the aortic arches at this stage.[4] The third aortic arches begin to elongate at about the 35th day of gestation. The common carotid arteries are derived from the proximal portions of the third arches; the distal portions of these arches form the internal carotid arteries. The left intersegmental artery forms the left subclavian artery. The right intersegmental artery forms the distal aspect of the right subclavian artery. The distal transverse arch and proximal descending thoracic aorta are formed by the left dorsal aorta. The proximal portion of the right fourth arch forms the proximal right subclavian artery; the distal part of the right fourth arch disappears.

After birth, the left ductus arteriosus usually closes, forming the ligamentum arteriosus. The aorta has a "question mark" configuration, with the aortic root (leaflets and sinuses of Valsalva) arising from the center of the cardiac base in the case of a *d*-bulboventricle loop (the normal configuration). The aortic root is oriented parallel to the long axis of the left ventricle. This orientation can vary between 20 and 50 degrees from the body's long axis, depending on the position of the heart (horizontal or vertical). The aortic root is usually located at the level of the eighth vertebral body. It is positioned anterior to the left atrium, medial to the right atrium, and posterior to the infundibulum. The right coronary sinus is located just above the interventricular septum (see Fig. 47–1).

The ascending aorta rises superiorly and to the right before crossing back to the midline at the level of the innominate artery. The main pulmonary artery passes to the left of the ascending aorta. The right pulmonary artery passes behind the ascending aorta. The superior vena cava is located to the right of the ascending aorta. The ascending aorta and the transverse portion of the arch join at the level of the fourth thoracic vertebral body. The transverse arch passes to the left and anterior to the trachea before continuing posteriorly to join the descending thoracic aorta (left arch). The descending aorta is located in the posterior mediastinum and to the left of the spine. The anterior-to-posterior branching pattern most often encountered (70 percent) is innominate artery, left common carotid artery, and left subclavian artery. In approximately 25 percent of the population, the left common carotid artery is fused with the innominate artery to form a common trunk (bovine pattern). On occasion (17 percent), the left superior intercostal vein appears as a small "nipple" arising from the left lateral aspect of the transverse arch on the frontal chest radiograph.

The aorta is the largest vessel in the body, with an average diameter of 3.3 cm at the aortic sinus, 3.0 cm at the ascending aorta, 2.7 cm at the arch, and 2.4 cm at the proximal descending aorta.[5] The thoracic aorta is an elastic artery that comprises three layers: the inner layer, the intima, is composed of a thin layer of endothelial cells; spiraled layers of elastic tissue intermixed with muscle make up the media; the outer layer is the adventitia, a thin connective tissue containing the vasa vasorum, lymphatics, and nerves.

TECHNIQUES

MRI is a superb noninvasive imaging modality for evaluation of the pathoanatomy and pathophysiology of thoracic aortic anomalies and diseases, provided the technique is properly implemented. Attention to prescan setup and selection of proper pulse sequences and imaging parameters will maximize image quality and therefore the amount of information that can be gleaned from the examination. Motion, whether it be patient, respiratory, cardiac, or arterial pulsatility, has deleterious effects on the image quality. Overcoming image degradation caused by these sources of motion is perhaps the biggest challenge of cardiovascular MRI.

Most adults can remain quiet enough during the course of the MRI examination so as not to require sedation. However, many patients complain of back pain that is worsened by having to lie flat on the MRI table. They invariably move during the MRI examination if they do not receive some pain medication, preferably by intravenous administration. Children cannot be relied on to remain still during the MRI study, and we therefore routinely sedate infants and children. Although many sedation schemes have been advocated, we have found intravenous administration of Nembutal, 2 to 4 mg/kg of body weight, to be the most reliable and controllable means of sedation.

Respiratory motion can result in significant ghosting through the chest, thereby degrading the quality of the study by introducing artifacts within the aorta that can be erroneously interpreted as representing disease (e.g., dissection). This ghosting is caused by bright signal from subcutaneous chest wall fat that is propagated in the phase-encoding direction through the chest. The more erratic the patient's breathing, the worse the ghosting. This phenomenon can be limited to some degree through respiratory compensation schemes that try to average out the effects of respiratory motion.[6] Alternatively, the operator can attempt to null the signal from subcutaneous fat through the use of fat saturation or by placing a saturation band along the anterior chest wall. The former method increases the overall length of the MRI examination because fewer slices can be obtained per acquisition. The latter method is somewhat haphazard in its effect because the anterior chest wall does not always stay within the saturation band during the entire respiratory cycle. As a result, respiratory motion with subsequent ghosting remains a problem in the study of the cardiovascular system.

Cardiac motion has a direct effect on the ascending aorta and causes ghosting (from pericardial and epicardial fat) that may be transmitted onto the descending aorta. For these reasons and also because dynamic MRI imaging techniques require that leads be placed on the patient for "reference," we perform electrocardiographic (ECG) gating in all our thoracic aortic studies. Most difficulties encountered with ECG-gated MRI can be traced to poor implementation of the technique. The ECG patches should be grouped closely together on the chest or back but not on the extremities, where idle movement could degrade the ECG signal. With close grouping of the patches, the ECG vector signal is maximized, enhancing the chances of obtaining discrete QRS complexes, which in turn are used to gate pulse sequence application. The ECG leads should be coiled around one another and placed parallel to the bore of the magnet in order to negate the electric flux that can be generated around a looped wire within a magnetic field.

Whenever possible, some type of dedicated coil should be used, especially in infants and children. The small FOVs required to analyze the aorta for coarctation membranes, subaortic stenosis, and other aspects of this patient population result in poor signal-to-noise ratios (SNRs) with the body coil. For infants, this problem can be overcome with the use of a head coil or a knee coil. Prototype cardiac, chest, and torso coils are becoming commercially available and should be used in studies of children, adolescents, and adults, in lieu of the body coil.

After the patient is on the MRI table and the proper coil has been selected, the ECG leads are attached. With the patient outside the magnetic bore, the ECG tracing is checked to ensure the presence of a discrete QRS complex. It is the QRS complex that is used to trigger spin-echo (SE) sequences and that serves as a reference point for prospective or retrospective dynamic (cine or phase-mapping) sequences. If a discrete QRS complex is not present, the leads are rearranged and connected to the junction box until a good tracing is obtained. Occasionally, it is necessary to rearrange the patch placement in order to obtain a proper ECG tracing. The patient is placed in the magnetic bore and the QRS complex tracing is rechecked. The magnetic field can have a significant effect on the tracing, and either the lead or the patch placement may need to be rearranged once again. While scanning is actually taking place, there is significant disruption of the ECG pattern.[7] Therefore, the ECG tracing cannot be used to monitor the patient for ischemic changes during the course of the MRI examination.

The standard contraindications to MRI scanning (i.e., intracerebral aneurysm chip, metallic foreign body in the eye, pacemaker) apply to patients undergoing a cardiovascular MRI evaluation. Although some heart valves have been shown to be deflected in a 1.5-T MRI scanner, the stress placed on those valves by the beating heart is greater. Therefore, the presence of a cardiac valve is not a contraindication to MRI examination.

The typical evaluation of the thoracic aorta consists of ECG-gated multislice SE pulse sequences performed in the transaxial, coronal, and left anterior oblique (LAO) planes (Fig. 47–2) through the thoracic aorta. An SE sequence can be obtained in approximately 5 minutes. The SE sequence maximizes tissue contrast between the aortic lumen, the aortic wall, and periaortic structures. As a multislice technique, each individual slice is obtained at a different phase of the cardiac cycle. If the slices are obtained in an interleaved fashion to decrease crosstalk, adjacent slices will not represent sequential time delay intervals. As a result, some slices will demonstrate an intermediate signal within the aortic lumen owing to the presence of stagnant diastolic arterial blood flow. This phenomenon is more pronounced with in-plane blood flow (in which the orientation of the blood flow remains within the plane of acquisition) and with venous blood flow (Fig. 47–3). It can be erroneously interpreted as a thrombus, mass, or abscess, depending on the location of the finding. This is usually not a diagnostic problem because the time delay from the QRS complex is indicated on the image annotation, thereby establishing where in the cardiac cycle the image was obtained. On occasion, a dynamic study may be required to differentiate a mass lesion from slow-flowing blood.

The repetition time (TR) is determined by the patient's RR interval. An echo time (TE) of about 20 msec gives good contrast resolution on 1.5-T scanners. The FOV should be kept between 20 and 30 cm but can be varied, depending on what structures are

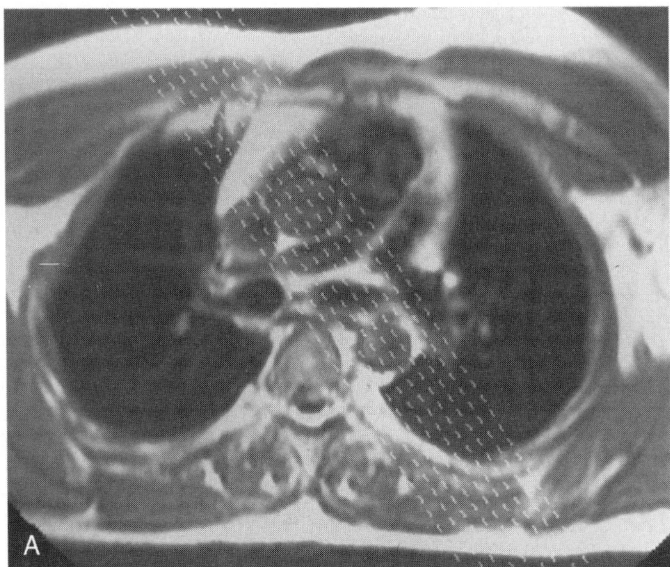

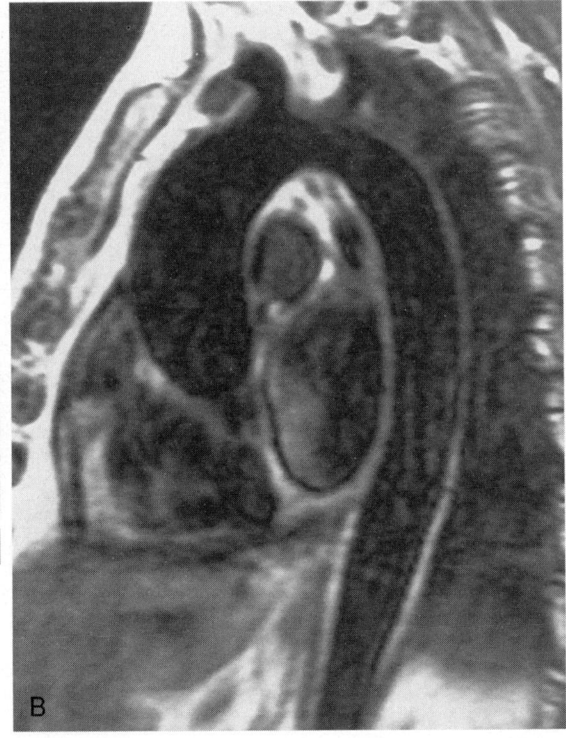

FIGURE 47–2. Left anterior oblique images through the thoracic aorta are obtained by scanning in a plane that bisects the ascending and descending aortas on a transaxial image (*A*). This view "unfolds" the thoracic aorta, resulting in images demonstrating the entire "question mark" configuration of the vessel (*B*).

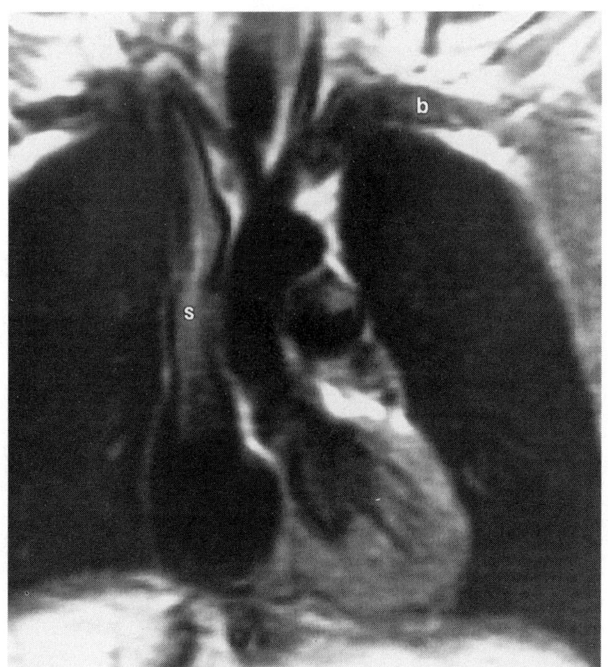

FIGURE 47–3. Electrocardiographically gated, 1-cm thick coronal image through the center of the heart. Note the intermediate signal within the superior vena cava (s) and the left brachycephalic vein (b) caused by slow in-plane blood flow.

being evaluated and on patient size. The authors recommend the use of a 128 by 256 matrix and 4 NEX. A slice thickness in children of 4 mm with a 1-mm gap and in adults of 8 mm with a 2-mm gap can usually answer most questions.

Although SE techniques can yield some indirect information regarding the pathophysiologic consequences of thoracic aortic anomalies and disease, dynamic MRI techniques have evolved for study of blood flow dynamics. Cine MRI refers to a gradient-refocused echo technique that acquires multiple phases of the cardiac cycle that can be played in a cine or movie format. The technique requires the use of low flip angles (30 to 60 degrees), short TEs (about 10 msec) and short TRs (20 to 50 msec).[8, 9] The low flip angle maintains SNR, and the short TE in the absence of a 180-degree pulse produces an image in which the blood pool is white instead of black, as it appears on SE images (Fig. 47–4).

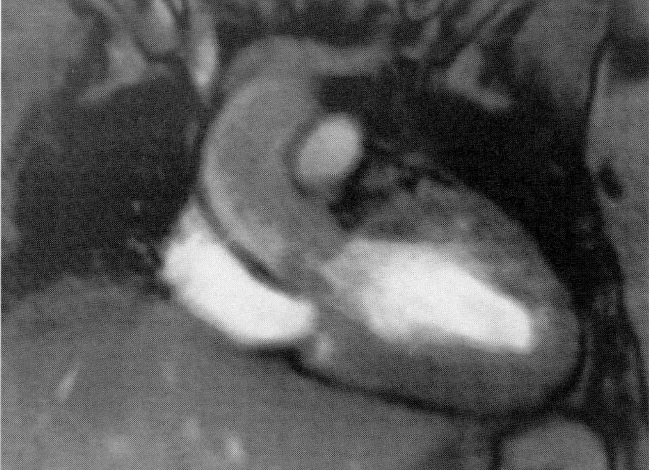

FIGURE 47–4. Electrocardiographically referenced coronal cine magnetic resonance imaging (MRI) through the center of the heart demonstrates the continuity of the aorta with the left ventricle. In contrast to spin-echo MRI, the blood pool is white on cine MRI.

Because the TR is so short, cine MRI is not gated. However, the QRS complex is used as a reference point from which acquisition information is reordered to produce the multiple images per heart cycle. Typically, 16 to 32 phases or frames are obtained during a cine MRI study, which takes about 3 minutes to obtain.

In addition to being able to image the blood pool (as with a catheter cine angiogram), cine MRI has the added advantage of being able to identify turbulent blood flow. Turbulent flow causes phase dispersion, which results in a signal void. This technique is therefore extremely accurate for detection of aortic valvular stenosis and regurgitation, subvalvular stenosis, and coarctation.[10–14]

The MRI signal has two components, a magnitude and a phase component. Standard MRI techniques make use of the magnitude component of the signal to produce images. The phase component of the MRI signal reflects the phase angle (and therefore the position) of a proton during the time course of the acquisition. The change in phase angle reflects proton motion over time, or a velocity.[15–20] These types of images are formed by mapping the change in phase angle on a voxel-by-voxel basis; hence the term phase- or velocity-mapping MRI. Stationary protons have a zero velocity or zero phase angle and are indicated by a signal assigned to the middle of a gray scale. Protons that move in one direction are indicated by an increasingly positive (white signal) phase angle, and those that move in an opposite direction by an increasing negative (black) phase angle, up to plus or minus 180 degrees[21] (Fig. 47–5). When studying normal blood flow states or a mild

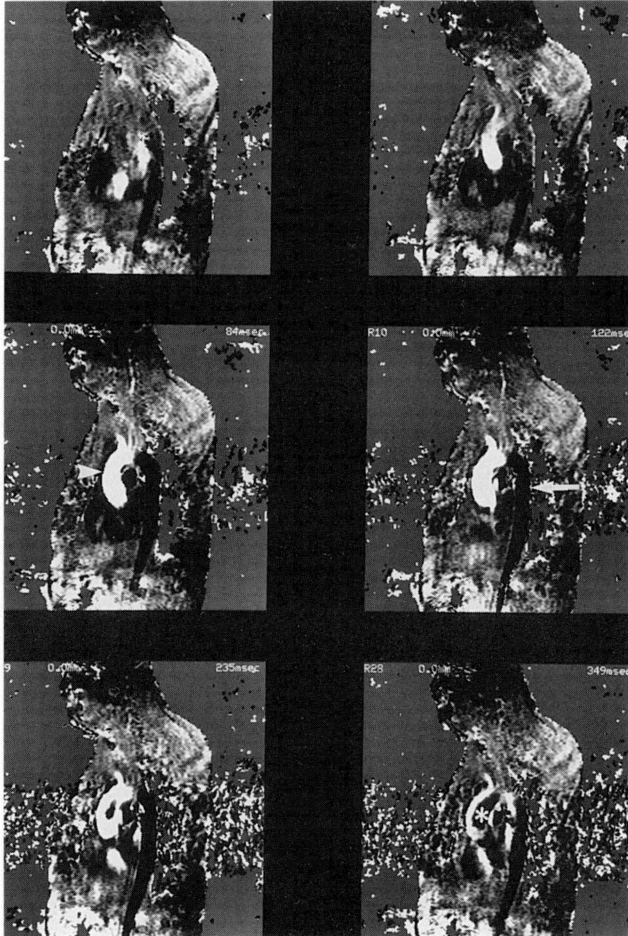

FIGURE 47–5. Electrocardiographically referenced left anterior oblique phase mapping study of the thoracic aorta. Stationary tissue is gray. Superior flow *(arrowhead)* is assigned an increasingly white signal, depending on its velocity. Inferior flow *(arrow)* is assigned an increasingly black signal, depending on its velocity. Note the normal retrograde posterolateral flow in the ascending aorta *(asterisk)*, which occurs during diastole. It is this flow that fills the sinuses of Valsalva and hence the coronary arteries.

stenosis, we use a velocity-encoded value of 200 cm/sec. With moderate to severe stenosis, we use 400 cm per second.[18, 22]

Phase-mapping techniques prove useful in cases in which there is a question of slow flow versus thrombosis, such as in the evaluation of aortic dissections and aortic aneurysms. The technique is also useful in evaluation of obstructive processes such as aortic stenosis, coarctation, and surgical anastomotic stenosis.[23] With a known blood velocity distal to an obstructive lesion, the pressure gradient across the lesion can be generated by use of a modified Bernoulli equation ($\Delta P = 4V^2$, where V is the velocity in meters per second).[24]

CONGENITAL ANOMALIES

There are a variety of congenital anomalies that involve the thoracic aorta. Those that result from maldevelopment of the conotruncus (i.e., persistent truncus arteriosus, transposition of the great arteries, and tetralogy of Fallot) are almost always present in conjunction with intracardiac defects. These anomalies are best viewed as congenital heart defects and are not discussed further here (see Chapter 46). The most common anomalies are discussed here with the Edwards hypothetical double aortic arch model used as an aid in understanding.[4]

Left Aortic Arch

The normal left aortic arch forms as a result of a break in the Edwards hypothetical double aortic arch distal to the right subclavian artery. The distal aspect of the right dorsal arch regresses. On occasion, it does not regress completely and forms an aortic diverticulum along the right lateral aspect of the descending aorta at its junction with the transverse arch. The proximal half of the right aortic arch migrates inferiorly to join the ascending aorta. In the process, the ostia of the right subclavian and common carotid arteries fuse to form the innominate artery. The left arch remains intact, with separate ostia for the left common carotid and left subclavian arteries. The right ductus is almost always obliterated, but the left ductus remains patent, supplying blood to the descending aorta.[4, 25]

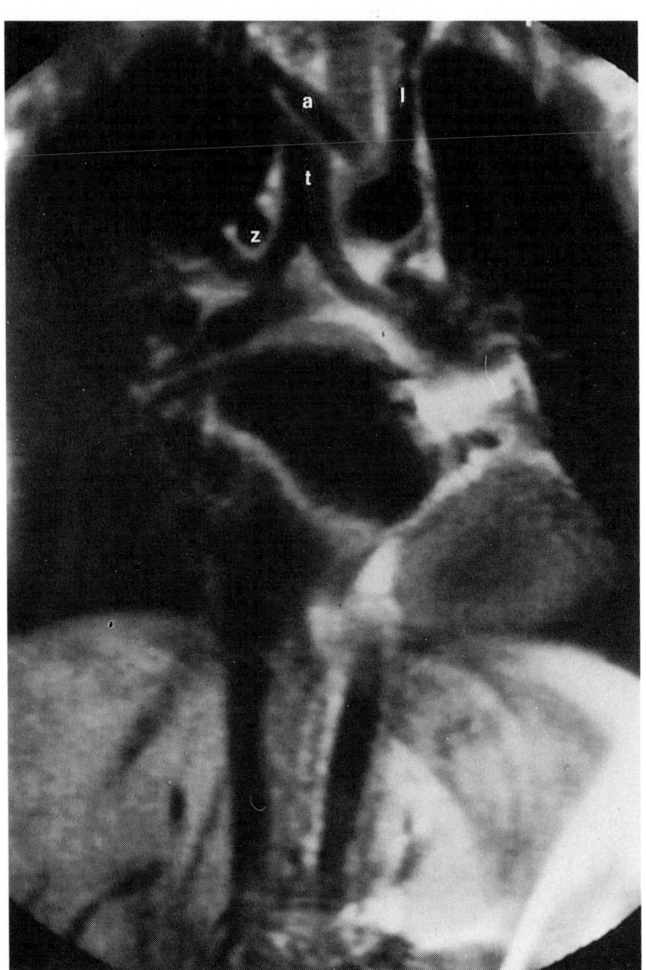

FIGURE 47–6. Electrocardiographically gated spin-echo coronal magnetic resonance image demonstrates an aberrant right subclavian artery (a). l = left subclavian artery; t = trachea; z = azygous vein. This study nicely demonstrates a situs solitus branching of the bronchial tree.

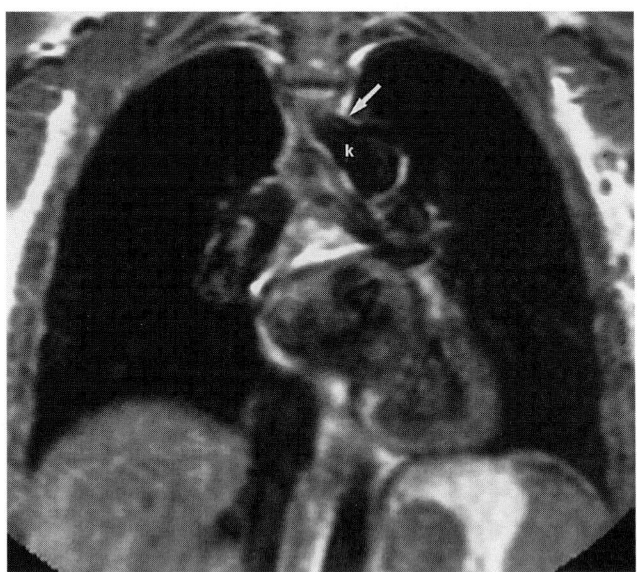

FIGURE 47–7. Electrocardiographically gated spin-echo coronal magnetic resonance image demonstrates an aberrant right subclavian artery *(arrow)* arising from a diverticulum of Kommerell (k).

The most common thoracic aortic arch anomaly, occurring in approximately 0.5 percent of the population, is the left aortic arch with an aberrant right subclavian artery. It results from a break in the hypothetical double aortic arch between the right common carotid artery and the right subclavian artery. The right ductus is obliterated. The right subclavian artery is incorporated into the descending aorta at its junction with the transverse arch. The right subclavian can arise directly from the descending aorta (Fig. 47–6), or it can arise from an aortic diverticulum (the diverticulum of Kommerell; Fig. 47–7). The aberrant right subclavian artery courses posterior to the esophagus, but, because a vascular ring is not intact, there is no associated dyspnea or dysphagia.[4] Identification of an aberrant right subclavian artery is usually an incidental finding on MRI evaluation of the thoracic spine or the chest. If there is a clinical suspicion that needs to be confirmed, MRI is the imaging modality of choice. Thin-section (4-mm-thick slices with a 1-mm gap) SE transaxial images through the arch and proximal descending aorta demonstrate the origin and proximal aspect of the aberrant vessel as it passes posterior to the esophagus. Thin-section coronal SE MRI through the junction of the transverse and descending aortas demonstrates the origin and superior diagonal course of the aberrant vessel. Usually, the presence of a diverticulum of Kommerell can be determined with the use of the body coil. On occasion, a dedicated surface coil is required. In cases of coarctation with an associated aberrant subclavian artery, the location of the subclavian ostium relative to the coarctation site is best demonstrated with coronal or LAO SE MRI. In cases of juxtaductal coarctation, it may be difficult to determine whether the aberrant subclavian artery serves as a collateral vessel. In these cases, phase-mapping MRI can demonstrate the direction of blood flow within the aberrant artery.[26–30]

There is an increased incidence of an aberrant right subclavian artery with tetralogy of Fallot and coarctation. With regard to the latter, if the aberrant artery arises distal to the coarctation, it serves as a major collateral vessel. In this situation, rib notching, if present, involves only the left hemithorax.[4]

Right Aortic Arch

The right aortic arch passes to the right of the trachea and can descend either to the right or left of the thoracic spine. If the arch descends to the right of the spine, it usually recrosses the midline at the level of the diaphragm so as to be to the left of the lumbar spine. In almost all cases, there is obliteration of the right ductus arteriosus.[4]

The mirror-image right aortic arch is formed by a break in the left dorsal arch distal to the ductus arteriosus. The first artery to arise from the transverse arch is the left innominate artery. It is, in turn, followed by the right common carotid artery and then the right subclavian artery. The arch passes to the right of the trachea and descends on the right side of the spine. The left ductus arteriosus usually arises from the left subclavian artery, and there is no vascular ring. In rare cases, the break occurs between the left subclavian artery and left ductus arteriosus. In these instances, the ductus arises from an aortic diverticulum and passes posterior to the trachea and esophagus, thereby forming a vascular ring. Almost all cases of mirror-image right aortic arch occur in conjunction with cyanotic congenital heart disease (Fig. 47–8), most notably tetralogy of Fallot (about 25 percent of cases) and persistent truncus arteriosus (35 to 50 percent of cases). Because tetralogy of Fallot is a much more common congenital defect than persistent truncus arteriosus (10 to 12 percent versus 1.5 to 2 percent of congenital heart disease), the mirror-image right aortic arch is more commonly seen in association with tetralogy of Fallot.[4]

The most common type of right aortic arch anomaly is the right arch with an aberrant left subclavian artery, which occurs in approximately 0.1 percent of the population. There is only a slightly higher than normal (about 5 percent) incidence of associated congenital heart disease. The anomaly results from a break in the left dorsal arch between the left common carotid and left subclavian arteries. The left common carotid artery arises first from the arch and is followed by the right common carotid artery and then the right subclavian artery. The aberrant left subclavian artery arises from the proximal descending aorta at its junction with the transverse arch.[4]

Two types of right aortic arch with an aberrant left subclavian artery exist. In the more common type, the arch passes to the right of the trachea and descends on the right side of the thoracic spine. The left subclavian arises from the proximal descending aorta, and the left ductus arteriosus arises from the left subclavian artery, thereby creating a vascular ring (Fig. 47–9). With the other variety, the arch passes to the right of the trachea and turns to the left to pass behind the esophagus before descending to the left of the spine. The left subclavian artery and left ductus arteriosus usually arise from an aortic diverticulum, completing the vascular ring. This variety is also known as a "right circumflex retroesophageal arch"[4] (Fig. 47–10).

Right aortic arches are best evaluated with transaxial and coronal SE MRI. In mirror-image right aortic arches, these views also serve to assess the heart for the associated intracardiac defects. Phase mapping can be used to assess the degree of infundibular stenosis and to detect collateral vessels to the pulmonary arteries. Aberrant left subclavian arteries are evaluated in essentially the same manner as aberrant right subclavian arteries.[29, 31–34]

Double Aortic Arch

As its name implies, this thoracic aortic anomaly results from a persistent hypothetical double aortic arch model. The ascending aorta lies anterior to the trachea. It divides into two arches, which pass on either side of the trachea before fusing posterior to the esophagus to form the descending aorta. The descending aorta typically courses to the left of the spine. The right aortic arch is

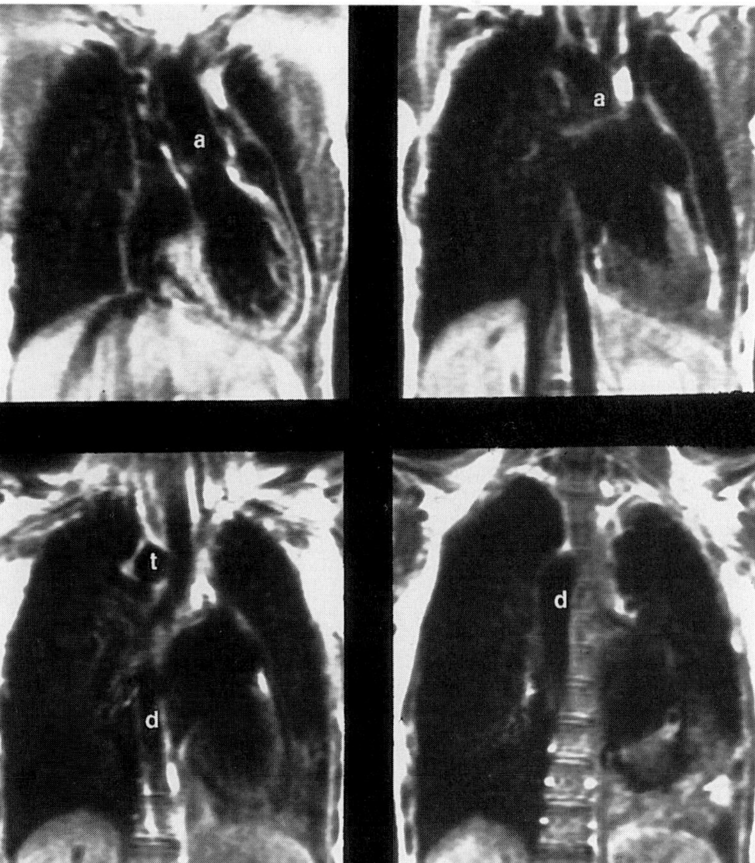

FIGURE 47–8. Sequential coronal electrocardiographically gated spin-echo magnetic resonance images in a patient with a mirror-image right aortic arch and double-outlet right ventricle. a = ascending aorta; t = transverse aorta; d = descending aorta.

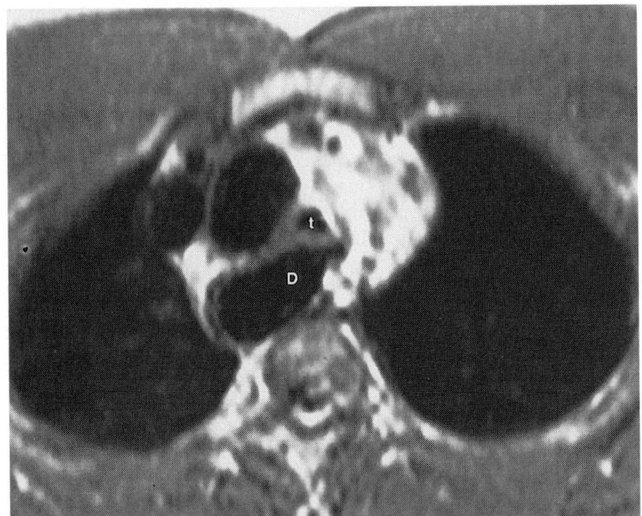

FIGURE 47–9. Transaxial electrocardiographically gated spin-echo magnetic resonance image through the junction of the transverse and descending aortas, demonstrating a right arch with an aberrant left subclavian artery arising from an aortic diverticulum (D). t = trachea.

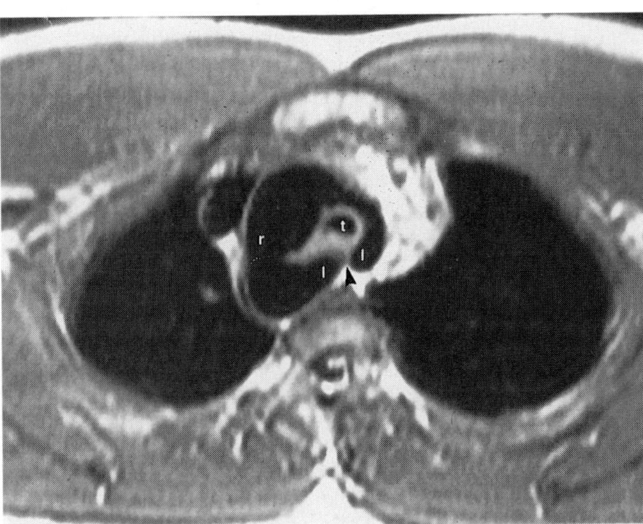

FIGURE 47–11. Transaxial electrocardiographically gated spin-echo magnetic resonance image through the inverted "U" of a type II double aortic arch. r = dominant right arch; l = left arch, interrupted by a focal atretic segment *(arrowhead)*; t = trachea.

usually the more dominant of the two arches. It is larger in caliber and more cephalad in position. A separate common carotid artery, subclavian artery, and ductus arteriosus arise from each arch. The right ductus is almost always obliterated. This configuration usually results in a tight vascular ring that almost always requires surgical intervention to alleviate symptoms of dyspnea and dysphagia.[4]

There are two varieties of double aortic arch. Type I, the most common type, has two patent aortic arches. In type II, the right arch is patent, but a portion of the left arch is atretic. It is uncommon for either type of double aortic arch to be found in conjunction with an intracardial defect.[4] Although the right aortic arch with an aberrant left subclavian artery is the most common cause of a vascular ring, the anatomical configuration typically results in a loose ring and rarely requires surgical intervention. Although much less common, the double aortic arch results in a tight ring that almost always necessitates surgical transection.

Double aortic arches are best studied with coronal and transaxial SE MRI and transaxial phase-mapping MRI. The coronal views demonstrate the larger-caliber dominant right aortic arch and its more cephalad location relative to the nondominant left aortic arch. The amount of esophageal and tracheal constriction caused by the vascular ring is graphically demonstrated by transaxial cine MRI at the level of the inverted "U" configuration of the double aortic arch[27, 32–34] (Fig. 47–11).

Coarctation

Coarctation is a common congenital anomaly that results from an abnormality in the aortic media.[35] Coarctation refers to a discrete infolding of the posterolateral wall of the aorta in the region of the ligamentum or ductus arteriosus. This is usually a discrete phenomenon that occurs just distal to the ductus; hence the term postductal coarctation. Because this form usually does not cause symptoms in the neonatal period, it is also referred to as adult coarctation.

The coarctation can occur proximal to the ductus and present itself shortly after birth. This variety has been termed preductal or infantile coarctation. It is less common than adult coarctation and is usually associated with hypoplasia of the arch between the left subclavian artery and the ductus of the aortic isthmus. In utero, during systole, blood from the ascending aorta passes preferentially into the branch arteries. Blood also passes from the left pulmonary artery into the descending aorta through the ductus arteriosus, and there is also reflux of blood into the isthmus. Because the coarctation is located proximal to the ductus, there is no reflux of blood into the segment of the aorta between the ductus and the left subclavian arteries. Hence, the aortic isthmus does not experience the necessary volume load needed for normal development. On the other hand, with the postductal variety, the coarctation forces

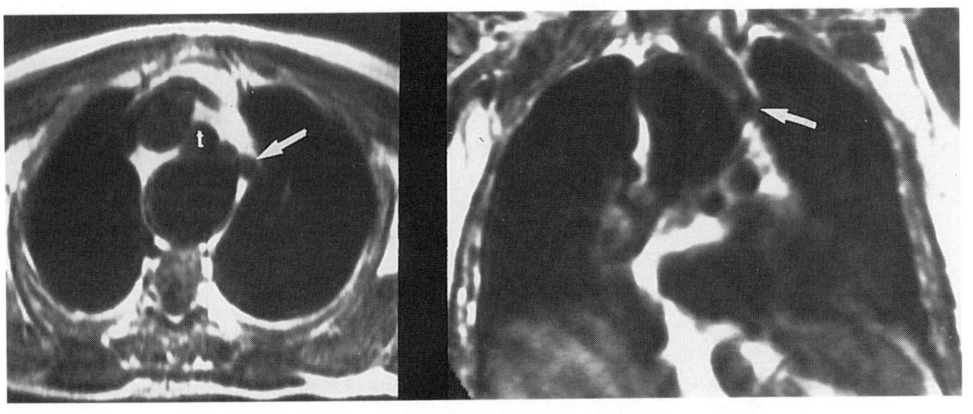

FIGURE 47–10. Transaxial and coronal electrocardiographically gated spin-echo magnetic resonance images demonstrate a right circumflex retroesophageal arch with an aberrant left subclavian artery *(arrow)*. The aorta crosses behind the esophagus and trachea (t).

blood from the ductus proximally into the distal arch and there is no hypoplasia. Occasionally, the coarctation site is found proximal to the left subclavian artery.[4]

With both forms, there is usually dilatation of the descending aorta distal to the coarctation. As a result of the obstruction caused by the coarctation, collateral vessels develop to increase flow into the descending aorta (Fig. 47–12). The intercostal arteries serve as a major source of collateral flow. The increased flow through these vessels results in their dilatation. This, in turn, can result in notching along the inferior aspect of the ribs, which usually takes 8 to 10 years to become significant enough to be observed on a chest radiograph. If there is an aberrant right subclavian artery that originates distal to the coarctation, it serves as a major collateral vessel, and rib notching only occurs on the left. If the left subclavian artery arises distal to the coarctation, it serves as a major collateral, and unilateral rib notching occurs on the right.[32]

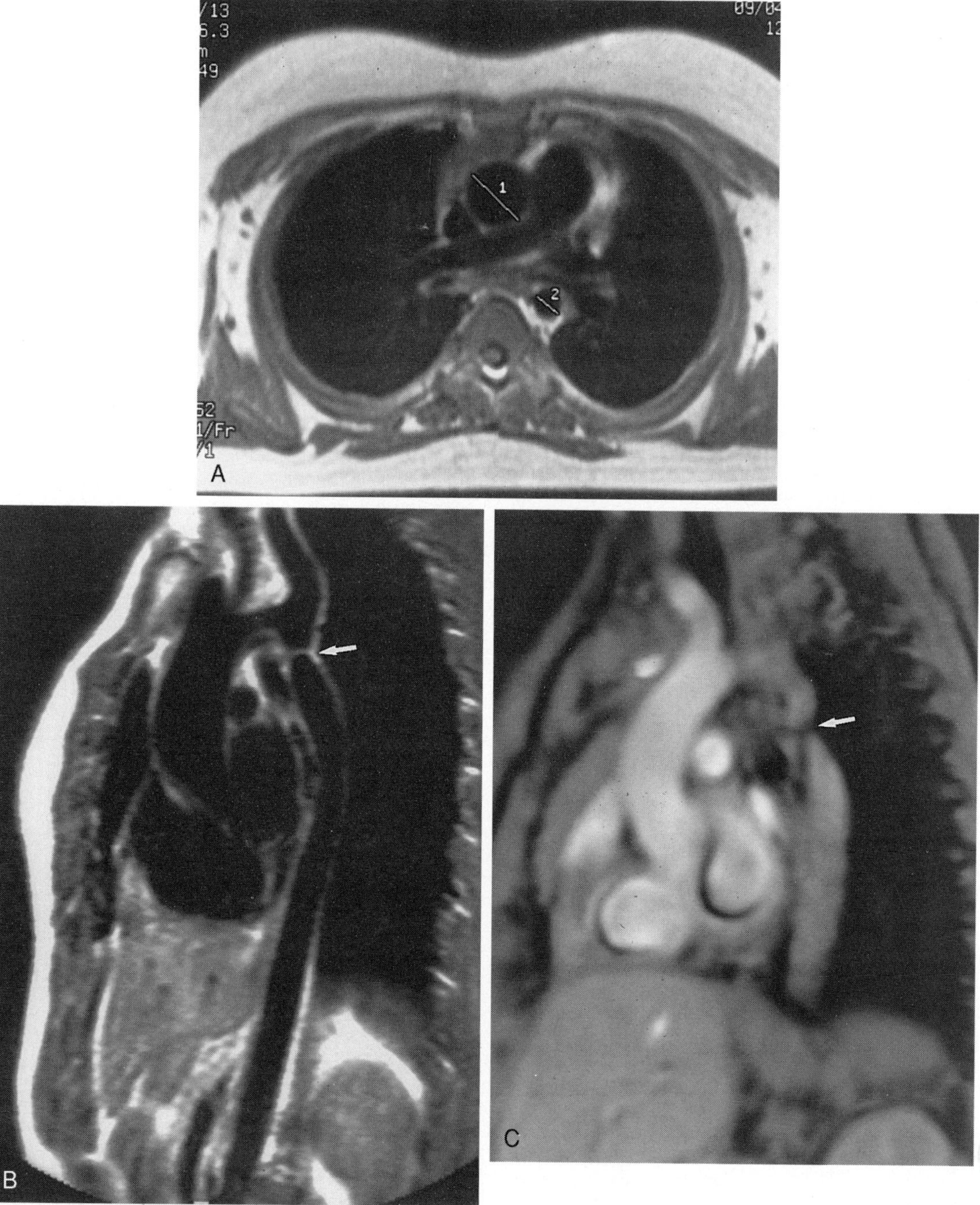

FIGURE 47–12. Postductal coarctation. Although the electrocardiographically gated spin-echo (SE) magnetic resonance image (MRI) demonstrates the marked decrease in diameter of the descending aorta (*A*), it is the left anterior oblique SE MRI that dramatically shows the actual coarctation membrane (*B*). The significance of the coarctation can be assessed with the magnitude component of a phase map study (*C*). 1 = ascending aorta; 2 = descending aorta; *arrow* = coarctation site.

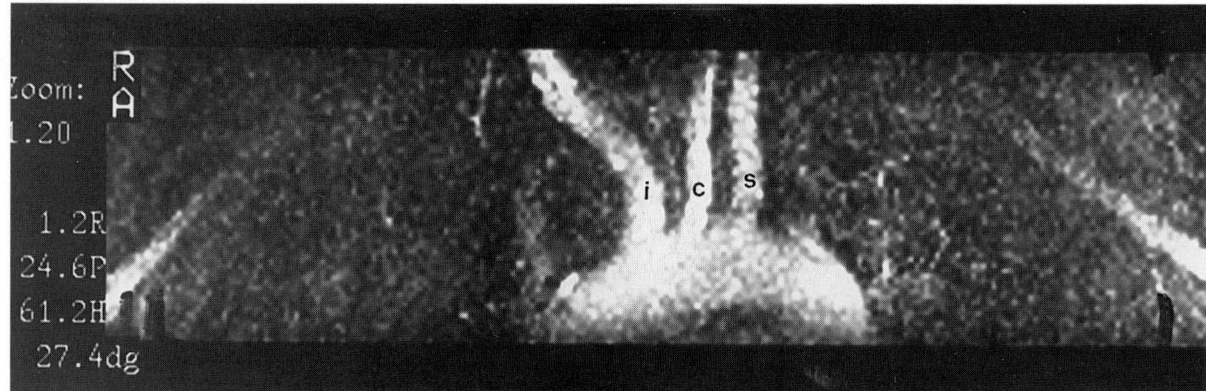

FIGURE 47–13. Three-dimensional time-of-flight magnetic resonance angiography of the transverse aorta demonstrates the proximal aspect of the innominate (i), the left common carotid (c), and the left subclavian (s) arteries.

With its multiplanar imaging, large FOV, and dynamic quantitative flow imaging, MRI is arguably the imaging modality of choice for evaluation of coarctation. The coarctation is most graphically demonstrated in the LAO plane centered on the middle of the ascending and descending aortas. MRI also demonstrates associated aortic stenosis, left ventricular hypertrophy, and ventricular septal defects, as well as their severity. This is important because there is a high association of bicuspid aortic valve and ventricular septal defects with coarctation.[27, 29, 32, 34, 36–38] The isthmus can be narrowed without any associated obstruction to blood flow. This entity is known as pseudocoarctation. In addition, there is usually elongation of the arch, which results in redundancy and kinking of the aorta. These features, as well as associated ventricular septal defects and bicuspid aortic valve, are easily diagnosed with coronal and LAO static and dynamic MRI.[39]

ACQUIRED DISEASES

MRI is effective for study of acquired diseases of the thoracic aorta. In fact, evaluation of the thoracic aorta for acquired diseases is the leading indication for cardiovascular MRI.[40] The large FOV, multiplanar imaging capability, and excellent contrast resolution, coupled with static anatomical and dynamic physiologic imaging techniques possible with this modality, provide for a complete evaluation of acquired aortic diseases. As clinical experience has increased, there is good evidence to suggest that MRI is the imaging modality of choice in hemodynamically stable patients with suspected or known thoracic aortic disease.[24] Although each study must be individualized, most examinations consist of a series of transaxial, coronal, and LAO SE images through the thoracic aorta. Depending on the results of these images and the question at hand, dynamic, preferably phase-mapping, MRI is performed, typically in the LAO and coronal planes. Phase mapping is preferable to cine MRI, especially in cases of aortic dissection, because it can better differentiate slow flow from thrombus.[9]

Magnetic resonance angiography may on occasion be useful in assessment of the branch vessels (Fig. 47–13). Usually, properly performed phase-mapping MRI is all that is needed to assess involvement of the branch vessels. Breath-hold fast dynamic imaging techniques have recently been introduced. These sequences depend on the acquisition of several lines of K-space per cardiac cycle, unlike the present ECG-referenced dynamic techniques, which collect a single line of K-space per cardiac cycle. The fast techniques suffer from a decreased temporal resolution, compared with standard dynamic imaging. Initial work with the fast techniques is encouraging, and, eventually, the standard examination may consist solely of these rapid acquisition sequences[41, 42] (Fig. 47–14).

Aortic Dissection

Dissection of the aortic wall is the result of repeated trauma to the media, most often from persistent hypertension. Untreated hypertension leads to the formation of an intramural hematoma, localized to the media (Fig. 47–15). The hematoma eventually

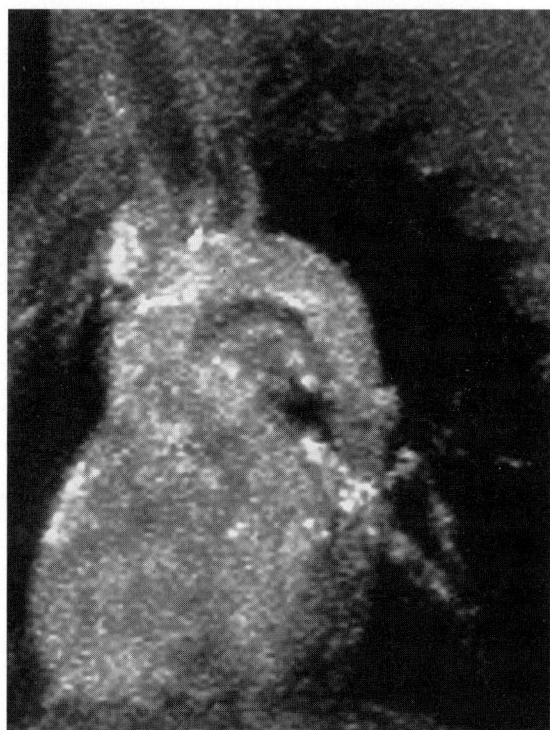

FIGURE 47–14. Left anterior oblique two-dimensional breath-hold fast magnetic resonance study of the thoracic aorta.

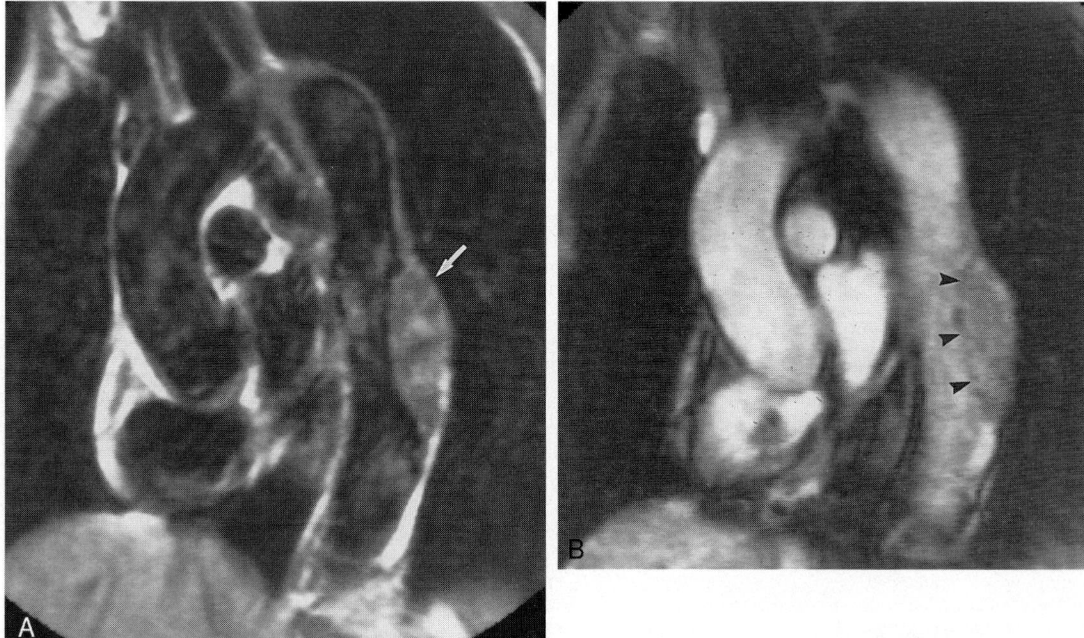

FIGURE 47–15. Intramural hematoma or nondissecting dissection. *A*, Left anterior oblique (LAO) spin-echo magnetic resonance image (MRI) demonstrates an elliptical intramural hematoma *(arrow)*. *B*, Cine LAO MRI of same patient. The intima is the dark line *(arrowheads)* between the hematoma and the aortic lumen.

forms a seroma; when this occurs, there is little structural support for the overlying intima. If the hypertension goes untreated, a rent or tear can form in the intima, with the subsequent development and propagation of a false lumen tracking along the media. There can be retrograde extension in addition to the typical antegrade involvement of the false lumen. Dissections commonly develop in aortas with underlying pathology, especially of the media, as in patients with Marfan syndrome or annuloaortic ectasia.[43]

If left untreated, aortic dissection can be rapidly fatal. Early surgical experiences demonstrated poor results with those dissections involving only the descending aorta. However, they do respond well to antihypertensive medication. Therefore, it is important to both detect and assess the degree of involvement as rapidly as possible. Dissection can be classified according to the DeBakey or Stanford classifications. Both schemes recognize the need to differentiate between involvement of the ascending aorta and involvement of only the descending aorta. Involvement of the ascending aorta constitutes a surgical emergency. Involvement localized to the descending aorta is best treated medically. A DeBakey type I dissection involves the ascending aorta, the aortic arch, and the descending aorta (Fig. 47–16). Type II dissections are confined to the ascending aorta (Fig. 47–17). Type III dissections begin distal to the left subclavian artery (Fig. 47–18). Both types I and III can extend for variable distances.[44, 45] The Stanford type A dissection involves the ascending aorta, regardless of its degree of extension; a type B dissection is confined to the descending aorta.[46]

Dissections can also be classified according to the nature of the false lumen. In 90 percent of cases, there is both an entrance and an exit site to the false lumen. This is referred to as a complete dissection (see Fig. 47–16*C*). In 10 percent of cases, there is an entrance site but no exit site; hence the term, "incomplete" dissection. A nondissecting dissection is a dissection without an entrance or exit site (see Fig. 47–15). This is usually considered to be an intramural hematoma or the precursor to the formation of a dissection.[47] The ascending aorta is involved in approximately 60 percent of dissections, and the descending aorta in 40 percent.[48]

In addition to identifying and classifying an aortic dissection, it is imperative to identify complications. With dissections involving the ascending aorta, complications can include aortic valve insufficiency, aortic rupture with development of hemopericardium and cardiac tamponade, and involvement of the branch vessels of the arch. Dissections limited to the descending aorta can form aneurysms of the false lumen, and they can rupture, form periaortic hematomas, and involve the abdominal branch vessels.[48]

Magnetic resonance imaging is quickly assuming the role of primary imaging modality for patients with suspected or known aortic dissection. Reported MRI accuracies vary from 90 to 100 percent.[49–52] Direct and indirect signs of aortic dissection are similar to those seen with angiography, echocardiography, and CT. Pathognomonic findings include a double lumen and the presence of an intimal flap. Indirect evidence may include compression of the true lumen, thickening of the aortic wall, branch vessel abnormalities, aortic insufficiency, or an ulcer-like projection beyond the aortic wall.[49]

MRI provides excellent contrast resolution and tissue differentiation for the aortic lumen, vessel wall, and adjacent soft tissues. Flowing blood has little or no signal intensity on SE MRI but high signal intensity with cine and phase-mapping sequences. However, slowly moving blood and turbulent flow may cause signal loss on cine studies and increased signal intensity on SE images. Spin echo MRI provides graphic images of the pathoanatomy. Dynamic techniques are mandatory for assessment of the aortic valve, for evaluation of the significance of pericardial fluid collections on cardiac function, and for a more precise determination of regions of suspected thrombosis. Generally speaking, if there is a patent false lumen, blood flow is fast enough to outline the intimal flap and false lumens with both SE and dynamic imaging techniques. However, if there is very slow flow in the false lumen, it can be

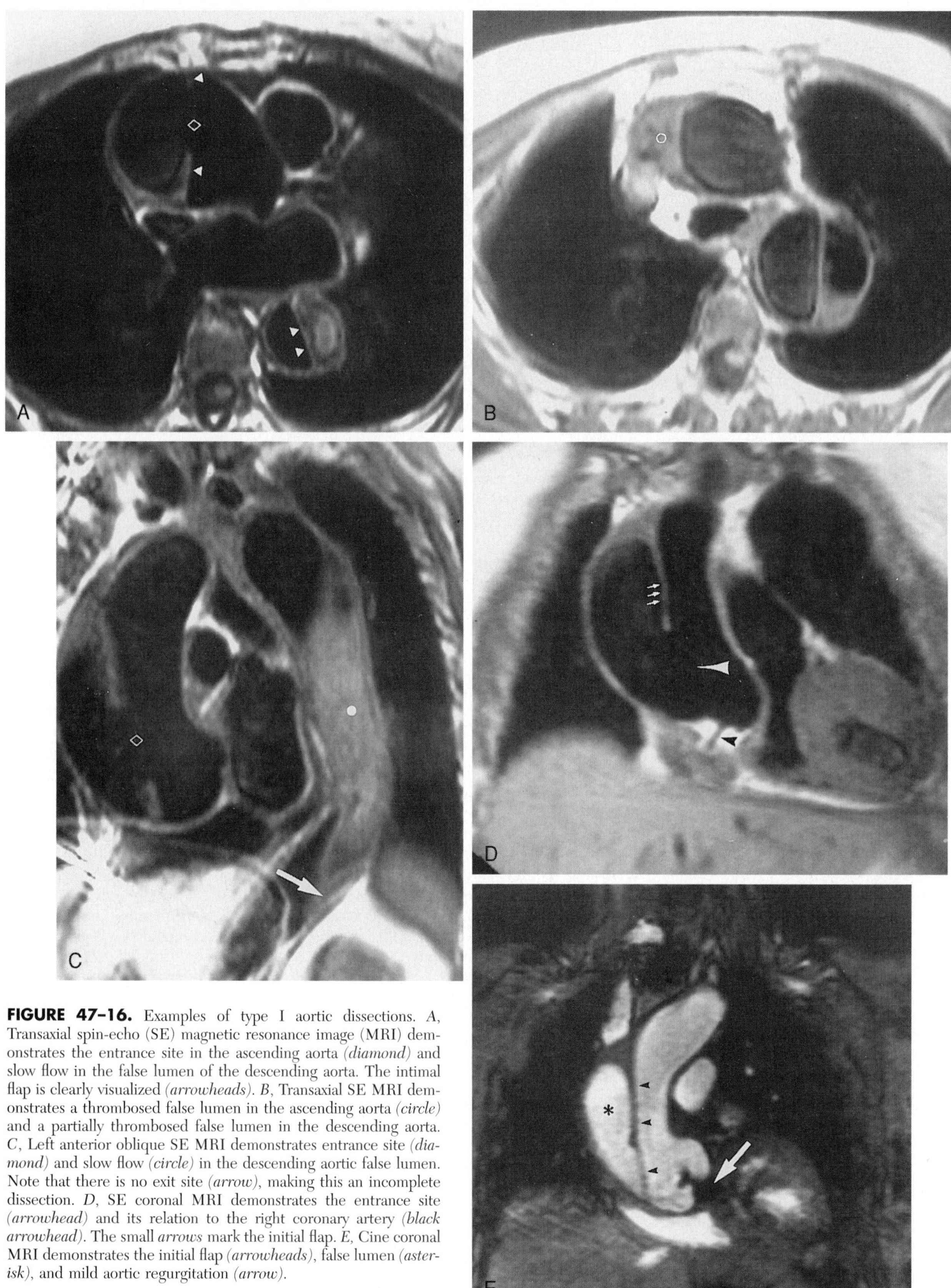

FIGURE 47–16. Examples of type I aortic dissections. *A*, Transaxial spin-echo (SE) magnetic resonance image (MRI) demonstrates the entrance site in the ascending aorta *(diamond)* and slow flow in the false lumen of the descending aorta. The intimal flap is clearly visualized *(arrowheads)*. *B*, Transaxial SE MRI demonstrates a thrombosed false lumen in the ascending aorta *(circle)* and a partially thrombosed false lumen in the descending aorta. *C*, Left anterior oblique SE MRI demonstrates entrance site *(diamond)* and slow flow *(circle)* in the descending aortic false lumen. Note that there is no exit site *(arrow)*, making this an incomplete dissection. *D*, SE coronal MRI demonstrates the entrance site *(arrowhead)* and its relation to the right coronary artery *(black arrowhead)*. The small *arrows* mark the initial flap. *E*, Cine coronal MRI demonstrates the initial flap *(arrowheads)*, false lumen *(asterisk)*, and mild aortic regurgitation *(arrow)*.

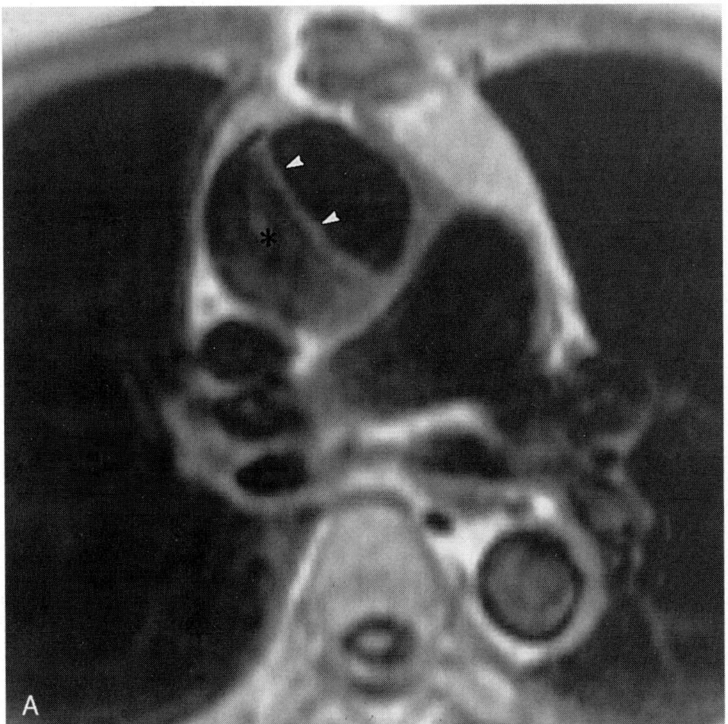

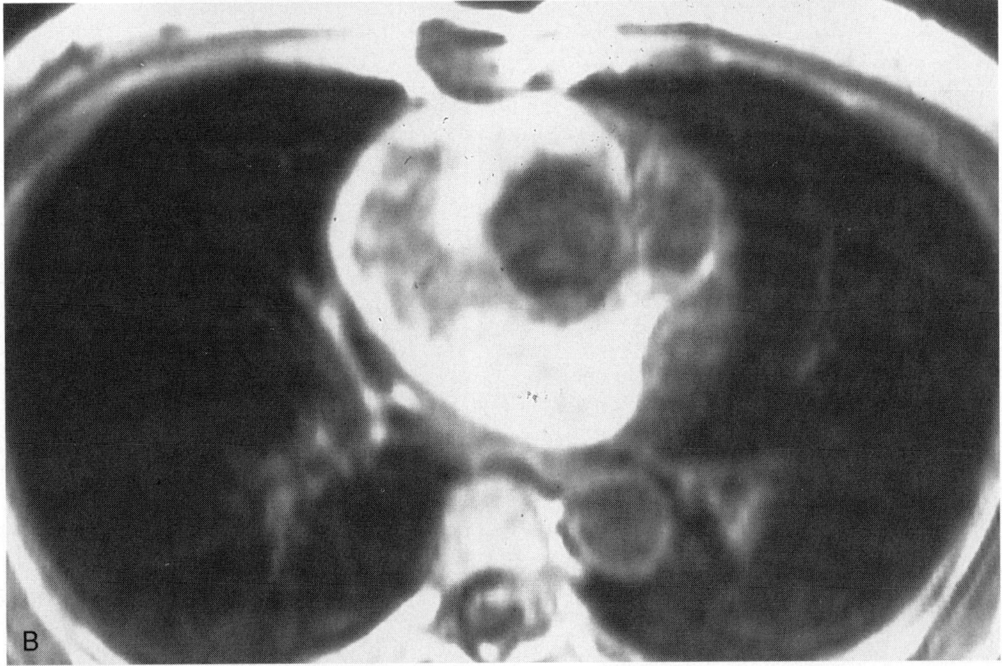

FIGURE 47–17. Type II aortic dissections. *A*, Spin-echo (SE) transaxial magnetic resonance image (MRI) demonstrates the intimal flap *(arrowheads)* and slow flow in the false lumen *(asterisk)*. *B*, SE transaxial MRI demonstrates a large, thrombosed false lumen. The different signal intensities represent various ages of thrombosis.

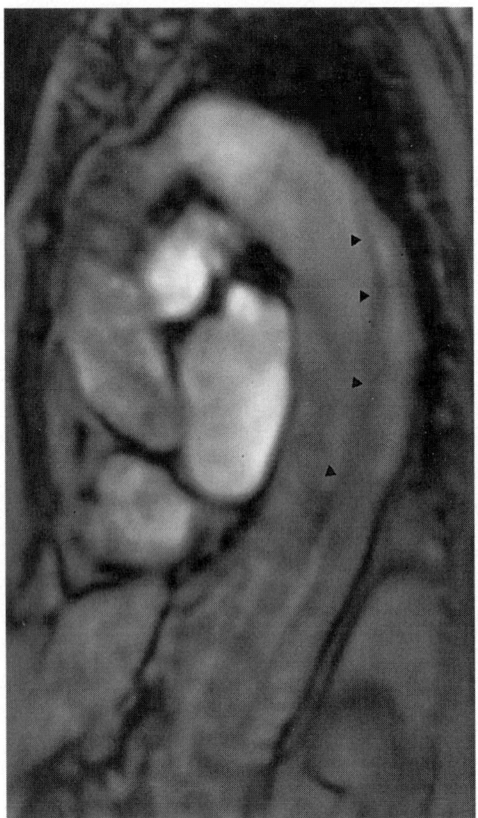

FIGURE 47–18. Cine left anterior oblique magnetic resonance image demonstrates the intimal flap *(arrowheads)* in this type III dissection.

difficult to distinguish from partial thrombosis. In these cases, phase-mapping techniques can play an important role (Fig. 47–19). However, a thrombosed dissection flap can be difficult to distinguish from thrombosis in the aorta or in an aneurysm, whether with SE, cine, or phase-mapping imaging.[53–55]

Another important attribute is MRI's ability to evaluate the thoracic aorta in its entirety, like to an angiogram, in the LAO imaging plane. This view is also used to study the ostia of the branch vessels of the arch. The coronal plane is better for assessment of aortic valve competency.

With the rapid advancement of imaging modalities, it is difficult to assess the role of each in the evaluation of patients with suspected aortic dissection, especially in light of the near-perfect published diagnostic accuracies by proponents of each modality. As a result, the workup of patients varies from institution to institution. Nienaber and colleagues[56] evaluated 110 patients with suspected aortic dissections by MRI, CT, transthoracic echocardiography (TTE), and transesophageal echocardiography (TEE). Comparison was with angiography (n = 64), surgical findings (n = 62), and autopsy findings (n = 7). The sensitivities and specificities were as follows: MRI, 98.3 and 97.8 percent; TEE, 97.7 and 77 percent; CT, 93.8 and 87.1 percent; and TTE, 59.3 and 83.0 percent. The authors concluded that MRI is the test of choice in hemodynamically stable patients and TEE in unstable patients suspected of having an aortic dissection.

Magnetic resonance imaging is very useful for following patients under medical management or after surgical intervention.[57, 58] With regard to the latter, it is important to know which surgical interventions took place (e.g., valve replacement, conduit placement). In most patients who have had surgery for a dissection involving the ascending and descending aorta, there continues to be a false lumen in the descending aorta. Competency of the aortic valve or replacement valve, integrity of a surgical graft, periaortic or perigraft hematoma or infection, cardiac tamponade, and aneurysm

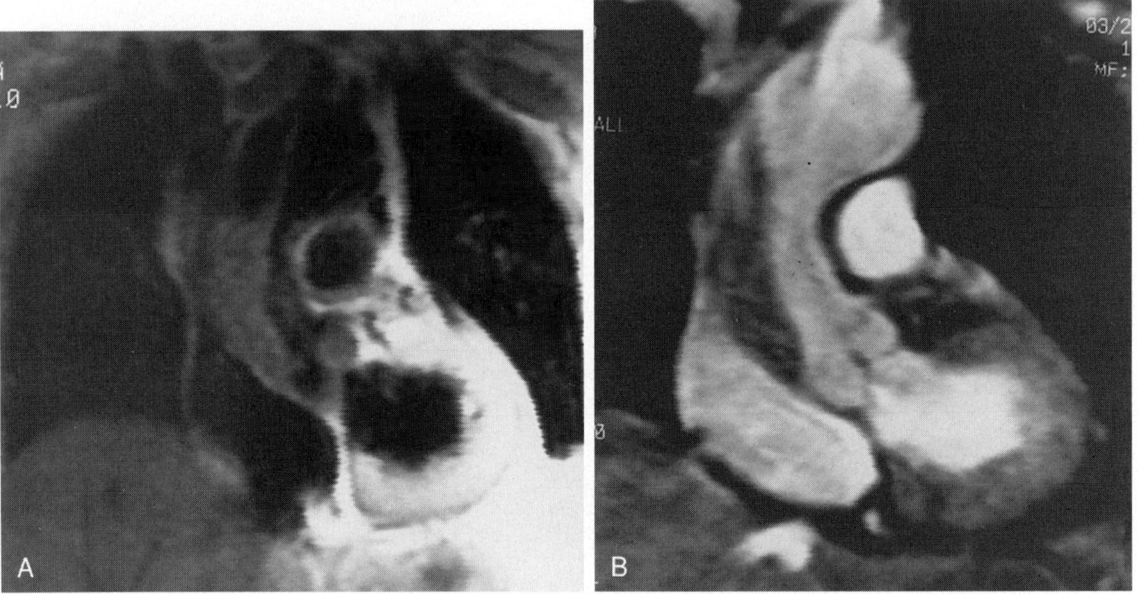

FIGURE 47–19. Partially thrombosed false lumen. Spin-echo (SE) coronal magnetic resonance image demonstrates a type I dissection. The false lumen may be thrombosed or have slow flow *(A)*. The phase map *(B)* demonstrates that the intermediate signal on the SE image within the false lumen is caused by a large thrombus.

formation in residual false lumen are some of the postoperative concerns that are easily answered with SE and dynamic MRI.

Thoracic Aortic Aneurysm

Limited dilatation of a blood vessel can be of two types: true aneurysm and false aneurysm. True aneurysms involve all layers of the aortic wall and result from the degeneration of the elastin fibers within the media. As its name implies, false aneurysms, or pseudoaneurysms, are not true aneurysms. With pseudoaneurysms, there is a contained perforation of the vessel wall. There is penetration of the intima and media. The adventitia and perivascular connective tissue contain the process, thereby preventing exsanguination. Pseudoaneurysms, therefore, have a narrow "neck" leading to the "aneurysm" (Fig. 47–20). These "structures" represent the point of penetration and the area of containment, respectively.[59]

Seventy percent of the aneurysms located in the thoracic aorta are caused by atherosclerosis. Almost all true aneurysms are the result of the atherosclerotic process of infiltration and damage to the aortic media. Pseudoaneurysms are typically some type of focal penetration of the intima and media, such as may be caused by trauma (20 to 25 percent of thoracic aneurysms) or infection (about 5 percent of thoracic aneurysms). The overwhelming number of aneurysms are caused by atherosclerosis, and this process can result in the formation of pseudoaneurysms if a true aneurysm ruptures and is contained by the adventitia and periaortic tissues.[59] It is important to characterize the lesion in order to establish its cause, the patient's prognosis, and the need for surgery. Important to this end is establishment of an aneurysm's location, extent, and shape, its relation to branch vessels and adjacent structures, and its associated complicating factors, such as rupture, periaortic hematoma or infection, hemopericardium, or aortic valve insufficiency.

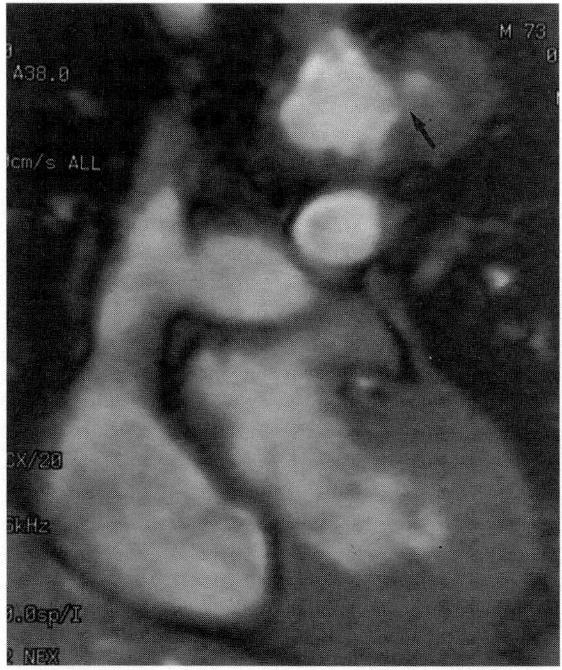

FIGURE 47–20. Cine magnetic resonance image demonstrates a contained pseudoaneurysm arising from the transverse portion of the aortic arch *(arrow)*. The isointense signal represents the periaortic hematoma that contained the pseudoaneurysm.

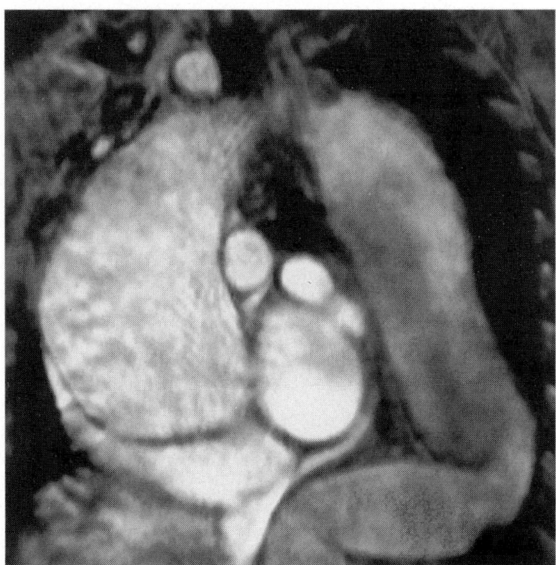

FIGURE 47–21. Left anterior oblique cine magnetic resonance image demonstrates the various findings of atherosclerotic disease of the thoracic aorta. These include tortuosity and kinking of the aorta, diffuse fusiform dilatation, and saccular dilatation of the ascending aorta.

Thoracic aortic aneurysms are common, occurring in about 10 percent of autopsies. Aneurysms have been classified according to their shape as either fusiform, saccular, or cylindroid (Fig. 47–21). Atherosclerotic aneurysms are usually fusiform, involving long segments of the aorta. It is not uncommon to find normal-appearing aorta between two fusiform aneurysms. Saccular aneurysms are less common, but, like fusiform aneurysms, they are most often the result of atherosclerosis. Infection, trauma, and degenerative disease also result in saccular aneurysms.[59]

The location of an aneurysm is another aid in establishing etiology, prognosis, and the need for surgery. Atherosclerosis rarely involves only the ascending aorta. It is a diffuse process that tends to involve the arch and descending aorta whenever the ascending aorta is involved, even if normal aorta is interposed. Aneurysms involving solely the ascending aorta tend to be saccular in shape. Most often they are caused by annuloaortic ectasia (Fig. 47–22), Marfan syndrome (Fig. 47–23), syphilis, or poststenotic dilatation resulting from aortic stenosis. The sinotubular junction is preserved in cases of aortic stenosis but effaced in the other entities. Pseudoaneurysms can be seen superimposed on poststenotic true aneurysms because of the incidence of infective endocarditis of the aortic valve and subsequent seeding of the aorta (Fig. 47–24). If isolated to the descending aorta, saccular aneurysms may be traumatic or infective, but atherosclerosis remains the leading cause (Fig. 47–25). Saccular aneurysms in the aortic root very often have associated aortic insufficiency.

MRI is effective in identification and characterization of thoracic aortic aneurysms as well as in evaluation of their pathophysiologic consequences.[60, 61] The entire thoracic aorta is demonstrated on the LAO plane, allowing for assessment of location and extent of aneurysms. In contrast to transaxial imaging, the oblique plane allows precise determination of lumen diameter. The relation of the branch vessels to the aneurysm is easily demonstrated with this imaging plane. The coronal plane graphically delineates ascending aortic aneurysms and associated aortic insufficiency (Fig. 47–26) or hemopericardium (Fig. 47–27) with the use of SE and phase-mapping techniques.[54, 62]

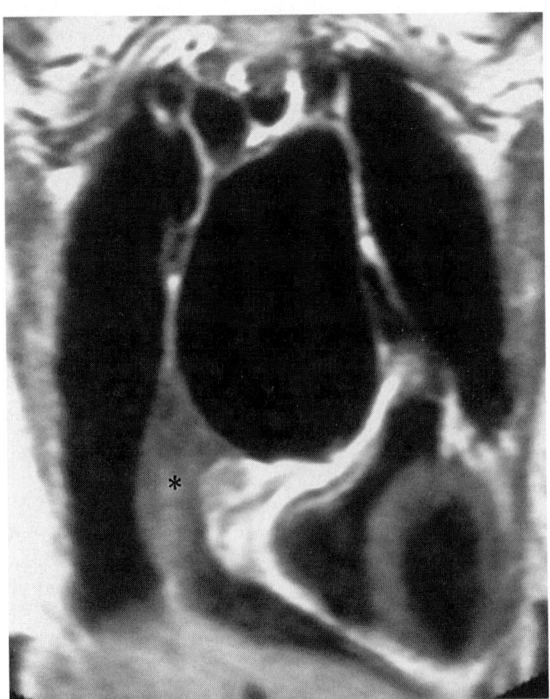

FIGURE 47–22. Coronal spin-echo magnetic resonance image demonstrates a large saccular aneurysm of the ascending aorta caused by annuloaortic ectasia. The intermediate signal intensity in the right aspect of the pericardial sac represents a hemopericardium *(asterisk)*.

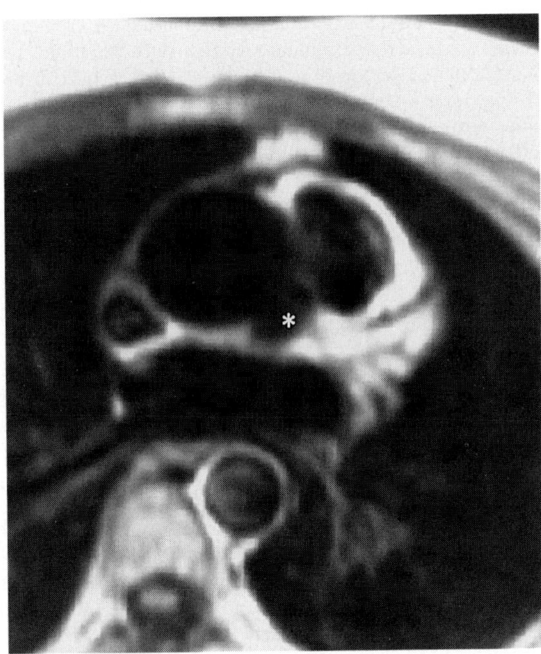

FIGURE 47–24. Transaxial spin-echo magnetic resonance image in a patient with bicuspid aortic valve demonstrates a pseudoaneurysm *(asterisk)*, the result of seeding from an infected valve leaflet.

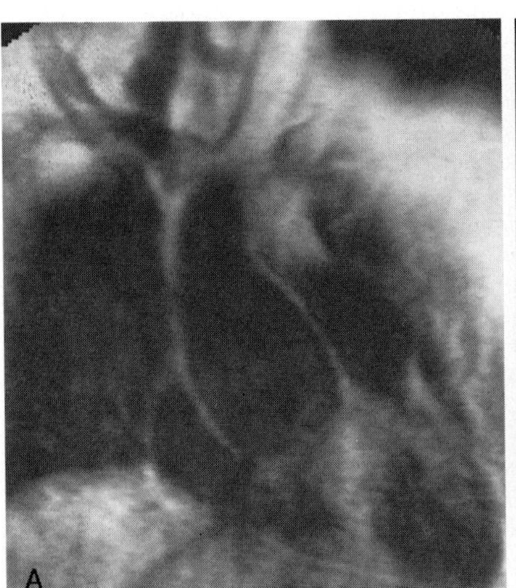

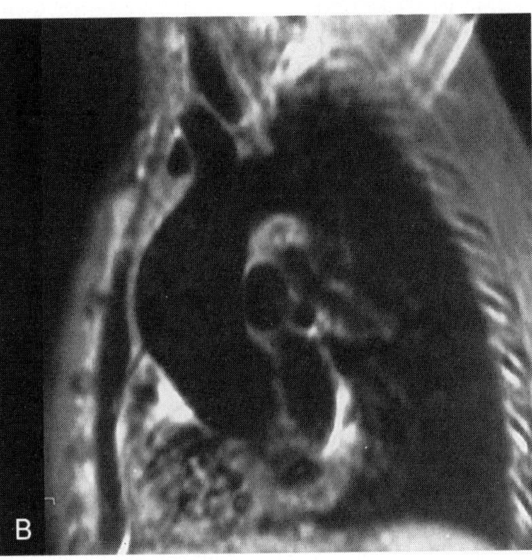

FIGURE 47–23. Coronal spin-echo (SE) magnetic resonance image (MRI) of a saccular ascending aortic aneurysm caused by Marfan syndrome *(A)*. The left anterior oblique SE MRI demonstrates a saccular aneurysm caused by postaortic valvular stenosis. In contrast to annuloaortic ectasia, in Marfan syndrome the sinuses are not effaced *(B)*.

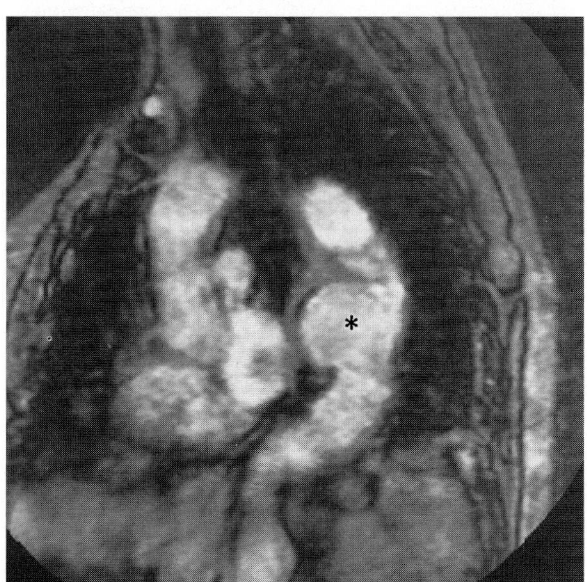

FIGURE 47–25. Cine left anterior oblique magnetic resonance image demonstrates a saccular mycotic aneurysm *(asterisk)* in the descending aorta.

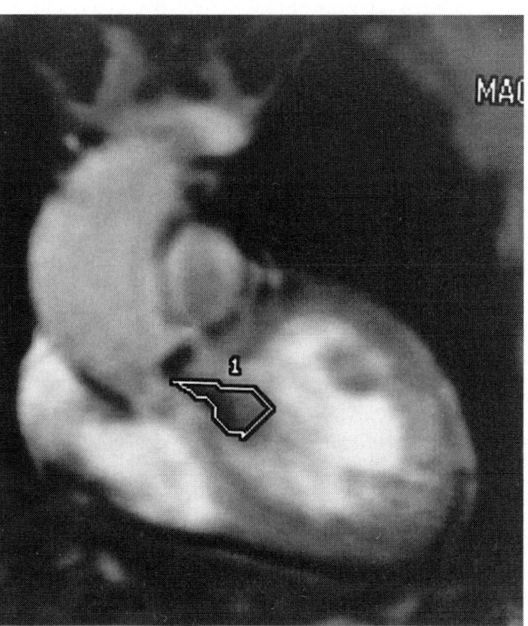

FIGURE 47–26. Coronal cine magnetic resonance image demonstrates aortic insufficiency *(outlined)* in this patient with a saccular aneurysm of the ascending aorta.

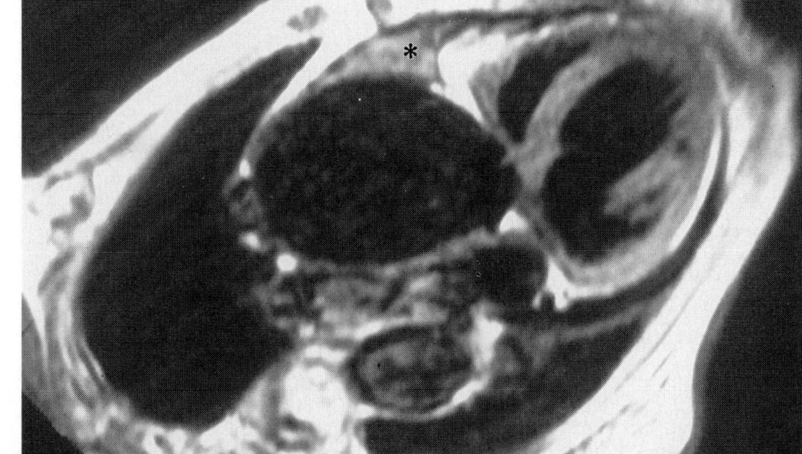

FIGURE 47–27. Long-axis spin-echo magnetic resonance image demonstrates a large saccular aneurysm of the ascending aorta that resulted in a hemopericardium *(asterisk)*.

Traumatic Tear

An aortic tear is a separate entity and should not be described in terms referring to dissections or aneurysms. As its name implies, an aortic tear is a shearing of the aorta, unlike the focal penetration of a pseudoaneurysm. This devastating event results in immediate death in approximately 90 percent of cases. In those fortunate enough to survive, the adventitia is usually intact and prevents exsanguination. If left untreated, 90 percent of these survivors will die. Therefore, it is imperative to establish the diagnosis quickly. Because aortic tears are usually caused by serious motor vehicle accidents, these patients typically have other life-threatening injuries that make MRI impractical. However, MRI is an appropriate technique in patients suspected of having a chronic or missed aortic tear. The tear is usually found in the area of the ligamentum arteriosus. It has the configuration of a localized saccular aneurysm, usually with an associated periaortic hematoma. The LAO and coronal planes graphically demonstrate the tear. Susceptibility artifacts are commonly present on cine MRI, owing to the high association with calcification at the site of injury (Fig. 47–28).

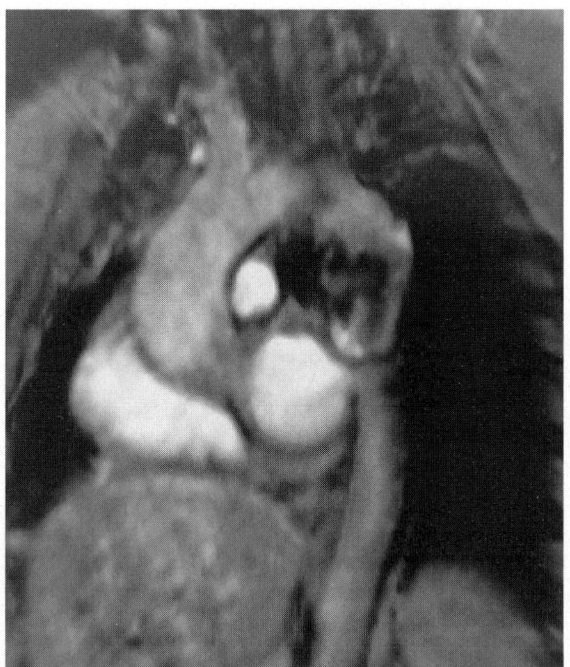

FIGURE 47–28. Left anterior oblique cine magnetic resonance image of a patient with a chronic transection. Note the saccular appearance of the aorta in the region of the ligamentum. The dark signal is caused by the presence of calcium.

Aortitis

Although there are many causes of aortitis, Takayasu arteritis is the type most often studied with MRI because of the diffuse stenotic nature of the disease, which often makes vascular access impossible by catheterization.[63] MRI typically demonstrates diffuse scattered stenosis of the thoracic and abdominal aorta as well as stenosis and occlusion of the branch vessels. There is often asymmetric thickening of the aortic wall that is caused by fibrosis. This can lead to the erroneous diagnosis of pseudoaneurysm on aortography, because the technique provides only a laminogram and is blind to the actual wall itself. Patients with aortitis are best studied by SE and dynamic MRI in the LAO, transaxial, and coronal planes (Fig. 47–29). Magnetic resonance angiography is often useful for evaluation of the branch vessels.

VALVULAR DISEASE

With advances in pulse sequence design and coil development, MRI can now be used to assess the pathoanatomy and pathophysiologic consequences of cardiac valvular disease. Given that MRI can be coupled with two-dimensional echocardiography with Doppler and color mapping, there are few indications for invasive evaluation of valvular disease.[64] Recent reports have demonstrated MRI as an alternative to echocardiography in the evaluation of valvular heart disease.[65, 66] In addition to being able to identify and quantify the severity of valvular disease, MRI provides a three-dimensional data set that can quantify ventricular function in the face of valvular disease.[67] These same attributes make MRI an excellent technique for monitoring the effects of surgical and medical intervention.

Technique

Until recently, SE techniques have been of little benefit in the assessment of valvular disease, other than being used to assess the cardiac chambers for hypertrophy or dilatation. With the introduction of dedicated cardiac or chest coils, SE MRI has become useful for visualization of the cardiac valves, especially for the presence of valvular vegetations and perivalvular abscesses. SE imaging is performed in a manner similar to that described for the thoracic aorta. ECG-gated scans are performed in planes specific to each valve, with as small an FOV as possible while still maintaining SNR. Slice thickness is typically 5 mm, with a 1-mm gap.[7]

The transaxial plane is well suited to study of the tricuspid valve, especially the anterior and septal leaflets. It is therefore the primary imaging plane for patients with Ebstein anomaly or tricuspid atresia. An oblique transaxial plane oriented perpendicular to the long axis of the main pulmonary artery and oblique sagittal imaging through the right ventricular outflow tract are the best planes for study of the pulmonic valve. An oblique transaxial plane oriented perpendicular to the aortic root, the coronal plane through the aortic root, and the horizontal long-axis view are the best imaging planes for study of the aortic valve (see Fig. 47–29). Although the transaxial view may be used to identify the mitral valve, it is best demonstrated on the horizontal and vertical long-axis views.[67]

Until the advent of phase-mapping techniques, cine MRI was the best method for identification and assessment of valvular disease.[7, 12] It is an ECG-referenced technique that demonstrates valvular motion outlined against a white blood pool background. The blood pool is white because of the implementation of a low flip angle (30 degrees) and short TE (5 to 12 msec) and TR (30 to 50 msec) times. Disturbances in blood flow are indicated by a loss of signal, referred to as a signal void. If caused by valvular disease, this results in what has been termed a signal void jet. It can be used to identify the valvular abnormality and to qualitatively assess its severity, based on the size of the signal void jet. Multiple images (usually 16) taken throughout the cardiac cycle at a single slice level are obtained and played back in a cine loop fashion. In this way, valvular function can be assessed throughout the cardiac cycle.[9–14]

The most recent dynamic imaging technique that can be used to study valvular disease is "fast" cine imaging.[68] The "fast" refers to very rapid image acquisition, typically accomplished within a single breath-hold. It has been used predominantly with cine sequences, although it also has been applied to phase-mapping techniques. With better gradients, very short TR (4 to 10 msec) and TE (2 to 4 msec) can be achieved. Instead of being able to collect a single line of K-space per heart beat, as with standard cine MRI, multiple lines (typically 8) can be acquired, thereby decreasing the scan duration to 16 heartbeats. This time is short enough to allow a patient to hold his or her breath during the entire acquisition,

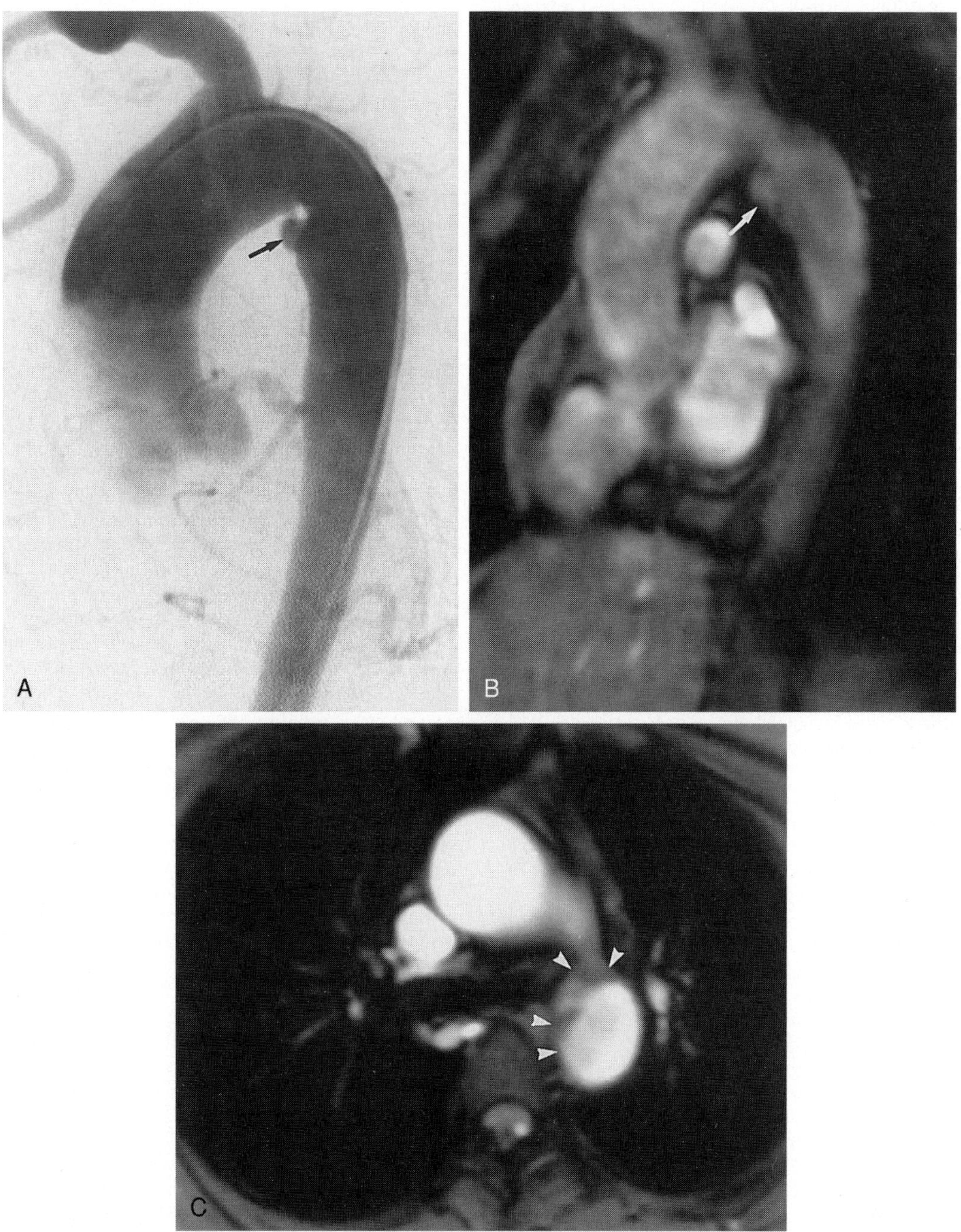

FIGURE 47–29. *A*, Digital left anterior oblique (LAO) angiogram demonstrates what appears to be a pseudoaneurysm *(arrow)*. *B*, LAO cine magnetic resonance image (MRI) looks just like the angiogram, demonstrating a presumed pseudoaneurysm *(arrow)*. *C*, Transaxial cine MRI shows that there has been encroachment on the aortic lumen by fibrosis *(arrowheads)*, giving the appearance of a pseudoaneurysm in this patient with Takayasu arteritis.

thereby decreasing respiratory motion artifacts. The major limitation of this technique is the decreased number of phases of the cardiac cycle that can be acquired. The temporal resolution is limited, and peak systolic and diastolic flow may be missed.

As previously discussed, phase or velocity mapping techniques allow for the measurement of proton motion over time, based on changes in the proton's phase angle, thereby yielding a velocity measurement.[15–23] This information in turn can be used to generate velocity-time and volume-time analysis curves. As a result, pressure gradients and regurgitant volumes across the cardiac valves can be determined. Oblique in-plane imaging through the center of the vena contracta of the signal void jet is best for determinations of velocity and calculations of pressure gradient with the modified Bernoulli equation. Oblique through-plane imaging performed parallel to the valve plane is best for measurement of the area of a great artery or cardiac chamber, and, coupled with velocity measurement, it is used to calculate flow, both forward stroke volume and regurgitant flow.

Stenosis and Regurgitation

Qualitative assessment of the severity of valvular stenosis and regurgitation is possible with cine MRI. Unsaturated flowing blood has bright signal under normal flow conditions except for predictable patterns of signal loss. However, abnormal flow patterns cause spin dephasing, which results in signal loss.[69, 70] Typically, this is caused by high-velocity turbulent flow, the type of pattern that results from valvular stenosis and regurgitation.

In valvular stenosis, turbulent flow causes a signal void jet that appears in the downstream great artery or cardiac chamber. It is important to use as short a TE value as possible in order to reduce dephasing so that the central vena contracta and the peripheral components of the jet may be recognized. The vena contracta corresponds to the area in which there is fast but stable flow. The peripheral component of the signal void jet reflects turbulent swirling blood flow, eddy currents, and countereddy currents (Fig. 47–30). It is important to differentiate between the two so that phase mapping can be performed along the vena contracta of the jet. Valvular regurgitation is recognized by a signal void jet forming retrograde to the valve in question. With mitral and tricuspid regurgitation, the signal void jet appears during ventricular systole. The signal void jet appears during ventricular diastole with aortic and pulmonic regurgitation.

The information gained from cine MRI is qualitative. The area and appearance of the signal void jet are greatly influenced by the TE time and flip angle as well as by how the image is windowed and leveled.[69, 71, 72] In addition, the jets are complex, three-dimensional phenomena that can change direction, shape, and location during the course of the cardiac cycle. Therefore, only a portion of the jet may be visualized in a particular imaging plane. The severity of the process can be greatly underestimated. Very often, dilatation of the aortic root can exacerbate the size of a signal void jet caused by a stenosis because of the turbulent flow generated by the anatomical configuration of the aortic dilatation. Similar problems exist with the signal void jets associated with regurgitation. Those methods that hope to assess the severity of valvular disease based on the area of signal void jets are only semiquantative, corresponding to the qualitative measurements obtained with Doppler echocardiography.[73]

Quantification of valvular disease is more difficult in that it requires the use of volumetric data, in the case of regurgitation, or of phase-mapping techniques, for either regurgitation or stenosis (see Chapter 50). MRI is the gold standard for calculation of ventricular volumes.[74–80] Multislice, multiphasic (either cine or SE) tomographic images through the entire extent of the ventricles are used to calculate end-diastolic and end-systolic volumes. In the normal heart, the stroke volumes are the same for the left and right ventricles, so the difference in stroke volume between the regurgitant and the normal ventricle equals the regurgitant volume. The forward stroke volume plus the regurgitant volume is equal to the total stroke volume of the regurgitant ventricle. The regurgitant fraction is the regurgitant volume divided by the total stroke volume of the regurgitant ventricle. This technique of planimetric calculation of regurgitant volume is time-consuming, in terms of image acquisition and postimage processing, requiring analysis of end-diastole and end-systole at approximately eight slice levels. However, it has the added benefit of allowing calculation of the cardiac mass and assessment of global and focal systolic wall thickening.[9]

Another method for quantification of valvular regurgitation is the use of phase mapping to measure the regurgitant flow.[81–84] If the imaging plane is located parallel to the annulus of the valve, flow across the valve can be determined by calculating the area and velocity profiles throughout the cardiac cycle. Phase mapping can differentiate antegrade from retrograde flow. In normal patients, there is virtually no retrograde flow during the diastolic phase of the cardiac cycle, whereas varying amounts of diastolic retrograde flow occur in cases of valvular regurgitation. If a flow-time graph is plotted, the area under the retrograde curve is equal to the regurgitant volume.

Multivalvular left-sided regurgitation can be assessed with a combination of phase mapping of the aorta and cine MRI ventricular volumetric measurements. The total regurgitation volume is calculated by planimetric measurements of the right and left ventricles in end-diastole and end-systole, performed in the short-axis plane through the extent of the ventricles. The total regurgitant volume is the difference between the left and right ventricular stroke volumes, provided that there is no significant right-sided regurgitation. The aortic regurgitation component of the total regurgitant volume can be measured by calculation of the retrograde flow in the aorta with phase mapping. The mitral regurgitant component is the difference between the total regurgitant volume and the aortic regurgitant volume.

There are fewer published reports dealing with quantification of valvular stenosis, although identification of stenoses with cine MRI is quite accurate.[85–88] Planimetric volumetric calculations do not play a role in the assessment of stenotic lesions as they do with regurgitant lesions. Stenoses are much more difficult to evaluate with phase-mapping MRI because of the very high velocities and turbulent flow associated with these lesions. Both of these factors lead to phase dispersion, subsequent loss of signal, and errors in velocity measurements. Recent work indicates that these obstacles can be overcome with the use of extremely short TE times (less than 4 msec) and by performing the scan in an in-plane orientation through the vena contracta of the jet.[87, 88] This technique provides accurate velocity measurements at multiple phases of the cardiac cycle, which can then be plotted on a graph of velocity versus time. The peak systolic velocity can be used in the modified Bernoulli equation to calculate a pressure gradient.

Evaluation of patients with valvular heart disease would be incomplete without an assessment of the amount of left ventricular dysfunction. Short-axis cine MRI performed from the cardiac base to its apex provides a three-dimensional data set that is used to measure left ventricular end-diastolic and end-systolic volumes, stroke volume, ejection fraction, and ventricular mass.[65, 74, 77, 79, 80] Similar measurements can be obtained of the right ventricle in cases of right-sided valvular disease.[75, 77] Mass determinations are especially important in relation to stenotic disease. Studies suggest that MRI is the gold standard for measuring left ventricular mass.[89, 90] Excellent interstudy reproducibility for MRI measurements of volumes and mass has been demonstrated.[68] Therefore, MRI is an excellent mechanism for monitoring changes in left ventricular function after therapy as well as for determining changes in the degree of valvular dysfunction.

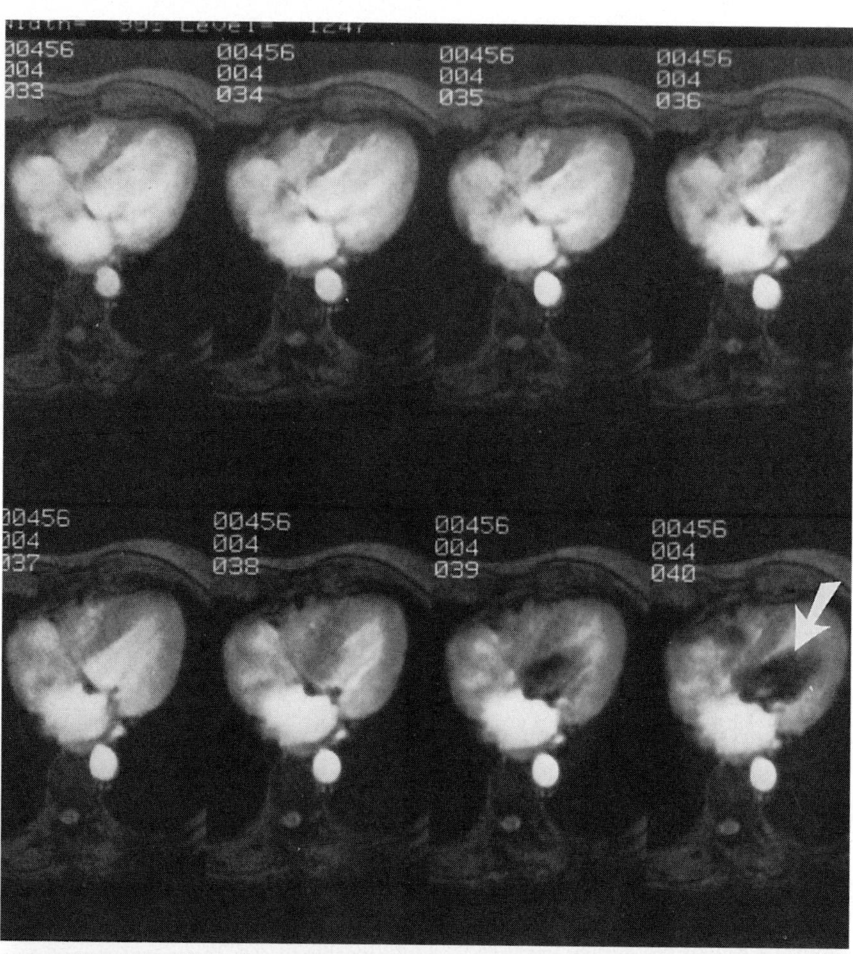

FIGURE 47–30. A series of 16 cine gradient-recalled axial images through the aortic valve, top of mitral valve, and left ventricle, beginning at the QRS. The dramatic signal loss from aortic insufficiency and mitral stenosis can be seen on the diastolic images *(arrow)*.

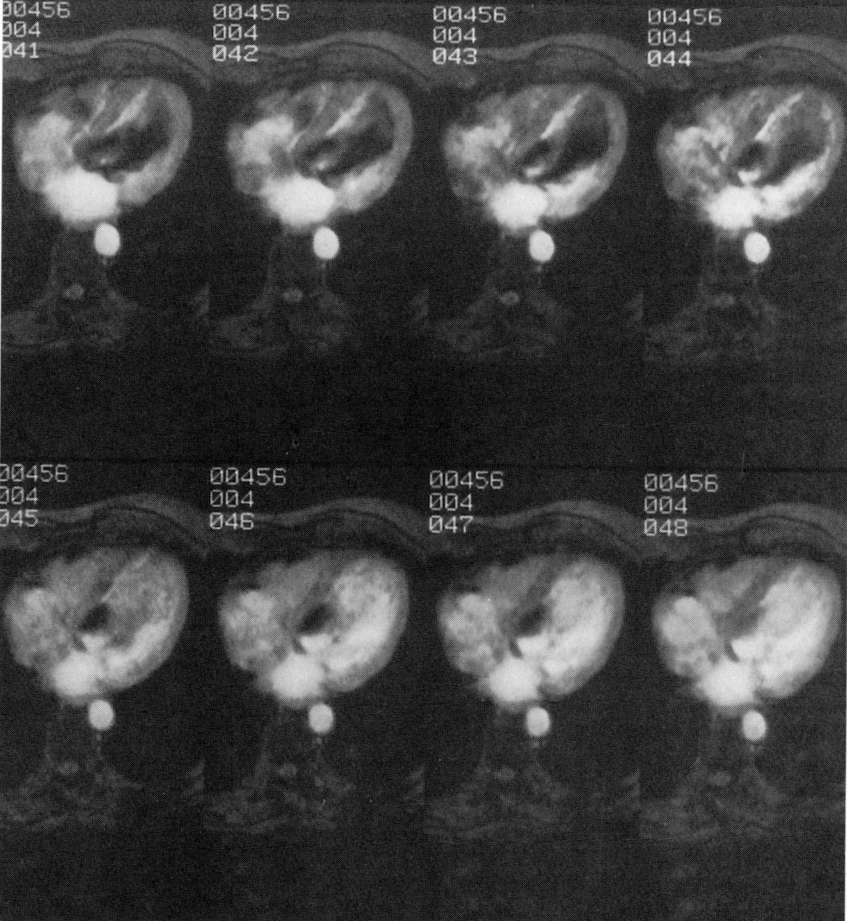

Specific Valvular Lesions

Pulmonary Valve

Isolated pulmonic stenosis is usually caused by a "dome-shaped" pulmonic valve and uncommonly by pulmonary valve dysplasia.[91] There is usually poststenotic dilatation of the main pulmonary artery, which may extend into the left pulmonary artery. Concentric right ventricular hypertrophy is present in varying degrees of severity, reflecting the degree of pulmonary stenosis. As the degree of hypertrophy progresses, secondary muscular infundibular stenosis may develop. Pulmonary stenosis may be seen in association with an anomalous muscle bundle of the right ventricle, the so-called double chamber right ventricle.[92] There may also be associated focal stenoses of the pulmonary arteries. Pulmonary stenosis is a very common congenital heart disease, accounting for approximately 10 percent of all cases.[93, 94]

Cine MRI is useful in identification of the presence of the dome-shaped valve, poststenotic dilatation, and degree of right ventricular hypertrophy. The valve is best shown on the oblique sagittal view through the right ventricular outflow tract. In-plane phase mapping performed through the center of the vena contracta is used to calculate a pressure gradient. MRI can subsequently be used to monitor the patient for worsening of the pressure gradient. Right ventricular hypertrophy is assessed by planimetric measurement of the endocardial and epicardial surfaces, as demonstrated on sequential short-axis cine MRI scans.

Tricuspid Valve

Tricuspid atresia is a rare congenital defect, accounting for approximately 1.5 percent of overall cardiac cases.[93, 94] There is a mandatory atrial septal defect and a ventricular septal defect to ensure that blood flows to the pulmonary arteries. The right ventricle is hypoplastic and hypertrophied. The former condition results from the lack of the normal blood flow pattern during embryonic development, the latter from the systemic pressures to which it is exposed as a result of the ventricular septal defect. The classic MRI presentation of tricuspid atresia is a thick, high-signal band in the right atrioventricular groove, the expected location of the valve plane, on standard transaxial images. This is caused by the epicardial fat herniae into the atrioventricular groove as the atria and ventricle "pinch-in" toward one another as a result of the absent tricuspid valve annulus.

Ebstein anomaly is a malformation of the tricuspid valve leaflets.[93, 94] The annulus remains in place at the right atrioventricular groove. The anterior leaflet has a normal proximal attachment to the annulus, but its middle and distal portions are dysplastic. The end of the leaflet is not free but is attached to a muscular ridge in the apex of the right ventricle. The septal and posterior leaflets are dysplastic and are displaced from their normal proximal attachment to the annulus. As a result, the leaflets encroach on the inflow and muscular portions of the right ventricle. This process has been termed the atrialization of the right ventricle. The infundibulum is usually spared from this encroachment and becomes the contracting portion of the right ventricle.[95] The pathoanatomy of this lesion is best demonstrated on transaxial and coronal imaging.[96] Tricuspid regurgitation may be associated and can be demonstrated by transaxial cine MRI and quantified either by planimetric volumetric calculations or by phase-mapping determination of regurgitant volume.

Tricuspid regurgitation that results from an isolated intrinsic valvular anomaly is rare, although it may be seen in conjunction with Ebstein anomaly.[97, 98] The most common cause of tricuspid regurgitation is right ventricular dilatation and failure. It can also result if there is left ventricular failure or pulmonary hypertension. The most common cause of isolated tricuspid regurgitation is infectious endocarditis in intravenous drug users. Transaxial SE MRI, performed with a dedicated coil, can usually identify abnormalities of the tricuspid valve. Valve leaflet tumors, fibroelastomas, and myxomas can also cause tricuspid regurgitation and can usually be differentiated from infection, especially with an accurate clinical history. Regurgitation is best identified by use of transaxial cine MRI to demonstrate a regurgitant signal void jet (Fig. 47–31). Quantification of the regurgitant volume can be made with cine MRI volumetric analysis or phase-mapping flow measurements.

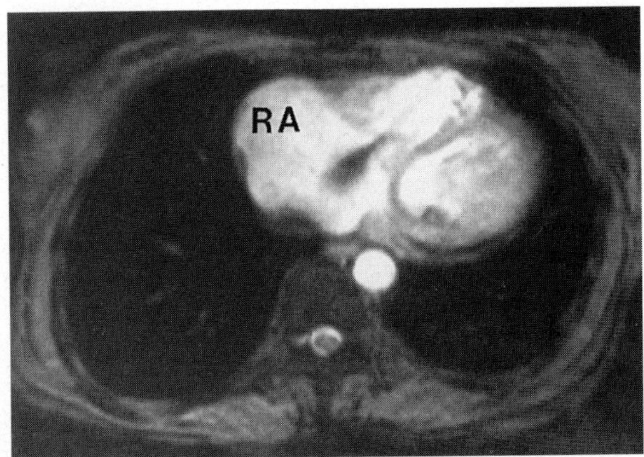

FIGURE 47–31. Systolic image shows a dilated right atrium (RA) in a patient with rheumatic valvular disease. A signal void caused by tricuspid regurgitation diverges after crossing the tricuspid valve plane.

The most common cause of tricuspid stenosis is rheumatic fever. Isolated rheumatic involvement of the tricuspid valve is uncommon; it is almost always seen in conjunction with mitral valve involvement and mitral stenosis.[99, 100] A slightly oblique transaxial cine MRI oriented parallel to a line from the middle right atrium to the apex of the left ventricle (as viewed from a coronal scout view) can usually demonstrate the signal void jets from both the tricuspid and mitral valves. In-plane phase mapping through the vena contracta of each jet provides peak systolic velocities that can be used to calculate peak systolic pressure gradients by the modified Bernoulli equation.

Mitral Valve

Although there are many causes of mitral stenosis, including congenital stenosis, atrial myxoma, and bacterial endocarditis, rheumatic fever remains the most common cause.[101] Recurrent rheumatic valvulitis results in scarring and retraction of the valve leaflets and chordae tendineae. If these processes cause the leaflets to be

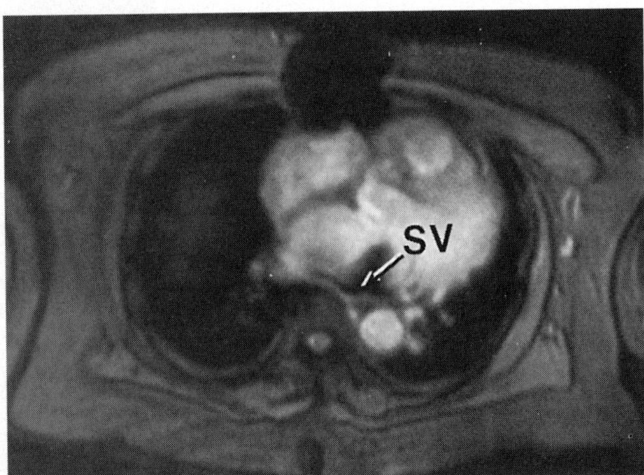

FIGURE 47–32. Large signal void (SV) in left atrium in systole results from mitral regurgitation. Connection to the valve plane does not appear in this section. The signal void diverges as it extends toward the posterior left atrium. The large signal void appearing anteriorly in the chest wall is an artifact caused by sternal wire sutures from a prior median sternotomy.

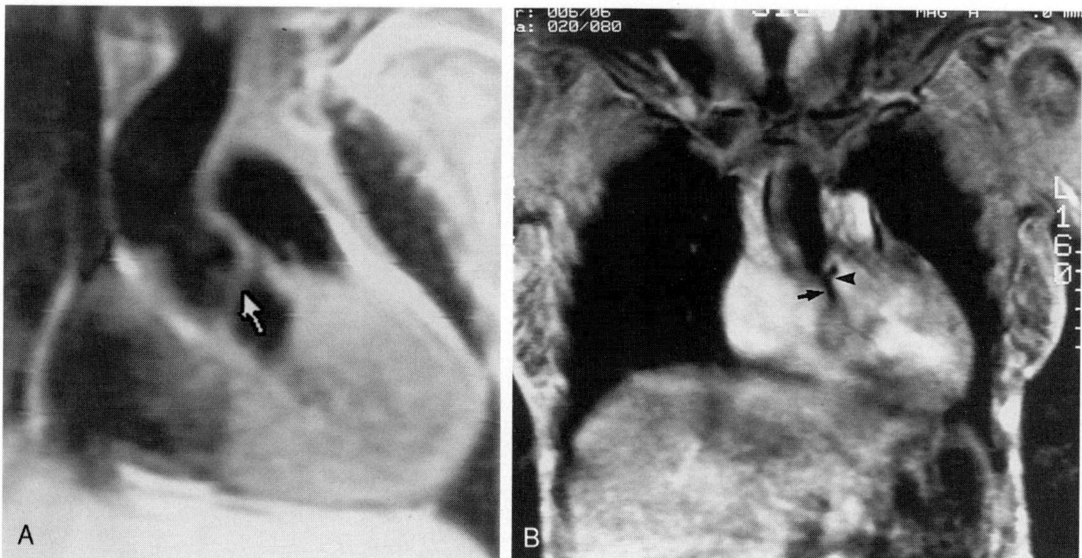

FIGURE 47–33. Electrocardiographically-gated spin-echo (SE) *(A)* and cine *(B)* magnetic resonance images through the aortic annulus demonstrate a membranous subvalvular stenosis. The membrane appears as an intermediate-signal, linear structure in the annulus on the SE image *(arrow)*. The cine study demonstrates the signal void jet arising inferior to the valve leaflets, which is caused by the membrane *(arrowhead)*. Note the retrograde signal void jet, indicating regurgitation across the membrane *(arrow)*.

fused in a closed position, mitral stenosis occurs. Typically, the leaflets form a funnel-shaped valvular apparatus that is pulled downward by the retracted chordae tendineae.[102] Mitral stenosis causes a pressure gradient between the left atrium and the left ventricle. The amount of the gradient depends on the area of the valve orifice and the amount of diastolic flow, which in turn depends on the cardiac output and the duration of ventricular diastole. As the process worsens, the increased atrial pressure and volume result in left atrial enlargement, pulmonary venous hypertension, and right ventricular hypertrophy.[103] SE MRI can demonstrate the degree of left atrial enlargement and, with the proper receiver coil, the valvular anatomy. Cine MRI aligned in the vertical and horizontal long-axis views is performed to identify the location and configuration of the signal void jet (see Fig. 47–30). In-plane phase mapping is then performed through the center of the vena contracta. From the velocity-time plot, the peak atrial systolic velocity is used in the modified Bernoulli equation to calculate the peak atrial systolic pressure.[88]

Rheumatic fever can also result in mitral regurgitation. The basic underlying valvulitis is the same as that in mitral stenosis.[104] Instead of the leaflets being scarred and contracted in the closed position, they are fused in the open position. A more common cause of mitral regurgitation is coronary artery disease. Myocardial infarction causing left ventricular dilatation can result in enlargement of the valvular orifice and distortion of the chordae tendineae.[105] Infarction or rupture of a papillary muscle also results in mitral regurgitation. The most common cause of mitral regurgitation in adults is mitral valve prolapse.[106] The valve and chordae tendineae undergo myxomatous degeneration and deterioration, which, in turn, leads to redundancy of the valve and chordae, improper coaptation of the leaflets, prolapse, and regurgitation.[107]

Regardless of its cause, mitral regurgitation results in left ventricular and left atrial volume overload and elevated left atrial systolic pressure. To accommodate the increased volume load, the left ventricle dilates in an effort to maintain forward systemic stroke volume.[108] In order to maintain adequate contractility, concomitant left ventricular hypertrophy develops. The mitral valve apparatus is best visualized in the vertical and horizontal long-axis views. Cine MRI performed in these planes is best for identification of the presence of regurgitation (Fig. 47–32). Regurgitant volume is calculated by either the planimetric method or the flow method, as has been outlined. Associated ventricular hypertrophy or dysfunction is best evaluated by short-axis cine MRI performed through the entirety of the ventricle.

Aortic Valve

Presumably the result of abnormalities in the conotruncal apparatus, congenital aortic stenosis can occur in three separate locations and can exist as an isolated anomaly or in conjunction with other thoracic aortic anomalies or intracardiac anomalies. Subvalvular stenosis occurs most commonly in pediatric and adolescent patients, with a male-to-female ratio of 2.5:1. There are three types of subvalvular aortic stenosis: the membranous type (Fig. 47–33); the fibromuscular type, involving a thick band of tissue that forms a subvalvular collar (Fig. 47–34); and the tunnel type.[32]

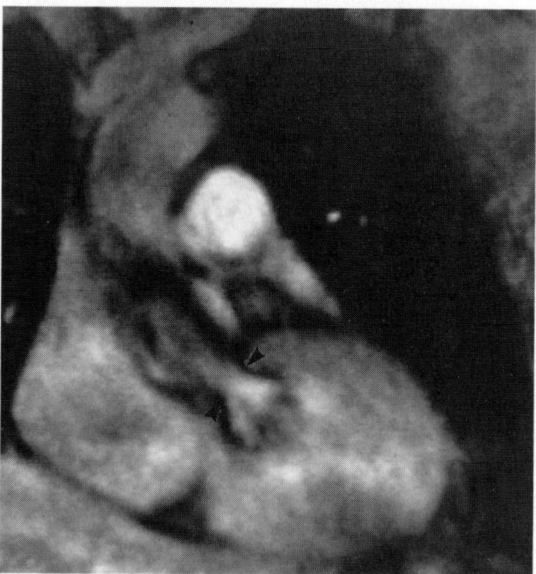

FIGURE 47–34. Electrocardiographically referenced coronal cine magnetic resonance image demonstrates a collar-type subvalvular stenosis *(arrowheads)*.

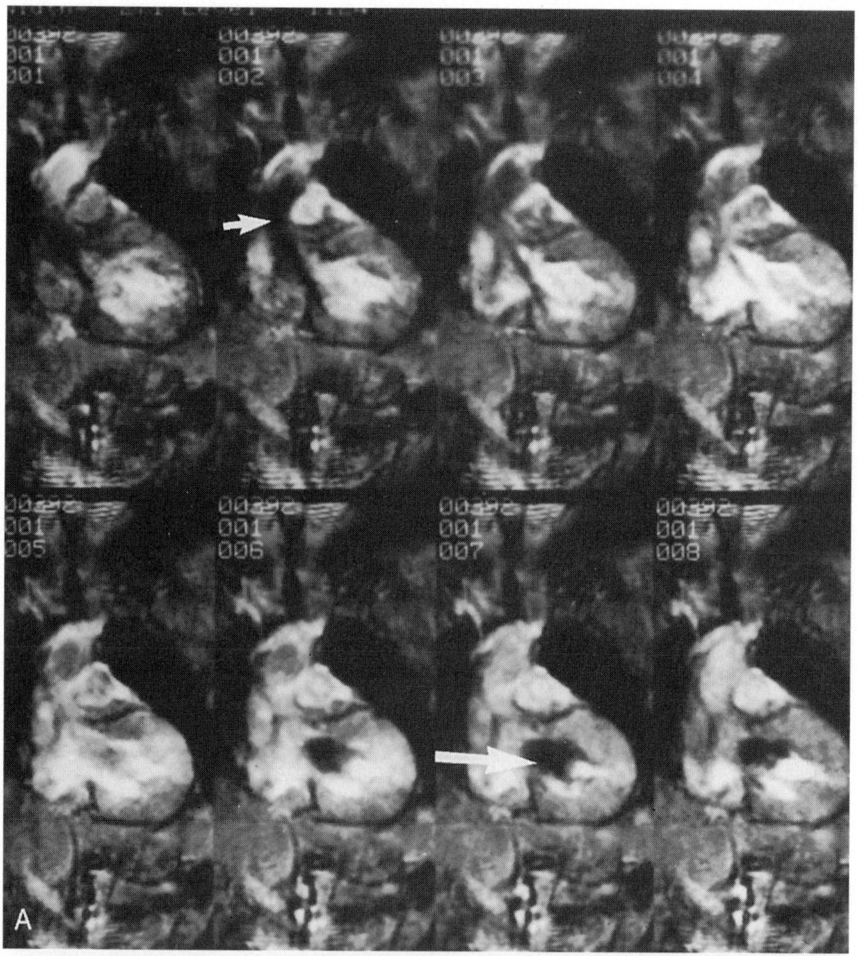

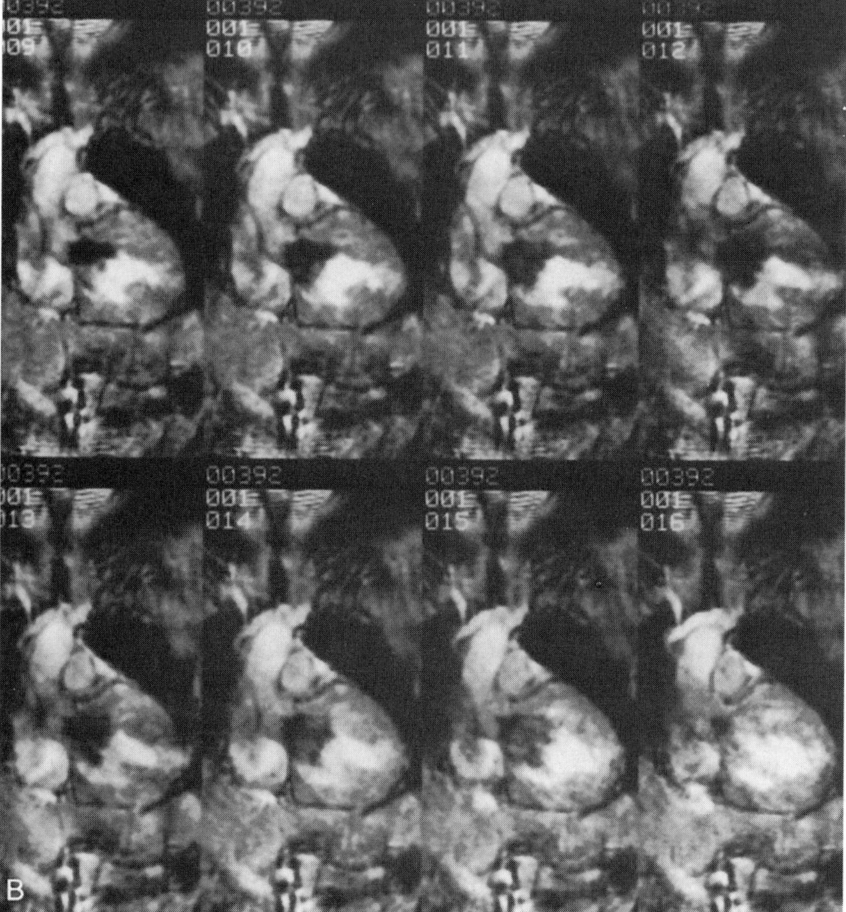

FIGURE 47–35. A series of 16 cine gradient-recalled coronal images through the aortic valve and left ventricle, beginning at the QRS. Note the loss of signal during systole, which is seen in the ascending aorta *(small arrow)* from relative aortic stenosis. The dominant lesion is aortic insufficiency, causing a diastolic loss of signal *(large arrow)* originating from the aortic valve and extending into the left ventricular cavity.

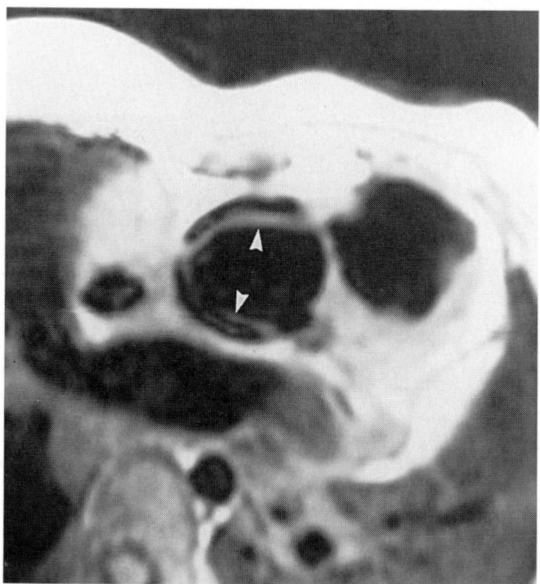

FIGURE 47–36. Electrocardiographically gated transaxial magnetic resonance image demonstrates the two thickened aortic valve leaflets *(arrowheads)* of a bicuspid aortic valve.

If used in conjunction with a chest coil, SE MRI can usually depict the anatomic anomaly. Cine MRI graphically demonstrates the pathophysiologic consequences of the anomaly as a signal void jet caused by the turbulent flow resulting from the stenosis (Fig. 47–35). With phase-mapping MRI, the degree of stenosis can be quantified. Phase mapping calculates the velocity of flow, which can then be used in the modified Bernoulli equation to generate a pressure gradient. Left ventricular hypertrophy can be quantitated, as can the left ventricular ejection fraction, with short-axis multislice cine MRI.[85–88]

Congenital bicuspid aortic valve is usually the cause of congenital valvular stenosis. If severe enough, the bicuspid aortic valve can cause critical stenosis in the newborn. However it usually takes 20 to 30 years before the bicuspid valve has undergone enough thickening, decreased mobility, and calcification to result in stenosis severe enough to warrant intervention (Fig. 47–36). These patients do, however, need to be closely monitored for secondary problems, especially infective endocarditis and valvular abscess[32] (Fig. 47–37). The stenosis is usually severe when symptoms develop in the newborn. Patients can deteriorate rapidly, and death is not uncommon if intervention is delayed. The classic chest radiograph demonstrates a rounded cardiac apex caused by left ventricular hypertrophy and a bulge above the right atrium caused by poststenotic aortic root dilatation. Calcification of the bicuspid valve is rarely present on a chest radiograph in newborns, children, or adolescents.[32]

Angiography, echocardiography with Doppler, and MRI can all be used to identify and quantify the severity of aortic valvular stenosis. They can all identify the classic doming of the aortic valve, the eccentric jet of blood flow distal to the narrow fishmouth deformity of the bicuspid valve, and the eccentric right-sided dilatation of the ascending aorta[24] (Fig. 47–38). Typically, the evaluation starts with echocardiography in children, followed by MRI if the echocardiogram is inconclusive. In older children, where the acoustic window is limited, MRI is the initial imaging modality. MRI is better at assessing the patient for associated ventricular septal defects and coarctation. Spin-echo MRI and phase mapping can identify and quantitate the severity of stenosis and associated coarctation and allow calculation of any shunt ratio in patients with septal defects. Angiography is used as a last resort if the two noninvasive modalities prove unsuccessful.

The rarest of the aortic stenosis anomalies is the supravalvular variety. This anomaly involves the tubular portion of the aorta just distal to the coronary artery ostia. The most common type is the hourglass deformity (Fig. 47–39). Less common are the fibrous diagram and tubular hypoplasia types.[32] Supravalvular stenosis is probably the result of abnormal fusion of the truncal ridges that divide the truncus arteriosus. This variety of aortic stenosis can occur as an isolated lesion or as part of the supravalvular aortic stenosis syndrome or Williams syndrome. It can be familial, and it is associated with idiopathic hypercalcemia, mental and physical retardation, peripheral pulmonary artery stenosis, and elfin faces.[32] Coronal SE MRI and phase mapping demonstrate the aortic narrowing and can be used to calculate the pressure gradient across the stenosis. Associated left ventricular hypertrophy and left ventricular ejection fractions are assessed with dynamic MRI imaging performed in the short-axis plane.

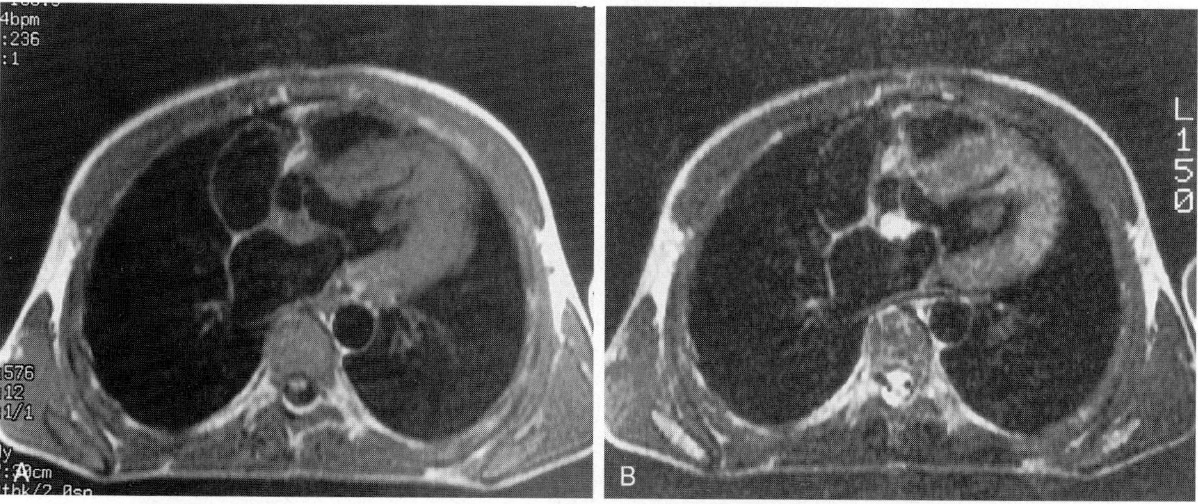

FIGURE 47–37. Paravalvular abscess in a patient with bicuspid aortic stenosis. T1-weighted image *(A)* demonstrates an intermediate signal mass that is increased in signal on the T2-weighted image *(B)*.

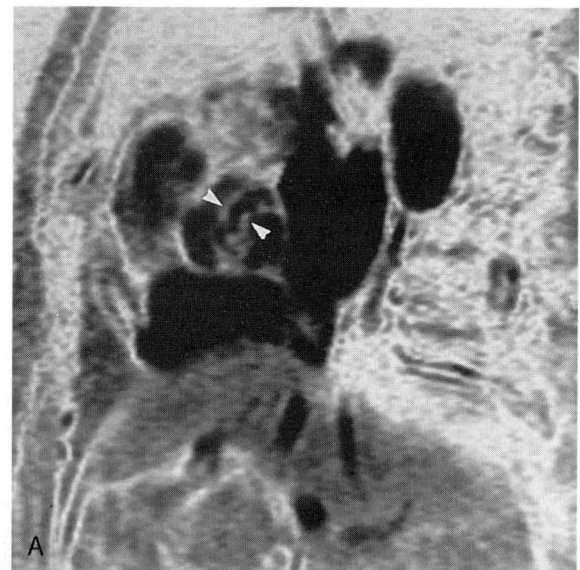

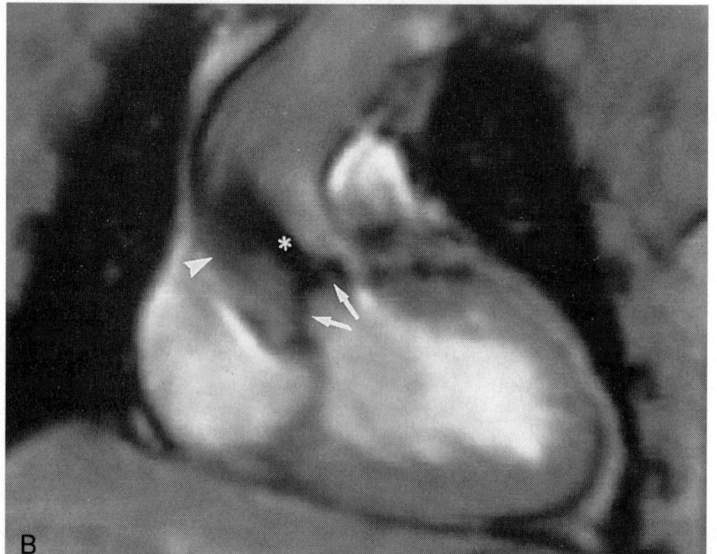

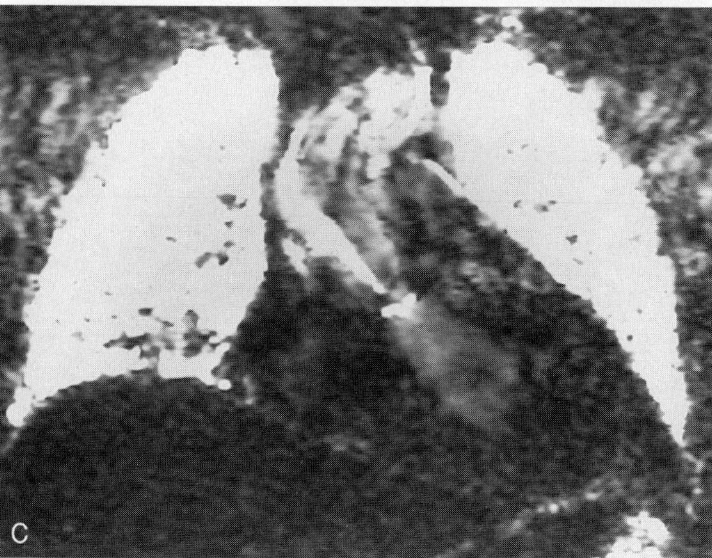

FIGURE 47–38. Dynamic magnetic resonance imaging (MRI) of bicuspid aortic valvular stenosis. *A*, Electrocardiographically referenced short-axis cine MRI (video reversed) demonstrates a fish-mouth *(small arrowheads)* bicuspid valve. *B*, Cine coronal MRI demonstrates a domed *(arrows)* stenotic bicuspid valve, a signal jet void *(asterisk)* caused by the stenosis, and asymmetric poststenotic dilatation of the ascending aorta *(large arrowhead)*. *C*, Coronal phase map used to calculate the pressure gradient across the stenotic bicuspid valve.

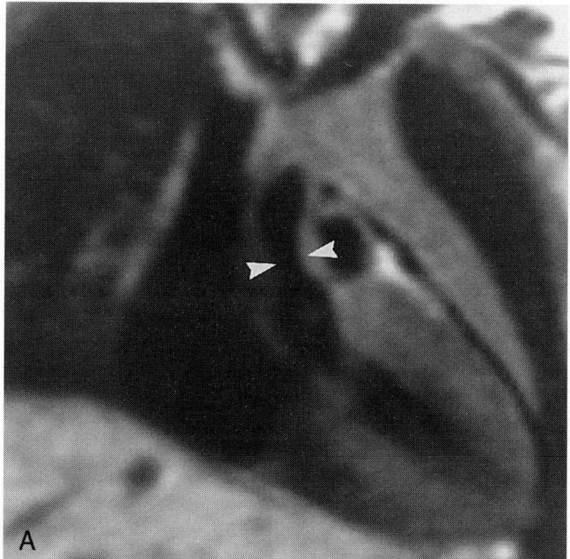

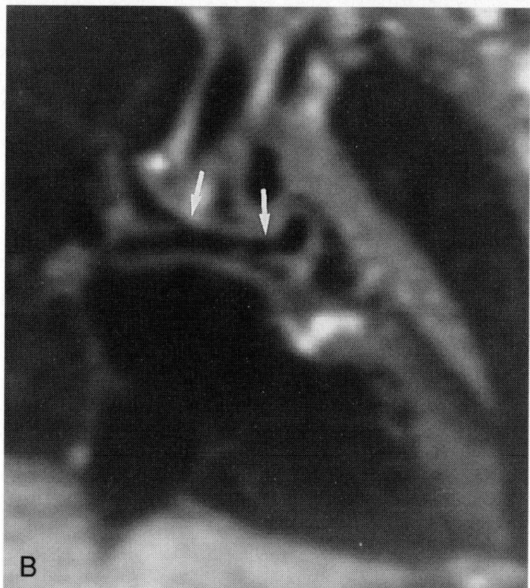

FIGURE 47–39. Electrocardiographically gated coronal spin-echo magnetic resonance images demonstrate hourglass supravalvular stenosis *(A, arrowheads)* and hypoplasia of the pulmonary arteries *(B, arrows)* in a patient with Williams syndrome.

Acknowledgments

We are indebted to Carla Muller and Miriam Vernon for their help in the preparation of this manuscript.

References

1. Eidemiler, L.R., and Keane, J.M.: Development of the heart. *In* Pearson, A.A. (ed.): The Development of the Cardiovascular System. Portland, University of Oregon Medical School Printing Department, 1968.
2. Moore, K.L.: The Circulatory System: The Cardiovascular and Lymphatic Systems. 2nd ed. Philadelphia, W.B. Saunders Co., 1977.
3. Netter, F.H.: Embryology. *In* Yonkman, F.F. (ed.): The CIBA Collection of Medical Illustrations. West Caldwell, N.J., CIBA, 1978.
4. Stewart, J.R., Kincaid, O.W., and Edwards, J.E.: An Atlas of Vascular Rings and Related Malformations of the Aortic Arch System. Springfield, Ill., Charles C. Thomas, 1964.
5. Kersting-Sommerhoff, B., Higgins, C.B., White, R.D., et al.: Aortic dissection: Sensitivity and specificity of MR imaging. Radiology 166:651, 1988.
6. Bailes, D.R., Gilderdale, D.J., Bydder, G.M., et al.: Respiratory ordered phase encoding (ROPE): A method for reducing respiratory motion artifacts in MR imaging. J. Comput. Assist. Tomogr. 9:835, 1985.
7. Link, K.M., and Lesko, N.M.: Cardiac MR: Techniques and normal anatomy. Contemp. Diagn. Radiol. 14:1, 1991.
8. Haase, A., Frahm, J., Matthaei, D., et al.: FLASH imaging: Rapid NMR imaging using low flip angle pulses. J. Magn. Reson. 67:258, 1986.
9. Pettigrew, R.I.: Dynamic magnetic resonance imaging of acquired heart disease. Semin. Ultrasound CT MR 12:61, 1991.
10. Herfkens, R., Utz, O.R., and Oeisimer, J.A.: A new technique that produces rapid dynamic nuclear magnetic resonance images of the heart in the assessment of valvular dysfunction. Circulation 74(Suppl 2):319, 1986.
11. Higgins, C.B.: MR of the heart anatomy, physiology and metabolism. AJR 151:239, 1988.
12. Pettigrew, R.I.: Dynamic cardiac MR imaging techniques and applications. Radiol. Clin. North Am. 27:1183, 1989.
13. Schiebler, M., Axel, L., Reichek, N., et al.: Correlation of cine MR imaging with two-dimensional pulsed Doppler echocardiography in valvular insufficiency. J. Comput. Assist. Tomogr. 11:627, 1987.
14. Sechtemm, U., Pfugfelder, P.W., Cassidy, M.M., et al.: Mitral or aortic regurgitation: Qualification of regurgitant volumes with cine MR imaging. Radiology 167:425, 1988.
15. Byrant, D.J., Payne, J.A., Firmin, D.N., and Longmore, D.B.: Measurement of flow with NMR imaging using a gradient pulse and phase difference technique. J. Comput. Assist. Tomogr. 8:588, 1994.
16. Firmin, D.N., Kilpstein, R.H., Hounsfield, G.L., et al.: Echo-planar high-resolution flow velocity mapping. Magn. Reson. Med. 12:316, 1989.
17. Firmin, D.N., Mayler, F.I., Kilpstein, R.H., et al.: In vivo validation of MR velocity imaging. J. Comput. Assist. Tomogr. 11:751, 1987.
18. Meier, D., Maier, S., and Bösiger, P.: Quantitative flow measurements on phantoms and on blood vessels with MR. Magn. Reson. Med. 8:25, 1988.
19. Moran, P.R.: A flow velocity zeugmatographic interface for NMR imaging in humans. Magn. Reson. Imaging 1:197, 1983.
20. Nayler, F.L., Firmin, D.N., and Longmore, D.B.: Blood flow imaging by cine magnetic resonance. J. Comput. Assist. Tomogr. 10:715, 1986.
21. Edelman, R.R., Mattle, H.P., and Atkinson, D.J.: MR angiography. AJR 154:937, 1990.
22. Ku, D.N., Biancheri, C., Pettigrew, R.I., et al.: Evaluation of magnetic resonance velocimetry. J. Biomech. Eng. 112:464, 1990.
23. Rumancik, W.M., Naidich, D.P., Chandra, R., et al.: Cardiovascular disease: Evaluation with MR phase imaging. Radiology 166:63, 1988.
24. Link, K.M.: Great vessels. *In* Stark, D.D., Bradley, W.G., Jr. (eds.): Magnetic Resonance Imaging. 2nd ed. St. Louis, Missouri, Mosby-Year Book, 1991, p. 1490.
25. Oelrich, T.M.: The cardiovascular system. *In* Anson, B.J. (ed.): Human Anatomy: A Complete Systematic Treatise. New York, Blakiston, 1966.
26. Barkovich, A.J.: Techniques and methods in pediatric magnetic resonance imaging. Semin. Ultrasound CT MR 9:186, 1988.
27. Burrows, P.E.: Magnetic resonance imaging of the aorta in children. Semin. Ultrasound CT MR 11:221, 1990.
28. Didier, D., Higgins, C.B., Fisher, M.R., et al.: Congenital heart disease: Gated MR imaging in 72 patients. Radiology 158:227, 1986.
29. Fletcher, B.D., and Jacobstein, M.D.: MRI of congenital abnormalities of the great arteries. AJR 146:941, 1986.
30. Kersting-Sommerhoff, B.A., Sechtem, U.P., Schiller, N.B., et al.: MR imaging of the thoracic aorta in Marfan patients. J. Comput. Assist. Tomogr. 11:633, 1987.
31. Bisset, G.S.: Pediatric applications of magnetic resonance imaging. J. Thorac. Imag. 4:51, 1989.
32. Gomes, A.S., Lois, J.F., George, B., et al.: Congenital abnormalities of the aortic arch: MR imaging. Radiology 165:691, 1987.
33. Jaffe, R.B.: Magnetic resonance imaging of vascular rings. Semin. Ultrasound CT MR 11:206, 1990.
34. Link, K.M.: Cardiovascular MR imaging: Present status. Radiology Syllabus. Chicago, IL, Radiological Society of North America, 1990, p. 123.
35. Freedom, R.M., Culham, J.A.G., and Moes, C.A.F.: Angiocardiography of Congenital Heart Disease. New York, Macmillan, Inc., 1984.
36. Bank, E.R., Aisen, A.M., Rocchini, A.P., et al.: Coarctation of the aorta in children undergoing angioplasty: Pretreatment and posttreatment MR imaging. Radiology 162:235, 1987.
37. Boxer, R.A., LaCorte, M.A., Singh, S., et al.: Nuclear magnetic resonance imaging in evaluation and follow-up of children treated for coarctation of the aorta. J. Am. Coll. Cardiol. 7:1095, 1986.
38. Von Schulthess, G.K., Higashino, S.M., Higgins, S.S., et al.: Coarctation of the aorta; MR imaging. Radiology 158:469, 1986.
39. LePage, J.R., Szezchenyi, E., and Ross-Duggan, J.W.: Pseudocoarctation of the aorta. Magn. Reson. Imaging 6:65, 1988.
40. Link, K.M., and Lesko, N.M.: The role of MR imaging in the evaluation of acquired diseases of the thoracic aorta. AJR 158:1115, 1992.
41. Atkinson, D.J., Burstein, D.D., and Edelmann, R.R.: First-pass cardiac perfusion: Evaluation with ultrafast MR imaging. Radiology 174:757, 1990.
42. Frahm, J., Merboldt, K.D., Bruhn, H., et al.: 0.3 second FLASH MRI of the human heart. Magn. Reson. Med. 13:150, 1990.
43. Anagnostopoulos, C.E., Prabahakar, M.J.S., and Little, C.F.: Aortic dissections and dissecting aneurysms. Am. J. Cardiol. 30:263, 1972.
44. DeBakey, M., Henley, W., and Cooley, D.: Surgical management of dissecting aneurysms of the aorta. J. Thorac. Cardiovasc. Surg. 49:130, 1965.
45. DeBakey, M., Cooley, D.A., and Creech, O.J.: Surgical considerations of dissecting aneurysm of the aorta. Ann. Surg. 142:586, 1955.

46. Daily, P.O., Trueblood, H.W., Stinson, E.B., et al.: Management of acute aortic dissections. Ann. Thorac. Surg. 10:237, 1970.
47. Yamada, T., Tada, S., and Harada, J.: Aortic dissection without intimal rupture: Diagnosis with MR imaging and CT. Radiology 168:347, 1988.
48. Roberts, W.C.: Aortic dissection: Anatomy, consequences, and causes. Am. Heart J. 101:195, 1981.
49. Kersting-Sommerhoff, B.A., Higgins, C.B., White, R.D., et al.: Aortic dissection: Sensitivity and specificity of MR imaging. Radiology 166:651, 1988.
50. Amparo, E.G., Higgins, C.B., Hoddick, W., et al.: Aortic dissection: Magnetic resonance imaging. Radiology 155:399, 1985.
51. Dinsmore, R.E., Wedeen, V.J., Miller, S.W., et al.: MRI of dissection of the aorta: Recognition of the intimal tear and differential flow velocities. AJR 146:634, 1987.
52. Geisinger, M.A., Risius, B., O'Donnell, J.A., et al.: Thoracic aortic dissections: Magnetic resonance imaging. Radiology 155:407, 1985.
53. Underwood, S.R., Firmin, D.N., Klipstein, R.H., et al.: Magnetic resonance velocity mapping: Clinical application of a new technique. Br. Heart J. 57:404, 1987.
54. Von Schulthess, G.K., and Augustiny, N.: Calculation of T2 values versus phase imaging for the distinction between flow and thrombus in MR imaging. Radiology 164:549, 1987.
55. White, E.M., Edelman, R.R., Wedeen, V.J., et al.: Intravascular signal in MR imaging: Use of phase display for differentiation of blood-flow signal from intraluminal disease. Radiology 161:245, 1986.
56. Nienaber, C.A., von Kodolitsch, Y., Nicolaws, V., et al.: The diagnosis of thoracic aortic dissection of noninvasive imaging procedures. N. Engl. J. Med. 328:1, 1993.
57. White, R.D., Ullyot, D.J., and Higgins, C.B.: MR imaging of the aorta after surgery for aortic dissection. AJR 150:87, 1988.
58. Auffermann, W., Olofsson, P., Stancy, R., et al.: MR imaging of complications of aortic surgery. J. Comput. Assist. Tomogr. 11:982, 1987.
59. Joyce, J.W., Fairbairn, J.F., Kincaid, O.W., et al.: Aneurysms of the thoracic aorta: A clinical study with special reference to prognosis. Circulation 29:176, 1964.
60. Amparo, E.G., Higgins, C.B., Hoddick, W.K., et al.: Magnetic resonance imaging of aortic disease: Preliminary results. AJR 143:1203, 1984.
61. Dinsmore, R.E., Liberthson, R.R., Wismer, G.L., et al.: Magnetic resonance imaging of thoracic aortic aneurysms: Comparison with other imaging methods. AJR 146:309, 1986.
62. Dinsmore, R.E., Wedeen, V.J., Rosen, B., et al.: Phase-offset technique to distinguish slow blood flow and thrombus on MR images. AJR 148:634, 1987.
63. Miller, D.L., Reinig, J.W., and Volkman, D.J.: Vascular imaging with MRI: Inadequacy in Takayasu's arteritis compared with angiography. AJR 146:949, 1986.
64. Cheitlin, M.: Valvular heart disease: Management and intervention. Circulation 84(Suppl):259, 1991.
65. Cranney, G., Lotan, C., and Pohost, G.: Nuclear magnetic resonance imaging for assessment and follow-up of patients with valve disease. Circulation 84(Suppl I):216, 1991.
66. Higgins, C., Wagner, S., Kondo, C., et al.: Evaluation of valvular heart disease with cine gradient echo magnetic resonance imaging. Circulation 84(Suppl I):198, 1991.
67. Burbank, S., Parrish, D., and Wexler, L.: Echocardiographic-like angled views of the heart by MR imaging. J. Comput. Assist. Tomogr. 12:181, 1988.
68. Atkinson, D., and Edelman, R.: Cineangiography of the heart in a single breath hold with a segmented turboFLASH sequence. Radiology 178:357, 1991.
69. Mirowitz, S., Lee, J.K.-T., Gutierrez, F., et al.: Normal signal-void patterns in cardiac cine MR imaging. Radiology 176:49, 1990.
70. Utz, J., Herfekens, R., Heinsimer, J., et al.: Valvular regurgitation: Dynamic MR imaging. Radiology 168:91, 1988.
71. Spielman, R.P., Schneider, O., Thiele, F., et al.: Appearance of poststenotic jets in MRI: Dependence on flow velocity and on imaging parameters. Magn. Reson. Imaging 9:67, 1991.
72. Suzuki, J.-I., Caputo, G., Kondo, C., et al.: Cine MR imaging of valvular heart disease: Display and imaging parameters affect the size of the signal void caused by valvular regurgitation. AJR 155:723, 1990.
73. Globits, S., Frank, H., Mayr, H., et al.: Quantitative assessment of aortic regurgitation by magnetic resonance imaging. Eur. Heart J. 13:78, 1992.
74. Debatin, J., Nagel, S., Sostman, H., et al.: Magnetic resonance imaging: Cardiac ejection fraction measurements. Phantom study comparing four different methods. Invest. Radiol. 27:198, 1992.
75. Doherty, N., Fujita, N., Caputo, G., et al.: Measurement of right ventricular mass in normal and dilated cardiomyopathic ventricles using cine MRI. Am. J. Cardiol. 69:1223, 1992.
76. Dulce, M.C., Mostbeck, G.H., Friese, K.K., et al.: Quantification of the left ventricular volumes and function with cine MR imaging: Comparison of geometric models with three-dimensional data. Radiology 188:371, 1993.
77. Sechtem, U., Pflugfelder, P., Gould, R., et al.: Measurements of right and left ventricular volumes in healthy individuals with cine MR imaging. Radiology 163:697, 1987.
78. Semelka, R., Tomei, E., Wagner, S., et al.: Normal left ventricular dimensions and function: Interstudy reproducibility of measurements with cine MR imaging. Radiology 174:763, 1990.
79. Utz, J.A., Herfkens, R.J., Heinsimer, J.A., et al.: Cine MR determination of left ventricular ejection fraction. AJR 148:839, 1987.
80. Van Rossum, A.C., Visser, F.C., Sprenger, M., et al.: Evaluation of magnetic resonance imaging for determination of left ventricular ejection fraction and comparison with angiography. Am. J. Cardiol. 62:628, 1988.
81. Mohiaddin, R.A., Amanuma, M., Kilner, P.J., et al.: MR phase-shift velocity mapping of mitral and pulmonary venous flow. J. Comput. Assist. Tomogr. 15:237, 1991.
82. Dulce, M., Mostbeck, G., O'Sullivan, M., et al.: Severity of aortic regurgitation: Interstudy reproducibility of measurements with velocity-encoded MR imaging. Radiology 185:235, 1992.
83. Honda, N., Machida, K., Hashimoto, M., et al.: Aortic regurgitation: Quantitation with MR imaging velocity mapping. Radiology 186:189, 1993.
84. Sondergaard, L., Thomsen, C., Stahlberg, F., et al.: Mitral and aortic valvular flow: Quantification with magnetic resonance phase mapping. J. Magn. Reson. Imaging 2:295, 1992.
85. Casolo, G.C., Zampa, V., Rega, L., et al.: Evaluation of mitral stenosis by cine magnetic resonance imaging. Am. Heart J. 123:1252, 1992.
86. deRoos, A., Reichek, N., Axel, L., et al.: Cine MR imaging in aortic stenosis. J. Comput. Assist. Tomogr. 13:421, 1989.
87. Kilner, P.J., Firmin, D.N., Rees, R.S.O., et al.: Valve and great vessel stenosis: Assessment with MR jet velocity mapping. Radiology 178:229, 1991.
88. Kilner, P.J., Monzara, C.C., Mohiuddin, R.H., et al.: Magnetic resonance jet velocity mapping in mitral and aortic valve stenosis. Circulation 87:1239, 1993.
89. Caputo, G., Suzuki, J.-I., Kondo, C., et al.: Determination of left ventricular volume and mass with use of biphasic spin-echo MR imaging: Comparison with cine MR. Radiology 177:773, 1990.
90. Shapiro, E., Rogers, W., Beyer, R., et al.: Determination of left ventricular mass by nuclear magnetic resonance imaging in hearts deformed by acute infarction. Circulation 79:706, 1989.
91. Edwards, J.E.: Classification of congenital heart disease in the adult. *In* Roberts, W.C. (ed.): Congenital Heart Disease in Adults. (Cardiovasc. Clin. Sciences 10/1). Philadelphia, F.A. Davis, 1979, p. 1.
92. Lucas, R.V., Jr., Varco, R.L., Lillehei, C.W., et al.: Anomalous muscle bundle of the right ventricle: Hemodynamic consequences and surgical considerations. Circulation 25:443, 1962.
93. Mitchell, S.C., Korones, S.B., Berendes, H.W.: Congenital heart disease in 56,109 births: Incidence and natural history. Circulation 43:323, 1971.
94. Hoffman, J.I.E., and Christianson, R.: Congenital heart disease in a cohort of 19,502 births with long-term follow up. Am. J. Cardiol. 42:641, 1978.
95. Lev, M., Liberthson, R.R., Joseph, R.H., et al.: The pathologic anatomy of Ebstein's disease. Arch. Pathol. 90:334, 1970.
96. Link, K.M., Herrera, M.A., D'Souza, V.J., and Formanek, A.G.: MR Imaging of Ebstein anomaly: Results in four cases. AJR 150:363, 1988.
97. Bharati, S., and Lev, M.: Congenital poly-valvular disease. Circulation 47:575, 1973.
98. Becker, A.E., Becker, M.J., and Edwards, J.E.: Pathologic spectrum of dysplasia of the tricuspid valve: Features in common with Ebstein's malformations. Arch. Pathol. 91:167, 1971.
99. Perloff, J.K., and Harvey, W.P.: Clinical recognition of tricuspid stenosis. Circulation 22:346, 1960.
100. Flammang, D., Juamin, P., and Kremer, R.: Organic tricuspid pathology in rheumatic valvulopathies. Acta Cardiol. 30:155, 1975.
101. Buchbinder, N.A., and Roberts, W.C.: Left-sided valvular active infective endocarditis: A study of forty-five necropsy patients. Am. J. Med. 53:20, 1972.
102. Bonnabeau, R.V. Jr., Stevenson, J.E., and Edwards, J.E.: Obliteration of the principal orifice of the stenotic mitral valve: A rare form of "re-stenosis." J. Thorac. Cardiovasc. Surg. 49:264, 1965.
103. Selzer, A., and Cohn, K.E.: Natural history of mitral stenosis: A review. Circulation 45:878, 1972.
104. Levy, M.J., and Edwards, J.E.: Anatomy of mitral insufficiency. Prog. Cardiovasc. Dis. 5:119, 1962.
105. Vlodaver, Z., and Edwards, J.E.: Rupture of ventricular septum or papillary muscle complicating myocardial infarction. Circulation 55:815, 1977.
106. Barlow, J.B., and Pocock, W.A.: The problem of nonejection systolic clicks and associated mitral systolic murmurs: Emphasis on the billowing mitral leaflet syndrome. Am. Heart J. 90:636, 1975.
107. Guthrie, R.G., and Edwards, J.E.: Pathology of the myxomatous mitral valve: Its nature, secondary changes and complications. Minn. Med. 59:637, 1976.
108. Rackley, C.E., and Hood, W.P. Jr.: Quantitative angiographic evaluation and pathophysiologic mechanisms in valvular heart disease. *In* Sonnenblick, E. J., and Lesch, M. (eds.): Valvular Heart Disease. New York, Grune & Stratton, 1975, p. 109.

CHAPTER

48 Magnetic Resonance Imaging Assessment of Ischemic Heart Disease

Warren J. Manning, M.D.
Robert R. Edelman, M.D.

Despite advances in both prevention and treatment, ischemic heart disease caused by coronary atherosclerosis remains a leading cause of morbidity and mortality in the western world. In the United States, more than a million myocardial infarctions and almost 600,000 deaths are attributed to coronary artery disease each year.[1] Magnetic resonance imaging (MRI), with its ability to acquire both static and dynamic images of the heart in double-oblique, true tomographic planes, offers a unique opportunity to provide a comprehensive, noninvasive cardiac evaluation of the patient with known or suspected coronary artery disease. Although the clinical potential of MRI for evaluation of the cardiovascular system has been recognized for more than a decade, the method was technically limited for many years because of the requirement for electrocardiographic (ECG) gating and lengthy acquisition times, often longer than 60 minutes to acquire complete anatomical or functional images of the heart. Despite this limitation, cardiovascular applications of MRI in patients with known or suspected coronary artery disease have increased considerably over the past 10 years. Many of these applications overlap those of more conventional and currently more cost-effective imaging technologies, such as echocardiography and radionuclide perfusion imaging or ventriculography. MRI, however, offers several unique features not available with these competing techniques, including superior spatial resolution, the capacity for three-dimensional imaging of cardiac function and perfusion, quantitative evaluation of valvular function, and noninvasive coronary angiography.

Since the first edition of this text, rapid MRI cardiac imaging techniques have been developed, including breath-hold K-space segmentation techniques, during which complete ECG-gated images are obtained in less than 20 seconds, and MRI echo planar imaging (EPI) of the heart, during which data for an entire image is acquired in less than 100 msec.[2] These faster imaging techniques have allowed for the further evolution of MRI applications in the evaluation of ischemic heart disease, including assessment of regional myocardial perfusion and noninvasive magnetic resonance coronary angiography (MRCA).

Although the development of MRI applications for the evaluation of ischemic heart disease continues to advance rapidly, clinically accepted MRI applications remain to be defined. Better hardware and software must be developed for both data acquisition and analysis. Validation of the utility and cost-effectiveness of these cardiac MRI applications in large, double-blind, multicenter trials also needs to be done. Nevertheless, the unique noninvasive and flexible attributes of MRI will probably make cardiac MRI the diagnostic technique of choice for the evaluation of patients with known or suspected ischemic heart disease.

IDENTIFICATION AND QUANTIFICATION OF ACUTE MYOCARDIAL INFARCTION

Noncontrast Animal Studies of Infarction

Investigators have capitalized on differences in T1 and T2 relaxation times between viable and infarcted myocardium (and resultant signal changes) to identify and quantify the size of myocardial infarctions by MRI. Early investigations of cardiovascular applications of MRI focused on models of acute myocardial infarction, a condition in which local edema leads to changes in T1 and T2 relaxation times, recognizable as regional signal intensity changes on ECG-gated spin-echo images. In 1980, Williams and colleagues[3] studied a canine model of myocardial infarction and reported that T1 relaxation times are increased after 30 minutes of coronary occlusion. Subsequent canine MRI studies by Higgins and colleagues[4] demonstrated that regional myocardium with acute infarction resulted in prolongation of both T1 and T2 relaxation times. These changes were detected 3 to 6 hours after coronary occlusion, with maximal contrast between normal and infarcted myocardium present approximately 4 hours after coronary occlusion (Fig. 48–1). Canine studies have also demonstrated increased signal intensity corresponding to the site of infarction on T2-weighted images,[5,6] with enhanced signal persisting for up to 3 weeks after coronary occlusion.[7] Similar findings of prolonged T2 relaxation have also been reported in a swine model of chronic infarction by Checkley and co-workers.[8]

Serial changes in T1 and T2 in a nonreperfused canine model of infarction were reported by Tscholakoff and colleagues.[9] These investigators found an initial increase in T1 at 5 minutes after occlusion, with a subsequent decrease in T1 relaxation time over the succeeding 5 hours of observation (Table 48–1). Four to fourteen days after infarction, T1 measurements were again greater than baseline. T2 measurements demonstrated a progressive increase in the area of infarction (Table 48–2). Initial hypoperfusion, followed by evolving edema in the infarct and the surrounding region, probably plays a significant role in producing the transient changes in T1 and T2 relaxation times.

Canine studies of varying durations of occlusion, either with or without reperfusion, showed that T1 changes did not correlate well with infarct zone until 3 weeks after occlusion, again highlighting the complex nature of changes in relaxation times during acute infarction[10] with resulting edema and cellular necrosis. Quantification of infarct size based on changes in T2 relaxation rates has been more successful. With the use of a 6-hour canine model of infarction, Rokey and colleagues[11] found prolongation of T2 relaxation in the area of infarction, with good correlation between MRI and triphenyltetrazolium chloride (TTC) estimates of infarct size over the range of 3 to 29 percent of left ventricular mass. Bouchard and colleagues,[12] using a closed-chest canine model of infarction with both in vivo and ex vivo T2-weighted MRI 1 week after infarction, found a good correlation between MRI estimate of infarct size and the results of radiolabeled microsphere injection, although both MRI studies resulted in a slight overestimation. Johnston and co-workers[13] studied serial changes in T2 relaxation over a 6-month period in a rabbit model of infarction and found that quantitation of infarct size based on changes in T2 relaxation measured 3 and 21 days after coronary ligation had a good correlation with histopathology. Caputo and colleagues[14] also obtained very accurate measurements with a canine coronary occlusion infarct model in animals subjected to anterior wall infarcts 3 to 21 days before MRI study. Infarct size did not change on T2-weighted images between the third and 21st day of study.

Particularly intriguing are animal data demonstrating that hypokinetic reperfused viable myocardium may be differentiated from hypokinetic reperfused infarcted myocardium. Ryan and colleagues[15] reported on 16 mongrel dogs who underwent transient occlusion of the left anterior descending artery or a diagonal artery for 30, 60, or 180 minutes, followed by reperfusion, and were examined by spin-echo MRI 12 to 14 hours later. Comparison was made with two-dimensional echocardiography and histology. All animals had depressed wall thickening and abnormal wall motion by two-dimensional echocardiography. Seven of eight dogs with histologic evidence of infarction had an increased signal intensity corresponding to the area of infarction, with MRI data overestimating the size of the infarct in the seven abnormal MRI studies (Fig.

TABLE 48–1. T1 RELAXATION TIMES (MSEC) OF INFARCTED MYOCARDIUM (ANTERIOR) AND NORMAL MYOCARDIUM (POSTERIOR)

Time After Occlusion	Anterior		Posterior	
	Mean	*SD*	*Mean*	*SD*
Preocclusion	613.5	165.9	681.5	237.2
5 min	831.2	367.1	703.2	254.1
30 min	790.5	366.8	746.2	492.2
1 hr	771.8	437.9	689.1	219.6
2 hr	617.7	250.5	631.8	285.2
3 hr	632.1	342.4	650.0	308.1
4 hr	649.3	192.5	565.0	143.0
5 hr	573.0	133.1	613.7	296.4
4–14 days	704.7	220.8	751.5	163.0

SD = standard deviation.
From Tscholakoff, D., et al.: Early-phase myocardial infarction evaluation by MR imaging. Radiology 159:667, 1986, with permission.

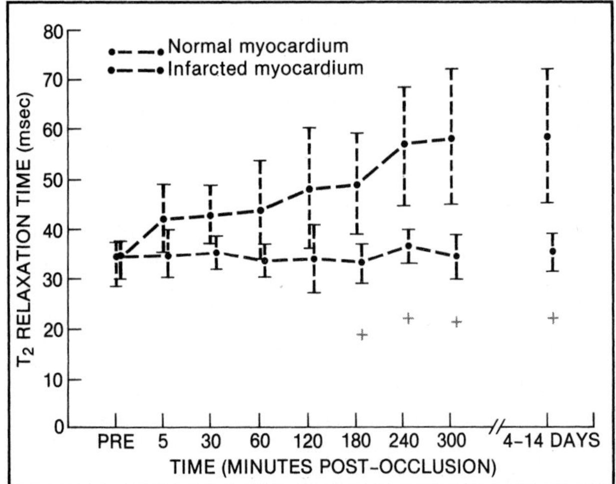

FIGURE 48–1. Mean T2 relaxation times for normal and infarcted myocardium during the first 6 hours and at several days after acute occlusion of the left anterior descending coronary artery. Significant increases in T2 relaxation time of infarcted myocardium were present at 3 hours after occlusion. Crosses indicate the time intervals during which there were significant differences between normal and infarcted myocardium. (From Higgins, C.B.: Overview of MR of the heart—1986. AJR 146[3]:907–918, 1986, with permission.)

TABLE 48–2. T2 RELAXATION TIMES (MSEC) OF INFARCTED MYOCARDIUM (ANTERIOR) AND NORMAL MYOCARDIUM (POSTERIOR)

Time After Occlusion	Anterior		Posterior	
	Mean	*SD*	*Mean*	*SD*
Preocclusion	33.3	4.6	34.1	3.8
5 min	42.3	6.9	35.2	5.0
30 min	43.2	5.6	35.4	3.5
1 hr	44.0	9.8	34.0	3.3
2 hr	48.3	11.8	34.3	6.8
3 hr*	49.2	9.9	33.6	3.7
4 hr*	57.1	11.6	37.1	3.3
5 hr*	58.8	13.6	35.0	4.4
4–14 days*	59.0	13.1	36.0	3.6

SD = standard deviation.
*$P < .01$.
From Tscholakoff, D., et al.: Early-phase myocardial infarction evaluation by MR imaging. Radiology 159:667, 1986, with permission.

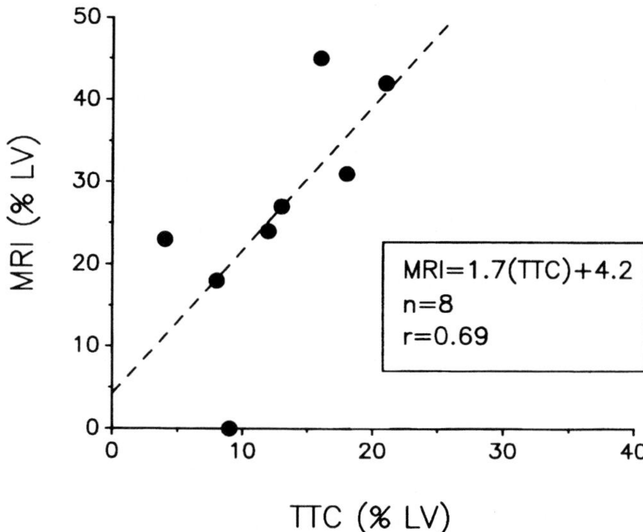

FIGURE 48–2. Infarct size versus extent of increased signal intensity. Infarct size is presented as a percentage of left ventricular (LV) mass as determined by triphenyltetrazolium chloride staining of short-axis slices. The size of the area of increased signal intensity was measured by planimetry of corresponding short-axis, TE 60-msec images. Despite the positive correlation, significant overestimation by magnetic resonance imaging is apparent. If the dog with the false-negative magnetic resonance imaging result is excluded, the degree of overestimation is approximately 12 percent. (From Ryan, T., Tarver, R.D., Duerk, J.L., et al.: Distinguishing viable from infarcted myocardium after experimental ischemia and reperfusion by using nuclear magnetic resonance imaging. J. Am. Coll. Cardiol. 15:1362, 1990. Reprinted with permission from the American College of Cardiology.)

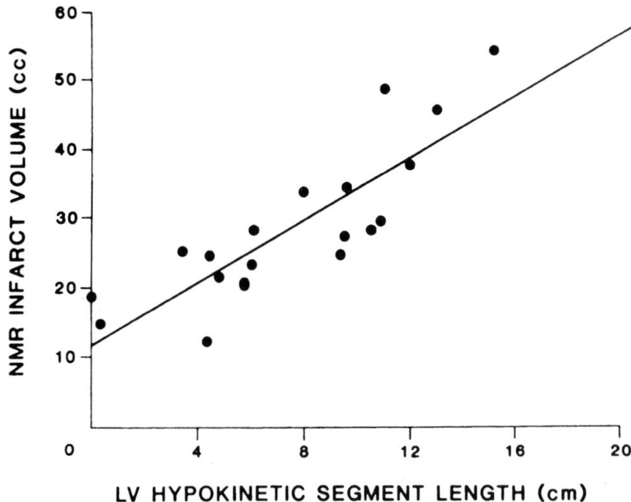

FIGURE 48–3. Correlation between the infarct volume computed by magnetic resonance imaging and the quantitative left ventricular (LV) hypokinetic segment length. (From Johns, J.A., Leavitt, M.B., Newell, J.B., et al.: Quantitation of acute myocardial infarct size by nuclear magnetic resonance imaging. J. Am. Coll. Cardiol. 15:148, 1990. Reprinted with permission from the American College of Cardiology.)

48–2). None of the eight dogs without infarction had visually apparent change in signal intensity, despite regional systolic dysfunction documented by echocardiography. If these data, with or without the use of a contrast agent, can be confirmed in human studies, they would offer the potential for infarct quantification among patients presenting with acute ischemia who undergo treatment with thrombolysis or angioplasty. MRI may allow for differentiation between infarcted and stunned myocardium in this population.

Noncontrast Human Studies of Infarction

Studies in patients with acute myocardial infarction have also demonstrated enhanced signal intensity with prolongation of T1 and T2 relaxation times in the area of infarction. McNamara and colleagues[16] studied nine patients 5 to 12 days after acute infarction and reported T2 prolongation and increased signal intensity within the infarct zone. A subsequent study by this same group[17] in a series of 29 patients confirmed the prior findings but also reported that increased myocardial signal intensity on T2-weighted images may be difficult to differentiate from slowly moving intraventricular blood flow immediately adjacent to the infarct zone. In the healthy heart, rapidly moving blood within the left ventricular cavity produces little or no signal on spin-echo imaging because of egress of excited protons out of the imaging plane between initial proton stimulation and subsequent data acquisition. Such rapid blood flow may not occur in areas adjacent to severely hypokinetic or akinetic myocardium, and the result is a more intense signal, similar to that of stationary blood.[18]

Postema and co-workers[19] compared thallium perfusion defects and regional T2 prolongation among 20 patients studied 8 days after acute myocardial infarction. These investigators found a good correlation in more than 80 percent of subjects. Johns and col-

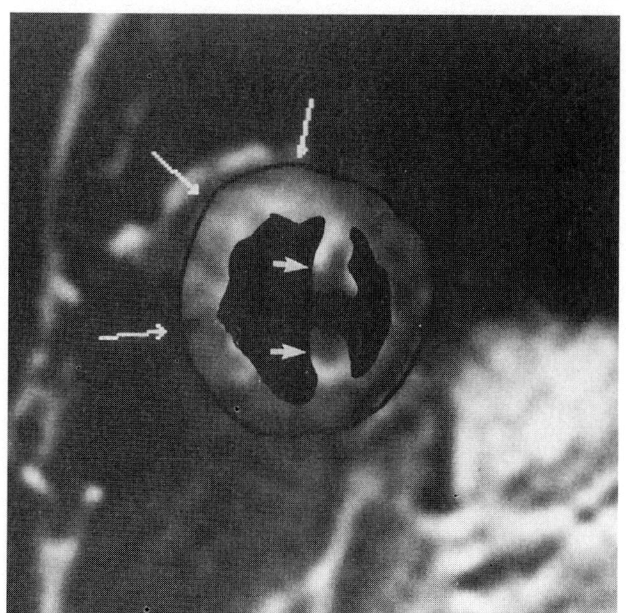

FIGURE 48–4. Anterior and septal wall infarction *(long arrows)*. There is a heterogeneous increase in signal intensity in both papillary muscles *(short arrows)*. (From Johnston, D.L., Wendt, R.E., III, Mulvagh, S.L., et al.: Characterization of acute myocardial infarction by magnetic resonance imaging. Am. J. Cardiol. 69:1294, 1992, with permission.)

leagues[20] studied 20 patients 9 days after acute infarction and reported a very good correlation between increased signal intensity and regional wall motion abnormalities on left ventriculography. There was also a good correlation between infarct volume and quantitated left ventricular hypokinetic segment (Fig. 48–3). Johnston and colleagues[21] studied 18 patients, 3 to 30 days after infarction, with ECG-gated spin-echo MRI. The images were satisfactory in 14 (78 percent) of the 18, and all demonstrated an increase in myocardial signal intensity consistent with acute myocardial infarction; in contrast, increased signal intensity was found in only 1 of 9 volunteers. Krauss and co-workers[22] studied 19 patients with acute infarction at discharge and 13 of these 4 to 7 months later. They found that the site and size of the infarct did not change in 77 percent of patients at both intervals, and T2 relaxation times remained prolonged, particularly among patients with anterior infarctions. More recently, Johnston and colleagues[23] reported on 17 acute myocardial infarction patients and 6 normal subjects studied with spin-echo MRI. The location of the infarction was identified in all patients, with near-doubling of the mean myocardial signal intensity in the area of the infarction. Patients often had a mixture of transmural and nontransmural injury (Fig. 48–4). Heterogeneous distribution of signal intensity within the infarction suggested the presence of hemorrhage.

Although these data are encouraging, other reports suggest the technique may not be as robust as initially suggested. Ahmad and colleagues,[24] in a study of 26 patients with unstable angina, acute myocardial infarction, and stable angina, showed that regional T2 prolongation was similar in both unstable angina and acute myocardial infarction, suggesting that such a finding may not be specific for myocardial infarction. Filipchuk and colleagues[25] reported spin-echo MRI data on 45 patients, including 27 patients studied 2 weeks after acute infarction and 18 asymptomatic volunteers. In this blinded study, these investigators found increased signal intensity in 88 percent of patients with infarction, but they also found focal areas of increased myocardial signal in 83 percent of asymptomatic volunteers. Regional wall thinning was seen in 67 percent of patients with infarction but in only 11 percent of volunteers. They concluded that wall thinning was the more predictive and specific indication of acute myocardial infarction.

Wisenberg and co-workers[26] performed MRI studies 3 weeks after infarction in 66 patients presenting with symptoms of acute myocardial infarction and randomly assigned to receive thrombolytic therapy with streptokinase or placebo. Although both groups had similar peak creatine kinase values and similar resting and exercise ejection fractions, there was a significant reduction in infarct volume, as measured by magnetic resonance imaging, for the streptokinase group.

Role of Magnetic Resonance Contrast Agents—Animal Studies

Administration of paramagnetic MRI contrast agents such as gadolinium–diethylenetriamine penta-acetic acid (Gd-DTPA) has been shown to improve contrast enhancement and thereby allow for better definition of infarcted myocardium. The utility of contrast-enhanced MRI has been studied in many animal models of coronary artery occlusion and ischemia with the use of agents such as Gd-DTPA, manganese gluconate, ferritic particles, or dysprosium (see Chapter 44). Although numerous MRI contrast agents

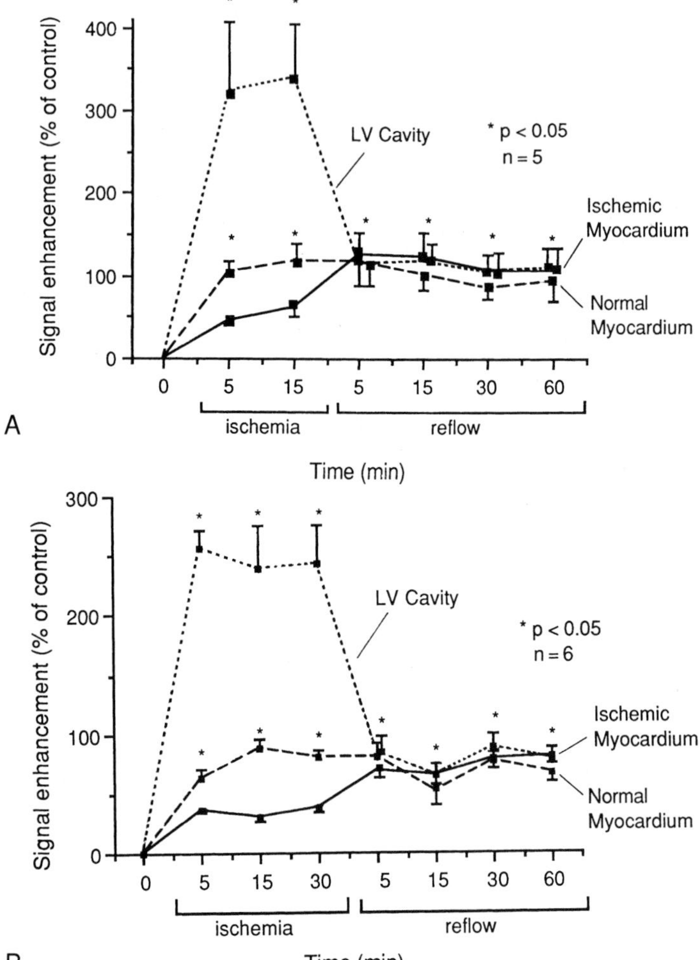

FIGURE 48–5. Magnetic resonance imaging enhancement of ischemic and nonischemic myocardium on T1-weighted images during various periods of ischemia and reperfusion. *A*, Sixteen minutes of ischemia followed by 60 minutes of reperfusion. Albumin–gadolinium–diethylenetriamine penta-acetic acid (albumin–Gd-DTPA) was given immediately after onset of ischemia. There was significant enhancement of normally perfused myocardium during ischemia. Ischemic myocardium was not significantly enhanced. There was marked enhancement within the left ventricular (LV) cavity adjacent to ischemic myocardium during coronary occlusion. After reflow, ischemic and nonischemic zones had uniform enhancement. *B*, Thirty minutes of ischemia followed by 60 minutes of reperfusion. Normal myocardium was enhanced significantly during coronary occlusion, whereas ischemic myocardium was not. The LV cavity adjacent to ischemic myocardium showed marked enhancement during coronary occlusion. After reflow, enhancement of ischemic and nonischemic myocardium was uniform.

have been investigated, most contrast media consist of paramagnetic ions such as gadolinium (Gd), dysprosium (Dy), or manganese (Mn). Of these MRI contrast agents, Gd-DTPA has received the most attention, and it has been approved by the U.S. Food and Drug Administration for human use. Gd-DTPA is rapidly cleared from normally perfused tissues, with 50 percent first-pass clearance. However, although Gd-DTPA is an extracellular agent with a tissue distribution similar to that of conventional iodinated contrast agents, there is a very complex and nonlinear relation between MRI regional signal intensity and local Gd-DTPA concentration.[27] Accumulation of Gd-DTPA in tissue depends not only on perfusion but also on the size of the interstitial space and surrounding edema. Both T1 and T2 relaxation times are shortened by Gd-DTPA in ischemic myocardium after experimental coronary artery occlusion. The effect on T1 relaxation time predominates at lower concentrations, with T1-weighted images demonstrating enhanced signal intensity in ischemic myocardium after Gd-DTPA administration.

Nishimura and colleagues[28] measured infarct size by MRI 24 hours after ligation of the left anterior descending coronary artery, using 0.5 mmol/kg Gd-DTPA, and compared the results with those obtained with the use of indium-111–labeled antimyosin. They found significant contrast enhancement within the infarct zone on MRI, though MRI data slightly overestimated indium-111 infarct size.

Wesbey and co-workers[29] subjected dogs to 24-hour coronary occlusions followed by Gd-DTPA injection. Ninety seconds after injection of 0.35 mmol/kg of Gd-DTPA, lower T1 and T2 relaxation times were found in normal myocardium, but there was minimal effect in infarcted regions. Five minutes after injection, however, Gd-DTPA had largely "washed out" of normal myocardium, and lower T1 relaxation times were then seen in the infarcted regions. Lesser effects were noted on T2 relaxation rate between normal and infarcted regions.

Finally, Wolfe and colleagues[30] reported on the use of albumin–Gd-DTPA, a macromolecular paramagnetic contrast agent largely confined to the intravascular space, in a rat model of reversible and irreversible myocardial injury, using a T1-weighted spin-echo sequence (Fig. 48–5). After 16 or 30 minutes of ischemia followed by reflow, they found uniform MRI signal intensity in both ischemic and normal (control) myocardium, and TTC staining revealed only small, nontransmural myocardial infarction in 2 of 11 of these hearts. In contrast, hearts subjected to 60 or 90 minutes of ischemia followed by reflow demonstrated marked enhancement of the ischemic zone compared with control regions, and transmural infarction was demonstrated in all these hearts by TTC staining. The data suggest that signal enhancement produced by intravascular agents such as albumin–Gd-DTPA, compared with extracellular agents such as Gd-DTPA, may be related to capillary permeability.

Role of Magnetic Resonance Contrast Agents—Human Studies

Although changes in T1 and T2 associated with edema and infarction should provide "natural" MRI contrast sufficient to delineate areas of infarction, the use of an MRI contrast agent has been studied as a means of improving the sensitivity of MRI for detection of infarction in humans. Gd-DTPA appears to be most beneficial in myocardial infarction if the patient is studied within the first few weeks after infarction. This result is probably related to the extensive edema that is initially present in the infarct zone, which is subsequently replaced by fibrosis and scar tissue.

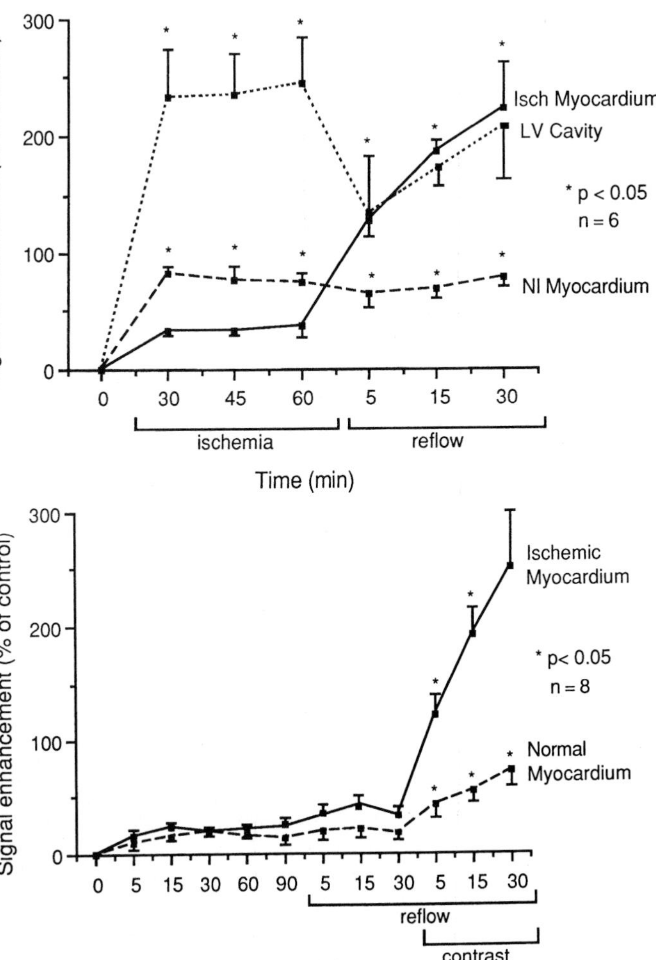

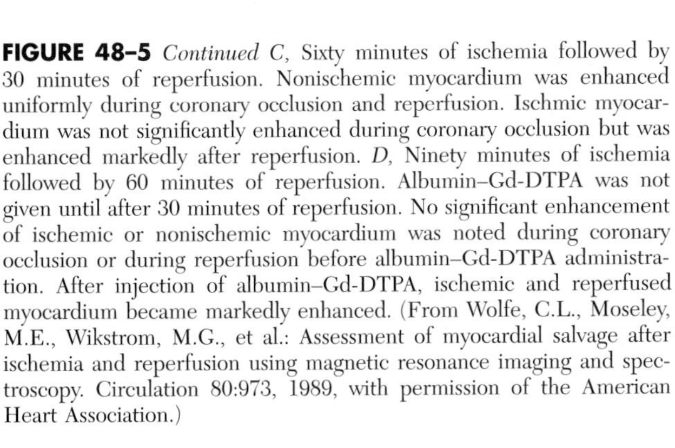

FIGURE 48–5 *Continued C,* Sixty minutes of ischemia followed by 30 minutes of reperfusion. Nonischemic myocardium was enhanced uniformly during coronary occlusion and reperfusion. Ischmic myocardium was not significantly enhanced during coronary occlusion but was enhanced markedly after reperfusion. *D,* Ninety minutes of ischemia followed by 60 minutes of reperfusion. Albumin–Gd-DTPA was not given until after 30 minutes of reperfusion. No significant enhancement of ischemic or nonischemic myocardium was noted during coronary occlusion or during reperfusion before albumin–Gd-DTPA administration. After injection of albumin–Gd-DTPA, ischemic and reperfused myocardium became markedly enhanced. (From Wolfe, C.L., Moseley, M.E., Wikstrom, M.G., et al.: Assessment of myocardial salvage after ischemia and reperfusion using magnetic resonance imaging and spectroscopy. Circulation 80:973, 1989, with permission of the American Heart Association.)

Van Dijkman and colleagues[31] studied 20 patients with acute myocardial infarction at baseline and at 10, 20, 30, and 40 minutes after injection of intravenous Gd-DTPA. These investigators found maximal contrast enhancement of infarcted myocardium approximately 20 minutes after Gd-DTPA injection. Van Dijkman and colleagues[32] subsequently reported on 84 patients studied at less than 1 week, 1 to 6 weeks, or more than 6 weeks after myocardial infarction with Gd-DTPA–enhanced MRI. They found that Gd-DTPA improved spin-echo MRI visualization of myocardial infarctions in more than 80 percent of patients examined less than 1 week after infarction, but in only 50 to 60 percent of those studied 1 to 6 weeks later, and in only a small minority (12 percent) of those studied more than 6 weeks after infarction. In a more recent report from this group,[33] in which 24 patients were studied 4 days after their first myocardial infarction with administration of 0.15 mmol/kg Gd-DTPA and T1-weighted spin-echo MRI, an excellent correlation was found with infarct size as assessed by serum α-hydroxybutyrate dehydrogenase.

Eichstaedt and co-workers[34] described the use of Gd-DTPA in 26 patients after acute (5 to 10 days), subacute (10 to 21 days), or chronic (more than 21 days) infarction and unsuccessful acute revascularization. Images were obtained immediately after injection of 0.1 to 0.2 mmol/kg Gd-DTPA and at 10, 25, and 45 minutes. They found a 70 percent enhancement of infarcted tissue in the acute infarction group (versus 20 percent for normal tissue). No difference was found in signal intensity between normal and infarcted tissue in the chronic infarction group. An intermediate, nonsignificant result was noted in the subacute group, possibly related to the small sample size (n = 3). These data were corroborated by Nishimura and colleagues,[35] who studied 17 patients at 5, 12, 30, and 90 days after acute infarction. Increased signal intensity corresponding to the infarct zone was seen at 5 and at 12 days, but not on later studies. These data are consistent with the previously mentioned hypothesis that the contrast-enhancing effect of Gd-DTPA is related to the increase in extracellular volume associated with edema at the site of infarction and subsequent delayed washout of Gd-DTPA. As the edema declines and the infarcted myocardium is replaced by fibrous scar, contrast enhancement is minimized.

In contrast to the aforementioned studies, de Roos and colleagues[36] reported on 45 patients with suspected acute myocardial infarction who received thrombolytic therapy and underwent coronary angiography. MRI was performed before and up to 30 minutes after administration of 0.1 mmol/kg of Gd-DTPA. These investigators found that signal intensity ratios increased between normal myocardium and both reperfused and nonreperfused myocardium. There was substantial overlap between groups, suggesting that Gd-DTPA–enhanced MRI did not differentiate between reperfused and nonreperfused infarcted tissue.

These studies all employed conventional, ECG-gated spin-echo imaging sequences, which typically require several minutes to acquire. These averaged or "steady-state" techniques fail to provide dynamic information. Gradient-echo MRI sequences, in which a complete ECG-gated image is acquired in less than 1 second (turboFLASH), have now been developed. Although lower in spatial resolution, these sequences permit sequential ECG imaging (every 2 to 4 heartbeats) during first passage of Gd-DTPA.[37] Because Gd-DTPA is a T1 agent at low concentrations, a 180-degree prepulse is typically applied to make the sequence T1-weighted and to null the signal from unenhanced myocardium (see section on myocardial perfusion techniques). Van Rugge and colleagues[38] studied 19 patients with chronic myocardial infarction at baseline, all of whom had evidence of regional wall motion abnormalities by two-dimensional echocardiography. TurboFLASH MRI was performed with the patient at rest after intravenous injection of 0.04 mmol/kg Gd-DTPA with single-level, short-axis imaging. After Gd-DTPA injection, there was progressive signal enhancement in both infarcted and normal myocardium (Figs. 48–6 and 48–7), with significantly faster and greater enhancement of normal myocardium compared with infarcted regions.

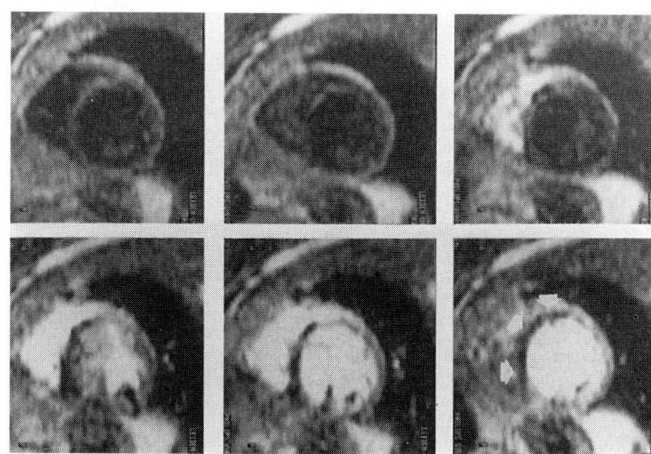

FIGURE 48–6. Series of six sequential, ultrafast, short-axis magnetic resonance images after bolus administration of gadolinium–diethylenetriamine penta-acetic acid (Gd-DTPA) in a patient with a healed myocardial infarction of the anteroseptal wall. Ultimately, a decreased signal intensity is observed in the infarcted anteroseptal myocardial area *(arrows)*, compared with the normal posterolateral region. (From van Rugge, F.P., van der Wall, E.E., van Dijkman, P.R.M., et al.: Usefulness of ultrafast magnetic resonance imaging in healed myocardial infarction. Am. J. Cardiol. 70:1235–1236, 1992, with permission.)

Finally, MRI in combination with Gd-DTPA may have a role in the identification of hibernating myocardium. Fedele and colleagues[39] studied 19 patients with prior anterior myocardial infarction and residual severe stenoses (90 percent diameter or greater) of the left anterior descending coronary artery, using spin-echo MRI, at 4, 8, 12, and 20 minutes after administration of 0.4 mmol/kg Gd-DTPA. Comparison was made with left ventricular segments of regional perfusion and metabolism determined by iodine-123–phenylpentadecanoic acid (IPPA) scintigraphy. Approximately half the segments were normal, and the remaining segments were split between hibernating and necrotic tissue. Regional MRI peak intensity data and time of maximum postcontrast enhancement were significantly different among the three groups, suggesting that this technique may have a role in differentiating viable from necrotic myocardium in postinfarction patients.

Cine Magnetic Resonance Imaging to Identify Regional Myocardial Infarction

Inasmuch as alterations in T1 and T2 relaxation alone do not reflect underlying myocardial function, investigators have used the inherent contrast between the moving blood pool and the relatively stationary myocardial wall on cine gradient-echo MRI to evaluate myocardial wall thickening in short-axis, tomographic sections. Typically, 5 to 9 contiguous 5- to 10-mm sections are used to cover the entire ventricles, with up to 25 frames per cardiac cycle to isolate end-systole and end-diastole. Both left and right ventricular systolic function can be studied qualitatively in a cine format or quantitatively by outlining endocardial borders on end-diastolic and end-systolic images (see Chapter 50). Automated methods for assessment of regional and global function are being developed and tested,[40] but much of the quantitative data currently require very tedious, manual identification and outlining of endocardial borders. Conventional cine MRI, in which several minutes are needed to complete data acquisition for multiphase images depicting a single slice, has been studied most extensively, and the technique has been validated against left ventriculography,[41] radionuclide ventriculography, and echocardiography.[42] More recently, breath-hold segmentation cine MRI techniques have been introduced[43] that allow for single-level data to be acquired within a single 15-second breath-hold.

Short-axis cine MRI studies have been used to demonstrate the

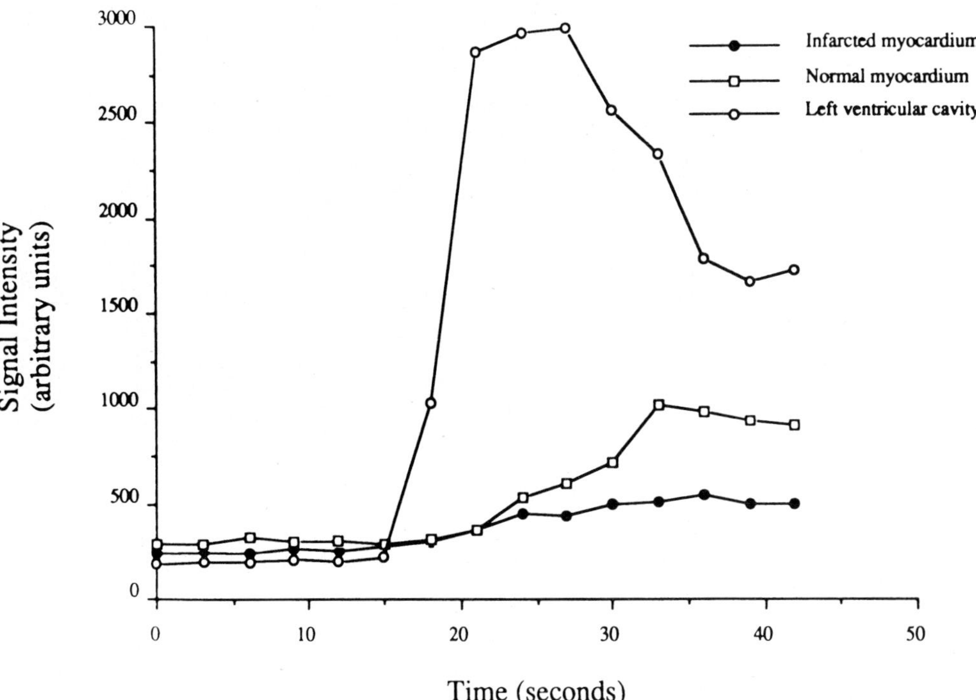

FIGURE 48–7. Alterations in regional myocardial signal intensities over time in 15 consecutive images obtained at intervals of 3 seconds in the same patient as shown in Figure 48–6. Bolus intravenous injection of gadolinium–diethylenetriamine penta-acetic acid (Gd-DTPA) was completed at time = 0 second. The upslope of the curve and the peak signal intensity of the infarcted region are markedly lower than those of the normal myocardial region. (From van Rugge, F.P., van der Wall, E.E., van Dijkman, P.R.M., et al.: Usefulness of ultrafast magnetic resonance imaging in healed myocardial infarction. Am. J. Cardiol. 70:1235–1236, 1992, with permission.)

extent of wall thickening throughout the cardiac cycle. The normal range for percent wall thickening and absolute extent of wall thickening during systole have been described for the left ventricle.[44] In normal young adult volunteers, the maximum wall thickening during systole is 60 percent. Reduction in percent wall thickening and in focal areas of wall thinning have been observed at sites of prior myocardial infarction, corresponding to areas of focal hypokinesis or akinesis on contrast left ventriculography.[44] Akins and colleagues[45] identified resting wall motion abnormalities in 16 of 17 patients with a prior Q-wave myocardial infarction who had undergone biplane left ventriculography demonstrating wall motion abnormalities. Left ventricular wall thickness at the site of infarction was significantly less than at adjacent noninfarcted myocardium, and the ratio of systolic wall thickness in the area of the infarction to that in the adjacent normal wall was depressed. Meese and co-workers[46] studied 25 patients with cine gradient-echo MRI 1 week after thrombolytic therapy for acute myocardial infarction. There was good concordance between regional wall motion analysis results obtained by MRI and those obtained by left ventriculography (Fig. 48–8). Two thirds of patients had evidence of more than 50 percent decrease in wall thickness within the infarcted region. Twenty patients had both an absolute decrease in myocardial signal and a matched regional wall motion abnormality on cine MRI study.

Although abnormal wall motion and wall thinning do appear to identify patients with healed myocardial infarction,[45] wall motion alone does not serve to differentiate infarcted from dysfunctional hibernating myocardium. Perrone-Filardi and co-workers[47] found evidence of viability on thallium reinjection or positron emission tomography (PET) in areas that were judged "nonviable" by spin-echo MRI. In their study of 25 patients with ischemic left ventricular dysfunction, end-diastolic wall thickness was greater in akinetic regions with evidence of ^{18}F-fluorodeoxyglucose uptake than in those without evidence of uptake, but there was poor correlation between ^{18}F-fluorodeoxyglucose uptake and either end-diastolic wall thickness or wall thickening. The poor correlation found by these investigators may be related to their use of transverse-plane MRI (rather than true short-axis images) and acquisition of spin-echo data at fixed time intervals rather than by the cine gradient-echo techniques used by others.

Johnston and colleagues[48] studied 24 patients 6 days after myocardial infarction with both T2-weighted spin-echo MRI and cine gradient-echo MRI. Viable myocardium was defined by MRI as a segment with increased signal intensity and preserved wall thickening. Data were compared with adenosine thallium single-photon emission computed tomographic (SPECT) images, with nonviable myocardium defined as a fixed defect without absence of redistribution at 4 hours. Of 11 patients with viable myocardium on SPECT imaging, 10 (91 percent) had evidence of wall thickening in the infarct area. Of 13 patients with fixed defects on SPECT, 6 (46 percent) had evidence of wall thickening in the same region on cine MRI. Therefore, the sensitivity of MRI was relatively good, but the specificity was poor, compared with adenosine-thallium SPECT imaging.

Finally, Baer and co-workers[49] compared ^{18}F-fluorodeoxyglu-

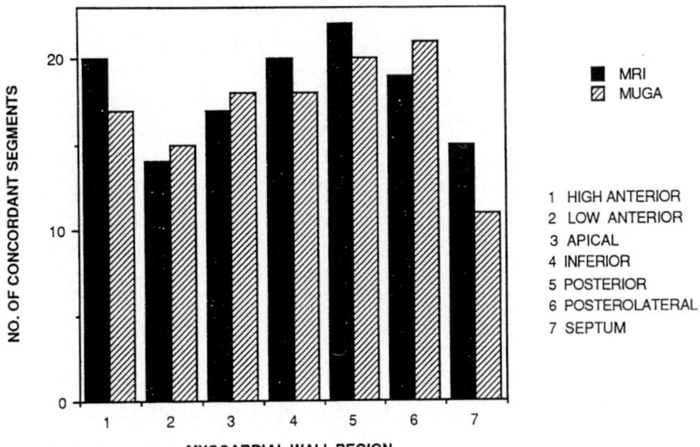

FIGURE 48–8. Regional wall motion, as determined by magnetic resonance imaging (MRI) and radionuclide angiography, compared with cardiac catheterization. The ordinate axis displays the number of concordant segments by either MRI or radionuclide angiography compared with cardiac catheterization. (From Meese, R.B., Spritzer, C.E., Negro-Vilar, R., et al.: Detection, characterization and functional assessment of reperfused Q-wave acute myocardial infarction by cine magnetic resonance imaging. Am. J. Cardiol. 66:8, 1990, with permission.)

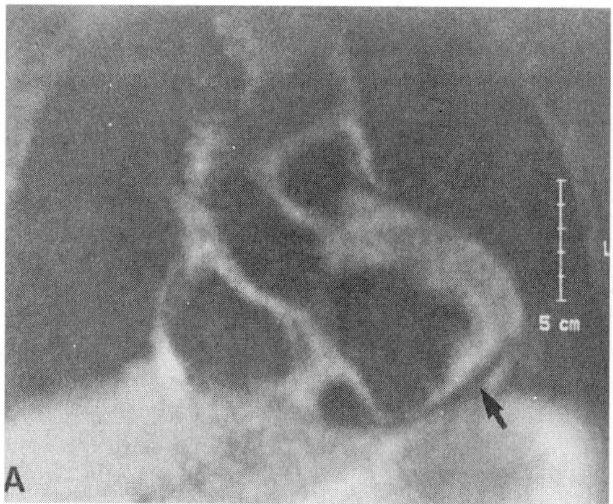

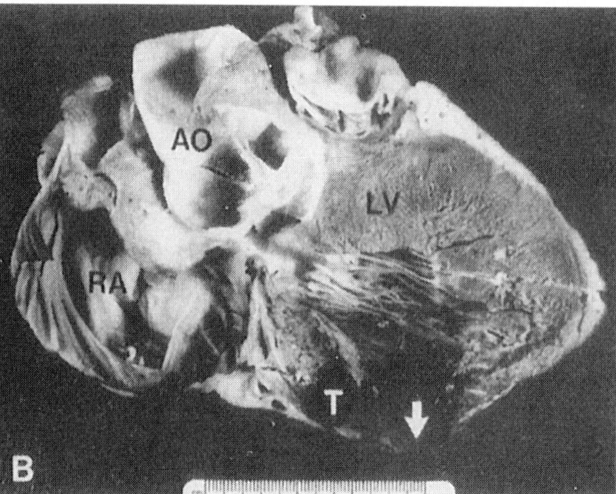

FIGURE 48–9. Correlation of autopsy pathology with results from cardiac magnetic resonance scanning. *A*, T1-weighted coronal magnetic resonance image showing defect in inferior left ventricle (LV) communicating with pericardial effusion *(arrow)*. *B*, Coronal section of heart showing pseudoaneurysm rupture point *(arrow)* and intramyocardial thrombus (T). AO = aorta; RA = right atrium. (From Harrity, P., Patel, A., Bianco, J., et al.: Improved diagnosis and characterization of postinfarction left ventricular pseudoaneurysm by cardiac magnetic resonance imaging. Clin. Cardiol. 14[7]:603–606, 1991. Copyrighted and reprinted with the permission of Clinical Cardiology Publishing Co., Inc., and/or Foundation for Advances in Medicine and Science, Inc., Mahwah, NJ 07430, USA.)

cose–PET with low-dose dobutamine cine MRI for the detection of viable myocardium in 35 patients with healed myocardial infarction. MRI data were analyzed by comparison of systolic wall thickening of 1 mm or more induced by administration of 10 μg/kg per minute dobutamine and resting preserved end-diastolic wall thickness of 5 mm or more. Preserved end-diastolic wall thickness in akinetic regions was found in 48 percent of patients, and rest and functional recovery within the infarct region were found in 54 percent of patients with dobutamine stimulation. PET data demonstrated viability in 66 percent of patients, with diagnostic agreement with MRI in 89 percent of patients studied.

Complications of Myocardial Infarction

In addition to delineating areas of myocardial wall thinning and regional hypokinesis, MRI is also helpful for the identification of complications of myocardial infarction. Left ventricular aneurysm may be recognized on MRI images as severe wall thinning (less than 2 mm) and diastolic bulging of the left ventricular free wall.[50] Left ventricular pseudoaneurysms may also be readily identified on MRI images.[51] The false aneurysm is characterized by a relatively small neck connecting the left ventricular chamber and the body of the aneurysm, with lack of myocardium in the wall of the aneurysm (Fig. 48–9). Left ventricular mural thrombus may be identified on spin-echo images as a density (mass) filling the left ventricular apex, especially in an area corresponding to a left ventricular aneurysm.[50, 52] Signal intensity of a thrombus varies with its age and organization. Although differentiation of thrombus from tumor may be difficult, evaluation of underlying myocardial anatomy (e.g., aneurysm, thinning related to infarction) and function (e.g., dyskinesis) usually allows for such discrimination. Intramyocardial hemorrhage may also be identified by MRI as a focal area of signal loss[53] (Fig. 48–10).

EVALUATION OF INDUCIBLE MYOCARDIAL ISCHEMIA

Brief periods of myocardial ischemia that do not result in myocardial infarction are not associated with significant changes in T1 or T2 relaxation times. For the detection of inducible ischemia, investigators have studied the use of cine MRI to identify regional myocardial systolic dysfunction and ultrafast MRI techniques in combination with MRI contrast agents to identify regional perfusion heterogeneity.

Transient Ischemia Detected by Wall Motion Abnormalities—Cine Magnetic Resonance Imaging

Exercise stress testing is commonly used to demonstrate inducible myocardial ischemia in patients with chest pain, but ST segment depression and angina are relatively late manifestations of myocardial ischemia and therefore would not be expected to be highly sensitive or specific for the detection of ischemia. An increase in left ventricular diastolic pressure and regional left ventric-

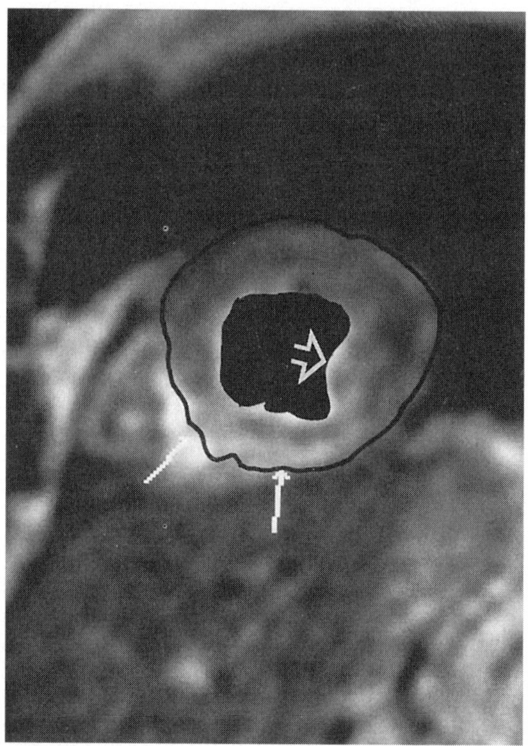

FIGURE 48–10. Acute inferior myocardial infarction. Signal intensity in this T2-weighted spin-echo systolic image is increased in the inferior wall *(solid white arrows)* and extends into the endocardium of the posterior wall. An area of decreased signal intensity in the midmyocardium inferiorly is consistent with intramyocardial hemorrhage. (From Johnston, D.L.: Myocardial tissue characterization with magnetic resonance imaging techniques. Am. J. Card. Imaging 8:141, 1994, with permission.)

ular systolic dysfunction are the first indicators of ischemia. Stress-induced regional left ventricular systolic dysfunction is an early and reliable sign of significant coronary artery disease.[54] Two-dimensional echocardiography has been used as a technique to identify regional ventricular asynergy (see Chapters 27 to 29), but adequate visualization of left ventricular endocardium may be difficult with transthoracic echocardiography because of chest wall or pulmonary interference. In theory, MRI should provide superior assessment of left ventricular systolic function because of its ability to acquire true tomographic short- and long-axis images of the heart and greater success at identifying endocardial borders. As mentioned previously, gradient-echo cine MRI provides high spatial resolution images and excellent contrast between the blood pool and left ventricular endocardium because of the inherent contrast between moving blood within the left ventricular cavity and the relatively stationary adjacent myocardium. MRI offers the ideal opportunity to identify regional myocardial asynergy after pharmacologic stress. Robust software for automated analysis of myocardial wall thickness and rate of thickening are currently lacking, and much of the published data is based on visual assessment or tedious manual tracings of endocardial borders from end-diastolic and end-systolic images.

Although space restriction and motion artifacts usually preclude physical exercise during MRI examination, hand grip and foot exercises[55] have been described. Much easier to adapt to the confines of current magnet platforms is pharmacologic stress with β-agonists such dobutamine or coronary vasodilators such as dipyridamole. Progressive β-agonist stimulation with dobutamine increases myocardial demand and is generally superior to primary coronary vasodilation for causing a new or worsening left ventricular systolic dysfunction. Low-dose β-agonist stimulation may also be helpful in differentiating stunned or hibernating myocardium from infarcted myocardium.[56] The primary mode of dipyridamole is to create a flow maldistribution without increased myocardial oxygen demand,[57] resulting in myocardial perfusion abnormalities. In normal coronary arteries, blood flow may increase fourfold with dipyridamole, whereas the increase in blood flow through diseased vessels is more limited, resulting in heterogeneity in perfusion. Regional ischemia and resulting hypokinesis related to a coronary "steal" phenomenon may sometimes occur in areas perfused by vessels with severe stenosis.[58]

Data from cine MRI studies that have employed pharmacologic stress with dobutamine or dipyridamole parallel two-dimensional echocardiographic pharmacologic stress data. Pennell and colleagues[59] were the first to report on the use of dobutamine-stress cine MRI for the detection of coronary artery disease in a group of 25 patients with chest pain and abnormal exercise stress tests. Dobutamine-stress cine MRI results were compared with dobutamine planar thallium imaging and with coronary angiography. Twenty-two patients in their series had significant coronary artery disease on angiography. Of these, 21 had evidence of reversible myocardial ischemia on dobutamine thallium imaging, and 20 had wall motion abnormalities on dobutamine cine MRI in a blinded qualitative wall motion analysis. Almost all patients experienced chest pain with dobutamine infusion, and abnormal wall motion was induced in 3 patients in their series who were free of angiographically significant coronary stenoses.

Van Rugge and co-workers[60] examined the clinical value of dobutamine-stress cine MRI for the detection of coronary artery disease in 45 patients with chest pain referred for coronary angiography, 37 of whom had significant coronary artery disease (50 percent diameter stenosis or greater). Cine MRI was performed in six adjacent short-axis planes at rest and after maximal pharmacologic stress with 20 μg/kg per minute dobutamine (Fig. 48–11). Dobutamine infusion was continued after MRI, and a 12-lead ECG was obtained outside the magnet environment. Dobutamine-stress cine MRI images were analyzed qualitatively by display of images in cinematographic loops; wall motion was assessed by two blinded observers, with any new or worsening wall motion abnormality indicative of a "positive" test. Comparison was made with dobutamine echocardiography, symptom-limited exercise-stress ECG, and coronary angiography. Thirty patients had new or worsening wall motion abnormalities by MRI examination, compared with 19 patients with such findings on dobutamine echocardiography and 26 patients with ischemia by maximal exercise ECG. The sensitivity of dobutamine MRI for the detection of coronary artery disease in patients with one-, two-, and three-vessel disease was 75, 80, and 100 percent, respectively. Overall sensitivity of dobutamine-stress cine MRI for the detection of coronary artery disease was 81 percent, and specificity was 100 percent. These data compared favorably with those obtained with ECG (51 percent sensitivity and 63 percent specificity) and with exercise echocardiography (70 percent sensitivity and 63 percent specificity).

More recently, van Rugge[61] reported on the use of dobutamine stress in combination with cine MRI for the detection and localization of coronary artery disease by quantitative rather than visual analysis of cine loops. Short-axis cine images were quantitatively analyzed at 100 equally-spaced chords constructed perpendicular to a centerline drawn midway between the end-diastolic and end-systolic contours (Fig. 48–12). Wall thickening was expressed as percent systolic wall thickening according to the following formula:

$$\% \text{ thickening} = [(ES - ED) \div ED] \times 100$$

where ES is end-systolic wall thickness and ED is end-diastolic wall thickness. Thirty-nine consecutive patients with clinically suspected coronary artery disease and 10 healthy adult volunteers were studied at rest and during stress with 20 μg/kg per minute dobutamine. Dobutamine-stress MRI results were considered positive for coronary disease if the percent wall thickening of at least four adjacent chords was less than 2 standard deviations below the mean obtained from normal volunteers. Sensitivity and specificity of dobu-

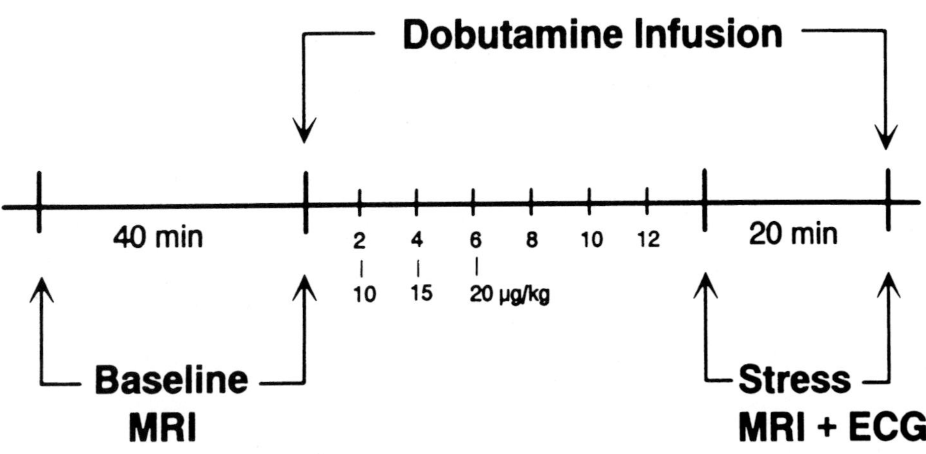

FIGURE 48–11. Time diagram of a dobutamine infusion protocol, with baseline and stress magnetic resonance imaging followed by electrocardiographic imaging under stress outside the magnetic environment. (From van Rugge, F.P., van der Wall, E.E., de Roos, A., et al.: Dobutamine stress magnetic resonance imaging for detection of coronary artery disease. J. Am. Coll. Cardiol 22[2]:431–439, 1993. With permission from the American College of Cardiology.)

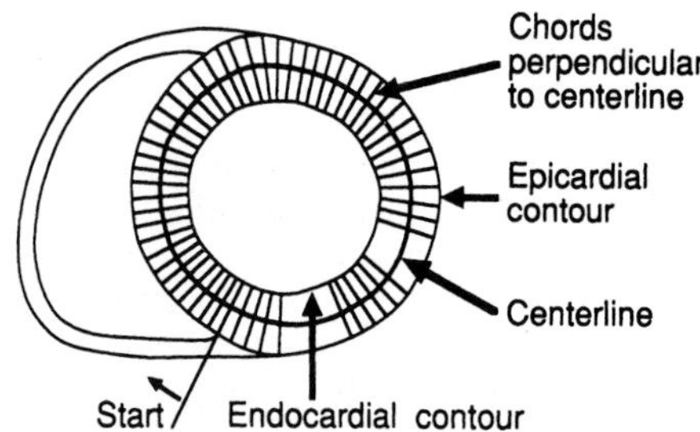

FIGURE 48–12. Schematic representation of a modification of the centerline method. The short-axis magnetic resonance images are analyzed at 100 equidistant chords constructed perpendicular to a centerline drawn midway between the end-diastolic and end-systolic contours to calculate wall thickness at both time frames. (From van Rugge, F.P., van der Wall, E.E., Spanjersberg, S.J., et al.: Magnetic resonance imaging during dobutamine stress for detection and localization of coronary artery disease: Quantitative wall motion analysis using a modification of the centerline method. Circulation 90[1]:127–138, 1994. With permission from the American College of Cardiology.)

tamine-stress MRI for the detection of significant coronary disease (50 percent diameter stenosis or greater) were 91 and 80 percent, respectively. Sensitivities for one-, two-, and three-vessel disease were 88, 91, and 100 percent, respectively. Although the number of patients studied was small, these data suggest improved sensitivity with the quantitative approach, especially for patients with one- or two-vessel disease. Their data suggest a lower specificity, possibly related to regional contractile heterogeneity in normal subjects.

Finally, Baer and colleagues[62] reported on 35 consecutive patients, with normal resting left ventricular systolic function and without a history of myocardial infarction, who had angiographically documented coronary artery disease (23 in the left anterior descending, 15 in the left circumflex, 16 in the right coronary artery). Patients underwent both multilevel short-axis cine MRI and thallium SPECT tomographic imaging at rest and during 10 to 20 μg/kg per minute dobutamine infusion. Three patients (9 percent) had uninterpretable MRI data because of motion artifacts or ECG-trigger problems. New wall motion abnormalities were observed in 27 (84 percent) of 32 patients during MRI, compared with 28 (87 percent) of 32 patients for SPECT examinations. Of the five patients in whom coronary artery disease was not suggested by cine MRI, three had single-vessel disease. The cine MRI rate of detection for severe stenoses (70 percent diameter or greater) was 90 percent, compared with 50 percent for moderate stenoses (50 to 70 percent diameter stenosis).

Pharmacologic stress with intravenous dipyridamole in combination with cine MRI has also been studied in humans as a means of identifying patients with coronary artery disease. As with two-dimensional echocardiographic stress with dipyridamole-stress, cine MRI data have not been as encouraging as dobutamine-stress cine MRI, possibly related to the minimal increase in myocardial oxygen demand with dipyridamole testing. Pennell and colleagues[63] studied 40 patients who had a history of angina and an abnormal exercise ECG with vertical long-axis, horizontal long-axis, and basal-apical short-axis cine MRI before and after a 4-minute infusion of 0.142 mg/kg per minute intravenous dipyridamole. Twenty-three patients had a history of prior myocardial infarction. Comparison was made with coronary angiography and with dipyridamole planar thallium-201 imaging. After dipyridamole, visually apparent reversible wall motion abnormalities were seen in 24 (62 percent) of 39 patients with angiographic evidence of coronary artery disease and in 24 (67 percent) of 36 patients with reversible thallium defects. Among those with abnormal wall motion on cine MRI studies, the site of reversible wall motion abnormality always corresponded to the site of a reversible thallium defect.

Baer and co-workers[64] performed basal and midventricular short-axis cine MRI before and during 0.75 mg/kg, 10-minute intravenous dipyridamole infusion. Twenty-three patients with at least one significant (70 percent diameter or greater) coronary stenosis on angiography but without prior myocardial infarction were studied. A test was considered indicative for coronary artery disease if a visually apparent worsening of wall motion was present with dipyridamole infusion. These investigators found a 78 percent sensitivity of dipyridamole-stress cine MRI for the identification of coronary artery disease, with 69 and 90 percent sensitivity for one- and two-vessel disease, respectively.

A limitation on current cine MRI stress studies has been the use of conventional cine MRI sequences, which require several minutes for data acquisition. This prolonged time interval for data acquisition severely limits the number of data sets that can be acquired, especially if patients are experiencing chest pain. Usually, two or four cine data sets are acquired during a 3- to 8-minute time period. The development of breath-hold cine MRI,[43] in which an entire cine data set may be completed within a single 15-second breath-hold, offers the opportunity to acquire more complete information (more levels) within a markedly abbreviated time frame. The optimal number of levels and slice orientations also remains to be identified.

Myocardial Perfusion Techniques With Gadolinium–Diethylenetriamine Penta-acetic Acid

Although cine MRI with pharmacologic stress suggests abnormal myocardial perfusion in areas of reversible regional systolic dysfunction, more direct assessment of myocardial perfusion is also possible. As previously mentioned, Gd-DTPA is a paramagnetic contrast agent of very low toxicity approved for human use (see Chapter 44). Because of the rapid dynamics of Gd-DTPA, it was not until the development of ultrafast MRI sequences that analysis of its first-pass effects were possible. Standard ECG-gated spin-echo and gradient-echo cine MRI sequences typically require several minutes to complete data acquisition. These averaged or "steady-state" techniques fail to provide dynamic information because Gd-DTPA equilibrates during the relatively long acquisition period. Ultrafast MRI techniques such as turboFLASH or EPI may be combined with intravenous administration of an MRI contrast agent to identify regional myocardial perfusion heterogeneity. An MRI approach offers the advantage of superior spatial resolution, compared with current radionuclide and PET techniques, with minimal interference related to overlying breast shadow, high diaphragms, and so on. Although Gd-DTPA has an extracellular distribution similar to that of iodinated contrast agents, there is a very complex and nonlinear relation between MRI signal intensity and local Gd-DTPA concentration. Canine turboFLASH studies by Wilke and colleagues[65] and EPI studies by Wendland and co-workers,[66] however, suggest that the MRI technique may eventually allow for quantification of regional myocardial perfusion. For an in-depth discussion of myocardial perfusion and factors related to signal intensity changes with Gd-DTPA, readers are referred elsewhere.[27, 67]

Typically, to assess first passage of Gd-DTPA through the left ventricular myocardium, an inversion recovery approach is used for turboFLASH sequences to make the image T1-weighted. A 180-degree inversion pulse serves to null the signal from unenhanced (precontrast and hypoperfused) myocardium, with myocardium perfused by Gd-DTPA displaying regional signal enhancement during first passage of the agent (Fig. 48–13). After gating off the R wave, spins are first inverted by a nonselective 180-degree pulse with imaging initiated 400 to 700 msec later, resulting in a nulling of signal from resting myocardium at baseline. On arrival of Gd-

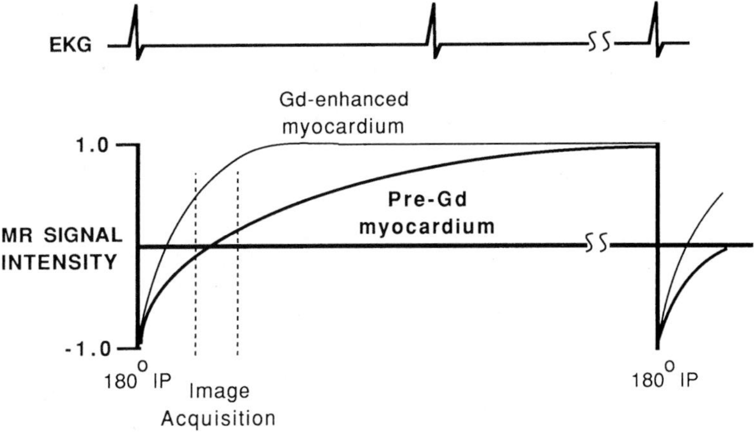

FIGURE 48–13. Schematic diagram of the effects of paramagnetic agents on signal intensity and timing of the inversion pulse and data acquisition portion of the ultrafast sequence. Refer to text for details. EKG = electrocardiogram; IP = inversion pulse. (From Manning, W.J., Atkinson, D.J., Grossman, W., et al.: First-pass nuclear magentic resonance imaging studies using gadolinium-DTPA in patients with coronary artery disease. J. Am. Coll. Cardiol. 18[4]:959–965, 1991. With permission from the American College of Cardiology.)

DTPA, there is shortening of T1 and enhanced (faster) relaxation, resulting in a shift in the signal-intensity–time curve upward and to the left. With the same acquisition time delay after R wave, this shift results in a positive signal for regional myocardium that is related (in a nonlinear fashion) to the local concentration of Gd-DTPA. In contrast, focal myocardium that is relatively hypoperfused has decreased local Gd-DTPA delivery, with less pronounced T1 shortening and lower signal enhancement.[68] Hypoperfused myocardium may also display prolonged signal enhancement owing to depressed Gd-DTPA washout. Because the T1 relaxation rate of myocardium is relatively long and the pulse sequence must allow for magnetization recovery, serial images are usually acquired every two to four heartbeats. In theory, one could image at multiple short-axis levels by sacrificing temporal resolution. This is likely to be acceptable in situations of severe coronary stenoses or occlusions, but the technique remains to be fully investigated.

Atkinson and co-workers[37] first described first-pass cardiac perfusion in humans with the use of Gd-DTPA injected into an antecubital or jugular vein. Subsequent resting human studies performed in our laboratory exemplified the clinical potential of this technique. We studied a group of 17 patients with chest pain who were referred for cardiac catheterization, including 12 with severe proximal coronary artery disease (more than 80 percent diameter stenoses).[68] Double-oblique, short-axis, ultrafast imaging was performed at the level of the papillary muscles (Fig. 48–14) after intravenous injection of 0.04 mmol/kg of Gd-DTPA, with repetitive images obtained every fourth heartbeat. Before injection there was almost undetectable signal from the left ventricular myocardium, consistent with the desired T1 nulling (see Fig. 48–14*A*). After injection of Gd-DTPA, signal intensity was easily detectable within the right ventricular cavity, and normal systemic recirculation could be characterized (see Fig. 48–14*A* through *G*). Semiautomated

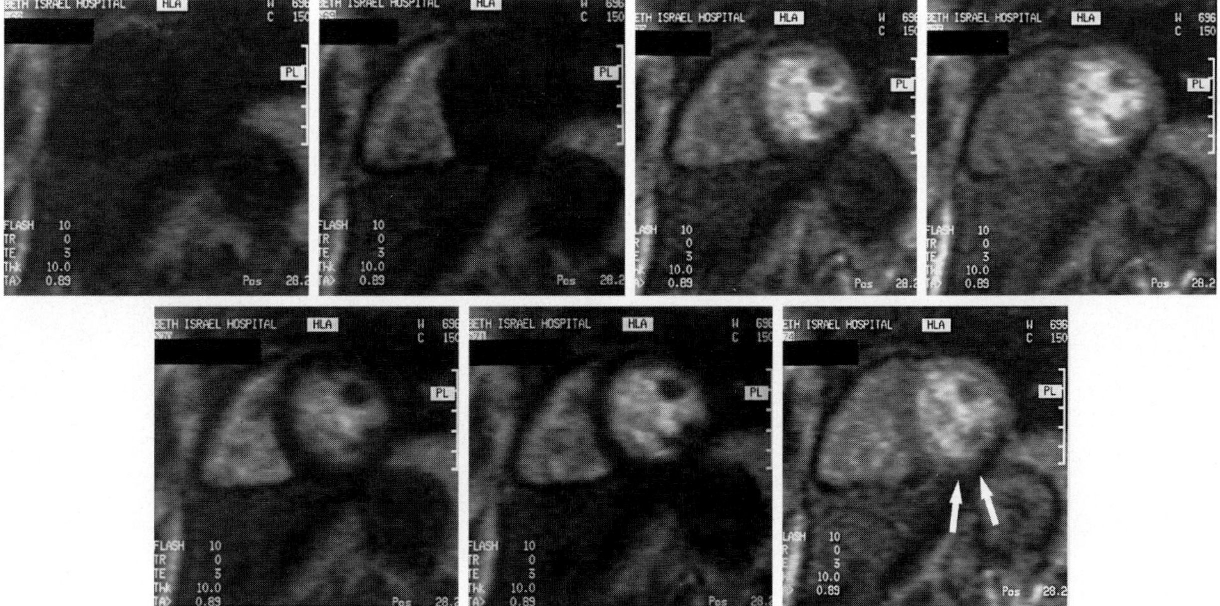

FIGURE 48–14. *A* through *G*, Series of seven sequential, electrocardiographically gated, ultrafast turboFLASH, short-axis magnetic resonance images after injection of gadolinium–diethylenetriamine pentaacetic acid (Gd-DTPA) in a patient with a 90 percent stenosis of the right coronary artery. Note the sequential appearance of increased signal in the right ventricular cavity, left ventricular myocardium with recirculation to the right ventricular cavity (*G*). Less enhancement is seen in the posterior wall (*arrows*). (From Manning, W.J., Atkinson, D.J., Grossman, W., et al.: First-pass nuclear magnetic resonance imaging studies using gadolinium-DTPA in patients with coronary artery disease. J. Am. Coll. Cardiol. 18[4]:959–965, 1991. With permission from the American College of Cardiology.)

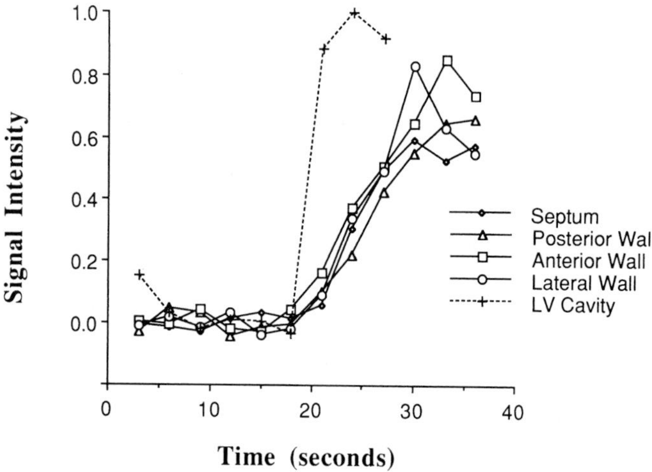

FIGURE 48–15. Regional myocardial signal intensities obtained from a subject with angiographically normal coronary arteries. Note that signal intensities from all myocardial regions demonstrate a prompt and coherent increase, with similar peak signal intensities. (From Manning, W.J., Atkinson, D.J., Grossman, W., et al.: First-pass nuclear magnetic resonance imaging studies using gadolinium-DTPA in patients with coronary artery disease. J. Am. Coll. Cardiol. 18[4]:959–965, 1991. With permission from the American College of Cardiology.)

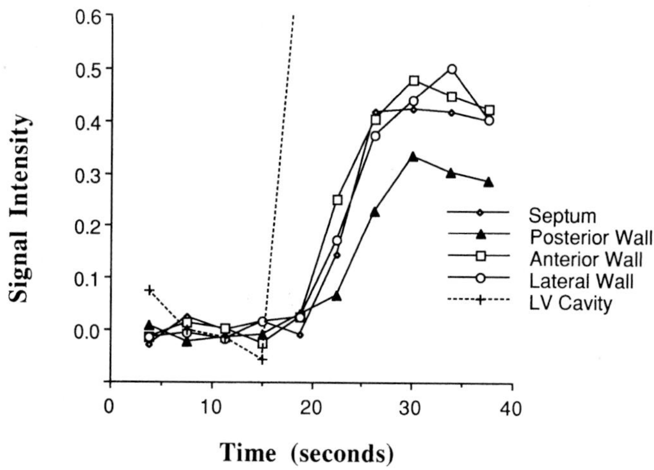

FIGURE 48–16. Regional myocardial signal intensities obtained from a subject with a 90 percent stenosis of the proximal right coronary artery (same patient as in Figure 48–14). Note that signal intensities from all myocardial regions demonstrate a prompt and coherent increase, with similar peak signal intensities. (From Manning, W.J., Atkinson, D.J., Grossman, W., et al.: First-pass nuclear magnetic resonance imaging studies using gadolinium-DTPA in patients with coronary artery disease. J. Am. Coll. Cardiol. 18[4]:959–965, 1991. With permission from the American College of Cardiology.)

analysis of regional myocardium from patients with normal left ventricular systolic function and angiographically normal coronary arteries displayed a rapid and homogeneous signal enhancement (Fig. 48–15), compared with delayed upslope and lower peak signal intensity in regional myocardium perfused by vessels with coronary stenoses (Fig. 48–16). Peak signal intensity (related to peak Gd-DTPA concentration) and upslope (rate of Gd-DTPA delivery) were significantly depressed in regional myocardium supplied by diseased vessels. After revascularization with percutaneous coronary angioplasty, there was normalization of signal enhancement profiles; patients undergoing coronary artery bypass grafting demonstrated persistent depression of upslope but normalization of peak signal intensity. We hypothesized that this persistent delay was related to delivery of contrast through bypass grafts rather than through the native coronaries.

As previously mentioned, van Rugge and colleagues[38] studied 19 patients with chronic myocardial infarction with resting single-level short-axis turboFLASH MRI. After Gd-DTPA injection, there was progressive signal enhancement in both infarcted and normal myocardium (see Fig. 48–7), with significantly faster and greater enhancement of normal myocardium in comparison with infarcted regions.

Limited human data are available on the use of pharmacologic stress in combination with bolus administration of an MRI contrast agent. Schaefer and co-workers[69] reported on six patients with coronary artery disease and four healthy subjects who underwent dipyridamole-stress Gd-DTPA turboFLASH MRI perfusion studies. Data were compared with the results of dipyridamole thallium scintigraphy and coronary angiography. TurboFLASH MRI was performed at the level of the base of the papillary muscles, with 12 contiguous regions of interest (Fig. 48–17). Nine myocardial regions supplied by diseased arteries showed diminished levels of

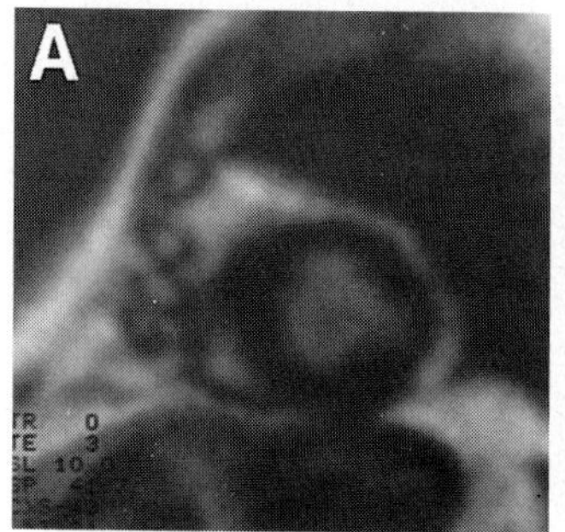

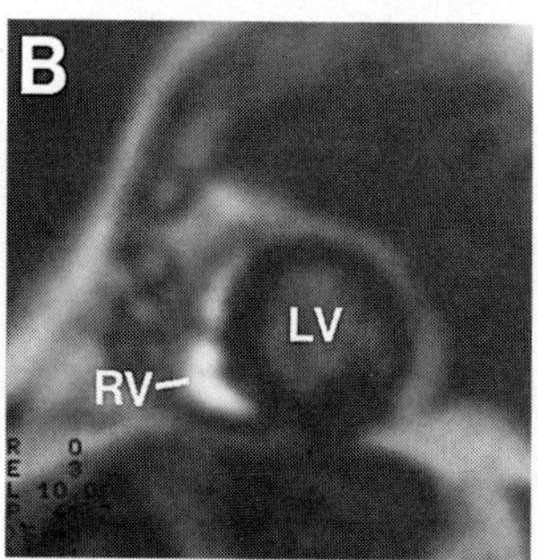

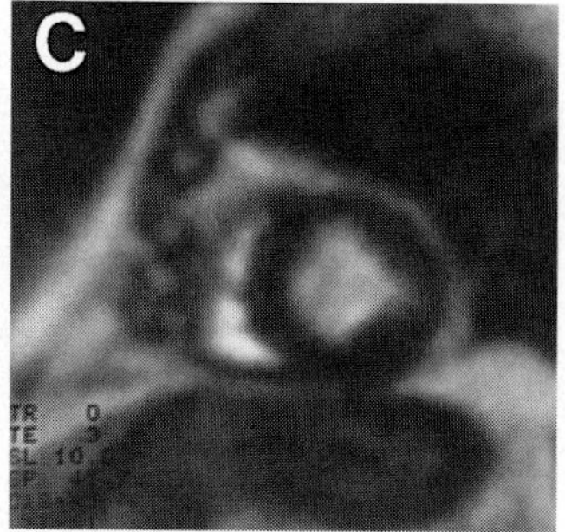

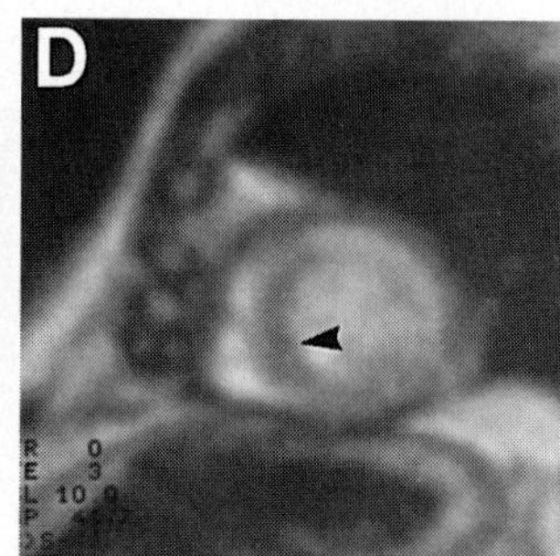

FIGURE 48–17. Short-axis magnetic resonance images from a patient after administration of dipyridamole and gadolinium–diethylenetriamine penta-acetic acid. *A,* Image obtained immediately before administration of contrast, with uniform nulling of myocardium. *B* and *C,* Image obtained after enhancement of blood in the left ventricular cavity. *D,* Passage of contrast into the myocardium causes nonuniform signal enhancement of the myocardium at 23 seconds, with decreased signal intensity in the septum and inferior wall *(arrowheads).* (From Schaefer, S., van Tyen, R., and Saloner, D.: Evaluation of myocardial perfusion abnormalities with gadolinium-enhanced snapshot MR imaging in humans: Work in progress. Radiology 185:795–801, 1992, with permission.)

regional enhancement, and these results were in agreement with those of both thallium and coronary angiography.

Common limitations of these turboFLASH imaging studies have included the poor temporal resolution (which results from the need to allow several seconds for complete T1 relaxation of myocardium) and the ability to acquire data at only one tomographic level. Because only a small amount of Gd-DTPA is used, repeat injections are theoretically possible to allow for analysis of multiple levels, but this may result in an impaired signal-to-noise ratio as the baseline T1 shortens after each Gd-DTPA injection because of residual Gd-DTPA within the myocardium. Software enhancement in the future may allow for tomographic sections to be acquired at different levels (i.e., base, middle, and apex) with each heartbeat, maintaining a similar temporal resolution. In addition, contrast agents providing enhanced signal-to-noise ratio such as gadobenate dimeglumine (Gd-BOPTA)[70] and intravascular agents such as Gd-DTPA–polylysine[71] are being studied and appear promising.

Rather than using a turboFLASH sequence inversion recovery, which is sensitive to T1 shortening, Saeed and colleagues[70] reported on a rat model of reperfused reversible and irreversible myocardial injury that employed both inversion recovery (T1-weighted) and gradient-recalled EPI (T2-sensitive) after administration of Gd-BOPTA–dimeglume, a novel paramagnetic agent that reduces both T1 and T2. Inversion recovery EPI studies displayed enhancement analogous to that obtained with the turboFLASH studies previously mentioned, whereas standard EPI imaging led to signal loss in regional myocardium supplied by normal vessels, with attenuated signal loss in reversibly injured myocardium (Fig. 48–18). Results with T2-weighted perfusion studies are generally inferior to those obtained on T1-weighted studies because of susceptibility effects extending out of the blood pool and also because of artifacts at the heart-lung interface intrinsic to a T2-sequence. Larger doses of Gd-DTPA are also needed for T2-weighted compared with T1-weighted imaging.

More recently, we have begun to investigate EPI for the evaluation of regional myocardial perfusion in human studies. With the use of an inversion-recovery EPI sequence (to make it T1-weighted) in combination with Gd-DTPA injection,[2] lack of enhancement was seen in the distal septum and apex in a patient with a severe stenosis of the left anterior descending coronary artery (Fig. 48–19). Significant advantages of EPI include the potential for complete image acquisition in less than 100 msec and the ability to acquire data at multiple levels during the same heartbeat. Although Gd-DTPA may be used as the contrast agent, the requirement for much larger doses of Gd-DTPA for T2 effects makes the use of dysprosium-DTPA or similar T2 agents more appealing.

It is premature to identify the exact role MRI perfusion studies will play in the evaluation of the patient with suspected or known coronary artery disease. As previously mentioned, regional MRI signal enhancement or intensity is related to multiple variables, including edema, fibrosis, fiber orientation, and cellular integrity.[27] Many of these variables may be affected by the same disease state, with contrasting effects on regional signal intensity and local T1 or T2. Prolonged "washin," caused by spreading of the peripherally injected bolus in the arm veins, represents a major problem in human studies, especially in patients with significant valvular regurgitation or depressed cardiac output. The development of intravascular agents may help minimize many of the complex relations between signal intensity and regional perfusion that are present for extracellular agents, although this remains to be fully investigated. Kraitchman and co-workers have investigated the use of novel agents such as polylysine–Gd-DTPA[71] as intravascular perfusion agents in canine models of controlled myocardial ischemia. As with cine MRI studies, analyses of regional signal intensity changes remain operator dependent. Finally, the potential use of MRI for the evaluation of regional myocardial diffusion without a contrast agent, using magnetization transfer, has been described.[72]

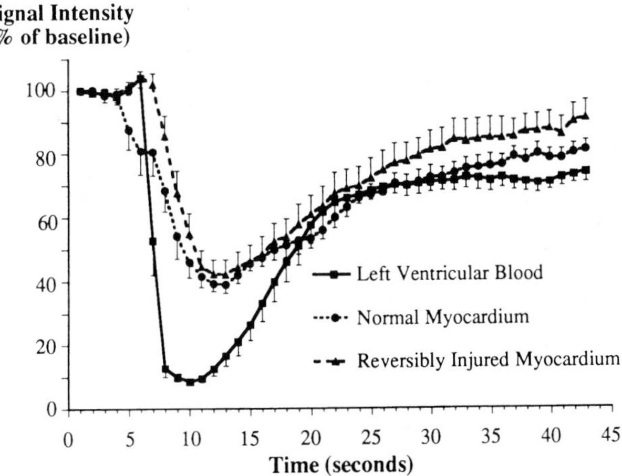

FIGURE 48–18. Plot of time course of changes in signal intensities in left ventricular (LV) chamber blood and in normal and reperfused reversibly injured myocardium during the passage of 0.25 mmol/kg Gd-BOPTA–dimeglume, as visualized by magnetic resonance echo planar imaging. Calculated signal intensities show the absence of differential signal and no time difference in the enhancement of normal and reperfused reversibly injured myocardium. (From Saeed, M., Wendland, M.F., Yu, K.K., et al.: Identification of myocardial reperfusion with echo planar magnetic resonance imaging: Discrimination between occlusive and reperfused infarctions. Circulation 90[3]:1492–1501, 1994, with permission of the American Heart Association.)

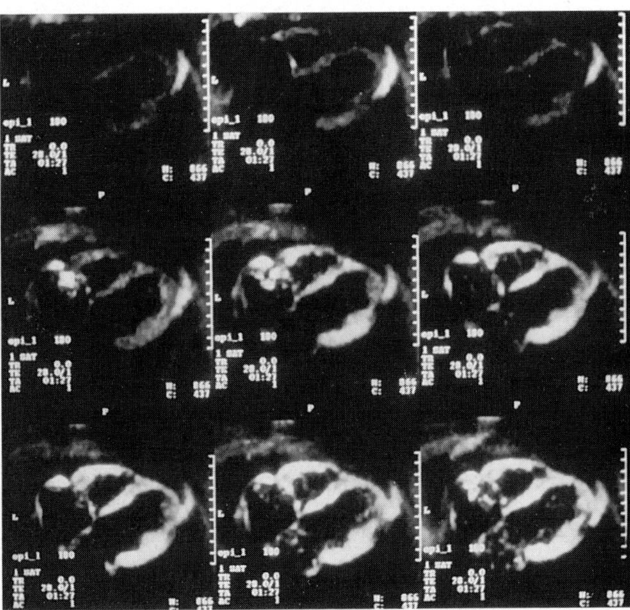

FIGURE 48–19. First-pass, T1-weighted inversion recovery echo planar imaging study after 10 mL of gadolinium–diethylenetriamine penta-acetic acid was given as a rapid intravenous bolus in a patient with a severe stenosis of the left anterior descending coronary artery. Note the lack of enhancement of the distal septum and left ventricular (LV) apex. (From Edelman, R.R., Wielopolski, P., and Schmitt, F.: Echo-planar MR imaging. Radiology 192[3]:600–612, 1994, with permission.)

MAGNETIC RESONANCE CORONARY ANGIOGRAPHY

MRI has proved to be highly accurate for the assessment of cardiac anatomy and ventricular function, but clinical cardiac MRI studies are rarely performed because other noninvasive imaging techniques, primarily echocardiography and radionuclide ventriculography, give similar anatomical and functional information at lower cost and with easier patient access. Similarly, despite enhanced spatial and temporal resolution, MRI perfusion data have yet to be proved superior to more conventional and less costly radionuclide and echocardiographic stress data. In today's era of medical economics and cost constraints, it no longer is sufficient to provide "better" information. Large trials documenting the clinical impact and cost-effectiveness of MRI, compared with ultrasound and radionuclide studies, need to be conducted. Nevertheless, because reliable noninvasive imaging of the coronary arteries and direct identification of significant coronary stenoses has yet to be accomplished by other noninvasive imaging technologies, the development of MRCA will probably have the greatest impact on the clinical practice of cardiology and will probably serve as the driving force for cardiac MRI.

The current "gold standard" for the evaluation of the coronary arteries is contrast angiography. More than 1 million diagnostic coronary angiograms are performed annually in the United States alone.[1] Information derived from such angiograms provides the basis on which diagnoses and mechanical interventions such as coronary artery bypass graft surgery or percutaneous transluminal coronary angioplasty, as well as pharmacologic therapies, are planned. In addition, prognostic information is also gained from data regarding coronary anatomy. The high cost ($3500 to $6000 per study) and associated risks make routine coronary angiography inappropriate for use as a screening test, even in high-risk groups. Moreover, although semiquantitative techniques exist for estimating the flow restriction caused by a coronary artery stenosis based on the conventional contrast angiogram,[73] conventional angiography does not provide a quantitative measure of coronary artery blood flow.

Although MRI is considered the premier noninvasive technique for imaging of the thoracic aorta,[74] the coronary arteries have diameters that are 10 times smaller than that of the ascending thoracic aorta. In addition, the coronary vessels are tortuous and there is extensive motion, both during the cardiac cycle and with normal respiration. Finally, there is extensive MRI signal from surrounding epicardial fat, which obscures visualization of the underlying coronary vessels.

Early Attempts at Magnetic Resonance Coronary Angiography of Native Coronaries

With conventional ECG-gated spin-echo techniques, images of the proximal aorta occasionally include the proximal portions of the major epicardial coronary arteries (Fig. 48–20). Paulin and colleagues[75] reported on the ability of ECG-gated, multislice, multiphase spin-echo imaging to identify the anatomy of the aortic root and coronary ostia in six patients who had recently undergone conventional contrast angiography. Despite data acquisition over several minutes and lack of respiratory gating, the presence and location of both coronary artery ostia were successfully identified in four patients. In the remaining two patients, the left but not the right coronary artery orifice was identified. Identification of a coronary stenosis was not achieved in any patient, but all stenoses were distal to the visualized coronary segment.

Advances in Magnetic Resonance Coronary Angiography

Although MRCA is not expected to fully supplant diagnostic coronary angiography or to allow for quantitation of focal stenoses for several years to come, the field is advancing very quickly. Success at visualization of the native coronary arteries has been achieved with MRI subtraction methods,[76] three-dimensional techniques[77] (Fig. 48–21), spiral scanning[78] (Fig. 48–22), and segmentation gradient-echo sequences.[79] In addition, EPI MRCA has been described[80, 81] and offers great promise. Common themes of most of these MRCA techniques are the use of multiple, 10- to 20-second breath-holds to minimize respiratory motion artifacts (blurring) and the performance of imaging during mid-diastole, a period of relative diastasis, so as to minimize the artifacts related to bulk cardiac motion. A review of the merits and detractions of each technique is beyond the scope of this chapter, and readers are referred elsewhere.[82]

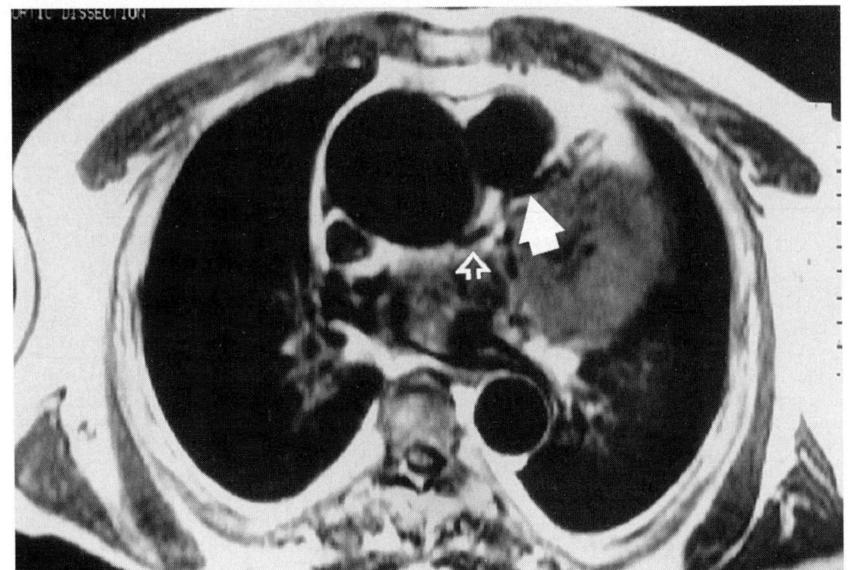

FIGURE 48–20. Conventional electrocardiographically gated, multiphase spin-echo axial section at the proximal aorta in a patient referred for evaluation of a dilated ascending aorta. Note the left main coronary artery *(open white arrow)* and extension into the left anterior descending (LAD) coronary artery *(solid white arrow)*. (From Manning, W.J., and Edelman, R.R.: MR coronary angiography. Magn. Reson. Q. 9[3]:131–151, 1993, with permission.)

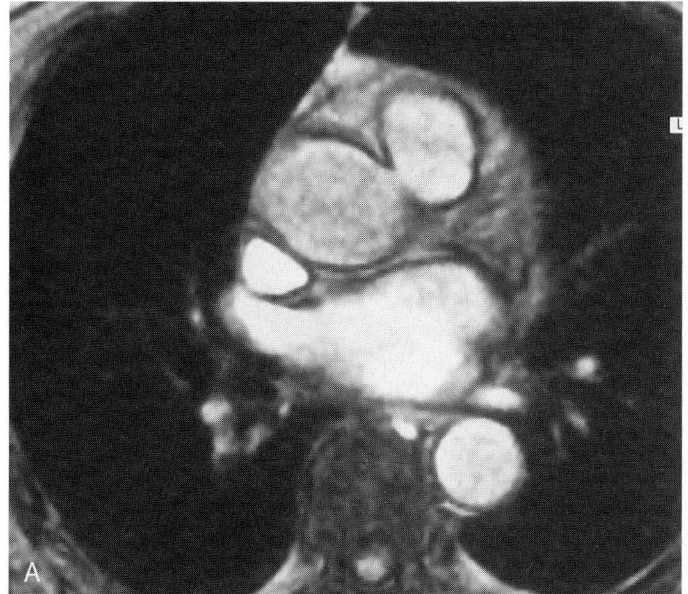

FIGURE 48–21. Three-dimensional, rapid-acquisition gradient-echo imaging with fat saturation (FS) and magnetization transfer contrast (MTC) to suppress myocardial signal. TR = 8.5 msec; TE = 2.9 msec; 15-degree flip angle; 32 partitions with central reordering of the three-dimensional section-encoding steps, slab thickness 64 mm; 150 × 256 matrix; four averages with electrocardiographic triggering and data acquisition in diastole. *A,* Single-partition magnetic resonance image from a three-dimensional image without FS. The coronary is buried in strong fat signal. *B,* Same section position, with FS. The fat signal is greatly suppressed, allowing delineation of the left anterior descending (LAD) artery *(white arrow)* and the left circumflex (LCX) artery *(short black arrow)*. *C,* After reformatting of the original transverse images with FS, the proximal portion of each major artery is depicted in one image. 1 = right coronary artery (RCA); 2 = left main coronary artery; 3 = LCX; 4 = LAD. (From Manning, W.J., and Edelman, R.R.: MR coronary angiography. Magn. Reson. Q. 9[3]:131–151, 1993, with permission.)

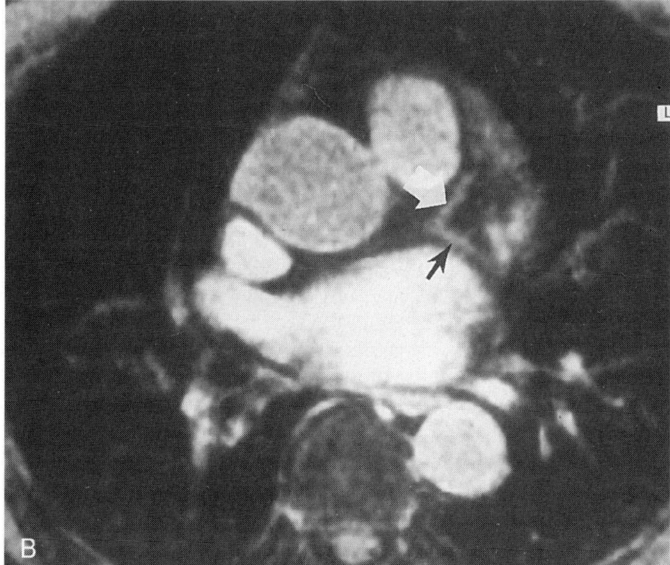

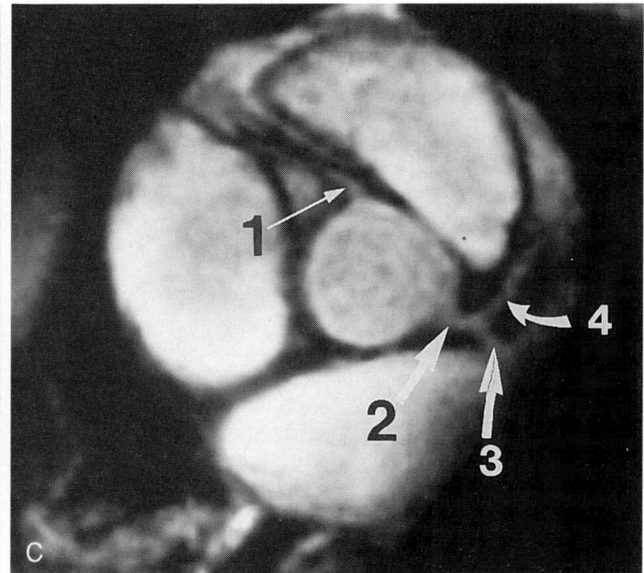

The greatest amount of investigation has been performed with two-dimensional, segmented K-space, gradient-echo MRCA approaches, first reported by Burstein.[83] With this method, multiple phase-encoding steps are acquired during the brief period of mid-diastole in each of a series of heartbeats.[79] Typically, 160 phase-encoding steps (matrix 160 × 256) are acquired (8 per heartbeat for 20 beats) with a field of view of 240 × 240 mm, resulting in a spatial resolution of 1.5 × 0.9 mm. Each two-dimensional image may be acquired with a slice thickness of 3 to 4 mm. Thirty or more breath-hold images are usually needed to define the major coronary anatomy. As with other gradient-echo sequences, rapidly-moving, laminar blood flow produces a bright signal because of the inflow of unsaturated protons, and stagnant blood (or tissue) appears dark because of saturation effects caused by repeated proton stimulation. Focal areas of turbulence within blood vessels also appear dark because of proton dephasing.

Typically, the coronary ostia are identified in the transverse plane (Fig. 48–23). An example of a transverse MRI image at the level of the right coronary artery is shown in Figure 48–23*A*, with a more inferior section depicted in Figure 48–23*B*. Taking advantage of the unique ability of MRI to directly acquire images in any orientation, these initial images may be followed by obliquely oriented images acquired along the major or minor axis of the vessels. Oblique images along the major axis of the right coronary artery are shown in Figure 48–23*C*, with adjacent sections delineating portions of the vessel that deviated into adjoining imaging sections (see Fig. 48–23*D* to *F*). The left main coronary artery may also be visualized in transverse section (Fig. 48–24), with superior and inferior sections delineating the left anterior descending and left circumflex coronary arteries. The left main and left circumflex coronary arteries are also frequently seen with oblique images. Double-oblique images may also be obtained along the axis of the left main and left anterior descending coronary arteries, allowing identification of large portions of the left coronary artery within a single section (Fig. 48–25). A cine variation of the sequence with double-oblique imaging planes may also allow for visualization of long segments of the left anterior descending and right coronary arteries.[84]

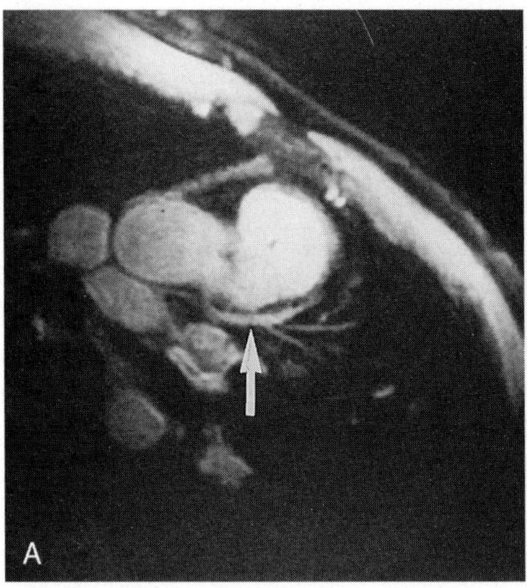

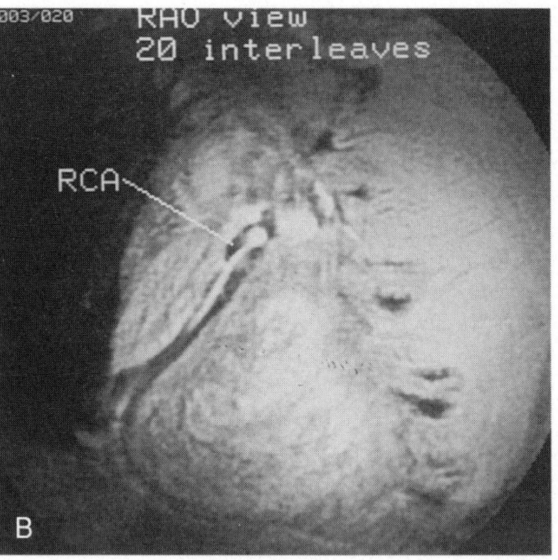

FIGURE 48–22. Spiral scan imaging. Each image was acquired during a single breath-hold (20 heartbeats, 17.5-msec readout, 90-degree flip angle). *A*, Oblique view of the left coronary artery of a normal volunteer. The left main coronary artery and the left anterior descending artery *(white arrow)*, including several branches (diagonals), are well seen. *B*, Right anterior oblique (RAO) image of the right coronary artery (RCA) in a normal volunteer. Approximately 8 cm of the RCA is visible. Both images were acquired 335 msec after a plethysmography trigger using a slice thickness of 5 mm *(A)* or 7 mm *(B)*. (From Manning, W.J., and Edelman, R.R.: MR coronary angiography. Magn. Reson. Q. 9[3]:131–151, 1993, with permission.)

Using this approach in a series of young adult volunteers,[79] we were able to identify the left main coronary artery in 96 percent of subjects, the left anterior descending and right coronary arteries in 100 percent of subjects, and the left circumflex coronary artery in 76 percent of subjects. In addition to these major vessels, diagonal branches of the left anterior descending coronary artery were identified in 80 percent of subjects and the great cardiac vein in 88 percent of subjects. The average vessel diameter and average length of contiguously observed coronary artery were as shown in Table 48–3. With this approach, quantitative contrast angiography of normal proximal vessel lumens has shown a good correlation with diameter data obtained by quantitative MRCA[84] (Fig. 48–26). Similar success has been described by others,[85, 86] with identification of acute marginal branches as well.[85] The obtuse marginal branches of the left circumflex coronary artery are more difficult to visualize with current two-dimensional approaches,[85–87] a problem that is probably related to their oblique orientation and that is potentially overcome by three-dimensional or cine approaches. Similar success has also been reported with three-dimensional MRCA techniques.[88]

Identification of Coronary Artery Stenoses by Magnetic Resonance Coronary Angiography

The small caliber of the native coronary arteries (3 to 4 mm) and the relatively limited spatial resolution of current MRCA techniques (1.5 × 0.9 mm), makes quantitative MRCA improbable with current approaches. The development of stronger gradient systems and specialized surface coils[89] may permit quantitative MRCA in the future. Though quantitative MRCA is not currently possible, we have used the sensitivity of gradient-echo MRCA to assess laminar and absent or turbulent blood flow. Laminar blood flow is depicted as a bright signal, and regions of turbulent, markedly diminished, or absent blood flow as signal "voids" that correspond to focal coronary stenoses. A total occlusion or severe stenosis with poor distal blood flow may be expected to appear as an abrupt loss of signal (Fig. 48–27), and arteries with severe stenoses but significant antegrade blood flow may be expected to demonstrate a focal loss of signal, corresponding to an area of turbulence at the stenotic site, followed by bright signal depicting laminar flow in the more distal lumen (Fig. 48–28).

We reported on a group of 39 patients referred for elective coronary angiography who also underwent MRCA examination, either immediately before or after conventional contrast angiography.[90] Individual major coronary arteries were graded as "normal or having minimal disease" if there were minimal or no luminal irregularities, or as having "substantial disease" if there was marked attenuation of the luminal diameter or a signal void. MRCA images of 98 percent of the major arteries were adequate for evaluation. In a blinded analysis, overall sensitivity and specificity of the two-dimensional MRCA technique for correctly classifying individual vessels as being with disease (i.e., 50 percent diameter stenosis, or greater, on conventional contrast angiography) or without disease were 90 and 92 percent, respectively. The corresponding positive and negative predictive values were 0.85 and 0.95, respectively. Data for individual vessels are shown in Table 48–4. The sensitivity and specificity of the MRCA technique for correctly classifying individual patients as having or not having significant coronary disease, in this population with a prevalence of coronary disease of 0.74, were 97 and 70 percent, respectively.

With the use of a similar approach, Pennell and co-workers chose to grade MRCA data as representing severe (complete signal loss), moderate (partial signal loss), or mild (wall irregularity only) stenoses.[91] These investigators found a significant relation between angiographic diameter stenoses and these classifications. Preliminary data from Rogers and co-workers,[92] however, suggest that computer-assisted measurement of coronary flow signal intensity does not correlate with severity of stenosis. Duerinckx and Urman,[93] as well as Post and colleagues,[85] have had more limited success with two-dimensional segmented MRCA for identification of coronary stenoses. This may be related to the relatively poor temporal resolution of their sequence,[93] shorter echo time,[85] poor patient cooperation with breath-holding, or irregular rhythm, all of which contribute to image degradation.

Although breath-hold methods used by these investigators appear successful for imaging the coronary arteries and identifying stenoses, such techniques do require significant patient cooperation. A novel method for respiratory gating has been described by Sachs and co-workers,[94] in which navigator echoes are used to assess the position of the diaphragm in real time. Frames of data with motion are rejected and may be reacquired with the next heartbeat. Such a technique is particularly exciting in that it may be combined with three-dimensional approaches, allowing for acquisition of comprehensive cardiac function and coronary data with minimal patient respiratory cooperation. Combined respiratory or navigator gating with ECG gating will allow for the use of non–breath-hold MRCA techniques. Other advantages include improved signal-to-noise ratio and improved spatial resolution (Fig. 48–29).

Magnetic Resonance Coronary Angiography in Patients With Intracoronary Stents

The widespread use of intracoronary stents, typically made from stainless steel or tantalum, has raised a concern regarding the effects of very strong magnetic fields on these devices and possible stent motion. Despite the absence of published complications,

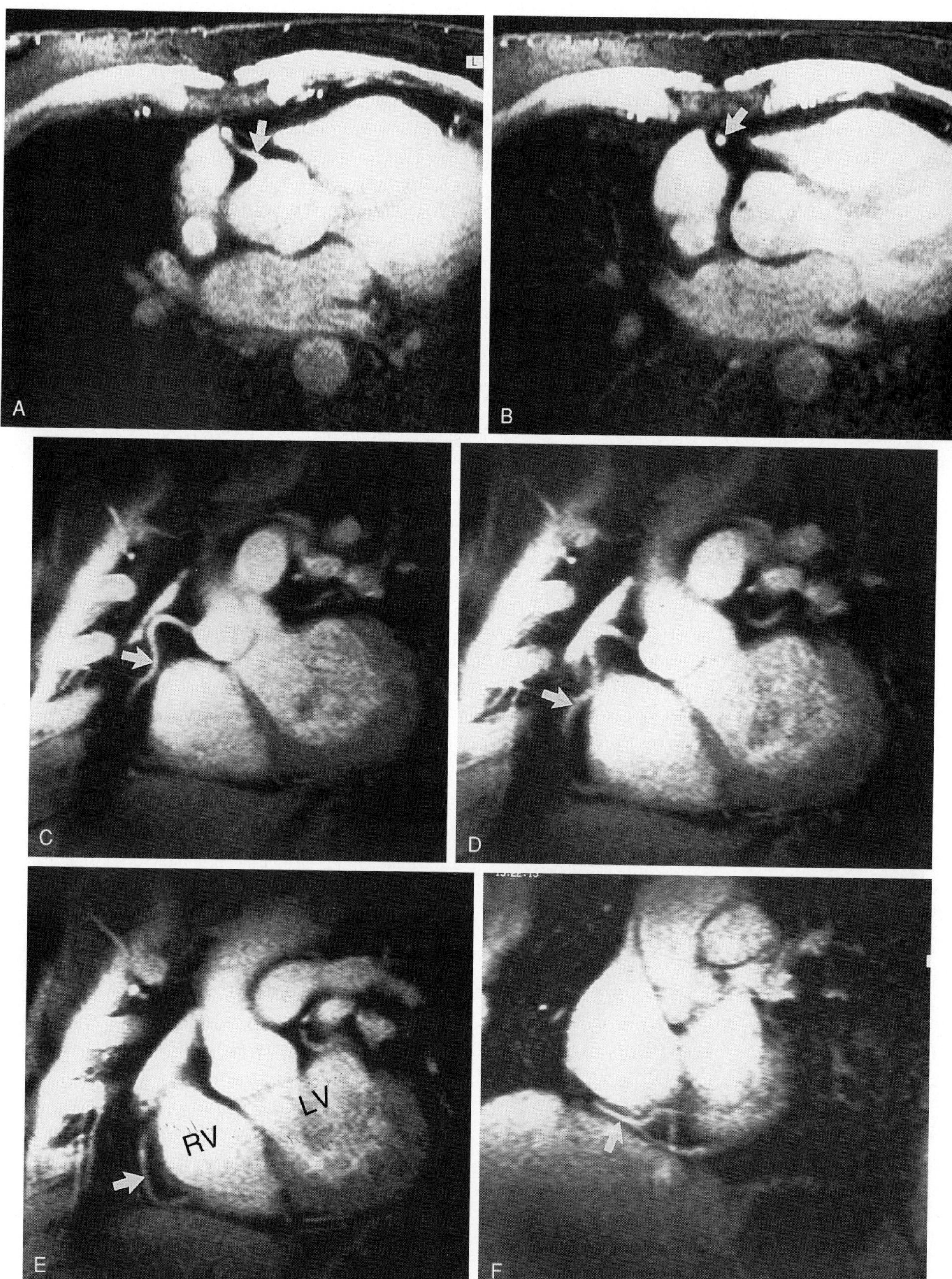

FIGURE 48–23. Breath-hold axial magnetic resonance sections of 3-mm thickness in a healthy volunteer. *A,* Transverse section at the level of the proximal right coronary artery (RCA; *solid white arrow*). *B,* Subsequent transverse section of the RCA at a more inferior level *(white arrow),* identifying the vessel in cross-section. *C,* Oblique section taken along the major axis of the vessel as defined by *A. D* through *E,* Adjacent sections depicting the middle RCA *(arrows). F,* Bifurcation of the distal RCA *(solid white arrow).* LV = left ventricular cavity; RV = right ventricular cavity; AO = aortic root. (From Manning, W.J., Li, W., Boyle, N.G., et al.: Fat-suppressed breath-hold magnetic resonance coronary angiography. Circulation 87[1]:94–104, 1993, with permission of the American Heart Association.)

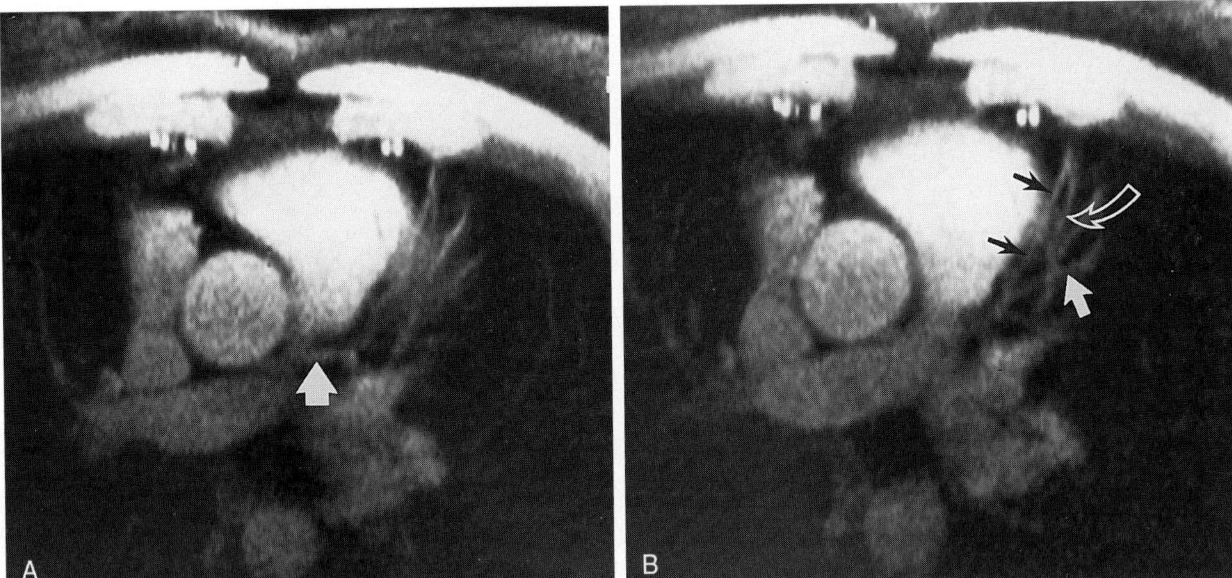

FIGURE 48–24. *A*, Axial magnetic resonance section of the left main coronary artery *(solid white arrow)*, continuing on into the left anterior descending (LAD) coronary artery *(B; black arrows)*. Note the diagonal branches off the LAD *(solid white arrow)* and the great cardiac vein *(open white arrow)*. (From Manning, W.J., Li, W., Boyle, N.G., et al.: Fat-suppressed breath-hold magnetic resonance coronary angiography. Circulation 87[1]:94–104, 1993, with permission of the American Heart Association.)

manufacturers have typically recommended against MRI for several months after intracoronary stent placement. Scott and Pettigrew[95] studied intracoronary stents ex vivo and found they were not significantly influenced by the magnetic fields currently used for clinical imaging (1.5 tesla or less). Imaging of the vessel lumen along the length of the stent, however, does result in a local image artifact, precluding evaluation of this portion of the vessel (Fig. 48–30).

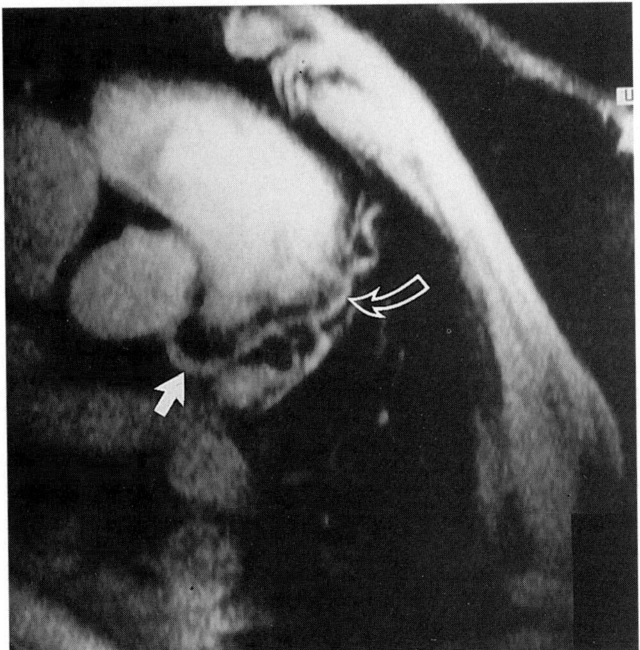

FIGURE 48–25. Oblique section depicting the left main coronary artery *(solid white arrow)* and left anterior descending (LAD) artery *(open white arrow)* in another subject. (From Manning, W.J., and Edelman, R.R.: MR coronary angiography. Magn. Reson. Q. 9[3]:131–151, 1993, with permission.)

Magnetic Resonance Coronary Angiography Assessment of Coronary Artery Blood Flow Velocity

In addition to imaging of the coronary arteries, MRI also offers the potential for assessment of coronary artery blood flow velocity. Currently, such assessment is limited to invasive techniques such as intracoronary Doppler flow probes[96] or semi-invasive transesophageal echocardiography.[97] Phase-contrast MRI techniques, in which signal intensity is proportional to blood flow velocity, have been validated for the assessment of ventricular stroke volume and cardiac output and for quantification of intracardiac shunts by assessment of blood flow within the great arteries.[98] Sequences analogous to the segmented two-dimensional turboFLASH approach for MRCA have been developed for phase-contrast assessment of coronary artery blood flow.[99, 100] This method has presently been described only in volunteers, with in vivo quantification of blood flow velocity at sites of coronary stenoses yet to be described. Although, in theory, the cross-sectional area of the coronary artery could also be assessed so as to measure coronary flow (e.g., in milliliters per minute of blood flow), the previously-mentioned relative spatial

TABLE 48–3. MRCA ASSESSMENT OF PROXIMAL CORONARY DIAMETER AND LENGTH OF VESSEL VISUALIZED

Vessel	Proximal Diameter (mean)	Proximal Diameter (range)	*Length (mean)*	*Observed (range)*
RCA	3.7	(2.7–5.1)	58	(24–22)
LM	4.8	(3.4–6.0)	10	(8–14)
LAD	3.6	(3.0–4.0)	44	(28–93)
LCX	3.5	(3.0–4.0)	25	(9–42)

MRCA, magnetic resonance coronary angiography; RCA, right coronary artery; LM, left main coronary artery; LAD, left anterior descending coronary artery; LCX, left circumflex coronary artery.

From Manning, W. J., Li, W., Boyle, N. G., and Edelman, R. R.: Fat-suppressed breath-hold magnetic resonance coronary angiography. Circulation 87:94–104, 1993, with permission from the American Heart Association, Inc.

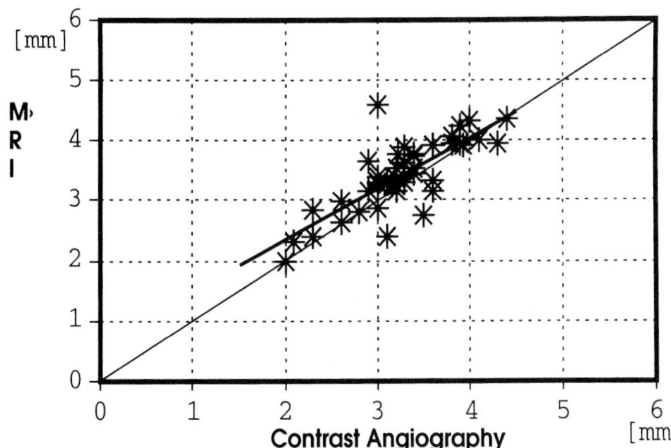

FIGURE 48–26. Scatterplot comparing results of assessment of normal proximal vessel diameter by magnetic resonance coronary angiography with results from quantitative (digital caliper) contrast angiography in a subset of patients who underwent both procedures. (From Scheidegger, M.B., Vassalli, G., Hess, O.M., et al.: Validation of coronary artery MR angiography: Comparison of measured vessel diameters with quantitative contrast angiography. *In* Book of Abstracts. Berkeley, CA, Society of Magnetic Resonance, 1994, p. 497, with permission of the American Heart Association.)

TABLE 48–4. SENSITIVITY, SPECIFICITY, POSITIVE/NEGATIVE PREDICTIVE VALUE OF MAGNETIC RESONANCE CORONARY ANGIOGRAPHY

	No. (%) with Disease	Sensitivity (%)	Specificity (%)	PV (+)	PV (−)
LM	2 (5)	100	100	1.00	1.00
LAD	23 (64)	87	92	0.95	0.80
LCX	7 (20)	71	90	0.63	0.93
RCA	20 (53)	100	78	0.83	1.00
Patients	29 (74)	97	70	0.90	0.88

PV (+), predictive value positive; PV (−), predictive value negative. Other abbreviations as in Table 48–3.

Modified from Manning, W. J., Li, W., and Edelman, R. R.: A preliminary report comparing magnetic resonance coronary angiography with conventional angiography. N. Engl. J. Med. 328:828–832, 1993, with permission.

resolution limitations of current MRCA approaches preclude accurate measurement of native coronary artery cross-sectional area at the present time.

After administration of intravenous adenosine, a fourfold increase in diastolic right coronary artery velocity has been found (Fig. 48–31). A study using time-of-flight EPI to measure coronary artery flow reserve documented a 52 percent increase in left anterior descending artery flow velocity among volunteers during isometric exercise.[101] Although few data involving patients with coronary disease, either at rest or after pharmacologic stress, have been published, this technique holds particular promise for assessment of the physiologic significance of a coronary artery stenosis and assessment of coronary artery flow reserve. Should this technique prove successful at identifying a particular resting flow profile that is characteristic for those with significant coronary stenosis, then it would be a particularly valuable adjunct to noninvasive MRCA, because both techniques could be performed in the absence of intravenous access or medication.

Magnetic Resonance Coronary Angiography of Anomalous Coronary Arteries

The ability of MRCA to acquire data in double-oblique orientations is uniquely suited for the evaluation of anomalous coronary arteries. Although rare, occurring in only 0.6 to 1.2 percent of adults referred for coronary angiography[102] and usually not associated with impaired myocardial perfusion, hemodynamically significant anomalies with abnormalities of myocardial perfusion are seen and may be associated with sudden death.[103] These hemodynamically significant lesions include origin of the left coronary artery from the right sinus of Valsalva with subsequent passage of the vessel between the aorta and right ventricular infundibulum. Although the diagnosis of anomalous coronary arteries is easily made by contrast angiography, definition of the subsequent course of these vessels (anterior or posterior to the right ventricular outflow tract) is often difficult. Such information is important, because it is the course directed posteriorly to the pulmonary artery and anterior to the ascending aorta that is associated with a poor prognosis. Both

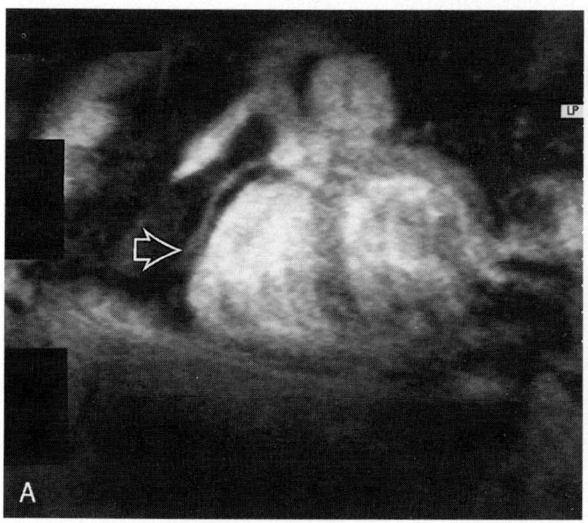

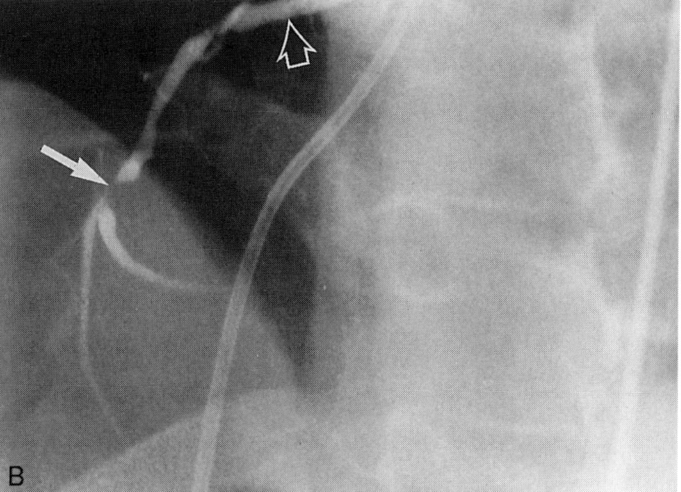

FIGURE 48–27. *A,* Oblique sections of the proximal right coronary artery (RCA). Note the abrupt loss of signal in the proximal artery *(open white arrow)*. The more distal artery was not visualized in adjacent sections. *B,* Corresponding conventional angiogram demonstrates the subtotal occlusion of the proximal RCA *(solid white arrow)* and the catheter in the right coronary ostium *(open white arrow)*. (From Manning, W.J., Li, W., and Edelman, R.R.: A preliminary report comparing magnetic resonance coronary angiography with conventional angiography. N. Engl. J. Med. 328[12]:828–832, 1993, with permission of the New England Journal of Medicine.)

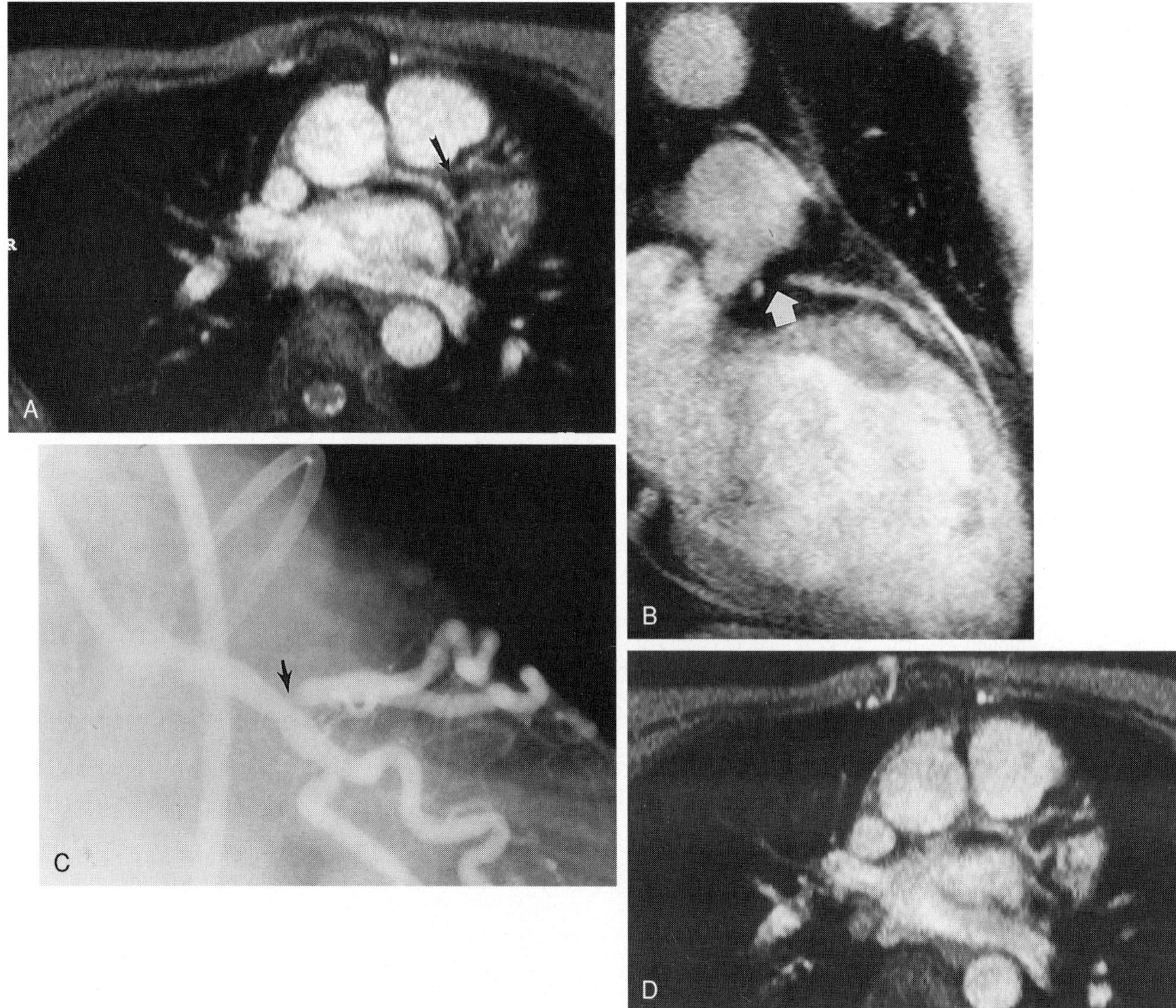

FIGURE 48–28. *A,* Axial section demonstrating the left main and left circumflex (LCX) arteries, with a signal void *(black arrow)* in the proximal left anterior descending (LAD) artery. Also, the more distal LAD and the diagonal *(white arrow)* can be seen. *B,* Single-oblique magnetic resonance coronary angiography image depicts signal void in the proximal LAD *(solid white arrow)*. *C,* Corresponding right anterior oblique (RAO) caudal conventional angiogram confirms the tight proximal LAD stenosis *(black arrow)*. *D,* Axial section after successful percutaneous transluminal coronary angioplasty and an exercise test that demonstrated no evidence of myocardial ischemia. Note that the proximal LAD is now well visualized *(open white arrow)*. (*A* and *C* from Manning, W.J., and Edelman, R.R.: Magnetic resonance coronary angiography. Magn. Reson. Q. 9:131, 1993.)

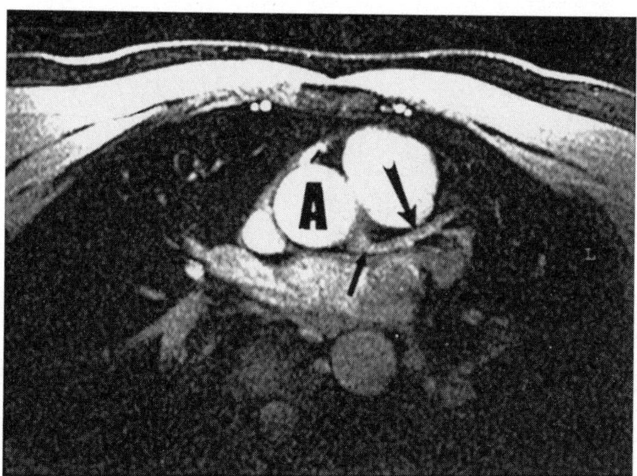

FIGURE 48–29. Transverse MRCA image acquired with fat saturation prepulse, K-space segmentation, and respiratory gating. This allows the use of a 256 × 512 matrix, two averages, and better spatial resolution. Note the enhanced resolution of the left main coronary artery *(short arrow)* and left anterior descending coronary artery *(long arrow)*. A = ascending aorta.

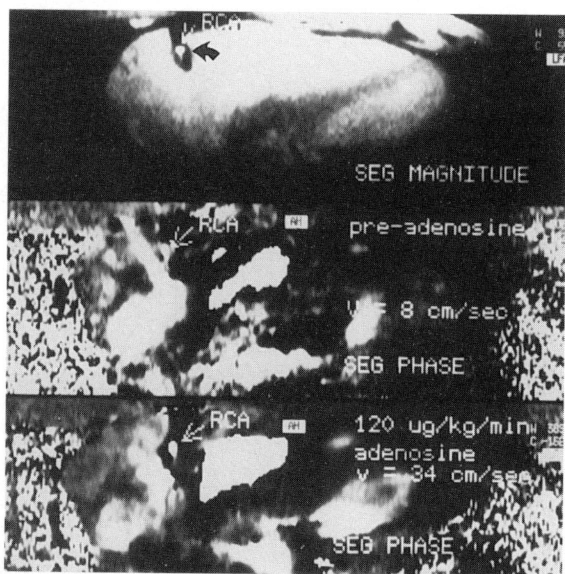

FIGURE 48–31. Top panel, Axial magnitude (anatomical) identifying the right coronary artery *(black arrow)*. Bottom two panels show phase-difference (flow) images obtained by the velocity quantification method during a single breath-hold. Phase-difference image gives flow velocity of 8 cm per second at rest *(middle panel)* and 34 cm per second after administration of adenosine at 120 μg/kg per minute *(bottom panel)*. (From Manning, W.J., and Edelman, R.R.: Magnetic resonance coronary angiography. Magn. Reson. Q. 9:131, 1993, with permission.)

conventional gradient-echo[104] and the two-dimensional segmented approaches[105] have been described as techniques to visualize the course of these vessels (Fig. 48–32). Although large series have not been reported, MRCA is considered the noninvasive technique of choice for delineation of the anatomical relations of these anomalous vessels.[106]

Echo Planar Imaging Magnetic Resonance Coronary Angiography

Advances in gradient hardware and software have led to the development of EPI sequences capable of imaging the coronary arteries. Very exciting is the development of segmented EPI techniques.[107] Such an approach offers the ability to acquire complete three-dimensional data sets encompassing the entire heart in one or two breath-holds (Fig. 48–33). Although the spatial resolution is relatively limited, this method does allow for the rapid identification of cardiac anatomy (takeoff and orientation of the coronary artery) and also provides the capacity for multiplanar reconstruction of three-dimensional data sets. However, the very short echo time (TE) may preclude identification of stenoses.

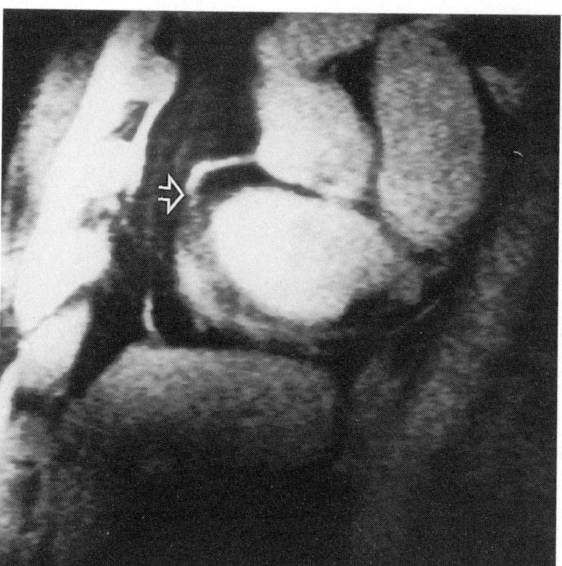

FIGURE 48–30. Segmented turboFLASH single-oblique magnetic resonance coronary angiography in a patient with an intracoronary stent in the proximal right coronary artery that was widely patent on contrast angiography. Note the abrupt loss of signal corresponding to the stent *(open white arrow)*.

Magnetic Resonance Coronary Angiography of Coronary Artery Bypass Grafts

Reverse saphenous vein and internal mammary coronary artery bypass grafts are easier to image by conventional MRI techniques than native coronary arteries are, because of their larger size (typically 5 to 10 mm in diameter) and more limited mobility with cardiac and respiratory motion. Conventional spin-echo[108, 109] and gradient-echo[110, 111] techniques have both been used to assess bypass graft patency. For most of these investigations, transverse images are obtained at a level corresponding to that expected for the bypass graft. The graft is then characterized as "patent" if the normal signal void (spin-echo) or bright signal (gradient-echo) of laminar blood flow (Fig. 48–34) is seen in at least two anatomical levels in the expected region of the bypass graft. If a signal void is seen at only one level, a graft is considered "indeterminate," and if no signal voids are identified, the graft is considered to be occluded. Data from several studies comparing MRI with contrast angiography are summarized in Table 48–5.

Major obstacles to imaging of bypass grafts are the local signal loss and artifacts associated with hemostatic clips or sternal wires. The avoidance of these clips would probably improve MRCA results, but it may be premature to advocate their exclusion in all patients based on the future potential of MRCA. Such a recommendation may be reasonable for younger patients, who are likely to need repeated angiographic data as their bypass grafts age and become diseased. Signal voids induced by these clips may be difficult to differentiate from those related to blood flowing rapidly through the bypass graft. In addition, grafts with very tight stenoses, in which blood flow would be expected to be low, often produce insufficient contrast to identify the graft as patent.[108]

Although both the spin-echo and standard gradient-echo techniques appear promising as noninvasive methods for assessment of bypass graft patency, it would also be helpful to be able identify saphenous vein grafts that are patent but have significant stenoses.

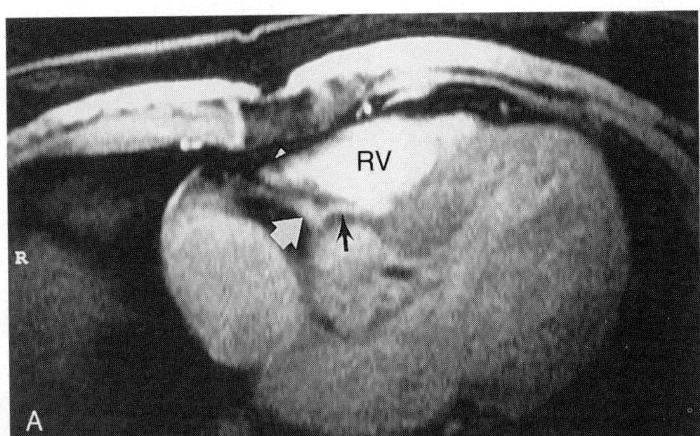

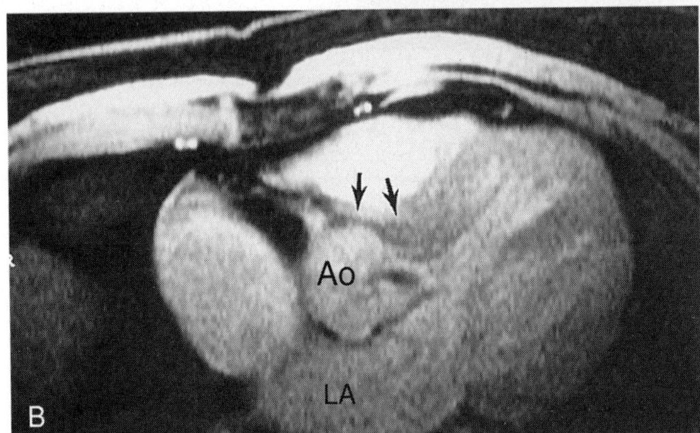

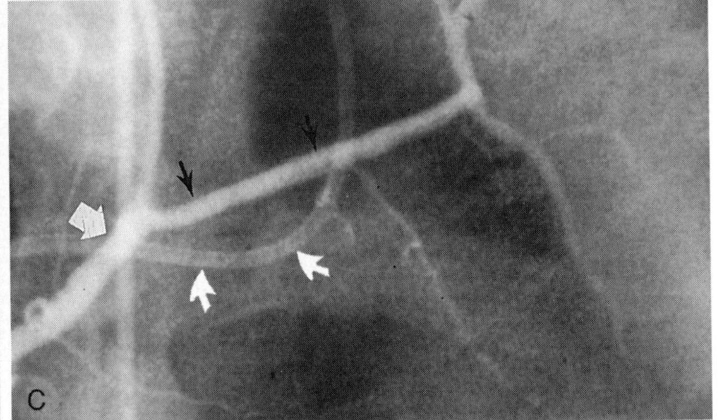

FIGURE 48–32. *A,* Transverse magnetic resonance coronary angiographic image at the level of the right coronary artery ostium *(solid white arrow)* and the origin of the anomalous left coronary artery *(black arrow). B,* Succeeding transverse image depicts the course *(black arrows)* of the left coronary artery. *C,* Contrast coronary angiogram obtained after contrast injection into the right coronary ostium *(large solid white arrow)* demonstrates the anomalous left coronary artery *(black arrows).* The pulmonary artery catheter is also visualized *(curved white arrows).* AO = ascending aorta; LA = left atrium; RV = right ventricular outflow tract. (From Manning, W.J., Li, W., Cohen, S.I., et al.: Improved definition of anomalous left coronary artery by magnetic resonance coronary angiography. Am. Heart J. 130:615, 1995.)

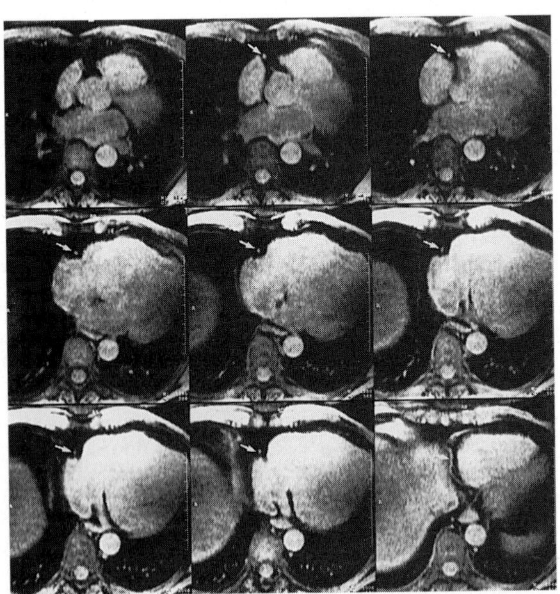

FIGURE 48–33. Nine 4-mm thick slices displaying the right coronary artery *(arrows)* from its origin to the apex of the heart. (From Wielopolski, P.A., Manning, W.J., and Edelman, R.R.: Single breath-hold volumetric imaging of the heart using magnetization prepared three-dimensional segmented echo planar imaging. J. Magn. Reson. Imaging 4:403, 1995.)

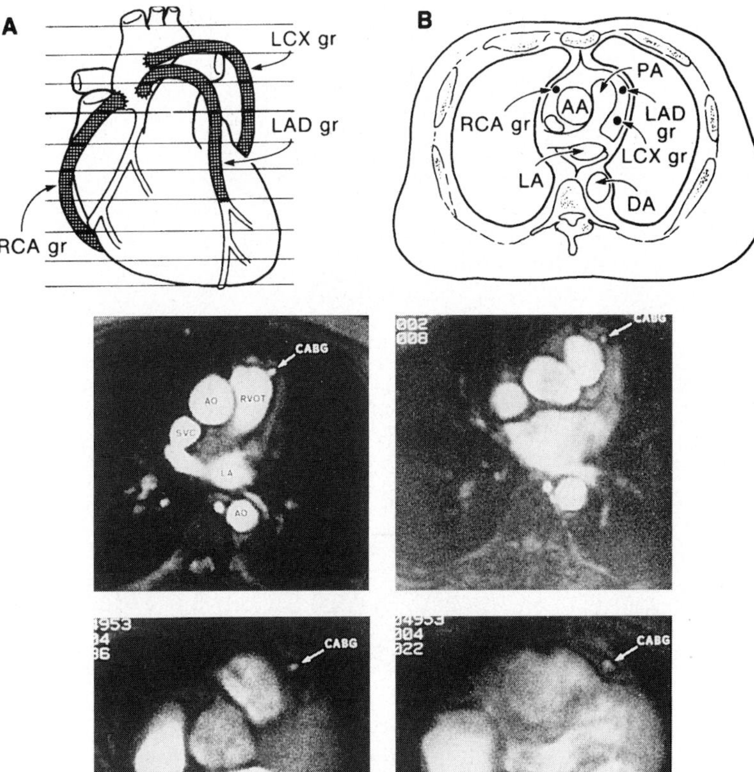

FIGURE 48–34. *A*, Typical location of bypass grafts coming off the proximal ascending aorta and anastomosing with the distal native coronaries with location of contiguous transaxial slices. *B*, The grafts as they might appear *(white arrows)* in a single transaxial slice. AA = ascending aorta; CABG = coronary artery bypass graft; DA = descending thoracic aorta; PA = pulmonary artery; RCA gr = graft to the right coronary artery (RCA); LAD gr = graft to the LAD; LCX gr = graft to the left circumflex coronary artery (LCX). (Top sketches from Rubinstein, R.I., Askenase, A.D., Thickman, D., et al.: Magnetic resonance imaging to evaluate patency of aortocoronary bypass grafts. Circulation 76:786–791, 1987. Bottom studies from Aurigemma, G.P., Reichek, N., Axel, L., et al.: Noninvasive determination of coronary artery bypass graft patency by cine magnetic resonance imaging. Circulation 80[6]:1595–1602, 1989, with permission of the American Heart Association.)

Such stenoses may certainly be the cause of ongoing myocardial ischemia, but, for the studies reported to date, a bypass graft with a significant stenosis would be "correctly" classified as patent by conventional spin-echo or gradient-echo imaging. Very preliminary data have been reported on the use of segmented gradient-echo techniques (similar to those used for imaging of the native vessels) for imaging of vein grafts,[112] but stenoses have not been described (Fig. 48–35).

Analogous to the technique reported for native coronary arteries, phase-velocity mapping has also been used to measure blood flow in native and grafted internal mammary arteries[113] and in reverse saphenous vein grafts.[114] Graft flow is characterized by a biphasic pattern, with average flow of 80 mL per minute. Indicators of graft dysfunction appear to be flow of less than 20 mL per minute and absence of normal biphasic flow pattern.[114]

CONCLUSION

In conclusion, we are now witnessing the evolution and early clinical application of novel MRI approaches to evaluate the patient with suspected ischemic heart disease. Ongoing clinical and animal studies will help further define the clinical role of many of the techniques described here. Further advances are needed in hardware (e.g., cardiac surface coils, faster and stronger gradient coils), in software (e.g., sequence optimization, automated data analysis, and image presentation), and in cardiac-specific contrast agents. Intravascular contrast agents may greatly improve signal-to-noise ratio for coronary imaging and allow for greater spatial resolution. The use of "navigator echoes" to monitor diaphragmatic motion appears very promising as a technique to minimize respiratory motion without the need for breath-holding. An ideal MRI perfu-

TABLE 48–5. SENSITIVITY/SPECIFICITY OF MAGNETIC RESONANCE FOR CHARACTERIZING CORONARY ARTERY BYPASS GRAFTS AS PATENT OR OCCLUDED

Author (ref.)	Technique	No. of Patients	No. of Grafts	% SVG	% Patent	Sensitivity	Specificity
White (108)	Spin-echo	25	72	88	69	0.86	0.72
Rubinstein°	Spin-echo	20	47	100	62[a]	0.90	0.72
Jenkins (109)	Spin-echo	16[b]	41	100	63	0.89	0.73
White (110)	cine gradient-echo	10	28	96	52	0.93	0.86
Aurigemma (111)	cine gradient-echo	20	45	91	73	0.88	1.00

SVG, reverse saphenous vein bypass graft.
[a]Graft with 99% diameter stenosis was considered occluded.
[b]Number of patients who had comparison angiograms.
°See Circulation 76:786, 1987.
Modified from Manning, W. J., and Edelman, R. R.: Magnetic resonance coronary angiography. Magn. Reson. Q. 9(3):136, 1993, with permission.

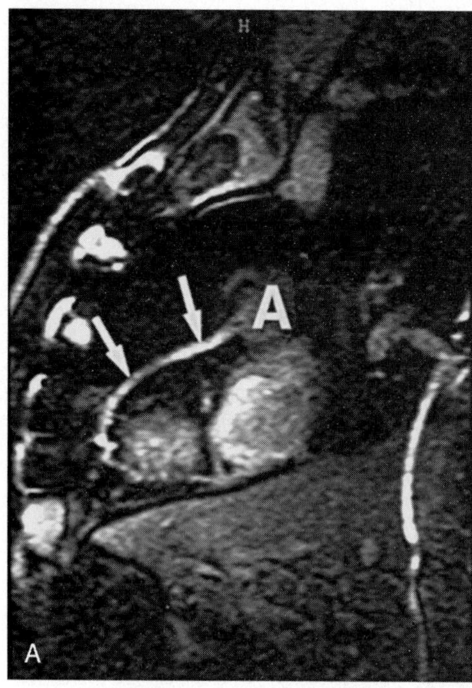

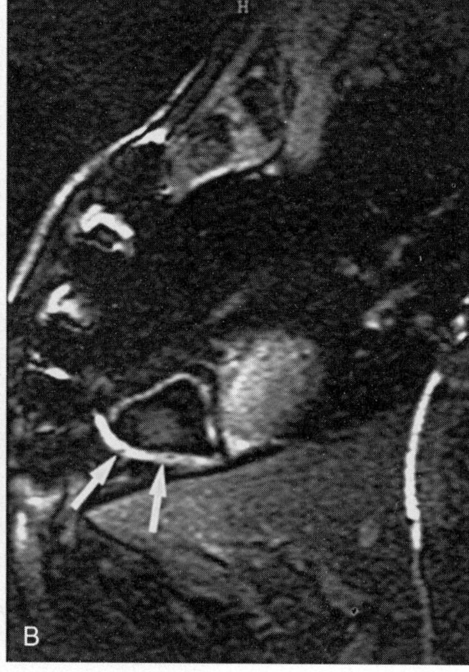

FIGURE 48–35. *A*, Oblique MRCA using breath-hold, K-space segmentation, and fat saturation prepulse, demonstrating the proximal half of an angiographically normal reverse saphenous vein graft *(arrows)*. The graft originates at the ascending aorta, and the first anastomosis is to an acute marginal coronary artery. *B*, Extension of the graft to the final anastomosis with the posterior descending coronary artery *(arrows)*.

sion agent may be one that "freezes" perfusion after injection. Such an agent could be injected during peak exercise or pharmacologic stress outside the magnet, with the patient electively imaged at a later time. EPI techniques for myocardial perfusion and MRCA are especially exciting, and the advance into "open" platforms opens the doorway to MRI-guided coronary intervention. Tremendous strides have been taken during the past 10 years, and we are optimistic that MRI will be able to provide a comprehensive, noninvasive cardiac evaluation, including precise data regarding cardiac anatomy, left ventricular systolic function, myocardial perfusion, myocardial viability, and coronary anatomy and blood flow.

References

1. 1993 Heart and Stroke Facts Statistics. Dallas, American Heart Association, p. 8.
2. Edelman, R.R., Wielopolski, P., and Schmitt, F.: Echo-planar MR imaging. Radiology 192:600, 1994.
3. Williams, E.S., Kaplan, J.I., Thatcher, F., et al.: Prolongation of proton spin lattice relaxation times in regionally ischemic tissue from dog hearts. J. Nucl. Med. 21:449, 1980.
4. Higgins, C.B., Herfkens, R., Lipton, M.J., et al.: Nuclear magnetic resonance imaging of acute myocardial infarction in dogs: Alterations in magnetic relaxation times. Am. J. Cardiol. 52:184, 1983.
5. Pflugfelder, P.W., Wisenberg, G., Prato, F.S., et al.: Early detection of canine myocardial infarction by magnetic resonance imaging in vivo. Circulation 71:587, 1985.
6. Wesbey, G., Higgins, C.B., Lanzer, P., et al.: Imaging and characterization of acute myocardial infarction in vivo by gated nuclear magnetic resonance. Circulation 69:125, 1984.
7. Pflugfelder, P.W., Wisenberg, G., Prato, F.S., et al.: Serial imaging of canine myocardial infarction by in vivo nuclear magnetic resonance. J. Am. Coll. Cardiol. 7:843, 1986.
8. Checkley, D., Loveday, B.E., Waterton, J.C., et al.: Detection of myocardial infarction in the mini-pig using NMR imaging. Magn. Reson. Med. 5:201, 1987.
9. Tscholakoff, D., Higgins, C.B., McNamara, M.T., et al.: Early-phase myocardial infarction: Evaluation by MR imaging. Radiology 159:667, 1986.
10. Wisenberg, G., Prato, F.S., Carroll, S.E., et al.: Serial nuclear magnetic resonance imaging of acute myocardial infarction with and without reperfusion. Am. Heart J. 115:510, 1988.
11. Rokey, R., Verani, M.S., Bolli, R., et al.: Myocardial infarct size quantification by MR imaging early after coronary artery occlusion in dogs. Radiology 158:771, 1986.
12. Bouchard, A., Reeves, R.C., Cranney, G., et al.: Assessment of myocardial infarct size by means of T2-weighted ^{1}H nuclear magnetic resonance imaging. Am. Heart J. 117:281, 1989.
13. Johnston, D.L., Homma, S., Liu, P., et al.: Serial changes in nuclear magnetic resonance relaxation times after myocardial infarction in the rabbit: Relationship to water content, severity of ischemia, and histopathology over a six-month period. Magn. Reson. Med. 8:363, 1988.
14. Caputo, G.R., Sechtem, U., Tscholakoff, D., et al.: Measurement of myocardial infarct size at early and late time intervals using MR imaging: An experimental study in dogs. AJR 149:237, 1987.
15. Ryan, T., Tarver, R.D., Duerk, J.L., et al.: Distinguishing viable from infarcted myocardium after experimental ischemia and reperfusion by using nuclear magnetic resonance imaging. J. Am. Coll. Cardiol. 15:1355, 1990.
16. McNamara, M.T., Higgins, C.B., Schechtmann, N., et al.: Detection and characterization of acute myocardial infarction in man with the use of gated magnetic resonance. Circulation 71:717, 1985.
17. Fisher, M.R., McNamara, M.T., and Higgins, C.B.: Acute myocardial infarction: MR evaluation in 29 patients. AJR 148:247, 1987.
18. Higgins, C.B., and McNamara, M.T.: Magnetic resonance imaging of ischemic heart disease. Prog. Cardiovasc. Dis. 28:257, 1986.
19. Postema, S., De Roos, A., Dornbos, J., et al.: Recent myocardial infarction: Detection and localization by magnetic resonance imaging and thallium scintigraphy. J. Med. Imaging 3:68, 1989.
20. Johns, J.A., Leavitt, M.B., Newell, J.B., et al.: Quantitation of acute myocardial infarct size by nuclear magnetic resonance imaging. J. Am. Coll. Cardiol. 15:143, 1990.
21. Johnston, D.L., Thompson, R.C., Liu, P., et al.: Magnetic resonance imaging during acute myocardial infarction. Am. J. Cardiol. 57:1059, 1986.
22. Krauss, X.H., van der Wall, E.E., van der Laarse, A., et al.: Long-term follow-up of regional myocardial T2 relaxation times in patients with myocardial infarction evaluated with magnetic resonance imaging. Eur. J. Radiol. 11:110, 1990.
23. Johnston, D.L., Wendt, R.E. 3rd, Mulvagh, S.L., et al.: Characterization of acute myocardial infarction by magnetic resonance imaging. Am. J. Cardiol. 69:1291, 1992.
24. Ahmad, M., Johnson, R.F., Fawcett, H.D. Jr., et al.: Magnetic resonance imaging in patients with unstable angina: Comparison with acute myocardial infarction and normals. Magn. Reson. Imaging 6:527, 1988.
25. Filipchuk, N.G., Peshock, R.M., Malloy, C.R., et al.: Detection and localization of recent myocardial infarction by magnetic resonance imaging. Am. J. Cardiol. 58:214, 1986.
26. Wisenberg, G., Finnie, K.J., Jablonsky, G., et al.: Nuclear magnetic resonance and radionuclide angiographic assessment of acute myocardial infarction in a randomized trial of intravenous streptokinase. Am. J. Cardiol. 62:1011, 1988.
27. Donahue, K.M., Burstein, D., Manning, W.J., et al.: Studies of Gd-DTPA relaxivity and proton exchange rates in tissue. Magn. Reson. Med. 32:60, 1994.
28. Nishimura, T., Yamada, Y., Hayashi, M., et al.: Determination of infarct size of acute myocardial infarction in dogs by magnetic resonance imaging and gadolinium-DTPA: Comparison with indium-111 antimyosin imaging. Am. J. Physiol. Imaging 4:83, 1989.
29. Wesbey, G.E., Higgins, C.B., McNamara, M.T., et al.: Effect of gadolinium-DTPA on the magnetic relaxation times of normal and infarcted myocardium. Radiology 153:165, 1984.
30. Wolfe, C.L., Moseley, M.E., Wikstrom, M.G., et al.: Assessment of myocardial salvage after ischemia and reperfusion using magnetic resonance imaging and spectroscopy. Circulation 80:969, 1989.
31. van Dijkman, P.R.M., Doornbos, J., de Roos, A., et al.: Improved detection of acute myocardial infarction by magnetic resonance imaging using gadolinium-DTPA. Int. J. Cardiac Imaging 5:1, 1989.
32. van Dijkman, P.R., van der Wall, E.E., de Roos, A., et al.: Acute, subacute, and chronic myocardial infarction: Quantitative analysis of gadolinium-enhanced MR images. Radiology 180:147, 1991.

33. Holman, E.R., van Jonbergen, H.-P.W., van Dijkman, P.R.M., et al.: Comparison of magnetic resonance imaging studies with enzymatic indexes of myocardial necrosis for quantification of myocardial infarct size. Am. J. Cardiol. 71:1036, 1993.
34. Eichstaedt, H.W., Felix, R., Dougherty, F.C., et al.: Magnetic resonance imaging (MRI) in different stages of myocardial infarction using contrast agent gadolinium-DTPA. Clin. Cardiol. 9:527, 1986.
35. Nishimura, T., Kobayashi, H., Ohara, Y., et al.: Serial assessment of myocardial infarction by using gated MR imaging and Gd-DTPA. AJR 153:715, 1989.
36. de Roos, A., van Rossum, A.C., van der Wall, E., et al.: Reperfused and nonreperfused myocardial infarction: Diagnostic potential of Gd-DTPA–enhanced MR imaging. Radiology 172:717, 1989.
37. Atkinson, D.J., Burstein, D., and Edelman, R.R.: First-pass cardiac perfusion: Evaluation with ultrafast MR imaging. Radiology 174:757, 1990.
38. van Rugge, F.P., van der Wall, E.E., van Dijkman, P.R.M., et al.: Usefulness of ultrafast magnetic resonance imaging in healed myocardial infarction. Am. J. Cardiol. 70:1233, 1992.
39. Fedele, F., Montesano, T., Ferro-Luzzi, M., et al.: Identification of viable myocardium in patients with chronic coronary artery disease and left ventricular dysfunction: Role of magnetic resonance imaging. Am. Heart J. 128:484, 1994.
40. Fleagle, S.R., Thedens, D.R., Stanford, W., et al.: Multicenter trial of automated border detection in cardiac MR imaging. J. Magn. Reson. Imaging 3:409, 1993.
41. Cranney, G.B., Lotan, C.S., Dean, L., et al.: Left ventricular volume measurement using cardiac axis nuclear magnetic resonance imaging: Validation by calibrated ventricular angiography. Circulation 82:154, 1990.
42. Mogelvang, J., Stokholm, K.H., Saunamaki, K., et al.: Assessment of left ventricular volumes by magnetic resonance in comparison with radionuclide angiography, contrast angiography and echocardiography. Eur. Heart J. 13:1677, 1992.
43. Atkinson, D.J., and Edelman, R.R.: Cineangiography of the heart in a single breath hold with a segmented turboFLASH sequence. Radiology 178:357, 1991.
44. Peshock, R.M., Rokey, R., Malloy, G.M., et al.: Assessment of myocardial systolic wall thickening using nuclear magnetic resonance imaging. J. Am. Coll. Cardiol. 14:653, 1989.
45. Akins, E.W., Hill, J.A., Sievers, K.W., et al.: Assessment of left ventricular wall thickness in healed myocardial infarction by magnetic resonance imaging. Am. J. Cardiol. 59:24, 1987.
46. Meese, R.B., Spritzer, C.E., Negro-Vilar, R., et al.: Detection, characterization and functional assessment of reperfused Q-wave acute myocardial infarction by cine magnetic resonance imaging. Am. J. Cardiol. 66:1, 1990.
47. Perrone-Filardi, P., Bacharach, S.L., Dilsizian, V., et al.: Metabolic evidence of viable myocardium in regions with reduced wall thickness and absent wall thickening in patients with chronic ischemic left ventricular dysfunction. J. Am. Coll. Cardiol. 20:161, 1992.
48. Johnston, D.L., Gupta, V.K., Wendt, R.E., et al.: Detection of viable myocardium in segments with fixed defects on thallium-201 scintigraphy: Usefulness of magnetic resonance imaging early after acute myocardial infarction. Magn. Reson. Med. 11:949, 1993.
49. Baer, F.M., Voth, E., and Schneider, C. A.: Comparison of low-dose dobutamine gradient-echo magnetic resonance imaging with positron emission tomography with [^{18}F] fluorodeoxyglucose in patients with chronic coronary artery disease: A functional and morphological approach to the detection of residual myocardial viability. Circulation 91:1006, 1995.
50. McNamara, M.T., and Higgins, C.B.: Magnetic resonance imaging of chronic myocardial infarctions in man. AJR 146:315, 1986.
51. Harrity, P., Patel, A., Bianco, J., et al.: Improved diagnosis and characterization of postinfarction left ventricular pseudoaneurysm by cardiac magnetic resonance imaging. Clin. Cardiol. 14:603, 1991.
52. Higgins, C.B., Lanzer, P., Stark, D., et al.: Imaging by nuclear magnetic resonance in patients with chronic ischemic heart disease. Circulation 69:523, 1984.
53. Lotan, C.S., Miller, S.K., Bouchard, A., et al.: Detection of intramyocardial hemorrhage using high-field proton (^{1}H) nuclear magnetic resonance imaging. Cathet. Cardiovasc. Diagn. 20:205, 1990.
54. Upton, M.T., Rerych, S.K., Newman, G.E., et al.: Detecting abnormalities in left ventricular function during exercise before angina and ST-segment depression. Circulation 62:341, 1980.
55. Quistorff, B., Nielsen, S., Thomsen, C., et al.: A simple calf muscle ergometer for use in a standard whole-body MR scanner. Magn. Reson. Med. 13:444, 1990.
56. Smart, S.C., Sawada, S., Ryan, T., et al.: Low-dose dobutamine echocardiography detects reversible dysfunction after thrombolytic therapy of acute myocardial infarction. Circulation 88:405, 1993.
57. Gould, K.L., Westcott, R.J., Albro, P.C., et al.: Noninvasive assessment of coronary stenoses by myocardial imaging during coronary vasodilation: II. Clinical methodology and feasibility. Am. J. Cardiol. 41:279, 1978.
58. Fung, A.Y., Gallagher, K.P., and Buda, A.J.: The physiologic basis of dobutamine as compared with dipyridamole stress interventions in the assessment of critical coronary stenosis. Circulation 76:1103, 1987.
59. Pennell, D.J., Underwood, S.R., Manzara, C.C., et al.: Magnetic resonance imaging during dobutamine stress in coronary artery disease. Am. J. Cardiol. 70:34, 1992.
60. van Rugge, F.P., van der Wall, E.E., de Roos, A., et al.: Dobutamine stress magnetic resonance imaging for detection of coronary artery disease. J. Am. Coll. Cardiol. 22:431, 1993.
61. van Rugge, F.P., van der Wall, E.E., Spanjersberg, S.J., et al.: Magnetic resonance imaging during dobutamine stress for detection and localization of coronary artery disease: Quantitative wall motion analysis using a modification of the centerline method. Circulation 90:127, 1994.
62. Baer, F.M., Voth, E., Theissen, P., et al.: Coronary artery disease: Findings with GRE MR imaging and ^{99m}Tc–methoxyisobutyl-isonitrile SPECT during simultaneous dobutamine stress. Radiology 193:203, 1994.
63. Pennell, D.J., Underwood, S.R., Ell, P.J., et al.: Dipyridamole magnetic resonance imaging: A comparison with thallium-201 emission tomography. Br. Heart J. 64:362, 1990.
64. Baer, F.M., Smolarz, K., Jungehülsing, M., et al.: Feasibility of high-dose dipyridamole-magnetic resonance imaging for detection of coronary artery disease and comparison with coronary angiography. Am. J. Cardiol. 69:51, 1992.
65. Wilke, N., Simm, C., Zhang, J., et al.: Contrast-enhanced first-pass myocardial perfusion imaging: Correlation between myocardial blood flow in dogs at rest and during hyperemia. Magn. Reson. Med. 29:485, 1993.
66. Wendland, M.F., Saeed, M., Masui, T., et al.: First pass of an MR susceptibility contrast agent through normal and ischemic heart: Gradient-recalled echo-planar imaging. J. Magn. Reson. Imaging 3:755, 1993.
67. Wilke, N., Jerosch-Herold, M., Stillman, A.E., et al.: Concepts of myocardial perfusion imaging in magnetic resonance imaging. Magn. Reson. Q. 10:249, 1994.
68. Manning, W.J., Atkinson, D.J., Grossman, W., et al.: First-pass nuclear magnetic resonance imaging studies using gadolinium-DTPA in patients with coronary artery disease. J. Am. Coll. Cardiol. 18:959, 1991.
69. Schaefer, S., van Tyen, R., and Saloner, D.: Evaluation of myocardial perfusion abnormalities with gadolinium-enhanced snapshot MR imaging in humans: Work in progress. Radiology 185:795, 1992.
70. Saeed, M., Wendland, M.F., Yu, K.K., et al.: Identification of myocardial reperfusion with echo planar magnetic resonance imaging: Discrimination between occlusive and reperfused infarctions. Circulation 90:1492, 1994.
71. Kraitchman, D.L., Wilke, N., Hexeberg, E., et al.: Integrated comparison of myocardial perfusion and function in dogs with coronary stenosis. (Abstract.) *In* Book of Abstracts. Berkeley, CA, Society of Magnetic Resonance, 1994, p. 1478.
72. Prasad, P.V., Burstein, D., and Edelman, R.R.: MRI evaluation of myocardial perfusion without a contrast agent using magnetization transfer. Magn. Reson. Med. 30:267, 1993.
73. Gould, K.L.: Detecting and assessing severity of coronary artery disease in humans. Cardiovasc. Intervent. Radiol. 13:5, 1990.
74. Nienaber, C.A., von Kodolitsch, Y., Nicolas, V., et al.: The diagnosis of thoracic aortic dissection by noninvasive imaging procedures. N. Engl. J. Med. 328:1, 1993.
75. Paulin, S., von Schulthess, G.K., Fossel, E., et al.: MR imaging of the aortic root and proximal coronary arteries. AJR 148:665, 1987.
76. Wang, S.J., Hu, B.S., Macovski, A., et al.: Coronary angiography using fast selective inversion recovery. Magn. Reson. Med. 18:417, 1991.
77. Li, D., Paschal, C.B., Haacke, E.M., et al.: Coronary arteries: Three-dimensional MR imaging with fat saturation and magnetization transfer contrast. Radiology 187:401, 1993.
78. Meyer, C.H., Hu, B.S., Nishimura, D.G., et al.: Fast spiral coronary artery imaging. Magn. Reson. Med. 28:202, 1992.
79. Manning, W.J., Li, W., Boyle, N.G., et al.: Fat-suppressed breath-hold magnetic resonance coronary angiography. Circulation 87:94, 1993.
80. Börnert, P., and Jensen, D.: Coronary artery imaging at 0.5 T using echo planar imaging. *In* Book of Abstracts. Berkeley, CA, Society of Magnetic Resonance, 1994, p. 372.
81. Edelman, R.R.: Cardiac angiography. *In* Book of Abstracts. Berkeley, CA, Society of Magnetic Resonance, 1994, p. 104.
82. Manning, W.J., and Edelman, R.R.: MR coronary angiography. Magn. Reson. Q. 9:131, 1993.
83. Burstein, D.: MR imaging of coronary artery flow in isolated and in vivo hearts. J. Mag. Reson. Imaging 1:337, 1991.
84. Sakuma, H., Caputo, G.R., Steffens, J.C., et al.: Breath-hold MR cine angiography of coronary arteries in healthy volunteers: Value of multiangle oblique imaging planes. AJR 163:533, 1994.
85. Post, J.C., van Rossum, A.C., Hofman, M.B.M., et al.: Current limitations of two-dimensional breath-hold MR angiography in coronary artery disease. *In* Book of Abstracts. Berkeley, CA, Society of Magnetic Resonance, 1994, p. 508.
86. Pennell, D.J., Keegan, J., Firmin, D.N., et al.: Magnetic resonance imaging of coronary arteries: Technique and preliminary results. Br. Heart J. 70:315, 1993.
87. Post, J.C., van Rossum, A.C., Hofman, M.B.M., et al.: Current limitations of two-dimensional breath-hold MR angiography in coronary artery disease. *In* Book of Abstracts. Berkeley, CA, Society of Magnetic Resonance, 1994, p. 508.
88. Post, J.C., van Rossum, A.C., Hofman, M.B.M., et al.: Respiratory-gated three-dimensional MR angiography of coronary arteries and comparison with X-ray contrast angiography. *In* Book of Abstracts. Berkeley, CA, Society of Magnetic Resonance, 1994, p. 509.
89. Chien, D., and Anderson, C.: Breathhold magnetic resonance angiography of coronary arteries using a circularly polarized phased array system. *In* Book of Abstracts. Berkeley, CA, Society of Magnetic Resonance, 1994, p. 502.
90. Manning, W.J., Li, W., and Edelman, R.R.: A preliminary report comparing magnetic resonance coronary angiography with conventional angiography. N. Engl. J. Med. 328:828, 1993.
91. Pennell, D.J., Bogren, H.G., Keegan, J., et al.: Assessment of coronary artery stenosis by magnetic resonance imaging. Br. Heart J. 1995 (in press).
92. Rogers, W.J., Kramer, C.M., Simonetti, O.P., et al.: Quantification of human coronary stenoses by magnetic resonance angiography. *In* Book of Abstracts. Berkeley, CA, Society of Magnetic Resonance, 1994, p. 370.
93. Duerinckx, A.J., and Urman, M.K.: Two-dimensional coronary MR angiography: Analysis of initial clinical results. Radiology 193:731, 1994.
94. Sachs, T.S., Meyer, C.H., Hu, B.S., et al.: Real-time motion detection in spiral MRI using navigators. Magn. Reson. Med. 32:639, 1994.

95. Scott, N.A., and Pettigrew, R.I.: Absence of movement of coronary stents after placement in a magnetic resonance imaging field. Am. J. Cardiol. 73:900, 1994.
96. Yamagishi, M., Hotta, D., Tamai, J., et al.: Validity of catheter-tip Doppler technique in assessment of coronary flow velocity and application of spectrum analysis method. Am. J. Cardiol. 67:758, 1991.
97. Iliceto, S., Marangelli, V., Memmola, C., et al.: Transesophageal Doppler echocardiography evaluation of coronary blood flow velocity in baseline conditions and during dipyridamole-induced coronary vasodilation. Circulation 83:61, 1991.
98. Brenner, L.D., Caputo, G.R., Mostbeck, G., et al.: Quantification of left to right atrial shunts with velocity-encoded cine nuclear magnetic resonance imaging. J. Am. Coll. Cardiol. 20:1246, 1992.
99. Edelman, R.R., Manning, W.J., Gervino, E., et al.: Flow velocity quantification in human coronary arteries using fast, breath-hold MR angiography. J. Magn. Reson. Imaging 3:699, 1993.
100. Keegan, J., Firmin, D., Gatehouse, P., et al.: The application of breath-hold phase velocity mapping techniques to the measurement of coronary artery blood flow velocity: Phantom data and initial in vivo results. Magn. Reson. Med. 31:526, 1994.
101. Poncelet, B.P., Weisskoff, R.M., Wedeen, V.J., et al.: Time-of-flight quantification of coronary flow with echo-planar MRI. Magn. Reson. Med. 30:447, 1993.
102. Kimbiris, D., Iskandrian, A.S., Segal, B.L., et al.: Anomalous aortic origin of coronary arteries. Circulation 58:606, 1978.
103. Cheitlin, M.D., Decastro, C.M., and McAllister, H.A.: Sudden death as a complication of anomalous left coronary origin from the anterior sinus of Valsalva: A not-so-minor congenital anomaly. Circulation 50:780, 1974.
104. Doorey, A.J., Wills, J.S., Blasetto, J., et al.: Usefulness of magnetic resonance imaging for diagnosing an anomalous coronary artery coursing between aorta and pulmonary trunk. Am. J. Cardiol. 74:198, 1994.
105. Manning, W.J., Li, W., Cohen, S.I., et al.: Improved definition of anomalous left coronary artery by magnetic resonance coronary angiography. Am. Heart J. 130:615, 1995.
106. McConnell, M.V., Ganz, P., Selwyn, A.P., et al.: Identification of anomalous coronary arteries and their anatomic course by magnetic resonance coronary angiography. Circulation 1995 (in press).
107. Wielopolski, P.A., Manning, W.J., and Edelman, R.R.: Single breath-hold volumetric imaging of the heart using magnetization prepared 3D segmented echo planar imaging. J. Magn. Reson. Imaging 4:403, 1995.
108. White, R.D., Caputo, G.R., Mark, A.S., et al.: Coronary artery bypass graft patency: Noninvasive evaluation with MR imaging. Radiology 164:681, 1987.
109. Jenkins, J.P.R., Love, H.G., Foster, C.J., et al.: Detection of coronary artery bypass graft patency as assessed by magnetic resonance imaging. Br. J. Radiol. 61:2, 1988.
110. White, R.D., Pflugfelder, P.W., Lipton, M.J., et al.: Coronary artery bypass grafts: Evaluation of patency with cine MR imaging. AJR 150:1271, 1988.
111. Aurigemma, G.P., Reichek, N., Axel, L., et al.: Noninvasive determination of coronary artery bypass graft patency by cine magnetic resonance imaging. Circulation 80:1595, 1989.
112. Pennell, D.J., Keegan, J., Firmin, D.N., et al.: Magnetic resonance coronary angiography: Early experience in coronary artery disease and visualization of vein grafts. *In* Book of Abstracts. Berkeley, CA, Society Magnetic Resonance Medicine, 1993, p. 219.
113. Debatin, J.F., Strong, J.A., Sostman, H.D., et al.: MR characterization of blood flow in native and grafted internal mammary arteries. J. Magn. Reson. Imaging 3:443, 1993.
114. Hoogendoorn, L.I., Pattynama, P.M.T., Buis, B., et al.: Noninvasive evaluation of aortocoronary bypass grafts with magnetic resonance flow mapping. Am. J. Cardiol. 75:845, 1995.

CHAPTER

49 Cardiomyopathies, Cardiac Masses, and Pericardial Disease: Value of Magnetic Resonance in Diagnosis and Management

George J. Hunter, M.D.
Eléonore Paquet, M.D.

CARDIAC MAGNETIC RESONANCE

In the investigation of heart disease, the identification of a definite cause and determination of a specific diagnosis may require the use of multiple diagnostic techniques of varying complexity. Rarely does a single modality yield the definitive answer; usually, several tests are performed and the results are interpreted together to arrive at a final diagnosis. Magnetic resonance imaging (MRI) is a method for the investigation of the heart that has been increasingly used over the last 10 years.[1–5] It is relatively noninvasive, it delivers high tissue contrast resolution with extremely good anatomical information in virtually any imaging plane, and, with recent advances in technology, it may provide high temporal resolution image sets with which to study cardiovascular dynamics.[6–9]

Another potentially important role of MRI is in the demonstration of metabolic abnormalities by magnetic resonance spectroscopy (MRS).[4] The use of MRS is, as yet, limited to a few research centers, and it has not become a routinely applied investigation in the diagnosis and management of heart disease. This situation is expected to change as more experience is obtained regarding the value of MRS in a clinical setting. Rapid imaging techniques now include, among others, turbo FLASH, segmented turbo FLASH, and echo planar imaging (EPI).[6, 10] These fast imaging methods allow global and regional ventricular function to be evaluated noninvasively and enable physiologic parameters of blood flow and valvular function to be included in the overall assessment of the cardiac patient.

Earlier methods for tissue characterization, based on T1 and T2 relaxation rates and proton densities, are being superseded by high-resolution EPI sequences that can provide the data necessary for yielding pixel-by-pixel maps of these parameters within short periods of time (about 10 minutes).[7, 11] However, the clinical utility of these data is still limited owing to the nonspecific nature of the information.

From a practical, clinical viewpoint, the typical MRI study for the investigation of heart disease uses a combination of T1-weighted spin-echo, T2-weighted spin-echo, and fast gradient-echo sequences. In all cases, gating to the electrocardiogram (ECG) is necessary for reducing and, if possible, eliminating motion artifact. A secondary value of gating, particularly with fast gradient-echo sequences in cine mode, is to allow the acquisition of image sets at well-defined times throughout the cardiac cycle. These data permit review of cardiac dynamics in the form of a cine loop, and they have value in identifying subtle areas of regional dysfunction. Calculation of ventricular volumes is possible from these dynamic cine data sets, as is estimation of regional wall thickening and wall motion.[7, 9–14] Respiratory movement may cause degradation in image quality, and in some cases gating to respiration may be necessary.[15] As with any radiologic imaging procedure, images in at least two planes are necessary for full diagnostic accuracy; this requirement is usually easily achieved with MRI.[16]

As research progresses, many new applications of MRI in heart disease have become possible. Nevertheless, despite the large array of uses of cardiac MRI, only a relatively small subset of MRI investigations are routinely used for clinical diagnosis. The feature of MRI that is so useful in the clinical arena is its superb tissue contrast resolution and ability to demonstrate anatomy in any plane. Of slightly less importance is the ability to demonstrate physiologic function. MRS is rarely used for routine clinical diagnosis, although this situation may alter with time.

CARDIOMYOPATHIES

Introduction

The literal meaning of the term cardiomyopathy is muscular pathology of the heart. As such, it encompasses almost every disease process that can afflict the heart. After many years of diverse usage, the World Health Organization and the International Society and Federation for Cardiology arrived at a consensus definition of cardiomyopathy, limiting the term to disease of the myocardium of unknown cause.[17] Based on the pioneering work of John Goodwin, three major classes of cardiomyopathy were included in the definition: dilated, hypertrophic, and restrictive.[18–22] Originally, this collection of miscellaneous diseases was divided into the three categories based on clinical and hemodynamic features: (1) congestive cardiomyopathy, with clinical features of cardiac enlargement, increased cardiac volume, and symptoms and signs of congestive cardiac failure with reduced pump function[23]; (2) hypertrophic cardiomyopathy, with clinical features of dyspnea, chest pain or palpitations, and signs of cardiac hypertrophy or cardiac failure[24–27]; and (3) restrictive cardiomyopathy, which was considered to be primarily an infiltrative myocardial disease associated with endomyocardial fibrosis, amyloid disease, scleroderma, hemochromatosis, and other disorders that interfere with cardiac filling and emptying.[28–34] This classification is principally descriptive of the final pathologic expression of many causes of heart disease.

Strictly speaking, if a specific cause for the cardiomyopathy can be identified, then the disease is not a cardiomyopathy by definition. However, in the initial stages of investigation, a working diagnosis of cardiomyopathy may be used and refined into a definitive diagnosis if possible. For instance, myocardial infarction, viral myocarditis, excessive alcohol intake, and cobalt ingestion, among other causes, may all lead to chronic dilatation of the left ventricle and a dilated cardiomyopathy.[35–41] Similarly, cardiac muscular hypertrophy may result from identifiable causes such as systemic hypertension or aortic valve stenosis, but only the idiopathic group is properly known as hypertrophic cardiomyopathy (HCM), and this disease is believed to occur in both sporadic and familial forms. Finally, restrictive cardiomyopathy proper is characterized by endomyocardial scarring of unknown origin that affects either or both ventricles and leads to restricted ventricular filling and cavity obliteration in the later stages of the disease process. Only after primary causes have been excluded should the term restrictive cardiomyopathy be used.

In practical terms, MRI is part of a range of tests used to classify a patient's heart disease. The specific value and limitations of MRI are presented here as they apply to the diagnosis and management of diverse cardiomyopathies, the term being used in this case loosely to include both known and unknown causes of cardiac disease.

Hypertrophic Cardiomyopathy

Anatomy

Cardiac morphology has been demonstrated by ECG-gated spin-echo MRI techniques. Typically, images are acquired gated to each R wave, with a echo time (TE) of 20 to 30 msec for T1-weighted images. The effective TR varies with the patient's heart rate; at a resting rate of 70 beats per minute, the repetition time (TR) is 857 msec. Increased heart rates yield shorter repetition times with more T1 weighting, and slower heart rates increase the TR and yield images that are less T1-weighted. To obtain T2 weighting, images must be acquired every two or three heartbeats, thus prolonging the TR beyond 1800 msec, with a TE of 60 to 90 msec.

ECG-gated MRI can identify the presence and extent of hypertrophy in patients in whom the disease has already been diagnosed by other means. The value of MRI under these circumstances is in the provision of additional information. For instance, assessment of the distribution of hypertrophy is essential in order to subdivide the diagnosis of HCM into different patterns, each of which may have a different prognosis or treatment strategy.[24] In order to adequately assess the wall thickness and the pattern of thickening, two orthogonal plane views are usually necessary. Furthermore, the images in the two planes need to be obtained at both end-systole and end-diastole. Care must be taken in the interpretation, because slight angles of obliquity in the planes imaged may lead to erroneous conclusions. A complete anatomical study should therefore include a true short-axis stack of images from apex to base and a four-chamber, double oblique stack from inferior wall to anterior wall. Parasagittal, vertical long-axis scans may be substituted for the four-chamber views, but a more complete study would also include this orientation. Figure 49–1 demonstrates concentric hypertrophy in both the short and long axis. Notice the classic pinpoint left ventricular cavity on the short-axis view at end-systole.

MRI has been of particular value in identifying the site of hypertrophy and any asymmetry that is present.[25, 42] Figure 49–2 shows asymmetric septal hypertrophy in short- and long-axis projection. In comparison with two-dimensional echocardiography, MRI is less operator dependent and is able to demonstrate with equal fidelity the anterior and inferior walls as well as the apex (areas of possible uncertainty with echocardiography). In particular, MRI is able to demonstrate the true distribution of hypertrophy in cases in which echocardiography has underestimated the extent

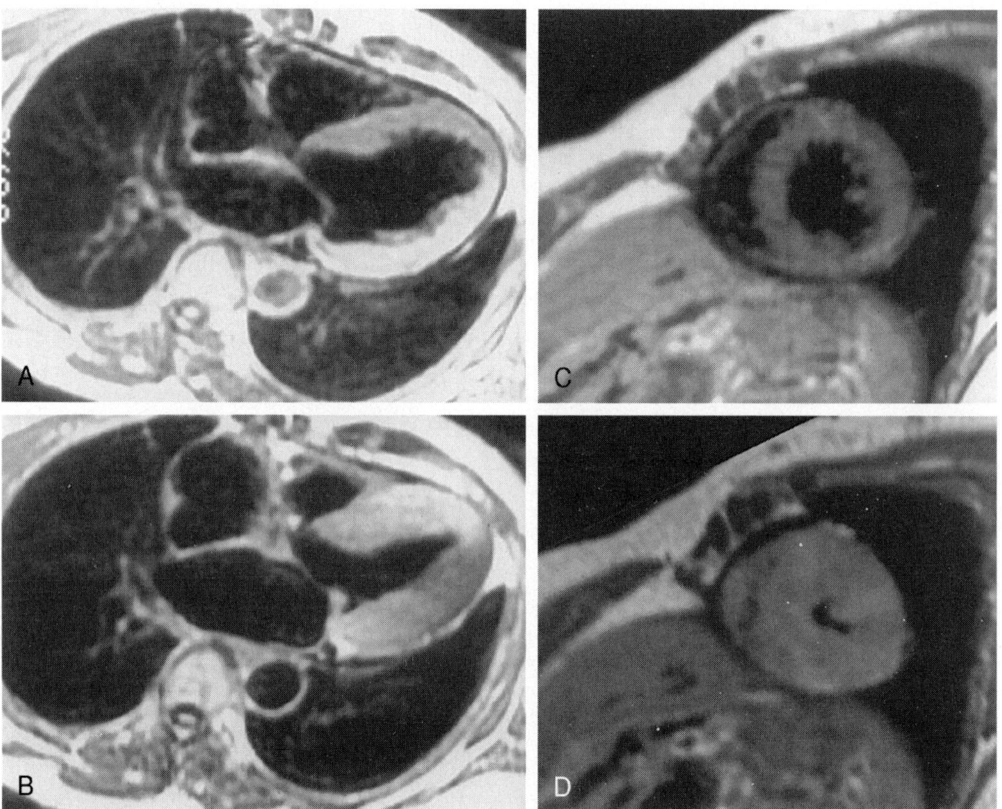

FIGURE 49–1. T1-weighted spin-echo (TR/TE = 938/20 msec) images of the heart in horizontal long-axis (*A* and *B*) and short-axis (*C* and *D*) projections, taken from the midportion of the left ventricle. End-diastolic (*A* and *C*) and end-systolic (*B* and *D*) images are shown at the same level. Note the concentric hypertrophy at end-systole. The left ventricular cavity is almost a pinpoint, a feature of hypertrophic cardiomyopathy.

of posterior or apical disease. Figure 49–3 shows severe apical hypertrophy with relative preservation of the basal parts of the left ventricle. Finally, assessment of the right ventricular myocardium is possible with MRI, and any hypertrophy at this site can easily be demonstrated (see Fig. 49–3*D*).

Physiology

Assessment of physiologic factors and their alteration from normal values has been an area of some interest in HCM. In this respect, MRI with a cine gradient-echo technique has been used to investigate wall thickening dynamics both globally and by region. Figure 49–4 shows typical cine acquisitions in short- and long-axis views. The brightness of the signal from blood in the ventricles can be compared with the dark blood seen on spin-echo sequences (see Fig. 49–1). With either technique, the myocardium can easily be differentiated from blood. With this method, the *percentage* thickening in hypertrophied segments has been shown to be less than in normal myocardium.[43] Similarly, assessment of wall thickness by MRI has been shown to be highly correlated with results from echocardiography. Alternative sequences can be used for assessment of wall thickening. In particular, recent work has shown that spin-echo EPI can produce an image set with individual images distributed through the cardiac cycle at 50-msec intervals[7] (Fig. 49–5). This allows good visualization of wall dynamics yet limits typical scan times to the order of 1 minute. The measurement of ejection fraction by MRI has also been shown to correlate strongly with left ventriculography.

Mitral regurgitation is often a component of HCM. Assessment of the degree of regurgitation can be difficult with simple ausculta-

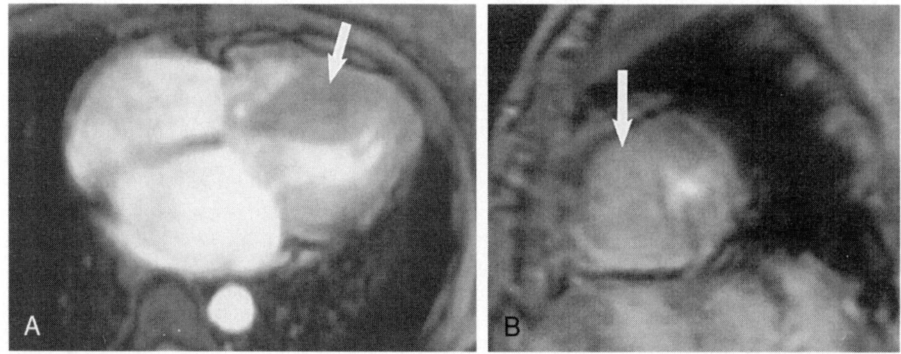

FIGURE 49–2. Gradient-echo (TR/TE/flip = 48 msec/10 msec/30 degrees) images of the left ventricle in four-chamber (*A*) and short-axis (*B*) projections. Note the relative asymmetry of hypertrophy, with the septum being particularly large. This is a classic case of asymmetric septal hypertrophy.

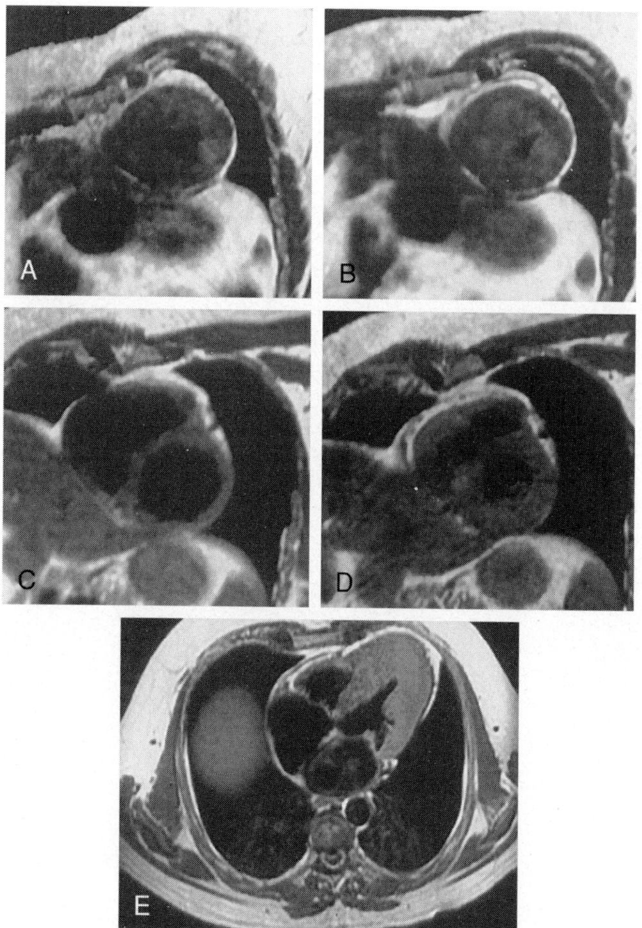

FIGURE 49–3. T1-weighted spin-echo (TR/TE = 1200/20 msec) images of the heart in two projections. End-systolic (*B* and *D*) and end-diastolic (*A* and *C*) frames are shown at the base (*C* and *D*) and apex (*A* and *B*) of the heart. The long-axis view (*E*) is shown at end-systole. Note the relative thickness of the muscle at the apex compared with the base of the heart. Note also the increased right ventricular wall thickness (18 mm) at the base (*D*).

tion. Although echocardiography with color flow Doppler may be of value, cine MRI has been found to be both sensitive and specific for this complication.[44–49] The regurgitation is seen as a signal void projecting into the left atrium, and its severity may be assessed by comparing right and left ventricular stroke volumes. This latter measurement is particularly well made with the use of breath-hold echo planar MRI, wherein images from which total ventricular volumes may be measured are acquired in about 15 seconds. In those patients with severe disease, the reduction in scan times is clearly a useful benefit, and motion artifact is limited to acceptable levels.[7] Figure 49–6 presents a set of end-systolic and end-diastolic slices obtained through the heart showing marked hypertrophy. The total imaging time for this acquisition was 13 seconds. Measurement of total cardiac mass may also be made with sequential short-axis images, and good correlation with echocardiographic measurements has been recorded. Finally, diastolic filling rates and other parameters have been shown to correlate well with traditional radionuclide techniques.

Tissue Characterization

In most patients, hypertrophic myocardium exhibits homogeneous signal intensity on high-quality MRI images. There is some evidence that in patients with HCM perfusion is not normal in the hypertrophied segments.[50] Differences in perfusion may result in relative ischemia and alteration in T1 relaxation rates consistent with ischemic injury and even localized fibrosis. Other studies have demonstrated alteration of signal intensity during the cardiac cycle in normal myocardium but no change in the hypertrophied muscle. These studies suggest that characterization of HCM may be possible with the use of relaxation rates to map underlying muscle variation. The value of this approach is as yet untested.

Dilated Cardiomyopathy

Introduction

Although dilated cardiomyopathy (IDC) is a disease of unknown cause, pathologically it represents a common end result of several factors that may initiate this disorder. Alcohol, peripartum cardiomyopathy, toxins, ischemia, hereditary factors, diabetes, hypertension, obesity, and viral disease may all lead to a grossly dilated ventricle with reduced pumping ability and heart failure.[35, 38, 39, 51–58] Magnetic resonance imaging is useful in identifying underlying causes and has a role similar to that in HCM.

Anatomy

The pathologic features of IDC are well described. By definition, coronary atherosclerosis, valve disease, and other specific cardiac abnormalities are absent. Perhaps surprisingly, the myocardium may be hypertrophied, weighing up to 1 kg, with ventricles that are dilated. Even with the hypertrophy, the ventricular walls are often thinned.[59] The left ventricle is grossly dilated and may be globular in shape, with a smooth endocardial surface caused by trabecular stretching. The atria and right ventricle may also be dilated.[59] Microscopic analysis usually shows hypertrophied myocytes interspersed with patchy areas of fibrosis; these appearances

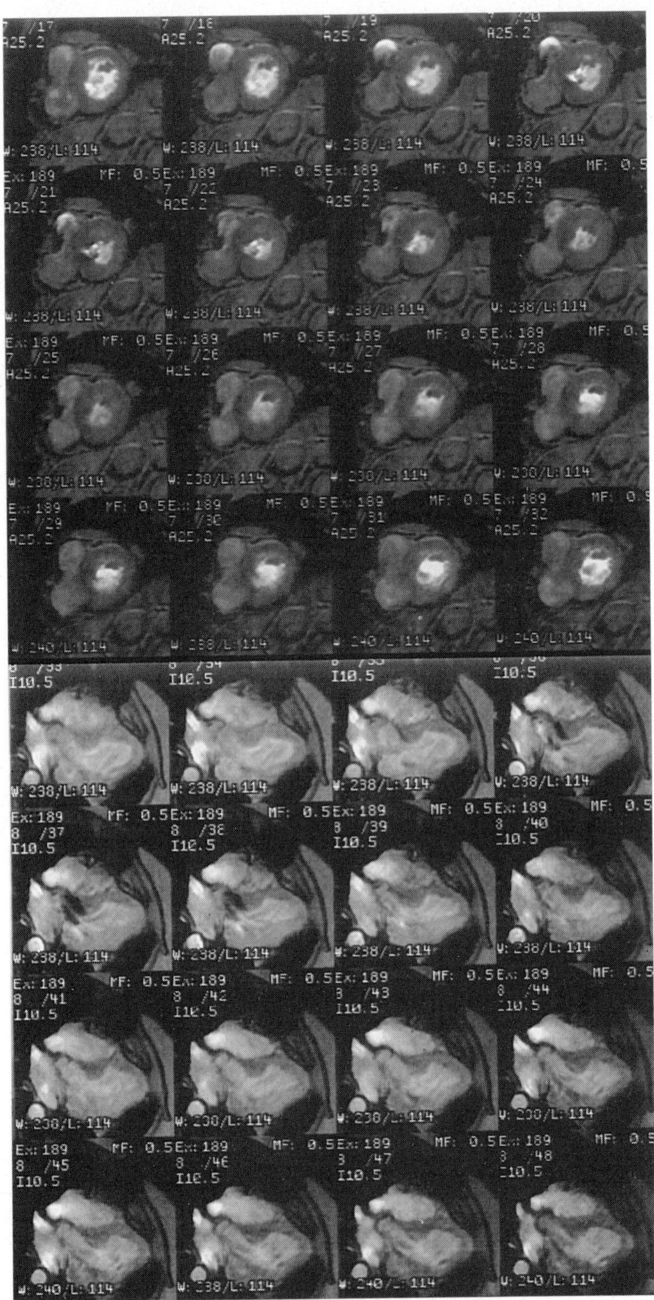

FIGURE 49–4. Sixteen frames spanning a single cardiac cycle from R wave to R wave are provided in the short- and long-axis orientations. This is a cine acquisition (TR/TE/flip = 40 msec/10 msec/30 degrees) and shows septal hypertrophy together with myocardial thickening regionally. Sets of images such as these may be used to calculate diastolic and systolic filling and emptying rates as well as regional wall dynamics.

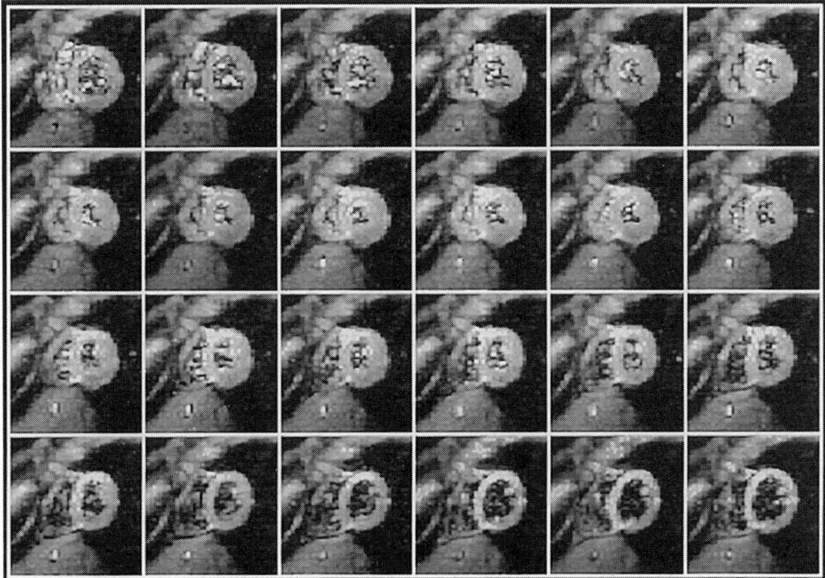

FIGURE 49–5. Twenty-four frames, acquired one per heartbeat at a progressively increased time from the R wave of each cycle. The effective interval between the frames is 50 msec. A spin-echo echo planar imaging sequence was used (TR/TE = 730/25 msec), which resulted in "black" blood.

account for the apparently paradoxical combination of increased muscle bulk with an associated decrease in contraction.

MRI is a useful imaging method for the demonstration of cardiac anatomy in suspected cases of IDC. Its primary value is in the exclusion of identifiable causes of dilatation, the most common of which is probably infarction. If other modalities, such as echocardiography or plain film radiography, suggest dilated myopathy, MRI may be able to show a localized dilatation consistent with previous occlusion of a clearly defined vessel.[60] For instance, the left anterior descending artery supplies the septum, among other areas, and an occlusion there may lead to septal thinning (Fig. 49–7) with preservation of the other parts of the left ventricle; clearly, this is not IDC. Another cause of cardiac dilatation is local aneurysm formation; again, MRI can differentiate this condition from the global dilatation of IDC.

Pathology of the right ventricle may be very difficult to demonstrate with other imaging methods.[61] Right coronary ischemia or infarction can be seriously underdiagnosed. Dilatation of the right ventricle with preservation of the left ventricle implies an ischemic event rather than IDC; however, even MRI may have difficulty in separating early IDC from localized right ventricular pathology (Figs. 49–8 and 49–9). Studies with MRI have enabled some more details of the internal anatomy of the heart in IDC to be documented. For instance, left atrial and right ventricular dilatation has been reported less frequently than expected, and in some patients heterogeneity within the left ventricular myocardium has been identified, with disproportionate thinning of the ventricular septum but relative preservation of normal architecture in the inferior and anterior left ventricular walls.[59]

Physiology

Cine MRI in a short-axis view may be used to demonstrate left ventricular wall thickness and thickening during the cardiac cycle.[60, 62–64] Stroke volumes may also be calculated, together with indices of diastolic and systolic function, by cine MRI or multiple-gated spin-echo sequences. Furthermore, the presence of valvular regur-

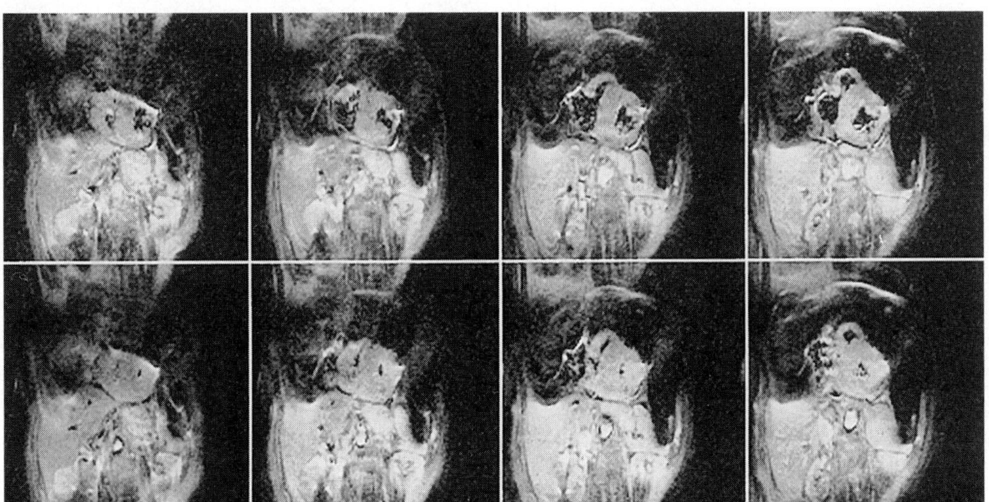

FIGURE 49–6. Four paired end-diastolic *(top row)* and end-systolic *(bottom row)* images are provided, spanning the midportion of the left ventricle. A spin-echo echo planar sequence (TR/TE = 638/20 msec) was used to obtain these frames. Total muscle bulk can be assessed in this manner, as can global and regional ejection fractions. Note the diffuse hypertrophy.

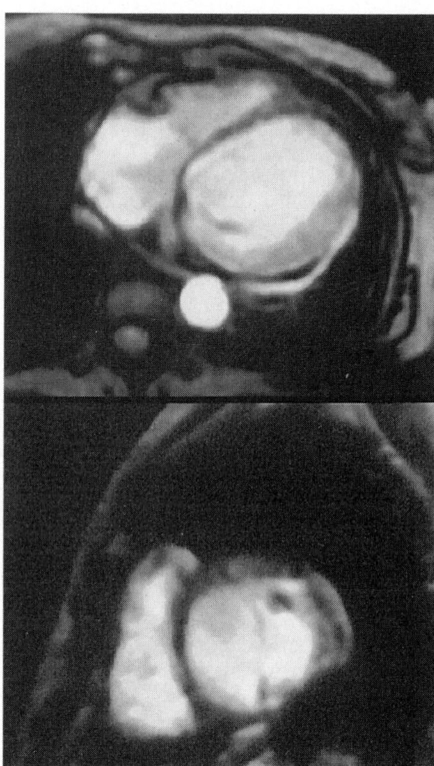

FIGURE 49–7. A pair of gradient-echo images (TR/TE/flip = 50 msec/12 msec/30 degrees) in early diastole show marked thinning of the septum compared with the left ventricular free wall. This was the end result of a previous occlusion of the left anterior descending artery.

gitation may be identified[48] (Fig. 49–10). Together, these parameters can define the severity of the cardiomyopathy. Comparison between normal volunteers and patients with IDC has shown significant differences in ejection fraction and left ventricular mass-to-volume ratios (Fig. 49–11). Also, left ventricular systolic wall thickening has been shown to be more heterogeneous in patients with IDC than in normal volunteers, with the pattern of left ventricular wall thickening significantly different in the two groups (Fig. 49–12).

A more objective method of characterizing left ventricular function in this disease is the measurement of myocardial wall stress.[9] This is usually an invasive procedure. However, with simultaneous

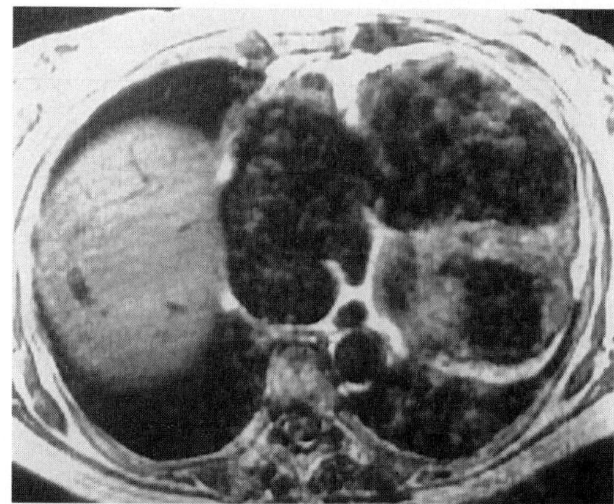

FIGURE 49–8. A single four-chamber view of the heart taken with a spin-echo sequence (TR/TE = 400/20 msec). Note the gross right ventricular enlargement with relative preservation of the left ventricle. These appearances are not entirely specific but imply localized right ventricular pathology rather than dilated cardiomyopathy. The patient was found to have right ventricular dysplasia at autopsy.

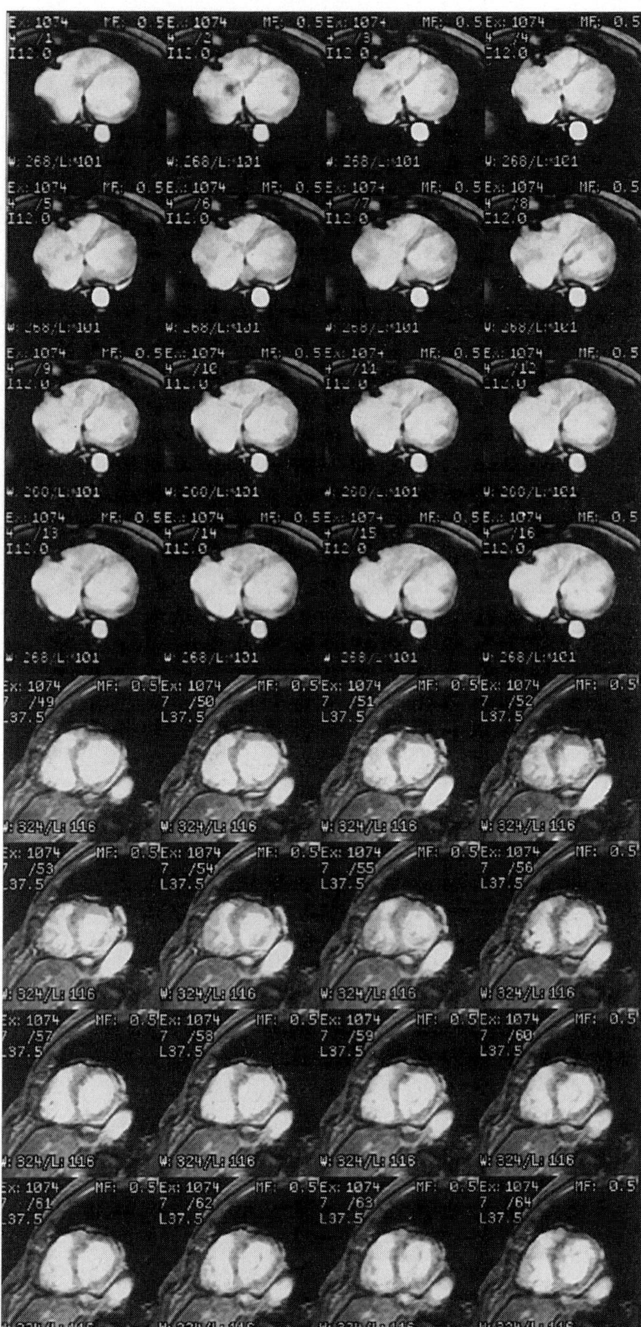

FIGURE 49–9. Short- and long-axis cine gradient-echo image sets (TR/TE/flip = 50 msec/12 msec/30 degrees) show virtually no contraction of the right ventricle, with reduction in left ventricular inferior wall contraction and dilatation of the left ventricle. These appearances suggest coronary pathology rather than dilated cardiomyopathy.

measurement of blood pressure throughout the investigation and indices of left ventricular end-systolic diameter and end-systolic wall thickness obtained with MRI, wall stress may be calculated with minimal invasiveness.[9] Because it has been shown that wall stress is elevated in dilated cardiomyopathy, this parameter may provide a reproducible method for monitoring patients and their response to treatment in this condition.

Tissue Characterization

Relaxation rates of tissues measured in vitro have indicated differences in normal myocardium compared with myocardium suffering toxic injury (e.g., from doxorubicin or as a result of viral infection). Calculation of relaxation rates in a clinical setting is

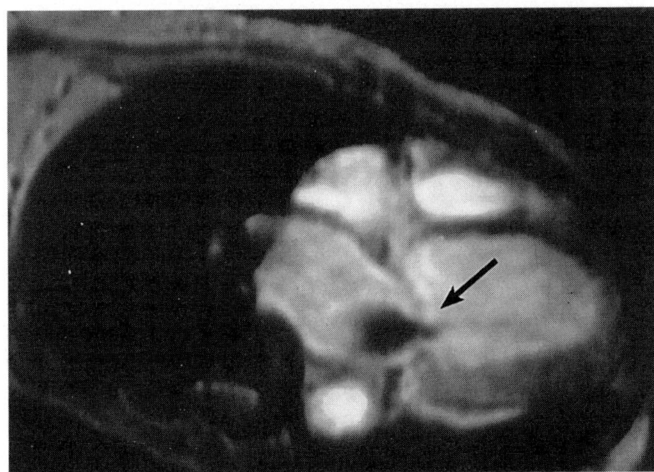

FIGURE 49–10. A single long-axis gradient-echo (TR/TE/flip = 50 msec/12 msec/30 degrees) image shows a flow void in the left atrium extending across the mitral valve *(black arrow)*. The appearances are those of mitral regurgitation resulting from gross dilatation of the left side of the heart and of the mitral valve ring in particular.

feasible with echo planar MRI, but as yet this technique is not routinely available. In patients who have undergone heart transplantation, assessment of the integrity of the transplanted myocardium is possible with MRI with minimal risk to the patient. Rejection episodes may manifest as dilatation of the left ventricle, heart failure with pulmonary edema, or both.[65]

In addition to the anatomical demonstration of left ventricular dilatation, MRI is able to show an alteration in T2 relaxation rates in areas of the myocardium that are undergoing rejection. The mechanism of this change is thought to be simply an increase in edema resulting from increased numbers of lymphocytes, which leads to, and is part of, an inflammatory reaction. Normal T2 values range between 25 and 40 msec; rejection is likely if the T2 increases above 50 msec and very likely if it rises above 80 msec. In this relatively rare but well defined situation, MRI may provide a unique, noninvasive method of monitoring the status of the heart and its response to treatment during a rejection episode. Because the technique is nonspecific, it becomes useful only after the acute inflammatory changes associated with the transplantation itself have subsided. Therefore, evaluation of tissue relaxation rates is not usually undertaken in the first 4 weeks after operation.

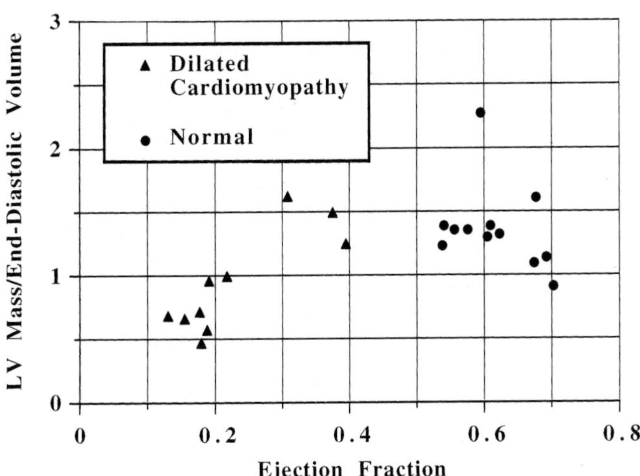

FIGURE 49–11. Plot of the ratio of left ventricular mass to end-diastolic volume versus the ejection fraction in normal subjects and in patients with dilated cardiomyopathy. There is a clear separation between the two groups. Cine gradient-echo imaging was used to provide the image sets from which the parameters were calculated.

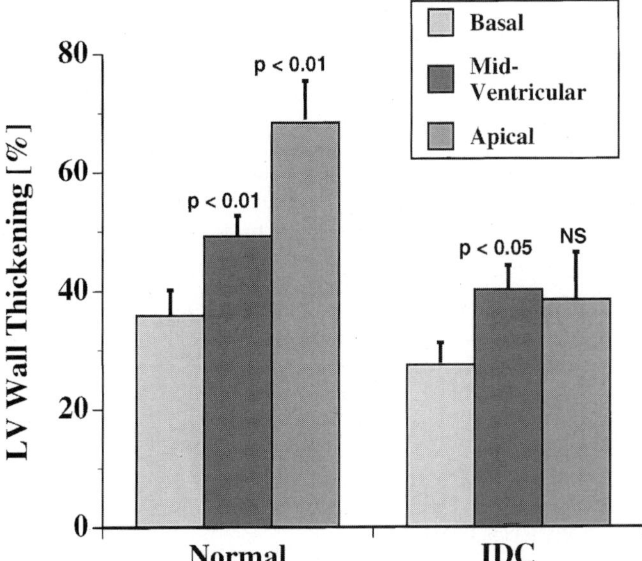

FIGURE 49–12. Bar diagram of percentage systolic wall thickening for various regions of the heart extending from apex to base of the left ventricle in normal subjects (n = 10) and in patients with dilated cardiomyopathy (IDC; n = 10). In normal subjects, there is a gradient in wall thickening from base to apex. This gradient is absent in patients with IDC. (Modified from Buser, P.T., Auffermann, W., Holt, W.W., et al.: Noninvasive evaluation of global left ventricular function with use of cine nuclear magnetic resonance. J. Am. Coll. Cardiol. 13:1294, 1989, with permission of the American College of Cardiology.)

Other causes of an IDC are similarly amenable to definitive investigation by MRI, for instance, hemochromatosis.[30, 66] In this condition, the relaxation rates are markedly reduced because of increased iron present in the myocardium. Not only can the diagnosis be made, but reduction in tissue iron may be monitored during therapy.

Restrictive Cardiomyopathy

This is a relatively rare condition, and there has been little experience with MRI in such cases. In general terms, MRI is capable of characterizing tissue relaxation rates and identifying a

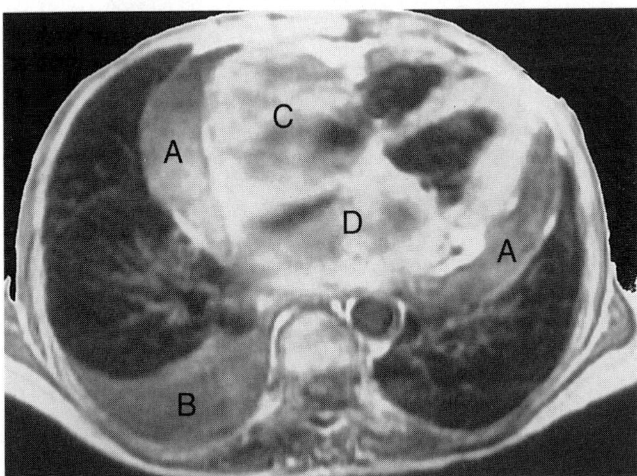

FIGURE 49–13. Single four-chamber slice taken with a spin-echo sequence (TR/TE = 1000/20 msec). Note the normal-sized ventricles with the large pericardial effusion (A) and bright blood in the atria (C and D), indicating relative stasis. The atria are also enlarged. There is no pericardial thickening, and the picture is that of a restrictive cardiomyopathy with associated pericardial effusion.

potential infiltrative process leading to myocardial stiffness and restriction.[33, 67, 68] Otherwise, the most important role of MRI in restrictive cardiomyopathy is to demonstrate the pericardium in order to exclude constrictive pericardial disease.[28, 31, 34]

MRI may demonstrate the anatomical changes of infiltrative myocardial diseases in a noninvasive fashion. Characteristic of restrictive cardiomyopathy is enlargement of the atria, with relatively normal-sized ventricles and prominent intracavitary signal caused by stasis and slow movement of blood in the chambers, particularly the atria (Fig. 49–13). On the other hand, a thickened pericardium with right ventricular narrowing and disproportionately dilated right atrium and caval veins is a feature of constrictive pericardial disease (Fig. 49–14), although not all cases of thickened pericardium indicate constriction.[29, 32, 69, 70] MRI offers a straightforward method of making the distinction between pericardial constriction and ventricular restriction; the treatments are very different for these two causes of essentially the same clinical picture.

THE PERICARDIUM

Anatomy

The pericardium is a specialized organ with complex physiology. It consists of a mesothelial sac, the serosa, which is closely applied to the heart and the immediately adjacent great vessels. The serosa continues as a lining to the outer layer of the pericardium, the fibrosa. The fibrosa is attached to the central tendon of the diaphragm and loosely joined to the xiphoid and manubrium. There are therefore three layers to the pericardium: the monocellular layer of the serosa applied to the heart is the visceral pericardium, and the rest of the serosa and its outer covering of fibrosa form the parietal pericardium. There is a variable amount of fat between the pericardium and the myocardium that surrounds the coronary vessels. This should be differentiated from mediastinal fat, which may surround the pericardium in obese patients.[71–74]

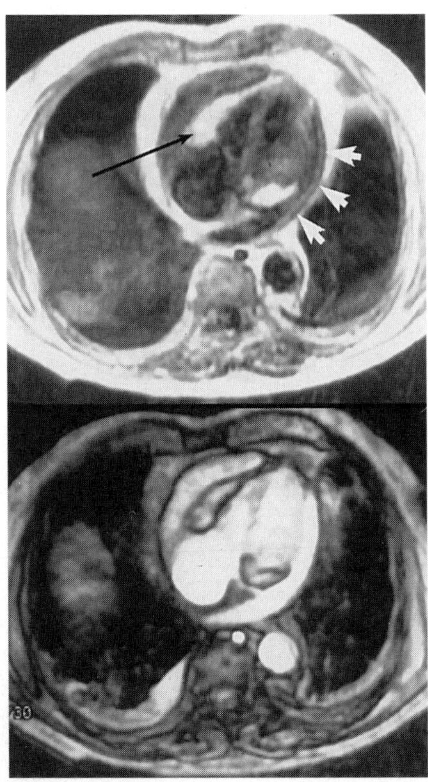

FIGURE 49–14. Two images in the four-chamber orientation through the heart. The top image was acquired by a T1-weighted spin-echo technique (TR/TE = 750/20 msec) and shows marked pericardial thickening *(white arrows)*. The black arrow indicates subpericardial fat. Note the small right and left ventricles. The bottom image, which is a gradient-echo study (TR/TE/flip = 50 msec/12 msec/30 degrees), confirms the presence of a pericardial effusion. The pericardium is less reliably assessed on gradient-echo images because of artifactual increase in the thickness. Dilatation of the superior caval vein is very clearly shown. Incidental note of a pleural effusion is made. These appearances are features of constrictive pericarditis rather than restrictive cardiomyopathy.

Physiology

The pericardium has a surprising number of physiologic functions. As a mechanical envelope, it promotes cardiac efficiency, particularly during hemodynamic overload. Because the envelope is relatively inelastic, it limits excessive cardiac dilatation and maintains normal ventricular compliance. The Starling mechanism is able to operate at all intraventricular pressures because of the pericardium. These and other functions maintain cardiocirculatory regulation by means of pericardial neuroreceptors and mechanoreceptors. As a membrane, the pericardium reduces friction, allowing smooth motion of the heart during contraction and relaxation; it acts as a barrier to inflammation from adjacent structures and strengthens the thinner portions of the heart, such as the atria and the right ventricle. The pericardium also acts as an external support, limiting the movement of the heart within the thorax by its attachments to the diaphragm and sternum.[75]

Imaging

Until relatively recently, assessment of the pericardium has been at best indirect. Plain film radiography, ventriculography, and conventional tomography are all of limited value.[76] Echocardiography provides an improvement over these imaging methods, although it cannot usually identify subtle changes within the layers themselves. Computed tomography (CT) can be useful because it allows separation of the pericardium and endocardium in some cases. In general, however, CT suffers from poor tissue contrast and is of limited usefulness.[77–79] MRI has become the imaging method of choice for evaluation of the pericardium. MRI has very high tissue contrast and is able to visualize the pericardium in multiple planes. Different sequences can be used to enhance tissue characteristics and to separate simple from complex effusions and pericardial fat from pathological thickening; they can also identify breaches of the pericardium secondary to myocardial or mediastinal pathology.[80–83]

MRI of the pericardium requires ECG gating; ungated scans are of limited value and usually can demonstrate only fixed pericardial masses or large effusions. Intrinsic abnormalities, such as thickening, can be demonstrated reliably only with ECG gating. Double-echo techniques with TE values in the range of 20 to 70 msec are useful in defining anatomy and separating tissue type in a single examination. Currently used sequences and equipment allow a comprehensive examination of the pericardium to be made in a reasonably short time, typically 45 minutes. Usually, fully diagnostic images can be obtained without compromise on the total imaging time.

On both T1- and T2-weighted MRI, the normal pericardium appears as a low-intensity signal sandwiched between high-intensity mediastinal tissues and medium-intensity epicardium (Fig. 49–15, *black arrows*). Even though the pericardium is thin, it can be reliably demonstrated with MRI in almost all patients. The visibility of the pericardium is enhanced by fat adjacent to it. In areas that have a paucity of fat, such as lung parenchyma, the pericardium is less well visualized (see Fig. 49–15, *white arrows*). Sechtem and associates assessed the value of MRI in the investigation of the pericardium.[84, 85] The sensitivity for visualization of the pericardium in any region of the heart is given in Table 49–1. The average pericardial thickness is 1.2 mm in diastole and 1.7 mm in systole, with a maximum thickness of 2.6 mm; these data are in keeping with previous CT observations.

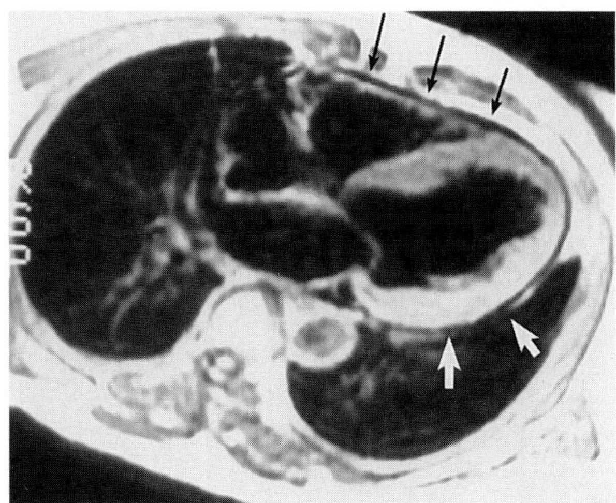

FIGURE 49–15. A single slice from a T1-weighted spin-echo (TR/TE = 938/20 msec) sequence shows the normal anatomy of the pericardium *(black arrows)*. Where there is less tissue with which to form contrast, the pericardium is less well seen *(white arrows)*.

Care must be taken in interpreting increased pericardial thickness in some regions. Caudal sections close to the diaphragm may show thicknesses of up to 7 mm. This is normal and results from the ligamentous insertion of the fibrosa into the diaphragm. Furthermore, the plane of imaging may cut tangentially through the pericardium, falsely recording increased thickness because of geometric factors. The most reliable estimation of pericardial morphology is made from sections acquired at anatomical levels that contain the right atrium and both ventricles. A four-chamber, horizontal long-axis view in the midventricle is ideal in this respect, although the vertical long-axis and even the short-axis view may be of value in some cases. Essentially, each investigation should be tailored to the needs of an individual situation, and this is something to which MRI is particularly amenable.[80, 81, 86–88]

Other components of the pericardium as a whole are also easily visualized with MRI. For instance, the transverse sinus is much more readily evaluated with MRI than with CT.[89, 90] Overall, the sensitivity of MRI in axial and sagittal planes is about 80 percent with gating and 50 percent without gating. On coronal images, sensitivity is slightly reduced, to about 70 percent. Not surprisingly, gated studies produce the greatest sensitivity, ranging from 67 to 100 percent. These sensitivities compare favorably with those of CT, which range from 24 to 49 percent.[91]

The pericardial signal is better visualized on first- than on second-echo images. Movement artifact may lead to blurring of the pencil-thin pericardial line and misinterpretation of normal thickness on the second-echo images. However, second-echo images may have improved tissue contrast resolution. These findings suggest that anatomy of the pericardium is best evaluated on the first-echo image, whereas the second echo may yield valuable tissue-discriminating information and may help to classify pathology.[80–82, 84, 85]

TABLE 49–1. SENSITIVITY OF GATED MAGNETIC RESONANCE IMAGING FOR VISUALIZATION OF THE PERICARDIUM AT VARIOUS REGIONS OF THE HEART

Region	Sensitivity* (%)
Right atrium	78
Right ventricle—right of sternum	100
Right ventricle—left of sternum	100
Left ventricle—apex	83
Left ventricle—lateral wall	61

*Number visualized divided by total number of subjects; n = 18 subjects.
Modified from Sechtem, U., Tscholakoff, D., and Higgins, C. B.: MRI of the normal pericardium. AJR 147:239, 1986. © by the American Roentgen Ray Society.

Diseases

As with disease of any organ or tissue in the body, pericardial disease may be classified as congenital or acquired. If acquired, it may be infective, inflammatory, invasive, or traumatic.

Congenital anomalies of the pericardium are rare. They include localized defects, cysts, diverticula, and benign teratoma.[86, 92] The underlying embryologic anomaly leading to such pathology is unclear; it may result from alteration of the pericardial blood supply in utero. The primary importance of such lesions is that they may mimic more serious pathology, such as malignancy or pulmonary artery dilatation.

Acquired pericardial disease may be expressed in one or more of three common ways: thickening of the pericardium, pericardial effusion, and localized pericardial mass. Depending on the cause, the natural history of the disease process, and the treatment, the outcome may be complete resolution with a normal end result, persistent thickening with or without constriction of the underlying ventricles, or replacement of the pericardium with fibrous tissue or calcification.[87, 93–96]

Viral pericarditis may lead to diffuse thickening and may be associated with effusion. Gross thickening is illustrated in Figure 49–16; the thickening is heterogenous, varying between 5 mm and 8 mm in different parts of the pericardium. Even quite extensive thickening may require computer-aided measurement to determine its presence. Comparison between Figures 49–15 and 49–16 gives some feel for the subtlety of the disease in Figure 49–16, even though a 5 mm pericardium is grossly abnormal. The noninvasive nature of MRI allows repeated, accurate estimation of response to treatment and resolution of this disease.

A relatively common complication of pericarditis with effusion is constriction of the ventricles, leading to engorged caval and hepatic veins with possible anasarca. Figure 49–14 shows a very large effusion with associated atrial enlargement and ventricular constriction. There is an extensive amount of fat in the mediastinum; separation of fat, effusion, and myocardium is achieved by acquiring both spin-echo and gradient-echo image sets and comparing the signals obtained from each.

MRI may also be very useful in monitoring treatment noninvasively. In Figure 49–17, for instance, a middle-aged woman complained of dyspnea and was found to have a large pericardial effusion without associated thickening or mass lesion. Note the extent of obesity seen throughout the mediastinum and thorax in this image. After treatment for myxedema, the effusion resolved

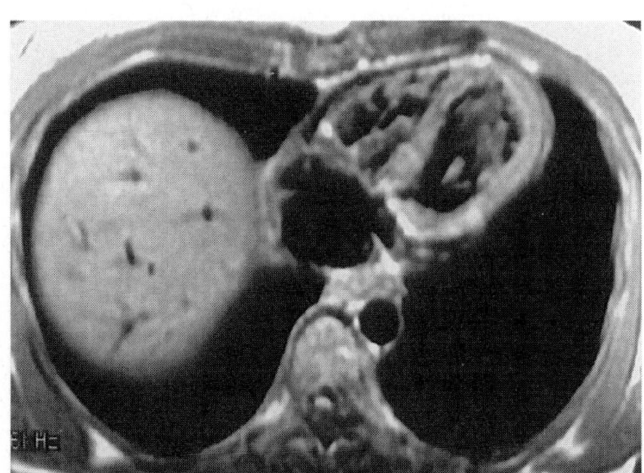

FIGURE 49–16. A single four-chamber view taken from a spin-echo (TR/TE = 400/20 msec) sequence. Note the thickened pericardium, particularly over the right ventricular free wall. Measurement of pericardial thickness yielded values between 5 and 8 mm.

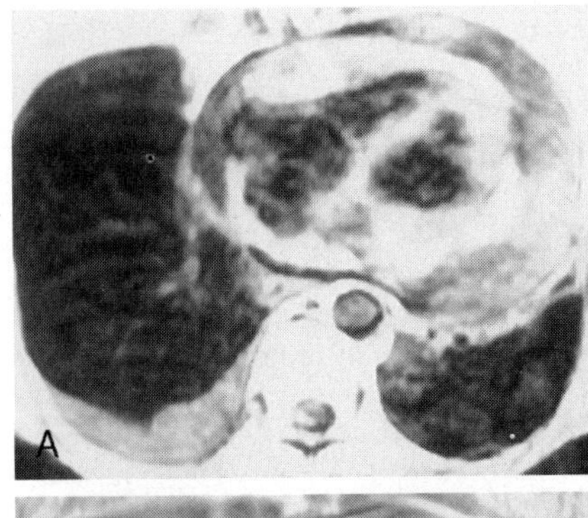

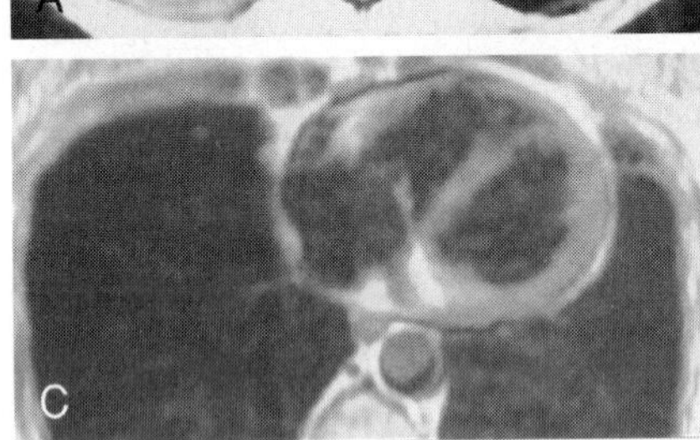

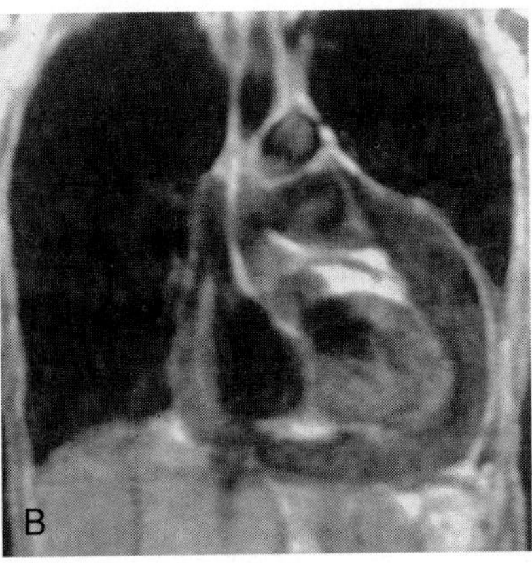

FIGURE 49–17. Axial and coronal (*A* and *B*) slices of the heart in a patient with gross pericardial effusion. After treatment for myxedema, the effusion resolved, leaving normal cardiac anatomy (*C*).

completely. Before MRI, the patient had been thought to have a malignant effusion. However, no nodules were found and there was no pericardial thickening, prompting a medical review of the case and leading to the diagnosis of thyroid-related pericardial effusion.

MRI has truly revolutionized surgical management of thoracic and mediastinal disease or complications after surgery. With MRI, the surgeon may plan the approach to the operation secure in the knowledge that there will be no surprises. This is especially true if focal pericarditis exists or if there is adherence of the pericardium to tissues disturbed by sternotomy or to fixed mediastinal contents. With this information, the surgeon may decide on a thoracotomy instead of a sternal approach and avoid potential complications such as hematoma resulting from unwanted pericardial rupture.[82, 97]

CARDIAC TUMORS

Primary cardiac neoplasia is relatively rare, occurring in 0.001 to 0.5 percent of unselected postmortem studies.[98–103] Despite their low incidence, it is important to diagnose and treat cardiac tumors promptly, because more than 80 percent are benign and are cured with resection. Secondary tumors are somewhat more common.[104] Disseminated malignancy may seed in the pericardium, leading to effusion. Atrial thrombus is common in patients with atrial fibrillation, and mural thrombus may form in akinetic or hypokinetic regions of the ventricle after myocardial infarction. Indeed, any region of the ventricular cavity is prone to thrombus formation if there is marked stasis of blood. Miscellaneous tumors include rhabdomyomas, rhabdomyosarcomas, ectopic endocrine tissue, fibromas, and secondary malignant melanoma.[104–108] Sometimes, tumors extrinsic to the heart may be mistakenly diagnosed as arising from the myocardium or pericardium.[109–111]

In general, symptoms and signs are nonspecific, and a high index of suspicion is required in order to seek the appropriate tests and make a diagnosis.[111–113] MRI, with its multiplanar capability and superb tissue contrast, offers improvements over echocardiography that outweigh the slightly lower convenience of the procedure.[108, 114–117] With MRI, tissue characterization can be undertaken, and in some cases this test alone may provide an unequivocal diagnosis. For instance, the signal characteristics of evolving hematoma are well known. In Figure 49–18, two images are shown. These are the first and second echoes, respectively, of a T2-weighted coronal study of the heart ($TR/TE_1/TE_2$ = 2250/20/70 msec). On the second-echo image, a bright area arising from the pericardium is seen. The first-echo image shows this same area as being almost isointense with myocardium. These appearances are diagnostic of an acute or semiacute hematoma and are caused by the relatively long T2 of fresh blood.

Of the true cardiac neoplasms, myxoma is the most common, accounting for some 50 percent of reported cases of mass lesions within the heart. Approximately 75 percent of myxomas are found in the left atrium (Fig. 49–19), and 20 percent in the right atrium.[118–121] The remainder are found in the ventricles. Myxomas present in various ways and may mimic lymphoma (night sweats), mitral stenosis (intermittent occlusion of the mitral valve caused by prolapsing tumor), stroke, coronary embolization or thoracic outlet

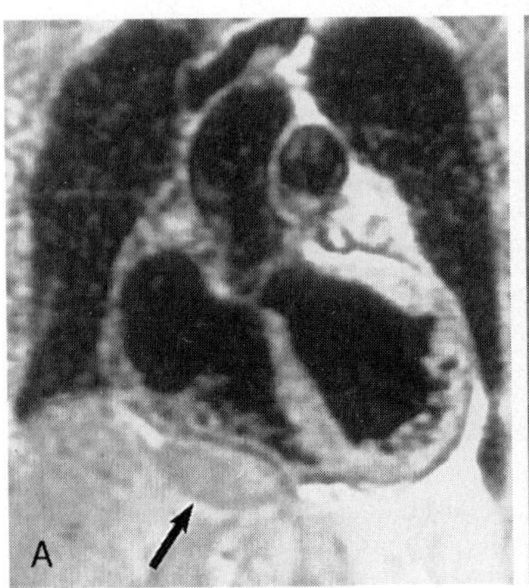

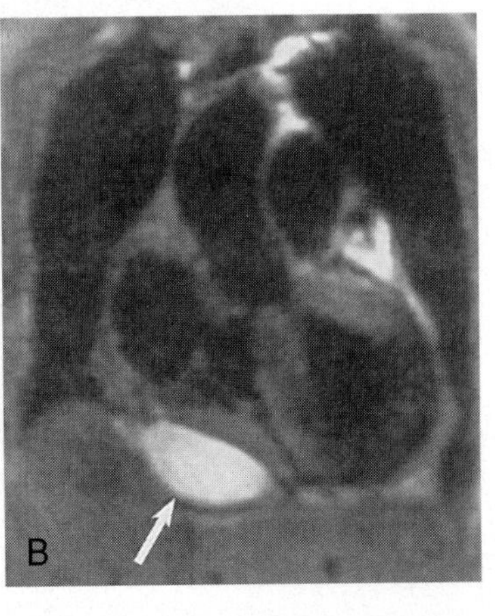

FIGURE 49–18. The first-echo (*A*) and second-echo (*B*) images from a T2-weighted spin-echo (TR/TE/TE = 2250/30/70 msec) image set. Note the localized pericardial collection *(arrows)*, which is much brighter than the myocardium on the second-echo image. These appearances are consistent with an acute or subacute hemorrhage.

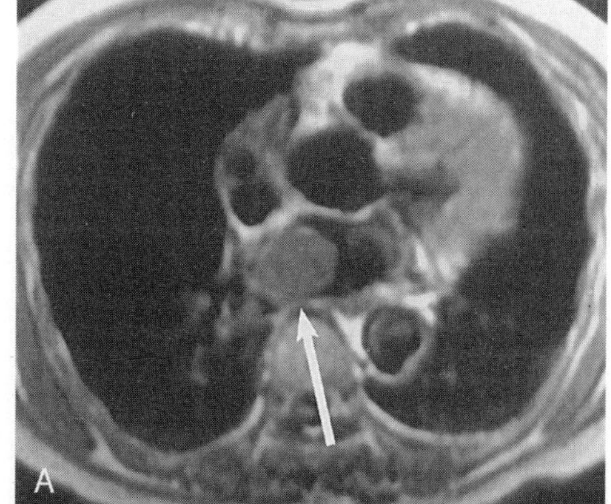

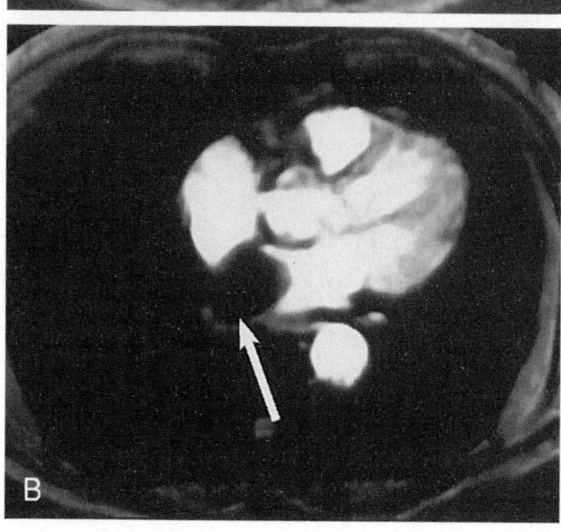

FIGURE 49–19. Spin-echo (*A*) (TR/TE = 952/20 msec) and gradient-echo (*B*) (TR/TE/flip = 50 msec/12 msec/30 degrees) four-chamber images show a left atrial mass. This proved to be a myxoma at surgery.

syndrome (distal embolization), malignancy (weight loss, finger clubbing) and many other conditions.[108, 120, 122–128] Differentiation from thrombus is important and can be made absolutely if the characteristic stalk of this pedunculated tumor is demonstrated. In contrast, the right ventricular mass in Figure 49–20 has intermediate signal intensity on T1-weighted spin-echo imaging, like a myxoma, but shows a broad base instead of a narrow pedicle. This tumor was diagnosed, after removal, as ectopic thyroid tissue. It may be appreciated from these examples that simple examination of the signal observed with MRI is insufficient to form a definitive tissue diagnosis in most cases of cardiac tumor.[129]

Collections in the myocardium arising from bleeding after valve replacement may be indistinguishable from collections arising as a result of infection and embolization. Figure 49–21 shows an organized hematoma compressing the infundibulum after mitral valve replacement and tricuspid annuloplasty. Compare this with the signal appearances of a mycotic abscess, also compressing the infundibulum, in a patient with bacterial endocarditis secondary to spinal myelography (Fig. 49–22). MRI is able to elegantly demonstrate such deep-seated mass lesions with virtually no risk to the patient. Furthermore, because MRI is not operator dependent, its interpretation may be more reliable than that of echocardiography.

Some mediastinal tumors are so adherent to the heart that echocardiography and CT scanning may not be able to identify their true nature. With judicious choice of sequences, external compression may be differentiated from invasion. This may be an important distinction to make in terms of treatment choice and prognosis.[109, 110, 123, 130–132] Figure 49–23 shows a large mass in the mediastinum involving the left atrium. On echocardiography, it was thought that this mass was invading the pericardium and myocardium. MRI was able to demonstrate a clear, smooth separation between the flowing blood in the left atrium and the mass. The coronal study also showed a pattern of smooth external compression rather than irregular invasion into and through the myocardium.

MRI is almost indispensable in the treatment of these tumors. Surgical planning makes it possible to choose the safest approach, and evaluation of invasion or penetration of myocardium or pericar-

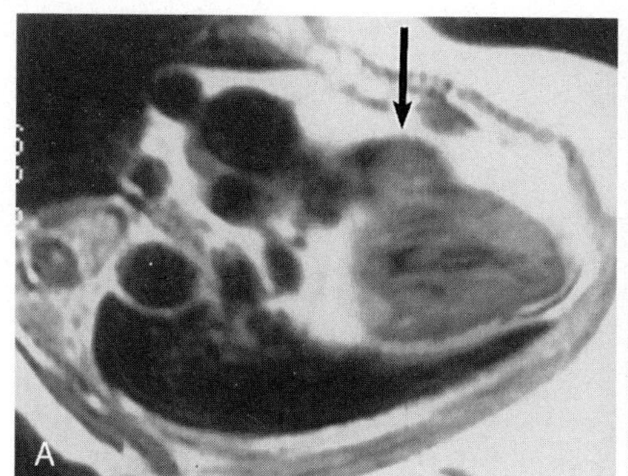

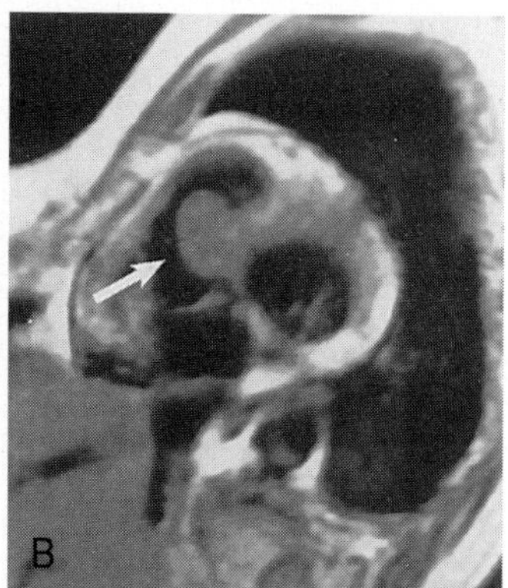

FIGURE 49–20. Long-axis (*A*) and short-axis (*B*) spin-echo (TR/TE = 857/20 msec) images of the heart show a broad-based mass in the right ventricular infundibulum. This proved to be ectopic thyroid tissue. (From Maillette S., Paquet, E., and Carrier, L.: Asymptomatic heterotopic thyroid tumor in the right ventricular infundibulum. Can. J. Cardiol. 10:37–40, 1994, with permission.)

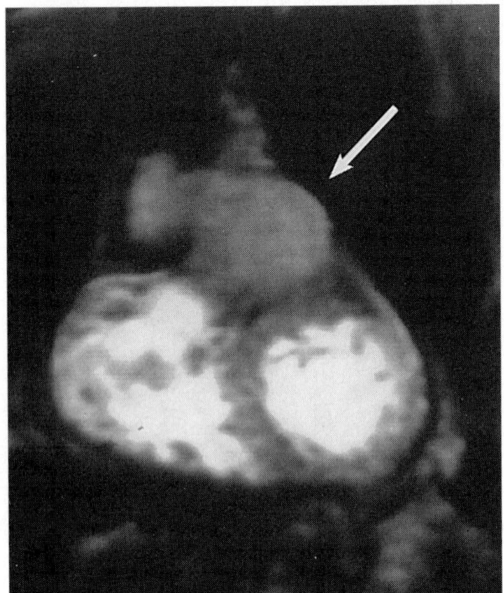

FIGURE 49–21. A coronal gradient-echo (TR/TE/flip = 50 msec/12 msec/30 degrees) image shows a collection compressing the right ventricular infundibulum after mitral valve replacement. The appearances are not specific. This was found to be an organized hematoma.

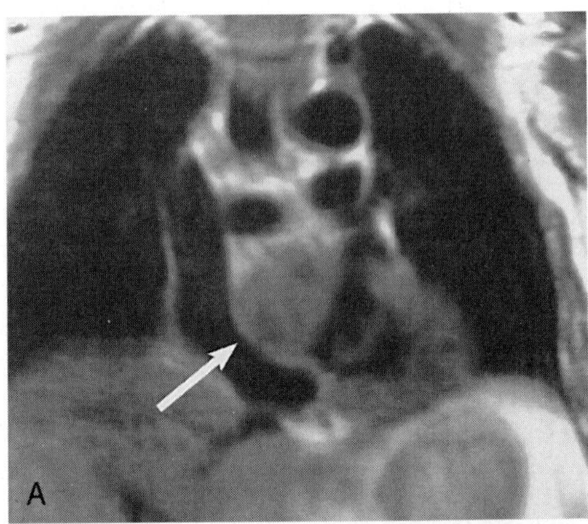

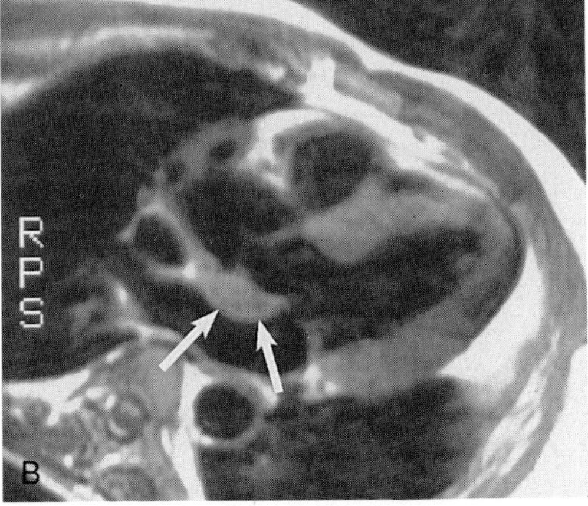

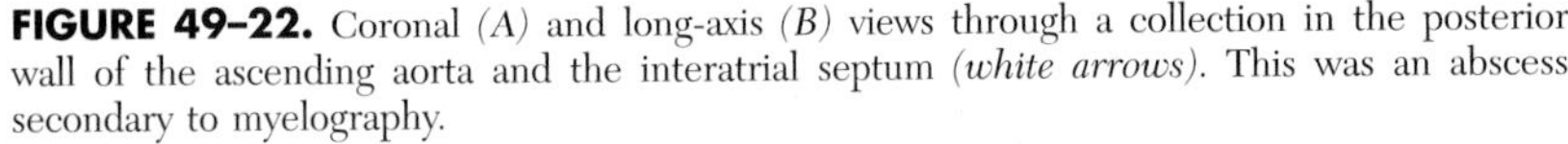

FIGURE 49–22. Coronal *(A)* and long-axis *(B)* views through a collection in the posterior wall of the ascending aorta and the interatrial septum *(white arrows)*. This was an abscess secondary to myelography.

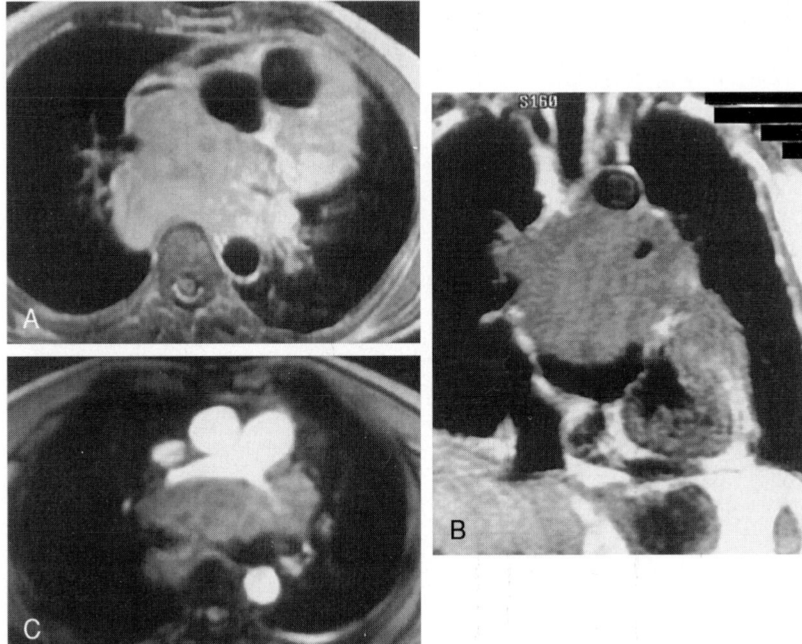

FIGURE 49–23. Coronal and axial views of the heart (*A* and *C*) from a spin-echo sequence (TR/TE = 2382/20 msec) show a large mass in the mediastinum displacing the left atrium but not invading it. The gradient-echo (TR/TE/flip = 50 msec/12 msec/30 degrees) axial slice (*B*) confirms a smooth transition between flowing blood *(bright)* and the mass, consistent with displacement without invasion.

dium is important in the choice of treatment. Furthermore, identification of possible vascular extension into the pulmonary veins may influence the treatment choices.[116]

CONCLUSION

MRI is a very versatile imaging modality that has been shown to provide useful and unique diagnostic information in the cardiac patient. This chapter has focused on the predominantly anatomical value of MRI in the investigation of cardiomyopathy, pericardial disease, and cardiac masses. Experience in these areas continues to be gained, and with it the realization that in many instances MRI alone may be sufficient to provide the correct diagnosis with which to manage and treat the patient. Coupled with the possibility of contrast studies to assess perfusion and drug pharmacokinetics, cardiac MRI could form the basis of a single investigation simultaneously evaluating anatomy and physiology. This has significant implications for delivery of cost-effective and well-tolerated treatment to the patient with heart disease.

References

1. Baer, F.M., Theissen, P., Schneider, C.A., et al.: Magnetic resonance tomography imaging techniques for diagnosing myocardial vitality. (Review.) (German.) Herz 19:51, 1994.
2. Edelman, R.R., and Warach, S.: Magnetic resonance imaging. (Review.) N. Engl. J. Med. 328:708, 1993.
3. Wendland, M.F., Saeed, M., Masui, T., et al.: Echo-planar MR imaging of normal and ischemic myocardium with gadodiamide injection. Radiology 186:535, 1993.
4. Hartiala, J., Sakuma, H., and Higgins, C.B.: Magnetic resonance imaging and spectroscopy of the human heart. (Review.) Scand. J. Clin. Lab. Invest. 53:425, 1993.
5. Council on Scientific Affairs: Magnetic resonance imaging of the cardiovascular system: Present state of the art and future potential. Report of the Magnetic Resonance Imaging Panel. (Review.) J.A.M.A. 259:253, 1988.
6. Pearlman, J.D., and Edelman, R.R.: Ultrafast magnetic resonance imaging: Segmented turboflash, echo-planar, and real-time nuclear magnetic resonance. (Review.) Radiol. Clin. North Am. 32:593, 1994.
7. Hunter, G.J., Hamberg, L.M., Weisskoff, R.M., et al.: Measurement of stroke volume and cardiac output within a single breath hold with echo-planar MR imaging. J. Magn. Reson. Imaging 4:51, 1994.
8. Gottdiener, J.S.: Left ventricular mass, diastolic dysfunction, and hypertension. (Review.) Adv. Intern. Med. 38:31, 1993.
9. Fujita, N., Duerinekx, A.J., Higgins, C.B., et al.: Variation in left ventricular regional wall stress with cine magnetic resonance imaging: Normal subjects versus dilated cardiomyopathy. Am. Heart J. 125(5 Pt. 1): 1337, 1993.
10. Pelc, N.J., Herfkens, R.J., Shimakawa, A., et al.: Phase contrast cine magnetic resonance imaging. (Review.) Magn. Reson. Q. 7:229, 1991.
11. Sakuma, H., Fujita, N., Foo, T.K., et al.: Evaluation of left ventricular volume and mass with breath-hold cine MR imaging. Radiology 188:377, 1993.
12. Dulce, M.C., and Higgins, C.B.: Evaluation of ventricular dimensions and function with magnetic resonance imaging. (Review.) Am. J. Card. Imaging 8:168, 1994.
13. Yu, K.K., Saeed, M., Wendland, M.F., et al.: Comparison of T1-enhancing and magnetic susceptibility magnetic resonance contrast agents for demarcation of the jeopardy area in experimental myocardial infarction. Invest. Radiol. 28:1015, 1993.
14. Dulce, M.C., Mostbeck, G.H., Friese, K.K., et al.: Quantification of the left ventricular volumes and function with cine MR imaging: Comparison of geometric models with three-dimensional data. Radiology 188:371, 1993.
15. Ehman, R.L., McNamara, M.T., Pallack, M., et al.: Magnetic resonance imaging with respiratory gating: Techniques and advantages. AJR 143:1175, 1984.
16. Dinsmore, R.E., Wismer, G.L., Levine, R.A., et al.: Magnetic resonance imaging of the heart: Positioning and gradient angle selection for optimal imaging planes. AJR 143:1135, 1984.
17. Report of the WHO/ISFC task force on the definition and classification of cardiomyopathies. Br. Heart J. 44:672, 1980.
18. Goodwin, J.F.: The nonobstructive cardiomyopathies. Acta Cardiol. 21:272, 1966.
19. Goodwin, J.F.: Obstructive cardiomyopathy. Cardiology 52:69, 1968.
20. Goodwin, J.F., and Oakley, C.M.: The cardiomyopathies. (Review.) Br. Heart J. 34:545, 1972.
21. Goodwin, J.F.: Cardiomyopathies and specific heart muscle diseases: Definitions, terminology, classifications and new and old approaches. (Review.) Postgrad. Med. J. 68(Suppl. 1):S3, 1992.
22. Goodwin, J.F.: Overview and classification of the cardiomyopathies. (Review.) Cardiovasc. Clin. 19:3, 1988.
23. Goodwin, J.F.: Congestive cardiomyopathy: Introduction, problems and aims of the Multicentre Research Project. Postgrad. Med. J. 54:431, 1978.
24. Webb, J.G., Sasson, Z., Rakowski, H., et al.: Apical hypertrophic cardiomyopathy: Clinical follow-up and diagnostic correlates (see comments). J. Am. Coll. Cardiol. 15:83, 1990.
25. Sasson, Z., Rakowski, H., and Wigle, E.D.: Hypertrophic cardiomyopathy. (Review.) Cardiol. Clin. 6:233, 1988.
26. Wigle, E.D.: Hypertrophic cardiomyopathy: A 1987 viewpoint. Circulation 75:311, 1987.
27. Goodwin, J.F.: Review of hypertrophic cardiomyopathy. (Review.) Ergebnisse der Inneren Medizin und Kinderheilkunde 55:41, 1987.
28. Shabetai, R.: Controversial issues in restrictive cardiomyopathy. Postgrad. Med. J. 68(Suppl. 1):S47, 1992.
29. Masui, T., Finck, S., and Higgins, C.B.: Constrictive pericarditis and restrictive cardiomyopathy: Evaluation with MR imaging. Radiology 182:369, 1992.
30. Steudel, A., Krahe, T., Becher, H., et al.: Cardiomyopathy in idiopathic hemo-

chromatosis: Diagnostic possibilities using proton spin tomography. (German.) Dtsch. Med. Wochenschr. 112:590, 1987.
31. Sechtem, U., Higgins, C.B., Sommerhoff, B.A., et al.: Magnetic resonance imaging of restrictive cardiomyopathy. Am. J. Cardiol. 59:480, 1987.
32. Isner, J.M., Carter, B.L., Bankoff, M.S., et al.: Differentiation of constrictive pericarditis from restrictive cardiomyopathy by computed tomographic imaging. Am. Heart J. 105:1019, 1983.
33. Meaney, E., Shabetai, R., Bhargava, V., et al.: Cardiac amyloidosis, contrictive pericarditis and restrictive cardiomyopathy. Am. J. Cardiol. 38:547, 1976.
34. Ziady, G.M., Oakley, C.M., Raphael, M.J., et al.: Proceedings: Primary restrictive cardiomyopathy. Br. Heart J. 37:1975.
35. Regan, T.J.: Alcoholic cardiomyopathy. (Review.) Prog. Cardiovasc. Dis. 27:141, 1984.
36. Goodwin, J.F.: Alcohol and the heart: Alcoholic cardiomyopathy. J. R. Coll. Physicians Lond. 12:5, 1977.
37. Alexander, C.S.: Alcoholic cardiomyopathy. Postgrad. Med. 58:127, 1975.
38. Burch, G.E., and Giles, T.D.: Viral cardiomyopathy. (Review.) Recent Advances in Studies on Cardiac Structure and Metabolism 2:121, 1973.
39. Alexander, C.S.: Cobalt-beer cardiomyopathy: A clinical and pathologic study of twenty-eight cases. Am. J. Med. 53:395, 1972.
40. Burch, G.E., and Giles, T.D.: Ischemic cardiomyopathy: Diagnostic, pathophysiologic, and therapeutic considerations. Cardiovasc. Clin. 4:203, 1972.
41. Burch, G.E., and Giles, T.D.: Alcoholic cardiomyopathy: Concept of the disease and its treatment. (Review.) Am. J. Med. 50:141, 1971.
42. Higgins, C.B., Byrd, B.F., III, Stark, D., et al.: Magnetic resonance imaging in hypertrophic cardiomyopathy. Am. J. Cardiol. 55:1121, 1985.
43. Sechtem, U., Sommerhoff, B.A., Markiewicz, W., et al.: Regional left ventricular wall thickening by magnetic resonance imaging: Evaluation in normal persons and patients with global and regional dysfunction. Am. J. Cardiol. 59:145, 1987.
44. Lederbogen, F., Rottbauer, W., Krahe, T., et al.: Noninvasive quantification of aortic and mitral insufficiency: Comparison of dynamic magnetic resonance imaging and Doppler color echocardiography. (German.) Dtsch. Med. Wochenschr. 119:611, 1994.
45. Fujita, N., Chazouilleres, A.F., Hartiala, J.J., et al.: Quantification of mitral regurgitation by velocity-encoded cine nuclear magnetic resonance imaging (see comments). J. Am. Coll. Cardiol. 23:951, 1994.
46. Suzuki, J., Caputo, G.R., Kondo, C., et al.: Cine MR imaging of valvular heart disease: Display and imaging parameters affect the size of the signal void caused by valvular regurgitation. AJR 155:723, 1990.
47. Pflugfelder, P.W., Landzberg, J.S., Cassidy, M.M., et al.: Comparison of cine MR imaging with Doppler echocardiography for the evaluation of aortic regurgitation. AJR 152:729, 1989.
48. Sechtem, U., Pflugfelder, P.W., Cassidy, M.M., et al.: Mitral or aortic regurgitation: Quantification of regurgitant volumes with cine MR imaging. Radiology 167:425, 1988.
49. Utz, J.A., Herfkens, R.J., Heinsimer, J.A., et al.: Valvular regurgitation: Dynamic MR imaging. Radiology 168:91, 1988.
50. Farmer, D., Higgins, C.B., Yee, E., et al.: Tissue characterization by magnetic resonance imaging in hypertrophic cardiomyopathy. Am. J. Cardiol. 55:230, 1985.
51. Regan, T.J., and Weisse, A.B.: Diabetic cardiomyopathy. (Editorial; Comment.) J. Am. Coll. Cardiol. 19:1165, 1992.
52. Regan, T.J., and Lyons, M. M.: Diabetic cardiomyopathy. (Letter; Comment.) Circulation 83:1830, 1991.
53. Homans, D.C.: Peripartum cardiomyopathy. (Review.) N. Engl. J. Med. 312:1432, 1985.
54. Julian, D.G., and Szekely, P.: Peripartum cardiomyopathy. (Review.) Prog. Cardiovasc. Dis. 27:223, 1985.
55. Alexander, J.K.: The cardiomyopathy of obesity. Prog. Cardiovasc. Dis. 27:325, 1985.
56. Goodwin, J.F.: Cardiomyopathy and ischaemic heart disease. Arch. Inst. Cardiol. Mex. 50:267, 1980.
57. Regan, T.J., Lyons, M.M., Ahmed, S.S., et al.: Evidence for cardiomyopathy in familial diabetes mellitus. J. Clin. Invest. 60:884, 1977.
58. Demakis, J.G., and Rahimtoola, S.H.: Peripartum cardiomyopathy. Circulation 44:964, 1971.
59. Higgins, C.B., Byrd, B.F., II, McNamara, M.T., et al.: Magnetic resonance imaging of the heart: A review of the experience in 172 subjects. Radiology 155:671, 1985.
60. Fujita, N., Hartiala, J., O'Sullivan, M., et al.: Assessment of left ventricular diastolic function in dilated cardiomyopathy with cine magnetic resonance imaging: Effect of an angiotensin converting enzyme inhibitor, benazepril. Am. Heart J. 125:171, 1993.
61. Doherty, N., III, Fujita, N., Caputo, G.R., et al.: Measurement of right ventricular mass in normal and dilated cardiomyopathic ventricles using cine magnetic resonance imaging. Am. J. Cardiol. 69:1223, 1992.
62. Hartiala, J.J., Mostbeck, G.H., Foster, E., et al.: Velocity-encoded cine MRI in the evaluation of left ventricular diastolic function: Measurement of mitral valve and pulmonary vein flow velocities and flow volume across the mitral valve. Am. Heart J. 125:1054, 1993.
63. Buser, P.T., Auffermann, W., Holt, W.W., et al.: Noninvasive evaluation of global left ventricular function with use of cine nuclear magnetic resonance. J. Am. Coll. Cardiol. 13:1294, 1989.
64. Pflugfelder, P.W., Sechtem, U.P., White, R.D., et al.: Quantification of regional myocardial function by rapid cine MR imaging. AJR 150:523, 1988.
65. Aherne, T., Tscholakoff, D., Finkbeiner, W., et al.: Magnetic resonance imaging of cardiac transplants: The evaluation of rejection of cardiac allografts with and without immunosuppression. Circulation 74:145, 1986.
66. Blankenberg, F., Eisenberg, S., Scheinman, M.N., et al.: Use of cine gradient echo (GRE) MR in the imaging of cardiac hemochromatosis. J. Comput. Assist. Tomogr. 18:136, 1994.
67. Mitchell, M.A., Horneffer, M.D., and Standiford, T.J.: Multiple myeloma complicated by restrictive cardiomyopathy and cardiac tamponade. Chest 103:946, 1993.
68. Carroll, J.D., Gaasch, W.H., McAdam, K.P., et al.: Amyloid cardiomyopathy: Characterization by a distinctive voltage/mass relation. Am. J. Cardiol. 49:9, 1982.
69. Gasperetti, C.M., Sarembock, I.J., Feldman, M.D., et al.: Usefulness of dynamic hand exercise for developing maximal separation of left and right ventricular pressures at end-diastole and usefulness in distinguishing restrictive cardiomyopathy from constrictive pericardial disease. Am. J. Cardiol. 69:1508, 1992.
70. Gerson, M.C., Colthar, M.S., Fowler, N.O., et al.: Differentiation of constrictive pericarditis and restrictive cardiomyopathy by radionuclide ventriculography. Am. Heart J. 118:114, 1989.
71. Holt, J.P.: The normal pericardium. (Review.) Am. J. Cardiol. 26:455, 1970.
72. Spodick, D.H.: The pericardium: Structure, function, and disease spectrum. Cardiovasc. Clin. 7:1, 1976.
73. Ishihara, T., Ferrans, V.J., Jones, M., et al.: Histologic and ultrastructural features of normal human parietal pericardium. Am. J. Cardiol. 46:744, 1980.
74. Spodick, D.H.: The normal and diseased pericardium: Current concepts of pericardial physiology, diagnosis and treatment. (Review.) J. Am. Coll. Cardiol. 1:240, 1983.
75. Shabetai, R., Mangiardi, L., Bhargava, V., et al.: The pericardium and cardiac function. (Review.) Prog. Cardiovasc. Dis. 22:107, 1979.
76. Hipona, F.A., and Paredes, S.: The radiology of pericardial disease. Cardiovasc. Clin. 7:91, 1976.
77. Doppman, J.L., Rienmuller, R., Lissner, J., et al.: Computed tomography in constrictive pericardial disease. J. Comput. Assist. Tomogr. 5:1, 1981.
78. Silverman, P.M., and Harell, G.S.: Computed tomography of the normal pericardium. Invest. Radiol. 18:141, 1983.
79. Solomon, A., Weiss, J., Stern, D., et al.: Computerized tomography in pericardial disease. Heart Lung 12:513, 1983.
80. Reinmuller, R., Gurgan, M., Erdmann, E., et al.: CT and MR evaluation of pericardial constriction: A new diagnostic and therapeutic concept. J. Thorac. Imaging 8:108, 1993.
81. Soulen, R.L.: Magnetic resonance imaging of great vessel, myocardial, and pericardial disease. Circulation 84:I311, 1991.
82. Hoit, B.D.: Imaging the pericardium. (Review.) Cardiol. Clin. 8:587, 1990.
83. Miller, S.W.: Imaging pericardial disease. (Review.) Radiol. Clin. North Am. 27:1113, 1989.
84. Sechtem, U., Tscholakoff, D., and Higgins, C.B.: MRI of the normal pericardium. AJR 147:239, 1986.
85. Sechtem, U., Tscholakoff, D., and Higgins, C.B.: MRI of the abnormal pericardium. AJR 147:245, 1986.
86. Fowler, N.O.: Pericardial disease. (Review.) Heart Disease and Stroke 1:85, 1992.
87. Maisch, B.: Pericardial diseases, with a focus on etiology, pathogenesis, pathophysiology, new diagnostic imaging methods, and treatment. (Review.) Curr. Opin. Cardiol. 9:379, 1994.
88. Kastler, B., Germain, P., Dietemann, J.L., et al.: Spin echo MRI in the evaluation of pericardial disease. Comput. Med. Imaging Graph. 14:241, 1990.
89. Levy, R.M., Auh, Y.H., Rubenstein, W.A., et al.: CT of the pericardial recesses. AJR 144:707, 1985.
90. Im, J.G., Rosen, A., Webb, W.R., et al.: MR imaging of the transverse sinus of the pericardium. AJR 150:79, 1988.
91. McMurdo, K.K., Webb, W.R., von Schulthess, G.K., et al.: Magnetic resonance imaging of the superior pericardial recesses. AJR 145:985, 1985.
92. Tierney, R.C.: Pericardial disease in children. Paediatrician 7:52, 1978.
93. Wefuan, J., and Aaron, S.L.: Pericardial disease in scleroderma: prognosis and clinical associations. (Letter.) Clin. Exp. Rheumatol. 11:582, 1993.
94. Wenger, N.K.: Pericardial disease in the elderly. Cardiovasc. Clin. 22:97, 1992.
95. Hancock, E.W.: Neoplastic pericardial disease. (Review.) Cardiol. Clin. 8:673, 1990.
96. Schiavone, W.A., and Rice, T.W.: Pericardial disease: Current diagnosis and management methods. Cleve. Clin. J. Med. 56:639, 1989.
97. Moncada, R., Kotler, M.N., Churchill, R.J., et al.: Multimodality approach to pericardial imaging. Cardiovasc. Clin. 17:409, 1986.
98. Grande, A.M., Ragni, T., Vigano, M., et al.: Primary cardiac tumors: A clinical experience of 12 years. Tex. Heart Inst. J. 20:223, 1993.
99. Lam, K.Y., Dickens, P., Chan, A.C., et al.: Tumors of the heart: A 20-year experience with a review of 12,485 consecutive autopsies. Arch. Pathol. Lab. Med. 117:1027, 1993.
100. Blondeau, P.: Primary cardiac tumors: French studies of 533 cases. (Review.) Thorac. Cardiovasc. Surg. 2:192, 1990.
101. Van, D.W.H., Fritschy, W.M., Skotnicki, S.H., et al.: Primary cardiac tumors. Acta Chir. Belg. 88:74, 1988.
102. Silverman, N.A.: Primary cardiac tumors. Ann. Surg. 191:127, 1980.
103. Arciniegas, E., Hakimi, M., Farooki, Z.Q., et al.: Primary cardiac tumors in children. J. Thorac. Cardiovasc. Surg. 79:582, 1980.
104. Smith, L.H.: Secondary tumors of the heart. (Review.) Rev. Surg. 33:223, 1976.
105. Cirri, G.P., and Andretta, O.: Secondary tumors of the heart: Reticulosarcoma and clear-cell carcinoma of the adrenal cortex. (Italian.) Arch. Ital. Patol. Clin. Tumori 11:95, 1968.
106. Gutierrez, L.Z., Rochegiani, H.A., and Martin, A.: Malignant secondary tumor of the heart. (Spanish.) Prensa Medica Argentina 53:1666, 1966.
107. Heath, D.: Pathology of cardiac tumors. Am. J. Cardiol. 21:315, 1968.
108. Sutsch, G., Jenni, R., von Schulthess, G.K., et al.: Heart tumors: incidence,

distribution, diagnosis. Exemplified by 20,305 echocardiographies. (German.) Schweiz. Med. Wochenschr. 121:621, 1991.
109. von Schulthess, G.K., McMurdo, K., Tscholakoff, D., et al.: Mediastinal masses: MR imaging. Radiology 158:289, 1986.
110. Dooms, G.C., Hricak, H., Sollitto, R.A., et al.: Lipomatous tumors and tumors with fatty component: MR imaging potential and comparison of MR and CT results. Radiology 157:479, 1985.
111. Bartecchi, C.E.: Primary cardiac tumors: Historically elusive lesions. South. Med. J. 75:1249, 1982.
112. Harvey, W.P.: Clinical aspects of cardiac tumors. Am. J. Cardiol. 21:328, 1968.
113. Selzer, A., Sakai, F.J., Popper, R.W., et al.: Protean clinical manifestations of primary tumors of the heart. Am. J. Med. 52:9, 1972.
114. Fujita, N., Caputo, G.R., and Higgins, C.B.: Diagnosis and characterization of intracardiac masses by magnetic resonance imaging. Am. J. Card. Imaging 8:69, 1994.
115. Krahe, T., Landwehr, P., Leibold, G., et al.: The determination of myocardial mass by cardiac magnetic resonance tomography: The effect of section alignment and section distance. (German.) Rofo Fortschr. Geb. Rontgenstr. Neuen Bildgeb. Verfahr. 157:439, 1992.
116. Seelos, K.C., Caputo, G.R., Carrol, C.L., et al.: Cine gradient refocused echo (GRE) imaging of intravascular masses: Differentiation between tumor and nontumor thrombus. J. Comput. Assist. Tomogr. 16:169, 1992.
117. Funari, M., Fujita, N., Peck, W.W., et al.: Cardiac tumors: Assessment with Gd-DTPA enhanced MR imaging. J. Comput. Assist. Tomogr. 15:953, 1991.
118. MacGowan, S.W., Sidhu, P., Aherne, T., et al.: Atrial myxoma: National incidence, diagnosis and surgical management. (Review.) Ir. J. Med. Sci. 162:223, 1993.
119. St. John Sutton, M.G., Mercier, L.A., Giulliani, E.R.,, et al.: Atrial myxomas: A review of clinical experience in 40 patients. Mayo Clin. Proc. 55:371, 1980.
120. Zitnik, R.S., and Giuliani, E.R.: Clinical recognition of atrial myxoma. Am. Heart J. 80:689, 1970.
121. Talley, R.C., Baldwin, B.J., Symbas, P.N., et al.: Right atrial myxoma: Unusual presentation with cyanosis and clubbing. Am. J. Med. 48:256, 1970.
122. Radermecker, M.A., Lavigne, J.P., Defraigne, J.O., et al.: Primary cardiac tumors: myxoma of the left auricle. (French.) Rev. Med. Liege 45:99, 1990.
123. Tillmanns, H.: Clinical aspects of cardiac tumors. Thorac. Cardiovasc. Surg. 2:152, 1990.
124. Dapper, F., Gorlach, G., Hoffmann, C., et al.: Primary cardiac tumors: Clinical experiences and late results in 48 patients. Thorac. Cardiovasc. Surg. 36:80, 1988.
125. Byrd, W.E., Matthews, O.P., and Hunt, R.E.: Left atrial myxoma presenting as a systemic vasculitis. Arthritis Rheum. 23:240, 1980.
126. Huston, K.A., Combs, J.J., Lie, J.T., et al.: Left atrial myxoma simulating peripheral vasculitis. Mayo Clin. Proc. 53:752, 1978.
127. Kaminsky, M.E., Ehlers, K.H., Engle, M.A., et al.: Atrial myxoma mimicking a collagen disorder. Chest 75:93, 1979.
128. Peters, M.N., Hall, R.J., Cooley, D.A., et al.: The clinical syndrome of atrial myxoma. J.A.M.A. 230:695, 1974.
129. Pflugfelder, P.W., Wisenberg, G., Boughner, D.R., et al.: Detection of atrial myxoma by magnetic resonance imaging. Am. J. Cardiol. 55:242, 1985.
130. Sechtem, U., and Jungehulsing, M.: Noninvasive imaging of cardiac masses. (Review.) Curr. Opin. Radiol. 2:575, 1990.
131. Brown, J.J., Barakos, J.A., and Higgins, C.B.: Magnetic resonance imaging of cardiac and paracardiac masses. J. Thorac. Imaging 4:58, 1989.
132. Amparo, E.G., Higgins, C.B., Farmer, D., et al.: Gated MRI of cardiac and paracardiac masses: Initial experience. AJR 143:1151, 1984.

CHAPTER 50 Quantitative Magnetic Resonance Imaging of the Heart

Ronald M. Peshock, M.D.
W. Gregory Hundley, M.D.
DuWayne L. Willett, M.D.
Dany E. Sayad, M.D.
Michael P. Chwialkowski, Ph.D.

Perhaps more than in any other area in medicine, quantitation is an essential element in the practice of cardiology. To completely evaluate the patient with heart disease, the clinician needs answers to a number of critical questions: (1) Are the chambers of normal size? (2) Are global and segmental function normal? (3) Is the myocardial tissue normal, or is there evidence of injury? (4) Are blood flow and tissue perfusion normal? and (5) Has the metabolic function of the tissue been altered? As evidenced in this book, a wide variety of approaches have been utilized in attempts to answer these questions.

The ideal cardiac imaging technique would allow one to address all the clinical questions posed above. Recently, nuclear magnetic resonance techniques have emerged as useful tools in the evaluation of the heart. Notably, magnetic resonance imaging (MRI) has several features that make it particularly applicable in addressing the critical questions enumerated above.

Thus, the purpose of this chapter is (1) to examine the general problem of cardiac quantitation, (2) to describe the MRI techniques available, and (3) to review the present status of MRI in the quantitation of cardiac size and function.

GENERAL PROBLEM OF CARDIAC QUANTITATION

To obtain quantitative information regarding the heart and its function, one must address several problems. First, the heart is a complex three-dimensional structure whose position and orientation in the chest is variable. In addition, its geometry can be significantly altered by common disease processes, such as ischemic heart disease or cardiomyopathy. This variability in geometry cannot be ignored when one attempts to measure chamber size. Second, structures of interest in the heart vary from millimeters to several centimeters in size. Thus, the spatial resolution of the ideal imaging method should span this entire range. Third, the heart is constantly in motion. Imaging methods used to evaluate cardiac motion must deal with this changing geometry. Thus, the temporal resolution, or time between images, must be small enough to provide an accurate representation of the multiple events that take place during the cardiac cycle. Finally, the method should be flexible enough to provide assessments of structure, function, and flow, as required during a single study.

Magnetic resonance imaging addresses many of these issues. First, MRI is fundamentally a three-dimensional imaging technique. It is not constrained by problems of acoustic window or attenuation. Hence, images can be obtained in virtually any orientation with knowledge of the exact location of the imaging plane. This ability permits a direct approach to the analysis of the complex shape and motion of the heart. Second, spatial resolution in MRI is easily varied over a wide range. Relatively simple changes in the imaging sequence lead to dramatic changes in image resolution and contrast. Thus, MRI can be uniquely tailored to specific problems in cardiac evaluation. Third, recent improvements in fast scanning techniques have improved temporal resolution and reduced total scan times, so that adequate temporal resolution is readily available. Finally, MRI is a remarkably flexible technique. It is inherently sensitive to motion, thus allowing differentiation of chamber lumen and wall without the use of contrast agents. Moreover, this sensitivity to motion can be used to directly measure cardiac motion and blood flow.

Magnetic resonance imaging of the heart must be tailored to the patient and the clinical question to be answered. The goal is to obtain an image with appropriate spatial and temporal resolution in an amount of time appropriate to the physiologic state under evaluation. To achieve this goal requires that the clinician (1) choose from the available MRI techniques available, (2) obtain the appropriate spatial and temporal resolution, (3) meet conditions for accurate measurement, and (4) avoid potential sources of error. Each of these aspects is discussed in more detail later.

Magnetic Resonance Imaging Techniques Available

A wide variety of MRI sequences can be used for quantitation of cardiac size and function:

Multislice Spin-Echo

Gated multislice spin-echo imaging is typically used to generate "black-blood" images, which provide high contrast between the blood pool, myocardium, and pericardium, facilitating quantitation. Typically, the RR interval is used as the repetition time (TR), and only one sample is obtained per cardiac cycle, so that the total imaging time is directly related to heart rate. Imaging time can be reduced by using fast spin-echo imaging, in which multiple samples are obtained with each cardiac cycle at the expense of some image degradation due to cardiac motion.

A fundamental limitation of multislice spin-echo MRI from the standpoint of quantitation is that the images of different slices are acquired at different points in the cardiac cycle. The clinician must know the timing of the slice in the cycle to correctly interpret measurements made on multislice spin-echo images (Fig. 50–1*A*).

Multislice Multiphase Spin-Echo

In this technique a multislice spin-echo sequence is repeated, permuting the order of slice acquisition so that each slice is imaged at each point in the cardiac cycle. This approach has been used extensively in the measurement of myocardial mass, stroke volume, and ejection fraction.[1] Although the images show excellent contrast, the technique is limited by its relatively poor temporal resolution (typically, 50 to 100 msec) and long imaging time (20 to 40 minutes). Total imaging time can be reduced by acquiring images only at end-diastole and end-systole for each slice (biphasic spin-echoes).[2, 3] This approach permits more efficient spin-echo imaging for determination of volumes and ejection fraction but is not widely available. In addition, predicting the timing of end-diastole and end-systole may be difficult.

Cine Magnetic Resonance Imaging

This method generates "white-blood" images with good contrast between myocardial chambers and walls. Short repetition time (TR, 20 to 33 msec), short echo time (TE, 4 to 20 msec), and partial flip (flip angle, 35 to 60 degrees) gradient echo images are obtained in a single slice (see Fig. 50–1*B*). The number of frames per cardiac cycle corresponds to the number of pulses delivered within one RR interval.[4] The images can then be displayed in a cine loop to evaluate function and blood flow.

Because cine MRI can rapidly provide multiple frames in a single slice, this technique has largely replaced multislice multiphase spin-echo imaging in the evaluation of function. The accuracy of cine MRI in quantitation has been shown to be comparable to spin-echo imaging. However, cine MRI is more prone to artifacts related to chemical shift and magnetic susceptibility as detailed below.

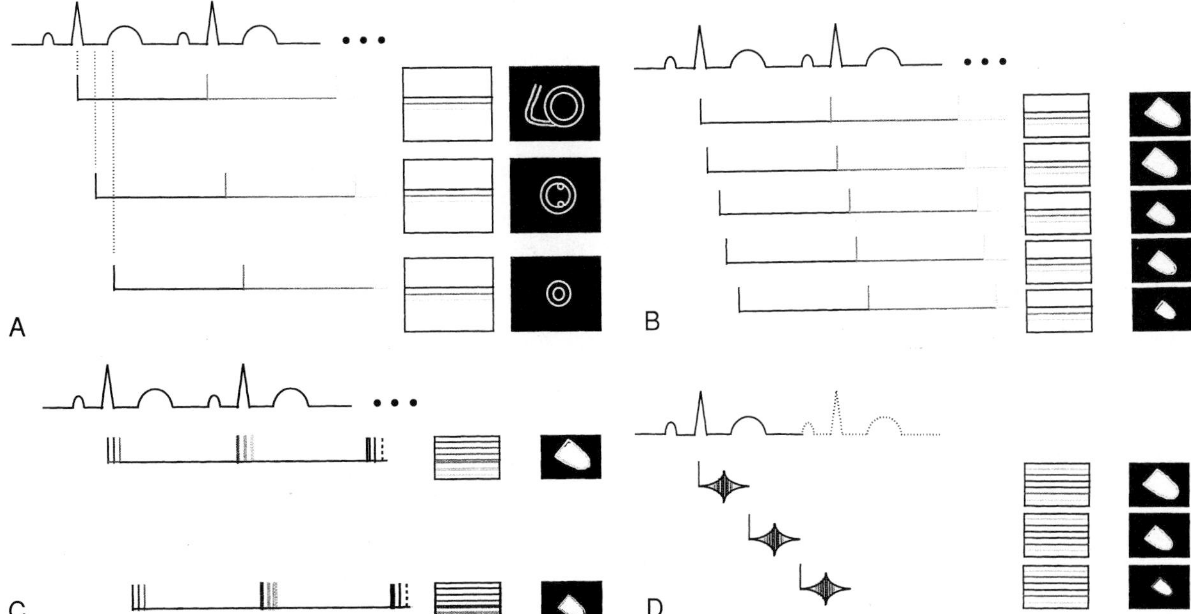

FIGURE 50–1. Diagrams illustrating specific pulse sequences. In each panel the electrocardiogram is shown to illustrate the timing of events. The vertical lines indicate the timing of data acquisition with respect to the cardiac cycle. The middle column of squares represents the K-space, or data that must be acquired to form a complete image. The column of squares to the right schematically represents the images obtained. *Panel A,* Gated multislice spin-echo imaging. In standard gated multislice spin-echo imaging, one phase-encoding step for each slice is acquired with each cardiac cycle. Note that this implies that information for each slice is at a different point in the cardiac cycle. Therefore, to correctly interpret wall thickness and chamber size in a gated multislice spin-echo image, the timing of the slice with respect to the cardiac cycle must be known. *Panel B,* Cine MRI. In cine MRI a short TR, short TE, partial-flip angle-field echo sequence is used to obtain multiple frames in a single slice. In standard cine MRI, one phase-encoding step for each frame in the cine is acquired with each cardiac cycle. As compared to gated multislice spin-echo, cine MRI provides information at multiple points in the cardiac cycle in a single slice. Typical temporal resolution of this sequence is in the range of 50 (TR, 20 msec) to 100 (TR, 10 msec) frames per second, with total acquisition times of 2 to 6 minutes. *Panel C,* Phase-encoding grouping (breath-hold imaging). This is a variation of cine MRI in which multiple phase-encoding steps are acquired with each cardiac cycle. In this illustration, three phase-encoding steps *(vertical lines)* are acquired, with each cardiac cycle reducing the total acquisition time by a factor of 3, which occurs at the expense of reducing the number of frames in the cine and thus reducing the temporal resolution. This approach is the basis for breath-hold imaging. Typical temporal resolution is in the range of 40 msec per frame to 100 msec per frame, with total acquisition times of 15 to 40 seconds. *Panel D,* Echo-planar imaging. In EPI all the phase-encoding steps required to construct the image (indicated by the *vertical lines* within the curved envelope) are obtained with a single pulse. Thus, images can be obtained in essentially real time. Typical temporal resolution is 60 to 100 msec per frame, with a total acquisition time for each frame equal to the temporal resolution.

Breath-Hold Cine Magnetic Resonance Imaging (Phase-Encoding Grouping, K-space Segmentation)

Breath-hold cine MRI is a variation of cine MRI in which multiple phase-encoding steps are acquired with each cardiac cycle.[5] By increasing the phase-encoding group size, the scan time can be dramatically decreased at the expense of increasing the time per frame and, thus, decreasing the temporal resolution. When coupled with a breath-hold technique, this method provides cine imaging without respiratory motion artifacts (see Fig. 50–1*C*).

Echo-Planar Imaging

As discussed in Chapter 43, echo-planar imaging (EPI), in which all of the information required for the image is obtained by using a single pulse, is the most rapid method of MRI[6] (see Fig. 50–1*D*). Typical total imaging times for EPI are on the order of 30 to 100 msec, thus raising the potential for real-time MRI. At present, EPI requires special hardware, has some limitations in regard to spatial resolution, and is not widely available. However, initial reports indicate that it can be used effectively for measures of cardiac chamber size and function.[7, 8]

Obtaining Appropriate Spatial and Temporal Resolution

In using any of these MRI techniques it is essential to choose the correct spatial and temporal resolution. As with many cardiac imaging techniques, the exact definition of spatial resolution in MRI is difficult.[9] Several concepts are important when defining spatial resolution in MRI:

Voxel Size

The tissue is the source of the signal used in MRI. This implies that the fundamental determinant of image quality in MRI is the amount of tissue in each volume element in the image, termed the voxel size (Fig. 50–2). As voxel size is decreased, smaller structures can be imaged without blurring. However, as voxel size is decreased, the signal is also decreased, reducing the signal-to-noise ratio. For example, magnetic resonance images with voxel sizes of 0.3 × 0.3 × 3 mm can easily be obtained, but the signal-to-noise ratio may be so poor that it precludes interpretation. Thus, the goal is to match the voxel size to the size of the structure of interest to obtain the necessary resolution with the best possible signal-to-noise ratio.

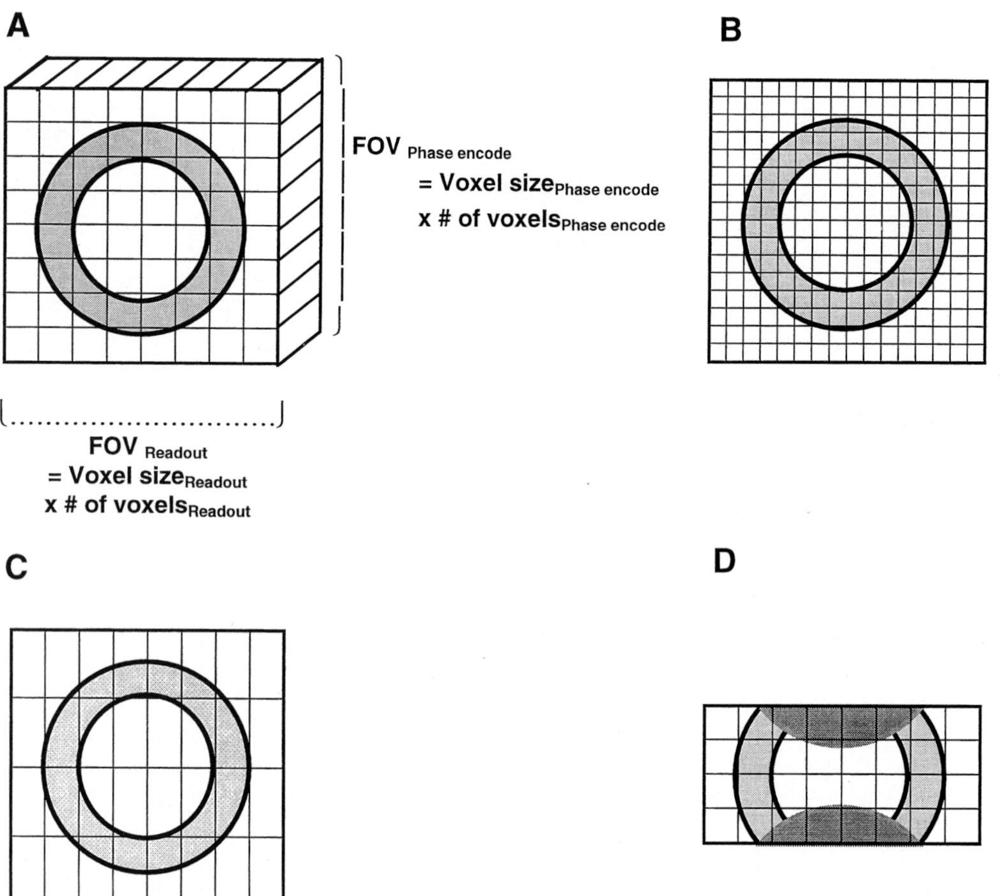

FIGURE 50–2. Diagram illustrating the effects of voxel size, matrix, and field of view. In each panel the left ventricular wall is represented by a gray ring, and the voxel size in the plane of the image is illustrated by the gridlines. The third dimension of the voxel size (slice thickness) is shown in panel *A* but is not shown in the other panels for simplicity. *Panel A,* Square field of view with square voxels. In this illustration the voxels have equal dimensions in the readout and phase-encoding directions. Multiplying the voxel dimension in each direction by the matrix size in that direction yields the field of view in that direction. *Panel B,* Square field of view with smaller square voxels. In this case the dimensions of the voxels have been reduced by a factor of 2 in both directions, which improves the resolution but at the expense of (1) reducing voxel volume and the signal per voxel by a factor of 2 × 2 = 4 and (2) doubling the total scan time by doubling the number of phase-encoding steps required. *Panel C,* Square field of view with rectangular voxels. Here, the dimension of the voxel in the phase-encoding direction has been increased by a factor of 2, which increases signal per voxel and decreases the total time required for the scan by a factor of 2. This approach has been widely applied to decrease scan time, which occurs at the expense of decreasing the resolution in the phase-encoding direction, resulting in decreased edge sharpness in that direction in the image. *Panel D,* Rectangular field of view with square voxels. Here the number of phase-encoding steps has been decreased while keeping the voxel square in the imaging plane, which results in a smaller field view in the phase-encoding direction. When the size of the body exceeds the field of view in the phase-encoding direction, aliasing, or "wraparound," occurs (darker gray regions), degrading image quality and complicating interpretation.

A reasonable goal is to strive for voxel sizes on the order of 1.0 to 1.5 mm × 1.0 to 1.5 × 8 mm (8 to 18 mm^3 voxel) at 1.5 Tesla (T). At 0.5 T or below, a voxel size of 1.7 × 1.7 × 10 mm (28.9 mm^3 voxel) is generally reasonable, but the exact values depend on the quality of the radiofrequency coil used for signal acquisition. On most MRI systems the voxel size desired is not directly entered. Instead, voxel size is determined by three factors: slice thickness, field of view (FOV), and matrix size.

Slice Thickness

It is desirable to minimize slice thickness to reduce partial volume effects; however, doing so reduces signal. The majority of studies that used MRI in cardiac quantitation have relied on a slice thickness between 8 and 10 mm in adults. Although the existing body of experience in pediatric cardiac MRI is more limited, it appears that thinner slices (5 to 7 mm) are desirable.

Field of View

For a given matrix size, decreasing the FOV reduces voxel size and, hence, improves resolution at the expense of the signal-to-noise ratio. In addition, reducing FOV frequently leads to aliasing or wraparound, which degrades images. Wraparound can be addressed by increasing matrix size in the phase-encoding direction, but at the cost of increasing imaging time. An FOV between 25 and 38 cm is generally used in chamber and great vessel imaging, with smaller FOV generally reserved for coronary artery imaging.

Matrix

Matrix size refers to the number of voxels acquired in the frequency-encoding and phase-encoding directions. Increasing matrix size while keeping field of view constant results in smaller voxels, less signal per voxel and, hence, a lower signal-to-noise ratio. On modern magnetic resonance devices, the matrix size and

FOV can be chosen independently. Thus, it is possible to increase matrix size in the phase-encoding direction while keeping voxel size constant. The cost of this strategy is typically an increase in imaging time, because the matrix size in the phase-encoding direction (in other words, the number of phase-encoding steps) determines the number of radiofrequency pulses required to construct an image. For example, in conventional spin-echo MRI an image with 256 phase-encoding steps would typically take twice as long as an image with 128 phase-encoding steps, all other factors being equal. Typical matrix size for cardiac quantitation is 128 or 256 in the frequency-encoding direction and 128 to 256 in the phase-encoding direction.

Temporal Resolution

In all MRI techniques a series of events—radiofrequency pulses, gradient pulses, and signal acquisition—occur over a period of less than 10 msec to potentially hundreds of milliseconds. The duration of these events sets an "imaging frame duration," which determines the eventual effective framing rate. For example, a very high temporal resolution cine MRI sequence would typically use an imaging frame duration of less than 10 msec, yielding an effective framing rate of 100 frames per second. The study would take several minutes to acquire all the phase-encoding steps necessary to create each image in the cine. In comparison, a cine EPI sequence may require 100 msec per frame but acquire all the information necessary for that image during that period. In this case, the framing rate would be only 10 frames per second, but the total imaging time would be 1 cardiac cycle.

Conditions for Accurate Measurement

Regardless of the approach used, several fundamental requirements must be met to make meaningful measurements from an MRI study:

First, the *spatial resolution* must be adequate for the structure being imaged. Typically, in-plane resolution on the order of 1 to 2 mm is necessary for most cardiac imaging. However, for coronary imaging, submillimeter resolution is required. Also, it is important to realize that it is possible to adjust the voxel dimensions independently, that is, the resolution in one direction can be different from the resolution in the other perpendicular directions. This difference in resolution is not necessarily obvious on qualitative examination of the image but must be considered in measurements made with MRI.

Second, *partial volume effects* must be minimized. Partial volume effects occur because each pixel in an image reflects the average composition of the tissue from which the signal is acquired. When a structure is imaged with the use of large voxels (i.e., low resolution), the edges of the structure are blurred because of the averaging of the change in signal intensity across the edge. When the same structure is imaged with the use of small voxels (i.e., high resolution), the edges are less blurred.

The largest dimension of the volume element is typically defined by the slice thickness, so maximum blurring of the image occurs in this direction. Thus, when a slice is perpendicular to the border between two tissues, the resulting edge is sharp; however, when the border is parallel to the slice, blurring of the edge is prominent. Thus, to minimize partial volume effects, it is important not only to use small volume elements but also to optimize their orientation with respect to the structures of interest. The significance of partial volume effects on the measurement of ventricular volume and mass has been examined.[10–13] Both slice thickness and orientation of the slice relative to the structure of interest are important.

Third, the *distortion* of the images must be small. MRI uses the local magnetic field to define position in the object; therefore, anything that distorts the magnetic field distorts the image and introduces errors in measurement.

Fourth, the *contrast-to-noise ratio* must be adequate to define tissue boundaries. Poor choice of acquisition parameters, such as TR, TE, and flip angle, can lead to an inability to define edges despite adequate voxel size, which is most frequently an issue in cine MRI that uses phase-encoding groups. Luckily, flow has such a major effect on contrast in these images that there is considerable latitude in choosing a flip angle. At 1.5 T, typical acquisition parameters would be TR of 10 to 20 msec, TE of 5 to 10 msec, and flip angle 35 to 60 degrees, although optimal choices would depend on the specific imaging device. In addition there is interest in using magnetization preparation techniques, such as magnetization transfer, to enhance contrast between myocardium and blood pool.[14, 15]

Fifth, *proper gating* is currently required for routine imaging of the heart and is essential for accurate and reproducible quantitation. Electrocardiographic gating provides the most reproducible signal for timing of intracardiac events and is readily obtainable when proper electrode positioning is used.[16] Even with adequate cardiac gating, images can be degraded by respiratory motion.[17] The use of respiratory gating improves image quality at the expense of increasing image-acquisition time.[18] The use of breath-hold imaging can also eliminate respiratory artifacts,[19] but matrix size is limited, to some degree, by the ability of patients to hold their breath.[20]

Potential Sources of Error in Magnetic Resonance Quantitation

Given its potential for high-contrast and excellent spatial and temporal resolution, it is easy to appreciate the potential of MRI in quantitative assessment of cardiac physiology. However, it is important to realize that there are a number of potential sources of error (Table 50–1).

Magnetic Field Distortion

Magnetic resonance imaging fundamentally determines the location of a structure on the basis of the local magnetic field strength. Thus, when there is alteration of the local magnetic field for any reason, image distortion takes place, and the potential for errors in

TABLE 50–1. SOURCES OF ERROR IN MAGNETIC RESONANCE QUANTITATION

Magnetic Field Distortion

Patient-Related

- Ferromagnetic materials
- Chemical shift

System-Related

- Main magnetic field inhomogeneity
- Magnetic gradient field inhomogeneity

Reconstruction Artifacts

Patient-Related

- Aliasing (wraparound)
- Partial volume averaging

System-Related

- Truncation
- Quadrature

Noise-Induced Errors

Patient-Related

- Voluntary motion
- Arrhythmia
- Respiration
- Blood flow

System-Related

- Extraneous radiofrequency

Modified from Bushong, S.C.: Magnetic Resonance Imaging: Physical and Biological Principles. New York, Pergamon Press, 1988, Vol. 16, pp. 308–309. With permission from Elsevier.

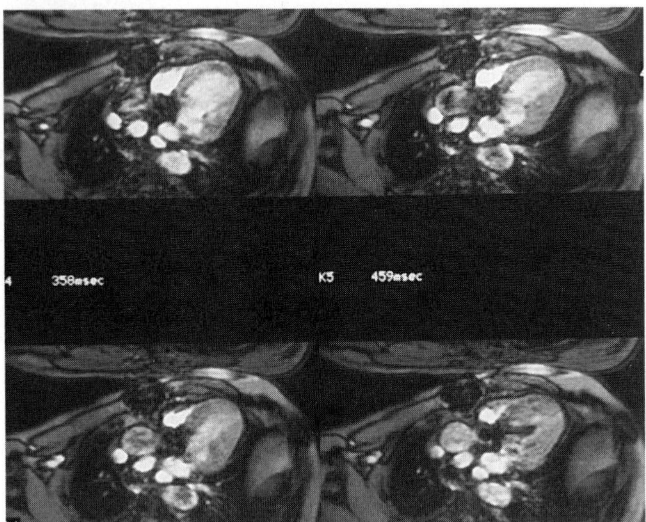

FIGURE 50–3. Sequential frames from a cine MRI study in a patient with a prosthetic aortic valve. There are signal loss and distortion in the area of a prosthetic aortic valve. The artifact from sternal wires is present anteriorly, as is evidence of slight aliasing, or wraparound.

measurement increases. Metallic structures, such as sternal wires and prosthetic valves, can cause localized alterations of field strength, even when they are not made from ferromagnetic materials (Fig. 50–3). Small currents and related magnetic fields are induced by the pulsed magnetic fields used in MRI; however, these effects are usually localized and minimally affect quantitation.

The local magnetic field is also affected by whether the hydrogen nuclei being imaged are in fat or water molecules. In the water molecule, the proximity of the oxygen atom to the hydrogen nucleus being imaged alters its local magnetic field, as compared to that of a hydrogen nucleus next to a carbon atom in fat, causing misregistration of fat in the body, as compared to water. Typically, imaging sequences are designed to minimize this effect. However, the so-called "India-ink" effect, in which a dark line is apparent at fat-water interfaces, may be seen in gradient echo images. Spin-echo imaging is relatively resistant to these effects, whereas cine MRI, which uses gradient echo imaging, is more sensitive to these inhomogeneities in the local magnetic field.

It is also important to realize that the main magnetic field and gradient magnetic fields become less homogenous toward the periphery of the magnet. Given the central location of the heart, this is less of a problem in cardiac imaging than in MRI in other portions of the body.

Reconstruction Artifacts

As described earlier, aliasing or wraparound occurs when the FOV in the phase-encoding direction is inadequate. Image degradation and confusion regarding positioning of structures results but can be readily avoided by increasing the FOV. The use of excessively large voxels can lead to a number of "ringing" artifacts at sharp edges, which can affect the measurements taken from magnetic resonance images.[21]

Noise-Induced Errors

Motion is an important potential source of error in magnetic resonance quantitation. Supraventricular and ventricular arrhythmias can lead to ghosting, degrading image quality and compromising quantitation. Slowly flowing blood within a cardiac chamber can produce an intraluminal signal that must be differentiated from intracardiac thrombus. This artifact must be recognized, or errors in the assessment of ventricular size and function will result.[22]

Comparison With Other Methods

In comparing quantitative measures obtained with MRI to other methods, it is customary to present the results in terms of regression equations, intraobserver and interobserver variability, and reproducibility. However, regression analysis and correlation coefficients do not necessarily address the key issues important in evaluating the clinical accuracy of a new test. Difference analysis, as described by Bland and Altman,[23] offers certain advantages, and is emphasized. In the discussion of magnetic resonance quantitation that follows, data that are compared to independent reference methods are emphasized whenever possible. However, both conventional linear regression and the Bland-Altman analysis are limited by the quality of the reference "gold standard." It is well known that many established, routine measures used in clinical cardiology are prone to substantial errors in even the best laboratories.[24–28]

ASSESSMENT OF CARDIAC SIZE AND SHAPE

Measurement of Cardiac Dimensions

Despite their known limitations, single linear measurements are frequently used to describe the size of cardiac chambers in all cardiac imaging techniques. Magnetic resonance imaging is a valuable tool for the assessment of cardiac dimensions because of its combination of excellent spatial resolution and the ability to obtain tomographic images in any plane.[29, 30] Using a gated, spin-echo pulse sequence, Kaul and associates found good correlation between MRI and two-dimensional echocardiography in determining left atrial and ventricular dimensions (Table 50–2).[31] Other studies have compared cardiac dimensions in transverse planes to two-dimensional echocardiography.[32–36] In addition there was excellent agreement between echocardiography and MRI in the measurement of aortic root size in Marfan's syndrome.[37]

Using cine MRI, Semelka and co-workers demonstrated a small interstudy variability[38] and close correlation with previous literature values for normals from cine computed tomography[39] and echocardiography.[40] Thus, it is clear that, given comparable views, both spin-echo and cine MRI provide accurate measures of cardiac dimensions.

Measurement of Chamber Volume

Left Ventricular Volume

Left ventricular volume is an important diagnostic and prognostic factor in patients with valvular regurgitation[41] and after myocardial

TABLE 50–2. NORMAL LEFT VENTRICULAR DIMENSIONS IN 16 SUBJECTS

Dimension: Location	Diastole	Systole
Left ventricular cavity diameter (mm)		
Chordal level	46.4 ± 5.5	33.6 ± 3.8
Papillary muscle level	43.4 ± 4.4	29.9 ± 4.8
Septum thickness (mm)		
Chordal level	10.3 ± 0.5	15.5 ± 1.4
Papillary muscle level	10.4 ± 1.8	15.6 ± 2.5
Posterior wall thickness (mm)		
Chordal level	10.2 ± 0.5	15.7 ± 1.0
Papillary muscle level	10.3 ± 1.2	15.4 ± 1.4
Left atrial diameter (mm)		
Anteroposterior	25.6 ± 4.2	—

Note: Left ventricular measurements were made at midpapillary muscle level and midway between the aortic valve and papillary muscle (chordal level). Measurements of the same structure from different planes are consolidated in this table.

Modified from Kaul, S., Wismer, G.L., Brady, T.J., et al.: Measurement of normal left heart dimensions using optimally oriented MR images. Am. J. Roentgenol. 146:7S, 1986, with permission.

infarction.[42] The ability of MRI to obtain images in any plane raises the potential for approaches to the assessment of left ventricular volumes. Although axial planes were used in early volume studies, approaches today use the standard imaging planes familiar to cardiologists, Simpson's rule, and a variety of formulas based on assumptions regarding left ventricular geometry (Fig. 50–4).

Simpson's rule refers to a method of volume calculation based on cutting the ventricular volume into a series of slices, thus minimizing geometric assumptions regarding ventricular shape. The technique requires the acquisition of a series of parallel image slices, all obtained at the same point in the cardiac cycle. The blood pool area of each slice is added and then multiplied by the interslice distance to calculate ventricular volume.

Rehr and associates showed an excellent correlation between MRI volume measurements and cast volume displacement, using this method (r = .99, standard error of the estimate [SEE] = 4.9 cm^3) (Fig. 50–5).[43] Validating MRI in humans in vivo is more difficult because there is no universally accepted gold standard.[44] Comparisons with nonsimultaneous contrast ventriculography are good, with correlation coefficients of 0.84 to 0.98.[45, 46] Semelka and colleagues used cine MR with short-axis slices in 11 normal volunteers and demonstrated excellent interstudy reproducibility.[47] Variability for measurement of left ventricular end-diastolic volume for two separate imaging sessions was 3.6 and 3.8 percent for two different observers. Similarly, variability for measurement of end-systolic volume was 9.7 and 9.0 percent. They performed further studies in morphologically abnormal left ventricles in patients with dilated cardiomyopathy and left ventricular hypertrophy.[48] Both left ventricular end-diastolic volumes (variability of less than 5 percent between studies) and end-systolic volumes continued to be highly reproducible (with variability of less than 5 percent in dilated cardiomyopathy and less than 8.5 percent in patients with left ventricular hypertrophy).

Pattynama and co-workers have carefully examined the basis for this variability in two subjects who underwent 20 repeated studies each, using the Simpson-rule approach with both multislice multiphase spin-echo and cine MRI.[49] There was no significant difference in reproducibility between spin-echo and cine MRI. Using variance component analysis, they found that interexamination variability was the most important contributor to the total variance and that further improvement in the already low interobserver and intraobserver variability would likely not reduce overall variance. They suggested that the most effective means of improving reproducibility is to average the results of two or more repeated imaging studies.

Thus, the available studies indicate that the Simpson-rule approach is highly accurate on the basis of studies that used ventricular casts, has low interobserver and intraobserver variability, and

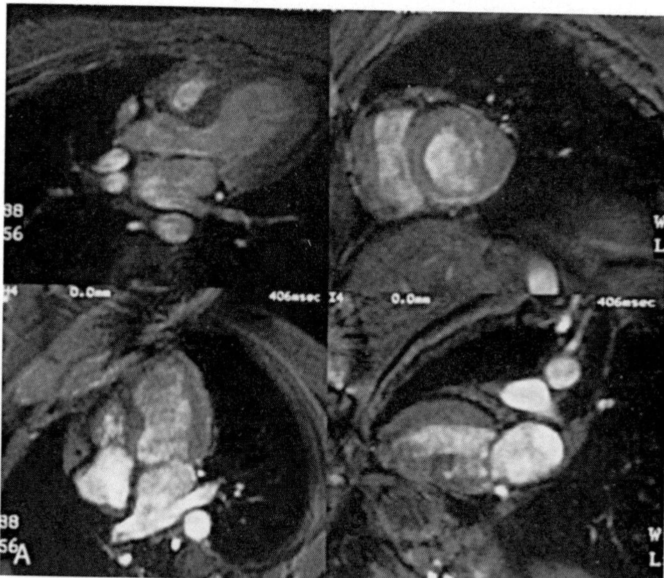

FIGURE 50–4. Standard imaging planes used in quantitation of left ventricular volumes. *Panel A,* Long-axis, short-axis, four-chamber, and two chamber imaging planes, obtained with cine MRI. *Panel B,* Short-axis slices to be acquired for a measurement of ventricular volume, using the Simpson rule, are indicated by the white lines on the long-axis reference image.

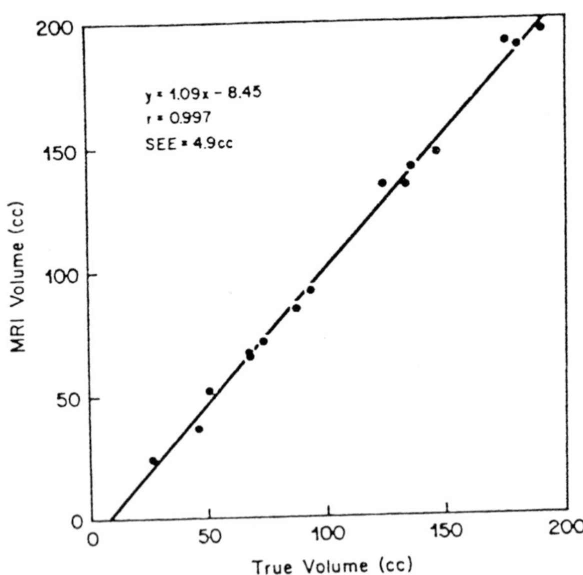

FIGURE 50–5. Correlation between MRI and displacement volume for left ventricular casts. There is excellent correlation between calculated volume and actual displacement volume. (From Rehr, R.B., Malloy, C.R., Filipchuk, N.G., et al.: Left ventricular volumes measured by MR imaging. Radiology 156:717, 1985, with permission.)

has a level of variability between repeated studies that appears to be dominated by interexamination variability. Although biphasic spin-echo[50] or breath-hold MRI[51] has been used to shorten long acquisition times, analysis of the images remains time consuming, limiting the clinical applicability of the Simpson-rule approach.

An alternative approach to reducing the image acquisition and analysis time is to use geometric assumptions to model the ventricle. The most commonly used form of geometric assumption involves modeling the left ventricle as an ellipsoid. This assumption is the basis for the familiar area-length methods used in contrast ventriculography and other forms of cardiac imaging.

Briefly, the simplification rests on calculating the volume of an ellipsoid from the lengths of its three axes. The general formula for volume of an ellipsoid is:

$$V = \frac{4\pi}{3} \cdot \frac{L}{2} \cdot \frac{M}{2} \cdot \frac{N}{2}$$

where V is the volume, and L, M, and N are the diameters of the ellipsoid along each of its three axes.

In the single plane area-length method, the ventricle is assumed to be a prolate ellipsoid,[52] which means that the minor axis of the ventricle in the image plane is assumed to equal the minor axis in the orthogonal plane. Ventricular length, L, is measured along its long axis from the apex to the base. Using the standard geometric formula for the area of an ellipse as a function of its major and minor axis:

$$A = \pi \cdot \frac{L}{2} \cdot \frac{M}{2} \quad \text{or} \quad M = \frac{4A}{\pi L}$$

Assuming that the ventricle is a prolate ellipse, M will be equal to N. Then:

$$V = \frac{\pi}{6} \cdot L \cdot M \cdot M = \frac{\pi}{6} \cdot L \cdot \frac{4A}{\pi L} \cdot \frac{4A}{\pi L} = \frac{8A^2}{3\pi L} = 0.85 \frac{A^2}{L}$$

In the biplane method the left ventricle is approximated by an ellipsoid and the major and minor axes are determined from two orthogonal images.[53] The volume V is given by the following equation:

$$V = \frac{\pi}{6} \cdot L \cdot M \cdot N = \frac{\pi}{6} \cdot L_{MIN} \cdot \frac{4A_{RAO}}{\pi L_{RAO}} \cdot \frac{4A_{LAO}}{\pi L_{LAO}} = 0.85 \frac{A_{RAO} \cdot A_{LAO}}{L_{MIN}}$$

where A_{RAO} and A_{LAO} are the areas in the RAO and LAO views, respectively, L_{RAO} and L_{LAO} are the long-axis length in the RAO and LAO images, and L_{MIN} is the minimum of the long-axis length in the two orthogonal images.

The major advantages of these methods are that the images are easy to acquire, the method of analysis is simple, and the approach is familiar to cardiologists. The major disadvantages are that (1) the volume measurement relies on geometric assumptions, which may be less accurate in the distorted ventricle; (2) errors in positioning the long-axis plane lead to "foreshortening" and an underestimation of the true volume; and (3) the presence of trabeculations and papillary muscles makes the endocardial edges less defined, introducing error into the calculations.

Using spin-echo MRI, Underwood and associates compared single-plane and biplane area-length methods with multislice imaging in the determination of left ventricular volume.[54] Long-axis and four-chamber views were obtained for comparison. In normal subjects there was good agreement between the results obtained from the single-plane and multislice approaches, with a mean difference of 2.0 ± 6.6 mL. The agreement between single-plane measurements made with the use of the long-axis and four-chamber views was good, indicating that either plane would be suitable for rapid single-plane measurement. Agreement was not as good in patients with prior infarction (mean difference, 4.5 ± 18.1 mL) and was greatest for patients with pronounced abnormalities of wall motion and decreased function, again indicating that the geometric assumptions used may not be appropriate for the abnormal ventricle.

In 21 patients Cranney and colleagues compared biplane cine MRI (perpendicular four-chamber and two-chamber views), short-axis multislice multiphase spin-echo MRI, and calibrated biplane contrast ventriculography[55] (Fig. 50–6). Both long-axis cine MRI and short-axis spin-echo MRI correlated well with ventriculography ($r > .90$ in all), with no systematic differences between the two strategies. Both forms of MRI measurement tended to underestimate end-diastolic volumes, as compared with contrast ventriculography, which led to a consistently lower ejection fraction from MRI than from ventriculography. This may be due to several factors: (1) underestimation of end-diastolic volume on MRI due to slowly moving blood near the endocardium being interpreted as wall, (2) underestimation of volume on MRI due to difficulty in defining the base in short-axis images, and (3) overestimation of volume on the contrast ventriculogram due to dye filling the space between trabeculae. Dell'Italia and co-workers used the bullet formula developed in echocardiography in the measurement of left ventricular volume by MRI.[56] There was excellent correlation ($r = .97$) between left ventricular end-systolic volumes derived by means of the bullet formula and those obtained using Simpson's rule during steady-state and altered loading conditions in six anesthetized intact dogs.

Recently, Dulce and associates used cine MRI to compare the modified Simpson-rule, the hemisphere cylinder, and the modified Teichholz models with the methods described earlier for the assessment of left ventricular volume in normal subjects and in subjects with left ventricular hypertrophy (Fig. 50–7).[57] Volumes calculated with each geometric model were compared with the volume determined with the use of the full Simpson-rule (or three-dimensional reconstruction) technique. In most cases the different models yielded comparable results in these subjects (Table 50–3). However, the use of the hemispheric cylinder and modified Teichholz models resulted in significantly different values.

Right Ventricular Volume

Assessing right ventricular volume is difficult with the use of most imaging techniques. The variability in the geometry and position of the right ventricle make application of geometric assumptions in contrast ventriculography difficult. The position of

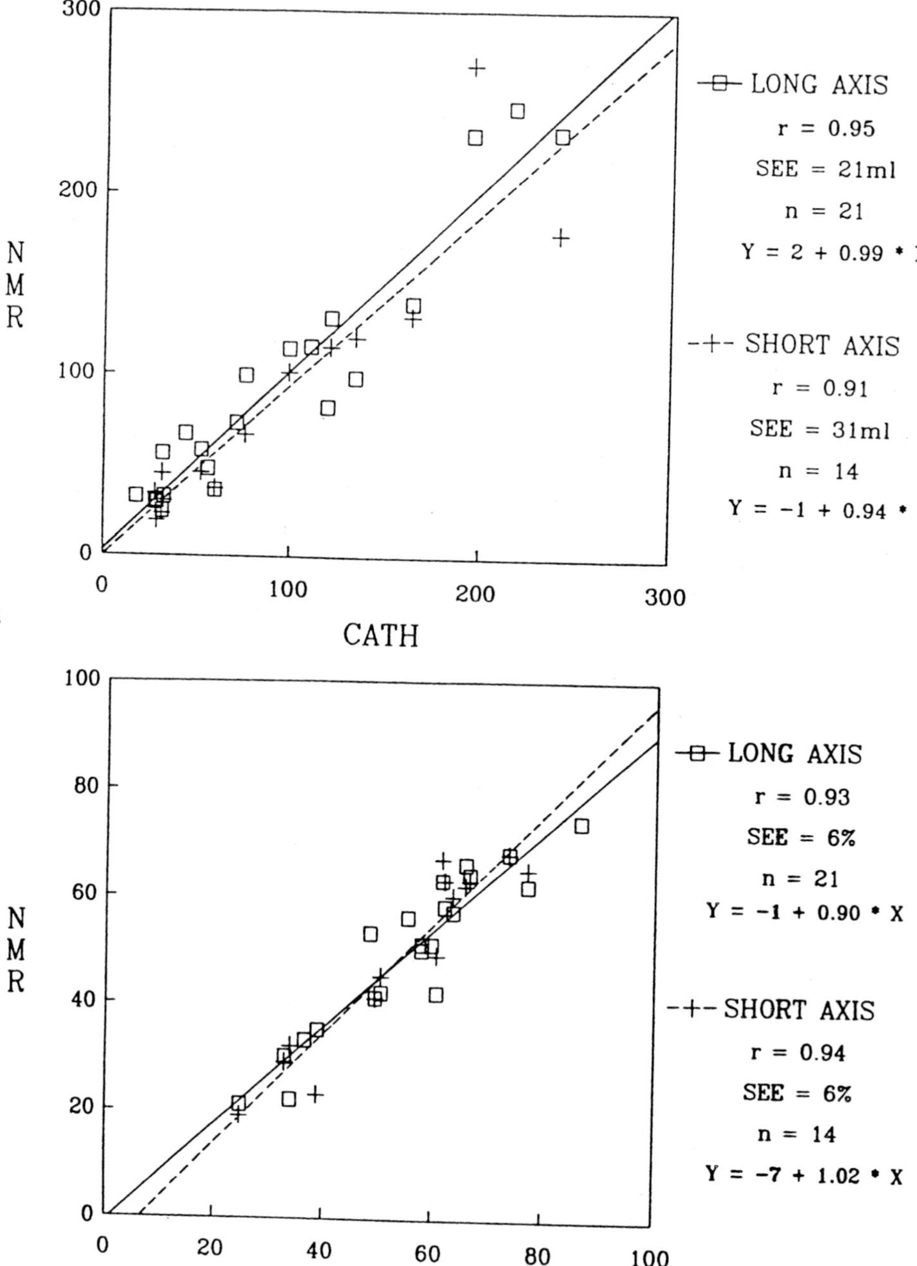

FIGURE 50–6. Linear regression analysis of NMR versus contrast ventriculography in assessment of ventricular volume. *Panel A,* Linear regression analysis, comparing both multislice, multiphase spin-echo and long-axis cine MRI with catheterization in the determination of left ventricular end-systolic volume. *Panel B,* Linear regression analysis, comparing both multislice, multiphase spin-echo and long-axis cine MRI with catheterization in the determination of ejection fraction. (From Cranney, G.B., Lotan, C.S., Dean, L., et al.: Left ventricular volume measurement using cardiac axis nuclear magnetic resonance imaging: Validation by calibrated ventricular angiography. Circulation 82:154, 1990, with permission. Copyright 1990, American Heart Association.)

the right ventricle relative to the anterior chest wall and sternum complicate the use of echocardiography. There is increasing evidence that MRI may be the optimal tool for the evaluation of right ventricular geometry and function. Boxt examined the usefulness of multislice, multiphase spin-echo MRI in the assessment of right ventricular volume.[58] When the Simpson-rule approach was used, there was excellent correlation between MRI and water displacement for right ventricular casts (MRI volume = 1.09 × true volume + 2.87, r = .98, SEE = 5.8 mL). In patients they found that this method had low intraobserver and interobserver variability and permitted evaluation of right ventricular volumes, mass, and function in patients with pulmonary hypertension.

Atrial Volumes

Järvinen and co-workers recently described the use of cine MRI in the measurement of atrial volume.[59] In right atrial casts MR assessment of right atrial volume correlated well with cast volume displacement (r = .99); however, MRI tended to underestimate right atrial volume, probably because of difficulty in defining the border of the atrial appendage. In in vivo studies they found that right atrial volumes were consistently larger than left atrial volumes. This method also provides a means of assessing right atrial phasic function.

In summary, MRI has been shown to be a highly accurate and reproducible method for the determination of ventricular volume. Calculations based on geometric assumptions are quite accurate but suffer from some of the same limitations as other imaging techniques. The exact positions of the imaging planes in space with MRI make the application of Simpson-rule approaches straightforward. The above aforementioned suggest that MRI that uses the Simpson-rule technique should be considered the reference method for the determination of ventricular volume, particularly in patients with distorted left ventricular geometry and in the evaluation of the right ventricle.

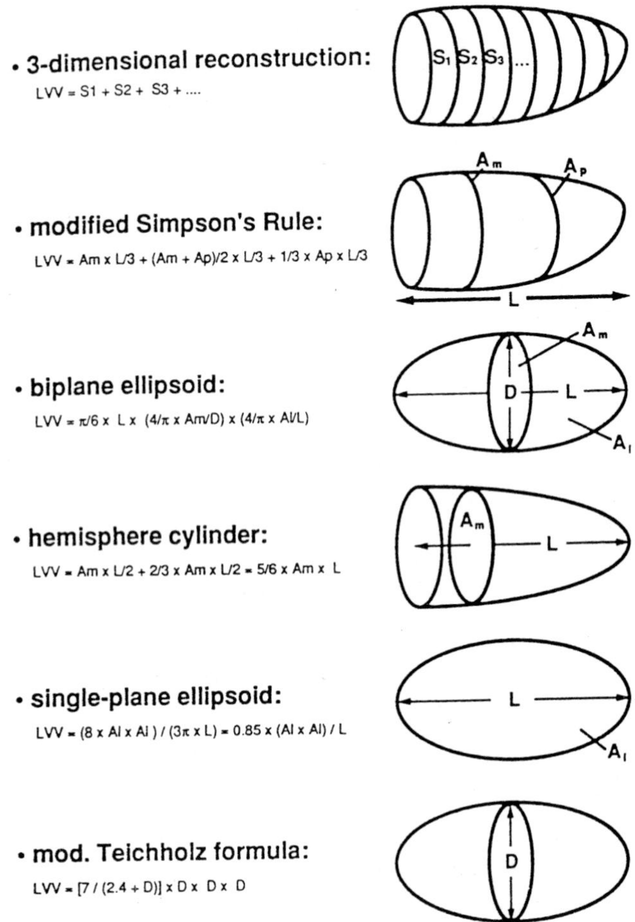

FIGURE 50–7. Different geometric models used in the determination of left ventricular volume. (From Dulce, M.C., Mostbeck, G.H., Friese, K.K., et al.: Quantification of the left ventricular volumes and function with cine MR imaging: Comparison of geometric models with three-dimensional data. Radiology 188:371, 1993, with permission.)

Myocardial Mass

The importance of MRI as a tool for quantitation is also evident in the assessment of left ventricular mass. An acoustic window is not required, which makes MRI particularly useful in making estimates of mass that require more complete measurements of the heart, such as the Simpson-rule method. Myocardial mass is estimated by multiplying the muscle volume by the specific gravity of myocardium, 1.05 g/cm^3. The effectiveness of this approach has been verified extensively in animal models and in humans.

Florentine and co-workers demonstrated an excellent correlation with actual postmortem mass (r = .95, SEE = 13.1 g), using transaxial slices 10 mm thick.[60] Keller and associates used short-axis, end-diastolic images and obtained an additional improvement in the estimation of mass (r = .98, SEE = 6.1).[61] Magnetic resonance imaging slightly overestimated left ventricular mass, which was attributed to partial volume effects and difficulties in proper border definition, owing to signal from slowly moving blood in the ventricular cavity.

In extensive studies, Maddahi and colleagues examined the effects of slice orientation and corrections for partial volume effects on the determination of myocardial mass, using Simpson's rule, in the dog model.[62] These studies indicated that in vivo estimates of left ventricular mass are most accurate when the images are obtained in the short-axis plane of the heart. Correction for partial volume effects at the apex when the short-axis plane was used for imaging led to only a small improvement in the correlation coefficient and standard error of the estimate (uncorrected, r = .989, SEE = 4.93, versus corrected, r = .996, SEE = 3.14). Images obtained in the transaxial and vertical long-axis planes were associated with larger errors, regardless of the method used to correct for partial volume effects. Hence, the optimal approach on the basis of animal studies appears to use short-axis images.

This approach has been used in the measurements of myocardial mass with acute aortic insufficiency and myocardial infarction. Manning and colleagues assessed in vivo left ventricular mass in both healthy adult rats and in animals subjected to cardiac volume overload by aortic leaflet disruption.[63] Linear regression analysis showed an excellent correlation between MR-estimated mass and autopsy-measured left ventricular mass (r = .98, SEE = 39 mg). An increase in left ventricular mass was detected within 5 days of aortic valve disruption and was complete at 3 weeks. The increase

TABLE 50–3. MEAN AND STANDARD DEVIATION OF GLOBAL LEFT VENTRICULAR VOLUMES AND FUNCTIONS IN BOTH GROUPS

Group and Method	EDV (mL)	ESV (mL)	SV (mL)	EF (%)
Healthy volunteers (n = 10)				
3D	122 ± 26.3	42 ± 12.2	80 ± 16.4	66 ± 4.7
SR	121 ± 26.3	43 ± 14.1	78 ± 15.2	65 ± 5.9
BP	118 ± 25.2	41 ± 11.3	77 ± 15.1	65 ± 4.1
HC	151 ± 32.2°	57 ± 19.0°	94 ± 17.6°	63 ± 7.0°
SP	123 ± 32.2	38 ± 11.2	84 ± 22.8	69 ± 4.7
TF	127 ± 27.1	49 ± 18.3	77 ± 15.5	62 ± 8.9
Patients with left ventricular hypertrophy (n = 10)				
3D	90 ± 14.7	25 ± 4.8	65 ± 12.4	72 ± 4.2
SR	88 ± 13.5	24 ± 5.7	64 ± 11.4	73 ± 5.3
BP	88 ± 13.1	26 ± 4.5	62 ± 10.6	70 ± 3.9
HC	113 ± 21.7°	32 ± 8.3°	81 ± 20.2°	71 ± 7.1
SP	90 ± 9.3	36 ± 8.5°	54 ± 13.4	61 ± 11.8°
TF	101 ± 22.6°	36 ± 7.2°	65 ± 22.2	63 ± 10.7°

Note: Values were obtained with geometric models and a three-dimensional data set of cine MR images. BP = biplane ellipsoid model; 3D = analysis with a three-dimensional data set; HC = hemisphere cylinder model; SP = single-plane ellipsoid model; SR = modified Simpson-rule model; TF = modified Teichholz model.

°Significant differences compared with a three-dimensional data set were $P < .05$.

Modified from Dulce, M.C., Mostbeck, G.H., Friese, K.K., et al.: Quantification of the left ventricular volume and function with cine MR imaging: Comparison of geometric models with three-dimensional data. Radiology 188:371, 1993.

averaged 40 percent (range, 19 to 64 percent) over the 44 days (range, 5 to 77 days) of observation. In another study, gated MRI was performed in 15 dogs before and after infarction.[64] There was excellent correlation between actual mass and mass after infarction estimated from end-diastolic images (r = .97, SEE = 6.6 g) and end-systolic images (r = .95, SEE = 6.5 g). Thus, MRI permits accurate determination of left ventricular mass, even in severely deformed hearts.

Human studies also have demonstrated an excellent correlation.[65, 66] Katz and associates performed imaging of cadaver hearts and examined intraobserver and interobserver variability in volunteers.[67] Cadaver heart studies were used to establish a linear regression equation for human hearts: True left ventricular weight (grams) = 7.14 + 0.91 × MR mass estimate (grams). The correlation coefficient was 0.99, with an SE of 6.8 g. Using 10 short-axis slices through the heart at end-diastole, they observed that the intraobserver variability (r = .96, SEE = 11.1 g) and the interobserver variability (r = .91, SEE = 17.8 g) were excellent (Fig. 50–8).

Germain and co-workers compared the interstudy reproducibility of left ventricular mass measurements by multislice, spin-echo, short-axis MRI, and by M-mode echocardiography in normal volunteers.[68] On repeat studies performed within 4 days, MRI was more reproducible. The correlation for repeated M-mode echocardiographic estimates of left ventricular mass was .89 (SEE = 22.7 g), whereas for MRI the correlation between repeated measures was .96 (SEE = 11.2 g).

Magnetic resonance imaging has also been used in the estimation of mass in clinical studies. Magnetic resonance imaging has been used to evaluate hypertrophy in competitive athletes[69] and to monitor the response to therapy in patients with hypertension[70] and dilated cardiomyopathy.[71] Allison and co-workers studied left ventricular mass in hypertrophic cardiomyopathy by means of MRI. Normalized left ventricular mass in normal subjects had a mean value of 1.8±0.20 g/kg, whereas in subjects with hypertrophic cardiomyopathy it had a mean value of 3.77±0.86 g/kg.[72] An added advantage of MRI in the measurement of myocardial mass is that the Simpson-rule method can be used to measure left and right ventricular mass simultaneously.[73, 74]

In summary, MRI that uses the Simpson-rule approach with short-axis images provides the most accurate and reproducible noninvasive estimate of myocardial mass.

ASSESSMENT OF CARDIAC FUNCTION

Ejection Fraction

Measurement of cardiac volumes at end-diastole and end-systole by multislice multiphase spin-echo or by cine MRI allows determination of left and right ventricular ejection fractions. Left ventricular ejection fraction can be measured most accurately with the Simpson-rule approach with multiple tomographic slices.[75] Excellent agreement is achieved between right ventricular and left ventricular stroke volumes in normal subjects with this method (left ventricular/right ventricular stroke volume ratio = 0.97±0.06; correlation coefficient r = .95). Although accurate, lengthy image analysis time limits its general clinical applicability.

As discussed previously, assumptions about left ventricular geometry can be used to reduce the number of images required to describe the ventricle, simplifying and reducing the time required for calculations of ejection fraction. Good results have been obtained with a biplane area-length method, with the use of orthogonal four-chamber and two-chamber views.[55] This method has been validated against left ventriculography (r = .93) and has excellent interstudy reproducibility (mean absolute difference in ejection fraction on two studies in the same patient = 1.9±1.4 percent).[76] Other geometric assumptions used previously in echocardiography also provide reasonable results when compared with the MRI method of three-dimensional reconstruction with the use of multiple short-axis slices in both healthy volunteers and patients with left ventricular hypertrophy (r = .87 to 0.97 for comparisons of the modified Simpson-rule, biplane ellipsoid, or hemisphere cylinder models with a three-dimensional MRI data set reference standard).[77]

Cardiac Output

Left ventricular volume data and the heart rate can be used to calculate stroke volume and cardiac output. Comparisons of MRI cardiac output with the clinical reference standards of cardiac catheterization (thermodilution, Fick method) and radionuclide ventriculography are complicated by the known assumptions and limitations of these accepted techniques. In general, comparisons of MRI with these measures have yielded results within the confidence limits of the reference techniques themselves.[78, 79] Stroke-volume determination with EPI has been demonstrated during a 15-second breath-hold (12 heartbeats) (Fig. 50–9).[80] Although not compared directly with an alternative reference standard, this method yielded excellent agreement between right and left ventricular stroke volumes in normal subjects (r = .995). In addition, there was excellent agreement with conventional MRI measurements of left ventricular stroke volume with the use of multiple short-axis images for volumetric reconstruction (r = .98), with no significant difference from the line of identity. Volume measurements of cardiac output by MRI correlate well with phase-contrast measurements of flow (r = .97 to .98, SEE for the left ventricular stroke volume = 3.2 to 3.7 mL).[81, 82]

Segmental Wall Motion

Many myocardial disease processes affect the heart nonuniformly. Although this nonuniformity is most clearly true for ischemic disease, regional nonuniformity also exists in hypertrophic cardiomyopathies and nonischemic, dilated cardiomyopathies. In addition, in mitral regurgitation the regional geometry and function of the left ventricle have been shown to directly influence overall cardiac performance after mitral valve surgery.[83]

Left ventricular regional wall motion can be assessed by means of various methods, including projection (contrast left ventriculography, radionuclide ventriculography) and tomographic (echocardiography, computed tomography, MRI) techniques. The projection techniques image the blood pool and not the myocardium; accurate separation of the myocardial walls can sometimes pose a problem. The tomographic techniques require accurate alignment of the tomographic plane with the desired cardiac axis to provide meaningful results. Because the ventricle undergoes translation and rotation in space at the same time that it is contracting, all wall motion analysis techniques suffer from the problem of defining a left ventricular "center" as a reference point from which to measure motion.[84] Tethering of adjacent walls also occurs; for example, an akinetic segment may appear to move because it is "pulled" by a neighboring contracting segment, leading to interpretation errors.[85] Because of these problems, regional wall thickening is the preferred method for the assessment of segmental function.

Wall Thickening

Wall thickening is a more accurate indicator of myocardial ischemia than wall motion.[86, 87] Additionally, abnormalities in wall thickening occur very early in ischemia—prior to electrocardiographic changes or chest pain—providing a sensitive marker of ischemia.[88, 89] Echocardiographic assessment of wall thickening has provided useful information in patients with chronic ischemic heart disease, those with acute ischemic syndromes, including myocardial infarction, and during exercise or pharmacologic stress–induced ischemia for the diagnosis of coronary artery disease.[90] In addition, regional improvement in wall thickening with inotropic stimulation ("contractile reserve") has been shown to identify viable myocardium and predict recovery of function in both acute and chronic coronary artery disease.[91, 92]

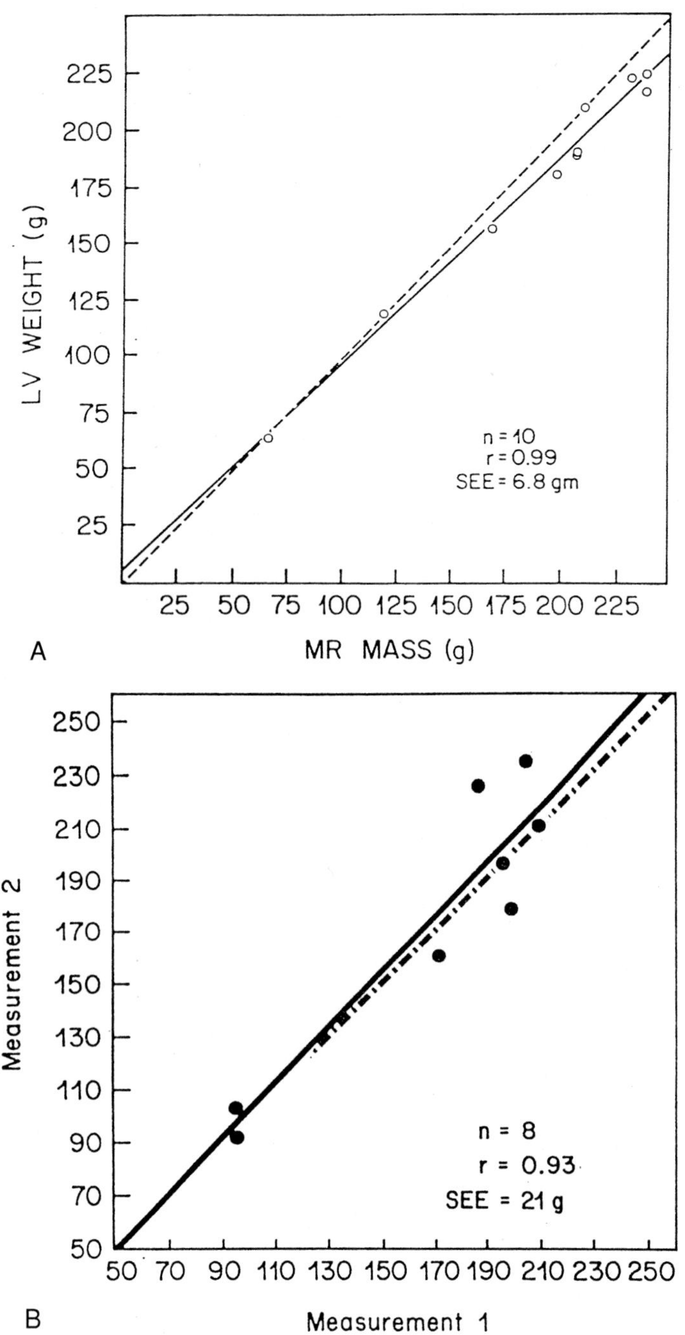

FIGURE 50–8. Correlation in estimation of myocardial mass. *Panel A,* Linear regression analysis for MRI in estimating myocardial mass, as compared to autopsy weight in cadaveric hearts. *Panel B,* Reproducibility analysis for repeated imaging sessions for estimation of myocardial mass in normal volunteers. There is excellent reproducibility in the measurement. (From Katz, J., Milliken, M.C., Stray-Gundersen, J., et al.: Estimation of human myocardial mass with MR imaging. Radiology 169:495, 1988, with permission.)

Echocardiographic measures of wall thickening have primarily been semiquantitative, using a visually derived wall-thickening score.[93] Wall thickening can be quantified with echocardiography, for example, with a centerline method[94]; however, this has not commonly been done, in part because of problems with border definition and difficulty in obtaining multiple parallel short-axis planes. Magnetic resonance imaging overcomes many of these difficulties. Regional wall thickening has been measured in normal subjects and in patients with ischemic wall motion abnormalities.[95] In the latter group, there was good correspondence with wall motion abnormalities.[95] In the latter group, there was good correspondence with wall motion abnormalities by biplane ventriculography (sensitivity of MRI = 0.94, specificity = 0.80).

Both dipyridamole and dobutamine have been used with MRI of regional wall motion for identification of stress-induced ischemia.[96, 97] Sensitivities and specificities for single-vessel and multivessel coronary disease have been comparable to other noninvasive imaging modalities; van Rugge found the sensitivity of dobutamine-MRI to be 88 percent (15 of 17) for detection of single-vessel disease, 91 percent (10 of 11) for two-vessel disease, and 100 percent (5 of 5) for three-vessel disease.[41] In their 39 consecutive patients, the overall sensitivity of dobutamine-MRI for detection of coronary disease was 91 percent and the specificity 80 percent.

Because the imaging plane is fixed, tomographic measures such as echocardiography, computed tomography, or traditional MRI cannot correct for through-plane myocardial motion during systole. Thus, during attempts at quantitation of wall thickening, the segment being measured at end-systole is not truly the same myocardium that was seen at end-diastole. Because of the curvature of the left ventricular surfaces, this through-plane motion (e.g., long-axis shortening through a short-axis imaging plane) can cause overestimation of wall thickening.[98] In-plane motion is also difficult to account for with tomographic methods, because there are few fixed internal landmarks in the left ventricle. It is well known that rotation (or torsion) occurs in the short-axis plane during left

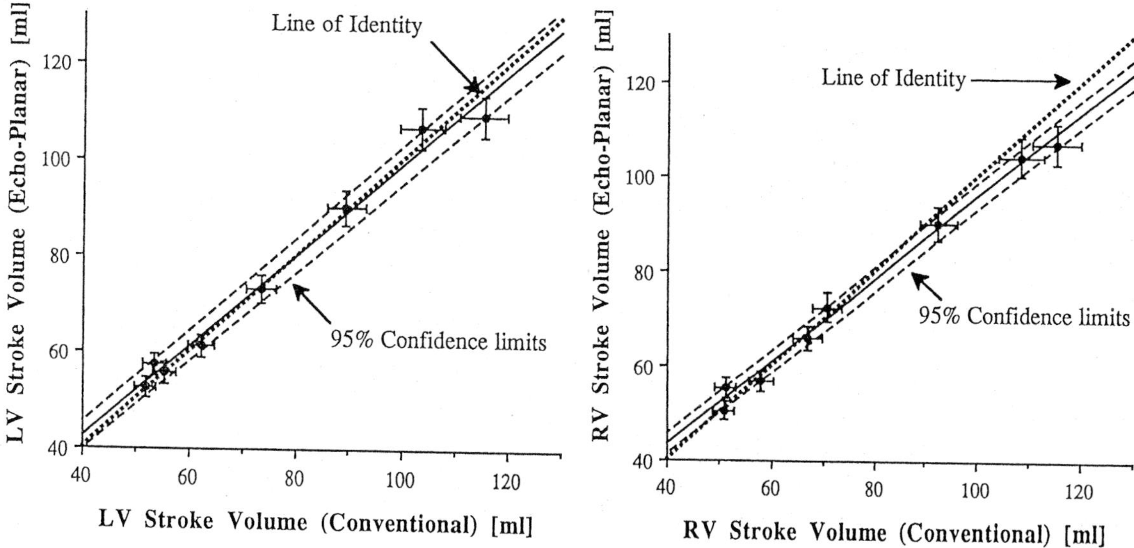

FIGURE 50–9. Echo-planar imaging and conventional MRI. Linear regression analysis, comparing EPI and conventional MRI in the determination of left ventricular and right ventricular stroke volumes. There is excellent correlation between the two techniques. (From Hunter, G.J., Hamberg, L.M., Weisskoff, R.N., et al.: Measurement of stroke volume and cardiac output within a single breath-hold with echo-planar MR imaging. J. Magn. Reson. Imaging 4[1]:51, 1994, with permission.)

ventricular contraction,[99] but this is difficult to measure and correct for with traditional noninvasive methods. Larger errors in wall-thickening measurements may be introduced when one changes the position or angle of the imaging plane when making comparisons between two points in time. MRI offers the advantage over echocardiography of imaging planes that are defined precisely in three-dimensional space.

Traditional MRI (along with echocardiography and computed tomography) cannot produce measurements in which the same segment of myocardium is imaged throughout the cardiac cycle. Until recently, the only approaches to this problem involved the use of surgically implanted radiopaque beads or sonomicrometers.[100] The highly invasive nature of these methods limits their use to animal models or a very few cardiac surgical patients. In addition, these approaches are significantly restricted in the amount of myocardium that can be evaluated, and the surgical attachment itself may alter the contractile behavior of the underlying myocardium in uncertain ways. However, MRI offers two novel, noninvasive approaches to the assessment of regional function and deformation: myocardial tagging and wall velocity encoding.

Myocardial Tagging

As is discussed in Chapter 45, myocardial tagging uses presaturation to "tag" regions of the myocardium, permitting tracking of segment motion. By appropriately choosing the imaging plane and tag orientation, one can evaluate regional and transmural differences in amount of wall thickening, torsion, long-axis shortening, or other contractile deformation. This method was originally described by Zerhouni in 1988,[101] and tagging of multiple regions with a single pulse was reported by Axel in 1989.[102] Since then, application of these methods has yielded important insights into the mechanics of myocardial contraction and regional myocardial stress and strain.

Measurements of wall thickening by MRI with tissue tagging have been shown to correlate well with sonomicrometer measurements in the dog.[103] Linear, area, and volume (three-dimensional) methods of calculating wall thickness were compared: the volume method correlated best with sonomicrometry ($r = .95$; regression equation: MRI percent wall thickening $= 0.19 + 1.49x$, where x is sonomicrometer percent wall thickening). All MRI methods consistently overestimated the sonomicrometer values, which has been a consistent finding in other MRI and echocardiographic studies.[104, 105] One possible explanation is that placement of the sonomicrometers affects (reduces) local contraction, possibly by means of entrainment of ventricular trabeculae, or by locally induced inflammation, hemorrhage, or fibrosis. Also, as the trabeculae converge at end-systole, apparent wall thickness increases, causing visual overestimation of wall thickening because of tomographic imaging methods. Because the sonomicrometer crystals are in the "valleys" of the trabeculae, their measurements are unaffected by this phenomenon.

Recently, the reproducibility of tagging was examined in a group of normal volunteers. Long-axis, four-chamber, and two-chamber views were obtained with single-axis tagging (Fig. 50–10).[106] There was excellent reproducibility of the imaging plane and the position of the tags in repeated images done the same day after repositioning and in repeated studies 4 weeks later. With the use of a Bland-Altman analysis, the mean differences in end-diastolic wall thickness, end-systolic wall thickness, and percent wall thickening mean between the baseline and the 4-week studies were -0.05 ± 0.69 mm, 0.00 ± 0.92 mm, and 0.98 ± 17.82 percent, respectively ($n = 108$ segments).

With the use of tagged cine MRI, hypertensive patients with left ventricular hypertrophy and normal ejection fractions have been shown to have reduced circumferential and longitudinal myocardial shortening (circumferential shortening $= 29 \pm 6$ percent in hypertensives versus 44 ± 6 percent in normals, $P = .0001$), suggesting the existence of contractile dysfunction in these patients despite overall "normal" pump performance.[107]

Left Ventricular Deformation

The left ventricle undergoes complex motion and shape changes during the cardiac cycle, complicating assessment of function. Translation and rotation of the ventricle as a whole occur (solid-body motion). Additionally, the left ventricular shape deforms, including torsion or twisting in the short-axis plane and shortening of the left ventricle in the long-axis plane, along with other deformations. Magnetic resonance imaging with tagging provides a unique noninvasive way of examining myocardial motion and deformation, with many more sample points than is possible with invasive methods.

The "wringing" motion of left ventricular systole has been con-

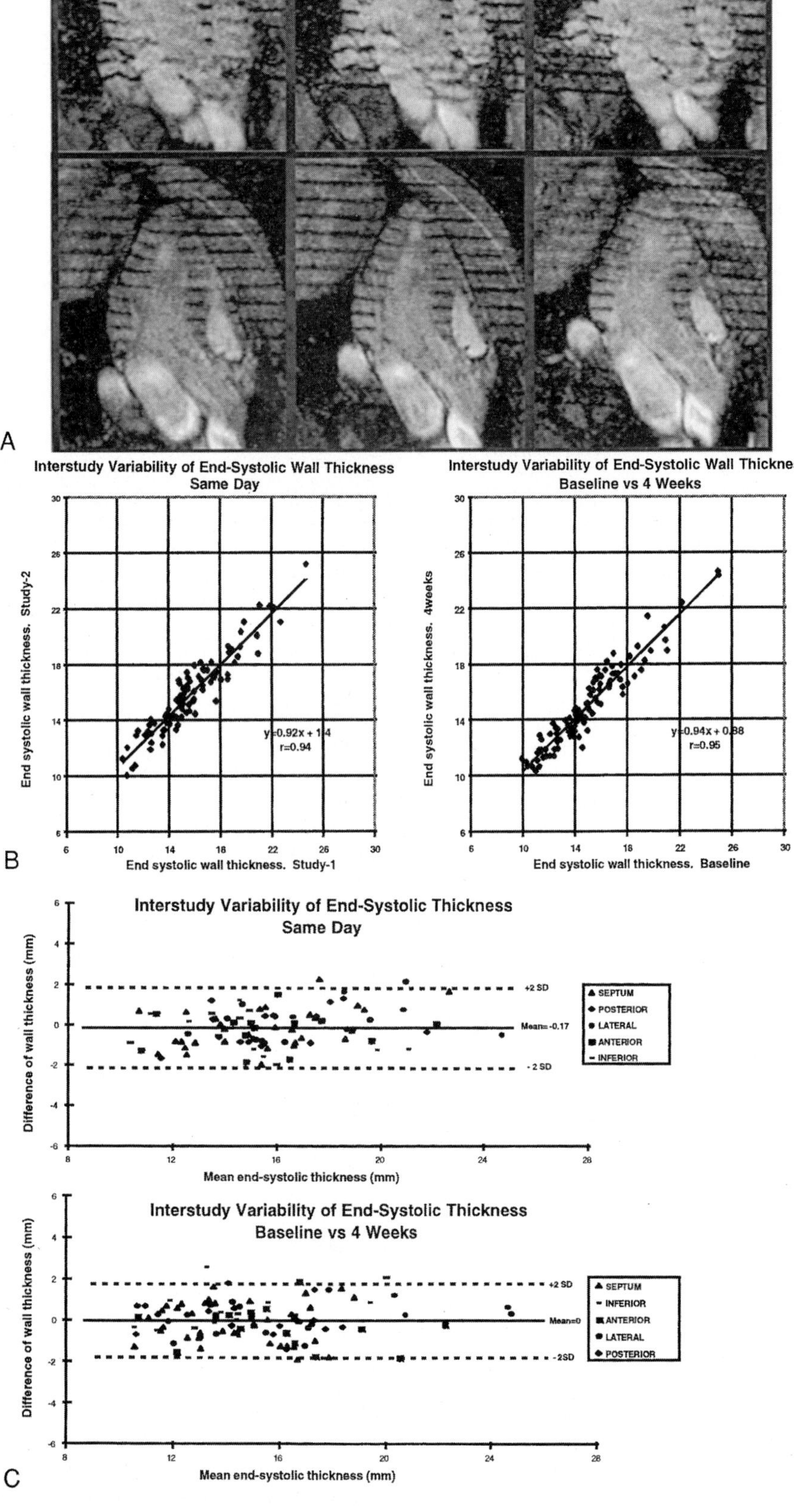

FIGURE 50–10. Reproducibility of tagging. *Panel A,* Tagged images obtained at baseline, after repositioning, and 4 weeks later in normal volunteers. The top row of images was taken 40 msec into systole, while the bottom row was obtained at end-systole. There is remarkable reproducibility in the images and the positioning of the tags. *Panel B,* Linear regression analysis for the end-systolic wall thickness from repeated imaging the same day and 4 weeks later. *Panel C,* Bland-Altman analysis of the difference in measurement of end-diastolic wall thickness for repeated imaging after repositioning the same day and repositioning 4 weeks later.

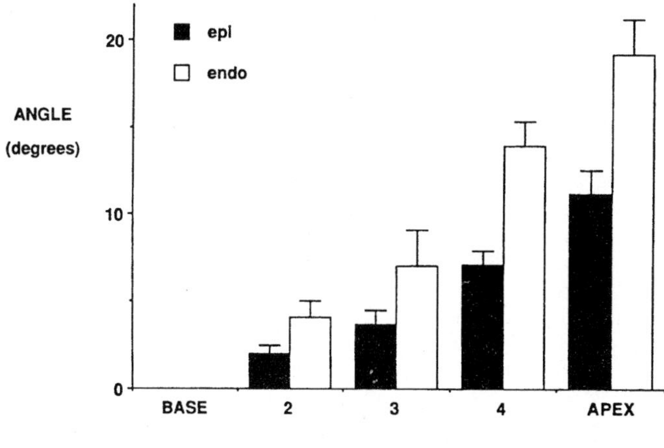

FIGURE 50–11. Torsion gradient across the ventricle. Measurement of epicardial and endocardial torsion with the use of myocardial tagging. It is apparent that the degree of torsion is greatest at the apex, and the twisting in the endocardial layers is greater than that in the epicardial layers. (From Lima, J.A., Jeremy, R., Guier, W., et al.: Accurate systolic wall thickening by nuclear magnetic resonance imaging with tissue tagging: Correlation with sonomicrometers in normal and ischemic myocardium. J. Am. Coll. Cardiol. 21[7]:1741, 1993. With permission of the American College of Cardiology.)

firmed with MRI myocardial tagging, with a slightly clockwise rotation of the base of the heart (5.0 ± 2.4 degrees, as viewed from the apex) and a more pronounced counterclockwise rotation of the apex (−9.6 ± 2.9 degrees).[108, 109] Torsion is greatest in the lateral wall and least in the interventricular septum. A transmural gradient of this twisting or torsion also exists, with the endocardium undergoing approximately twice as much torsion as the epicardium at any given level of the ventricle (Fig. 50–11). Ventricular torsion may represent a way of storing energy during systole. Most of this torsion is reversed in the isovolumic relaxation phase of diastole, prior to mitral valve opening, suggesting that it may be a mechanism for the generation of ventricular "suction" that promotes early diastolic filling (Fig. 50–12).[110] This process is substantially enhanced by catecholamine infusion—providing a possible mechanism for the increase in early diastolic filling and stroke volume that occurs during physiologic stress, despite a shorter diastolic filling interval.

As was previously known, myocardial tagging has shown that the apex of the heart remains virtually stationary during the cardiac cycle. During systole, as the long-axis shortens, the base of the heart moves toward the apex. This long-axis movement progressively increases with distance from the apex. As with torsion, regional variations exist, with more long-axis displacement of the lateral and posterior walls than of the septal and anterior walls at any level.[111] At the base of the heart, the posterior wall was shown to displace longitudinally 13.4 ± 2.2 mm, and the anterior wall 9.7 ± 1.8 mm ($P < .001$) in 12 normal human volunteers. Thus for a midventricular short-axis imaging plane, not only is different myocardium drawn into the imaging plane at end-systole, as compared to that at end-diastole, but also a greater amount of such through-plane translation occurs inferolaterally than anteroseptally. Magnetic resonance imaging with myocardial tagging offers the only current way of describing and accounting for such effects.

Regional Stress and Strain

Measures of forces experienced by the myocardium can be derived from regional wall-thickness and deformation measurements, including circumferential-longitudinal shear forces,[112] myocardial strain,[113, 114] and myocardial wall stress.[115] Elevated wall stress has been demonstrated with progressively worsening grades of mitral regurgitation and aortic regurgitation.[116] In addition, three-dimensional portrayals of left ventricular function can be generated with three axes, showing ejection fraction, left ventricular mass (by MRI), and peak systolic wall stress.[117] Important differences can be seen on such a plot between the hearts of normal persons and those with left ventricular hypertrophy, valvular regurgitation, or dilated cardiomyopathy (Fig. 50–13). In addition, regional wall stress analyses may provide helpful insights into the mechanisms and results of ventricular remodeling in the postmyocardial infarction patient.[118]

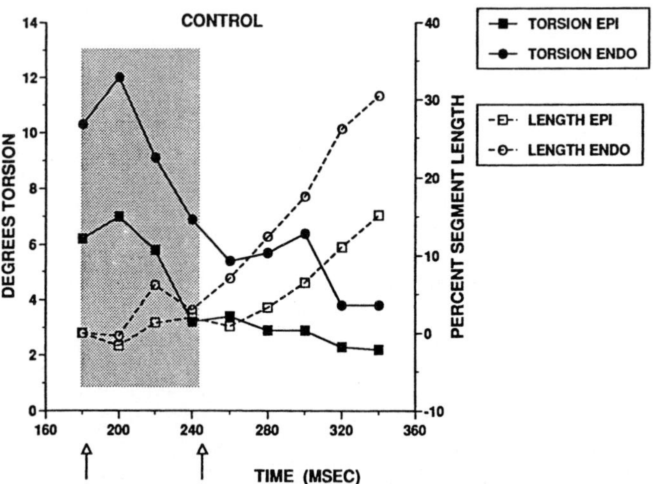

FIGURE 50–12. Evaluation of torsion and segment lengthening during diastole with myocardial tagging. There is evidence of important untwisting of the ventricle during isovolumic relaxation prior to mitral valve opening and prior to segment lengthening. (From Axel, L.: Blood flow effects in magnetic resonance imaging. Am. J. Radiol. 143:1157, 1984, with permission.)

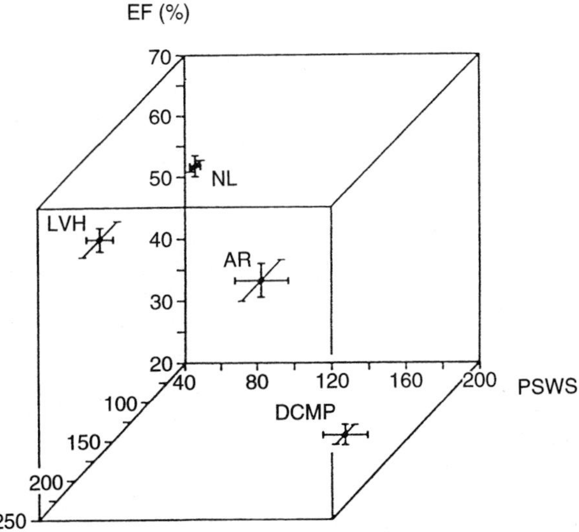

FIGURE 50–13. Three-coordinate plot of ejection fraction, left ventricular mass, and wall stress, determined from MRI data in patients with a variety of cardiac pathologies. EF = left ventricular ejection fraction; LV mass = left ventricular mass; PSWS = peak left ventricular wall stress; NL = normal; LVH = left ventricular hypertrophy; AR = severe aortic regurgitation; DCMP = dilated cardiomyopathy. (Modified from Higgins, C.B., Caputo, G., Wendland, M.F., et al.: Measurement of blood flow and perfusion in the cardiovascular system. Invest. Radiol. 27:S66, 1992, with permission.)

Wall Velocity Mapping

Myocardial tagging has three important limitations. First, because it uses presaturation, it reduces the signal in the image. This problem becomes more and more severe as the number of tagging lines is increased, placing a practical limit on the smallest piece of myocardial tissue that can be tracked. Second, the tags fade over the cardiac cycle because of the return of the tagged regions to equilibrium. With present techniques the practical limit for tracking the tags is 350 to 400 msec, limiting the portion of the cardiac cycle that can be examined with a single tag. Third, manual tracking of all of the tag lines is extremely time consuming, limiting the clinical use of the technique.

Recently, measuring myocardial wall velocity has been suggested as a means of addressing these problems.[119] MR images can be constructed from the phase of the received signal, as opposed to the signal magnitude (as with most magnetic resonance images). Such phase images can be made to be sensitive to velocity, so that the intensity of any resultant image point is proportional to the velocity of the structure at that point. The velocity of solid objects, including myocardial tissue, can be measured throughout the cardiac cycle, and the trajectory of small regions of myocardium can be calculated. This method is attractive because it has the potential to provide information on each point in the wall, to maintain signal, to be applied to the entire cardiac cycle, and to simplify the process of analysis of myocardial function.

There are two major limitations of this technique. First, it fundamentally measures wall velocity. Changes of the position or displacement of a point in the myocardial wall must be calculated by multiplying the velocity at that point by time. Thus, the accuracy of that calculated displacement is limited by the accuracy of the velocity measurement. Further, this error tends to accumulate over the course of the cardiac cycle. Second, this approach typically measures the velocity along a single axis, so measuring velocity in two or three dimensions requires multiple acquisitions, prolonging scan time. Although myocardial wall velocity mapping has not been used as extensively as myocardial tagging, regional inhomogeneities in left ventricular systolic and diastolic function have been demonstrated with this technique in healthy subjects[120] and in patients with hypertrophic cardiomyopathy.[121]

FLOW QUANTITATION

Basic Approaches

As described in Chapter 48, two methods are used to measure blood flow in the cardiovascular system: time-of-flight and phase-contrast (Fig. 50–14). In time-of-flight, radiofrequency pulses are used to "label" localized volumes of blood, which then can be tracked over time.[122–125] The principal advantage of this technique is that velocity measurements are straightforward (distance/time calculations). However, a contiguous and preferably straight segment of vessel is required to make the measurement. Other factors that affect signal amplitude can alter the measurement; it is difficult to assess velocity profiles, particularly in small vessels, and turbulent nonlaminar flow cannot be measured accurately.[126]

The phase-contrast technique measures the phase shifts that accumulate as hydrogen nuclei move through a magnetic field gradient.[127, 128] Typically, two scans are acquired when one performs velocity-encoded, phase-contrast MRI. In the first acquisition, the magnetic field gradients are adjusted so that there is no net phase change in the magnetic resonance signal because of flow (first-order, motion-compensated). In the second acquisition (velocity-sensitized scan), the gradient fields produce a phase change that has been calibrated to encode for a specific range of flow velocities. Velocity is calculated from the phase-contrast images by voxel-to-voxel subtraction of the velocity-sensitized and motion-compensated phase images and application of a correction algorithm designed to remove background phase error.[129]

The phase-contrast technique does not depend on the analysis of signal amplitude, such as that found with time-of-flight measurements, and bidirectional flows can be calculated.[130, 131] However, there are several disadvantages of the phase-contrast technique. First, one must encode a velocity range to include the peak velocities being sampled. Second, the vessel of interest must be properly aligned within the slice to avoid partial volume effects, because when the voxel length:vessel radius is less than 0.5, greater than 10 percent errors in flow measurements occur.[132] Third, a minimum of 8 to 12 voxels must be sampled within the vessel lumen to obtain accurate measurements.[133] Adequate spatial resolution may be difficult to accomplish in small-diameter vessels in which signal noise is limited. Fourth, two sequences are required, creating a potential for misregistration. Fifth, proper subtraction algorithms must be in place for good background correction to be performed. Sixth, precise gating is required for nonconstant pulsatile flow, so as to avoid artifacts caused by high orders of motion in the phase-encoding direction.[134]

Cardiac Output and Shunts

In three studies of normal volunteers, time-of-flight and phase-contrast MRI measurements of forward output in the proximal pulmonary artery and aorta in humans correlated well with pulsed Doppler ultrasound measurements (r = .86 to .98).[135–137] In addition, stroke volumes derived from phase-contrast flow measurements correlated well (r = .96 to .98) with stroke volume calculated from MRI multislice short-axis acquisitions of the left ventricle.[138, 139] In 18 patients referred for hemodynamic evaluation, cardiac output evaluated with MRI correlated well with Fick and thermodilution measurements made within 2 hours of the MRI study (Fig. 50–15).[140]

The ability to determine flow direction with flow direction with phase-contrast MRI can be useful in determining the entry and exit sites of flow within true and false channels in aortic dissection.[141] In six patients with type B aortic dissection, velocity mapping across the aortic lumen showed average spatial and temporal velocities of 13.4 ± 1.5 cm per second in the true channel and 3.1 ± 0.8 cm per second in the false channel ($P < .05$).[142]

In addition to determining cardiac output, MRI can detect differences in pulmonary and systemic flow in patients with left-to-right intracardiac shunting. Evans and co-workers found an average of 5 percent difference between measurements of flow in the aorta and pulmonary artery in 10 volunteers without intracardiac shunting.[143] In nine patients with large ostium secundum defects, MRI determinations of pulmonary-to-systemic flow ratios (Qp/Qs) correlated with oximetric determinations of Qp/Qs (r = .93).[144] Sieverding and colleagues measured Qp/Qs ratios in six children with phase-contrast MRI measurements of flow in the aorta and pulmonary artery, with gradient-echo stroke volume determinations in the right and left ventricles, and with oximetry during catheterization.[145] In all subjects MRI phase-contrast measurements of flow correlated with MRI volumetric assessments of cardiac output (r = .98), and in five of the children phase-contrast Qp/Qs measurements correlated well with those made by oximetry (r = .98). Hundley and associates measured Qp/Qs with MRI and within 2 hours with oximetry and indocyanine green in a prospective evaluation of 21 adults with and without intracardiac shunts of varying size and location.[146] Compared to invasive measurements, MRI accurately determined the magnitude of intracardiac left-to-right shunting (r = .94) and, importantly, discriminated which patients to consider for surgical correction of their intracardiac communication (Qp/Qs > 1.5) from those who could be managed medically (Qp/Qs ≤ 1.5) (Fig. 50–16).

Regurgitant Lesions

Turbulent flow associated with regurgitant lesions (likely due to intravoxel dephasing of spins with subsequent cancellation of net

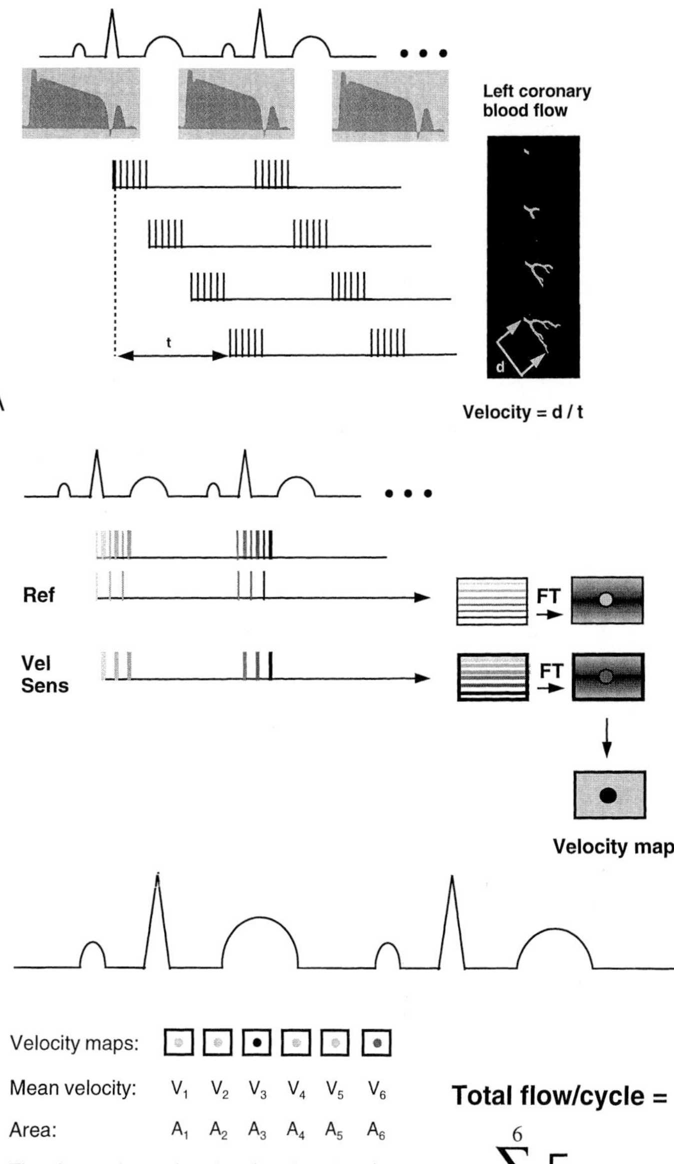

FIGURE 50–14. Illustration of time-of-flight and phase-contrast flow approaches. *Panel A,* Basic concept in time-of-flight measurement of flow. A tag or other presaturating pulse is applied at the beginning of QRS, as indicated by the heavy bar. The blood is allowed to flow with an image obtained at time t after the original tag. The distance d that the blood moves during time t can be used to calculate the average velocity. The limitations of this approach are discussed in the text. *Panel B,* Basic concept of phase-contrast flow measurement. Images are obtained with a reference sequence and one that is sensitized to motion. Subtracting these two images yields a velocity map. In the example shown here, the acquisitions of the reference and sensitized images are interleaved with the use of a phase-encoding grouping technique to decrease the total scan time. *Panel C,* Method for determining total vessel flow with velocity maps. The mean velocity for the vessel for each frame is multiplied by the area of the vessel in that frame to determine the volume flow per interval, which is then summed over the cardiac cycle to calculate the rate of flow per cycle.

signal)[147] causes signal voids on gradient echo images of the heart and therefore, allows detection of regurgitant lesions with sensitivity and specificity similar to those of Doppler echocardiography.[148, 149] The size of these signal voids correlates generally with color Doppler jet size.[150] However, measurement of regurgitation by the signal-void size appears to suffer from factors similar to those that limit quantitative use of color Doppler jets (substantial dependence on instrument type and settings, chamber wall effects, entrainment of nonregurgitant blood into jets, and nonlinear and complex relationships among jet size, regurgitant volume, and regurgitant orifice size). In addition, changes in TE, the degree of motion compensation, and orientation of the imaging plane relative to the regurgitant jet can alter the dimensions of the signal void.[151] Thus, accurate quantitation of valvular regurgitation is unlikely with this method.

To quantitate regurgitant volume, three approaches can be used. First, the difference in right and left ventricular stroke volumes in patients with isolated regurgitant lesions can be calculated.[152] For a single regurgitant valve, regurgitant volume and fraction can be derived by comparison of right and left ventricular stroke volumes by MRI.[153, 154] Although this has been shown to be accurate, long acquisition and analysis times complicate its general clinical use. In addition, multiple regurgitant lesions pose a problem for this method, as they do for assessment of regurgitant fraction by radionuclide, angiographic, or Doppler echocardiographic techniques. Second, the size and persistence of the proximal signal loss zone associated with convergence as flow accelerates proximal to the regurgitant orifice can separate grades of aortic regurgitation.[155] Although this technique has been shown to estimate regurgitant flow in phantom models, its use in patients has yet to be proved.

Third, regurgitant flow can be measured directly, measuring reverse flow across a valvular orifice, or indirectly, subtracting forward stroke flow from total stroke flow.[156] In patients with aortic regurgitation, estimates of regurgitant volume derived from phase-contrast sequences placed across the proximal aorta correlate (r = .8 to .9) with angiographic grades of aortic regurgitation.[157, 158] Similarly, in 19 patients with isolated mitral regurgitation, the severity of mitral regurgitation as determined by regurgitant fraction correlated (r = .87) with mild, moderate, and severe estimates of mitral regurgitation, as assessed by color Doppler echocardiography.[159]

Recent results directly comparing catheterization and magnetic

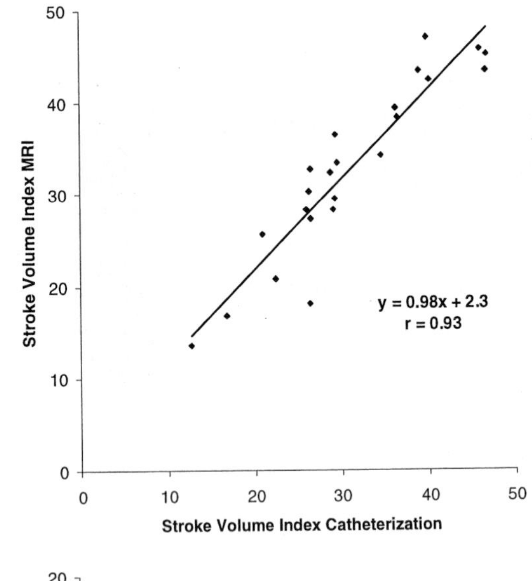

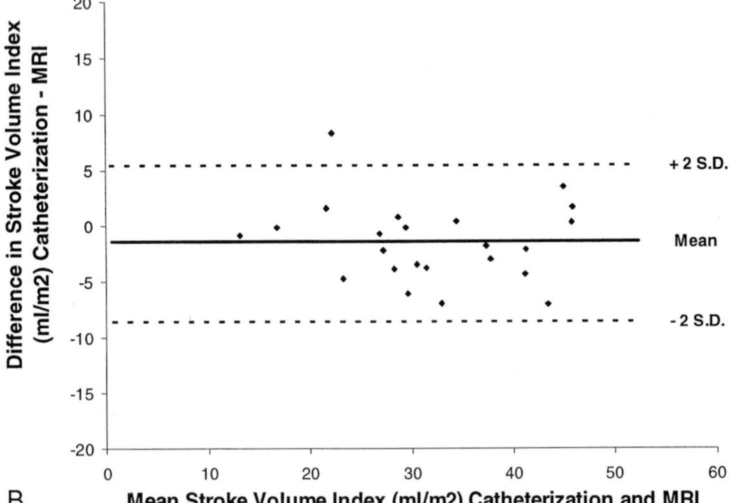

FIGURE 50–15. Comparison of stroke-volume index by phase-contrast velocity mapping MRI and catheterizaton. *Panel A,* Linear regression analysis, demonstrating an excellent correlation between stroke-volume index as measured by MRI and at catheterization. The slope of the line is essentially one with an intercept near zero. *Panel B,* Bland-Altman difference analysis comparing the difference in stroke-volume index by MRI and catheterization with the mean stroke-volume index from both techniques. Note that the dashed lines indicate two standard deviations on either side of the mean. This implies that 95 percent of the time the two measurements will be within this range of each other. In addition, the difference does not appear to increase with increasing stroke volumes. (From Hundley, W.G., Li, H.F., Hillis, L.D., et al.: Quantitation of cardiac output with velocity-encoded, phase-difference magnetic resonance imaging: Validation with invasive measurements. Am. J. Cardiol. 75:1250–1255, 1995, with permission.)

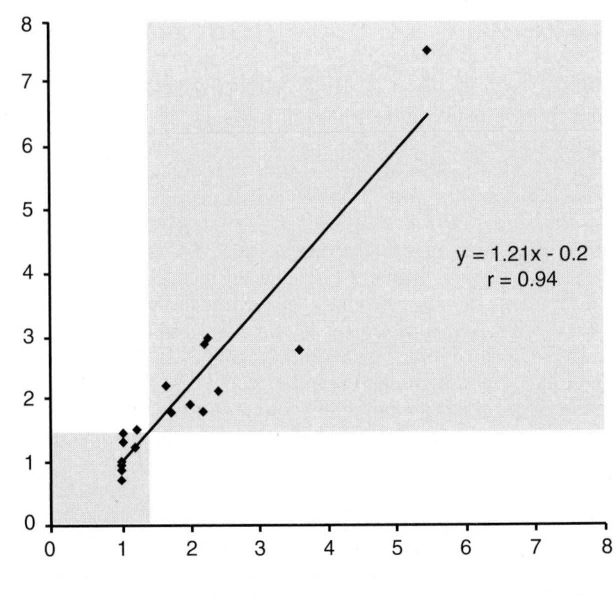

FIGURE 50–16. Comparison of Qp/Qs determined with phase-contrast MRI versus catheterization. Note that MRI was as effective as catheterization in distinguishing patients with significant shunts (Qp/Qs ≥ 1.5, shaded upper right-hand region) from those with insignificant shunts (Qp/Qs < 1.5, shaded lower left-hand corner). (Redrawn from Hundley, W.G., Li, H.F., Landau, C., et al.: Assessment of left-to-right intracardiac shunting by velocity-encoded, phase-difference magnetic resonance imaging: A comparison with oximetric and indicator dilution techniques. Circulation 91:2955–2960, 1995, with permission. Copyright 1995, American Heart Association.)

resonance flow quantitation indicate that they are comparable in determining regurgitant fraction (Fig. 50–17).[160, 161] In patients with regurgitant lesions, MRI can noninvasively detect the lesion, potentially quantitate regurgitant volume and fraction, and provide accurate assessments of end-diastolic and end-systolic volumes and thus of the hemodynamic consequences of valvular lesions on the ventricle.

Valvular Stenosis

Evaluation of patients with stenotic valvular lesions by MRI is similar to evaluation of such patients with echocardiography in that the pressure gradient across the valve is estimated with the modified Bernoulli equation, and the functional cross-sectional area imposed by the stenotic lesion is estimated with the continuity equation. Velocity-encoded MRI offers potential advantages in that (1) there are no limitations on pulse repetition frequency that limit maximum velocity measurements by ultrasound in deep structures and (2) MRI can potentially measure the true velocity vector by measuring the velocity along the three orthogonal axes, eliminating concerns about the true direction of the jet, as occurs with ultrasound. Unfortunately, up to this point these advantages have not been fully realized.

Signal voids occurring around areas of turbulent flow complicate estimates of transvalvular velocities with phase-contrast, velocity-encoded acquisitions that incorporate TE $\geq$ 10 msec.[162, 163] In two series of small numbers of patients, pressure gradients across mitral and aortic valves with marked stenoses correlated (r = .96 to .97) with catheterization and echocardiographic estimates of pressure gradient.[164] Determinations of valve area with MRI have been reported in 12 patients.[165] In this study MRI overestimated valve area compared to catheterization and underestimated valve area compared to Doppler echocardiography.

Several problems persist when one measures valve area or estimates pressure gradient with MRI. First, proper alignment of the velocity-encoded slice perpendicular to the direction of flow is difficult, especially in patients with eccentric jets, which can lead to flow artifacts that introduce errors in the velocity measurements. Second, positioning the velocity-encoded slice in relation to the site of stenosis is also difficult. When the slice is too far distal to the stenosis, spin incoherence and signal loss occur with increasing degrees of turbulence, whereas when the slice is too close to the stenotic valve, the leaflets move in and out of the imaging slice and interfere with the velocity profile. Third, acquisition and processing time has been long (45 to 80 minutes). The potential solutions to these problems include real-time, interactive positioning of the slices, rapid measurement of true vectoral velocity, and development of automated methods for processing and analyzing acquired data.[166]

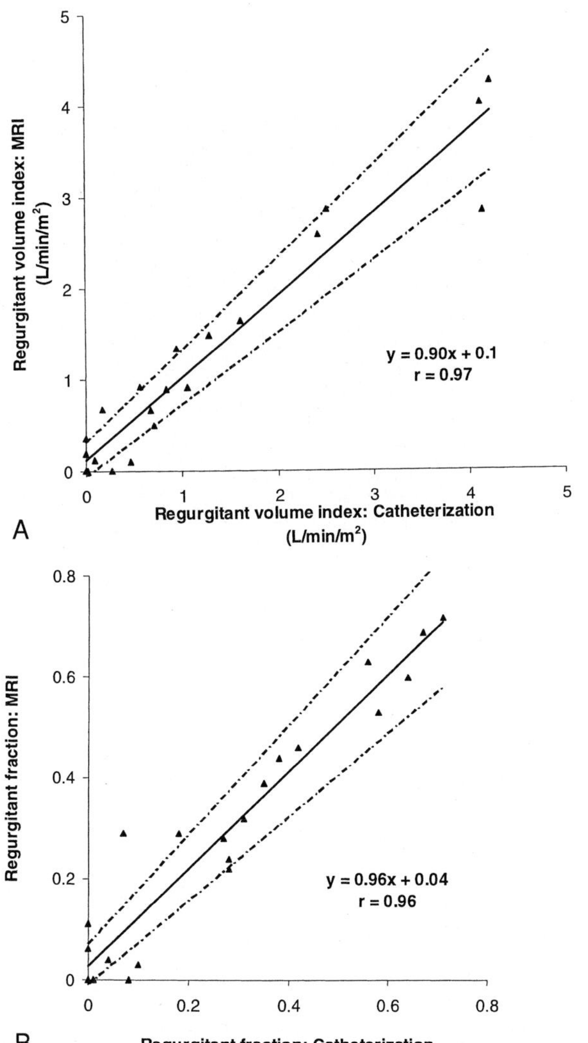

FIGURE 50–17. Comparison of MRI and catheterization in the assessment of regurgitant volume index and regurgitant fraction in patients with mitral regurgitation. *Panel A,* Linear regression analysis for the regurgitant volume index. The line of regression is indicated by the solid line, while the dashed lines indicate the 95 percent confidence limits. *Panel B,* Linear regression analysis for regurgitant fraction. The line of regression is indicated by the solid line, while the dashed lines indicate the 95 percent confidence limits. (From Hundley, W.G., Li, H.F., Willard, J.E., et al.: Magnetic resonance imaging of the severity of mitral regurgitation: A comparison with invasive techniques. Circulation 92:1151, 1995, with permission. Copyright 1995, American Heart Association.)

Right and Left Ventricular Inflow

MRI measurements of mitral inflow have been shown to correlate with Doppler echocardiographic measurements of E:A ratio in normal volunteers and those with evidence of mitral stenosis (r = .67 to .94).[167, 168] In an analysis of 10 normal volunteers and 5 patients with mitral stenosis, the contour of the peak velocities across the mitral valve was elevated continuously throughout diastole in the patients with mitral stenosis, whereas two distinct peaks were noted in the normal volunteers.[169] In patients with constrictive or restrictive heart disease, abnormal right ventricular inflow has been demonstrated with echocardiography. In 10 normal volunteers, phase-shift, velocity-encoded MRI correlated well with peak E- and A-wave velocities obtained with Doppler echocardiography.[170] In future studies these flow measurements may be combined with myocardial tagging studies of the ventricular chambers to provide insight into the mechanisms of disease processes that affect the diastolic phases of ventricular relaxation.

Coronary Flow and Flow Reserve

Time-of-flight MR coronary angiography can noninvasively visualize flow in the coronary arteries without the injection of contrast materials.[171] The sensitivity and specificity of MRI coronary angiography for correctly identifying stenosis of 50 percent or more were 90 and 92 percent, respectively, in a prospective study of 39 patients referred for cardiac catheterization and coronary angiography.[172] In 20 patients referred for catheterization after coronary artery bypass grafting, MRI was able to detect the presence or absence of flow with a sensitivity of 88 percent and a specificity of 100 percent.[173] In 18 patients consecutively referred for coronary angiography after sustaining a myocardial infarction, MRI correctly identified the presence or absence of antegrade flow in the infarct-related artery in all patients.[174]

Phase-contrast methods have been used to measure velocity and flow in coronary vessels in animal models and humans. Clarke and

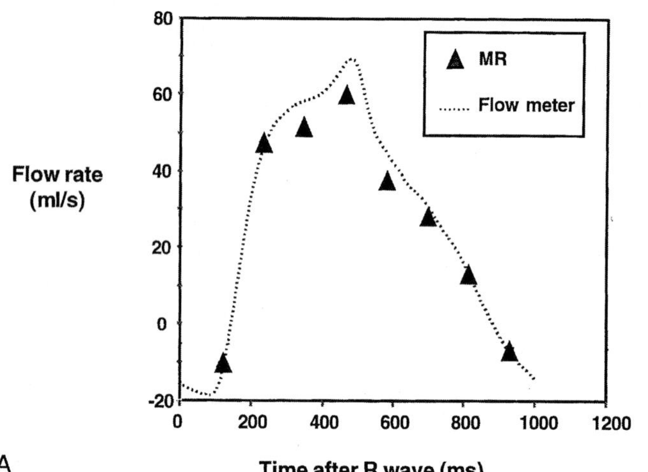

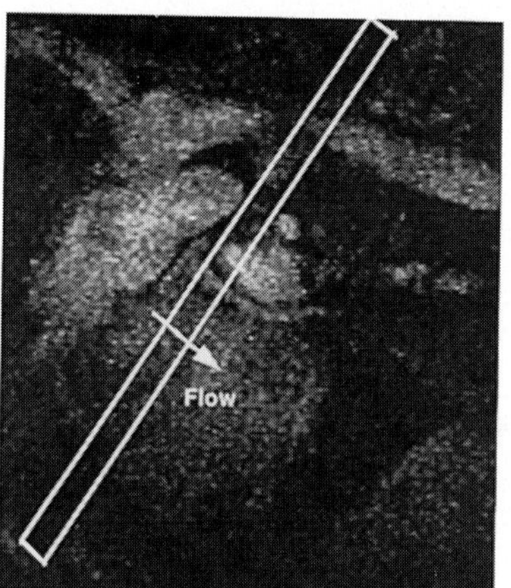

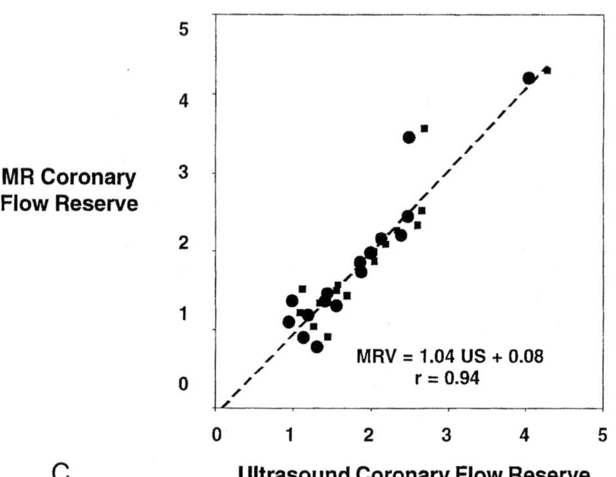

FIGURE 50–18. Comparison of MRI and ultrasonic flow probe in assessing coronary artery flow and flow reserve. *Panel A,* Comparison of pulsatile flow waveform determined with cine MR flow mapping and a perivascular transit time ultrasound probe. There is an excellent correlation between the measurements made with MR and those from ultrasound. *Panel B,* Positioning of the imaging plane for determination of circumflex coronary artery flow in an animal model. The left anterior descending artery is seen curving in the anterior interventricular groove. *Panel C,* Linear regression analysis of coronary flow reserve in response to dipyridamole in an instrumented animal model of partial coronary occlusion. There is an excellent correlation in the flow reserve, as assessed by transit time ultrasonic probe and MRI. (*A* from Li, W.H., Clarke, G.D., Liu, H., et al.: MRI k-space segmentation using phase-encoding groups: The accuracy of quantitative measurements of pulsatile flow. Med. Phys. 22:391–399, 1995; and *B* and *C* from Clarke, G.D., Eckels, R., Chaney, C. et al.: Measurement of absolute epicardial coronary artery flow and flow reserve using breath-hold cine phase contrast magnetic resonance imaging. Circulation 91:2627–2634, 1995, with permission. Copyright 1995, American Heart Association.)

colleagues used phase-contrast MRI to quantitate coronary flow and flow reserve in stenosed and normal coronary arteries in a closed-chest animal model.[175] Measurements of coronary flow and flow reserve correlated well (r = .96 and .94, respectively) with measurements made by perivascular ultrasound flow probes (Fig. 50–18). In humans, coronary velocity reserve has been measured in four subjects after infusion of intravenous adenosine.[176] In these four normal subjects, coronary velocity reserve was shown to increase by a factor of 4 during infusion. Debatin and associates measured internal mammary artery blood flow and velocity in 10 volunteers and 15 patients after bypass grafting.[177] The results suggest that the technique is feasible, but the measurements were not confirmed with invasive techniques. Although obstacles regarding technique must still be overcome, phase-contrast MRI may offer the first method of noninvasively measuring coronary flow and flow reserve in humans.

AUTOMATED ANALYSIS

Basic Approaches

As described previously, although it is well established that MRI can provide accurate measures of chamber volumes, segmental function, and flow, the routine clinical use of these methods has been limited because of, at least in part, the time required for data analysis. It is not unusual to obtain a magnetic resonance dataset for Simpson-rule determination of volume that consists of 8 to 10 slices obtained at 12 or more points in the cardiac cycle, resulting in more than 100 images for review and analysis. Thus, automated methods for data analysis must be developed for these studies to be clinically useful.

The task of automated processing of cardiac magnetic resonance images always revolves around automated image segmentation techniques, which view every point in the image as a measurement vector constructed of many local or region-related properties of that point. These local properties of various points in the image, often referred to as features, are used by the segmentation algorithm to cluster points in the image according to selected criteria that serve as a measure of similarity among the points that belong to the same physical organ.

Because of the astronomically high number of possible groupings that would have to be considered to find M objects contained within an image made of N points,[178] the realistic segmentation algorithm attempts to find a balance between processing speed and the reliability of results. This balance is achieved by taking advantage of the image context to introduce constraints resulting from spatial distribution of the candidate points or by using information about the local properties of the immediate neighborhoods of these points. Among the local regional properties, the gradients in local image intensity and the assessment of the textural properties of the region are the most frequently used vehicles for the segmentation of cardiac magnetic resonance images.

The evaluation of local intensity gradients in the image results in delineation of natural boundaries between different parts of the cardiac anatomy. Regional image filters may be designed in such a way that the presence of a transition from one image intensity to another results in high local intensity of the filtered image. Many particular edge-detection operators can be used for this purpose[179] (Laplace, Roberts, Sobel, Chen, and others), but without exception, all these methods produce a large number of false edges, which can be attributed to the presence of factors such as noise, motion artifacts, and tissue inhomogeneity. Therefore, a significant computational effort must be made to eliminate the unwanted edges and to ensure that the genuine edges and their continuity are preserved. The algorithms involved at this stage include various forms of digital erosion and thresholding. The erosion uses geometrically structured elements for morphologic elimination of the edges that do not possess suitable connectivity, span, curvature, or directionality. Thresholding operation removes edges that are poorly defined or exhibit inadequate change in the regional image intensity. Combined, edge thresholding and digital erosion reduce the incidence of false edges in the processed image and improve the overall delineation of the anatomy of interest. Once the cardiac anatomy is delineated, boundary closure algorithms are applied, which attempt to restore broken boundaries left by the previously described steps of the image segmentation process. The boundary closure can be accomplished either interactively, under operator supervision, or by an iterative process that uses geometric models of the segmented anatomy for finding the most probable position of the missing edges or relies on some form of continuity criteria for the completion of the detected edges.[180, 181]

An alternative method of image segmentation is based on exploiting differences in tissue intensity and texture. Statistical information, such as average intensity, standard deviation, and higher order statistical moments, are gathered for the small regions of the image.[182] These samples are then used to define the characteristics of each tissue of interest. Statistical information for each point in the image is then calculated and compared to the characteristics of the reference samples. In this way, points are classified on the basis of their degree of similarity to the reference regions. Although this method is attractive, it tends to be computationally intensive, is sensitive to small changes in image-acquisition parameters, and generally requires user definition of the characteristic regions.

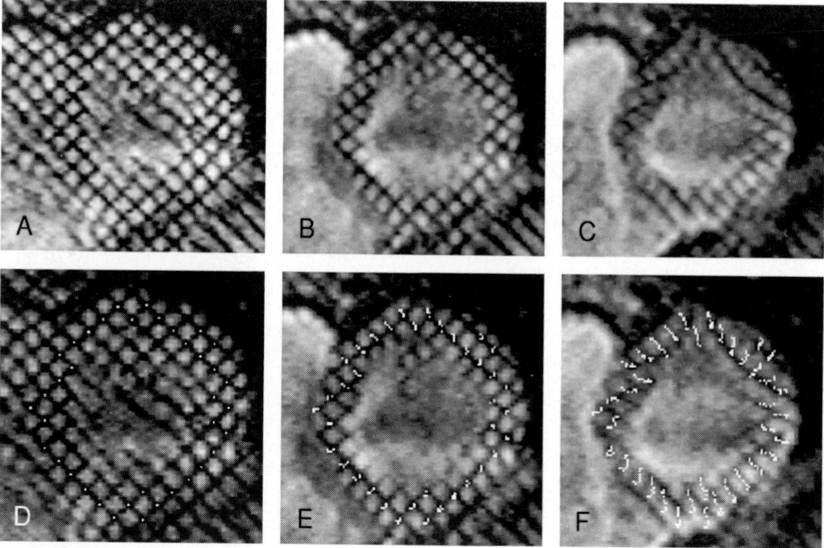

FIGURE 50–19. Automated tracking of myocardial tags. *Panels A, B, and C,* Short-axis images through the midventricle with grid tagging. Image A is at early systole, B is at midsystole, and C is at end-systole. The motion of the intersection of the tag points is apparent. *Panels D, E, and F,* The same short-axis images, with automated identification of the intersection points. Images E and F demonstrate the trace or path of motion of each intersection point during systole.

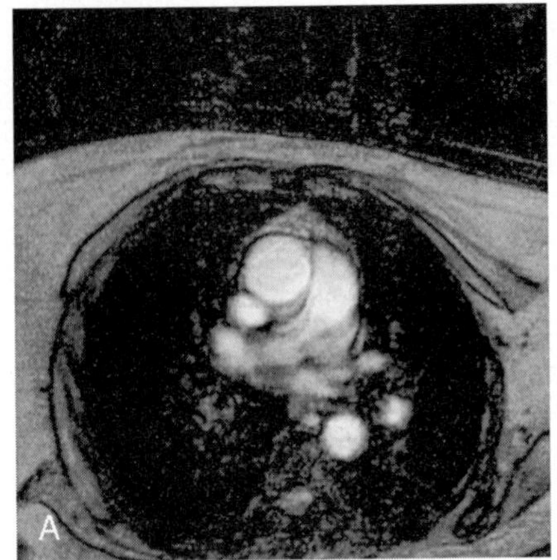

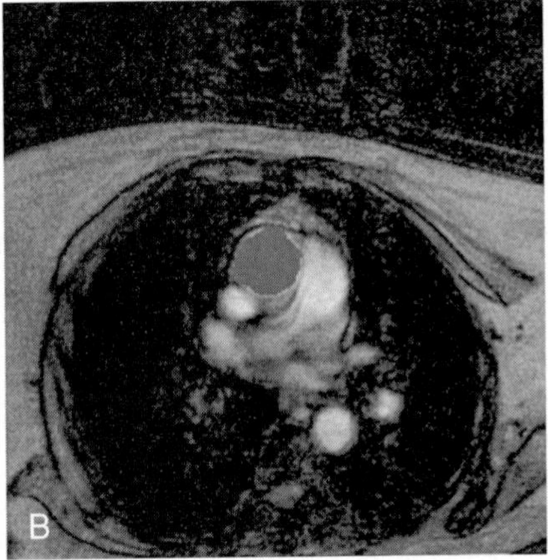

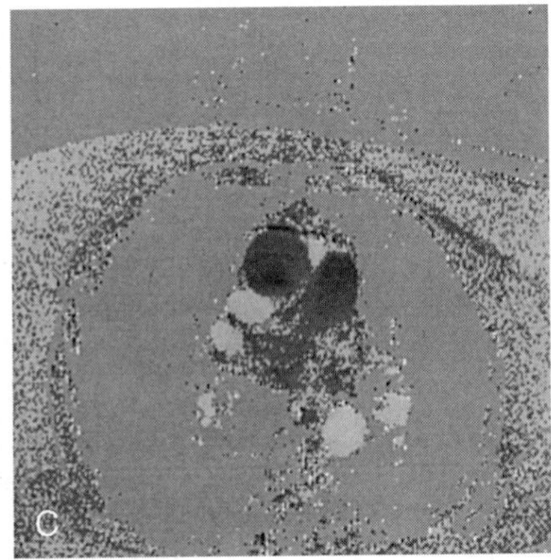

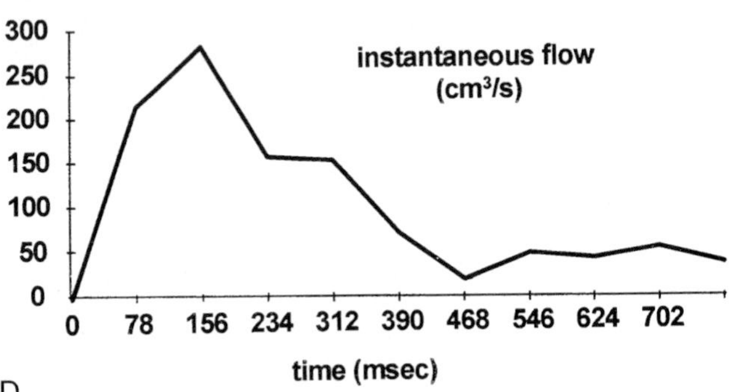

Time	Measured Velocity	Flow	Summary
78 ms	21.64 cm/s	215.67 cm^3/s	
156 ms	27.69 cm/s	282.74 cm^3/s	
234 ms	15.13 cm/s	157.37 cm^3/s	
312 ms	13.96 cm/s	152.29 cm^3/s	
390 ms	6.74 cm/s	70.51 cm^3/s	
468 ms	1.74 cm/s	17.98 cm^3/s	
546 ms	4.32 cm/s	46.87 cm^3/s	*Stroke Volume:*
624 ms	3.79 cm/s	40.45 cm^3/s	91.55 cm^3
702 ms	4.93 cm/s	52.17 cm^3/s	*Cardiac Output:*
1017 ms	3.35 cm/s	34.09 cm^3/s	5.401 L/min

E

FIGURE 50–20. Automated flow determination. *Panel A,* Transaxial magnitude image at the level of the ascending aorta. *Panel B,* Automated identification of the location and cross section of the ascending aorta. *Panel C,* Velocity map at the same level. *Panel D,* Automated graph of the ascending aortic flow over the cardiac cycle. *Panel E,* Automated determination of phasic flow and cardiac output.

Specific Applications

Fortunately, the high contrast available in MR images and their high reproducibility make automated processing feasible. Recently, Baldy and co-workers demonstrated good correlation between automated methods based on edge tracking and human measures of both ventricular volume and myocardial mass.[183] Fleagle and colleagues have reported the results of a multicenter trial of automated border detection.[184] Despite differences in the image-acquisition protocols, MRI systems, and field strengths, there was excellent agreement between manual and computer-derived endocardial and epicardial areas (correlation coefficients, .94 to .99).

As shown in this chapter and others, myocardial tagging offers a unique method for precisely and consistently evaluating segmental ventricular function. Manual analysis of grid-tagged images is extremely time consuming, severely limiting its clinical applicability. Recently, several groups have described computer-assisted or fully automated methods for analysis of tagged images (Fig. 50–19).[185]

Automated methods have also been applied to the problem of measuring flow.[186] The results of these studies suggest that the automated methods have less variability than manual measurements and may improve the precision of flow measurements. The initial results obtained with the use of a wavelet transform method for detecting the edge of the aorta and pulmonary artery for automated determination of cardiac output have been quite encouraging, demonstrating excellent correlation with manual measurements and a dramatic reduction in image-analysis time (Fig. 50–20).[187]

SUMMARY

MRI is well suited to cardiac quantitation because of its high contrast, its high spatial and temporal resolution, and its flexibility. There is now a well-established body of evidence that it is accurate, highly reproducible, and feasible, with the use of equipment available in most hospitals. In the areas of determination of myocardial mass, evaluation of right ventricular function, and quantitative measurements of flow in the great vessels and peripheral vasculature, there is growing evidence that MRI is, in fact, the reference method. With continuing improvements in imaging speed and automated quantitation, it appears that the role of MRI in characterizing cardiovascular structure and function will continue to grow.

References

1. Fisher, M.R., von Schulthess, G.K., and Higgins, C.B.: Multiphasic cardiac magnetic resonance imaging: Normal regional left ventricular wall thickening. AJR 145:27, 1985.
2. Caputo, G.R., Suzuki, J-I., Kondo, C., et al.: Determination of left ventricular volume and mass using biphasic spin-echo MR imaging: Comparison with cine MR. Radiology 177:773, 1990.
3. Forbat, S.M., Karwatowski, S.P., Gatehouse, P.D., et al.: Technical note: Rapid measurement of left ventricular mass by spin echo magnetic resonance imaging. Br. J. Radiol. 67:86, 1994.
4. Wagner, S., Buser, P., Auffermann, W., et al.: Cine magnetic resonance imaging: Tomographic analysis of left ventricular function. Cardiol. Clin. 7:651, 1989.
5. NessAvier, M.: Breathhold cines using phase encoding grouping. *In* Pohost, G.M. (ed.): Cardiovascular Applications of Magnetic Resonance. Mt. Kisco, NY, Futura, 1993, p. 133.
6. Pykett, I.L., and Rzedzian, R.R.: Instant images of the body by magnetic resonance. Magn. Reson. Med. 5:563, 1987.
7. Hunter, G.: Measurement of stroke volume and cardiac output within a single breath hold with echo-planar MR imaging. J. Magn. Reson. Imaging 4:51, 1994.
8. Rapid Dynamic Cardiac Imaging (SMR Poster No. 505, Debatin, J.F., Leung, D.A., Unterweger, M., et al.: Cardiac ejection fraction: comparison of echo planar and conventional cine MRI; and SM Poster No. 506, Leung, D.A. et al.: Cardiac imaging: Comparison of 2 Shot EPI with segmented k-space and conventional cine acquisitions). Milwaukee, General Electric Medical Systems HiSpeed Imaging, New Applications, August 1994.
9. Constable, R.T., and Henkelman, R.M.: Contrast, resolution, and detectability in MR imaging. J. Comput. Assist. Tomogr. 15(2):297, 1991.
10. Hoffman, E.A., and Ritman, E.L.: Shape and dimensions of cardiac chambers: Importance of CT section thickness and orientation. Radiology 155:739, 1985.

11. Harris, L.D.: Identification of the optimal orientation of oblique sections through multiple parallel CT image. J. Comput. Assist. Tomogr. 5:881, 1981.
12. Maddahi, J., Crues, J., Berman, D.S., et al.: Non invasive quantitation of left ventricular mass by gated proton magnetic resonance imaging. J. Am. Coll. Cardiol. 10:682, 1987.
13. Hunter, G.J., Hamberg, L.M., Weisskoff, R.M., et al.: Measurement of stroke volume and cardiac output within a single breathhold with echo-planar imaging. J. Magn. Reson. Imaging 4(1):51, 1994.
14. Haraldseth, O.: Early detection of regional myocardial ischemia in ex vivo piglet hearts: MR imaging with magnetization transfer. J. Magn. Reson. Imaging 4:603, 1994.
15. Wolff, S.D.: Magnetization transfer imaging: Practical aspects and clinical applications. Radiology 192:593, 1994.
16. Dimick, R.N., Hedlund, L.W., Herfkens, R.J., et al.: Optimizing electrocardiograph electrode placement for cardiac-gated magnetic resonance imaging. Invest. Radiol. 22:17, 1987.
17. Axel, L., Summers, R.M., Kressel, H.Y., et al.: Respiratory effect in two-dimensional Fourier transform MR imaging. Radiology 160:795, 1986.
18. Bailes, D.R., Gilderdale, D.J., Bydder, G.M., et al.: Respiratory ordered phase encoding (ROPE): A method for reducing respiratory motion artifacts in MR imaging. J. Comput. Assist. Tomogr. 9:835, 1985.
19. NessAvier, M.: Breathhold cines using phase encoding grouping. *In* Pohost, G.M. (ed.): Cardiovascular Applications of Magnetic Resonance. Mt. Kisco, NY, Futura, 1993, p. 133.
20. Gay, S.B., Sistrom, C.L., Holder, C.A., et al.: Breath-holding capability of adults: Implications for spiral computed tomography, fast-acquisition magnetic resonance imaging, and angiography. Invest. Radiol. 29:848, 1994.
21. Haacke, E.M., Liang, Z.P., and Boada, F.: Image reconstruction using projection onto convex sets, model constraints, and linear prediction theory for the removal of phase, motion, and Gibbs artifacts in magnetic resonance and ultrasound imaging. Optical Eng. May 29(5):555, 1990.
22. Brown, J.J., Barakos, J.A., and Higgins, C.B.: Magnetic resonance imaging of cardiac and paracardiac masses. J. Thorac. Imaging 4(2):58, 1989.
23. Bland, J.M., and Altman, D.G.: Statistical methods for assessing agreement between two methods of clinical measurement. Lancet 307, 1986.
24. Hillis, L.D., Firth, B.G., and Winniford, M.D.: Comparison of thermodilution and indocyanine green dye in low cardiac output or left-sided regurgitation. Am. J. Cardiol. 57:1201, 1986.
25. Hillis, L.D., Firth, B.G., Winniford, M.D.: Analysis of factors affecting the variability of Fick versus indicator dilution measurements of cardiac output. Am. J. Cardiol. 56:764, 1985.
26. Brogan, W.C., Glamann, D.B., Lange, R.A., et al.: Comparison of single and biplane ventriculography for determination of left ventricular volume and ejection fraction. Am. J. Cardiol. 69:1079, 1992.
27. Hillis, L.D., Winniford, M.D., Dehmer, G.J., et al.: Left ventricular volumes by single-plane cineangiography: In vivo validation of the Kennedy regression equation. Am. J. Cardiol. 53:1159, 1984.
28. Higgins, C.B.: Which standard has the gold? (Editorial.) J. Am. Coll. Cardiol. 19:1608, 1992.
29. Jacicki, J.S., Weber, K.T., Gochman, R.F., et al.: Three-dimensional myocardial and ventricular shape: A surface representation. Am. J. Physiol. 10:H1, 1981.
30. Sandler, H.: Dimensional analysis of the heart: A review. Am. J. Med. Sci. 260:56, 1970.
31. Kaul, S., Wismer, G.L., Brady, T.J., et al.: Measurement of normal left heart dimensions using optimally oriented MR images. AJR 146:75, 1986.
32. Friedman, B.J., Waters, J., Kwan, O.L., et al.: Comparison of nuclear magnetic resonance imaging and echocardiography in determination of cardiac dimensions in normal subjects. J. Am. Coll. Cardiol. 5:1369, 1985.
33. Fisher, M.R., von Schulthess, G.K., and Higgins, C.B.: Multiphasic cardiac magnetic resonance imaging: Normal regional left ventricular wall thickening. AJR 145:27, 1985.
34. Byrd, F.B., Schiller, N.B., Botvinick, E.H., et al.: Normal cardiac dimensions by magnetic resonance imaging. Am. J. Cardiol. 55:1440, 1985.
35. Buser, P.T., Auffermann, W., Holt, W.W., et al.: Non invasive evaluation of the global left ventricular function using cine MR imaging. J. Am. Coll. Cardiol. 13:1294, 1989.
36. Longmore, D.B., Underwood, S.R., Hounsfield, G.N., et al.: Dimensional accuracy of magnetic resonance imaging in studies of the heart. Lancet i:1360, 1985.
37. Schaefer, S., Peshock, R.M., Malloy, C.R., et al.: Nuclear magnetic resonance imaging in Marfan's syndrome. J. Am. Coll. Cardiol. 9:70, 1987.
38. Semelka, R.C., Tomei, E., Wagner, S., et al.: Normal left ventricular dimensions and function: Interstudy reproducibility of measurements with cine MR imaging. Radiology 174:763, 1990.
39. Feiring, A.J., Rumberger, J.A., Reiter, S.J., et al.: Sectional and segmental variability of left ventricular function: Experimental and clinical studies using ultrafast computed tomography. J. Am. Coll. Cardiol. 12:415, 1988.
40. de Simone, G., Moccia, D., Buonissimo, S., et al.: Normal left ventricular quantitative analysis of physical and functional determinants of geometry and performance. Am. J. Noninvas. Cardiol. 2:217, 1988.
41. Borow, K.M., Green, L.H., Mann, T., et al.: End-systolic volume as a predictor of post operative left ventricular performance in volume overload from valvular regurgitation. Am. J. Med. 68:655, 1980.
42. White, H.D., Norris, R.M., Brown, M.A., et al.: Left ventricular end-systolic volume as a major determinant of survival after recovery from myocardial infarction. Circulation 76:44, 1987.
43. Rehr, R.B., Malloy, C.R., Filipchuk, N.G., et al.: Left ventricular volumes measured by MR imaging. Radiology 156:717, 1985.
44. Pattynama, P.M.T., de Roos, A., Van der Wall, E.E., et al.: Evaluation of cardiac function with magnetic resonance imaging. Am. Heart J. 128:595, 1994.
45. Just, H., Holubarsch, C., and Friedburg, H.: Estimation of left ventricular volume and mass by magnetic resonance imaging: Comparison with quantitative biplane angiography. Cardiovasc. Intervent. Radiol. 10:1, 1987.
46. MacMillan, R.M., Murphey, J.L., Kresh, J.Y., et al.: Left ventricular volumes using cine-MRI: Validation with catheterization ventriculography. Am. J. Cardiac. Imaging 4:79, 1990.
47. Semelka, R.C., Tomei, E., Wagner, S., et al.: Normal left ventricular dimensions and function: Interstudy reproducibility of measurements with cine MR imaging. Radiology 174:763, 1990.
48. Semelka, R.C., Tomei, E., Wagner, S., et al.: Interstudy reproducibility of dimensional and functional measurements between cine magnetic resonance studies in the morphologically abnormal left ventricle. Am. Heart J. 119:1367, 1990.
49. Pattynama, P.M.T., Lamb, H.J., van der Velde, E.A., et al.: Left ventricular measurements with cine and spin-echo MR imaging: A study of reproducibility with variance component analysis. Radiology 187:261, 1993.
50. Caputo, G.R., Suzuki, J.I., Kondo, C., et al.: Determination of left ventricular volume and mass with use of biphasic spin-echo MR imaging: Comparison with cine MR. Radiology 177:773, 1990.
51. Sakuma, H., Fujita, N., Foo, T.K., et al.: Evaluation of left ventricular volume and mass with breath-hold cine MR imaging. Radiology 188:377, 1993.
52. Sandler, H., and Dodge H.T.: The use of single plane angiocardiograms for the calculation of left ventricular volume in man. Am. Heart J. 75:325, 1968.
53. Dodge, H.T., Sandler H., Ballew, D.W., et al.: The use of biplane angiocardiography for the measurement of left ventricular volume in man. Am. Heart J. 60:762, 1960.
54. Underwood, S.R., Gill, C.R.W., Firmin, D.N., et al.: Left ventricular volume measured rapidly by oblique magnetic resonance imaging. Br. Heart J. 60:188, 1988.
55. Cranney, G.B., Lotan, C.S., Dean, L., et al.: Left ventricular volume measurement using cardiac axis nuclear magnetic resonance imaging: Validation by calibrated ventricular angiography. Circulation 82:154, 1990.
56. Dell'Italia, L.J., Blackwell, G.G., Pearce, W.J., et al.: Assessment of ventricular volumes using cine magnetic resonance in the intact dog: A comparison of measurement methods. Invest. Radiol. 2:162, 1994.
57. Dulce, M.C., Mostbeck, G.H., Friese, K.K., et al.: Quantification of the left ventricular volumes and function with cine MR imaging: Comparison of geometric models with three-dimensional data. Radiology 188:371, 1993.
58. Boxt, L.M., Katz, J., Kolb, T., et al.: Direct quantitation of right and left ventricular volumes with nuclear magnetic resonance imaging in patients with primary pulmonary hypertension. J. Am. Coll. Cardiol. 19:1508, 1992.
59. Järvinen, V.M., Kupari, M.M., Hekali, P.E., et al.: Right atrial MR imaging studies of cadaveric atrial casts and comparison with right and left atrial volumes and function in healthy subjects. Radiology 191:137, 1994.
60. Florentine, M.S., Grosskreutz, C.L., Chang, W., et al.: Measurement of left ventricular mass in vivo using gated nuclear magnetic resonance imaging. J. Am. Coll. Cardiol. 8:107, 1986.
61. Keller, A.M., Peschock, R.M., Malloy, C.R., et al.: In vivo measurement of myocardial mass using nuclear magnetic resonance imaging. J. Am. Coll. Cardiol. 8:113, 1986.
62. Maddahi, J., Crues, J., Berman, D.S., et al.: Noninvasive quantification of left ventricular myocardial mass by gated proton nuclear magnetic resonance imaging. J. Am. Coll. Cardiol. 10:682, 1987.
63. Manning, W.J., Wei, J.Y., Fossel, E.T., et al.: Measurement of left ventricular mass in rats using electrocardiogram-gated magnetic resonance imaging. Am. Physiol. Society 258:H:1181, 1990.
64. Shapiro, E.P., Rogers, W.J., Beyar, R., et al.: Determination of left ventricular mass by magnetic resonance imaging in hearts deformed by acute infarction. Circulation 79:706, 1989.
65. Devereux, R.B., and Reicheck, N.: Echocardiographic determination of left ventricular mass in man—anatomic validation of the method. Circulation 55:613, 1977.
66. Ostrzega, E., Maddahi, J., Honma, H., et al.: Quantification of left ventricular myocardial mass in humans by nuclear resonance imaging. Am. Heart J. 2:444, 1989.
67. Katz, J., Milliken, M.C., Stray-Gundersen, J., et al.: Estimation of human myocardial mass with MR imaging. Radiology 169:495. 1988.
68. Germain, P., Roul, G., Kastler, B., et al.: Inter-study variability in left ventricular mass measurement: Comparison between M-mode echocardiography and MRI. Eur. Heart J. 13:1011, 1992.
69. Milliken, M.C., Stray-Gunderson, J., Peshock, R.M., et al.: Left ventricular mass as determined by magnetic resonance imaging in male endurance athletes. Am. J. Cardiol. 62:301, 1988.
70. Eichstaedt, H., Danne, O., Langer, M., et al.: Regression of left ventricular hypertrophy under ramipril treatment by nuclear resonance imaging. J. Cardiovasc. Pharmacol. 13:S75, 1989.
71. Doherty, N.E., Seelos, K.C., Suzuki, J., et al.: Application of cine nuclear magnetic resonance imaging for sequential evaluation of response to angiotensin-converting enzyme inhibitor therapy in dilated cardiomyopathy. J. Am. Coll. Cardiol. 19:1294, 1992.
72. Allison, J.D., Flickinger, F.W., Wright, J.C., et al.: Measurement of left ventricular mass in hypertrophic cardiomyopathy using MRI: Comparison with echocardiography. Magn. Reson. Imaging 11:329, 1993.
73. Katz, J., Whang, J., Boxt, L.M., et al.: Estimation of right ventricular mass in normal subjects and in patients with primary pulmonary hypertension by nuclear magnetic resonance imaging. J. Am. Coll. Cardiol. 21:1475, 1993.

74. McDonald, K.M., Parrish, T., Wennberg, P., et al.: Rapid, accurate and simultaneous noninvasive assessment of right and left ventricular mass with nuclear magnetic resonance imaging using the snapshot gradient method. J. Am. Coll. Cardiol. 19:1601, 1992.
75. Sechtem, U., Plugfelder, P.W., Gould, R.G., et al.: Measurement of right and left ventricular volumes in healthy individuals with cine MR imaging. Radiology 163:697, 1987.
76. Benjelloun, H., Cranney, G.B., Kirk, K.A., et al.: Interstudy reproducibility of biplane cine nuclear magnetic resonance measurements of left ventricular function. Am. J. Cardiol. 67:1413, 1991.
77. Dulce, M.C., Mostbeck, G.H., Friese, K.K., et al.: Quantification of the left ventricular volumes and function with cine MR imaging: Comparison of geometric models with three-dimensional data. Radiology 188(2):371, 1993.
78. Utz, J.A., Herfkens, R.J., Heinsimer, J.A., et al.: Cine MR determination of left ventricular ejection fraction. AJR 148:839, 1987.
79. Culham, J.A.G., and Vince, D.J.: Cardiac output by MR imaging: An experimental study comparing right ventricle and left ventricle with thermodilution. J. Can. Assoc. Radiol. 39:247, 1988.
80. Hunter, G.J., Hamberg, L.M., Weisskoff, R.M., et al.: Measurement of stroke volume and cardiac output within a single breath hold with echo-planar MR imaging. J. Magn. Reson. Imaging 4:51, 1994.
81. Kondo, C., Caputo, G.R., Semelka, R., et al.: Right and left ventricular stroke volume measurements with velocity-encoded cine MR imaging: In vitro and in vivo validation. AJR 157:9, 1991.
82. Firmin, D.N., Nayler, G.L., Klipstein, R.H., et al.: In vivo validation of MR velocity imaging. J. Comput. Assist. Tomogr. 11:751, 1987.
83. Sarris, G.E., Cahill, P.D., Hansen, D.E., et al.: Restoration of left ventricular systolic performance after reattachment of the mitral chordae tendineae. J. Thorac. Cardiovasc. Surg. 95:969, 1988.
84. Zoghbi, W.A., Charlat, M.L., Bolli, R., et al.: Quantitative assessment of left ventricular wall motion by two-dimensional echocardiography: Validation during reversible ischemia in the conscious dog. J. Am. Coll. Cardiol. 11:851, 1988.
85. Feigenbaum, H.: Coronary artery disease. 5th ed. *In* Echocardiography, Philadelphia, Lea & Febiger, 1994, p. 447.
86. Lieberman, A.L., Weiss, J.L., Jugdutt, B.I., et al.: Two-dimensional echocardiography and infarct size: Relationship of regional wall motion and thickening to the extent of myocardial infarction in the dog. Circulation 63:739, 1981.
87. Hecschke, C.I., Risser, T.A., Sandor, T., et al.: Quantitative computer-assisted analysis of left ventricular wall thickening and motion by 2-dimensional echocardiography in acute myocardial infarction. Am. J. Cardiol. 52:960, 1983.
88. Tennant, R., and Wiggers, C.J.: The effect of coronary occlusion on myocardial contraction. Am. J. Physiol. 112:351, 1935.
89. Upton, M.T., Rerych, S.K., Newman, G.E., et al.: Detecting abnormalities in left ventricular function during exercise before angina and ST-segment depression. Circulation 62:341, 1980.
90. Sawada, S.G., Segar, D.S., Ryan, T., et al.: Echocardiographic detection of coronary artery disease during dobutamine infusion. Circulation 83:1605, 1991.
91. Smart, S.C., Sawada, S., Ryan, T., et al.: Low-dose dobutamine echocardiography detects reversible dysfunction after thrombolytic therapy of acute myocardial infarction. Circulation 88:405, 1993.
92. Cigarroa, C.G., deFilippi, C.R., Brickner, M.E., et al.: Dobutamine stress echocardiography identifies hibernating myocardium and predicts recovery of left ventricular function after coronary revascularization. Circulation 88:430, 1993.
93. Bourdillon, P.D.V., Broderick, T.M., Sawada, S.G., et al.: Regional wall motion index for infarct and noninfarct regions after reperfusion in acute myocardial infarction: Comparison with global wall motion index. J. Am. Soc. Echocardiogr. 2:398, 1989.
94. McGillem, M.J., Mancini, G.B.J., DeBoe, S.F., et al.: Modification of the centerline method for assessment of echocardiographic wall thickening and motion: A comparison with areas of risk. J. Am. Coll. Cardiol. 11:861, 1988.
95. Peshock, R.M., Rokey, R., Malloy, C.M., et al.: Assessment of myocardial systolic wall thickening using nuclear magnetic resonance imaging. J. Am. Coll. Cardiol. 14(3):653, 1989.
96. Pennell, D.J., Underwood, S.R., Ell, P.J., et al.: Dipyridamole magnetic resonance imaging: a comparison with thallium-201 emission tomography. Br. Heart J. 64:362, 1990.
97. van Rugge, F.P., van der Wall, E.E., Spanjersberg, B.S., et al.: Magnetic resonance imaging during dobutamine stress for detection and localization of coronary artery disease. Quantitative wall motion analysis using a modification of the centerline method. Circulation 90:127, 1994.
98. Beyar, R., Shapiro, E.P., Graves, W.L., et al.: Quantification and validation of left ventricular wall thickening by a three-dimensional volume element magnetic resonance imaging approach. Circulation 81:297, 1990.
99. Hansen, D.E., Daughters, G.T., Alderman, E.L., et al.: Torsional deformation of the left ventricular midwall in human hearts with intramyocardial markers: Regional heterogeneity and sensitivity to the inotropic effects of abrupt rate changes. Circ. Res. 62:941, 1988.
100. Mitchell, J.H., Wildenthal, K., and Mullins, C.B.: Geometrical studies of the left ventricle using biplane cinefluorography. Fed. Proc. 28(4):1334, 1969.
101. Zerhouni, E.A., Parish, D.M., Rogers, W.J., et al.: Human heart: Tagging with MR imaging—a method for noninvasive assessment of myocardial motion. Radiology 169(1):59, 1988.
102. Axel, L., and Dougherty L.: MR imaging of motion with spatial modulation of magnetization. Radiology 171:841, 1989.
103. Lima, J.A., Jeremy, R., Guier, W., et al.: Accurate systolic wall thickening by nuclear magnetic resonance imaging with tissue tagging: Correlation with sonomicrometers in normal and ischemic myocardium. J. Am. Coll. Cardiol. 21:1741, 1993.
104. Yeon, S.B., Reichek, N., Palmon, L.C., et al.: Validation of circumferential shortening by magnetic resonance tagging. (Abstr.) Circulation 82 (Suppl. III):III-488, 1990.
105. Pandian, N.G., and Kerber, R.E.: Two-dimensional echocardiography in experimental coronary stenosis. I. Sensitivity and specificity in detecting myocardial dyskinesis: Comparison with sonomicrometers. Circulation 66:597, 1982.
106. Sayad, D., Willet, D.W., Chwialkowski, M., et al.: Rapid, noninvasive quantitation of regional left ventricular function using gradient-echo MRI with myocardial tagging: Interstudy reproducibility. Am. J. Cardiol. 76:985, 1995.
107. Palmon, L.C., Reichek, N., Yeon, S.B., et al.: Intramural myocardial shortening in hypertensive left ventricular hypertrophy with normal pump function. Circulation 89(1):122, 1994.
108. Maier, S.E., Fischer, S.E., McKinnon, G.C., et al.: Evaluation of left ventricular segmental wall motion in hypertrophic cardiomyopathy with myocardial tagging. Circulation 86:1919, 1992.
109. Buchalter, M.B., Weiss, J.L., Rogers, W.J., et al.: Noninvasive quantification of left ventricular rotational deformation in normal humans using magnetic resonance imaging myocardial tagging. Circulation 81(4):1236, 1990.
110. Rademakers, F.E., Buchalter, M.B., Rogers, W.J., et al.: Dissociation between left ventricular untwisting and filling. Accentuation by catecholamines. Circulation 85(4):1572, 1992.
111. Young, A.A., Imai, H., Chang, C.N., et al.: Two-dimensional left ventricular deformation during systole using magnetic resonance imaging with spatial modulation of magnetization. Circulation 89:740, 1994.
112. Buchalter, M.B., Weiss, J.L., Rogers, W.J., et al.: Noninvasive quantification of left ventricular rotational deformation in normal humans using magnetic resonance imaging myocardial tagging. Circulation 81:1236, 1990.
113. Rademakers, F.E., Rogers, W.J., Guier, W.H., et al.: Relation of regional cross-fiber shortening to wall thickening in the intact heart: Three-dimensional strain analysis by NMR tagging. Circulation 89:1174, 1994.
114. McVeigh, E.R., and Zerhouni, E.A.: Noninvasive measurement of transmural gradients in myocardial strain with MR imaging. Radiology 180:677, 1991.
115. Auffermann, W., Wagner, S., Holt, W.W., et al.: Noninvasive determination of left ventricular output and wall stress in volume overload and myocardial disease by cine MRI. Am. Heart J. 121:1750, 1992.
116. Carabello, B.A., Green, L.H., Grossman, W., et al.: Hemodynamic determinants of prognosis of aortic valve replacement in critical aortic stenosis and advanced congestive heart failure. Circulation 62:42, 1980.
117. Wagner, S., Auffermann, W., Buser, P., et al.: Functional description of the left ventricle in patients with volume overload, pressure overload and myocardial disease using cine nuclear magnetic resonance imaging (NMRI). Am. J. Cardiac. Imaging 5:87, 1991.
118. Lima, J.A., Reichek, N., Ferrari, V.A., et al.: Regional differences in function within noninfarcted myocardium during left ventricular remodeling. Circulation 88:1279, 1993.
119. Pelc, L.R., Sayre, J., Kwok, Y., et al.: Evaluation of myocardial motion tracking with cine-phase contrast magnetic resonance imaging. Invest. Radiol. 29:1038, 1994.
120. Karwatowski, S.P., Mohiaddin, R., Yang, G.Z., et al.: Assessment of regional left ventricular long-axis motion with MR velocity mapping in healthy subjects. J. Magn. Reson. Imaging 4(2):151, 1994.
121. Beache, G.M., Wedeen, V.J., Weisskoff, R.M., et al.: MRI derived myocardial strain-rates in hypertrophic cardiomyopathy. NY Soc. Magn. Reson. Med. 1:266, 1993.
122. Axel, L.: Blood flow effects in magnetic resonance imaging. Am. J. Radiol. 143:1157, 1984.
123. Higgins, C.B., Caputo, G., Wendland, M.F., et al.: Measurement of blood flow and perfusion in the cardiovascular system. Invest. Radiol. 27:S66, 1992.
124. Wehrli, F.W.: Time-of-flight effects in MR imaging of flow. Magn. Reson. Med. 14:187, 1990.
125. Nishimura, D.G.: Time-of-flight MR angiography. Magn. Reson. Med. 14:194, 1990.
126. Edelman, R.R., Mattle, H.P., Kleefield, J., et al.: Quantification of blood flow with dynamic MR imaging and presaturation bolus tracking. Radiology 171:551, 1989.
127. Pelc, L.R., Pelc, N.J., Rayhill, S.C., et al.: Arterial and venous blood flow: Noninvasive quantitation with MR imaging. Radiology 185:809, 1992.
128. Mostbeck, G.H., Caputo, G.R., and Higgins, C.B.: MR measurement of blood flow in the cardiovascular system. Am. J. Radiol. 159:453, 1992.
129. Boesiger, P., Maier, S.E., Kecheng, L., et al.: Visualization and quantification of the human blood flow by magnetic resonance imaging. J. Biomech. 25:55, 1992.
130. Stahlberg, F., Sondergaard, L., Thomsen, C., et al.: Quantification of complex flow using MR phase imaging: A study of parameters influencing the phase/velocity relation. Magn. Reson. Imaging 10:13, 1992.
131. Spritzer, C.E., Pelc, N.J., Lee, J.N., et al.: Rapid MR imaging of blood flow with a phase-sensitive, limited-flip-angle, gradient recalled pulse sequence: Preliminary experience. Radiology 176:255, 1990.
132. Tang, C., Blatter, D.D., and Parker, D.L.: Accuracy of phase-contrast flow measurements in the presence of partial volume effects. J. Magn. Reson. Imaging 3:377, 1993.
133. Tang, C., Blatter, D.D., and Parker, D.L.: Accuracy of phase-contrast flow measurements in the presence of partial volume effects. Magn. Reson. Med. 3:377, 1993.
134. Buonocore, M.H., and Bogren, H.: Factors influencing the accuracy and precision of velocity-encoded phase imaging. Magn. Reson. Med. 26:141, 1992.
135. Matsuda, T., Shimizu, K., Sakurai, T., et al.: Measurement of aortic blood

flow with MR imaging: Comparative study with Doppler ultrasound. Radiology 162:857, 1987.
136. Maier, S.E., Meier, D., Boesiger, P., et al.: Human abdominal aorta: Comparative measurements of blood flow with MR imaging and multigated Doppler ultrasound. Radiology 171:487, 1989.
137. VanRossum, A.C., Sprenger, M., Visser, F.C., et al.: An in vivo validation of quantitative blood flow imaging in arteries and veins using magnetic resonance phase-shift techniques. Eur. Heart J. 12:117, 1991.
138. Firmin, D.N., Mayler, G.L., Klipstein, R.H., et al.: In vivo validation of MR velocity imaging. J. Comput. Assist. Tomogr. 11:751, 1987.
139. Kondo, C., Caputo, G.R., Semelka, R., et al.: Right and left ventricular stroke volume measurements with velocity-encoded cine MR imaging: In vitro and in vivo validation. Am. J. Radiol. 157:9, 1991.
140. Hundley, W.G., Li, H.F., Hillis, L.D., et al.: Quantitation of cardiac output with velocity-encoded, phase-difference magnetic resonance imaging: Validation with invasive measurements. J. Am. Coll. Cardiol. 7S:1250, 1995.
141. Iwai, F., Sostman, H.D., Evans, A.J., et al.: Cine phase-contrast magnetic resonance imaging for analysis of flow phenomena in experimental aortic dissection. Invest. Radiol. 26:1071, 1991.
142. Chang, J.M., Friese, K., Caputo, G.R., et al.: MR measurement of blood flow in the true and false channel in chronic aortic dissection. J. Comput. Assist. Tomogr. 15:418, 1991.
143. Evans, A.J., Iwai, F., Grist, T.A., et al.: Magnetic resonance imaging of blood flow with a phase subtraction technique: In vitro and in vivo validation. Invest. Radiol. 28:109, 1993.
144. Brenner, L.D., Caputo, G.R., Mostbeck, G., et al.: Quantification of left to right atrial shunts with velocity-encoded cine nuclear magnetic resonance imaging. J. Am. Coll. Cardiol. 20:1246, 1992.
145. Sieverding, L., Jung, W.I., Klose, U., et al.: Noninvasive blood flow measurement and quantification of shunt volume by cine magnetic resonance in congenital heart disease. Pediatr. Radiol. 22:48, 1992.
146. Hundley, W.G., Li, H.F., Lange, R.A., et al.: Assessment of left-to-right intracardiac shunting by velocity-encoded, phase-difference magnetic resonance imaging: A comparison with oximetric and indicator dilution techniques. Circulation 91:955, 1995.
147. Cranney, G.B., Lotan, C.S., and Pohost, G.M.: Nuclear magnetic resonance imaging for assessment and follow-up of patients with valve disease. Circulation 84 (Suppl I):216, 1991.
148. Utz, J.A., Herfkens, R.J., Heinsimer, J.A., et al.: Valvular regurgitation: Dynamic MR imaging. Radiology 168:91, 1988.
149. Pflugfelder, P.W., Landzberg, J.S., Cassidy, M.M., et al.: Comparison of cine MR imaging with Doppler echocardiography for the evaluation of aortic regurgitation. AJR 152:729, 1989.
150. Wagner, S., Auffermann, W., Buser, P., et al.: Diagnostic accuracy and estimation of the severity of valvular regurgitation from signal void on cine MRI. Am. Heart J. 118:760, 1989.
151. Suzuki, J.-I., Caputo, G.R., Kondo, C., et al.: Cine MR imaging of valvular heart disease: Display and imaging parameters affect the size of the signal void caused by valvular regurgitation. AJR 155:723, 1990.
152. Underwood, S.R., Klipstein, R.H., Firmin, D.N., et al.: Magnetic resonance assessment of aortic and mitral regurgitation. Br. Heart J. 56:455, 1986.
153. Underwood, S.R., Klipstei, R.H., Firmin, D.N., et al.: Magnetic resonance assessment of aortic and mitral regurgitation. Br. Heart J. 56:455, 1986.
154. Sechtem, U., Plugfelder, P.W., Cassidy, M.M., et al.: Mitral and aortic regurgitation: Quantification of regurgitant volumes with cine MR imaging. Radiology 167:425, 1988.
155. Walker, P.G., Cape, E.G., Pohost, G.M., et al.: Regurgitant orifice isovelocity contour mapping using NMR velocity encoding. (Abstract.) Circulation 82 (Suppl. III):44, 1990.
156. Higgins, C.B., and Caputo, G.R.: Magnetic resonance imaging of valvular heart disease. *In* Pohost, G.M. (ed.): Cardiovascular Applications of Magnetic Resonance, Mt. Kisco, NY, Futura, 1993.
157. Honda, N., Machida, K., Hashimoto, M., et al.: Aortic regurgitation: Quantitation with MR imaging velocity mapping. Radiology 186:189, 1993.
158. Sondergaard, L., Lindvig, K., Hildebrandt, P., et al.: Quantification of aortic regurgitation by magnetic resonance velocity mapping. Am. Heart J. 125:1081, 1993.
159. Fujita, N., Chazouilleres, A.F., Hartiala, J.J., et al.: Quantification of mitral regurgitation by velocity-encoded cine nuclear magnetic resonance imaging. J. Am. Coll. Cardiol. 23:951, 1994.
160. Hundley, W.G., Li, H.F., Willard, J.E., et al.: Magnetic resonance imaging assessment of the severity of mitral regurgitation: Comparison with invasive techniques. Circulation 92:1151, 1995.
161. Cranney, G.B., Lotan, C.S., and Pohost, G.M.: Part III: Evaluation of aortic regurgitation by nuclear magnetic resonance imaging. Curr. Probl. Cardiol. 2:87, 1990.
162. Adler, R.S., Chenevert, T.L., Fowlkes, J.B., et al.: Calculation of pressure gradients from MR velocity data in laminar flow model. J. Comput. Assist. Tomogr. 15:483, 1991.
163. Spielman, R.P., Schneider, O., Thiele, F., et al.: Appearance of poststenotic jets in MRI: Dependence on flow velocity and on imaging parameters. Magn. Reson. Med. 9:67, 1991.
164. Kilner, P.J., Manzara, C.C., Mohiadin, R.H., et al.: Magnetic resonance jet velocity mapping in mitral and aortic valve stenosis. Circulation 87:1239, 1993.
165. Sondergaard, L., Hildebrandt, P., Lindvig, K., et al.: Valve area and cardiac output in aortic stenosis: Quantification by magnetic resonance velocity mapping. Am. Heart J. 127:1156, 1993.
166. Evans, A.J., Richardson, D.B., Tien, R., et al.: Poststenotic signal loss in MR angiography: Effects of echo time, flow compensation and fractional echo. Am. J. Neuroradiol. 14:721, 1993.
167. Engels, G., Muller, E., Reynen, K., et al.: Evaluation of left ventricular inflow and volume by MR. Magn. Reson. Imaging 11:957, 1993.
168. Hartiala, J.J., Mostbeck, G.H., Foster, E., et al.: Velocity-encoded cine MRI in the evaluation of left ventricular diastolic function: Measurement of mitral valve and pulmonary vein flow velocities and flow volume across the mitral valve. Am. Heart J. 125:1054, 1993.
169. Mohaiddin, R.H., Amanuma, M., Kilner, P.J., et al.: MR phase-shift velocity mapping of mitral and pulmonary venous flow. J. Comput. Assist. Tomogr. 15:237, 1991.
170. Mostbeck, G.H., Hartiala, J.J., Foster, E., et al.: Right ventricular diastolic filling: Evaluation with velocity-encoded cine MRI. J. Comput. Assist. Tomogr. 17:245, 1993.
171. Debiao, L., Paschal, C.B., Haacke, E.M., et al.: Coronary arteries: Three dimensional MR imaging with fat saturation and magnetization transfer contrast. Radiology 187:401, 1993.
172. Manning, W.J., Li, W., and Edelman, R.R.: A preliminary report comparing magnetic resonance coronary angiography with conventional angiography. N. Engl. J. Med. 328:828, 1993.
173. Aurigemma, G.P., Reicheck, N., Axel, L., et al.: Noninvasive determination of coronary artery bypass graft patency by cine magnetic resonance imaging. Circulation 80:1595, 1989.
174. Hundley, W.G., Clarke, G.D., Landau, C., et al.: Noninvasive determination of infarct artery patency by cine magnetic resonance angiography. Circulation 91:1347, 1995.
175. Clarke, G.D., Eckels, R., Chaney, C., et al.: Measurement of absolute epicardial coronary artery flow and flow reserve using breath-hold cine phase contrast magnetic resonance imaging. Circulation 91:2627, 1995.
176. Edelman, R.R., Manning, W.J., Gervino, E., et al.: Flow velocity quantification in human coronary arteries with fast, breath-hold MR angiography. J. Magn. Reson. Imaging 3:699, 1993.
177. Debatin, J.F., Strong, J.A., Sostman, H.D., et al.: MR characterization of blood flow in native and grafted internal mammary arteries. J. Magn. Reson. Imaging 3:443, 1993.
178. Duda, R.O., and Hart, P.E.: Pattern Classification and Scene Analysis. New York, Wiley, 1973.
179. Frei, W., and Chen, C.C.: Fast boundary detection: A generalization and a new algorithm. IEEE Trans. Comput. 26:988, 1977.
180. Chu, C.H., Delp, E.J., and Buda, A.J.: Detecting left ventricular endocardial and epicardial boundaries by digital 2-D echocardiography. I.E.E.E. Trans. Med. Imaging 7:81, 1988.
181. Feng, J., Lin, W.C., and Chen, C.T.: Automatic left ventricular boundary detection in digital 2-D echocardiography using fuzzy reasoning techniques. Proc. SPIE Conference on Biomedical Image Processing 1245:19, 1990.
182. Tou, J.T., and Gonzalez R.C.: Pattern Recognition Principles. Redding, MA, Addison-Wesley, 1974.
183. Baldy, C., Doueck, P., Croisille, P., et al.: Automated myocardial edge detection from breath-hold cine-MR images: Evaluation of left ventricular volumes and mass. Magn. Reson. Imaging 12:589, 1994.
184. Fleagle, S.R., Thedens, D.R., Stanford, W., et al.: Multicenter trial of automated border detection in cardiac MR imaging. J. Magn. Reson. Imaging 3:409, 1993.
185. Ibrahim, Y., Chwialkowski, M.P., Templeton, G., et al.: Three-dimensional myocardial motion assessment from MR SPAMM images. Radiology 181(P):253, 1991.
186. Burkart, D.J., Felmlee, J.P., Johnson, C.D., et al.: Cine phase-contrast MR flow measurements: Improved precision using an automated method of vessel detection. J. Comput. Assist. Tomogr. 18(3):469, 1994.
187. Ibrahim, Y., Chwialkowski, M., Li, H.F., et al.: A method for fully automated quantitative analysis of arterial flow using flow-sensitized MR images. 1995 (submitted for publication).

CHAPTER

51 Cardiac Magnetic Resonance Spectroscopy: Principles and Applications

Robert G. Weiss, M.D.
Paul A. Bottomley, Ph.D.

Nuclear magnetic resonance of the hydrogen nuclei (^{1}H) in tissue and vessel water can be used in imaging applications to define cardiac anatomy, function, and perfusion. The same principles are used in magnetic resonance spectroscopy studies to noninvasively evaluate the chemistry and metabolism of tissues under physiologic conditions. Magnetic resonance spectroscopy (MRS)—specifically phosphorus (^{31}P) magnetic resonance spectroscopy—is unique in its ability to noninvasively quantify and monitor the high-energy phosphate compounds, such as adenosine triphosphate (ATP) and creatine phosphate (PCr), that fuel ongoing myocardial contractile function and are necessary for the viability of cardiac tissues. This chapter provides an overview of the current methods, findings, and potential clinical applications of human cardiac magnetic resonance spectroscopy studies. In addition to a review of spectroscopic techniques for spatial localization and quantification of metabolic information, we shall examine recent insights into human myocardial energy metabolism that have been provided by magnetic resonance spectroscopy in normal and several pathologic conditions, including coronary artery disease, heart failure, and transplant rejection.

PRINCIPLES AND METHODS

The Heart Spectrum

A magnetic resonance spectrum is a plot of the nuclear magnetic resonance signal intensity as a function of magnetic resonance frequency, standardly measured in units of parts per million (ppm) relative to the resonance frequency of a reference compound, such as PCr in ^{31}P studies in vivo or tetramethyl silane for ^{1}H or carbon (^{13}C) magnetic resonance spectroscopy. The spectrum is commonly obtained by mathematical Fourier transformation of a transient, time-dependent magnetic resonance signal, recorded in the absence of any spatial localization or imaging magnetic-field gradients. Each peak, or multiple of peaks, in a spectrum derives from a different chemical moiety in the sample, and its integrated signal or area is proportional to the concentration of that moiety.

Thus, the normal human cardiac ^{1}H spectrum is dominated by a water resonance at about 4.7 ppm, which is usually suppressed by various magnetic resonance methods to permit observation of less abundant moieties, and (CH_2) and CH_3 peaks from lipids at 1.3 and 0.9 ppm, likely dominated by pericardial fat. Because the total creatine pool is routinely quantified in brain ^{1}H spectra at 3.0 ppm and the creatine concentration is higher in myocardium, its detection in the heart by ^{1}H spectroscopy is anticipated as well. Resonances associated with deoxymyoglobin and oxymyoglobin at 75 ppm and −2.8 ppm that correlate with intracellular Po_2 have been reported in rat hearts,[1] but this work has not yet been extended to the human heart.

The normal human ^{31}P cardiac spectrum typically exhibits a single sharp PCr peak at 0 ppm; three phosphate peaks from ATP at about −2.7 ppm (γ-ATP), −7.8 ppm (α-ATP), and −16.3 ppm (β-ATP); variable amounts of phosphodiester at 2 to 3 ppm; inorganic phosphate (Pi), whose chemical shift varies from 3.9 to 5.1 ppm, depending on the intracellular pH; two blood 2,3-diphosphoglycerate (DPG) peaks at 5.4 and 6.3 ppm, often as a contaminant from the ventricular chamber; and phosphomonoester resonances at 6.3 to 6.8 ppm.[2, 3] Calibration curves permit intracellular pH measurements from the Pi chemical shift.[4] The pseudo–first-order forward rate constant for the creatine kinase reaction can also be measured by selectively exciting the γ-ATP resonance and noting the decrease in the PCr peak (known as the saturation transfer method) as a consequence of the flux of the moiety throughout the reaction.[5]

Like the ^{1}H spectrum, the natural-abundance ^{13}C spectrum from the human heart is dominated by fat resonances: (CH_2) at about 30 ppm, CH=CH at about 19 ppm, glycerol and carboxyl (CO) resonances at about 171 ppm when ^{1}H decoupling is used (decoupling involves irradiation of the sample at the ^{1}H magnetic resonance frequency during ^{13}C acquisition). A glycogen resonance at about 101 ppm may also be discerned.[6] Moreover, interest in cardiac ^{13}C spectroscopy has focused on the use of substrates such as glucose, whose ^{13}C isotopic abundance has been enhanced, thereby permitting the progress of an infusion to be monitored through glycolysis and the citric acid cycle.[7] Although ^{13}C-labeled substrates have been used extensively in animal models, human cardiac applications are yet to come.

Figure 51–1 shows examples of localized ^{1}H, ^{31}P, and natural-abundance ^{13}C magnetic resonance spectra from the normal human heart. Because the bulk of human spectroscopy studies and all those involving patients have employed ^{31}P magnetic resonance

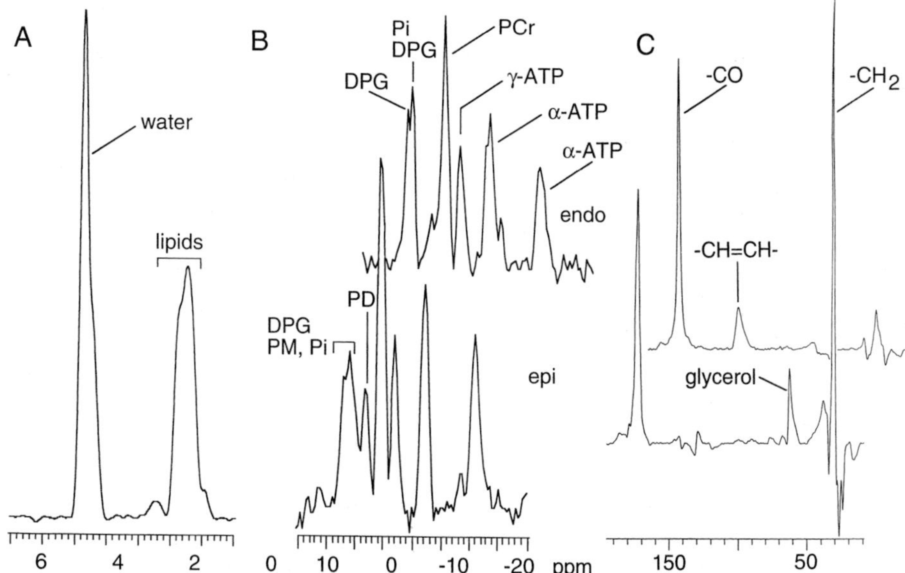

FIGURE 51–1. Localized surface coil magnetic resonance spectra from the normal human heart obtained on a General Electric 1.5-T MRI system. *A*, Fully relaxed cardiac-gated ^{1}H spectrum from a three-dimensional resolved, 6-mL voxel in the lateral left ventricular wall, localized by a stimulated echo sequence (three slice-selective 90-degree pulses, without water suppression, 30 msec echo time). *B*, Cardiac-gated ^{31}P spectra acquired from coronal slices 1 cm thick, endocardially (*top*) and epicardially (*bottom*) displaced in the anterior left ventricle, in about 10 minutes. *C*, ^{1}H-decoupled, Overhauser-enhanced, cardiac-gated natural-abundance ^{13}C spectra acquired from coronal slices, 2-cm thick, from the septum and anterior wall in about 7 minutes. Spectra in *B* and *C* were localized by the one-dimensional CSI and DRESS methods, respectively (see text). PM = phosphomonoester; DRESS = depth-resolved surface-coil spectroscopy. (Adapted from Bottomley, P.A., Hardy, C.J., Roemer, P.B., et al.: Proton-decoupled, Overhauser-enhanced, spatially localized carbon-13 spectroscopy in humans. Magn. Reson. Med. 12:348, 1989, with permission.)

imaging (MRI), we shall now focus our attention on that phenomenon.

Protocols

The typical human cardiac spectroscopy examination lasts about 1 hour. It uses ^{31}P detection coils with a 6 to 12-cm in diameter surface, located on the chest closest to the myocardium of interest, to optimize magnetic resonance sensitivity. A separate, larger magnetic resonance transmitter coil is used to provide a substantially uniform excitation field over the sensitive volume of the surface coil when imaging gradients are used for spatial localization, or a substantially linear gradient is used in the radiofrequency excitation field when rotating frame zeugmatography localization techniques are used.[8] The patient is preferably positioned prone in the magnetic resonance magnet to minimize the distance between the myocardium and the detection coil, as well as motion artifacts from respiration.[9] An electrocardiogram is established for patient monitoring and for gating magnetic resonance acquisitions synchronous to the cardiac cycle. Conventional magnetic resonance images are acquired to identify the region of interest and verify the desired coil placement, which is critical for small detection coils whose fields of view are very limited. The patient is repositioned, if necessary. Spectroscopy is initiated, and the magnetic-field homogeneity is shimmed over the region of interest to maximize peak height and minimize the width of the H_2O peak in a ^{1}H surface coil spectrum. The ^{31}P resonance is selected, the magnetic resonance flip-angle adjusted, and a spectroscopic data set acquired. Acquisitions may be repeated with stress or other stimuli.

Generally, the depth in the myocardium from which ^{31}P magnetic resonance spectra may be acquired will be limited to the anterior wall and perhaps several centimeters of septum, because of the decline in surface-coil sensitivity with depth. Three technical enhancements that promise some relief of the sensitivity problem are the uses of nuclear Overhauser enhancement, phased arrays of surface detection coils, and higher magnetic-field strengths. Nuclear Overhauser enhancement involves irradiating a sample at the ^{1}H resonance frequency during the course of a ^{31}P experiment, which causes a transfer of nuclear magnetization to the ^{31}P nuclei from nearby protons. The enhancement is about 60 percent (1.6-fold) for PCr and 30 to 40 percent for ATP resonances.[10, 11] Second, phased arrays of ^{31}P surface coils can provide an additional improvement of up to about 40 percent, compared with the best-positioned surface coil of the same diameter, just as they have done for conventional MRI. Moreover, their extended fields of view alleviate the positioning problem by enabling more myocardium to be optimally positioned relative to any coil; therefore, sensitivity enhancements of much more than 40 percent can, in practice, result for regions of myocardium that are not optimally positioned in the single-coil experiment.[12] Third, while most clinical MRI machines capable of spectroscopy operate at 1.5 to 2 Tesla (T), whole-body research machines operating at 3 T and 4 T offer potential increases in signal-to-noise ratio or reductions in the size of the spectroscopy volume element (voxel) that are roughly linear with field strength, or reductions in acquisition time in proportion to the square of the field, assuming sample dominant coil-noise conditions.[5, 13, 14]

The ^{31}P spectrum from a surface coil on the chest is usually dominated by signals from chest wall muscle immediately beneath it. Signals from the heart are commonly discriminated by any of five localization schemes illustrated in Figure 51–2.[8] All methods, except rotating frame zeugmatography, incorporate MRI gradients: one-dimensional localization to a single plane is afforded by slice-selective excitation in depth-resolved surface-coil spectroscopy,[2] or to a discrete voxel in the heart by slice selection in all three dimensions in the ISIS (image selected in vivo spectroscopy) method.[15] The one-dimensional chemical-shift imaging (CSI) method[16] and the rotating frame zeugmatography method[17] spatially encode magnetic resonance signals to multiple contiguous planes through the chest and heart with phase-encoding MRI gradient

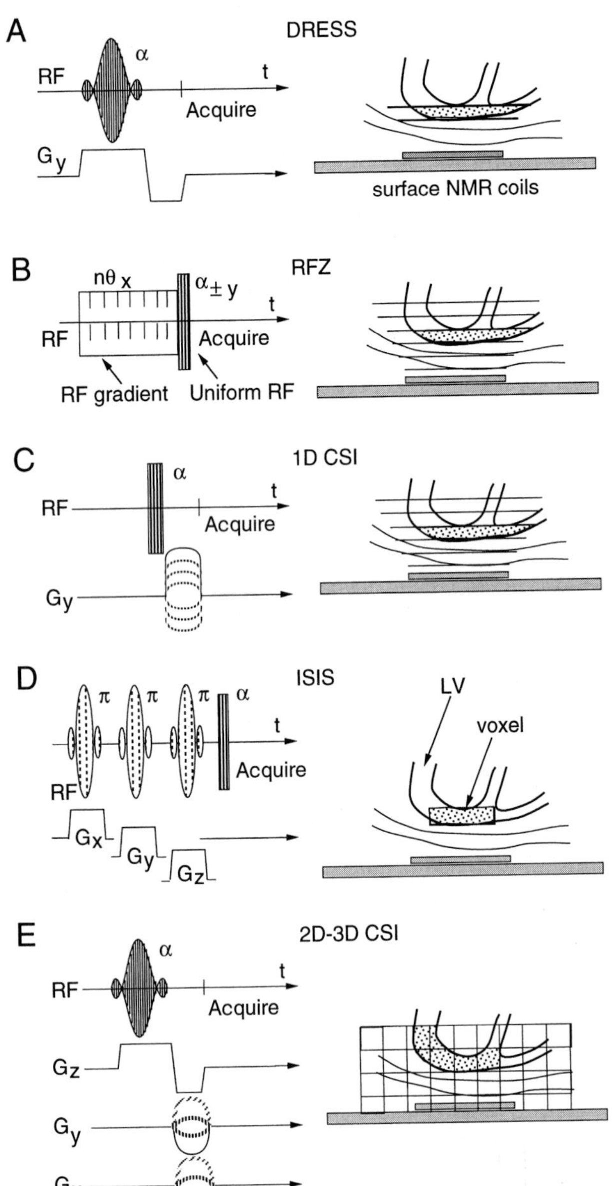

FIGURE 51–2. The DRESS (*A*), RFZ (*B*), one-dimensional CSI (*C*), ISIS (*D*), and slice-selective three-dimensional CSI magnetic resonance pulse sequences (*left*), localizing magnetic resonance spectroscopy signals to various voxels in the heart (*right*). G_x, G_y, and G_z are imaging gradients, and magnetic resonance pulses with flip angles of α or π are applied on the radiofrequency channel. With DRESS, a plane is selectively excited with a single-sequence application (*A*). With RFZ, localization results from encoding the magnetic resonance signal by using a different flip-angle pulses applied with a nominally linear gradient in the excitation field, which precedes the normal excitation pulse. The spatial information is obtained by FT of the signal with respect to the flip angle (*B*). The one-dimensional CSI method does essentially the same but uses an imaging gradient whose amplitude is varied (*C*). The ISIS sequence selectively excites a single volume when the signals from all eight combinations of the x, y, and z selective excitation pulses, being applied and not applied, are properly added (*D*). *E*, An axial slice through the chest is selectively excited, and the remaining two dimensions encoded by the other two gradients. The sequence is repeated $n = n_x \cdot n_y$ times, where $n_x \cdot n_y$ is the array size, and a two-dimensional FT with respect to gradient amplitude yields the spatial information. DRESS = depth-resolved surface-coil spectroscopy; RFZ = rotating-frame zeugmatography; ISIS = image selected in vivo spectroscopy. (Adapted from Bottomley, P.A.: MR spectroscopy of the human heart: The status and the challenges. Radiology 191:593–612, 1994, with permission.)

pulses and radiofrequency excitation-field gradient, respectively. Three-dimensional CSI extends the phase-encoding gradients of the one-dimensional CSI method to all three dimensions, generating a contiguous image array of multiple fully resolved voxels, from which images of a particular moiety may be reconstructed.[12, 18] The encoding methods and ISIS require repeated applications of the excitation sequence, with different encoding gradients or slice selection, to complete a spectral localization procedure. As this process can prove to be lengthy for three-dimensional CSI, hybrid methods, such as slice selection, followed by two-dimensional phase-encoding,[19] or two-dimensional ISIS, followed by one-dimensional phase encoding,[14, 20] are useful options. For one-dimensional methods, the spatial selectivity of the surface coils limits the extent of the selected planes in the other two dimensions.[2] An example of a three-dimensional resolved ^{31}P spectral data set acquired with a phased array of detection coils is shown in Figure 51–3.[12]

Metabolite Quantification

Often, metabolite quantification is complicated by overlapping contributions from neighboring peaks, which must be deconvolved for accurate measurements of peak areas. This is usually achieved by best-fitting curves to the peaks in the spectrum and by measuring the areas of those curves or, analogously, by fitting signal decay curves to the raw, time-dependent signal. Ratios of metabolites calculated from the ratios of areas can ultimately be converted to concentrations when the signal from a known concentration standard is also measured, and when the signals are carefully corrected for sample volume, inhomogeneity in the sensitivity of the magnetic resonance coils, and other distortions, for example, those from magnetic resonance relaxation effects.[19]

Systematic errors from relaxation effects are probably responsible for the bulk of the scatter in reported normal myocardial PCr:ATP ratios, which, to date, range from about 0.9 ± 0.3[18] to 2.1 ± 0.4.[21] This effect occurs through the use of MRI pulse-sequence repetition periods (TR) shorter or comparable to the spin-lattice relaxation times (T1) of PCr and ATP, which are about 4.4 ± 0.5 seconds and 2.3 ± 0.5 seconds (mean $\pm$ 95 percent confidence intervals), respectively.[22] The difference in T1 values means that a PCr signal acquired synchronous to the heart rate is differentially reduced by a factor of up to almost two-fold, relative to the ATP signal, depending on the pulse sequence flip angle (α).[8] To correct for the distortion, the observed PCr:ATP ratio must be multiplied by a factor

$$F = \frac{[1 - \exp(\frac{-y}{x})][1 - \cos\alpha \exp(\frac{-1}{x})]}{[1 - \exp(\frac{-1}{x})][1 - \cos\alpha \exp(\frac{-y}{x})]}$$

where x = T1 (PCr)/TR and y = T1(PCr)/T1(ATP), and the relative T1s are usually assumed to be unaltered in patients.[23] It is also practical to measure F directly from the ratio of short TR to fully relaxed unlocalized surface-coil signals on each subject.[23] The correction, and errors resulting from it, are minimized by keeping α small.[8]

Another source of intergroup variability in PCr:ATP ratios is contamination from blood, especially when voxels intersect the ventricular cavities. Blood contains ATP but no PCr and hence may reduce the observed PCr:ATP ratio. The amount of blood ATP contaminant can be estimated and subtracted from the spectrum by measuring the blood 2,3-diphosphoglycerate (DPG) peak. Because [ATP]/[DPG] ≅ 0.3 in blood and DPG has two phosphates, the ATP contaminant is approximately 15 percent of the DPG signal.[8, 24] The correction typically increases the T1-corrected PCr:ATP ratio by about 13 percent.[8] Potential sources of error for this correction are T1 effects and contamination of the DPG measurement by PM or Pi, or both. Blood corrections for other metabolites, such as phosphodiester, may also be important for comparing different study groups.[20]

Normal Metabolite Levels

When only the published studies that correct for T1 distortion and account for blood contamination are considered, a consensus for a normal myocardial PCr:ATP ratio of 1.83 ± 0.12 emerges[8, 14, 20, 24–26] (Table 51–1). This should be the best current estimate of the true value, because the metabolites appear to be 100 percent MR-visible,[27] and biochemical assays of biopsies taken at surgery[28] may result in some metabolite loss. Concentration measurements

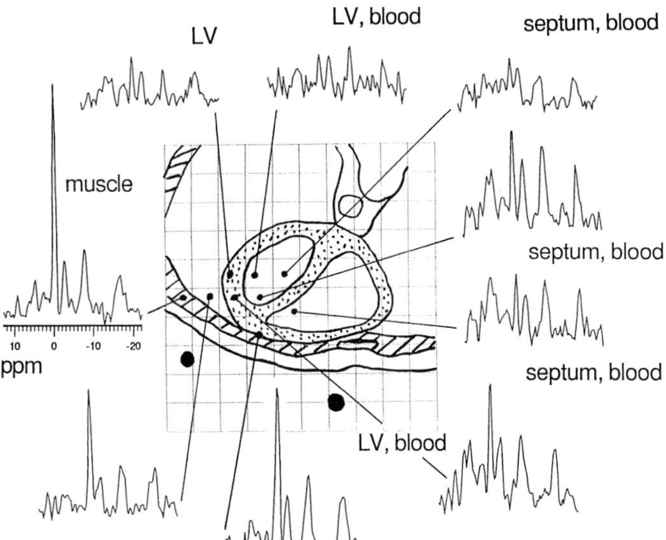

FIGURE 51–3. Three-dimensional resolved, cardiac-gated, ^{31}P CSI spectra acquired with a phased array of four 6.5-cm surface coils with 2 cm × 2 cm × 4 cm resolution in about 15 minutes from the heart of a normal volunteer. The CSI grid is overlaid on a tracing from a transaxial scout image. Note the difference in the PCr:ATP ratio between voxels intersecting myocardium and voxels intersecting chest muscle. The signal-to-noise ratio of (recombined) phased-array spectra was, on average, 30 percent higher than the best spectrum from any one coil in the array. LV = left ventricle. (From Hardy, C.J., Bottomley, P.A., Rohling, K.W., et al.: An NMR phased array for human cardiac ^{31}P spectroscopy. Magn. Reson. Med. 28:54, 1992, with permission.)

TABLE 51–1. INDICES OF NORMAL HUMAN CARDIAC PHOSPHATE METABOLISM MEASURED BY ^{31}P MRI

Parameter	Value*	Reference Number
PCr:ATP	1.80 ± 0.211.93 ± 0.21	24
	1.8 ± 0.1	25
	1.95 ± 0.45	14
	1.65 ± 0.26	26
		20
(mean:	*1.83 ± 0.12)*	
[PCr]	11 ± 3 μmol/g wet wt	19
	11.3 ± 3.7 μmol/g wet wt	29
	10.2 ± 4.6 μmol/g wet wt	30
[ATP]	6.9 ± 1.6 μmol/g wet wt	19
	7.4 ± 1.6 μmol/g wet wt	29
	7.0 ± 1.8 μmol/g wet wt	30
Pi:PCr	<0.25	3
	0.14 ± 0.06	20
pH	7.15 ± 0.2	3
	7.15 ± 0.03	20
CK forward rate	0.5 ± 0.2/sec	5
CK forward flux	6 ± 13 μmol/g wet wt per second	5

CK = creatine kinase reaction.
*Values are means ± SD.

obtained with the use of a reference signal, after correcting for tissue volumes, are about 11 μmol/g wet weight for PCr and 7 μmol/g wet weight for ATP.[19, 29, 30] Pi is very difficult to quantify in normal heart, as it often overlaps DPG and phosphomonoester resonances, and may be undetectable in many subjects[20]: the normal Pi:PCr ratio appears to be less than 0.25.[3] The Pi chemical shift corresponds to a pH of about 7.15, which is most likely intracellular, as blood Pi is imperceptible in ^{31}P blood spectra.[31, 32] The pseudo–first-order forward creatine kinase reaction rate for the human heart, estimated at 4 T with the saturation transfer method, is about 0.5 per second corresponding to a PCr flux of about 5 to 6 μmol/g wet wt per second.[5]

CLINICAL STUDIES

Ischemia and Infarction

In animal hearts, myocardial ischemia rapidly inhibits oxidative metabolism, which results in increased Pi from the rapid depletion of PCr and a subsequent, slower decline of ATP. Therefore, the metabolic consequences of ischemia are a decline in the PCr:ATP and PCr:Pi ratios. In humans, myocardial high-energy phosphates have been studied during transient stress-induced ischemia and after chronic ischemic damage and infarction. Myocardial stress has been induced inside magnetic resonance scanners by the administration of pharmacologic agents, such as the β-adrenergic agent dobutamine,[33] and by lower-extremity aerobic exercise[34, 35] and isometric handgrip exercise.[16, 36]

Transient, exercise-induced ischemia was evaluated with ^{31}P one-dimensional CSI in 16 patients with critical coronary disease involving the anterior left ventricular wall.[16] These subjects were studied before, during, and after continuous isometric handgrip exercise, and metabolic information obtained from the anterior left ventricular wall, as determined with ^{1}H magnetic resonance images obtained at that time. The mean cardiac PCr:ATP ratio at rest was 1.45 ± 0.31, slightly lower than in normal subjects at rest (P = .05). During exercise this mean cardiac PCr:ATP ratio fell significantly to a mean of 0.91 ± 0.24 (P < .001; Figs. 51–4 and 51–5), while that from the more superficial skeletal muscle was unchanged. This finding was associated with ischemic symptoms in only three patients. The myocardial PCr:ATP ratio recovered toward baseline levels shortly after exercise. Stress-induced declines in the cardiac

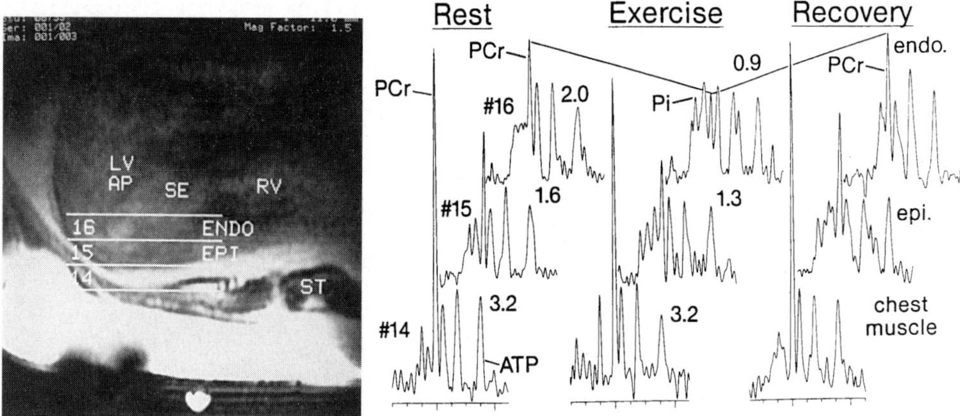

FIGURE 51–4. Hand-grip exercise ^{31}P stress-test data from a patient with coronary artery disease involving 70 to 90 percent stenosis of the left anterior descending coronary artery and near total occlusion of the first diagonal. Phosphorus-31 spectra derive from the three sections annotated in the ^{1}H surface coil image at left. During exercise, the PCr:ATP ratio in the predominantly endocardial spectrum (*16*) decreased from 2.0±0.2 to 0.9±0.2, consistent with ischemia. Spectral data were acquired in 14, 7, and 7 minutes during rest, exercise, and recovery phases, respectively. (From Weiss, R.G., Bottomley, P.A., Hardy, C.J., et al.: Regional myocardial metabolism of high-energy phosphates during isometric exercise in patients with coronary artery disease. N. Engl. J. Med. 323:1593–1600, 1990, with permission.)

PCr: ATP ratio were not detected in 11 age-matched control subjects or in 9 patients with valvular or myopathic disease in the absence of coronary artery disease, even though a similar heart rate–blood pressure product was obtained. These findings suggest that these stress-induced metabolic changes are specific for ischemic disease. The absence of change in the cardiac PCr:ATP ratio in normal subjects confirmed earlier findings during leg exercise.[34] In addition, stress-induced declines in cardiac PCr:ATP ratio were not detected in five subjects with coronary disease when they were restudied after revascularization with percutaneous balloon angioplasty or bypass surgery.[16] This study demonstrated that transient changes in myocardial high-energy phosphates characteristic of reversible myocellular ischemia in humans can be detected with magnetic resonance spectroscopy.

These observations were recently confirmed and extended in a study of 27 individuals with coronary disease of the anterior left ventricular wall and 11 normal control subjects.[36] The PCr:ATP ratio in 11 normal subjects also did not change during isometric stress from that at rest (1.85±0.29 versus 1.90±0.23, P = not significant). The patients with coronary disease were divided into two groups, based on a reversible or fixed thallium-201 (^{201}Tl) defect in that myocardial region. During isometric handgrip exercise in 15 subjects with critical coronary disease and a reversible ^{201}Tl defect, the PCr:ATP ratio fell significantly from 1.60±0.19 at rest to 0.96±0.28 ($P < .001$). In contrast, the PCr:ATP ratio in 12 subjects with a fixed ^{201}Tl defect was low at rest (1.24±0.30) and did not change significantly during exercise stress (1.19±0.28, P = not significant). The findings support the notion that ^{31}P magnetic resonance spectroscopy with isometric stress may be a sensitive and specific method for detecting reversible cardiac ischemia. Thus, stress-induced declines in the PCr:ATP ratio may constitute a marker for viable myocardium in a region supplied by a stenosed coronary artery.

Severe prolonged ischemic injury can lead to infarction, with loss of high-energy phosphate metabolism and stores. Reduced myocardial PCr:Pi ratios at rest, in the absence of any detectable changes in myocardial PCr:ATP ratio, were first observed in patients with recent anterior myocardial infarctions, using spatially localized ^{31}P magnetic resonance spectroscopy.[3] More recently, efforts to quantify the amounts of high-energy phosphates, rather than just ratios, have demonstrated a significant reduction in the myocardial levels of PCr (50 percent reduction) and ATP (65 percent reduction) in subjects with Q-wave infarctions.[37] In addition, there was a negative correlation between ^{201}Tl scintigraphy extent score and ATP amount in a subset of these patients.[37] Although it is clear that improved spatial resolution and depth of detection would enhance the ability of ^{31}P MRI to evaluate the consequences of prior ischemic injury, the available clinical evidence is consistent with prior basic findings that high-energy phosphates are absent in infarcted, irreversibly injured myocardium. The scientific appeal of using ^{31}P MRI detection of preserved high-energy phosphates for characterizing reversibly injured myocardium over the more established approach of detecting uptake of an administered metabolic tracer[38] is that the former quantifies the

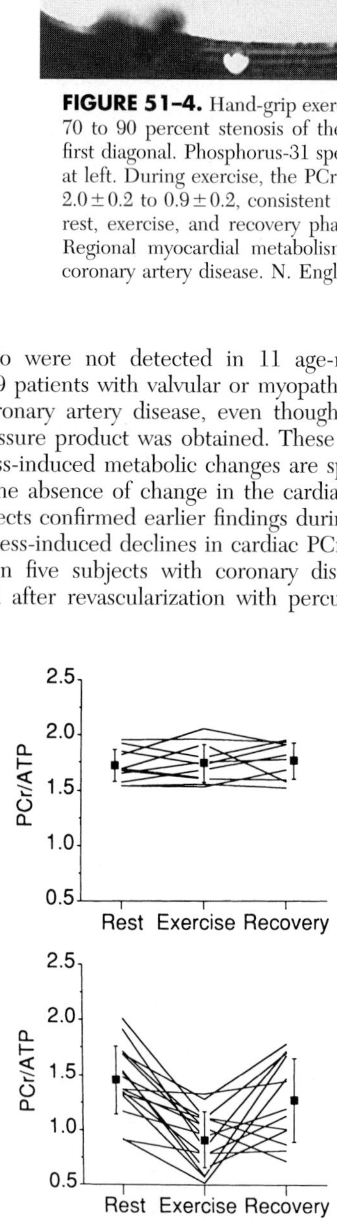

FIGURE 51–5. Cardiac PCr:ATP ratios for individuals with significant coronary artery disease (*bottom*) and age-matched normal control subjects (*top*), acquired at rest (*left*), during isometric handgrip exercise (*center*), and during early postexercise recovery (*right*). A significant decline in the myocardial PCr:ATP ratio was observed during isometric exercise in subjects with coronary disease ($P < .001$), which recovered partially during early recovery. No significant changes in the PCr:ATP ratio were observed in normal control subjects during the same exercise protocol. (From Weiss, R.G., Bottomley, P.A., Hardy, C.J., et al.: Regional myocardial metabolism of high-energy phosphates during isometric exercise in patients with coronary artery disease. N. Engl. J. Med. 323:1593–1600, 1990, with permission.)

metabolites essential for myocellular viability and is not confounded by questions of tracer availability under partial and no-flow conditions.

Cardiomyopathy and Congestive Heart Failure

Because cardiac contractile function is closely related to, and dependent on, oxidative metabolism, it has been hypothesized that contractile dysfunction in heart failure, at least in part, is due to chronically decreased high-energy phosphate metabolism or reserve.[39, 40] In the first report from a patient with left ventricular hypertrophy and heart failure symptoms studied with localized spectroscopy, the cardiac PCr:ATP ratio was reduced compared with that of normal individuals.[41] However, subsequent studies of patients with dilated cardiomyopathy and heart failure have produced conflicting results. Normal levels or nonsignificant reductions in the myocardial PCr:ATP ratio at rest have been reported in patients with dilated cardiomyopathy.[18, 42] Inotropic stress with dobutamine also did not significantly alter the mean PCr:ATP ratio in eight patients with dilated cardiomyopathy.[33] Other groups have observed significant reductions of about 20 percent in the nonstressed myocardial PCr:ATP ratios in subjects with dilated cardiomyopathy.[24, 26] Another study of six patients with dilated cardiomyopathy reported mean PCr:ATP ratios similar to those of control subjects but significantly higher Pi:PCr ratios in subjects with heart failure.[21]

Differences in the severity of heart failure in subjects among these studies may be an important factor contributing to the heterogeneity of the findings. Several lines of evidence suggest that subjects with more severe heart failure exhibit the most severe metabolic abnormalities.[24, 26] In general, studies reporting lower PCr:ATP ratios tended to enroll subjects with more severe heart failure findings and symptomatology. When subjects with the most severe symptoms or the lowest left ventricular ejection fractions in the latter studies are excluded, the significance of the reduction in PCr:ATP ratio in cardiomyopathy, compared to that of normals, decreases.[24, 26] Correlations of PCr:ATP ratios with heart failure symptoms were not specifically examined in most studies, including those showing unchanged PCr:ATP ratios in heart failure.[18, 42] In a more recent study of 19 subjects with dilated cardiomyopathy, the resting PCr:ATP ratio was reduced in those with severe heart failure (1.4 ± 0.5 versus 2.0 ± 0.5) and correlated negatively with the New York Heart Association class of failure severity[26] (Fig. 51–6). Moreover, a subset of individuals were restudied after clinical improvement with medical therapy for heart failure and demonstrated normalization of cardiac PCr:ATP ratios.[26] Because the total creatine pool measured with the use of classic techniques in biopsy samples obtained from failing hearts (class IV) is reduced by about 50 percent,[43] it is likely that the PCr content is decreased as well. One could conclude from all these studies that altered cardiac high-energy phosphates occur in subjects with heart failure but are most prominent in those with severe cardiac dysfunction and symptomatology. Larger, serial studies with homogeneous patient populations and careful hemodynamic and functional measures are needed to elucidate whether altered high-energy phosphate metabolism contributes mechanistically to the contractile dysfunction. Studies of high-energy phosphate turnover (e.g., that measured by the magnetization transfer experiment[5]), rather than just levels or ratios, may be more sensitive markers of altered metabolism or reduced reserve.

Some investigators reported an increase in the intensity of the phosphodiester resonances in patients with dilated cardiomyopathy.[18, 42] It was postulated that this change in the magnetic resonance spectrum reflected membrane damage. More recent studies provide evidence suggesting that the phosphodiester resonances may arise predominantly from blood, rather than from myocardium.[26, 32, 44] The contribution of intraventricular blood to a voxel typically increases with progressive left ventricular cavity dilation and wall thinning, as in dilated cardiomyopathy.

Left ventricular hypertrophy (LVH) can occur as the result of several conditions and can evolve in some patients, after a number of years, into a dilated cardiomyopathy with heart failure symptoms. One could hypothesize a role for altered high-energy metabolism contributing to the progression from normal or hypercontractile LVH over a prolonged period of time to a hypocontractile cardiomyopathy in some settings. Normal myocardial PCr:ATP ratios have been reported in apparently asymptomatic subjects with LVH by several groups.[18, 21] In other subjects characterized as having hypertrophic cardiomyopathy, however, reduced cardiac PCr:ATP ratios have been observed in at least three different studies.[21, 31, 44] In a subset of these patients in whom Pi was detectable, intracellular pH was significantly lower than in control subjects.[44] In patients with LVH due to aortic valvular disease, subjects with heart failure symptoms had lower resting PCr:ATP ratios than those without heart failure.[45] The data are superficially consistent with the hypothesis that metabolic abnormalities may contribute to the progression of cardiomyopathy in LVH, but larger studies with serial measures of high-energy phosphates over time in the same subjects, especially in the presence and absence of interventions that cause regression of LVH, are likely to expand our understanding of this pathophysiology.

Heart Transplantation and Transplant Rejection

Phosphorus-31 magnetic resonance spectroscopy studies of animals with nonworking, heterotopically implanted hearts show sig-

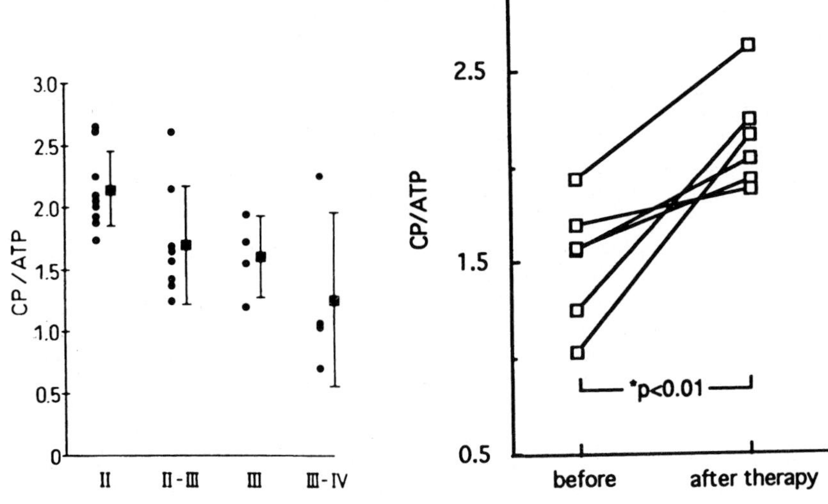

FIGURE 51–6. Myocardial PCr:ATP ratios versus New York Heart Association Heart Failure Classification in subjects with cardiomyopathy (*left panel*). The PCr:ATP ratio correlated inversely with heart failure severity ($r = .60$, $P < .005$). In six subjects with cardiomyopathy treated with medical therapy for approximately 3 months, the cardiac PCr:ATP ratio increased significantly ($P < .01$) (*right panel*). (Adapted from Neubauer, S., Krahe, T., Schindler, R., et al.: ^{31}P magnetic resonance spectroscopy in cardiomyopathy and coronary artery disease. Circulation 86:1810–1818, 1992, with permission.)

nificant decreases in myocardial PCr:Pi and PCr:ATP ratios in the first weeks after transplantation, that precede histologic evidence for allograft rejection.[46–49] This finding raised the possibility that ^{31}P indices may usefully predict rejection in heart transplant patients. The presence and severity of rejection is currently assessed by repeated endomyocardial biopsies obtained with a transvenous right-heart bioptome. Many heart transplants are often histologically classified as nonrejecting or mildly rejecting, and all patients receive chronic immunosuppressive medication. A decision to augment immunosuppressive therapy for moderate or severe rejection is typically based on the histologic appearance of myocyte necrosis. Therefore, patient management critically depends on the ability to characterize the severity of rejection and to detect rejection involving myocyte necrosis early.

Phosphorus-31 magnetic resonance studies of transplant patients have generally confirmed that myocardial PCr:ATP or PCr:Pi ratios are reduced in transplanted human hearts. Although initially some findings provided hope that ^{31}P MRI might predict histologic status,[50–51] subsequent work has indicated that ^{31}P MRI is not a reliable predictor of histologic rejection involving myocyte necrosis in many patients.[25, 52, 53] Thus, although the anterior myocardial PCr:ATP ratio was significantly lower in transplanted hearts for up to 5.5 years after transplantation (1.6 ± 0.5 versus 1.9 ± 0.2, $P < .01$), ^{31}P MRI measures were poorly correlated with histologic indices for rejection and agreement between abnormalities in ^{31}P spectra, and histologic evidence for necrosis could be achieved in only about 60 to 70 percent of cases.[25] Reduction in PCr:ATP ratio could not be linked to hypertrophy or coronary artery disease,[25] but some data suggest that reductions are more prevalent early after transplantation, perhaps because of ischemia and reperfusion injury during transplantation or subsequent edema, or both.[53]

The differences between metabolic and histologic findings probably reflect fundamental differences in the properties measured. Dead cells are depleted of high-energy phosphates, so a PCr:ATP ratio cannot index myocyte necrosis. A lower PCr:ATP ratio could warn of impending damage, however, if it were manifested by a myocyte population large enough to be observable with ^{31}P MRI.[25] However, when this lower PCr:ATP ratio does not progress to cell death or resolves in response to the chronic immunosuppressive medication, the ^{31}P indices register as false-positive predictions of rejection when compared to the histologic standard. Elevated Pi levels could index necrosis better if the problems of its quantification could be overcome, but even here the animal data do not lend strong support to the view that Pi measurements may permit differentiation of rejection involving necrosis from milder forms.[8] Although causes and applications remain unclear, the reduced energy reserve measured by the altered PCr:ATP ratio in transplant patients is a source of concern meriting further investigation.

THE FUTURE OF CARDIAC MAGNETIC RESONANCE SPECTROSCOPY

In recent years considerable advances have been made in implementing cardiac magnetic resonance spectroscopy and performing studies in relatively small numbers of patients with important clinical conditions. Despite the unique scientific insights into cardiac metabolism that ^{31}P magnetic resonance spectroscopy can provide, it is not currently used in the general clinical evaluation of heart disease. The reasons for this phenomenon include the relatively recent development of spatially localizing spectroscopic techniques, the limited spatial resolution and the low sensitivity at distances remote from the anterior chest surface, and the limited number of published clinical trials. Recent strategies for minimizing the sensitivity problems have been noted earlier and remain an active and important area of research. The ultimate role of cardiac magnetic resonance spectroscopy in clinical cardiology will probably depend on the success in minimizing these weaknesses as well as the outcomes of further studies in larger patient populations. Until then, ^{31}P magnetic resonance spectroscopy promises to provide a unique window for the noninvasive study of cardiac high-energy phosphate metabolism under physiologic conditions and thereby may provide insights into the pathophysiology of many common clinical cardiac diseases.

References

1. Kreutzer, U., Wang, D.S., and Jue, T.: Observing the ^{1}H NMR signal of the myoglobin Val-Ell in myocardium: An index of cellular oxygenation. Proc. Natl. Acad. Sci. U.S.A. 89:4731, 1992.
2. Bottomley, P.A.: Noninvasive study of high-energy phosphate metabolism in human heart by depth-resolved ^{31}P NMR spectroscopy. Science 229:769, 1985.
3. Bottomley, P.A., Herfkens, R.J., Smith, L.S., et al.: Altered phosphate metabolism in myocardial infarction: P-31 MR spectroscopy. Radiology 165:703, 1987.
4. Gadian, D.G.: Nuclear Magnetic Resonance and Its Applications to Living Systems. New York, Oxford University Press, 1982, pp. 30–34.
5. Bottomley, P.A., and Hardy, C.J.: Mapping creatine kinase reaction rates in human brain and heart with 4 Tesla saturation transfer ^{31}P NMR. J. Magn. Reson. 99:443, 1992.
6. Bottomley, P.A., Hardy, C.J., Roemer, P.B., et al.: Proton-decoupled, Overhauser-enhanced, spatially localized carbon-13 spectroscopy in humans. Magn. Reson. Med. 12:348, 1989.
7. Weiss, R.G., Chacko, V.P., Glickson, J.D., et al.: Comparative ^{13}C and ^{31}P NMR assessment of altered metabolism during graded reductions in coronary flow in intact rat hearts. Proc. Natl. Acad. Sci. U.S.A. 86:6426, 1989.
8. Bottomley, P.A.: MR spectroscopy of the human heart: The status and the challenges. Radiology 191:593, 1994.
9. Bottomley, P.A., and Hardy, C.J.: Strategies and protocols for clinical ^{31}P research in the heart and brain. Philos. Trans. R. Soc. Lond. A 333:531, 1990.
10. Bottomley, P.A., and Hardy, C.J.: Proton Overhauser enhancements in human cardiac phosphorus NMR spectroscopy at 1.5T. Magn. Reson. Med. 24:384, 1992.
11. Kolem, H., Sauter, R., Friedrich, M., et al.: Nuclear Overhauser enhancement and proton decoupling in phosphorus chemical shift imaging of the human heart. *In* Pohost, G.M. (ed.): Cardiovascular Applications of Magnetic Resonance. Mt. Kisco, NY, Futura, 1993, pp. 417–426.
12. Hardy, C.J., Bottomley, P.A., Rohling, K.W., et al.: An NMR phased array for human cardiac ^{31}P spectroscopy. Magn. Reson. Med. 28:54, 1992.
13. Hardy, C.J., Bottomley, P.A., Roemer, P.B., et al.: Rapid ^{31}P spectroscopy on a 4-T whole-body system. Magn. Reson. Med. 8:104, 1988.
14. Menon, R.S., Hendrich, K., Hu, X., et al.: ^{31}P NMR spectroscopy of the human heart at 4T: Detection of substantially uncontaminated cardiac spectra and differentiation of subepicardium and subendocardium. Magn. Reson. Med. 26:368, 1992.
15. Schaefer, S., Gober, J., Valenza, M., et al.: Nuclear magnetic resonance imaging-guided phosphorus-31 spectroscopy of the human heart. J. Am. Coll. Cardiol. 12:1449, 1988.
16. Weiss, R.G., Bottomley, P.A., Hardy, C.J., et al.: Regional myocardial metabolism of high-energy phosphates during isometric exercise in patients with coronary artery disease. N. Engl. J. Med. 323:1593, 1990.
17. Blackledge, M.J., Rajagopalan, B., Oberhaensli, R.D., et al.: Quantitative studies of human cardiac metabolism by P-31 rotating frame NMR. Proc. Natl. Acad. Sci. U.S.A. 84:4283, 1987.
18. Schaefer, S., Gober, J.R., Schwartz, G.G., et al.: In vivo phosphorus-31 spectroscopic imaging in patients with global myocardial disease. Am. J. Cardiol. 65:1154, 1990.
19. Bottomley, P.A., Hardy, C.J., and Roemer, P.B.: Phosphate metabolite imaging and concentration measurements in human heart by nuclear magnetic resonance. Magn. Reson. Med. 14:425, 1990.
20. de Roos, A., Doornbos, J., Luyten, P.R., et al.: Cardiac metabolism in patients with dilated and hypertrophic cardiomyopathy: Assessment with proton-decoupled P-31 MR spectroscopy. J. Magn. Reson. Imaging 2:711, 1992.
21. Masuda, Y., Tateno, Y., Ikehira, H., et al.: High-energy phosphate metabolism of the myocardium in normal subjects and patients with various cardiomyopathies: The study using ECG gated MR spectroscopy with a localization technique. Jpn. Circ. J. 56:620, 1992.
22. Bottomley, P.A., and Ouwerkerk, R.: Optimum flip-angles for exciting NMR with uncertain T1 values. Magn. Reson. Med. 32:137, 1994.
23. Bottomley, P.A., Hardy, C.J., and Weiss, R.G.: Correcting human heart ^{31}P NMR spectra for partial saturation: Evidence that saturation factors for PCr/ATP are homogeneous in normal and disease states. J. Magn. Reson. 95:341, 1991.
24. Hardy, C.J., Weiss, R.G., Bottomley, P.A., et al.: Altered myocardial high-energy phosphate metabolites in patients with dilated cardiomyopathy. Am. Heart J. 122:795, 1991.
25. Bottomley, P.A., Weiss, R.G., Hardy, C.J., et al.: Myocardial high-energy phosphate metabolism and allograft rejection in patients with heart transplants. Radiology 181:67, 1991.
26. Neubauer, S., Krahe, T., Schindler, R., et al.: ^{31}P magnetic resonance spectroscopy in dilated cardiomyopathy and coronary artery disease. Circulation 86:1810, 1992.
27. Humphrey, S.M., and Garlick, P.B.: NMR-visible ATP and Pi in normoxic and reperfused rat hearts: A quantitative study. Am. J. Physiol. 260:H6, 1991.
28. Swain, J.L., Sabina, R.L., Peyton, R.B., et al.: Derangements in myocardial purine and pyrimidine nucleotide metabolism in patients with coronary artery disease and left ventricular hypertrophy. Proc. Natl. Acad. Sci. U.S.A. 79:655, 1982.
29. Okada, M., Mitsunami, K., Yabe, T., et al.: Quantitative measurements of phospho-

rus metabolites in normal and diseased human hearts by ^{31}P NMR spectroscopy. (Abstract.) Proc. Soc. Magn. Reson. Med. 2:2305, 1992.

30. Yabe, T., Mitsunami, K., Okada, M., et al.: Quantitative measurements of phosphorus metabolites in coronary artery diseases by ^{31}P slice-selected one-dimensional chemical shift imaging. (Abstract.) Proc. Soc. Magn. Res. Med. 3:1220, 1994.
31. Sakuma, H., Takeda, K., Tagami, T., et al.: ^{31}P MR spectroscopy in hypertrophic cardiomyopathy: Comparison with Tl-201 myocardial perfusion imaging. Am. Heart J. 125:1323, 1993.
32. Horn, M., Neubauer, S., Bomhard, M., et al.: ^{31}P-NMR spectroscopy of human blood and serum: First results from volunteers and patients with congestive heart failure, diabetes mellitus and hyperlipidaemia. Magn. Reson. Materials Physic. Biol. Med. 1:55, 1993.
33. Schaefer, S., Schwartz, G.G., Steinman, S.K., et al.: Metabolic response of the human heart to inotropic stimulation: In vivo phosphorus-31 studies of normal and cardiomyopathic myocardium. Magn. Reson. Med. 25:260, 1992.
34. Conway, M.A., Bristow, J.D., Blackledge, M.J., et al.: Cardiac metabolism during exercise measured by magnetic resonance spectroscopy. Lancet 861:692, 1988.
35. Conway, M.A., Bristow, J.D., Blackledge, M.J., et al.: Cardiac metabolism during exercise in healthy volunteers measured by ^{31}P magnetic resonance spectroscopy. Br. Heart J. 65:25, 1991.
36. Yabe, T., Mitsunami, K., Okada, M., et al.: Detection of myocardial ischemia by ^{31}P magnetic resonance spectroscopy during handgrip exercise. Circulation 89:1709, 1994.
37. Mitsunami, K., Okada, M., Inoue, T., et al.: In vivo ^{31}P nuclear magnetic resonance spectroscopy in patients with old myocardial infarction. Jpn. Circ. J. 56:614, 1992.
38. Tillisch, J.H., Brunken, R., Marshall, R.C., et al.: Reversibility of cardiac wall-motion abnormalities predicted by positron tomography. N. Engl. J. Med. 314:884, 1986.
39. Krause, S.M.: Metabolism in the failing heart. Heart Failure 1:267, 1988.
40. Ingwall, J.S.: Is cardiac failure a consequence of decreased energy reserve? Circulation 87:VII-58, 1993.
41. Rajagopalan, B., Blackledge, M.J., McKenna, W.J., et al.: Measurement of phosphocreatine to ATP ratio in normal and diseased human heart by ^{31}P magnetic resonance spectroscopy using the rotating frame-depth selection technique. Ann. N.Y. Acad. Sci. 508:321, 1987.
42. Auffermann, W., Chew, W.M., Wolfe, C.L., et al.: Normal and diffusely abnormal myocardium in humans: Functional and metabolic characterization with P-31 MR spectroscopy and cine MR imaging. Radiology 179:253, 1991.
43. Nascimben, L., and Ingwall, J.S.: Decreased energy reserve may cause pump failure in human dilated cardiomyopathy. (Abstract.) Circulation 84:II-563, 1991.
44. deRoos, A., Doornbos, J., Luyten, P.R., et al.: Cardiac metabolism in patients with dilated and hypertrophic cardiomyopathy: Assessment with proton-decoupled P-31 MR spectroscopy. J. Magn. Reson. Imaging 2:711, 1992.
45. Conway, M.A., Allis, J., Ouwerkerk, R., et al.: Detection of low phosphocreatine to ATP ratio in failing hypertrophied human myocardium by ^{31}P magnetic resonance spectroscopy. Lancet 338:973, 1988.
46. Canby, R.C., Evanochko, W.T., Barrett, L.V., et al.: Monitoring the bioenergetics of cardiac allograft rejection using in vivo P-31 nuclear magnetic resonance spectroscopy. J. Am. Coll. Cardiol. 9:1067, 1987.
47. Haug, C.E., Shapiro, J.L., Chan, L., et al.: P-31 nuclear magnetic resonance spectroscopic evaluation of heterotopic cardiac allograft rejection in the rat. Transplantation 44:175, 1987.
48. Fraser, C.D., Chacko V.P., Jacobus, W.E., et al.: Metabolic changes preceding functional and morphological indices of rejection in heterotopic cardiac allografts. Transplantation 46:346, 1988.
49. Fraser, C.D., Chacko, V.P., Jacobus, W.E., et al.: Early phosphorus-31 nuclear magnetic bioenergetic changes potentially predict rejection in heterotopic cardiac allografts. J. Heart Transplant. 9:197, 1990.
50. Herfkens, R.J., Charles, H.C., Negro-Vilar, R., et al.: In vivo phosphorus-31 NMR spectroscopy of human heart transplants. (Abstract.) Proc. Soc. Magn. Reson. Med. 2:827, 1988.
51. Evanochko, W.T., Bouchard, A., Kirklin, J.K., et al.: Detection of cardiac transplant rejection in patients by ^{31}P NMR spectroscopy. (Abstract.) Proc. Soc. Magn. Reson. Med. 1:246, 1990.
52. Evanochko, W.T., den Hollander, J.A., Luney, D.J.E., et al.: ^{31}P MRS in human heart transplants: A clinical update. (Abstract.) Proc. Soc. Magn. Reson. Med. 3:1092, 1993.
53. van Dobbenburgh, J.O., de Jonge, N., Klopping, C., et al.: Altered myocardial energy metabolism in heart transplant patients: Consequence of rejection or a postischemic phenomenon? (Abstract.) Proc. Soc. Magn. Reson. Med. 3:1093, 1993.

PART 6

FAST COMPUTED TOMOGRAPHY

CHAPTER

52 Ultrafast Computed Tomography: Principles and Instrumentation

Cynthia H. McCollough, Ph.D.
Richard A. Robb, Ph.D.

The discovery of x-rays in 1895 heralded a new era in the practice of medicine: visualization into the body without painful and often life-threatening surgery. The discovery was almost immediately recognized and accepted for its potential as a new medical diagnostic technique. During the subsequent 100 years, there have been numerous improvements in this field of medicine, which has come to be known as diagnostic radiology.

X-ray imaging is essentially noninvasive. Although modest risks are incurred owing to the ionizing effect of x-rays,[1] these risks are usually acceptable because of the diagnostic benefits provided when such examination is indicated by illness and associated symptoms.

However, conventional x-ray imaging techniques (radiography and fluorography) have several important limitations: much detail is lost in the radiographic process because of superposition of three-dimensional structural information onto a two-dimensional detector; small differences (1 to 2 percent) in x-ray attenuation by various body tissues are not readily detectable on x-ray film or fluoroscopic screen displays; and a large percentage of the radiation detected is scattered within the patient, thus reducing the signal-to-noise ratio of the recorded information. The development of x-ray computed tomography (CT) in the 1970s had a revolutionary impact on diagnostic imaging because it eliminated or greatly minimized these problems, providing the physician with a capability for noninvasive examination of internal structures of the body with an accuracy and specificity previously unavailable.

HISTORY

The mathematical basis for CT is known as image reconstruction. The goal of image reconstruction as applied to medical imaging is to create a two-dimensional quantitative map (image) of the contents within a thin anatomical section (slice) of a three-dimensional object (patient) using multiple one-dimensional projections of the object's contents. In other words, in x-ray CT, the reconstruction process creates a cross-sectional view of an object from multiple projections about the object.

The concept of mathematical image reconstruction existed long before its application to medical imaging. In 1917, an Austrian mathematician, Radon, published an exact analytic solution to the problem of reconstructing an object from its projections.[2] This knowledge remained theoretical for many years, in part because of the difficulty of solving Radon's equation for discrete, finite, and noisy data sets. In the 1950s, mathematical image reconstruction techniques began to be independently developed and applied in a variety of scientific investigations. These included solar radioastronomy[3,4] and electron microscopy.[5,6]

The application of mathematical image reconstruction techniques to radiographic medical imaging was first published in the early 1960s, quite independently, by Oldendorf and by Cormack.[7, 8] Cormack's early studies led to a mathematically accurate method of reconstructing images from x-ray projections (radiographs), for which work he received the Nobel Prize in 1979.[9, 10]

In 1963, Kuhl and Edwards[11] developed the first practical, clinically-applied gamma-emission (not x-ray transmission) CT scanner, which detected the transaxial distribution of radionuclides in the brain. The reconstruction method used, known as backprojection, distributed the signal at any point along the projection uniformly "backward," along the path traveled by the emerging photon (a gamma ray, in this case). For a bright point object in a dark background, this technique produced an image having bright "tails" emanating in a radial fashion away from the bright central point. For objects composed of many points, it produced a blurred representation of the original object.

In 1967, Bracewell and Riddle[12] proposed the mathematical basis for a direct approximation of Radon's formula, which came to be known as filtered backprojection. This approach was also discovered by Ramachandran and Lakshminarayanan,[13] who derived a numerically implementable formulation. Filtered backprojection, modified and refined by several investigators, has become the method of choice for most commercial x-ray CT scanners and overcomes the limitations of the simple backprojection method.

In the late 1960s, British scientist Godfrey Hounsfield was independently developing his ideas that mathematical techniques could be used to reconstruct the internal structure of the body from a number of different x-ray measurements.[14] His efforts eventually resulted in construction of the first clinical x-ray CT scanner, the EMI Mark I (model) brain scanner (EMI, Ltd. Great Britain), which was installed at Atkinson Morleys Hospital, Wimbledon, England, in 1971. The results from the EMI brain scanner were presented in 1972, followed by the now classic publications in 1973[15, 16] that heralded the revolutionary era of diagnostic x-ray CT. Hounsfield accomplished the remarkable synthesis that resulted in a successful clinical machine: recognizing the diagnostic need, developing a numerically implementable mathematical solution to the image reconstruction problem, and organizing electromechanical and x-ray technology into a precisely engineered instrument that resulted in a successful clinical machine. The award to Hounsfield in 1979 of the Nobel Prize,[10, 14] which was shared with Cormack, recognized perhaps the greatest advance in diagnostic imaging in more than 75 years and provided significant scientific credibility to the field of computed medical imaging.

With the successful introduction of the EMI brain scanner into the clinical arena, an explosive era of development and marketing of CT scanners by a variety of manufacturers followed. Notable was the development by Robert Ledley[17] of the first CT scanner for the body as well as the head, called the ACTA scanner (Pfizer Medical Systems, Inc.). This development was significant in opening the door to a variety of designs of CT scanners directed at improving scan speed and accuracy while maintaining patient comfort and safety.

By 1976, more than 20 companies were producing one or more models of x-ray CT scanners for commercial purposes. By 1980, this number had decreased significantly, as smaller companies realized they could not compete with major radiographic equipment manufacturers. The decade of the 1980s saw CT scanners installed in more than 1000 medical institutions throughout the world, with a prodigious accumulation of published data.[18] In the 1990s, the introduction of spiral (helical) CT has produced a renewed interest in CT equipment design and the emergence of several new clinical applications, including CT angiography.[19–31]

BASIC PRINCIPLES

Fundamental Radiation Physics

A beam of x-rays passing though the body is differentially absorbed and scattered by structures in the beam path. The amount of absorption depends on the physical density and atomic composition of these structures and on the energy of the x-ray beam. For equivalent x-ray energy, a more dense structure attenuates the beam more than a less dense structure. This differential absorption pattern is carried by the transmitted x-ray beam and recorded by the x-ray detector, usually film.

Even though two separate x-ray beams of equal energy may be recorded by the detector as having almost equal total attenuation, they may have passed through entirely different materials. This is because attenuation is dependent on path length through an object as well as on its physical density and atomic composition. In such cases, it is impossible to "see" or determine from the detector (film) the different materials through which the beam has passed. The attenuations at different points along the beam path accumulate and are superimposed on the detector, as illustrated in the left panel of Figure 52–1, with the result that only in those regions where large density and elemental composition differences exist between adjacent structures can details be clearly discerned on the film, as in the case of the ribs (bone) against the lungs (air).

Conventional (blurring) tomography, which was developed in the 1930s,[32, 33] attempts to overcome the superposition problem, as illustrated in the center panel of Figure 52–1. However, the problem of superposition is not eliminated. Small density differences are difficult to detect in conventional tomograms, owing to superposition and scattering, even under the favorable conditions of small field size and low x-ray energy.[33]

In computed (transaxial) tomography, scatter is minimized by collimation of the beam, and superposition is eliminated by scanning around a transaxial plane, as shown in the right-hand panel of Figure 52–1. The x-ray beam transmitted through the plane or slice is measured with detectors that can record intensity differences less than 0.1 percent, and the individual attenuation coefficients of structures in the beam path are determined from these measurements by image reconstruction.

Techniques to calculate the cross-sectional distribution of attenuation coefficients are based, in part, on a well-known law of radiation physics (the Lambert-Beer law),[34] which states that when a monoenergetic x-ray beam (i.e., a beam with a single x-ray wavelength) passes through an object of varying densities, it is attenuated according to the following exponential relation:

$$I_t = I_o e^{-\int \mu dl} \tag{1}$$

where I_O is the incident intensity, I_t is the transmitted intensity, dl is the differential path length of the beam through the object, and μ is the linear attenuation coefficient of the object along the beam path. These values of μ are determined by the physical density and atomic composition of the object and are dependent on the energy (voltage or wavelength) of the x-ray beam.[35]

In CT, I_O and I_t are measured from many different angles of view by x-ray detectors, and dl is mathematically defined to be arbitrarily small. These measurements give multiple equations in the same unknowns, the individual attenuation coefficients, which are solved by various mathematical approaches called image reconstruction.

This description is idealized relative to the practical situation, because monoenergetic x-ray sources of sufficient intensity to irradiate the body are not available, and photon interaction within the body may alter beam direction, resulting in the detection of scattered as well as directly-transmitted x-rays. However, the latter problem is significantly reduced in CT by appropriate collimation of the x-ray beam at the source and at the detector.

Problems caused by changes in the x-ray spectrum changes during irradiation of an object with a polyenergetic x-ray source (often called "beam hardening")[36, 37] are minimized by mathematical corrections[38, 39] to the measured projection data before image reconstruction. Ideally, the beam attenuation is directly proportional to the thickness of the body traversed by the beam. However, because the x-ray beam is polyenergetic (i.e., possessing a distribution of energies), lower-energy x-rays are preferentially absorbed

CONVENTIONAL RADIOGRAPHY CONVENTIONAL TOMOGRAPHY COMPUTED TOMOGRAPHY

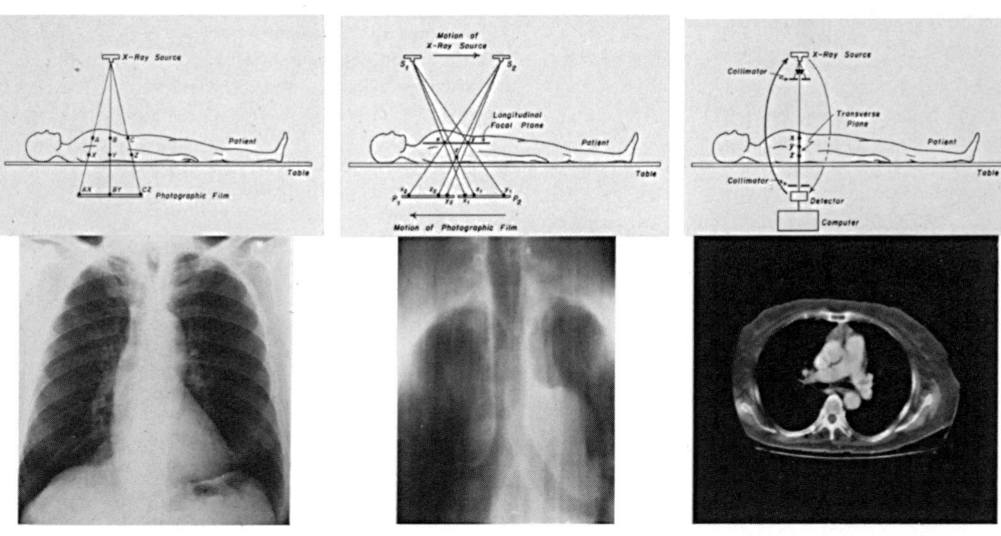

FIGURE 52–1. *Left Panel,* Conventional x-radiographic technique. All points in the path of any ray (e.g., A and X) are projected onto the same point on the film (e.g., AX), resulting in superimposition of structures on the photographic images. This phenomenon is demonstrated in the conventional chest radiograph, on which the ribs, heart, and spine are superimposed on one another, rendering detailed visualization of these separate structures difficult. *Center Panel,* Conventional tomographic technique. X-ray source and detector (film) are moved in opposite directions at appropriate relative speeds so that only points in a longitudinal plane (e.g., X) are projected onto the same points (e.g., $X_1 = X_2$) on the photographic film. The result is that structures within the plane are in sharper focus on the film than structures not within the plane (e.g., point Z). The tracheal tomogram shown illustrates the sharpened features of the trachea, which lie within the focal plan, but structures outside of this plane, whose projections degrade image quality, are also superimposed on the film. *Right Panel,* Computed tomography technique. The x-ray source and detector are collimated to define a beam that passes through only a transverse plane or "slice" of the body and is rotated about the body so that x-ray absorption patterns are recorded from many different directions about the transverse plane. These recordings are used by the computer to accurately determine the correct distribution of attenuation values at all points within the plane. The computed tomographic transverse image of the thorax shows the sternum, heart, spine, and ribs in correct position, permitting visualization of anatomical detail without superimposition of these structures. (From Robb, R.A.: X-ray computed tomography: An engineering synthesis of multi-scientific principles. Crit. Rev. Biomed. Eng. 74:265, 1982, with permission.)

as the beam passes through the object. The continuing x-ray beam is more penetrating because of its increasing average energy, causing the object to appear less dense than if a monoenergetic beam equivalent to the average incident energy of the polyenergetic beam were used. Relative to the average energy in the incident beam, the average energy of the transmitted beam is increased more for longer pathways through the body than for shorter pathways, and thus the relationship of transmitted energy to body thickness becomes nonlinear.

The problem of beam hardening has been well described for x-ray CT,[35–37] with several approaches proposed and implemented to correct it.[38–41] The approach with the first CT scanner[16] was to use a waterbag around the head to serve as a "compensating" filter.[35] The waterbag made all beam path lengths similar, so that beam hardening was made linear. A similar linear correction can be obtained by mathematical processing[39, 40] of the measured transmission data within the computer, eliminating the need for and inconvenience of the waterbag. However, more sophisticated mathematical approaches[38, 41] are required to adequately correct the substantial nonlinear beam hardening caused by dense material within the body, such as compact bones, x-ray contrast agents, or prosthetic implants.

In general, these more exact methods for correction of beam hardening involve an iterative approach to first approximate the distribution and amount of dense material (e.g., bone) in the scan region and then correct the absorption measurements relative to the known (assumed or measured) x-ray energy spectrum before performing the final reconstruction. These procedures increase the computational time required to reconstruct a CT image, but this is usually an acceptable tradeoff for obtaining improved image quality and quantitative accuracy.

Image Reconstruction From Projections

Figure 52–2 diagrammatically illustrates the concept of generating projections of a slice of an object by scanning an x-ray beam and detector across and around the object. Several different schemes and geometries for scanning have been implemented, with various advantages for speed and calibration, as discussed in the next section. Two of these schemes are known as parallel-beam geometry and fan beam geometry. For intuitive simplicity, the parallel scanning geometry scheme, as illustrated in Figure 52–2, is used here to describe the basic mathematical approach to reconstruction. Fan beam geometry can be reduced to parallel-beam geometry,[42] or appropriate geometric calculations can be used to perform fan beam reconstructions directly.[43, 44]

Conventional image reconstruction algorithms require that during data acquisition the x-ray source and detector lie in the same plane as the slice to be reconstructed. X-ray transmission measurements, called projection data, are made at many different discrete positions of the x-ray source and detector relative to the body. The set of projection data collected at each angular setting of the x-ray source and detector is often called a profile or view (the terms projection, profile, and view are used interchangeably). The dis-

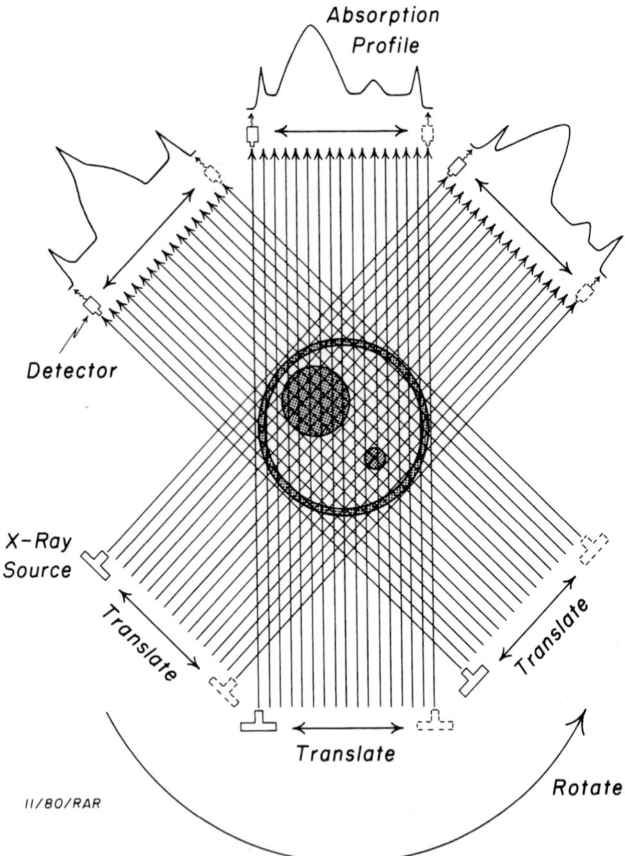

FIGURE 52–2. The procedure for generation of multidimensional x-ray attenuation profiles. The x-ray source and detector are translated across the body as transmitted x-radiation is measured at successive points. These measurements, when divided by (or logarithmically subtracted from) the amount of x-radiation measured incident on the body, can be expressed as profiles of absorption versus position. The amplitude at each point on the absorption profile is proportional to the total absorption along the corresponding ray path through the object. These absorption profiles are recorded for many directions of x-rays passing through the body by incremental rotation of the x-ray source and detector in tandem about the body. (From Robb, R.A.: X-ray computed tomography: An engineering synthesis of multi-scientific principles. Crit. Rev. Biomed. Eng. 74:265, 1982, with permission.)

crete data samples along a projection are called line-integral values or ray sums (the terms profile sample, line-integral value, and ray sum are used interchangeably).

The image reconstruction algorithm implemented on a computer specifies a finite region within the irradiated plane that contains all structures of interest to be reconstructed. Attenuation of the beam outside of this region is assumed to be zero. This planar region is usually bounded by a square or a circle and is partitioned into a matrix (grid) of small, nonoverlapping regions (usually square) called pixels (for picture elements), each of which is assumed to have a uniform x-ray attenuation coefficient. The number and size of pixels is based on the spatial resolution desired in the picture and on the spatial resolution that is practically achievable for a given scanner geometry.[45, 46] Because the detected x-ray beam has finite width, the pixels are really small volume elements (voxels), and the reconstruction plane is really a slice or slab.

The task of the reconstruction algorithm is to geometrically determine the paths of the x-ray beams passing through the voxels of the reconstruction matrix and to mathematically relate the measured ray sums (total attenuation) from many different views to the fractional attenuation by each voxel. The result is a map of the attenuation coefficients within the object that can be displayed as an image by assigning brightness values to each pixel in proportion to the attenuation values determined at each point throughout the matrix.

The value of each pixel in an image is known as the CT number and is given in Hounsfield units (HU):

$$\text{CT number (in HU)} = \frac{\mu_{\text{material}} - \mu_{\text{water}}}{\mu_{\text{water}}} \cdot 1000 \qquad (2)$$

The CT number of a given pixel is defined as the difference between the linear attenuation coefficient of the material represented and that of water normalized to the attenuation coefficient of water. By definition, water has a CT number of 0 HU, air (no attenuation) has a CT number of −1000 HU, and dense bone (highly attenuating) has a large positive CT number. Figure 52–3 details typical CT numbers for a variety of biologic tissues.

The CT number for each pixel is stored digitally and can range in magnitude from −1000 HU to +3000 HU. However, the number of gray scale levels that can be displayed on a cathode ray tube is limited (typically to 8 bits, or 256 levels). Specific CT

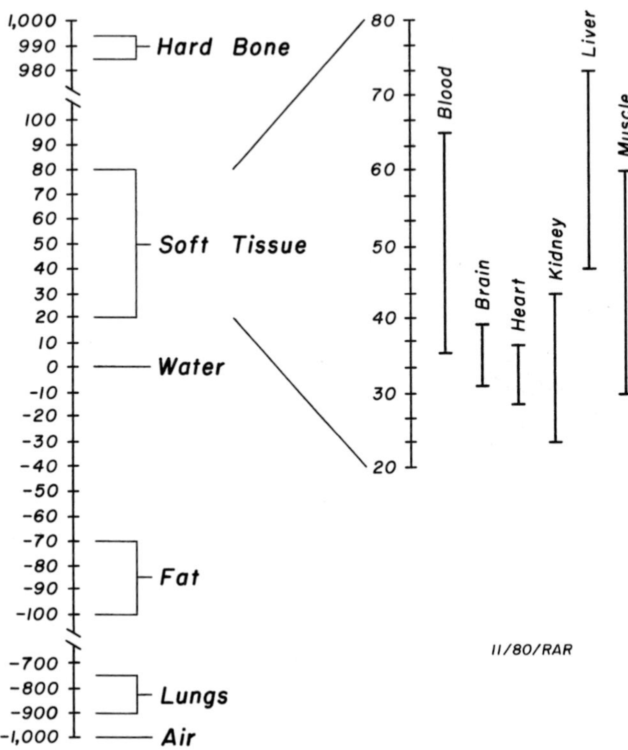

FIGURE 52–3. Typical computed tomographic number scale and values for various body tissues. Values are based on measurements with effective x-ray energy of 72 KeV. The range of values for a given tissue reflects both measurement errors and actual attenuation differences among samples. The data include both in vitro measurements made with monoenergetic sources and in vivo measurements made with actual computed tomography scanners. (From Robb, R.A.: X-ray computed tomography: An engineering synthesis of multi-scientific principles. Crit. Rev. Biomed. Eng. 74:265, 1982, with permission.)

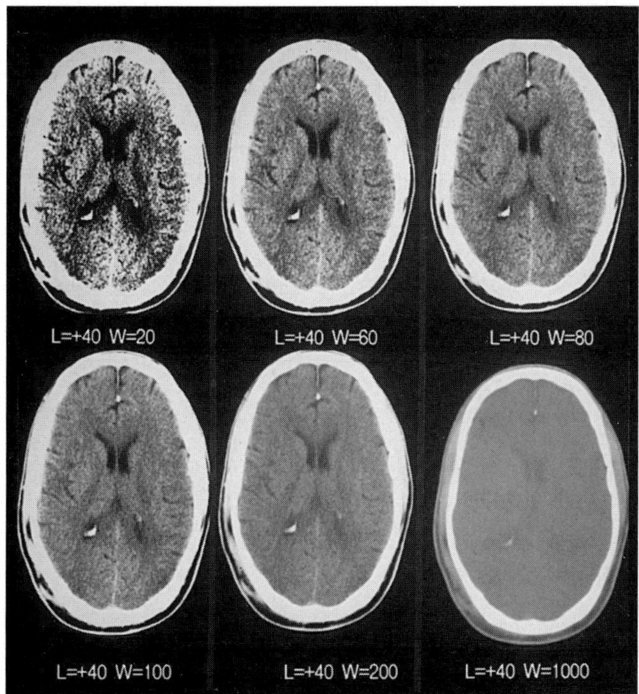

FIGURE 52–4. The same computed tomographic image data set displayed at six different window widths (20, 60, 80, 100, 200, and 1000 HU) and the same window level (40 HU).

numbers within the image must therefore be mapped to a smaller range of gray scale levels for cathode ray tube display. The window width and window level parameters are used to define this transformation. The window width is the total range of CT numbers in the original image to be represented by the various shades of gray on the viewing device; the window level is the center of this range. For example, in an image displayed with a window width of 500 and a window level of 200, CT numbers in the image with values below −50 HU are displayed as completely black, and CT numbers with values above +450 HU are displayed as completely white. Only the CT numbers between the range of −50 to +450 HU are mapped to the available shades of gray on the cathode ray tube display device. Changes in the window width and window level change only the mapping of the digital image data to the display device; they do not change the digital values of the CT numbers themselves. Figure 52–4 shows the same CT data, an image of the brain, displayed at six different window widths, with the same window level in each case.

A wide variety of mathematical approaches to the reconstruction problem have been developed.[13, 47–51] The most common approaches can be classified into one of the following categories: summation methods (e.g., simple backprojection), iterative methods (e.g., algebraic reconstruction technique [ART]), transform methods (e.g., Fourier transform), and direct analytic methods (e.g., filtered backprojection or convolution).

Filtered backprojection is the method most used in commercial x-ray CT scanners for image reconstruction from projections. As the name suggests, it is related to the simple backprojection method, but with an important difference: it corrects the blurring produced when the projections are simply overlapped[49] by appropriate prefiltering of the projection data before the backprojection process. The two basic steps for this method are readily implemented on a computer: filtration (convolution) of the projection data with a function selected to negate the blurring effect of the summation process, and summation (backprojection) of the filtered projections. Filtered backprojection is computationally efficient with parallel processing because projections can be filtered and backprojected independently of each other.

Figure 52–5 shows two examples of commonly used convolution filter functions.[13, 52] The purpose of the "negative side lobes" in each filter is to compensate for the positive side lobes or spokes of the point spread distribution introduced by backprojection. If the filter is carefully chosen, these negative and positive side lobes

TWO CONVOLUTION KERNEL FUNCTIONS USED IN FILTERED BACK PROJECTION METHOD OF IMAGE RECONSTRUCTION

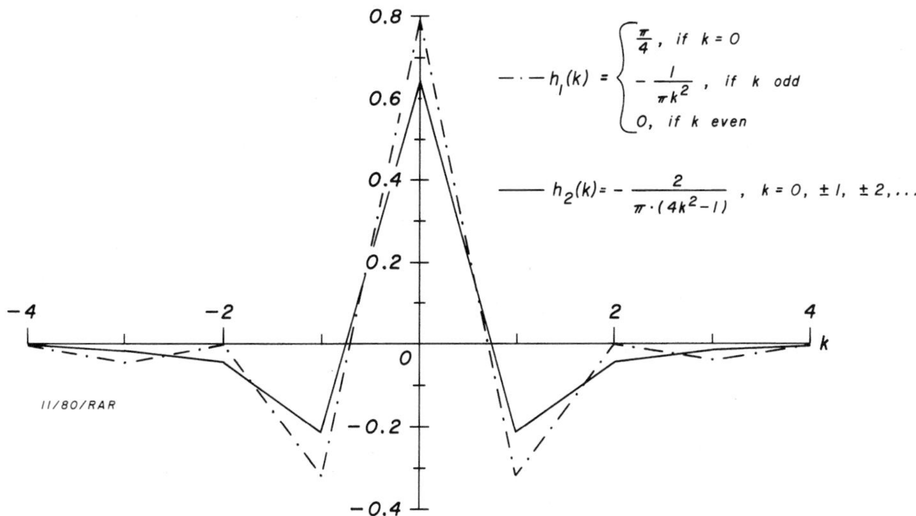

FIGURE 52–5. Two convolution filter functions used in the filtered backprojection method of image reconstruction. The width of $h_1(k)$, often called the Ram-Lak filter, and the width of $h_2(k)$, often called the Shepp-Logan filter, are almost the same for the central lobe, so that image resolution for noiseless data is similar with the use of either filter. However, the side lobes of $h_2(k)$ are more damped, producing greater attenuation of higher frequencies than $h_1(k)$. (From Robb, R.A.: X-ray computed tomography: An engineering synthesis of multi-scientific principles. Crit. Rev. Biomed. Eng. 74:265, 1982, with permission.)

cancel each other when the filtered projections are summed, resulting in an unblurred image of the original object. This result, in effect, is a "deconvolution" of the blurred picture that would be obtained by simple backprojection.[53]

Equipment Design and Performance

X-ray CT scanners are complex, precisely-engineered machines that create noninvasive, clinical diagnostic transaxial images of the body. Many papers and proceedings of workshops have been published[31, 54–58] that provide detailed information regarding the evolution and current status of engineering accomplishments in x-ray CT.

X-ray CT systems include a variety of components, which can be categorized into four major subsystems: the gantry, which includes the x-ray source and collimation assembly (with associated power supplies and cooling systems) and the detector/collimation system (with associated data acquisition electronics); the subject table or "couch"; the reconstruction computer system; and the image display and analysis consoles.

Conventional Computed Tomography

In conventional CT, the x-ray tube, alone or in combination with a detector array, must be rotated about the patient to obtain the necessary projections. This involves the precise movement of large mechanical and electrical devices. Since the introduction of x-ray CT in the early 1970s, the scanning geometry of CT gantries has evolved through four distinct geometries, as illustrated in Figure 52–6. (Alternative geometries are discussed in the section on ultrafast CT systems.) These changes have been motivated primarily by the need for faster scan times, in order to reduce blurring and eliminate streak artifacts caused by biologic motion,[59] and they have resulted in improved detection efficiency, calibration techniques, and image quality.[60]

Until recently, conventional CT scanner designs necessitated a time delay between scans to reverse rotation direction and unwind the high voltage and data acquisition cabling. State-of-the-art conventional CT scanners have eliminated this cabling restriction by the use of slip-ring technology, which allows voltage and data transmission across a circular metal track on which the x-ray tube rotates.[61–63] The tube is able to rotate continuously about the subject, and a 360-degree data acquisition can be acquired in times as short as 0.75 second. The use of continuous table motion during data acquisition further allows continuous spiral (helical) scanning of a patient volume, which is briefly described in the next section.[19–22, 31, 64] Regardless of gantry design, the motion of the gantry is subject to strict mechanical tolerances (e.g., less than 0.1 mm wobble) during scanning to ensure precise alignment of the x-ray source and detectors relative to the body section being imaged.

Typical x-ray tubes in first- and second-generation CT scanners were oil-cooled, fixed-anode, continuous-operation x-ray sources. The x-ray tubes used in current third- and fourth-generation CT scanners operate between 80 to 140 kV peak voltage at up to 200 to 400 mA of tube current. Rotating anodes and sophisticated anode and bearing designs are used to provide very high anode and tube housing heat capacities (3.5 million heat units or more). The emergent photon spectrum is polyenergetic, with an average

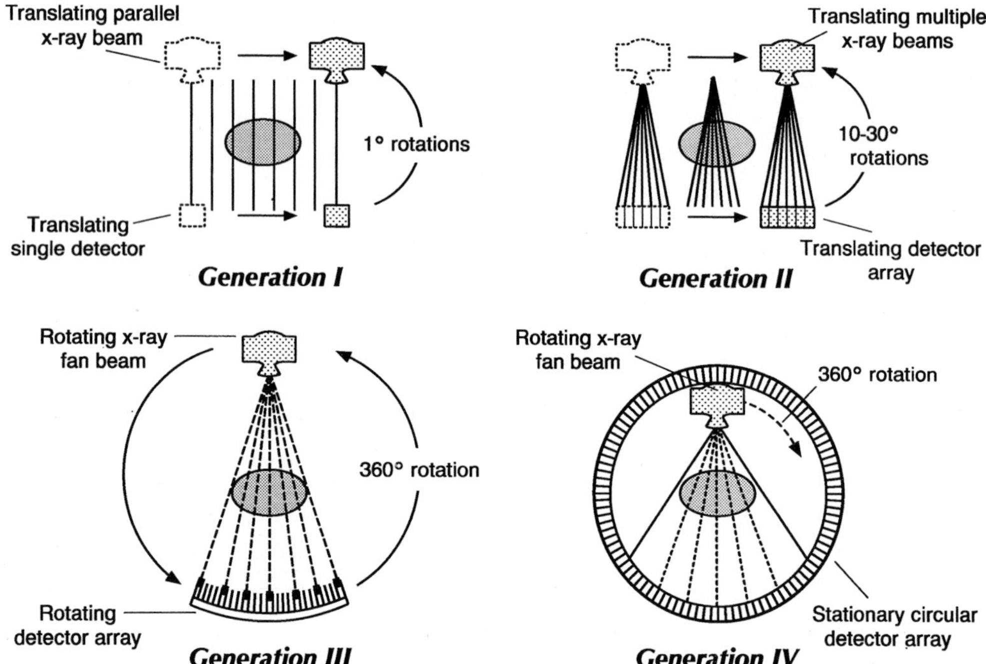

FIGURE 52–6. Diagram of the evolution of computed tomography (CT) scanner geometries. First-generation CT scanners used a pencil beam defined by a well-collimated x-ray source and a single detector. The source and detector were first translated in tandem in a rectilinear pattern, with successive beam measurements parallel to each other. Then, the source and detector are rotated through a small angle, and the rectilinear scan is repeated. This translate-rotate procedure continues for 180 degrees. Second-generation scanners used a small linear array of detectors, instead of a single detector, to speed up data acquisition with the use of fan beam geometry. A translation and rotation of source and detectors were still required. Third-generation systems use a larger array of detectors so that the entire body is subtended by the x-ray fan beam, and the source and detector array are rotated in tandem to obtain the readings for image reconstruction. Fourth-generation systems use a fixed circular array of many detectors and a rotating x-ray source inside (or outside) of the detector ring. In this geometry, each detector position defines the apex of the fan beam as x-rays are recorded from the various source positions. The geometry considerations for image reconstruction are the same, however, as those for third-generation systems, where the source position defines the apex of the fan beam. (From McCollough, C.H., and Morin, R.L.: The technical design and performance of ultrafast computed tomography. Radiol. Clin. North Am. 32:521, 1994, with permission.)

energy of approximately 70 keV.[31] Focal spot sizes, which directly influence the limiting resolution of the system, are typically 0.6 to 1.2 mm in width, with target angles of 15 to 30 degrees.[31, 56] Aluminum filters of at least 2.5 mm thickness (and typically more) are used to preharden the x-ray spectrum. X-ray beam collimation on the source side of the patient restricts the radiation exposure along the longitudinal axis of the scanner so as to irradiate only the scan plane of interest. The beam is also "shaped" to compensate for body size and the dynamic range of the detector. One commonly-used compensating filter is the "bowtie" filter, so called for its characteristic shape. The resulting beam has less intensity at the body periphery and greater intensity at the center of the body.

The detectors used in x-ray CT play a fundamental role in the formation of quality medical images. Important detector characteristics include high detection and geometric efficiencies, short afterglow, stability, and uniformity. Commercially, one of two detector types is used: gas ionization (xenon) detectors or solid-state scintillators. The solid-state detectors are available in two variations: cadmium tungstate crystals or rare earth–doped ceramic compounds. Although each detector type has its own strengths and weaknesses, the industry trend is toward solid-state detectors, in part because of their higher detection efficiency, which results in lower patient doses for comparable image quality.[31]

The size of the detector aperture on x-ray CT scanners ranges from 0.5 to 2.0 mm. This, along with x-ray source focal spot size (0.6 mm to 1.2 mm), defines the reconstruction beam width used for image reconstructions and generally dictates the maximum absolute spatial resolution attainable. In fourth-generation systems, spatial resolution is determined by the frequency of data samples during the continuous rotation of the x-ray source. In such systems, the spatial resolution is a function of the width of the fan beam at the center of the scan region and the number of samples recorded across the fan. Ray spacing can be as small as 0.1 mm. However, this does not necessarily mean that 0.1 mm spatial resolution is produced in a CT system with 0.1 mm sampling precision. Other factors, such as the modulation transfer function of the overall imaging system, the accuracy of analog-to-digital conversion, and the reconstruction algorithm used, also influence spatial resolution.

X-ray beam collimation is performed on the detector side of the subject as well as on the source side. The purpose of detector collimation is to reject scattered radiation, and careful design and alignment of the collimator is critically important to overall image quality. Collimators also help determine the aperture size of the detector. Pixel sizes in the reconstruction matrix may be two, three, or four times smaller than the detector aperture size in order to ensure true aperture resolution and to produce a more aesthetically pleasing effect in the reconstructed image.[60]

The electronic signal from the detector, after appropriate amplification, is converted to digital form by an analog-to-digital converter. To maintain the incident contrast resolution after image reconstruction and to accurately capture the full dynamic range of the detector signal, current CT scanners use up to 22 bits (4×10^6 unique digital levels) in the analog-to-digital conversion.[56]

The Couch

The patient couch is designed to move the subject in and out of the scan plane of the CT gantry. Special devices are often added to facilitate subject positioning, such as a laser beam that illuminates a line on the surface of the body indicating the section of anatomy to be scanned. Angulation of the couch (typically ± 20 degrees) and tilting of the gantry (typically ± 30 degrees) provide the capability for scanning of sections oblique to the long axis of the body. The couch is made of radiotranslucent material so as not to significantly interfere with the transmission of the x-ray beam through the body. To assist in localizing the scan plane to the anatomy of interest, a scanned projection (digital) radiograph can be acquired by moving the couch continuously through the gantry while the x-ray source and detection system acquire data at a fixed angular position. This image, sometimes called a "scout view," facilitates the selection of the range and spacing of the scan levels desired for a particular examination.

The Reconstruction Computer

The computational capabilities of the modern computer have played a major role in the development and maturation of x-ray CT. Images with a total number of pixels ranging from 65,536 (256 × 256) to 262,144 (512 × 512) may be reconstructed from 500,000 to more than 5,000,000 measurements. Current minicomputers, aided by special-purpose, high-speed arithmetic hardware (often called array processors) can perform such reconstructions in seconds. With filtered backprojection, which can be performed during data collection, some systems can have the reconstructed image available in less than 1 second after the scan is finished.

The computer software on most current x-ray CT computer systems permits the user to select one of several different reconstruction parameters, including matrix size, pixel size, and the reconstruction algorithm used (this refers to different convolution or field-of-view filter functions or corrections for such problems as beam hardening). In addition to reconstruction and storage of the images, the computer system also controls the scanning process, including tracking the positions of the x-ray source and detectors, monitoring voltage and tube current, converting detector signals to digital values, and correcting for variations in detector response. Multiple computers may be used within a single CT system to support simultaneous scanning, reconstruction, and display.

The Display and Analysis Console

The display console of a modern x-ray CT system provides a wide variety of operator-interactive image display and analysis capabilities. Images can be displayed with up to 256 gray levels (or colors) on 512 × 512 or 1024 × 1024 screens, with alphanumeric and graphic information displayed on the same screen, either adjacent to or superimposed on the image. Simple keystrokes invoke complex image processing and analysis functions of advanced software programs. Rapidly positioned cursors provide identification of specific points in the image or outlining of desired regions of interest. For these selected regions, mean values, histograms, standard deviations, magnified images, or distance measurements can be obtained. Sagittal and coronal sections can be computed and displayed from a series of transaxial slices stored in the computer memory. The image data is stored on large magnetic discs (usually 1 gigabyte or more of data storage) for rapid retrieval, manipulation, display, and analysis. The data can also be recorded for archival storage on a variety of peripheral storage media (e.g., analog or digital magnetic tape, optical disks or platters). Permanent hard copy records of the CT images can be recorded on film in a variety of sizes and formats by special imaging devices attached to the display console.

Spiral (Helical) Computed Tomography

Spiral CT scanning differs from conventional CT scanning in that data is acquired for a given volume of interest by simultaneously translating the patient couch through the gantry during the x-ray exposure. Instead of traversing concentric circular rings along the longitudinal axis of the patient, the incident x-rays follow a spiral or helical path along the patient's surface. The resulting projection data do not lie in any single transaxial plane, and an interpolation algorithm must be employed to reconstruct an image representative of a given transaxial plane.[21, 22, 24, 30, 31, 64]

To produce high-quality images in x-ray CT, the patient must remain stationary during the data acquisition process. Patient motion can produce both image unsharpness and image artifacts. Motion artifacts occur when the image reconstruction algorithm is presented with an inconsistent data set because the object has moved during the data acquisition.[21, 22] Short scan times are highly desirable to limit motion artifacts. In the case of spiral CT, in which the patient is continuously moved throughout the gantry, motion artifacts (including motion blurring and increased partial volume effects) can be significant. However, appropriate modifications of the original projection data can be applied to minimize these effects. These modifications are made with the use of different interpolation algorithms, which transform the raw data sets (which relate to angled sections of anatomy) into projections corresponding to transaxial slices at specific locations.[20–22, 31, 64]

When spiral CT was first introduced, interpolation of the projection data was accomplished using projections that were separated by one complete rotation of the x-ray tube (360 degrees).[21, 22] This significantly reduced the effect of patient motion (couch translation) but produced significant blurring along the direction of the table motion. Subsequent interpolation algorithms used data points separated by one-half rotation of the x-ray tube (180 degrees) and either a linear or a higher-order interpolation scheme. These 180-degree interpolation algorithms have resulted in a substantial increase in the longitudinal resolution of the reconstructed spiral images and are the current industry standard.[65, 66] Because the projection data for spiral CT is acquired in a continuous manner, scans can be retrospectively reconstructed at any given longitudinal position or spacing. Multiple overlapping transaxial images can be generated from a single data set, and high-quality two- and three-dimensional reformations can be produced from these overlapping images (which are generated without an increase in patient dose).[25, 27, 28, 31, 64]

Since the introduction of spiral CT in the early 1980s, there has been considerable investigation of its advantages for conventional CT applications.[19, 20, 23, 25–31, 64] Commercial spiral CT scanners are now available from all major CT vendors and offer a variety of sophisticated data acquisition and image reconstruction protocols.[64] However, optimal utilization of spiral CT scanning capabilities requires the careful selection of several inter-related technical parameters, including scan collimation, table speed, reconstruction interval, interpolation algorithm, and x-ray technique. In addition, optimal visualization of contrast media requires careful consideration of injection timing and rate.[64]

Finally, the volumetric data acquisition offered by spiral CT provides a significant advantage over conventional CT imaging and is sure to play an important role in the practice of medical diagnostic imaging. However, even the fastest of current spiral scanners offer minimum scan times on the order of 0.75 to 1.0 second and acquire at most two simultaneous anatomical slices.[64] In addition, the continuous x-ray exposure required in spiral scanning, coupled with the high tube currents required for short scan times, places a great demand on conventional x-ray tube technology and, in many instances, can limit the amount of data that can be acquired in a single acquisition. Therefore, although spiral CT will continue to play an important role in CT imaging of the head and body and offers substantial promise for many angiographic applications, its role in cardiac imaging has not been well established.[64]

ULTRAFAST COMPUTED TOMOGRAPHY: THE NEED FOR SPEED

The function and performance of the heart, lungs, and circulatory system are intrinsically related to their motion in three dimensions. Direct simultaneous measurement of the changes in size, shape, and perfusion of the heart and lungs over their entire anatomical extent is required to accurately and comprehensively assess their normal physiologic or pathophysiologic status.[67] Several investigations[68–78] have described the potential use of x-ray CT for dynamic studies of the heart, lungs, and circulation. However, most approaches using conventional CT systems are inadequate for true dynamic structural or functional studies of moving organs, because they either ignore the motion and thereby suffer the inevitable deleterious effects on image resolution or they use gating techniques[72, 74, 75] in an attempt to reduce motion artifacts, which also cause image degradation.

In retrospective gating, the projections at various angles of view are assembled for reconstruction after the scan on the basis of the ECG recorded during the scan. In prospective gating, the scan is performed at preselected points within the cardiac cycle. In both methods, collection of enough angles of view to achieve reasonable resolution in the reconstructed transaxial image requires data acquisition over several cardiac cycles and during several rotations of the x-ray source.

The advantage of retrospective gating is that different sets of projection data can be assembled after the continuous data acquisition to reconstruct the same cross section of the heart at different points within the cardiac cycle. The advantage of prospective gating is the reduced dose to the patient; x-ray exposure is required only during the portion of the cardiac cycle that is of interest during successive heartbeats. However, even though these cardiac gating techniques may provide improved CT images of regions of the body that are contiguous to the heart (and therefore subject to displacement by its motion), both techniques suffer a serious disadvantage for CT imaging of the heart itself. This is because ECG-gated scanning requires that there be physiologic stationarity—that is, exact reproducibility of the position of the thorax and the intrathoracic position, shape, dimensions, and contrast opacification of the heart during the several heartbeats required for the scan, and that the heart rate, function, and position of the heart be independent of respiratory effects. These conditions are usually not true for extended periods of time, even in the presence of cardiac pacing. This represents a difficult paradox for gated scanning of the heart: to improve resolution in the CT images, more views must be collected, which means that more heartbeats need to be used, which in turn may degrade resolution because of the lack of physiologic stationarity.

Further, gated scanning cannot be used for angiographic imaging of vascular anatomy or circulatory function, because the transient distribution pattern and concentration of the contrast medium during and after its injection varies in a continuous and nonreproducible manner. Moreover, the pharmacologic effect of the contrast medium alters the hemodynamic and cardiodynamic status considerably, so that beat-to-beat constancy of the heart cannot be achieved during or for a considerable period after the injection of contrast materials.

The capability to measure cardiac, pulmonary, and circulatory dynamics using x-ray CT required the development of high-temporal-resolution, three-dimensional imaging systems. Two different approaches have been developed and are often referred to as "ultrafast" CT: electron-beam CT (EBCT) a commercially available x-ray CT scanner originally developed at the University of California, San Francisco, and the dynamic spatial reconstructor (DSR), a biomedical research system developed at the Mayo Clinic.

Electron-Beam Computed Tomography

The progression of conventional CT scanner geometries and the introduction of slip-ring technology have allowed scan times for a single slice to drop dramatically (Fig. 52–7). However, acquisition times on the order of one tenth of a second (or less) are necessary to avoid image artifacts caused by patient or involuntary organ motion, particularly those involving the heart. EBCT was developed by Boyd and associates during the early 1980s in an effort to produce a CT scanner capable of imaging cardiac structures with adequate temporal and spatial resolution.[79–81] The EBCT technology has been described using a variety of terms, including scanning-electron-beam CT, ultrafast CT, cine-CT, and fifth-generation CT. The term EBCT is used throughout this discussion. An additional goal for the EBCT scanner was to obtain near-simultaneous images at multiple anatomical levels, for example, to scan the entire left ventricle without moving the patient table. To obtain such subsecond scan times, the EBCT design eliminated the mechanical movement of both the x-ray source and the detector array. The details of the design are presented in the following section. Figure 52–8 provides two cross-sectional views of an EBCT scanner.

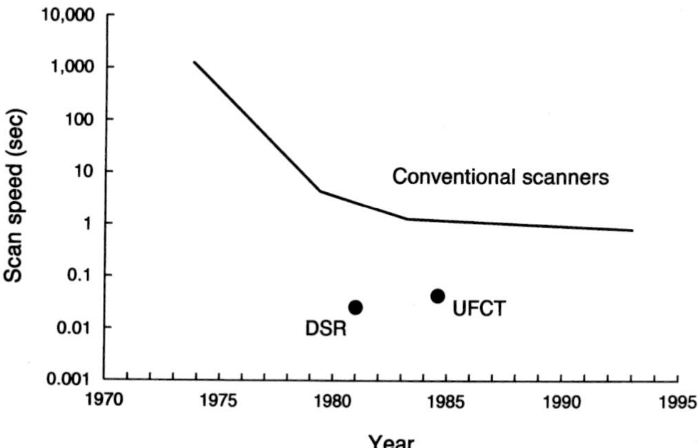

FIGURE 52-7. Since the inception of x-ray computed tomography (CT) in the early 1970s, the time required to image one transaxial slice has decreased dramatically. State-of-the-art conventional CT scanners can now acquire one image slice in as little as 0.75 second (360-degree data acquisition). Two unique CT devices, the Dynamic Spatial Reconstructor (DSR) and the ultrafast computed tomography (UFCT) scanner, provide an order of magnitude reduction in scan acquisition time, which is necessary for cross-sectional imaging of rapidly moving organs such as the heart. (From McCollough, C.H., and Morin, R.L.: The technical design and performance of ultrafast computed tomography. Radiol. Clin. North Am. 32:521, 1994, with permission.)

X-Ray Production

In conventional CT systems, bremsstrahlung x-rays are produced when energetic electrons are decelerated by striking a tungsten target. In EBCT, bremsstrahlung x-rays are also produced by deceleration of energetic electrons in a tungsten target. However, the distance between the source of electrons (cathode) and the point of x-ray production (target anode) is on the order of several meters. The moving source of x-rays is produced by steering an electron beam (600 to 650 mA) around a semicircular tungsten target. The 210-degree target ring is centered below the patient at a radius of 90 cm from scanner isocenter. The voltage difference between the electron gun (ground) and the tungsten target (positive potential) is 130,000 V. The electromagnetic deflection system used to control the path of the electron beam must precisely steer the beam onto the target in a consistent manner. The high-voltage supply must operate within 0.1 percent of the nominal voltage. The prehardening of the x-ray beam spectrum is also considerably greater for EBCT scanners (10.5 mm aluminum half-value-layer) compared with conventional CT scanners (4 to 7 mm aluminum half-value-layer).

At the energies used in diagnostic imaging, only about 1 percent of the energy from the electron beam is converted to x-rays; the remainder produces heat in the target and surrounding tube housing. In EBCT, the massive size of the tungsten target ring distributes the heat produced by the electron beam over a large area, and a direct-contact water cooling system behind the target rings removes heat quickly from the target assembly, allowing the rapid acquisition of many scans without overheating of the tungsten target rings. The EBCT scanner is also equipped with four target rings, which further distribute the heat delivered to the targets. This is a substantial benefit over conventional CT, in which volume scanning can be limited by tube-heating constraints.

X-Ray Detection

A stationary detector ring is centered above the patient and forms a 216-degree arc opposite the target ring. The radius from isocenter is 67.5 cm, so a portion of the detector ring lies between the target ring and the patient. This overlap requires that the two rings be placed in slightly different planes to allow the x-ray source to pass uninhibited through the patient on its way to the detector ring. This geometric configuration limits the amount of z-axis collimation that can be employed and results in a cone-shaped x-ray beam.

The EBCT scanner uses cadmium tungstate detectors that are optically coupled to silicone photodiodes. These solid-state detectors are extremely efficient and have rapid decay times such that the signal quickly returns to baseline after each exposure. These detectors are well suited for short scan times. The detector ring is composed of two detector arrays, one having 432 detector elements and the other having 864 detector elements. The combination of two detector arrays and four x-ray source positions allows eight anatomical levels to be scanned without movement of the patient table. This mode of operation is referred to as the multislice or cardiac mode. Both detector rings can be used for cardiac imaging with any combination of the four target rings. In this mode, the signal from two elements of the high-density ring are summed, so that it effectively also has 432 elements.

In CT, spatial resolution is in part determined by the physical size of the detector elements. The high-density (864-element) detector ring is referred to as the high-resolution detector ring and is used for conventional (radiology) CT applications requiring a 512 × 512 pixel matrix. The high-resolution scan mode uses an additional collimator ring surrounding the patient to restrict the x-ray beam to the high-resolution detector. In this single-slice mode, only one x-ray target and the high-density detector ring are used.

Data Handling

The rapid scan speeds and multiple-level acquisition capabilities produce an enormous volume of data in a very short time and therefore require a very fast data acquisition system. Preamplifiers directly coupled to each detector element amplify and scale the detector signal, which is then converted into digital values by an

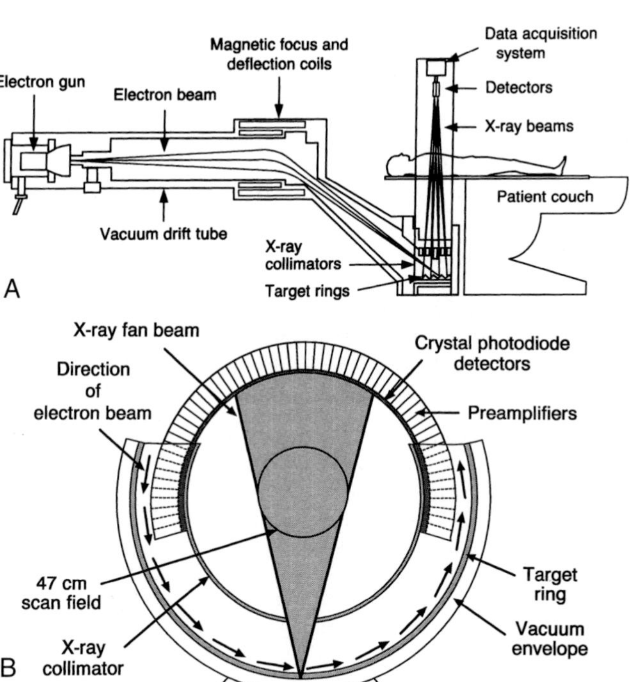

FIGURE 52-8. Illustration of an electron beam computed tomography scanner. *A,* This side view emphasizes the distance between the electron gun and the tungsten target rings. Magnetic coils focus and steer the electron beam through the evacuated drift tube. *B,* This cross-sectional view of the gantry is seen from the perspective of the incoming electron beam. The electrons strike the tungsten target at the upper left and are circularly scanned over 210 degrees. An opposing detector array acquires patient transmission information as the 30-degree fan beam rotates about the lower half of the scan circle. (From McCollough, C.H., and Morin, R.L.: The technical design and performance of ultrafast computed tomography. Radiol. Clin. North Am. 32:521, 1994, with permission.)

analog-to-digital converter at the rate of 14.4 megabytes per second. The raw digital data is transferred by fiberoptic connections to the solid-state memory, which acts as a temporary storage area. This scan cache memory can accommodate the data from as many as 160 scans in multislice mode or 63 scans in single-slice mode.

Image Reconstruction

Image reconstruction is performed by a filtered backprojection technique similar to that used in conventional CT scanners. The system computer allows image reconstruction to be prioritized by the user (e.g., the user may wish to view the first, middle, and last scans of a large sequence before reconstructing the remainder of the images). Reconstruction of a 512 × 512 matrix image requires approximately 12 seconds on the C-100, C-150, C-150L (Imatron Inc., South San Francisco, California) and Evolution (Siemens Medical Systems, Iselin, New Jersey) models. The newest model (Evolution XP, Siemens) offers parallel data processing to yield an average reconstruction rate of 3.5 seconds per image. A reconstruction algorithm that compensates for the cone-beam geometry is available but requires overlapping scans (which doubles the dose) and longer reconstruction times.

Image Processing and Display

The reconstruction process results in a matrix of digital values, each representing the attenuation properties corresponding to a specific volume element, or voxel, of anatomy. Matrix sizes of 256 × 256, 360 × 360, or 512 × 512 can be used. The CT number for each pixel is stored digitally and can range in magnitude from −1000 to +3000 HU. As with conventional CT, the number of gray scale levels that can be displayed on a cathode ray tube viewing device is limited, so specific values within the image must be mapped to a smaller range of gray scale levels for CRT display. The window width and window level parameters are used to define this transformation.

As in conventional CT, the digital nature of the data provides the user with the opportunity to perform quantitative analysis or postprocessing of the original image. Specific regions of anatomy can be outlined with digital cursors and an area or volume calculated. Distance measurements along a line, a plot of CT number versus distance, mean and standard deviation calculations, and multiplanar reformations are all possible with the use of digital data and appropriate software tools. However, the user interface, image review and filming tools, and speed of both the physician and operator consoles are limited by the outdated computer system (LSI 11/23 hardware running under an RT-11 operating system). Because EBCT scanners can scan large volumes of anatomy in relatively short times (less than 1 minute), the data is well suited for CT angiographic applications.

Because of the increased temporal resolution of EBCT compared with conventional CT, quantitative analysis of the image data is useful for a variety of clinical applications, particularly for those applications involving cardiovascular anatomy.[82] The area of the left ventricle can be estimated at different scan levels throughout the cardiac cycle, and these area measurements can be summed to determine end-diastolic and end-systolic volumes, ejection fractions, and stroke volumes. The rate of contrast enhancement of tissue can be measured to estimate myocardial perfusion, or the transit time of a contrast bolus can be estimated. Time-density analysis can be performed using both gamma-variate and bimodal curve fitting routines. Software tools to perform many of these postprocessing functions are available on the scanner's physician console.

Modes of Operation

Single-Slice Mode

The single-slice mode of operation uses one of the four tungsten targets and the high-resolution (864-element) detector ring in conjunction with additional collimation to yield image scan widths of 1.5, 3, or 6 mm. A 10-mm scan width can be obtained by using the 6-mm collimator and moving the table during the scan acquisition. In the single-slice mode, each sweep of the target ring occurs in 100-msec (0.1 second). Successive 100-msec sweeps of the target ring can be integrated to provide higher radiation exposures, thus decreasing image noise. A 16-msec delay between consecutive 100-msec scans is needed, so the maximum scan rate is 9 scans per second. Multiple 100-msec scans are averaged before image reconstruction so that the integration of additional scans does not increase reconstruction time. The maximum cumulative scan time is 2.0 seconds.

Multislice Mode

In the multislice mode of operation, the four tungsten target rings and two detector arrays can be used to acquire two, four, six, or eight slices without movement of the patient table. The data from two consecutive detector elements of the high-density ring are summed to provide 432 effective detector elements to match the low-density array. Each traverse of the target ring by the electron beam occurs in 50 msec (0.05 second) and produces an image for each of the two detector rings. Thus, scans at two independent levels can be acquired in 50 msec. An 8-msec delay exists between subsequent sweeps of the same or another target ring, allowing an 8-cm volume to be imaged in just under one quarter of a second (224 msec).

Acquisition Sequences

In both the single-slice and multislice acquisition modes, the rapid scan acquisition times can be used in a variety of ways, depending on the clinical application. Four different data acquisition protocols can be employed and are referred to as the movie, flow, step-volume, and continuous-volume scanning modes.

In the movie mode, the first scan is triggered either manually or at a specific point of the cardiac cycle, and subsequent scans of the same target are acquired continuously at the highest scan rate available. Consecutive images are acquired at very short time intervals such that playback of the image data displays the motion of the anatomical region of interest. In cardiac imaging, the scan is typically initiated at the R wave of the ECG signal, and one target is scanned at the maximum rate throughout the entire cardiac cycle. At subsequent R waves, the sequence is repeated for each of the remaining targets. In this manner, the entire left ventricle is imaged throughout the cardiac cycle within several heartbeats.

In the flow mode, the first scan is initiated manually, and subsequent images of the same level or levels are collected at regular intervals. Alternatively, the first scan can be initiated at a particular point in the cardiac cycle and subsequent images of the same levels collected at the same point in the cardiac cycle. At playback, a given level is displayed at the same point in the cardiac cycle over several seconds. This scan sequence is used to track the characteristics of flowing contrast media through vascular anatomy or to note changes in anatomy at a specific point in the cardiac cycle over many heartbeats. The difference between the movie and flow acquisition modes is demonstrated in Figure 52–9.

Finally, the use of table movement allows acquisition of a volume of data in a very short time. In the single-slice mode, this acquisition sequence acquires cross-sectional images at various levels throughout a volume of anatomy in a manner that is completely analogous to the operation of conventional CT. Contiguous scans are acquired when the table increment equals the image scan width. Alternatively, gaps between scans occur when the table increment is greater than the image scan width. In the single-slice step-volume mode, the table is moved in discrete steps between scan acquisitions, imposing an interscan delay on the order of 1 second. In step-volume mode, 40 contiguous 6-mm scans (400 msec exposure) of the chest or abdomen can be acquired in 52 seconds. For shorter exposures (100 msec), the time required to scan 40 contiguous scans drops to only 38 seconds. A factor of 4 reduction in overall acquisition time is not realized when the exposure time is reduced by a factor of 4 because the primary time constraint is the table motion and not the scan time.

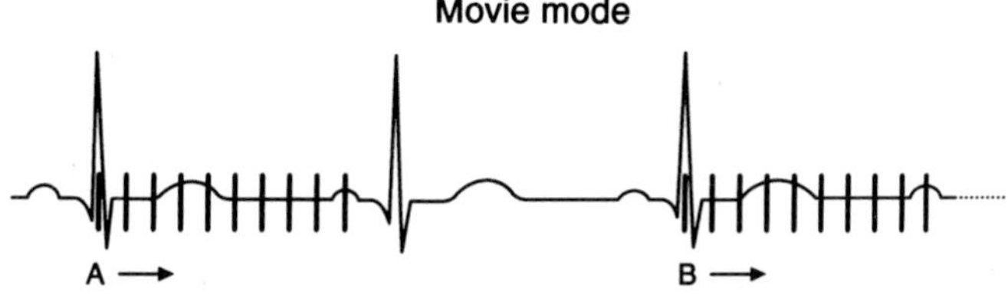

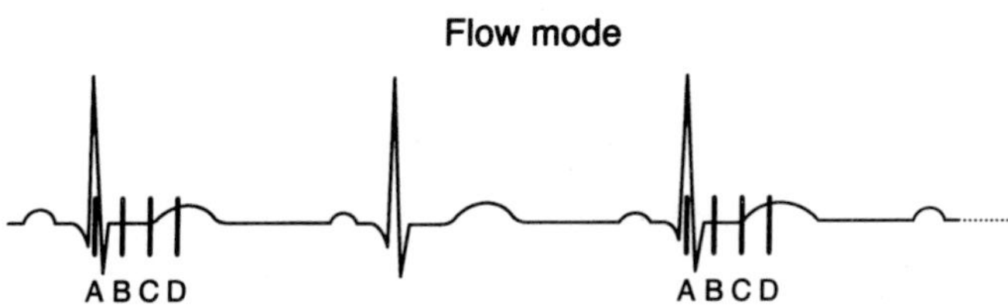

FIGURE 52–9. Both the movie and the flow modes of data acquisition are illustrated. In the movie mode, scans are produced throughout the cardiac cycle, beginning at the R wave, one target at a time. Thus, images are produced throughout the cardiac cycle at two levels of anatomy. Often, one heartbeat transpires while the high-voltage system is reset and the sequence is repeated on subsequent targets. Within seven heartbeats, multiple images for each of eight levels can be acquired. In the flow mode, each target is scanned in quick succession, beginning with the R wave. A heartbeat often transpires during the recovery of the high-voltage system, and the sequence is repeated. In this manner, eight levels of the heart are imaged at a specific point in the cardiac cycle over many heartbeats. (From McCollough, C.H., and Morin, R.L.: The technical design and performance of ultrafast computed tomography. Radiol. Clin. North Am. 32:521, 1994, with permission.)

In order to further reduce the acquisition time for volume scanning, the table is moved continuously during data acquisition. This mode is referred to as the continuous-volume scanning mode. The continuous-volume scanning mode is analogous to spiral (helical) CT in that the table is in constant motion during data acquisition. In spiral CT, the patient table usually moves a distance of one to two times the scan width during one scan. Interpolation algorithms are used before image reconstruction to modify the projection data so that they correspond to a single z-axis position. In the continuous-volume scanning mode of EBCT, the table moves a distance of approximately 0.3 times the scan width during the extremely short scan time (100 msec). Each individual 100-msec scan is essentially free from motion artifact, and interpolation algorithms are not needed before image reconstruction. To reduce image noise for body imaging applications, three or four 100-msec scans are typically averaged. Averaging of several scans from different discrete locations can produce a stroboscopic motion artifact (see the section on temporal resolution). When multiple continuous-volume scanning mode scans are averaged, the slice sensitivity profile is wider than that obtained with the step-volume acquisition mode.

Nonorthogonal image planes can be acquired in EBCT by tilting the patient table (because of the scanner design, the gantry cannot be tilted). Table tilt (up-down angulation) and slew (left-right angulation) are often combined in cardiac examinations to obtain short- and long-axis views of the left ventricle.

Performance Characteristics

In EBCT, the peak voltage and current are fixed at 130 kV and 600 to 650 mA, respectively. To specify the x-ray technique, one need know only the exposure time, scan width, and acquisition mode (multislice or single-slice). EBCT can be used in the same manner as conventional CT for examinations of the chest, abdomen, and pelvis. The very short scan times are beneficial in reducing overall examination time and in reducing the amount of motion artifact caused by patient or involuntary organ motion. The use of EBCT in pediatric and trauma examinations is particularly advantageous. A direct comparison of image quality and dose between EBCT and conventional CT scanners can be made for conventional body CT applications; however, direct comparison to conventional CT equipment is not possible for the variety of cardiac imaging applications available only with EBCT.

EBCT body examinations are typically performed in the single-slice mode, using a 6-mm scan width and a 0.4 second exposure (which is the average of four 100-msec exposures). Studies of the coronary arteries for the detection of calcified lesions require high temporal and spatial resolution and thin scan widths. For this application, the single-slice mode with a 3-mm scan width and 100-msec exposure is used. Examinations used to determine the anatomy and function of cardiac structures are performed in the multislice mode with 50-msec exposures. The scan width in this mode is nominally 8 mm. The following sections provide quantitative measures of dose and image quality for each of these three clinical applications and comparisons to conventional CT performance, if applicable.[83]

Radiation Dose

A CT study usually consists of multiple scans through the anatomy of interest using a prescribed scan width at a prescribed interval. The radiation dose to a specific location is delivered by the scan positioned at that location and by neighboring scans. Averaged over one scan interval, this dose is known as the multiple-scan average dose (MSAD). Because the tails of the dose profile extend several millimeters beyond the image scan width, in a multiple-scan examination there is some overlap of radiation dose profiles and the value of the MSAD exceeds the peak radiation dose from a single scan, often by a factor of 2 or 3.[84, 85]

A quantity known as the CT dose index (CTDI) allows estimation of the MSAD based on a single ionization chamber measurement.[85, 86] The CTDI is the exposure from a single scan integrated along the axial direction and divided by the nominal scan width. If the scan interval equals the scan width, the MSAD equals the CTDI; otherwise, it is equal to the ratio of the scan width to the scan interval times the CTDI.

In practice, the integrated exposure is conveniently measured using a CT (pencil) ionization chamber, which has a length of 10 cm. However, if the radiation dose profile from a single scan extends beyond the chamber length, the CTDI will underestimate the MSAD. This is the case for EBCT systems, where the radiation dose profiles have extensive "tails" and can be substantially broader than the nominal scan width (Fig. 52–10).[87, 88] The 3-mm single-slice mode is the only mode for which the full-width at half-maximum (FWHM) of the radiation dose profile is approximately equal to the nominal scan width. In the 6-mm single-slice mode, the FWHM of the radiation profile is about 10 mm at the 6:00 position and about 30 mm at the center of the phantom; thus, a substantial amount of radiation is not utilized in the image formation process. This is also the case in the multislice mode, where the FWHM of the radiation profiles from an individual target range from 21 to 26 mm but only 16 mm of anatomy is represented in the image data. This extraneous radiation outside of the imaging volume is caused by collimation restrictions imposed by the cone-beam geometry and makes the scanner less dose-efficient than those employing conventional x-ray sources and geometries.

The CTDI values provided by CT scanner manufacturers use the Center for Devices and Radiologic Health integration limits (14 times the nominal scan width), which may or may not equal the length of the ionization chamber. They also use the exposure-to-dose conversion for acrylic (0.78 rad/R) instead of that for muscle or water (0.94 or 0.98 rad/R, respectively). Thus, the manufacturer's CTDI values tend to underestimate the actual doses delivered to patients, particularly in the case of narrow scan widths. The magnitude of the error depends on the shape of the radiation dose profile, but it is at least 20 percent owing to the use of the acrylic conversion factor.

In the single-slice mode of operation, calculating the MSAD using the ionization chamber CTDI underestimates the MSAD by 15 to 32 percent.[87] The unique clinical use of the multislice mode,

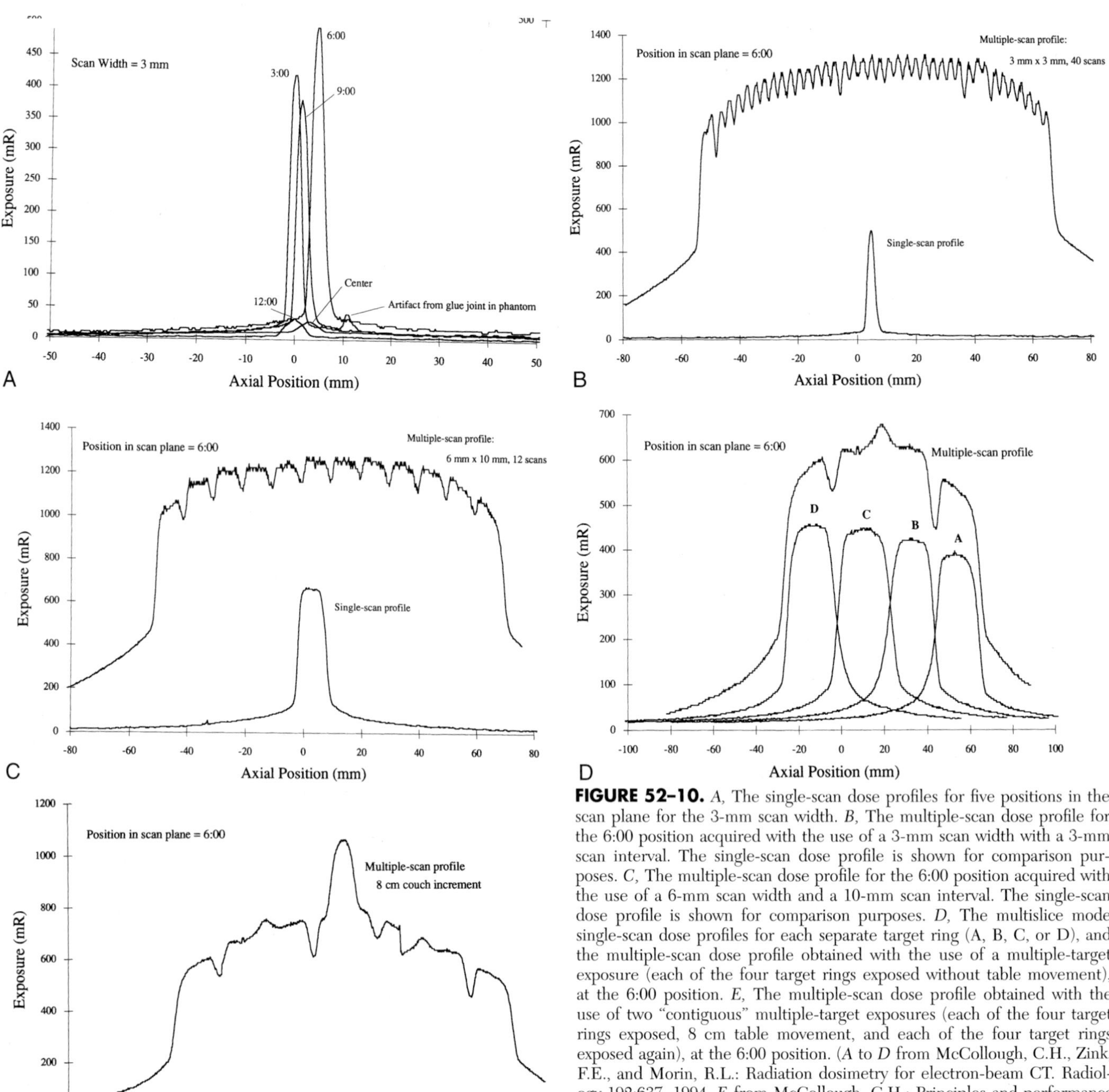

FIGURE 52–10. *A*, The single-scan dose profiles for five positions in the scan plane for the 3-mm scan width. *B*, The multiple-scan dose profile for the 6:00 position acquired with the use of a 3-mm scan width with a 3-mm scan interval. The single-scan dose profile is shown for comparison purposes. *C*, The multiple-scan dose profile for the 6:00 position acquired with the use of a 6-mm scan width and a 10-mm scan interval. The single-scan dose profile is shown for comparison purposes. *D*, The multislice mode single-scan dose profiles for each separate target ring (A, B, C, or D), and the multiple-scan dose profile obtained with the use of a multiple-target exposure (each of the four target rings exposed without table movement), at the 6:00 position. *E*, The multiple-scan dose profile obtained with the use of two "contiguous" multiple-target exposures (each of the four target rings exposed, 8 cm table movement, and each of the four target rings exposed again), at the 6:00 position. (*A* to *D* from McCollough, C.H., Zink, F.E., and Morin, R.L.: Radiation dosimetry for electron-beam CT. Radiology 192:637, 1994. *E* from McCollough, C.H.: Principles and performance of electron-beam CT. *In* Goldman, L.W., and Fowlkes, J.B. [eds.]: Medical CT and Ultrasound: Current Technology and Applications. Madison, WI, Advanced Medical Publishing, 1995, p. 422.)

in which multiple-scan exposures are performed without table movement, makes the MSAD dose descriptor difficult to apply. The ionization chamber CTDI (for a single target) overestimates the MSAD by 25 to 50 percent in the multislice mode (no table increment).[87] Occasionally, additional levels of anatomy are imaged in the multislice mode after incremental 8-cm movement of the patient couch. For this case, superposition of the measured MSAD multiple-scan profiles produces a very nonuniform profile, with a maximum and average exposure (over the 16-cm imaged volume) at the 6:00 position of about 1100 mR and about 700 mR, respectively. With an 8-cm table increment, the ionization chamber CTDI (for a single target) overestimates the MSAD by 7 to 29 percent in the multislice mode.[87] In addition, eight levels of anatomy are often imaged multiple times throughout the cardiac cycle, thereby increasing the patient dose by the number of multiple exposures.

Table 52–1 provides CTDI and MSAD values for a variety of EBCT clinical applications, as well as a comparison to conventional CT scanners, where applicable. The MSAD values shown in Table 52–1 for EBCT were determined with the use of film dosimetry techniques.[87, 88]

The data in Figure 52–10 illustrate the nonuniform dose distribution within a CTDI phantom caused by the partial (210-degree) irradiation of the subject. The maximum dose (100 percent) is delivered to the posterior surface of a supine patient (6:00 position), and the minimum dose (15 percent) is delivered to the anterior surface (12:00 position). The dose to the center of the patient is approximately 25 to 30 percent of the dose to the 6:00 position. This dose distribution differs significantly from that of conventional CT, as demonstrated in Figure 52–11. For anatomy with less attenuation than the CTDI phantom (such as within the

TABLE 52–1. RADIATION DOSE

Scanner/Mode	Scan Width (mm)	Scan Interval (mm)	Time (sec)	Body CTDI* (rad)	MSAD† (rad)
Adult Body Examinations					
Imatron C-100/SS (130 kVp, 250 mAs)	6	6	0.4	6.9	8.4
Imatron C-100/SS (130 kVp, 250 mAs)	6	10	0.4	6.9	5.0
Picker PQ2000§ (120 kVp, 200 mAs)	10	10	1.0	2.9	2.9
GE HiSpeed Advantage‖ (120 kVp, 280 mAs)	10	10	1.0	1.6	1.6
Cardiac Examinations					
Imatron C-100/SS (130 kVp, 62.5 mAs)	3	3	0.1	1.0	1.2
Imatron C-100/MS (130 kVp, 31.3 mAs)	8	—	0.05	≈0.9	0.6
Imatron C-100/MS (130 kVp, 31.3 mAs)	8	80	0.05	≈0.9	0.7

kVp = peak kilovoltage; mAs = tube current × time in milliamperes • seconds; SS = single slice; MS = multislice.
*Radiation absorbed dose to water (0.984 rad/R) at 6:00 position, measured with ionization chamber.
†MSAD = CTDI • scan width/scan interval; EBCT data from McCollough, C. H., Zink, F. E., and Morin, R. L.: Radiation dosimetry for electron-beam CT. Radiology 192:637, 1994.
Imatron, South San Francisco, CA; Picker International, Cleveland, OH; General Electric Medical Systems, Milwaukee, WI.

chest), the dose to the anterior surface of a supine patient is higher. The average breast dose for a single-slice multiple-scan examination using EBCT is about 25 percent of the dose delivered to the posterior surface of a supine patient.[89]

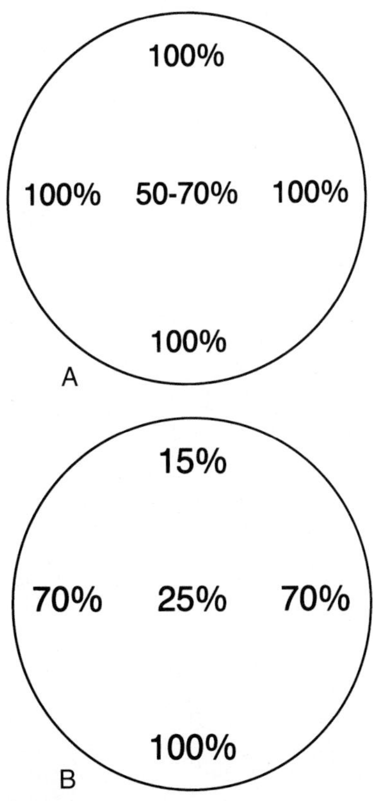

FIGURE 52–11. Radiation dose distribution within a circular acrylic phantom 32 cm in diameter. *A,* In conventional computed tomography (CT), the maximal radiation dose is imparted to the periphery of a circular object and is uniform about the periphery. *B,* In electron-beam CT, the maximal radiation dose is imparted to the edge of the object closest to the radiation source (tungsten targets). The radiation dose decreases substantially toward the top of the object and is symmetrical from left to right. (*A* from McCollough, C.H., and Morin, R.L.: The technical design and performance of ultrafast computed tomography. Radiol. Clin. North Am. 32:521, 1994; *B* from McCollough, C.H.: Principles and performance of electron-beam CT. *In* Goldman, L.W., and Fowlkes, J.B. [eds.]: Medical CT and Ultrasound: Current Technology and Applications. Madison, WI, Advanced Medical Publishing, 1995, p. 424, with permission.)

Temporal Resolution

To freeze anatomical motion, a very short exposure time is required. Because the radiation exposure entering and exiting the patient scales linearly with the exposure time, short exposures result in a decrease in the number of photons measured by the detectors. This results in an increase in image noise levels. Thus, a tradeoff between image noise (which affects contrast resolution) and temporal resolution (which can affect spatial resolution) is necessary, and the choice depends on the specific clinical application. The relation between radiation dose and temporal resolution is demonstrated in Figure 52–12.

High-Contrast (Spatial) Resolution

One method of characterizing the spatial resolution of a scanner is to examine the limiting high-contrast resolution, defined as the highest spatial frequency that is resolvable. Limiting resolution is typically measured by examining a phantom with line-pair patterns of varying spatial frequency to determine which spatial frequency is "just resolvable." Table 52–2 details the spatial resolution of both EBCT and conventional scanners. Images of a spatial resolution phantom for the 6-mm single-slice, 3-mm single-slice, and 8-mm multislice modes are shown in Figure 52–13.

The significant reduction in spatial resolution in the multislice mode compared with the single-slice mode results from the fact that the detector aperture is doubled (432 detector elements are used to span the 216-degree detector ring in the multislice mode, and 864 detector elements are used in the single-slice mode). In either single-slice or multislice mode, the limiting spatial resolution of the EBCT scanner is reduced slightly at very short exposure times because of increased image noise (Fig. 52–14). This effect is of little clinical relevance for rapidly moving objects, because increasing the exposure time provides only a small increase in spatial resolution, but it may decrease the visibility of small objects as a result of motion artifacts.

Low-Contrast Resolution

The low-contrast resolution of an imaging system represents the ability of the device to image objects of very low contrast (i.e., when the CT number of an object differs by only a small amount from that of the surrounding background material). To measure low-contrast resolution, (0.6 percent) objects of varying sizes are embedded in a phantom and imaged. The low-contrast resolution is defined as the diameter of the smallest low-contrast object visualized. Table 52–3 gives data for both conventional and EBCT systems.

The statistical fluctuation of CT numbers in the image of a uniform object (noise) depends on radiation exposure and strongly

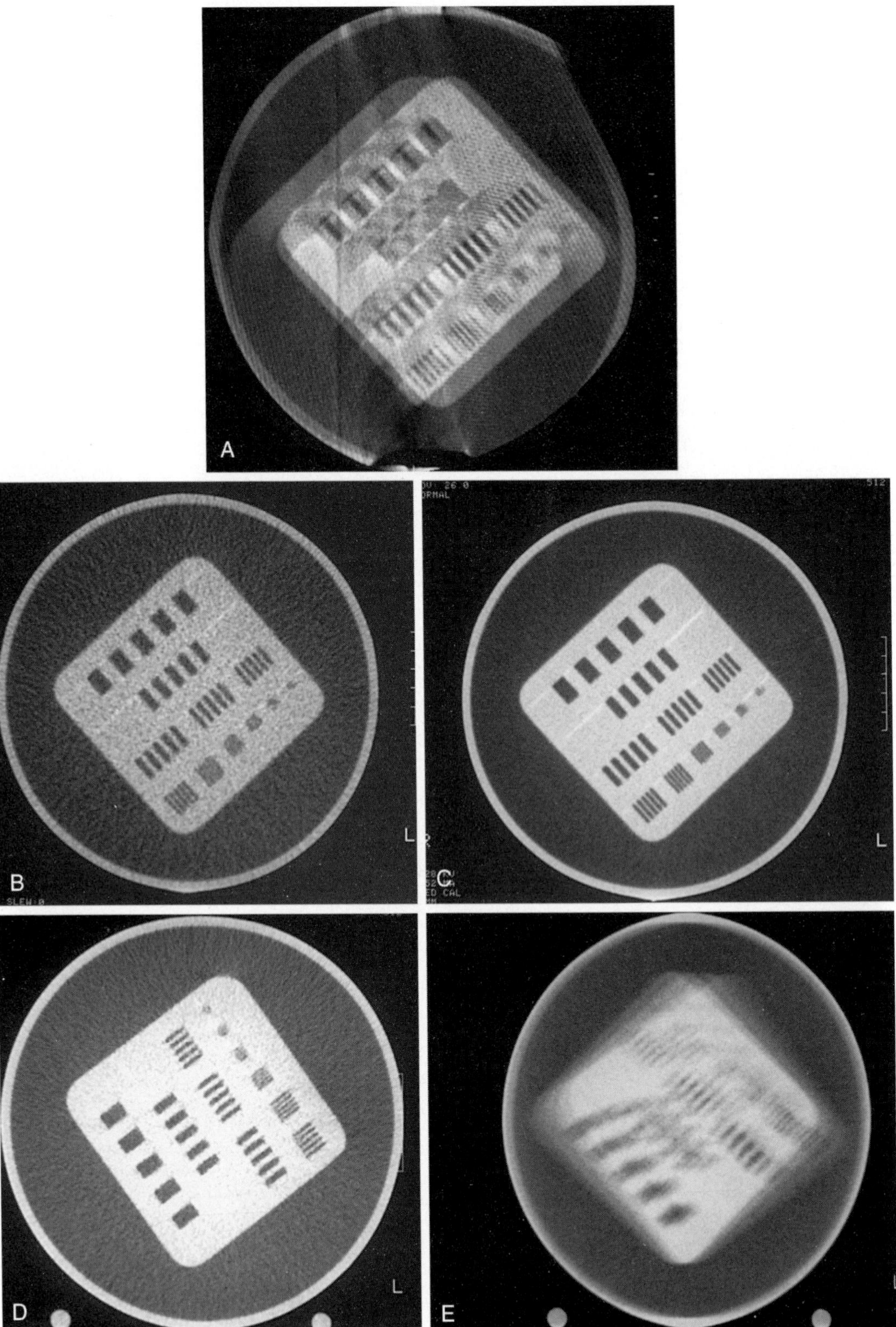

FIGURE 52–12. Computed tomography (CT) images of a spatial resolution target, both at rest and when spinning about the z-axis. *A,* 2-second exposure acquired with the use of a conventional CT scanner, phantom rotating. Note the degradation in image quality caused by motion artifacts. In conventional CT, motion artifacts produce streaks and ghosting throughout the image. *B,* 100-msec exposure with electron-beam CT, phantom at rest. *C,* 1.4-second exposure with electron-beam CT, phantom at rest. Notice the significant decrease in image noise as the exposure time is increased by a factor of 14. *D,* 100-msec exposure with electron-beam CT, phantom rotating. *E,* 1.4-second exposure with electron-beam CT, phantom rotating. The stroboscopic motion artifact occurs because the 1.4-second image is a summation of 14 individual 0.1-second images, each of which stops the motion of the target at a slightly different point in the rotation. This stroboscopic motion artifact, which is limited in its spatial extent and allows the motion of the object to be tracked, differs significantly from that seen with the use of conventional scanners. (From McCollough, C.H., and Morin, R.L.: The technical design and performance of ultrafast computed tomography. Radiol. Clin. North Am. 32:521, 1994, with permission.)

TABLE 52–2. SPATIAL RESOLUTION

Scanner/Mode*	Scan Width (mm)	Time (sec)	Spatial Resolution† (lp/cm)
Adult Body Examinations			
Imatron C-100/SS (130 kVp, 250 mAs)	6	0.4	5.0
Picker PQ2000 (120 kVp, 200 mAs)	10	1.0	7.9
GE HiSpeed Advantage (120 kVp, 280 mAs)	10	1.0	6.3
Cardiac Examinations			
Imatron C-100/SS (130 kVp, 62.5 mAs)	3	0.1	3.9
Imatron C-100/MS (130 kVp, 31.3 mAs)	8	0.05	1.9

*Equipment manufacturers are listed in Table 52–1.
†Using "normal" or "standard" reconstruction algorithm; values reported in number of line pairs resolvable per centimeter.

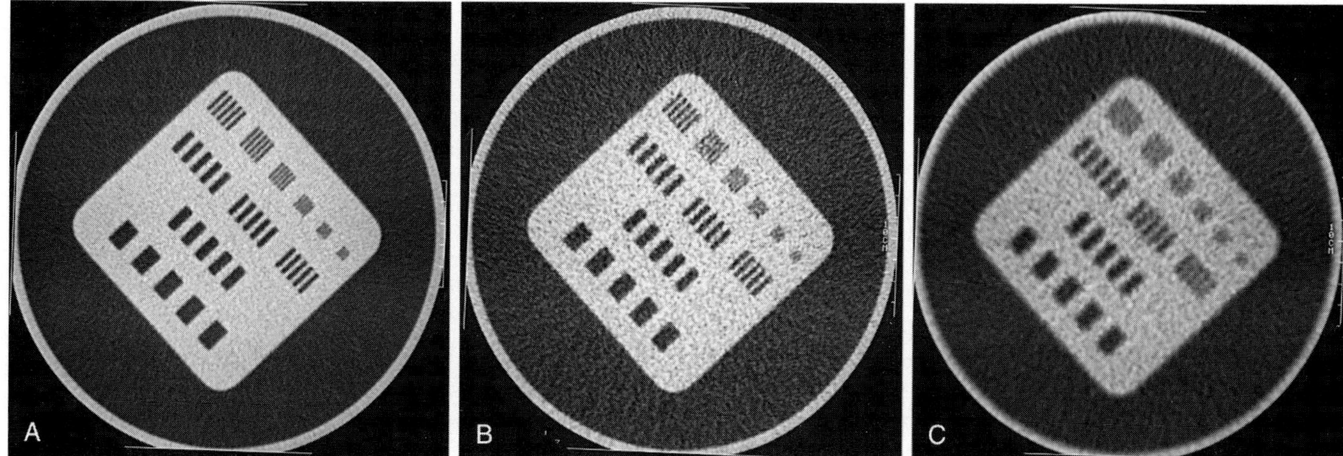

FIGURE 52–13. *A*, Electron-beam computed tomography (EBCT) image of a spatial resolution phantom acquired using a 400-msec exposure, 6-mm scan width, normal reconstruction algorithm, and the single-slice acquisition mode. This technique is typically used for body imaging and has a limiting spatial resolution of approximately 5 line pairs per centimeter (lp/cm). *B*, EBCT image of a spatial resolution phantom acquired with a 100-msec exposure, 3-mm scan width, normal reconstruction algorithm, and the single-slice acquisition mode. This technique is typically used for high-spatial-resolution cardiac imaging and has a limiting spatial resolution of approximately 4 lp/cm. *C*, EBCT image of a spatial resolution phantom acquired with the use of a 50-msec exposure, 8-mm scan width, normal reconstruction algorithm, and the multislice acquisition mode. This technique is typically used for high-temporal-resolution cardiac imaging and has a limiting spatial resolution of approximately 2 lp/cm. The significant reduction in spatial resolution in the multislice mode compared with the single-slice mode occurs because the detector aperture is doubled (half the number of detectors are used to span the same distance). (From McCollough, C.H., and Morin, R.L.: The technical design and performance of ultrafast computed tomography. Radiol. Clin. North Am. 32:521, 1994, with permission.)

TABLE 52–3. LOW-CONTRAST RESOLUTION

Scanner/Mode*	Scan Width (mm)	Time (sec)	Low-Contrast Resolution† (mm)
Adult Body Examinations			
Imatron C-100/SS (130 kVp, 250 mAs)	6	0.4	4.5
Picker PQ2000 (120 kVp, 200 mAs)	10	1.0	3.0
GE HiSpeed Advantage (120 kVp, 280 mAs)	10	1.0	3.0
Cardiac Examinations			
Imatron C-100/SS (130 kVp, 62.5 mAs)	3	0.1	20
Imatron C-100/MS (130 kVp, 31.3 mAs)	8	0.05	20

*Equipment manufacturers are listed in Table 52–1.
†0.6 percent contrast.

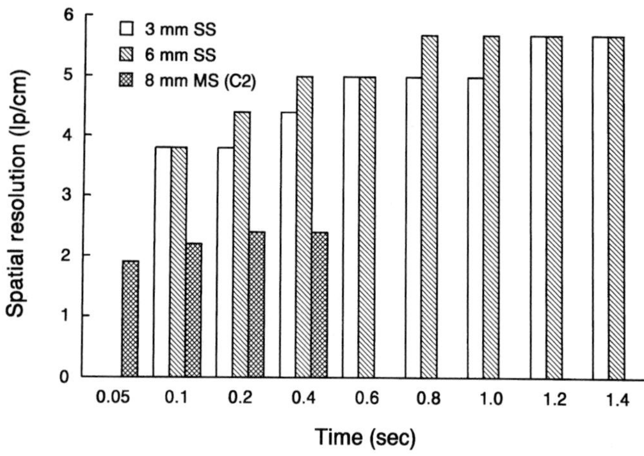

FIGURE 52–14. In either the single-slice (SS) or the multislice (MS) mode, the limiting spatial resolution of the electron-beam CT scanner is reduced slightly at very short exposure times owing to increased image noise. This effect is of little clinical relevance for rapidly moving objects, where adequate spatial resolution can be maintained because of the improved temporal resolution (see Fig. 52–12). (From McCollough, C.H., and Morin, R.L.: The technical design and performance of ultrafast computed tomography. Radiol. Clin. North Am. 32:521, 1994, with permission.)

influences the low-contrast resolution of a system. Figure 52–15 shows the improvement in contrast resolution obtained by increasing the exposure time. This increase in contrast resolution must be weighed against an increase in motion blurring and patient dose.

Noise

The statistical fluctuation of CT numbers in the image of a uniform object is directly related to the number of photons used to create the image. This random fluctuation of CT numbers, or noise, is measured as the standard deviation of pixel values within a region of interest located at the center of a uniform object (32 cm diameter, water-filled acrylic cylinder). The noise values for both conventional and EBCT systems are shown in Table 52–4. Figure 52–16 shows the measured relationship between noise and exposure time for an EBCT system.

Uniformity

Various physical phenomena, including the hardening of the x-ray beam that occurs as it traverses an attenuating object and the

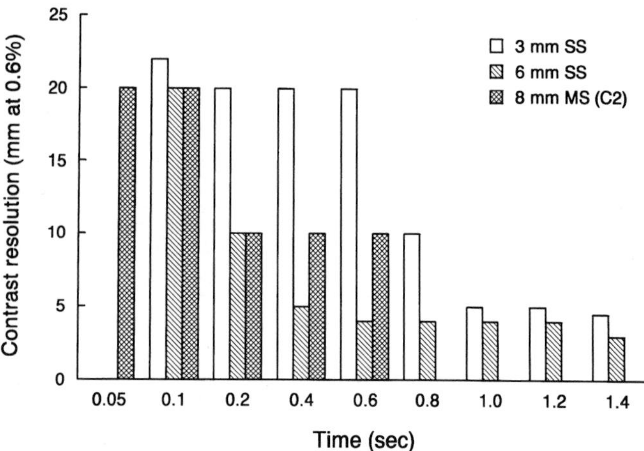

FIGURE 52–15. Low-contrast resolution of an electron-beam computed tomography scanner is measured as the diameter of the smallest visible low-contrast object. As the exposure time increases, smaller low-contrast objects can be visualized. (From McCollough, C.H., and Morin, R.L.: The technical design and performance of ultrafast computed tomography. Radiol. Clin. North Am. 32:521, 1994, with permission.)

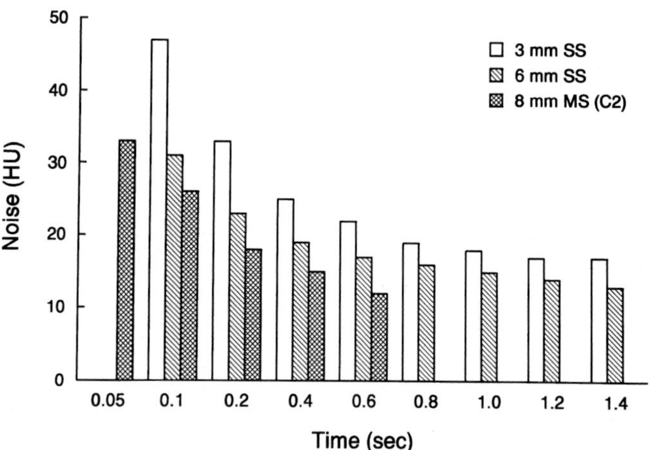

FIGURE 52–16. Noise is measured as the standard deviation of pixel values in the center of a uniform object. As the exposure time increases, more photons reach the detector and a better estimate of each pixel value can be made. Although images acquired with the use of longer exposure times exhibit less noise, motion blurring can limit the ability to resolve anatomical detail. As demonstrated in Figure 52–12, images using short exposure times are free from motion artifacts and provide superior spatial resolution of moving objects, despite higher noise levels. (From McCollough, C.H., and Morin, R.L.: The technical design and performance of ultrafast computed tomography. Radiol. Clin. North Am. 32:521, 1994, with permission.)

detection of x-ray scatter, can cause nonuniformities in the image of a uniform object. Software corrections made during reconstruction attempt to compensate for these effects so that the mean CT number within a specific-size region of interest is as similar as possible between the center of an object and around its periphery. These corrections are typically based on physical measurements of phantoms of various sizes.

An image is taken of a uniform object (32 cm diameter, water-filled acrylic cylinder) to measure both image noise and image uniformity. Images of a water uniformity phantom for the 6-mm single-slice, 3-mm single-slice, and 8-mm multislice modes are shown in Figure 52–17. The difference in mean CT numbers within a region of interest at the image center and at the edge is used to represent the absolute nonuniformity of the image. Data for conventional and EBCT systems are provided in Table 52–5. Brightness nonuniformity between the edge and center regions is greater for EBCT than for conventional CT scanners, particularly in the multislice mode of operation. This may result from differences in the uniformity corrections applied by the vendors and the greater amount of x-ray scatter detected by an EBCT scanner.

Computed Tomography Number Linearity

In order to identify the composition of materials based on their CT numbers, the relation between measured CT numbers and known x-ray attenuation must be linear and consistent over the full range of CT numbers measured. To measure CT number linearity, a test object consisting of materials having different known CT numbers was imaged, and the mean CT number of each of the objects is measured. Table 52–6 shows the slope and y-intercept of a linear regression between measured CT numbers and known CT numbers. The relation is linear over the measured range of −100 to +1000 HU for all EBCT modes. The intercept of the line differs from 0 HU when the calibrations are not suited to the test phantom. Note that for EBCT applications using the 3- or 6-mm single-slice modes, the CT number calibration is very similar to that for conventional scanners. In the multislice mode, the increased level of x-ray scatter caused by the decreased collimation changes the CT number calibration significantly.

Geometrical Accuracy

Software tools provided by the manufacturer allow distance and area measurements to be performed. The accuracy of these mea-

TABLE 52–4. NOISE

Scanner/Mode*	Scan Width (mm)	Time (sec)	Noise† (HU)
Adult Body Examinations			
Imatron C-100/SS (130 kVp, 250 mAs)	6	0.4	14
Picker PQ2000 (120 kVp, 200 mAs)	10	1.0	11.2
GE HiSpeed Advantage (120 kVp, 280 mAs)	10	1.0	7.7
Cardiac Examinations			
Imatron C-100/SS (130 kVp, 62.5 mAs)	3	0.1	30
Imatron C-100/MS (130 kVp, 31.3 mAs)	8	0.05	19

*Equipment manufacturers are listed in Table 52–1.
†Standard deviations, using "standard" or "normal" reconstruction algorithms.

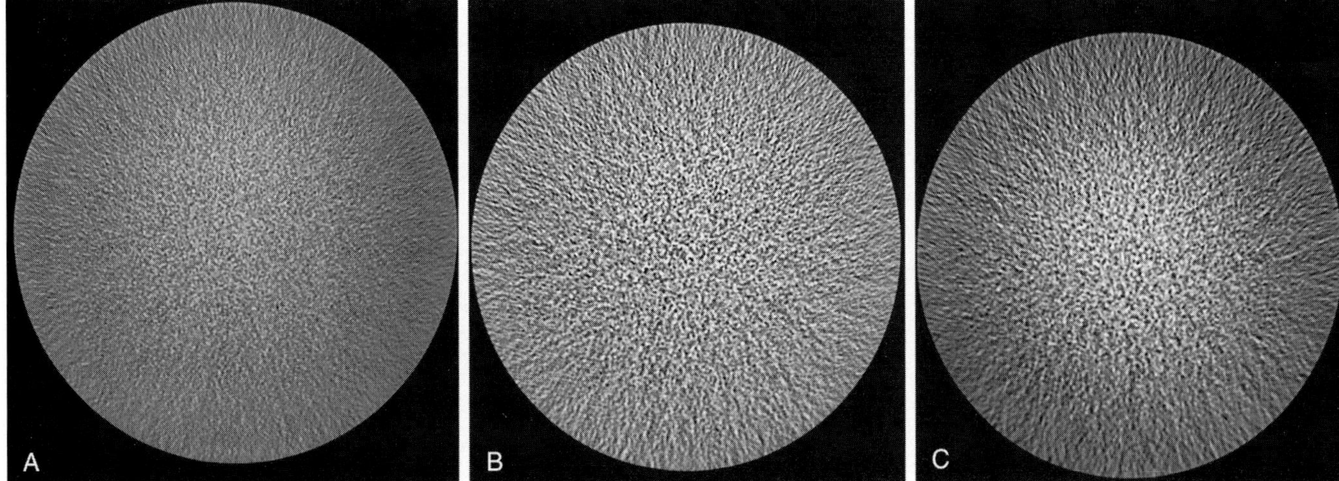

FIGURE 52–17. Electron-beam computed tomography (EBCT) images of a uniform acrylic phantom 32 cm in diameter. Both the uniformity of pixel brightness and the amount of image noise can be measured from these images. *A*, 400-msec exposure, 6-mm slice width, single-slice acquisition. *B*, 100-msec exposure, 3-mm slice width, single-slice acquisition. *C*, 50-msec exposure, 8-mm slice width, multislice acquisition. Note the increased noise for images having shorter exposure times and the increased nonuniformity of image brightness for the multislice mode. Brightness uniformity between the edge and the center regions is somewhat less than that of conventional CT scanners in the single-slice mode of operation. (From McCollough, C.H., and Morin, R.L.: The technical design and performance of ultrafast computed tomography. Radiol. Clin. North Am. 32:521, 1994, with permission.)

TABLE 52–5. UNIFORMITY

Scanner/Mode*	Scan Width (mm)	Time (sec)	Center-to-Edge Difference (HU)
Adult Body Examinations			
Imatron C-100/SS (130 kVp, 250 mAs)	6	0.4	5–14
Picker PQ2000 (120 kVp, 200 mAs)	10	1.0	0–5
GE HiSpeed Advantage (120 kVp, 280 mAs)	10	1.0	0–5
Cardiac Examinations			
Imatron C-100/SS (130 kVp, 62.5 mAs)	3	0.1	4–10
Imatron C-100/MS (130 kVp, 31.3 mAs)	8	0.05	−24–8

*Equipment manufacturers are listed in Table 52–1.

TABLE 52–6. COMPUTED TOMOGRAPHY NUMBER LINEARITY

Scanner/Mode*	Scan Width (mm)	Time (sec)	Computed Tomography Number Linearity† (y-intercept and slope)	
Adult Body Examinations				
Imatron C-100/SS (130 kVp, 250 mAs)	6	0.4	≈0	0.96
Picker PQ2000 (120 kVp, 200 mAs)	10	1.0	≈0	1.0
GE HiSpeed Advantage (120 kVp, 280 mAs)	10	1.0	≈0	1.0
Cardiac Examinations				
Imatron C-100/SS (130 kVp, 62.5 mAs)	3	0.1	1	0.97
Imatron C-100/MS (130 kVp, 31.3 mAs)	8	0.05	−14	0.84

*Equipment manufacturers are listed in Table 52–1.
†Measured computed tomographic number versus known computed tomographic number.

surements is verified by imaging an object with known dimensions. As with conventional CT, the accuracy of geometric measurements within the plane of the image (x and y axes) is excellent. Volume measurements require a knowledge of the image scan width. In the 3-mm and 6-mm single-slice modes, the measured image scan width is approximately 3.0 ± 0.5 mm and 6.0 ± 0.5 mm, respectively. However, in the multislice mode, the image scan widths are not necessarily uniform, nor are images from different targets contiguous. A diagram of the nominal spacing of multislice images from the four targets and two detectors is shown in Figure 52–18.

At isocenter, each multislice image is nominally 8 mm wide with a 4-mm gap between images acquired from different target rings. Measurements show that both the image scan width and image gap width vary at isocenter from nominal values, by ±1 mm and ±2 mm, respectively. In addition, because the detector and target rings do not lie within the same plane, the image scan width widens at the periphery of an object. Thus, volume measurements should be made in the center portion of the image with an understanding of the uncertainty associated with the image scan width.[90]

Equipment Considerations

Technical Strengths

The ability of the EBCT scanner to acquire cross-sectional x-ray images in times as short as 50 or 100 msec is unmatched by any other commercially available CT scanner. (The DSR, which is described in the following section, is capable of acquisition times of the same order of magnitude but is not commercially available.)[91, 92] State-of-the-art conventional CT scanners employing slip-ring technology can acquire partial-view images (less than a 360-degree rotation of the x-ray tube) in 0.45 or 0.6 second. The multislice acquisition mode of the EBCT scanner offers the order-of-magnitude decrease in exposure time (0.05 to 0.1 second) that is necessary for cardiac imaging. In addition, the multiple x-ray targets and dual detector arrays allow for the near-simultaneous scanning of eight unique anatomical levels. Thus, EBCT can be successfully used for a variety of cardiac imaging tasks to measure both anatomy and function.

EBCT systems can also be used to perform cross-sectional imaging of the chest, abdomen, and pelvis in a manner that is clinically comparable to that of conventional CT systems. For such applications, the image quality measured with static phantoms is slightly reduced compared with that of state-of-the-art conventional CT scanners. However, the short scan times decrease the degradation of image quality caused by patient or involuntary organ motion. This is particularly advantageous for pediatric and trauma patients. With the use of the single-slice (high-resolution) mode, large anatomical volumes can be scanned very rapidly (in the continuous-volume-scanning mode, 40 cm can be scanned in as little as 13.8 seconds). This technology also provides the ability to perform large volume acquisitions without concern for anode heat storage and dissipation.

Technical Weaknesses

The geometry used in the EBCT scanner causes the x-ray beam to map out a conical volume through the patient instead of a thin cylindrical volume. This phenomenon, known as cone-beam geometry, causes the image scan width to increase at the periphery of an object.[90] The effect is particularly pronounced in the multislice mode, where the image scan width varies several percent throughout the field of view. This geometry also fails to fully utilize the radiation exposing the patient.[87, 93]

Although the very short exposure time allows moving structures

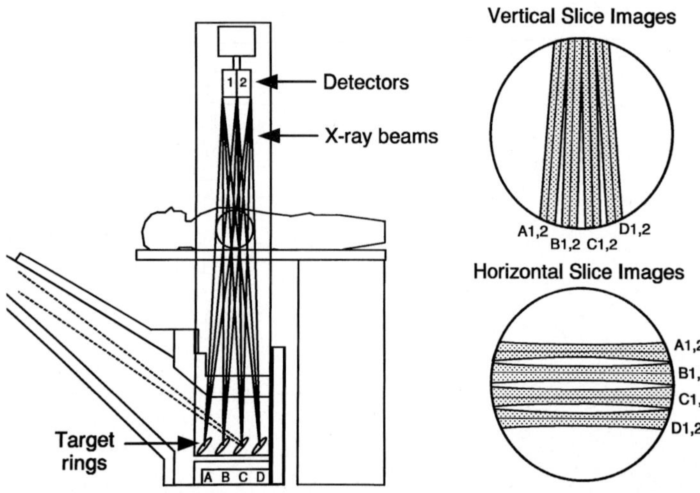

FIGURE 52–18. Geometric configuration of the eight scan levels obtained in the multislice mode of operation. The targets are labeled with the letters A through D, and the detectors with the numbers 1 and 2. The irradiation of an individual target produces an x-ray beam wide enough to cover both detector rings and produces two nominally 8-mm-wide images. A physical gap between target rings causes a nominally 4-mm gap to exist between scans obtained with the use of different targets. In the multislice mode, the eight image levels encompass a volume of approximately 76 mm. Nominal scan and gap widths are quoted at isocenter. Variations in scan and gap width occur throughout the field-of-view owing to the cone-beam geometry of the electron-beam computed tomography scanner. Widening of the image scan width is most significant at the periphery of the image along the horizontal axis. Along the vertical axis, the gaps between the scans are widest at the bottom of the object and narrower toward the top of the object. (From Goldman, L.W., and Fowlkes, J.B. [eds.]: Medical CT and Ultrasound: Current Technology and Applications. Madison, WI, Advanced Medical Publishing, 1995, p. 433.)

to be imaged with minimal blurring or motion artifact, the limited photon flux for such short time intervals produces lower radiation exposures than conventional scanners and results in noisier images. For most applications, an appropriate tradeoff between temporal resolution (motion blurring) and contrast resolution (noise) can be achieved.

EBCT scanners are technically complex. Vacuum systems, magnetic focus and deflection coils, and high-current electron guns are components not found in conventional CT systems. This increased complexity results in an increased need for preventive maintenance, quality control, and corrective maintenance. The installed base of EBCT scanners worldwide is relatively small, with approximately 30 scanners in the United States and about 60 scanners worldwide (David King, Imatron Inc., personal communication, March 1995). Thus, the growth of clinical applications and the maturation of the technology have moved forward at a relatively slow pace. Finally, the space requirements for an EBCT scanner are considerably greater than for conventional CT scanners. For example, a Siemens Evolution EBCT scanner (with operator and physician consoles and laser imager) requires approximately 800 square feet, whereas a Picker PQ2000 (Picker International, Cleveland, Ohio) spiral CT scanner (with operator console and laser imager) requires approximately 300 square feet (actual space requirements depend on room layout).

Product Evolution

A partnership between Imatron, previously the sole manufacturer of EBCT technology, and Siemens, a major vendor of radiographic equipment, has resulted in the release of new models of EBCT scanners. The original model (C-100) had changed little since its introduction in the mid-1980s. A decade later, a second model was made available (C-150). The C-150 scanner is marketed in the United States and Europe by Siemens under the name "Evolution." Some of the features of this new model include a thinner scan width (1.5 mm), the continuous-volume-scanning acquisition mode, smaller site requirements (the length of the drift tube vacuum chamber was reduced from 9 feet to approximately 5 feet), more self-diagnostic software programs, and additional cache memory. Collaborative development work continues to focus on replacing the outdated computer systems, increasing component reliability, providing more modern workstations and consoles, and improving the reconstruction algorithms. The image quality and radiation dose are not significantly different from those of the original model (C-100).

The Mayo Dynamic Spatial Reconstructor

A second unique geometry for dynamic volume CT, the DSR, was developed beginning in 1975 in the Biodynamics Research Unit of the Mayo Clinic.[92, 94–100] Figure 52–19 is a diagram of the multisource, multiple detector scanning concept on which the DSR system is based. The design is different from that of other x-ray CT systems in two major respects: first, data from many angles of view are rapidly (almost simultaneously) acquired from an "electronic scan" by multiple x-ray tubes placed around a 160-degree arc of a circular gantry that mechanically rotates about the patient; and second, a continuous, curved fluorescent screen viewed by multiple video imaging systems is used to record two-dimensional projection images for each x-ray source, providing the data for reconstruction of dynamic three-dimensional volumes of the body.

Even though the DSR is based on both the physics and mathematical principles of x-ray CT, it is designed to achieve *dynamic volume scanning*, in contrast to the static cross-sectional scanning performed by conventional x-ray CT scanners. The DSR can simultaneously scan up to 240 adjacent, 1-mm-thick cross sections at rates up to 60 per second. Desired tradeoffs between temporal, spatial, and density resolution can be achieved by retrospective selection and processing of appropriate subsets of the total data recorded during a DSR scan sequence. This capability permits high-spatial- and high-contrast-resolution imaging of nonmoving structures or high-temporal-resolution imaging of moving organs such as the heart, lungs, or circulatory system.

The Scanner

The DSR collects two-dimensional data at high temporal resolution to generate dynamic images of selected volumes of the body. As illustrated in Figure 52–20, 14 x-ray tubes and 14 television

ELECTRONIC WHOLE-BODY CYLINDRICAL SCANNING SYSTEM

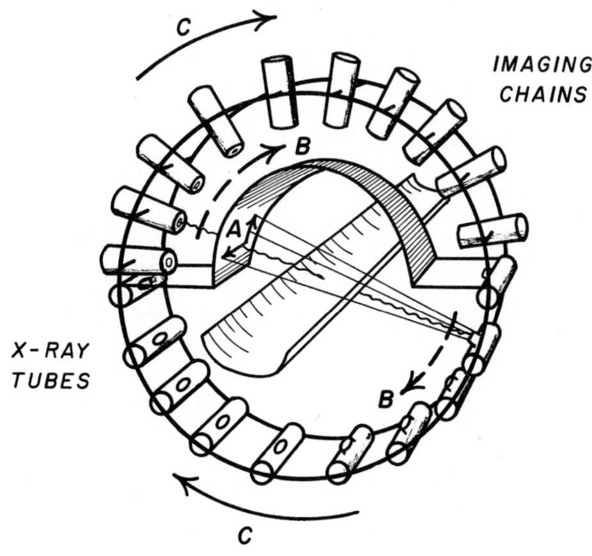

A = Electronic Planar Scan
B = Electronic 180° Circumferential Scan for Maximum Temporal Resolution
C = Accessory 180° Mechanical Rotation for Maximum Spatial and Density Resolution, 360° Circumferential Scanning

FIGURE 52–19. Scanning geometry concept for high-temporal-resolution volume computed tomographic scanning system. A two-dimensional detector simultaneously records projection data (A) for reconstruction of multiple cross sections. Multiple x-ray sources perform high-speed electronic scan (B) for stop-action high-repetition-rate reconstructions, and mechanical rotation of the entire system (C) provides more data for high-spatial- and high-density-resolution reconstructions. (From Ritman, E.L.: Quantitative transaxial imaging of the heart. Eur. J. Cardiol. 53:203, 1977, with permission.)

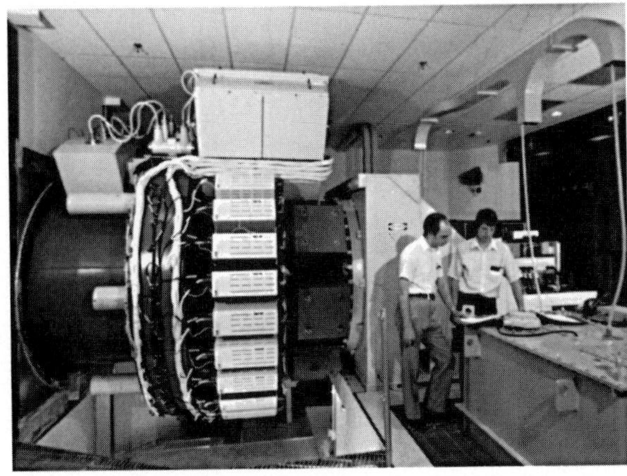

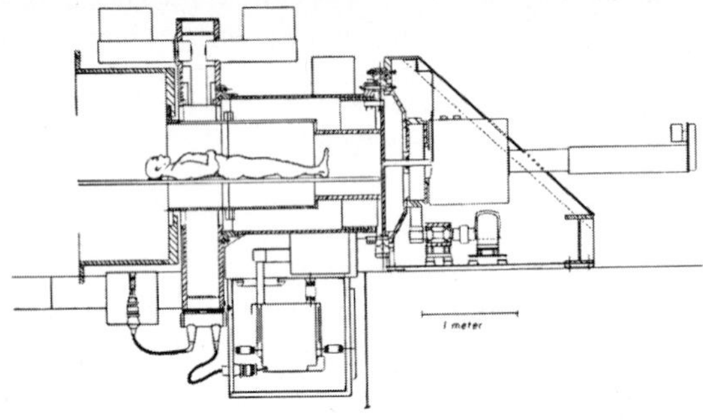

FIGURE 52–20. *Upper Panel,* Dynamic spatial reconstructor scanner assembly. The entire structure to the left of the men is cantilevered from the triangular base. Multiple television cameras and corresponding x-ray sources are arranged along a vertical plane. Rotation of the cantilevered section increases the number of angles of view per scan in proportion to the programmed duration of the scan. *Lower Panel,* Midline longitudinal section of the scanner shows the relation of the human subject lying on table and the surrounding gantry. (From Behrenbeck, T., Sinak, L.J., Robb, R.A., et al.: Some imaging characteristics of the dynamic spatial reconstructor x-ray scanner system. *In* Reba, R.C., Goodenough, D.J., [eds.]: Diagnostic Imaging Medicine. NATO ASI Series, Series E: Appl. Sciences—No. 61. Norwell, MA, Kluwer Academic, 1981, with permission.)

cameras (of the 28 for which it is designed) are attached to the scanner. The x-ray tubes are arranged 12 degrees apart along a semicircular array, with television cameras positioned opposite each x-ray source. As each x-ray tube is pulsed for 350 msec, a 30 cm × 30 cm image is generated on a portion of the curved fluorescent screen. The corresponding television camera is gated on for 762 msec to read out the fluoroscopic image. The subject scanned is positioned inside the machine at the center of rotation, as indicated in the schematic in Figure 52–20. The 14 television images of the fluoroscopic screens, generated in one scan by the 14 x-ray pulses over a period of 11 msec, are recorded on seven videodisc channels at a repetition rate of 60 scans per second. Each television image consists of 240 horizontal lines, but because only seven recording channels are available, sets of two views are recorded on each channel by combining every other line in each view into one video field. Therefore, up to 120 horizontal scan lines of each of the 14 video fields can be used to reconstruct the image of a corresponding anatomical cross section.

The DSR simultaneously scans a cylindrical volume, 22 cm in axial height and 22 to 38 cm in transaxial diameter. Using the 14 x-ray source system, the 22-cm-diameter volume can be scanned in 0.011 second for a 14-view reconstruction, 0.127 second for a 112-view reconstruction, or 2.244 seconds for a 240-view reconstruction from a complete 360-degree range of views. The 38-cm-diameter volume is scanned in 0.06 second for a 16-view reconstruction or 0.57 second for a 135-view reconstruction. (In this mode, three adjacent cameras are simultaneously exposed and subsequently combined to provide a "wide angle" view, so that only four total angles of view are recorded every 1/60 second.)

The volume can be scanned repetitively at selected rates, ranging between 60 scans per second and 1 scan in 2.2 seconds. If desired, the sequential scans can be retrospectively selected so as to overlap in time. The repetitive scans can continue for up to 20 total seconds—the recording capacity of the video discs. The DSR can produce 300 volumes of 120 cross sections each in 5 seconds.

An Alderson Rando phantom was used to evaluate DSR x-ray exposure.[98] At 100 kV peak voltage and 1000 mA current for each x-ray pulse, the radiation entrance exposure for the 14 x-ray tube system was 0.9 R/sec in the thoracic region of interest. The thyroid region was exposed to less than 300 mR/sec, the eye 7 mR/sec, and the gonads less than 1 mR/sec. Consequently, for a 4- to 5-second scan encompassing the several heart cycles required to evaluate cardiac function during the passage of contrast agent through the myocardium and lung, a total entrance exposure of 4 to 5 R may be delivered. This is of similar magnitude to the radiation exposure delivered by conventional CT. In clinical cardiac angiography, patient entrance exposures may be up to 5 to 10 times this amount.

A special-purpose reconstruction program has been developed to produce DSR volume images.[44] This program allows the user to interactively select (after the DSR scan) the time increments and spatial extent of recorded projection data to be processed. Options are available to combine recorded time points (to obtain more views per reconstruction) or adjacent lines (for thicker cross sections) in each view to obtain the temporal, spatial, or contrast resolution desired in the reconstructed volume image. This capability for retrospective recombining of the reconstructed volume images is possible because the projection data acquisition and image reconstruction processes are linearly dependent.[99, 100] The program provides a special feature for "zoom" or "target" reconstructions to obtain high spatial resolution images of selected regions of interest within the scan volume. If specified, the program will also calculate the volume images in cubic dimensions. This is accomplished by appropriately interpolating between sections (usually, the spacing between adjacent sections, 0.9 mm, is greater than the pixel size within sections). This feature capitalizes on the intrinsic capability of the DSR to scan many adjacent thin cross sections of the body and facilitates efficient and accurate computation of arbitrarily-oriented (oblique) sections without loss of spatial resolution.

Analysis and Display

The quantitative analysis of four-dimensional DSR image data (three spatial dimensions plus one temporal dimension) requires multidimensional display methods, primarily because the tremendous amount of image data generated by the DSR must be edited and quantitatively analyzed in order to extract useful information, and because the structures and processes studied with the DSR are most often four-dimensional by nature. Multidimensional displays facilitate quantitative analysis of these data by providing direct visualization of three-dimensional shapes and spatial relations among imaged structures. This direct visual feedback in turn facilitates the detection of the presence or absence of imaged features, cognition (understanding) of three-dimensional shapes, identification of the optimal orientation of oblique cross-sectional images, and measurement of organ shape and dimensions. A special software package, called ANALYZE, for multidimensional image display and analysis is described in a subsequent section.

Basic Imaging Performance

When DSR image data recorded under practical conditions are appropriately manipulated so that the signal-to-noise ratio is maximized and the partial volume effect is minimized, the characteristic imaging capabilities of the DSR may be summarized as follows:[91]

- Maximum spatial resolution of high-contrast, stationary structures is 8 lp/cm in both transaxial (transverse) and axial (cephalocaudal) directions.

- For the 14 x-ray tube configuration, the spatial resolution of a high-contrast structure moving at 80 mm/sec is 4 lp/cm in the transverse and cephalocaudal directions.
- For a 112-view (i.e., 0.127-second duration) scan of a 10-cm diameter water-equivalent test phantom, the contrast resolution (defined as the smallest resolvable difference between the reconstructed linear attenuation coefficients of a structure of given size and its uniformly dense surroundings) is 100 percent of the linear attenuation coefficient of water in a 1 mm^3 volume (i.e., average data from 100 voxels). Contrast resolution of 3 percent in 1 mm^3 can be achieved in images produced from 2.24-second scans of 240 views around 360 degrees.
- The small increments of volume occurring in a balloon during successive 0.06-second DSR scans produced by injection of 100 mL contrast agent into the balloon at the rate of 150 mL/sec were estimated correctly from reconstructed images of the balloon to within 3 percent of the known values.
- Lung volume (air plus parenchyma) and total heart muscle mass estimated from DSR images of intact anesthetized experimental animals is correct to within 3 and 5 percent of postmortem measurement, respectively.
- Estimates of blood flow in carotid arteries of anesthetized dogs from dynamic DSR images is correct to within 10 percent of electromagnetic flow meter measurements. Similarly, the relative cardiac output of anesthetized dogs calculated from dynamic DSR images is correct to within 10 percent of the outputs estimated with conventional techniques such as dye dilution curves.[67]
- Stenoses (constrictions or blockages) as small as 0.6 mm diameter by 1.5 mm long, placed in 3.2-mm diameter plastic tubing sutured to the heart of an anesthetized dog, were calculated correctly from DSR images of the intact thorax.

These imaging performance capabilities are decreased somewhat as the size of the subject being scanned is increased. This is primarily a result of the limited sensitivity and dynamic range of the fluoroscopic video detector system.[92, 97] Therefore, the DSR in its present form has limited applicability for large adults.

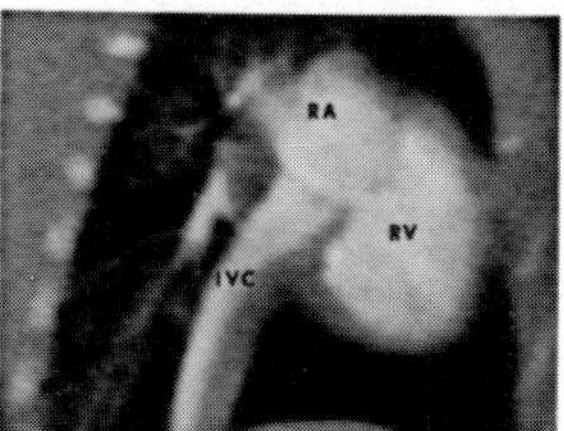

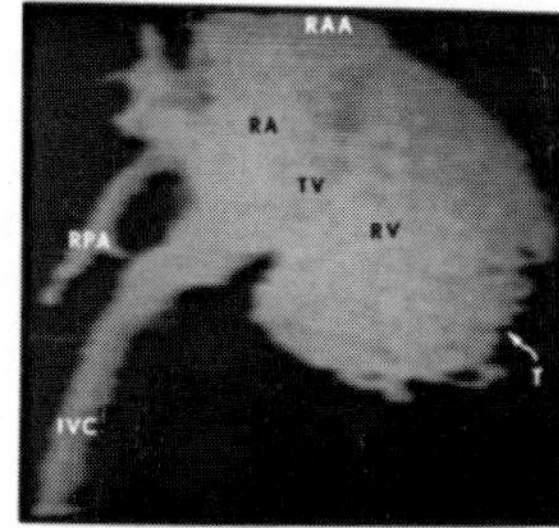

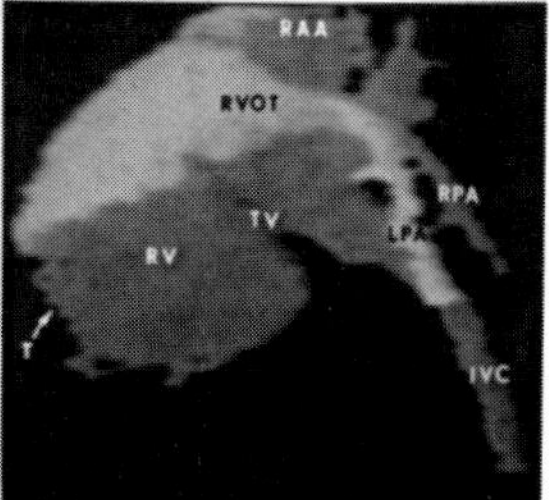

FIGURE 52–21. Visualization of right heart chambers and major vessels. The top panel is an 8-mm-thick sagittal section reconstructed from a 240-view DSR scan, viewed from the right side of the 12-kg, supine, anesthetized dog after contrast injection into the inferior vena cava (IVC). Because of the slow heart rate (produced by vagal stimulation), dye settled into the dorsal portion of the IVC. Also visible are the right atrium and ventricle (RA and RV). Right and left lateral aspects of a shaded surface display of the right heart chambers and associated vessels of the same dog is shown in the lower panels. Structures of interest are the RA and RV, the tricuspid valve region (TV), the right atrial appendage (RAA), the right ventricular outflow track (RVOT), the right and left pulmonary arteries (RPA and LPA), the IVC, and a negative cast of trabeculae (T). (From Robb, R.A., Hoffman, E.A., Sinak, L.J., et al.: High-speed three-dimensional x-ray computed tomography: The dynamic spatial reconstructor. Proceedings of the IEEE 713:308, 1983. © 1983 IEEE.)

Applications

The DSR offers unique capabilities for cognitive visualization and accurate measurement of shapes and dimensions of the thoracic contents, such as cardiac chambers, pleural surfaces, airways (down to three levels of branching), diaphragm, kidneys, and pulmonary and systemic blood vessels. Such measurements obtained throughout a cardiac and respiratory cycle, in conjunction with simultaneous recording[101] of various physiologic parameters such as blood pressures, pleural pressure, and ECG, can yield new insights into the function of the heart and lungs and their interaction. Experience with the DSR has shown that adequate delineation of these structures can be achieved from images reconstructed with as few as 56 views. With the present 14 x-ray imaging chain system, 56 views are obtained for every successive 1/15 second of scanning time. These 56-view reconstructions are obtained by adding together four successive 14-view reconstructions. Alternatively, each 14-view reconstruction can be obtained during a specific physiologic event, such as a specific point in the cardiac cycle (as determined from the ECG), before summation. This latter method is similar to "gated" imaging.

Images obtained from the DSR require no assumptions about size and shape of organs. True three-dimensional structure of the heart and cardiac chambers can be detected by imaging radiopaque contrast agent, injected peripherally, as it passes through the various chambers and vascular structures, as illustrated in Figure 52–21. A 12-kg anesthetized dog was placed supine in the DSR and scanned during injection of radiopaque contrast (Renovist; 1.2 mL/kg) into the inferior vena cava. In the upper panel, an 8-mm-thick sagittal section selected from the reconstructed volume image is shown in which the right atria, right ventricle, and inferior vena cava are clearly visible. Employing a computer-aided three-dimensional surface detection and shaded surface display algorithm,[102, 103] the three-dimensional surface of the contrast agent detected within the right heart chambers can be displayed, as shown in the lower panels of Figure 52–21.

Figure 52–22 illustrates the capability of the DSR for rapid three-dimensional imaging of the heart and circulation for study of the dynamic distributions of blood flow to, within, and from the heart using circulatory contrast agents. The entire heart was dynamically imaged using successive 0.067-second DSR volume scans for one complete heartbeat (about 0.7 second) during infusion of contrast material into the superior vena cava.

Figure 52–23 shows images of midline sagittal, coronal, and transverse sections from one point in time during the injection of contrast material in a patient scanned with the DSR. The volume image may also be used to create planar images at oblique angles to the transverse scanning plane.[104] The right-most panels of Figure 52–23 show oblique sections passing through the main course of the pulmonary arteries. This figure demonstrates how the operator-interactive sectioning program works to retrospectively select a plane through a structure of interest. The leftmost three of the panels are midsagittal, midcoronal, and midtransverse orientation sections. The bright line intersecting these orientation images indicates the location of the oblique section shown at the right of the figure.

Figure 52–24 is an example of a projection display of the left main, left anterior descending, and left circumflex coronary arteries

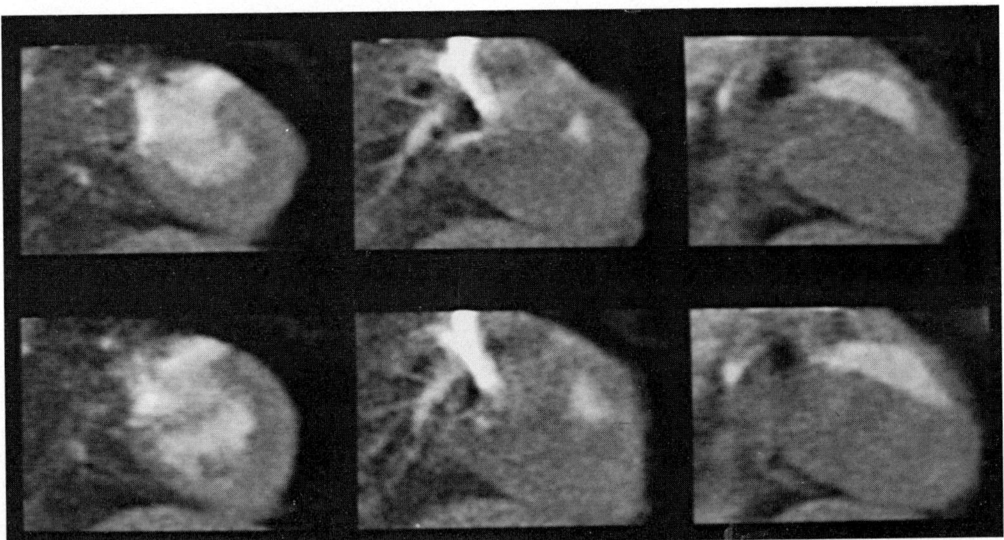

FIGURE 52–22. Dynamic images of sagittal sections of a dog's heart obtained from 15-per-second synchronous volume scans performed by the DSR throughout one complete cardiac cycle during injection of x-ray contrast material into the superior vena cava. The top row shows three different 1-mm-thick sagittal sections, each 8 mm apart, all in the right half of the heart. These sections were obtained at an instant in the cardiac cycle near end-systole (minimal volume of chambers). The bottom row shows the same three sagittal sections obtained at an instant near end-diastole (maximal volume of chambers) of the same heartbeat. The left-hand images show the right atrium and a small part of the right ventricle filled with contrast material. The center images show the superior vena cava and pulmonary artery with small branching vessels. The right-hand images show more of the right ventricular chamber and demonstrate a marked difference in chamber area between systole (*top*) and diastole (*bottom*). (From Robb, R.A.: X-ray computed tomography: An engineering synthesis of multi-scientific principles. Crit. Rev. Biomed. Eng. 74:265, 1982, with permission.)

of a dog scanned with the DSR during an aortic root injection. Note the blurring of the left anterior descending coronary artery relative to the left circumflex coronary artery. This blurring is reduced when 0.9 mm thick slices are scanned (as compared with 1.8 mm thick slices) and if the dog is scanned in the 30-degree head-up (supine) position. The prone image is not different from the supine image. These images suggest that viscosity and specific gravity of the contrast medium are not major causes of this blurring.[104]

DIGITAL IMAGE DISPLAY AND ANALYSIS

The ability to extract objective and quantitatively accurate information from three-dimensional images produced by x-ray CT (and other medical imaging devices) has not kept pace with the ability to produce the images themselves. What is required is efficient capabilities to display, manipulate, and measure the intrinsic and relevant information contained in the multidimensional image data produced by these three-dimensional modalities (i.e., the true morphologic, pathologic, biologic, physiologic, and metabolic "meaning" of the numbers).

The process of forming an image involves mapping some properties of an object or set of objects into or onto what is called image space. This space is used to visualize an object and its properties and may be used to quantitatively characterize its structure or function. Imaging science may be defined as the study of these mappings and the development of ways of better understanding them, improving them, and productively using them. Generally, the steps involved in imaging procedures include image-data acquisition, image display and analysis (including evaluation of image quality), and image observation (i.e., perception, cognition, and interpretation). Most modern imaging devices are digital computer-based and produce an image in the form of an array of picture elements (pixels). Emerging imaging modalities produce three-dimensional images of volume elements (voxels), and even four-dimensional images of volume-time elements (voxtels), like the DSR.[105] The numbers associated with these pixels and voxels represent the mappings of object properties that can be detected and localized spatially and they quantitatively characterize these properties.

The challenge of imaging science is to define and facilitate development of advanced capabilities for acquisition, processing, visualization, and quantitative analysis of images in order to significantly increase the faithful extraction of the scientific, educational, and clinical information they contain. This is a formidable task, and continued advances are required to address it effectively. The need for new approaches to image analysis has become increasingly important and pressing as advances in imaging technology enable more complex objects and processes to be imaged and simulated.

The complementary nature of many of the three-dimensional medical imaging modalities, including x-ray CT, magnetic resonance imaging, radionuclide imaging (including single-photon emission tomography and positron emission tomography), and ultrasound imaging, has given rise to the era of multimodality imaging and provided a new emphasis in imaging science. This emphasis may be referred to as the "calculus of imaging"—namely, the differentiation and integration of three-dimensional images. Arguably the most important challenges and the most profound promises of three-dimensional imaging in biology and medicine are automatic segmentation and classification (i.e., differentiation) of tissues and tissue properties and, conversely, the registration and "fusion" (i.e. integration) of the complementary information provided by different imaging modalities into a single multivalued image. The synthesis of multimodal, multidimensional images into an integrated multispectral image provides capabilities for truly synergistic measurements.

Imaging science and biomedical visualization have benefited by the significant advances in the microelectronics industry during the last two decades. The capabilities of the supercomputers of yesterday are now available in desktop workstations for a fraction of the

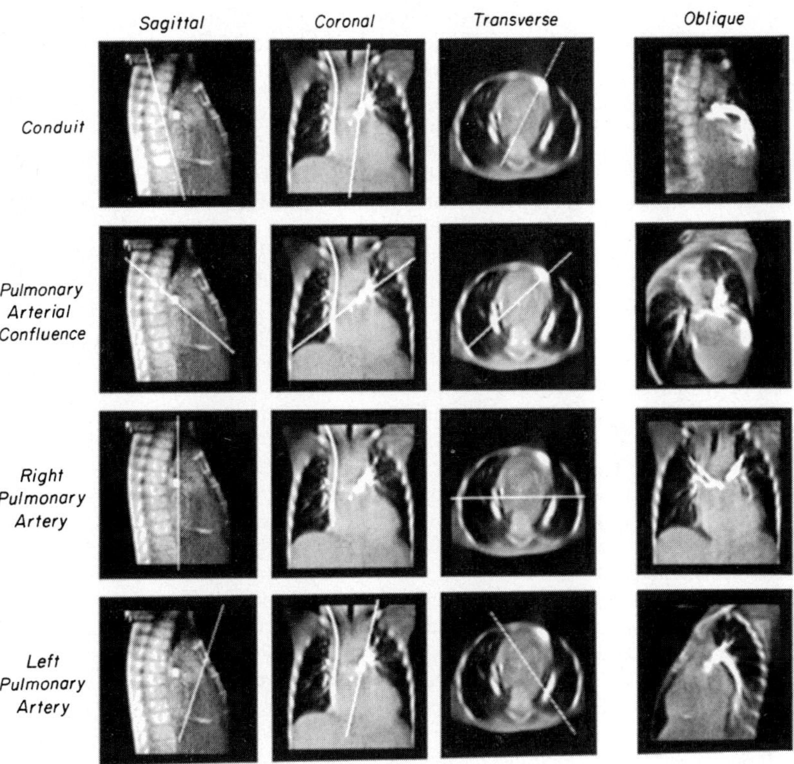

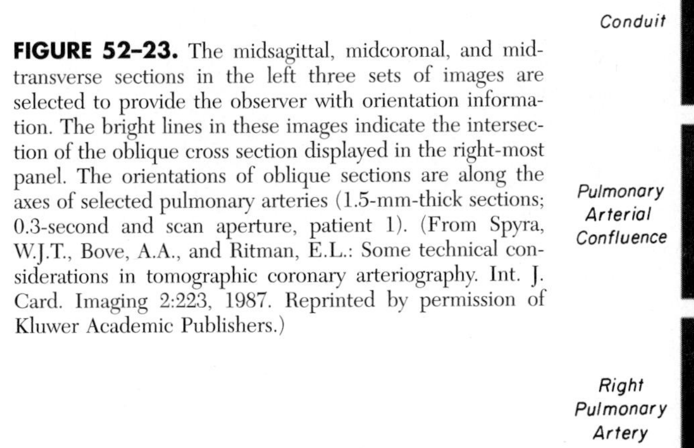

FIGURE 52–23. The midsagittal, midcoronal, and midtransverse sections in the left three sets of images are selected to provide the observer with orientation information. The bright lines in these images indicate the intersection of the oblique cross section displayed in the right-most panel. The orientations of oblique sections are along the axes of selected pulmonary arteries (1.5-mm-thick sections; 0.3-second and scan aperture, patient 1). (From Spyra, W.J.T., Bove, A.A., and Ritman, E.L.: Some technical considerations in tomographic coronary arteriography. Int. J. Card. Imaging 2:223, 1987. Reprinted by permission of Kluwer Academic Publishers.)

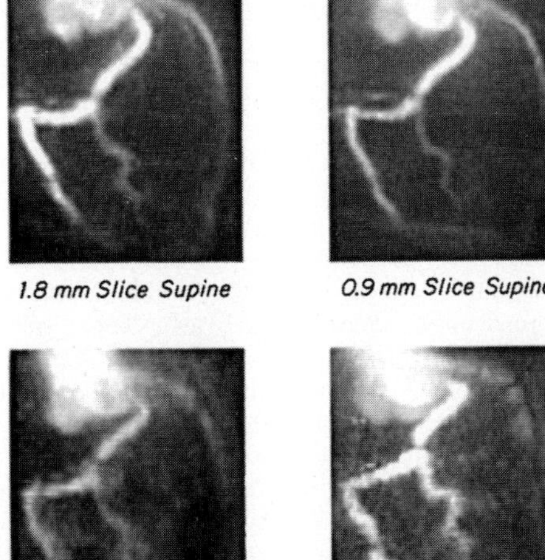

FIGURE 52–24. A computer-generated projection display of the coronary arteries of a dog during an aortic root injection of contrast medium. In this instance, the left anterior descending (LAD) coronary artery is blurred relative to the left circumflex (LCx) coronary artery. This blurring was somewhat diminished when the DSR was programmed to scan with 0.9-mm-thick slices (*right upper panel*) instead of 1.8-mm-thick slices (*left upper panel*). The lower two panels show no significant difference in blurring of the LAD coronary artery when the dog is scanned in the prone or 30-degree head-up supine orientation. (From Liu, Y.H., Hoffman, E.A., Hagler, D.J., et al.: Accuracy of pulmonary vasculature dimensions estimated with the dynamic spatial reconstructor. Am. J. Physiol. Imaging 1:201, 1986, with permission. © 1986 Munksgaard International Publishers Ltd., Copenhagen, Denmark.)

cost. These powerful computers made available at modest cost have liberated programmers and software developers to be more creative and to develop and test algorithms without spending significant time and effort in optimizing code or compromising functionality to achieve acceptable performance. Concomitantly, the quality of images produced by medical and biological imaging systems has improved dramatically in the last decade, providing faithful high-resolution recordings of three- and even four-dimensional objects. The combination of high-quality three-dimensional images and high-performance low-cost computing provides an ideal opportunity for the development of powerful yet practical software for useful biomedical image visualization, manipulation, and measurement.

The algorithms and processes required for useful display and analysis of multidimensional, multimodality biomedical images have been synthesized into a variety of commercially available software packages. One comprehensive software system, ANALYZE, is produced by the Biomedical Imaging Resource of the Mayo Clinic.[105, 106] It is written entirely in the C programming language and contains approximately 400,000 lines of source code. The system comprises more than 55 individual programs, each representing a specific function or class of functions, all of which are built on a base of a dozen libraries providing common input and output, graphics, and other basic operations. ANALYZE features integrated, complementary tools for fully interactive display, manipulation, and measurement of multidimensional image data. It has been applied to data from many different imaging modalities. The software runs efficiently on standard UNIX workstations without the need for special-purpose hardware. It utilizes several features of the UNIX operating system to facilitate and complement its modular architecture.

The ANALYZE software incorporates many functions for solving the calculus of imaging and for exploring, developing, testing, and applying solutions to real problems. It is readily extensible so that new approaches and paradigms can be tested, evaluated, and documented. Indeed, ANALYZE functions and features have approximately doubled every year over its lifetime. This significant growth has been facilitated by concomitant improvements in workstation performance, software development aids, and network environment support tools. Even though many of the new functions have incorporated more and more sophisticated algorithms and procedures requiring increased computation, the performance of ANALYZE has still increased and improved. The program is highly interactive, and some functions are accomplished almost in real time.

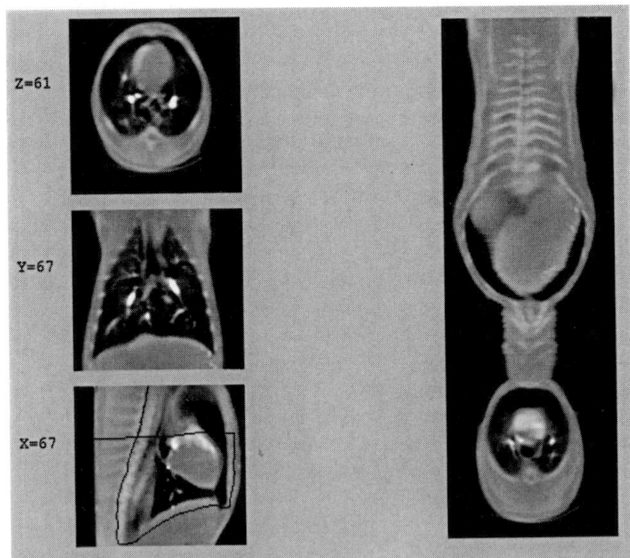

FIGURE 52–26. An example of interactive curved sectioning in ANALYZE, wherein a trace (*lower left*) along an arbitrary path on any section (*left column*) generates a curved planar image (*right*). A curved image is computed and displayed during tracing on any of the three orthogonal reference images. (From ANALYZE: A software system for biomedical image analysis. *In* Proceedings of the First Conference on Visualization in Biomedical Computing. May 22–25, 1990, Atlanta, GA. Atlanta, IEEE Computer Society Press, 1990, pp. 507–518. © 1990 IEEE.)

The various functions available with such analysis packages provide the capabilities required for detailed display and analysis of the data provided by fast CT scanning systems. Figures 52–25 through 52–29 are examples of DSR data visualization and analyses produced by ANALYZE. Both ANALYZE and the DSR have made significant contributions in establishing three-dimensional imaging as a powerful new technology in the study and treatment of health and disease.[107]

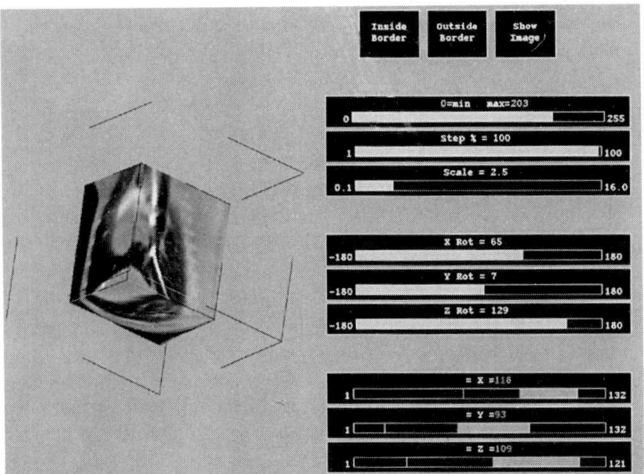

FIGURE 52–25. Interactive orthogonal sectioning and three-dimensional visualization of DSR image of thorax with the use of ANALYZE. The volume image can be dissected in real time along orthogonal axes and rotated and scaled to view orthogonal planes within the volume. (From ANALYZE: A software system for biomedical image analysis. *In* Proceedings of the First Conference on Visualization in Biomedical Computing. May 22–25, 1990, Atlanta, GA. Atlanta, IEEE Computer Society Press, 1990, pp. 507–518. © 1990 IEEE.)

CONCLUSION

The trend in development of x-ray CT systems has been toward faster and faster scanners, with concomitant improvement in image quality. However, conventional CT systems do not scan rapidly enough to eliminate motion blurring in images of moving organs like the heart and circulation, and they produce only one or two two-dimensional image slices for each scan. The results from the EBCT and DSR scanners suggest the advent of two new, powerful dimensions in x-ray CT: high temporal resolution and synchronous volume scanning. Such imaging capabilities, coupled with powerful computer workstations and comprehensive display and analysis software, promise to make possible new basic investigative and clinical studies of the relations between structure and function in moving organ systems like the heart and lungs, and of the circulation in any organ of the body. This state-of-the-art CT technology holds the promise of exciting new clinical and research capabilities, such as quantitative analysis of regional blood flow and perfusion, simultaneous measurement of physiologic function and anatomical structure, and differential diagnosis of disease based on determination of tissue composition and dynamics in any organ or region of the body.

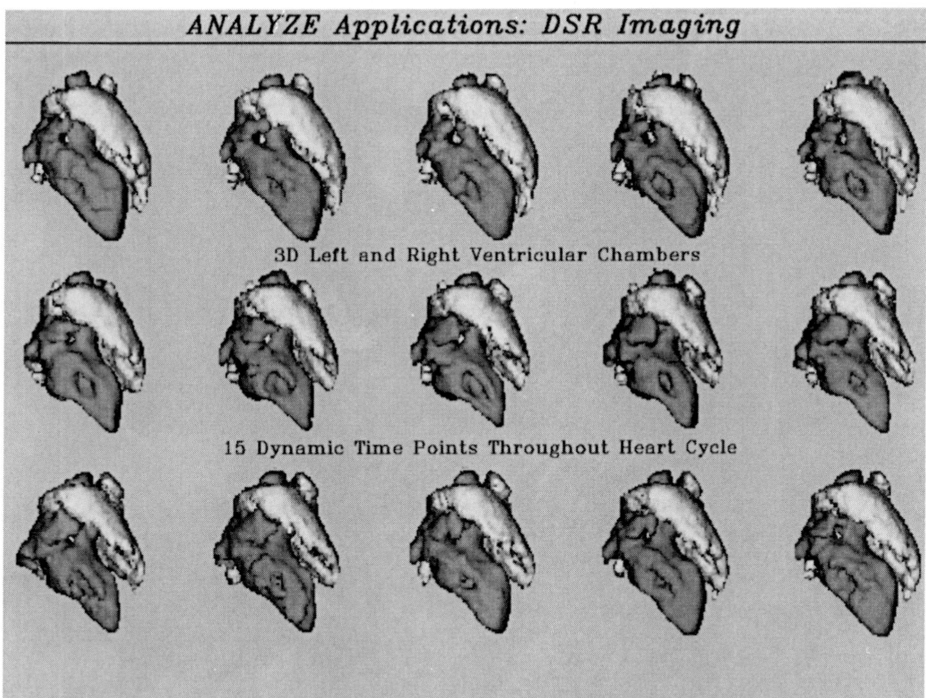

FIGURE 52–27. Time sequence of three-dimensional rendered volume displays of heart chambers throughout one heart cycle computed and displayed in ANALYZE from dynamic spatial reconstructor image data. Such images comprise four-dimensional data sets made up of vectors of volume-time elements (voxtels). Filling and emptying of the chambers can readily be appreciated. (From ANALYZE: A software system for biomedical image analysis. *In* Proceedings of the First Conference on Visualization in Biomedical Computing. May 22–25, 1990, Atlanta, GA. Atlanta, IEEE Computer Society Press, 1990, pp. 507–518. © 1990 IEEE.)

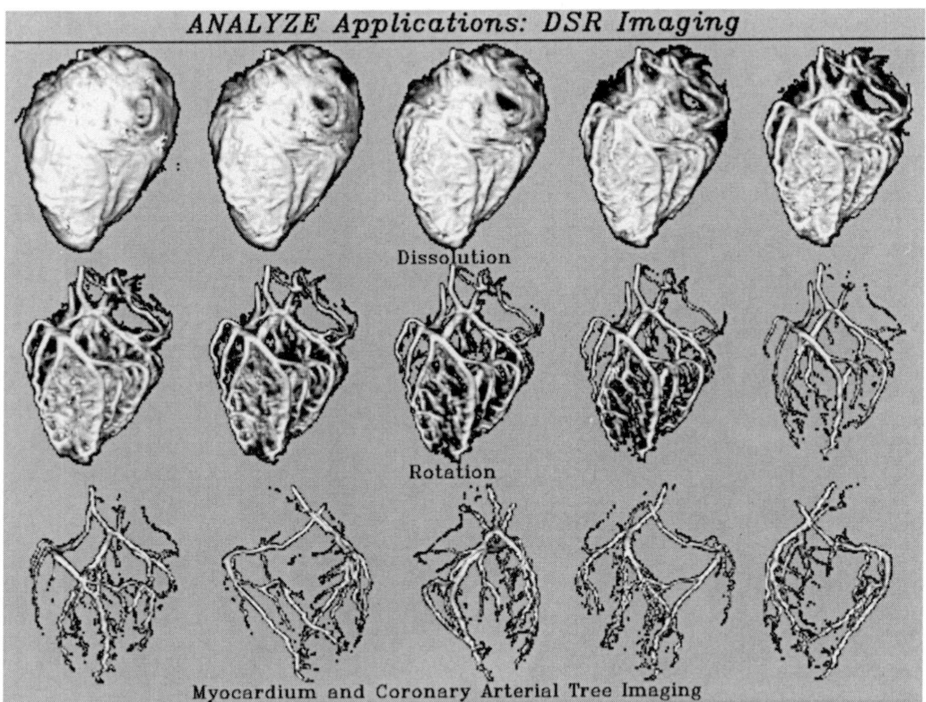

FIGURE 52–28. Volume-rendered images of the myocardium and coronary arterial tree from dynamic spatial reconstructor images, demonstrating successive tissue dissolution and rotation with the use of ANALYZE. The coronary tree can then be subjected to further quantitative analysis functions in ANALYZE to compute segment lengths, branching angles, and cross-sectional areas to detect and measure potential stenoses. (From ANALYZE: A software system for biomedical image analysis. *In* Proceedings of the First Conference on Visualization in Biomedical Computing. May 22–25, 1990, Atlanta, GA. Atlanta, IEEE Computer Society Press, 1990, pp. 507–518. © 1990 IEEE.)

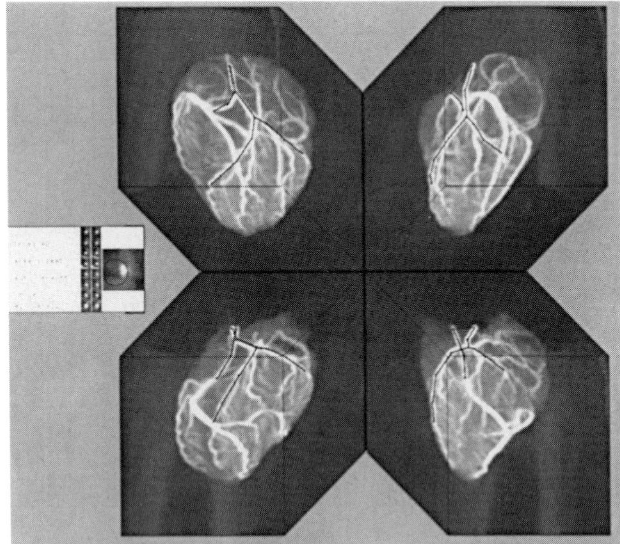

FIGURE 52–29. The four brightest voxel projection images computed from the trace program in ANALYZE to give an unambiguous view of three-dimensional vessel structures, such as the coronary arterial tree shown here, rendered from a dynamic spatial reconstructor scan. Tracing or pointing can be performed on any view and reflected in the other views to facilitate accurate delineation of branches and selection of branching points. Oblique images perpendicular to any traced line segment can be computed and displayed (*left center*) to show a cross section of the vessel structure from which the brightness-area-product is computed to estimate blood flow through the vessel or classification of stenotic lesions. (From Robb, R.A.: A software system for interactive and quantitative analysis of biomedical images. *In* Hohne, K.H., Fuchs, H., and Pizer, S.M. [eds.]: Three-Dimensional Imaging in Medicine. NATO ASI Series, Vol. F. New York, Springer-Verlag, 1990, 60:333–361, with permission.)

Acknowledgments

The authors would like to thank Dr. Richard L. Morin for his significant contributions to the previous edition of this chapter, much of which has been incorporated into the present version. We also wish to thank Cindy E. Lyon, Betty J. James, and Darlene M. Bernard for their expert assistance in the preparation of this manuscript.

References

1. Federal Drug Administration: Symposium on Biological Effects, Imaging Techniques, and Dosimetry of Ionizing Radiations: Publ. No. 80–8126. Washington, DC, U.S. Department of Health and Human Sciences, 1980.
2. Radon, J.: Uber die bestimmung von funktionen durch ihre integralwerte langs gewisser manningfaltigkeiten. Bu. Succss. Akad. Wiss. Leipzig Math. Phys. K. 69:262, 1917.
3. Bracewell, R.N.: Strip integration in radioastronomy. Aust. J. Phys. 9:198, 1956.
4. Christiansen, W.N., and Warburten, J.A.: The distribution of radio brightness over the solar disk at a wavelength of 21 centimeters: III. The quiet sun: Two-dimensional observations. Aust. J. Phys. 8:474, 1955.
5. Crowther, R.A., deRosier, D.J., and Klug, A.: The reconstruction of three-dimensional structure from projections and its application to electron microscopy. Proc. R. Soc. Lond. A 317:319, 1970.
6. DeRosier, D.J., and Klug, A.: Reconstruction of three-dimensional images from electron micrographs. Nature (Lond.) 217:130, 1968.
7. Oldendorf, W.H.: Isolated flying spot detection of radio-density discontinuities displaying the internal structural pattern of a complex object. I.R.E. Trans. Bio-Med. Elect. B.M.E. 8:68, 1961.
8. Cormack, A.M.: Representation of a function by its line integrals, with some radiological applications. J. Appl. Phys. 34:2722, 1963.
9. Cormack, A.M.: Early two-dimensional reconstruction (CT scanning) and recent topics stemming from it: Nobel Lecture, December 8, 1979. J. Comput. Assist. Tomogr. 4:658, 1980.
10. DiChiro, G., and Brooks, R.A.: The 1979 Nobel Prize in physiology and medicine. J. Comput. Assist. Tomogr. 4:241, 1980.
11. Kuhl, D.E., and Edwards, R.Q.: Rapid brain scanner with self contained computer and CRT display for both rectilinear and transverse section viewing. J. Nucl. Med. 9:332, 1968.
12. Bracewell, R.N., and Riddle, A.C.: Inversion of fan-beam scans in radioastronomy. Astrophys. J. 150:427, 1967.
13. Ramachandran, G.N., and Lakshminarayanan, A.V.: Three-dimensional reconstruction from radiographs and electron micrographs: Application of convolutions of Fourier transforms. Proc. Natl. Acad. Sci. U.S.A. 68:2236, 1971.
14. Hounsfield, G.N.: Computed medical imaging: Nobel Lecture, December 8, 1979. J. Comput. Assist. Tomogr. 4:665, 1980.
15. Ambrose, J.: Computerized transverse axial scanning (tomography): II. Clinical application. Br. J. Radiol. 46:1034, 1973.
16. Hounsfield, G.N.: Computerized transverse axial scanning (tomography): I. Description of system. Br. J. Radiol. 46:1016, 1973.
17. Ledley, R.S., DiChiro, G., Leussenhop, A.J., et al.: Computerized transaxial x-ray tomography of the human body. Science 186:207, 1974.
18. Dwyer, S.J. III, Brenner, D.J., Takasugi, S., et al.: Annotated Bibliography of Computed Tomography; Special Publication Series UMC-HCTC/E-001. Columbia, University of Missouri, 1979.
19. Vock, P., Soucek, M., Daepp, M., et al.: Lung: Spiral volumetric CT with single-breath-hold technique. Radiology 176:864, 1990.
20. Rigauts, H., Marchal, G., Baert, A.L., et al.: Initial experience with volume CT scanning. J. Comput. Assist. Tomogr. 14:675, 1990.
21. Kalender, W.A., Seissler, W., Klotz, E., et al.: Spiral volumetric CT with single-breath-hold technique, continuous transport, and continuous scanner rotation. Radiology 176:181, 1990.
22. Crawford, C.R., and King, K.F.: Computed tomography scanning with simultaneous patient translation. Med. Phys. 17:967, 1990.
23. Costello, P., Anderson, W., and Blume, D.: Pulmonary nodule: Evaluation with spiral volumetric CT. Radiology 179:875, 1991.
24. Kalender, W.A., and Polacin, A.: Physical performance characteristics of spiral CT scanning. Med. Phys. 18:910, 1991.
25. Fishman, E.K., Wyatt, S.H., Ney, D.R., et al.: Spiral CT of the pancreas with multiplanar display. AJR 159:1209, 1992.
26. Hacking, J.C., and Dixon, A.K.: Spiral versus conventional CT in soft tissue diagnosis. Eur. J. Radiol. 15:224, 1992.
27. Napel, S., Marks, M.P., Rubin, G.D., et al.: CT angiography with spiral CT and maximum intensity projection. Radiology 185:607, 1992.
28. Ney, D.R., Fishman, E.K., Kawashima, A., et al.: Comparison of helical and serial CT with regard to three-dimensional imaging of musculoskeletal anatomy. Radiology 185:865, 1992.
29. Remy-Jardin, M., Remy, J., Wattinne, L., et al.: Central pulmonary thromboembolism: Diagnosis with spiral volumetric CT with the single-breath-hold technique—comparison with pulmonary angiography. Radiology 185:381, 1992.
30. Zeman, R.K., Fox, S.H., Silverman, P.M., et al.: Helical (spiral) CT of the abdomen. AJR 160:719, 1993.
31. Goldman, L.W., and Fowlkes, J.B. (eds.): Medical CT and Ultrasound: Current Technology and Applications. Madison, Advanced Medical Publishing, 1995.
32. Kieffer, J.: The laminagraph and its variations: Applications and implications of the planigraphic principle. AJR 39:497, 1938.
33. Edholm, P.: The tomogram: Its formation and content. Acta Radiol. Suppl. 193:1, 1960.
34. Bursch, J., Johs, R., and Heintzen, P.H.: Validity of Lambert-Beer's Law in roentgen-densitometry of contrast material using continuous radiation. *In* Thieme, G. (ed.): Roentgen-Cine and Videodensitometry. Stuttgart, George Thieme Verlag, 1971, p. 81.
35. McCullough, E.C., Baker, H.L., Houser, O.W., et al.: An evaluation of the quantitative and radiation features of a scanning x-ray transverse axial tomography: The EMI scanner. Radiology 111:709, 1974.
36. Brooks, R.A., and DiChiro, G.: Beam hardening in x-ray computed tomography. Phys. Med. Biol. 21:390, 1976.
37. Zatz, L.M., and Alvarez, R.G.: An inaccuracy in computed tomography: The energy dependence of CT values. Radiology 124:91, 1977.
38. Joseph, P.M., and Spital, R.A.: A method for correcting bone induced artifacts in computed tomography scanners. J. Comput. Assist. Tomogr. 2:100, 1978.
39. McDavid, W.D., Waggener, R.G., Payne, W.H., et al.: Correction for spectral artifacts in cross-sectional reconstructions from x-rays. Med. Phys. 4:54, 1977.
40. Herman, G.T., and Simmons, R.: Illustrations of a beam hardening correction method in computerized tomography. Appl. Opt. Instrumen. Med. III, SPIE 173:264, 1979.
41. Ruegsegger, P., Hangartner, T., Keller, H.U., et al.: Standardization of computed tomographic images by means of material-selective beam hardening correction. J. Comput. Assist. Tomogr. 2:184, 1978.
42. Drieke, P., and Boyd, D.: Convolution reconstruction of fan beam projections. Comput. Graphics Image Proc. 5:459, 1976.
43. Herman, G.T., Lakshminarayanan, A.V., and Naparstek, A.: Convolution reconstruction techniques for divergent beams. Comput. Biol. Med. 6:259, 1976.
44. Robb, R.A., Greenleaf, J.F., Ritman, E.L., et al.: Three-dimensional visualization of the intact thorax and contents: A technique for cross-sectional reconstruction for multiplanar x-ray views. Comput. Biomed. Res. 7:395, 1974.
45. Glover, G.H., and Eisner, R.L.: Theoretical resolution of computed tomography systems. J. Comput. Assist. Tomogr. 3:85, 1979.
46. Huesman, R.H.: The effects of a finite number of projection angles and finite lateral sampling of projections on the propagation of statistical errors in transverse section reconstruction. Phys. Med. Biol. 22:511, 1977.
47. Cho, Z.H., Ahn, I., Bohm, C., et al.: Computerized image reconstruction methods with multiple photon/x-ray transmission scanning. Phys. Med. Biol. 19:511, 1974.
48. Gilbert, P.F.C.: Iterative methods for the reconstruction of three-dimensional objects from projections. J. Theor. Biol. 36:105, 1972.
49. Gordon, R., and Herman, G.T.: Three-dimensional reconstruction from projects: A review of algorithms. Int. Rev. Cytol. 38:111, 1974.

50. Shepp, L.A., and Kruskal, J.B.: Computerized tomography: The new medical x-ray technology. Am. Math. Mo. 85:420, 1978.
51. Vainshtein, B.K.: Finding the structure of objects from the projections. Kristallografiya 15:894, 1970.
52. Shepp, L.A., and Logan, E.C.: The Fourier reconstruction of a head section. IEEE Trans. Nucl. Sci. 21:21, 1974.
53. Budinger, T.F., and Gullberg, G.T.: Three-dimensional reconstruction in nuclear medicine imaging. IEEE Trans. Nucl. Sci. 21:2, 1974.
54. Kinlaks, J.R.: Computer tomographic equipment survey. Appl. Radiol. 4:81, 1976.
55. Boyd, D.P., Korbin, M.T., and Moss, A.: Engineering status of computerized tomographic scanning. Opt. Eng. 16:37, 1977.
56. Waggener, R., and McDavid, W.: Transmission computed tomographic system components. *In* Fullerton, G. (ed.): Medical Physics of CT and Ultrasound Tissue Imaging Characteristics. AAPM Med. Phys. Monogr. 6:94, 1980.
57. Workshop on Physics and Engineering in Computerized Tomography. IEEE Trans. Nucl. Sci. NS-262, 1979.
58. Robb, R.A.: X-ray computed tomography: An engineering synthesis of multiscientific principles. CRC Crit. Rev. Biomed. Eng. 74:265, 1982.
59. Alfidi, R.J., MacIntyre, W.J., and Haager, J.R.: The effects of biological motion on CT resolution. AJR 127:11, 1976.
60. Hounsfield, G.N.: Picture quality of computed tomography. AJR 127:3, 1976.
61. Filipczak, P.A.: Slip ring assembly for high voltages. U.S. Patent Number 2,979,685, 1961.
62. Slavin, P.E.: X-ray helical scanning means for displaying an image of an object within the body being scanned. U.S. Patent Number 3,432,657, 1969.
63. Dinwiddie, K.L., Friday, R.G., and Rascz, G.A.: Tomographic scanning apparatus having detector signal digitizing means mounted to rotate with detectors. U.S. Patent Number 4,190,772, 1980.
64. Zeman, R.K., Brink, J.A., Costello, P., et al. (eds.): Helical/Spiral CT: A Practical Approach. New York, McGraw-Hill, 1995.
65. Polacin, A., Kalender, W.A., and Marchal, G.: Evaluation of section sensitivity profiles and image noise in spiral CT. Radiology 185:29, 1992.
66. Polacin, A., and Kalender, W.A.: Measurement of slice sensitivity profiles in spiral CT. Med. Phys. 21:133, 1994.
67. Wood, E.H., Ritman, E.L., Sturm, R.E., et al.: The problem of determination of the roentgen density, dimensions and shape of homogeneous objects from biplane roentgenographic data with particular reference to angiocardiogrpahy. Proc. San Diego Biomed. Symp. 2:3, 1972.
68. Robb, R.A., and Ritman, E.L.: High-speed synchronous volume computer tomography of the heart. Radiology 133:655, 1979.
69. Ritman, E.L., Robb, R.A., Johnson, S.A., et al.: Quantitative imaging of the structure and function of the heart, lungs, and circulation. Mayo Clin. Proc. 53:3, 1978.
70. Guthaner, D.F., Wexler, L., and Harell, G.: Computed tomography demonstration of cardiac structures. AJR 133:75, 1979.
71. Gur, D., Drayer, B.P., Borovetz, H.S., et al.: Dynamic computed tomography of the lung: Regional ventilation measurements. J. Comput. Assist. Tomogr. 3:749, 1979.
72. Harell, G.S., Guthaner, D.F., Brieman, R.S., et al.: Stop-action cardiac computed tomography. Radiology 123:515, 1977.
73. Heinz, E.R., Dubois, P.J., Drayer, B.P., et al.: A preliminary investigation of the role of dynamic computed tomography in renovascular hypertension. J. Comput. Assist. Tomogr. 4:63, 1980.
74. Sagal, S., Weiss, E.S., Gillard, R.G., et al.: Gated computed tomography of the human heart. Invest. Radiol. 12:554, 1977.
75. Beringer, W.H., Redington, R.W., Doherty, D., et al.: Gated cardiac scanning: Canine studies. J. Comput. Assist. Tomogr. 3:155, 1979.
76. Taber, P., Chang, L.W.M., and Campion, G.M.: Left brachycephalic vein simulating aortic dissection on computed tomography. Radiology 133:562, 1979.
77. Lipton, M.J., Brundage, B.H., Doherty, P.W., et al.: Contrast medium-enhanced computed tomography for evaluating ischemic heart disease. J. Comput. Assist. Tomogr. 4:571, 1980.
78. Young, S.W., Noon, M.A., Nassi, M., et al.: Dynamic computed tomography body scanning. J. Comput. Assist. Tomogr. 4:168, 1980.
79. Boyd, D.P., Gould, R.G., Quinn, J.R., et al.: A proposed dynamic cardiac 3-D densitometer for early detection and evaluation of heart disease. IEEE Trans. Nucl. Sci. 26:2724, 1979.
80. Boyd, D.P.: Future technologies, transmission CT. *In* Newton, T.H., and Potts, D.G. (eds.): Radiology of the Skull and Brain. Chap. 5. St. Louis, Mosby, 1981.
81. Boyd, D.: Computerized transmission tomography of the heart using scanning electron beams. *In* Higgins, C.B. (ed.): CT of Heart and the Great Vessels: Experimental Evaluation in the Clinical Application. Mt. Kisco, NY, Futura, 1983.
82. Stanford, W., and Rumberger, J. (eds.): Ultrafast Computed Tomography in Cardiac Imaging. Mt. Kisco, NY, Futura, 1992.
83. McCollough, C.H., and Morin, R.L.: The technical design and performance of ultrafast computed tomography. Radiol. Clin. North Am. 32:521, 1994.
84. McCullough, E.C., and Payne, J.T.: Patient dosage in computed tomography. Radiology 129:457, 1978.
85. Shope, T.B., Gagne, R.M., and Johnson, G.C.: A method for describing the dose delivered by transmission x-ray computed tomography. Med. Phys. 8:488, 1981.
86. Suzuki, A., and Suzuki, M.N.: Use of a pencil-shaped ionization chamber for measurements of exposure resulting from a computed tomography scan. Med. Phys. 5:536, 1978.
87. McCollough, C.H., Zink, F.E., and Morin, R.L.: Radiation dosimetry for electron-beam CT. Radiology 192:637, 1994.
88. Zink, F.E., and McCollough, C.H.: The measurement of radiation dose profiles for electron-beam computed tomography using film dosimetry. Med. Phys. 8:1287, 1994.
89. McCollough, C.H., and Lui, H.H.: Breast dose during electron-beam CT: Measurement with film dosimetry. Radiology 196:153, 1995.
90. Chang, W.: Slice characteristics of the Imatron cine-CT scanner. J. Comput. Assist. Tomogr. 11:554, 1987.
91. Behrenbeck, T., Kinsey, J.H., Harris, L.D., et al.: Three-dimensional spatial, density and temporal resolution of the DSR. J. Comput. Assist. Tomogr. 6:1138, 1982.
92. Ritman, E.L., Kinsey, J.H., Robb, R.A., et al.: Physics and technical considerations in the design of the DSR: A high temporal resolution volume scanner. AJR 134:369, 1980.
93. Gould, R.G.: Patient dose considerations from an ultrafast CT scanner. Radiology 181:112, 1991.
94. Robb, R.A., Ritman, E.L., Gilbert, B.K., et al.: The DSR: A high-speed three-dimensional x-ray computed tomography system for dynamic spatial reconstruction of the heart and circulation. I.E.E.E. Trans. Nucl. Sci. NS-26:2713, 1979.
95. Ritman, E.L., Kinsey, J.H., Robb, R.A., et al.: Three-dimensional imaging of heart, lungs, and circulation. Science 210:273, 1980.
96. Robb, R.A., and Gilbert, B.K.: Description and evaluation of a system for high-speed three-dimensional computed tomography of the body: The dynamic spatial reconstructor. NCC-80. National Computer Conference, American Federation of Information Processing Society, Las Vegas, 1980. 49:427, 1980.
97. Kinsey, J.H., Robb, R.A., Ritman, E.L., et al.: The DSR: A high temporal resolution volumetric roentgenographic CT scanner. Herz 5:177, 1980.
98. Kinsey, J.H., and Orvis, A.L.: High repetition rate volumetric x-ray CT scanning. I.E.E.E. Trans. Nucl. Sci. NS-28:1732, 1981.
99. Robb, R.A., Lent, A.H., Gilbert, B.K., et al.: The dynamic spatial reconstructor: A computed tomography system for high-speed simultaneous scanning of multiple cross sections of the heart. J. Med. Syst. 4:253, 1980.
100. Robb, R.A., Hoffman, E.A., Sinak, L.J., et al.: High-speed three-dimensional x-ray computed tomography: The dynamic spatial reconstructor. Proc. IEEE 713:308, 1983.
101. Sturm, R.E., Ritman, E.L., Hansen, R.J., et al.: Recording of multichannel analog data and video images on the same video tape or disc. J. Appl. Physiol. 36:761, 1974.
102. Artzy, E., Frieder, G., and Herman, G.: The theory, design, implementation and evaluation of a three-dimensional algorithm. Comput. Graphics Image Proc. 15:1, 1981.
103. Liu, Y.H., Hoffman, E.A., Hagler, D.J., et al.: Accuracy of pulmonary vascular dimensions estimated with the dynamic spatial reconstructor. Am. J. Physiol. Imaging 1:201, 1986.
104. Spyra, W.J.T., Bove, A.A., and Ritman, E.L.: Some technical considerations in tomographic coronary arteriography. Int. J. Card. Imaging 2:223, 1987.
105. Robb, R.A.: A software system for interactive and quantitative analysis of biomedical images. *In* Hohne, K.H., Fuchs, H., and Pizer, S.M. (eds.): 3D Imaging in Medicine. Berlin, Springer-Verlag, F 60, 1990, p. 333.
106. Robb, R.A.: ANALYZE™: Visualization and analysis of biomedical images. Proceedings of the IS&T/SPIE Symposium on Electronic Imaging: Science and Technology, San Jose, CA, 1993. Vol. 1905.
107. Robb, R.: Three-Dimensional Biomedical Imaging: Principles and Practice. New York, VCH Publishers, 1994.

CHAPTER

53 Evaluation of Cardiovascular Structure and Function with Electron-Beam Computed Tomography

Robert M. Weiss, M.D.
William Stanford, M.D.

X-ray computed tomography, first conceived by Hounsfield,[1] revolutionized the field of medical diagnostic imaging. This genre was further developed for dynamic study of the heart by Robb and coworkers[2] in the form of the dynamic spatial reconstructor—a device that produces images from an array of image intensifiers. Boyd and associates[3] proposed a novel device for image acquisition that used magnetically guided electron bombardment of stationary semicircular tungsten targets to produce a plane of x-rays that are detected by a stationary array of detectors. A device based on these principles was commercially introduced in the 1980s and has since been referred to in the literature as electron-beam computed tomography (EBCT), cine CT, rapid-acquisition computed axial tomography (RACAT), fast CT, and Ultrafast CT (a registered trademark of the Imatron Corp., South San Francisco, CA). Because the device does not rely on any mechanical moving parts, images with very high spatial and density resolution can be acquired rapidly enough to portray cardiac motion. These features have been capitalized on so that EBCT has become a tool for the precise evaluation of cardiac structure and function. The purposes of this chapter will be to describe the general techniques for cardiovascular imaging using EBCT, to review the extensive quantitative experimental and clinical validation, and to discuss its practical applications.

TECHNICAL CONSIDERATIONS

Image Acquisition

Cardiac evaluation with EBCT is performed in one of two modes: a normal-resolution multislice mode or a higher resolution single-slice mode. The scanning features of each are shown in Table 53–1. In both scanning modes, images may be obtained serially throughout a single cardiac cycle or, alternatively, at the same point (e.g., at end-diastole) in successive cardiac cycles. The choice of scanning mode generally depends on the diagnostic questions being asked. For precise definition of static cardiac and thoracic anatomy, the single-slice mode is usually preferred because of its higher resolution. Images of the field of interest are obtained during suspended respiration by moving the patient through the scanner in the time between acquisition of serial images, which are electrocardiographically triggered. For precise quantitation of cardiac function, the multislice mode is usually selected because of its more rapid acquisition. The scanner can acquire a series of images at eight tomographic locations, with a total span of 8 cm. Thus, two complete imaging sequences are required to span the entire heart. Scanning in planes parallel to the cardiac short or long axis is accomplished by positioning the patient with respect to the imager, which is fixed in the vertical position. Because blood and cardiac muscle have similar x-ray absorption properties, administration of iodinated contrast medium is necessary to delineate specific cardiac structures. When transit of blood is to be visualized (e.g., for indicator-dilution measurement of cardiac output or determination of bypass graft patency), contrast material is administered as a brisk bolus (Fig. 53–1). When the goal is assessment of ventricular function, contrast medium is administered as a constant infusion so that dye is distributed approximately equally among all cardiac chambers during image acquisition (Fig. 53–2).

Image Analysis

After image acquisition, images are synthesized and stored for later analysis. Standardized image-analysis hardware and software

TABLE 53–1. IMAGE FEATURES FOR MULTISLICE AND SINGLE-SLICE SCANNING MODES

	Multislice	Single Slice
Maximum number of slices	8	1
Slice thickness	8 mm	1.5 or 3 mm
Acquisition time per image	50 msec	100 msec
Nominal in-plane resolution	<2 mm	~0.7 mm
ECG-triggered	+	+

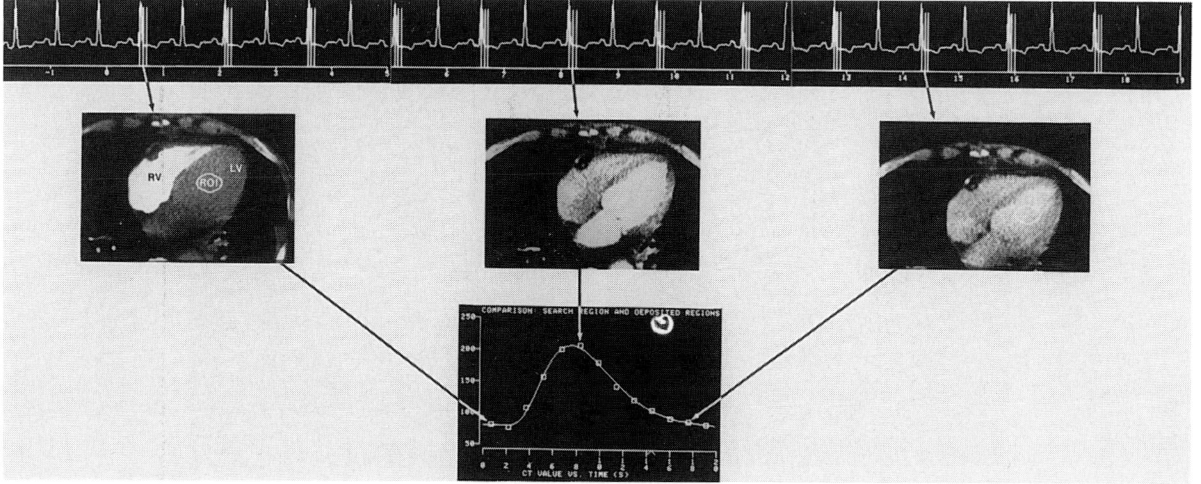

FIGURE 53–1. ECG-triggered scans acquired in the "flow" mode. In this sequence, pairs of parallel tomograms are repetitively acquired during successive cardiac cycles. Tomograms are shown before dye arrival in the left ventricle (LV, *left*), during peak opacification (*center*), and during dye washout (*right*). A left ventricular time intensity curve is shown, from which cardiac output may be determined. RV = right ventricle; ROI = region of interest.

are available from the manufacturer. Alternatively, several off-line customized image-analysis packages have been adapted for use with EBCT.[4, 5] To perform indicator-dilution analysis, the operator first draws a region of interest in one or more cardiac or vascular structures (see Fig. 53–1). The standardized image-analysis software then reports a time-versus-radiodensity plot for each region. Radiodensity is reported in Hounsfield numbers, frequently abbreviated as "CT#." Baseline radiodensity values for body structures correspond approximately to those reported for conventional x-ray CT, which are periodically confirmed by calibration against reference standards of known density. The change in radiodensity after contrast injection is proportional to the change in concentration of contrast material within the region of interest. Thus, the time-versus-radiodensity plot can be considered a time-versus-concentration plot and can be curve-fitted for quantitative calculations.

Quantitation of cardiac chamber size, mass, or function requires meticulous attention to location of the borders between adjacent structures (e.g., epicardium and lung). The actual border may not

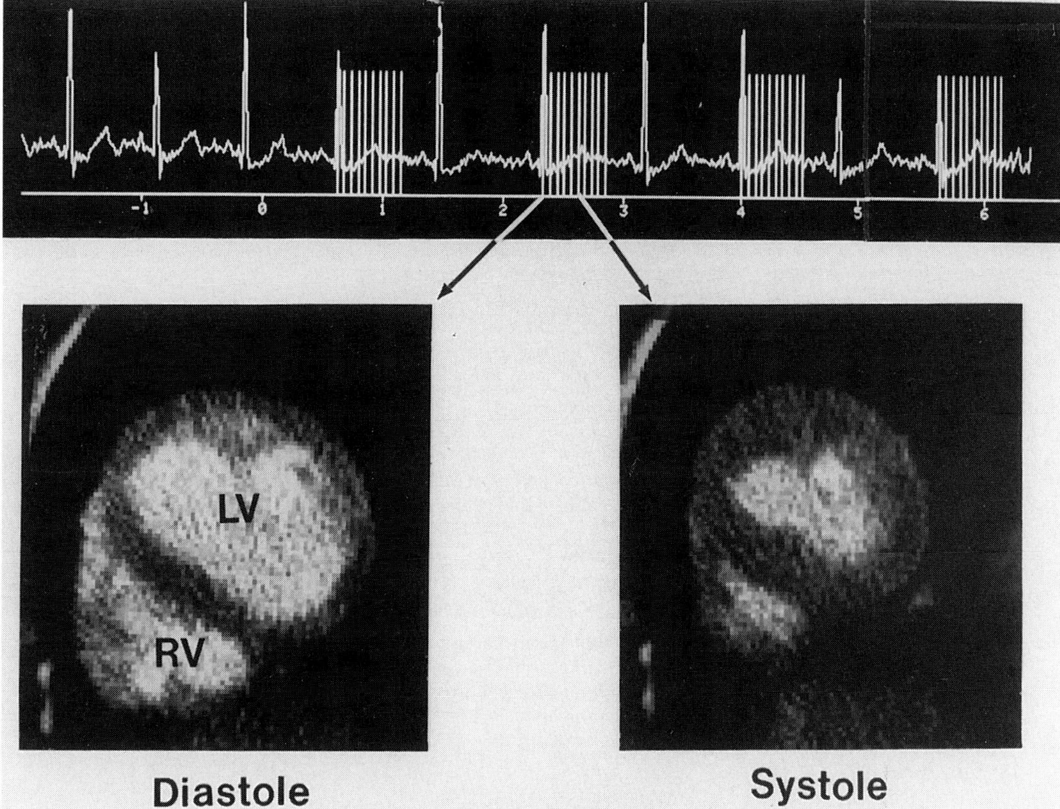

FIGURE 53–2. ECG-triggered scans acquired in "movie" mode. Each vertical line superimposed on the ECG tracing represents acquisition time for a pair of images in contiguous tomographic planes. Representative images from diastole and systole are shown.

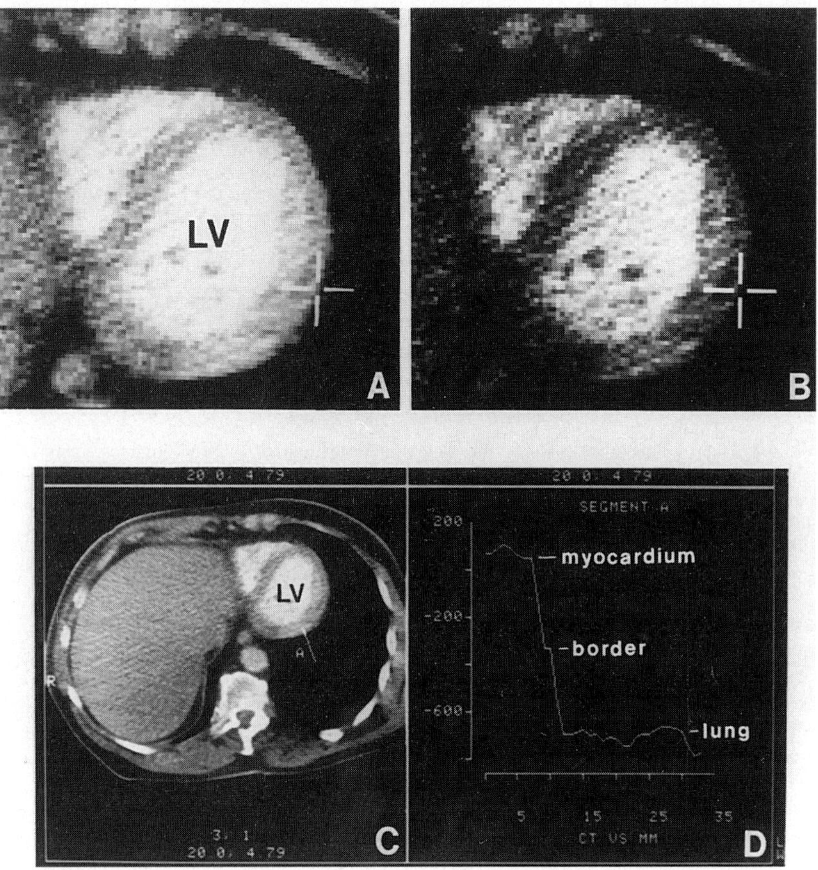

FIGURE 53–3. Border detection method. *A and B*, The same short-axis midventricular tomogram is shown, using two different video display settings. A "+" is placed at identical locations in both pictures to demonstrate the degree to which the visually determined border is dependent on chosen display parameters. *C*, A line is drawn from midmyocardium to lung. *D*, A graph depicting radiodensity (CT #) along that line. The border is determined by finding the point at which radiodensity is the arithmetic mean of the two adjacent structures (myocardium and lung) LV = left ventricle. (From method described by Feiring and associates.[6])

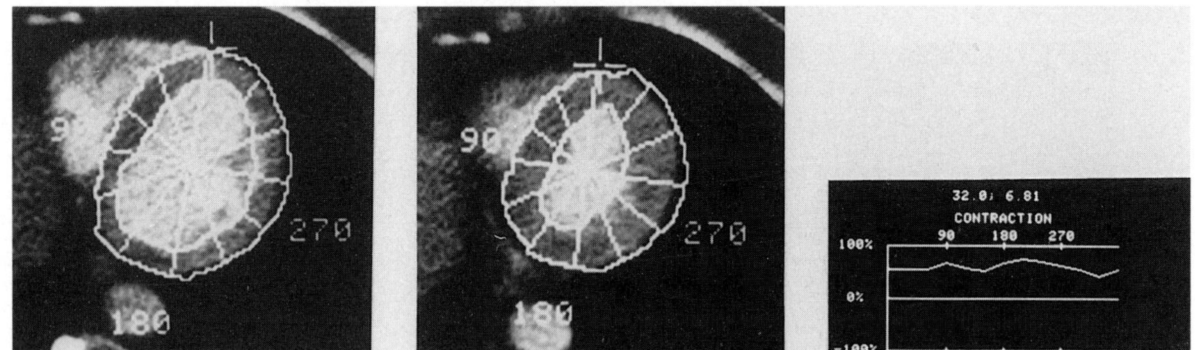

FIGURE 53–4. Assessment of regional left ventricular function within a tomographic slice. End-diastolic and end-systolic frames are each divided into 12 "pie-slice" segments, each representing 30 degrees of the endocardial circumference. In this analysis, a fixed center of mass is employed. A floating reference point, located on the anterior interventricular septum, is used to correct for cardiac systolic rotation. A map of segmental ejection fraction is shown at right.

be visually apparent, depending on the operator-selected video display parameters. Feiring and colleagues developed a computer-assisted algorithm that was applied to the task of left ventricular mass quantitation.[6] The border between structures is located by finding the picture element (pixel) with a radiodensity that is the arithmetic mean of the densities of the two adjacent structures (Fig. 53–3). Fortunately, automated computer border-detection has been developed and validated, making this task much less laborious.[4, 5, 7] This procedure produces a measurement of the area that a given structure occupies in a single tomogram. Tomographic volume is calculated by multiplying by slice thickness. Subsequently, mass is determined by multiplying the volume of the structure by its presumed mass density (1.05 g/mL for myocardium). Finally, the total volume or mass of a given structure is calculated by means of summing values obtained from all tomographic slices, with the use of a modification of Simpson's rule, which compensates for interslice gaps (either 0 or 4 mm in the multislice mode[6]). Image acquisition and analysis throughout the cardiac cycle allow calculation of stroke volumes, systolic ejection rate, and diastolic filling rates.

After endocardial and epicardial borders are identified, regional ventricular function analysis is facilitated by image-analysis software that divides the ventricle into segments that incorporate 10 or 30 degrees of its circumference, relative to its center of mass (Fig. 53–4). Selection of a floating reference point (e.g., the left anterior descending artery in cross section) can be used to correct for cardiac rotation during the cardiac cycle. Regional function is reported as the "segmental ejection fraction," which portrays endocardial motion, or alternatively as the regional change in ventricular wall thickness.

PRECISION OF QUANTITATIVE MEASUREMENTS

EBCT methods have undergone extensive experimental and clinical validation and now may be considered a "gold standard" for in vivo quantitation of cardiac structure and function. Before undertaking quantitative assessment of cardiac structure or function, one must ensure that the process of measurement does not significantly perturb the parameters to be measured. Iodinated contrast medium has been reported to have hemodynamic and direct cardiac effects.[8, 9] Reiter and colleagues[10] demonstrated that peripheral venous injection of ionic contrast material produces substantial perturbation of cardiovascular function. However, at doses commonly given, nonionic contrast media have negligible effects on blood pressure, heart rate, coronary flow, or ventricular stroke volume.[10]

Ventricular Mass

Feiring and co-workers[6] were able to demonstrate the precision with which left ventricular mass can be quantitated, using EBCT (Fig. 53–5, *left*). This method is superior to conventional planar determinations, because it makes no presumptions about ventricular shape, which may be distorted in some disease states. A similar degree of accuracy has been achieved in quantitation of right ventricular mass in experimental animals[11] (see Fig. 53–5, *right*) and in postmortem casts of human hearts.[12] This algorithm capitalizes on the special capabilities of the high-resolution scanning mode. Once again, the method does not rely on any presumptions about the shape of the right ventricle.

Cardiac Chamber Volume

Instantaneous measurements of ventricular volume are difficult to validate for lack of a practical reference standard. However, Reiter and associates[10] were able to demonstrate precise measurements of both right and left ventricular stroke volumes in laboratory animals, using simultaneous measurements made by the thermodilution method or by electromagnetic flow probes as the validation standard (Fig. 53–6). Oren and co-workers[13, 14] were able to demonstrate a similar degree of accuracy in human subjects, using simultaneous thermodilution measurements as the reference standard (r = .98, standard error of the estimate [SEE] = 4.5 mL). Because the researchers calculated EBCT assessment of stroke volume using measurement of end-diastolic and end-systolic volumes, this study lends strong support to the contention that instantaneous ventricular volume measurements are accurate as well. Both left and right atria are clearly delineated by EBCT scanning in both normal- and high-resolution scanning modes. Because an in vivo reference standard is not available to validate these measurements,

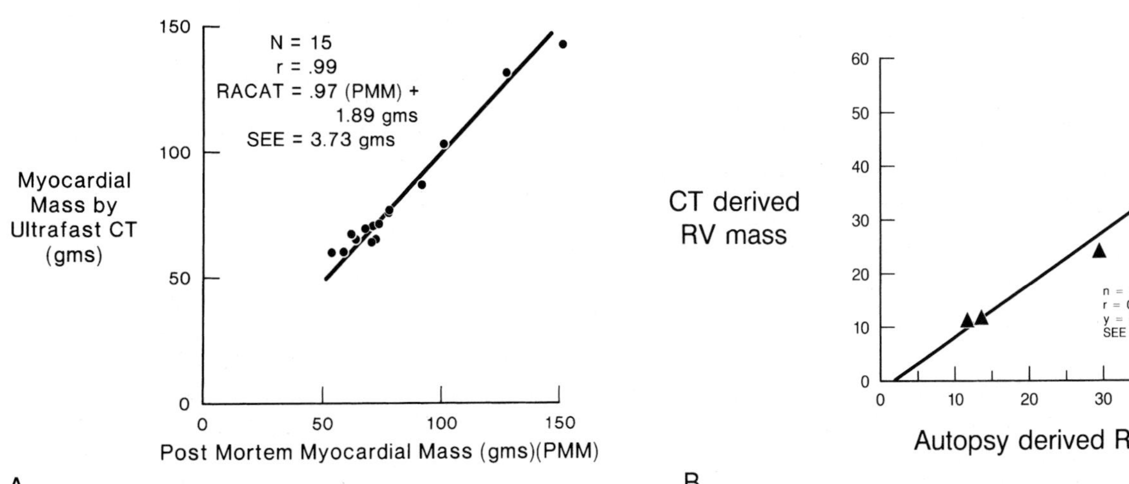

FIGURE 53–5. *A*, The very close agreement between left ventricular mass determined by EBCT (Ultrafast CT) and actual postmortem mass is shown. *B*, Agreement between EBCT-determined right ventricular mass and actual postmortem mass. (*A* from Feiring, A.J., Rumberger, J.A., Reiter, S.J., et al.: Determination of left ventricular mass in dogs with rapid-acquisition cardiac computed tomographic scanning. Circulation 72:1355, 1985; with permission of the American Heart Association. *B* from Hajduczok, Z.D., Weiss, R.M., Stanford, W., et al.: Determination of right ventricular mass in humans and dogs with Ultrafast cardiac computed tomography. Circulation 82:202, 1990; with permission of the American Heart Association.)

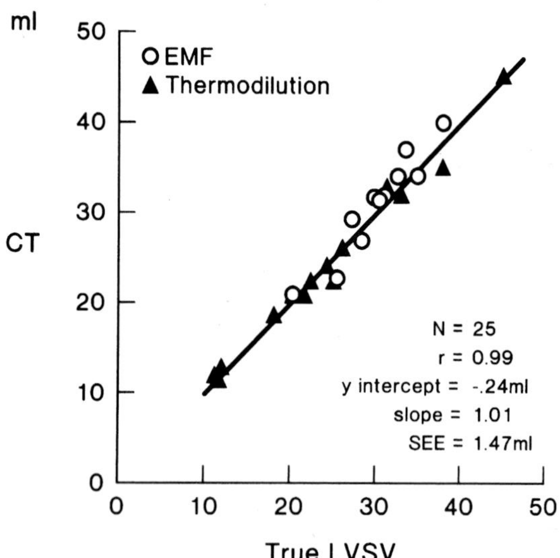

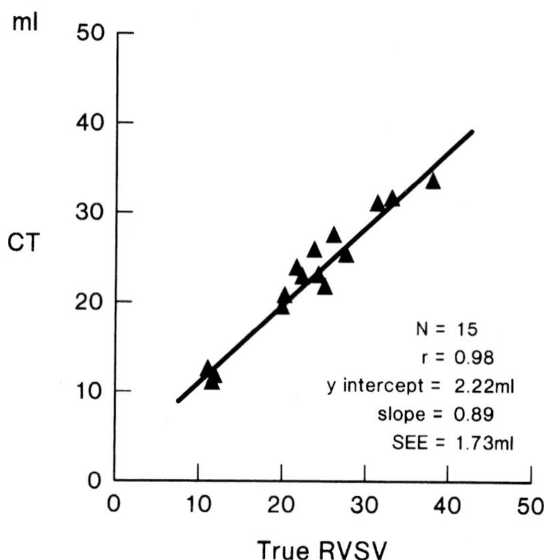

FIGURE 53–6. The precision with which stroke volumes of left and right ventricles (LVSV and RVSV) can be measured with EBCT. These studies were performed in laboratory animals, with the use of measurements of stroke volume by the thermodilution method or with chronically implanted electromagnetic flow (EMF) probes as the reference standard. (From Reiter, S.J., Rumberger, J.A., Feiring, A.J., et al.: Precision of measurements of right and left ventricular stroke volume by cine computed tomography. Circulation 74:890, 1986; with permission of the American Heart Association.)

Vandenberg and associates[15] used radiopaque casts of postmortem hearts. There was reasonable agreement between EBCT measurements of left atrial volume and the actual water displacement volumes (r = .99, SEE = 2 mL).

Ventricular Function

The data above indicate that ventricular volume can be measured with precision. It is a simple matter to calculate ejection fractions for both ventricles. This technique has shown reasonable agreement with more established methods, such as radionuclide angiography (Fig. 53–7). Ventricular diastolic function is determined with the use of a method previously reported for radionuclide angiography.[16] Ventricular volume is determined for each time throughout the cardiac cycle. The early diastolic portion of the time-versus-volume curve is fitted to a third-order polynomial. Peak filling rate is calculated by finding the inflection point of this fitted curve. EBCT measurements of diastolic function have shown very good agreement with the radionuclide method[17] (Fig. 53–8). Oren and colleagues[18] have reported a simplification of this method: measurement of early diastolic filling fraction (%FF), which is the fraction of total diastolic filling that occurs in the first 174 msec after end-systole. This time interval is dictated by the fixed framing rate of the EBCT device. This parameter has demonstrated usefulness in identifying patients with constrictive pericarditis—a disease characterized by diastolic dysfunction (see later text).

TABLE 53–2. NORMAL VALUES*

	LV	RV	LA	RA
EDVI (mL/m^2)	72±9	86±12	14±3	22±8
ESVI (mL/m^2)	21±5	37±9	31±5	44±11
SVI (mL/m^2)	51±6	49±7		
EF (%)	70±5	57±6		
Mass index (g/m^2)	80±10	25±3		

*Mean±SD. Values were obtained from nine normal volunteers, age 23±4 years.

LV = left ventricle; RV = right ventricle; LA = left atrium; RA = right atrium; EDVI = end-diastolic volume/body surface area; ESVI = end-systolic volume/body surface area; SVI = stroke volume/body surface area; EF = ejection fraction.

Indicator-Dilution Measurements

As noted previously, indicator concentration-versus-time plots can be generated for any cardiovascular region of interest after bolus injection of contrast material. Data from each selected region are fitted to a gamma-variate curve with the use of standardized image-analysis software. The Stewart-Hamilton equation[19] is then applied to determine flow through that structure. This procedure involves nonlinear manipulation of time-density data. The relationship between contrast concentration and radiodensity is highly linear, but with a slope that varies slightly from patient to patient because of differences in beam characteristics caused by body attenuation. Thus, for precise indicator-dilution measurements, an "in vivo calibration" must be performed by placing vials of known dye concentration on the patient's chest during scanning.

Calculation of flow through the pulmonary circuit is performed after peripheral venous bolus injection by placing a region of

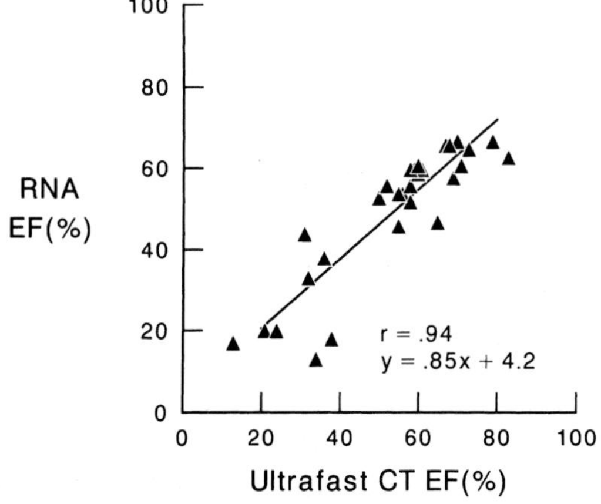

FIGURE 53–7. Comparison of measurements of left ventricular ejection fraction (EF) with radionuclide angiography (RNA) and with EBCT (cine CT). These measurements were made in human subjects several days apart.

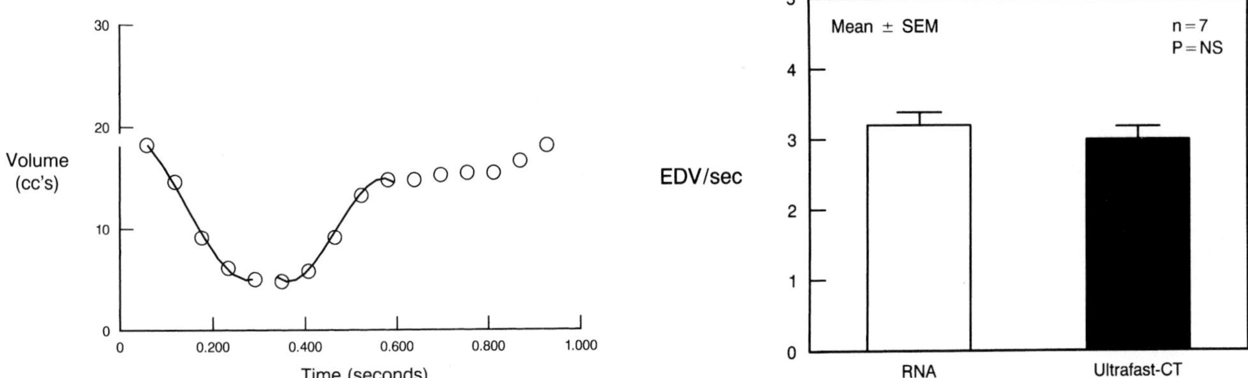

FIGURE 53–8. *Left Panel,* Plot of cavity area versus time for a single tomographic slice, using EBCT. Third-order polynomial curves are fitted to peak-ejection and peak-filling segments. *Right Panel,* Global left ventricular peak filling rate, normalized to end-diastolic volume (EDV/sec), using EBCT (ultrafast-CT) and radionuclide angiography (RNA) in seven normal human subjects. Measurements with the two techniques were made several hours apart. (From Rumberger, J.A., Weiss, R.M., Feiring, A.J., et al.: Patterns of regional diastolic function in the normal human left ventricle: An Ultrafast CT study. J. Am. Coll. Cardiol. 14:119, 1989, with permission of the American College of Cardiology.)

interest in the pulmonary artery, which allows for adequate mixing of dye. Systemic circuit flow is determined by placing a region of interest in a left heart chamber. Reiter and associates[20] used this method to demonstrate very precise measurements of cardiac output in laboratory animals (Fig. 53–9). This technique has been applied to humans by Ludman and colleagues.[21] By comparing outputs in pulmonary and systemic circuits, quantitative evaluation of intracardiac shunts may be performed (see Chapter 58).

SPECIAL CLINICAL APPLICATIONS

At centers where the device is available, EBCT can provide a minimally invasive, quantitatively reliable, comprehensive assessment of cardiac structure and function in virtually every patient. Table 53–2 depicts normal values obtained by comprehensive assessment of normal human subjects. The very high reproducibility of data obtained[22] facilitates the use of serial examinations for assessment of the progression of disease or response to therapeutic interventions.[23] The device lends itself to application of special

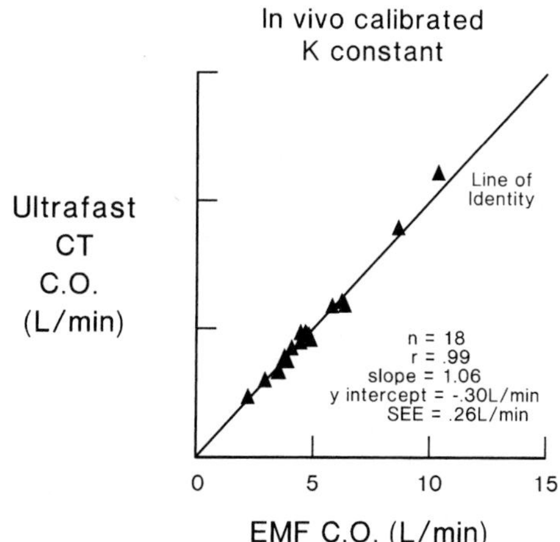

FIGURE 53–9. Measurements of cardiac output (C.O.), using indicator-dilution analysis, made by EBCT (Ultrafast CT) compared with simultaneous measurements using electromagnetic flow (EMF) probes. These studies were performed in laboratory animals. (Adapted from Reiter, S.J., Feiring, A.J., Stanford, W., et al.: Precise measurements of contrast clearance curve cardiac outputs using cine computed tomography. [Abstract.] J. Am. Coll. Cardiol. 9:161A, 1987.)

clinical problems of interest to the clinical cardiologist. A series of demonstrative examples follow.

Constrictive Pericarditis

The diagnosis of constrictive pericarditis can be problematic for the clinician. The disease syndrome results from limitation of cardiac filling by chronically inflamed or scarred pericardium. The clinical presentation is characterized by overt systemic venous congestion and the inability to raise cardiac output during stress. These features are common to a number of cardiac and noncardiac conditions.[24, 25] A clinical history and physical examination often fail to elicit the inciting event (i.e., pericardial trauma, infection, or inflammation) because it is often temporally remote. Conventional imaging techniques do not reliably image pericardium, particularly in the absence of dense calcification.[26] An invasive hemodynamic study can reveal characteristic findings, but even these data may be misleading.[27] These difficulties were highlighted by Seifert and co-workers,[28] who found that a substantial number of patients referred for surgical treatment of constrictive pericarditis were ultimately found to have normal pericardium at the time of thoracotomy. EBCT, by virtue of imaging with superior spatial and temporal resolution, is a very useful diagnostic tool in this setting. Grover-McKay and associates[29] demonstrated the very high accuracy of pericardial thickness measurements in an animal model of pericarditis. Oren and colleagues[18] studied a series of 12 patients who were suspected of having constrictive pericarditis on the basis of complete clinical evaluation, including invasive hemodynamic study. For each patient, there was histopathologic confirmation of the status of the pericardium by surgery or autopsy. EBCT assessment was able to demonstrate definitively both the abnormal anatomy (thickened pericardium) and physiology (abnormally rapid early diastolic right ventricular filling) in patients with constriction and to clearly distinguish them from the patients who were ultimately found to have histopathologically normal pericardium (Fig. 53–10). It is critically important for the clinician to ascertain both the abnormal anatomy and physiology in this setting because some patients can present with grossly thickened pericardium in the absence of functional sequelae.[30]

Valvular Regurgitation

Clinical decision-making in the setting of mitral or aortic regurgitation may hinge on quantitative assessment of left ventricular function. EBCT provides the clinician with this information, as

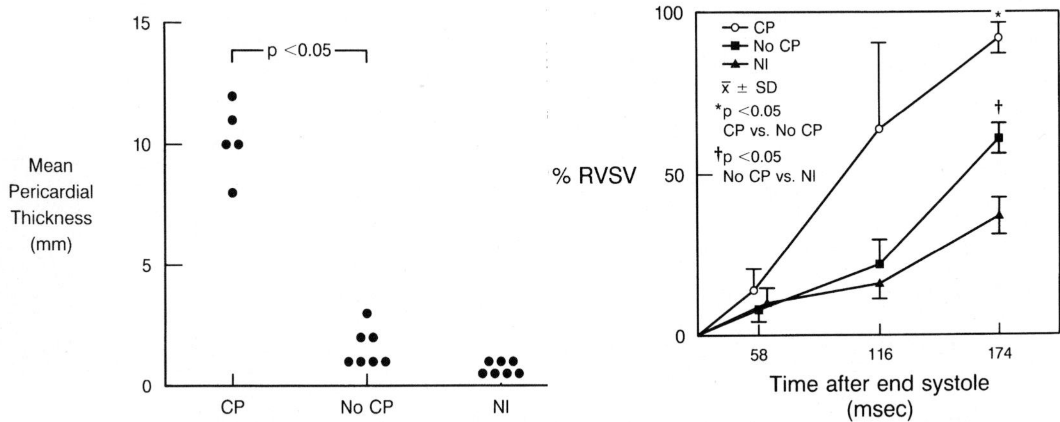

FIGURE 53–10. *Left Panel,* Measurements of pericardial thickness with the use of EBCT in patients with constrictive pericarditis proved by histopathologic examination (CP); in patients with constrictive pericarditis suspected on clinical and hemodynamic examination, in whom histopathologic examination disclosed a normal pericardium (No CP); and in normal subjects (NI). *Right Panel,* Right ventricular filling patterns in these same groups of patients. Patients with histopathologically proven constrictive pericarditis demonstrated markedly more rapid early diastolic filling. %RVSV = the cumulative fraction of total diastolic right ventricular filling that has occurred at each designated time. (From Oren, R.M., Grover-McKay, M., Stanford, W., et al.: Accurate preoperative diagnosis of pericardial constriction using cine computed tomography. J. Am. Coll. Cardiol. 22:832, 1993, with permission of the American College of Cardiology.)

well as absolute quantitation of the amount of valvular regurgitation. The latter is based on comparison of right and left ventricular stroke volumes. Figure 53–11 shows the accuracy with which determinations of regurgitant volume were confirmed in an animal model of aortic regurgitation.[31] The clinical importance of this capability is demonstrated in Figure 53–12, which graphically depicts EBCT findings in nine patients for whom aortic valve replacement was being considered on the basis of complete clinical evaluation, including cardiac catheterization.[32] Two of these patients actually had very mild valvular dysfunction; ventricular systolic dysfunction and dilation were ultimately ascribed to other causes.

Coronary Artery Disease

Assessment of ventricular systolic function can play a role in clinical decision-making in patients with coronary artery disease. Roig and associates[33] have used analysis of EBCT images obtained at rest and during stress as a functional test for identification of physiologically important coronary stenoses. This technique has been found to be useful in stratifying patients after myocardial infarction, by virtue of its sensitivity in identifying patients with multivessel disease. Weiss[34] has used regional systolic function analysis to quantitate ischemic zone size after coronary occlusion. This technique, when applied clinically, can be used to foretell the process of ventricular "remodeling" in the months and years after myocardial infarction.[35] Therapeutic modification of this process, which is a key predictor of clinical morbidity and mortality,[36] has been identified as a target for aggressive intervention.[37]

Coronary artery bypass graft patency status can be reliably assessed with EBCT (see Chapter 54). More recently, a number of preliminary studies have shown promise of the potential to visualize the native coronary arteries with EBCT. The presence of coronary mural calcification, an indicator of atherosclerosis, has been used as a screening technique (see Chapter 54). High-resolution images have been employed to evaluate coronary artery lumen status in experimental[38, 39] and clinical[40] settings. Improvements in image-acquisition and image-analysis techniques may bring clinical applicability to EBCT coronary angiography in the near future.

The examples given earlier, taken with capabilities for assessment of myocardial perfusion (Chapter 55), identification of cardiac mural thrombi and tumors (Chapter 57), assessment of aortic and pulmonary arterial anatomy (Chapter 56), and quantitative assessment of simple and complex congenital heart disease (Chapter 58), demonstrate the clinical applicability of EBCT for truly comprehensive cardiac assessment.

Noncardiac Conditions

Patients who undergo cardiac evaluation for common symptoms of dyspnea or chest pain may have noncardiac conditions that

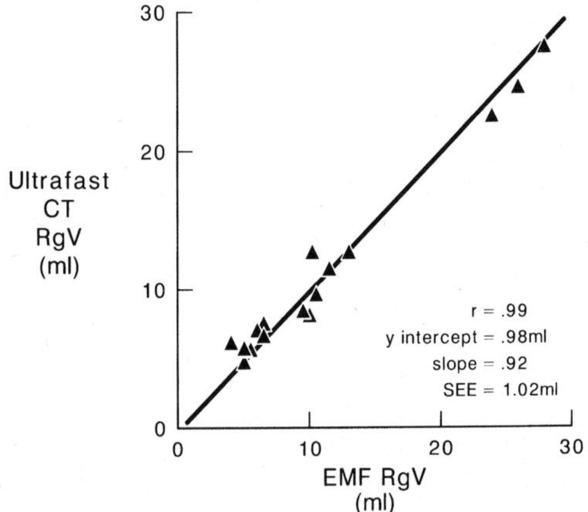

FIGURE 53–11. Measurement of regurgitant volume (RgV) in an experimental model of aortic regurgitation. EBCT (ultrafast CT) measurements are compared to simultaneous measurements made with the use of implanted electromagnetic flow (EMF) probes. (From Reiter, S.J., Rumberger, J.A., Stanford, W., et al.: Quantitative determination of aortic regurgitant volumes in dogs by Ultrafast computed tomography. Circulation 76:728, 1987, with permission of the American Heart Association.)

TABLE 53–3. RELATIVE COST* OF IMAGING STUDIES FOR ASSESSMENT OF CARDIAC FUNCTION

Study	Relative cost
Transthoracic echocardiography	1.0
Electron-beam CT	1.2
Transesophageal echocardiography	1.4
Magnetic resonance imaging	1.8
Radionuclide ventriculography	1.9
Contrast ventriculography (invasive)	1.9

*Charges to the patient, including physician's fees, for complete examination at the University of Iowa Hospitals and Clinics.

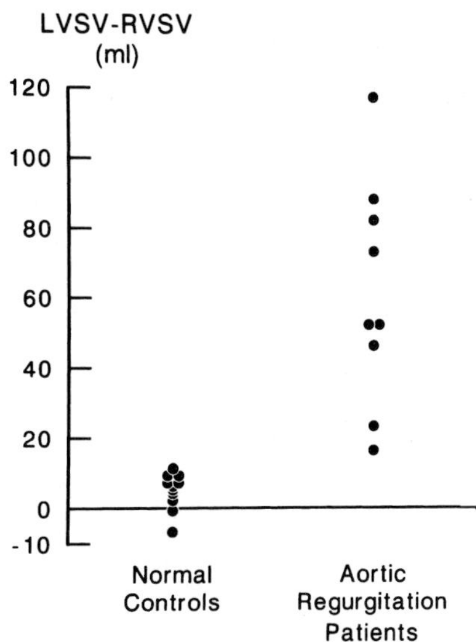

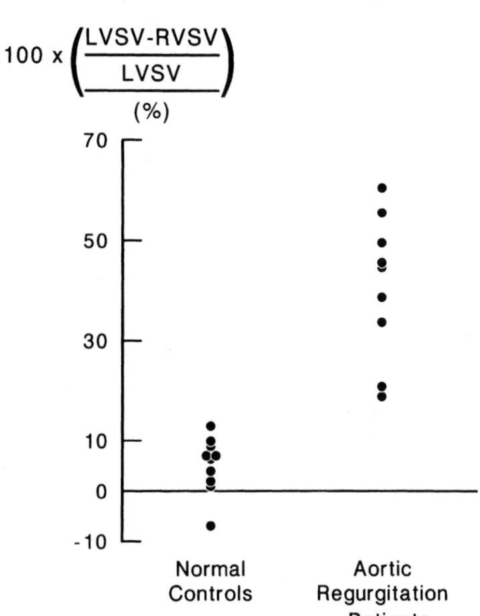

FIGURE 53–12. Measurements of regurgitant volume (*top panel;* left ventricular stroke volume − right ventricular stroke volume) and measurements of regurgitant fraction *(bottom panel)* in normal subjects and in patients with clinical evidence of aortic regurgitation. (Adapted from Stark, C.A., Rumberger, J.A., Reiter, S.J., et al.: Use of cine CT in assessing the severity of aortic regurgitation in patients. [Abstract.] Circulation 74:II-4, 1986; with permission of the American Heart Association.)

contribute to their clinical presentation. EBCT has demonstrated usefulness in the evaluation of interstitial lung disease,[41] chest wall deformities, airway anatomy,[42] sleep apnea,[43] esophageal dysfunction, and pulmonary vascular function.[44]

SUMMARY

Advantages of Electron-Beam Computed Tomography

The principal advantage of imaging with EBCT is the ability to obtain high-quality tomograms in virtually every patient. This advantage is not universally shared. For example, a study by Love and co-workers[45] evaluated the utility of EBCT and transthoracic echocardiography for evaluation of the presence of cardiac mural thrombus in patients presenting with stroke. They found that conventional two-dimensional echocardiographic images were technically inadequate to enable physicians to make this determination in roughly one third of cases, whereas EBCT provided adequate images 97 percent of the time. Vigneswaran and colleagues[46] found a similar degree of difficulty in obtaining adequate visualization of the right ventricle, using echocardiography in a series of patients undergoing cardiac evaluation before lung transplantation, whereas EBCT provided high-quality images in all cases. The validated precision of quantitative measurements of cardiac structure and function is unsurpassed and has been used as a clinical gold standard for validation of other methods.[15, 47] Image quality and image-acquisition techniques are essentially identical at all centers and are calibrated with the use of universal standards, which facilitates sharing of analysis techniques and clinical applications between institutions.

Disadvantages

The principal disadvantage of EBCT is its limited availability. There are roughly 60 scanners currently in operation, half of which are in the United States. The device requires substantial initial investment, although the cost per individual study is comparable to that of other cardiac imaging modalities (Table 53–3). The procedure exposes the patient to ionizing radiation and iodinated contrast media, with their attendant risks.[8] Finally, the technique is relatively new. Thus, the prognostic value of EBCT findings is not as well established as that for more conventional techniques.

CONCLUSIONS

EBCT is a relatively new cardiac imaging device with a very impressive record of image reliability and quantitative validation. Future developments in image acquisition and analysis are expected to broaden the application of this novel device for the comprehensive assessment of patients with known or suspected cardiac disease.

References

1. Hounsfield, G.N.: Computerized transverse axial scanning (tomography): Description of the system. Br. J. Radiol. 46:1016, 1973.
2. Robb, R.A., Ritman, E.L., Gilbert, B.K., et al.: The DSR: A high-speed three-dimensional x-ray computed tomography system for dynamic spatial reconstruction of the heart and circulation. I.E.E.E. Trans. Nucl. Sci. 26:2713, 1979.
3. Boyd, D.P., Gould, R.G., Quinn, J.R., et al.: A proposed dynamic cardiac 3-D densitometer for early detection and evaluation of heart disease. I.E.E.E. Trans. Nucl. Sci. NS-26:2724, 1979.
4. Hoffman, E.A., Gnanaprakasam, D., Gupta, K.B., et al.: VIDA: An environment for multidimensional image display and analysis. S.P.I.E. Proc. 1660:694, 1992.
5. Robb, R.A., Hanson, D.P., Karowski, R.A., et al.: ANALYZE™: A comprehensive operator-interactive software package for multidimensional medical image display and analysis. Comput. Med. Imaging Graph. 13:433, 1989.
6. Feiring, A.J., Rumberger, J.A., Reiter, S.J., et al.: Determination of left ventricular mass in dogs with rapid-acquisition cardiac computed tomographic scanning. Circulation 72:1355, 1985.
7. Dove, E.L., Philip, K., Gotteiner, N.L., et al.: A method for automatic edge detection and volume computation of the left ventricle from Ultrafast computed tomographic images. Invest. Radiol. 29:945, 1994.
8. Hessel, S.J., Adams, D.F., and Abrams, J.L.: Complications of angiography. Radiology 138:273, 1981.
9. Friedman, J.Z., DeBoe, S.F., McGillem, M.J., et al.: The immediate effects of iohexol on coronary blood flow and myocardial function in vivo. Circulation 74:1416, 1986.
10. Reiter, S.J., Rumberger, J.A., Feiring, A.J., et al.: Precision of measurements of right and left ventricular volume by cine computed tomography. Circulation 74:890, 1986.
11. Hajduczok, Z.D., Weiss, R.M., Stanford, W., et al.: Determination of right ventricular mass in humans and dogs with Ultrafast cardiac computed tomography. Circulation 82:202, 1990.
12. Cutrone, J.A., Georgiou, D., Khan, S.U., et al.: Right ventricular mass measurement by electron beam computed tomography. Invest. Radiol. 30:64, 1995.
13. Oren, R.M., Schobel, H.P., Hill, G.A., et al.: Precise assessment of ventricular stroke volume with cine tomography utilizing the long axis in humans. Circulation 86:II-483, 1992.

14. Oren, R.M., Schobel, H.P., Weiss, R.M., et al.: Importance of left atrial baroreceptors in the cardiopulmonary baroreflex of normal man. J. Appl. Physiol. 74:2672, 1993.
15. Vandenberg, B.V., Weiss, R.M., Kinzey, J., et al.: Left atrial volume measurement from two-dimensional echocardiography: Validation by cine computed tomography. Am. J. Cardiol. 75:754, 1995.
16. Bonow, R.O., Vitole, D.F., Bacharach, S.L., et al.: Asynchronous left ventricular regional function in impaired global diastolic filling in patients with coronary artery disease: Reversal after coronary angioplasty. Circulation 71:297, 1985.
17. Rumberger, J.A., Weiss, R.M., Feiring, A.J., et al.: Patterns of regional diastolic function in the normal human left ventricle: An Ultrafast CT study. J. Am. Coll. Cardiol. 14:119, 1989.
18. Oren, R.M., Grover-McKay, M., Stanford, W., et al.: Accurate preoperative diagnosis of pericardial constriction using cine computed tomography. J. Am. Coll. Cardiol. 22:832, 1993.
19. Stewart, G.N.: Researches on the circulation time and on the influences which affect it. IV: The output of the heart. J. Physiol. 22:159, 1897.
20. Reiter, S.J., Feiring, A.J., Stanford, W., et al.: Precise measurements of contrast clearance curve cardiac outputs using cine computed tomography. J. Am. Coll. Cardiol. 9:116A, 1987.
21. Ludman, P.F., Coats, A.J.S., Poole-Wilson, P.A., et al.: Measurement accuracy of cardiac output in humans: Indicator-dilution technique versus geometric analysis by Ultrafast computed tomography. J. Am. Coll. Cardiol. 21:1482, 1993.
22. Roig, E., Georgiou, D., Chomka, E.V., et al.: Reproducibility of left ventricular volume and mass measurements by Ultrafast computed tomography. J. Am. Coll. Cardiol. 18:990, 1991.
23. Grover-McKay, M., Weiss, R.M., Vandenberg, B.F., et al.: Assessment of cardiac volumes and left ventricular mass by cine computed tomography before and after mitral balloon commissurotomy. Am. Heart J. 128:533, 1994.
24. Meany, E., Shabetai, R., Bhargava, V., et al.: Cardiac amyloidosis, constrictive pericarditis and restrictive cardiomyopathy. Am. J. Cardiol. 38:547, 1976.
25. Vaitkus, P.T., and Kussmaul, W.G.: Constrictive pericarditis versus restrictive cardiomyopathy: A reappraisal and update of diagnostic criteria. Am. Heart J. 122:431, 1991.
26. Pandian, N.G., Skorton, D.J., Kieso, R.A., et al.: Diagnosis of constrictive pericarditis by two-dimensional echocardiography: Studies in a new experimental model and in patients. J. Am. Coll. Cardiol. 4:1164, 1984.
27. Shabetai, R., Fowler, N.O., Guntheroth, W.G., et al.: The hemodynamics of cardiac tamponade and constrictive pericarditis. Am. J. Cardiol. 47:791, 1981.
28. Seifert, F.C., Miller, C.D., Oesterle, S.N., et al.: Surgical treatment of constrictive pericarditis: Analysis of outcome and diagnostic error. (Abstract). Circulation 72:II-264(Suppl.):1985.
29. Grover-McKay, M., Burke, S., Thompson, S.A., et al.: Measurement of pericardial thickness by cine computed tomography. Am. J. Card. Imaging 5:98, 1991.
30. Weiss, R.M., Otoadese, T., and Oren, R.M.: Differentiation of constrictive pericarditis from restrictive cardiomyopathy: The case for high-resolution dynamic tomographic imaging. S.P.I.E. Proc., 1995 (in press).
31. Reiter, S.J., Rumberger, J.A., Stanford, W., et al.: Quantitative determination of aortic regurgitant volumes in dogs by ultrafast computed tomography. Circulation 76:728, 1987.
32. Stark, C.A., Rumberger, J.A., Reiter, S.J., et al.: Use of cine CT in assessing the severity of aortic regurgitation in patients. Circulation 74:II-4, 1986.
33. Roig, E., Chomka, E.V., Castaner, A., et al.: Exercise Ultrafast computed tomography for the detection of coronary artery disease. J. Am. Coll. Cardiol. 12:1073, 1989.
34. Weiss, R.M.: The extent of left ventricular systolic dysfunction during acute coronary occlusion is load-dependent. S.P.I.E. Proc. 2168:162, 1994.
35. Rumberger, J.A., Behrenbeck, T., Breen, J.R., et al.: Nonparallel changes in global left ventricular chamber volume and muscle mass during the first year after transmural myocardial infarction in humans. J. Am. Coll. Cardiol. 21:673, 1993.
36. Pfeffer, M.A., Lamas, G.A., Vaughan, D.E., et al.: Effect of captopril on progressive ventricular dilatation after anterior myocardial infarction. N. Engl. J. Med. 319:80, 1988.
37. Nidorf, S.M., Siu, S.C., Galambos, G., et al.: Benefit of late coronary reperfusion on ventricular morphology and function after myocardial infarction. J. Am. Coll. Cardiol. 21:683, 1993.
38. Napel, S., Rutt, B.K., and Pflugfelder, P.: Three-dimensional images of the coronary arteries from Ultrafast computed tomography: Method and comparison with two-dimensional angiography. Am. J. Card. Imaging 3:237, 1989.
39. Weiss, R.M., and Grover-McKay, M.: Assessment of coronary artery patency with cine computed tomography in a dog model of occlusion-reperfusion. Invest. Radiol. 29:168, 1994.
40. Moshage, W.E., Achenbach, S., Seese, B., et al.: Contrast-enhanced electron beam tomography for 3-D reconstruction of coronary arteries: Detection of stenoses and documentation of angioplasty success. J. Am. Coll. Cardiol. 25:134A, 1995.
41. Galvin, J.R., Mori, M., and Stanford, W.: High-resolution computed tomography and diffuse lung disease. Curr. Prob. Diagn. Radiol. 21:33, 1992.
42. Woodring, J.H.: Pulmonary artery-bronchus ratios in patients with normal lungs, pulmonary vascular plethora, and congestive heart failure. Radiology 179:115, 1991.
43. Galvin, J.R., Rooholamini, S.A., and Stanford, W.: Obstructive sleep apnea: Diagnosis with Ultrafast CT. Radiology 171:775, 1989.
44. Hoffman, E.A., Tajik, J.K., Petersen, G., et al.: Perfusion deficit versus anatomic visualization in detection of pulmonary emboli via electron-beam CT: Validation in swine. SPIE Proc., 1995 (in press).
45. Love, B.B., Struck, L.K., Stanford, W., et al.: Comparison of two-dimensional echocardiography and Ultrafast cardiac computed tomography for evaluating intracardiac thrombi in cerebral ischemia. Stroke 21:1033, 1990.
46. Vigneswaran, W.T., McDougall, J.C., Olson, L.J., et al.: Right ventricular assessment in patients presenting for lung transplantation. Transplantation 55:1051, 1993.
47. Kircher, B., Abbott, J.A., Pau, S., et al.: Left atrial volume determination by biplane two-dimensional echocardiography: Validation by cine computed tomography. Am. Heart J. 121:864, 1991.

CHAPTER

54 Evaluation of Coronary Artery Disease by Electron-Beam Computed Tomography

Stuart Rich, M.D.
Christopher J. Wolfkiel, Ph.D.

Coronary artery disease remains the major source of morbidity and mortality of adults in the United States. For decades, attention has been devoted to the treatment of patients with advanced coronary artery disease, including development of antianginal drugs, drugs that reduce the likelihood of recurrent myocardial infarction, and advances in coronary bypass graft surgery and in coronary angioplasty. Trials focused toward the secondary prevention of coronary events with antithrombotic agents, β-blockers, and lipid-lowering medications have also been successful. Unfortunately, attempts at primary prevention through risk factor modification in patients believed to be at increased risk for coronary events have not been widely successful. This problem stems from the fact that although risk factors may identify a population likely to experience an increased number of coronary events, they are nonspecific in identifying individuals at risk for a coronary event.[1]

Exercise testing has been the traditional screening modality for asymptomatic patients believed to be at increased risk for coronary artery disease. Unfortunately, exercise electrocardiogram (ECG) testing has not been shown to be effective in asymptomatic adults,[2] largely because the most common mechanism for acute coronary events is plaque rupture and coronary thrombosis, which often occurs in plaques that are not flow limiting and thus are nondetectable with stress testing.[3]

Electron-beam computed tomography (EBCT) holds the promise of allowing the quick and accurate identification of patients with asymptomatic coronary artery disease by providing high-resolution images of the coronary arteries and identification of atherosclerotic plaques by virtue of their calcium content.[4]

ASSOCIATION OF CORONARY ARTERY CALCIUM WITH ATHEROSCLEROSIS

The fact that calcium deposition occurs in the intima of coronary arteries with atherosclerosis has been known for decades.[5–8] Calcification rarely occurs in the media of coronary arteries as a result of the aging process, even in the setting of marked intimal atherosclerosis.[9] The prevalence of coronary arterial calcification increases with age, which is a reflection of the fact that atherosclerosis of the coronary arteries is also related to age.[8]

Calcium deposits are usually associated with more advanced coronary lesions.[9] Coronary plaque composition ranges from fatty streaks that appear early in life to complex lesions that include lipid-laden foam cells, a fibrous cap, and calcium deposits.[10] The deposition of calcium in atherosclerotic plaques results from a cascade of events that is initiated from endothelial injury and progresses through successive plaque ruptures. The time interval from the initiation of plaque growth to the deposition of calcium is unknown but is probably influenced by local factors. Coronary calcification is formed from hydroxyapatite, which crystallizes and proliferates in physiologic extracellular concentrations. The initial deposits occur in extracellular vesicles, which provide a matrix that includes calcium-binding acidic phospholipids and phosphatases that promote mineralization.[11] When exposed to extracellular fluid, the subsequent calcification is regulated by local pH, proteoglycan aggregates, osteonectin, and polyphosphate molecules, which inhibit deposition, and by collagen, which promotes nucleation. It is presumed that the initial matrix is formed from degenerative smooth muscle cells from the atherosclerotic process. Although plaque regression has been demonstrated in animals and humans by alterations in lipid content, it is unlikely that calcified crystals will regress.

ELECTRON-BEAM COMPUTED TOMOGRAPHY AND CORONARY ARTERY SCANNING

The traditional approach to screening patients at risk for coronary events has included risk factor stratification and the use of exercise testing. The value of identifying asymptomatic patients with modifiable risk factors, such as elevated cholesterol, cigarette smoking, or hypertension, with the goal of reducing subsequent coronary events has had only modest success.[1] The use of exercise ECG testing in these patients has not been shown to be useful, as the majority of the patients who will subsequently experience coronary events and sudden coronary death are those most likely to have negative test results.[12] These negative findings are due to the fact that acute coronary events most often result from the rupture of coronary plaque that may not be flow limiting.[3, 13, 14] The use of radionuclide perfusion agents, such as thallium, or of other strategies that involve echocardiographic imaging is not likely to yield better results in screening asymptomatic individuals for the same reasons. The circumstances that trigger coronary plaque rupture and thrombosis are not well understood and have not been linked to easily identifiable signs, such as cholesterol level and blood pressure.

The association of coronary calcium with coronary events has been shown with fluoroscopic detection.[5] In one study, patients with detectable coronary calcium had greater cardiovascular mortality than patients without coronary calcium, irrespective of the severity of coronary disease by angiography. EBCT is more sensitive than fluoroscopy for detection of calcific deposits,[15] as the coronary arteries can be easily visualized without contrast medium because of the contrast differential between the arteries and the surrounding fat (Fig. 54–1). Tomographic imaging allows potential false-positive results from mitral and aortic calcifications to be easily distinguished. A coronary screening with EBCT is a quick, noninvasive procedure that exposes the subject to a maximum of approximately 12 mGy of x-ray radiation posteriorly and 2 mGy anteriorly.[16] The procedure typically involves the acquisition of 20 3-mm-thick slices, ECG gated to 80 percent of every second RR interval during a single breath hold. Scanning time averages about 30 to 40 seconds. A complete study can usually be acquired in less than 10 minutes.

The presence of coronary calcium is defined as coronary pixels with a CT density greater than 130 Hounsfield units.[4] Although somewhat arbitrary, it represents a density that is two to three times higher than that of the surrounding myocardial tissue and appears to reliably identify calcium deposition. A quantification scheme initially proposed by Agatston and colleagues[4] is the most widely accepted standard. According to that scheme, the calcium score for a calcific deposit is equal to the area of the deposit multiplied by a scaling factor based on the peak pixel attenuation: 1 (130 to 199), 2 (200 to 299), 3 (300 to 499), and 4 (400+). Scores for each artery (left main, left anterior descending, circumflex, and right coronary) are the sums of each set of deposit scores, and the total score for the patient is the sum of the arterial scores.

Validation Studies

An autopsy study performed at the Mayo Clinic investigated the amount of coronary calcification and the corresponding luminal area.[17] The presence of coronary calcium was virtually 100 percent specific for atherosclerosis but not for the degree of stenosis. The range of percent stenosis and luminal area for a given calcium score was large. The absence of coronary calcium was associated with the absence of obstructive disease, as only 2.5 percent of nonsignificantly stenotic lesions were without detectable calcium. Mautner and associates compared the amount of coronary calcium from EBCT to that of histomorphometric calcium in hearts from symptomatic and asymptomatic patients.[18] They showed an excellent correlation between calcium score and histomorphometric calcium (r = .92), with a sensitivity of 94 percent and specificity of 76 percent. Thus, EBCT is an accurate method for the detection and measurement of coronary artery calcium in vitro, although the relationship between coronary artery calcium and coronary arterial stenosis is limited.

In studies comparing the presence of coronary artery calcium with that of angiographically defined disease in patients, the sensitivity for coronary calcification to be associated with flow-limiting disease was excellent (95 to 100 percent); however, the specificity was low (44 to 59 percent).[19] More recent work suggests that this excellent sensitivity may be reduced in subjects younger than 50 years of age[20] and in women younger than 60 years of age.[21] These studies may reflect biases related to the high prevalence of coronary disease in the sample population, although a study of patients with a reduced prevalence of disease found similar measures of sensitiv-

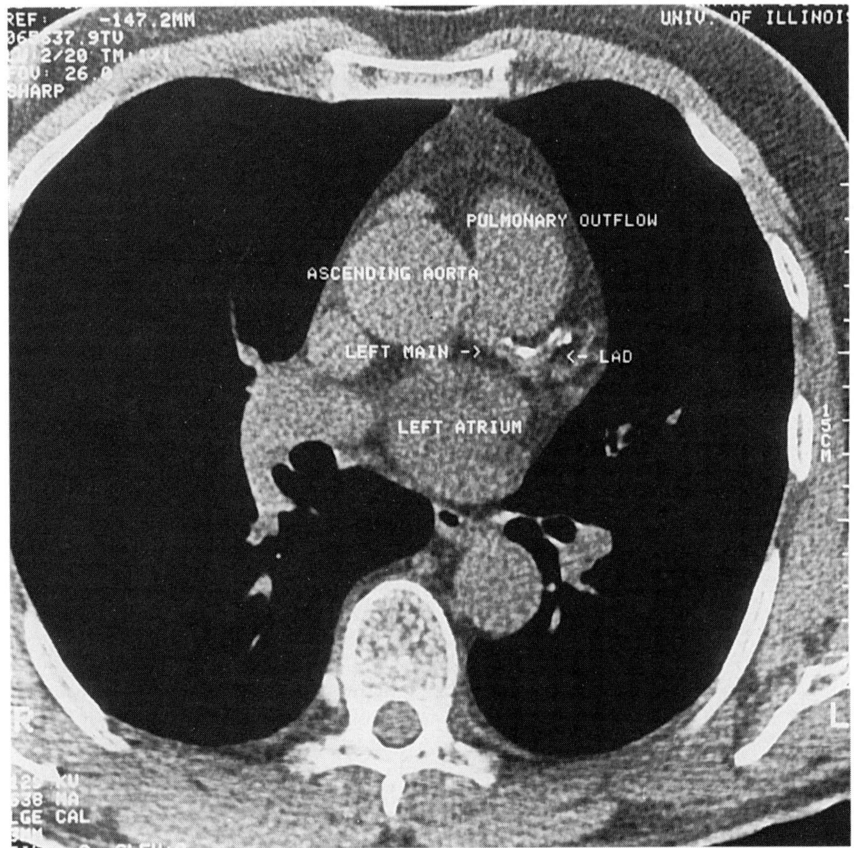

FIGURE 54–1. Electron-beam CT scan through the base of the aorta. The left main and left anterior descending coronary arteries are identified. The increased density in the left anterior descending artery (LAD) represents coronary artery calcium.

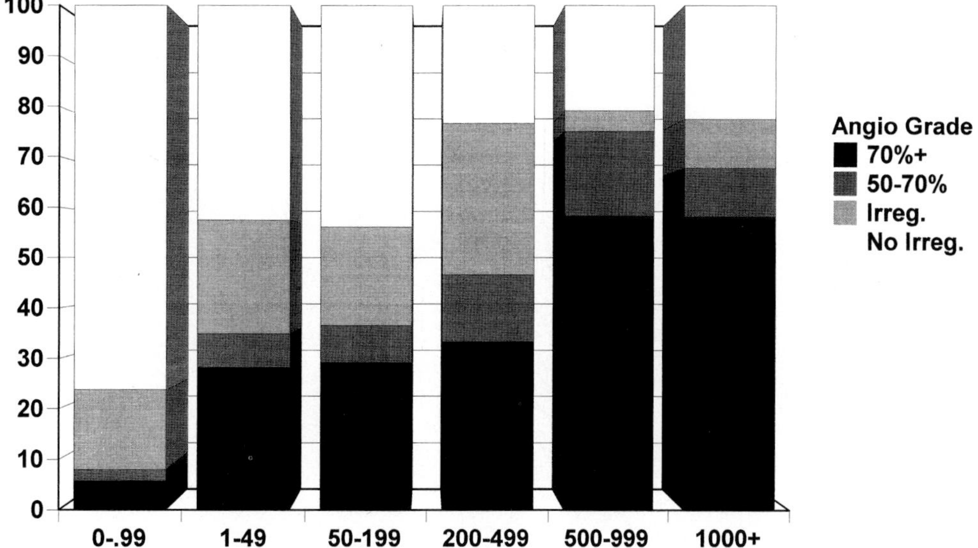

FIGURE 54–2. The relationship between severity of coronary artery stenosis by angiography and coronary artery calcium score. These data are based on 140 patients who underwent coronary angiography and EBCT coronary artery calcification scans. Higher coronary artery calcium scores are associated with increased likelihood of coronary stenosis.

ity and specificity.[22] Nonetheless, the data suggest that higher amounts of coronary calcium are more likely to be associated with higher degrees of stenosis (Fig. 54–2). In addition, the likelihood of a patient having a significant coronary lesion is related to the number of calcified vessels, as well as to the total calcium score for the entire coronary bed.

The prevalence and amount of coronary calcification in asymptomatic subjects is influenced by age and gender.[23] Women have a 10-year time lag in both the prevalence and the amount of coronary calcification when compared with men (Figs. 54–3 and 54–4), presumably because of protective effects associated with estrogen. This fact implies that there may be a cutoff or threshold calcium score, influenced by age and gender, that separates dormant coronary disease from disease that may progress to a level of clinical significance.

Limitations of Coronary Artery Screening

Because the calcium deposits imaged are usually smaller than the thickness of the slice (3 mm), the accuracy in imaging the calcium is often influenced by a partial volume effect. Inconsistencies in ECG gating or breath-holding can result in areas of the coronary arteries being missed or multiply imaged. The reproducibility of the technique has been evaluated in several studies by immediately repeating the scanning procedure.[24–26] These studies show that 4 to 10 percent of patients may have false-negative results with a single scanning sequence. The correlation between scans was excellent over the wide range of calcium scores (0 to 3000), whereas the variability of scores was greater in lower scores, up to 200 percent in scores less than 20, compared with 20 to 50 percent in scores above 100. Although sources of observer-based variability include incorrect inclusion of ostial or annular calcifications, incorrect identification of suprathreshold pixels, and inappropriate inclusion of multiple deposits for scoring purposes, interobserver variability was determined to be 2.5 ± 5 percent.[4]

A strategy for reducing false-negative results uses a second scan covering the proximal coronary arteries, which would detect small amounts of calcium missed by the initial scan. Preliminary results suggest that this may be useful.[27] These results suggest that the lower sensitivity of coronary screening in younger subjects may be

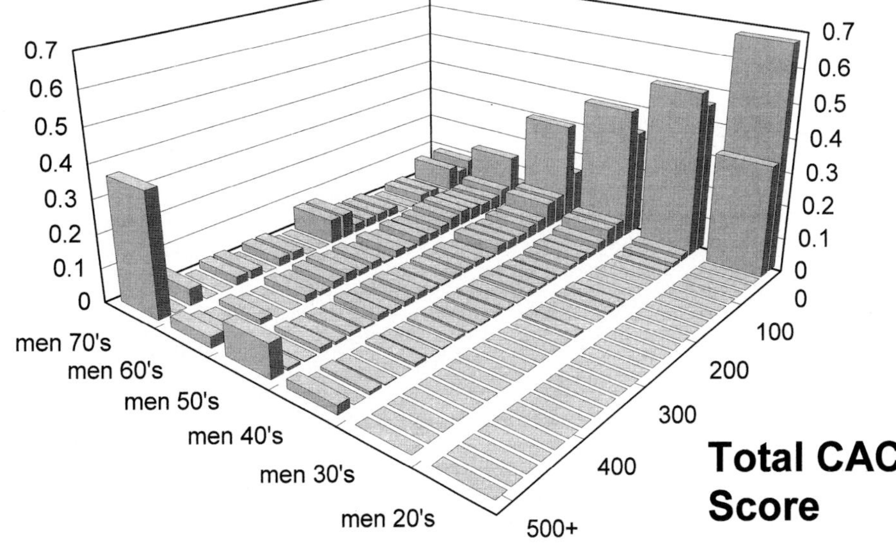

FIGURE 54–3. The prevalence of coronary artery calcium in 1317 asymptomatic men. With age, men are more likely to have positive scans and scans with higher coronary artery calcium scores.

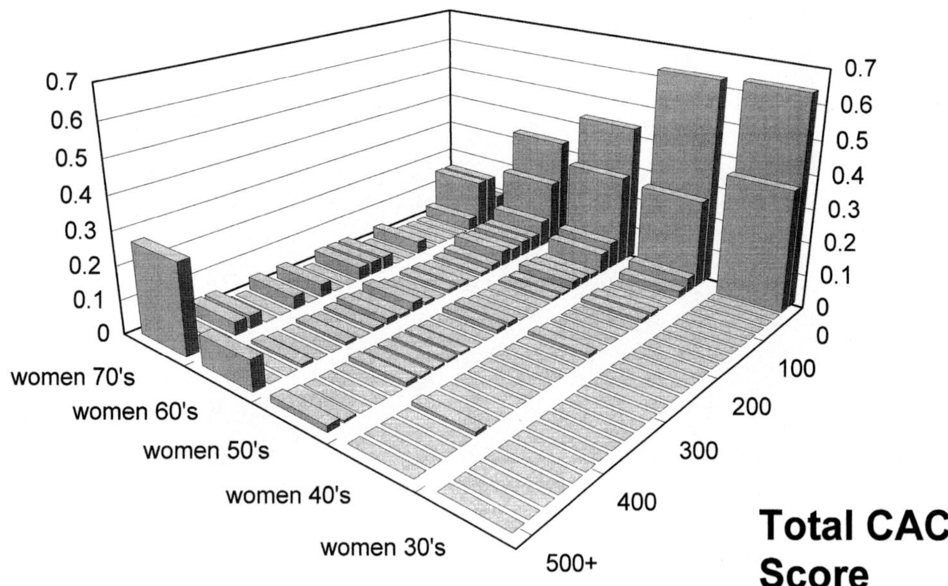

FIGURE 54–4. The prevalence of coronary artery calcium in 413 asymptomatic women. As with their male counterparts, the likelihood of having a positive scan increases with age, as does the total calcium score. However, compared with their male counterparts, the prevalence and extent of coronary calcium at a given age is less in women than in men.

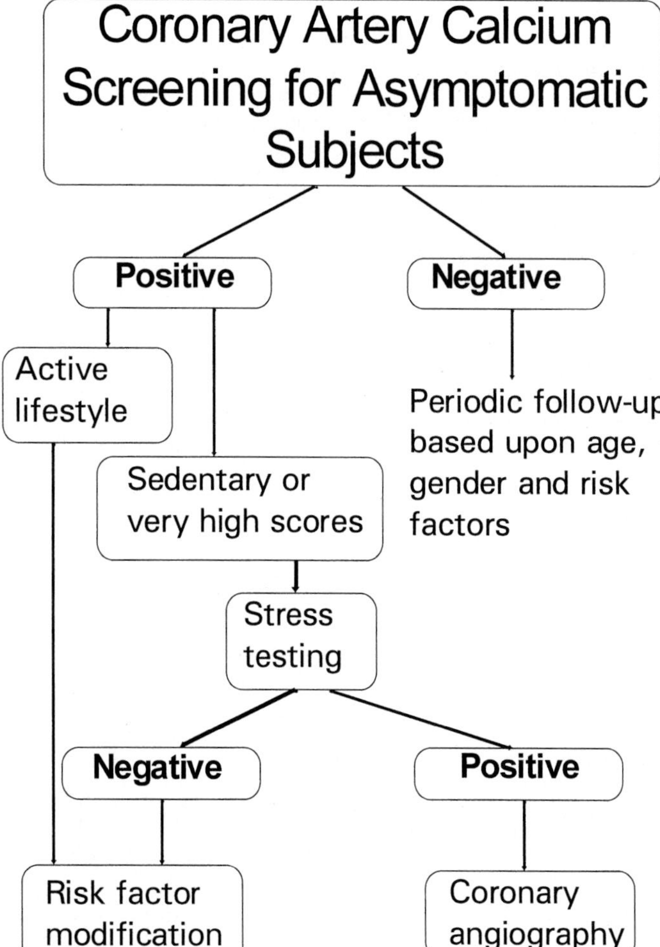

FIGURE 54–5. An algorithm for the use of coronary artery calcium screening in asymptomatic patients. The use of coronary artery calcium screening as the initial test is intended to limit the use of exercise testing and angiography only to individuals who have coronary artery calcium.

due to the fact that smaller deposits have a greater likelihood of being missed with a one-pass scanning protocol.

Clinical Applications

EBCT detection of coronary artery calcification currently appears to be the most reliable and precise way of detecting the presence of coronary atherosclerosis noninvasively. As a screening test, it should not be applied to patients with known coronary artery disease, such as those who have had previous myocardial infarction or interventional procedures, because it is not likely to yield new or useful information about the presence of atherosclerosis. However, a negative test result in an asymptomatic individual expected to have a high likelihood of coronary disease appears highly specific for the absence of atherosclerosis, and thus should be expected to be associated with a very low likelihood of the development of coronary events in the near future. In younger subjects with reduced prevalence of coronary disease, a negative test result may not be as powerful a predictor of a lack of risk for coronary events. Confusion about the clinical implications of a positive scan relate to the notion that only flow-limiting stenoses confer a risk of coronary events. It is now established that the extent of disease, rather than percent stenosis, is a more important feature.[28]

It has not been possible to determine the amount of calcium that predisposes an individual to experiencing a coronary event. Because the presence of calcium is related to both age and gender, it may be that there are threshold values of calcification, whereby small amounts of coronary atherosclerosis in defined subgroups do not represent a marked risk of coronary events, whereas larger amounts do. Interestingly, an intravascular ultrasound study performed in patients who underwent coronary angioplasty noted that the site of intimal dissection created by balloon dilation was usually adjacent to areas of intimal calcification.[29] Thus, calcium may serve as a nidus for focal weakening of the fibrous cap, which may predispose an individual to plaque rupture and subsequent thrombosis. If this is the case, it may be that calcium could be an independent risk factor for coronary events and that the amount of calcium present in an individual may be indicative of the level of risk.

At the present time it is reasonable to recommend risk factor modification, such as cessation of smoking and control of blood pressure, in asymptomatic individuals who have coronary artery calcium. The aggressive use of lipid-lowering therapy in this subset of asymptomatic individuals to reduce cardiac morbidity and mortality is promising but remains unproved. Preliminary studies, however, do show that asymptomatic individuals with extremely high levels of coronary artery calcium appear to be at a markedly increased risk for having coronary events in the subsequent 12 months.[30]

Coronary artery screening may also be useful in patients with atypical chest pain and a low likelihood of having coronary artery disease, whereas other tests are often inconclusive, such as in women with mitral valve prolapse. In this setting, a negative test should be supportive of the absence of a flow-limiting coronary lesion and thus may circumvent the need for further testing, including coronary angiography. Coronary artery screening may also be useful in patients presenting in an emergency room with chest pain that may be inconclusive for cardiac origin. Although the presence of coronary calcium may not clearly indicate that the chest pain is of cardiac etiology, a negative test result in an individual expected to have a high likelihood of disease would render the presence of coronary stenosis and subsequent angina unlikely.

Preliminary studies also show that serial coronary artery screening studies may be useful in following the progression of plaque growth noninvasively. One study showed that patients with symptomatic coronary artery disease have a much greater growth rate in plaque volume than asymptomatic individuals followed over 14 months.[31] Although the idea remains untested, it is intriguing that plaque growth rates may be a better indicator of the risk of coronary events. In that regard, therapies directed toward reducing plaque growth rate may be able to be linked to a reduction of future coronary events.

Based on currently available data, it is a reasonable strategy to use coronary artery screening as a tool to identify asymptomatic patients with coronary atherosclerosis who may be at increased risk for subsequent events. In this regard, coronary artery screening, by virtue of its low cost and easy application, may be the ideal initial screening test (Fig. 54–5). Patients who have active life styles and are truly symptom free but have positive scans are unlikely to have positive exercise tests, and thus no further testing may be indicated, unless the level of coronary calcification is unusually high. These latter patients, or patients with positive coronary scans who are sedentary or unable to exercise, may benefit from stress testing to determine whether a potential flow-limiting lesion exists that is not clinically apparent. Coronary angiography may then be indicated for the very small subset of asymptomatic patients who have positive stress tests. Patients without inducible ischemia should have risk factor modification using proven modalities, such as stopping cigarette smoking and blood pressure control. It is also reasonable to use aspirin as a preventive measure in this subset.[32] The use of pharmacologic agents for lipid modification may also seem reasonable.

OTHER APPLICATIONS OF ELECTRON-BEAM COMPUTED TOMOGRAPHY FOR CORONARY ARTERY DISEASE

Electron-beam computed tomography has many other applications in assessing the status of patients with coronary artery disease. In addition to the high-resolution, single-slice mode used for coronary calcification screening, a multislice lower resolution mode is capable of cine studies of 17 frames per second at eight levels of approximately 1 cm thickness each. Dynamic scanning over time with ECG gating allows assessments of bypass graft patency by direct visualization of contrast-enhanced grafts. The premise is that when the graft is patent, it is enhanced by the peripheral injection of contrast medium as it flows through the circulation. The accuracy of using contrast-enhanced EBCT to determine graft patency has been evaluated in several studies, with excellent results.[33, 34] A multicenter study showed a 93 percent sensitivity and an 89 percent specificity, which included saphenous veins and internal mammary arteries.

Attention to the technique used is important, as there are many possible sources of error. A sufficient bolus of contrast material must be injected, with the scanning timed to estimate the contrast appearance in the aorta. The scan itself must cover all levels, including the takeoff of the grafts, and should begin at the thoracic inlet when the internal mammary artery is used. As in all studies, patient cooperation and adequate breath-holding are essential. Operative reports are necessary if one is to know the number and placement of grafts to be detected.

One clinical limitation in the assessment of bypass graft patency is that it provides an answer only as to whether there is flow through the graft, and it does not address the issue of inherent stenosis. Although strategies for determining bypass graft flow rate have been proposed,[35] the very broad range of flows that exists in clinical situations makes the application of this technique extremely problematic.

Exercise With Electron-Beam Computed Tomography for Coronary Artery Disease

It has been well established that the coupling of contrast medium administration with EBCT allows the accurate measurement of ventricular mass, ejection fraction, and wall motion. The use of semisupine bicycle ergometry with the EBCT has allowed rest and exercise studies in patients with suspected coronary disease, with good clinical results.

The cardiovascular response to exercise is typically manifested by an increase in left ventricular ejection fraction, which becomes impaired in patients with exercise-induced ischemia. In one clinical study, patients with three-vessel coronary disease were shown to have a reduction in resting left ventricular ejection fraction with exercise, whereas patients with no disease or single-vessel disease had a left ventricular ejection fraction that either stayed the same or increased.[36] Regional wall motion can also be evaluated both qualitatively and quantitatively with a computer-assisted program that divides the short axis of the left ventricle into multiple radii.[37] It has been reported that patients who do not have coronary disease have relatively uniform contraction of segmental function at rest and with exercise, whereas patients with coronary disease have a marked widening of the distribution of normalized subsegmental ejection fractions with exercise.[37] The studies that utilized EBCT with exercise for the assessment of left ventricular function and wall motion are comparable to the experience obtained with nuclear imaging and echocardiography that used exercise to detect coronary disease with respect to changes in left ventricular function and wall motion.

References

1. Yanowitz, F.G., and Charlton, G.A.: Arguments for prevention. *In* Yanowitz, F. G. (ed.): Coronary Heart Disease Prevention. New York, Marcel Dekker, 1992.
2. Epstein, S.E., Quyyumi, A.A., and Bonow, R.O.: Sudden cardiac death without warning: Possible mechanisms and implications for screening asymptomatic populations. N. Engl. J. Med. 321:320, 1989.
3. Ambrose, J.A., Tannebaum, M.A., Alexopoulus, D., et al.: Angiographic progression of coronary artery disease and the development of myocardial infarction. J. Am. Coll. Cardiol. 52:56, 1988.
4. Agatston, A.S., Janowitz, W.R., Hildner, F.J., et al.: Quantification of coronary artery calcium using ultrafast computed tomography. J. Am. Coll. Cardiol. 15:827, 1990.
5. Margolis, J.R., Chen, J.T., Kong, Y., et al.: The diagnostic and prognostic significance of coronary artery calcification. A report of 800 cases. Radiology 137:609, 1980.
6. Blankenhorn, D.H.: Coronary calcification: A review. Am J Med Sci 242:1, 1961.
7. McCarthy, J.H., and Palmer, F.J.: Incidence and significance of coronary artery calcification. Br. Heart J. 36:499, 1974.
8. Uretsky, B.J., Rifkin, R.D., Sharma, S.C., et al.: Value of fluoroscopy in the detection of coronary stenosis: Influence of age, sex and the number of vessels calcified on diagnostic efficacy. Am. Heart J. 115:323, 1988.
9. McGill, H.C.: Basic biology and pathophysiology of vessel wall and plaque. *In* Zaret, B.L., Kaufman, L., Berson, A.S., et al. (eds.): Frontiers in Cardiovascular Imaging. New York, Raven Press, 1993.
10. Ross, R., and Glomset, J.: The pathogenesis of atherosclerosis. N. Engl. J. Med. 295:369, 1976.
11. Tanimura, A., McGregor, D.H., and Anderson, H.C.: Calcification in atherosclerosis. I. Human studies. J. Exp. Pathol. 2:261, 1986.
12. Sox, H., Litenburg, G., and Garber, A.M.: The role of exercise testing in screening for coronary artery disease. Ann. Intern. Med. 110:456, 1989.
13. Davies, M.J., and Thomas, A.: Thrombosis and acute coronary artery lesions in sudden cardiac ischemic death. N. Engl. J. Med. 310:1137, 1984.
14. Ambrose, J.A., Winters, S.L., Stern, A., et al.: Angiographic morphology and the pathogenesis of unstable angina pectoris. J. Am. Coll. Cardiol. 5:609, 1985.
15. Stanford, W., Thompson, B., and Weiss, R.M.: Coronary artery calcification: Clinical significance and current methods of detection. AJR 161:1139, 1993.
16. McCollough, C.H., Zumbe, F.E., and Morin, R.L.: Radiation dosimetry for electron beam CT. Radiology 192:637, 1994.
17. Simons, D.B., Schwartz, R.S., Edwards, W.D., et al.: Noninvasive definition of anatomic coronary artery disease by ultrafast computed tomography scanning: A quantitative pathologic study. J. Am. Coll. Cardiol. 20(5):1118, 1992.
18. Mautner, G.C., Mautner, S.L., Froehlich, J., et al.: Coronary artery calcification: Assessment with electron beam CT and histomorphometric correlation. Radiology 192:619, 1994.
19. Breen, J.F., Sheedy, P.F., Schwartz, R.S., et al.: Coronary artery calcification detected with ultrafast CT as an indication of coronary disease. Radiology 185:435, 1992.
20. Fallavotta, J.A., Brody, A.S., Bunnell, I.L., et al.: Fast computed tomography detection of coronary calcification in the diagnosis of coronary artery disease comparison with angiography in patients less than 50 years old. Circulation 89:285, 1994.
21. DeVries, S., Wolfkiel, C.J., Fusman, B., et al.: The influence of age and gender on the presence of coronary calcium detected by ultrafast computed tomography. J. Am. Coll. Cardiol. 25:76, 1995.
22. Wong, N.D., Vo, A., Abrahamson, D., et al.: Detection of coronary artery calcium by UFCT and its relation to clinical evidence of coronary disease. Am. J. Cardiol. 73:223, 1994.
23. Janowitz, W.R., Agatston, A.S., Kaplan, G., et al.: Differences in prevalence and extent of coronary artery calcium detected by UFCT in asymptomatic men and women. Am. J. Cardiol. 73:223, 1994.
24. Shah, V., Claudio, J., Wolfkiel, C.J., et al.: Reproducibility of coronary artery calcium scoring with UFCT. J. Am. Coll. Cardiol. 19:189A, 1992.
25. Kajinami, K., Seki, H., Takekoshi, H., et al.: Quantification of coronary artery calcification using ultrafast computed tomography: Reproducibility of measurements. Coronary Art. Dis. 4:1103, 1993.
26. Bielak, L.F., Aufmann, R.B., Moll, P.P., et al.: Small lesions in the heart identified at electron beam CT: Calcification or noise. Radiology 192:631, 1994.
27. Eusebio, J., Rich, S., and Wolfkiel, C.: Overlap scanning in coronary artery calcium screening with ultrafast computed tomography. Am. J. Card. Imaging 8(Suppl. 1):10, 1994.
28. Kragel, A.H., Reddy, S.G., Wittes, J.T., et al.: Morphometric analysis of the composition of atherosclerotic plaques in the four major epicardial coronary arteries in acute myocardial infarction and in sudden coronary death. Circulation 20:1747, 1989.
29. Fitzgerald, P.J., Ports, T.A., and Yock, P.G.: Contribution of localized calcium deposits to dissection after angioplasty. Circulation 86:64, 1992.
30. Brundage, B.H., Rich, S., Rassman, W., et al.: Follow-up of asymptomatic individuals with high coronary calcium scores on UFCT scans. J. Am. Coll. Cardiol. 161a:901, 1994.
31. Janowitz, W.R., Agatston, A.S., and Viamonte, M.: Comparison of serial quantitative evaluation of calcified coronary artery plaque by ultrafast computed tomography in persons with and without coronary artery disease. Am. J. Cardiol. 68:1, 1991.
32. Ridker, P.M., Manson, J.E., Buring, J.E., et al.: Circadian variation of acute myocardial infarction and the effect of low dose aspirin in a randomized trial of physicians. Circulation 82:897, 1990.
33. Bateman, T.M., Gray, R.J., Whiting, J.S., et al.: Prospective evaluation of ultrafast computed tomography for determination of coronary bypass graft patency. Circulation 75:1018, 1987.
34. Stanford, W., Brundage, B.H., MacMillan, R., et al.: Sensitivity and specificity of assessing bypass graft patency with ultrafast computed tomography: Results of a multicenter study. J. Am. Coll. Cardiol. 12:1, 1988.
35. Whiting, J.S., Bateman, T.M., Sethra, D.H., et al.: Quantitation of saphenous vein bypass graft flow using intravenous contrast ultrafast CT. Circulation 74(Suppl. II):41, 1986.
36. Roig, E., Chomka, E.V., Castaner, A., et al.: Exercise ultrafast computed tomography for the detection of coronary artery disease. J. Am. Coll. Cardiol. 13:1073, 1989.
37. Feiring, A.J., Rumberger, J.A., Reiter, S.J., et al.: Sectional and segmental variability of left ventricular function: Experimental and clinical studies using ultrafast computed tomography. J. Am. Coll. Cardiol. 12:415, 1988.

CHAPTER

55 Measurement of Myocardial Perfusion Using Electron-Beam (Ultrafast) Computed Tomography

John A. Rumberger, Ph.D., M.D.
Malcolm R. Bell, M.B.B.S.

Routine clinical quantification of regional myocardial perfusion by a safe, reliable, repeatable, and accurate noninvasive methodology would significantly aid in diagnosis and assessment of therapy in patients with cardiac disease. For instance, in patients with known or suspected coronary artery disease the physiologic significance of coronary artery stenoses could be quantified by definition of absolute regional flow and/or relative flow reserve.[1] This quantification would provide a firm foundation for the need to identify coronary anatomy via selective angiography and/or direct the application of specific therapeutic options (e.g., percutaneous coronary angioplasty, bypass grafting, pharmacologic manipulations) in patients after angiography.

Two general methods may be applied to studies of coronary-myocardial blood flow in humans: direct and indirect measurement techniques. Direct techniques are invasive and require either selective cardiac catheterization or coronary flow determination during cardiac surgery. Examples of direct measurement techniques include application of a Doppler ultrasonic probe[1] or flow-velocity catheter,[2] as well as the electromagnetic flowmeter.[3, 4]

Indirect techniques are divided into internal- or external-type detection methods. All require intravascular administration of a surrogate "indicator" for definition of blood-flow transit kinetics. Internal-type detection techniques include coronary sinus thermodilution,[5] whereas external-type techniques include thallium-201 (^{201}Tl) scintigraphy,[6, 7] two-dimensional echocardiography,[8, 9] inert gas clearance,[10, 11] digital-substraction angiography,[12, 13] positron emission tomography,[14–16] magnetic resonance imaging,[17, 18] and high-speed computed tomography (CT). Of these, ^{201}Tl scintigraphy, positron emission tomography, magnetic resonance imaging, and high-speed CT do not require direct cardiac catheterization and thus share the potential for widespread outpatient determination of regional myocardial perfusion. Intravenous contrast agents for application to perfusion imaging with the use of transthoracic two-dimensional echocardiography have been developed but have a limited application to clinical studies at present. Thallium-201 scintigraphy is routinely employed for the evaluation of myocardial blood-flow distribution in patients with coronary heart disease but offers only a qualitative assessment with limited applicability to patients with triple-vessel disease or extensive prior infarction. Positron emission tomography requires assessment of regional uptake kinetics and partition coefficients for diffusible indicators, whereas magnetic resonance imaging and CT have traditionally used methods based on classical indicator transit kinetics. At the present time, only positron emission tomography, magnetic resonance imaging, and CT have been sufficiently developed to offer the promise of quantitation of absolute regional myocardial perfusion noninvasively.

Thallium-201 scintigraphy, positron emission tomography, and magnetic resonance imaging are discussed in detail in other chapters. This chapter reviews the application of CT and presents past and current studies that have used this external detection method for quantitation of regional myocardial perfusion. As the techniques are discussed, the promise of applications to humans and the potential pitfalls or limitations of these applications will be specifically examined.

HIGH-SPEED COMPUTED TOMOGRAPHIC SCANNERS

The majority of studies presented in this chapter were performed with an "electron-beam" computed tomographic scanner. Traditional computed tomographic scanners employ mechanical rotation of a single x-ray source about the patient in concert with a stationary or rotating collimator-detector combination; however, scan speeds on the order of 1 to 2 seconds for conventional scanners and even 250 to 600 msec for the new spiral technology are still too slow to freeze cardiac motion or evaluate the fine details of cardiac anatomy, function, and flow.

Boyd[19] introduced the use of a scanning electron beam that could be swept rapidly across one or more parallel tungsten target rings, thus functioning as a "stationary" x-ray source, coupled to a fixed detector array. Rapid, serial, and consecutive imaging of the beating heart and vascular system could then be performed, as polytomographic images were acquired within milliseconds of an electrocardiographic "trigger."

Terminology separating "conventional" CT from the Boyd scanner has been varied, and it often has been referred to by the proprietary name (Ultrafast CT®) or variations of this name, which relate to the speed of imaging (e.g., fast CT). "Cine-CT" is a term commonly used by clinicians and researchers to refer to this method of cardiac imaging; however, radiologists object to the use of this term because it refers to only one of several means by which the device can obtain images of the body. At present, there is only one manufacturer of the electron-beam CT scanning technology (Imatron Inc., San Francisco, CA). Recently, there has been a trend to refer to all these names by a common label.[20] Because this CT technology is sufficiently distinct, "electron-beam computed tomography" (EBCT) has been suggested as the most appropriate description. This term encompasses many facets of this application to imaging of the heart, great vessels, thorax, and abdomen into a single descriptor and thus is used throughout the remainder of the discussion, in preference to "ultrafast computed tomography."

This fourth-generation geometry instrument has no moving parts aside from the patient scanning table. Tomographic images are obtained by magnetic deflection of an electron beam swept rapidly across one to four semicircular (210-degree) tungsten targets that surround the subject. Current EBCT scanning options include an electrocardiographically triggered, rapid-sequence, polytomographic (2- to 12-level), 50 msec per scan acquisition for studies requiring information from temporal sequences (e.g., cardiac function and myocardial perfusion) and a single-slice, 100 msec per scan acquisition for studies requiring improved density and spatial resolution from static images (e.g., coronary artery calcium). Tomographic slice thicknesses are nominally 0.8 cm for the 50-msec images and 0.3 cm for the 100-msec cardiac images. Sequential scan repetition rate is 17 frames per second in the polytomographic (cine) mode, in which up to 8 cm of the myocardium can be scanned in as little as 7 cardiac cycles and up to 80 scans can be taken in rapid sequence.

Imaging for assessment of myocardial perfusion is done in the traditional radiographic transaxial plane or, with the use of tilt and/or slew of the imaging table, in both the cardiac "short" (transverse cardiac) and the "long" (modified, horizontal long) axes. Electrocardiographic triggering at a designated time during each cardiac cycle (nominally every other cardiac cycle) allows for stop-action scans obtained as an indicator (iodinated contrast material) traverses the left ventricular cavity, proximal aorta, and myocardium. Sophisticated off-line image analysis software allows for evaluation of arterial (input) and myocardial (response) indicator transit curves within any operatively defined tomographic region of interest.[21]

The remainder of the studies that use high-speed CT discussed in this chapter were derived from the Mayo Clinic's "Dynamic Spatial Reconstructor" (DSR). This unique, solely research-based instrument allows for simultaneous volumetric imaging of the heart, as has been described elsewhere.[22]

THEORETICAL CONSIDERATIONS

Historical Aspects of Indicator-Dilution Methods

The earliest report on the use of an indicator to determine circulation times in vivo was made by Haller (cited in reference 23), who, in 1761, reported injection of a colored liquid into the vena cava of an animal to compare pulmonary circulation times through inflated versus collapsed lungs. However, it was Stewart[24–26] who first applied the indicator-dilution technique to the determination of cardiac output and the "central blood volume." Additionally, he devised the first method of permitting the continuous detection of indicator concentration (hypertonic saline) at the sampling site.

In 1913, Henriques[27] used sodium thiocyanate as an indicator because it was easily quantitated colorimetrically. He was the first to note the presence of indicator recirculation by observing the failure of the downslope (or washout) of the dilution curve to return to baseline in the systemic circulation. He also devised an application for measuring coronary blood flow, using the simultaneous injection of two indicators into different sites in the systemic circulation. Koch[28] first applied indicator-dilution principles to measurements in humans, using fluorescein as an indicator. In 1927, Blumgart and Yens[29] reported the first application of external detection methods that used radioactive tracers.

Hamilton and co-workers[29, 30] extended the original work of Stewart by using a sudden, single injection of indicator. They subsequently increased the overall accuracy of the method to determine cardiac output by extracting the contribution of recirculated indicator through semilogarithmic replotting and linear extrapolation of the downslope of the original curve, recorded in the systemic circulation. This landmark contribution cannot be overemphasized and amply justifies the name "Stewart-Hamilton technique," as applied to classic indicator-dilution theory. However, to Meier and Zierler[31, 32] goes the credit for presentation of an organized and mathematically sound theory for the general application of indicator-dilution concepts to estimation of physiologic flows.

Prinzmetal and colleagues[33, 34] developed an original application of external detection techniques to the measurement of cardiac flow in humans, using radioactive tracers and a technique termed "angiocardiography." Additional data derived from external detection methods were provided from the Mayo Clinic laboratories of E. H. Wood and associates,[35, 36] who used an ear oximeter to continuously evaluate the concentration of methylene blue in blood. These studies were the first to describe the systemic patterns of circulation for an indicator in the presence of right-to-left and left-to-right shunting, as compared with the normal intact circulation. Henley and colleagues[37] used iodinated serum albumin to make the first measurements of myocardial blood flow in intact dogs, but Love and Burch[38] and Nolting and colleagues[39] first reported the use of external counting methods for measuring coronary blood flow with radioactive rubidium. These foundations underlie the future developments of ^{201}Tl scintigraphy (a potassium analog with distribution similar to that of rubidium) and positron emission tomography. As can be appreciated from the above discussion, the development and application of indicator-dilution methods to the calculation of cardiac blood flow was widely known 30 to 50 years ago.

A general discussion of the physical principles of CT, in general, and EBCT, in particular, is beyond the scope of this review but can be found elsewhere in Chapter 52 by R.L. Robb; however, an important principle of CT paramount to its application to myocardial perfusion is that the Hounsfield "density"[40] of any object or field within the tomogram be directly proportional to the true roentgen attenuation coefficient of tissue within that area. The use of iodinated contrast material with an x-ray attenuation factor significantly greater than soft tissue as a marker for the passage of blood allows for ready separation of blood vessels from soft tissue and also provides a surrogate marker for the flow of blood across any designated tissue-perfusion field. The magnitude of the changes in contrast density and the time course of these changes as one follows the transit of contrast medium through any designated region of interest within the tomogram provides a relative index of blood flow and perfusion via direct application of indicator-dilution theory.

Assumptions of Indicator-Dilution Theory as Applied to Computed Tomography

The general assumptions of classic indicator-dilution theory as extended to application of external detection techniques were first discussed by Newman and colleagues in 1951.[41] These assumptions also directly influence the application of high-speed CT to the analysis of contrast clearance data from the myocardium, as modified and discussed below. In this instance, the indicator is iodinated contrast medium, administered into either the venous or the arterial circulation.

Assumption 1: Complete Mixing of the Indicator

When applied to computed tomographic measurement of myocardial blood flow with the use of an intravenous injection of contrast material, the assumption that the indicator is well mixed with the blood is generally true because it will have traversed at least two cardiac mixing chambers (right and left ventricles) prior to entry into the coronary ostia. For central (aortic root) injection, this assumption is less secure because the contrast entering into the coronary system would not have previously traversed a true mixing chamber; however, external sampling of arterial input from the coronary ostia or proximal aortic root should provide an accurate characterization of the input to the myocardium. Incomplete mixing of the contrast indicator, either at the site chosen for characterization of the input function or at the tissue site, yields erroneous values for regional myocardial perfusion.

Assumption 2: The Volume of Indicator Injected Is Negligible

In practice for intravenous (and presumably systemic) injection routes, the amount of contrast material required per study is between 0.5 and 1.0 mL/kg.[21, 42–44] This volume is negligible, compared to the central circulating blood volume (or total volume of distribution). Roughly, 5 percent of this injected volume enters the coronary circulation, and this amount (0.025 to 0.05 mL/kg) can be assumed to be negligible, compared to the total myocardial blood volume.

Assumption 3: The Indicator Does Not Perturb Hemodynamic and Vascular Equilibrium During Its Transit

Measurements of regional myocardial perfusion with high-speed CT are made by sampling contrast-clearance data during the first pass of the indicator through the circulation. Such measurement requires that flow be at steady state at least during the determination and mandates that not only the baseline hemodynamics remain invariate during the passage of the indicator but also the volume of distribution of the indicator (vascular blood volume) remain constant during the measurement.

The intravascular administration of conventional ionic contrast agents, such as meglumine sodium diatrizoate, is associated with a variety of significant hemodynamic perturbations that may occur within seconds of injection. Thus, myocardial flow and vascular blood volume could be dynamically changing during the first pass of such an indicator, violating assumption 3. However, studies that use nonionic contrast agents, when compared directly with conventional agents, have demonstrated little or no changes in coronary flow or systemic hemodynamics after intravenous administration,[21, 45] as illustrated in Figure 55–1. Significant changes in systemic and coronary hemodynamics are seen within a few seconds after injection of the ionic agent but not after injection of the nonionic contrast agent. Nonionic contrast agents are the indicator of choice for studies of regional myocardial perfusion that use high-speed CT.

Assumption 4: No Extravascular Loss of Indicator During Measurement

Implicit in the assumption of complete mixing of the indicator with the blood (assumption 1) is that the distribution volume of the indicator be identical to the distribution volume of blood; however, iodinated contrast medium has both an intravascular and an extravascular volume of distribution. Several studies have suggested that during the first pass of contrast agent it remains primarily (95 percent) intravascular.[46, 47] However, a recent study by Canty and co-workers[48] has indicated that in its transit through the myocardium, there may be substantial extravasation of nonionic iodinated contrast media during the first pass, potentially violating this assumption. Extravasation, which according to Canty and his team appears during the latter phase of the first pass of the iodinated contrast media through the tissue, may cause the externally recorded time course of the contrast material through the region (i.e., the indicator-clearance curve) to be artificially prolonged; thus, flow algorithms that require information on the area under the entire contrast-clearance curve within the myocardium (see later section on theoretical concepts) may yield erroneous results.

Because first-pass regional indicator contrast-clearance curves are used in the determination of regional myocardial perfusion by high-speed CT, careful considerations of the potential for extravascular loss of contrast material during this time period must be taken into account during data analysis. To substantially attenuate the effect of contrast extravasation on the calculation of myocardial perfusion during the first pass through the myocardium, algorithms that use only the information determined from the peak opacification within the myocardium may be more applicable in a general sense. If under certain circumstances, substantial extravasation of contrast medium occurs prior to peak myocardial opacification, then this assumption (using theoretical constructs presented later) may also be violated. Wolfkiel and Brundage[49] have suggested that values of perfusion representing maximum coronary vasodilation in normal areas (blood flow up to sixfold greater than that of resting values) obtained with the use of EBCT may underestimate myocardial perfusion by as much as 50 percent because of contrast extravasation into the myocardium.

Assumption 5: Indicator Recirculation Can Be Ignored

Recirculation of indicator occurs in intact, closed circulation and is routinely observed from contrast-clearance data in both the central circulation and the myocardium with the use of high-

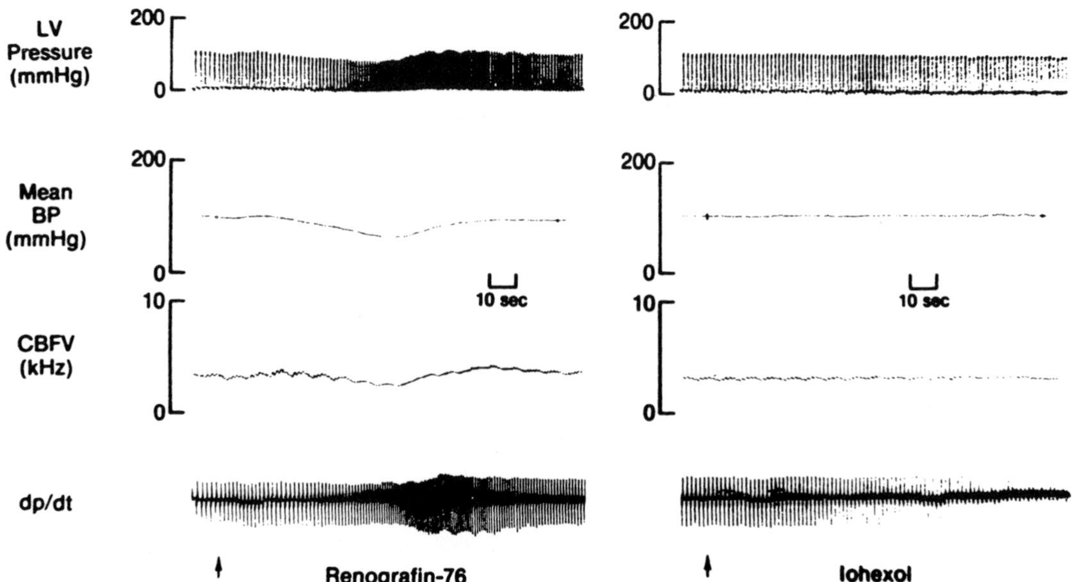

FIGURE 55–1. Canine study demonstrating high-fidelity left ventricular (LV) pressure, mean aortic pressure, coronary blood flow velocity (CBFV, Doppler probe), and dP/dt after injection of iodinated contrast material into the inferior vena cava (1 mL/kg over 3 seconds). Left panel is after injection of conventional ionic contrast (Renografin-76), while right panel is after injection of nonionic contrast medium (Iohexol). Note the significant changes seen after ionic contrast injection, where no change in systemic hemodynamics is noted after injection of nonionic contrast. (From Rumberger, J.A., Feiring, A.J., Lipton, M.J., et al.: Use of ultrafast computed tomography to quantitate regional myocardial perfusion: A preliminary report. J. Am. Coll. Cardiol. 9:59–69, 1987, with permission.)

speed CT. However, in most cases the "recirculation" peak can be eliminated directly from the final analysis either by semilogarithmic extrapolation of the washout portion of the curve or by application of a gamma variate curve fit[50] to the rising, peak, and initial falling portions of the measured regional indicator-dilution curve.

Assumption 6: Appropriate Coronary Input Function

This assumption relates to the overall shape and character of the indicator input function to the coronary ostia. The nature of this phenomenon has far-reaching implications and may underlie one of the pitfalls of the computed tomographic technique with respect to application across the entire physiologic range of values for myocardial perfusion. Intravenous contrast material cannot be administered as an ideal bolus (or impulse "input" function). The contrast agent must be given rapidly enough to avoid overlap with recirculation, but at a rate that does not alter the subsequent characteristics of the coronary (aortic root) input function.

Burbank and co-workers[51] have shown that characteristics of intra-aortic digital subtraction contrast-clearance curves (e.g., mean transit time and peak opacification) after intravenous contrast administration are not altered by the bolus input kinetics, provided that the injection time is less than one half the subsequent aortic contrast mean transit time. Contrast injection times of 2 to 3 seconds or less in the central venous circulation probably satisfy this requirement (see later text). Tacitly assumed with this assumption for application to studies of myocardial perfusion is that the mean transit time of the indicator through the vascular-tissue volume is greater than the mean transit time for the indicator input function to that vascular-tissue space. For central aortic contrast administration, the input to the coronary system can more precisely mimic a true bolus but may suffer from lack of complete mixing, as discussed under assumption 1. The potential limitations of both the intravenous injection and the central aortic (systemic) injection methods for this application are considered in a later section.

Assumption 7: Intravascular and Intramyocardial Contrast Density Can Be Accurately Measured Externally

This assumption requires that the CT device (acting as an external videodensitometer) accurately record the time-dependent contrast densities from baseline across a defined dynamic range. This assumption mandates that the system response be known and that imaging artifacts be minimal. Under certain conditions, this assumption may not be completely satisfied (see later section on imaging and reconstruction artifacts), although in most instances EBCT and the DSR provide reliable and linear system responses for assessment of computed tomographic density values across the range of contrast concentrations generally encountered in vivo (Fig. 55–2).

Derivation of Basic Flow Algorithms

Classic indicator-dilution theory (Stewart-Hamilton principle), as elegantly described by Meier and Zierler,[31, 32] denotes the absolute

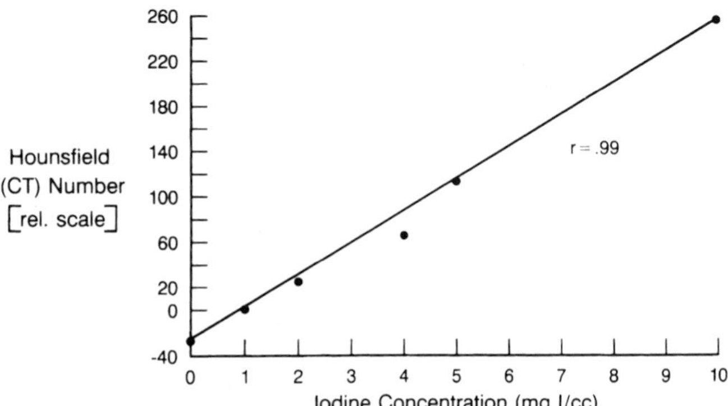

FIGURE 55–2. Study performed in a phantom with the use of EBCT comparing the results of iodine study using concentration with computed tomography (Hounsfield number) above baseline, which demonstrates the linear system response and the use of computed tomographic values (relative scale *above* baseline) to substitute for videodensitometric values to define flow phenomena after injection of iodinated contrast medium. (From Rumberger, J.A., Bell, M.L., Feiring, A.J., et al.: Quantitation of myocardial perfusion using fast computed tomography. *In* Marcus, M.L., Skorton, D.J., Schelbert H., et al. (eds.): Cardiac Imaging. Philadelphia, W.B. Saunders, 1991, pp. 688–702, with permission.)

flow rate in the central systemic circulation (or forward cardiac output from the left ventricle), F_{LV}, as the ratio of the absolute amount of indicator injected into that vascular volume, q, divided by the area under the indicator-clearance curve in the systemic circulation, A_{LV}. The subscript "LV" designates the calculation made in the left ventricular cavity, as may be made after intravenous injection of iodinated contrast material, but the same concept holds true for systemic injection of contrast with the use of using data from contrast clearance in the central aortic root. Thus:

$$F_{LV} = q/A_{LV} \quad (1)$$

Figure 55–3 is a schematic of the left ventricular cavity–aorta–coronary artery system. Here K = a + b + c (where K is the fraction of total indicator injected, q, that enters the coronary system from the input [left ventricular cavity]). Thus q°a, q°b, and q°c represent the amount of indicator delivered to each of the three major coronary branches individually, as illustrated. However, the sum of contrast material delivered to the coronary system (K°q) remains small compared to q itself; that is, the fraction of total indicator delivered to the coronary system is much less than the amount of indicator remaining in the systemic circulation: (q − K°q) ≅ q.

The absolute blood flow through any coronary artery (or region) is directly proportional to the fraction of total indicator delivered to that region, which underlies the principle initially proposed by Sapirstein[52] and is the basis for the commonly used radiolabeled microsphere technique used experimentally to determine regional organ flow. Therefore:

$$F_a = a^*F_{LV},\ F_b = b^*F_{LV},\ F_c = C^*F_{LV}$$

This equation, by analogy, should hold true for any "myocardial" region, f. Thus:

$$F_f = f^*F_{LV} \quad (2)$$

Whereby f represents the fraction of total indicator injected (either intravenously or systemically) that enters that myocardial region. However, the question remains: What is the value of f?

Figure 55–4 is a schematic of an indicator-dilution curve recorded in the systemic circulation after intravenous injection of indicator. For such a curve as recorded, for example, in the left ventricular cavity, the area under the curve can be approximated as follows[31]:

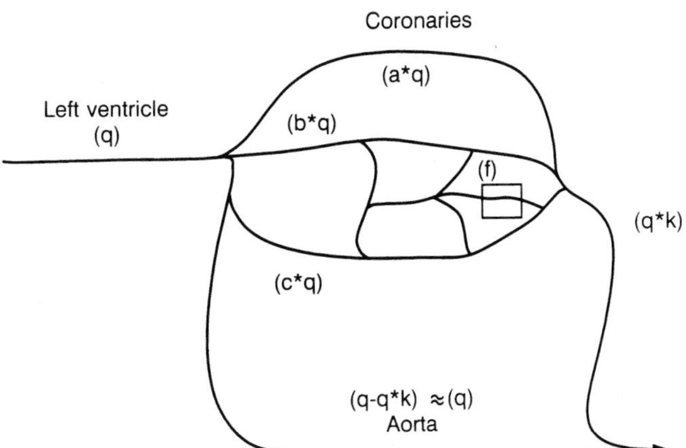

FIGURE 55–3. Schematic illustration of coronary artery-aorta system. Note that the portion of contrast material entering the coronary system (k) is only a small portion of the total amount injected at the source (q). The portions (fractions of k) that enter each coronary artery are designated as a, b, and c. The portion that enters a given myocardial region is designated as f. (From Rumberger, J.A., Feiring, A.J., Lipton, M.J., et al.: Use of ultrafast computed tomography to quantitate regional myocardial perfusion: A preliminary report. J. Am. Coll. Cardiol. 9:59–69, 1987, with permission.)

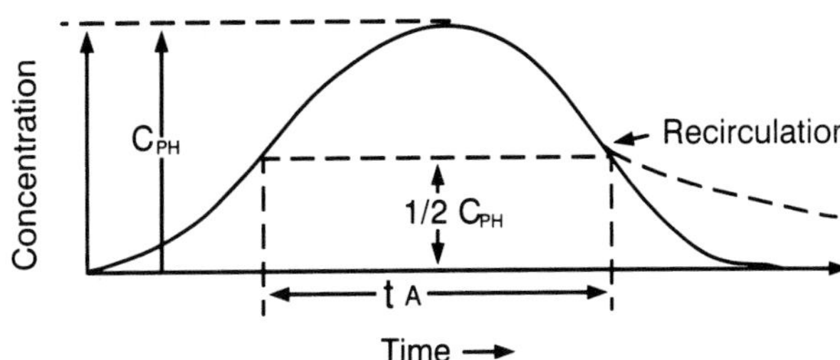

FIGURE 55–4. Schematic of an indicator-dilution curve, as recorded in the systemic circulation after an intravenous injection of indicator (iodinated contrast). C_{PH} is the peak concentration (height) above baseline; t is the "full width half-maximum time" (see text for details); and A is the area under the curve. (From Rumberger, J.A., Feiring, A.J., Lipton, M.J., et al.: Use of ultrafast computed tomography to quantitate regional myocardial perfusion: A preliminary report. J. Am. Coll. Cardiol. 9:59–69, 1987, with permission.)

$$A_{LV} = C_{PH}{}^*t_A \quad (3)$$

Here, C_{PH} is the peak indicator concentration (or density above baseline) and t_A is the "full width–half maximum time," a characteristic of the time spread of the curve. Both of these parameters can be determined from a straightforward analysis of the curve.

From classic indicator-dilution theory,[31] the following equation is valid:

$$F_{LV}/V_{LV} = 1/MTT_A \quad (4)$$

Here, V_{LV} is the central blood volume (volume of distribution of the indicator) and MTT_A is the "mean transit time" of the indicator-dilution curve for an impulse-type input function. The mean transit time is equal to the centroid, or first moment of the indicator curve, when appearance time and injection time are considered to be simultaneous (i.e., impulse injection at time t = 0). Equation 4 then simply states that the cardiac output per unit distribution (blood) volume is inversely proportional to mean transit time.

Now, consider that t_A and MTT_A (both of which describe the time spread of the clearance curve) to be related by the nondefined parameter, ξ_A, as:

$$t_A = \xi_A{}^*MTT_A \quad (5)$$

For a true bolus (impulse) type input function (satisfying assumption 6), t_A is exactly equal to MTT_A.[31, 32]

Combining equations 1, 3, 4, and 5:

$$q = C_{PH}{}^*V_{LV}{}^*\xi_A \quad (6)$$

By direct analogy, the contrast-clearance curve in the myocardium, f, can be described as:

$$A_f = C_f{}^*t_f \quad (7)$$

Again, by analogy from the equations that describe the indicator kinetics in the systemic circulation, and equation 2:

$$f^*q = C_f{}^*V_f{}^*\xi_f \quad (8)$$

Therefore,

$$f = \xi_f{}^*C_f{}^*V_f/q \quad (9)$$

Here, A_f is the area under the myocardial indicator clearance curve; C_f is a "characteristic" concentration (density above baseline) for the clearance curve (e.g., the "peak concentration," by analogy with the systemic circulation); t_f is the full width–half maximum time for the myocardial indicator curve; ξ_f is analogous to ξ_A but remains undefined at present; and MTT_f is the myocardial (tissue) mean transit time. As before, V_f is the volume of distribution of the indicator in the region (in this case, the myocardium, i.e., the regional myocardial volume), which, a priori, is unknown.

The flow (absolute) in the myocardial region f is given by direct substitution into equation 2 as:

$$F_f = C_f{*}\xi_f{*}V_f{*}F_{LV}/q \tag{10}$$

Combining equation 10 with equation 1:

$$F_f = C_f{*}V_f{*}\xi_f/A_{LV} \tag{11}$$

Although V_f is not known a priori, the absolute flow (perfusion) per unit volume of myocardium can be given as:

$$F_f/V_f = C_f{*}\xi_f/A_{LV} \tag{12}$$

From the previous discussion, there are two obvious values for C_f (setting $\xi_f = 1.0$, thus satisfying assumption 6):

$$C_f = A_f/t_f \tag{13}$$

or

$$F_f/V_f = (A_f/A_{LV}){*}1/t_f \tag{14}$$

and

$$C_f = C_{PH} \tag{15}$$

or

$$F_f/V_f = C_{PH}/A_{LV} \tag{16}$$

Here, C_{PH} refers to the peak concentration (CT density above baseline, or "peak height") of the indicator-dilution curve within the myocardial region f. Equation 14 is the equation put forward by Axel[53] for studies of regional cerebral perfusion that use CT, and equation 16 was used by Mullani and co-workers[54] for analysis of regional myocardial perfusion using ^{82}Rb.

STUDIES THAT USED INTRAVENOUS CONTRAST INJECTION

In Vitro Studies

Investigations in models of the circulation to evaluate the application of CT for studies of vascular flow serve three purposes: to test theoretical constructs, to evaluate the dynamic range of the measuring device, and to reveal limitations of the method that are seen even under ideal conditions.

Tonge and colleagues[55] and Guthaner and associates[56] used conventional CT devices (1 to 3-second scan acquisition) for studies of cardiac output and direct application of the Stewart-Hamilton principle; however, Jaschke and co-workers[57] were the first to perform an in vitro (phantom) study of tissue perfusion with the use of EBCT. The flow phantom consisted of a system of tubes to simulate vessels and a central cylinder packed with small, irregularly shaped plastic parts to simulate tissue. Saline was pumped into the cylinder via a single tube downstream of a mixing chamber, to which the indicator (iodinated contrast material) was added as a bolus (1 to 3 seconds in duration to simulate intravenous injection techniques). Recirculation of contrast medium was avoided by directing the outflow into a collecting tank. The total volume of the "central" input tubing and the "tissue" equivalent cylinder was fixed and known.

Using the above injection technique, Jaschke and associates found a mean transit time of the "input" to the tissue equivalent that ranged from 6 to 20 seconds as flow within the cylinder (timed collections) was varied from a high of 1.45 L per minute to a low of 0.4 L per minute. Calculations of regional tissue flow by EBCT were made with equation 16. Here, the distribution volume, V_f, was known, so absolute flow through the tissue equivalent could be calculated. Figure 55–5 shows results from their study. Note that the estimation of flow by EBCT is very linear over a range of flows that could be expected in vivo in a system such as the coronary arteries. However, they were aware of assumption 6 and thus kept the input flow rate high enough to allow for no outflow of contrast medium from the sampled region prior to complete entry of the indicator from the input.

Ludman and co-workers[58] studied the application of EBCT to quantification of continuous and pulsatile flow in large tubes and in a tissue-equivalent phantom. As in the study by Jaschke and associates, recirculation of iodinated contrast media was eliminated, and the distribution volume of contrast material was known, so absolute tissue flow could be estimated. Evaluating flow studies in both the 50- and 100-msec imaging modes, they found that in general, the 100-msec imaging model provided for less noise and better statistical correlations. Under these rather ideal circumstances and using first-pass kinetics (equation 16), they found absolute flow to be linearly related to EBCT-calculated flow across a range of 2 to 8 L per minute. The standard deviation of the differences between measured and calculated flows varied between 0.2 and 0.6 L per minute (about 10 percent of the mean).

In Vivo Studies

Studies in Animals

The potential of EBCT to measure regional myocardial perfusion was first reported by Rumberger and colleagues.[21] In this study from six dogs, serial computed tomographic scans were taken during rapid injection of nonionic contrast material into the inferior vena cava under resting conditions and various degrees of coronary vasodilation. For comparison, quantitation of regional myocardial perfusion per unit mass was determined during simultaneous injection of radiolabeled microspheres into the left atrium.

Figure 55–6 shows a representative example of the time-dependent contrast density data obtained from the left ventricular cavity and myocardium at a resting flow state (*left panel*) and after coronary vasodilation (*right panel*). Note that the peak left ventricular cavity opacification is significantly greater than that observed in the adjacent myocardium and that peak myocardial opacification occurs

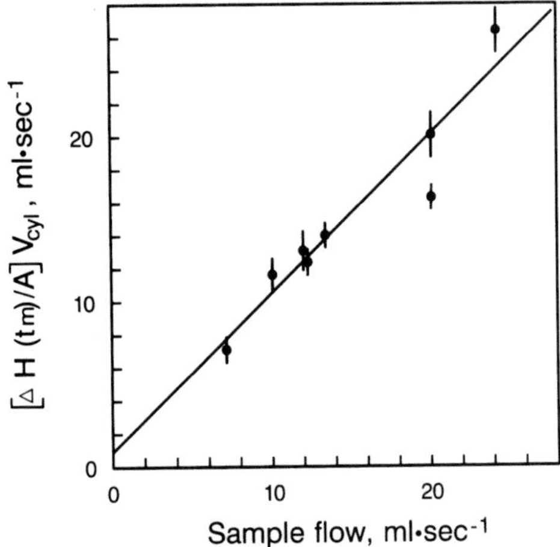

FIGURE 55–5. Comparison of flow per unit volume in a flow phantom, compared to metered flow measurement. This study by Jasche and associates demonstrates a very linear relationship across an expected physiologic range. In this study the volume of distribution (analogous to vascular volume) was fixed and known. [ΔH (tm)/A]V_{cyl} = change in Hounsfield number over area of input function within the volume of the cylinder. (From Jaschke, W., Gould, R.G., Assimakopoulos, P.A., et al.: Flow measurements with a high-speed computed tomography scanner. Med. Phys. 14(2):238–243, 1987, with permission.)

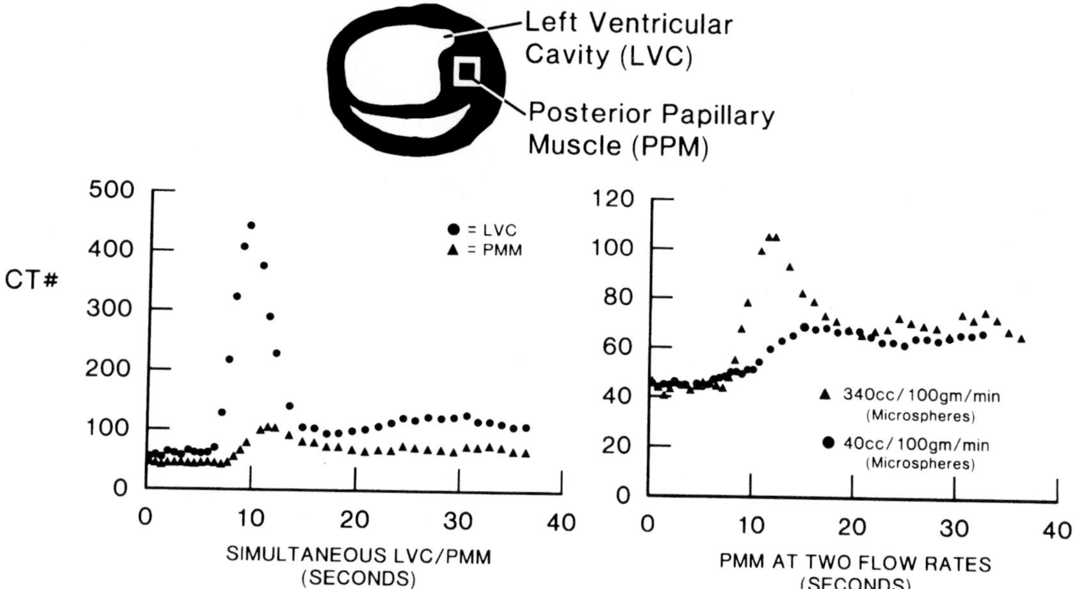

FIGURE 55–6. *Top*, Schematic illustration of a cardiac short-axis tomogram in a dog at the posterior papillary muscle area (PPM) in the middle left ventricle. *Left Panel*, Simultaneous indicator (contrast) clearance versus time within the left ventricular cavity (LVC) and posterior myocardial muscle (PMM) regions after bolus inferior vena cava injection of nonionic contrast material. *Right Panel*, Posterior myocardial muscle contrast density versus time from a dog at a high regional myocardial perfusion rate (340 mL min/100 g) and a low resting perfusion state (40 mL min/100 g). See text for details. (From Rumberger, J.A., Feiring, A.J., Lipton, M.J., et al.: Use of ultrafast computed tomography to quantitate regional myocardial perfusion: A preliminary report. J. Am. Coll. Cardiol. 9:59–69, 1987, with permission.)

well after that observed in the left ventricular cavity (*left panel*). In the right panel, quantitative differences are readily apparent with regard to peak opacification above baseline, the area inscribed by the myocardial time-density curve, and the overall contrast transit time of the curves when the high myocardial perfusion state is compared to the resting perfusion state. These observations are consistent with the theoretical considerations previously stated, which indicated that for values of flow per unit volume above baseline, as compared to control, the peak concentration above baseline increases and the mean transit time decreases.

A total of 13 scan and microsphere pairs were judged technically adequate for analysis. Absolute regional myocardial perfusion values as assessed by the microsphere technique ranged from 30 to 450 mL/min/100 g (mean 167 ± 125). Regional myocardial flow per unit mass by EBCT was calculated by multiplying the flow per unit volume by the density of the myocardium (1.05 g/mL. Individual time-density (contrast-clearance) data were displayed simultaneously from the left ventricular cavity and the region of the posterior myocardium for each flow state in each animal. Parameters derived from the computed tomographic studies involved the use of a gamma variate fit to the left ventricular cavity and myocardial data,[50] calculation of the peak concentrations (CT densities) above baseline, areas under the curves, and the full width–half maximum transit time for the myocardium.

Calculated myocardial flow per unit mass ranged from 30 to 390 mL/min/100 g (mean 150 ± 140, not significantly different from the microsphere data). A comparison of the regional myocardial flow per unit mass by microspheres (abscissa) and EBCT (ordinate) is shown in Figure 55–7, using Equation 16. The correlation was statistically significant ($r = .72$; SEE = 65 mL/min/100 g; $P < .01$).

Wolfkiel and colleagues[44] performed a similar study in a group of 16 dogs, in whom ionic contrast material was administered from a distal venous site (femoral vein) and data analysis was performed in a fashion similar to that noted earlier. Intravenous chromonar was administered to produce variable degrees of coronary vasodilation in 10 dogs, whereas temporary occlusion of the left anterior descending coronary artery was done prior to scanning in a separate group of six dogs. Radiolabeled microspheres again were employed to allow for comparison to flow rates calculated with CT. In this study, three separate flow algorithms were evaluated, but the best fit to the microsphere data used the formulation given previously by equation 16.

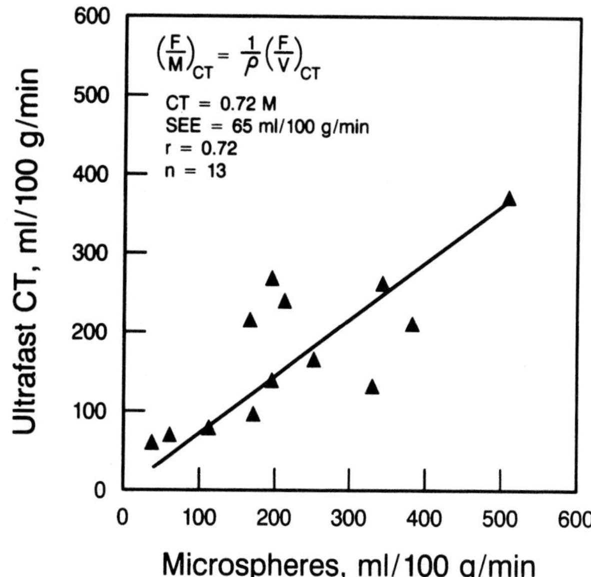

FIGURE 55–7. Comparison of myocardial perfusion (flow per unit mass, F/M) in the posterior papillary muscle region of the dog, as assessed by radiolabeled microspheres and EBCT, using equation 16 (see text for details). In this instance, flow per unit volume F/V, as assessed by EBCT (ultrafast CT), is converted for comparison to flow per unit myocardial mass, as determined by radiolabeled microspheres. (From Rumberger, J.A., Bell, M.L., Feiring, A.J., et al.: Quantitation of myocardial perfusion using fast computed tomography. *In* Marcus, M.L., Skorton, D.J., Schelbert, H., et al. (eds.): Cardiac Imaging. Philadelphia, W.B. Saunders, 1991, pp. 688–702, with permission.)

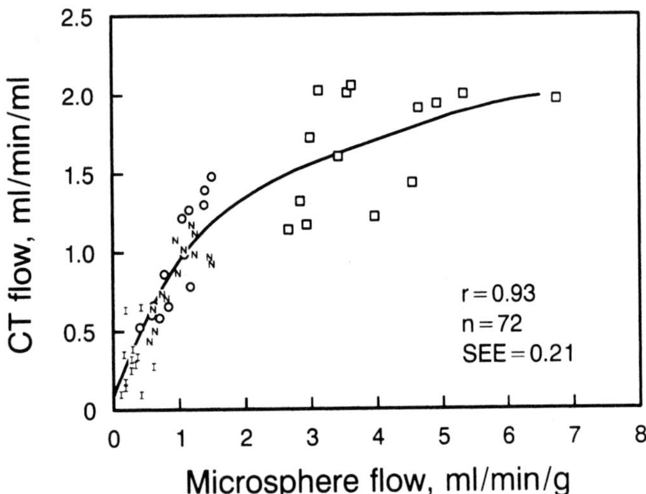

FIGURE 55–8. Regional myocardial perfusion (flow per unit mass) versus regional perfusion as measured by radiolabeled microspheres in a series of dog experiments. Data are taken from Wolfkiel and associates, who used a femoral vein injection of contrast material. Note the plateau in the relationship at approximately 1.3 mL/min/g (130 mL/min/100 g). Computed tomographic calculations were made with equation 14. (From Wolfkiel, C.J., Ferguson, J.L., Chomka, E.V., et al.: Measurement of myocardial blood flow by ultrafast computed tomography. Circulation 76:1262–1273, 1987, with permission.)

A composite of data from this initial study by Wolfkiel is shown in Figure 55–8. Note that the calculation of regional flow per unit mass by EBCT is nearly linear from zero up to values of approximately 150 mL/min/100 g. Above this range, computed tomographic estimates of flow significantly underestimated microsphere flow; in fact, the calculation reached a "plateau" at the higher flow rates.

Gould and colleagues[42] reported on additional studies of regional myocardial perfusion that used EBCT in the canine model. The animal model and methods of contrast injection were similar to the two previous in vivo studies; however, in this study they modified the basic flow algorithm (equation 16), after noting some difficulties with the linearity of the standard calculation at high flow rates. This modification consisted of adding an empiric term to account for the difference between the time of peak contrast opacification in the left ventricle and that noted in the myocardium. This modification added a parameter related to the "effective" mean transit time from the input (aorta) to the myocardium. Addition of this factor allowed for a first-order estimate for deconvolution between the input and the (tissue) response contrast-clearance curves. However, their approach was empiric, and although the results suggested that this method might allow extension of the calculation by EBCT to high flow rates, they were inconclusive.

Studies in Patients

There are limited clinical validation data available obtained with the use of EBCT to estimate absolute and relative myocardial perfusion in patients. Rumberger and co-workers[43] presented preliminary data from six normal patients before and after intravenous injection of dipyridamole.[59]

Nonionic contrast (0.33 mL/kg) was injected as a rapid bolus into an antecubital vein just prior to computed tomographic scanning in the baseline (resting) state and after administration of dipyridamole (0.56 mg/kg over 4 minutes, with maximum effect at 9 minutes after infusion). Data analysis was performed on the subsequent images from the middle left ventricle in a fashion identical to that previously described for the animal studies.

Figure 55–9 shows simultaneous left ventricular cavity and regional myocardial time-density curves from the same subject at rest (*left*) and after intravenous infusion of dipyridamole (*right*). The myocardial curve during maximum vasodilation demonstrated a greater peak concentration (density above baseline) and a shorter contrast transit time, compared to the data from the control state. These qualitative observations with respect to the shape and character of the indicator-dilution curves in humans are in accord with the observations in animals (see Fig. 55–6).

For each patient, the areas under the left ventricular cavity and regional myocardial contrast-clearance curves were determined. The mean contrast transit times through the myocardial region of interest were calculated and the values of flow per unit mass determined using equation 14. Individual resting regional myocardial flow ranged from 55 to 141 mL/min/100 g (104 ± 30), whereas perfusion rates after dipyridamole infusion ranged from 128 to 389 mL/min/100 g (277 ± 88; $P < .01$, compared to baseline). Regional flow reserve was calculated for each subject as the ratio of flow per unit mass during maximum vasodilation, compared to baseline. This parameter ranged from 2.23 to 3.5 (2.67 ± 0.50) (Fig. 55–10).

Bell and colleagues[60] reported a preliminary investigation in 14 normal subjects at rest and in 10 of these 14 during maximum coronary vasodilation produced with intravenous infusion of adenosine (140 μg per minute). Intravenous nonionic contrast material was administered in the superior vena cava at 10 mL per second for 2 seconds, and EBCT scanning was done over approximately 30 seconds. Global resting flow (mean ± SE), as estimated by EBCT, was 106 ± 7 mL/min/100 g and increased to 301 ± 25 mL/min/100 g during adenosine infusion (global flow reserve 3.1 ± 0.3). They also attempted to define regional absolute flow and flow reserve. Resting flows in the anterior, lateral, and septal myocardial walls were relatively uniform at rest and showed similar increases in flow during adenosine administration. Flow reserve varied from 2.7 ± 0.3 in the anterior wall to 3.3 ± 0.4 in the septal wall. Imaging was done in the transaxial plane in this study, unlike imaging in the ventricular "short-axis" (transverse cardiac axis), as had been done in prior animal studies. Thus, flow could not be assessed in the inferior wall, which was out of the imaging plane. In addition, a

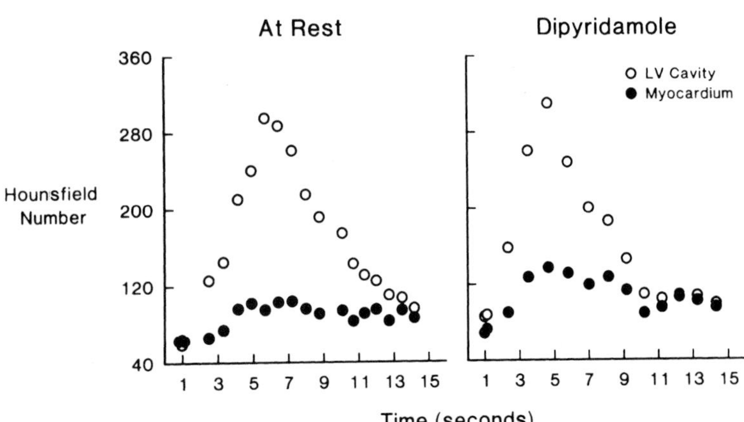

FIGURE 55–9. Simultaneous left ventricular (LV) cavity and regional myocardial time-density curves from the same patient at rest (*left panel*) and after intravenous injection of dipyridamole (*right panel*) (0.56 mg/kg). Note that these data resemble the data from the same dog as in Figure 55–6. (From Rumberger, J.A., Stanford, W., and Marcus, M.L.: Quantitation of regional myocardial perfusion by ultrafast-CT: Promises and pitfalls. Am. J. Card. Imaging 1[4]:336–343, 1987, with permission.)

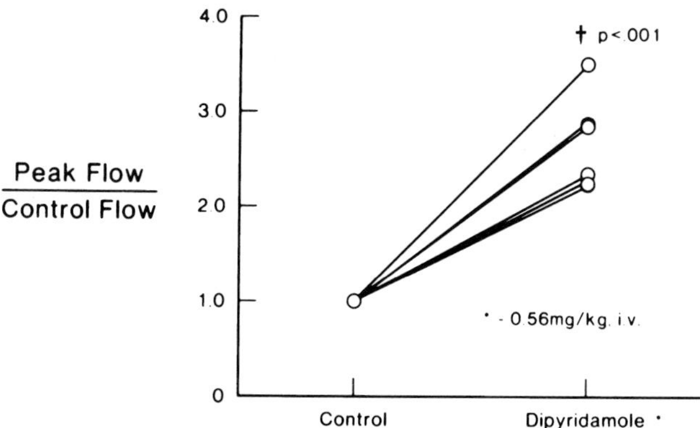

FIGURE 55–10. Regional myocardial flow reserve in the posterior myocardium, as assessed by EBCT in normal patients (n = 6). The average flow reserve calculated in this group was 2.67 to 1. (From Rumberger, J.A., Stanford, W., and Marcus, M.L.: Quantitation of regional myocardial perfusion by ultrafast-CT: Promises and pitfalls. Am. J. Card. Imaging 1[4]:336–343, 1987, with permission.)

modification of equation 16 was used to define myocardial perfusion by factoring in changes in intramyocardial blood volume during vasodilation. This addition to the classic theory will be more fully discussed later in this chapter.

Ludman and colleagues[61] recently reported on validation studies in 14 patients with known coronary disease in which they compared perfusion with EBCT and intravenous contrast injection in a single short-axis slice with perfusion data from a similar image obtained with the use of ^{201}Tl single-photon emission computed tomography at rest and during adenosine infusion. Additionally, reproducibility of EBCT was assessed in 10 patients at rest and in 6 patients during adenosine infusion. All patients had both EBCT and ^{201}Tl imaging done on the same day. EBCT scans were done, using the 100-msec scan mode triggered at end-diastole in accord with their prior phantom studies.[58] They calculated absolute myocardial perfusion by means of EBCT, using equation 16, and compared qualitatively the regional blood flow distribution and relative correlations between normal and reduced perfusion from the EBCT versus that from ^{201}Tl scans. Using a 32-segment model for regional perfusion around the short-axis slices, they found a moderate degree of similarity between the regional blood flow distribution by ^{201}Tl and EBCT (Fig. 55–11).

They found no consistent differences in the repeatability of the EBCT scans; however, the variability was less in the lateral and posterior walls, as compared to that in the anterior and septal walls, which could represent the results of heterogeneous imaging artifacts. The mean values for perfusion increased as a whole in the segments during pharmacologic vasodilation, but the flow in segments judged to be normal on ^{201}Tl scanning ranged from 52 mL/min/100 g (range 20 to 83) at rest to only 84 mL/min/100 g (range 18 to 177) with adenosine. These values at supposed maximum flow are significantly less than what would be expected, suggesting some problems with methodology or further limitations in the maximum flow calculations possible with the use of EBCT. Unlike the case with the study by Bell and colleagues[60] noted above, no attempt was made to correct for underestimations of maximum blood flow by accounting for dynamic changes in intramyocardial vascular volume during vasodilation.

STUDIES THAT USED INTRA-ARTERIAL (SYSTEMIC) CONTRAST INJECTION

Animal Studies

The data set defined by Wolfkiel and colleagues[44] with the use of a femoral vein injection of contrast material (Fig. 55–8) demonstrated a plateau for EBCT quantitation of myocardial perfusion around 200 mL/min/100 g where the data set defined by Rumberger and co-workers,[21] using a more central venous injection of contrast medium into the inferior vena cava (Fig. 55–7) suggested a plateau in perfusion quantitation around 300 to 350 mL/min/100 g. Using the Mayo Clinic DSR *and* an aortic root injection of nonionic contrast, Wang and associates[62] determined that regional myocardial perfusion could be quantitated by high-speed CT techniques at flow rates up to 1000 mL/min/100 g. This later study

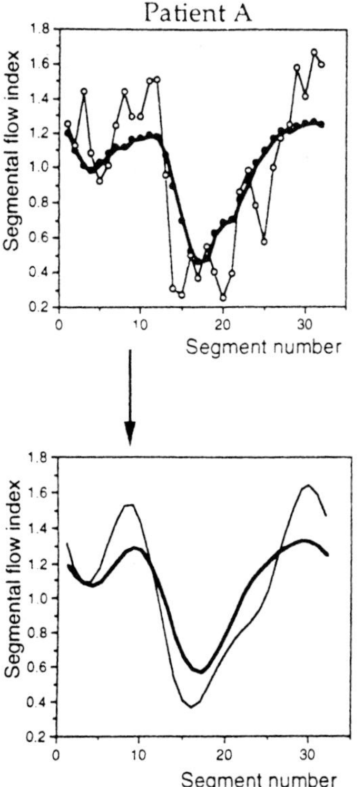

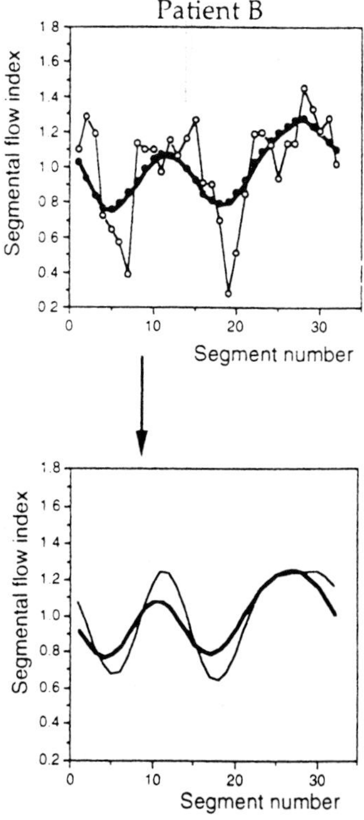

FIGURE 55–11. Comparison of results from regional myocardial perfusion (relative) from a single slice ^{201}Tl tomograph (●) with (relative) regional myocardial perfusion from a single-slice electron-beam CT scan (○) from the same anatomical level in two different patients (*A* and *B*). Segment number refers to circumferential position around the short-axis slice (32-segment model). The top panels show the raw data, and the bottom panels show the same data after Fourier analysis, used to fit a curve to each data set. Note that there is relative agreement with respect to magnitude and regional flow between these two different models. (From Ludman, P.F., Coast, A.J.S., Burger, P., et al.: Validation of measurement of regional myocardial perfusion in humans by ultrafast x-ray computed tomography. Am. J. Card. Imaging 7:267–279, 1993, with permission.)

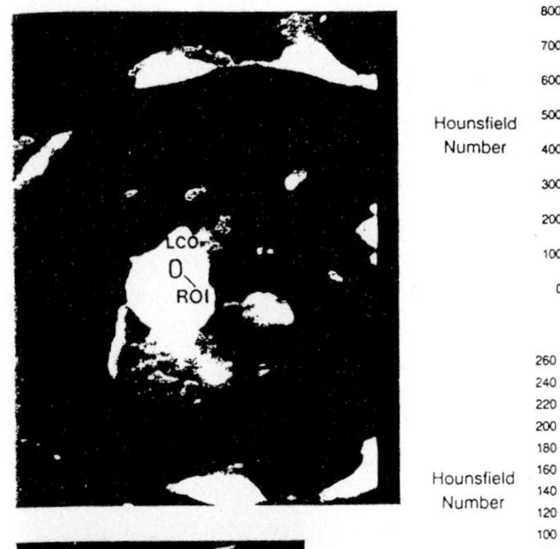

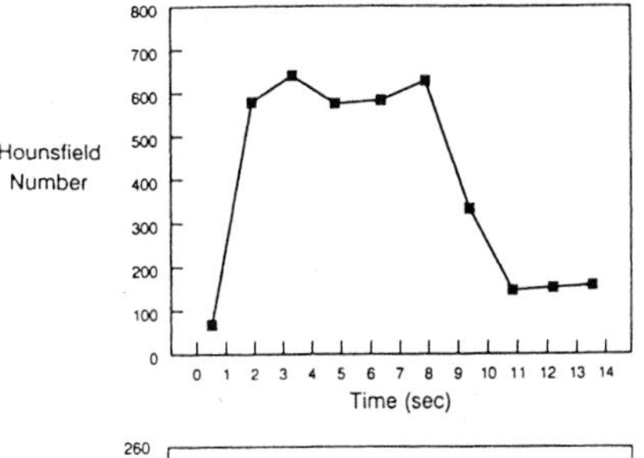

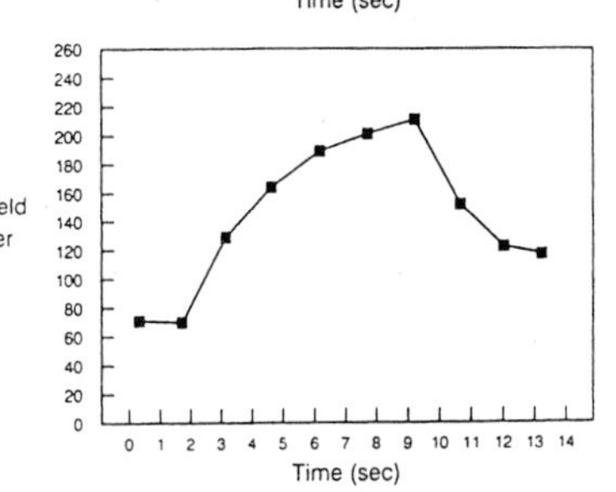

FIGURE 55–12. Computed tomographic density (Hounsfield number) versus time data from EBCT in the left sinus of Valsalva (*top*) and the anterior myocardial wall (*bottom*) after aortic root injection of iodinated contrast. LCO = left coronary artery; LV = left ventricle; RV = right ventricle. (From Weiss, R.M., Otoadese, E.A., Noel, M.P., et al.: Quantitation of absolute regional myocardial perfusion using cine computed tomography. J. Am. Coll. Cardiol. 23:1186–1193, 1994. Reprinted with permission from the American College of Cardiology.)

used the principles of classic indicator-dilution theory, as discussed previously, and also included (as was done by Bell and colleagues[60]) a flow algorithm accounting for changes in regional myocardial blood volume during vasodilation. For this study, they placed a region of interest in the image of the left coronary ostia and sampled the contrast-clearance curve there as the coronary input function. Interestingly, they used a variation of equation 14 for their analysis and thus obtained information from the entire regional myocardial contrast-clearance curve to determine its area. Theoretical underestimations of myocardial blood flow due to significant extravasation of contrast material during the first pass, as predicted by Canty and co-workers,[48] did not appear to limit their quantitative estimates, which would indirectly suggest that contrast extravasation may not play a major role in limiting applications of high-speed CT, at least with systemic injection of contrast media.

Weiss and colleagues[63] have recently published a study in eight dogs, using a "square-wave" injection method into the ascending aorta (7.5 mL per second, for 8 seconds). During this time they used EBCT to define the coronary input function characteristics (left coronary cusp) and the subsequent time course of opacification in the anterior, septal, lateral, and inferior myocardial walls. This method differs from the classic indicator-dilution methods used by other investigators. Here, the inverse of the initial portions of the myocardial time versus CT density curve (roughly over 4 to 6 cardiac cycles) were fit to a model that assumed that the myocardial flow curve behaved initially as a monoexponential. Absolute flow per unit volume of myocardium is then given as the calculated slope of this curve (termed the "turnover rate" by Weiss) multiplied by an estimation of myocardial blood volume fraction within that region of myocardium. A typical aortic input and myocardial response curve from this study are given on Figure 55–12. Correlations were made to estimations of regional myocardial perfusion by EBCT with simultaneously injected radiolabeled microspheres during infusion of dipyridamole (vasodilation) as well as instances during regional ischemia produced by a coronary occluder. Regional perfusion rates from 26 mL/min/100 g to 613 mL/min/100 g were evaluated, where the slope of the regression line and coefficient of correlation in 32 paired comparisons between EBCT and microspheres were both nearly in unity (Fig. 55–13). Additionally, in situations of unrestricted flow, there were no differences in blood flow distribution, as determined by EBCT, between the four myocardial regions. These data, and the data of Wang and associates,[62] noted above, confirm that EBCT, in principle, can estimate myocardial perfusion in vivo over the complete dynamic range of possible blood flow rates and also point out some of the limitations of intravenous contrast injection, as compared with intra-arterial contrast injection.

Weiss and co-workers[64] have extended these applications to investigations of myocardial perfusion and flow reserve in patients as well as suggested that with the use of their approach, transmural myocardial perfusion estimations are possible by means of EBCT.[65]

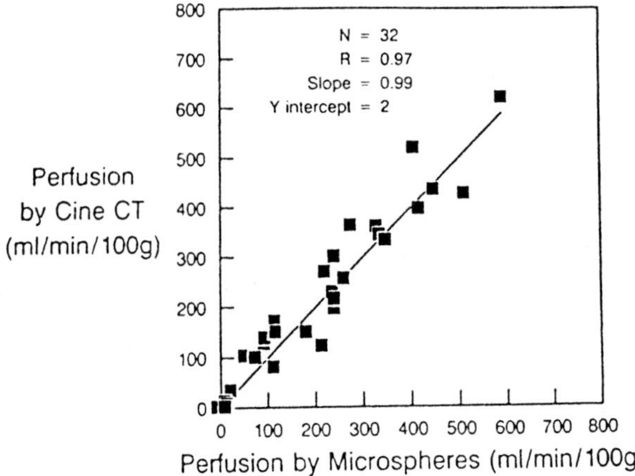

FIGURE 55–13. Scatterplot of paired data from quantifying myocardial perfusion from electron-beam CT (*Cine CT, ordinate*) versus radiolabeled microspheres (*abscissa*). (From Weiss, R.M., Otoadese, E.A., Noel, M.P., et al.: Quantitation of absolute regional myocardial perfusion using cine computed tomography. J. Am. Coll. Cardiol. 23:1186–1193, 1994. Reprinted with permission from the American College of Cardiology.)

Questions Raised From Studies Using Intravenous Contrast Administration, as Compared to Systemic Contrast Administration

It is evident from the work done in tissue-equivalent phantoms that the theoretical constructs of classic indicator-dilution theory and application of EBCT to quantitation of cardiovascular flow phenomena validate this approach and suggest that extension to assessment of physiologic flow phenomena in vivo should be possible. However, in some aspects, the applicability in animals and in humans has fallen short of these goals, thus resulting in modifications of these applications by some investigators, as it relates to scanning procedures and analysis of the data.

Prior studies done by Wolfkiel and associates,[66] Garrett and colleagues,[67] and Rumberger[68] have demonstrated that absolute cardiac output can be quantitated with EBCT after intravenous contrast injection by direct application of classic indicator-dilution theory. Similarly, the studies shown above indicate that EBCT can be used to evaluate regional myocardial perfusion, but there remain shortcomings with respect to scatter of the data about any given regression line, regional variability of blood flow even in normal subjects, and potential limitations of the theory or contrast administration methods, or both, during coronary vasodilation. In particular, the calculated values of regional myocardial flow per unit mass in the resting or baseline state totally agree with data available from other sources in normal patients[5, 10, 69]; however, the calculated maximum flow reserve ratio was found to be on the order of 2.5 to 3.3:1. This flow reserve calculation in normal subjects falls significantly short of the expected value of 5:1 to 7:1 from direct Doppler coronary artery flow measurements reported by Wilson and associates.[2, 59]

The causes of these errors, as well as of other errors noted in the animal studies, are multifactorial but can be divided into three categories:

1. Imaging or reconstruction artifacts
2. Failure to account for changes in intramyocardial vascular volume during vasodilation
3. Failure to characterize or completely understand the limitations related to the input function to the myocardium when contrast material is administered intravenously

These problems and limitations are more fully discussed in the following sections.

IMAGING AND RECONSTRUCTION ARTIFACTS

Scanner- and Patient-Related Artifacts

Significant image artifacts may result from the computed tomographic system or from the patient. Artifacts from the system may arise secondary to instability, imbalance, and misalignment of the detector–x-ray system. However, developments in scanner tuning and digital evaluation of the systems on a regular basis make basic alignment and hardware problems minimal and predictable; thus, these potential sources of artifacts are not expected to contribute significantly to imaging artifacts when EBCT is used.

EBCT acquires data through an arc of 210 degrees, whereas conventional scanners acquire source-detector data through a complete 360-degree arc. Although only 180 degrees of scan information are necessary (because of symmetry) for the reconstruction of a tomogram with the use of filtered-back projection methods, the uniformity of noise and thus the precision of Hounsfield density values tend to improve with increasing scan angles, which is partly because of a more uniform radiation scatter distribution by the patient's body and smoothing of this scatter across the entire series of x-ray detectors. As a consequence of the scanning architecture, the patient radiation dose, radiation scatter, and stochastic (random, statistical) noise distributions of EBCT scans are radially asymmetric. Although these phenomena have not been examined in detail, such limitations of scanning arc, which are necessary to allow for the rapid speed of scanning, may also introduce scan reconstruction artifacts that then alter the contrast-clearance curves and thus confound calculations of absolute and relative myocardial perfusion. Quantitative computed tomographic densities from scanning with EBCT depend on the location of the object being scanned within the scanning circle. These types of problems can be compounded when dynamic scanning is involved, especially when one is attempting to follow a bolus of contrast medium through various cardiac chambers. In effect, the object being imaged, high-density iodinated contrast medium, is moving in spatial location from image to image.

Patient-related artifacts arise from motion during scanning and include peristaltic, muscular, respiratory, and cardiac movements. Of these potential sources of artifacts, respiratory and cardiac motions during scanning are among the most important for high-speed computed tomographic images. Multilevel EBCT scanning in patients for analysis of regional myocardial perfusion, using intravenous techniques, can be accomplished in about 20 seconds. Patients are asked to suspend respiration during scanning at approximately one half of tidal volume.[43] Except in unusual circumstances, most patients can maintain a breath-hold for this period of time without difficulty; thus, artifacts caused by respiratory motion may be kept to a minimum during EBCT scanning.

Cardiac motion is complex and represents three-dimensional conformational changes that occur with each cardiac cycle. There is no agreement as to which portion of the cardiac cycle is best for scans intended to evaluate mean (time-averaged) regional myocardial perfusion; however, consistency in maintaining a stable position for the region of interest during data analysis is of paramount concern. Electron-beam computed tomography images are acquired within a time frame of 50 to100 msec; that is, 1/10 to 1/20 of a second. Dynamic spatial reconstructor studies are acquired in only 1/60 of a second. During this short acquisition time, very little cardiac motion occurs except during the most rapid phases of ejection and early diastolic filling. Imaging confined to either end-diastole or end-systole should avoid confounding problems related to cardiac motion during scanning. The authors prefer to scan at end-diastole to ensure a more reliable time index (peak of the R wave on the electrocardiogram) and anatomical location for the region of interest. However, a variable region of interest can be used for each image to allow for changes in anatomical position of the region of interest between scans acquired during end-systole, as has been used by Wolfkiel and co-workers.[44]

Volume-Averaging Artifacts

A computed tomographic image is a composite or grid (matrix) of picture elements or "pixels" displayed on a video monitor. During "reconstruction" of the x-ray data, each pixel is assigned an x-ray attenuation (or density) value compared, by convention, to the attenuation coefficient of water; generally, this represents 2000 "gray levels" or densities (10-"bit" data), with scaling as follows: bone = 1000; water = 0; and air = −1000. Although one evaluates the image as a two-dimensional data set, in reality the tomogram has a finite thickness. Thus, the computed tomographic densities are actually representative densities within a volume element or "voxel." Averaging of true Hounsfield densities across the voxel may produce a "partial volume" artifact.

A "partial volume" artifact can pose a problem with EBCT by falsely altering the actual computed tomographic tissue density; however, by careful examination of the region chosen for data analysis (both within the myocardium and within the left ventricular cavity-aorta), by viewing of the voxel above and below the tomographic region of interest, and by avoidance of analysis near the border of the cavity or lung with the myocardium, one can in practice substantially reduce or virtually eliminate this problem.

Beam Hardening and Photon Scatter

Subtle artifacts may result from alterations of the x-ray beam not dependent on the configuration of the scanning device. The CT density (or Hounsfield unit) for a given material (regardless of the partial volume effect) may be highly variable, depending on what structures are surrounding that material. For instance, it had originally been advocated that one could determine the benign nature of a given pulmonary nodule if its Hounsfield number was above a certain value[70] (presumably then indicating the presence of calcium); however, it subsequently has been shown that the "density" of pulmonary nodules is highly variable between patients. This variability is an "artifact" of the variable beam energy as it traverses patients of different physiognomy, because the beam energy spectrum is polychromatic, rather than, ideally, monochromatic.

As this polychromatic x-ray beam traverses the body, the lower energies attenuate preferentially, so the "effective" beam energy increases (or the beam "hardens"). These "spectral" or "beam-hardening" changes then artificially reduce the Hounsfield density of the object on which the beam is incident.[71] All manufacturers of CT devices are aware of these problems, and specific reconstruction algorithms have been designed to account for this problem[72]; however, the subsequent effect on the final images has not been totally eliminated.

Photon scatter is also a problem. Ideally, the detector should receive only x-ray information directly in-line with the incident beam through the object; however, scatter of photons through a patient alters its path, and the detector may receive x-ray information from nonparallel sources. For computed tomographic imaging and for random geometry of the object being scanned, the effect of photon scatter is reduction of the "density" of a given object, analogous to that seen with beam hardening. To significantly reduce this problem, manufacturers of computed tomographic devices install collimators external to the detectors to substantially reduce x-ray information from scattered photons not directly parallel with the incident beam-detector pair.

Artifacts caused by beam hardening or photon scatter, or both, as contrast material travels from the right side to the left side of the circulation are apparent on some EBCT images and may specifically affect calculations of absolute regional myocardial perfusion during intravenous contrast administration. Regional blood flow within the normal myocardium (and thus indicator-clearance data) should be relatively uniform in character[73]; however, regional variation in the contrast-clearance curve in the myocardium can be seen with EBCT in the absence of regional differences in true myocardial perfusion.[21] The most striking artifactual alterations in the contrast-clearance curves are manifested as a distinct "dip" in the data prior to maximal opacification of the myocardium during the first pass.

It may be theoretically anticipated[74] that artificial (artifactual) reduction of the myocardial computed tomographic densities would occur in proportion to the changing computed tomographic density within the adjacent left ventricular cavity during the first passage of the contrast bolus. This "shadow phenomenon" (which may result from beam hardening, photon scatter, and/or a variety of undefined reconstruction artifacts, including those related to scanning angle, as discussed above) results in the artificial reduction of peak tissue contrast density and an artificial prolongation of the true contrast transit time. For example, Figure 55–14 shows contrast-clearance curves from the anterior myocardium in a dog simultaneous with the contrast-clearance curve within the left ventricular cavity after bolus intravenous injection of indicator. Note that the "dip" in computed tomographic density within the myocardium is simultaneous with the initial rise of computed tomographic density within the adjacent left ventricular cavity. As more contrast material enters the myocardium from the aortic input, a more positive (above baseline) density deflection is observed.

Figure 55–15 demonstrates one method of accounting for the imaging artifacts noted above and thus a means of minimizing (but, not necessarily, eliminating) their effects on quantification of

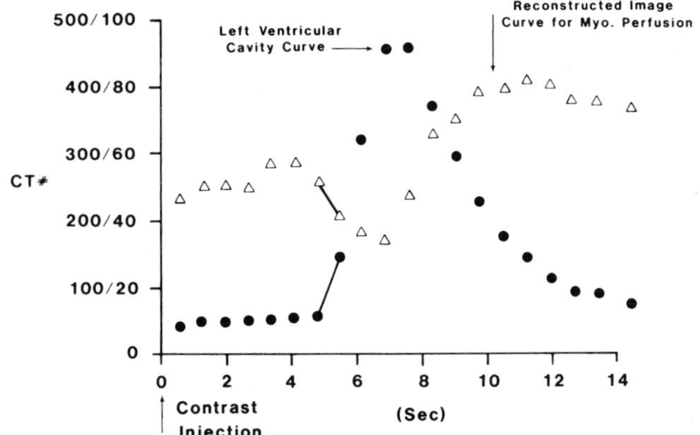

FIGURE 55–14. Simultaneous left ventricular cavity and anterior myocardial time-density curves from a dog after intravenous bolus contrast administration (1 mL/kg). Note the significant "dip" in the myocardial contrast-density data, coincident with the appearance of the iodinated contrast into the adjacent left ventricular cavity ("shadow phenomenon"; see text for details). As the contrast enters the myocardium; the positive deflection in the myocardial contrast density is subsequently observed. (From Rumberger, J.A., Stanford, W., and Marcus, M.L.: Quantitation of regional myocardial perfusion by ultrafast-CT: Promises and pitfalls. Am. J. Card. Imaging 1[4]:336–343, 1987, with permission.)

perfusion by EBCT with the use of intravenous contrast injection. If one considers a situation in which there is no regional distribution of indicator (contrast material) within a myocardial region, then the computed tomographic time-density curve from that myocardial region will reflect only the artifactual "shadow phenomenon" resulting from time-varying changes in densities in the adjacent left ventricular cavity after rapid intravenous contrast administration. During the first pass, this theoretical "no-perfusion" curve would demonstrate a time-dependent decrease and subsequent return to baseline of densities in unison with time-dependent increases and decreases in densities in the adjacent left ventricular cavity. Thus, the "reconstructed" time-density curve in any perfused region of the myocardium is a combination of the "no-perfusion" (artifact) curve and the "true" perfusion curve. As a

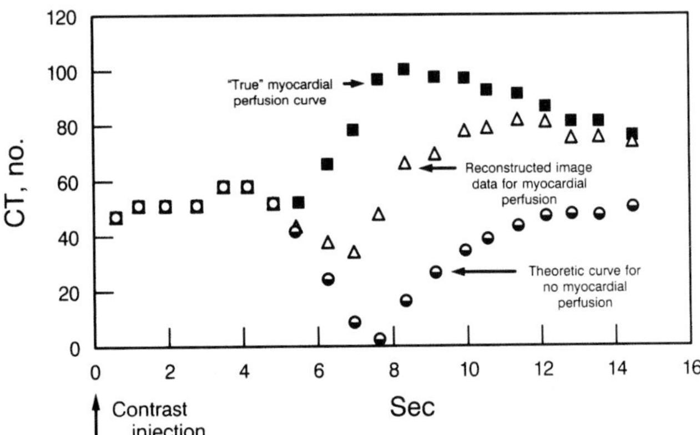

FIGURE 55–15. Construct of a possible method (first-order approximation) of eliminating the "dip" in the myocardial contrast curve noted in the myocardium as a result of increasing contrast density within the adjacent left ventricular cavity after intravenous injection of iodinated contrast. Here, the "true" myocardial perfusion curve is the sum of the reconstructed (raw) contrast-clearance curve and the "no-perfusion" curve (which characterizes the extent of the artifact over time). Imaging artifacts (see text for details) after the shape and character of the contrast-clearance data within the myocardium. (From Rumberger, J.A., Bell, M.L., Feiring, A.J., et al.: Quantitation of myocardial perfusion using fast computed tomography. *In* Marcus, M.L., Skorton, D.J., Schelbert, H., et al. (eds.): Cardiac Imaging. Philadelphia, W.B. Saunders, 1991, pp. 688–702, with permission.)

first-order approximation to extraction of the true perfusion curve from the reconstructed perfusion curve, estimation of the magnitude of the artifact in any given region can be derived from noting the amplitude of the initial decreases in reconstructed regional myocardial densities recorded before contrast material actually reaches the myocardium in proportion to the simultaneous initial increases in left ventricular cavity contrast densities (see Fig. 55–14). Assuming that the magnitude of the regional myocardial "shadow" is a linear proportion of the computed tomographic time-dependent densities in the ventricular cavity, the theoretical "no-perfusion" curve can be generated. A convolution of the reconstructed computed tomographic time-density curve with the "no-perfusion" curve yields the final (true) curve, as shown on Figure 55–15. This true curve resembles that noted in the posterior myocardium of Figure 55–6, which did not demonstrate obvious imaging artifacts. Using the areas under this true myocardial contrast-clearance curve and the ventricular input curve in equation 14 yielded an estimation of regional flow by EBCT in this canine study of 173 mL/min/100 g; the actual flow per unit mass from the regional microsphere data was 190 mL/min/100 g, representing a subsequent underestimation of less than 10 percent. Using the data from the original reconstructed time-density curve would have yielded a measure of myocardial perfusion on the order of 120 mL/min/100 g, an underestimation of nearly 40 percent.

The theoretical constructs above imply that a reduction in the computed tomographic density within the left ventricular cavity after intravenous injection of contrast reduces the myocardial "shadow" artifacts. A reduction of the amount of indicator administered intravenously (i.e., total iodine load) reduces the concentration in the left ventricular cavity and the subsequent imaging artifact seen within the adjacent myocardium. This assumption has been preliminarily validated in vivo in the authors' laboratory and is probably the reason that Wolfkiel and colleagues[44] failed to note the above "shadow" artifacts (the dose of contrast given was 0.33 mL/kg versus 1.0 mL/kg, as reported in reference 21). A final way of reducing shadow artifacts in the myocardium is to inject contrast material into the aortic root. This approach avoids several problems by eliminating overlapping simultaneous opacifications of the left ventricular cavity and myocardium, which occur during intravenous contrast injections.

REGIONAL INTRAMYOCARDIAL VASCULAR VOLUME

Derivations of the classic indicator-dilution theory, as discussed previously, and as applied in the early in vivo studies,[21, 43, 44, 56] assumed that the "distribution" volume for the contrast, V, within the myocardium was defined as the ratio of muscle density, ρ, to muscle mass, m (i.e., V = m/ρ). Thus, one could use this simple relationship to compare flow per unit mass determined by CT to flow per unit mass determined by radiolabeled microspheres. However, EBCT actually measures flow per unit myocardial volume in vivo, whereas microspheres measure flow per unit mass as estimated in exsanguinated tissue ex vivo. One must then account for the additional volume of the blood-filled vasculature, b, as separate from the volume of the muscle mass present in vivo, before making such direct comparisons. In effect, the myocardial volume of blood flow distribution in vivo (V) to be used in equations 14 and 16 is not simply {m/ρ} but is more properly {m/ρ + b}.

The physiologic determinants of regional myocardial perfusion are multifactorial; classic theory, as noted previously, defines flow as directly proportional to vascular blood volume and inversely proportional to mean transit time (equation 4). However, regional vascular volume is not a static parameter but changes in response to physiologic demand for increased regional flow.

In a review of coronary pressure-flow relationships, Spaan[75] quoted a value of 1.6 mL/100 g of myocardium for the entire volume of the coronary arterial tree at baseline (normal, resting) flow (vessels larger than 200 μm, at a perfusion pressure of 100 mm Hg). Studies from the laboratory of Schaper and associates,[76] using postmortem barium angiography, noted an average vascular volume of the left ventricular free wall of 3.6 mL/100 g under control conditions, which is roughly twice the value quoted by Spaan.

No direct measurements of myocardial or venous vascular volumes exist. However, Weiss and Winbury[77] examined the volume of blood in the small (<100 μm) vessels. Here, they found the small vessel vascular volume to be approximately 7 mL/100 g at rest; this increased to 14 mL/100 g during asphyxia. Unfortunately, although they assumed that maximum coronary vasodilation was achieved during asphyxia, no direct comparison was made between regional small-vessel vascular volume and absolute regional flow.

Total intramyocardial vascular volume has been examined by several investigators. Eliasen and associates[78] calculated total red cell and plasma volume within regions of canine left ventricle, using radioactive tracers at basal levels of regional myocardial flow (70 to 95 mL/min/100 g). Corresponding values for vascular volume ranged from 3.6 to 4.9 mL/100 g of myocardium. Both Ziegler and Goretsky[79] and Morgenstern and co-workers[80] evaluated total regional myocardial volume as it related to regional values for myocardial flow per unit mass. Both groups indicated a linear relationship between vascular volume and perfusion. Ziegler and Goretsky noted a value of 8 mL/100 g at baseline and an increase to 12 mL/100 g at 220 mL/min/100 g. Morgenstern and co-workers noted a value of 11 mL/100 g at rest, which increased to 14 mL/100 g at a regional value for perfusion of 130 mL/min/100 g. If one were to extrapolate their data to a maximum myocardial flow of 400 mL/min/100 g (normal flow reserve of at least 4:1), then estimates of regional intramyocardial vascular volume at maximum vasodilation would range from 20 to 29 mL/100 g. Although the shape of the vascular volume versus regional flow relationship is more likely curvelinear, as will subsequently be suggested, it is apparent that regional vascular volume is not necessarily inconsequential, especially at high values for regional myocardial flow.

If one substitutes V = m/ρ + b into equation 16, then:

$$F_f/m_f = (1/\rho + b/m) * C_{PH}/A_{LV} \tag{17}$$

The question remaining is how to calculate b/m.

In their initial studies evaluating regional myocardial perfusion with the DSR at the Mayo Clinic, Wang and associates[62] and Wu and co-workers[81] noted the need to account for changes in regional intramyocardial vascular volume and added a nonlinear factor to equation 16 by theoretically assuming that {b/m} was proportional to the ratio of the areas under the regional myocardial and aortic input contrast-clearance curves. However, an estimation of {b/m} can be made directly from the indicator "concentration" data derived from the myocardial CT data, in comparison to the indicator "concentration" derived from a purely vascular segment, such as the aorta or left ventricular cavity.

The computed tomographic "densities" of myocardium and blood are nearly identical, as are their specific gravities. Therefore, iodinated contrast material must be used to separate structures of similar densities. For example, consider two regions within a given computed tomographic image where the densities were noted before and after administration of contrast, one that is totally vascular (e.g., the aorta or ventricular cavity) and another that is exactly one-half nonvascular and one-half vascular. The ratio of the mean concentration (or Hounsfield density) in the mixed region above baseline to that within the purely vascular region, again above baseline, should be 0.5; that is, exactly, one-half vascular and one-half avascular. The estimation of intramyocardial (or "tissue") vascular blood volume is shown schematically in Figure 55–16. In the limit that the mixed region becomes totally vascular, the ratio approaches 1.0 (the left ventricular cavity or aorta, as shown in Fig. 55–16). In the limit that the mixed region becomes less and less vascular, the ratio becomes diminishingly smaller. The ratio of the densities (above baseline) within the mixed tissue-blood

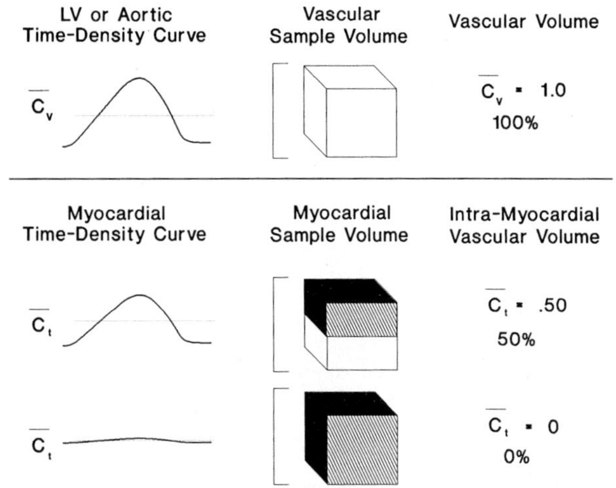

FIGURE 55–16. Schematic of calculation of intramyocardial vascular volume from time-density (or contrast-clearance) curves, using EBCT. $\overline{C}_v$ = mean "concentration" of contrast material as it passes through the left ventricular (LV) cavity or aorta (purely vascular segment) during the first pass; $\overline{C}_t$ = mean "concentration" of contrast medium passing through the myocardial region of interest during the first pass. The purely "vascular" sample volume is 100 percent blood volume. The myocardial sample volumes, however, contain variable mixtures of myocardial muscle (*shaded*) and blood-filled vasculature. In the limit of 100 percent muscle volume and no vascular volume, the myocardial time-density curve is flat. See text for details.

myocardial region, compared to that of a purely vascular region, then defines the ratio of tissue vascular volume per unit total volume (i.e., b/V). This may be more easily understood as a "partial volume parameter," which notes the dilution of the purely vascular region by nonopacified tissue within the region of interest.

The above paradigm is analogous to determining the activity of combined red blood cell and plasma markers (total vascular volume) within the myocardium, compared to the activity within the aorta, as defined by Eliasen[78] to calculate the microvascular blood content in the canine myocardium. This same principle has also been used by Iida and associates[69] to define the partitioning of $H_2{}^{15}O$ within the myocardial vasculature, as applied to quantitation of regional myocardial perfusion by positron emission tomography.

The parameter, b/V, may be defined as the ratio of mean computed tomographic density (above baseline) in the myocardium ($\overline{C}_t$) to the mean computed tomographic density (above baseline) in the ventricular cavity ($\overline{C}_{LV}$) determined by EBCT after intravascular contrast administration (one could also use the density in the aorta, rather than that in the ventricular cavity, particularly in the case of systemic contrast injection). If one assumes negligible extravasation of contrast material during the first pass, homogeneous mixing of indicator with the blood, and no perturbation of the vascular volume by the contrast medium (assumptions 1 to 4), then:

$$b/V = \overline{C}_t/\overline{C}_{LV} \tag{18}$$

however,

$$V = m/\rho + b \tag{19}$$

Therefore,

$$\frac{b}{m} = \frac{1}{\rho}\left[\frac{(\overline{C}_t/\overline{C}_{LV})}{(1 - (\overline{C}_t/\overline{C}_{LV})}\right] \tag{20}$$

The original data from reference 21 were reanalyzed, taking into account the potential for significant changes in regional intramyocardial vascular volume during pharmacologic vasodilation. In this model the calculation of {b/V} was made directly from the contrast-clearance data in the left ventricular cavity and posterior myocardium by determining the mean (time-averaged) density above baseline, noted during the passage of the contrast material through each region.

Figure 55–17 shows the intramyocardial vascular volume, {b/V}, versus regional flow per unit mass (defined, as before, directly from the regional microsphere data). Values of regional intramyocardial vascular volume at baseline (normal regional flow of 100 mL/min/100 g) are on the order of 0.05 (i.e., 4.9 mL/100 g myocardium, using a density of 1.05 g/mL). These results are in general agreement with data reported by others; however, note that as regional perfusion increases, regional intramyocardial vascular volume increases rapidly but asymptotically approaches a maximum toward the end of the physiologic range. These data for changes in intramyocardial vascular volume during vasodilation, obtained with EBCT, are quantitatively in agreement with data obtained with the DSR and systemic contrast injection, as reported by Wu and associates.[81]

The maximum value for regional intramyocardial vascular volume estimated by EBCT may be on the order of 0.20 (24 mL/100 g), as noted in Figure 55–17, and this value is not inconsequential. Figure 55–18 shows a correlation of regional myocardial perfusion, estimated by EBCT versus radiolabeled microspheres, that uses the same computed tomographic data derived and presented in Figure 55–7, but the flow algorithm employed was equation 17, which incorporated an estimation of intramyocardial vascular blood volume for each individual flow rate. Note that although EBCT still underestimates flow per unit mass at the higher values for regional perfusion, the slope of the regression line across the range of flows examined now approaches unity. A failure to account for changes in regional intramyocardial vascular volume during vasodilation results in artifactual underestimation of regional myocardial perfusion by CT. This principle is not confined to EBCT but applies to other methods that use vascular indicators (digital subtraction angiography, two-dimensional echocardiography, positron emission tomography, magnetic resonance imaging, and myocardial scintigraphy).

KINETICS OF THE INPUT FUNCTION TO THE MYOCARDIUM

Assumption 6 (see the section on theoretical considerations above), which related the application of classic indicator-dilution

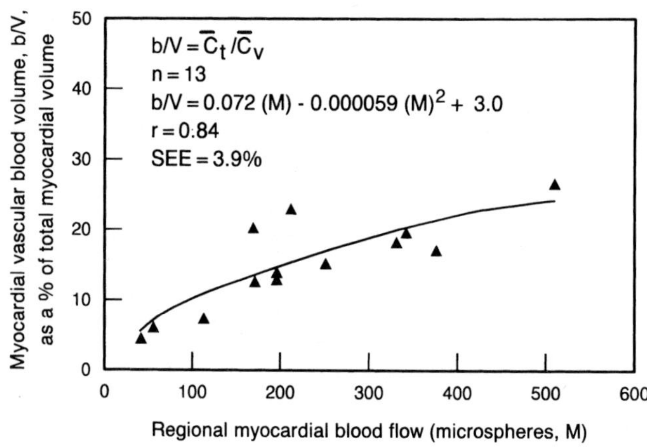

FIGURE 55–17. Myocardial vascular blood volume (b/V) as a percentage of total myocardial volume within a region of the myocardium. See text for details. Abbreviations defined same as in Figure 55–16. (From Rumberger, J.A., Bell, M.L., Feiring, A.J., et al.: Quantitation of myocardial perfusion using fast computed tomography. *In* Marcus M.L., Skorton, D.J., Schelbert, H., et al. (eds.): Cardiac Imaging. Philadelphia, W.B. Saunders, 1991, pp. 688–702, with permission.)

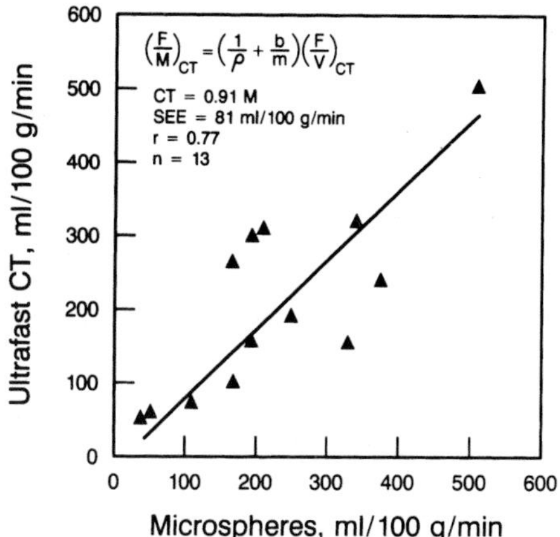

FIGURE 55–18. Regional myocardial perfusion (flow per unit mass [F/M_{CT}]) versus radiolabeled microspheres, as calculated by EBCT, using the modified algorithm noted in equation 17. The data constitute a reanalysis of the data shown in Figure 55–8. Here, the algorithm incorporates the concept of changes in regional intramyocardial vascular volume during vasodilation. See text for details. (From Rumberger, J.A., Bell, M.L., Feiring, A.J., et al.: Quantitation of myocardial perfusion using fast computed tomography. *In* Marcus, M.L., Skorton, D.J., Schelbert, H., et al. (eds.): Cardiac Imaging. Philadelphia, W.B. Saunders, 1991, pp. 688–702, with permission.)

theory to EBCT, required that the mean transit time of the indicator from the input to the coronary ostia be less than the mean transit time for that indicator to traverse the vascular-tissue space within the myocardium. This concept is not new but was initially applied to an external detection system by Mullani and associates[54] for studies using the positron emitter ^{82}Rb. This fact may account, in part, for the underestimations of myocardial flow made by Wolfkiel and co-workers,[44] using EBCT, because the contrast input function to the coronary ostia was severely splayed after contrast injection distally from the femoral vein, rather than centrally, as was done in some animal and patient studies.

Figure 55–19 puts forward a schematic whereby the quantitation of regional myocardial perfusion, given satisfaction of all other assumptions, is limited by the injection site of the contrast or indicator. As contrast material is administered closer to the coronary ostia, the dynamic range of quantitation or regional flow for CT is expanded. The characterization of the transit of the bolus to the input then is a function of the actual initial injection time and the site of injection.

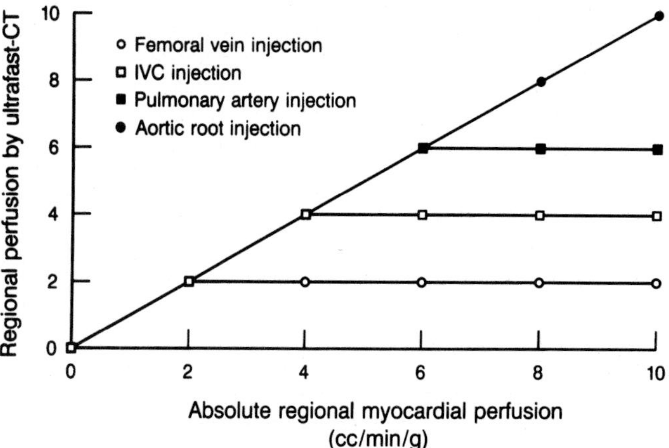

FIGURE 55–19. Theoretical construct relating the absolute value of regional myocardial perfusion versus that determined by means of EBCT for various contrast injection sites. Note that as contrast material is administered closer and closer to the systemic circulation, the plateau reached by the calculations using EBCT extends further into the physiologic range of known myocardial perfusion values. IVC = inferior vena cava. (From Rumberger, J.A., Stanford, W., and Marcus, M.L.: Quantitation of regional myocardial perfusion by ultrafast-CT: Promises and pitfalls. Am. J. Card. Imaging 1[4]:336–343, 1987, with permission.)

As stated earlier, the data set defined by Wolfkiel and co-workers,[44] using a femoral vein injection of contrast material (Fig. 55–8), demonstrated a plateau above 200 mL/min/100 g where the data set defined by Rumberger and co-workers,[21] using an injection into the inferior vena cava (Figs. 55–7 and 55–18), suggested a significant underestimation above 300 to 350 mL/min/100 g. Using an aortic root injection of contrast material, Wang and associates[62] and Weiss and colleagues[63] suggested that regional myocardial perfusion can be quantitated by high-speed computed tomographic techniques (after accounting for dynamic changes in intramyocardial vascular volume during vasodilation) at flow rates of up to 600 mL/min/100 g. Thus, it appears that EBCT may be used to quantitate resting and ischemic myocardial flows and myocardial flow reserve of up to about 3:1 to 4:1, using an intravenous injection of contrast; however, examination of the full dynamic range of possible values for perfusion appears to require an aortic root injection of iodinated contrast medium.

RECOMMENDED METHODS FOR ASSESSING MYOCARDIAL PERFUSION IN PATIENTS WITH ELECTRON-BEAM COMPUTED TOMOGRAPHY

Intravenous Contrast Administration

The methods of performing studies of regional myocardial perfusion with EBCT using intravenous injection of iodinated-contrast media are straightforward. Central venous access is probably the most appropriate so that the contrast media may be administered rapidly, as a bolus, with attempts to satisfy assumption 6 (see section on theoretical considerations) as closely as possible. In the authors' laboratory for studies in patients, they insert a small 5-Fr., multiple side-hole catheter directly through an intravenous cannula placed in a cephalic vein in the antecubital fossa. This catheter can then be placed directly into the superior vena cava or the superior portion of the right atrium with or without fluoroscopic guidance.

In patients, an assessment of circulation time is done to assist with timing of the contrast bolus.[82] After a noncontrast localization scan is taken, the subject is positioned in the scanner gantry to facilitate acquisition of multilevel images through the midsection of the left ventricular cavity and myocardium. For measurements of myocardial perfusion, 20 mL of nonionic contrast medium can be administered through the central venous catheter at a rate of 10 mL per second. Multilevel electrocardiogram-triggered imaging is performed on consecutive heartbeats, commencing after contrast injection at a time roughly one half the measured circulation time, which ensures registration of contrast material entering and leaving the systemic circulation (i.e., the first pass) during the time of the scan series (generally requiring 10 to 20 seconds for completion). Throughout this brief time period, the subject is instructed to suspend spontaneous respiration.

For assessment of maximal myocardial perfusion and myocardial flow reserve, a second scan series is performed with the same protocol during intravenous administration of either dipyridamole (0.56 mg/kg per minute)[43] or adenosine (140 μg/kg per minute).[60, 61] A second intravenous site (usually in the contralateral antecubital fossa) is required for administration of these drugs. Both of these drugs have been previously shown to provide for maximum coronary vasodilation and to be useful in assessing myocardial perfusion.

After completion of the imaging protocols, accomplished generally in less than 30 minutes, the intravenous lines are removed, and the subject is allowed to leave the scanner area.

Off-line analysis of contrast-clearance data can be performed rapidly by displaying the data from selected regions of interest on the display console and applying a gamma variate curve fit to obtain the data required for the flow algorithms, as previously discussed in detail.

Intra-arterial (Systemic) Contrast Administration

It would appear that both the methods of Wang and co-workers[62] and Weiss and associates[63] may be used for analysis of perfusion data obtained with EBCT using intra-arterial contrast injection. However, neither has published in detail the proposed methods in patients. The most likely method would be to insert a small 5- or 6-Fr. pigtail catheter by means of the Seldinger method into the central aorta retrogradely from the left brachial artery or either femoral artery. The method of Wang and co-workers would involve administration of approximately 10 to 20 mL of dilute, nonionic contrast material into the central aorta as a bolus (over a period of approximately 2 to 3 seconds). Contrast injection into the central aorta by the method of Weiss and associates would involve about 60 mL of dilute (2:1) nonionic contrast in less than 10 seconds during simultaneous scanning with EBCT on every to every-other cardiac cycle. Caution must be taken, however, because central injection of even these small amounts of nonionic contrast medium can result in transient and significant perturbations in hemodynamics, potentially violating assumption 3. Weiss and associates, in their report in canine studies, specifically addressed this issue and stated that the hemodynamic alterations do not appear for 10 seconds or longer after contrast injection; by that time, the imaging data for calculation of the "transfer function" (or ingress of contrast material into the regional myocardium) have been recorded, and thus subsequent transient changes in central aortic hemodynamics may not alter the practical application of this method.

REGIONAL TRANSFER FUNCTION

High-speed computed tomographic scanning may also be useful in providing data related to the fractional distribution of myocardial flow in various physiologic, pathologic, or pharmacologically altered flow states. Segmental, spatial, and temporal nonuniformity of regional perfusion has been described in the normal mammalian heart.[83] Nonuniformity of flow may be important if one is attempting to accurately quantitate the transport of nondiffusible substrates or metabolites through the myocardium or to assess the efficacy of therapeutic interventions aimed at normalizing flow distribution.

If one assumes a steady-state flow situation during the first pass of contrast, the studies presented will have demonstrated the potential for high-speed CT to determine segmental differences in myocardial perfusion. However, the fractional distribution of the regional blood flow among microvessels of differing path lengths is not apparent from the analysis of the regional contrast-clearance data because the "response" curve in the myocardium depends on the input bolus kinetics of the indicator (e.g., intravenous versus aortic root injection), the intravascular dispersion due to velocity gradients between microvessels, and the spatial uniformity (or nonuniformity) of the microvasculature.

If one assumes a hypothetical instantaneous (impulse) input function, the response (output function) would reflect the inherent impulse response of the regional vasculature and describe any spatial nonuniformity within the system. The relationship between input and output is referred to as the "transfer function"[84] and is derived by deconvolving the recorded input and response functions (contrast-clearance or time-density data) to yield an idealized response for that system, based on an idealized step input.

Such a deconvolution model has been described in the canine heart by Knopp and co-workers,[85] who attempted to define a transcoronary transfer function by analysis of indocyanine green dye injected into the left atrium and sampled in the coronary sinus. Using the DSR, Bell and colleagues[86] employed the same deconvolution method and were able to evaluate the regional transfer function of the myocardium at rest and after maximum vasodilation. Eigler and associates[87] measured myocardial transfer function in dogs, using direct coronary contrast injections and digital angiography. They found the transfer function to be independent of bolus kinetics and superior to conventional contrast-clearance analysis for determination of coronary flow and flow reserve.

Transfer function or deconvolution analysis that uses high-speed CT may be helpful in the characterization of the microvasculature in a variety of conditions known to alter small vessels (e.g., left ventricular hypertrophy[88] and aortic stenosis[89]) and may allow for further insight into the functional significance of coronary collateral vessels.

SUMMARY AND CONCLUSIONS

Clinical quantitation of regional myocardial perfusion with the use of a minimally invasive and easily applied technique could allow for ready quantitation of the physiologic significance of coronary disease, allow for further understanding of flow reserve in various cardiomyopathic and overload (pressure versus volume) conditions, and possibly provide firm concepts regarding the development and clinical significance of coronary collateral vessels.

This chapter has demonstrated the development of the concept of classic indicator techniques for use by an external detection system such as EBCT. Initial and preliminary studies in vitro and in vivo have been presented, and the potential limitations of the techniques as applied to humans have been discussed. These potential limitations are not insurmountable. Significant attenuation of imaging artifacts can be accomplished via a reduction in total amount of contrast material administered for intravenous injection techniques or implementation of appropriate computed tomographic hardware and software modifications developed to address this issue. An approach to accounting for changes in regional intramyocardial vascular volume has been demonstrated, and a more general theoretical approach that incorporates this concept was presented.

A limitation remains regarding input function kinetics if the entire dynamic range of possible regional myocardial perfusion is to be studied. However, the use of a less invasive central venous injection for contrast injection, as compared to the more invasive aortic root injection, may depend on the question posed in a given subject. The data presented from the original animal study using an inferior vena cava injection,[21] and the preliminary work by Bell and associates[60] in normal subjects, suggested that absolute regional myocardial perfusion (after accounting for changes in regional vascular volume) can be quantitated up to about 40 mL/min/100 g. If normal resting flow is approximately 100 mL/min/100 g, then this would imply that studies could be done with intravenous injection methods for characterization of regional myocardial perfusion up to 4:1. Flow reserve above this value would be underestimated by EBCT. Studies by Wilson and co-workers,[2, 59] using a unique intracoronary Doppler catheter, have shown that "normal" flow reserve (in the absence of hypertrophy) is 3.7:1 or greater and that patients with physiologically significant coronary artery disease have reserve, usually, of less than 3:1. The EBCT method in patients with coronary artery disease may then be adequate to separate significant lesions from insignificant coronary ones. In a practical sense, therefore, an aortic root contrast injection may be necessary only for research purposes, when more precision as to the total range of flow reserve in a subject is required. Even then a 5-Fr. catheter-sheath system (as is currently used for coronary angiography) may be all that is required, and the study can be completed on an outpatient basis.

Electron-beam computed tomography offers a unique avenue for quantitating regional myocardial perfusion in both the clinical and the research setting.

References

1. Marcus, M., Wright, C., Doty, D., et al.: Measurements of coronary velocity and reactive hyperemia in the coronary circulation of humans. Circ. Res. 49:877, 1981.
2. Wilson, R.F., Laughlin, D.E., and Ackell, P.H.: Transluminal subselective measurement of coronary artery blood flow velocity and vasodilator reserve in man. Circulation 72:82, 1985.
3. Marston, E.L., Barefoot, C.A., and Spencer, M.P.: Non-cannulating measurements of coronary blood flow. Surg. Forum 10:636, 1959.
4. Mills, C.J.: Measurement of pulsatile flow and flow velocity. *In* Bergel, D.H. (ed.): Cardiovascular Fluid Dynamics. Vol. 1. London, Academic Press, 1970, pp. 71–77.
5. Ganz, W., Tamura, K., Marcus, H.S., et al.: Measurement of coronary sinus blood flow using continuous thermodilution in man. Circulation 44:181, 1971.
6. Rigo, P., Baley, I.K., Griffith, L.S.C., et al.: Value and limitations of segmental analysis of stress thallium myocardial imaging for localization of coronary artery disease. Circulation 61:973, 1980.
7. Ritchie, J.L.: Myocardial perfusion imaging. Am. J. Cardiol. 49:1341, 1982.
8. Feinstein, S.B.: Myocardial perfusion imaging: Contrast echocardiography today and tomorrow. J. Am. Coll. Cardiol. 8:251, 1986.
9. Mor-Avi, V., David, D., Akselrod, S., et al.: Myocardial regional blood flow: Quantitative measurement by computer analysis of contrast enhanced echocardiographic images. Ultrasound Med. Biol. 19:619, 1993.
10. Canon, P.J.: Measurement of coronary blood flow in evaluation of regional myocardial perfusion by intracoronary injection techniques. *In* Donath, A., and Righetti, A. (eds.): Cardiovascular Nuclear Medicine. Vol. 6. New York, Karger, 1980, pp. 85–95.
11. Klocke, F.J., Bunnell, I.L., Green, E.D.G., et al.: Average coronary blood flow per unit weight of the left ventricle in patients with and without coronary artery disease. Circulation 50:547, 1974.
12. Vogel, R., LeFree, M., and Bates, E.: Application of digital techniques to selective coronary arteriography: Use of myocardial contrast clearance time to measure coronary flow reserve. Am. Heart J. 107:153, 1984.
13. Legrand, V., Mancini, G.B.J., Le Free, M.T., et al.: Clinical value of digital radiographic coronary quantification: Comparison with visual assessment and coronary flow reserve. Eur. Heart J. 13:95, 1992.
14. Shah, A., Shelbert, H., and Schwaiger, M.: Measurement of regional myocardial blood flow with N-13 ammonia and positron emission tomography in intact dogs. J. Am. Coll. Cardiol. 5:92, 1985.
15. Weisenberg, G., Shelbert, H.R., and Hoffman, E.J.: In-vivo quantitation of regional myocardial blood flow by positron emission computed tomography. Circulation 63:1248, 1981.
16. Rechavia, E., Araujo, L.I., De Silva, R., et al.: Dipyridamole vasodilator response after human orthotopic heart transplantation: Quantification by oxygen-15-labeled water and positron emission tomography. J. Am. Coll. Cardiol. 19:100, 1992.
17. Tong, C.Y., Prato, F.S., Wisenberg, G., et al.: Measurement of the extraction efficiency and distribution volume for Gd-DTPA in normal and diseased canine myocardium. Magn. Reson. Med. 30:337, 1993.
18. Wilke, N., Simm, C., Zhang, J., et al.: Contrast-enhanced first pass myocardial perfusion imaging: Correlation between myocardial blood flow in dogs at rest and during hyperemia. Magn. Reson. Med. 29:485, 1993.
19. Boyd, D.B.: Computerized transmission tomography of the heart using scanning electron beams. *In* Higgins, C.H. (ed.): Computed Tomography of the Heart and Great Vessels. Mt. Kisco, NY, Futura, 1983, pp. 45–52.
20. Siegelman, S.S.: Editor's page. Radiology 186:36, 1993.
21. Rumberger, J.A., Feiring, A.J., Lipton, M.J., et al.: Use of ultrafast computed tomography to quantitate regional myocardial perfusion: A preliminary report. J. Am. Coll. Cardiol. 9:59, 1987.
22. Ritman, E.L., Kinsey, J.H., Robb, R.A., et al.: Physics and technical considerations in the design of the DSR: A high-temporal resolution volume scanner. Am. J. Radiol. 134:369, 1980.
23. Dow, P.: Estimations of cardiac output in central blood volume by dye dilution. Physiol. Overview 36:77, 1956.
24. Stewart, G.N.: Researches on the circulation time and the influences which affect it. I. Preliminary paper. II. The time of the lesser circulation. III. The circulation time in the thyroid gland and the effect of secretion and stimulation of nerves upon it. J. Physiol. (Lond.): 1:2, 1893.
25. Stewart, G.N.: Researches on the circulation time and on the influences which affect it. IV. The output of the heart. J. Physiol. 22:159, 1897.
26. Stewart, G.N.: Researches on the circulation time and on the influences which affect it. Circulation time of the spleen, kidney, intestine, heart (coronary circulation), and retina, with observations on time of lesser circulation. Am. J. Physiol. 58:278, 1921.
27. Henriques, V.: Uber die Verteilung des, Blutes vom, linken, Herzenzwischen dem Herzen und dem ubrigen Organismus. Biochem. Zeitschr. 56:230, 1913.
28. Koch, E.: Die Stromgeschwindigkeit des Blutes: Ein Beitrag zur Arbeitsprufung des Kreislaufes. Arch. Klin. Med. 140:39, 1922.
29. Blumgart, H.L., and Yens, O.C.: Studies on the velocity of blood flow. I. The method utilized. J. Clin. Invest. 4:1, 1927.
29. Hamilton, W.F., Moore, J.W., Kinsman, J.M., et al.: Studies on the circulation. IV. Further analysis of the injection method and of changes in hemodynamics under physiological and pathological conditions. Am. J. Physiol. 99:534, 1932.
30. Moore, J.W., Kinsman, J.M., Hamilton, W.F., et al.: Studies on the circulation. II. Cardiac output determinations: Comparison of the injection method with the direct Fick procedure. Am. J. Physiol. 89:331, 1929.
31. Meier, P., and Zierler, K.L.: On theory of indicator-dilution method for measurement of blood flow and volume. J. Appl. Physiol. 6:731, 1954.
32. Zierler, K.R.: A simplified explanation of the theory of indicator-dilution for measurement of fluid flow and volume and other distributive phenomena. Bull. Johns Hopkins Hosp. 103:199, 1958.
33. Prinzmetal, M., Corday, E., Bergman, H.C., et al.: Radiocardiography: A new method for studying blood flow through the chambers of the heart in human beings. Science 108:340, 1948.
34. Prinzmetal, M., Corday, E., Spritzler, R.J., et al.: Radiocardiography and its clinical applications. JAMA 139:617, 1949.
35. Knutson, J.R.B., Taylor, B.E., Ellis, E.J., et al.: Studies on circulation time with the aid of the oximeter. Mayo Clin. Proc. 25:405, 1950.
36. Wood, E.H., and Geraci, J.E.: Photoelectric determination of arterial oxygen saturation in man. J. Lab. Clin. Med. 34:387, 1949.
37. Henley, W.S., Creech, O., Couves, C.M., et al.: Determination of myocardial blood flow utilizing iodinated (^{131}I) human serum albumin. Surg. Forum 8:237, 1957.
38. Love, W.D., and Burch. G.E.: A study in dogs of methods suitable for estimating the rate of myocardial uptake of ^{86}Rb in man and the effect of L-norepinephrine and pitressin on ^{86}Rb uptake. J. Clin. Invest. 36:468, 1957.
39. Nolting D., Mack, R., Luthy, E., et al.: Measurement of coronary blood flow and myocardial rubidium uptake with Rb-86. J. Clin. Invest. 37:921, 1958.
40. Hounsfield, G.N.: Picture quality of computed tomography. AJR 127:3, 1976.
41. Newman, E.V., Merrell, M., Genecin, A., et al.: The dye dilution method for describing the central circulation: An analysis of factors shaping the time-concentration curves. Circulation 4:735, 1951.
42. Gould, R.G., Lipton, M.J., McNamara, M.T., et al.: Measurement of regional myocardial blood flow in dogs by ultrafast-CT. Invest. Radiol. 23:348, 1988.
43. Rumberger, J.A., Stanford W., and Marcus, M.L.: Quantitation of regional myocardial perfusion by ultrafast-CT: Promises and pitfalls. Am. J. Cardiac Imaging 1(4):336, 1987.
44. Wolfkiel, C.J., Ferguson, J.L., Chomka, E.V., et al.: Measurement of myocardial blood flow by ultrafast computed tomography. Circulation 76:1262, 1987.
45. Reiter, S.J., Rumberger, J.A., Feiring, A.J., et al.: Precision of measurements of right and left ventricular volumes by cine computed tomography. Circulation 74:890, 1986.
46. Newhouse, J.H.: Fluid compartment distribution of intravenous iothalamate in the dog. Invest. Radiol. 12:346, 1977.
47. Newhouse, J.H., and Murphy, R.X.: Tissue distribution of soluble contrast: Effective dose variation and changes with time. AJR 136:436, 1981.
48. Canty, J.M., Judd, R.M., Brody, A.S., et al.: First-pass entry of nonionic contrast agent into the myocardial extravascular space. Effects on radiographic estimates of transit time and blood volume. Circulation 84:2071, 1991.
49. Wolfkiel, C.J., and Brundage, B.H.: Measurement of myocardial blood flow by UFCT: Towards clinical applicability. Int. J. Cardiac Imaging 7:89, 1991.
50. Thompson, H.K., Starmer, C.F., Waylon, R.F., et al.: Indicator transit time considered as a gamma variate. Cir. Res. 14:502, 1964.
51. Burbank, F.H., Brody, W.R., and Bradley, B.R.: Effective volume and rate of contrast medium injection on intravenous digital subtraction angiographic contrast median curves. J. Am. Coll. Cardiol. 4:308, 1984.
52. Sapirstein, L.A.: Regional blood flow by fractional distribution of indicators. Am. J. Physiol. 193:161, 1958.
53. Axel, L.: Cerebral blood flow determination by rapid-sequence computed tomography: Theoretical analysis. Radiology 137:679, 1980.
54. Mullani, N., Goldstein, R.A., Gould, K.L., et al.: Myocardial perfusion with rubidium-82. I. Measurements of extraction fraction and flow with external detectors. J. Nucl. Med. 24:898, 1983.
55. Tonge, R.A., Wright, C.H., Mathew, J., et al.: Flow rate determination using computed tomography. Br. J. Radiol. 53:946, 1980.
56. Guthaner, D.F., Nassi, M., and Bradley, B.: Validation of a CT method for flow determination. Radiology 151:429, 1984.
57. Jaschke, W., Gould, R.G., Assimakopoulos, P.A., et al.: Flow measurements with a high-speed computed tomography scanner. Med. Phys. 14(2):238, 1987.
58. Ludman, P.F., Darby, M., Tomlinson H., et al.: Cardiac flow measurement by ultrafast CT: Validation of continuous and pulsatile flow. J. Comput. Assist. Tomogr. 16:795, 1992.
59. Wilson, R.F., Laughlin, D.E., Hartley, C.G., et al.: Selective measurements of coronary blood flow velocity and vasodilator reserve in man. J. Am. Coll. Cardiol. 3:529, 1984.
60. Bell, M.R., Rumberger, J.A., Stanson A.W., et al.: Rapid and minimally invasive measurement of myocardial flow reserve in man with ultrafast CT. Circulation 84:II-678, 1991.
61. Ludman, P.F., Coast, A.J.S., Burger, P., et al.: Validation of measurement of regional myocardial perfusion in humans by ultrafast x-ray computed tomography. Am. J. Cardiac Imaging 7:267, 1993.
62. Wang, T., Wu, X., Chung, N., et al.: Myocardial blood flow quantitated by synchronous, multi-slice, high-speed computer tomography. IEEE Trans. Med. Imaging 8:70, 1989.
63. Weiss, R.M., Otoadese, E.A., Noel, M.P., et al.: Quantitation of absolute regional myocardial perfusion using cine computed tomography. J. Am. Coll. Cardiol. 23:1186, 1994.
64. Weiss, R.M., Grover-McKay, M., Quillen, J.E., et al.: Why does coronary flow reserve vary so widely among patients without evidence of cardiac disease? J. Am. Coll. Cardiol. 19:322A, 1992.
65. Weiss, R.M., Grover-McKay, M., Rossen, J.D., et al.: Direct quantitation of the subendocardial-to-subepicardial perfusion ratio in man. Circulation 86:I-164, 1992.
66. Wolfkiel, C.J., Ferguson, J.L., Chomka, E.V., et al.: Determination of cardiac output by ultrafast computed tomography. Am. J. Cardiac Imaging 1:117, 1986.
67. Garrett, J.S., Lanzer, P., Janchke W., et al.: Measurement of cardiac output by cine computed tomography. Am. J. Cardiol. 56:657, 1985.
68. Rumberger, J.A., Stanford, W., and Marcus, M.L.: Quantitation of regional myo-

cardial perfusion by ultrafast computed tomography: Promises and pitfalls. Am. J. Card. Imaging 1:336, 1987.
69. Iida, H., Kanno, I., Takahashi, A., et al.: Measurement of absolute myocardial blood flow with H_2O^{15} and dynamic positron-emission tomography: Strategy for quantification in relation to the partial-volume effect. Circulation 78:104, 1988.
70. Siegelman, S.S., Zerhouni, E.A., Leo, F.P., et al.: CT of the solid solitary pulmonary nodule. Am. J. Radiol. 135:1, 1980.
71. Herman, G.T.: Correction for a beam hardening in computed tomography. Phys. Med. Biol. 24:81, 1979.
72. Herman, G.T.: Demonstration of beam hardening correction in computed tomography of the head. J. Comput. Assist. Tomogr. 3:373, 1979.
73. Cobb, F.R., Bache, R.J., and Greenfield, J.C., Jr.: Regional myocardial blood flow in awake dogs. J. Clin. Invest. 53:H1618, 1974.
74. Joseph, B.M.: Artifacts in computed tomography. *In* Newton, P.M., and Potts, D.G. (eds.): Radiology of the Skull and Brain, Technical Aspects of Computed Tomography. St. Louis, C.V. Mosby, 1980, pp. 39–80.
75. Spaan, J.A.E.: Coronary diastolic pressure-flow relation in 0 flow pressure explained on the basis of intramyocardial compliance. Circ. Res. 56:293, 1985.
76. Wusten, B., Buss, D.D., Deist, H., et al.: Dilatory capacity of the coronary circulation and its correlation to the arterial vasculature in the canine left ventricle. Basic Res. Cardiol. 72:636, 1977.
77. Weiss, H.R., and Winbury, M.M.: Nitroglycerin and chromonar on small-vessel blood content of the ventricular wall. Am. J. Physiol. 226:838, 1974.
78. Eliasen, P., Amtorp, O., Tondevold, E., et al.: Regional blood flow, microvascular blood content, and tissue hematocrit in canine myocardium. Cir. Res. 16:593, 1982.
79. Ziegler, W.H., and Goresky, C.A.: Transcapillary exchange in the working left ventricle of the dog. Circ. Res. 24:181, 1971.
80. Morgenstern, C., Holjes, U., Arnold, G., et al.: The influence of coronary pressure and coronary flow on intracoronary blood volume angiometry of the left ventricle. Pflugers Arch. 340:101, 1973.
81. Wu, X., Ewert, D.L., Liu, Y.H., et al.: In vivo relation of intramyocardial blood volume to myocardial perfusion: Evidence supporting microvascular site for autoregulation. Circulation 85:730, 1992.
82. Rumberger, J.A., Behrenbeck, T., Sheedy, P.F., et al.: Ultrafast computed tomography. *In* Giuliani, et al. (eds.): Cardiology: Fundamentals and Practice. 2nd ed. St. Louis, Mosby–Year Book, 1991, pp. 387–397.
83. Yipintsoi, T., Dobbs, W.A., Jr., Scanlon, P.D., et al.: Regional distribution of diffusible tracers and carbonized microspheres in the left ventricle of isolated dog hearts. Circ. Res. 33:573, 1973.
84. Bassingthwaighte, J.B.: Circulatory transport and the convolution integral. Mayo Clin. Proc. 42:137, 1967.
85. Knopp, T.J., Dobbs, W.A., Greenleaf, J.F., et al.: Transcoronary intravascular transport functions obtained via a stable deconvolution technique. Ann. Biomed. Eng. 4:44, 1976.
86. Bell, M.R., Spyra, W.J.T., Thomas, P.J., et al.: A method for characterizing the spatial distribution of regional transcoronary transfer-function using fast-CT. Physiology 31:A64, 1988.
87. Eigler, N., Schuhlen, H., Whiting, J.S., et al.: Digital angiographic impulse response analysis of regional myocardial perfusion: Estimation of coronary flow, flow reserve, and distribution volume by compartmental transit time measurement in a canine model. Circ. Res. 68:870, 1991.
88. Wangler, R.D., Peters, K.G., Marcus, M.L., et al.: Effects of duration and severity of arterial hypertension in cardiac hypertrophy and coronary vasodilator reserve. Circ. Res. 51:10, 1982.
89. Marcus, M.L., Doty, D.B., Hiratzka, L.F., et al.: Decreased coronary reserve—a mechanism for angina pectoris in patients with aortic stenosis and normal coronary arteries. N. Engl. J. Med. 307:1362, 1982.

CHAPTER 56 The Great Vessels: Imaging by Electron-Beam Computed Tomography

William Stanford, M.D.
Brad H. Thompson, M.D.

Diseases of the great vessels, especially aortic aneurysms and dissections, are associated with significant morbidity and mortality, which make it imperative to have imaging techniques that can quickly and accurately diagnose these pathologic conditions. At present, such techniques include aortography, chest radiography, magnetic resonance (MR) techniques, transthoracic and transesophageal echocardiography, conventional computed tomography (CT), spiral CT, and electron-beam computed tomography (EBCT) (ultrafast CT).

The gold standard has long been angiography, but this method is invasive and associated with potential morbidity and high radiation exposure. Although aortography has proved itself capable of demonstrating aneurysms and dissections and identifying pulmonary emboli, it is not without drawbacks.[1] Aortography can show the longitudinal lumen of the vessel only—not the cross-sectional anatomy, and it does not have the ability to visualize the surrounding tissues. Thrombosed lumina may be missed. Yet, because aortography is preferred by many vascular surgeons, it continues to be popular at many hospitals.

Chest radiographs are relatively insensitive. They can show mediastinal widening, vessel tortuousity, pleural effusions and, at times, abnormal calcifications. Generally, the chest film is not reliable in making a definitive diagnosis. In cases of pulmonary embolism, however, the chest film may show the characteristic Hampton hump.

Magnetic resonance techniques have assumed a preeminent role at many institutions in demonstrating aortic and pulmonary disease. Features such as multiplanar imaging, freedom from ionizing radiation, and dynamic imaging are attractive. Recent technologic advances such as MR angiography and phase contrast studies have further enhanced the versatility of MR in vascular imaging. However, standard sequences such as conventional spin-echo imaging tend to be time-consuming. Potential drawbacks include the requirement for cardiac gating, poorer resolution, cost, and increased susceptibility to artifacts. Claustrophobia and the inability to image patients with pacemakers or those on respirators are additional problems unique to MR techniques.

Echocardiography, and especially transesophageal echocardiography, are useful in assessing the aorta and proximal pulmonary arteries; however, echocardiography also has limitations and relies heavily on satisfactory acoustic windows and operator skill.

All things considered, CT may be the ideal imaging method for interrogating the aorta and pulmonary arteries. Conventional CT can produce high-quality axial images of both vessels and surrounding structures with reliability and only moderate expense. Furthermore, when a diagnosis of vessel injury or thrombus is questionable, CT may reveal an unexpected pathologic condition that may mimic the suspected disease process. Besides providing anatomical information about the great vessels, CT is capable of assessing the lung parenchyma and showing any complications attendant to dissection or vessel rupture.

With the development of EBCT, or ultrafast CT, tomographic imaging of the aorta and pulmonary arteries has been further refined. By virtue of millisecond image acquisition times, EBCT images are superior to conventional CT. First, faster scan times help minimize patient and respiratory motion artifact, which can be especially problematic in injured and very ill patients who are unable to suspend respiration. Second, fast image acquisition times enable scans to be completed during contrast bolus optimization, thereby providing superior vascular enhancement. The latter is often not possible with conventional scanners. Furthermore, since EBCT can scan the entire aorta and pulmonary arterial tree in seconds, delays in treatment and diagnosis are minimized. This chapter provides an overview of EBCT imaging of great vessels.

SCANNER CHARACTERISTICS

The C-150 electron-beam scanner, which is the updated version of the C-100, is the model currently in use at our institution, where we have scanned several thousand patients. Both versions incorporate electron-beam technology, whereby moving electrons are bent electromagnetically onto one of four tungsten target rings lying in the gantry below the patient (Fig. 56–1).[2] The x-rays generated from the bombardment of the target ring are tightly collimated and pass through the patient onto a double ring of sodium iodide detectors lying in the gantry above the patient. Electron bombardment of the target ring can occur in as little as 50 msec and can produce two contiguous images 8 mm thick. There is a 4-mm gap between images from adjacent target rings and an 8-msec delay to reset the electron beam. The newer C-150 scanner has two imaging options: step volumetric scanning (SVS) and continuous volumetric scanning (CVS), both of which are applicable in great vessel imaging.

Volume Mode

The SVS mode is the most commonly used sequence for the evaluation of the aorta and great vessels. The C-100 scanners have only SVS capabilities. In this sequence, volumetric data are acquired by firing electrons at one target ring at a rate of 100 msec per sweep. This produces sequential axial sections 6 or 10 mm in thickness and requires 300 or 400 msec (depending on the number of averages) for each slice. A complete 40-slice study of the entire aorta requires approximately 76 seconds. Improved resolution is possible by taking thinner slices (3 mm), but this is rarely required for most aortic studies.

The C-150 scanner has CVS capabilities, permitting considerably faster image acquisition than is possible with SVS. This is primarily a result of improvements in software, table speed, and bulk memory storage. Although the time required for the electron-beam sweep stays the same (100 msec), these improvements allow 40 slices (10 mm thick) to be obtained in 17 seconds. Slice thickness options are also expanded from 6 through 10 mm. If thinner slices are required, the C-150 can be operated in the SVS mode. This mode enables slices as thin as 1.5 mm to be obtained. Both modes

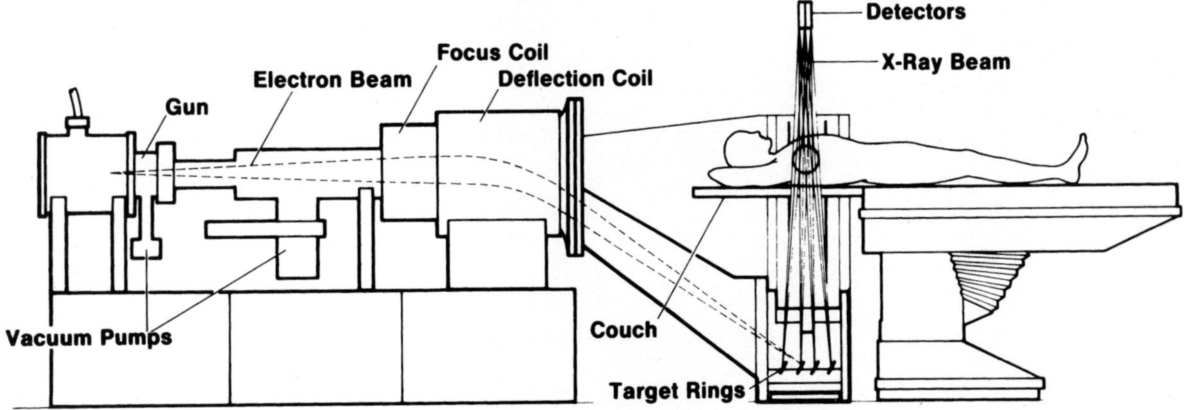

FIGURE 56–1. C-150 electron-beam computed tomography (EBCT) scanner. Electrons emitted from the gun are magnetically deflected onto one of four tungsten target rings. The x-rays generated from the sweep of the target rings pass through the patient and are detected by a double bank of sodium iodide detectors lying in the gantry above the patient. Each sweep of the electron beam requires 50 msec for completion. (Courtesy of Imatron, Inc., San Francisco, CA.)

allow image manipulation such as reformatting and region-of-interest density measurements.

Flow Mode

In the flow-mode sequence, each target ring is sequentially swept once every 50 msec with imaging triggered off the R wave of the electrocardiogram. Four images, 8 mm in thickness, are produced in 224 msec. After a programmed delay, the sequence can be repeated. Since scanner memory is limited to 80 images, an eight-level, 10-image sequence is typically programmed. If additional temporal resolution is desired, 13 or 20 images can be acquired at six or four levels, respectively. When imaging is performed during contrast injection, the images will show progressive vascular enhancement followed by eventual washout as the contrast bolus traverses the great vessels (Fig. 56–2).[3] With this technique, time-density curves can be generated that, in effect, graphically depict the pattern and rate of enhancement of a particular vessel. This is most useful in characterizing differential flow between the true and false lumina of aortic dissection; however, time-density curves can help confirm dissection when the results from the volume study are equivocal (see Fig. 56–2). The flow mode can also be used to evaluate perfusion to organs such as the brain, kidney, or spleen, and it is useful in documenting blood flow across aortovenous fistulas. The flow-mode sequences in both the C-100 and C-150 scanners operate identically.

Movie Mode

Although the movie-mode sequence is not routinely used in great vessel imaging, it has potential applications in the evaluation of aortic dissections and right ventricular function in patients with pulmonary hypertension secondary to pulmonary emboli. In this mode, the scanner is programmed to sweep a single target ring at a rate of 17 times (images) per second (50 msec per sweep). Imaging is performed with electrocardiographic gating and can produce a series of consecutive images throughout the cardiac cycle that can be viewed as a closed-loop movie or as individual frames. In aortic imaging, the movie mode would show the aortic wall movement or dissection flap, or both, in nearly real time.

CONTRAST ADMINISTRATION

Volumetric studies of the great vessels are almost always performed with the use of contrast administration, since the rapid image acquisition times of both the SVS and the CVS modes ensure superior vascular enhancement of each slice throughout the entire study. Because of slower scan times, comparable vascular enhancement may not always be possible with conventional CT.

In imaging the great vessels, the majority of patients undergo a 40-slice volume study during intravenous injection of 76 percent iodine nonionic contrast material. The use of nonionic contrast in great vessel imaging is preferred for two reasons: (1) improved patient tolerance because of fewer constitutional symptoms such as burning and nausea and (2) a higher contrast dose limit, which may be important when additional imaging, such as angiography or a flow study, is needed to confirm the diagnosis. For a volume study, approximately 180 mL of contrast material is administered with a power injector through an 18- or 20-gauge 1 to 1.5-inch antecubital catheter at a rate of 1 to 1.5 mL per second. To ensure optimal vascular enhancement, the timing of the initiation of scan-

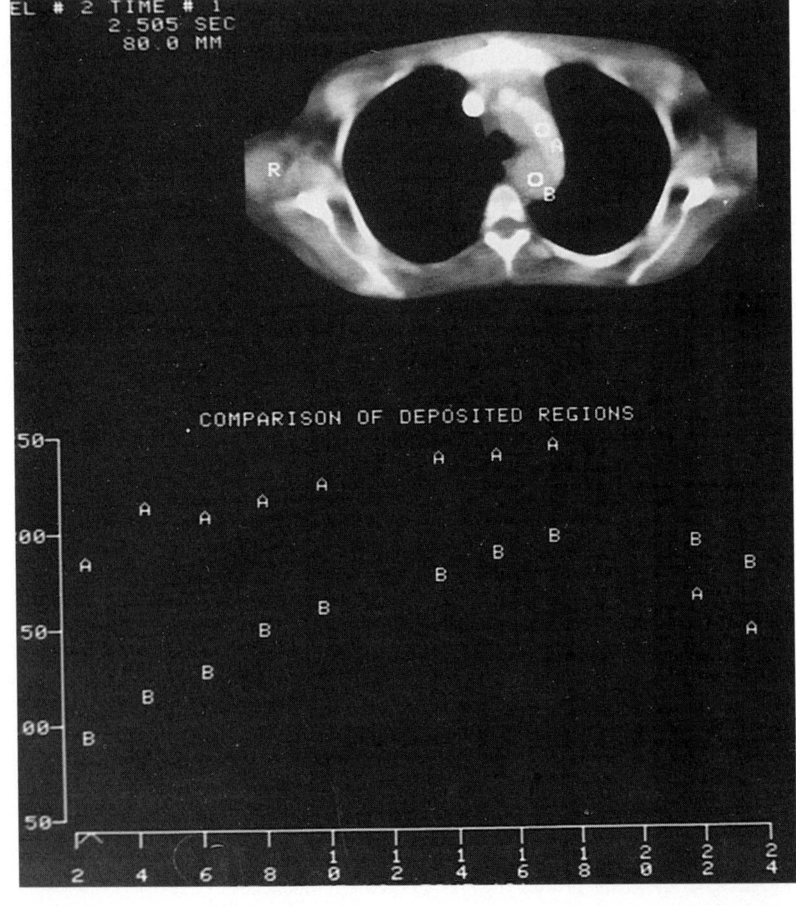

FIGURE 56–2. An EBCT flow study. A representative image of the aortic arch in a patient with type I dissection shows immediate opacification of the true lumen *(A)*, with later enhancement of the larger false lumen *(B)*. The time-density analysis with regions of interest placed over the true and false lumina shows progressive enhancement and washout of contrast media from both lumina. This enhancement of the false lumen indicates patency. (From Stanford, W., Rooholamini, S.A., and Galvin, J.R.: Ultrafast computed tomography in the diagnosis of aortic aneurysms and dissections. J. Thorac. Imaging 5:32, 1990, with permission.)

ning is critical. Because of EBCT's millisecond acquisition times, circulation times are usually measured and scanning is delayed until one half of the total contrast dose is infused.

In a flow study, 40 mL of 76 percent iodine contrast material is usually administered at a rate of 10 mL per second. This speed of injection is needed to achieve a tight contrast bolus. Usually, it is necessary to insert a large (18 gauge or greater) intravenous catheter to accommodate the 10 mL per second flow rate.

The movie sequence usually requires approximately 60 mL of 76 percent iodine contrast material given at 1 to 1.5 mL per second. This rate of injection ensures optimal opacification of the heart and great vessels. Commonly, there is a programmed delay until half of the total contrast dose has been administered.

RADIATION DOSAGE

The radiation dose for the EBCT scanner is markedly less than that for conventional CT. This difference is primarily due to faster image acquisition times. The entrance dose for a volume study that uses a slice thickness of 10 mm and an exposure time of 100 msec is 0.9 cGy per slice. This compares with 2 to 4 cGy per slice for conventional CT. Multislice studies (flow or movie) deliver a dose of 0.58 cGy per image using a scan time of 50 msec; a dose of 1.17 cGy is required when a 100-msec scan time is used (actual measurements from our scanner). This can be compared with the radiation exposure for a thoracic angiogram, which is approximately 8 to 10 cGy for a typical 12-image cut film run.

Because the photon target source is located underneath the patient, the calculated exit doses anteriorly are approximately 17 percent of the entrance dose. This has important implications regarding breast and thyroid exposure. Characteristic EBCT thyroid exposures are 0.06 cGy per slice.

AORTIC ANEURYSMS

Aortic aneurysms without dissection occur in 2 to 4 percent of the adult population, with a commensurate increase in frequency with age.[4] The incidence of thoracic aneurysm rupture has been reported to be as high as 44 percent in patients not treated surgically.[5] Aortic dissection occurs in 5 to 10 cases per million population annually, or approximately 1 per 10,000 hospital admissions,[6] and has a higher rate of rupture (estimated as high as 77 percent). Many of these ruptures (60 percent) occur within days of the diagnosis.[4] This high morbidity and mortality rate make it imperative to have an imaging modality that can quickly and accurately detect aortic pathology.

Anatomy

The normal diameter of the aorta progressively decreases as it travels from the heart to the iliac bifurcation. The normal ascending aortic caliber is approximately 3 cm near the root, tapering to approximately 2.5 cm near the arch. The descending aorta tapers gradually from a diameter of 2 cm at the level of the diaphragm to less than 1.5 cm at the bifurcation.[7] The diagnosis of an aneurysm of the aorta can be made radiographically when the diameter exceeds 3 to 4 cm; however, there will be a commensurate increase in the aortic caliber with age. A diameter of 3 cm for the descending thoracic aorta may be viewed as within normal limits in an 80-year-old patient but as abnormal in a 30-year-old individual. It is also important to remember that for every thoracic aortic aneurysm, there is a 25 percent likelihood of a concomitant abdominal aneurysm.[5] Aneurysms of the thoracic aorta tend to be less common than their abdominal counterparts; however, they typically have a poorer overall prognosis, especially those involving the ascending and transverse portions of the aorta.

Classification

Aneurysms are commonly classified according to location, type, and shape and can involve the ascending, transverse, or descending aorta, or any combination of these locations. Thoracic aortic aneurysms are caused by atherosclerosis, Marfan syndrome–cystic medial necrosis, trauma, poststenotic dilatation, or by infectious-mycotic causes.

Further classification of aneurysms can be based on type (true or false), depending on vessel wall integrity. A true aneurysm is characterized by an intact aortic wall, that is, all layers of the wall enclose the aneurysmal segment. In contrast, when there is disruption of the wall, the aneurysm is classified as false because the blood column is usually contained by the adventitia or surrounding tissues, which results in a thin, fibrous sac. Aneurysms can be further classified according to their shape: fusiform or saccular. Fusiform aneurysms represent a generalized enlargement of the entire aortic circumference and are commonly due to atherosclerosis (Fig. 56–3). False aneurysms, in contrast, are commonly saccular. They appear as focal areas of outpouching and usually arise as a complication of surgery, infection, or atherosclerotic disease. They are most commonly located in the ascending aorta and may present radiographically as an anterior mediastinal mass (Fig. 56–4). Traumatic aneurysms generally have a localized dilatation and are typically located at the level of the ligamentum arteriosum.

Both types of aneurysm can have associated mural thrombus; however, the saccular variety is more often filled with clot, and this may explain its lower frequency of rupture compared with the fusiform variety. Importantly, the thrombus contained within the aneurysm may result in a substantial underestimation of its true size by angiography (Fig. 56–5).

Regardless of their location, aortic aneurysms typically enlarge over time. Although many are detected incidentally, some patients may present only when the aneurysm becomes large enough to produce symptoms attributable to compression of adjacent structures such as the trachea or recurrent laryngeal nerve. Progressive enlargement also places the patient at increased risk for catastrophic rupture. According to the Laplace law, an increase in the radius of a fluid-filled cylinder results in an increase in mural pressure. Therefore, the walls of larger aneurysms experience a

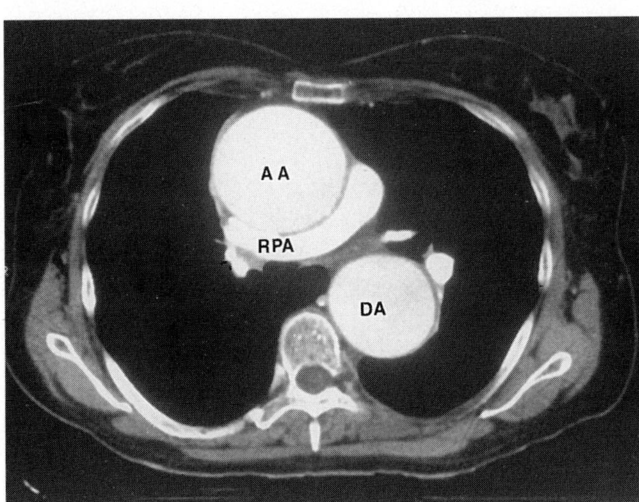

FIGURE 56–3. A fusiform thoracic aortic aneurysm imaged with EBCT. An axial image at the level of the right pulmonary artery (RPA) shows generalized enlargement of the ascending (AA) and descending (DA) portions of the thoracic aorta. Note that the ascending aortic enlargement is compressing the right pulmonary artery. (From Stanford, W., Rooholamini, S.A., and Galvin, J.R.: Ultrafast computed tomography in the diagnosis of aortic aneurysms and dissections. J. Thorac. Imaging 5:32, 1990, with permission.)

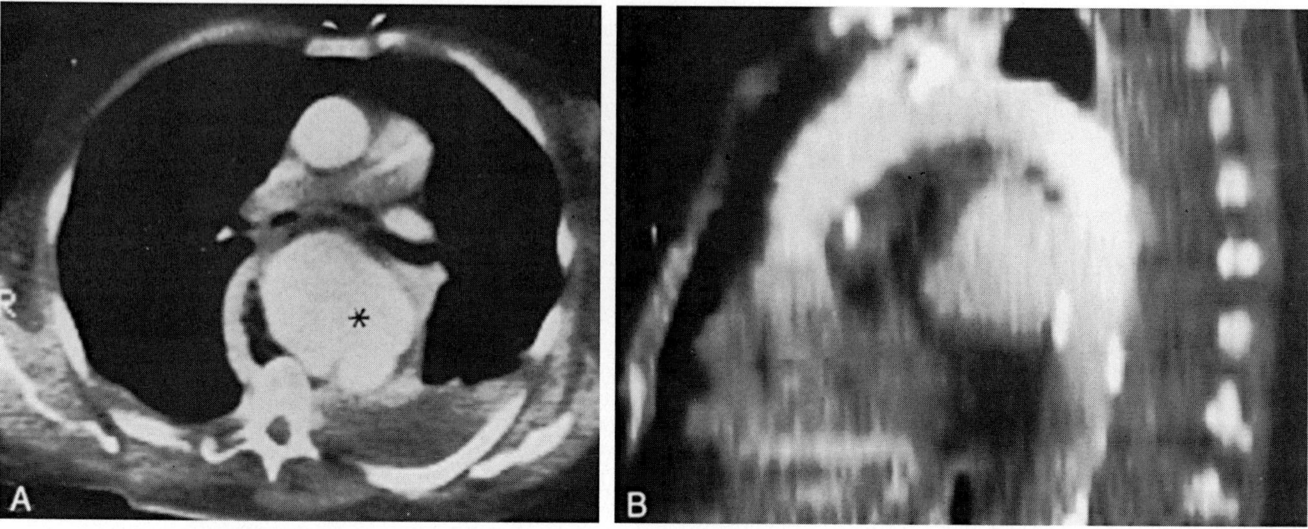

FIGURE 56–4. A saccular aortic aneurysm. *A,* An axial image of a saccular aneurysm of the descending aorta. Note that the contrast material extends beyond the aortic lumen in the area of the aneurysm neck *(asterisk)*. *B,* The reformatted image shows the saccular configuration.

markedly greater pressure, and this translates into a concomitant increased likelihood of rupture.

AORTIC DISSECTION

Classically, patients with aortic dissection complain of acute "ripping" or "tearing" back pain. Others may complain of severe chest pain that mimics myocardial infarction. Regardless of the cause, aortic dissection represents the dissection of blood through the vessel wall from a small tear in the intima. Once initiated, the dissection usually is completed within minutes, commonly involving the aorta distal to the tear, unless its pathway is interrupted by a branch vessel or by pre-existing vascular disease. The jet of blood results in a separation of the tunica media, thus creating two or more parallel channels: the true channel (actual aortic channel) and one or more false channels (Fig. 56–6). The false channel may either become thrombosed or remain patent and demonstrate variable blood flow velocities. The false lumen is often large in diameter and may cause deformity and effacement of the true lumen. False lumina of dissections can terminate by re-entering

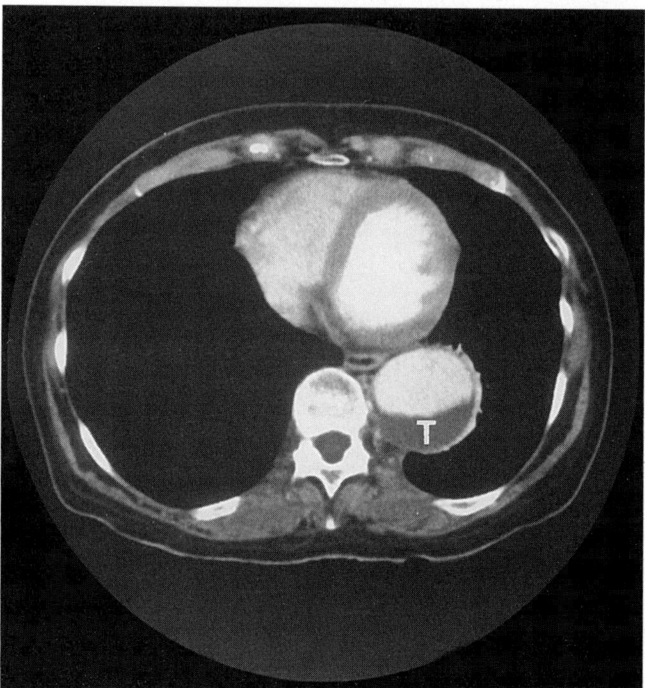

FIGURE 56–5. This is the same patient as in Figure 56–3. The wall of the descending aortic aneurysm is calcified, and there is a large intraluminal thrombus (T) within the aneurysm. The patient was followed clinically. (From Stanford, W., Rooholamini, S.A., and Galvin, J.R.: Ultrafast computed tomography in the diagnosis of aortic aneurysms and dissections. J. Thorac. Imaging 5:32, 1990, with permission.)

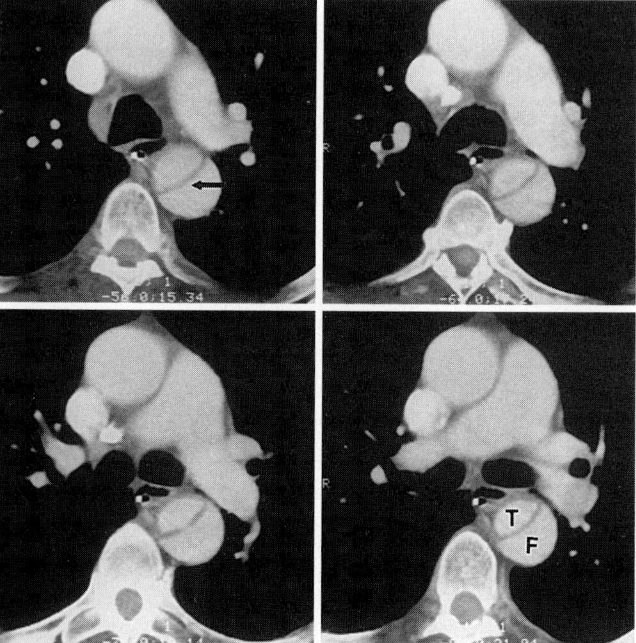

FIGURE 56–6. Aortic dissection involving the descending thoracic aorta and extending into the abdominal aorta in a 65-year-old man who presented with a cold, paralyzed right leg. EBCT images show a type III dissecting aneurysm with an intimal flap *(arrow)* and true (T) and false (F) lumina. This patient underwent surgery solely on the basis of the EBCT findings. (From Stanford, W., Rooholamini, S.A., and Galvin, J.R.: Ultrafast computed tomography in the diagnosis of aortic aneurysms and dissections. J. Thorac. Imaging 5:32, 1990, with permission.)

the true lumen through another intimal tear or end blindly. Lateral termination along a branch vessel is also possible.

Although the cause of nontraumatic dissections appears multifactorial, the true cause is unknown. It is currently accepted that the formation of a dissection relies on a mix of precipitating factors, such as elevated blood pressure and turbulent blood flow superimposed on an underlying intrinsic abnormality in the tunica media. Specifically, dissections have a high association with systemic hypertension (70 to 94 percent) and occur in older individuals (50 years or older). They are three to four times more likely to occur in males than in females.[8–10] Besides hypertension, cystic medial necrosis, aortic coarctation, and bicuspid aortic valve all appear to have a causal relationship with dissection, with the predisposing medial disease process likely related to some form of cystic medial necrosis. The pathogenesis does not appear to be histologically related to or to result from atherosclerosis.

Patients with dissection are often clinically unstable, especially when aortic rupture has occurred. If the dissection involves branch vessels, the patients may present with a wide array of signs such as stroke or syncope. Some are found to have discrepancies in extremity blood pressures or they complain of abdominal pain resulting from visceral infarction. Besides the risks inherent in branch vessel occlusion, rupture makes dissection a potentially catastrophic disease process.

Dissections involving both the ascending and the descending thoracic aorta are classified as DeBakey type I, dissections involving only the ascending aorta are classified as DeBakey type II or Stanford type A, and dissections limited to the descending aorta are classified as DeBakey type III or Stanford type B. The locations are important because type II dissections usually require immediate surgery, whereas type III dissections are often managed medically.

The path of the dissection tends to be predictable. In dissections involving the entire aorta (DeBakey type I), the intimal tear usually occurs just above the sinuses of Valsalva near the sinotubular junction. It typically begins along the right side of the ascending aorta and courses superiorly and posteriorly along the transverse portion of the aorta, at which point extension superiorly into the great vessels can occur (Fig. 56–7). Interruption of blood flow through critically important branch vessels such as the carotid arteries by the dissecting hematoma can result in serious medical consequences. Type I dissections usually arise de novo. It is distinctly uncommon to have retrograde dissection from a distal entry site involve a long proximal segment of the aorta. Type I dissections can terminate anywhere along the ascending, transverse, or distal segments of the thoracic aorta.

Type I and type III dissections both involve the descending aorta. In these instances, the false channel typically runs along the left side of the vessel. Any branch vessel originating from the false lumen is at increased risk for occlusion or eventual thrombosis, or both. Subdiaphragmatic extension, which is common, is associated with an increased risk of occlusion of the celiac, superior mesenteric, or renal arteries. Inferior extension may occlude the iliac arteries and result in claudication. Impaired visceral perfusion or infarction is often well seen with EBCT (Fig. 56–8), and it is important that the integrity of all branch vessels be established.

The radiologic detection of aortic dissection is generally straightforward on CT. The CT signs include (1) inward displacement of intimal calcification by the false lumen (Fig. 56–9), (2) an intimal flap separating the true and false lumina, (see Fig. 56–6), (3) differential contrast opacification between patent true and false lumina (see Fig. 56–2), and (4) presence of clot within a thrombosed false lumen. Typically, the intimal tear signifying the entry or exit site is not visualized on CT, and diagnostic difficulties may arise when thrombosis of the false lumen has occurred. Care must also be taken not to confuse a periaortic atelectatic lung with a dissection (Fig. 56–10). Acutely, dissection does not usually produce aneurysmal dilatation of the aorta. Only with time does the aortic diameter enlarge as the thin adventitial covering of the false lumen enlarges. In a study of EBCT in aortic dissection, Stanford and associates[7] evaluated 50 patients suspected of having aortic aneurysms or dissections. The CT diagnosis was confirmed by angiography or surgery in 95.8 percent of cases.

COMPLICATIONS OF THORACIC ANEURYSMS AND DISSECTIONS

It is primarily the associated life-threatening complications that make vascular lesions of the aorta potentially catastrophic. One potential complication has already been discussed, namely, impaired perfusion of critical organs resulting from branch vessel occlusion (see Fig. 56–8). The most catastrophic complication of an aortic aneurysm or dissection is related to rupture (Fig. 56–11). It has been shown that approximately 90 percent of untreated patients with aortic dissection will eventually die as a result of rupture,[11] and it has been reported that 35 percent of the ruptures occur within 15 minutes after the onset of symptoms.[12]

ELECTRON-BEAM COMPUTED TOMOGRAPHY PROTOCOL FOR IMAGING THE THORACIC AORTA

Patients with a known or suspected aneurysm or dissection of the aorta initially undergo a volume study consisting of contiguous

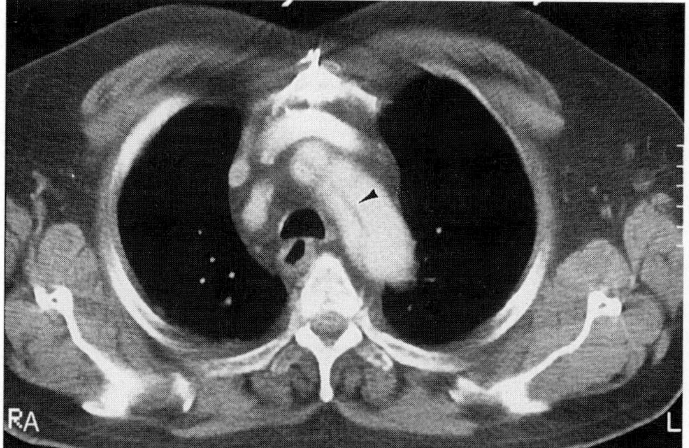

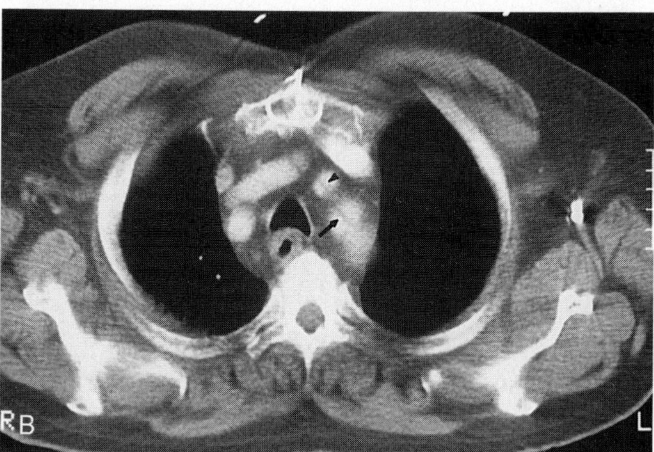

FIGURE 56–7. Aortic dissection with great vessel involvement. *A,* An axial image through the aortic arch shows an intimal flap *(arrowhead),* indicating a type I dissection. *B,* An image more superior to *A* shows extension of the dissection flap into the left subclavian artery *(straight arrow)* and the left carotid artery *(arrowhead).*

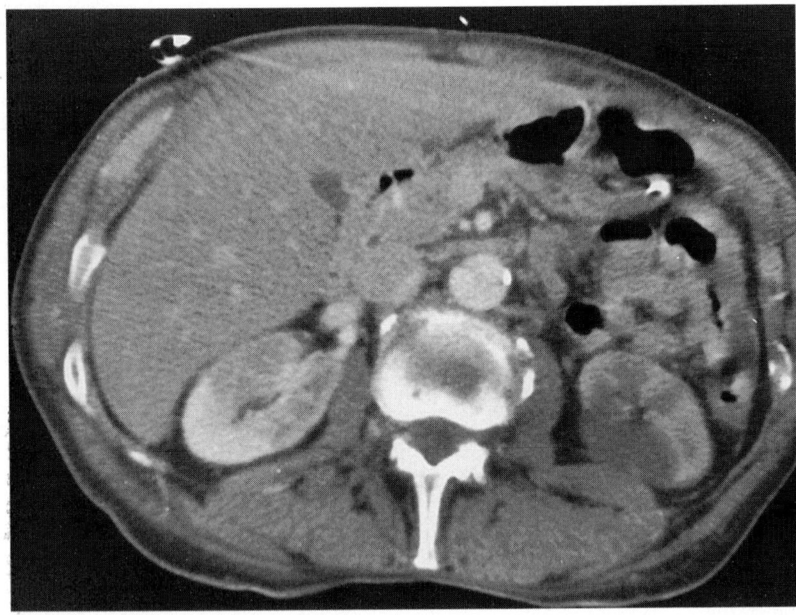

FIGURE 56–8. Acute renal infarction secondary to aortic dissection. An axial image through the kidneys shows diminished enhancement in the ventral half of the right kidney and poor enhancement of the entire left kidney.

axial 6- or 10-mm-thick slices. This can be performed with the use of either the SVS or the CVS modes. As part of our standard protocol, imaging is begun approximately 2 cm cephalad to the top of the aortic arch so that the proximal great vessels are included. If carotid dissection is suspected, imaging can begin at even higher levels to include the thoracic inlet or midneck. When one evaluates the aorta, it is generally advantageous to interrogate the entire length of the vessel, and this is easily and quickly performed with EBCT. Inferiorly, the images usually encompass the aortic bifurcation and routinely extend into the common iliac arteries. In dissection, it is imperative to document the course and extent of the tear as well as to look for branch vessel involvement and associated periaortic complications. Routine imaging with a 30- to 35-cm field of view (FOV) provides sufficient inclusion of periaortic tissues and abdominal viscera for adequate evaluation of these areas. This FOV would show any nonuniform enhancement of an organ, which would suggest impaired perfusion and thus provide indirect evidence of branch vessel involvement. A larger FOV would allow detection of possible nonvascular abnormalities that, on occasion, may explain the patient's symptomatology.

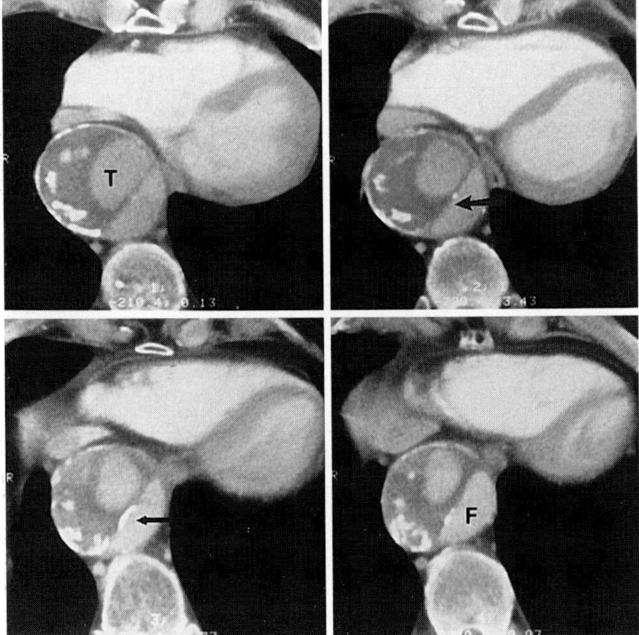

FIGURE 56–9. Type I aortic dissection. An axial computed tomography (CT) image obtained at the level of the carina shows the inward displacement of intimal calcification *(arrow)* characteristic of aortic dissection. Contrast material opacifies both the true (T) and the false (F) lumina. (From Stanford, W., Rooholamini, S.A., and Galvin, J.R.: Ultrafast computed tomography in the diagnosis of aortic aneurysms and dissections. J. Thorac. Imaging 5[4]:32, 1990, with permission.)

ADVANTAGES AND DISADVANTAGES OF ELECTRON-BEAM COMPUTED TOMOGRAPHY IMAGING

Faster imaging time equates to faster patient throughput, thereby limiting delays in patient treatment and management. The

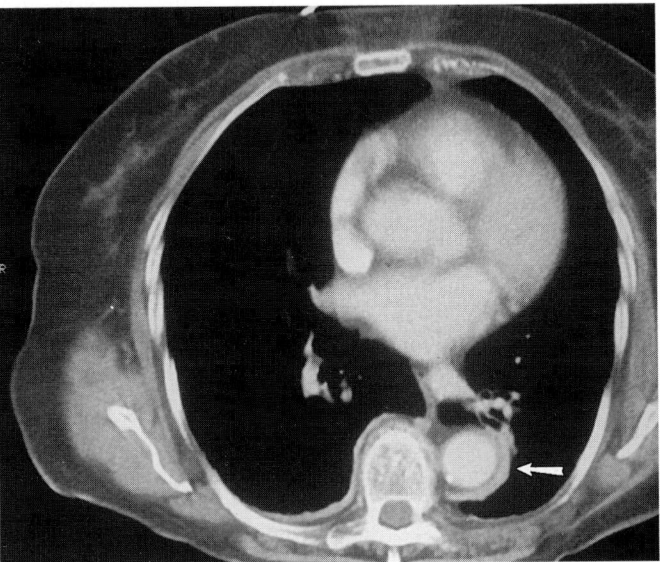

FIGURE 56–10. A periaortic atelectatic lung *(arrow)*. On enhanced images, the atelectatic lung may have the appearance of a dissection. (From Thompson, B.H., and Stanford, W.: Electron beam computed tomography imaging of aortic aneurysms and dissections. J. Invasive Cardiol. 6:213, 1994, with permission.)

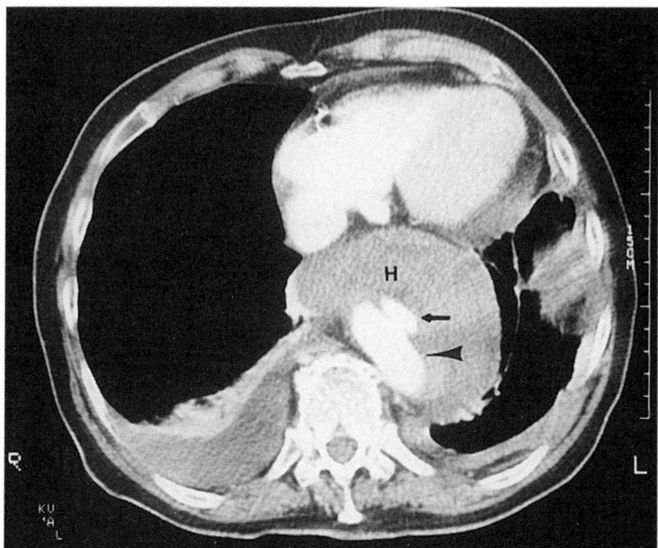

FIGURE 56–11. Ruptured aortic dissection. Axial image obtained at the level of the heart shows large periaortic hematoma (H) in this patient with type III dissection. Contrast material opacifies both the true *(arrowhead)* and the false *(arrow)* lumina. The transit of blood into the pleural spaces is indicated by the presence of bilateral pleural effusions. (From Thompson, B.H., and Stanford, W.: Utility of ultrafast computed tomography in the detection of thoracic aortic aneurysms and dissections. Semin. Ultrasound CT MR 14:117, 1993, with permission.)

speed of the EBCT scanner and its ability to image during maximal contrast opacification provide unparalleled vascular enhancement throughout the entire length of the aorta, a feature that is often not possible with conventional CT. The additional versatility of time-density analysis and flow-mode imaging increases its usefulness. In dissections, the ability to visualize the dissection flap and the periaortic tissues is an important attribute.

Disadvantages of both conventional CT and EBCT include suboptimal demonstration of the aortic valvular apparatus. Although EBCT can provide quantitative evidence of valvular regurgitation, such information cannot be ascribed to any specific valve.

In cases of dissection, limited image resolution may preclude an accurate assessment of involvement of smaller branch vessels. Neither CT nor EBCT can reliably show the site of intimal tears, and artifacts from calcium or surgical clips may produce linear streaks that may be mistaken for a dissection flap. Fortunately, these artifacts infrequently pose a problem with image interpretation.

IMAGING OF THE PULMONARY ARTERIES AND GREAT VEINS

Structural abnormalities and disease processes involving the pulmonary arteries and great veins are also important and at times difficult to diagnose. In the pediatric population, pulmonary artery stenoses and abnormalities in pulmonary vein sites are not uncommon entities. In the adult population, pulmonary embolism is the most frequent concern, although other abnormalities such as pulmonary artery aneurysms and obstructions of the superior vena cava need to be evaluated, especially in the differential diagnosis of mediastinal masses. Arteriovenous fistulas or venous developmental abnormalities can be the cause of peripheral pulmonary parenchymal masses. Because congenital abnormalities of the great vessels will be considered in Chapter 58, the present section focuses on pulmonary embolism and disease processes involving the great vessels other than the aorta.

PULMONARY EMBOLI

Pulmonary thromboembolism has an estimated incidence in the United States of 630,000 cases per year[13]; it is fatal in up to 30 percent of untreated cases.[14] Since antemortem diagnosis of pulmonary embolism is made in fewer than one third of patients,[15, 16] there are approximately 100,000 deaths per year that might be preventable with early diagnosis.[13] Treatment is provided primarily by anticoagulants, which lower mortality to approximately 8 percent; however, this treatment is not without risk and has an estimated 15 percent complication rate.[17] Hence, the diagnosis of pulmonary embolism needs to be rapid and accurate.

Imaging modalities currently being used in the diagnosis of pulmonary embolism include chest radiography, ventilation-perfusion (V/Q) scanning, and pulmonary arteriography. Each has advantages and disadvantages, and each has different sensitivities and specificities; unfortunately, there is no single imaging modality that appears appropriate in every patient. In the chest film and the radionuclide scan, pulmonary embolism is inferred from associated findings without direct visualization of the embolus.[18] Pulmonary angiography and CT show a cutoff or filling defect of the contrast-enhanced pulmonary artery. Because CT is relatively noninvasive, however, it is becoming increasingly popular as an ideal method for the diagnosis of pulmonary embolism. This is especially true with EBCT[3, 19] and spiral CT imaging.[20]

Central Pulmonary Emboli

The volume mode of the EBCT scanner is the sequence most commonly used in the identification of pulmonary thromboembolism. Scanning generally encompasses an area 1 to 3 cm cephalad to the main pulmonary artery and extends 3 to 6 cm caudally. Slices (3 mm, 100 to 400 msec) are obtained while the patient either holds the breath or breathes. This sequence gives excellent visualization of the main, left, and right proximal pulmonary arteries as well as the first and second divisions of the pulmonary arteries. Scanning is performed during maximal contrast opacification, and only 27 seconds is required to scan 20 slices. Although the image quality is improved when the patient is able to hold the breath, the inability to hold one's breath does not markedly detract from the images. Contrast needs to be maximized, and most diagnosticians use approximately 100 mL of 76 percent iodine contrast material injected at a rate of 1 to 1.5 mL per second through an antecubital vein catheter. The circulation time is obtained before the injection. Scanning is initiated at a time delay equal to or slightly after the circulation time to allow maximal opacification of the pulmonary arteries before scanning is initiated. A typical examination takes approximately 10 to 15 minutes.

Emboli are seen as filling defects in the contrast-enhanced pulmonary arteries (Fig. 56–12). Because of the scanner's ability to obtain cross-sectional slices without the interference of overlying structures, which sometimes pose a problem in angiography, CT has the advantage of generating high-resolution images with great detail, and this enhances the diagnosis (Fig. 56–13). As in any scanning modality, there are pitfalls. One area that causes interpretive difficulty is at the branching of the left and right pulmonary arteries. On the right, the pulmonary artery divides into the truncus anterior, which travels superiorly, and the descending pulmonary artery. At this branching, there is often tissue that may contain lymph nodes. This nonopacified tissue can have an appearance similar to that of an embolus. In excluding emboli, it is helpful to visualize slices at several levels to see whether there is a lack of vessel opacification. Pulmonary emboli are commonly bilateral, so other filling defects seen in either of the pulmonary arteries add credence to the diagnosis, as does a lack of opacification extending over more than one slice. Better resolution can be achieved with 3-mm-thick slices; however, adequate visualization is provided with 6-mm slices, and this slice thickness allows more of the pulmonary arterial tree to be encompassed during a single scan sequence.

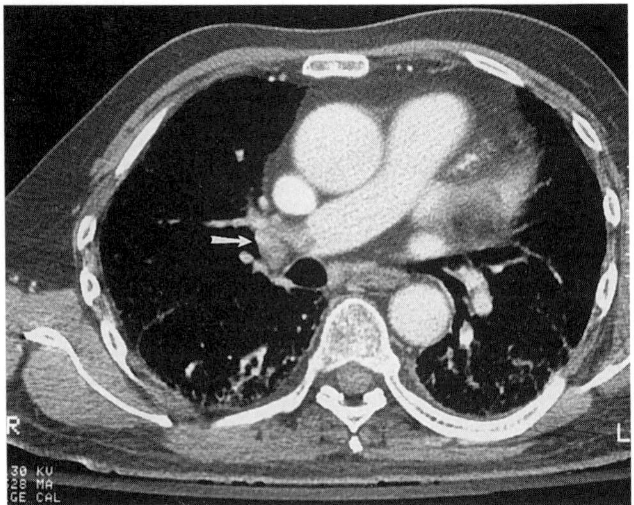

FIGURE 56–12. A large pulmonary embolus *(arrow)* occluding the right main pulmonary artery. The embolus was confirmed by angiography.

Whenever pulmonary emboli are suspected, it is important to visualize the right-sided cardiac chambers. At times, filling defects consistent with intracardiac thrombus are seen within the apex or body of the right ventricle. Also, it is not uncommon for patients undergoing a CT examination for another reason to have an unsuspected thromboembolism. At times, the movie- or flow-mode imaging sequences, or both, are helpful. In the flow-mode sequence, a bolus of contrast traverses the pulmonary artery, and this can optimize vessel opacification and aid in demonstrating filling defects. The movie-mode sequences can demonstrate ventricular contraction and can help identify filling defects within the ventricle. Both sequences aid in the identification of thromboemboli.

Occasionally, pulmonary emboli are calcified and therefore identifiable on nonenhanced scans (Fig. 56–14). If calcification is seen, the pulmonary embolus is probably long-standing. The chest film usually cannot detect this calcification, unless it is relatively dense and located in an area that is well visualized without the overlapping structures that tend to mask its identification.

Peripheral Pulmonary Emboli

EBCT studies have shown peripheral pulmonary emboli both in experimental animals and in clinical cases. Experimental studies in the dog[19] and the pig[21] have shown that EBCT scanning has the capability to identify emboli in small third- and fourth-division pulmonary arteries (7-mm vessels).

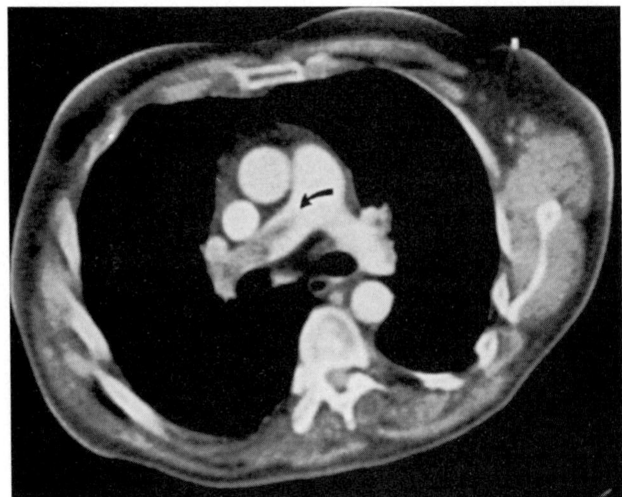

FIGURE 56–13. A flame-shaped pulmonary embolus *(arrow)* in a patient presenting with syncopal attacks. The embolus was an unexpected finding.

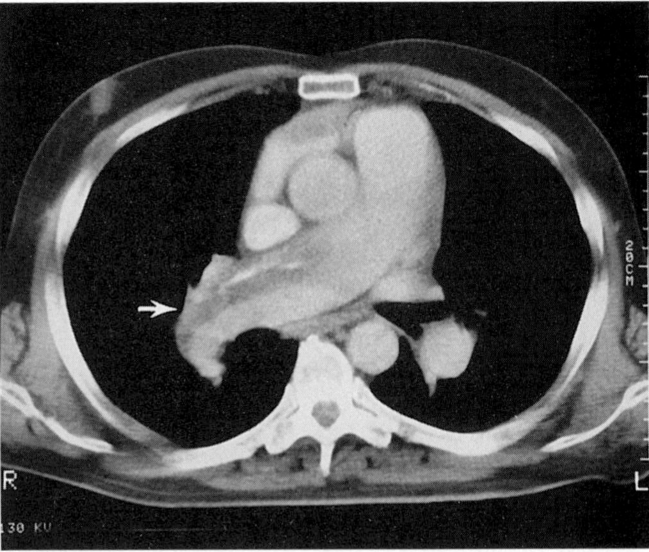

FIGURE 56–14. A pulmonary embolus with calcification *(arrow)*. Calcification may be seen in thrombi of long duration.

Stanford and colleagues[21] reported visualization of autologous emboli introduced in eight pigs via the superior vena cava and confirmed by sectioning the frozen chest. On these scans, emboli were identified as filling defects occluding the vessel or presenting with a surrounding rim of contrast material. The emboli were best seen on cross-sectional images (Fig. 56–15). In clinical studies, Stanford and associates[22] were able to identify pulmonary emboli verified by angiocardiography or autopsy. Teigen and coworkers[23]

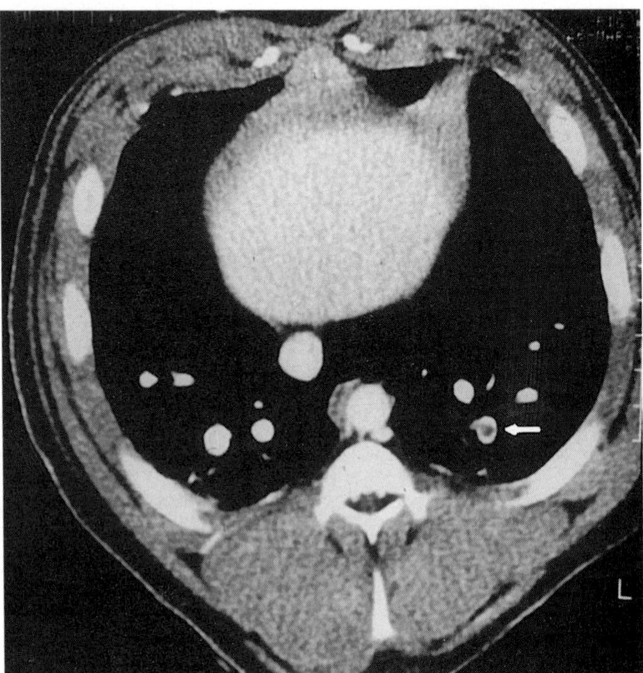

FIGURE 56–15. An ultrafast CT image of an autologous embolus in a 7-mm left lower lobe pulmonary artery of a pig *(arrow)*. This was a 100-msec scan of a 3-mm-thick slice. (From Stanford, W., Reiners, T.J., Thompson, B.H., et al.: Contrast-enhanced thin-slice ultrafast computed tomography for the detection of small pulmonary emboli: Studies using autologous emboli in the pig. J. Invest. Radiol. 29:184, 1994, with permission.)

conducted the largest clinical series. They studied 86 patients suspected of having a pulmonary embolism and reported thromboembolic material in 39 of these individuals. In 25 patients, both EBCT and angiographic confirmation or pathologic confirmation, or both, was possible. Nineteen of the EBCT scans proved positive by both EBCT and angiography, four proved negative, and there was one false-positive and one false-negative scan. EBCT findings were correlated with angiography on a zone-by-zone basis in 21 patients. Thromboembolic disease was seen in 88 vascular zones. In 53 zones, both CT and angiography showed evidence of thromboembolic disease, whereas 18 zones showed angiographic findings for thromboembolic disease, but the CT scan was negative. In 17 zones, the CT scan was positive, whereas the angiographic studies were negative; 143 zones were considered negative on both the angiogram and CT. With EBCT, the interobserver agreement was 95 percent and the intraobserver agreement was 96 percent.

Because V/Q nuclear scans cannot directly visualize emboli, the current practice in many medical centers is to perform a V/Q scan as an initial screening procedure and, if entirely negative, to perform no other studies.[18] Conversely, if there was a high probability of pulmonary embolism, additional imaging studies also would not be performed. In the 75 percent of indeterminate studies, however, other imaging modalities would be needed.[18, 24] The necessity of introducing a catheter into the right atrium or pulmonary artery, or both, in patients who are extremely ill and prone to arrhythmias, coupled with the problems of injecting contrast material into patients with high pulmonary artery pressures, makes angiography less desirable.[25] Digital subtraction angiography[26] and MR[27] techniques have also been used, but each has drawbacks. Digital subtraction angiography can visualize filling defects within the pulmonary arteries. The advantages are that less contrast material is needed. The disadvantages are that a catheter often needs to be positioned in the superior vena cava or right side of the heart for optimal contrast material injection and, because of the necessity for subtraction of images, any motion will significantly degrade the images. With MR techniques, the ability to characterize the vessel wall and the embolus is helpful. With the newer MR techniques, flow can also be measured and vessel visualization can be enhanced with MR angiography.[27] Magnetic resonance techniques, however, have poorer resolution than CT. Other imaging modalities such as plethysmography and Doppler examination of the lower limbs may also help identify a source for the embolus, but again these are indirect tests that may or may not be suggestive of deep venous thrombosis. The ability to visualize an embolus has considerable appeal, and for this reason EBCT scanning is increasing in importance. Other imaging modalities such as spiral CT[20] and CT angiography have also reported high accuracy in identifying pulmonary emboli.

OTHER PULMONARY ARTERY DISEASES

At times, pulmonary artery enlargement can be problematic and masquerade as a mediastinal mass lesion. Pulmonary artery hypertension secondary to obstructive lung disease can cause enlargement of the proximal pulmonary arteries, as can Eisenmenger physiology secondary to intracardiac shunts. Again, EBCT has importance in the visualization of pulmonary vessels. This imaging often confirms the diagnosis of the pulmonary artery as a source of the mass.

Pulmonary parenchymal mass lesions can also have a vascular cause. Arteriovenous fistulas can be diagnosed by visualizing large vessels entering and exiting a parenchymal mass. These vessels are readily identified with enhanced CT. Individuals with arteriovenous malformations secondary to Osler-Weber-Rendu disease may show enhancing vascular masses. In these individuals, there is opacification of a peripheral mass secondary to contrast accumulation in venous lakes. These tumors are less striking than arteriovenous fistulas, but again CT is useful in making the diagnosis.

OTHER ARTERIAL AND VENOUS LESIONS AND MALFORMATIONS

EBCT is extremely useful in identifying obstructions of the superior vena cava and in verifying the locations of the aberrant veins draining into the heart. Superior vena cava obstruction is identified by the formation of collateral vessels, especially when there is associated blockage of either the right or the left brachiocephalic or azygos system. Because of the cross-sectional nature of CT, tumors and granulomatous inflammatory processes constricting the superior vena cava can usually be identified. Collateral vessels can be seen as opacified columns draining into the right or left brachiocephalic or azygos system. The volume study is used most frequently and allows adequate opacification of all of the vessels, including the collateral vessels. Flow studies can also be helpful; however, interpretive problems sometimes arise because unopacified blood comes into the superior and inferior vena cava from other sources such as the azygos vein and collateral intercostal or

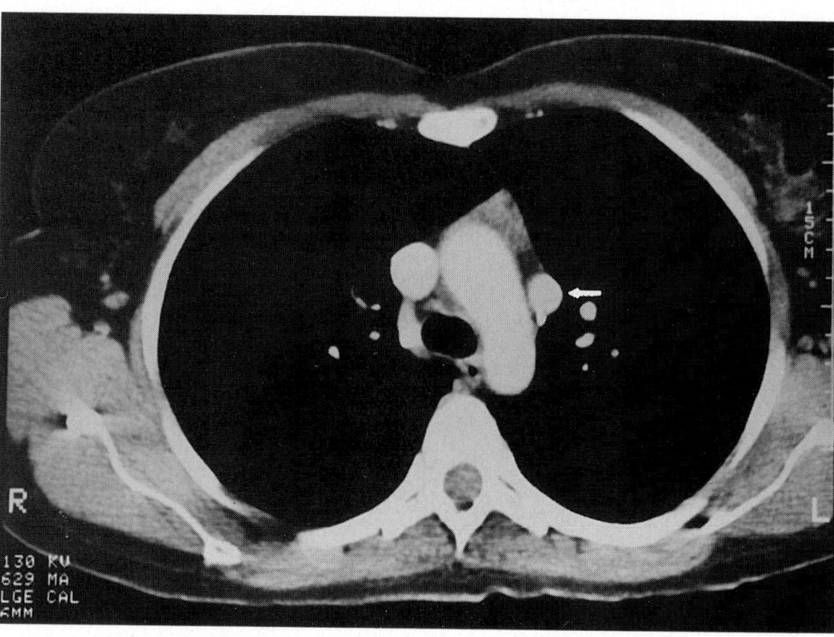

FIGURE 56–16. An aberrant left superior vena cava *(arrow)*. Blood flow was into the coronary sinus.

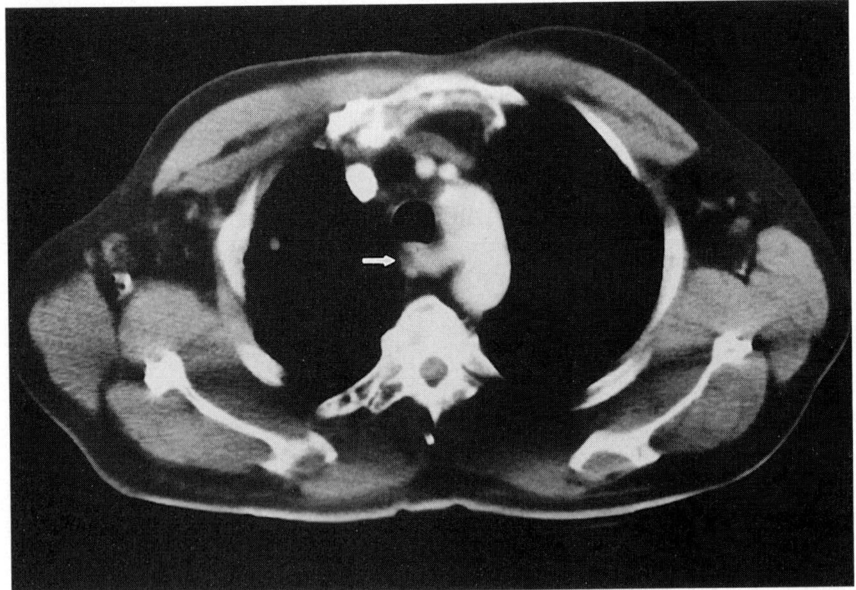

FIGURE 56–17. An aberrant right subclavian artery (*arrow*). The aberrant right subclavian artery came off the aorta in the area of the ligamentum arteriosum and coursed behind the trachea before going toward the right arm.

hepatic vessels. These can cause filling defects in the otherwise opacified contrast column. The unopacified blood needs to be excluded as a source of the filling defects.

Other vessels such as aberrant superior venae cavae and aberrant subclavian arteries are also readily identified with CT. An aberrant superior vena cava is identified on the CT images as a contrast-enhanced column running along the left border of the heart (Fig. 56–16). It is better visualized with left arm injections because contrast material from a right arm injection may not extend sufficiently in a lateral direction to opacify an aberrant left superior vena cava. Aberrant right subclavian arteries are commonly identified as contrast-enhanced vessels running behind the trachea from the aorta cephalad toward the right arm (Fig. 56–17).

CONCLUSIONS

EBCT has important applications in the identification of structural abnormalities of the great arteries and veins, in the diagnosis of pulmonary emboli, and in the diagnosis of aortic aneurysms and dissections. The speed of the scanner, the excellent resolution and vessel opacification, and the lack of overlying structures have made CT an important imaging modality in evaluating the great vessels of the thorax.

References

1. Shuford, W.H., Sybers, R.G., and Weens, H.S.: Problems in the aortographic diagnosis of dissecting aneurysm of the aorta. N. Engl. J. Med. 280:225, 1969.
2. Stanford, W., Galvin, J.R., Weiss, R.M., et al.: Ultrafast computed tomography in cardiac imaging: A review. Semin. Ultrasound CT MR 12:45, 1991.
3. Thompson, B.H., and Stanford, W.: Utility of ultrafast computed tomography in the detection of thoracic aortic aneurysms and dissections. Semin. Ultrasound CT MR 14:117, 1993.
4. Pasch, A.R., Ricotta, J.J., May, A.G., et al.: Abdominal aortic aneurysm: The case for elective resection. Circulation 70:1, 1984.
5. Bickerstaff, L.K., Pairolero, P.C., Hollier, L.H., et al.: Thoracic aortic aneurysms: A population-based study. Surgery 92:1103, 1982.
6. Athanasuleos, C.L., Anagnostapoulos, C.E., and Resnekov, L: Acute aortic dissection: Introduction and medical therapy. *In* Anagnostapoulos, C.E. (ed.): Lethal Disease of the Ascending Aorta. Baltimore, University Park Press, 1976, p. 98.
7. Stanford, W., Rooholamini, S.A., and Galvin, J.R.: Ultrafast computed tomography in the diagnosis of aortic aneurysms and disssections. J. Thorac. Imaging 5:32, 1990.
8. Spencer, F.C.: Diseases of great vessels. *In* Schwartz, S.I. (ed.): Principles of Surgery. 4th ed. New York, McGraw-Hill, 1984, p. 883.
9. Stanford, W., and Thompson, B.H.: Evaluation of the great heart vessels and pulmonary vasculature. Curr. Opin. Radiol. 3:533, 1991.
10. Kumar, V., Cotran, R.S., and Robbins S.L.: Basic Pathology. Philadelphia, W.B. Saunders, 1979, p. 294.
11. Kadir, S.: Diagnostic Angiography. Philadelphia, W.B. Saunders, 1986, p. 140.
12. Pressler, V., and McNamara, J.J.: Thoracic aortic aneurysm, natural history and treatment. J. Thorac. Cardiovasc. Surg. 79:489, 1980.
13. Dalen, J.E., and Alpert, J.S.: Natural history of pulmonary embolism. Prog. Cardiovasc. Dis. 17:259, 1975.
14. Hermann, R.E., Davis, J.H., and Holden, W.D.: Pulmonary embolism: A clinical and pathologic study with emphasis on the effect of prophylactic therapy with anticoagulants. Am. J. Surg. 102:19, 1961.
15. Chintapalli, K., Thorsen, M.K., Olson, D.L., et al.: Computed tomography of pulmonary thromboembolism and infarction. J. Comput. Assist. Tomogr. 12:553, 1988.
16. Goldhaber, S.Z., Hennekens, C.H., Evans, D.A., et al.: Factors associated with the current antemortem diagnosis of major pulmonary embolism. Am. J. Med. 73:822, 1982.
17. Mant, M.J., Thong, K.L., Birtwhistle, R.V., et al: Hemorrhagic complications of heparin therapy. Lancet 1:1133, 1977.
18. Hanson, M.W., and Coleman, R.E.: Pulmonary nuclear medicine evaluation of thromboembolic disease. J. Thorac. Imaging 4:40, 1989.
19. Geraghty, J.J., Stanford, W., and Galvin, J.R.: Ultrafast computed tomography in experimental pulmonary embolism. Invest. Radiol. 27:60, 1992.
20. Remy-Jardin, M., Remy, J., Wattinne, L., et al.: Central pulmonary thromboembolism: Diagnosis with spiral volumetric CT with the single-breath-hold technique: Comparison with pulmonary angiography. Radiology 185:381, 1992.
21. Stanford, W., Reiners, T.J., Thompson, B.H., et al: Contrast enhanced thin slice ultrafast computed tomography for the detection of small pulmonary emboli: Studies using autologous emboli in the pig. J. Invest. Radiol. 29:184, 1994.
22. Stanford, W., Rooholamini, S.A., and Galvin, J.R.: Ultrafast computed tomography in the detection of intracardiac masses and pulmonary artery thromboembolism. *In* Stanford, W., and Rumberger, J.A. (eds.): Ultrafast Computed Tomography in Cardiac Imaging: Principles and Practice. Mt. Kisco, NY, Futura Publishing, 1992, p. 248.
23. Teigen, C.L., Maus, T.P., Sheedy, P.F., et al.: Pulmonary embolism: Diagnosis with electron beam CT. Radiology 188:839, 1993.
24. PIOPED Investigators: Value of the ventilation perfusion scan in acute pulmonary embolism: Results of the prospective investigation of pulmonary embolism diagnosis (PIOPED). JAMA 263:2753, 1990.
25. Mills, S.R., Jackson, D.C., Older, P.A., et al.: The incidence, etiologies and avoidance of complications of pulmonary angiography in a large series. Radiology 136:295, 1980.
26. Musset, D., Rosso, J., Petitpretz, D., et al.: Acute pulmonary embolism: Diagnostic volume of digital subtraction angiography. Radiology 166:455, 1988.
27. Schiebler M.L., Holland G.A., Hatabu H., et al: Suspected pulmonary embolism: Prospective evaluation with pulmonary MR angiography. Radiology 189:125, 1993.

CHAPTER

57 Cardiac Masses and Pericardial Disease: Imaging by Electron-Beam Computed Tomography

William Stanford, M.D.
Brad H. Thompson, M.D.

Electron-beam computed tomography (EBCT) is an extremely useful imaging modality in evaluating intracardiac masses and pericardial disease. The 0.75 to 1.5-mm^2 resolution, superb vessel opacification, reduced motion artifact, and decreased radiation dose make the electron-beam scanner ideal for cardiac and pericardial imaging. This chapter deals with the imaging of cardiac masses and pericardial disease. The characteristics of the EBCT (ultrafast CT) scanner have been described elsewhere (see Chapter 52).

IMAGING SEQUENCES

The sequences used to image cardiac masses and pericardial disease are the volume mode, flow mode, and movie (cine) mode.

Volume Mode

The step volumetric scanning mode is the most commonly used sequence for the evaluation of cardiac masses. In this sequence, volumetric data are acquired by firing electrons at one target ring at a rate of 100 msec per sweep. This produces sequential axial sections 3, 6, or 10 mm in thickness and requires 100- to 400-msec scan time, depending on the number of averages, for each slice. A complete 40-slice study of the heart requires approximately 76 seconds. Improved resolution is possible when one is obtaining thinner slices (3 mm).

The scanner has continuous volumetric scanning capabilities, which permit a considerably faster image acquisition than step volumetric scanning. This capacity is a result primarily of improvements in software, table speed, and bulk memory storage. Although the time required for the electron-beam sweep remains the same (100 msec), these improvements allow 40 slices (10 mm thick) to be obtained in 17 seconds. The slice-thickness options are 6 through 10 mm. If thinner slices are required, the scanner can be operated in the step volumetric scanning mode. This mode enables one to obtain slices as thin as 1.5 mm. Both modes permit image manipulation, such as reformatting and region-of-interest density measurements.

Flow Mode

In the flow-mode sequence, each target ring is sequentially swept once every 50 msec with imaging triggered off the R wave of the electrocardiogram. Eight images 8 mm in thickness are produced in 224 msec. After a programmed delay, the sequence can be repeated. Because scanner memory is limited to 80 images, an eight-level, 10-image sequence is typically programmed. If additional temporal resolution is desired, 13 or 20 images can be acquired at six or four levels, respectively. When imaging is performed during contrast injection, the images show progressive vascular enhancement, followed by eventual washout as the contrast bolus traverses the great vessels. With this technique, time-density curves can be generated to depict the pattern and rate of enhancement of a particular vessel.

Movie Mode

The movie-mode sequence is routinely used in cardiac imaging. In this mode, the scanner is programmed to sweep a single target ring at a maximum rate of 17 times (images) per second (50 msec per sweep). Imaging is triggered from electrocardiographic gating, which produces a series of consecutive images throughout the cardiac cycle. These resultant images can be viewed as a closed-loop cine sequence or as individual frames.

Advantages and Disadvantages of Particular Sequences

Because opacification is usually greater in the flow mode and because the structures are stationary, the definition of mass lesions is often better than that in the movie mode. The flow mode also has the advantage of defining arrival times of the contrast bolus within the chambers, and by determining this arrival time, one can reduce the amount of contrast material required for subsequent sequences. It is preferable to obtain these images with the patient in the neutral position (transaxial views).

The flow mode, however, does not show movement relationships, and because these are especially important in intracardiac tumor imaging, scanning in the movie mode is commonly added. The scan sequence that best shows the lesion should be performed first, in the event that scanning has to be discontinued. Because contrast material is administered via a peripheral vein, a catheter does not have to be manipulated in the vicinity of an intracardiac tumor.

CONTRAST ADMINISTRATION

Volumetric studies of the thorax are almost always performed with contrast administration because the rapid image-acquisition times of both the step volumetric scanning and the continuous volumetric scanning modes ensure superior vascular enhancement of each slice throughout the entire study. Because of slower scan times, comparable vascular enhancement may not always be possible with conventional CT.

In imaging of the heart and the great vessels, the majority of patients undergo a 40-slice volume study of the chest during the intravenous injection of 76 percent iodine nonionic contrast material. Nonionic contrast material is preferred in cardiac imaging for two reasons: (1) improved patient tolerance due to fewer constitutional symptoms, such as burning and nausea, and (2) higher contrast dose limit, which may be important when additional imaging sequences are required. In addition, ionic contrast material causes perturbations of the heart rate, and when quantification of ventricular function is desired, nonionic contrast material must be used. For a volume study, approximately 150 mL of contrast material is administered with a power injector through an 18- or 20-gauge 1.5-inch antecubital venous catheter at a rate of 1 to 2 mL per second. To ensure optimal vascular enhancement, correct timing of the initiation of scanning is critical. Because of EBCT's millisecond acquisition times, circulation times are usually performed with scanning delayed until one half of the total contrast dose is infused.

RADIATION DOSAGE

The radiation dose for the EBCT scanner is significantly less than that for conventional CT, primarily because of the faster image-acquisition times. The entrance dose for a volume study that uses a slice thickness of 10 mm and an exposure time of 100 msec is 0.9 cGy per slice, compared with 2 to 4 cGy per slice for conventional CT. Multislice studies (flow or movie) deliver a dose of 0.58 cGy per image with the use of a scan time of 50 msec; the patient receives a dose of 1.17 cGy when a 100-msec scan time is used (these are actual measurements from the authors' scanner). This dose can be compared with the radiation exposure for a cardiac catheterization study, which is approximately 47 cGy. Because the target source is located posterior to the patient, the calculated exit doses anteriorly are approximately 17 percent of the entrance dose.

INTRACARDIAC TUMORS

Atrial Myxomas

Atrial myxomas account for 50 percent of intracardiac tumors. They generally arise within the left atrium in the area in and around the limbus of the fossa ovalis, average 4 to 8 cm in diameter,[1] and are often pedunculated. The pedunculation allows the myxoma to prolapse through the mitral valve in diastole; in systole, the tumor usually lies within the atrium. The second most common site of origin is the right atrium. Here, myxomas tend to be more solid and have a flat or sessile configuration. The third site is within the right ventricle. The size, location, attachment, and configuration of the myxoma can be demonstrated by means of EBCT imaging, as can any movement occurring during the cardiac cycle. With its axial orientation, CT does not have the superimposition of other tissues and therefore is very useful for defining myxomas.

Electron-Beam Computed Tomography Appearance of Atrial Myxomas

Intracavitary tumor masses appear as filling defects within the opacified blood pool. Myxomas may be sessile but more often are pedunculated, and this pedunculation allows the tumor to prolapse through the mitral valve. When this occurs, the tumor may abut the anterior leaflet of the mitral valve and thicken or deform the valve (Fig. 57–1). Sessile tumors are more commonly seen on

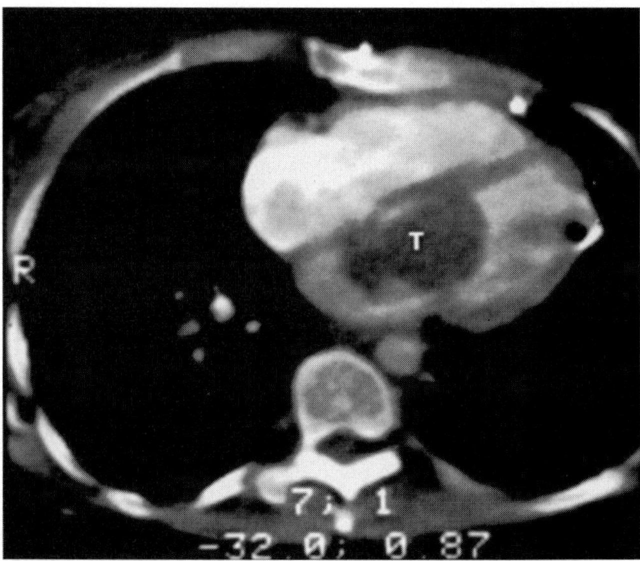

FIGURE 57–1. Long-axis view of a left atrial myxoma (T) prolapsing through the mitral valve in diastole. The tumor often abuts the anterior leaflet of the mitral valve. A left atrial myxoma was found at operation. R = right. (From Scholtz, T.D., Boskis, M., Roust, L., et al.: Noninvasive diagnosis of recurrent familial left atrial myxoma: Observations with echocardiography, ultrafast computed tomography, nuclear magnetic resonance imaging, and in vitro relaxometry. Am. J. Card. Imaging 3:142–145, 1989, with permission.)

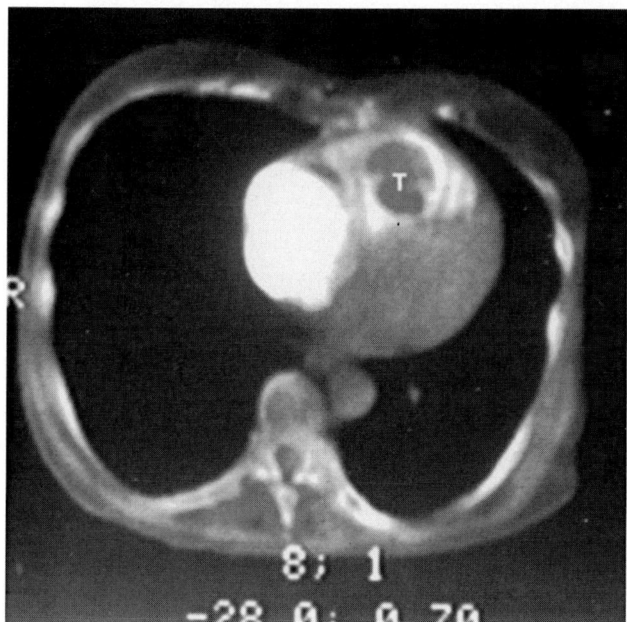

FIGURE 57–2. Right ventricular myxoma (T) arising from a papillary muscle of the tricuspid valve. This was confirmed at operation. (From Stanford, W., and Galvin, J.R.: The radiology of right heart dysfunction: Chest roentgenogram and computed tomography. J. Thorac. Imaging 4(3):7–19, 1989, with permission.)

EBCT images as a thickening of the intra-atrial septum. Right ventricular myxomas have a more rounded appearance and are usually attached to the right ventricular free wall, the interventricular septum, or a papillary muscle of the tricuspid valve (Fig. 57–2). The Hounsfield numbers of these tumors often approximate those of the myocardium, but this phenomenon does not usually interfere with the diagnosis. The tumors may be multiple.

Less Common Primary Cardiac Tumors

Rhabdomyomas, fibromas, and lipomas constitute a group of less common benign cardiac tumors. Rhabdomyomas usually occur in children and are associated with tuberous sclerosis.[2] They frequently arise within the ventricular free wall or septum and are seen as deformities of the contrast-filled ventricular cavity. Fibromas may present a similar appearance. The densities of both tumors are the same as that of the myocardium, which may preclude separation of the tumor from normal myocardium. Fibromas, however, may calcify. Lipomas tend to arise within the atrial septum and cause deformity of the septum on CT images. Their density is considerably less than that of the myocardium, and they are readily identifiable without contrast enhancement.

The imaging sequences used for the less common primary cardiac tumors are similar to those used for myxomas.

Metastatic Tumors and Intracardiac Extensions of Infradiaphragmatic Tumors

Melanomas and lung and breast carcinomas are the most frequent tumors to metastasize to the heart.[1] They appear either as mass lesions within the cardiac chambers or as nodules on the epicardial surface. Lymphomas and renal carcinomas may grow intraluminally within the inferior vena cava and, at times, may extend into the right atrium and ventricle (Fig. 57–3). If an intracavitary extension is suspected, the flow mode is the better sequence to use, because it can both define tumor location and show the route of contrast material as it passes around the tumor. A movie sequence may also be helpful in showing tumor movement and defining wall motion irregularities. Both sequences show the extent of tumor involvement and define the presence of tumor extending outside the cardiac chambers. Similarly, conventional and spiral CT images can show the extent of the tumor, but movement artifact and poor opacification may degrade images.

INTRACARDIAC THROMBI

Intracardiac thrombi are responsible for 15 percent of all ischemic strokes. The risk is increased in patients with nonrheumatic atrial fibrillation (45 percent), ischemic heart disease (25 percent), rheumatic mitral stenosis (10 percent), and prosthetic cardiac valve replacement (10 percent).[3]

Since the presence of an intracardiac thrombus usually requires treatment, the early identification of thrombus is important. Because of the morbidity and mortality associated with anticoagulation, a definitive diagnosis is often required before therapy is instituted.

Thrombi may be solitary or multiple. Within the heart they are seen as filling defects within the opacified cardiac chambers (Fig. 57–4). The thrombi may be sessile or pedunculated. In the ventricle, they usually lie adjacent to areas of infarcted myocardium. Because thrombus identification may be difficult, it is the authors' practice to image patients in both short- and long-axis projections, which allows viewing in different orientations and helps identify and differentiate structures such as aberrant muscle bands and papillary muscles. Axial images provide excellent visualization of the left atrial appendage and of the entrance of the pulmonary veins.

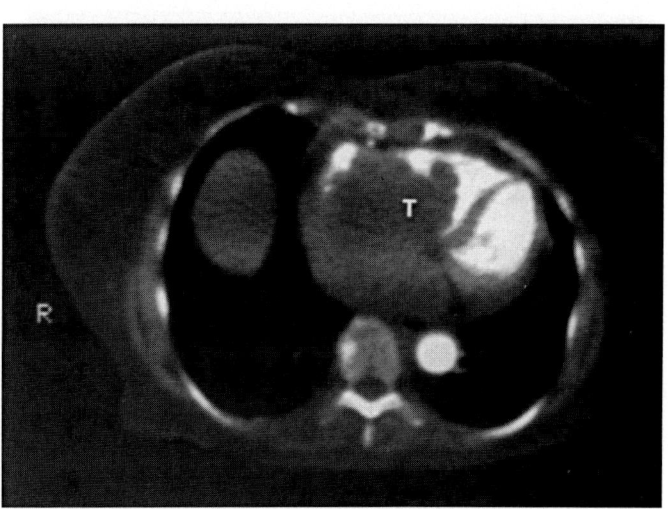

FIGURE 57–3. Histiocytic lymphoma (T) arising from the liver and growing up the inferior vena cava into the right atrium and ventricle. The tumor is infiltrating the wall of the right atrium. (From Stanford, W., and Galvin, J.R.: The radiology of right heart dysfunction: Chest roentgenogram and computed tomography. J. Thorac. Imaging 4(3):7–19, 1989, with permission.)

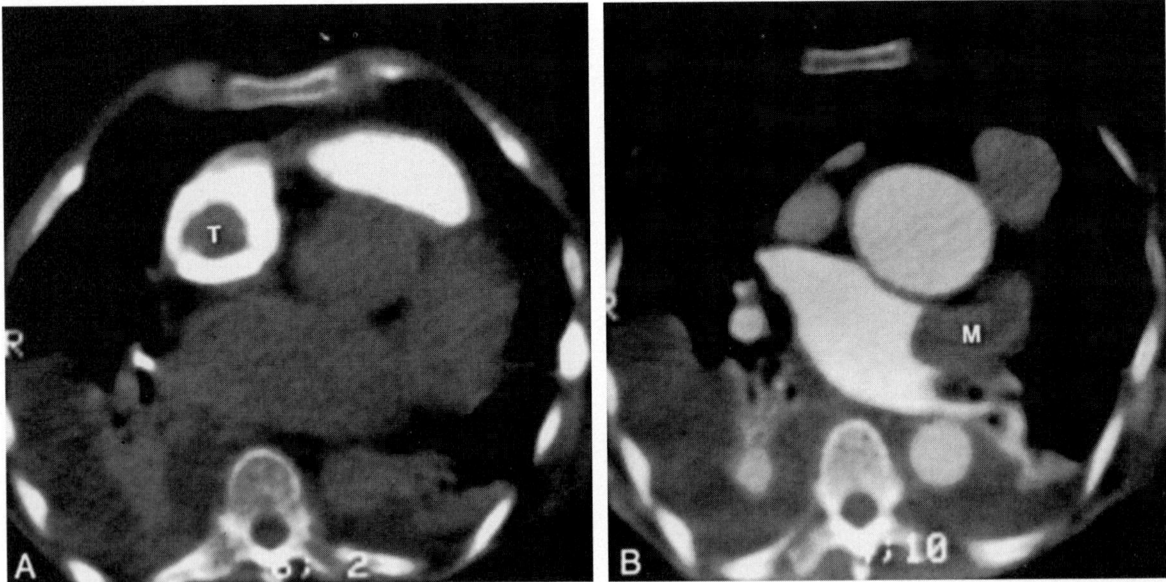

FIGURE 57–4. Probable right *(A)* atrial (T) and left *(B)* atrial appendage (M) thrombi in a patient with breast carcinoma. The patient was anticoagulated but was lost to follow-up. Metastatic tumor could not be excluded completely.

Electron-Beam Computed Tomography Appearance of Thrombi

Sessile or flat, laminated thrombi are more difficult to diagnose than the pedunculated variety. Characteristically, they present as curvilinear filling defects along the wall of the contrast-opacified ventricle. Alternatively, they may present as an oval-shaped filling defect projecting into the ventricular cavity.[4] There is usually an associated wall motion abnormality, and, if this is not present, one should be cautious in diagnosing thrombus. Occasionally, cases are seen in which thrombi project a considerable distance into the ventricular cavity. However, in these instances, the thrombus can often be seen moving or swirling within the ventricular chamber during cardiac contraction (Fig. 57–5).

The differentiation of thrombus from papillary muscle may be difficult. The most helpful technique is acquiring a thorough knowledge of the location and configuration of the papillary muscles. In the left ventricle, the anterior papillary muscle arises from the anterior wall lateral to the apex and away from the interventricular septum. The location of the posterior papillary muscle is somewhat more variable. It is usually seen along the posterolateral aspect of the ventricle on both the long- and short-axis images. Both muscles appear as smooth, oval filling defects approximately 1 cm in diameter. A problem arises when the papillary muscles are prominent and there is thickening or conglutination of the subchordal structures, as is sometimes the case in mitral stenosis. In these instances, the thickening may extend almost to the valve leaflet. Thrombi, on the other hand, often lie adjacent to the apex of the left ventricle and septum and are commonly associated with abnormalities of wall motion. An alternative site is the inferior aspect of the left ventricle. Inferiorly located thrombi are best seen on short-axis views.

Atrial thrombi may be present in patients with mitral stenosis, especially when there is associated atrial fibrillation. The tip of the left atrial appendage has the highest incidence of thrombus formation.[5] EBCT shows the left atrial appendage in cross section, thereby providing information better than that available with transthoracic echocardiography. Fibrous tissue ingrowth can occur in long-standing thrombi, as can calcification. Calcifications are readily seen on EBCT (Fig. 57–6). Since the density of thrombus is

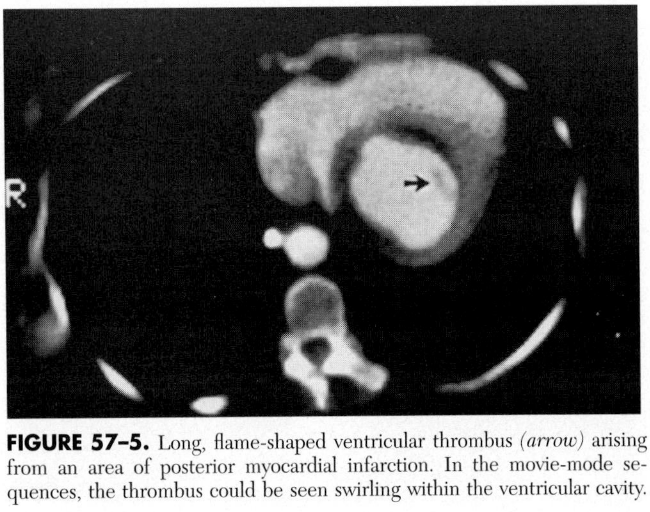

FIGURE 57–5. Long, flame-shaped ventricular thrombus *(arrow)* arising from an area of posterior myocardial infarction. In the movie-mode sequences, the thrombus could be seen swirling within the ventricular cavity.

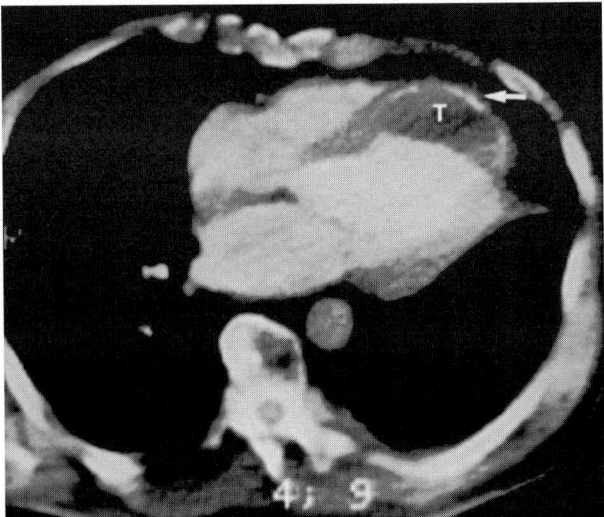

FIGURE 57–6. Calcification in the wall of the left ventricle *(arrow)* in a patient with a previous myocardial infarction. There is a large thrombus (T) adjacent to the infarct.

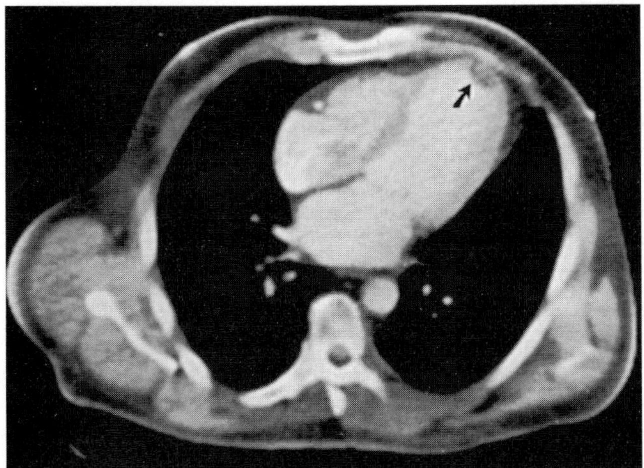

FIGURE 57–7. Thrombus *(arrow)* in the apex of the left ventricle in a patient with syncopal attacks. The patient had a history of myocardial infarction.

similar to that of myocardium, Hounsfield numbers may not help differentiate thrombus from normal myocardium or from papillary muscle.

Indications for Electron-Beam Computed Tomography Imaging in Suspected Thrombi

Patients with recent cerebrovascular accidents or emboli, or both, are candidates for scanning; however, during scanning for various indications a number of patients will be identified in whom thrombus is an unexpected finding (Fig. 57–7). In the evaluation of intracavitary thrombi, the usual practice is to scan in both the short- and the long-axis projections. If a thrombus is identified, anticoagulation therapy is often instituted, and EBCT is a useful technique for following the results of the anticoagulation treatment (Fig. 57–8).

Scanning Sequences

In patients with suspected thrombi, the movie mode is the most informative sequence, because the images show associated abnormalities of wall motion. The use of both short- and long-axis movie sequences allows imaging of the cardiac chambers in two projections and gives excellent visualization of ventricular movement throughout a full cardiac contraction. These sequences require only slightly more scan time and only small amounts of additional contrast material.

Accuracy of Electron-Beam Computed Tomography in Detecting Intracavitary Thrombi

In a study comparing EBCT with two-dimensional transthoracic echocardiography in the detection of intracardiac thrombi in 41 stroke patients, Love and associates[6] found agreement between the techniques in 86 percent of patients (both were negative in 76 percent, both positive in 10 percent). In the six patients (14 percent) about whom there was disagreement, echocardiography was positive and tomography equivocal in four patients, echocardiography was equivocal and tomography negative in one patient, and echocardiography was equivocal and tomography positive in one patient (the latter patient had autopsy confirmation of left ventricular thrombus). Love and associates concluded that EBCT was an important imaging technique for detecting intracardiac thrombi, especially in patients for whom two-dimensional echocardiography was difficult or equivocal. Helgason and colleagues[7] also found EBCT to be more sensitive than echocardiography in detecting intracardiac thrombi.

THE PERICARDIUM

EBCT images provide excellent detail of the pericardium, especially when 1.5- or 3-mm, high-resolution axial images are obtained. These images consistently show pericardial thickening, calcification, intrapericardial tumors, and fluid collections. The scanner has the additional capability to evaluate chamber volumes, measure ventricular filling, and define wall motion, all of which are important when evaluating pericardial constriction.

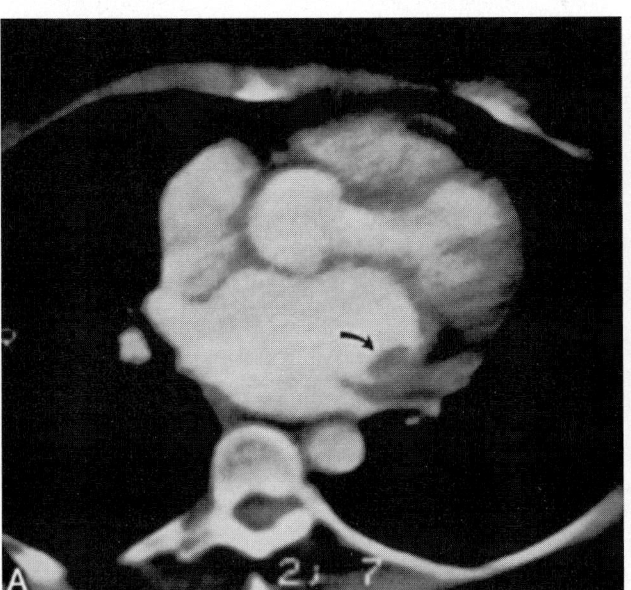

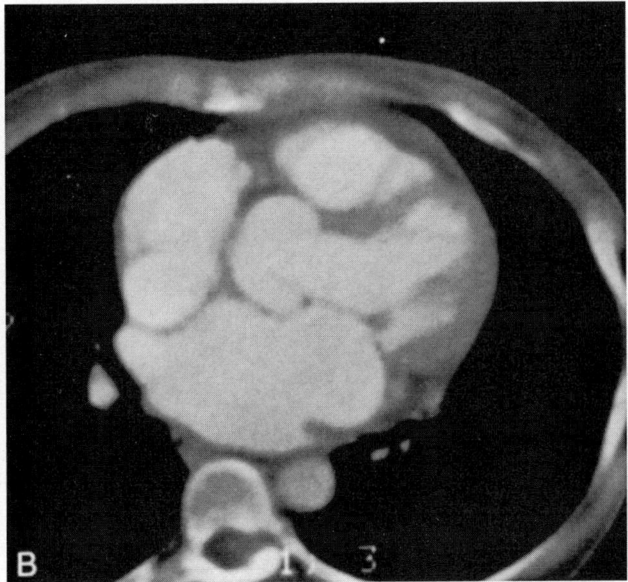

FIGURE 57–8. Images from a patient with mitral stenosis and a normal atrial echo examination. *A*, On EBCT study, there was a small thrombus *(arrow)* attached to the lateral wall of the left atrium just below the orifice of the superior pulmonary vein. *B*, Six weeks later, after the patient had been treated with anticoagulants, the thrombus disappeared.

Pericardial Computed Tomography Anatomy

The pericardium is a fibrous sac that surrounds the heart. It attaches to the great vessels at the level of the aortic and pulmonary valves and to the central tendon of the left hemidiaphragm.[8, 9] It has two layers, parietal and visceral, which are separated by a potential space containing approximately 25 mL of serous fluid.[9, 10] The parietal pericardium is usually separated from the sternum by mediastinal fat and from the myocardium by a layer of epicardial fat, which makes the pericardium visible on CT, especially in the area anterior to the right ventricle.

The pericardium is seen as a 1- to 2-mm, linear soft-tissue density lying between mediastinal fat ventrally and epicardial fat dorsally (Fig. 57–9).[11] Inferiorly, at its insertion into the diaphragm, it thickens to 3 or 4 mm.[12] Although the ventral pericardium is usually visualized, the posterior pericardium is seen only about 25 percent of the time. There is little fat superiorly, so the pericardium is often not seen in this area. Only when the pericardial cavity is distended by air, fluid, or mass lesions is the posterior pericardium visualized with CT.[12]

There can be problems in imaging the pericardium. Thickening at the attachment to the diaphragm is commonly seen and should not be confused with an infiltrative process. Similarly, nodular thickenings over the right atrium and ventricle are common. Superoposteriorly, at its attachment to the aorta, there is a recess that can sometimes be mistaken for adenopathy. However, EBCT has proved very accurate in assessing pericardial thickness.[13]

Imaging Sequences

The most frequently used imaging sequence for evaluation of the pericardium is a volume-mode sequence consisting of contiguous axial images 6- or 10-mm thick. Forty slices can be acquired in 76 seconds, which is usually sufficient to encompass the entire chest and upper abdomen. Additional 1.5- or 3-mm cuts to define further the pericardial anatomy are also taken. In patients with pericardial disease, it is often important to evaluate ventricular function and the pattern of left and right ventricular filling.[14, 15] The cine sequence allows the accurate calculation of left and right ventricular end-diastolic and end-systolic volumes, stroke volume, ejection fraction, left ventricular mass, and cardiac output. Playing the images back in a closed-loop cine sequence allows the viewer to observe global and regional contraction and the pattern of ventricular filling.

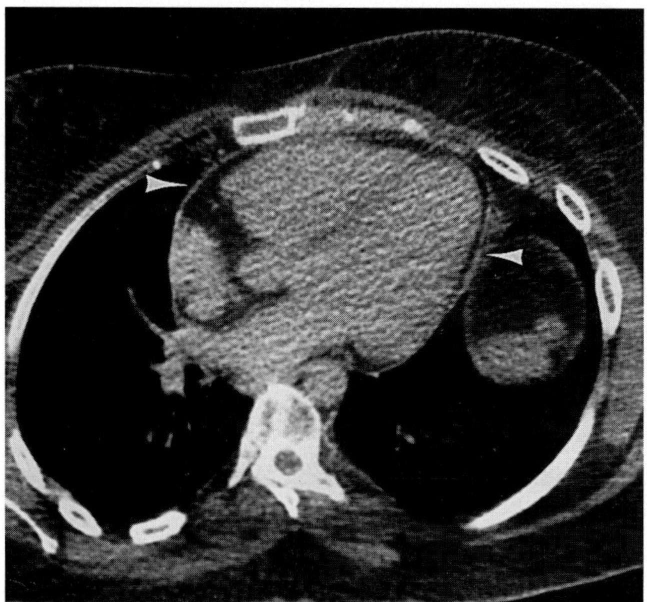

FIGURE 57–9. Neutral-axis image of a patient with a normal pericardium. The pericardium is seen as a 2-mm, linear soft-tissue density *(arrowheads)*, lying between the anterior mediastinal and the epicardial fat.

Positional Considerations

In the imaging of pericardial disease, the neutral axis with the patient lying supine is the preferred position. This position allows the image sequences to be taken through the chest and upper abdomen without moving the patient. It also allows slices 1.5 to 3 mm thick to be taken for better anatomical definition. In the volume-mode program, the image sequences can be merged, and sagittal reconstruction is possible; however, these projections are rarely needed. If ventricular function or right ventricular filling, or both, are to be calculated, the patient needs to be placed in a short-axis configuration. Because measurement of the functional parameters in patients suspected of having constrictive physiology is common, the short-axis movie sequence is frequently used. In this sequence, either eight-level 10-image or six-level 13-image short-axis movie sequences are obtained. The latter sequence allows the measurement of the rate of diastolic filling.[14, 15] It usually requires two runs to encompass the entire left and right ventricles and atria. After the short-axis sequence, the patient is moved into a neutral position, and several 1.5- to 3-mm unenhanced high-resolution images are taken to define further the pericardial anatomy and to detect possible pericardial calcification or fluid.

Contrast Considerations

Non–contrast-enhanced images commonly show pericardial anatomy, especially when there is a moderate amount of epicardial and mediastinal fat to accentuate the fat-pericardial interface. With non–contrast-enhanced images, pericardial calcification is readily apparent, and cysts and effusions are readily appreciated. Tissue density measured in Hounsfield units is helpful in defining the composition of any pericardial mass or effusion.

Contrast enhancement has certain advantages. In the majority of protocols, as much as 150 mL of 76 percent iodine contrast medium are administered through an 18- to 20-gauge catheter, 1 to 1.5 inches in length, inserted into an antecubital vein. The contrast is delivered at a rate of 1.5- to 2.0 mL per minute via a power injector, which is sufficient to outline cardiac chambers, determine pericardial enhancement in inflammatory states, and differentiate between pericardial thickening and adjacent atelectatic lung. Highly vascular tumors are generally better defined with contrast material, which also aids in visualizing the pericardium in patients with minimal amounts of epicardial fat. Contrast material, of course, is contraindicated in patients with allergies and those with renal compromise.

Radiation Considerations

A 10-image short-axis cine sequence delivers 5.4 cGy of radiation to the skin of the patient's back. If a 3-mm high-resolution image is also required, the additional radiation exposure is 1.17 cGy. If only a 10-mm axial image and a 3-mm high-resolution image are taken, the radiation exposure is 2.1 cGy. By comparison, conventional CT high-resolution images of the chest would give single-image exposures of 2 to 5 cGy and 10-image exposures of 20 to 50 cGy. Both CT sequences give much less radiation exposure than cardiac catheterization. Because of the distance from the pericardium, gonadal exposure is nil. Thyroid exposure from a movie frame would be 0.04 cGy.

Pericardial Imaging Techniques and Protocols

EBCT imaging sequences vary. The most frequently used sequence consists of movie-mode images in the short and long axes. Several 3-mm cuts with the patient in the neutral position are often added for better definition of the anatomy.

Examinations can be done either with or without contrast material. When there is a moderate amount of epicardial and mediastinal fat, the non–contrast-enhanced images show the pericardial anatomy with great clarity. Low-density cysts, effusions, and pericardial calcification can be visualized without contrast, and Hounsfield numbers can be used to characterize the composition of fluid collections.

Contrast enhancement is useful in delineating cardiac chambers, assessing wall motion abnormalities, defining inflammatory and vascular lesions, and differentiating pericardial thickening from adjacent atelectatic lung.

Pericardial Effusions

The pericardium reacts to injury by fluid production, fibrin formation, and cellular proliferation.[16] These reactions may occur together or independently. When an effusion is present, it initially accumulates in the caudal portion of the pericardium and appears as a thin, elliptical, low-density collection lying dorsal to the left ventricular myocardium. As the effusion increases, it extends up and over the ventral surface of the right atrium and ventricle and may even surround the origins of the great vessels (Fig. 57–10). Loculated small effusions are more commonly seen inferiorly and dorsolaterally to the left ventricle as well as in pericardial recesses such as the transverse sinus, the area surrounding the ascending aorta and pulmonary trunk, the oblique sinus, and the pulmonary recess.[17, 18]

The amount of fluid and its physiologic effects vary. A normal pericardium can become markedly distended yet cause little hemodynamic alteration. Conversely, if the fluid accumulates rapidly or in an area in which a thickened pericardium limits its distensibility, it may produce cardiac tamponade (Fig. 57–11).

Fluid composition may be serous or proteinaceous. Effusion with a high-protein content may have CT numbers that approach those of soft tissue and hence may be difficult to distinguish from thickened pericardium.

Pericardial Thickening

Pericardial thickening is seen as a response to trauma, inflammation, or tumor and as a sequela of pericardiotomy and radiation injury. The thickening may be localized or generalized and may extend in excess of 6 cm. Both the parietal and the visceral pericardia are commonly involved, and the process may additionally infiltrate the myocardium.

When identification of an effusion is difficult, placing the patient in a decubitus position may change the configuration of the effusion and help define its location. This change does not occur in fibrous thickening, a difference that may be useful in differentiating fluid from thickening. Atelectatic lung usually enhances with contrast material, which may help differentiate this entity from pericardial thickening.

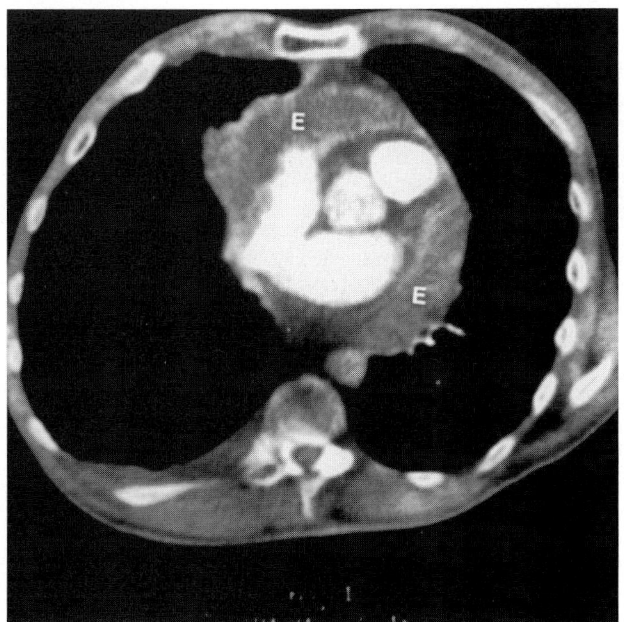

FIGURE 57–10. Large pericardial effusions (E) lying anterior to the right atrium and posterior to the left atrium. (From Stanford, W., and Galvin, J.R.: The radiology of right heart dysfunction: Chest roentgenogram and computed tomography. J. Thorac. Imaging 4(3):7–19, 1989, with permission.)

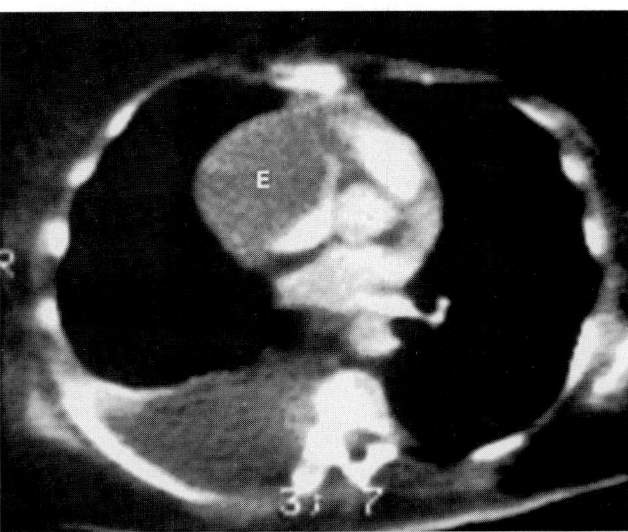

FIGURE 57–11. Loculated effusion (E) compressing the right atrium in a postoperative coronary artery bypass patient. The patient presented with low cardiac output. After the collection was drained, her cardiac output immediately returned to normal. (From Stanford, W., and Galvin, J.R.: The radiology of right heart dysfunction: Chest roentgenogram and computed tomography. J. Thorac. Imaging 4(3):7–19, 1989, with permission.)

Malignant Disease

Breast and lung carcinomas commonly metastasize to the pericardium. Malignant mesothelioma may also invade the pericardium. The latter may present as a solitary mass or form diffuse plaques that encase the parietal pericardium (Fig. 57–12). Lymphoma may present as a diffuse pericardial infiltration.

Constrictive Pericarditis

Tuberculosis, mediastinal fibrosis, tumor infiltration, and infection may result in pericardial fibrosis and constriction. The fibrosis may prevent diastolic filling and result in a low cardiac output. The extent of pericardial involvement can usually be identified with EBCT (Fig. 57–13).

EBCT can also differentiate restrictive cardiomyopathy from constrictive pericarditis. In normal ventricles, 44 percent of the left ventricular filling occurs by the third frame after systole. In ventricles with restrictive cardiomyopathy, 63 percent of the filling has occurred by the third frame, and in constrictive pericarditis 83 percent.[14, 15] In addition, in patients with restrictive cardiomyopathy, the pericardium is normal in thickness, whereas in pericardial constriction it is thickened. In dilated myocardiopathy, the ventricular chambers are enlarged and systolic function is greatly impaired; however, the pericardium is normal.

Less Common Pericardial Lesions

Pericardial cysts are less common pericardial lesions; however, they are readily identifiable with CT. This lesion appears as a mass

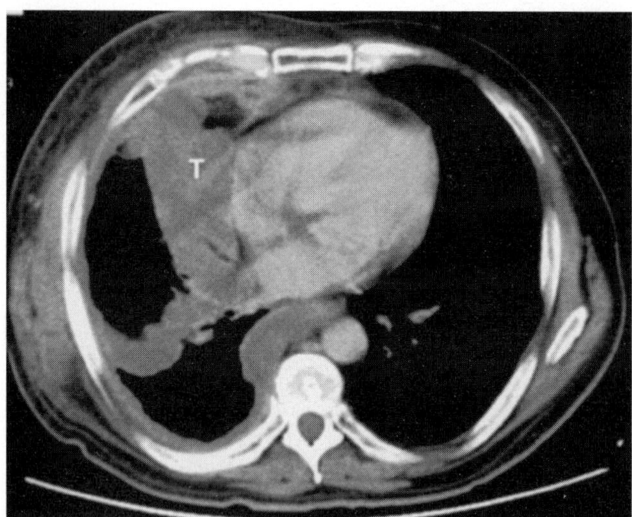

FIGURE 57–12. A mesothelioma (T) involving the parietal pericardium. (From Stanford, W., and Galvin, J.R.: The radiology of right heart dysfunction: Chest roentgenogram and computed tomography. J. Thorac. Imaging 4(3):7–19, 1989, with permission.)

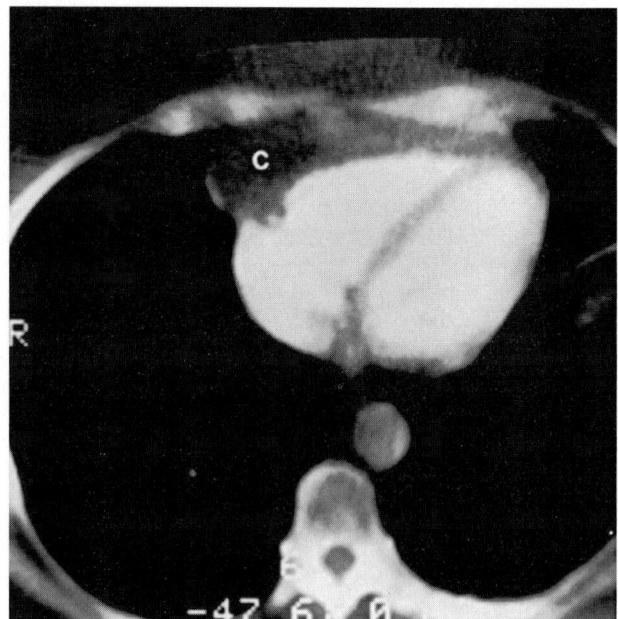

FIGURE 57–14. Pericardial cyst (C) located in the right pericardiophrenic angle. The cyst contents had Hounsfield numbers similar to those of water.

in the right or, occasionally, the left pericardiophrenic angle. The cysts are filled with a clear, low-density fluid and have Hounsfield numbers approaching those of water density (Fig. 57–14).[12]

Congenital partial absence of the left hemipericardium often presents as a lack of pericardial continuity in association with herniation of the left atrial appendage through the defect.[19] If the entire left hemipericardium is absent, one may see direct apposition between the heart and the lung tissue.

Benign tumors of the pericardium include teratomas, bronchogenic cysts, leiomyomas, hemangiomas, and lipomas.[11, 20] Lipomas have densities ranging from −55 to −120 Hounsfield units and are readily identifiable. Hemangiomas may be enhanced markedly with contrast material and are generally easy to identify. Bronchogenic cysts with high-protein fluid and leiomyomas have CT numbers similar to those of soft tissue, and therefore malignancy often cannot be excluded. In teratomas, both fat and tooth calcifications may be seen.

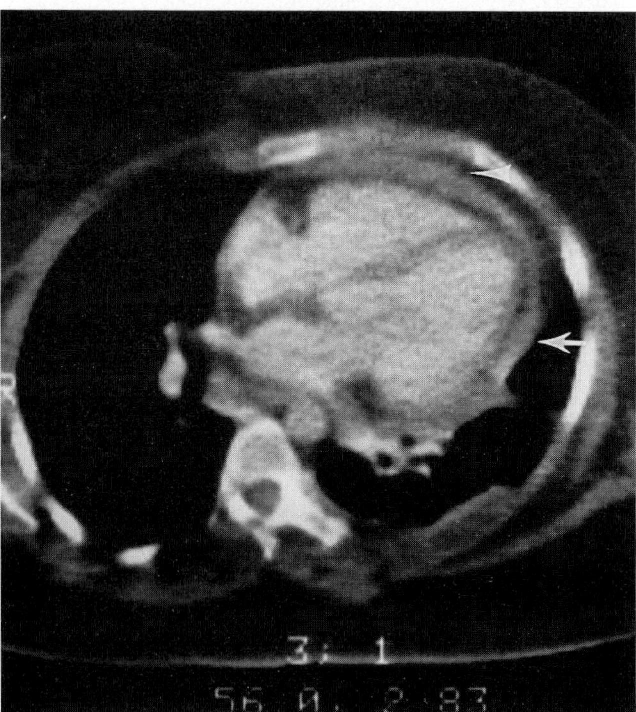

FIGURE 57–13. Thickened pericardium encases the right *(arrowhead)* and left ventricles *(arrow)*, producing constriction. The cause of the constriction was thought to be an inflammatory process. (From Stanford, W.: Computed tomography and ultrafast computed tomography in the diagnosis of pericardial disease. *In* Elliott, L.P. [ed]: The Fundamentals of Cardiac Imaging in Infants, Children, and Adults. Philadelphia, J.B. Lippincott, 1991, p. 418, with permission.)

Advantages and Disadvantages of Electron-Beam Computed Tomography in Pericardial Disease

EBCT is a useful adjunct to echocardiography. The CT images show loculations and thickening better than do those of echocardiography. In addition, the images are reproducible and allow the assessment of ventricular function, as well as the composition of any effusion. The ability to calculate functional parameters is an additional advantage. The technique is particularly useful in assessing loculated effusions and compressive hematomas as causes of postoperative low cardiac output.

EBCT is not suitable in the agitated patient who cannot lie still or who is too ill to be transported to the imaging suite. It cannot be used in patients with renal compromise or those with allergies to contrast agents. However, it is suitable in patients who cannot hold their breath.

SUMMARY

EBCT retains the advantages of conventional CT in showing cardiac and pericardial anatomy. Its ability to assess wall motion is especially helpful in the evaluation of cardiac masses. An important attribute of EBCT imaging is its capacity to visualize overlying structures while at the same time assessing wall motion. The ability to determine left and right ventricular end-diastolic and end-systolic volumes, stroke volume, ejection fraction, left ventricular mass, cardiac output, and diastolic filling, which is important in patients suspected of having pericardial constriction, is an additional advantage.

References

1. Colucci, W.S., and Braunwald, E.: Cardiac tumors, cardiac manifestations of systemic disease, and traumatic cardiac history. *In* Harrison, T.R. (ed.): Principles of Internal Medicine. 12th ed. New York, McGraw-Hill, 1991, p. 988.
2. Stanford, W., Abu-Yousef, M.M., and Smith, W.: Intracardiac tumor (rhabdomyoma) diagnosed by in utero ultrasound: A case report. J. Clin. Ultrasound 15:337, 1987.
3. Cerebral Embolism Task Force: Cardiogenic brain embolism. Arch. Neurol. 43:71, 1988.
4. Stanford, W., Rooholamini, S.A., and Galvin, J.R.: Ultrafast computed tomography in the detection of intracardiac masses and pulmonary artery thromboembolism. *In* Stanford, W., and Rumberger, J.A. (eds.): Ultrafast Computed Tomography in Cardiac Imaging: Principles and Practice. Mt. Kisco, NY, Futura, 1992, p. 240.
5. Braunwald, E.: Valvular heart disease. *In* Harrison, T.R. (ed.): Principles of Internal Medicine. 12th ed. New York, McGraw-Hill, 1991, p. 940.
6. Love, B.B., Struck, L.K., Stanford, W., et al.: Comparison of two dimensional echocardiography and ultrafast computed tomography for evaluating intracardiac thrombi in cerebral ischemia. Stroke 21:1033, 1990.
7. Helgason, C.M., Chomka, E., Louie, E., et al.: The potential for ultrafast cardiac computed tomography in patients with stroke. Stroke 20:467, 1989.
8. Moncada, R.: Pericardium. *In* Naidich, D.P., Zerhouni, E.A., and Siegelman, S.S. (eds.): Computerized Tomography of the Thorax. New York, Raven Press, 1984, pp. 269–289.
9. Williams, P.L., Warwick, R., Dyson, M., et al. (eds.): Gray's Anatomy. Edinburgh, Churchill-Livingstone, 1989, p. 694.
10. Holt, J.P.: The normal pericardium. Am. J. Cardiol. 26:455, 1970.
11. Higgins, C.B.: Heart and pericardium. *In* Moss, A.A., Gamsu, G., and Genant, H.K. (eds.): Computed Tomography of the Body with Magnetic Resonance Imaging. Philadelphia, W.B. Saunders, 1992, p. 306.
12. Moncada, R., Demos, T.C., and Hammer, R.: Computed tomography in pericardial heart disease. *In* Taveras, J.M., and Ferruci, J.T. (eds): Radiology: Diagnosis, Imaging, Intervention. Philadelphia, J.B. Lippincott, 1994, pp. 1–19.
13. Grover-McKay, M., Burke, S., Thompson, S.A., et al.: Measurement of pericardial thickness by cine computed tomography. Am. J. Card. Imaging 5:98, 1991.
14. Oren, R.M., Grover-McKay, M., Stanford, W., et al.: Accurate preoperative diagnosis of pericardial constriction using cine computed tomography. J. Am. Coll. Cardiol. 22:832, 1993.
15. Rumberger, J.A., Weiss, R.M., Feiring, A.J., et al.: Patterns of regional diastolic function in the normal human left ventricle: An ultrafast computed tomographic study. J. Am. Coll. Cardiol. 14:119, 1989.
16. Roberts, W.C., and Spray, T.L.: Pericardial heart disease: A study of its causes, consequences and morphologic features. Cardiovasc. Clin. 7:11, 1976.
17. Levy-Ravetch, M., Auh, Y.H., Rubenstein, W.A., et al.: CT of pericardial recesses. A.J.R. 144:707, 1985.
18. Aronberg, D.J., Peterson, R.R., Glazer, H.S., et al.: The superior sinus of the pericardium: CT appearance. Radiology 153:489, 1984.
19. Nasser, W.K.: Congenital absence of the left pericardium. Am. J. Cardiol. 26:466, 1970.
20. Sagel, S.S.: Lung, pleura, pericardium and chest wall. *In* Lee, J.K., Sagel, S.S., and Stanley, R.J. (eds.): Computed Body Tomography. New York, Raven Press, 1983, p. 124.

CHAPTER

58 Ultrafast Computed Tomography Evaluation of Congenital Cardiovascular Disease in Children and Adults

Tarek S. Husayni, M.D.

In the past 3 decades, there have been significant advances in the medical and surgical management of congenital heart disease (CHD), resulting in dramatic improvement in patient survival and in quality of life. Lesions such as transposition of the great vessels, which were uniformly fatal in the past, are now successfully repaired in the newborn period with low mortality and morbidity. Of the estimated 25,000 babies born annually with congenital heart disease, approximately 85 percent survive to adulthood. It is estimated that in the United States alone, there are currently 500,000 to 600,000 adults with congenital heart disease,[1] many of whom will require at least periodic cardiac evaluations. Hence, the management of patients with CHD is no longer limited to the domain of pediatric cardiologists. Adult medicine specialists, especially cardiologists, radiologists, and obstetricians, are being called on with increasing frequency to lend their expertise in the care of these patients.

Improvements in the management of CHD have been facilitated by parallel advances in diagnostic procedures. Cardiac catheterization was formerly the only laboratory procedure through which anatomical and hemodynamic information could be obtained in the

TABLE 58–1. CONTRAST INJECTION PROTOCOLS FOR PATIENTS WITH CONGENITAL HEART DISEASE

Imaging Mode	Dose	Infusion Rate	Scan Delay
Flow	0.3–0.5 mL/kg, maximum 24 mL	Deliver contrast in ≤2 sec, followed by NS for 3–4 sec, (total injection 5–6 sec)	1–2 sec before injection
Cine (function)	Children: 1–2 mL/kg Adults: 60–90 mL	Total dose divided by Circ. T* 2–3 mL/sec	Circ. T (usually 16 to 20 sec) Circ. T (usually 18 to 24 sec)
Hi Res (anatomy)	Children: 2.0 mL/kg Adults: 90–100 mL	Dose divided by [Circ. T + imaging time] (total time usually 45–55 sec) 2–3 mL/sec	Same as cine

*Circ. T = circulation time from IV to aorta, calculated from flow study or magnesium sulfate injection; NS = normal saline solution; Hi Res = high resolution.

past. With the advent of echocardiography, nuclear imaging, and magnetic resonance imaging, all of which are to a large extent noninvasive, initial evaluation and long-term follow-up of CHD has been greatly facilitated.

Ultrafast computed tomography (UFCT) is a relatively new modality in the area of noninvasive cardiac imaging. It possesses several attributes that make it attractive for imaging CHDs. The spatial resolution is excellent, with image acquisition times short enough to minimize artifacts resulting from cardiac motion (50 to 100 msec per image). The image is tomographic, eliminating the uncertainties produced by overlapping and superimposition of anatomical structures, and it is minimally affected by surrounding tissues, such as bones and lungs, or by patient size, except in small infants. In addition to the exceptional ability of UFCT to define cardiac anatomical structures even in the most complex lesions, blood flow disturbances caused by shunting defects, and obstructive lesions can be characterized. Cardiac performance and ventricular functional reserve can be evaluated with the use of multislice imaging modes that define changes in ventricular volumes over time, at rest, and during stress maneuvers. UFCT imaging is accomplished with minimum discomfort to the patient, using iodinated contrast-material injections and ionizing radiation exposures well within the medically accepted range.

IMAGING PROTOCOLS

The basic image acquisition characteristics of the UFCT scanner that make it useful in CHD are multislice acquisition of 8-mm-thick, 50-msec images synchronized to the patient's electrocardiogram (ECG). As many as 80 images can be acquired, distributed evenly over two to four pairs of slices (see Chapter 52 for full description of the technical aspects of the scanner). Specific iodinated contrast injections (Table 58–1) and specific image synchronization to the patient's ECG are combined to provide information on blood flow and cardiac function.

In the *flow imaging mode*, imaging is started before injection of contrast material and is continued, one set of slices per cardiac cycle, until the contrast bolus passes through the central circulation. The images are acquired preferentially at end-diastole to allow for maximum contrast mixing. The contrast material injected in 2 seconds or less is followed by an injection of normal saline for 3 to 4 seconds to ensure rapid delivery of contrast material into the central circulation (see Table 58–1). The site of injection depends on whether abnormalities of systemic veins are suspected, that is, left arm injection in suspected left superior vena cava or foot injection in suspected obstructed inferior vena cava or in patients with concomitant Glenn and Fontan repairs. The images are viewed in a closed-loop cine format to assess qualitatively anatomical and flow disturbances.[2] Then, time-density curves are generated in multiple anatomical structures to study disturbances of blood flow, as will be described later.

In the *cine imaging mode*, images are obtained rapidly at 17 images per second over several slices, starting at the R wave of the patient's ECG. Iodinated contrast is infused continuously before and during imaging to provide adequate blood pool opacification in both ventricles. Qualitative examination of the cine images in motion provides information about relative chamber size, function, and regional wall motion abnormalities. Alternatively, quantitation of slice volume and its changes in systole and/or diastole, slice muscle mass, wall thickness, and thickening during contraction and segmental changes in volume can be carried out with the use of semiautomatic edge-detection techniques.[3] Global ventricular function is obtained by summing the values of individual slices.

Single-slice *high-resolution imaging* uses 6-, 3- or, more recently, 1.5-mm-thick, 100-msec acquisition time, with 512 × 512 matrix images. As many as 20 contiguous images can be obtained, synchronized to the patient's ECG to acquire diastolic or systolic images. Here also, a continuous contrast-infusion technique is used (see Table 58–1). The transverse images are studied to evaluate the anatomy of central veins, the heart, and great arteries. Oblique planes can be reformatted a posteriori to reveal abnormalities not well defined on transverse images.

UFCT imaging requires patient cooperation to minimize motion between slice acquisitions. Hence, babies and uncooperative children require sedation. The intravenous catheter size is chosen, depending on the maximum rate of infusion (usually, the flow study). Injection rates that are comfortable to the patient and minimize extravasation are shown in Table 58–2. Nonionic contrast material is used to minimize complications and hemodynamic perturbations. Most complete studies are done with less than 4 mL/kg.

ANALYSIS OF BLOOD FLOW

Evaluation of blood flow by UFCT is based on its ability to measure changes in blood density after intravenous injections of iodinated contrast material. Because of UFCT's tomographic nature, the course of contrast passage through the central circulation can be characterized simultaneously in multiple chambers and vessels after a single peripheral injection. This is a major advantage over the traditional dye dilution analysis performed extensively during cardiac catheterization in the past.[4, 5] In addition to the need for invasive instrumentation, the dye dilution studies from cardiac catheterization were based on dye dilution curves obtained one at a time from each cardiac site of interest requiring repeat injections. The process was cumbersome when multiple sites were examined,[5] and hence it has fallen into disfavor. UFCT's "dye dilution curves," called time-density curves (TDCs), represent x-ray attenuation over time as measured in CT numbers (CT No), also called Hounsfield units (Hu). The CT No relates tissue attenu-

TABLE 58–2. MAXIMUM INFUSION RATES

IV Gauge	Rate (mL/sec)
24	1
22	3
20	5
18	12

ation to that of water. One CT No equals 0.1 percent the attenuation of water.

Two contrast-injection techniques can be used to generate indicator-dilution curves.[6,7] The first technique uses constant rate infusion of an indicator until a plateau concentration is reached in the great vessels.[8,9] The relative magnitude of contrast concentrations in the pulmonary artery and aorta will primarily be a function of their respective flow volumes, thus facilitating estimation of pulmonary-to-systemic flow ratios. Cardiac output has also been measured, based on the rate of indicator infusion and its maximum aortic concentration.[9] The constant rate injection technique has not been used in UFCT, and its value in evaluating patients with CHD is not known.

The second injection technique delivers a compact volume of an indicator into a vein in 2 seconds or less. The indicator reaches the heart as a compact bolus, forming single-peak curves. Deformation of the curves downstream, as the indicator flows in the central circulation, provides important information about practical clinical application in CHD.

In the normal circulation, the TDCs obtained successively in the various cardiac chambers and great vessels from systemic venous inflow to systemic arterial outflow show progressive delay in the time of contrast appearance and peaking. The peak of the curve also becomes progressively lower, and the curve wider. The typical TDC shows its upslope to be steeper than its downslope, and the trailing limb returns to baseline levels. After variable delay, a second and much smaller peak may be occasionally seen in the right heart, representing the contrast returning from the systemic circulation (Fig. 58–1).

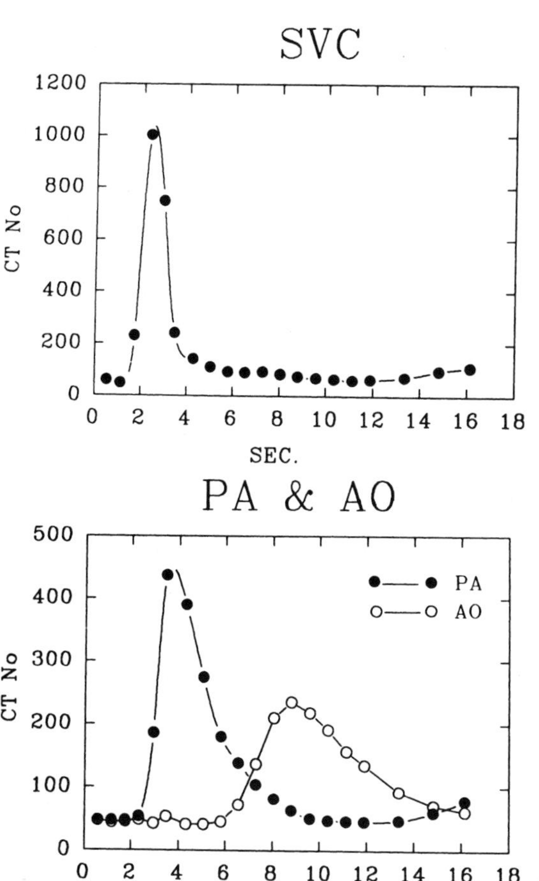

FIGURE 58–1. Normal time-density curves. The superior vena cava curve (SVC) examines the adequacy of contrast injection. The pulmonary artery (PA) and aortic (AO) curves rule out the presence of shunting (Reprinted with permission from the American College of Cardiology, Heart House *Learning Center Highlights*, Vol. 6, No. 4, Summer 1991, pp. 1–7.)

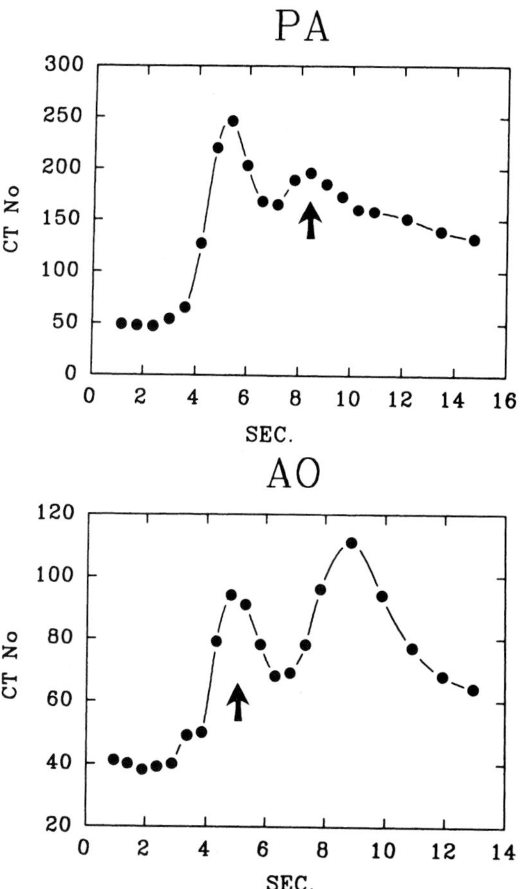

FIGURE 58–2. The effect of shunting on time-density curves. *Top*, A left-to-right shunt causes a second peak (*arrow*) in the pulmonary artery (PA) curve and elevation of the tail. *Bottom*, A right-to-left shunt causes an early peak (*arrow*) in the aortic (AO) curve. (Reprinted with permission from the American College of Cardiology, Heart House *Learning Center Highlights*, Vol. 6, No. 4, Summer 1991, pp. 1–7.)

The following blood flow parameters can be obtained to detect flow abnormalities in patients with CHD.

Cardiac Output

Cardiac output has been determined accurately and validated by several authors,[10–12] provided that the K constant relating iodine concentration to x-ray attenuation is calculated on a patient-by-patient basis.

Cardiac and Great Vessels Shunting

In patients with intracardiac shunting or shunting between the great vessels, the TDCs can be analyzed to determine the presence, direction, localization, and magnitude of shunting.

When left-to-right shunting is present, the curves obtained in the chambers and vessels receiving shunted blood show a second distinct peak or a notable change in the slope of the descending limb of the TDC, with variable elevation of the trailing limb above baseline levels (Fig. 58–2). Screening for most left-to-right shunt lesions can usually be accomplished by sampling the pulmonary artery. An exception is seen occasionally in patients with a single-ventricle equivalent after venopulmonary artery repair (Fontan-type surgery) or in patients with severe obstruction to pulmonary blood flow who have significant systemic-to-pulmonary collaterals, causing left-to-right shunting at the intrapulmonary level. The shunt effect here is not detected in the pulmonary artery but will be seen in the left heart. Such patients may benefit from transcatheter embolization of these abnormal arteries.

Localization of the site of shunting is provided by comparing the configurations of TDCs from the various chambers and vessels. The most proximal chamber or vessel to show shunt configuration is the probable site of shunting. It should be pointed out that in the presence of multiple levels of left-to-right or right-to-left shunting, only the most proximal site will be defined by this method. Demonstrative examples are discussed later in this chapter.

In lesions causing right-to-left shunting, the left heart chambers, or aorta at or distal to the shunt site, show early appearance of contrast material prior to the normal predominant peak caused by the normal flow through the lungs. The size of the early peak depends on the amount of shunting and on the site of sampling in the receiving chamber (see Fig. 58–2).

Bidirectional shunting causes both types of curve deformation: a left-to-right shunting effect in the descending limb of the right heart receiving structures and in downstream structures, and a right-to-left early peak in the ascending limb of the left heart receiving structures.

Quantitation of shunting by indicator dilution principles with the use of UFCT is feasible when the following conditions are satisfied: (1) x-ray attenuation measurements are linearly related to iodine concentrations in blood; (2) complete mixing of contrast and of the shunted blood has occurred in the sample site; and (3) there has been no significant change of hemodynamics or the amount of intravascular contrast material between the time of inscription of the primary curve and that of the shunt circulation. The first condition is largely satisfied by UFCT within the range of CT numbers encountered in shunt evaluation, because variations in the energy output of the scanner from image to image are minimal, and quantitation of primary and shunt flows are done at the same site. A mild effect of beam hardening due to passage of concentrated dye in the superior vena cava may be seen in the baseline portion of curves obtained from adjoining pulmonary artery, right upper pulmonary vein, and aorta. This effect is actually negligible because it accounts for only a few CT numbers, contrasted with those of the pulmonary artery and aortic peaks, which range between 100 and 300 CT No.

The second condition is satisfied by sampling distally from the shunt site to allow for complete mixing of blood. The sampling site, however, should not be situated too far distally, so as to preserve as much as possible the distinguishing characteristics of the curves. The pulmonary artery is generally an ideal sampling site for quantitating the left-to-right shunt in all patients, except in cases in which a ventricular septal defect is at the right ventricular outflow tract, in patients with a patent ductus arteriosus or surgical systemic-pulmonary shunts, or in some patients after venous switch repair for transposition of the great vessels. In these instances, mixing may not be complete in the pulmonary artery, and the left atrial curve can then be used for quantitative analysis. In right-to-left shunting, sampling at the ascending or descending aorta is adequate for almost all patients.

With regard to the third condition, the use of nonionic contrast material, as well as patient cooperation or sedation, minimize fluctuations in hemodynamics. Also, it is a well-known fact that iodinated contrast material is not a strictly intravascular agent. Loss to the extravascular space can occur, even during the first pass through an organ.[13, 14] The magnitude of nonionic contrast material lost to the pulmonary extravascular space in its first passage has, to the author's knowledge, not been determined. A significant loss would decrease the estimated left-to-right shunt and cause overestimation of the right-to-left shunt.

Several methods have been proposed to quantitate left-to-right shunting with the use of dye dilution techniques.[15–17] In UFCT, the most accepted method is to quantitate the areas under the curve that correspond to those of the pulmonary flow (primary curve) and those of the shunt flow, by applying a mathematical formula called a Gamma variate.[18] This formula helps separate the partially superimposed two components of the curve. Left-to-right shunting in the form of pulmonary-to-systemic flow ratio (QP/QS) equals the following:

$$QP/QS = \frac{A}{A - B}$$

where A is the area under the first peak (pulmonary flow) and B is the area under the second peak (shunt flow). Several published reports show the reliability of estimating left-to-right shunting by this method in clinical situations.[19–21] Vigorous validation studies, however, have not been done.

Quantitation of right-to-left shunting, with the use of ascending or descending aorta TDCs, is as follows:

$$QP/QS = \frac{B}{A + B}$$

where A is the area under the first peak (right-to-left shunt flow) and B is the area under the second peak (pulmonary flow reaching the aorta). Validation studies comparing shunt quantitation by UFCT with oximetry showed good correlation.[22] Figure 58–3 is an example of quantitation of a right-to-left shunt.

As in other shunt quantitation methods, the accuracy of UFCT can be affected by technical considerations, such as inadequate contrast injections, although curve deconvolution can correct for this problem,[23] and by hemodynamic factors, such as significant valvular insufficiency and spontaneous changes in hemodynamics during the curve registration.[24]

Vessel Obstruction

Certain forms of vascular obstruction can influence the passage of a bolus of contrast through them. In a branching system, obstruction to flow in one branch can delay the peaking of density in this branch in comparison to that of other unobstructed branches. For example, progressive stenosis of a coronary bypass graft produced by balloon occlusion in experimental animals produced progressive delay in the graft's peak TDC, compared to that of the aorta.[25] Conversely, when coronary vasodilation was induced, the time difference between the graft and aortic peaks shortened. The author has encountered this phenomenon in unilateral pulmonary vein stenosis in some patients after the Fontan repair for single-ventricle equivalent, venous switch repair for transposition of great vessels,[26] and repair of partial anomalous pulmonary venous return. Examples are discussed below.

Pulmonary Perfusion

Regional lung perfusion may be measured by UFCT with the use of dye dilution techniques. Postural changes in regional lung perfusion have been demonstrated by UFCT in experimental animals.[27] In human studies, detection of abnormal regional perfusion by UFCT flow imaging, combined with direct visualization of thrombi by high-resolution imaging, have ensured accurate diagnosis of pulmonary embolism in all patients studied.[28] Such analysis can be extremely useful in evaluating patients with CHD and stenosis or distortion of pulmonary arteries or veins. Unfortunately, this diagnostic test requires transient suspension of respiration during the measurements, which cannot be easily accomplished in young children.

Myocardial Perfusion

Assessment of regional myocardial perfusion and coronary flow reserve noninvasively greatly facilitates the task of evaluating and managing patients with coronary heart disease or other causes of myocardial ischemia. Patients with CHD benefit from such analysis

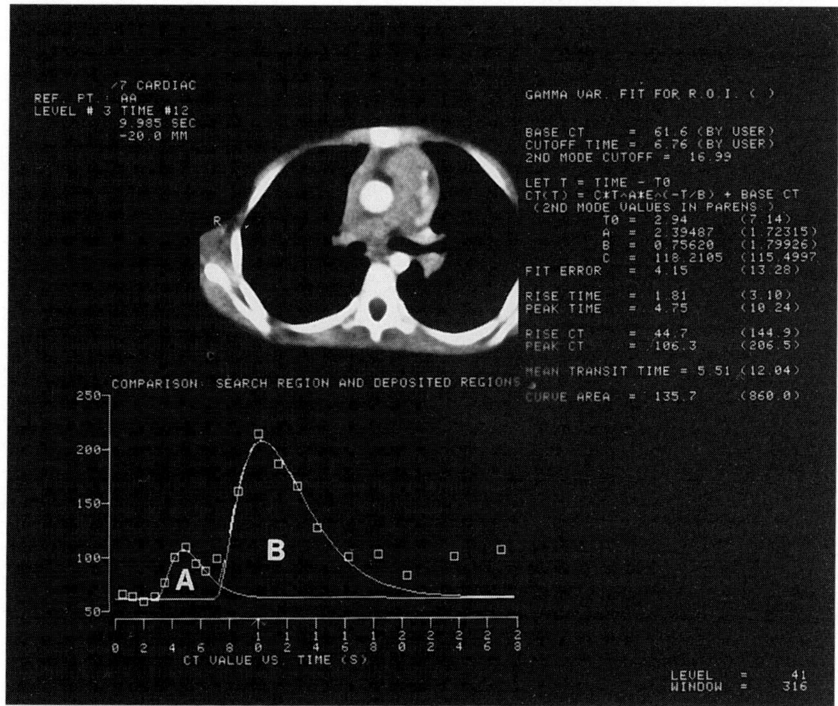

FIGURE 58–3. Quantitation of a right-to-left shunt from aortic time-density curve. Each peak is fitted to a gamma variate function to determine the areas under the curve. The first area (A), corresponding to shunt flow (*first column, upper right*), and the second (B), corresponding to pulmonary flow reaching the aorta (*numbers between parentheses*), are used to calculate the shunt, as described in the text. In this patient with residual atrial septal defect after tetralogy of Fallot repair, QP/QS = 860/(135.7 + 860) = 0.86. Other curve parameters derived from the formula are appearance times (To), rise and peak times, rise and peak CT values, and mean transit times.

when their physician is dealing with anomalous origin of coronary artery, coronary insufficiency after a vessel switch operation or Kawasaki disease, after ventriculotomy, and adults with concomitant CHD and coronary heart disease. The reader is referred to Chapter 55 for a full discussion of this subject.

Recognition of Vascular Structures

Occasionally, a vascular structure may not be identified from its anatomy alone. The timing of contrast passage through this structure in relation to other known structures aids in defining its nature. Such situations arise in some types of anomalous pulmonary veins, in unusual mediastinal vessels, and in crowded areas such as pulmonary hilum. Figure 58–4*A* shows an unusual right lung vessel (vessel X, *right upper image*) that is similar in appearance to a nearby pulmonary artery branch (*arrowhead*). Figure 58–4*B* demonstrates how this vessel is proved to be a pulmonary vein by comparing time-density curves.

ASSESSMENT OF VENTRICULAR FUNCTION

The high-resolution quality of UFCT images ensures accurate delineation of the endocardial and epicardial surfaces of both ventricles in most children and adults. Because as many as eight slices, each 8 mm in thickness, can be obtained at least throughout all of systole, the volume of the ventricle can be imaged to allow analysis of regional and global changes in volume and mass.[29, 30] Extending the imaging to diastole allows measurements of diastolic function parameters as well.[31–33] Validation studies have shown accurate determinations of ventricular end-diastolic volumes, end-systolic volumes, stroke volumes, and ejection fractions of the right and left ventricles at rest and during stress.[34–37] Sophisticated analyses of regional and global three-dimensional stress and systolic function parameters have been published about patients with anterior aneurysms of the left ventricle after myocardial infarction.[38] This study demonstrated that the systolic dysfunction extended beyond the aneurysmal region into the adjoining normal mycardium, identifying an area of dysfunction that was significantly larger than the aneurysm itself. This type of analysis may be applicable to patients with CHD who have undergone ventriculotomy as part of the repair, to some patients with extensive primary myocardial disease, or to patients with congenital or postsurgical abnormalities of coronary arteries.

Although measurements of ventricular functional parameters have not been validated in children, validation studies in animals suggest that this imaging modality can be helpful in patients whose weight is as low as 20 kg. In smaller subjects, the 8-mm-thick slices might be too thick to allow for such sophisticated studies.

CLINICAL APPLICATIONS

Management of patients with CHD requires optimal definition of cardiac morphology, hemodynamics, and cardiac function. This requirement is especially challenging when the cardiac lesions are complex, when extracardiac organs are also abnormal, or when one is evaluating residual defects after cardiac repair. In the pediatric population, transthoracic echocardiography done in the outpatient setting or at the patient's bedside frequently provides the necessary information with minimum discomfort and at reasonable cost. However, echocardiography has its limitations because of nontransmission of ultrasonic waves through air and bones and because of degradation of the image with increasing patient body size. Hence, the efficacy of transthoracic echocardiography becomes limited in large children and adults and in those with multiple complex cardiac defects or when extracardiac anomalies are present, such as visceroatrial heterotaxy syndromes and compression of airways

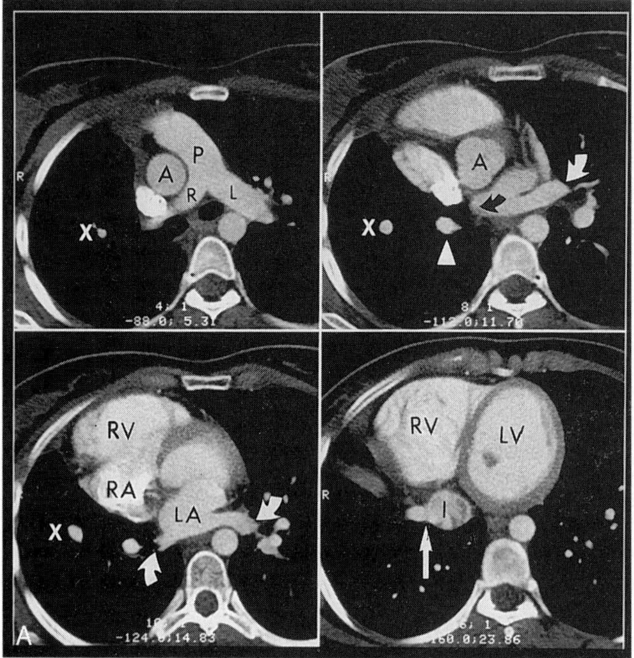

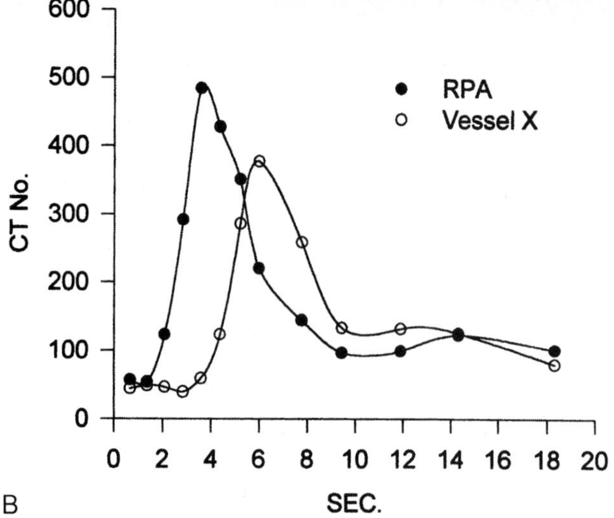

FIGURE 58–4. *A*, Selected tomograms from an adult with scimitar syndrome variant who has exertional dyspnea and wheezing. The right lung is hypoplastic, with the heart and great vessels shifted to the right. The right pulmonary artery (R) is smaller than the left (L). The lateral vessel (X) in the right lung is the right upper pulmonary vein draining to the inferior vena cava (*white straight arrow, lower right image*). The rest of the pulmonary veins (*curved white arrows*) return normally to the left atrium (LA). The black curved arrow in the upper right image shows the site of drainage of a normal right upper pulmonary vein. A = aorta; P = pulmonary artery; I = inferior vena cava; RV and LV = right and left ventricles. *B*, Time-density curves registered from vessel X and from the medial right pulmonary artery (RPA) branch (see *arrowhead, upper right image* in *A*). The two vessels are indiscernible on high-resolution images. The passage of contrast material through the medial RPA vessel matches that through the pulmonary artery, while vessel X flow is delayed, indicating that X is a pulmonary vein. The left-to-right shunt is small; hence, surgery was deemed unnecessary. UFCTs findings were confirmed on subsequent cardiac catheterization. QP/QS by oximetry was 1.2.

by vascular structures. Hyperinflation of the lungs from any cause limits the accuracy of echocardiography, especially in regard to the atrial septum and pulmonary arterial and venous anatomy.

In the past few years, other clinically useful noninvasive imaging systems have appeared. These include transesophageal echocardiography, magnetic resonance imaging, and UFCT, which can overcome many of the shortcomings of transthoracic echocardiography and, at the same time, obviate the need for frequent diagnostic cardiac catheterizations.

UFCT can be complementary to echocardiography by filling information gaps missed by the latter. Conversely, echocardiography may be complementary to UFCT for the same reason. In addition to providing the cardiac functional and blood flow parameters discussed above, UFCT's high-resolution imaging protocols provide exquisite anatomical details of the central veins, the heart, and the great vessels and main branches. The images are taken in the transverse plane, where the three spatial coordinates are well defined and can be used as a reference base for postimaging reconstruction in oblique planes to enhance critical anatomical structures. Tomographic slices that are 6-, 3-, or 1.5-mm-thick are acquired usually in diastole, to minimize motion artifacts. At least one flow mode study and one high-resolution study are performed whenever possible.

Abnormalities of Central Systemic Veins, the Atria, and Atrial Septum

The anatomy of abnormal central systemic veins can be well defined with UFCT. Superior and inferior vena cava obstruction from thrombi or after surgical interventions and anomalous drainage of a superior vena cava to the coronary sinus or directly to the left atrium with obligatory right-to-left shunt have been diagnosed.[21, 39] Figure 58–5 shows an anomalous right superior vein draining to the anatomical left atrium (the pulmonary venous atrium), causing obligatory right-to-left shunting in a patient with situs inversus. Details of numerous other lesions in this patient are nicely shown by UFCT's high-resolution images.

UFCT shows the anatomy of atriae with regard to size, morphology, and relationship to the atrioventricular valves and ventricles, and extracardiac structures as well. Recognition of the morphology of the atrial appendages helps define the visceroatrial situs. Defects of the atrial septum are easily diagnosed, based on the combined data from the multiple TDCs, together with the high-resolution images. Sinus venosus-type defects appear as defects in the posterior wall of the superior vena cava as it enters the right atrium. This lesion is frequently associated with abnormal drainage of one or more pulmonary veins into the cava or cava-atrial junction, which also can be determined by UFCT. The less frequent, inferiorly located sinus venosus defect near the entrance site of the inferior vena cava into the right atrium is also readily demonstrated. The most frequent type of atrial septal defects, the secundum atrial septal defect is also readily identified in virtually all patients, including adults. Because the thin membrane of the fossa ovalis may not be easily identifiable in some patients, careful evaluation of the time-density curves for presence or absence of left-to-right shunting is necessary. If present, the localization and relative magnitude of the shunt may be further derived from the curves. Also, a right-to-left shunt at rest or during Valsalva maneuver can be detected while one is investigating suspected paradoxical embolization in patients with unexplained systemic embolic disease.

Primum-type atrial septal defects are also easily diagnosed, usually as large defects at the inferior margin of the atrial septum.

Patients with transposition of the great vessels who have undergone a venous switch operation (Mustard or Senning procedures) may present as a difficult imaging problem. Echocardiography may fail to determine the patency of systemic and/or pulmonary venous channels or the presence of residual atrial shunting, especially in large patients. UFCT is exceptionally useful in these patients because the complex systemic and pulmonary venous pathways can be imaged in their entirety, and flow disturbances as well as residual shunting can be detected.[21, 26, 39, 40]

In UFCT studies in these patients, the author has identified superior and inferior vena cava obstruction isolated or with baffle disruption causing right-to-left shunting, intra-atrial baffle disruption causing left-to-right shunting, and pulmonary venous obstruction.[21, 26, 39]

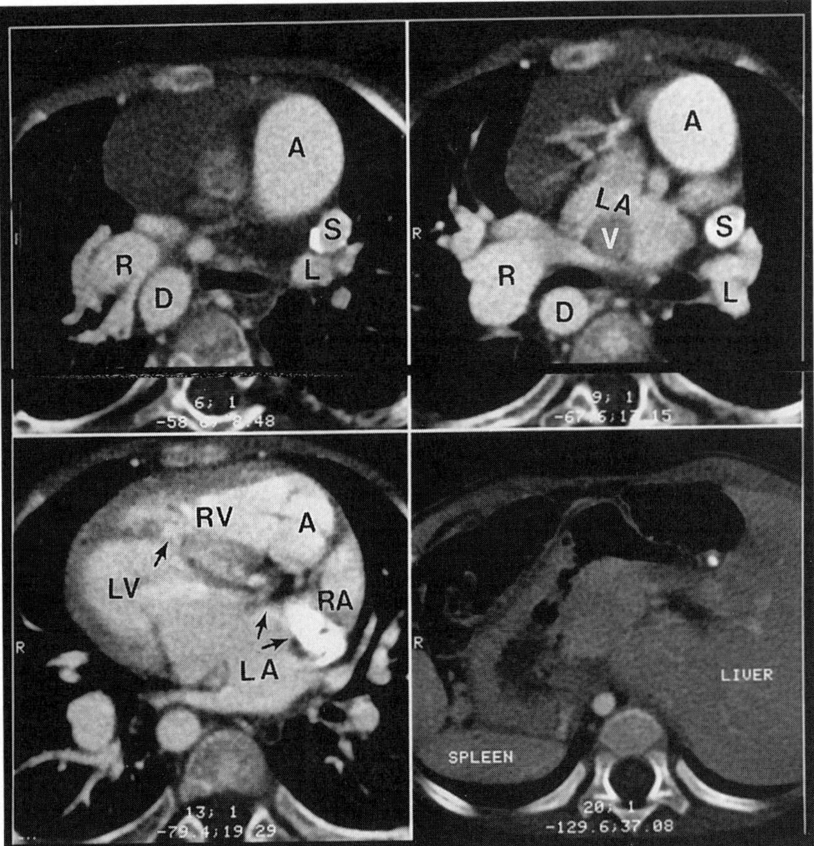

FIGURE 58–5. Selected images from a child with situs inversus, arterial transposition, pulmonary atresia, atrial and ventricular septal defects (*black arrows, lower left image*), and anomalous drainage of a right superior vein (V) to the anatomical left atrium (LA). The vein (V) flow causes an area of low contrast in the LA (*upper right image*). The superior vena cava (S) draining to the anatomical right atrium (RA) is on the patient's left, and the LA on the right. The anterior aorta (A) arises from the right ventricle (RV). The main pulmonary artery is atretic with a wide gap between right (R) and left (L) pulmonary arteries. Lower left image shows dextrocardia, and the lower right (from another patient) shows inversion of abdominal viscerae. LV = left ventricle; D = descending aorta. (Reprinted with permission from the American College of Cardiology, Heart House *Learning Center Highlights*, Vol. 6, No. 4, Summer 1991, pp. 1–7.)

Figures 58–6 and 58–7 are images from two patients with transposition of the great vessels who underwent multiple surgical procedures and whose residual complex cardiac lesions were identified only with UFCT imaging, whereas transthoracic and transesophageal echocardiography and cardiac catheterization failed to provide the complete diagnosis.

Abnormalities of the Ventricles, Valves, and Ventricular Septum

High-resolution UFCT images enable assessment of ventricular morphology and volume, even in severely hypoplastic ventricles. Inversion of the ventricles in corrected transposition (L-TGV) is recognized by the typical morphologic features particular to each ventricle; prominent trabeculae and a moderator band in the right ventricle and smooth intracavitary surface in the left ventricle (Fig. 58–8). Absolute ventricular volumes can be calculated.[41] Although atrioventricular valve anomalies, such as atresia, hypoplasia, and straddling, are readily recognized by CT imaging, the fine anatomical details of valve leaflets and chordae are not well defined because of the nature of their CT signal (a void of signal in a sea of high-density contrast). The information from echocardiography and UFCT is complementary in these situations. One can quantitate solitary valvular insufficiency by measuring regurgitant fraction and regurgitant volume.[42] Unlike echocardiography, UFCT is not very helpful in assessing atrioventricular and semilunar valve stenosis because no pressure data can be determined. However, it provides reliable information about annular size and ventricular muscle mass.

Ventricular septal defects of all types and locations are well defined by UFCT.[43] Incorporating flow information derived from time-density curves enhances the UFCT diagnosis, especially when dealing with the thin area of the membranous septum, where identification of a small septal defect can be quite deceptive.

Quantitation of the shunt is important because it is one of the major determinants of surgical feasibility after the functional size of the defect, for example, if it is getting smaller, and may aid in determining pulmonary vascular reactivity to vasodilators in long-standing defects with pulmonary hypertension.

Anomalies of Pulmonary Arteries and Veins

Definition of the anatomy of pulmonary arteries and veins is one of the most useful contributions of UFCT to the study of patients with CHD. The pulmonary trunk, right and left main branches, and lobar arteries, especially to the lower lobes, are well identified in the vast majority of patients, regardless of vessel size or etiology of vessel abnormality. Native and postoperative stenosis, occlusion, and distortion of pulmonary arteries have been described.[21, 26, 39] In pulmonary obstruction caused by embolism, UFCT is almost as accurate as pulmonary angiography for clinically significant obstruction and is superior to nuclear ventilation-perfusion scanning.[44] In another study,[28] identification of emboli by high-resolution imaging, combined with regional lung perfusion, determined by UFCT time-

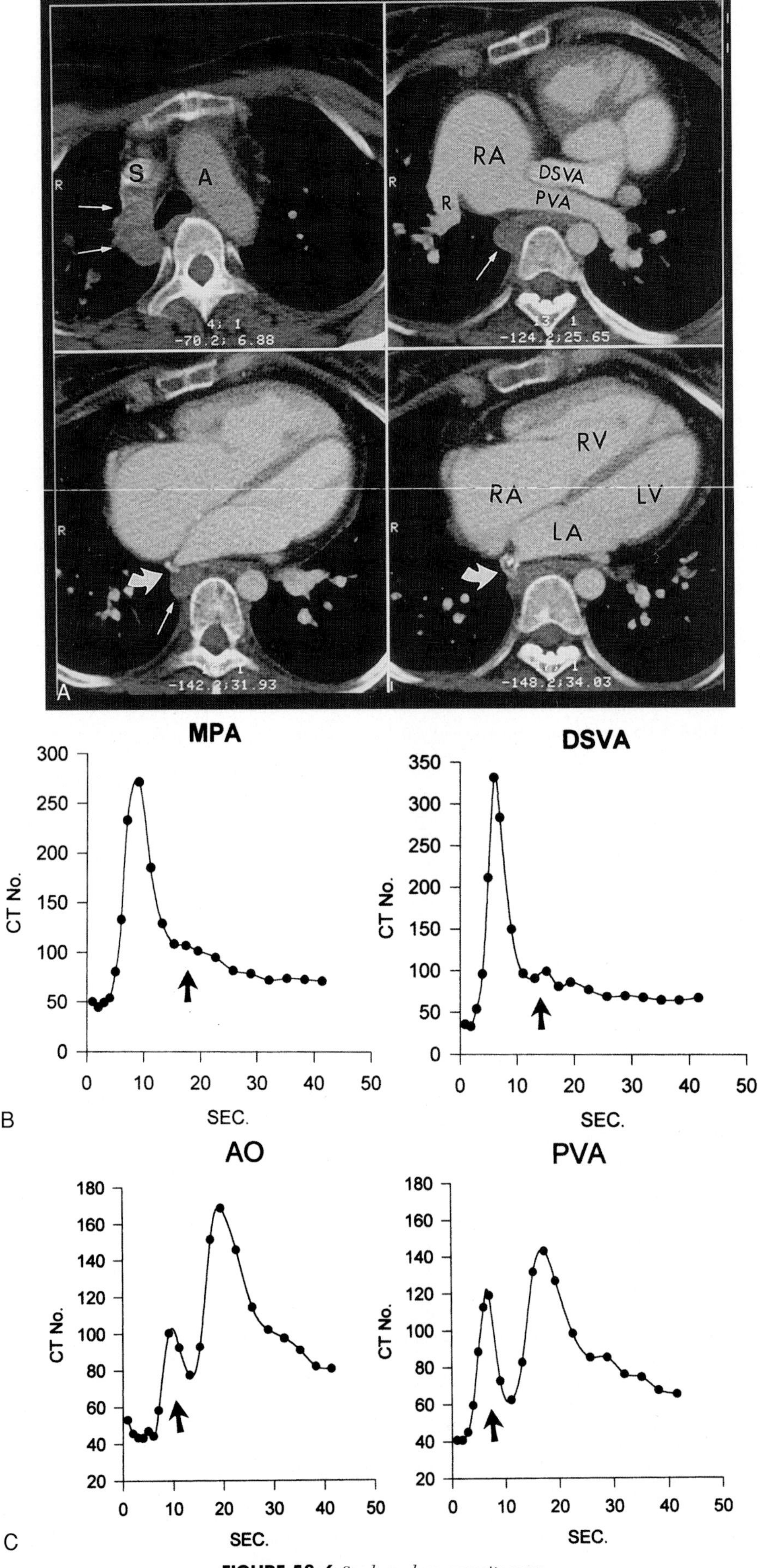

FIGURE 58–6 *See legend on opposite page*

density curves allowed demonstration of obstruction from main pulmonary artery to the fourth segmentation branches. Figures 58–5, 58–9, 58–10, and 58–12 are examples of the exquisite anatomical and flow information UFCT obtained on very abnormal pulmonary arteries.

Partial anomalous pulmonary venous drainage of all types, whether isolated or in combination with an atrial septal defect or other lesions, have been well demonstrated by UFCT at The Heart Institute for Children, Christ Hospital & Medical Center, Oak Lawn, IL.[21, 26, 39, 45] Figure 58–11 shows detailed anatomy of a patient with partial anomalous venous return to the superior vena cava preoperatively and postoperatively, revealing abnormal hemodynamics that is very difficult to demonstrate with other imaging techniques or pressure measurements. Several patients with total anomalous pulmonary venous return, in the context of asplenia syndrome and postoperative pulmonary venous stenosis, have also been diagnosed by means of this technique.

Abnormalities of the Aorta

Anomalies of the aorta such as malposition, hypoplasia, dilation, and dissection are readily identified by UFCT. Coarctation of the aorta and airway compression caused by vascular rings have also been diagnosed, including clear demonstration of the components of the ring and the extent of airway compression.[2, 46]

Evaluation of the Postoperative Patient

In the long-term follow-up of postoperative patients, in which echocardiography is somehow unable to provide complete information, UFCT may be the imaging system of choice before proceeding to cardiac catheterization. This obviates the need for repeated cardiac catheterizations. UFCT readily provides information about residual shunting, systemic and pulmonary venous obstruction, localization of site of narrowing in obstructed right ventricle-to-pulmonary artery conduits or systemic-to-pulmonary artery shunts. The patency and blood flow characteristics of patients with cavopulmonary repair for single ventricular equivalent (Glenn and Fontan operations) and baffle obstructions after venous switch repair for d-transposition of the great vessels (Mustard and Senning procedures) are also easily diagnosed.

THREE-DIMENSIONAL RECONSTRUCTION

Treatment of patients with congenital heart disease demands full understanding of the cardiac anatomy, specifically of the cardiac defects to be repaired, in three dimensions. The original cardiac imaging systems, such as angiography, produced projection images in two dimensions, necessitating mental reconstruction of the displayed images to formulate a three-dimensional format. However, this system, although still the most popular imaging system for routine clinical work, suffers from overlapping of structures, not to mention its invasive nature. Now, three-dimensional imaging systems, namely, magnetic resonance, volumetrically acquired echocardiography, and computed tomography, are available and can provide truly three-dimensional data. Although conventional CT can provide adequate three-dimensional images of vascular structures such as the aorta, carotid, and renal arteries, three-dimensional images of the heart can be provided only by means of a rapid acquisition machine, such as UFCT and the digital spatial reconstructor.[47, 48]

With the use of dedicated software,[49] the reconstruction process involves realigning the tomograms in relation to a fixed reference system in the imaging field. Two reconstruction techniques appear to be the most informative, especially for studying congenital cardiac defects. *Surface reconstruction* highlights the boundaries of the anatomical structures in question and can be shown either as a "cast" (i.e., an intraluminal cavity) or as a "shell" (i.e., cardiac and vascular walls).[47] Figure 58–12*A* and *B* shows three-dimensional reconstructions of the pulmonary arterial tree in an adolescent with complex native anatomy and further distortion after multiple surgeries.

The second reconstruction technique, called *maximum intensity projection*, is used in magnetic resonance and CT angiography to study the anatomy of blood vessels. Voxels with the highest density are isolated to reconstruct the vascular anatomy, which can be viewed from any projection. The three-dimensional image can be electronically dissected to highlight anatomical interrelationships or sliced by flat or curved planes to expose the anatomy in question. The routine use of three-dimensional reconstruction is likely to improve greatly our assessment of patients with congenital heart disease through the application of new parameters of cardiac function that may be more predictive of cardiac overload and decompensation and new surgical techniques that optimize the use of remaining native tissues.

At this time, the three-dimensional reconstruction process is still labor-intensive and cannot be done on a routine basis. However, rapid improvements in software and computer technology, complemented by increasing interest in the subject, are likely to make this technology increasingly available for clinical use in the near future. It will undoubtedly improve the diagnosis and management of CHD in the future.

CONCLUSIONS AND FUTURE DEVELOPMENTS

The major obstacles to CT imaging in CHD at present are the long imaging time of the ubiquitous conventional scanners and the limited number of UFCT scanners available (only 57 worldwide, as compared with more than 1000 magnetic resonance imaging scanners in the United States alone), with only a handful involved in the diagnosis or study of congenital heart disease. This situation may change, however, because the scanner can be used also for routine extracardiac studies. Moreover, the cost of the equipment is likely to decrease as more scanners are produced, making them affordable for many centers.

Text continued on page 886

FIGURE 58–6. *A*, Selected images from an adult with transposition of the great arteries who underwent Baffe's palliation in infancy (translocation of right pulmonary veins to right atrium, ligation of proximal inferior vena cava and homograft interposition between distal inferior vena cava and left atrium), followed a few years later by Mustard venous switch repair. High contrast in the superior vena cava (S) is washed out by low contrast flow from a markedly enlarged azygous vein (*straight arrows*) caused by inferior vena cava homograft calcification and occlusion (*curved arrows, lower images*). The patient had large varicose veins and hepatic dysfunction. The distal systemic venous tunnel (DSVA), draining to the anatomical left ventricle (LV), is widely patent. The right pulmonary veins (R) and the tunnel from the left pulmonary veins (PVA) to the anatomical right atrium (RA) are also widely patent. Compare these images with those of the patient in Figure 58–7. LA, RA, LV, and RV = left and right atria and ventricles. *B*, Time-density curve from main pulmonary artery (MPA) of patient in *A* shows a small left-right shunt (*arrow*) that is traced back to the distal systemic venous atrium (*arrow, DSVA*). *C*, A right-left shunt is detected in the aorta (AO) in patient in *A*. The pulmonary venous atrium (PVA, right upper image, in *A*) is the first site to show shunt effect. There was a baffle leak in this area that caused bidirectional shunting.

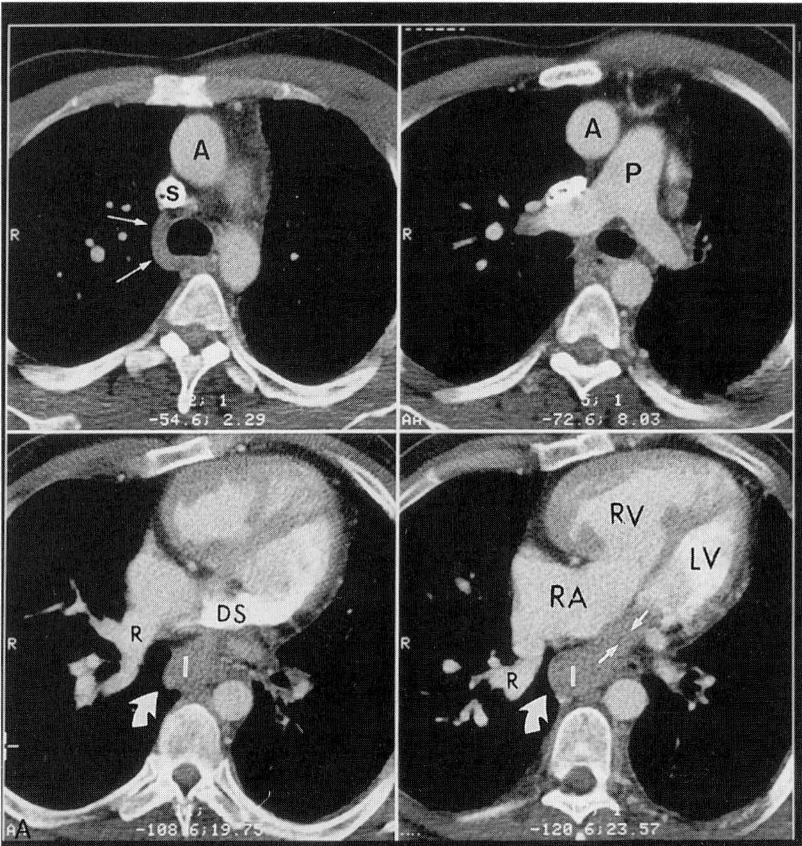

FIGURE 58–7. *A*, Selected images from an adult with transposition of the great vessels (*upper right* image) who underwent the same surgical procedures as the patient in Figure 58–6. The high contrast in the superior vena cava (S) is preserved with normal-sized azygous vein (*long straight arrows, upper left* image). The distal portion of systemic venous tunnel (DS, *lower left* image) is widely patent, with contrast washout at lower levels (*short straight arrows, lower right image*) caused by low contrast flow from inferior vena cava (I). The right pulmonary veins (R) are widely patent, whereas the left are obstructed (compare with those of patient in Figure 58–6). Note right ventricular (RV) hypertrophy in both patients and thicker left ventricular (LV) walls in patient in Figure 58–7 due to pulmonary hypertension. (Abbreviations as in previous figures.) RA = right atrium; P = main pulmonary artery.

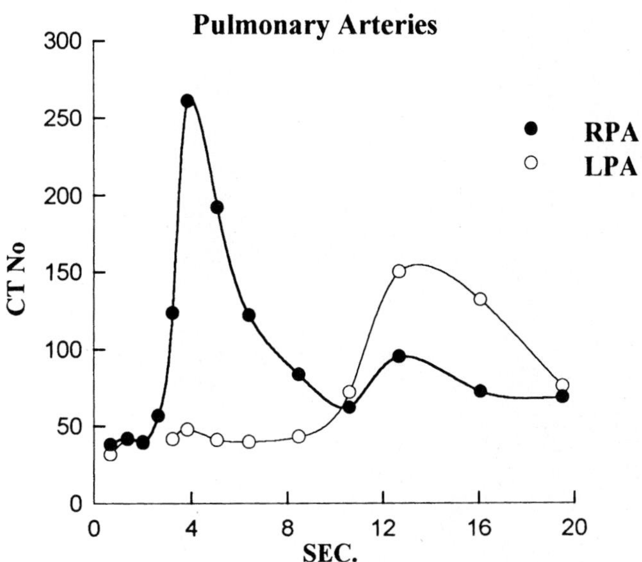

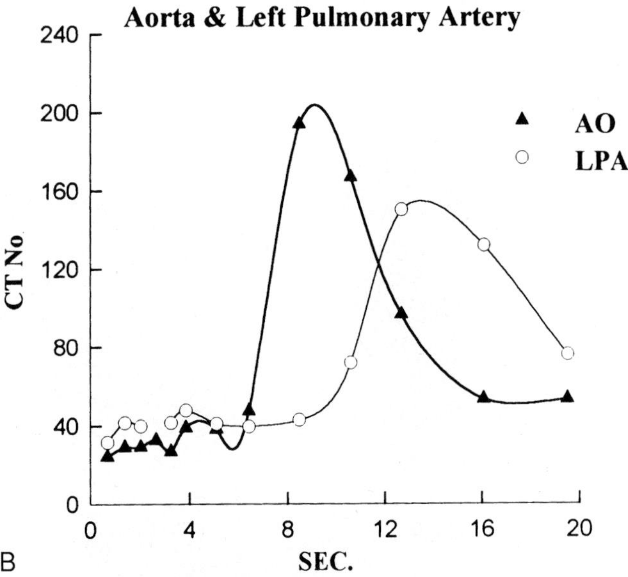

FIGURE 58–7 *Continued B*, Time-density curves in pulmonary arteries of patient in *A* show marked delay in contrast appearance and peaking in the left pulmonary artery (LPA), as compared with the right (RPA), despite a widely patent LPA (*upper right image* in *A*). LPA contrast appears even later than that in the aorta (AO) (lower curves, *B*). Subsequent cardiac catheterization showed no forward LPA flow on pulmonary angiography and retrograde LPA opacification via bronchial collaterals on aortography. The reversed flow from LPA to RPA caused by severe left pulmonary vein obstruction accounts for the second RPA peak. (*B* From Emmanouilides, G. C., Riemenschneider, T. A., Allen, H. D., et al. [eds.]: Moss & Adams' Heart Disease in Infants, Children, and Adolescents, Including the Fetus and Young Adult. 5th ed. Baltimore, Williams & Wilkins, 1995, p. 204, with permission.)

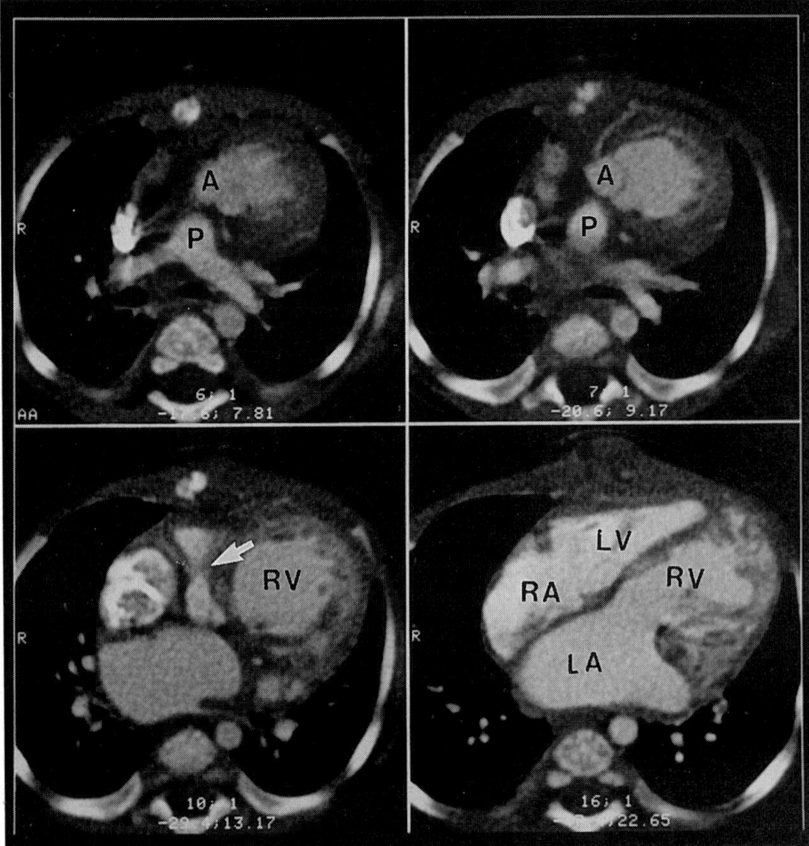

FIGURE 58–8. A 9-month-old child with ventricular inversion (congenitally corrected or levotransposition of great arteries) subpulmonic stenosis, and Ebstein malformation of the tricuspid valve, after valvuloplasty and annuloplasty. The aorta (A) with the left coronary artery is anterior and to the left of the pulmonary artery (P) (*upper images*). There is a muscular subaortic conus (*upper right image*) and subpulmonary obstruction (*arrow, lower left image*). The left-sided ventricle is anatomically a right ventricle with its valve inserted more apically than its counterpart. There is marked enlargement of the left chambers. LA, RA, LV, and RV = anatomical left and right atria and ventricles.

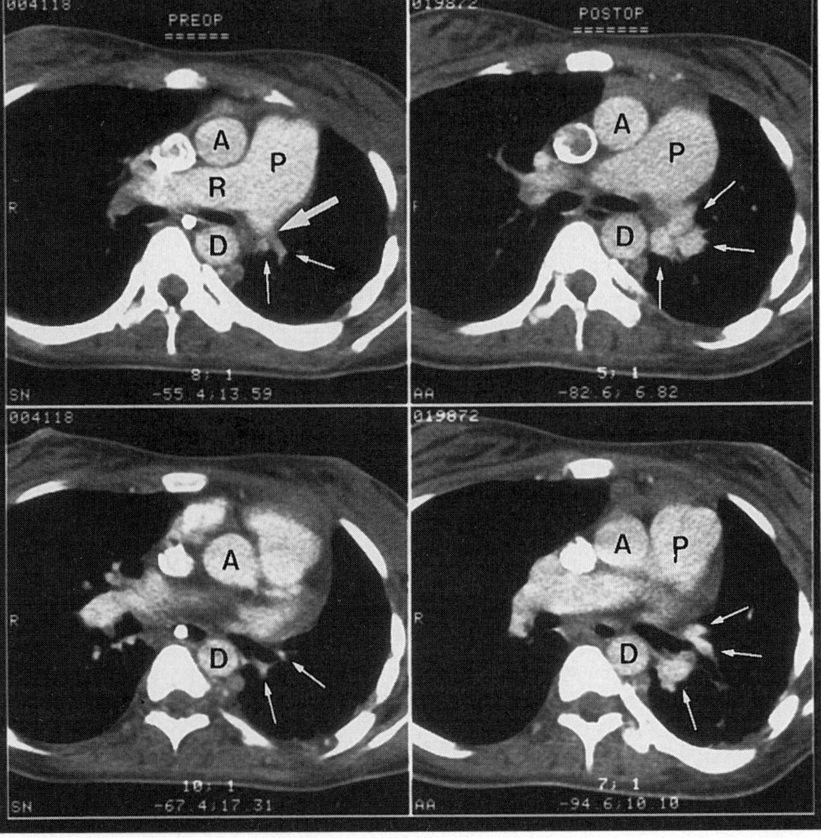

FIGURE 58–9. A 15-year-old patient 14 years after accidental ligation of the left pulmonary artery (LPA) instead of a large patent ductus arteriosus (PDA) done at another institution. Left images taken before surgical left pulmonary artery angioplasty show the site of that artery's ligation (*thick arrow, upper left image*) and severe hypoplasia of its distal branches (*thin arrows, left images*). Postoperative slices almost at the same levels (*right images*) show marked enlargement of central and peripheral left pulmonary artery branches (*thin arrows, right images*). A and D = ascending and descending aorta; P = main pulmonary artery; R = right pulmonary artery.

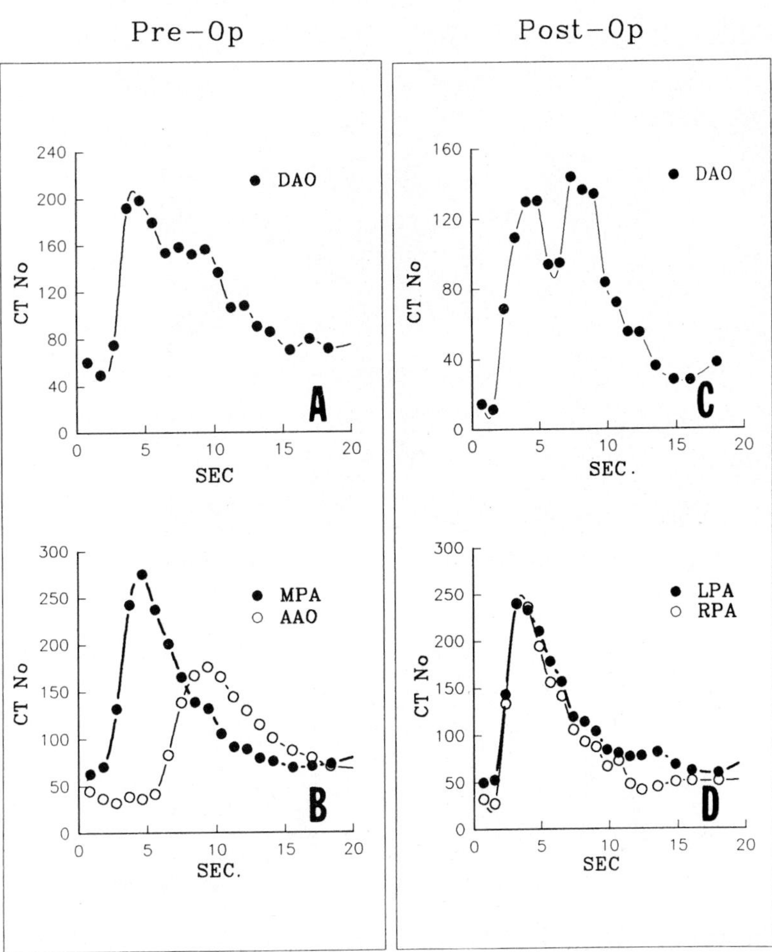

FIGURE 58–10. Selected time-density curves from the patient in Figure 58–9 before (Pre-Op) and after (Post-Op) surgical left pulmonary artery (LPA) enlargement. *A*, The descending aorta (DAO) curve preoperatively has two peaks, the origins of which are clarified by examining main pulmonary artery (MPA) and ascending aorta (AAO) curves in *B*. The first peak in *A* is caused by a large right-to-left shunt of MPA blood shunted via the PDA because of pulmonary hypertension. The second peak in *A* is caused by contrast material traversing the lungs and reaching the descending aorta via the ascending aorta. Postoperatively, the second DAO peak is significantly higher (*C*) because of increased flow to the left lung. LPA flow, not detectable preoperatively, matches that of the right pulmonary artery (RPA) (*D*). DAO oxygen saturation increased by 8 percent postoperatively.

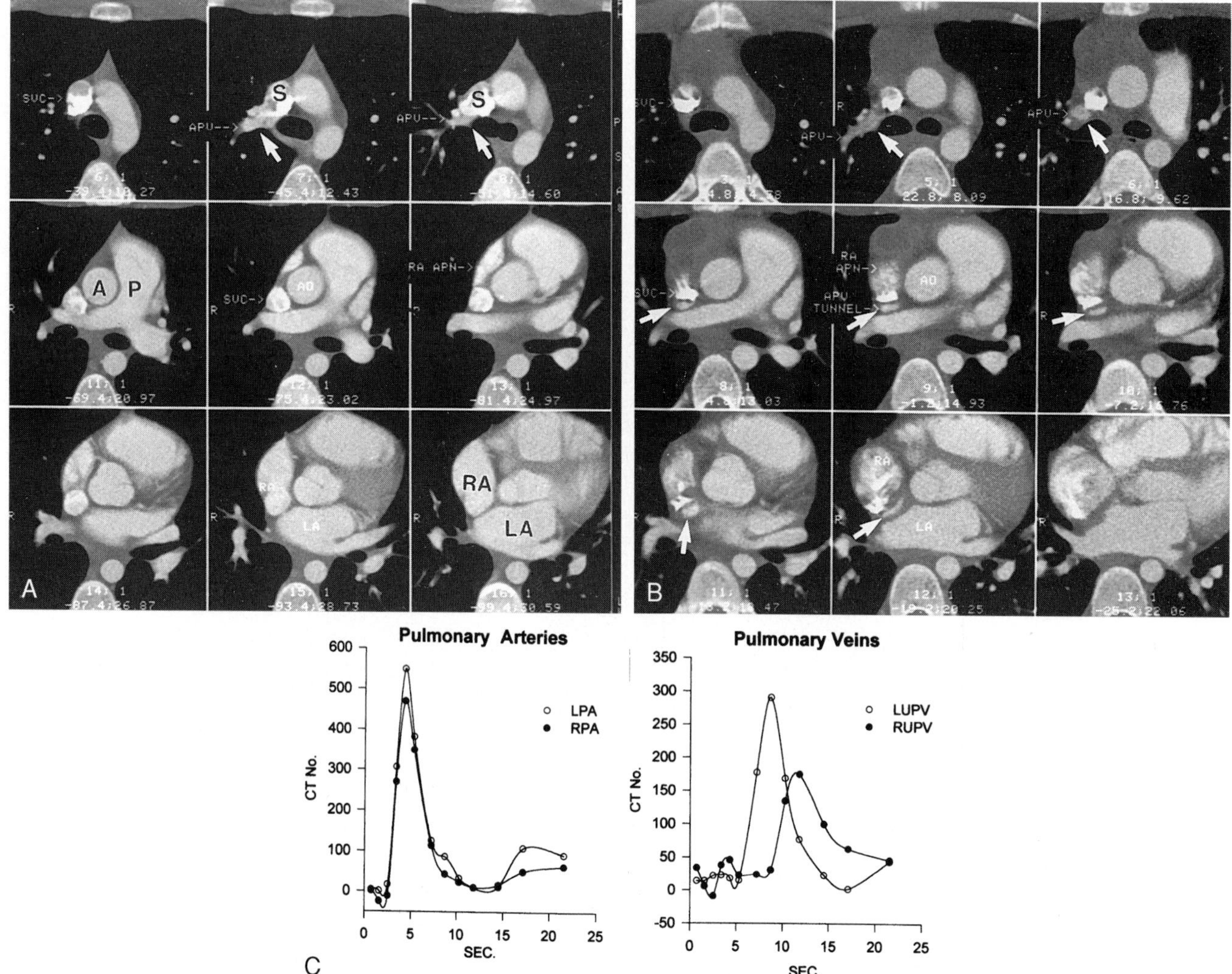

FIGURE 58–11. *A*, Preoperative tomograms from an adolescent with right upper pulmonary vein (*white arrows*) draining to the superior vena cava (S) and a ventricular septal defect. A = aorta; P = pulmonary artery; RA APN = right atrial appendage; RA and LA = right and left atria. *B*, Postoperative images almost at the same level as in *A*. The ventricular septal defect was patched, and APV was tunneled inside the superior vena cava (*arrows*) to the left atrium. To avoid SVC obstruction, the right atrium appendage was used to enlarge the superior vena cava anteriorly (*middle images*). *C*, Postoperative, simultaneous time-density curves obtained in pulmonary arteries (LPA and RPA) and upper pulmonary veins (RUPV and LUPV) of patient in *B*. Although the RUPV tunnel is patent (*arrows* in *B*), contrast flow in the RUPV is much delayed and, when it is compared with that in LUPV, indicates obstruction to flow. The variations in baseline data points 2 to 5 in RUPV curve are due to passage of high-density contrast in the adjoining superior vena cava. The baseline stabilizes thereafter (points 6 to 8). There is no residual left-to-right shunt.

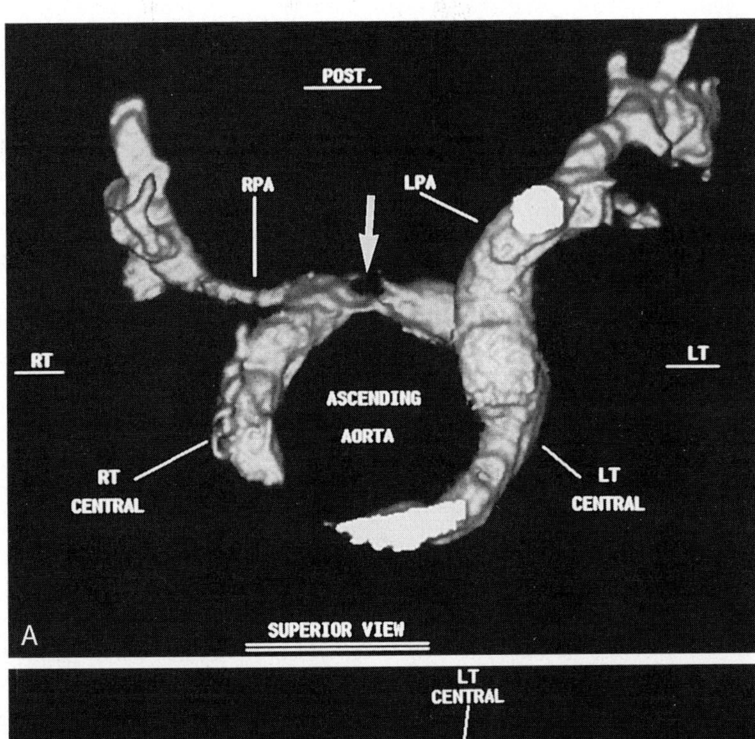

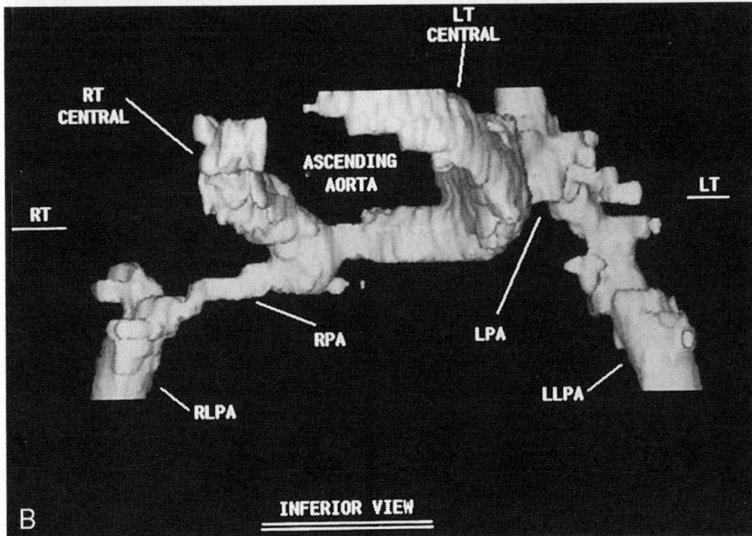

FIGURE 58–12. *A and B*, Three-dimensional reconstructions of the pulmonary arterial system in an adolescent with pulmonary atresia and ventricular septal defect after multiple surgical systemic-pulmonary shunts. *A* approximates the surgical view, showing widely patent left central aorta (LT central) to native main pulmonary artery shunt and adequately sized left pulmonary artery (LPA). Both *A* and *B* show also widely patent right central shunt (RT central), discrete severe proximal stenosis (*white arrow* in *A*) and long-segment distal right pulmonary artery (RPA) stenosis. The lower lobe branches (RLPA and LLPA in *B*) are of normal size. Post = posterior.

Because transthoracic echocardiography provides the diagnostic information needed in most patients with CHD, UFCT is currently used only when the echocardiographic data are incomplete for a variety of reasons, including complexity of anatomical structures. The latter situation arises in large patients with hyperinflated lungs and in patients who require evaluation of central pulmonary arteries and major intrapulmonary branches, where there is a need to assess regional pulmonary flow and perfusion in the presence of arterial or venous stenosis or occlusion. It also occurs in anomalies of pulmonary veins, shunt lesions, investigation of complex lesions involving extra cardiac organs, and when there is a need to assess shunt lesions through multiple dye-dilution curves as discussed previously.

The disadvantages of UFCT include the need for intravenous injections of iodinated contrast, the need for sedation in small children, exposure to ionizing radiation, the inability to measure pressures directly, and equipment that is not portable. UFCT does not show anatomical details of the valves, and the high-resolution, thin-image slices are static in systole or diastole. Ongoing improvements in the UFCT scanner, such as a greater number of slices per study, faster acquisition of high-resolution images, and respiratory gating,[50] in addition to ongoing research in the areas of x-ray generation and data processing, the search for new contrast agents with more predictable physiologic properties, and improvements in computer technology and software,[51] are likely to increase the usefulness of computed tomography for the evaluation of children and adults with CHD.

References

1. Perloff, J. K.: Congenital heart disease in adults. Circulation 84:1881, 1991.
2. Eldredge, W. J.: Comprehensive evaluation of congenital heart disease using ultrafast computed tomography. *In* Marcus M. (ed.): Marcus' Cardiac Imaging: A Companion to Braunwald's Heart Disease. Philadelphia, W. B. Saunders, 1990, p. 714.
3. Rumberger, J. A.: Principles and practice of cardiac edge-detection and border definition using ultrafast computed tomography. *In* Stanford, W., and Rumberger, J. A. (eds.): Ultrafast Computed Tomography in Cardiac Imaging: Principles and Practice. Mt. Kisco, N.Y., Futura, 1992, p. 25.
4. Zierler, K.: Theoretical basis of indicator-dilution methods for measuring flow and volume. Circ. Res. 10:393, 1962.
5. Wood, E.: Diagnostic applications of indicator-dilution techniques in congenital heart disease. Circ. Res. 10:531, 1962.
6. Antman, S.: Foundations of indicator-dilution theory. *In* Bloomfield, D. A. (ed.): Dye Curves: The Theory and Practice of Indicator Dilution. Baltimore, University Park Press, 1974, p. 21.
7. Meier, P., and Zierler, K. L.: On the theory of the indicator-dilution method for measurement of blood flow and volume. J. Appl. Physiol. 6:731, 1954.
8. Hamilton, W. F., Moore, J. W., Kinsman, J. M., et al.: Studies on the circulation. IV. Further analysis of the injection method and of changes in hemodynamics under physiological and pathological conditions. Am. J. Physiol. 99:534, 1932.
9. Stewart, G. N.: Researches on the circulation time and on the influences which affect it. IV. The output of the heart. J. Physiol. 22:159, 1897.
10. Reiter, S. J., Feiring, A. J., Rumberger, J. A., et al.: Precise measurement of contrast clearance curve cardiac outputs by cine CT. (Abstract.) J. Am. Coll. Cardiol. 9:161, 1987.
11. Rumberger, J. A., and Bell, M. R.: Measurement of myocardial perfusion and cardiac output using intravenous injection methods by ultrafast (cine) computed tomography. Invest. Radiol. 27:S40, 1992.
12. Ludman, P., Darby, M., Tomlinson, N., et al.: Cardiac flow measurement by ultrafast CT: Validation of continuous and pulsatile flow. J. Comput. Assist. Tomogr. 16(5):795, 1992.
13. Ritman, E. L.: Myocardial capillary permeability to iohexol evaluation with fast x-ray computed tomography. Invest. Radiol. 29:612, 1994.
14. Canty, J., Judd, R., Brody, A., et al.: First-pass entry of nonionic contrast agent into the myocardial extravascular space: Effects on radiographic estimates of transit time and blood volume. Circulation 84:2071, 1991.
15. Krovetz, L. J.: Detection and quantification of intracardiac and great vessel shunts. *In* Bloomfield, D. A. (ed.): Dye Curves: The Theory and Practice of Indicator Dilution. Baltimore, University Park Press, 1974, p. 119.
16. Parker, J., and Treves, S.: Radionuclide detection, localization, and quantitation of intracardiac shunts and shunts between the great vessels. Prog. Cerebrovasc. Dis. 20(2):121, 1977.
17. Alderson, P.: Basic principles of shunt quantitation by radionuclide angiography. Appl. Radiol./NM, Nov.–Dec. 1980, pp. 162–170.
18. Thompson, H. K., Starmer, F. C., Whalen, R. E., et al.: Indicator transit time considered as a gamma variate. Circ. Res. 14:502, 1964.
19. MacMillan, R., Rees, M., Eldredge, W. J., et al.: Quantitation of shunting at the atrial level using rapid acquisition computed tomography with comparison with cardiac catheterization. J. Am. Coll. Cardiol. 7:946, 1986.
20. Skotnicki, R., MacMillan, R., Rees, M., et al.: Detection of atrial septal defect by contrast-enhanced ultrafast computed tomography. Cathet. Cardiovasc. Diagn. 12:103, 1986.
21. Husayni, T.: Ultrafast computed tomographic imaging in congenital heart disease. *In* Stanford, W., and Rumberger, J. A. (eds.): Ultrafast Computed Tomography in Cardiac Imaging: Principles and Practice. Mt. Kisco, N.Y., Futura, 1992, p. 311.
22. Garrett, J., Jaschke, W., Aherne, T., et al.: Quantitation of intracardiac shunts by cine CT. J. Comput. Assist. Tomogr. 12:82, 1988.
23. Nakamura, M., Suzuki, Y., Nagasawa, T., et al.: Detection and quantitation of left-to-right shunts from radionuclide angiocardiography using the homomorphic deconvolution technique. IEEE Trans. Biomed. Eng. 29:192, 1982.
24. Sinclair-Smith, B. C.: Measurement of valvular insufficiency. *In* Bloomfield, D. A. (ed.): Dye Curves: The Theory and Practice of Indicator Dilution. Baltimore, University Park Press, 1974, p. 145.
25. Stanford, W., and Rumberger, J. A.: Assessment of bypass graft patency and flow. *In* Ultrafast Computed Tomography in Cardiac Imaging: Principles and Practice. Mt. Kisco, N.Y. Futura, 1992, p. 97.
26. Husayni, T.: Computed tomography. *In* Emmanouilides, G.C., Riemenschneider, T. A., Allen, H. D., et al. (eds.): Moss & Adams' Heart Disease in Infants, Children, and Adolescents, Including the Fetus and Young Adult. Baltimore, Williams & Wilkins 1995, p. 190.
27. Wolfkiel, C. J., and Rich, S.: Analysis of regional pulmonary enhancement in dogs by ultrafast computed tomography. Invest. Radiol. 27:211, 1992.
28. Aschauer, M., Groll, R., Pilger, E., et al.: Pulmonary embolism: Diagnosis and follow-up after fibrinolytic therapy with electron beam tomography. (Abstract.) Am. J. Card. Imaging 8(Suppl. 1):6, 1994.
29. Rumberger, J.: Quantifying left ventricular regional and global systolic function using ultrafast computed tomography. Am. J. Card. Imaging 5:29, 1991.
30. Roig, E., Georgiou, D., Chomka, E., et al.: Reproducibility of left ventricular myocardial volume and mass measurements by ultrafast computed tomography. J. Am. Coll. Cardiol. 18:990, 1991.
31. Rumberger, J., Bell, M., Sheedy, P., et al.: Use of ultrafast computed tomography to assess early diastolic filling of the left ventricle in humans. Am. J. Card. Imaging 4:130, 1990.
32. Rumberger, J., Weiss, R., Feiring, A., et al.: Patterns of regional diastolic function in the normal human left ventricle: An ultrafast computed tomographic study. J. Am. Coll. Cardiol. 14:119, 1989.
33. Marzullo, P., L'Abbate, A., and Marcus, M.: Patterns of global and regional systolic and diastolic function in the normal right ventricle assessed by ultrafast computed tomography. J. Am. Coll. Cardiol. 17:1318, 1991.
34. Reiter, S. J., Rumberger, J. A., Feiring, A. J., et al.: Precision of right and left ventricular stroke volume measurements by rapid acquisition cine computed tomography. Circulation 74:890, 1986.
35. Chomka, E., and Brundage, B.: Left ventricular evaluation by exercise ultrafast computed tomography. *In* Stanford, W., and Rumberger, J. A. (eds.): Ultrafast Computed Tomography in Cardiac Imaging: Principles and Practice. Mt. Kisco, N.Y., Futura, 1992, p. 139.
36. Hajduczok, A. D., and Weiss, R. M.: Right ventricular mass can be accurately assessed by ultrafast computed tomography. Clin. Res. 36:821A, 1988.
37. Rich, S., Chomka, E. V., Stagl, R., et al.: Determination of left ventricular ejection fraction using ultrafast computed tomography. Am. Heart J. 112:392, 1986.
38. Lessick, J., Sideman, S., Azhari, H., et al.: Regional three dimensional geometry and function of left ventricles with fibrous aneurysms: Cine computed tomography study. Circulation 84:1072, 1991.
39. Husayni, T.: Ultrafast CT imaging of congenital heart disease in children and adults. Heart House Learning Center Highlights 6:1, 1991.
40. Matherne, G. P., Frey, E. E., Atkins, D. L., et al.: Cine computed tomography for diagnosis of superior vena cava obstruction following the mustard operation. Pediatr. Radiol. 17:246, 1987.
41. Hajduczok, W., Weiss, R., Stanford, W., et al.: Determination of right ventricular mass in humans and dogs with ultrafast cardiac computed tomography. Circulation 82:202, 1990.
42. Reiter, S. J., Rumberger, J. A., Stanford, W., et al.: Quantitative determination of aortic regurgitant volumes in dogs by ultrafast computed tomography. Circulation 76:728, 1987.
43. Eldredge, W. J., Rees, M. R., Flicker, S., et al.: Cine CT scanning of the ventricular septum for the diagnosis of ventricular septal defect. (Abstract.) Circulation 72(Suppl. 3):27, 1985.
44. Sheedy, P. F., II: Mayo Clinic, diagnostic radiology. (Abstract.) Am. J. Card. Imaging 8(Suppl. 1):6, 1994.
45. DeLeon, S., Ilbawi, M., Husayni, T., et al.: Surgical techniques in partial anomalous pulmonary veins to the superior vena cava. Ann. Thorac. Surg. 55:1222, 1993.
46. Kao, S., and Kimura, K.: Utility of electron-beam computed tomograph (EBCT) in the dynamic assessment of pediatric trachea. (Abstract.) Am. J. Card. Imaging 8(Suppl 1):8, 1994.
47. Hoffman, E. A.: A historical perspective of heart and lung 3D imaging. *In*: 3D Imaging in Medicine, Vol. 11. Boca Raton, Fla., CRC Press, 1991, p. 285.
48. Liu, Y. H., Hoffman, E. A., and Ritman, E. L.: Measurement of three-dimensional anatomy and function of pulmonary arteries with high-speed x-ray computed tomography. Invest. Radiol. 22:28, 1987.
49. Hemmy, D. C., and Brigman, P. M.: A comparison of modalities. *In*: 3D Imaging in Medicine, Vol. 5. Boca Raton, Fla., CRC Press, 1991, p. 89.
50. Mori, M., Murata, K., Takahashi, M., et al.: Accurate contiguous sections without breath-holding on chest CT: Value of respiratory gating in ultrafast CT. (Abstract.) Am. J. Card. Imaging 8(Suppl. 1):7, 1994.
51. Ritman, E.: Fast computed tomography for quantitative cardiac analysis: State of the art and future perspectives. Mayo Clin. Proc. 65:1336, 1990.

PART 7

RADIONUCLIDE IMAGING

CHAPTER

59 Principles and Instrumentation

Ernest V. Garcia, Ph.D.
John R. Votaw, Ph.D.
S. James Cullom, Ph.D.
James R. Galt, Ph.D.
C. David Cooke, M.S.E.E.

PRINCIPLES OF RADIATION DETECTION

Radionuclide imaging is based on the ability to detect electromagnetic radiation emitted from an injected radioactive tracer that has been taken up by the myocardium or mixed in the cardiac blood pool. The electromagnetic radiation used is in the form of a γ-ray or an x-ray, depending on whether it originated in the nucleus or from transitions of the orbital electrons. Ideally, this radiation should not interact with the patient and should be totally absorbed by the detector, which is usually a sodium iodide (NaI) crystal. The main interactions of γ-rays (or x-rays) with matter are photoelectric absorption and Compton scattering. These interactions cause attenuation and scatter of the beam of γ-rays from the point at which the radiation was emitted in the patient. The result is tissue ionization and, ultimately, a small radiation absorbed dose (rad) deposited in the patient, roughly equivalent to that from a standard chest radiograph. The γ-rays that are not absorbed by the patient can potentially be detected by scintigraphic devices.

Scintillation Counter

The fundamental principles that govern how scintigraphic devices detect radiation can be explained by a description of the basic detector unit, called the scintillation counter. Two principles are used by this device: scintillation and photodetection.

Scintillation

A suitable material, such as a sodium iodide thallium–activated [NaI(Tl)] crystal, is used to stop the radiation to be measured. The γ-ray interacts with the crystal in the same manner as with the patient, that is, by photoelectric absorption and Compton scattering. The result of this interaction is the ejection of a high-speed electron from an atom in the crystal. This energetic electron disturbs other atoms in its path and creates pairs of ions in numbers proportional to its total kinetic energy. Within the NaI(Tl) crystal, an additional phenomenon takes place. The ion pairs migrate in the crystal until they are trapped by an impurity (such as thallium), which causes the emission of a photon of light for each ion pair. A large number of visible photons, directly proportional to the energy of the γ-ray, are emitted for each γ-ray absorbed by the crystal. This large number of visible photons gives rise to a burst of visible light known as a scintillation.

Photodetection

Although there are many visible photons emitted in each scintillation, their number is still not high enough to be seen by the naked eye. The burst of visible light (photons) is converted into an electrical pulse by a light-sensitive device known as a photomultiplier tube (Fig. 59–1). This device is coupled optically to the crystal in order to gather as many of the visible photons as possible. The photomultiplier detects the visible photons by means of a thin plate known as a photocathode, which releases electrons in proportion to the number of photons striking it. This signal is then amplified by acceleration of these released electrons through a series of plates, known as dynodes, which multiply the number of electrons striking them in proportion to the voltage difference between the plates. As this interaction is repeated through 10 plates and a voltage difference of hundreds of volts, the original number of electrons is amplified by a factor of approximately 1 million. The electrons are collected by a plate known as the anode and shaped by a preamplifier in order to generate an electrical pulse. The voltage (height) of this pulse, which is created by a single scintillation, is directly proportional to the amount of light released by the crystal, which in turn is directly proportional to the energy of the γ-ray that was absorbed by the crystal. Each of these pulses could be counted by a scaler, without regard for its energy, to measure the number of γ-rays absorbed by the crystal.

Determination of the energy of the γ-ray that was absorbed by the crystal is important because it allows selection of different radionuclides with different energies or elimination of the less energetic, scattered photons from the patient. A pulse height ana-

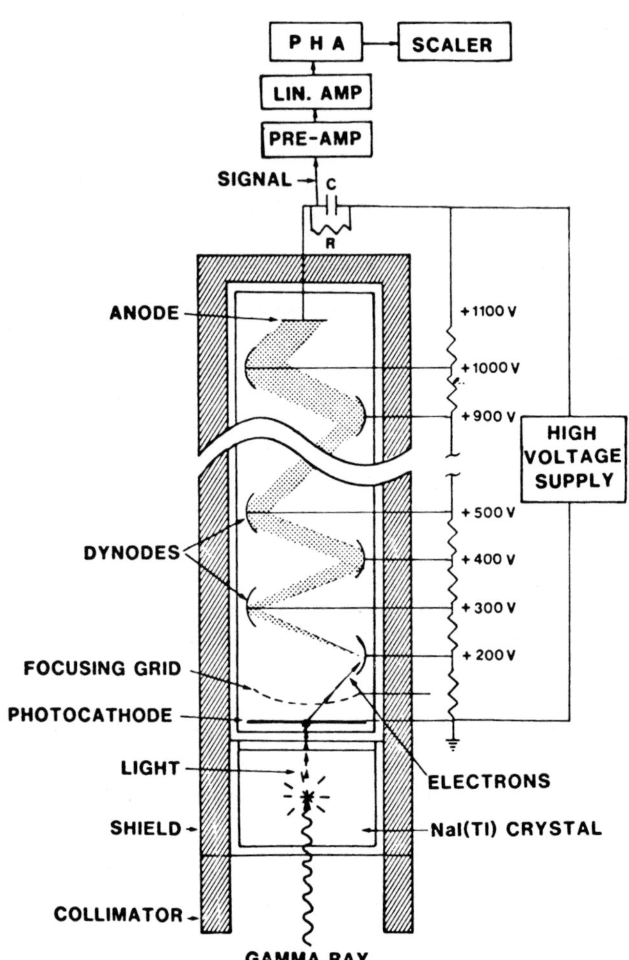

FIGURE 59–1. Schematic diagram of a sodium iodide thallium (NaI[Tl]) detector. PHA = pulse height analyzer. (From Patton, J.A., Rollo, F.D., and Freeman, L.M. [eds.]: Clinical Radionuclide Imaging. Orlando, Grune & Stratton, 1984, p. 48, with permission.)

This work was supported in part by grant RO1 HL42052 from the National Heart, Lung, and Blood Institutes, National Institutes of Health, and by grant R29-LM 04692 from the National Library of Medicine.

lyzer (PHA) is used to preselect from the distribution of available energies (energy spectrum) the range of energies to be counted (energy window), as shown in Figure 59–2. Pulses corresponding to γ-rays of energies outside this window are rejected. The combination of an NaI(Tl) crystal, a photomultiplier, a PHA, and a scaler makes up the scintillation counter (see Fig. 59–1), which may be used to count radioactive samples in vitro (well counter) or in vivo (probe).

The use of a PHA is particularly important for imaging with radiation, because a basic assumption of scintigraphy is that the γ-rays interacting with the crystal travel in a straight line from the emitting source. Therefore, the PHA, by rejecting energies below a certain threshold, eliminates γ-rays that have lost their original energy and direction during a Compton scatter event in the patient and yet continued on to strike the crystal. The pulses generated by unscattered γ-rays that strike the crystal are not all of the same amplitude; they are distributed around the amplitude that corresponds to the exact characteristic energy of the radionuclide (photopeak). The narrower the spread of energies around the photopeak, the better the energy resolution of the system and the better the inherent counting and imaging characteristics of the device.

IMAGING INSTRUMENTATION

Single-Crystal Gamma Camera

The most significant breakthrough in nuclear medicine instrumentation came in 1958, when Anger invented the conventional analog scintillation camera.[1] This device was able to both detect and localize scintillation events, thus providing the potential for imaging a radionuclide distribution with a stationary detector, without the necessity for scanning.

The scintillation camera uses a large (300 to 500 mm), flat (0.25 to 0.5 inch) NaI(Tl) crystal and an array of photomultipliers that range in number from 19 to 91. The photomultipliers are arranged in a specific array that covers the area of the crystal face (Fig. 59–3). The γ-rays are first collimated to preselect a desired direction from which to strike the crystal. A γ-ray that passes through the holes of the lead collimator is usually absorbed by the crystal, giving rise to a scintillation. The light (visible photons) from the scintillation is "seen" by all photomultipliers. Those photomultiplier tubes closer to the event gather more light than those farther away. The outputs of all tubes are fed into electronic computer circuitry (a positional analyzer) that is capable, by analysis of their outputs, of determining at which point beneath the array of photomultipliers each scintillation occurred and of assigning to each such event a pair of x and y coordinates. The output of all of the tubes is also summed to form an energy or z pulse.

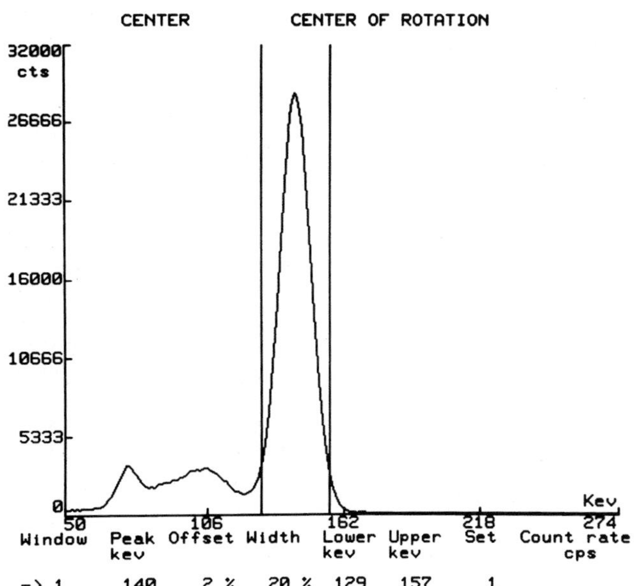

FIGURE 59–2. Technetium-99m energy spectrum. The superimposed energy window *(vertical lines)* surrounds the 140-keV photopeak. cts = counts; cps = counts per second.

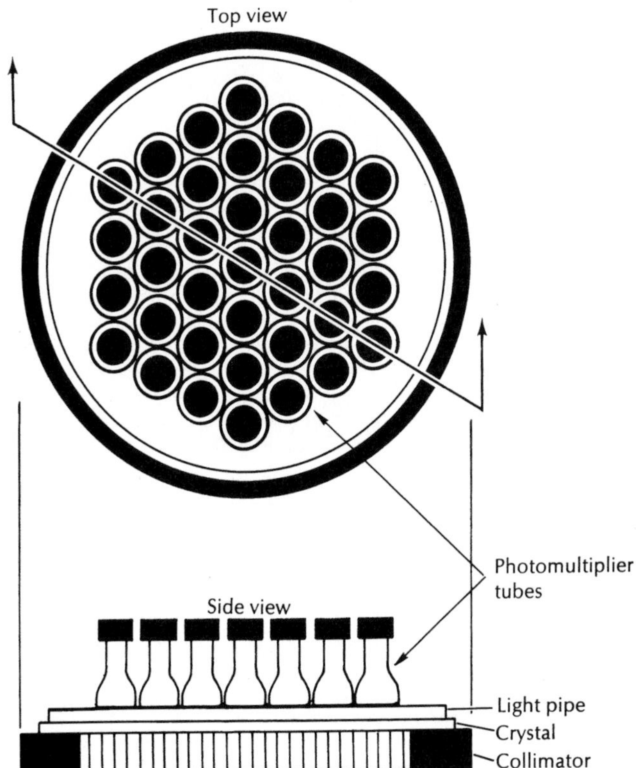

FIGURE 59–3. Relative placement of the photomultiplier tubes in a scintillation camera. (From Rollo, F.D. [ed.]: Nuclear Medicine Physics, Instrumentation, and Agents. St. Louis, Mosby, 1977, p. 234, with permission.)

Electronic Processing

For each γ-ray that interacts with the NaI crystal, the scintillation camera generates three information pulses. Two of these pulses correspond to the Cartesian coordinates of the scintillation, and the third is the z pulse, representing the total energy of the γ-ray that interacted with the crystal (Fig. 59–4A). The z pulse is sent to the PHA, which has been set to accept a preselected range of energies. After the z pulse has been accepted by the PHA, it becomes a trigger pulse, also known as a signal (s) pulse, signaling a scintillation event to be counted. The x, y, and z pulses are in analog format and are meant to be used in conjunction with the scope of a cathode ray tube. The word analog signifies that the information contained in these pulses is coded as a continuously variable voltage; in other words, a small deflection in the voltage implies a small change in the position of the scintillation.

The z pulse, or trigger pulse, is also known as the unblank signal when it is used to control a cathode ray tube. Each time this trigger pulse comes in, it allows the emission of electrons from the electron gun. The x and y positional pulses are fed to the horizontal and vertical plates to create a deflection in the path of the electrons corresponding to the scintillation coordinates (see Fig. 59–4A). The electrons then hit the phosphor screen of the cathode ray tube, creating a small scintillation that can be recorded on a photographic film as a dot. The analog nuclear medicine image is a collection of these dots, distributed according to the radioactivity in the patient.

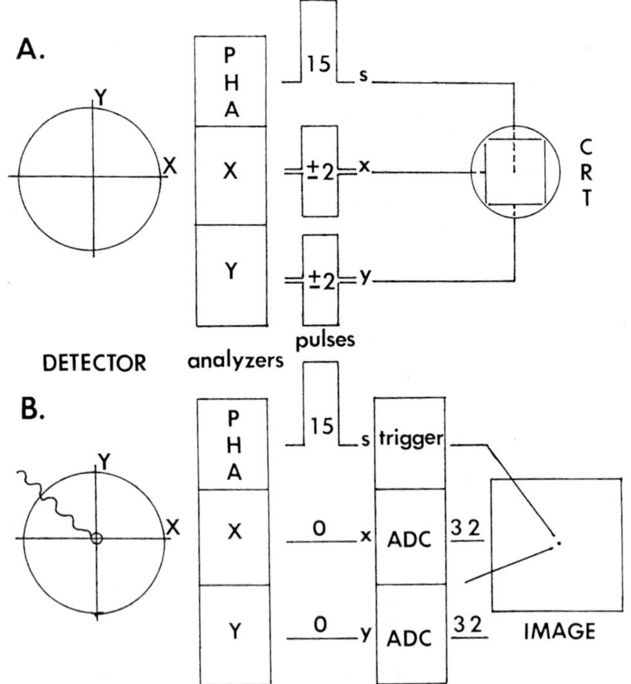

FIGURE 59–4. *A*, Block diagram of a scintillation camera shows how the x and y positional pulses and the s (or z) trigger pulse are generated to control the cathode ray tube (CRT). *B*, Block diagram of a computer interface illustrates how the x, y, and s (or z) pulses generated by the camera when the scintillation occurs in the center of the NaI crystal are used to update the digital image. PHA = pulse height analyzer; ADC = analog-to-digital converter.

Advanced Electronics

The basic electronic scheme developed by Anger to position the scintillation event has been improved by a number of correction circuitry additions, which are available in most state-of-the-art cameras. These cameras are able, in real time, to perform signal processing that corrects the position of the scintillation event before the event is recorded on film or on a digital matrix. In general, there are three different types of real-time correction electronics. They correct for tube drift, for energy variations, and for spatial nonlinearity.

The tube drift correction is used to automatically calibrate or "tune" the photomultipliers so that each tube generates the same pulse voltage when it gathers the same light from reference light sources that flash up to 1000 times per second during acquisition. This type of correction is particularly needed for rotational tomography, to correct for the differences in photomultiplier output as a function of angle that result from the influence of the earth's magnetic field. Mu metal shields around each photomultiplier tube have also been used to reduce this effect.[2]

The energy correction circuit corrects for the fact that each photomultiplier, even after being automatically tuned for its light sensitivity, generates a slightly different energy spectrum. These differences are caused by the response of the photomultiplier, by differences in the crystal, or by differences in the regional light-gathering properties. The correction circuit applies, in real time, a premeasured energy map that normalizes the relation of the energy window to the shape of the spectrum, effectively eliminating the variations in energy response. This correction requires the periodic acquisition of energy-specific field floods to generate the time-dependent energy maps.

The linearity correction circuit corrects for the fact that the Anger positioning scheme does not perfectly image straight radioactive line sources as straight lines. The correction consists of imaging a phantom of straight lines in the horizontal and vertical position and measuring and storing the displacement that will force the lines to appear perfectly straight in the image. These regional displacement correction factors are then applied in real time on an event-by-event basis.

Collimation

There are no known lenses that can gather and refract (bend) γ-rays as a photographic camera does with light rays. Instead, a collimator or lead disk with multiple holes is used to selectively interfere or block those γ-rays not traveling in the selected direction. The most commonly used collimator in nuclear cardiology is the parallel-hole collimator. This collimator consists of a large number of parallel holes perpendicular to the face of the crystal. The lead septa between holes are made thick enough to absorb most of the γ-rays of a preselected energy that are traveling in a straight line but at an off-angle. The larger the diameter of the holes, or the shorter the length of the holes, the greater the sensitivity of the detector, defined as the number of γ-rays counted per unit time (per γ-ray emitted). Improvements in sensitivity are usually accompanied by a deterioration of the spatial resolution of the system, that is, the ability to discern in the image two separate radioactive objects as distinct. Although the parallel-hole collimator is by far the most widely used, there are several other collimators available that may outperform the parallel-hole collimator for specific applications, including the pinhole, converging, diverging, and parallel-hole slant collimators.

Computer Interface Used by Analog Cameras

The same x, y, and z analog pulses that are sent to the cathode ray tube in analog cameras are also routed to the computer interface input. Interface is defined as the coupling between two instruments (anything needed to make one system understand the other). The computer cannot handle these pulses in their analog format. Before they can have meaning within the computer, they must be converted into digital information. (The word digital refers to a discrete number or a countable number such as an integer.) The computer must be equipped with an analog-to-digital converter. This instrument converts the pulse height into discrete numbers. The x and y pulses each have an analog-to-digital converter. The z pulse acts as a trigger, signaling the converters to convert the analog pulses into digital numbers (see Fig. 59–4*B*). Most computers have a direct memory access hardware device that updates the memory without any intervention by the software or the central processing unit, thus freeing up the computer while it is acquiring data. How the memory is updated depends on the preselected acquisition format (see the section on acquisition of scintigraphic images).

Digital Camera

When the computer hardware is an integral part of the scintillation camera system and is used for processing the scintillation event, the computer-camera system is called a "digital camera." In reality, there is no commercial system that is either totally analog or totally digital, so it is a confusing term. In general, manufacturers use the term to mean that they use advanced digital circuits (like those that have been described) to correct the photomultiplier output, energy, and position of the scintillation event. A more strict definition is that of a scintillation camera that generates only digital images in matrix format, without ever generating an analog image. One advantage of the digital camera, as implemented by one manufacturer, is that it can effectively reduce the dead time of the system by using distributed processing with multiple microprocessors and temporary memory storage (buffers) of pulse data. This type of digital camera implementation has allowed acquisition of count rates close to those of the multicrystal camera but with the use of a single, large crystal and Anger-type positioning. The manufacturers of one digital camera system claim that their detector has a count-rate capability of 200,000 counts per second with a loss of 10 percent.[3] More recently, digital cameras have been developed with ADCs corresponding to each photomultiplier tube.

Each tube generates a digital output per scintillation that can be processed in a more accurate, straight-forward manner. This configuration has many advantages, including improved energy resolution, scatter rejection, and spatial resolution.

Multicrystal Gamma Camera

In addition to the popular, single-crystal gamma camera, another camera design, known as the multicrystal or autofluoroscope camera, has also been used in nuclear cardiology. This camera, originally developed by Drs. Bender and Blau,[4] consists of a mosaic pattern of 294 NaI crystals (each 1 cm × 1 cm × 1 inch), arranged in an array of 14 rows by 21 columns, and 35 photomultipliers (one for each row and one for each column). Each crystal is coupled to two photomultiplier tubes (one for the row position and one for the column position) by means of fiber optics. The light from the scintillation emitted for each γ-ray absorbed by the crystal is detected by the corresponding horizontal and vertical photomultipliers, quickly identifying the crystal position. Because of the simplicity of the electronics, the time that it takes to process the necessary pulses, during which the system cannot respond to new events, is much shorter than in the conventional Anger camera. This shorter deadtime implies that, for an intense radioactive source (200,000 counts per second), a count rate much closer to the true rate can be observed with this system than with the conventional Anger camera.

Because of its potential for fast counting, the multicrystal camera has become the instrument of choice at many institutions for imaging the transit of the first pass of a radiotracer through the heart chambers. The ability to count fast has been exploited by the use of collimators with holes close to the dimensions of the crystals, which allows a higher γ-ray flux incident on the crystals. For example, a 25-mCi (925 MBq) dose of ^{99m}Tc imaged with a high-sensitivity collimator (1 inch thick) results in more than 400,000 counts per second in the overall image.[5] A newer version of this design, with improved fiber optics and newer electronics, performs even better.

Multiwire Gamma Camera

Single-photon imaging detectors based on multiwire proportional counters have been developed. One group in particular[6] has developed and applied in first-pass radionuclide angiography[7] a multiwire gamma camera with both high count-rate capability and high spatial resolution. The detector illustrated in Figure 59–5 consists of a drift region and a detection region contained within an aluminum pressure vessel having a thin aluminum entrance window of spherical shape. Photons entering through the aluminum window interact with xenon gas under moderate pressure in the drift region. The interaction causes the creation of ions, which are drifted to the detection region. The detection region consists of three parallel wire planes: a central anode plane and the two outer cathode planes. The drifted ionization is collected at the anode, where the charge is amplified by a gas avalanche. Position determination of the anode avalanche is obtained by detection of the signals induced in the two cathode grids, which are oriented perpendicular to each other. This detector is very compact, lightweight, and capable of portable operation. Because the stopping power of the pressurized xenon gas is low compared with that of NaI crystals, detection efficiency limits the application of the multiwire camera to energies below 100 keV. A generator-produced tracer, tantalum-178, which has a low energy (60-keV) and a short half-life (9.3 minutes), has been shown to be ideal[7] for performing first-pass angiography with this camera.

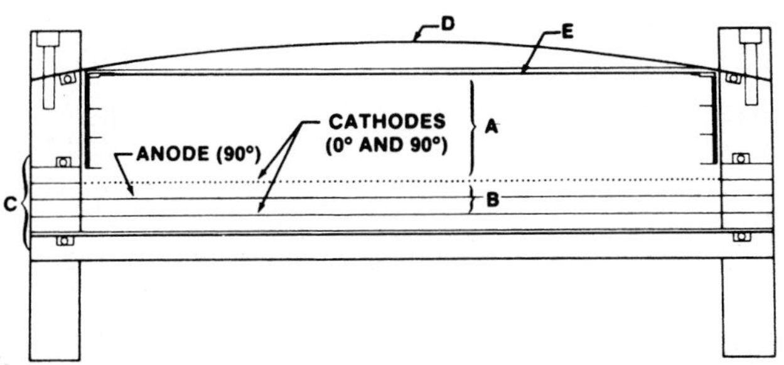

FIGURE 59–5. Longitudinal diagram of multiwire proportional counter gamma camera. A = Drift region; B = detection region; C = aluminum pressure vessel; D = aluminum entrance window; E = negative high-voltage collection electrode. (From Lacey, J.L., et al.: A gamma camera for medical applications, using a multiwire proportional counter. J. Nucl. Med. 25:1004, 1984, with permission.)

Because the duration of the signal in the multiwire proportional counter detector is one tenth that of NaI detectors, these devices can be designed for high count rates, similar to those of the multicrystal cameras. In particular, the multiwire gamma camera described has an intrinsic peak count rate of 850,000 counts per second, with an intrinsic spatial resolution of 2.5 mm.[6]

NONIMAGING DEVICES FOR RADIATION DETECTION

Nonimaging probes can be used to monitor radioactivity in the heart. In contrast to gamma cameras, these probes do not form an image of the heart but are used specifically to record count changes within their field of view. Because no image is generated by the system, detector design is as simple as that described for the scintillation counter. This simplicity in detector configuration makes the system portable, inexpensive, and count-efficient compared with gamma cameras.

Nuclear Stethoscope

The most popular nonimaging probe is the "nuclear stethoscope," which is used for measuring and monitoring left ventricular global function after labeling of the cardiac blood pool with ^{99m}Tc. The detector for this probe consists of an NaI crystal (2 inches in diameter by 1.5 inches thick), a photomultiplier, and a single-bore, flat-field converging collimator.[8] This detector is mounted on a 50-inch arm with two degrees of freedom and interfaced to a dedicated microprocessor. The microprocessor simultaneously samples and records in real time both the counts emanating within the field of view and the patient's electrocardiographic data. The microprocessor is also used to assist in the positioning of the detector for measurement of counts from a left ventricular region and a background region. The detector position for the left ventricular region is identified by the microprocessor as the point at which the ratio of stroke counts to average counts is highest. The detector position for the background region is identified by the microprocessor as that position immediately inferolateral to the left ventricular region which yields minimal stroke counts and at which the average count initially decreases.

After positioning of the probe, beat-to-beat left ventricular time-activity curves are displayed. After the time-activity curves have been filtered, left ventricular ejection fraction (EF) may be calculated on a beat-to-beat basis, or the cardiac cycle time-activity data may be summed for any length of time, usually 30 seconds to 2 minutes. Averaging significantly improves the statistical accuracy of the data, yielding high temporal resolution volume curves from which parameters of left ventricular function, such as EF and filling and emptying rates, may automatically be calculated.

Although the positioning of the detector is based on algorithms, accurate measurements still require considerable operator expertise in positioning. Because of this limitation, the best application of this probe is to use it to monitor changes in cardiac performance over an acquisition session with the detector in the same relative position. If the relative positioning geometry of the detector and the heart is carefully recorded and reproduced, this device is also useful for studying changes in cardiac performance from separate acquisition sessions.

VEST

More recently, new nonimaging probe systems have been made so small that the entire system can be worn like a vest. This device, which looks like a vestlike garment (hence the name VEST), allows for continuous, ambulatory monitoring of left ventricular performance during normal day-to-day activities that may cause ischemic events absent from or different from those seen during exercise testing. Like the nuclear stethoscope, the VEST simultaneously and continuously records the electrocardiographic data and the counts from the detector's field of view.

The VEST consists of a radionuclide detector, a molded plastic garment to hold the detector in place, and electronic devices to count the scintillations and record the events. In addition, the recorder contains an event marker and a real-time clock. The entire device weighs 3.1 kg. Positioning is done with the assistance of a gamma camera. After injection of 15 to 25 mCi (555 to 925 MBq) of ^{99m}Tc-radiolabeled red blood cells, the best-septal left anterior oblique (LAO) view of the left ventricle is identified. The VEST's detector is then positioned over the left ventricle with guidance from the shadow cast on the gamma camera display by the lead shield around the detector. After the VEST is fixed in place, monitoring of left ventricular function is performed while the patient is mentally or physically challenged or while the patient goes on with regular daily activities. Recording of cardiac performance may continue for up to 6 hours.

After the data recording session is ended, the stored data are replayed into a computer system for analysis and graphic display. Background activity is defined as 70 percent of the counts recorded at end-diastole. A patient's beat-to-beat, background-corrected left ventricular time-activity curve and corresponding electrocardiogram is available for display. The beat-to-beat time-activity curves may be added and filtered to yield high-resolution left ventricular time-activity curves. An EF decrease of greater than 6 percent units lasting 1 minute or longer is considered significant.[9] Preliminary validation[10] has shown the ability of the VEST to measure EF at rest with the same degree of accuracy as that obtained from gated blood pool imaging.

ACQUISITION OF SCINTIGRAPHIC IMAGES

Three basic considerations determine the format in which scintigraphic data should be collected. Of prime importance is appropriate matching of the speed of the physiologic event to that of image acquisition; this match determines the temporal resolution. A second important consideration is matrix resolution, which is based on matching of the spatial resolution of the imaging system to the number of pixels (picture elements) per frame. The third consideration is information density, which determines whether the number of counts per pixel is appropriate for the information intended to be extracted from the images. For cardiac blood pool imaging, the variables associated with these three acquisition formats are, respectively, the number of frames per cardiac cycle, the number of pixels per frame, and the number of bits per pixel. The required temporal resolution, matrix resolution, and information density vary with the specific cardiac study being acquired and the type of information being extracted. The formats also differ in how the incoming scintillation and physiologic events are handled by the computer. This section describes the options that most nuclear medicine computer systems have for handling data acquisition requirements.

Planar Imaging in Frame Mode

Almost all planar studies are acquired in frame (histogram) mode, in which a portion of computer memory is used to represent an image that has been acquired for either a predefined time or a total number of scintillations or counts. Each memory location allocated to this frame represents a digital counter of how many scintillations occurred at each pixel location during acquisition. In preset time mode, after the time of acquisition for that frame has elapsed, the frame is transferred to a peripheral device such as a disk for longer-term storage. In preset counts mode, the computer also updates a counter that keeps track of the total number of counts; after this counter reaches a preset number, the frame is transferred. Frame mode can be subdivided into static and dynamic forms of acquisition.

Static Imaging

Static image acquisition, either nongated or gated, is used when the radionuclide distribution is assumed not to change for a period of time. This applies to myocardial perfusion imaging with thallium-201, to acute myocardial infarction imaging with ^{99m}Tc-pyrophosphate, and, in a variation, to cardiac blood pool imaging.

Nongated Static Acquisition

Thallium-201 myocardial scintigrams of stress-redistribution or rest-redistribution are usually acquired for a preset time, such as 6 to 10 minutes per view. Sequential imaging optimally begins 5 to 6 minutes after ^{201}Tl injection in the anterior, middle LAO, and steep LAO views. The same views are repeated 3 to 6 hours later to study both washout and reversibility. A 128 × 128 matrix format is normally used as a tradeoff between derived spatial resolution and adequate information density per pixel. The field of view is usually about 8 × 8 inches, which allows an ample number of pixels to define the heart and to give an accurate representation of the background surrounding the heart. A 10-minute acquisition yields between 300,000 and 800,000 total counts in the image from a 2 mCi (74 MBq) ^{201}Tl dose.[11]

Multiple-Gated Acquisition

Multiple-gated acquisition employs from 14 to 100 frames, with a physiologic marker (the R wave) used as a synchronizing signal.[12] Corresponding frames are added together over a preset time or a preset number of counts, making this a form of static imaging. Scintigraphic data from the camera are channeled to a series of image frames located in the computer memory. Count allocations to particular frames are governed by the time delay between the R wave and the count event (Fig. 59–6). Immediately after the trigger, counts are placed in frame 1 for a fixed duration of time. After the desired sampling interval has elapsed, scintigraphic data are channeled to frame 2, and the process continues up to the last frame (frame N). After the time interval for the last frame has elapsed, the remaining data from the camera are discarded until the next trigger signal arrives. Data from successive beats are added into the appropriate frames until the desired total count is achieved or the preset time is reached.

The time interval of each frame can be shortened or lengthened according to the application and the number of frames available to represent the cardiac cycle. Approximately 20 frames per cycle are required for accurate measurement of left ventricular EF.[13] If the system is limited to a few frames, these should be divided over the initial two thirds of the cardiac cycle to maintain high-accuracy measurement of EF. For detailed analysis of the activity-time curve, and for accurate assessment of ejection and filling velocities, more frames per cardiac cycle are required (e.g., 64 to 100 frames).[14]

An important aspect of multiple-gated acquisition is that the gating signal must accurately represent the onset of systole (true end-diastole). Potential problems with achieving this include gating on "noise" rather than on the R wave, which results from faulty

PLATE 22

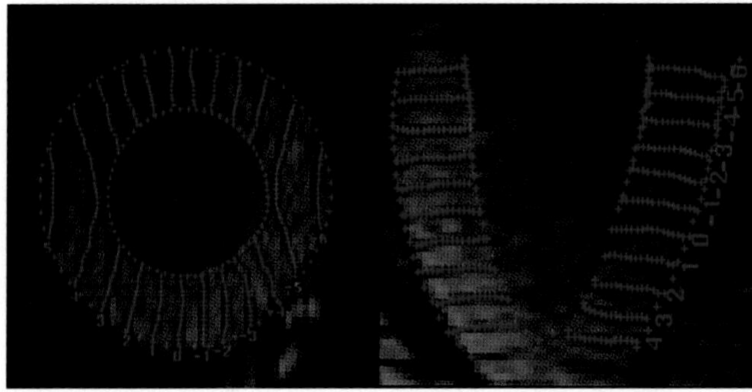

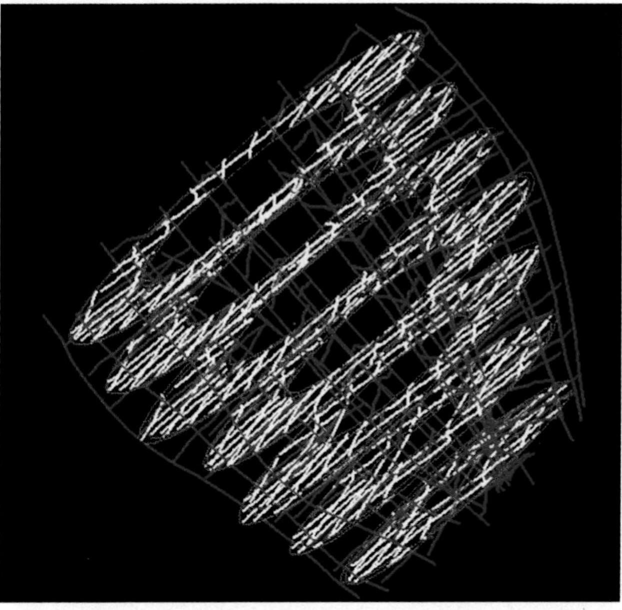

FIGURE 45–2. Computer analysis of tagged cine images. *Left,* Each image is automatically contoured, and each tag line identified and numbered for each image. *Right,* After segmentation of each image, a three-dimensional display of all tag lines and contours is obtained to ensure good registration of data.

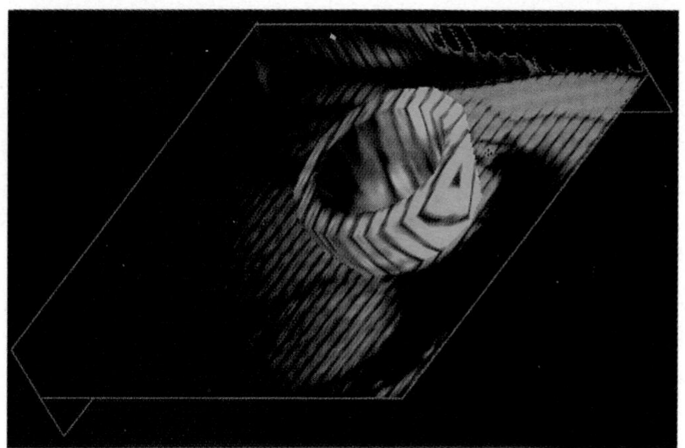

FIGURE 45–3. Fusion of anatomical and functional data. Using a high-speed graphics computer, the functional strain data can be superimposed on a dynamic three-dimensional display of the beating heart with perfect temporal and spatial coregistration.

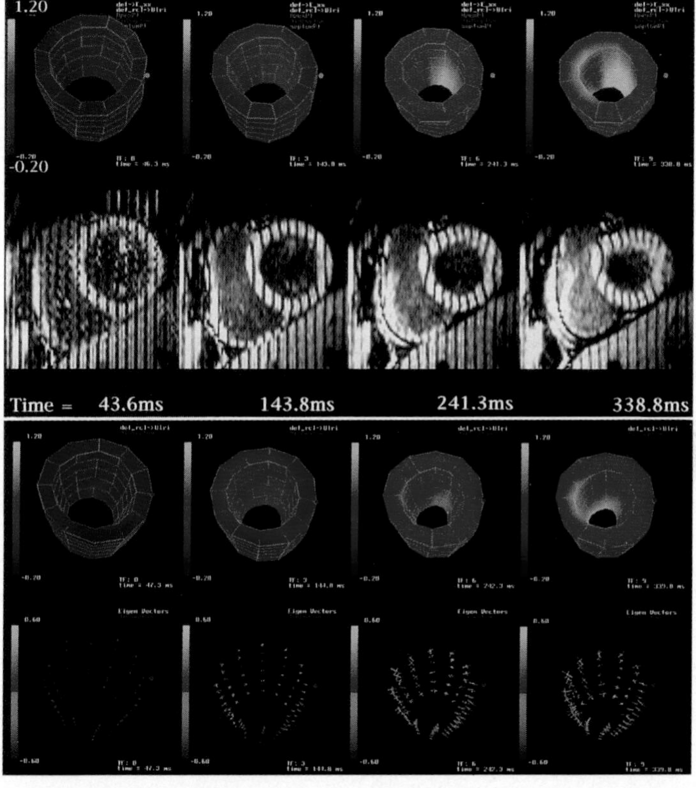

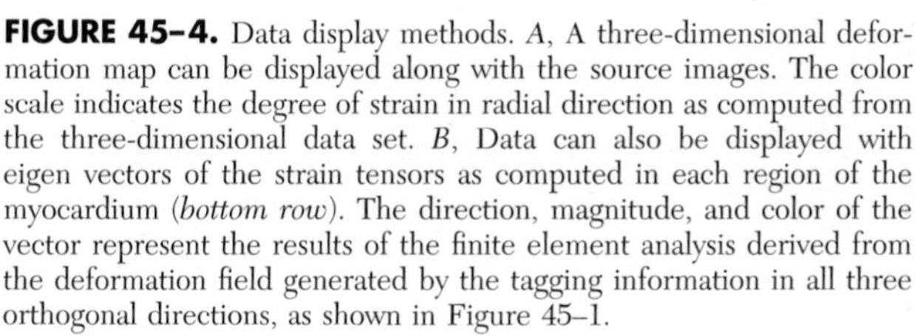

FIGURE 45–4. Data display methods. *A,* A three-dimensional deformation map can be displayed along with the source images. The color scale indicates the degree of strain in radial direction as computed from the three-dimensional data set. *B,* Data can also be displayed with eigen vectors of the strain tensors as computed in each region of the myocardium (*bottom row*). The direction, magnitude, and color of the vector represent the results of the finite element analysis derived from the deformation field generated by the tagging information in all three orthogonal directions, as shown in Figure 45–1.

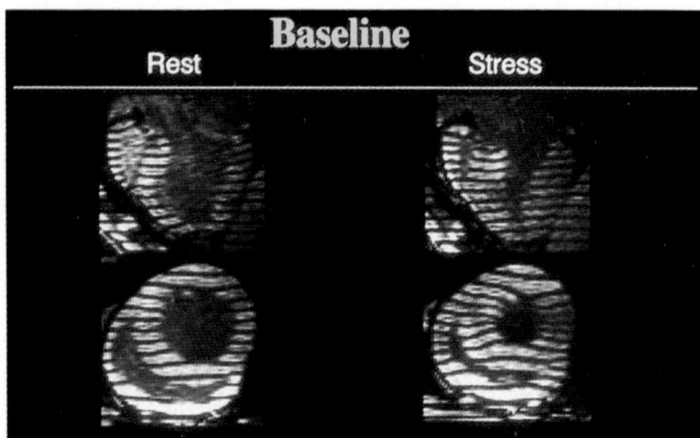

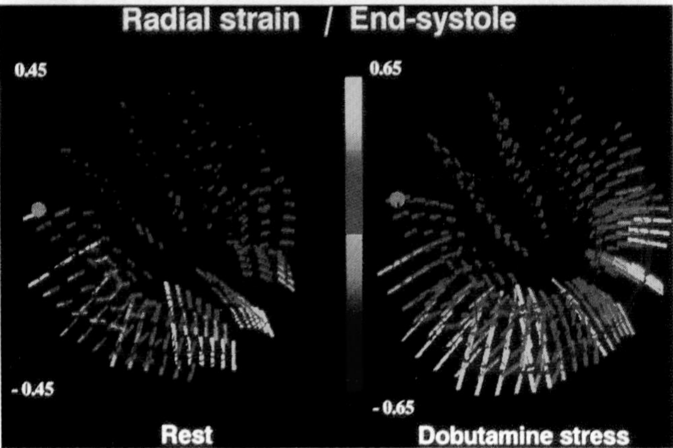

FIGURE 45–5. Cardiac function at rest and during stress. *Top,* Cine tagged magnetic resonance series at rest and after low-dose dobutamine stress in a canine model of infarction reperfusion. Note the overall change in shape of the myocardium between rest and stress conditions with reduction in left and right ventricular chamber size. Accurate correlation of changes in contraction at stress relative to rest conditions requires correction not only for the effect of in-plane and through-plane motion but also for the shape changes shown here. *Bottom,* Three-dimensional reconstruction of the radial strain vectors at rest and during stress demonstrates changes in strain in the remote regions (3 to 6 o'clock), increases in strain at stress in regions adjacent to the infarct zone suggestive of recovery in stunned myocardium (2, 3, and 10 o'clock), and regions with no recovery after stress in the infarcted regions (10 to 1 o'clock).

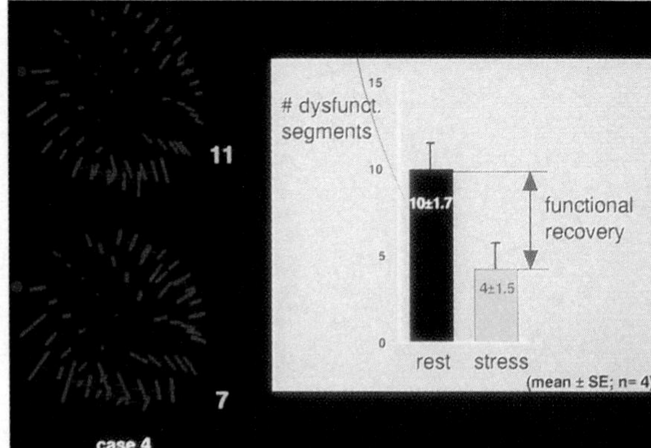

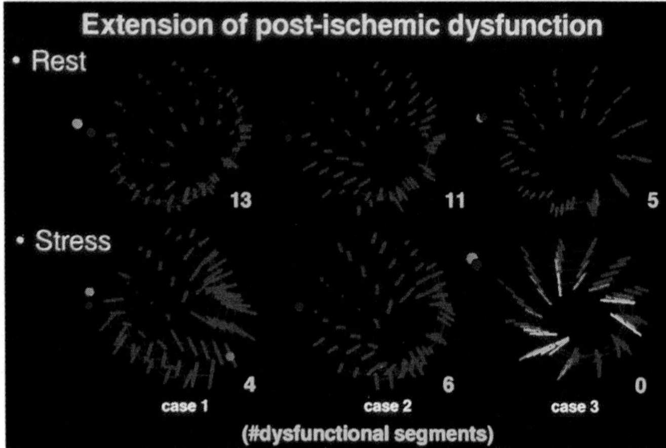

FIGURE 45–6. Stunned myocardium at rest and during low-dose dobutamine stress in a series of four dogs showing recovery of dysfunctional volume elements when comparing three-dimensional radial strain vector maps at rest *(top row)* against stress *(bottom row).* Note complete recovery in case 3, where no infarction was found at autopsy, but dysfunction was present at rest. Each vector represents radial strain in one volume element at end systole.

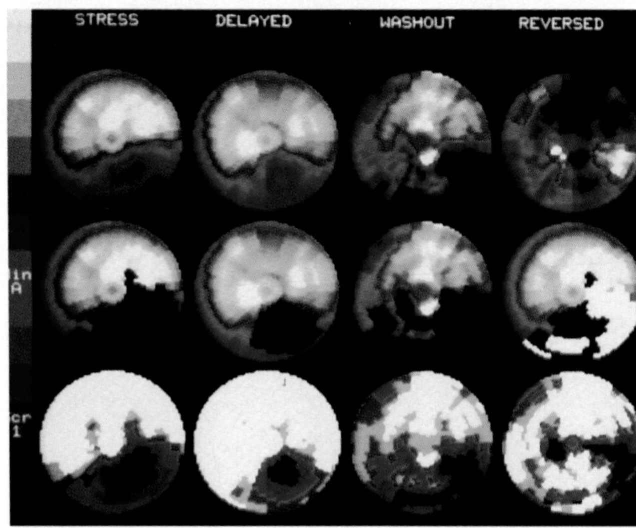

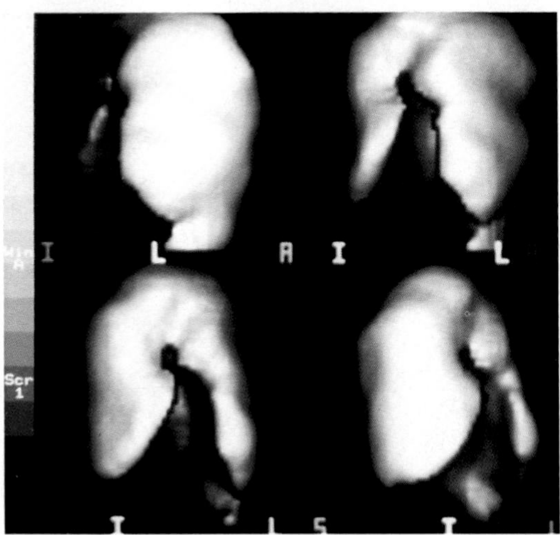

FIGURE 59–30. Surface rendering of three-dimensional thallium-201 perfusion distribution of a patient with left circumflex coronary artery disease. Each panel demonstrates a slightly different rotation (apex pointing up) of a hypoperfused inferolateral myocardial wall. Perfusion defect is demonstrated by the missing region between the inferior (I) and lateral (L) walls. [A = anterior wall, S = septal wall] (Results courtesy of David Nowak, General Electric Co.)

FIGURE 59–26. Bull's-eye polar representation of myocardial perfusion. Complete set of 12 bull's-eye polar maps for a patient with an inferolateral, reversible perfusion defect. Top four polar maps are the raw bull's eyes before comparison to normal limits. The four polar maps (blackout bull's eyes) in the middle row represent the raw data after a single threshold cut-off criterion for abnormality (2.5 standard deviations from the mean for the stress, delayed, and washout, 1.5 for reversibility). Note blacked out region in the inferolateral wall of the stress bull's eye corresponding to the perfusion defect. Although the defect appears to remain fixed in delayed bull's eye, the large whited out region in the reversibility map corresponds to significant reversibility. The four polar maps in the bottom row are the standard deviation bull's eyes in which the deviation of each pixel from the mean normal response is color coded from white (least) to black (most).

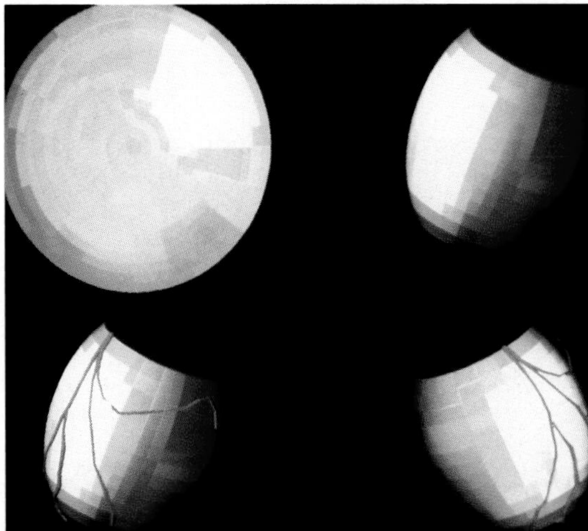

FIGURE 59–31. Three-dimensional heart models of a patient exhibiting hypoperfusion of the inferior and inferolateral myocardial walls. Top left panel illustrates the patient's bull's-eye polar map where the perfusion defect is represented by shades of blue. Top right panel represents the corresponding three-dimensional ellipsoidal model of the myocardium. Bottom panels show two different orientations of a unified model where the patient's own left coronary arteries have been registered onto the ellipsoidal perfusion model. Note on the bottom left panel a high-grade lesion at the midcourse of the left circumflex coronary artery. (Results generated by C. David Cooke and John Peifer.)

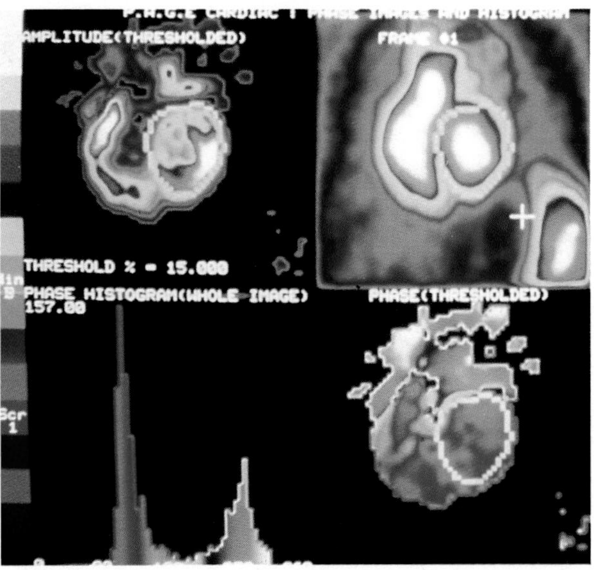

FIGURE 59–39. Phase-analysis of a normal Tc-99m multiple gated equilibrium study. Top right panel is a filtered end-diastolic frame. Top left panel is the stroke count or amplitude image. Bottom right panel is the phase image. Left-ventricular edge is superimposed in all three images. Bottom left panel illustrates a phase histogram where the color-coded phase (x-axis) is plotted vs. the number of pixels in the phase image with that phase. Note bimodal peaks corresponding to synchronous contractions of ventricles (blue-green) and atria (red-white). (Courtesy of John Almasi, General Electric Co.)

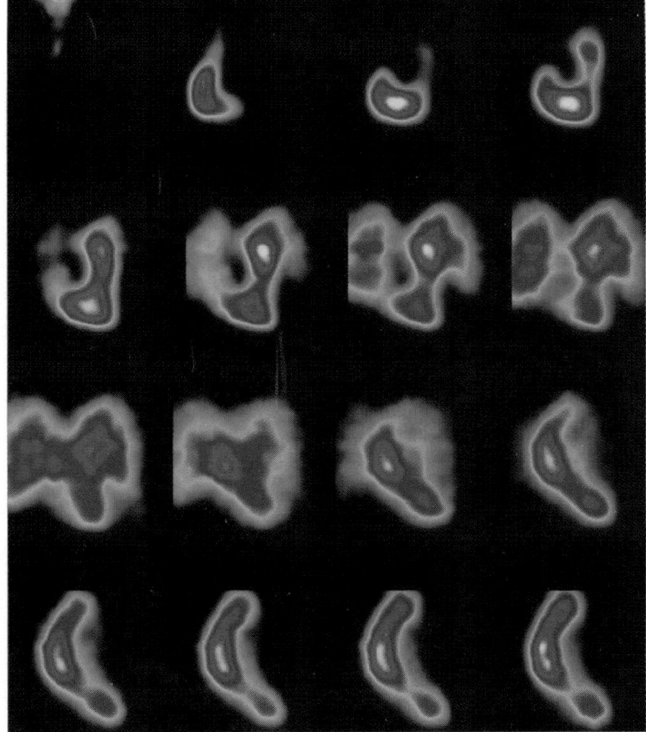

FIGURE 60–1. After acquisition at 25 to 50 msec per image, the data can be regrouped into 1-second images to display the transit of the injected radionuclide through the central circulation. *Left to Right,* Superior vena cava, right atrium and ventricle, pulmonary artery and lungs, and left ventricle and ascending aorta.

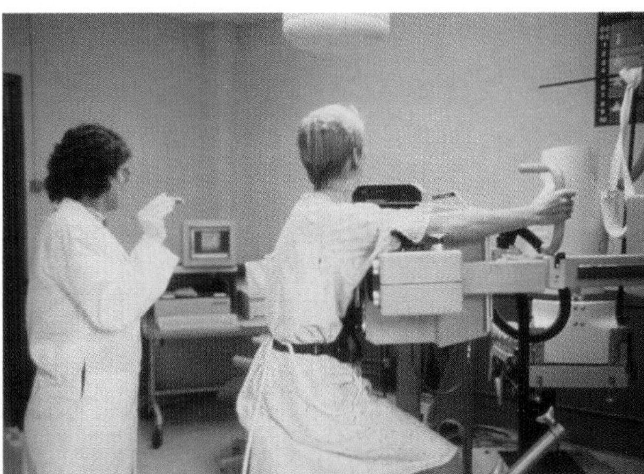

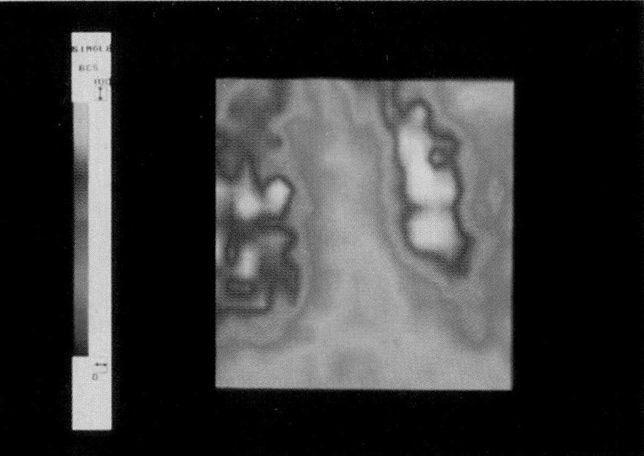

FIGURE 60–5. Because positioning for a first-pass study must be accurate before injection, it is helpful to use a syringe source *(top)* or a uniform flood source to generate an image of the lungs and mediastinum *(bottom)*, thereby localizing the heart in the field of view.

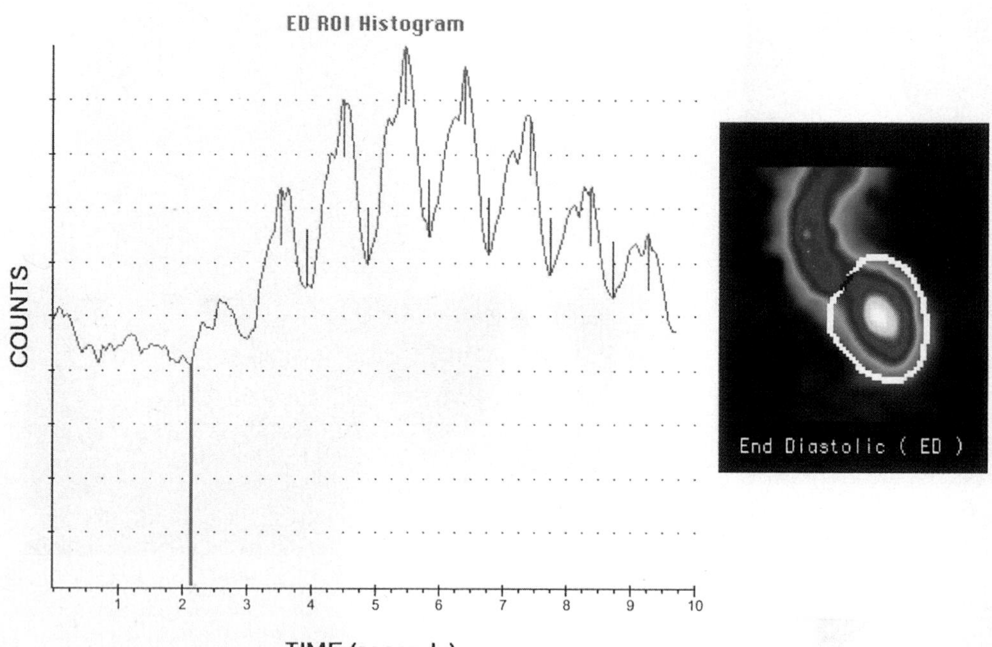

FIGURE 60–7. Data processing of first-pass studies begins with the identification of a frame of raw data that clearly displays the ventricle of interest, in this case the left ventricle (LV). A region of interest is manually drawn to represent the LV *(right)* and a time-activity curve is generated *(left)*. The curve displays the change in recorded radioactivity during the time that the bolus is traveling through the LV. The beat-to-beat changes from end-diastole *(peaks)* to end-systole *(valleys)* are easily appreciated. They represent stroke counts and, after background correction, are used to calculate the ejection fraction. ED ROI = end-diastole region of interest.

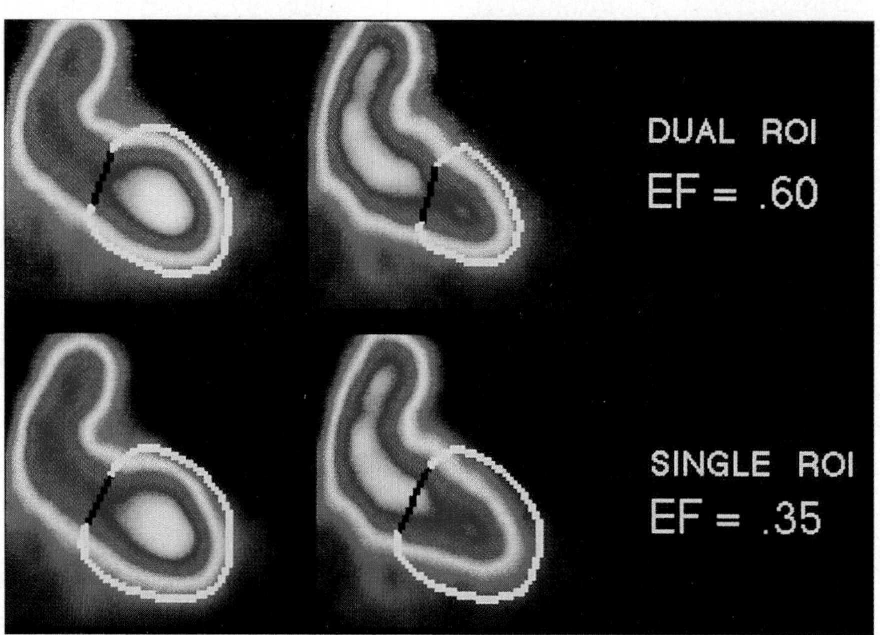

FIGURE 60–8. Final data processing of first-pass studies acquired in the anterior view should be performed with the use of separate regions of interest (ROIs) for end-diastole and end-systole. In the case example shown here, the same study is processed with separate end-diastolic and end-systolic ROIs *(top)* and with a single end-diastolic ROI *(bottom)*. In this case, chosen because of the magnitude of the discrepancy, the latter approach includes both aortic and left atrial activity at end-systole *(lower right)*, thus spuriously lowering the ejection fraction (EF). Careful drawing of a separate end-systole ROI *(upper right)* enables the operator to exclude nonventricular activity from the ROI. (From Murphy, P., and Port, S.: Radionuclide evaluation of left ventricular function. *In* Sandler, M.P., Patton, J.A., Coleman, A.E., et al. [eds.]: Diagnostic Nuclear Medicine. Baltimore, Williams & Wilkins, 1996, with permission.)

PLATE 26

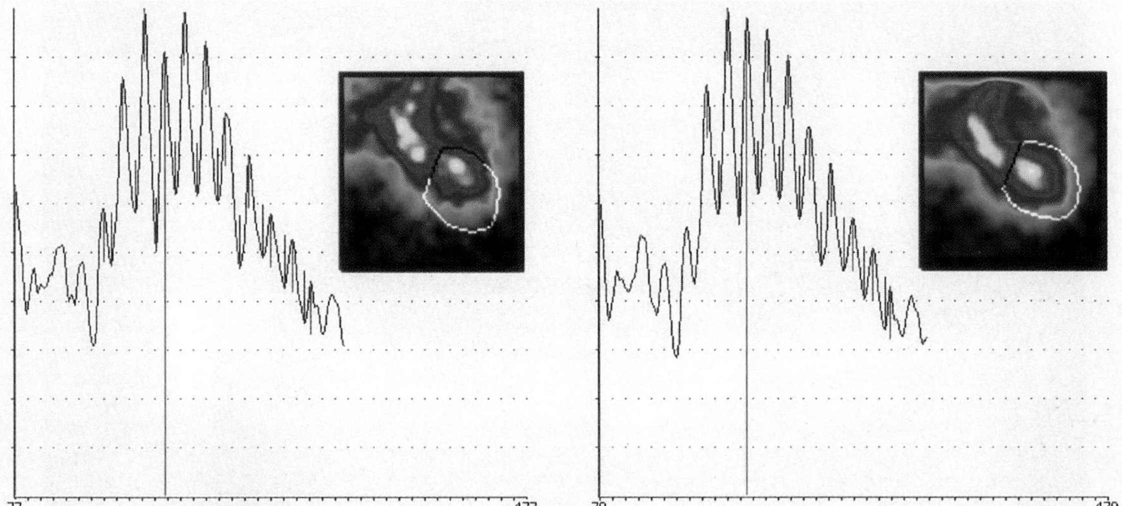

FIGURE 60–11. Motion during the left ventricular phase of a first-pass study is easily recognized by inspecting the time-activity curve or images of the ventricle. The curve should show a steady increase in counts up to a peak and then a steady decrease. In the absence of motion, all the individual peaks connected to each other would describe a monoexponential curve. In the example at the left, there is clearly a disruption of the usual sequence, with count rates rising and falling out of synch with the expected transit through the chamber. This is a result of motion that causes the cardiac activity to drift in and out of the region of interest used to generate the curve. The image insert shows an end-diastolic frame that is partially outside the region of interest. After motion correction *(right)*, the overall appearance of the time-activity curve is much improved, and the image insert now shows the end-diastolic activity well within the region of interest.

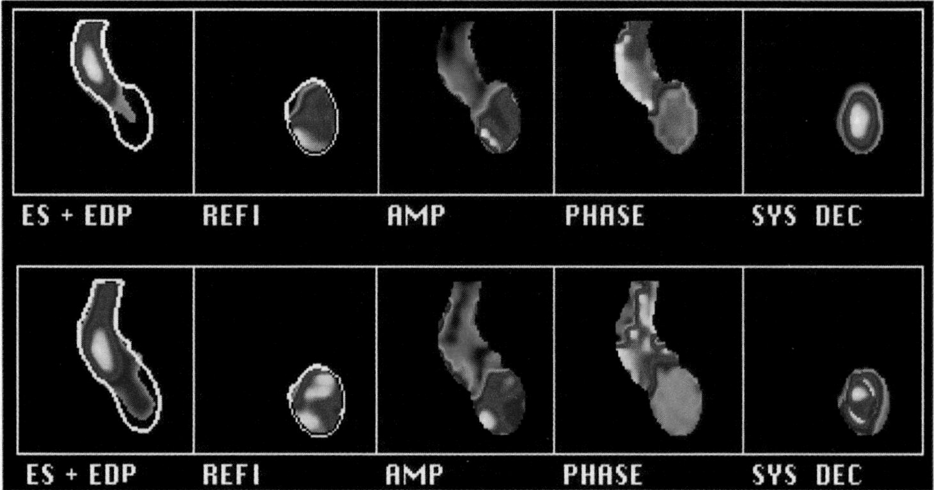

FIGURE 60–13. Some of the more commonly used parametric images generated from first-pass representative cycles at rest *(top row)* and during exercise *(bottom row)* in a patient with exercise-induced anteroapical dysfunction. The end-diastolic perimeter (EDP), defined by an arbitrary edge threshold, and the contained end-systolic (ES) volume are shown at the left. The regional ejection fraction image (REFI) displays the ejection fraction of each pixel in the left ventricle. The amplitude (AMP) image color-codes the height of the cosine wave that is mathematically fitted to the curve of the patient's representative cycle. The phase (PHASE) image color-codes the phase angle of each pixel and is useful for examination of the timing of contraction throughout the ventricle. The systolic decrease (SYS DEC) image color-codes the rate of decrease in counts during systole on a pixel-by-pixel basis. It is derived from a linear least squares fit to the systolic frames of the representative cycle.

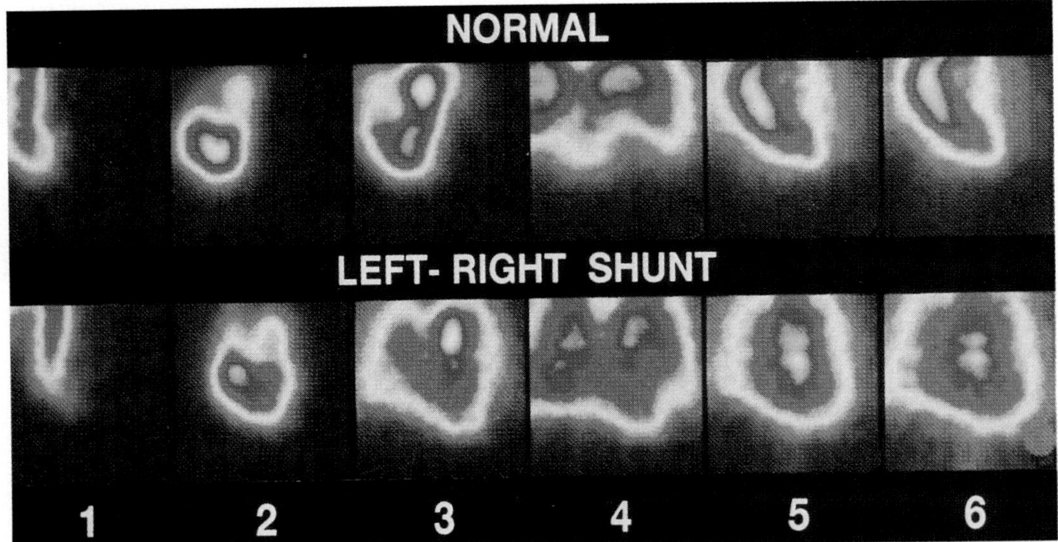

FIGURE 60–19. The presence of a significant intracardiac left-to-right shunt is easily confirmed by visual inspection of tracer transit. Contrast the image sequences from a normal subject with those of a patient with a left-to-right shunt. Images 1 through 4 show that initial transit through the right heart and lungs is similar, although the patient with the shunt has a dilated right heart. After the tracer reaches the left side of the heart (images 5 and 6), there is a clear difference between the two series. In the normal sequence, there is clear identification of the left ventricle and ascending aorta, free of any right ventricular activity or pulmonary activity. In the case of the shunt, the almost simultaneous appearances in the right and left sides of the heart preclude identification of a clear left ventricle or ascending aorta. A rather amorphous appearance of activity in both ventricles, the pulmonary circulation, and the aorta results. (From Port, S.C.: Recent advances in first-pass radionuclide angiography. Cardiol. Clin. 12:359, 1994, reprinted with permission.)

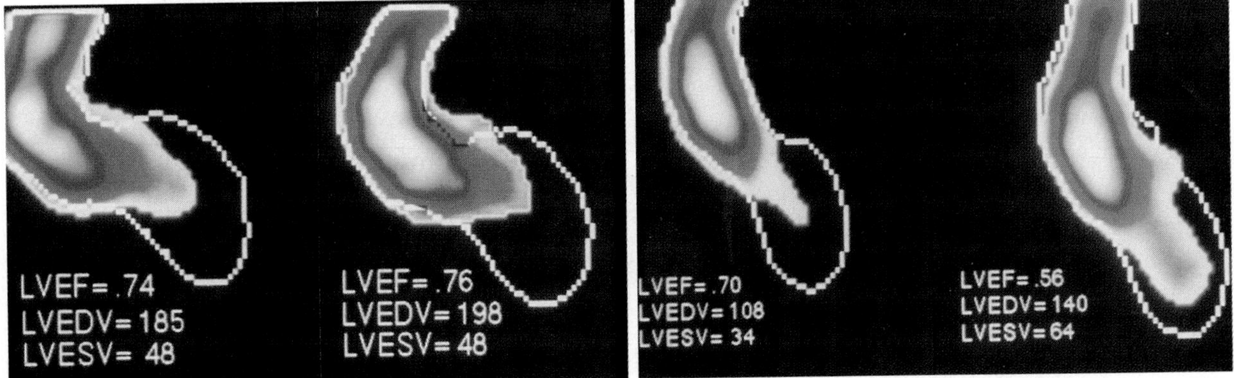

FIGURE 60–20. The classic ischemic response *(right)* during upright bicycle exercise is contrasted with the response of a normal volunteer *(left)*. During exercise-induced ischemia, there is an increase in end-diastolic volume (LVEDV), an increase in end-systolic volume (LVESV), a decrease in ejection fraction (LVEF), and appearance of a regional wall motion abnormality, in this case at the apex. (From Port, S.C.: Recent advances in first-pass radionuclide angiography. Cardiol. Clin. 12:359, 1994, reprinted with permission.)

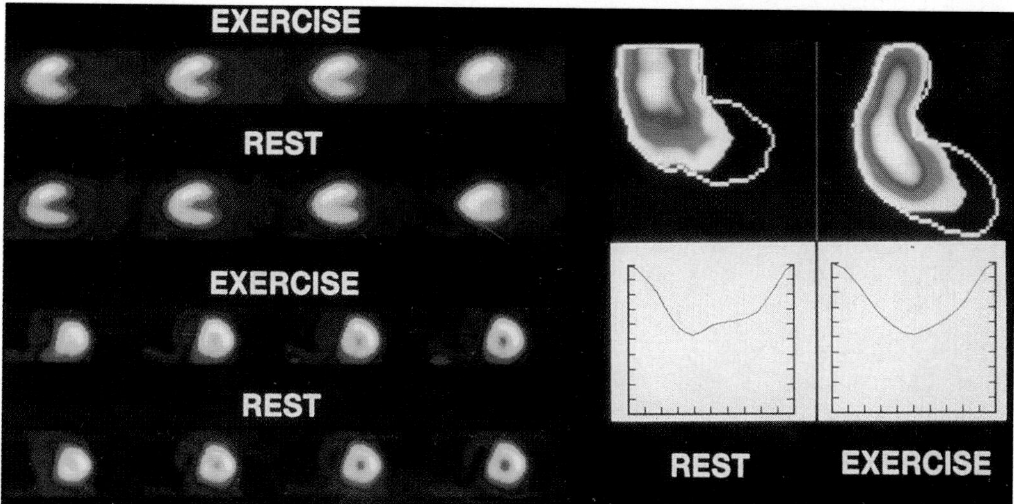

FIGURE 60–22. A benefit of combined function-perfusion imaging with first-pass radionuclide angiography is the ability to examine diastolic as well as systolic function. In this patient, coronary disease was suspected clinically, but neither the perfusion data nor the systolic ventricular function results supported that diagnosis. The marked diastolic dysfunction detected on the first-pass study had not been suspected. (From Port, S.C.: Recent advances in first-pass radionuclide angiography. Cardiol. Clin. 12:359, 1994, reprinted with permission.)

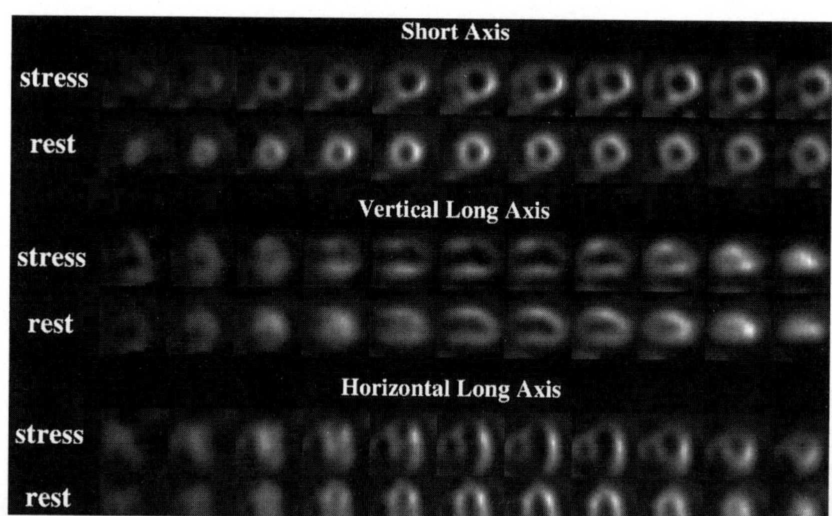

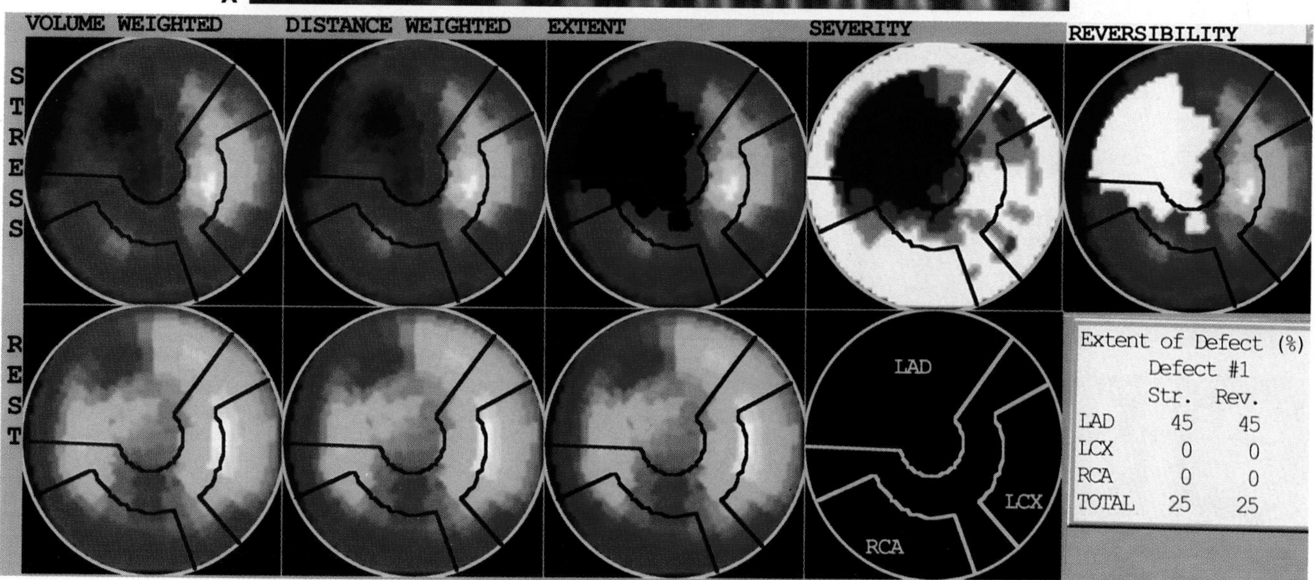

FIGURE 63–2. *Top,* An example of a stress-rest myocardial perfusion SPECT study in a patient with a 95 percent proximal LAD coronary artery stenosis. Reversible defects are noted in the middle and distal anterior, anteroseptal, and anterolateral walls, as well as the apex. *Bottom,* The "CEqual" quantitative analysis program shows a large reversible defect in the LAD territory.

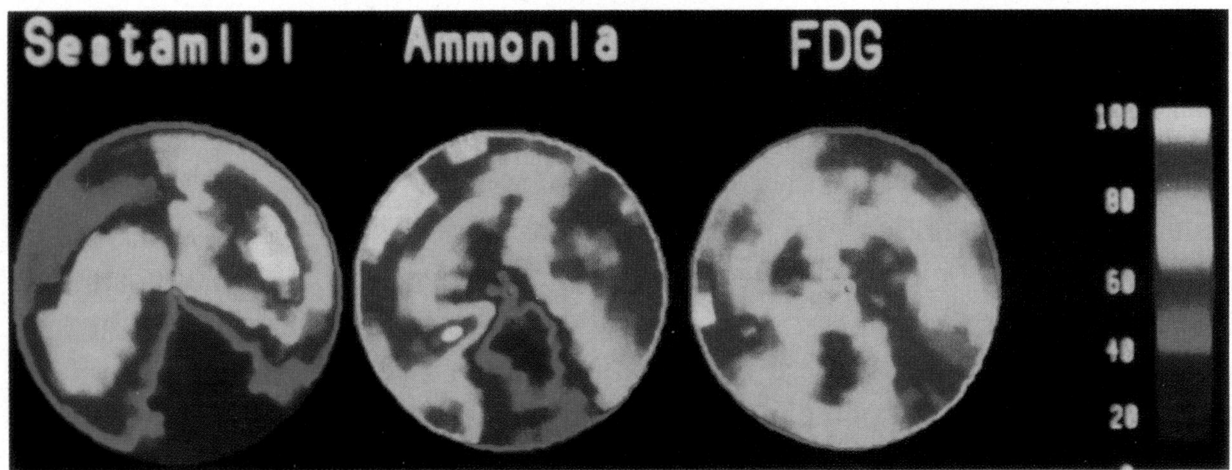

FIGURE 64–16. ^{99m}Tc-sestamibi (Sestamibi), ^{13}N-ammonia (Ammonia), and ^{18}F-2,deoxyglucose (FDG) polar maps in a patient with an inferior ^{99m}Tc-sestamibi defect. (From Sawada, S.G., Allman, K.C., Muzik, O., et al.: Positron emission tomography detects evidence of viability in rest technetium-99m sestamibi defects. J. Am. Coll. Cardiol. 23:92, 1994, with permission.)

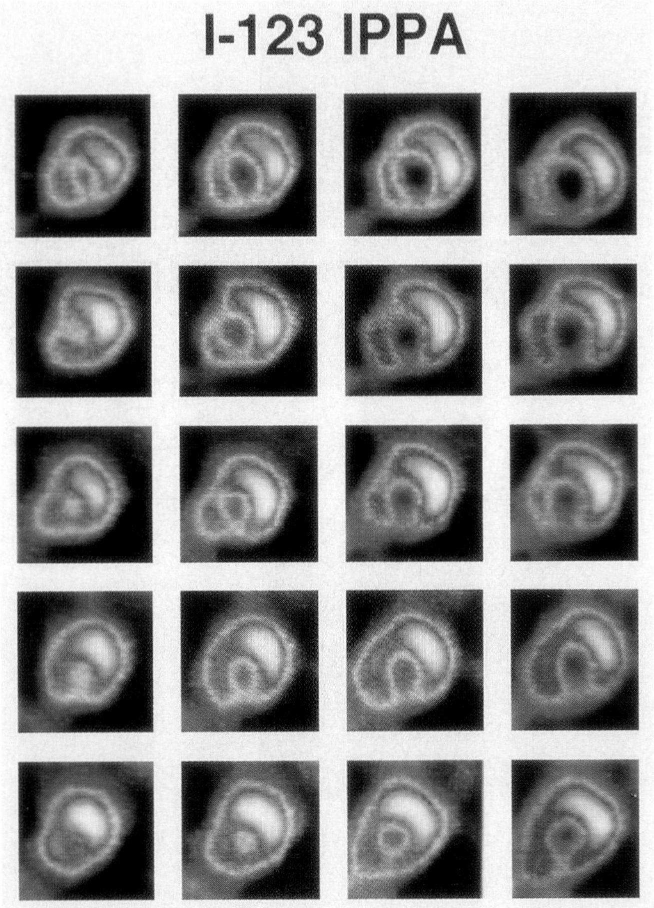

FIGURE 66–7. Serial 15-(*p*-[^{123}I]-iodophenyl)-pentadecanoic acid (IPPA) images from a patient with coronary artery disease. The five rows represent short-axis image sets obtained within 1 hour. The short-axis images are oriented from the apex (*left*) to the base (*right*). The interventricular septum is at the left, the anterior wall at the top, the lateral wall at the right, and the inferior wall at the bottom of each panel. Perfusion defects are noted in the septum, the inferior wall, and the inferolateral wall on the early images. The late images show considerable redistribution with improved tracer accumulation in the septum and inferior wall, suggesting myocardial viability. (From Iskandrian, A.S., Powers, J., Cave, V., et al.: Assessment of myocardial viability by dynamic tomographic iodine-123 iodophenylpentadecanoic acid imaging: Comparison with rest-redistribution thallium-201 imaging. J. Nucl. Cardiol. 2:101–109, 1995, with permission.)

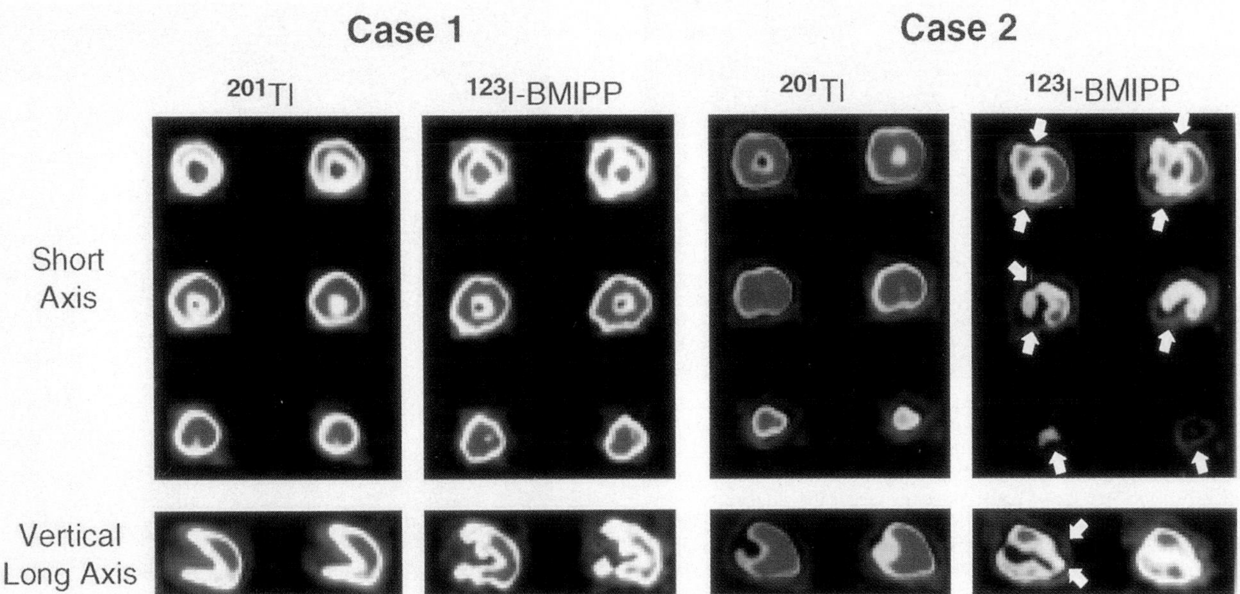

FIGURE 66–11. Thallium and 15-(*p*-[^{123}I]-iodophenyl)-3-methylpentadecanoic acid (BMIPP) tomograms from a patient with left ventricular hypertrophy and hypertension (case 1) and a patient with hypertrophic cardiomyopathy (case 2). Hypertensive heart disease was associated with a concordant pattern between ^{201}Tl and BMIPP distribution; in contrast, a mismatch between ^{201}Tl and BMIPP distribution was observed in the patient with hypertrophic cardiomyopathy. (From Hase, M., Nakata, T., Yonekure, S., et al.: Correlation of regional wall motion and fatty acid metabolism in coronary artery disease, hypertension and hypertrophic cardiomyopathy: Assessment by dual isotope SPECT with thallium-201 and iodine-123 β-methylfatty acid analogue. Kaku Igaku 30:529, 1993, with permission.)

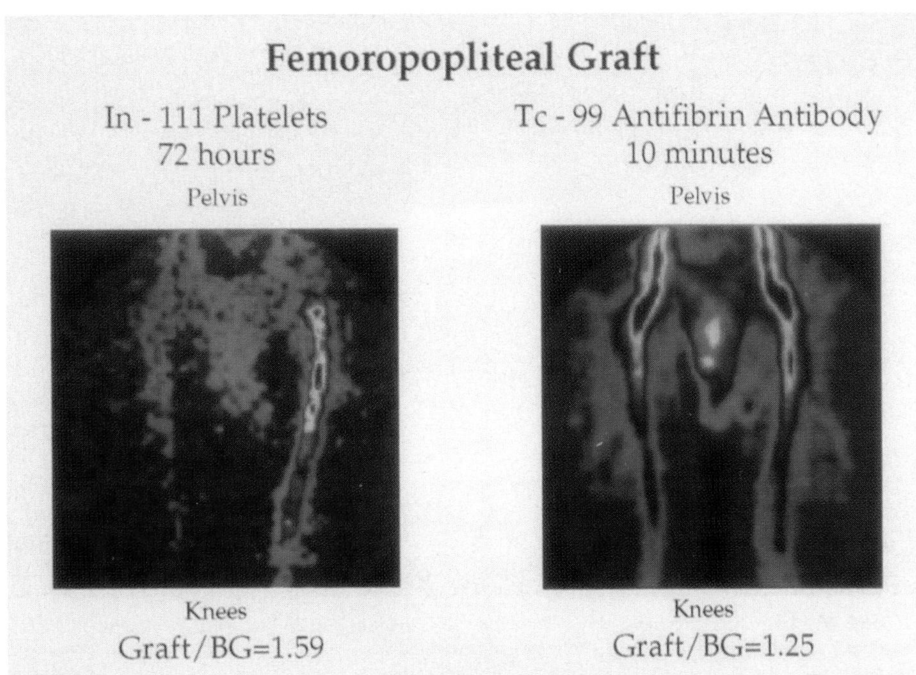

FIGURE 67–13. Comparison of ^{111}In platelet imaging and ^{99m}Tc antifibrin imaging in a patient with a polytetrafluoroethylene femoropopliteal graft. Intense uptake was present in several sections of the graft by ^{111}In platelet imaging (visual grade = 2). In contrast, antifibrin uptake in the grafted leg was more diffuse and even, compared with the contralateral leg (visual grade = 1). The graft-to-blood pool ratio was 1.59 by platelet imaging and 1.25 by antifibrin imaging.

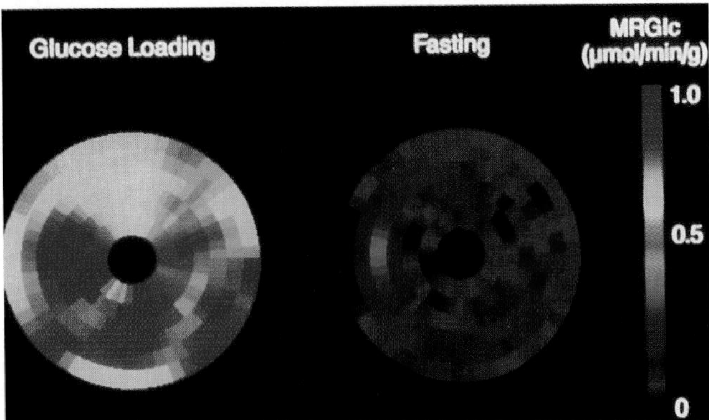

FIGURE 69–11. Parametric polar maps of myocardial glucose metabolic rates (MMRGlcs) in a normal volunteer obtained in the fasted state and again after an oral glucose loading 1 hour prior to the ^{18}F-2-deoxyglucose administration. The color code on the right side indicates the rate of glucose utilization in μmol/min/g. Note the low rates of glucose utilization in the fasted state when free fatty acid levels are high and glucose and insulin levels are on the low side of normal. Oral administration of 100 g of glucose is followed by an increase in plasma glucose and insulin levels and is associated with a decline in free fatty acid concentrations. In response, myocardium utilizes more glucose, as also seen on the parametric images.

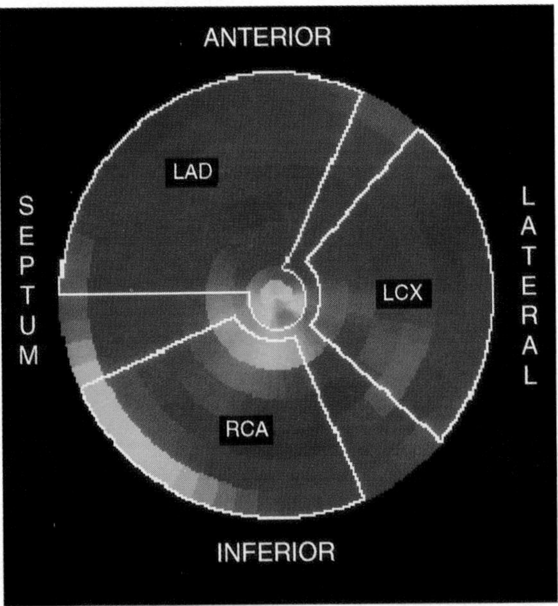

FIGURE 69–17. A polar map display of the myocardial ^{18}F-2-deoxyglucose uptake in a normal volunteer. The polar map depicts the three-dimensional distribution of tracer activities throughout the left ventricular myocardium in the form of a two-dimensional map. The polar map was obtained from the short-axis cuts in the study shown in Figure 69–16.

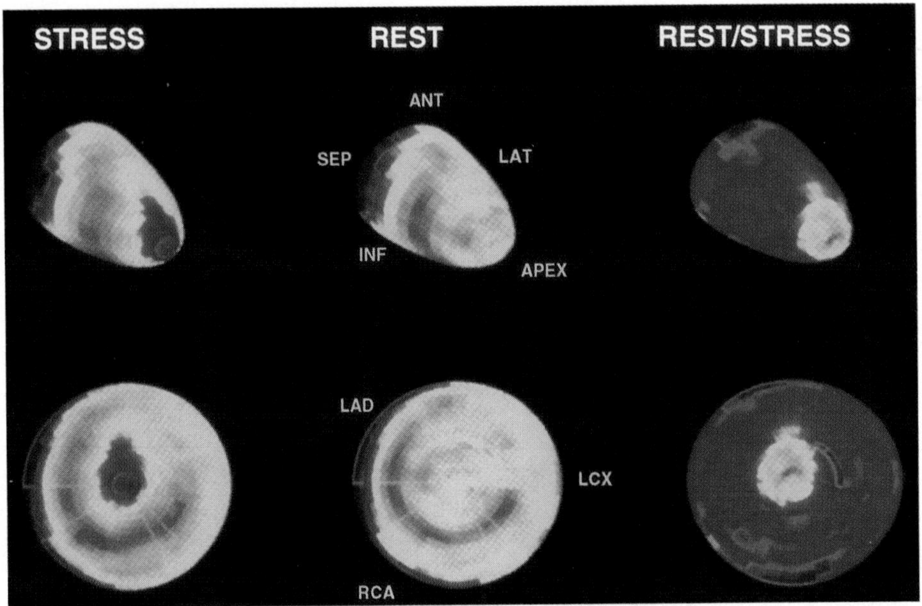

FIGURE 69–18. Three-dimensional display of the ^{13}N-ammonia activity distribution throughout the left ventricular myocardium in a patient with coronary artery disease. *Upper Panel,* Note the homogeneous distribution at rest and the dipyridamole-induced perfusion abnormality in the distal left anterior descending artery territory. The stress image shows again the defect in the distal left anterior descending artery territory. *Lower Panel,* Polar maps depict the tracer distribution in two dimensions and again indicate the stress-induced perfusion abnormality in the distal anterior wall. (Adapted from Laubenbacher, C., Rothley, J., Sitomer, J., et al.: An automated analysis program for the evaluation of cardiac PET studies: Initial results in the detection and localization of coronary artery disease using nitrogen-13 ammonia. J. Nucl. Med. 34:968, 1993, with permission.)

PLATE 32

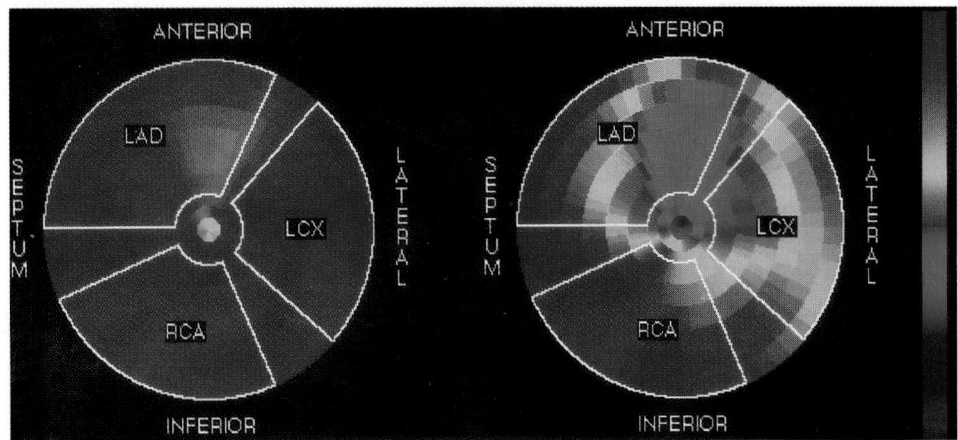

FIGURE 70–4. A two-dimensional display of the myocardial ^{13}N-ammonia uptake in the form of polar maps generated from the images shown in Figure 70–1. The polar map on the left shows the distribution of ^{13}N-ammonia uptake in the left ventricular myocardium at rest, and the polar map on the right was obtained after ^{13}N-ammonia was injected during hyperemia. Note the extensive uptake, and thus flow defect, in the anterior wall, as also seen on the short- and long-axis images in Figure 70–1.

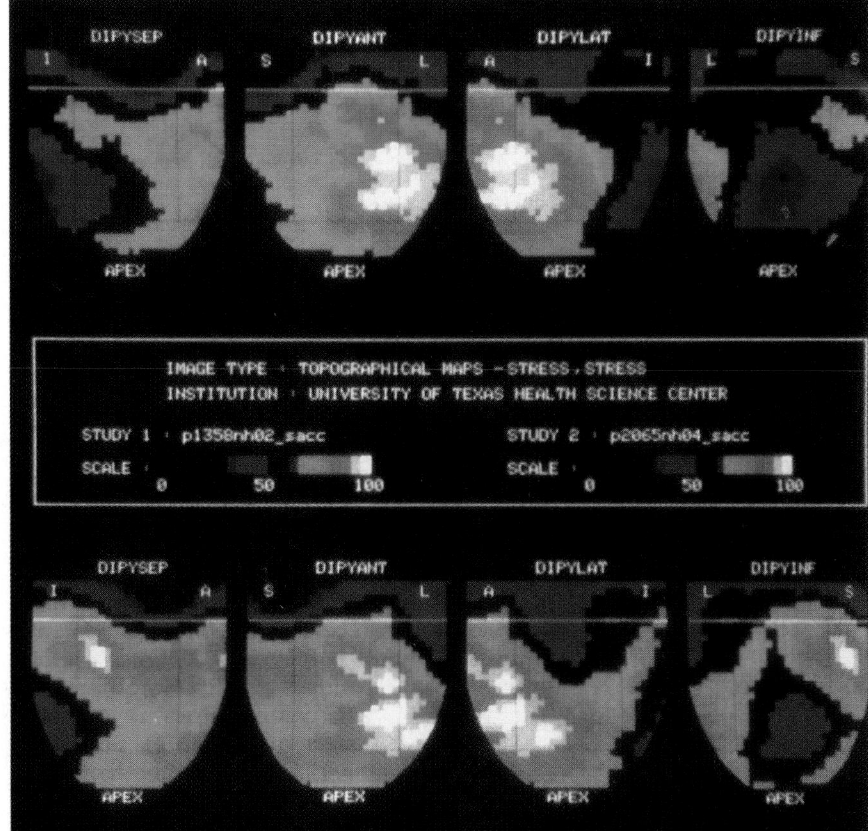

FIGURE 70–19. The effects of strict dietary and lifestyle changes on dipyridamole-induced myocardial blood flow defects are shown on a Mercator-type map of the left ventricular myocardium. Note the decrease in the size of the flow defect from the study taken before dietary and lifestyle changes *(top)* to the follow-up study *(bottom)*. Both image sets were obtained during dipyridamole-induced hyperemia. The change in defect size is seen best on the images on the very left (DIPYSEP) and on the very right (DIPYINF). (From Gould, K., Martucci, J., Goldberg, D., et al.: Short-term cholesterol lowering decreases size and severity of perfusion abnormalities by positron emission tomography after dipyridamole in patients with coronary artery disease: A potential noninvasive marker of healing coronary endothelium. Circulation 89:1530, 1994, with permission of the American Heart Association, Inc.)

PLATE 33

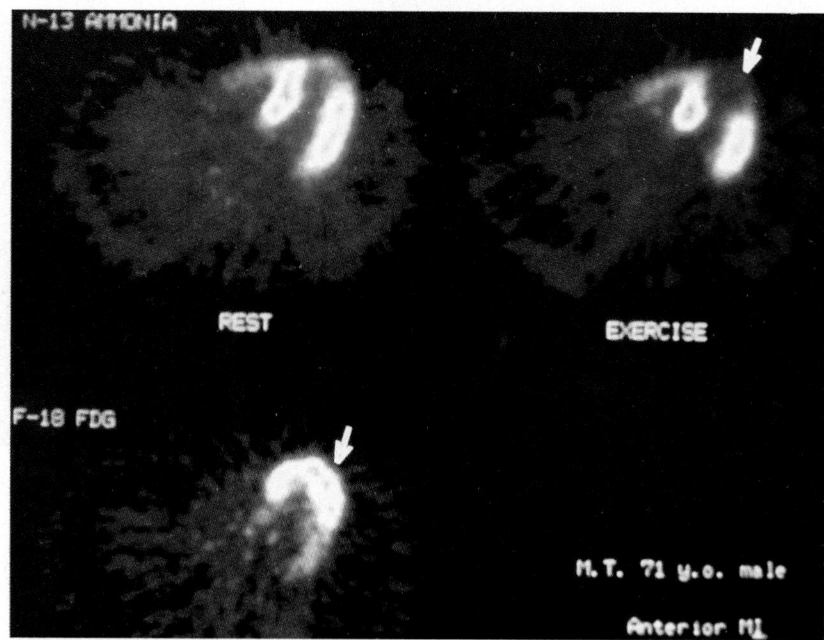

FIGURE 71–3. Representative resting and stress ^{13}N-ammonia perfusion images and resting ^{18}F-2-fluoro-2-deoxyglucose metabolic images in a patient 8 weeks after anterior myocardial infarction. The resting perfusion images demonstrate a decrease in relative myocardial perfusion in the anterior region of the ventricle. With exercise, the perfusion defect extends peripherally and is more pronounced. On metabolic imaging with ^{18}F-2-fluoro-2-deoxyglucose on a different day, augmented uptake of the glucose analog is identified in the anteroseptal and anterolateral regions of the ventricle, corresponding to the territory encompassed by the stress induced perfusion defect. (From Yonekura, Y., Tamaki, N., Kambara, H., et al.: Detection of metabolic alterations in ischemic myocardium by F-18 deoxyglucose uptake with positron emission tomography. Am. J. Card. Imaging 2:122, 1988, with permission.)

FIGURE 71–11. Patterns of myocardial blood flow and metabolism as observed on positron emission tomography in patients with coronary artery disease. The blood flow images were obtained with ^{13}N-ammonia and the glucose metabolic images were obtained with ^{18}F-2-fluoro-2-deoxyglucose. Each panel shows a short-axis *(left)*, a vertical long-axis *(center)*, and a horizontal long-axis cut *(right)*. *Panel A,* This patient with coronary artery disease had mild hypokinesis of the anterior wall. However, both myocardial blood flow and glucose use are normal (pattern A). *Panel B,* The blood flow images reveal a large area of decreased blood flow in the anterior apical and distal inferior wall. There is also a decrease in blood flow in the posterior septum. As noted on the metabolic images, however, glucose metabolism is homogeneous and therefore preserved in the dysfunctional and hypoperfused myocardial regions. Pattern B represents a blood flow–metabolism mismatch. *Panel C,* Again, images are shown from a patient with an inferior wall motion abnormality. The ^{13}N-ammonia images reveal an extensive blood flow defect in the inferior wall, whereas the metabolic images reveal a concordant decrease in ^{18}F-2-fluoro-2-deoxyglucose uptake. This pattern C represents a blood flow–metabolism match.

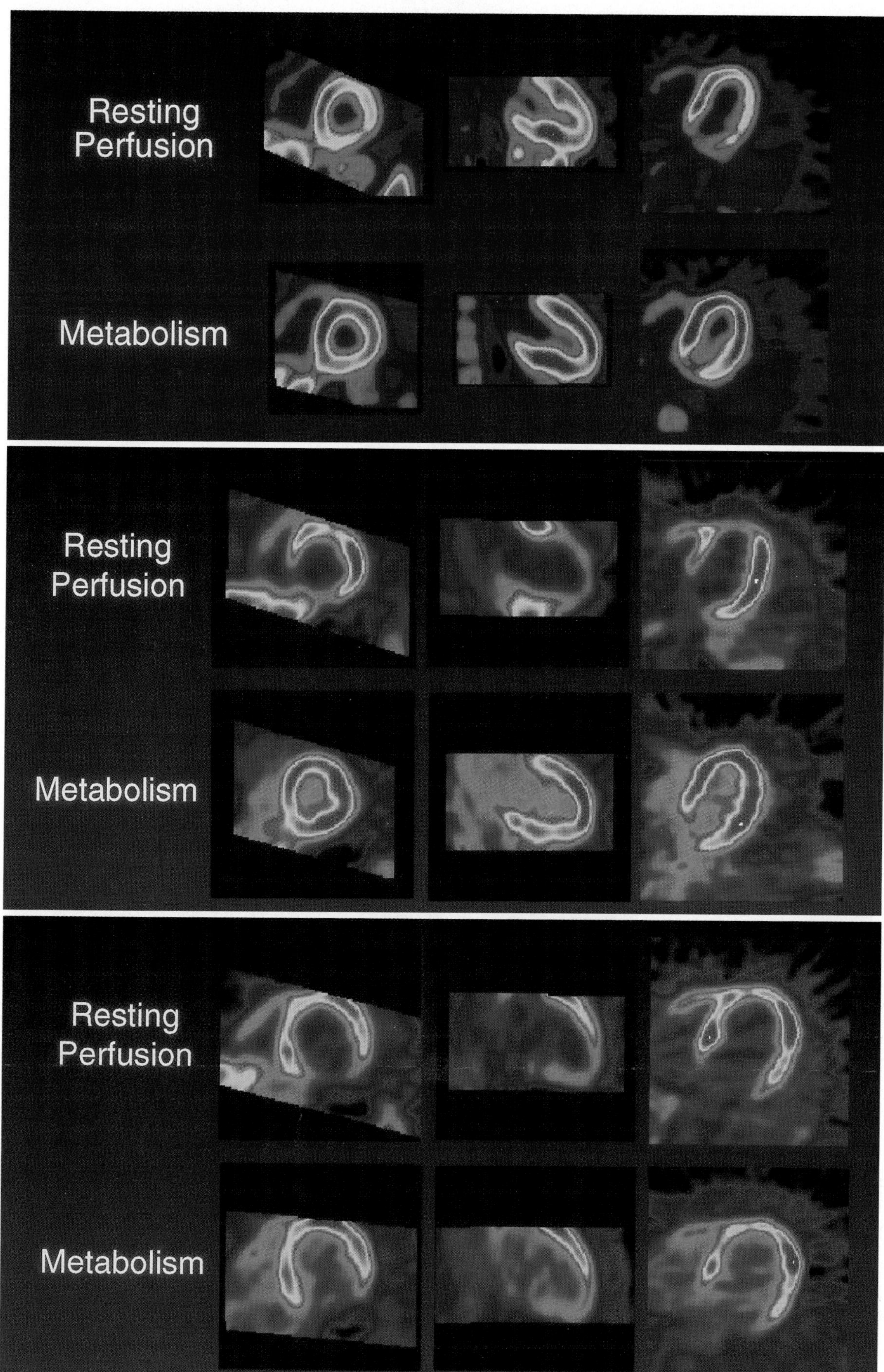

FIGURE 71–11 *See legend on opposite page*

PLATE 35

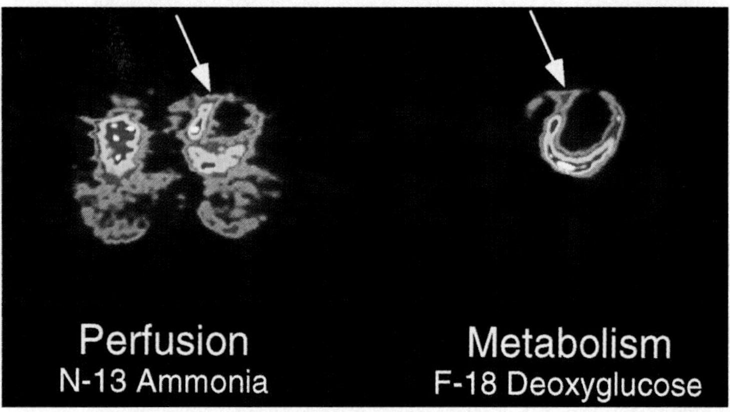

FIGURE 71–13. ^{13}N-ammonia and ^{18}F-2-fluoro-2-deoxyglucose metabolic images from a patient with ischemic cardiomyopathy. The arrows depict the intersection of the right ventricular free wall and the left ventricle, the starting point used for the circumferential profile analysis of the images. (From Berry, J.J., Hoffman, J.M., Steenbergen, C., et al.: Human pathologic correlation with PET in ischemic and nonischemic cardiomyopathy. J. Nucl. Med. 34:39–47, 1993, by permission).

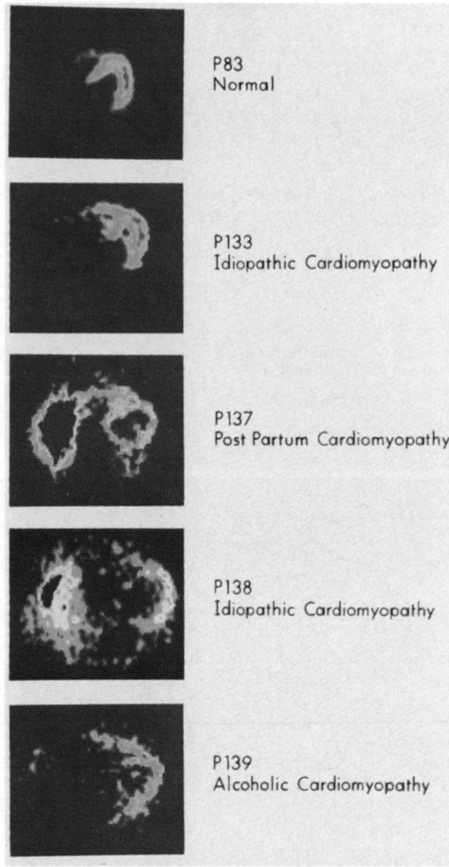

FIGURE 72–2. Positron emission tomographic images obtained after the intravenous (IV) administration of carbon-11–labeled palmitate (^{11}C-palmitate) at the midventricular level of a normal subject and patients with dilated cardiomyopathy from the causes indicated. The top of each image represents the patient's anterior; the right of each image represents the patient's left side. Areas in red represent areas of greatest accumulation of tracer, whereas areas in blue represent the least amount of tracer. The posterior discontinuity is due to the mitral valve apparatus and atria, which are below the spatial resolution of the instrument. Accumulation of radioactivity in the normal subject was homogeneous, with smooth transition between regions with intense accumulation to regions of only modest accumulation of tracer. Patients with cardiomyopathy demonstrate marked spatial heterogeneity in the accumulation of ^{11}C-palmitate. The regions of accumulation on the left of each image represent activity in the dome of the liver. (From Geltman, E.M., Smith, J.L., Beecher, D., et al.: Altered regional myocardial metabolism in congestive cardiomyopathy detected by positron tomography. Am. J. Med. 74:773, 1983, with permission.)

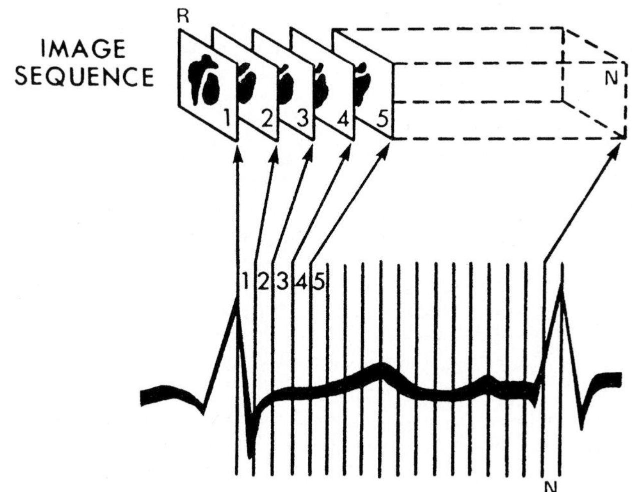

FIGURE 59–6. The method by which the computer generates multiple-gated images. The cardiac cycle is divided into a preselected number of frames of equal duration. Scintigraphic data from successive beats are placed into separate parts of the computer memory, depending on the temporal relation of the scintigraphic data to the R-wave marker (R). For each frame (numbered 1 through N), scintigraphic data from successive beats are accumulated, either until a preset time is reached (e.g., 2 minutes for exercise scintigraphy) or until the average cardiac image contains a predetermined number of counts (e.g., 200,000 counts for typical resting studies).

electrode connection or electrical interference; gating on the P or T wave, which in some disease states may be of larger amplitude than the R wave; gating on an atrial pacing spike; or delayed onset of mechanical systole caused by left bundle branch block. These problems can usually be prevented by evaluation of the resting electrocardiogram and the relation of the R wave to the gating signal before acquisition commences.

Constancy of the interval between gating signals is important for high temporal resolution. If the cardiac rhythm is not regular, the computer must compensate for fluctuations in the interval between successive R waves (the RR interval). At least two computer techniques can compensate for rhythm or rate changes. The first is directed toward the problem of changing heart rates, as seen during exercise. With this method, the time per frame automatically changes as a function of the average heart rate of the last few beats.[15] The second technique, which requires much more computer memory and sophistication, is designed to solve the problem of arrhythmia. In this method, part of the computer memory is used for transitory storage of the counts from only the last cardiac cycle. If the RR interval of this cycle is not within a preselected range, the counts are discarded. If it is within this interval, the counts are used to update the images recorded from previous beats.[16] A further development in this technique has been the use of multiple RR windows for each study. This allows the use of a narrow window to provide images with optimal temporal resolution at the same time that a broad window is used to provide images with the maximum number of counts. This technique also permits reconstruction of the cardiac cycles of arrhythmic and compensating beats as well as the standard beat.[17]

Another development that helps to maintain correct temporal sampling is synchronization of the acquisition of scintigraphic data, not only from the R wave forward in time, but also from the R wave backward in time (Fig. 59–7). Some form of beat rejection or backward gating is imperative for accurate synchronization of the last third of the cardiac cycle, as required for the measurement of diastolic events.[18]

Attention to the potential problems of gating is an important aspect of quality control for multiple-gated equilibrium scintigraphy (MGES). For assessment of RR interval constancy, a computer program that provides a beat-length histogram (plot of the number of beats versus their cycle length) should be used. An ideal study is represented on this histogram by a single narrow spike centered on the patient's cycle length, indicating little variation in RR interval (Fig. 59–8).

Proper selection of matrix type and size is another major consideration for acquisition and storage of MGES studies. In order to assess regional wall motion, the highest possible digital resolution with adequate counts per pixel should be sought. Nevertheless, the greater the number of pixels, the fewer the counts per pixel. As a general rule, a minimum matrix size of 64 × 64 pixels is recommended for accurate assessment of regional wall motion, whereas a matrix size of 32 × 32 may suffice for measurement of EF and other parameters derived from time-activity curves.

Dynamic Imaging

First-Pass Acquisition

Dynamic frame-mode acquisition is similar to filming a movie of the heart. It is used when the radionuclide distribution is rapidly changing. The frame rate for acquisition depends on the speed of this change and the frequency of the information that needs to be extracted. To analyze beat-to-beat changes from a first-pass study of a bolus of ^{99m}Tc, a fast frame rate is required. To analyze lower-frequency changes, such as the transit time between cardiac chambers of the same bolus of ^{99m}Tc, a slow frame rate can be employed.

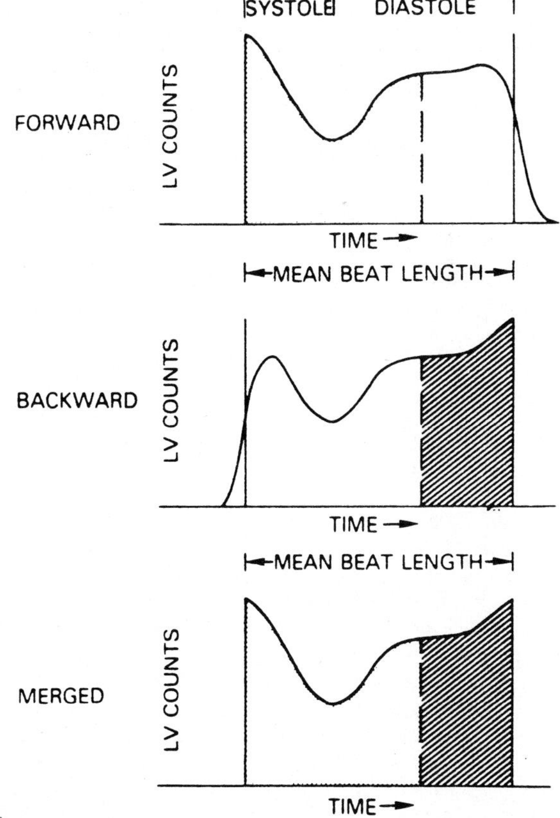

FIGURE 59–7. Reconstruction of the cardiac cycle by framing acquired count events both forward and backward in time from the R wave. *Top Panel,* A left ventricular (LV) volume-time curve created by forward gating exhibits a trail-off in late diastole owing to fluctuations in cardiac cycle length. *Middle Panel,* A volume-time curve created by backward gating exhibits a trail-off in the systolic region. *Bottom Panel,* Merging of the first two thirds of the top curve and the last one third of the middle curve yields a complete cardiac cycle with improved registration of the late-diastolic counts compared with standard forward gating alone. (From Bacharach, S., et al.: Instrumentation and data processing in cardiovascular nuclear medicine: Evaluation of ventricular function. Semin. Nucl. Med. 9:269, 1979, p. 269, with permission.)

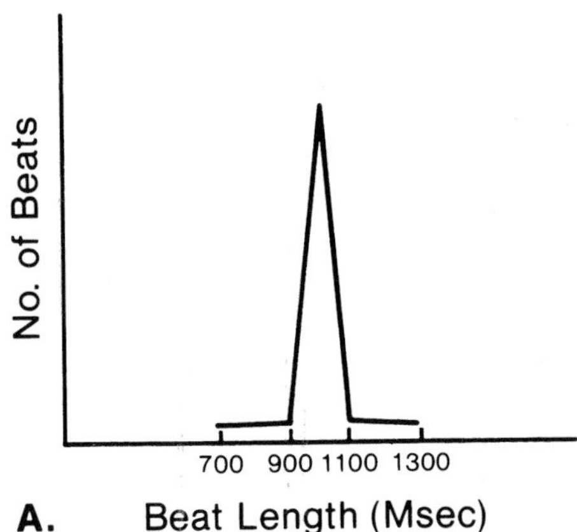

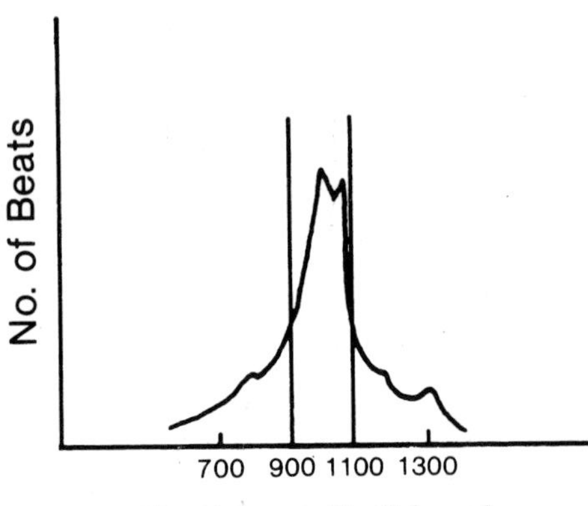

FIGURE 59–8. Examples of R-R histograms. *A*, An ideal R-R histogram of a patient with a very stable heart rate (approximately 1 beat per second). *B*, R-R histogram of a patient with significant beat-to-beat variations (between 800 and 1300 msec), which give rise to a poorly registered volume-time curve (not shown). The vertical lines through histogram B illustrate the potential in some systems of windowing the length of the beats accepted; this procedure results in a better registered (more accurate) volume-time curve at the cost of rejection of a significant number of beats.

The number of frames per second is preselected. For example, acquisition of the first pass of a radionuclide bolus through the heart for assessment of biventricular function should be acquired at a minimum of 20 frames per second for 25 seconds, and ideally at 25 to 100 frames per second for 60 seconds. This acquisition requires storage of at least 500 separate frames, necessitating a storage device other than computer memory. Magnetic disks can hold from hundreds to thousands of frames and can store the information rapidly, making them the storage medium of choice. If the acquisition is being performed at 20 frames per second, a frame is written to the disk every 50 msec.

After acquisition, the study is formatted into images of representative cardiac cycles for the right and left ventricles. The two ventricles are separated by identifying the anatomic configuration and temporal appearance of the bolus as it passes through the central circulation. Regions of interest are assigned for each ventricle. Preliminary time-activity curves are generated from each ventricular region of interest. These time-activity curves consist of multiple peaks and valleys that correspond to end-diastolic and end-systolic frames of individual beats. These curves are used to generate representative cardiac cycles by using the frames with the highest peaks as the starting points, summing all of them together, then summing together the next 50-msec frames of each cardiac cycle, and then the next, and so on until end-diastole is again reached. This is done for the time-activity curve from the right ventricle and left ventricle separately, generating "representative" cardiac cycles for both the right and left sides of the heart. Another technique used to generate representative cardiac cycles is to use the maxima of the first derivatives on the time-activity curves as points of alignment.

First-pass studies can also be acquired at a slower frame rate of 2 frames per second for adults in order to evaluate lower-frequency events. Such studies can be obtained either by acquiring the counts at that rate or by combining the frames from a study obtained at a higher frame rate. A first-pass study obtained at 20 frames per second for assessment of ventricular function can be converted to a study at 2 frames per second by combining every 10 frames into a single composite frame until an entire sequence of these 0.5-second composite frames is created.

Low-frequency time-activity curves can be extracted for regions of interest over the different cardiac chambers. These have found purpose for measurement of transit times between the different chambers and to indicate the relative volume and flow from each chamber. Combined with measurements of blood volume, these curves can approximate cardiac output. In addition, quantification of left-to-right shunts and of regurgitant fractions is possible.

First-Pass Multiple-Gated Acquisition

The most common cardiac function study is blood pool MGES, in which the imaging is performed over a period of several minutes. However, the same hardware and software can be applied to multiple-gated first-pass studies.[19] In this approach, a bolus of radionuclide is injected intravenously. The computer is manually started after the bolus is seen to have entered the right atrium and is stopped after the tracer clears the right ventricle. A similar process is repeated for the left ventricular phase. During the time of imaging, changes of tracer concentration are ignored; therefore this, too, is a form of static imaging. Because the right atrium overlaps the right ventricle in equilibrium studies, first-pass is the study of choice for measurement of right ventricular EF.[20]

Planar Imaging in List Mode

List (serial) mode is the alternative to frame mode acquisition. The principle here is that a portion of computer memory is reserved to keep a temporal list of each event that takes place. The list usually consists of one computer word (memory location) per event, and it records the *x-y* coordinates of each scintillation, physiologic markers indicating each R-wave trigger occurrence, and time markers every 1 to 10 msec as appropriate for the particular study. These data are reconstructed after acquisition, allowing the operator a choice of frame rate, matrix size, and dynamic or static format. The main advantage is the flexibility of what can be done with the data after acquisition, and the main disadvantages are the large storage requirements and the time needed for reconstruction of the cardiac images before a display is available or analysis can be performed.

Equilibrium Studies

The list mode can be used to reconstruct cardiac images similar to those obtained from MGES acquisition.[16] The reconstruction software program is similar to that of the acquisition program that formats the multiple-gated images. The operator selects the number of frames per cardiac cycle, and the reconstruction program divides the calculated RR interval by the number of frames to obtain the time per frame. Each R-wave marker triggers the program to incorporate the subsequent counts on the first frame until enough time markers have been counted to correspond to the calculated time per frame. The scintigraphic data obtained is then channeled to frame 2, and the process continues until the last time interval has elapsed or until the next R wave is encountered in the list. An advantage of this approach is that RR tolerance intervals can easily be assigned so that counts from ectopic beats outside of this "window" are not added to the cardiac cycle. This technique also allows for reconstruction of the cardiac cycle from the R wave both forward and backward in time. This option produces increased temporal resolution during the last third of the cardiac cycle, improving the calculations of diastolic events.

Because of these advantages, list mode acquisition with real-time reconstruction has been incorporated in some multiple-gated acquisition systems.[16] In this combined mode, counts from the most recent heart beat are acquired in list mode. These counts are examined in real time to see whether the last beat falls outside the preselected RR interval; if it does, the beat is rejected. If the beat falls inside the preselected interval, the list mode buffer is formatted into frames with both forward and backward gating, and the formatted frames are added to the composite cardiac cycle.

First-Pass Studies

List mode can also be used to acquire first-pass studies.[21] The incorporation of R-wave triggers, if acquired, enhances the temporal resolution of the reconstructed representative cardiac cycle. This method is theoretically superior to use of the ventricular time-activity curves themselves to synchronize the different beats, because the curves are contaminated by tissue crosstalk (background) and are affected by camera and computer performance. List mode acquisition of first-pass studies also allows the reformatting of the scintillation data into fast dynamic, slow dynamic, or gated first-pass studies.

SINGLE-PHOTON EMISSION COMPUTED TOMOGRAPHY

Tomographic imaging, in contrast to conventional planar imaging, yields slices of the heart without overlapping counts from radioactivity of neighboring slices or background tissue. This attribute results in an increase in contrast resolution, or the ability to discern differences in tracer concentration in neighboring tissues. This increase in contrast resolution is advantageous in thallium imaging, in which ischemic hypoperfused areas need to be differentiated from normally perfused myocardium. In circular rotational tomography, because the detector is forced to orbit at times far away from the patient, the increase in contrast resolution is accompanied by a decrease in spatial resolution. Figure 59–9 illustrates the difference between contrast and spatial resolution. In myocardial perfusion imaging, the increase in contrast resolution produced by tomographic imaging is preferred over the higher spatial resolution of planar imaging. Clinically, this improvement in contrast resolution translates into improved detection of less-ischemic perfusion defects. This improvement is realized at the cost of an increase in technical difficulty, which requires, among other things, that the center of rotation of the mechanical axis of the camera is aligned to the electronic axis representing the acquired projection, and that the plane defined by the camera's crystal remains parallel to the axis of rotation during scanning.[2]

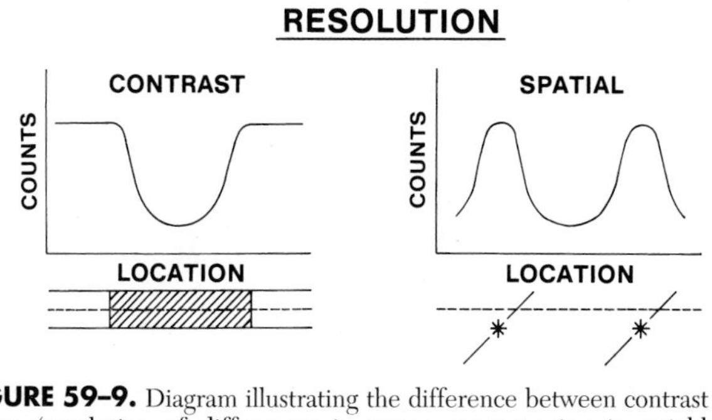

FIGURE 59–9. Diagram illustrating the difference between contrast resolution (resolution of differences in tracer concentration in neighboring myocardial walls) and spatial resolution (resolution of two separate radioactive line sources). Curves represent count profiles extracted from corresponding radioactive distributions.

Acquisition of Projections

Most nuclear medicine single-photon emission computed tomography (SPECT) is performed with one gamma camera mounted on a gantry. This gantry allows rotation of the detector around the patient for a full 360-degree angular sampling. The orbit of the detector can be either circular or elliptical. Elliptical orbits have the advantage of keeping the detector closer to the patient during rotation and thus preserving the spatial resolution that is lost by circular orbits when the detector is forced occasionally to image far from the patient.

The most widespread mode of tomographic acquisition is the step-and-shoot method. In this approach, the detector stops at preselected angles (32 to 128 stops covering 360 degrees). The detector acquires γ-rays (shoots) while the gantry is stationary for a preselected period of time. After the time for each projection has elapsed, the gantry steps to the next angular position. While it is stepping, it is not recording events. This process is repeated until the total number of preselected projections are acquired.

The angular range that should be used in tomographic scanning of cardiac studies remains a source of disagreement. Some investigators insist that accurate, artifact-free reconstruction necessitates acquisition of projections from a full 360-degree orbit.[22] Nevertheless, most of the groups using SPECT clinically point out that 180-degree orbits (45 degrees RAO to 45 degrees left posterior oblique [LPO]) yield, in half the acquisition time, higher contrast resolution than the 360-degree orbits, which are contaminated by noise from a significant amount of attenuation for the projections acquired through the patient's back.[23] This is particularly true for acquisition of the low-energy (80-keV) photons emitted by ^{201}Tl and acquired with the use of a single gamma camera system.

Multihead Cameras

The most obvious benefit of adding more camera heads to a SPECT system is the increase in sensitivity that comes from doubling or tripling the crystal area used to image the heart. Doubling the number of heads doubles the number of photons that may be counted in a given period of time, assuming that attenuation is neglected and that counts from all of the projections are used to reconstruct the final images. The increase in sensitivity may be used to shorten the imaging time, to acquire more counts, or to add higher-resolution collimation. In practice, the properties of the radiopharmaceutical and the clinical need determine which of these advantages should be emphasized. An increase in counts may result in much better image quality in a count-poor study. A shortened imaging time reduces the chance of patient motion during acquisition. Higher resolution allows the detection of smaller defects.

Many popular SPECT systems are configured with two large-field-of-view rectangular camera heads mounted opposite each other (180 degrees), which increases the throughput of whole-body bone imaging by allowing simultaneous acquisition of anterior and posterior images. These systems can also increase throughput for 360-degree SPECT imaging by halving the imaging time.

The addition of a second camera head opposite the first, however, is of no benefit for cardiac SPECT if a 180-degree orbit is preferred (Fig. 59–10). Furthermore, even if a 360-degree orbit is used, a second head at 180 degrees does not result in doubled sensitivity for cardiac imaging because counts in the posterior planar images are more severely attenuated than those of the anterior projections. For example, analysis of ^{99m}Tc-sestamibi SPECT images of a 170-pound, 31-year-old male normal volunteer shows that 65 percent of the total myocardial counts are collected between 45 degrees of RAO to 45 degrees of LPO.

The addition of a second camera head at a 90-degree angle to the first is a superior configuration for cardiac SPECT because it allows a true doubling of sensitivity for 180-degree orbits as well as 360-degree orbits. In order for the system to acquire a 180-degree orbit, each camera must move through only 90 degrees.

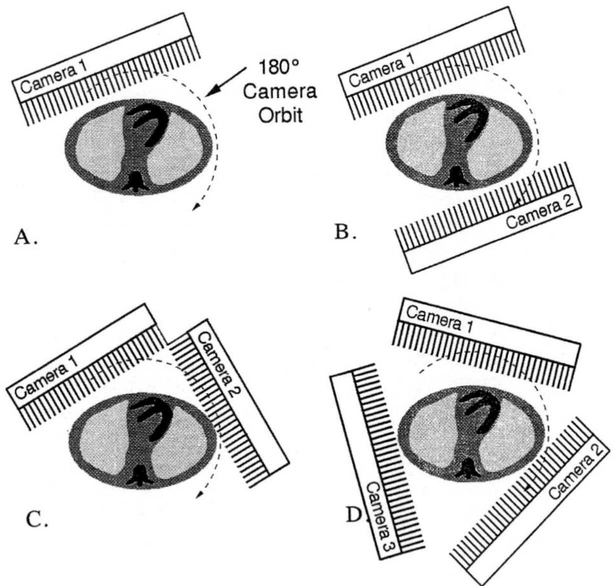

FIGURE 59–10. A, Standard single-head camera. The arc shows the 45-degree right anterior oblique to 45-degree left posterior oblique orbit used for 180-degree cardiac single-photon emission computed tomography. *B,* Addition of a second head doubles the sensitivity for 360-degree camera orbits but provides no increase in sensitivity if the 180-degree orbit is used. *C,* Addition of a second head at 90 degrees doubles the sensitivity for both 360- and 180-degree orbits and may be preferred for cardiac imaging. *D,* The use of three heads, evenly spaced at 120-degree intervals, increases the sensitivity by only 50 percent for 180-degree single-photon emission computed tomography but triples the sensitivity for 360-degree orbits.

The disadvantages of dual-head cameras with a 90-degree configuration is a loss of utility for noncardiac imaging and the fact that each head must orbit at least 270 degrees for a 360-degree orbit to be acquired. The use of camera heads in this configuration is not limited to SPECT but allows biplanar blood pool imaging (multiple-gated and first-pass acquisition). SPECT cameras are available that allow two camera heads to rotate from a 180-degree separation to a 90-degree configuration. These cameras give added flexibility at the cost of some additional complexity.

Triple-headed cameras are usually dedicated to SPECT imaging. The three heads give increased sensitivity compared with a single head, but if 180-degree orbits are used, the increase is not as great as for two camera heads mounted at 90 degrees. If 180-degree SPECT is required, the increase in sensitivity is only 50 percent: one head will not be used at all, and the other will be used for only half of its 120-degree orbit. Triple-headed SPECT systems are best suited for clinics that perform a large number of 360-degree SPECT studies and can afford to have a camera dedicated solely to that task.

It is possible to fit two of the camera heads with slant-hole collimators to better utilize a triple-head camera for 180-degree imaging. Fifteen-degree slant-hole collimators, combined with the 60 degrees between the cameras, results in a 90-degree view angle between the heads, doubling the sensitivity for 180-degree SPECT. The remaining camera is then freed for a different type of collimator. For example, a high-sensitivity parallel-hole collimator may be used for first-pass studies before the SPECT acquisition.

Drawbacks of multiheaded cameras include the increase in quality control required by the additional heads and the loss of flexibility. This may prevent these devices from being easily used for some types of planar imaging (e.g., gated blood pool imaging) for which it is often difficult to position the camera correctly.

Image Reconstruction

Backprojection

Tomographic projections are nothing more than a series of planar images taken at different angles around the patient. These images are then backprojected into transverse axial (or transaxial) images or slices inherently oriented perpendicular to the axis of rotation, which usually corresponds to the long axis of the patient. The transaxial images can then be reoriented to produce sagittal, coronal, or oblique angle images. The backprojection algorithm uses the fact that any photon that interacts with the camera crystal must have passed through one of the collimator holes, thus defining its direction. Because parallel-hole collimators are usually employed, the reconstruction algorithm backprojects or "sends back" the counts from the recorded location in the crystal along a line perpendicular to the face of the crystal.

These backprojected lines are recorded in the computer memory, which represents the three-dimensional space occupied by the object being imaged. Because it is not known exactly where the emissions took place along this backprojected line, the algorithm deposits the counts in each pixel traversed by the line. Tomograms are generated because the backprojected lines cross at the location at which the radiation originated. The parts of the lines that do not cross at the correct location give rise to a star pattern, which blurs the image and reduces its contrast (Fig. 59–11).

Filtered Backprojection

The goal of tomographic reconstruction is to provide a blur-corrected transaxial tomogram from processed planar projections. The solution to this problem in frequency space involves the application of a Ramp filter (Fig. 59–12) to the frequency components of each projection. Galt and colleagues[24] have provided an in-depth description of filtering in frequency space. After filtration, each projection is transformed back into the conventional spatial domain and then backprojected to form the blur-corrected transaxial tomograms.

The Ramp filter, as shown in Figure 59–12, is a high-pass filter

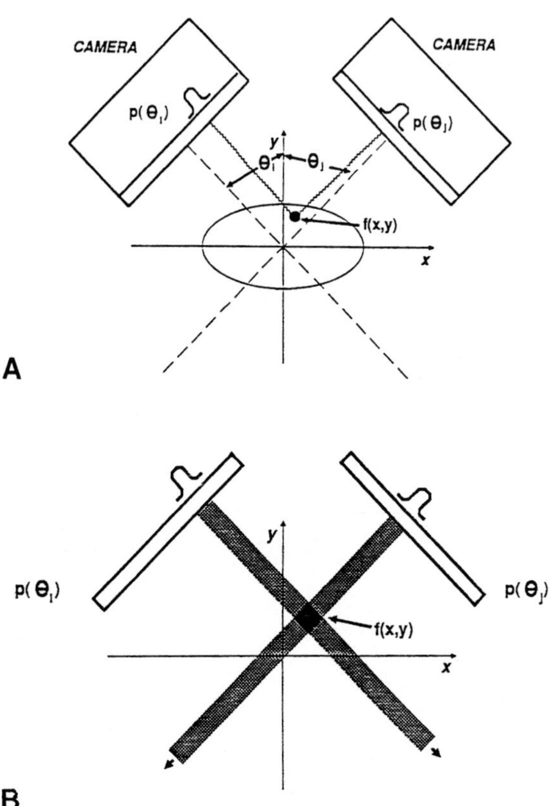

FIGURE 59–11. Principle of backprojection. *A,* The acquisition of two planar projections of a point source [f(x,y)] of radioactivity. *B,* The backprojection of these projections. The backprojected counts sum at the original source of activity, but counts are left in other parts of the image, resulting in a star artifact.

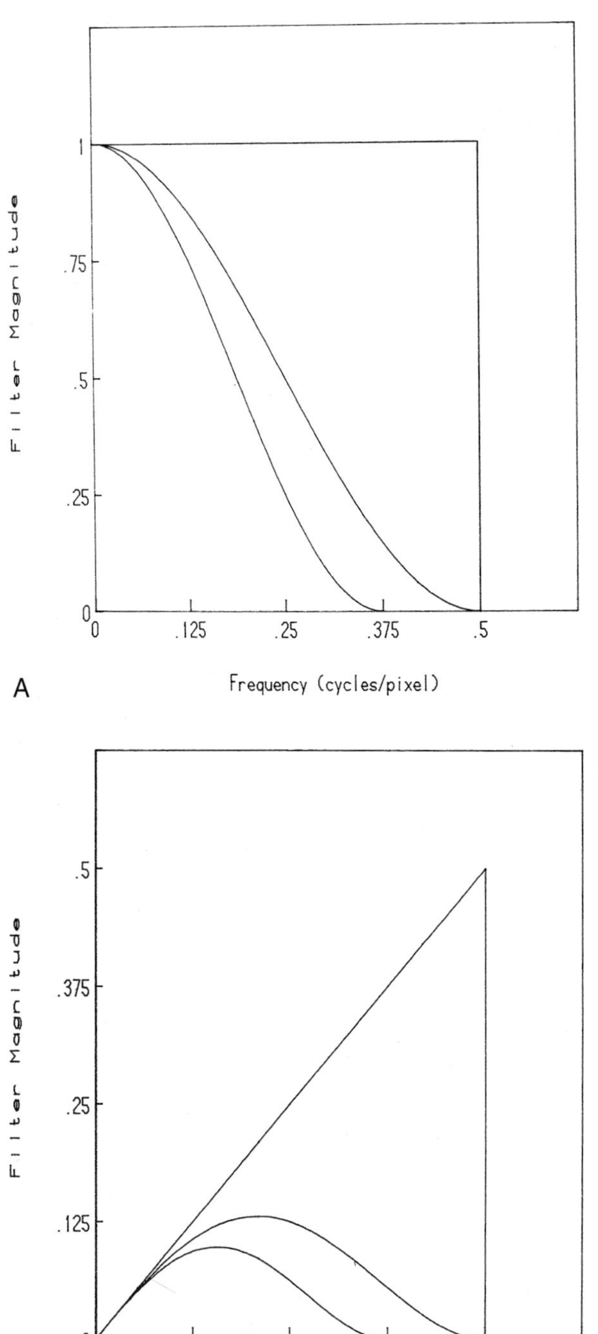

FIGURE 59–12. Curve representation of commonly used filters. *A,* Plot of filter amplitude versus frequency for a rectangular filter, a Hanning filter with filter window cutoff at 0.5 cycles per pixel, and a Hanning filter with cutoff at 0.375 cycles per pixel. *B,* The same filters were then multiplied by a Ramp filter and plotted as magnitude versus frequency.

that enhances the edges of the radioactive distribution in the image. Intuitively, the reconstruction process known as filtered backprojection (FBP) may be thought of as, first, extraction of the edges of a three-dimensional radioactive source from different angles and, second, backprojection of the edges from the different angles to generate the count distribution in a transaxial tomogram. The Ramp filter, being a high-pass filter that linearly enhances higher frequencies, yields the highest resolution possible in a reconstruction but also propagates, along the backprojected lines, the high-frequency noise associated with low-count statistics. This propagation of noise often results in clinically uninterpretable images.

Filtering

Modifications to the Ramp filter must be made to compensate for the undesirable noise. This is done by combining the Ramp characteristics with those of a low-pass (smoothing) filter or window. Hanning and Butterworth filters are two commonly used windows that can be multiplied by a Ramp filter to yield different degrees of tradeoff between reduction of statistical noise and degradation of spatial and contrast resolution.

Figure 59–12*A* illustrates examples of a rectangular filter and two Hanning filters that may be used to modify or "window" the Ramp filter. When these windows are multiplied by the Ramp, the filter function curves then become those shown in Figure 59–12*B*. After this is done, the filter is referred to as a Ramp-Hanning filter for clarification. Noise can also be removed from the final tomograms by application of the smoothing filters to the planar projections, either before backprojection or afterward by filtration of the transaxial slices. Filtering before backprojection may be more desirable for two reasons. First, it reduces the propagation of noise at an earlier stage in the image formation process, and second, it promotes the implementation of a filter that is symmetric in three dimensions (i.e., that has the same resolution in the x, y, and z directions). Proponents of postprocessing argue that the same results could be obtained by careful selection of filters applied to the transaxial tomograms.

Factors That Influence Clinical Interpretation

Clinicians who interpret tomograms from SPECT imaging procedures usually assume that the distribution of intensities (counts) that they observe is directly proportional to the radionuclide concentration. In interpretation of a ^{201}Tl myocardial short-axis slice, it may be naively assumed that, if the intensity of the septum is twice as bright as the lateral wall, then the septum has twice the concentration. Although this ability to extract counts (brightness) directly proportional to tracer concentration is the ultimate goal of SPECT imaging, there are several limiting physical and technical factors. These factors not only affect the quantitative aspects of the reconstructed tomograms but also degrade the overall quality of the image. Correction methodologies exist that compensate for these effects, some of which are commercially available and some which are being tested in experimental settings.

Scatter Correction

Scatter correction is the ability to compensate for photons that have undergone a Compton scatter event in the patient and have continued on to be recorded by the detector. These accepted scattered photons significantly degrade the image during the reconstruction process because they are backprojected along lines different from their original path.

Two main approaches are being investigated for determination of the amount of scatter that is present: use of a scatter mask calculated from the projections or tomograms,[25] and use of a scatter mask calculated from counts acquired with one or more additional PHA windows.[26] In the first approach, the scatter characteristics are measured a priori and used to predict the scatter contribution. In the second approach, two PHA windows are used, one on the photopeak and another below it, defining the Compton scatter component of the photopeak. After the scatter image mask is generated, its contribution is subtracted from the photopeak image, thus compensating for scattered photons.

These two methods have been shown to provide improvements to image contrast and quantification.[25, 26] Nevertheless, they remain largely investigational. The correction method that is used, although seldom in cardiac studies, is one that assumes a lower than actual linear attenuation coefficient during attenuation correction, so that the photons that are scattered but not absorbed are not overcompensated.

Attenuation Correction

The attenuation of photons in the patient can result from scatter or absorption interactions. The most common type of scatter for diagnostic nuclear medicine is Compton scattering, which results when a photon interacts with an orbital electron and is characterized by a decrease in the photon's energy and a change in direction. If the photon goes on to be detected, important information about its spatial origin is lost. When scatter occurs, image contrast resolution is decreased, which can lead to limited detection and quantitation of tracer concentration. Absorption results if a photon interacts with an orbital electron and ceases to exist. These photons are never detected, and tracer concentration is therefore inaccurately represented in the images. Both processes contribute to the presence of SPECT image artifacts that complicate image interpretation and diagnosis, particularly for cardiac studies.

The attenuation process is defined quantitatively by the linear attenuation coefficient (usually designated μ) and has two components, one describing the absorption process and one describing the scattering process. Both processes reduce the number of photons with the original emitted energy. If it is assumed that the system will correctly prevent the scattered photons from being counted in the photopeak window, then a narrow beam attenuation coefficient reflecting true attenuation is used. If these scattered counts are not removed then an artificially, lower broad beam attenuation coefficient is used to prevent overcorrection due to acquiring more counts than expected. Typical values for ^{99m}Tc are 0.15 cm^{-1} for the narrow beam and 0.12 cm^{-1} for the broad beam value. Both narrow and broad beam attenuation coefficients are exponential in nature. However, the smaller broad beam value results in a more rapid loss or "fall-off" of the number of photons with increasing depth of tissue.

Attenuation correction is the ability to compensate for photons that have been absorbed or scattered in the patient. Because activity located deeper in the body is attenuated more than activity near the surface, attenuation manifests itself in a transaxial slice by artifactually decreasing the counts near the center of the body. Moreover, in SPECT thallium tomograms, photon attenuation is responsible for generation of artifactual defects in the anterior wall of women with large breasts and in the inferior wall of men with elevated diaphragms. This effect can be less pronounced with ^{99m}Tc-sestamibi, owing to the greater photon energy of ^{99m}Tc relative to ^{201}Tl, but the potential for artifactual defects remains.[27]

Until recently, only methods that correct radionuclide distributions in a constant (or homogeneous) attenuating medium, such as the liver, were available clinically. The two most commonly used methods for homogeneous imaging are the Sorenson preprocessing method and the Chang postprocessing method.

In Sorenson's method, the length of the attenuating tissue traversed by each projection is either assumed or determined from the patient's transaxial body contour. A hyperbolic sine function of this attenuating length is then multiplied by the mean count value of the corresponding pixel of the 180-degree opposing projection.[28] Some groups have reported the use of this approach for correction of ^{201}Tl SPECT studies; the method requires acquisition of a 360-degree angular range.[22]

In Chang's method, the patient's transaxial body contour is used to define the length of medium that attenuates each pixel in each projection. Each voxel (volume element) from the transaxial slice is corrected for attenuation by multiplying its reconstructed count value by the inverse of the average attenuation of all projections, measured from the voxel location to the body contour at each projection.[29] A linear attenuation coefficient lower than actual is routinely used to help compensate for scatter. The original method proposed by Chang is an iterative process in which the attenuation-corrected reconstructions are reprojected into planar projections. The differences between these reprojected planar projections and the originally acquired projections are used as error calculations to improve the previous estimation.

However, these homogeneous imaging methods do not work well in the thorax because the heart is surrounded by tissue of varying density and, therefore, of different attenuation coefficients (e.g., lung, blood, spine). Accurate attenuation compensation in cardiac imaging requires that the methods used allow for the variable attenuation distribution surrounding the heart. Furthermore, these methods do not directly compensate for the scatter component of the attenuation process. Different attenuation coefficient values can be used from the range of narrow to broad beam values to indirectly (and inaccurately) compensate for the scatter component. Patient-specific scatter compensation is therefore especially important for the nonhomogeneous geometry of the thorax and is essential for the accurate quantitation of cardiac SPECT images.

Several manufacturers have introduced clinically feasible methods for obtaining the necessary variable attenuation information for use in correction of the reconstructed images of the heart. The feasibility of these methods is the result of new detector designs for simultaneous emission-transmission image acquisition and the dramatic increase in computer power needed for the necessarily complex algorithms to complete image reconstruction in an acceptable time frame. The attenuation information is obtained from the acquisition of transmission projection images, which are used to reconstruct a transmission tomogram and to estimate the variable attenuation coefficients in the thorax. The simultaneity is essential because the spatial alignment of the attenuation coefficient map with the emission distribution is critical for accurate correction of the images and to prevent the introduction of new artifacts. It also minimizes patient imaging time by eliminating the need for a separate transmission acquisition.

One approach to simultaneous emission-transmission image acquisition is to use a collimated scanning line source, which moves across the field of view at a constant rate and is electronically coupled to a moving window that allows energetic and spatial separation of the transmission and emission images (Fig. 59–13*A*).[30] This configuration has the advantage that it can be implemented on both single- and dual-detector systems oriented at either 90 or 180 degrees with respect to each other. With this configuration, scatter contamination is minimized by the overwhelming flux of transmission photons relative to the emission flux and by the energy and spatial discrimination of the moving electronic window.

Another technique for obtaining simultaneous emission-transmission images is to use a collimated line source placed at the focal point of a fan beam collimator in a triple-detector system; the other two detectors acquire the emission data (see Fig. 59–13*B*).[31] A potential problem related to this imaging geometry is that the patient's body can move out of the field of view for some angles, thereby producing a truncated attenuation coefficient map. Contouring orbits must also be used to keep the heart in the field of view. So-called "truncation artifacts" can result and are minimized by the use of special reconstruction algorithms that can partially compensate for the missing data. The detection of scattered transmission photons in the emission detectors is minimized by the angle of scatter required to reach the detectors and the effects of collimation and photon energy discrimination. Line sources consisting of technetium-99m, americium-241, and gadolinium-153 have been proposed for this application. Of these, ^{153}Gd, with its significant γ-ray photopeaks at 97 and 103 keV, is emerging as the most practical line source for both ^{99m}Tc and ^{201}Tl imaging. The 242-day half-life of this radionuclide requires its replacement approximately every 2 years, depending on the initial activity.

The commonly used FBP algorithm does not provide the mathematical framework to accommodate the necessary information to accurately correct the images for attenuation and the other physical factors that limit image quality in SPECT. Therefore, modified forms of this algorithm have evolved and are known as iterative FBP (IFBP) algorithms. These algorithms use the conventional FBP algorithm as the basis for reconstruction but include the postreconstruction application of an attenuation correction map

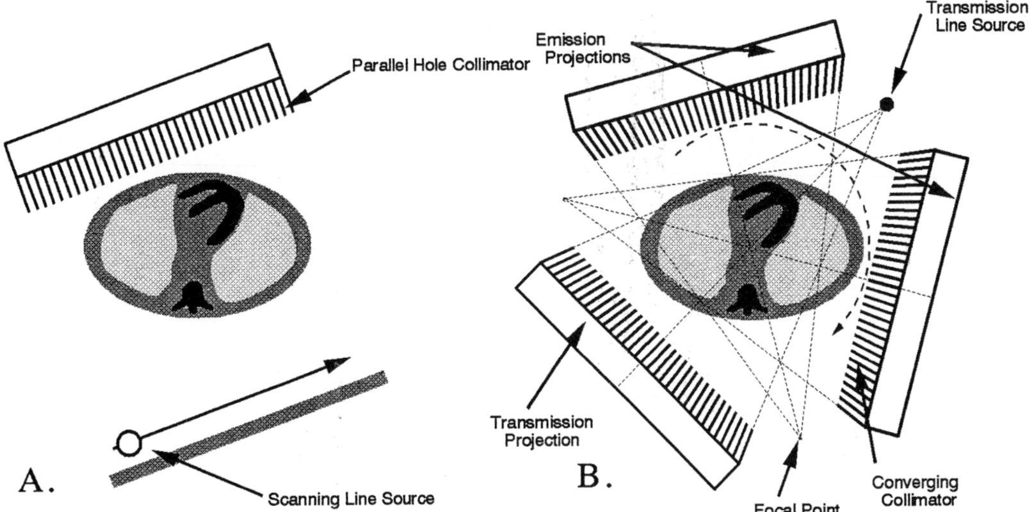

FIGURE 59–13. Two approaches for simultaneous acquisition of emission and transmission projections. *A,* A radioactive (transmission) line source with energy different from that of the tracer in the heart is scanned across each projection. *B,* Transmitted photons from a radioactive line source positioned at the focal point of the fan beam collimator are used to generate transmission scans, and two other detectors are used to acquire emission projections.

generated from the transmission images to correct the original reconstructions.[32, 33] So-called "statistical reconstruction algorithms," which employ a probabilistic approach, are also being developed for attenuation compensation. Both the modified FBP and statistical algorithms are referred to as iterative algorithms because they yield successively closer approximations to the true image until suitable accuracy is obtained. The most recent corrected estimate of the reconstruction is used with the attenuation coefficient map to generate reprojections of the radionuclide distribution. The differences between measured and estimated projection data are then used to refine the reconstructed image estimate.

The most common form of the statistical reconstruction algorithms, the maximum likelihood algorithm, is designed to give the most likely tracer distribution that would have produced the measured projection data.[34] The reconstructed image is obtained in an iterative manner and incorporates the attenuation coefficient map to generate the projection image estimates. Statistical algorithms have a theoretical advantage in that they can model the noise in the images that arises from radioactive decay more accurately than other algorithms. However, they require exceptionally long computation times and are only now becoming clinically realizable with the development of faster algorithms and more powerful computers. IFBP algorithms have the advantage in that they require much less computational time and yield significantly improved image quality and quantitation over FBP alone. Another advantage of the iterative algorithms over conventional FBP reconstruction is that they can use information about the spatial blurring that results from the limited and variable spatial resolution of the SPECT system to restore image accuracy; this is especially important for quantitation of cardiac structures because the dimensions of the myocardium are similar to the spatial resolution of the imaging system.[32, 35]

Object Size Correction

It has been shown for SPECT that even after scatter and attenuation correction, the counts recovered from reconstructed tomograms are dependent on the object size for objects smaller than two resolution elements (full width at half maximum) in any of its three dimensions.[14, 35] This dependence limits the accuracy with which regional radionuclide distributions can be derived from these objects. For example, in a thallium-201 myocardial short-axis slice, if the septal wall is significantly thicker than the lateral wall and the tracer is uniformly distributed, the septum in the image will appear hot in relation to the lateral wall. This may mislead the clinician into interpreting that the patient has a perfusion defect in the lateral wall.

Correction methods to date remain experimental and depend on either measurement or calculation of a recovery coefficient as a function of object size. The object size is then independently estimated. Correction consists of multiplying the voxel count value by the appropriate recovery coefficient.[14, 35]

Uniformity Correction

Most state-of-the-art gamma cameras correct for differences in energy response from the different photomultipliers and for nonlinearities. Although these corrections are important in reducing field uniformity errors in planar projections, uniformity requirements for SPECT are more stringent and require further correction. The greatest sources of image nonuniformities in SPECT imaging are "imperfect" collimators. A local nonuniformity from a collimator is propagated in the reconstructed transaxial slice in the form of a circular or "ring" artifact because the same nonuniformity is backprojected at each of the angles of acquisition. The higher the number of acquired counts for that slice, the more prominent the artifact, because it rides above the random noise error. This correction is less important in thallium SPECT, where the number of counts per slice is low compared with blood pool imaging. Also, the closer the local nonuniformity is to the axis of rotation, the higher the amplitude of the artifact, because the backprojected lines are closer together and there is more overlapping of the count values.

Uniformity correction for SPECT usually requires imaging of a cobalt-57 flood source for 30 million counts in order to reduce the error caused by nonuniformity to less than 1 percent.[36] (It is important that the flood source used have a variation in radionuclide concentration of less than 1 percent.) Normalization factors are determined from this image and applied to each of the projection views. The 30 million count rule assumes that a 64 × 64 matrix is used to reconstruct a 1 million count slice. A 128 × 128 matrix requires four times the 30 million count flood in order to maintain the same variation. It is usually suggested that these floods be acquired and new normalization matrices be generated once a week and also at any time a different collimator is used, although actual need may vary according to the stability of the specific detector.

Patient Motion Detection and Correction

Patient motion as small as half a voxel (3 mm) has been reported[37, 38] to create thallium-201 SPECT image artifacts that mimic perfusion defects. The larger the motion, the greater the defect, particularly if it is abrupt and occurs halfway through the scan. Another type of motion artifact that has been reported is "diaphragmatic creep."[37] This phenomenon occurs in patients under stress whose breathing pattern changes drastically from deep to shallow during acquisition, allowing the heart to gradually "creep" upward in the chest. Because this motion is more gradual and of small magnitude, it seldom leads to significant artifacts. It is also easily circumvented by delaying the start of acquisition for approximately 10 to 15 minutes after peak stress.

Patient motion of 3 mm is easily detected by inspection of the planar projections dynamically displayed in a movie format. Computer algorithms have been developed to automatically detect and correct for patient motion, particularly vertical motion.[38] These algorithms usually track either the entire myocardium or the center of mass of the myocardium from projection to projection. The shifts in heart position are then reported to the operator on a projection-by-projection basis. The operator decides whether to allow the computer to translate the image projections back to a fixed frame of reference. Although the motion detection algorithms are useful for flagging potential artifacts, the value of the motion correction methodology in elimination of artifacts is yet to be established.

Technetium-99m Versus Thallium-201

Another factor that influences image quality is the choice of radionuclide. Technetium-99m myocardial perfusion agents have been developed, most notably ^{99m}Tc-methoxyisobutyl isonitrile (^{99m}Tc-MIBI). A technetium perfusion agent has several imaging advantages over thallium-201. Compensation for variable attenuation in the thorax is more feasible with a monoenergetic, higher-energy technetium agent. Compensation for the myocardial ^{201}Tl distribution is difficult for two reasons. First, the 80-keV photopeak of ^{201}Tl, which is the most commonly used because of its high relative abundance compared with the other peaks, is associated with greater scattering, greater attenuation, and greater variability of attenuation coefficients across the thorax.[39] Second, the ^{201}Tl spectrum exhibits several photopeaks, including 135 and 167 keV, and down-scattered photons from these peaks that fall within the PHA window corresponding to the 80-keV photopeak make the attenuation compensation problem even more difficult.

In addition, the ideal energy of ^{99m}Tc for imaging yields both a higher spatial resolution and a more favorable radiation dosimetry. The higher spatial resolution not only improves image quality but also reduces the object size effect, which is a function of finite spatial resolution. The favorable radiation dosimetry, which in part is a result of the shorter half-life of ^{99m}Tc (6 hours, versus 73 hours for ^{201}Tl) allows the administration of up to 30 mCi (1110 MBq) of ^{99m}Tc-MIBI, compared with the 3.5-mCi (130 MBq) maximum dose of ^{201}Tl. This higher dose leads directly to more counts per image and thereby to reduced statistical image noise. Table 59–1 illustrates the imaging superiority of the ^{99m}Tc-MIBI perfusion agent over ^{201}Tl. Figure 59–14 shows the superior image quality of ^{99m}Tc-MIBI compared with ^{201}Tl tomograms in the same patient.

Multiple-Gated Single-Photon Emission Computed Tomography

Many commercial nuclear medicine computer systems now have the capability of acquiring and reconstructing multiple-gated tomographic studies. This feature has promoted studies investigating the use of SPECT for assessment of cardiac global and regional function, including assessment of myocardial wall thickening. Investigators have applied primarily ^{99m}Tc blood pool tomographic imaging[40] and tomographic imaging of the myocardial wall perfused by ^{99m}Tc-MIBI.[41]

TABLE 59–1. SPECT MYOCARDIAL IMAGING CHARACTERISTICS OF ^{201}Tl VERSUS ^{99m}Tc-MIBI

	^{201}Tl (3.5 mCi or 130 MBq)	**^{99m}Tc (22 mCi or 814 MBq)**
Spatial resolution (mm) and collimator type	19 (LEAP)	13 (high-resolution)
Relative sensitivity		
Stress	1.0	2.4
Delayed/Rest	0.5	2.2
Percent scattered counts	40	22
Average attenuation correction factor	4.9	3.8

LEAP = Low-energy all-purpose.

Acquisition consists of performing multiple-gated acquisition at each of the planar projections, for the same total time per projection. These acquisitions are usually obtained at 1 minute or less per projection so as to maintain the total study time at 30 to 60 minutes. Because of both the short acquisition time per projection and the reconstruction times, the number of frames per cardiac cycle is kept to a minimum (i.e., between 8 and 16). The reconstruction process is the same as that for nongated SPECT imaging, except that the frames must be shuffled so that individual projection sets are created for each frame of the cardiac cycle. If, for example, a multiple-gated SPECT study is acquired at eight frames per cardiac cycle, eight individual sets of projections are created and, subsequently, individually reconstructed. After it has been reconstructed into transaxial slices, each set is reconstructed along the same oblique angles in order to generate vertical, horizontal, and short-axis slices that have the same orientation from frame to frame. After the oblique slices have been generated, the program reshuffles each of the slices from each of the eight tomographic sets back into sets of eight frames, multiple-gated tomographic slices that may be displayed in a closed-loop cine format for assessment of cardiac function. This same procedure is performed for either blood pool imaging or imaging of the perfused myocardial walls (Fig. 59–15).

POSITRON EMISSION TOMOGRAPHY

A positron emission tomography (PET) scanner uses the same principles of radiation detection as those employed in single-photon

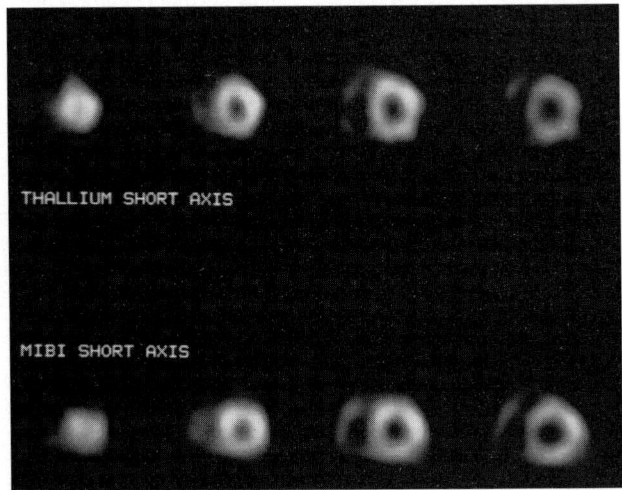

FIGURE 59–14. Comparison of ^{201}Tl myocardial short-axis slices *(above)* and corresponding ^{99m}Tc-MIBI slices *(below)* in the same normal patient. Notice the superior image quality of the ^{99m}Tc-MIBI tomograms. These four representative short-axis slices are arranged from apex *(left)* to base.

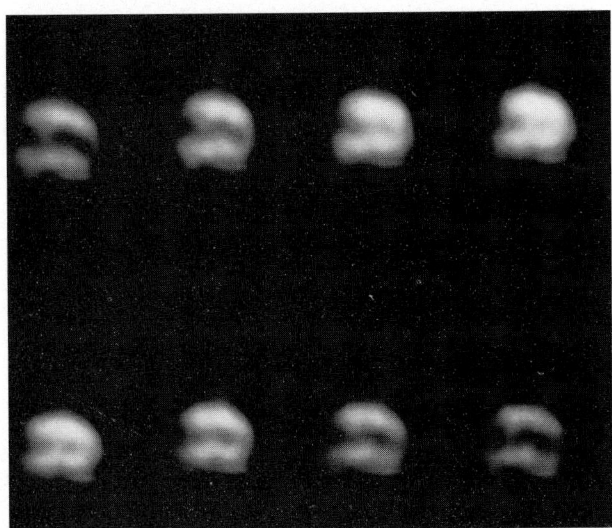

FIGURE 59–15. ^{99m}Tc-MIBI multiple-gated myocardial SPECT mid-vertical long-axis slices. Eight frames are displayed throughout the cardiac cycle from end-diastole *(top left)* to end-systole *(top right)* and back to end-diastole *(bottom right)*. Notice that the apical perfusion defect, which is obvious at end-diastole, disappears at end-systole. Also notice how the walls become brighter as the myocardium contracts and thickens.

detection, but the system is tuned for detection of the radiations that result from positron decay. The usual mode of decay for a positron is annihilation with an electron—they are antiparticles of each other. In the annihilation, the mass of the particles is converted into energy according to Einstein's famous formula, $E = mc^2$. Usually, this energy is carried away by two photons that are equal in energy and travel in opposite directions (Fig. 59–16).

The designers of the first PET scanners[42] took advantage of the 180-degree nature of the two photons to obviate the need for lead collimation. Because both of the annihilation photons are detected at the same time, the direction of travel for each photon is known, in complete analogy with the lead-collimated photons measured with a single-photon scintillation camera. This method of determining the direction of the photons has come to be known as "electronic collimation." Techniques for reconstruction of the source distribution of radioactivity from the primary data are identical for the two types of cameras.

In principle, PET and SPECT are similar, but they differ in several key details. Photons in PET have higher energy than those in SPECT. Therefore, the type and shape of detector materials that can be used and the energy and temporal resolution properties differ between the two techniques. Because of the use of electronic collimation, the geometry and electronics of the scanners are very different. Finally, the PET requirement that two photons reach the

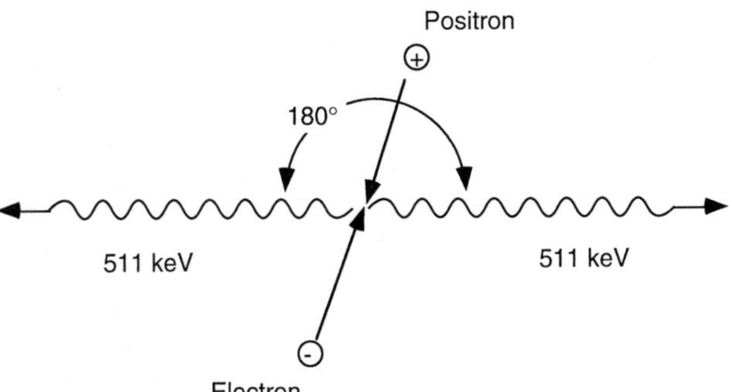

FIGURE 59–16. Positron emission tomography scanners detect the two 511-keV photons that result from the annihilation of a positron and an electron.

detector system, as opposed to only one in SPECT, implies that attenuation by the patient's body must be carefully considered. These areas are discussed in detail in the following sections.

Detectors

The detected photon energy in PET is always 511 keV, which is much greater than the typical single-photon γ-ray energy. Because higher-energy photons penetrate further into detector material, detectors used in PET must either be thicker or have greater stopping power than those used in SPECT, or both. Currently known detectors with greater stopping power have decreased energy resolution compared with NaI, causing the energy resolution of most PET scanners to be worse than that of single-photon cameras. This has implications for accurate rejection of scattered photons.

The mass attenuation coefficient for different detector materials is typically a factor of 2 less for 100-keV as opposed to 511-keV photons. Therefore, a detector must be approximately twice as thick to detect 511-keV photons with the same intrinsic efficiency as 100-keV photons. The designers of PET systems have two options: use thicker detectors, or use detectors that have greater attenuation properties. Commercial scanners have been produced for both options. The two most common detector materials for PET scanners are bismuth germanate ($Bi_4Ge_3O_{12}$, or BGO) and NaI. The mass attenuation for BGO is almost twice that of NaI.

Efficiency is only one criterion for choosing a detector. Others are the maximum count-rate capability and the energy resolution. The maximum count rate is determined by the decay constant for the visible photons (termed scintillation light) created in the scintillator. The smaller the decay constant, the faster the scintillation light can be collected and the more events can be counted per unit time. The decay constant for the major portion of the scintillation light in an NaI detector (0.23 μsec) is similar to that of BGO (0.30 μsec). However, approximately 9 percent of the overall scintillation light yield in NaI detectors decays with a constant of 0.15 seconds. Therefore, BGO is a superior detector for very high count-rate applications.

The energy resolution of a detector is determined by the total number of scintillation photons created in the scintillator after an interaction with a γ-ray. If more scintillation photons are created, then the accuracy of the energy measurement is greater. For a γ-ray of a given incident energy, the number of scintillation photons created in a BGO detector is only 8 percent of the number produced in an NaI detector. Because of this, the energy resolution of BGO is only 25 to 30 percent of the photopeak energy, compared with 7 to 9 percent for NaI. Therefore, NaI is superior to BGO for energy measurements. Energy resolution is important in PET scanning because it is the primary means of rejecting scattered photons. If one or both of the annihilation photons scatter in patient tissue before detection by the scanner, then the recorded directional information will be incorrect. Because a scattered photon has less energy than the original photon, an energy measurement can be used to determine whether a detected photon is the result of a scatter event. A more accurate energy measurement results in better scatter rejection.

Construction of a PET scanner with currently available detectors is a tradeoff between count-rate capability, efficiency, and energy resolution. In most PET scanning applications, the needs for greater efficiency and higher counting capability outweigh the need for scatter rejection through an energy measurement. Of importance here are errors caused by random radioactive decay and by acceptance of scattered photons. Images from a scanner constructed with a BGO detector, compared with those from an NaI-based scanner, have less error from decay statistics but more error from scatter events. Most PET applications are count-limited, so reducing the error caused by decay provides a greater payoff than reducing the error caused by scattering. Therefore, most current PET scanners are manufactured with BGO detectors.

Scanner Geometry and Electronic Collimation

PET scanners must include detectors on opposite sides of the field of view so that both of the annihilation photons can be detected. A single-photon camera usually has one to three detectors that rotate around the field of view, and it may be operated in planar or tomographic modes. A PET camera, on the other hand, is usually constructed with many separate detectors arranged in a circle that completely surrounds the field of view and is always operated in tomographic mode. A single-photon camera can acquire data along only one direction (view) at a time because of the lead collimator. In order to collect tomographic images, the detectors and collimators must rotate around the field of view. Substitution of electronic collimation for lead collimation in PET cameras enables collection of data along all of the different view angles simultaneously. This leads to much greater sensitivity (number of detected events for a given amount of radioactivity in the field of view) for PET, and tomographic data is always acquired.

The detector ring in a PET camera is constructed from smaller units of detectors, commonly called blocks.[43] Each block consists of detector material and several photomultiplier tubes. As with the single-photon camera, Anger-type logic is used to determine the location of the detected event. To improve the localization, deep cuts into the detector material are used to alter the distribution of scintillation light that is received by each photomultiplier (Fig. 59–17). The energy of the detected event is determined by summing all of the photomultiplier tube signals. This summed signal is also used to record the arrival time of the event.

Electronic collimation is achieved by recording the arrival times of each detected 511-keV γ-ray. If two events are recorded within a small time window, they are said to be in coincidence. A true event is defined as a coincident event in which both detected γ-rays originate from the same positron annihilation. If the detected γ-rays originate from separate positron annihilations, the coincident event is termed a random event. If more than two signals are recorded within the time window, it is impossible to determine which pair of signals (if any) represents a true event; this case is termed a multiple event and is discarded. As the duration of the time window is increased, the number of random coincident events also increases; therefore, the time window is made as small as possible. Typical time windows are 10 to 12 nsec in duration. These different terms are illustrated in Figure 59–18.

All PET scanners either estimate or measure the number of random coincident events. Then, the number of true events is calculated by subtracting the random from the total number of coincident events. The rate (R) can be estimated as $R = 2TN_aN_b$, where T is the time window and N_a and N_b are the detection rates for detectors a and b, respectively.[44] This is a very precise method for estimating random events if the radioactivity remains constant in the field of view during acquisition of the scan. However, normal physiologic metabolism almost always causes the activity to vary over the course of a scan. If this is the case, a "delayed coincidence" technique can be used to measure the random coincidence rate. A circuit that illustrates the electronic collimation and the random events measurement electronics is shown in Figure 59–19. The circuit is typical of the coincidence circuits in a PET scanner. An actual scanner would have many copies of these electronics—one circuit (or equivalent) for each pair of detectors in the scanner.

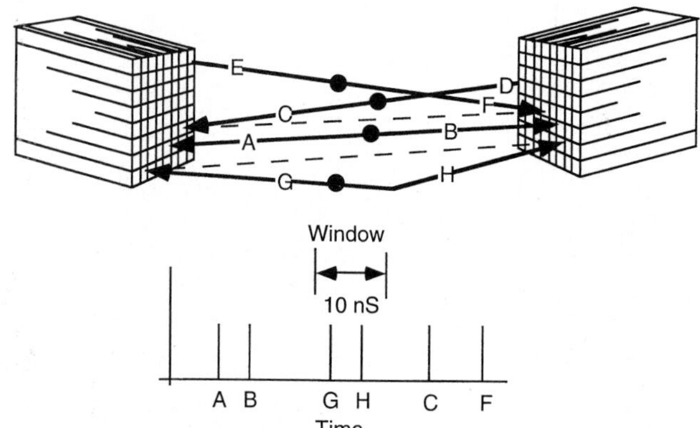

FIGURE 59–18. Four positron annihilations are depicted to illustrate coincident true, random, and scatter events in positron emission tomography. To simplify the drawing, only two of the blocks that constitute the detector ring are shown. Each positron annihilation results in production of two 511-keV photons, which may or may not be detected by the scanner. The graph shows the relative timing for each of the detected events. Events AB, GH, and CF occur within the time window duration and are coincident events. AB is a true coincident event because both A and B originate from the same positron annihilation. GH is a scatter event that gives the false impression of activity along the dashed line. CF is a random coincident event because C and F originate from different annihilations. Recording of the event CF causes the mistaken impression that radioactivity is present along its dashed line.

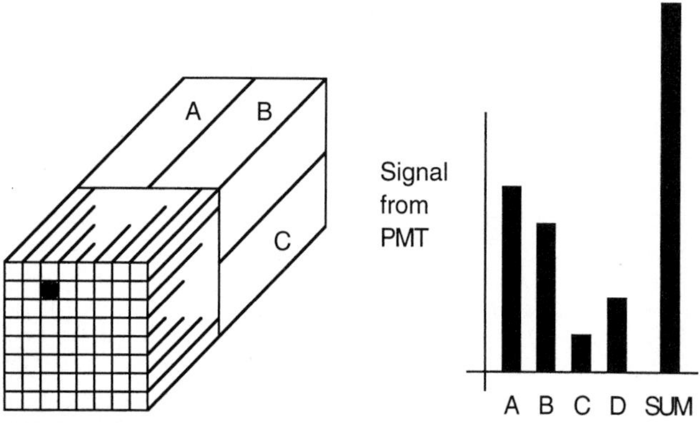

FIGURE 59–17. Typical detector block used in positron emission tomograms. The block of detector material is scored to different depths to alter the amount of scintillation light reaching each photomultiplier tube (*A* to *D*). An event occurring in the indicated detector produces signals from the four photomultiplier tubes, as shown. The different signal levels can be used to determine where the event took place. SUM is the sum of the four photomultiplier signals, which is used for energy and timing determinations.

A PET scanner is constructed by arranging blocks of detectors in a ring around the field of view and connecting a coincidence circuit between each pair of detectors. Typically, three or four rings of detector blocks (each approximately 80 cm in diameter) are set next to each other to provide for a 16- to 20-cm axial field of view. The detector blocks and Anger positioning circuits can record the position of an event to within approximately 5 mm. This accuracy is sufficient to produce images with 6-mm spatial resolution.

Historically, rings of lead (called septa) have been placed in front of the detector blocks at the position of the scored lines. Their purpose is to effectively isolate separate rings of detectors. If this is done, only data perpendicular to the axis of the scanner is collected. The two advantages of using septa are simplification of image reconstruction and elimination of between-plane scatter. The major disadvantage is that a tremendous amount of data containing image information is not collected. With the advent of faster and more powerful computers, the simplification of image reconstruction is diminishing in importance. The advantage of decreasing interplane scatter must be considered with respect to the lost information in the data that are not collected. Current state-of-the-art PET scanners have septa that can easily be removed by the user. This enables the acquisition protocol to be tailored to best suit each separate study. In applications that are decay statistics–limited, it is advantageous to remove the septa, but in applications that are not count-limited, it is often best to eliminate as much scatter as possible from the start by using the septa. This later approach yields data that are more quantitatively accurate.

Scanner Resolution

The intrinsic resolution of a PET scanner is determined by the positron range, the accuracy with which events are localized in the

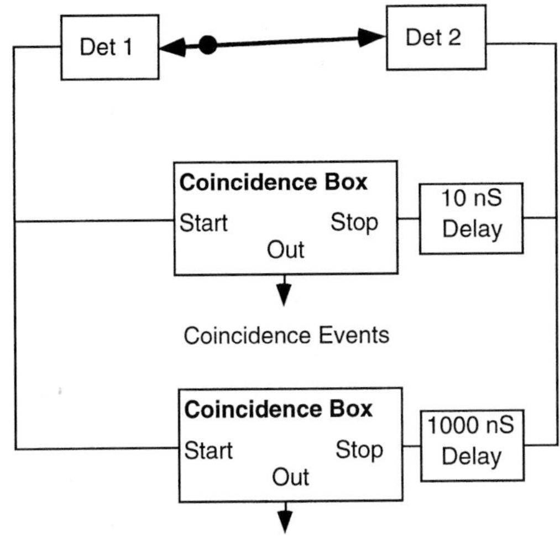

FIGURE 59–19. Circuit for detection of coincidence and random events in a positron emission tomograph with a timing window of 10 nsec. After a positron annihilation, 511-keV gamma rays enter detectors 1 and 2. In this example, detector 1 registers the event first because the decay occurred closer to this detector. The coincidence boxes work by starting a clock when a pulse arrives at the "start" input; if a pulse arrives within 20 nsec at the "stop" input, an output signal is generated. At the end of 20 nsec, the box resets itself and waits for the next start pulse. The 10-nsec delay and 20-nsec window are set so that it doesn't matter which detector registers a γ-ray first: as long as the two events are within 10 nsec of each other, an output is generated. The lower half of the circuit measures the random coincidence rate. The 1000-nsec delay ensures that the stop input signal from a true event will arrive long after the 20-nsec time window has elapsed. The only way a random event will be registered is if a second γ-ray happens to interact in the detector 1000 ± 10 nsec later by chance. The true coincidence rate equals the number of coincidence events minus the number of random events in a given time period.

detector system, and the noncolinearity of the two annihilation γ-rays. Intrinsic resolution is defined as the resolution that could be expected in an image that is reconstructed from a data set that has a very large number of detected events. If the data is count-limited, as many PET studies are, the realized resolution of the images will be worse.

Of primary interest in PET scanning is the distribution of the injected radiotracer. The distribution is inferred by the location of the annihilation γ-rays, and these rays originate at the location of the positron-electron annihilation. After the radionuclide in the tracer decays and emits a positron, the positron travels some distance before it meets an electron and annihilates. This range leads to a degradation in resolution in the images. The higher the positron energy, the greater the degradation. Therefore, the resolution is radionuclide-dependent. The common PET isotopes, arranged in order of increasing maximal positron energy, are fluorine-18 (0.64 MeV), carbon-11 (0.96 MeV), nitrogen-13 (1.2 MeV), and oxygen-15 (1.7 MeV). The range contributes 1 to 2 mm to the uncertainty in resolution, depending on the radionuclide.

The second factor that contributes to the resolution is the accuracy of localization of the individual 511-keV γ-rays in the detector blocks. The limit arises from the scoring of the detector material. Score lines that are closer together improve localization of the event, but at a price. As the cuts are put closer together, the thickness of the saw blade becomes a critical factor. The cuts must be more than several saw-widths apart to prevent loss of a substantial amount of detector material in the scoring process. Current technology limits the cuts to a separation of approximately 4 mm. With this limit, nearest neighbor rays are separated by 2 mm at the center of the field of view—degrading the resolution by approximately this factor.

Finally, the assumption that the two γ-rays are exactly 180 degrees apart is not strictly correct. If the positron and electron are moving when they annihilate, the γ-rays will be emitted slightly in the direction of the combined motion. Although this deflection is a fraction of a degree, by the time the rays are detected, the offset is 1 to 2 mm.

The resolution of a PET scanner is the combination of these three components. In state-of-the-art clinical scanners, the intrinsic resolution is approximately 4 mm. Special-purpose research scanners have been constructed with extremely small detectors in order to produce images with 2.6-mm resolution.[45] Because of the positron range and the noncolinearity of the annihilation γ-rays, the resolution of a PET camera is limited to approximately 2 mm.

Attenuation

In PET, each event requires that two photons be detected. Because of this, a greater fraction of events is absorbed by the patient during PET imaging, compared with SPECT. This seems to be a disadvantage because fewer events reach the detection system, however, it is a great advantage because the number of attenuated photons can easily be measured or calculated. In principle, this enables an exact correction to be applied to the data to remove all effects of attenuation.

Many of the positron annihilations are not recorded by the scanner because one or both of the resultant γ-rays are attenuated by patient tissues. This effect is most drastic at the center of the body. On average, γ-rays that originate from annihilations at the edge of the body pass through much less attenuating medium (tissue) before they are detected. At the center of the head, only about 15 percent of the events result in both γ-rays' reaching the detector ring. Images reconstructed from this data are greatly depressed at the center. Fortunately, these effects of attenuation can be either calculated or measured, and corrections can be applied to the data before reconstruction.

Figure 59–20 depicts the attenuation problem for both PET and SPECT imaging. In single-photon imaging, the probability that a γ-ray will be attenuated depends on the depth of the event within the patient. In PET, because the two γ-rays travel in opposite directions, the total amount of tissue that must be traversed is independent of the depth at which the annihilation occurs. Furthermore, because the same tissue must be traversed by one of the 511-keV γ-rays regardless of the annihilation position along the

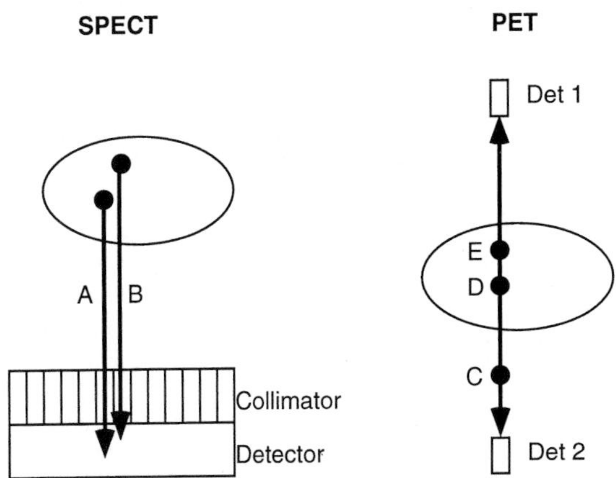

FIGURE 59–20. Comparison of attenuation in single-photon emission computed tomography (SPECT) and in positron emission tomography (PET). In SPECT imaging, the depth of the radioactive decay event within the patient is important. Gamma ray B has a greater probability of being attenuated than gamma ray A. In PET, because both γ-rays must be detected, the depth is unimportant. Whether the annihilation takes place at C, D, or E, the same tissue must be traversed by a 511 keV γ-ray. The probability of losing an event because of attenuation is therefore the same no matter where along the line the annihilation takes place—even if the annihilation takes place outside the body.

line, the attenuation probability is the same for every annihilation along the line. Likewise, if the annihilation takes place outside the patient, the probability of missing an event because of attenuation is still the same. This property can be exploited to measure or calculate an exact attenuation correction in PET. Measured corrections have the advantage of being more accurate, but they introduce additional random noise into the final images as a result of the statistics of radioactive decay. A calculated correction may be less accurate, but the random noise is eliminated. Often, a calculated correction proves superior for conveying essential information in the images.

To perform a measured attenuation correction, a source is placed outside the patient in a position analogous to that shown at C in Figure 59–20. Two scans are acquired before injection of the radionuclide. First, a scan is collected without the patient in the scanner; this is called the blank scan. Then, the patient is positioned in the scanner and a second scan is collected; this is called the transmission scan. During these scans, the source (at position C) is set to rotate around the scanner field of view. In this way, the source will be between every pair of detectors in the scanner at some time during the acquisition. The ratio of detected events in the transmission data to those in the blank scan represents the fraction of events that is lost to attenuation. The attenuation correction factor for any pair of detectors is simply the inverse of this fraction. To correct the radionuclide scan (termed the emission scan) for attenuation effects, the data from the emission scan is multiplied by the corresponding attenuation correction factor. An image reconstructed from the primary data after this correction will be free of attenuation effects.

A calculated attenuation correction involves estimation of the attenuation correction factors. This can be done if the path length through the body and the attenuation properties of the body are known. For example, in a brain scan it may be necessary to know the attenuation of a ray passing through 2 cm of bone and 20 cm of water (assuming that brain tissue has the attenuation properties of water). These values can easily be calculated; the difficult part is determining how much bone and tissue each ray passes through. The usual method for calculated attenuation correction in brain scans is as follows. The uncorrected data are reconstructed, producing an image of the brain that is depressed in the center. The edge of the brain is located on these images, and a constant thickness of bone is assumed to surround the brain. With this information, the path length through each tissue is determined for the rays that connect every pair of detectors, and the attenuation factors are calculated. The primary data are then corrected using these factors and reconstructed a second time. This reconstruction will be free of attenuation effects.

The accuracy of a calculated attenuation correction depends on the accurate identification of the various distinct tissues in the scanner field of view. This is relatively easy for brain scans, where the field of view can reasonably be considered to contain only bone and water in a simple geometry. (A head holder can easily be included because its position and attenuation properties are easily determined.) In the thorax, however, the position of bone, tissue, and lungs (at the minimum) must be known in a geometry that is much more complicated than the geometry of the brain. A satisfactory calculated attenuation correction does not currently exist for areas of the body other than the brain, although algorithms are being developed that combine measured and calculated techniques.[46] These new algorithms, termed segmentation routines, use a short transmission scan to define the geometry and then calculate the attenuation. In so doing, the accuracy of the measured correction is retained while the random noise is eliminated.

As with all aspects of imaging, there are tradeoffs to be considered with regard to the attenuation correction. Measured correction is the most accurate, but it is susceptible to random noise and to motion artifacts. If the patient is in different positions for the emission and transmission scans, then the attenuation correction will be in error. This error is manifested by asymmetries at the edge of the image and at boundaries between dissimilar attenuating tissues. For example, errors would be expected at the boundary between the heart and lungs if there is motion between the emission and transmission scans. The motion causes the heart attenuation correction to be applied to the lungs (or vice versa), which causes the reconstructed lung activity to be too large (or the heart activity to be too small). In either case, bright or dark rims at the boundaries between different attenuating tissues constitute the definitive sign of movement between the transmission and attenuation scans. With newer segmentation routines, total scanning time is much shorter and motion artifacts are kept to a minimum.

TECHNICAL ASPECTS OF QUANTIFICATION OF CARDIAC PARAMETERS

Assessment of cardiac performance is markedly enhanced by a quantitative description of the specific physiologic parameters evaluated by scintigraphic images. Quantification enables objective interpersonal comparison and objective assessment of cardiac status in a single patient over time or after intervention. Furthermore, computer algorithms that enhance the images, extract parameters of cardiac performance, and define criteria for normality and abnormality have the potential to be precisely described. These algorithms can then be widely disseminated to promote standardization of image interpretation. More importantly, these algorithms can stand as a foundation from which specific criticisms can be assessed and into which improvements can be readily incorporated.

Cardiovascular nuclear medicine techniques are inherently quantitative. This is because the pixel count value from within a cardiac region is related to some parameter of cardiac performance. In the case of planar equilibrium blood pool studies, in which the radionuclide concentration is assumed to be constant, the pixel count value from a region within the heart is related to chamber volume. In the case of myocardial perfusion imaging, in which the volume is assumed to be constant, the pixel count value from a region is related to the concentration of the radionuclide and thus to blood flow.

In this section, digital image processing techniques developed for quantification of myocardial perfusion and ventricular function are reviewed. Many of the techniques illustrated reflect computer methods developed at Cedars-Sinai Medical Center and at Emory University.

Quantification of Myocardial Perfusion

Sequential thallium-201 scintigraphy after injection at peak exercise is a useful noninvasive method for detection and evaluation of patients with significant coronary artery disease (CAD). Visual interpretation of analog ^{201}Tl images, even by experienced observers, is subject to substantial variability.[47] This approach is further limited by dependence on the quality of the hard copy output and inability to accurately compensate for background activity or attenuation. Finally, although the myocardial ^{201}Tl regional washout characteristics contain important diagnostic information, these can be difficult to detect by visual inspection.

Several approaches have provided significant contributions to the quantitation of initial distribution and washout of myocardial ^{201}Tl, both from planar scintigraphic projections[48–51] and from tomographic sections.[23, 52–54] The purpose of this section is to discuss the steps involved in quantitation of stress-redistribution ^{201}Tl planar and tomographic studies.

Planar Methods

Background Subtraction

Background is an important consideration because it degrades the contrast of perfusion defects and it contaminates the measurement of the washout of ^{201}Tl from the myocardium with the clearance from overlapping tissue.[51, 55, 56] Interpolative background subtraction provides the most satisfactory approach because it compensates for nonuniformity in background distribution, which changes spatially and as a function of time in the delayed images. Methods that do not correct for tissue crosstalk[50, 54] and those that use the subtraction of a constant background appear to be inadequate.

In the approach used by the Cedars-Sinai Quantitative Thallium Programs (Cedars), each image is compensated for tissue crosstalk by bilinear interpolative background subtraction, as described by Goris and colleagues.[55] For this purpose, a rectangular boundary enclosing the heart is positioned by the computer operator approximately four pixels away from the myocardium. The pixels defining the rectangle are used as the origin of background. Each pixel outside the rectangle is set to 0, and each one inside is corrected by subtracting from it the weighted average of the four pixels falling in the rectangle with a common Cartesian coordinate of the point being modified. The average is weighted in relation to how close to each of these four pixels the point being corrected is located. If the point is exactly equidistant from the four pixels, a simple average is used. The Cedars program uses a modification of this proximity-weighting function, first described by Watson and associates,[51] that produces a more rapid fall-off of the computed tissue crosstalk. Without this more rapid fall-off (and sometimes even with it), interpolative background subtraction tends to oversubtract in myocardial regions close to where the rectangle crosses areas of high uptake, such as the liver. This oversubtraction may result in artifactual perfusion defects or washout measurements.

Several investigators have reported on the use of different methods of interpolative background subtraction,[57] mostly designed for use in blood pool studies. There is no consensus that any one method is better than another. Nichols[58] reported on the use of irregular rather than rectangular regions as the source of background. Leidholdt and colleagues[57] reported on the use of polygonal matrices of 12 vertices surrounding the heart. Okada and colleagues[59] used all of the pixels outside a user-defined ellipse to correct each of the points inside the ellipse. All of the approaches that employ irregular regions are important improvements in cases in which a rectangle is forced to cross a high-count background away from the heart. This is particularly true for correction for tissue crosstalk in resting ^{201}Tl studies, in which the background counts are considerably higher than in stress studies.

Smoothing and Filtering

Smoothing serves two purposes. First, it improves statistical accuracy, which varies in low-information-density scintigraphic studies. Second, the algorithm, which searches radially for the myocardial sample, looks for one pixel with the maximum counts. In order for this pixel to be more representative of a larger segment of the myocardium, smoothing is necessary. The Cedars approach employs simple spatial smoothing by a nine-point weighted average that uses a 3 × 3 convolving kernel with weights of 4 in the center, 1 in the diagonals, and 2 elsewhere. Other investigators have also used unweighted five-point smoothing. Although the nine-point weighted smoothing approach has been found to be effective when applied to stress-redistribution images, it may not be enough for resting studies, which have even lower count densities. In such cases, the application of Fourier filtering[49] may offer better image enhancement.

Generation of Circumferential Profiles

Several methods have been developed for extraction of the regional count distribution from ^{201}Tl images. The Cedars program employs maximal count circumferential profiles. For this purpose, profiles are generated of the maximal counts per pixel along each of 60 radii spaced 6 degrees apart and plotted clockwise. These profiles quantitate the segmental activity as an angular function referenced from the visually located center of the left ventricular cavity (Fig. 59–21). This also could be located by automatic determination of the geometric center of the myocardium.[60] The operator also assigns the maximum and minimum radii to which the computer will search, to prevent the algorithm from searching outside the myocardium.

The choice of maximal rather than average or total counts was based on the work of Vogel and colleagues,[61] who determined that maximal count circumferential profiles provided the most accurate measure of abnormality. Furthermore, the use of average counts in circumferential profile analysis has been found to be less sensitive than visual interpretation.[50] Several available algorithms allow the user to choose different methods of assigning counts to the circumferential profile. Okada and co-workers used the mean counts in three (or more) pixels that define the myocardial regions.[59] These regions are defined as the area between an inner and an outer ellipse surrounding the myocardium.

The profiles are aligned so that the apex in each view is assigned to 90 degrees. Apex alignment is valuable[50] for partial correction of variation in heart position. This alignment is particularly important because the lower limits or normal profiles vary for the different angular locations in each view. For example, if in a normal study the apex were misaligned, this region, which characteristically has the fewest counts, could fall below the lower limits of normal, causing a falsely abnormal result. Methods that use lower limits of normal without proper alignment are therefore limited. Apex alignment is also important for washout or reversibility calculations, in which one curve is operated by another curve and each angle has to correspond region by region.

In the Cedars approach, the computer automatically shifts that point in the circumferential profile identified as the apex to coincide with 90 degrees. Profiles are subsequently plotted for each view at each time interval. These distribution curves are normalized to the maximum pixel value found in either the stress or delayed

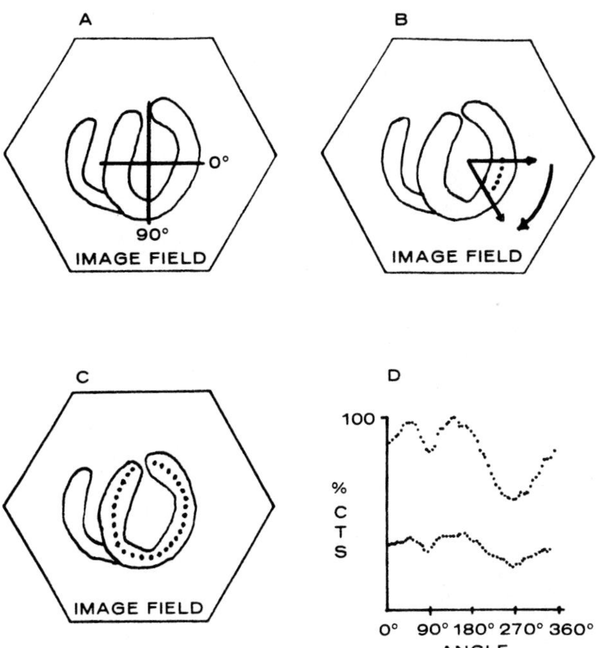

FIGURE 59–21. Method for obtaining circumferential profiles of the myocardium. *A*, The coordinate reference axis is shown. *B*, Image pixels for circumferential profile analysis are found by performing radial search for maximal count values (cts) at 6-degree intervals throughout 360 degrees. *C*, Maximal values, shown as black dots, are then plotted (in *D*) for each angle as a percentage of the maximum value for the circumferential profile. *D*, The top curve represents the circumferential profile from a stress thallium-201 image; the bottom curve shows the profile from the 4-hour delayed image.

profile (see Fig. 59–21*D*). Watson[51] and Okada[59] and their colleagues aligned the stress and redistribution images themselves rather than the count profiles. This is done by iterative translation of the position of the delayed images until the cross-correlation coefficient between the two images is maximized.

Generation of Washout Rate Profiles

Different methods have been developed to quantitatively assess change in regional myocardial ^{201}Tl content over time. The Cedars approach employs washout circumferential profiles, calculated as percentage washout from stress to the redistribution time of approximately 4 hours. Figure 59–22 demonstrates the manner in which each point on the washout rate profile is calculated. As shown, despite regional count variation at the time of stress and 4-hour redistribution, the percentage regional washout rate of ^{201}Tl is fairly uniform from all myocardial regions. The mean effective half-life of ^{201}Tl in the myocardium for stress-redistribution studies by this technique, assuming a monoexponential net washout (3.97 ± 1.3 hours), was in excellent agreement with the values reported by Watson and associates.[62]

The main difference between these methods is that the Cedars approach recommends imaging at 4 hours instead of at 2 hours after injection, allowing a greater degree of washout to occur, and that the algorithm automatically calculates washout for each 6-degree location in each view, as opposed to automatically sampling a limited number of preselected myocardial locations. By assuming a monoexponential washout, difficulty was encountered in extrapolation of the 4-hour percentage washout normal limit profile to less than 2.5 hours or longer than 6 hours. Patients with imaging delays of less than 2.5 hours tended to have falsely normal washout, and those with delays longer than 6 hours tended to have falsely abnormal washout. It has been shown that the normal patient population behaves as though it exhibited a multiexponential washout. These results indicate that, between 3 and 7 hours, the mean half-time is 12.2 hours.

The amount of washout that takes place in patients injected at rest has also been studied. Preliminary results suggest that regional myocardial percentage washout of ^{201}Tl is much slower than that observed after injection at peak exercise.[63]

Reversibility analysis is an additional technique that offers promise for better separation of infarcted and ischemic regions. Patients with significant CAD but no myocardial infarction usually demonstrate the pattern of reversible relative hypoperfusion (redistribution). In this phenomenon, a perfusion defect seen in the immediate poststress images "fills in" and disappears by the time of delayed imaging. Vogel and colleagues[54] implemented a quantitative method for analysis of reversibility. They normalized the highest point in each of the stress and delayed maximal count circumferential profiles. The patient showed reversibility if a profile that showed a defect at stress, below normal limits, significantly improved during delayed imaging. We have further developed this technique for planar analysis[64] by scaling the stress distribution to the delay profile so that the normal areas, defined by the stress distribution and washout, were superimposed. Watson[51] and Okada[59] and their co-workers also displayed functional images that help to assess reversibility visually. In Okada's approach, normal segments that show no change between initial and delayed images are displayed in red; abnormal segments that exhibit redistribution are shown in green and infarcted segments in black.

Washout and reversibility occur for the same physiologic reason: the amount of thallium leaving the myocardium compared with the amount going in (net washout) is less in an ischemic than in a normal myocardial segment. Nevertheless, the mechanisms for detection are technically quite different. Washout analysis is an absolute (spatially nonrelative) measurement that does not require a normal reference segment in the view to detect abnormality. Because it is an absolute measurement, it is associated with a wide variation of normal responses and thus a large standard deviation (SD) around the mean normal response. Reversibility analysis is a relative measurement that does require a normal reference segment in the view to detect abnormality. Because it is a relative measurement, it is associated with less variation in normal responses and therefore less error. Wackers and associates have pointed out that localized drops in the washout rate profiles are an indication[65] of a reversible segment. The incorporation of reversibility analysis to differentiate ischemic from infarcted myocardial segments may provide an improvement to such assessment.

Establishment of Normal Limits

After stress-redistribution regional count and washout profiles have been generated, some method of determining whether they are normal or abnormal has to be employed. The Cedars approach uses lower limits of normal circumferential profiles generated from patients with a less than 1 percent pretest likelihood of having CAD.[48] This method avoids the pitfalls of using patients with normal coronary arteriograms who may have nonatherosclerotic ischemic disease.[66, 67] Furthermore, it allows the use of age-matched controls, which, if attempted with "normal volunteers," could result in inclusion of an unacceptable proportion of patients with occult coronary disease. The mean value and SDs were established from the pooled data of these patients for each of the 60 angular locations for the anterior, 45-degree LAO, and steep LAO images for each time interval. The time between the stress and the redistribution imaging, if other than 4 hours, was used to extrapolate the washout profile to exactly 4 hours.[48] The lower limits of normal for the stress and washout profiles were established as the profile 2.5 SDs below the mean observed profiles. Alternative approaches have used a threshold[51] for detection of perfusion defects and the range of regional normal values as lower limit profiles.

Development of Quantitative Criteria for Abnormality

The next step in the development of a quantitative method is to determine which type of mechanism is significant in detecting abnormality and the extent to which this mechanism (profile) should fall below normal limits before the patient is considered abnormal. In the Cedars approach, a pilot group of normal and

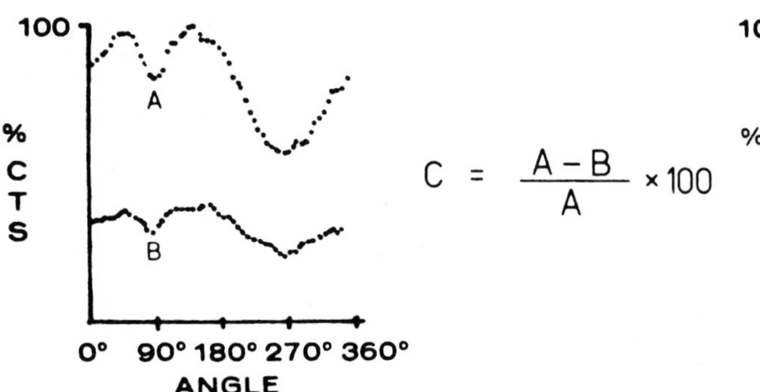

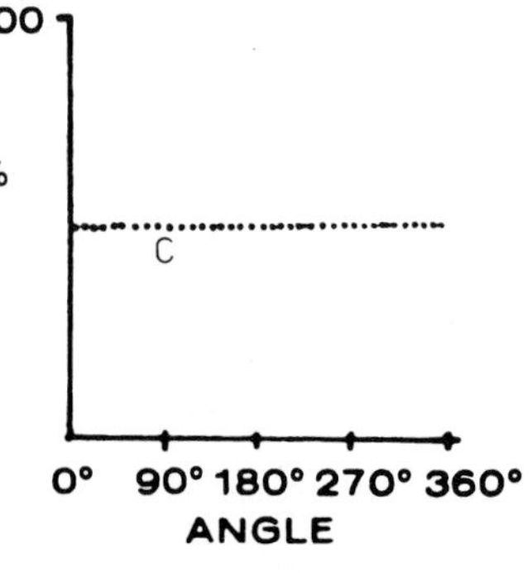

FIGURE 59–22. Percent washout calculation. The thallium-201 myocardial washout rate circumferential profile *(right)* is generated from the initial and 4-hour redistribution circumferential count profiles *(left top* and *left bottom*, respectively). Notice that despite interregional variations in thallium counts, the ^{201}Tl washout rate is fairly uniform throughout the myocardium. cts = counts.

CAD patients was used to establish these criteria.[48] This algorithm compared each patient's stress and washout profiles against the lower limits of normal. The program identified any arc of the profile that fell below normal limits. Different quantitative criteria for type and magnitude of abnormality were assessed in all patients in this pilot group for their ability to best discriminate normal from CAD patients. The following criteria best separated the populations:

1. A "stress defect" was defined as the occurrence of any segment of 18 degrees (three contiguous radii) of the stress profile falling below normal limits.
2. A "slow washout" abnormality was defined as the occurrence of any segment of 18 degrees of the washout profile falling below normal limits.
3. To be considered abnormal, the patient had to have at least two abnormal 18-degree arcs in the combined stress and washout rate profiles in three views.

Computerized Display of Results

After the patient's study has been analyzed, the results must be displayed in a concise but comprehensive report. Figure 59–23 demonstrates an example of the computerized quantitative display of the results that has been developed by Van Train and colleagues.[68] The stress and washout profiles in this patient with CAD were compared with the established normal limits. Using the above criteria, myocardial regions with stress perfusion defect or slow washout were identified. Findings were then displayed on concentric ellipses in all three planar views. In each view, the inner ellipse is the diagrammatic representation of the myocardium in that view, the border of different myocardial regions being shown as small break points on this ellipse. The missing portions of the middle ellipse demonstrate the presence of stress perfusion defects. The missing portions of the outer ellipse indicate the presence of a slow washout abnormality. These abnormalities are listed according to view and location in the written report at lower right. The concentric ellipse display not only facilitates interpretation of a given case as normal or abnormal but also aids in assignment of abnormalities to specific myocardial regions.

Another method for displaying quantitative results has been described by Reiber and associates.[60] With this method, the location, extent, and type of abnormality is presented in a functional image. For each radial line, it is determined whether the stress, redistribution, and washout profile values are normal or abnormal. The outcomes are then compared with the entries in a decision table to define the type of abnormality for that particular radial line.

Comprehensive computerized quantitative approaches to analysis of the regional stress myocardial distribution and washout rates of thallium-201 have been developed. These methods minimize many of the problems associated with the subjectivity of visual analysis of ^{201}Tl scintigrams. In addition, the quantitative techniques have been shown to be more accurate than visual image interpretation for detection and localization of CAD.[69]

Tomographic Methods for Thallium-201 Imaging

Rotational myocardial tomography after injection of thallium-201 at peak exercise offers significant improvement over planar scintigraphy for the detection and localization of myocardial ischemia.[70–72] Rotational ^{201}Tl tomography at rest has also been reported to be better than planar imaging for detection and localization of myocardial infarction and for estimation of the extent of infarcted myocardium.[73, 74] Several investigators[23, 52, 75] have used extensions of the planar quantitation concept to quantify the three-dimensional distribution of myocardial ^{201}Tl at stress and at redistribution from rotational tomograms. These algorithms express the percentages of myocardium that are involved with perfusion defect, washout abnormality, and reversible abnormality.

Protocol

In the approach implemented at Emory University,[52] the patient undergoes the same exercise protocol as for planar imaging, with the exception that a thallium dose of 3.5 mCi (130 MBq) is used.

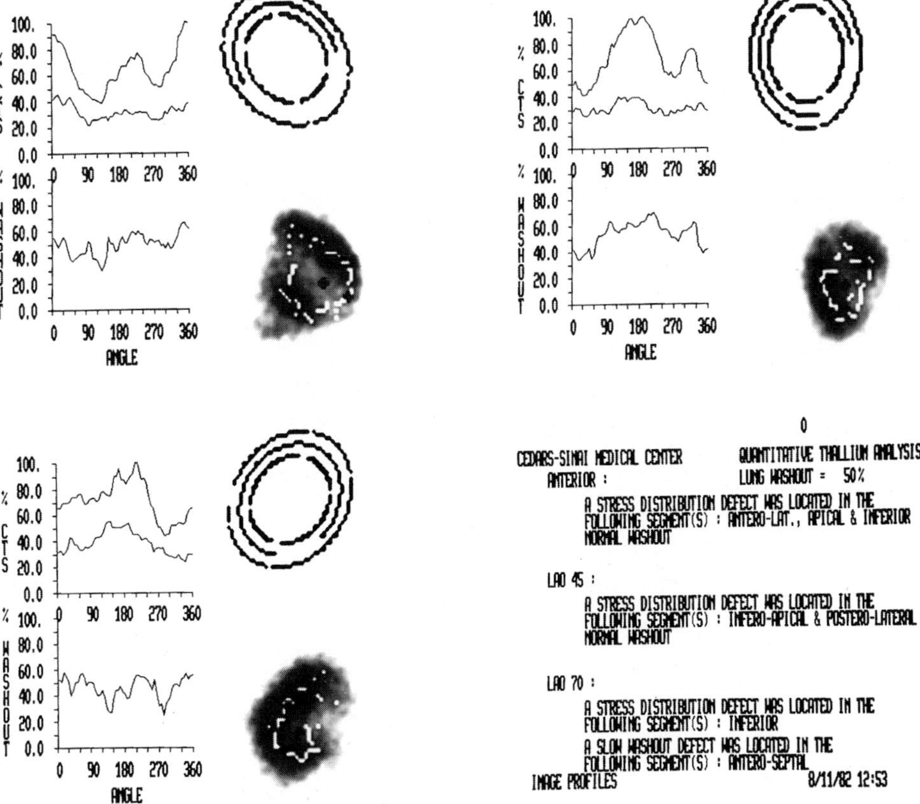

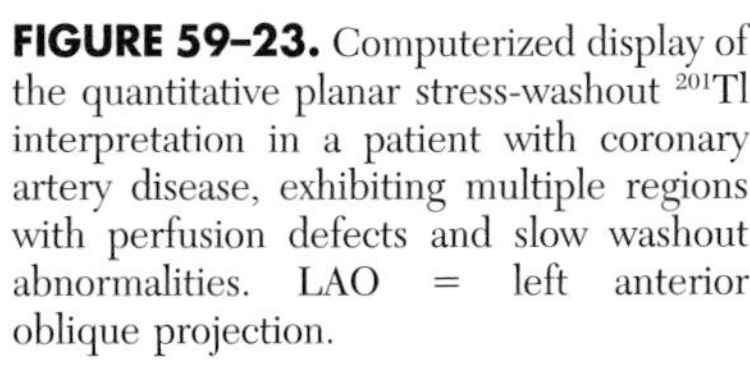

FIGURE 59–23. Computerized display of the quantitative planar stress-washout ^{201}Tl interpretation in a patient with coronary artery disease, exhibiting multiple regions with perfusion defects and slow washout abnormalities. LAO = left anterior oblique projection.

Acquisition consists of obtaining 32 projections for 40 seconds, each over the 180-degree arc extending from the 45-degree RAO to the 45-degree LPO projection. Each of the 32 projections is corrected for field nonuniformity and for misalignment of the mechanical center of rotation with respect to the reconstruction matrix. The projections are prefiltered before backprojection with the use of a Hanning filter with a cutoff frequency of 0.82 cycles per centimeter. FBP is then performed to reconstruct the transverse axial tomograms (of 6.25 mm each) encompassing the entire heart. Oblique tomograms parallel to the vertical and horizontal long axis and to the short axis of the left ventricle are extracted from the filtered transaxial tomograms by a coordinate transformation with appropriate interpolation.[76] The tomograms are reconstructed without scatter or attenuation correction because of the difficulties involved in correcting for the variable attenuation of ^{201}Tl 80-keV photons through the thorax. These effects are accounted for in part by comparison of each patient's thallium distribution to distribution files of normal patients exhibiting similar effects.

Three-Dimensional Quantification—Emory University Approach

The short slices to be quantified are selected by an operator according to a strict protocol. Using the long-axis slice with the largest cavity length, the operator selects the short-axis cuts for quantification to extend from the base of the left ventricle to the apical cap. On the short-axis cut that falls halfway between the apex and base, the operator then defines the center of the left ventricular cavity and the radius of search (Fig. 59–24*B*). The maximal count circumferential profiles for each short-axis cut are then generated automatically from the most apical to the most basal cut, as shown in Figure 59–18*A*. The actual raw counts are extracted and used without normalization. This procedure is performed for each stress and delayed tomographic study. Percent washout is also calculated, using the profiles of the corresponding anatomic cut at stress and at delayed tomography.

In Figure 59–24*A*, alternating short-axis slices of the left ventricle are displayed from base to apex. Approximately 12 slices are obtained from a normal-sized heart. In this example, there is a defect in the septum, which is highlighted in the middle slice. In Figure 59–24*B*, this slice has been divided into 40 sectors of 9 degrees each. The septum is represented by the sectors from 90 to 180 degrees. The maximal counts per pixel within each sector is determined. In Figure 59–25*A*, these 40 values have been plotted as a circumferential profile of the maximal counts per pixel versus angular location. A similar profile is constructed for each slice except for the first two, which contain the apex and are represented by a single value for maximal counts per pixel within the entire slice. To take into account variations in the number of slices per study, these curves are interpolated to produce a total of 15 profiles. Each of the rectangular coordinate profiles is translated into a polar coordinate profile (see Fig. 59–25*B*), which displays the curve as a circle composed of 40 pixels.

In Figure 59–25*C*, these data are displayed as a polar map called a bull's-eye plot, which consists of a series of 15 concentric circles with the apex at the center and the base at the periphery. Individual bull's-eye plots are constructed for the stress and delayed images as well as for percent washout. The bull's-eye plots from a patient with myocardial hypoperfusion in the inferior and inferolateral walls are displayed in Figure 59–26. In this display format, the stress and delay bull's eyes plots have been adjusted by multiplying each pixel in the delayed bull's eye by the ratio of the maximal counts per pixel in the stress bull's eye to maximal counts per pixel in the delay bull's eye. Notice the large anteroseptal defect at stress, which demonstrates marked redistribution in the delay bull's eye.

FIGURE 59–26. See Color Plate 23.

Normalization occurred only when the profiles were compared with the gender-matched normal files (developed from the group with low probability of disease) in which the mean values and SDs were established from the pooled data for each of the angular locations in each of the 15 profiles.[77] This was accomplished by dividing each bull's eye into four regions of 90 degrees each (anterior, septal, inferior, and lateral), from profiles 4 through 12, and determining the ratio of the average counts per pixel in each region of the patient's bull's eye to the same region in the appropriate normal file. The region with the highest ratio was assumed to be

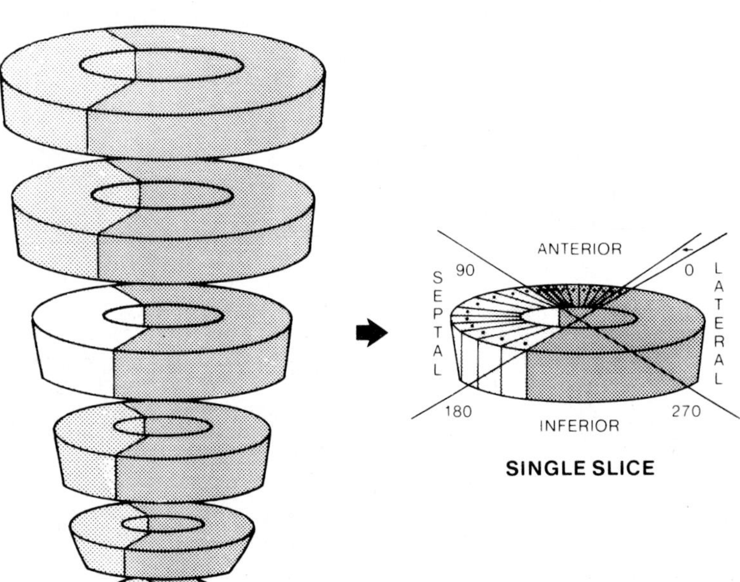

FIGURE 59–24. Method for obtaining circumferential profiles from tomographic slices. *A*, Alternating short-axis slices of the left ventricle are displayed. A septal defect is present from base to apex. *B*, The highlighted middle slice is divided into 40 sectors of 9 degrees each.

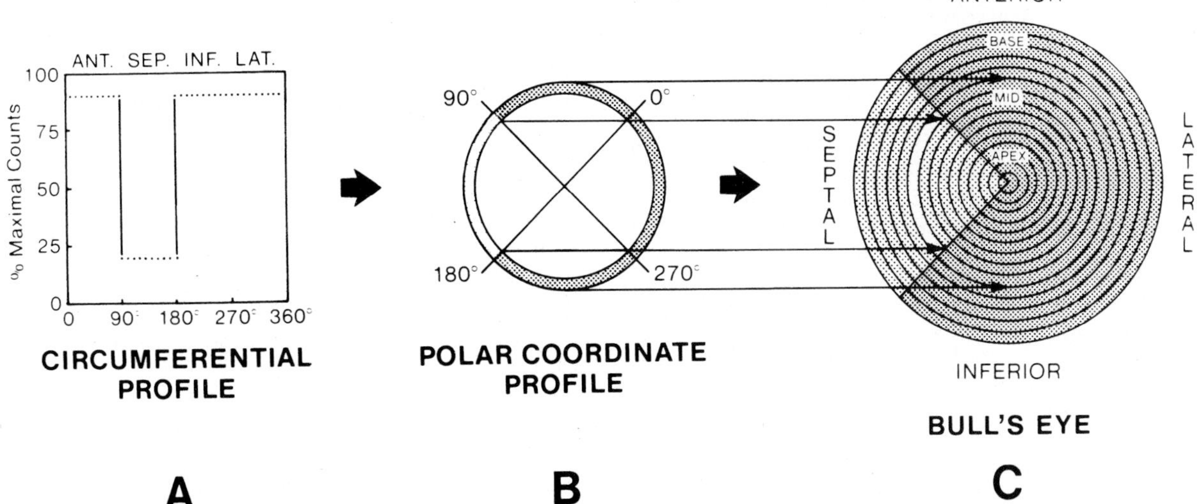

FIGURE 59–25. Method for obtaining bull's-eye polar maps. *A*, The maximal counts per pixel for each sector are plotted as a circumferential profile. Similar profiles are constructed for each slice. *B*, The rectangular coordinate profiles are converted into a polar coordinate profile, which displays the curve as a circle composed of 40 pixels. *C*, The polar coordinate profiles are displayed as a polar map (bull's-eye) plot with the apex at the center and the base at the periphery.

normal, and each pixel in the patient's bull's-eye polar map was multiplied by the reciprocal of this ratio.

The comparison of each individual patient's bull's-eye plot to a gender-matched normal file resulted in the conversion of the bull's eye into an SD map displaying pixels color-coded to the number of SDs below normal (see Fig. 59–26). The pixels that fell below normal limits were submitted to a clustering criterion that eliminated pixels without two adjacent abnormal neighbors from being displayed. These quantitative images were compared with the angiographic data of a pilot group of patients to determine the best criteria for identification of the presence and location of a significant coronary stenosis. This analysis resulted in establishing the profile curves representing 2.5 SDs below the mean normal responses as the threshold for defect detection. The clustered profile points falling below this established normal limit are plotted in a "blackout bull's eye," in which the black region within the bull's-eye plot defines the extent of the perfusion abnormality. The locations, sizes, and shapes of the blacked-out regions are used in conjunction with heuristic rules developed from a pilot group to identify the stenosed coronary artery associated with each specific pattern of perfusion abnormality. Figure 59–27 illustrates the approximate location on a bull's-eye plot of the regions perfused by specific coronary arteries.

Washout and reversibility bull's eyes are also generated. As with planar quantification, washout profiles are determined for each short-axis slice as the percent change in counts from stress to delayed imaging. Before comparison of the washout profiles with the corresponding normal profiles, the normal curves were adjusted to correspond to the same acquisition interval as the patient's study by moving the values in the normal curves along a monoexponential curve.

Reversibility bull's eyes are generated by subtraction of the stress profiles from the corresponding delay profiles after normalization to a 5 × 5 pixel maximal count reference area in the stress study. In addition to this reversibility bull's-eye polar plot and the reversibility SD bull's eye, a third polar plot is generated to easily display the application of the best single cutoff criterion determined (1.5 SDs). This plot duplicates the stress blackout bull's-eye plot but also includes the region that has reversed by the time of delayed imaging. This is displayed as a whited-out region and is determined from the application of the normal limits and criteria for reversibility that were developed[78, 79] (see Fig. 59–26).

A numerical report accompanies this reversibility whiteout bull's-eye map and includes, for each defect, the extent (number of pixels) of both the stress perfusion defect (blacked-out area) and the subregion within the defect that reverses within 4 hours (whited-out area). A severity score is also reported as the sum of the number of SDs from the mean of the pixels in the stress map that have been blacked out and those in the reversibility map that have been whited out. These scores are determined for each defect. A reversal of 15 percent or more of the original stress defect has been determined to be significant reversibility.[78, 79]

Other Approaches

Other investigators have also used circumferential profiles to extract the initial ^{201}Tl myocardial distribution and washout rates. Tamaki and associates[75] assessed the myocardium by using circumferential profiles from three short-axis sections and one middle RAO long-axis section. The main difference in other approaches has been in how the profiles are normalized. Caldwell and col-

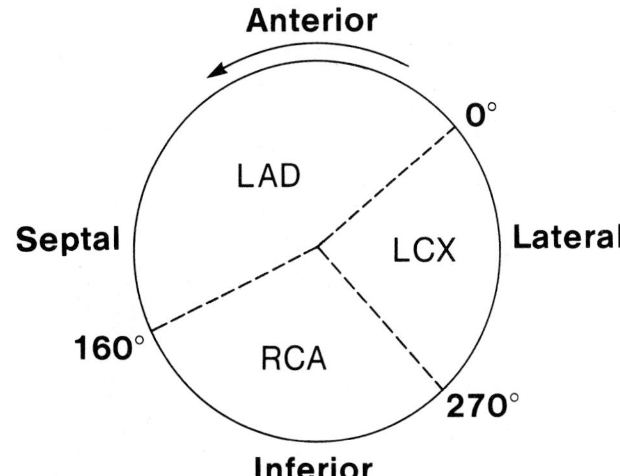

FIGURE 59–27. Coronary vascular territories corresponding to the bull's-eye polar map. LAD = left anterior descending artery; LCX = left circumflex artery; RCA = right coronary artery.

leagues[53] scaled the circumferential profiles to a percentage of maximal counts in the entire left ventricular region of interest. In the Cedars method,[23] each profile is normalized to the maximum pixel value for that profile.

In the Cedars approach, the circumferential profile arcs between 60 and 120 degrees of each ventricle long-axis cut are mapped into the central region of the display to depict the apical ^{201}Tl distribution. Immediately surrounding the apical region, the entire profile corresponding to the most apical short-axis slice is mapped, with all the subsequent short-axis profiles being mapped in increasingly larger circles until the most basal profile is reached. This approach helps to circumvent the partial volume effect at the apex that is inherent in the Emory University approach. In the two-dimensional Cedars polar map, the size of the display always remains the same, so the size of the left ventricle is reflected by the number of profiles that are mapped. In larger left ventricles, the band representing each slice is thinner compared with smaller left ventricles.

Assessment of Coronary Artery Disease

The severity of a perfusion defect in a thallium tomographic study may be judged objectively by comparison of patient data with gender-matched normal files. Through clinical experience and comparison with coronary angiography,[52] the investigators at Emory University have realized optimum accuracy in the diagnosis of CAD when only those bull's-eye abnormalities that are 2.5 SDs or more below normal limits are judged abnormal.

A number of important limitations and potential errors of this quantitative method must be emphasized. The bull's-eye plot is dependent on an observer's correct selection of the apex and the base of the left ventricle from oblique tomographic slices. If the slices extend too far past the actual base (or apex), there will be a rim of apparently decreased tracer concentration at the periphery of the bull's eye (or a localized central defect near the apex). Because the basal portion of the ventricle is relatively magnified in the bull's-eye plot and regions near the apex are minified, basal perfusion abnormalities appear larger than equivalent defects in the middle and distal portions of the left ventricle. Furthermore, image artifacts that result in decreased count density (e.g., attenuation by unusually large breasts or by an elevated left hemidiaphragm, patient motion, center of rotation errors) appear as defects in the bull's-eye plot and are represented as abnormalities in the thallium score. Alterations in myocardial anatomy and symmetry also create relative abnormalities in patient data as compared with normal gender-matched files. An artifact of this type is commonly encountered in patients with hypertrophic cardiomyopathy in whom there is a disproportionate increase in thickness of the septum in addition to concentric myocardial hypertrophy. Because the highest count density is in the septum, the remainder of the ventricle appears relatively decreased in intensity and may be judged to be abnormal when compared with normal files. Relative septal hypertrophy causes a marked abnormality in the thallium score in all regions of the myocardium, with the exception of the septum.

With due consideration of the limitations in the quantitative analysis of thallium bull's-eye plots, this method serves as a valuable tool for determination of the severity of myocardial ischemia and the amount of myocardium at jeopardy in patients with CAD. In the experience at Emory University, a thallium score greater than 40 SDs represents a true perfusion defect. Patients with more severe and extensive CAD demonstrate more markedly abnormal thallium scores.

Application of the Emory University bull's-eye quantitative technique to a prospective group of 210 patients (179 with and 31 without CAD) resulted in an overall sensitivity of 95 percent, a specificity of 74 percent, and an accuracy of 92 percent for detection of the presence or absence of CAD. The ability of this analysis to identify individual coronary stenoses is displayed in Figure 59–28 for each major coronary artery and for the left circumflex and right coronary arteries combined. The results of this prospective evaluation of the method demonstrate a high sensitivity and specificity for the detection of CAD and of individual coronary stenoses.[52]

Although these results are encouraging, they are based on the manual measurement of percent diameter stenosis with digital electronic calipers on the coronary arteriogram as a gold standard. Furthermore, they include patients taking antianginal medications and do not specifically exclude patients with prior myocardial infarction, left ventricular hypertrophy, or coronary collaterals, which could significantly interfere with the sensitivity and specificity of the procedure. In particular, the use of percent diameter stenosis

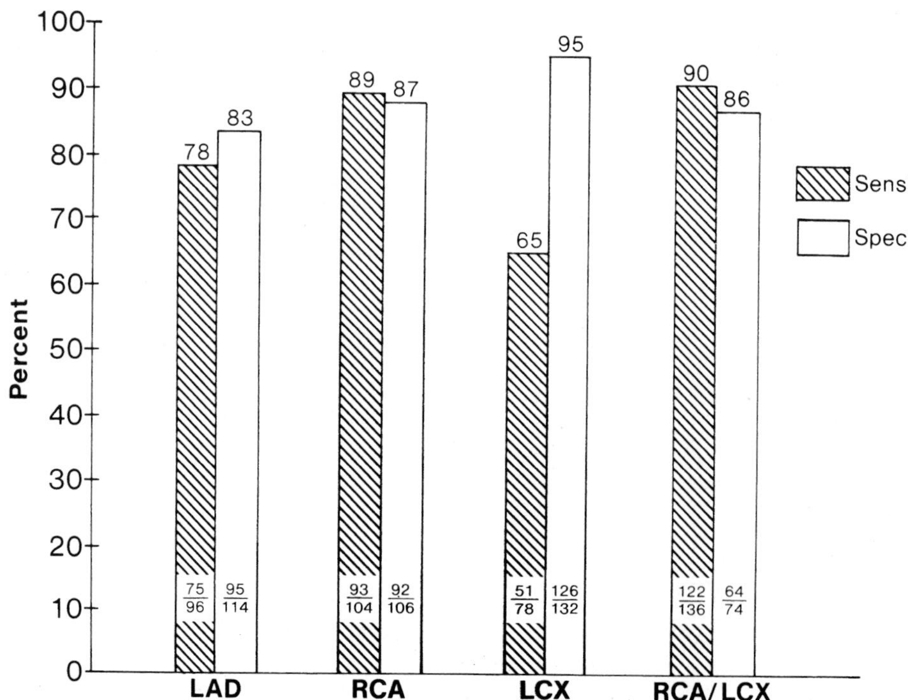

FIGURE 59–28. Sensitivity and specificity of quantitative ^{201}Tl tomography for detection of individual coronary artery stenoses. LAD = left anterior descending artery; LCX = left circumflex artery; RCA = right coronary artery.

as a gold standard for assessing the physiologic significance of a coronary obstructive region has been heavily criticized.[80] As consequence of these problems, additional studies using more sophisticated gold standards and more carefully defined patient populations are necessary to further define the specificity and sensitivity of SPECT thallium perfusion images.

Present Limitations of Sizing

It is possible to approximate the percentage of the myocardium that is abnormal by the methods that have been described. Of major prognostic importance is how accurately these calculations reflect the myocardium that is in jeopardy or infarcted. Accuracy of sizing the percentage of abnormal myocardium is somewhat affected by cardiac and thoracic motion. This motion has been reported to account for overestimation of defect activity during quantification of infarct size[81] or myocardial blood flow.[82] This motion has also been reported by Kirsch and colleagues[83] to be responsible for false-negative results in patients with small hearts and high EFs or hypertrophy. Kirsch and colleagues also reported cardiac motion to result in false-positive findings in large hypertrophic hearts and in patients with cardiomyopathy. This distortion caused by motion is nevertheless considered to be small compared with that caused by attenuation and scatter. As pointed out in previous sections, accuracy of sizing of the percentage of abnormal myocardium is also affected by spatial resolution. It is likely that this dependence on the system's spatial resolution would tend to mask small nontransmural perfusion defects while overestimating the size of transmural defects.

With respect to sizing of perfusion defects, Tamaki and colleagues[73] measured the infarct volume by applying manual planimetry of the normal and infarcted regions to tomographic cross sections. The results of this approach were compared with similar measurements made with the use of planar ^{201}Tl tomography with respect to the ability to correlate with the accumulated release of the myocardial component of creatine kinase (CK-MB). In spite of the limitations of ^{201}Tl tomography, they found a better correlation with CK-MB release with manual planimetry of the reconstructed tomograms than with planar measurements. Although encouraging, these results need further verification with gold standards that have fewer problems than those of CK-MB for prediction of infarct size.

Although polar map approaches offer the important attribute of objectivity over manual or visual assessment methods, some limitations in defect sizing are worthy of note. This approach gives equal weight to the contributions of small and large slices. Accurate measurement of the size of perfusion defects necessitates the development of methods that account for differences in myocardial mass contributed by slices of different sizes and of different endocardial-to-epicardial thicknesses.[84] Methods of calculating the severity of abnormality also become increasingly significant with the incorporation of true left ventricular mass.[85] Without corrections for scattering, attenuation, finite resolution, heart motion, and myocardial thickness, the error of measuring infarct size or perfusion defect size could be considerable.

Tomographic Methods for ^{99m}Tc-Sestamibi Imaging

Investigators at Emory University and at Cedars-Sinai Medical Center have collaborated to develop methods for quantifying myocardial perfusion from ^{99m}Tc-sestamibi studies.[39, 86, 87] This section describes the techniques.

Three-Dimensional Sampling

This approach was developed so that the myocardium could be sampled perpendicular to the myocardial wall; this type of sampling generates the best representation of the three-dimensional distribution.[39] Maximal count circumferential profiles are automatically generated from the short-axis slices with the use of a two-part three-dimensional sampling scheme (Fig. 59–29). First, the "apical hemisphere" is identified as those stacked short-axis slices that form a hemisphere; that is, the radius of the top slice of the stack is equal to the depth of the stack (left diagram of Fig. 59–29).

This apical hemisphere is then sampled in a spherical coordinate system, as seen in the bottom right diagram of Figure 59–29. Each point in the profile represents the maximal counts per pixel encountered along the radius of search for each ϕ (vertical angle) and θ (radial angle), as ϕ decreases from 180 to 90 degrees in 25.7-degree increments, producing eight equally spaced spherical rings, and as θ increases from 45 to 405 degrees in 9-degree increments, producing 40 equally spaced sectors. The remaining portion of the myocardium is relatively cylindrical in shape and is sampled slice by slice in a cylindrical coordinate system, as shown in the top right diagram of Figure 59–29. As before, each point in the profile represents the maximal counts per pixel encountered along the radius of search for increases from 0 to 360 degrees in 9-degree increments, producing 40 equally spaced sectors.

The radii of the extracted maximal counts are filtered in both depth and angle with a 3 × 3 low-pass filter kernel. The filtered radii are then fit to circles and transformed into Cartesian coordinates. These coordinates, along with their associated maximal counts, are recorded and used to generate the visualization models described in the following section.

Two-Dimensional Polar Maps

Two polar maps have been developed to take advantage of the more accurate information that is extracted from the short-axis slices by the two-part sampling scheme described. The first polar map, called the distance-weighted polar map, is constructed so that every ring in the polar map is the same width. The width is determined by dividing the radius of the polar map by the total number of sampled segments (spherical rings and cylindrical slices) in the patient data. The second polar map, called a volume-weighted polar map, is constructed in two parts. First, the volume of the apical hemisphere is determined, and its percentage of the total volume is calculated. The apical hemisphere is then mapped so that the area of the apical hemisphere occupies that same percentage of the total area of the polar map, with each ring within the apical hemisphere being equal in width. For the remainder of the myocardium, the area of each ring is proportional to the volume of the corresponding slice.

In a blinded evaluation of these two polar maps and the standard Emory University bull's eye by two experts, the distance-weighted polar map was judged to be the best for determining defect location, the volume-weighted polar map to be best for determining defect size, and both maps to be best for assessing apical distributions. The standard Emory University bull's eye was judged to be the worst of the three in all three categories. Although the distance-weighted and volume-weighted polar maps offer improvements in characterization of perfusion defects over standard maps, there are still distortions in the size, shape, and location of perfusion defects inherent in mapping three-dimensional data into two dimensions. These distortions can be greatly reduced if the perfusion data is visualized in three dimensions. The distortions are not inherent in the actual quantification procedure but only in the polar map representation.

Assessment of Coronary Artery Disease

As with the quantitative techniques for ^{201}Tl imaging, a gender-matched normal database and regional criteria for determining abnormality were developed for the 1-day rest-stress myocardial distribution of ^{99m}Tc-sestamibi.[86] This is done in order to objectify the detection and localization of CAD. This method and its corresponding normal database and abnormality criteria were evaluated in a multicenter trial comprising 161 patients from seven hospitals.[87] Quantitative analysis of data from these patients compared with coronary angiography results yielded a sensitivity for detection of CAD of 88 percent (90 of 102 patients), a specificity of 32 percent (7 of 22 patients), and a normalcy rate of 81 percent (30 of 37 patients) in persons with low likelihood of CAD. The sensitivi-

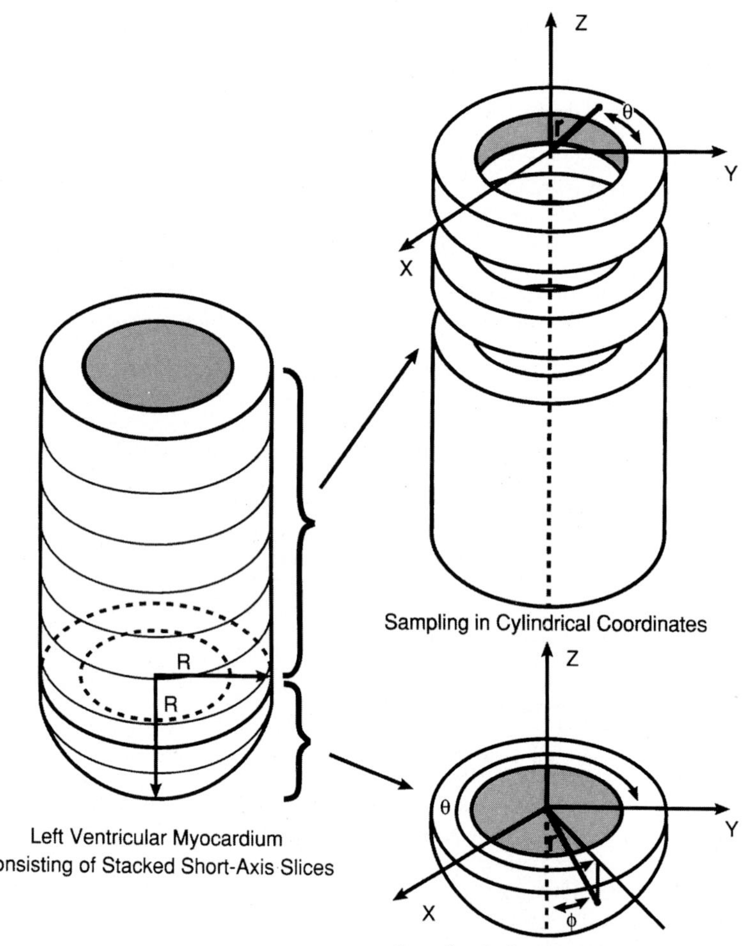

FIGURE 59–29. Two-part three-dimensional hybrid sampling scheme. (See text for details.)

ties for the vascular territories of the left anterior descending, left circumflex, and right coronary arteries were 67 percent (52 of 78 patients), 70 percent (35 of 50 patients), and 77 percent (44 of 57 patients), respectively, and the corresponding specificities were 76 percent (35 of 46 patients), 78 percent (58 of 74 patients), and 85 percent (57 of 67 patients), respectively. These results demonstrate that this objective quantitative analysis is clinically applicable for the accurate detection and localization of CAD.

Quantification of Myocardial Wall Thickening

Even though the spatial resolution in SPECT is too low to geometrically measure the distance between endocardium and epicardium to yield myocardial thickness, Galt and colleagues[35] have shown that the change in myocardial counts throughout the cardiac cycle is proportional to the change in myocardial thickness. If a region of the myocardium is followed throughout the cardiac cycle and the brightness in that region increases from end-diastole (when the heart is dilated and the walls are thin) to end-systole (when the myocardium thickens), it means that the wall is thickening and therefore that it is viable. Therefore, the change in counts throughout the cardiac cycle may be used as another marker of myocardial viability. In addition to the fact that gated acquisition is necessary for either SPECT or PET to freeze the motion of the heart in order to extract the accurate myocardial tracer quantification, a significant amount of clinically relevant functional information may also be obtained from these studies.

Quantification of myocardial function from gated perfusion SPECT has been pursued by use of this count-based approach, which assumes that the change in counts extracted from the same region of the left ventricular myocardium is proportional to the change in myocardial wall thickness. Galt and associates,[35] building on the concepts of Hoffman and co-workers,[14] have shown that the counts extracted along the center of a cardiac phantom of uniform tracer concentration and varying wall thickness vary in direct proportion to the thickness of the wall, up to a thickness that is about twice the spatial resolution of the imaging system (about 26 mm).

This relation between myocardial thickness and extracted counts has been quantified by Cooke and colleagues[88] with the use of the first harmonic of the fast Fourier transform to measure the amplitude and phase of the time-activity curve generated by extraction of the counts along the cardiac cycle from each of the three-dimensional myocardial samples. Twice the amplitude of this curve yields the difference in counts between the end-systolic sample and the end-diastolic sample. Percent systolic wall thickening is then measured by dividing twice the amplitude by the end-diastolic counts times 100 percent. The phase information, obtained as the offset of one time-activity curve in a given region of the left ventricular myocardium compared with another, is indicative of the onset of the wave of contraction. The three-dimensional mean normal response expected when measuring percent systolic wall thickening and phase has been generated and applied in selected patient groups. Algorithm optimization for speed and extensive clinical validation have yet to be reported; completion of these tasks is required before this technique is ready for clinical use.

Positron Emission Tomography Quantification and Polar Display

Polar maps have also been used in PET imaging to synthesize and display myocardial information. Two-dimensional polar map ("bull's-eye") approaches previously used for SPECT imaging[23] are now being implemented for the display and quantification of rubidium-82,[89, 90] carbon monoxide,[89] $^{13}NH_3$,[91, 92] and fludeoyglucose[91, 92] studies. A key aspect in generation of these displays is the method used to sample the myocardium. Older methods depended on sampling the short-axis slices on a slice-by-slice basis. Newer methods use a variety of three-dimensional sampling techniques that are more accurate,[39, 92] particularly around the apical region, because they tend to sample perpendicular to the myocardial wall. Extension of this polar map approach has resulted in three-dimensional surface models of the ventricle in which the actual shape and dimensions of the ventricle are preserved and the surface is color coded to represent the tracer distribution.[39, 92, 93]

Three-Dimensional Display

Methods are being developed to extend the functional two-dimensional polar map approaches to three dimensions. Three-dimensional representations of myocardial perfusion SPECT studies should aid physicians in the visualization and determination of the extent and severity of perfusion defects. At present, the investigated three-dimensional rendering methods code the myocardial perfusion information on a three-dimensional surface. These three-dimensional surface display approaches render either a surface that approximates the actual myocardial shape[94, 95] or a surface that models the shape of the myocardium, such as an ellipsoid.[96]

Surface Rendering

Methods that render the actual myocardial shape have in common their main processing steps, which originate in methods developed for three-dimensional display of bony surfaces from computed tomographic imaging.[97] The input is usually a set of contiguous two-dimensional tomographic slices, each made up of a matrix of voxels. From these sets of voxels, an algorithm generates a binary representation of the myocardium by determining whether a voxel is part of the myocardium (setting that voxel to 1) or outside the myocardium (setting that voxel to 0). Often, a single count threshold is used to determine this classification. After all the voxels have been classified as 0 or 1, another computer algorithm tracks the surface as the boundary between 0s and 1s. For representation of the myocardium, an outside (epicardial) and an inside (endocardial) surface may be generated, although present methods use a single surface to code the myocardial perfusion information.

After a three-dimensional surface has been created in the memory of the computer, it can be used to generate a set of multiple projections that may be animated in cinematic form to give the illusion of a moving three-dimensional surface. A number of common processing tricks are used to shade the surface in order to give this illusion a sense of reality. Each projection is coded so that areas of the surface that are "farther" from the viewer are shaded dimmer and the ones that are "closer" are brighter. If a far surface area falls behind a nearer portion of the surface along the viewer's line of sight, it is hidden from the display at that projection. A light source is assumed in these projections; areas of the surface that are perpendicular to the "rays" from the light source are shaded brighter, and areas that are parallel are dimmer. Figure 59–30 illustrates an application of this methodology as implemented by Nowak.[94]

FIGURE 59–30. See Color Plate 23.

Surface Modeling

A more direct approach to extending the two-dimensional polar maps (bull's-eye displays) to three dimensions is being developed in a joint project between Emory University and the Georgia Institute of Technology.[96] In this approach, the myocardial surface is modeled as a three-dimensional ellipsoid covered by small tiles of equal dimensions. The same maximal count circumferential profiles that are mapped onto the bull's-eye displays are now mapped onto the three-dimensional ellipsoidal surface with length and width relative to actual myocardial dimensions. Each circumferential profile count value that is used to assign a color to the bull's-eye map is also used to assign the same color to a "tile" on the ellipsoidal surface; the color represents the ^{201}Tl concentration in that region of the myocardium. In addition to this color coding, each tile is further shaded for each generated two-dimensional projection to give the illusion of a three-dimensional display, as described in the section on surface rendering. These projections are then animated to give the illusion of a left ventricular myocardium rotating about the patient's long axis. Figure 59–31*B* shows an example of this display.

Ideally, accurate assessment of the extent and severity of CAD requires integration of physiologic information derived from thallium SPECT and anatomic information derived from coronary arteriography. In order to accomplish this goal, the surface modeling method of representing myocardial perfusion can be enhanced by superimposition of the patient's own coronary arterial tree. The patient-specific coronary arterial tree is obtained from a three-dimensional geometric reconstruction performed on simultaneously acquired, digital biplane angiographic projections.[98] The coronary arterial tree is approximated by successive conical segments. After the arterial tree has been reconstructed in three dimensions, it is scaled, transformed (warped), and rotated to fit onto the myocardial ellipsoidal surface. The left and right coronary arteries are fixed onto the myocardial perfusion ellipsoidal model by registration of the proximal left anterior descending coronary artery onto the region corresponding to the anterior interventricular groove and the posterior descending artery onto the inferior interventricular groove. Figure 59–31 illustrates this unified display. Although the use of these three-dimensional images offers potential for a better understanding of CAD, they represent very preliminary results. Several years of development and evaluation are still needed to determine the true validity of this approach.

FIGURE 59–31. See Color Plate 24.

Quantification of Radionuclide Ventriculograms

Radionuclide ventriculography is important for the assessment of ventricular function at rest and during exercise. Background-corrected total counts extracted from a left ventricular region of interest provide a measurement of the relative volume of the ventricle at that instant of the cardiac cycle. To date, measurement of EF remains, for the most part, operator dependent. Moreover, assessment of regional function is usually performed by visual evaluation of closed-loop cine displays of the beating heart.

Manual assignment of regions of interest for calculation of EF and visual assessment of regional wall motion are imprecise because of observer variability. Expert observers are needed to perform these subjective tasks in order to obtain acceptable levels of inter-observer and intraobserver variability. Moreover, the operator time involved in preparation of studies for visual evaluation and for determination of EF is extensive. These limitations have prompted development of quantitative techniques for the automatic (or semi-automatic) determination of global and regional left ventricular function from either MGES or first-pass studies. In general, these quantitative techniques involve the following steps: preprocessing or filtering of the scintigraphic images, isolation of the left ventricular chamber, determination of background, edge detection of the left ventricle throughout the cardiac cycle, quantification of the parameter of regional function, establishment of normal limits, and development of a quantitative criterion for definition of abnormality. This section explains each of these steps as they apply to MGES studies.

Image Processing

Preprocessing of Images

Preprocessing is applied to the digital images of the cardiac cycle before any analysis is undertaken. It consists of space-time smoothing of the images in either the spatial or the frequency domain, as has been explained. It is performed mainly to minimize the statistical count fluctuations, which are random in space and time. This image enhancement is at the expense of both spatial and temporal resolution. Degradation of resolution gives rise to a blurred cardiac cycle. Nevertheless, because the counts at the edge of the ventricle determine the accuracy of assessment of regional wall motion[99] as well as the accuracy of definition of the left ventricular edge, it is imperative that preprocessing be performed before any quantitative or visual analysis of wall motion is attempted.

Left Ventricular Isolation

The next step in the quantitative process is to localize the left ventricular chamber with image segmentation techniques. An early implementation suggested by Burow and colleagues[100] consisted of manually assigning a box around the left ventricle. Other investigators locate the left ventricle by first identifying a pixel somewhere close to the center of the chamber. Douglass[101] and Reiber[102] and their associates use properties of profiles representing the column and row sums, either of the difference image (end-diastolic minus end-systolic counts) or of the first frame of the study.

Nelson and Verba[103] developed a novel approach by using a minimum pixel image to separate the atria from the ventricles. In this approach, for each pixel's Cartesian coordinates, the computer searches throughout the cardiac cycle and assigns the minimal count value of that location to a minimum image. This minimum image is then subtracted from each frame. Subtraction eliminates the structures that are not moving and results in stroke images with the isolated ventricles at end-diastole and the isolated atria at end-systole. The left ventricle is then found from the frame of the isolated ventricles as the counts to the left of the center of gravity of the entire cycle of stroke images. Links and colleagues[104] and the Cedars group[105–108] have used variations of these methods.

In the Cedars approach, stroke images, defined as described in the previous paragraph, are used to simplify identification of the moving structures. The four stroke images with the lowest center of mass (closest to the bottom) are summed to create a composite of ventricular end-diastole. The four images with the highest center of mass are summed to create a composite of ventricular end-systole. After subtracting the atrial image from the ventricular image to minimize problems with overlapping structures, thresholding of the column and row profiles is used to determine the location and size of a rectangle enclosing only the ventricles. The interventricular septum is located by scanning each horizontal profile inside the rectangle for a local minimum between two maxima.

Background Determination

In order to isolate the counts coming from the left ventricle, the computer algorithm must subtract the counts that fall on the region of the left ventricle from radioactivity in tissues in front of and behind the ventricle as well as radiation that is scattered into the region of the left ventricle from surrounding tissues. This type of background noise is also known as tissue crosstalk. Moreover, in order to isolate the left ventricle, the counts in the background that define the right ventricle, the atria, the great vessels, and the lungs must be eliminated.

Both of these background eliminations can be performed simultaneously with the use of interpolative background subtraction techniques. The Cedars approach uses a rectangle around the left ventricle to define the origin of background to be subtracted, using the same interpolative background scheme as that described for the analysis of planar ^{201}Tl scintigrams. The pixels outside the rectangle are set to 0. The subtraction is performed on a frame-by-frame basis. This not only is effective in eliminating the background counts but also serves to increase the image contrast, thus preparing the image for subsequent edge enhancement and detection.

Several investigators[57, 105–107] have reported on the utility of applying interpolative background subtraction to MGES studies and on the improvements to this technique. In particular, Stamm and colleagues[109] showed that wall motion from interpolative, background-subtracted, gated blood pool images compared well with contrast angiography results; Leidholdt and associates[57] have reported that EFs calculated by subtracting polygonal matrices of 12 vertices from the entire heart in MGES data showed good correlation with EFs determined by the standard measurement technique. The Cedars approach differs from these in that the left ventricle alone is identified as the matrix to be subtracted. Nichols[58] reported on the use of irregular regions and weights without arbitrary roll-off constants as improvements to the method that allow more accurate approximation of true ventricular background.

Other approaches require that the left ventricular edges be defined before background is determined. One of the first methods for semiautomated background determination was suggested by Burow and associates.[110] In their approach, a background region of interest is assigned a set distance to the left of the left ventricle. The region is defined as being a set number of pixels wide and extending from the apex through two thirds of the length of the left ventricular vertical axis. The method requires that the time-activity curve extracted from this region be confirmed by the operator to be flat or that the region be moved away from blood pool structures.

In another approach, described by Almasi and colleagues,[111] background activity is automatically subtracted on a pixel-by-pixel basis with the use of two perimeters or edges. The inner perimeter corresponds to the left ventricular edge. The outer perimeter corresponds to the septal border of the right ventricle to right of the left ventricle, or to the hepatic edge or lung elsewhere. The pixels outside of the outer perimeter are set to 0. The global background is determined from the pixels with the lowest count rate located around the 45-degree sector between the outer and inner perimeters. In addition to subtraction of global background, the counts extracted from the pixels in the region between the inner and outer perimeter are also adjusted to compensate for the contribution of tissue crosstalk from the left ventricle and surrounding chambers. This compensation is done regionally by interpolation of the counts between the inner and outer perimeters.

Edge Detection

Edge detection is needed to define the borders of the left ventricle throughout the cardiac cycle. These borders are used to define regions of interest from which counts are extracted for calculation of global or regional EF. The radial changes in these edges are also used to assess regional wall motion. The process of edge detection includes edge enhancement, boundary recognition, and edge tracking in both space and time. These techniques were covered in detail in the image processing section of this chapter.

An example of edge detection methodology used by the Cedars group is described here. A 3×3 Laplacian operator is applied to obtain nondirectional, second derivative images that are termed Laplacian images. These images are then smoothed in space and time. From the smoothed Laplacian images, the program searches radially out from the center for the highest pixel value, which is defined as the ventricular edge. The edge points are then connected, subject to threshold analysis with respect to radial length so as not to allow any one edge point to be too far away from its neighbors. After thresholding, the edge points are smoothed in space and time. This approach had a success rate of 100 percent in detecting the left ventricular edges from a training set of 80 2-minute MGES studies acquired in the best septal LAO projection (approximately 100,000 counts per frame).[107] Goris and co-workers[112] have also reported successful use of Laplacian algorithms for edge detection. Although there are other edge enhancement operators, such as the Sobel operator, that are less sensitive to noise and could work with MGES data, the implementation of those more sophisticated operators could slow down execution time considerably.

Global Function Calculations

Two parameters of left ventricular global function that can be evaluated from radionuclide ventriculographic studies are EF and absolute chamber volume.

Ejection Fraction

In the approach implemented at Cedars-Sinai Medical Center,[108] the regions of interest generated from edge detection of the left ventricle throughout the cardiac cycle are applied to the images of the MGES study. The total counts within each region are plotted against frame number to create a volume curve (time-activity curve), from which EF is calculated. The point in the volume curve with the highest value corresponds to the global end-diastolic frame, and that with the minimum value corresponds to the global end-systolic frame. As suggested by Burow and colleagues,[110] the outline of the end-systolic region is used to create a paraventricular background region that is located to the left of the left ventricular edge and follows the edge contour. An average background value in counts per pixel is calculated by summing the counts in the background region and dividing by the number of pixels in that region. This background value is used to correct the left ventricular volume curve after normalization for the number of pixels within the left ventricular region. EF is then calculated in the standard manner as the background-corrected end-diastolic counts minus the end-systolic counts, divided by the end-diastolic counts.

This automatic approach yielded a success rate of 100 percent for detection of the left ventricular edges from a training set of 80 MGES studies applied to 20 patients and resulted in a good correlation coefficient for left ventricular EF measurements when compared with manual techniques. Figure 59–32 illustrates an

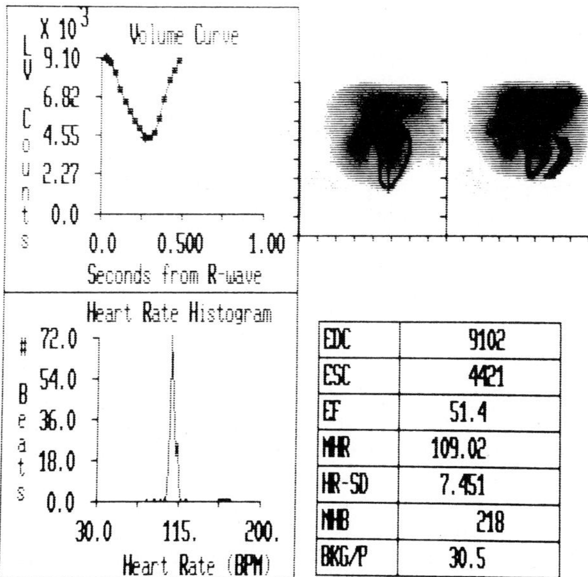

FIGURE 59–32. Global function report generated from a totally automatic analysis of a peak exercise multiple-gated equilibrium scintigraphic study from a patient with triple-vessel coronary artery disease. Shown are the left ventricular (LV) volume curve *(top left)*; the heart rate histogram *(bottom left)*; the automatically chosen end-diastolic, end-systolic, and background regions *(top right)*; and the measured parameters *(bottom right)*. BPM = beats per minute; EDC = end-diastolic counts; ESC = end-systolic counts; EF = ejection fraction; MHR = mean heart rate; HR-SD = heart rate standard deviation; NHB = number of heart beats; BKG/P = background counts per pixel.

example of a global function report generated from this automatic analysis.

Other investigators have also reported on the accuracy of automatic methods. Links and colleagues,[104] processing only the end-diastolic and end-systolic frames, reported a 90 percent operating success rate in 40 patients, with a correlation coefficient of .95 for left ventricular EF by manual techniques. Almasi and associates,[111] processing all frames of the cardiac cycle in 69 patients at rest, reported an 84 percent success rate and a correlation coefficient of .91 for manual left ventricular EF. Yuille and co-workers[113] reported on the use of a space-time smoothing algorithm followed by a high-emphasis filter to improve edge definition. These methods are significantly more successful in measuring left ventricular EF when they are applied to high-count density, high-resolution resting MGES, compared with low-count, low-resolution exercise MGES.

Volume Determinations

Automatic measurement of absolute left ventricular volume from MGES has not been described, but several manual approaches exist for geometric and nongeometric determination of left ventricular volume.

Geometric techniques, first described by Dodge and co-workers[114] for application in contrast ventriculography, have been applied to gated blood pool studies by Strauss and associates.[115] This method assumes the left ventricle to be either an ellipsoid or a prolate spheroid, which is not an accurate assumption for hearts with regional dysfunction. Geometric determination of absolute left ventricular volumes from MGES studies has been shown to give good correlation with angiographically determined volumes.[116, 117]

Nongeometric radionuclide techniques for the measurement of left ventricular volume were first described for tracer dilution curves[118, 119] and later for MGES studies.[120–122] In one method,[121] the count rate from the left ventricle is converted to arbitrary volume units by employing the activity measured from a small sample of the patient's blood. This approach, which does not account for photon attenuation through the chest wall, yields only an index rather than an absolute measurement of left ventricular volume. In nongeometric methods, a blood sample is withdrawn during imaging of the LAO view and counted on the collimator face after acquisition of patient data has been completed. Left ventricular volume at end-diastole is calculated as the ratio of the attenuation-corrected count rate in the LAO view to the count rate per milliliter from the blood sample. The left ventricular end-diastolic count rate is obtained by dividing the total background-corrected counts in the left ventricular end-diastolic region of interest by the product of the time per end-diastolic frame and the number of cardiac cycles acquired.

Other investigators, such as Links[120] and Schwaiger[122] and their associates, have pointed out the need to correct for attenuation and have developed preliminary methods for this correction. In the Schwaiger approach, the attenuation factor is calculated as the ratio of the deadtime-corrected counts obtained from the image of the bolus in the right ventricle to the counts derived from a reference activity image close to the collimator surface. In the Links approach, attenuation correction is made by dividing the left ventricular end-diastolic count rate by $e^{-\mu d}$. In this calculation, μ is the linear attenuation coefficient for water (0.15 cm^{-1}); d is the distance from a skin marker (which is placed on the skin over the left ventricle in the LAO view and imaged during the anterior view) to the center of the left ventricle in the anterior view, divided by the sine of 400 to yield the depth of the left ventricle in the LAO view.

Although the results of both techniques show excellent correlation for left ventricular end-diastolic volume with angiography results, in our experience both are cumbersome and prone to error. Schwaiger's approach requires a very tight bolus and the additional effort of acquiring and processing a first-pass study. Links' method, besides requiring additional acquisition and processing, uses a simple exponential equation that assumes the ventricle is a point source. This assumption tends to overcorrect for the attenuation from large ventricles and to undercorrect for the attenuation from small ventricles.

Regional Function Calculations

Although quantitation of global left ventricular and right ventricular EFs is a well-established clinical procedure, quantitative evaluation of regional function by radionuclide ventriculography is in a developmental stage, as it is for all cardiac imaging modalities. Extraction of regional myocardial function indices began in 1967 with the work on hemiaxis shortening from contrast ventriculographic studies by Herman and colleagues.[123] The literature in this field reveals a spectrum of unsolved problems ranging from which coordinate system to use[124, 125] to whether to use an area, chord, or radial method.[126, 127] The publication of hundreds of manuscripts on this subject and the multiplicity of approaches to the same problem indicate that there is no consensus as to which is the best approach. Radionuclide ventriculographic methods for evaluation of regional function include segmental wall motion (radial or area change), regional EF (count [volume] change), and regional phase analyses.

Segmental Wall Motion

In an early attempt to quantify segmental wall motion from MGES,[128] the ventricle was divided into 12 30-degree sectors originating at the center of area of the end-systolic 45-degree LAO image. (A similar approach was independently developed by Silber and colleagues.[129]) The change in area of these sectors between end-diastole to end-systole was expressed as a contraction fraction and compared with lower limits of normal values obtained from normal volunteers. The limitations were that the sectors were too large and masked both small regional abnormalities and abnormalities at boundaries between sectors. Lack of an alignment system led to improper comparison with normal limits in some cases. Even though left ventricular edge detection was semiautomatic, there was interoperator disagreement on what the correct edges should be. Furthermore, quantification of the regional area change gave no information regarding the walls if motion was perpendicular to the plane of the detector in this view.

This last limitation was partially circumvented by the work on regional EF that originated from the Johns Hopkins Medical Institutions and was reported separately by Burow and colleagues[110] and by Douglass and colleagues.[101] In their approach, the ventricle is divided into 45-degree sectors, each constructed from the end-diastolic region of interest about its geometric center. The EF from each of these eight regions is calculated from the curve of background-corrected counts (volume) versus time. Because the counts are proportional to volume if attenuation is disregarded, then the regional EF reflects the function of all of the walls contained within it, thus providing information regarding the motion of all ventricular segments from a single view. Burow and colleagues[130] and Douglass and colleagues[101, 131] have independently reported that regional EF is more accurate than global EF for the detection of CAD. Preliminary results from the Cedars group suggest that this approach is more sensitive than the contraction fraction technique.[107]

In the most recent Cedars approach for quantitation of regional wall motion and EF, 60 6-degree arcs are evaluated, letting observed data dictate the criterion for abnormality (i.e., how many contiguous areas will represent a significant abnormality). This approach has a major advantage over arbitrary segmental division of the left ventricle in that no matter how large the combined sector deemed the criterion for abnormal, it can move at 6-degree increments. This approach circumvents the problems inherent in undersampling.[132]

Cedars-Sinai Medical Center Approach

Segmental parameters are based on two composite edges rather than the actual edge determined for any one frame[105, 126] (Fig. 59–33). A composite end-diastolic edge represents the greatest relaxation of each angular position, not only in the global end-diastolic frame, but also in the frame before and the frame after that one. Likewise, a composite end-systolic edge represents the greatest contraction of each segment within one frame of global end-systole. The reason for the composite edge is the fact that all segments do not reach end-diastole and end-systole at the same point in time. On the other hand, constraining the definition of edges to be close to the global state precludes misinterpretation of dyskinesis as normal motion.

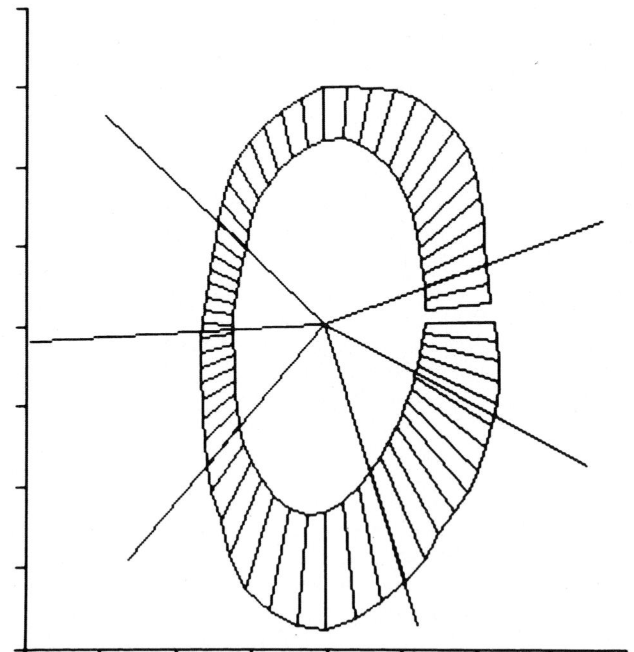

FIGURE 59–33. Graphical representation of segmental wall motion in a resting multiple-gated equilibrium scintigraphic study from a normal patient. The outer border corresponds to end-diastole and the inner one to end-systole. Zero degrees is aligned at 3 o'clock and proceeds clockwise.

The contraction fraction is used as a measure of regional wall motion. It is based solely on the composite end-diastolic and end-systolic edges. For each angular position, the contraction fraction is defined as (ED − ES)/ED, where ED is the end-diastolic length of that segment and ES is the end-systolic length, and it is plotted as a circumferential profile (Fig. 59–34).

The regional EF is based on the measured activity in small regions of the ventricular cavity. The end-diastolic length of a segment is divided in half, the inner half representing a volume that moves perpendicular to the detector face. The outer region is affected primarily by walls that move parallel to the detector face. A region representing the entire segment is also used (Fig. 59–35). For each segment, a search is made for the largest volume near end-diastole and the smallest volume near end-systole. In order to mitigate the effect of such small regions, the regions of interest used in these calculations are interpolated to 128 × 128 resolution. After the raw curves are created, they are smoothed to reduce the effect of low counting statistics (Fig. 59–36). Vitale and colleagues have also reported on a similar method of separating the left ventricle into an inner and outer regional EF.[133]

Burow and associates initially demonstrated,[50] and the Cedars group implemented in the planar thallium and regional function work, the alignment of the regional circumferential profiles to an anatomic landmark (the cardiac apex). This alignment is needed for two reasons: first, because the lower limits of normal exhibit regional variations, alignment of the apex to the 90-degree sector ensures that the correct segment will be compared with the lower normal limits; second, during comparison of changes in the response of a segment (i.e., between rest and exercise), this approach

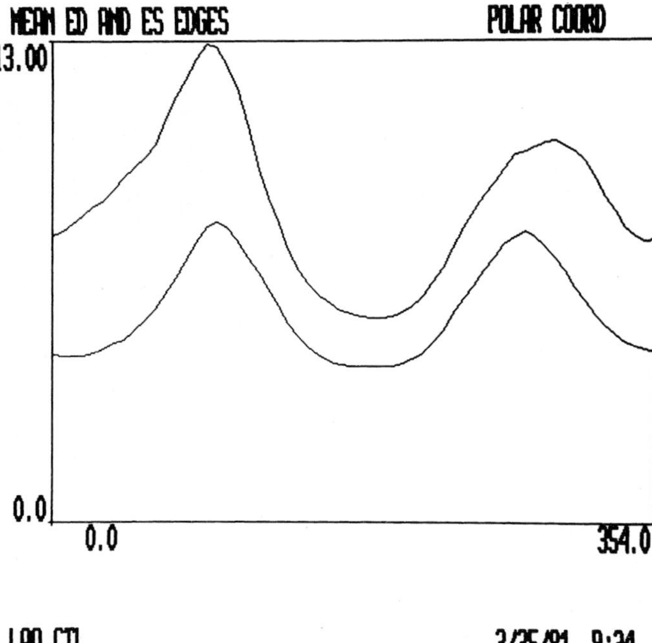

FIGURE 59–34. Circumferential profile representation of the segmental wall motion of the patient in Figure 59–33. Graph shows distance versus angle for each of 60 end-diastolic (ED; *top curve*) and end-systolic (ES; *bottom curve*) circumferential profile points. The first peak is the point chosen to represent the apex, which is then used to align the circumferential profiles to 90 degrees. The contraction fraction profile is determined on a point-by-point basis from these two profiles as the percent difference between ES and ED, similar to the determination of the myocardial ^{201}Tl washout profile shown in Figure 59–22. Polar Coord = polar coordinates (angle versus radius).

compensates for changes in heart orientation that could create miscalculation of the difference profiles.

The system used by the Cedars group since 1979 employs polar coordinates centered at the geometric end-systolic center in a fixed frame of reference (see Fig. 59–33). The end-systolic geometric centroid was chosen because, in the 45-degree LAO view at peak exercise, contraction of the normal ventricle often is such that the end-systolic silhouette lies outside the end-diastolic centroid. Use of the end-systolic centroid in that case would result in calculation of regional parameters more logical to the intuitive visual observation of the motion. Use of the end-diastolic centroid should result in similar accuracy but in less intuitive findings. This hypothesis needs further testing. Ingels and colleagues[124] reported that the end-systolic point would be the optimum position for the polar origin of a fixed external reference system. Because of the low-resolution matrices used in MGES studies, a fixed reference system is mandatory. The error that would result from trying to align the different frames of the cardiac cycle to anatomic landmarks would greatly outweigh any benefits. In regard to the choice for polar coordinates, Steckley and colleagues[134] have reported that there was a higher correlation coefficient for polar area reduction techniques than for rectangular areas.

Phase Analysis

In radionuclide ventriculographic studies, the combined time-activity curves from pixels within the left ventricle represent volume changes over time.[135, 136] The counts contributed by each pixel within the left ventricle represent the volume change behind their projected data. The volume-time curve from each pixel, because it resembles a sinusoidal wave, can be reasonably well approximated

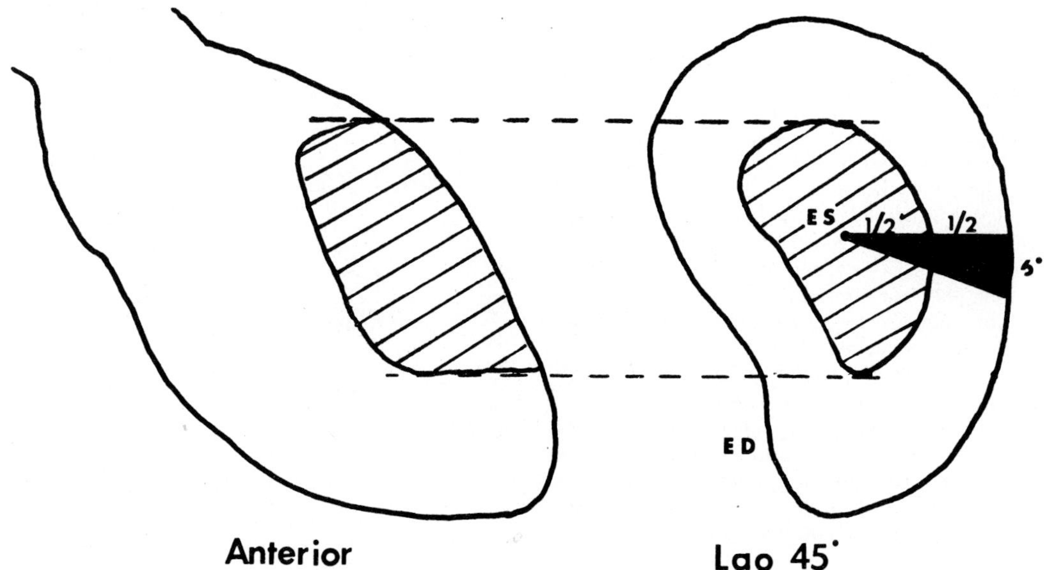

FIGURE 59–35. Schematic representation of division of a lateral region into inner, outer, and combined sectors for determination of regional ejection fraction. The inner and outer regions are arbitrarily defined as half the distance to the end-diastolic (ED) edge from the end-systolic (ES) center of mass. Notice that the inner region corresponds mostly to anterior wall function. Lao = left anterior oblique.

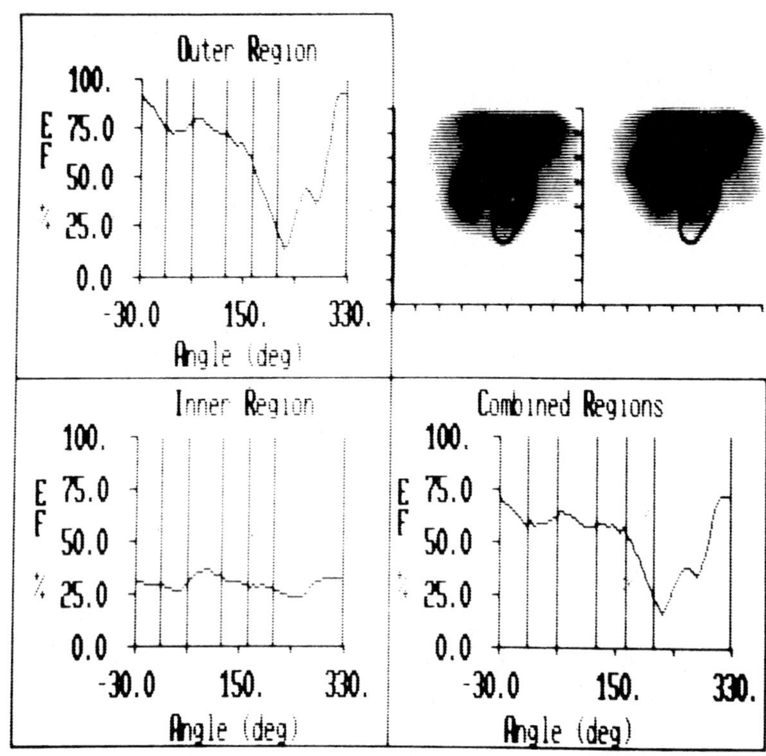

FIGURE 59–36. Regional ejection fraction (EF) report of a peak exercise multiple-gated equilibrium scintigraphic study in the same patient as in Figure 59–32. Comparison of the patient's regional EF profiles with normal limits profiles predicted abnormality of the posterolateral and inferoapical areas (from the outer EF) and in the anterior wall (from the inner EF), consistent with triple-vessel disease, which was documented by subsequent cardiac catheterization.

by a single cosine component with a frequency equal to that of the heart rate. Because this frequency is the lowest frequency extracted from the volume-time curve, it is known as the fundamental frequency; the cosine component of that frequency times the extracted amplitude is the first harmonic. The cosine component with the next higher frequency is known as the second harmonic. The counts in each pixel within the heart region located in cartesian coordinates (x, y) as a function of time (t) can then be expressed as a cosine wave with a frequency equal to the heart rate, aligned by a phase angle, times an amplitude:

$$\text{Counts } (x,y,t) = A_0 + \text{Amplitude } (x,y)\cos[\text{heart rate } (t) + \text{phase } (x,y)]$$

The constant A_0, known as the zero harmonic (divided by two) or the DC term, is given by the average value of counts at that pixel location. To a first approximation, the amplitude of the fundamental frequency is proportional to stroke volume, and the phase is related to the time in the cardiac cycle at which emptying begins[135] (Fig. 59–37). If two of the pixels defining the heart reach a maximum (end-diastole) or a minimum (end-systole) at the same time, then there is no phase difference between the two; otherwise, the difference in the times at which the two reach a maximum is given by the phase angle difference between them (Fig. 59–38). Given that a cycle is represented by 360 degrees and the normal ventricle reaches a maximum at the same time that the atrium reaches a minimum, the two are said to be 180 degrees out of phase. Functional cardiac images can be generated that display the values for the temporal average, stroke counts, and phase shift on a pixel-by-pixel basis (Fig. 59–39). Study of the differences in phase between one part of the ventricle and another, or between one chamber of the heart and another, gives information as to the pattern that the wave of contraction follows. This type of information extraction is helpful in studying the pattern of electrical activity of the heart and regional wall motion contraction patterns.

FIGURE 59–39. See Color Plate 24.

The accuracy of determining phase shifts has been reported[137] to improve when the first harmonic analysis is generalized to include the first three harmonics. This improvement is a result of better representation of the volume-time curve with continued maintenance of a marked degree of temporal filtering. Phase analysis can evaluate the temporal sequence of systolic ventricular wall motion from MGES studies in the modified LAO view.[135, 136, 138] In the preliminary approaches, the computer was used to perform Fourier transforms of the time-activity curve on a pixel-by-pixel basis, and only the first Fourier coefficients were used, as described in the image processing section.

There are two major limitations to the method as reported. First, as has been pointed out by Bacharach,[16] use of only the first Fourier coefficient results in significant errors in determination of the phase. Second, the current approach to assessing regional wall motion from this analysis is to visually assess the display of the wave of contraction in color or black and white. This visual assessment

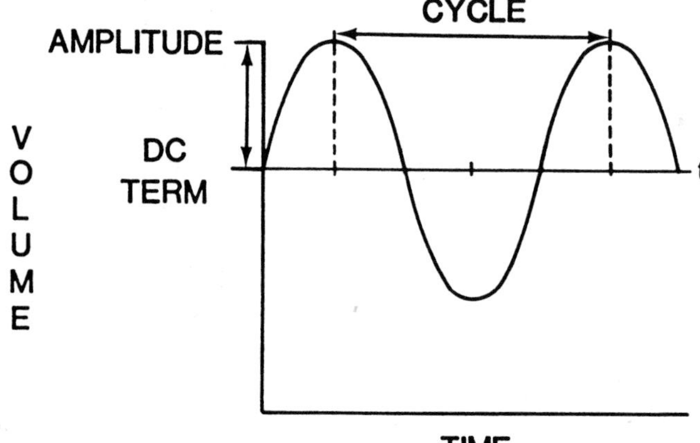

FIGURE 59–37. Cosine wave and phase analysis. The diagram illustrates the relation between a cosine wave and the definitions associated with phase analysis discussed in the text. The cosine function is used to approximate the volume-time curve of the cardiac cycle.

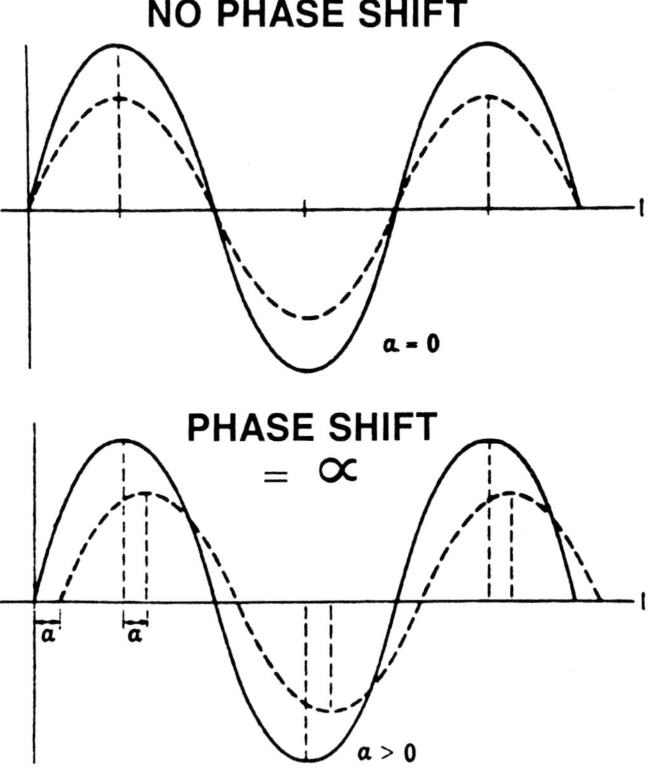

FIGURE 59–38. Cosine waveforms. The diagram illustrates two sets of cosine waveforms with ($\alpha > 0$; *bottom*) and without ($\alpha = 0$; *top*) a phase shift.

is again subjective, cumbersome, and imprecise. A method for overcoming this subjectivity has been reported by Ratib and coworkers,[139] who studied wall motion abnormalities resulting from stress-induced ischemia by assessing histograms of the entire left ventricular phase distribution. In this method, the SD from the mean of the distribution is calculated, and the change between rest and exercise is compared with the results from a group of normal patients. Although this is a significant contribution to quantification of phase distributions for the detection of regional wall motion abnormality, the method does not predict where the regional abnormality is and thus cannot be used for localization of disease.

It has also been demonstrated that the left ventricular phase histograms of patients with wall motion abnormalities exhibit asymmetries. Gerber and colleagues[140] suggested looking at the skewness of the distribution to detect disease. Asymmetry of the left ventricular histogram is probably caused by the superimposition of the phase distribution from normally contracting segments on that from abnormally contracting segments. In another approach, Yaron and associates[141] divided the ventricle into four regions (posterolateral wall, septum, inferoapical wall, and midventricular wall) and quantified the SD of the phase in each region. This method further proposed to separate the abnormal from the normal phase distribution by measuring the difference in angle between the onset of the contraction (emptying) of the entire left ventricle and the mean of the regional phase histogram in each of the four regions. One limitation of this method of dividing the ventricle into four regions is statistical. Because the regions are smaller, there are fewer pixels to form the phase distribution, which creates a source of statistical error in the calculation.

Normal Limits and Abnormality Criteria

Previous work[23, 48] has demonstrated the value of defining lower limits of normal for each mechanism of disease detection (e.g., stress defect and washout abnormality with thallium-201) and of comparing prospective patients against those limits for detection of regional abnormalities. Similarly, the mean value and SD can be established from the pooled data of low-likelihood normal patients for each of the 60 angular locations. In the Cedars approach, this is done for the contraction fraction profile and for the inner, outer, and combined regional EF profiles in the control condition and at maximum stress, as well as for the difference of each corresponding profile between one state and another (see Fig. 59–36). For all these profiles, normal limits are defined as the curves representing two SDs below the mean and are used as a threshold for detection of wall motion abnormalities. These curves are obtained by averaging the profile for each view, point by point, around the circumference of the left ventricle and calculating the SD from each point (Fig. 59–40).

The criterion for abnormality was developed for rest-exercise studies in a group of 20 CAD patients and 20 normal subjects.[107] The criterion for abnormality that best differentiated jeopardized regions from normal regions was defined as the occurrence of any segment of 30 degrees (five contiguous 6-degree arcs) of the inner or outer regional EF, or both, falling below the normal limits. Of 42 jeopardized regions in the CAD patients, 36 were detected by quantitative analysis and 35 by visual analysis. Of the 11 nonjeopardized regions, 4 were abnormal by combined quantitative analysis. The remaining 7 regions were apical and could not be ascribed to a specific vessel in this view alone. Among the 20 normal subjects, all 60 regions were normal by visual analysis, as were 56 by quantitative analysis. Furthermore, when the mechanism for detection of disease was assessed in the 36 regions detected by visual analysis, regional EF of the inner region or outer region, or of both regions, was present in all 36. No additional regions were identified by analysis of regional contraction fraction or by analysis of the combined inner and outer EF. This preliminary experience suggests that quantitative assessment is as accurate as the visual method for detection of regional dysfunction, that this accurate detection can be made primarily by regional EF measurement, and that no additional information appears to be gained through the automated assessment of contraction fraction. These data suggest that the approach described results in accurate objective assessment of regional function.

Preliminary results regarding regional phase analysis in 30 patients undergoing exercise radionuclide ventriculography have also been reported.[141] This population included 15 patients undergoing clinically indicated cardiac catheterization. Patients with prior myocardial infarction or conduction abnormalities were excluded. All of the catheterized patients had CAD. For the entire left ventricle, the rest-exercise variation of the SD and of the onset-mean interval was significantly different between normal and CAD populations. In addition, there was a significant difference between the normal subjects and the patients with CAD in the corresponding vessels for both the variation of the SD and the regional onset-mean interval between rest and exercise, except for the onset-mean interval of the posterolateral wall. Because of the small amount of data in this analysis, there was a significant overlap between patients with and without coronary disease and between regions with and without coronary disease, which limits its value for assessment of individual patients. Analysis was performed with only the first Fourier harmonic, and skewness was not evaluated. The question as to whether analysis of phase significantly adds to the other regional analyses described (outer and inner regional EF and regional wall motion) has not yet been evaluated.

FUTURE DEVELOPMENTS

Most progress in the next few years in the application of powerful computers to cardiovascular disease is expected to be in the area of image interpretation and decision-making. This advancement will entail the implementation of artificial intelligence techniques. Artificial intelligence is concerned with the design of systems that exhibit the characteristics of human behavior in interpreting images, learning, reasoning, solving problems, and so

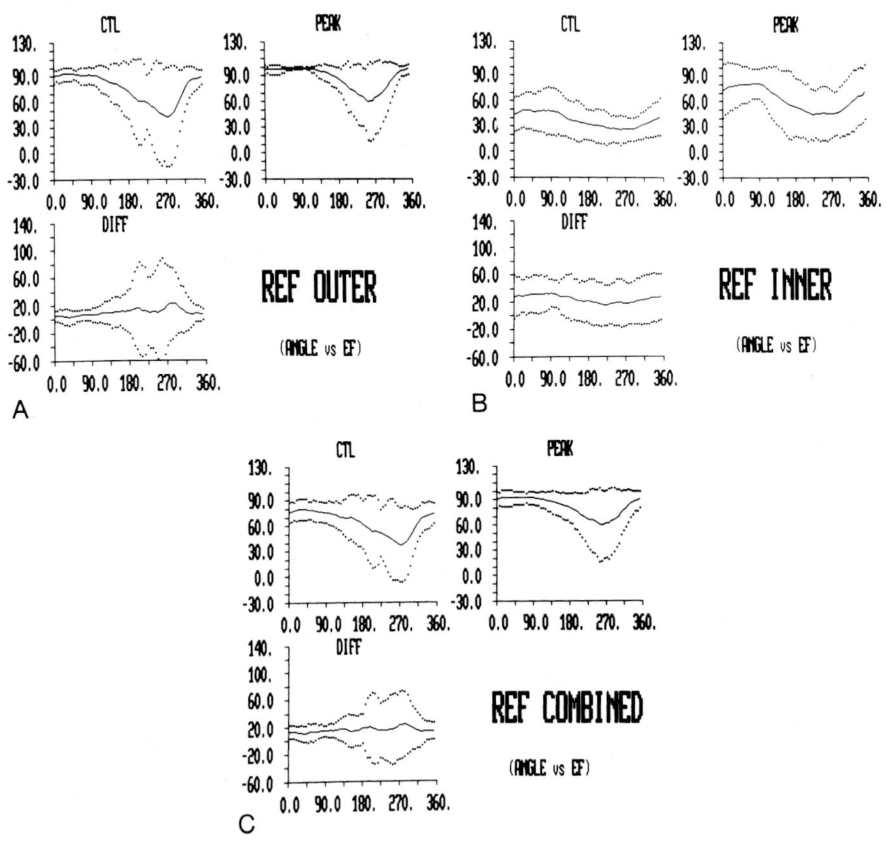

FIGURE 59–40. Normal limits of regional ejection fraction (EF). Preliminary normal limits from the automatic analysis of 20 patients with less than 5 percent likelihood of coronary artery disease. Each panel shows the mean value plus two standard deviations of a regional parameter, in the control condition (ctl) and at peak exercise (peak), and the difference between rest and exercise (diff) for the left anterior oblique view. Shown are the results of outer regional ejection fraction (REF), inner REF, and combined REF.

on. Expert systems use artificial intelligence techniques to allow the collection of "knowledge" from human experts, which can then be used by the computer at a later time. Other important attributes of expert systems are their ability to handle incomplete or noisy data, their ability to justify their results in English, and their ability to use certainty factors to assert their conclusions. Already, preliminary expert systems have been developed to automatically interpret tomographic thallium studies from processed polar maps.[142] Artificial intelligence techniques have also been used to help automate edge detection from ^{99m}Tc multiple-gated equilibrium studies[143, 144] and to quantify wall motion.

It should also be evident from this discussion that powerful computers with large, well-organized databases that can handle sophisticated image processing algorithms will soon play a significant role in aiding the physician in image interpretation and day-to-day clinical decision-making.

Acknowledgments

The author gratefully acknowledges the collaboration in the development of many of the described methods by Kenneth Van Train, Tracy Faber, Joseph Areeda, Robert Eisner, Norberto Ezquerra, John Peifer, Gordon DePuey, Jamshid Maddahi, Timothy Bateman, Alan Rosanski, and Daniel Berman.

References

1. Anger, H.O.: Scintillation camera. Rev. Sci. Instrument 29:27, 1958.
2. Williams, D.L., Ritchie, J.L., Harp, G.D., et al.: Preliminary characterization of the properties of a transaxial whole-body single-photon tomograph: Emphasis on future application to cardiac imaging. *In* Esser, P.D. (ed.): Functional Mapping of Organ Systems. New York, Society of Nuclear Medicine, 1981, p. 149.
3. Rollo, F.D., and Patton, J.A.: Instrumentation and information portrayal. *In* Freeman, L.M. (ed.): Freeman and Johnson's Clinical Radionuclide Imaging. Orlando, Grune & Stratton, 1984, p. 241.
4. Bender, M.A., and Blau, M.: The autofluoroscope. *In* Kniseley, R.M., Andrews, G.A., and Harris, C.C. (eds.): Progress in Medical Radioisotope Scanning, TID-7673. Washington, DC: United States Atomic Energy Commission, 1963, p. 151.
5. Berger, H.J., and Zaret, B.L.: Radionuclide assessment of cardiovascular performance. *In* Freeman, L.M. (ed.): Freeman and Johnson's Clinical Radionuclide Imaging. Orlando, Grune & Stratton, 1984, p. 418.
6. Lacy, J.L., LeBlanc, A.D., Babich, J.W., et al.: A gamma for medical applications, using a multiwire proportional counter. J. Nucl. Med. 25:1003, 1984.
7. Lacy, J.L., Verani, M.S., Ball, M.E., et al.: Improved first-pass radionuclide angiography in man using a new multiwire gamma camera and short-lived tantalum-178. J. Nucl. Med. 29:293, 1988.
8. Wagner, H.N. Jr., Wake, R., Nickoloff, E., et al.: The nuclear stethoscope: A simple device for generation of left ventricular volume curves. Am. J. Cardiol. 38:747, 1976.
9. Tamaki, N., Yasuda, T., Moore, R.H., et al.: Continuous monitoring of left ventricular function by an ambulatory radionuclide detector in patients with coronary artery disease. J. Am. Coll. Cardiol. 12:669, 1988.
10. Wilson, R.A., Sullivan, P.J., Moore, R.H., et al.: An ambulatory ventricular function monitor: Validation and preliminary results. Am. J. Cardiol. 52:601, 1983.
11. Berman, D.S., Garcia, E.V., and Maddahi, J.: Thallium-201 myocardial scintigraphy in the detection and evaluation of coronary artery disease. *In* Berman, D.S., and Mason, D.T. (eds.): Clinical Nuclear Cardiology. New York, Grune & Stratton, 1981, pp. 49–106.
12. Green, M.V., Ostrow, H.G., Douglas, M.A., et al.: High temporal resolution ECG gated scintigraphic angiocardiography. J. Nucl. Med. 16:95, 1975.
13. Hamilton, G.W., Williams, D.L., and Caldwell, J.H.: Frame-rate requirements for recording time-activity curves by radionuclide angiocardiography. *In* Nuclear Cardiology: Selected Computer Aspects. Proceedings of the 1978 Symposium sponsored by the Computer Council of the Society of Nuclear Medicine, Atlanta, GA, January 22–23, 1978, pp. 75–83.
14. Hoffman, E.J., Huang, S.C., and Phelps, M.E.: Quantitation in positron emission computed tomography: 1. Effect of object size. J. Comput. Assist. Tomogr. 3:299, 1979.
15. Bell, G.B., Spade, B.W., and Scheibe, P.O.: Cyclically gated cardiac studies with R-R interval dependent window widths. *In* Nuclear Cardiology: Selected

Computer Aspects. Proceedings of the 1978 Symposium sponsored by the Computer Council of the Society of Nuclear Medicine, Atlanta, GA, January 22–23, 1978, pp. 63–73.
16. Bacharach, S.L., Green, M.V., and Borer, J.S.: Instrumentation and data processing in cardiovascular nuclear medicine: Evaluation of ventricular function. Semin. Nucl. Med. 9:257, 1979.
17. Kalff, V., Chan, W., Rabinovitch, M., et al.: Radionuclide evaluation of post extrasystolic potentiation of left ventricular function induced by atrial and ventricular stimulation. Am. J. Cardiol. 50:106, 1982.
18. Bacharach, S.L., Green, M.V., Borer, J.S., et al.: ECG-gated scintillation probe measurement of left ventricular function. J. Nucl. Med. 18:1176, 1977.
19. Garcia, E.V., Sardi, E., Hammer, S., et al.: A method for isolating the left ventricle in the right anterior oblique projection from equilibrium gated blood pool radionuclide imaging. Circulation 56:11, 1977.
20. Berger, H.J., Matthay, R.A., Loke, J., et al.: Assessment of cardiac performance with quantitative radionuclide angiocardiography: Right ventricular ejection fraction with reference to findings in chronic obstructive pulmonary disease. Am. J. Cardiol. 41:897, 1978.
21. Jengo, J.A., Mena, I., Blaufuss, A., et al.: Evaluation of left ventricular function (ejection fraction and segmental wall motion) by single pass radioisotope angiography. Circulation 57:326, 1978.
22. Go, R.T., MacIntyre, W.J., Houser, T.S., et al.: Clinical evaluation of 360° and 180° data sampling techniques for transaxial SPECT thallium-201 myocardial perfusion imaging. J. Nucl. Med. 26:695, 1985.
23. Garcia, E.V., Van Train, K., Maddahi, J., et al.: Quantification of rotational thallium-201 myocardial tomography. J. Nucl. Med. 26:17, 1985.
24. Galt, J.R., Hise, L.H., Garcia, E.V., et al.: Filtering in frequency space. J. Nucl. Med. Tech. 14:152, 1986.
25. Axelsson, B., Msaki, P., and Israelsson, A.: Subtraction of scattered photons in single photon computerized tomography. J. Nucl. Med. 25:490,1984.
26. Jaszczak, R.J., Floyd, C.E., and Coleman, R.E.: Scatter compensation techniques for SPECT. IEEE Trans. Nucl. Sci. 32:786, 1985.
27. Galt, J. R., Cullom, S. J., and Garcia, E. V.: SPECT quantification: A simplified method of attenuation correction for cardiac imaging. J. Nucl. Med. 33:2232, 1992.
28. Sorenson, J.A.: Methods for quantitative measurement of radioactivity in vivo by whole body counting. *In* Hine, G.J., and Sorenson, J.A. (eds.): Instrumentation in Nuclear Science. Vol. 2. New York, Academic Press, 1974, pp. 311–348.
29. Chang, L.T.: A method for attentuation correction in radionuclide computed tomography. IEEE Trans. Nucl. Sci. NS 25:638, 1978.
30. Bailey, D.L., Hutton, B.F., and Walker, P.J.: Improved SPECT using simultaneous emission and transmission tomography. J. Nucl. Med. 28:844, 1987.
31. Tung, C.H., Gullberg, G.T., Zeng, G.L., et al.: Non-uniform attenuation correction using simultaneous transmission and emission converging tomography. IEEE Trans. Nucl. Sci. 39:1134, 1992.
32. Ye, J., Cullom, S.J., Kearfott, K.K., et al.: Simultaneous attenuation and depth-dependent resolution compensation for 180° myocardial perfusion SPECT. IEEE Catalog Number 92CH3232-6. IEEE Nuclear Sciences Symposium 2:1056–1058, 1992.
33. Liang, Z.: Compensation for attenuation, scatter, and detector response in SPECT reconstruction via iterative FBP methods. Med. Phys. 20:1097, 1993.
34. Tsui, B.M.W., Gullberg, G.T., Edgerton, E.R., et al.: Correction of nonuniform attenuation in cardiac SPECT imaging. J. Nucl. Med. 30:497, 1989.
35. Galt, J.R., Garcia, E.V., and Robbins, W.: Effects of myocardial wall thickness on SPECT quantification. IEEE Trans. Med. Imaging 9:144, 1990.
36. Rogers, W.L., Clinthorne, H.N., Harkness, B.A., et al.: Field-flood requirements for emission computed tomography with an Anger camera. J. Nucl. Med. 23:162, 1982.
37. Friedman, J., Berman, D.S., Van Train, K., et al.: Patient motion in thallium-201 myocardial SPECT imaging: An easily identified frequent source artifactual defect. Clin. Nucl. Med. 13:321, 1988.
38. Eisner, R.L., Noever, T., Nowak, D., et al.: Use of cross-correlation function to detect patient motion during SPECT imaging. J. Nucl. Med. 28:97, 1987.
39. Garcia, E.V., Cooke, C.D., Van Train, K.F., et al.: Technical aspects of myocardial SPECT imaging with technetium-99m sestamibi. Am. J. Cardiol. 66:23E, 1990.
40. Moore, M.L., Murphy, P.H., and Burdine, J.A.: ECG-gated emission computed tomography of the cardiac blood pool. Radiology 134:233, 1980.
41. Corbett, J.R., Henderson, E.B., Akers, M.S., et al.: Gated tomography with technetium-99m RP-30A in patients with myocardial infarcts: Assessment of myocardial perfusion and function. (Abstract.) Circulation 76(Suppl. 4):217, 1987.
42. Phelps, M.E., Hoffman, E.J., Mullani, M., et al.: Application of annihilation coincidence detection to transaxial reconstruction tomography. J. Nucl. Med. 16:210, 1975.
43. Casey, M.E., and Nutt, R. A multicrystal two-dimensional BGO detector system for PET. IEEE Trans. Nucl. Sci. 33:460, 1993.
44. Knoll, G.F.: Radiation Detection and Measurement. New York, John Wiley & Sons, 1979, p. 694.
45. Derenzo, S.E., Huesman, R.H., Cahoon, J.L., et al. A positron tomograph with 600 BGO crystals and 2.6 mm resolution. IEEE Trans. Nucl. Sci. NS 35:659, 1988.
46. Xu, E.Z., Mullani, N.A., Bould, K.L., et al. A segmented attenuation correction for PET. J. Nucl. Med. 32:161,1991.
47. Trobaugh, G.V., Wackers, F.J.T., Sokole, E.B., et al.: Thallium-201 myocardial imaging: An interinstitutional study of observer variability. J. Nucl. Med. 19:395, 1978.
48. Garcia, E.V., Maddahi, J., Berman, D.S., et al.: Space-time quantitation of thallium-201 myocardial scintigraphy. J. Nucl. Med. 22:309, 1981.
49. Meade, R.C., Bamrah, V.S., Horgan, J.D., et al.: Quantitative methods in the evaluation of thallium-201 myocardial perfusion images. J. Nucl. Med. 19:1175, 1978.
50. Burow, R.D., Pond, M., Schafer, A.W., et al.: "Cicumferential profiles": A new method for computer analysis of thallium-201 myocardial perfusion images. J. Nucl. Med. 20:771, 1979.
51. Watson, D.D., Campbell, N.P., Read, E.K., et al.: Spatial and temporal quantitation of plane thallium myocardial images. J. Nucl. Med. 22:577, 1981.
52. DePasquale, E., Nody, A., DePuey, G., et al.: Quantitative rotational thallium-201 tomography for identifying and localizing coronary artery disease. Circulation 77:316, 1988.
53. Caldwell, J., Williams, D., Harp, G.: Quantitation of size of relative myocardial perfusion defect by single-photon emission computed tomography. Circulation 70:1048, 1984.
54. Vogel, R.A., Kirch, D.L., LeFree, M.T., et al.: Thallium-201 myocardial perfusion scintigraphy: Results of standard and multi-pinhole tomgraphic techniques. Am. J. Cardiol. 43:787, 1979.
55. Goris, M.L., Daspit, S.G., McLaughlin, P., et al.: Interpolative background subtraction. J. Nucl. Med. 17:744, 1976.
56. Goris, M.L.: Nontarget activities can we correct for them? J. Nucl. Med. 20:1312, 1979.
57. Leidholdt, E.M., Watson, D.D., Read, M.E., et al.: Interpolative background subtraction using polygonal boundary regions for gated blood pool imaging. *In* Functional Mapping of Organ Systems and Other Computer Topics. New York, Society of Nuclear Medicine, 1981, pp. 91–101.
58. Nichols, K.: Interpolative background corrections for gated blood pool studies on low signal-to-noise ratios. *In* Esser, P. (ed.): Digital Imaging. New York, Society of Nuclear Medicine, 1982, pp. 227–240.
59. Okada, R.D., Lim, Y.L., Boucher, C.A., et al.: Clinical, angiographic, hemodynamic, perfusional and functional changes after one-vessel left anterior descending coronary angioplasty. Am. J. Cardiol. 55:347, 1985.
60. Reiber, J.H.C., Lie, S.P., Simoons, M.L., et al.: Computer quantitation location, extent and type of thallium-201 myocardial perfusion abnormalities. *In* Proceedings of the First International Symposium on Medical Imaging and Image Interpretation (ISMIII). IEEE Cat. No. CH 1804-4/82. New York, Institute of Electrical and Electronics Engineers, 1982, pp. 123–128.
61. Vogel, R.A., Kirch, K.L., LeFree, M.T., et al.: Improved diagnostic results of myocardial perfusion tomography using a new rapid inexpensive technique. (Abstract.) J. Nucl. Med. 19:730, 1978.
62. Watson, D.D., Campbell, N.P., Berger, B.C., et al.: Quantitation of thallium-201 myocardial distribution and washout: Normal standards for graded exercise studies. (Abstract.) Am. J. Cardiol. 45:480, 1980.
63. Murphy, F.L., Maddahi, J., Van Train, K., et al.: Thallium-201 uptake and washout of rest vs exercise in patients without coronary artery disease-implications for quantitation. (Abstract.) J. Am. Coll. Cardiol. 1:601, 1983.
64. Areeda, J., Van Train, K., Garcia, E., et al.: Improved analysis of segmental thallium myocardial scintigrams: Quantiation of distribution, washout, and redistribution. *In* Esser, P. (ed.): Digital Imaging. New York, Society of Nuclear Medicine, 1982, pp. 257–267.
65. Wackers, F.J., Bales, D., Fetterman, R.C., et al.: Nonuniform washout of thallium-201 (within normal range): Criterion for improved detection of single vessel coronary disease. (Abstract.) J. Nucl. Med. 24:46, 1983.
66. McKillop, J.H., Murray, R.G., Turner, J.G., et al.: Can the extent of coronary artery disease be predicted from thallium-201 myocardial images? J. Nucl. Med. 20:715, 1979.
67. Pohost, G.M., O'Keefe, D.D., Gewirtz, H., et al.: Thallium redistribution in the presence of severe fixed coronary stenosis. (Abstract.) Clin. Res. 26:260A, 1978.
68. Van Train, K., Garcia, E., Maddahi, J., et al.: Improved space-time quantitation of segmental thallium-201 myocardial scintigrams. Clin. Nucl. Med. 6:449, 1981.
69. Maddahi, J., Garcia, E.V., Berman, D.S., et al.: Improved noninvasive assessment of coronary artery disease by quantitative analysis of regional stress myocardial distribution and washout of thallium-201. Circulation 64:924, 1981.
70. Van Train, K.F., Garcia, E.V., Cooke, C.D., et al.: Quantitative analysis of SPECT myocardial perfusion. *In* DePuey, E.G., Berman, D.S., and Garcia, E.V. (eds.): Cardiac SPECT Imaging. New York, Raven Press, 1994.
71. Go, R.T., Cook, S.A., MacIntyre, W.J., et al.: Comparative accuracy of stress and redistribution thallium-201 cardiac single photon emission transaxial tomography and planar imaging in the diagnosis of myocardial ischemia. (Abstract.) J. Nucl. Med. 23:24, 1982.
72. Maddahi, J., Van Train, K.F., Wong, C., et al.: Comparison of thallium-201 SPECT and planar imaging for evaluation of coronary artery disease. (Abstract.) J. Nucl. Med. 27:999, 1986.
73. Tamaki, S., Nakajima, H., Murakami, T., et al.: Estimation of infarct size by myocardial emission computed tomography with thallium-201 and its relation to creatine kinase-MB release after myocardial infarction in man. Circulation 66:994, 1982.
74. Ritchie, J.L., Williams, D.L., Harp, G., et al.: Transaxial tomography with thallium-201 for detecting remote myocardial infarction. Am. J. Cardiol. 50:1236, 1982.
75. Tamaki, N., Yonekura, Y., Kadaa, S., et al.: Value of quantitative stress thallium-201 emission CT for localization of coronary artery disease: Comparison with qualitative analysis. J. Nucl. Med. 25:61, 1984.
76. Borello, J.A., Clinthorne, N.H., Rogers, W.L., et al.: Oblique-angle tomography: A restructuring algorithm for transaxial tomographic data. J. Nucl. Med. 22:471, 1981.
77. Eisner, R.L., Gober, A., Cerqueira, M., et al.: Quantitative analysis of normal thallium-201 tomographic studies. (Abstract.) J. Nucl. Med. 26:49, 1984.

78. Klein, L., Garcia, E., DePuey, E.G., et al.: Reversibility of stress induced SPECT Tl-201 myocardial perfusion defects. (Abstract.) J. Nucl. Med. 28:642, 1987.
79. Luna, E., Klein, L., Garcia, E., et al.: Reversibility bullseye polar map: Accuracy in detecting myocardial ischemia. J. Nucl. Med. 29:951, 1988.
80. Marcus, M.L., Skorton, D.J., Johnson, M.R., et al.: Visual estimates of percent diameter coronary stenosis: "A battered gold standard." J. Am. Coll. Cardiol. 11:882, 1988.
81. Keyes, J.W., Leionard, P.F., Brody, S.L., et al.: Myocardial infarct quantification in the dog by single photon emission computed tomography. Circulation 58:227, 1978.
82. Caldwell, J.H., Williams, D.L., Hamilton, G.W., et al.: Regional distribution of myocardial blood flow measured by single-photon tomography: Cmparison with in vitro counting. J. Nucl. Med. 23:490, 1982.
83. Kirsch, C.M., Doliwa, R., Buell, U., et al.: Detection of severe coronary heart disease with Tl-201: Comparison of resting single photon emission tomography with invasive arteriography. J. Nucl. Med. 24:76, 1983.
84. Prigent, F., Maddahi, J., Garcia, E., et al.: Comparative methods for quantifying myocardial infarct size by thallium-201 SPECT. J. Nucl. Med. 28:325, 1987.
85. Prigent, F., Maddahi, J., Garcia, E., et al.: Quantification of myocardial infarct size by thallium-201 single photon emission computerized tomography: Experimental validation in the dog. Circulation 74:852, 1986.
86. Van Train, K.F., Areeda, J., Garcia, E.V., et al.: Quantitative same-day rest-stress technetium-99m-sestamibi SPECT: Definition and validation of stress normal limits and criteria for abnormality. J. Nucl. Med. 34:1494, 1993.
87. Van Train, K.F., Garcia, E.V., Maddahi, J., et al.: Multicenter trial validation for quantitative analysis of same-day rest-stress technetium-99m-sestamibi myocardial tomograms. J. Nucl. Med. 35:609, 1994.
88. Cooke, C.D., Garcia, E.V., Cullom, S.J., et al.: Determining the accuracy of calculating systolic wall thickening using a fast Fourier transform approximation: A simulation study based on canine and patient data. J. Nucl. Med. 35:1185, 1994.
89. Miller, T.R., Starren, J.B., and Grothe, R.A.: Three-dimensional display of positron emission tomography of the heart. J. Nucl. Med. 29:530, 1988.
90. Hicks, K., Ganti, G., Mullani, N., et al.: Automated quantitation of three-dimensional cardiac positron emission tomography for routine clinical use. J. Nucl. Med. 30:1787, 1989.
91. Porenta, G., Kuhle, W., Czernin, J., et al.: Semiquantitative assessment of myocardial blood flow and viability using polar map displays of cardiac PET images. J. Nucl. Med. 33:1623, 1992.
92. Laubenbacher, C., Rothley, J., Sitomer, J., et al.: An automated analysis program for the evaluation of cardiac PET studies: Initial results in the detection and localization of coronary artery disease using nitrogen-13–ammonia. J. Nucl. Med. 34:968, 1993.
93. Garcia, E.V., and Cooke, C.D.: Computer methods in nuclear cardiology. *In* Zarel, B.L., and Beller, G.A. (eds.): Nuclear Cardiology: State of the Art and Future Directions. St. Louis, Mosby, 1993, pp. 97–108.
94. Nowak, D.J.: Three dimensional surface display of nuclear medicine images. (Course summary.) J. Nucl. Med. 29:967, 1988.
95. Miller, T.R., Starren, J.B., and Grothe, R.A.: Three-dimensional display of positron emission tomography of the heart. J. Nucl. Med. 29:530, 1988.
96. Cooke, C.D., and Garcia, E.V.: Three-dimensional display of cardiac single photon emission computed tomography. Am. J. Card. Imaging 7:179, 1993.
97. Herman, G.T.: Computerized reconstruction and 3-D imaging in medicine. Annu. Rev. Comput. Sci., 1:153, 1986.
98. Klein, J.L., Peifer, J.W., Garcia, E.V., et al.: Three-dimensional coronary angiography. Am. J. Card. Imaging 7:187, 1993.
99. Chapman, D.R., Garcia, E.V., Berman, D.S., et al.: Detection of one millimeter motion under conditions simulating equilibrium blood pool scintigraphy. J. Nucl. Med. 23:42, 1982.
100. Burow, R., Pond, M., Rehn, T., et al.: A semiautomatic edge detection program for the analysis of multiple-gated acquisition cardiac blood pool images. J. Nucl. Med. 18:608, 1977.
101. Douglass, K., Links, J., and Wagner, H.N.: Fully automated measurement of regional left ventricular ejection fraction. (Abstract.) J. Nucl. Med. 23:024, 1982.
102. Reiber, J.N.C.: Review of methods for computer analaysis of global and regional left ventricular function from equilibrium gated blood pool scintigrams. *In* Simon, M.L., and Reiber, J.N.C. (eds.): Nuclear Imaging in Clinical Cardiology. Boston, Martinus-Nijhoff, 1984, pp. 172–217.
103. Nelson, T.R., Perkins, G.C., Slutsky, R.A., et al.: Automated on-line analysis of all four cardiac chambers for rapid setup, data acquisition and reduction. (Abstract.) J. Nucl. Med. 22:P63, 1981.
104. Links, J., Brown, G., Hau, D., et al.: A new method of fully automatic processing of gated blood pool studies. (Abstract.) J. Nucl. Med. 23:85, 1982.
105. Areeda, J., Garcia, E., Van Train, K., et al.: Comprehensive analysis of rest/exercise segmental left ventricular function from radionuclide ventriculograms. *In* Computers in Cardiology. Long Beach, CA, IEEE Computer Society, 1982, pp. 109–112.
106. Garcia, E., Areeda, J., Van Train, K., et al.: A comprehensive method for quantitative analysis of rest/exercise ventricular function from radionuclide ventriculography. (Abstract.) Circulation 66(Suppl. II):127, 1982.
107. Garcia, E., Areeda, J., Rozanski, A., et al.: Clinical validation of a totally automated method for assessing regional left ventricular function from rest/exercise radionuclide ventriculography. (Abstract.) J. Nucl. Med. 24:53, 1983.
108. Areeda, J., Garcia, E., Van Train, K., et al.: A comprehensive method for automatic analysis of rest/exercise ventricular function from radionuclide ventriculography. *In* Esser, P. (ed.): Digital Imaging. New York, Society of Nuclear Medicine, 1982, pp. 241–256.
109. Stamm, R.B., Watson, D.D., and Taylor, G.: Comparison of two-dimensional echocardiography, gated heart pool scan, and left ventriculography in the detection of regional wall motion abnormalities. Am. J. Cardiol. 45:403, 1980.
110. Burow, R.D., Strauss, W.H., Singleton, R., et al.: Analysis of left ventricular function from multiple-gated acquisition cardiac blood pool imaging: Comparison to contrast angiography. Circulation 56:1024, 1977.
111. Almasi, J.J., DePuey, E.G., Eisner, R.L., et al.: Totally automated computer processing of gated blood pool studies. (Abstract.) J. Nucl. Med. 23:42, 1982.
112. Goris, M.L., McKillop, J.H., Fawcett, H.D.S., et al.: Edge tracing for the determination of the left ventricular projection area. J. Nucl. Med. 21:60, 1980.
113. Yuille, D.L.: Analysis of stress or nitroglycerin gated heart studies utilizing dimensional filtering and MUGG: A new program for automatic analysis of gated heart studies. (Abstract.) J. Nucl. Med. 21:47, 1980.
114. Dodge, H.T., Sandler, H., Ballew, D.W., et al.: The use of biplane angiocardiography for the measurement of left ventricular volume in man. Am. Heart J. 60:762, 1960.
115. Strauss, H.W., Zaret, B.L., Hurley, P.J., et al.: A scintiphotographic method for measuring left ventricular ejection fraction in man without cardiac catherization. Am. J. Cardiol. 28:575, 1971.
116. Pantaleo, N., Freeman, M., Van Train, K., et al.: A simple, objective method for measurement of absolute left ventricular end-diastolic volume with multiple-gated equilibrium scintigraphy. Clin. Nucl. Med. 5:S29, 1980.
117. Uren, R.F., Newman, H.N., Hutton, B.F., et al.: Geometric determination of left ventricular volume from gated blood-pool studies using a slant-hole collimator. Radiology 147:541, 1983.
118. Ishii, Y., and MacInTyre, W.I.: Measurement of heart chamber volumes by analysis of dilution curves simultaneously recorded by scintillation camera Circulation 44:37, 1971.
119. Van Kyke, D., Anger, H.O., Sullivan, H.W., et al.: Cardiac evaluation from radioisotope dynamics. J. Nucl. Med. 13:585, 1972.
120. Links, J.M., Becker, L.C., Shindledecker, J.C., et al.: Measurement of absolute left ventricular volume from gated blood pool studies. Circulation 65:82, 1982.
121. Slutsky, R., Karliner, J., and Ricci, D.: Left ventricular volume by gated equilibrum radionuclide angiography: A new method. Circulation 60:556, 1979.
122. Schwaiger, M., Henze, E., Ratib, O., et al.: Acurate determination of left ventricular volumes with gated blood pool studies using a direct measurement of photon attenuation. (Abstract.) J. Nucl. Med. 23:P70, 1982.
123. Herman, M.V., Heinie, R.A., Lein, M.D., et al.: Localized disorders in myocardial contraction. N. Engl. J. Med. 227:222, 1967.
124. Ingels, N.B., Daughters, G.T., Stinson, E.B., et al.: Evaluation of methods for quantitating left ventricular segmental wall motion in man using myocardial markers as a standard. Circulation 60:966, 1980.
125. Chaitman, B.R., Bristow, J.D., and Rahimtoola, S.H.: Left ventricular wall motion assessed using fixed external reference systems. Circulation 48:1043, 1973.
126. Gelberg, H.J., Brundage, B.H., Glantz, S., et al.: Quantitation of left ventricular wall motion analysis: A comparison of area, chord and radial methods. Circulation 59:991, 1979.
127. Daughters, G.T., Schwarzkopf, A., Merd, C.W., et al.: A clinical evaluation of five techniques for left ventricular wall motion assessment. *In* Computers in Cardiology. Long Beach, CA, IEEE Computer Society, 1981, pp. 249–252.
128. Garcia, E.V., Sardi, E., Hammer, S., et al.: A method for isolating the left ventricle in the right anterior oblique projection from equilibrium gated blood pool radionuclide imaging. Circulation 56:11, 1977.
129. Silber, S., Schwaiger, M., Klein, U., et al.: Quantitative beurteilung der linkens-ventrikularen funktion mit der radionuklid-ventrikulographie. Herz 5:146, 1980.
130. Burow, R.D., Wilson, M.F., Allen, E.W., et al.: Regional left ventricular time-activity curves from multiple-gated equilibrium scintigraphy: Correlation with contrast angiography. (Abstract.) J. Nucl. Med. 22:P61, 1981.
131. Douglass, F.H., Chen, D.C.P., Wond, D.F., et al.: Relative accuracy of automated analysis of regional wall motion in diagnosis of CAD. (Abstract.) J. Nucl. Med. 24:91, 1983.
132. Freeman, M., Garcia, E., Berman, D., et al.: An objective and quantitative method for assessment of regional left ventricular wall motion using multiple-gated equilibrium scintigraphy. (Abstract.) J. Nucl. Med. 21:62, 1980.
133. Vitale, D., Bacharach, S., Bonow, R., et al.: Assessment of regional left ventricular function by sector analysis: A method for objective evaluation of radionuclide blood pool studies. Am. J. Cardiol. 52:1112, 1983.
134. Steckley, R.A., Kronenbert, M.W., Born, M.L., et al.: Radionuclide ventriculography: Evaluation of automated and visual methods for regional wall motion analysis. Radiology 142:179, 1982.
135. Links, J.M., Douglas, K.H., and Wagner, H.N.: Patterns of ventricular emptying by Fourier analysis of gated blood-pool studies. J. Nucl. Med. 21:978, 1980.
136. Bacharach, S.L., de Graaf, C.N., Van Rijk, P., et al.: Fourier distribution map: Toward an understanding of what they mean. *In* Esser, P.D. (ed.): Functional Mapping of Organ Systems and Other Computer Topics. New York, Society of Nuclear Medicine, 1981, p. 139.
137. Bacharach, S.L., Green, M.V., Vitale, D., et al.: Optimum number of harmonics for fitting cardiac volume curves. (Abstract.) J. Nucl. Med. 24:17, 1983.
138. Adam, W.E., Tarkowski, A., Bitter, F., et al.: Equilibrium (gated) radionuclide ventriculography. Cardiovasc. Radiol. 2:161, 1979.
139. Ratib, O., Henze, E., Schon, H., et al.: Phase analysis of radionuclide ventriculograms for the detection of coronary artery disease. Am. Heart J. 104:1, 1982.
140. Gerber, K.H., Norris, S.L., Slutsky, R.A., et al.: Quantitative phase analysis of exercise radionuclide left ventriculography in normals and patients with coronary artery disease. Comput. Biomed. Res. 16:88, 1983.
141. Yaron, M., Garcia, E., Friedman, J., et al.: A new objective approach assessing

regional left ventricular function at rest and exercise using phase analysis of radionuclide ventriculography. (Abstract.) Circulation 66(Suppl. II):353, 1982.
142. Ezquerra, N., Mullick, R., Cooke, D., et al.: PERFEX: An expert system for interpreting 3D myocardial perfusion. *In* Expert Systems with Applications. 6:459, 1993.
143. Duncan, J.S.: Intelligent determination of left ventricular wall motion from multiple-view, nuclear medicine image sequences. *In* Proceedings of the International Symposium on Medical Images and Icons. New York, Institute of Electrical and Electronics Engineers, 1984, pp. 265–169.
144. Niemann, H., Bunke, H., Hofman, I., et al.: A knowledge based system for analysis of gated blood pool studies. IEEE Trans. Patt. An. Mach. Int., Vol. PAMI-7, 3:246–258, 1985.

CHAPTER

60 First-Pass Radionuclide Angiography

Steven Port, M.D.

First-pass radionuclide angiography (FPRNA) derives its name from the fact that all the data to be used for image processing and quantitation are acquired during the initial transit of a radionuclide bolus through the central circulation (Fig. 60–1). Unlike its counterpart, gated equilibrium imaging, the technique does not require any labeling of red blood cells and does not depend on the spatial separation of ventricular chambers in order to quantify ventricular function. Rather, the first-pass technique depends on the *temporal* separation of the cardiac chambers as the radionuclide bolus makes its way from one chamber to the next. Although the application of FPRNA to the evaluation of the cardiovascular system dates back to 1927, when Blumgart first measured the circulation time in a man,[1] it took another 42 years for the first imaging application to be reported.[2] But even after that report, first-pass imaging was practiced in only a small minority of clinical laboratories, including laboratories dedicated to cardiac imaging, because the detectors necessary for FPRNA were not suited for other types of radionuclide imaging. Recently, there has been a resurgence of interest in first-pass imaging because of the widespread application of the technetium-based myocardial perfusion imaging agents, which allow combined FPRNA and SPECT perfusion imaging from the same injection.

FPRNA has several advantages over gated equilibrium imaging. Because only the initial transit of a radionuclide bolus is required for imaging, the acquisition time is very short, in the order of seconds. That makes FPRNA ideal for the evaluation of ventricular function during exercise or during other transient phenomena. FPRNA can record the transit of an injected tracer through the central circulation, which permits detection and quantitation of left-to-right shunts and valvular insufficiency and identification of congenital abnormalities. Because individual beat information is stored, arrhythmic beats can be excluded easily or analyzed separately. Last, there is no dependence on a red blood cell tag.

In this chapter, the details of acquisition and processing, the results of the procedure, and the clinical applications of FPRNA are discussed.

FIGURE 60–1. See Color Plate 24.

DATA ACQUISITION

Injection Technique

Because the first-pass study depends on the temporal separation of cardiac chambers, the radionuclide must be injected as a discrete compact bolus into a large vein as close to the central circulation as possible. For routine clinical practice, only two sites are used, the antecubital and the external jugular veins. Injection into any veins distal to the elbow are likely to result in fractured or delayed boluses, yielding suboptimal images and inaccurate quantitation at best and uninterpretable data at worst. To ensure a rapid bolus injection, the radionuclide dose and a saline flush syringe should be attached to a three-way stopcock that is placed at the end of a short length of tubing connected to an intravenous cannula (Fig. 60–2). For external jugular veins, a 20-gauge, 1-inch long cannula is adequate; for the antecubital vein, an 18-gauge, 1.5-inch long cannula is preferred.

An exception to the general rule of rapidly injecting the bolus is the injection technique for right ventricular studies, in which it is helpful to reduce the speed of injection so that more right ventricular beats are available for analysis. However, this approach may compromise left ventricular analysis. If results for both ventricles are equally important, it may be necessary to perform two injections.

Radionuclides

For first-pass studies, the radionuclide must remain in the intravascular space for the duration of the transit through the central circulation, and it must be safe enough to inject in an amount sufficient to generate the high count rates required of FPRNA. Those requirements can be met by a variety of agents, but technetium-99m is the radionuclide used in almost all clinical studies. Technetium-99m has a primary photopeak of 140 KeV, which makes it very well suited to standard gamma cameras. It is used in many nuclear medicine procedures.

Technetium-99m is typically injected as either the pertechnetate salt or as ^{99m}Tc-DTPA (diethylenetetramine-pentaacetic acid). The latter is preferred because it enhances renal excretion, thus reducing radiation exposure. Technetium may be injected with a high specific activity, thereby keeping the bolus volume to a minimum. More recently, with the appearance of the technetium-based myocardial perfusion imaging agents, adequate FPRNA has been performed with the use of ^{99m}Tc-sestamibi,[3, 4] ^{99m}Tc-teboroxime,[5, 6] and ^{99m}Tc-tetrofosmin.[7] Because ^{99m}technetium has a relatively long physical half-life (6 hours), there is a limit to the amount that can be injected in one day. No more than three technetium first-pass studies are performed in one day, and typically only two. There are very short-lived radionuclides that have been used for FPRNA that permit multiple sequential studies.

Iridium-191m has an extremely short half-life of 4.9 seconds, which minimizes radiation exposure. It is particularly well suited to pediatric imaging. However, the ultrashort half-life requires that the subject be connected to the portable generator. Treves and colleagues have demonstrated its application for assessment of left ventricular function and for detection and quantitation of left-to-right shunts.[8]

Gold-195m has a half-life of 30.5 seconds. It can be produced with a portable generator that uses a mercury parent. First-pass left ventricular ejection fractions (LVEFs) have been validated with ^{195m}Au,[9] and because of ^{195m}Au's very short physical half-life, multiple studies in rapid sequence are possible. Unfortunately, problems with mercury breakthrough and the possibility of cyanide contamination from the thiocyanate column of the generator precluded clinical approval of the portable generator.

Tantalum-178m has a half-life of 9.3 minutes, making it easier to use than either iridium or gold. However, its primary photopeak energy of 55 to 65 KeV makes it unsuitable for standard gamma cameras. The development of a proportional wire detector that is well suited to such low energies and the approval of a portable generator have led to clinical validation of FPRNA using tantalum.[10–12]

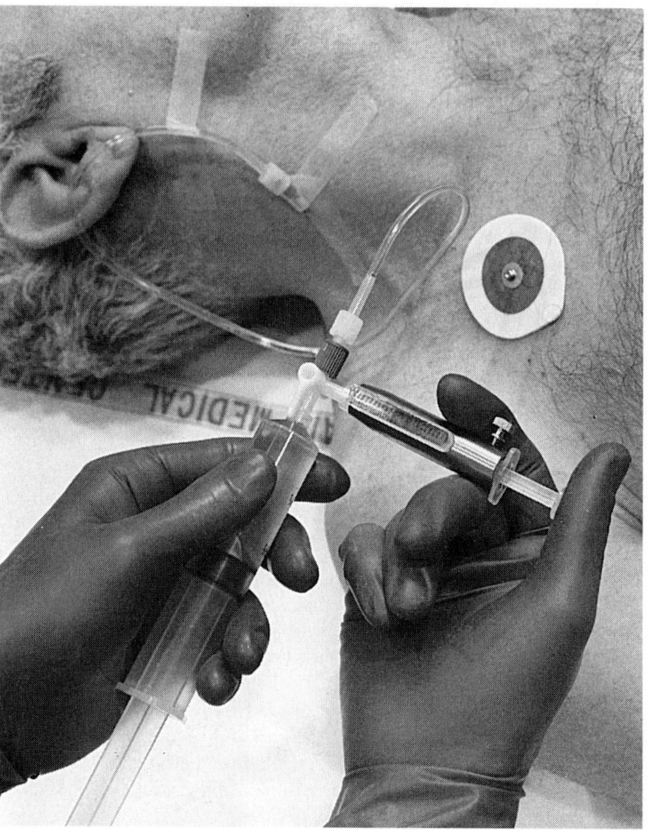

FIGURE 60–2. The typical approach to venous cannulation (in this case, the external jugular vein) for a first-pass study requires insertion of an 18- to 22-gauge, 1- to 1.5-inch long cannula attached by a length of tubing to a three-way stopcock that allows loading of the radionuclide into the tubing and flushing of the bolus with 10 to 20 mL of saline. (From Port, S.: First-pass RNA. *In* Early, P.J., and Sodee, D.B. [eds.]: Principles and Practice of Nuclear Medicine. St. Louis, Mosby–Year Book, 1996, p. 379, with permission.)

Radionuclide Dose

The required dose for a given injection depends on the size of the individual patient, the sensitivity of the detector, the number of injections to be made that day, and the specific radionuclide to be used. With the high sensitivity of the multicrystal gamma camera, doses as low as 8 to 10 mCi of technetium-99m may be used. However, 20 to 25 mCi is recommended to guarantee adequate count rates, especially in large patients or if few beats are expected to be available for analysis (e.g., in an exercise study). If two studies are being performed, such as rest and exercise studies, then two doses of 20 to 25 mCi are appropriate. If lower total doses are mandated by regulation, then the resting study can be performed with about 10 mCi and the exercise study with approximately 20 mCi. However, a 10-mCi dose may be suboptimal in large patients even with a multicrystal camera. For single-crystal systems in which the count-rate sensitivity is lower, doses of 20 to 25 mCi are recommended for all injections, although FPRNA has been performed successfully in patients at rest with doses as low as 10 mCi. If an ultrashort-lived radionuclide is used, then the dose may be considerably higher.

Instrumentation

During the initial transit of a radionuclide bolus through the left ventricle, there are, on average, only 6 to 10 beats at rest and 4 to

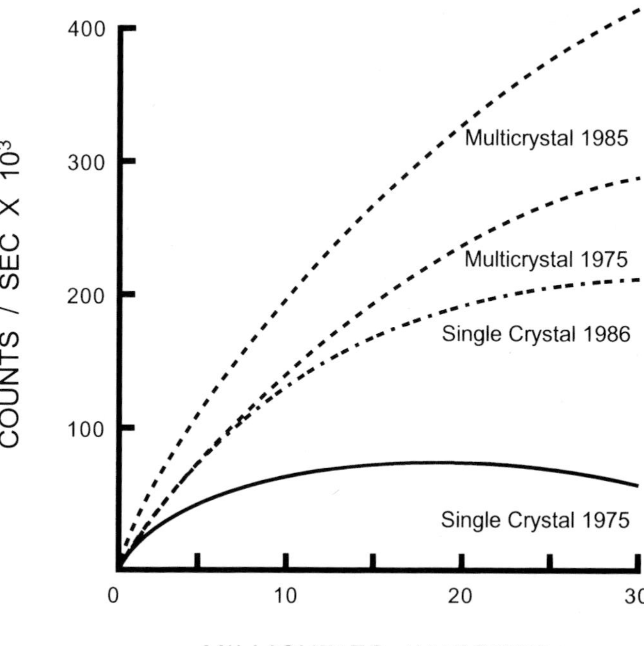

FIGURE 60–3. Count-rate capabilities of both single-crystal and multicrystal gamma cameras have evolved over the years. All the early and some current single-crystal systems were incapable of recording clinical count rates of 100,000 counts per second. Newer single-crystal cameras can record 200,00 counts per second. The latest generation of multicrystal camera can achieve clinical count rates (with a patient and a collimator) in excess of 350,000 counts per second.

8 beats during exercise that may be used for data analysis. Consequently, the imaging devices used for FPRNA must be capable of recording very high count rates in order to extract as much data as possible from each beat. Although ejection fractions can be calculated with total count rates as low as 100,000 per second, the error of the measurement is high and the image quality is marginal to unacceptable. Count rates should exceed 150,000 counts per second for the whole field of view during the right ventricular phase and, ideally, should be higher than 200,000 counts per second. The count rate capacities of available gamma cameras have slowly but steadily evolved over the past 20 years (Fig. 60–3).

The multicrystal gamma camera was the first instrument specifically designed for high-count-rate FPRNA. The first generation of multicrystal cameras was able to record count rates in excess of 250,000 counts per second while maintaining enough spatial resolution to produce clinically adequate images. However, there is always a tradeoff between count rates and resolution, and earlier instruments dedicated to FPRNA were therefore inadequate for other types of clinical imaging. To some degree, the latest generation of multicrystal camera has improved on both the spatial resolution and the count-rate capability. However, the spatial resolution is still not equivalent to that of a single-crystal camera. The newer multicrystal systems are smaller, more maneuverable, and truly portable (Fig. 60–4). The multicrystal camera remains the instrument of choice for FPRNA, especially for exercise studies.

Conventional single-crystal gamma cameras were designed more for resolution than for count-rate capability. Until recently, most examples of the genre were able to count linearly up to about 60,000 counts per second; at higher count rates, there was substantial data loss caused by system deadtime, and peak count rates rarely exceeded 100,000 counts per second. Those systems were inadequate for high-count-rate FPRNA. However, a new genera-

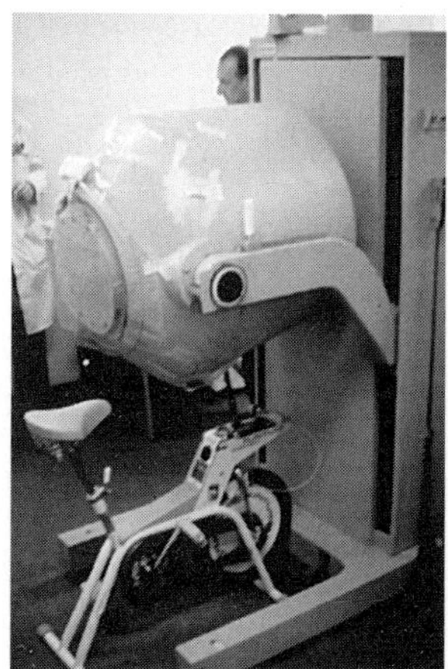

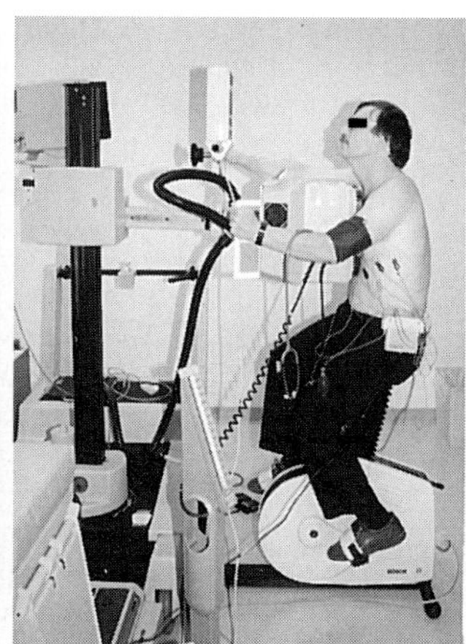

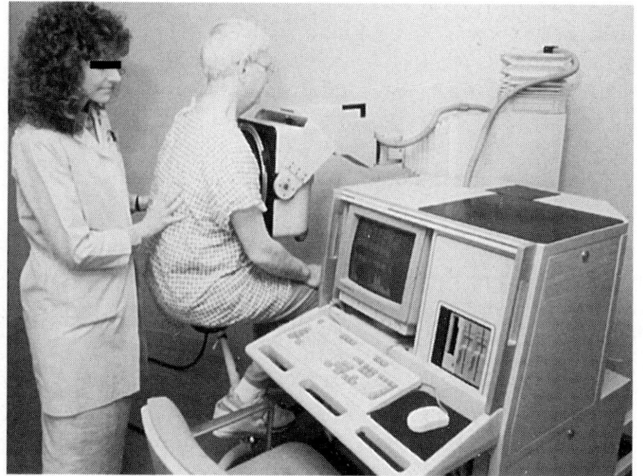

FIGURE 60–4. Cameras dedicated to first-pass imaging include the vintage Baird System 77 *(left)*, a heavy, immobile, multicrystal device; the latest Scinticor SIM-400 multicrystal camera *(middle)*, which is much smaller in configuration and portable; and the proportional wire counter *(right)*, which travels with an on-board generator for tantalum-178. (Photograph of proportional wire counter courtesy of Dr. Jeffrey Lacy, Baylor College of Medicine, Houston, TX. From Murphy, P., and Port, S.: Radionuclide evaluation of left ventricular function. *In* Sandler, M.P., Patton, J.A., Coleman, A.E., et al. [eds.]: Diagnostic Nuclear Medicine. Baltimore, Williams & Wilkins, 1996, with permission.)

tion of single-crystal cameras takes advantage of both integrated digital technology and newer collimation devices to reduce system deadtime and enhance count rates. Count rates of up to 200,000 counts per second have been recorded, and clinically adequate FPRNA studies have been performed and validated with these new single-crystal cameras.[13, 14] The high- or ultrahigh-sensitivity collimators that must be used on the single-crystal gamma cameras to achieve the requisite count rates result in lower spatial resolution.

Although it is not commercially available, the proportional wire camera has been used in clinical research to acquire FPRNA with ^{178}tantalum, an ultrashort-lived radionuclide.[10–12] The images appear to be of diagnostic quality, although no prospective trial is available that has tested the sensitivity and specificity of the results.

Positioning

The first-pass study can theoretically be acquired in any view because of the temporal separation of the cardiac chambers. However, either the anterior or a shallow right anterior oblique (RAO) view is recommended. FPRNA was widely applied to bicycle exercise studies for many years, and the straight anterior view was popular because it was a simple matter to stabilize the subject's chest against the detector while exercise continued (see Fig. 60–4). Because of its similarity to contrast angiographic ventriculography, a shallow RAO view was also popular. The shallow RAO view enhances separation between the atria and ventricles and between the left ventricle and the descending aorta. For right ventricular studies, the 30-degree RAO view is best for separating the right atrium from the right ventricle. The left anterior oblique (LAO) view may be used for interrogating the circumflex coronary distribution. However, left atrial activity tends to be rather high in a first-pass study, more so than during an equilibrium study, and therefore LAO views of 30 to 60 degrees may result in considerable left atrial–left ventricular overlap, which may compromise analysis of regional ventricular function and spuriously lower the LVEF. The left lateral view is better in that regard. For detection and quantitation of a left-to-right shunt, the straight anterior view is preferred, and as much of the lung fields as possible, especially the right lung, should be in the field of view.

After the desired imaging angle has been established, the detector must be positioned so that the entire heart is well within the field of view. In contrast to the equilibrium study, in which the angle can be adjusted repeatedly, positioning for a first-pass study must be correct before the bolus is injected. Use of a uniform flood source or an exposed dose syringe placed behind the subject allows identification of the lungs and mediastinum (Fig. 60–5). Alternatively, a test dose of 1 mCi may be injected for positioning. If two or more studies are to be performed, the background from the previous injection may be used to identify the location of the heart.

FIGURE 60–5. See Color Plate 24.

For most studies, the subject should be in the upright position. This is true for both rest and exercise acquisitions. The upright position minimizes pulmonary blood volume and therefore background activity, which results in better-quality images. Supine studies can be performed and may be particularly appropriate for studies acquired during inotropic or vasodilatory stimulation.

Frame Rate

First-pass studies are acquired by arbitrarily assigning timing intervals and then storing whatever image information appears during each interval. This is distinctly different from a typical frame-mode gated equilibrium study, in which each cardiac cycle is divided into a number of frames, so that each frame contains data from all beats, and no individual beat information is retained. The first-pass study is more akin to a list-mode equilibrium acquisition, but the temporal resolution is predetermined by the time assigned to each interval, the so-called frame time. In general, the frame time should vary inversely with the heart rate. At resting rates of 50 to 100 beats per minute, 50 msec (20 frames per second) is adequate to measure systolic and diastolic events. As the heart rate reaches 150 to 200 beats per minute (e.g., during exercise), frame times of 10 to 25 msec are necessary to adequately characterize the physiology of emptying and filling.[15] For practical reasons, most laboratories have compromised on a single frame time of 20 to 25 msec for all heart rates in order to avoid any confusion or errors from repeatedly changing the acquisition parameters.

The overall length of the acquisition must also be determined before the study begins. Enough time should be allowed for the bolus to completely clear the left ventricle, which at rest is 20 to 30 seconds and during exercise or inotropic stimulation is 10 to 20 seconds. To allow for the occasional, unintentional delay between the starting of the gamma camera and the injection of the radionuclide, and also for the markedly prolonged transit times in some patients, it is customary to acquire at least 30 seconds for all studies. Unnecessary frames may be discarded before the data are processed.

Electrocardiographic Recording

At very high count rates, the time-activity curves displaying the cyclic change in counts in the ventricle have sufficient resolution to clearly identify each end-diastole and end-systole without the aid of an electrocardiographic (ECG) signal. When count rates are consistently lower, as occurs with single-crystal gamma camera acquisitions, it is particularly helpful to record an ECG signal with the image data. The ECG can be used during processing to aid in identification of end-diastolic frames and in creation of a preliminary representative cycle (see the sections on data processing).

Bicycle Exercise

For many years, FPRNA and bicycle exercise were virtually synonymous. With so few heartbeats available for analysis during exercise, it was mandatory that any cardiac motion during the study be eliminated. During bicycle exercise, it is relatively easy to stabilize the chest against the detector while the subject continues to exercise. Initial work with FPRNA actually used supine exercise but upright bicycle ergometry proved better for stabilization of the chest and also decreased background activity.[16, 17] In addition, upright exercise was better tolerated, especially in deconditioned individuals. Although any graded exercise protocol is acceptable, we have found that starting at 12.5 to 25 W and increasing by 12.5 W every minute or 25 W every 2 minutes works well for most middle-aged and older adults. Younger patients or trained individuals may require a more aggressive protocol. Exercise should be continued and the chest should be stabilized against the detector until the radionuclide bolus has been seen to clear the left ventricle. For most clinical studies, resting and peak exercise acquisitions are sufficient. If additional exercise data are required or if a postexercise study is necessary, then the doses must be adjusted accordingly. Acquisitions may be repeated almost immediately as long as the computer software has the capability of correcting for background activity from a previous injection.

Treadmill Exercise

Until recently, FPRNA was never performed during treadmill exercise because there was so much chest motion. Now, however, there is one reported approach to detection and correction of cardiac motion during FPRNA that uses an external radioactive source attached to the chest (Fig. 60–6). The external marker must contain a gamma emitter that can be distinguished from the 140 KeV photon of the technetium study. Both americium-241 and iodine-125 have been used successfully. The camera is set for a dual energy acquisition. In essence, two first-pass studies are acquired simultaneously, one of the marker moving and one of the technetium bolus traveling through the central circulation. The movement of the marker is determined in each frame, and the technetium study is then spatially re-registered on a frame-by-frame basis according to the direction and magnitude of the marker motion. Clinically satisfactory FPRNA studies can be achieved during treadmill exercise with such a scheme.[4, 5]

This approach to motion correction does result in some image distortion. As a result, chamber volumes during treadmill exercise are larger than the volumes recorded in the same subjects during bicycle exercise. The ejection fraction measurements, however, are not significantly different.[18, 19]

Whether exercise is performed on a bicycle or a treadmill, it is paramount that images be acquired at the peak of exercise, not immediately after exercise is terminated. It is clear from the experience of laboratories performing first-pass or gated equilibrium imaging that there are rapid changes in ventricular function immediately after exercise is terminated. The first-pass literature suggests that exercise ejection fraction rapidly increases within 30 seconds of stopping exercise in both normal individuals and those with ischemic exercise responses.[71] The rapid changes in left ventricular function after a decrease in workload or cessation of exercise have been demonstrated only for upright exercise and may not be as dramatic during supine exercise.

DATA PROCESSING

First-pass data processing for ventricular function involves four basic routines: the creation of a time-activity curve displaying the cyclic changes in radioactivity within the ventricle; the selection of the beats to be included in the analysis; background correction; and the creation of the final representative cycle, from which all quantitative data and wall motion data are derived.[13, 20–26] A fifth routine is that of motion correction, which is crucial to treadmill exercise studies and occasionally is necessary for bicycle exercise studies.

Time-Activity Curve

The changes in radionuclide concentration of each beat during the ventricular phase of the study are displayed as a time-activity curve (Fig. 60–7). It is generated by outlining the region of interest (ventricle) on a raw data frame and displaying the entire ventricular phase of the study. An initial representative cycle can be created by cyclically adding together each beat of the time-activity curve. If counts are low and exact identification of end-diastolic frames is difficult, the R wave of an ECG signal may be used to identify end-diastole. The initial representative cycle can then be displayed and the preliminary ventricular region of interest modified on the now statistically stronger image of the chamber. The updated ventricular region of interest is then used to generate a new ventricular time-activity curve. Various parametric images, such as phase and stroke volume images, may be used to facilitate drawing of the ventricular region of interest and are recommended. Automated and semiautomated methods are also available for that purpose.

Either a single end-diastolic region of interest or both end-diastolic and end-systolic regions of interest may be used for the final representative cycle. For studies acquired in the anterior view, left atrial and aortic root activity are frequently contained within a single end-diastolic region of interest at end-systole, and a separate end-systolic region of interest is therefore necessary (Fig. 60–8). For studies acquired in the RAO view, two regions of interest may not be necessary, but the option should be available.

FIGURES 60–7 and 60–8. See Color Plate 25.

Beat Selection

During normal sinus rhythm, beat selection is a straightforward process. All beats whose counts are sufficient may be included in the final representative cycle. Any beat whose end-diastolic count equals 50 to 70 percent of the highest end-diastolic count in the left ventricular phase may be selected. Beats below that threshold should probably not be used unless there is a paucity of beats for analysis. Premature ventricular contraction (PVC) beats should be excluded, as should beats occurring after PVCs (Fig. 60–9). The latter have an ejection fraction that is significantly higher than that of a sinus beat.

Separate ejection fractions may be generated for sinus, premature, and post-PVC beats, if necessary. If there are frequent PVCs or ventricular bigeminy, an accurate ejection fraction cannot be determined. Every effort should be made to avoid first-pass acquisitions in subjects with such rhythm disturbances. If either frequent

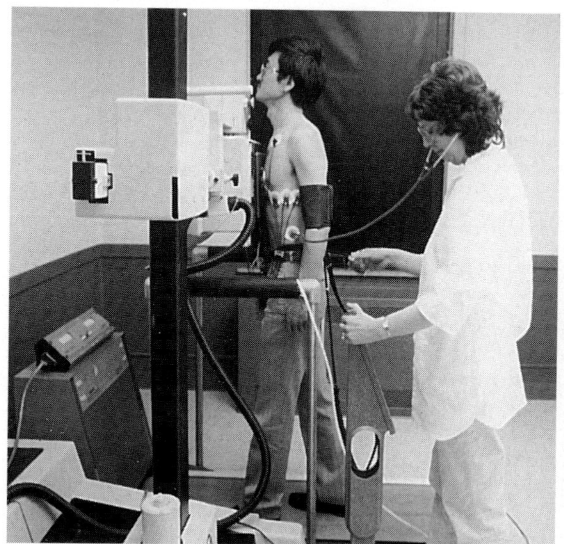

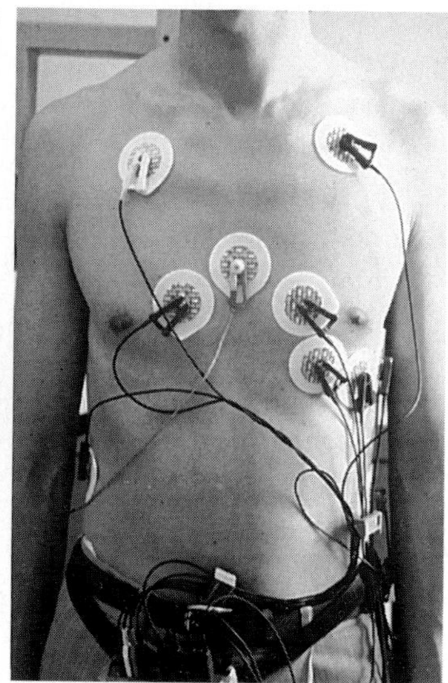

FIGURE 60–6. First-pass imaging has recently been adapted to treadmill exercise by application of a motion detection and correction scheme that requires an external marker placed on the subject's chest. What appears to be an electrode placed over the sternum of the subject on the right is actually a small, sealed source of americium-241 that will be used to track and subsequently correct for the movement of the chest throughout the study. The subject then exercises on the treadmill *(left)* as in any treadmill stress test, except that care must be taken to ensure that both the marker and the ventricles remain in the field of view especially at the time of image acquisition. (From Murphy, P., and Port, S.: Radionuclide evaluation of left ventricular function. *In* Sandler, M.P., Patton, J.A., Coleman, A.E., et al. [eds.]: Diagnostic Nuclear Medicine. Baltimore, Williams & Wilkins, 1996, with permission.)

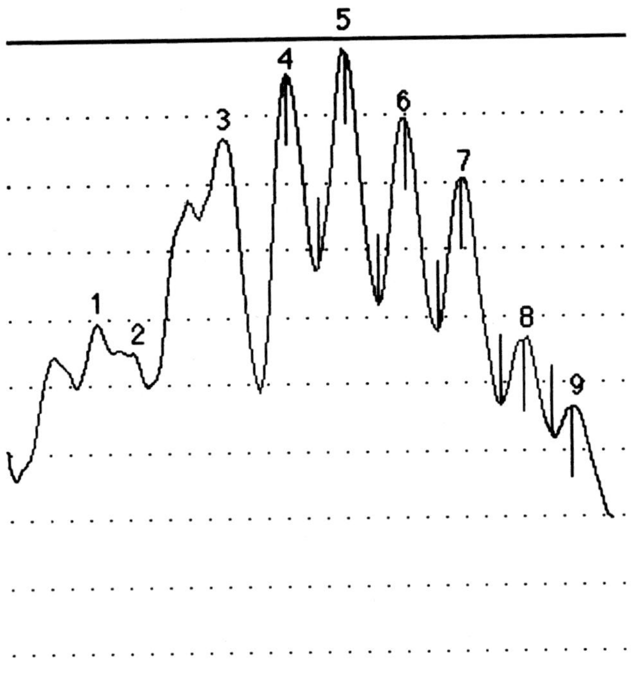

FIGURE 60–9. An important part of data processing is selection of the beats to be used for creation of the final representative cycle from which all quantitative data will be derived. In this example, beat number 2 is a premature ventricular contraction (PVC), and beat number 3 is a post-PVC beat. Beat 1 and beats 4 through 9 are sinus beats. Both beat 2 and beat 3 should be excluded from the final data processing. (From Murphy, P., and Port, S.: Radionuclide evaluation of left ventricular function. *In* Sandler, M.P., Patton, J.A., Coleman, A.E., et al. [eds.]: Diagnostic Nuclear Medicine. Baltimore, Williams & Wilkins, 1996, with permission.)

PVCs or bigeminy is noted before acquisition, the study should be postponed. Atrial fibrillation can also be problematic during FPRNA, much more so than during an equilibrium study, in which many RR intervals may be screened before beat acceptance. If atrial fibrillation is present, the calculated ejection fraction will obviously represent an average of the ejection fractions of the individual beats. If the atrial fibrillation is very irregular, the study probably should not be performed.

Background Correction

The purpose of background correction of the data is to isolate the true ventricular counts from those counts adjacent to the left ventricle, so that an accurate quantitative analysis of left ventricular function may be performed. All background methods are approximations, and no one method works in all situations. Of all the steps in data processing, the calculation of ejection fraction is most influenced by the operator through variation in the background estimate. The ejection fraction is calculated as follows:

$$EF = [(ED - BKGD) - (ES - BKGD)] / (ED - BKGD)$$

where EF is the ejection fraction and ED, ES, and BKGD are the end-diastolic, end-systolic, and background counts, respectively. Because the calculated background is virtually the same for ED and ES, the background term cancels out of the numerator and the above equation simplifies to

$$EF = (ED - ES) / (ED - BKGD)$$

The ejection fraction therefore varies directly with the background activity, because the higher the background, the smaller the denominator and the higher the EF.

Although several approaches to background correction of FPRNA have been described, the most accurate appears to be the lung-frame method.[24] The name lung-frame method is taken from the frame in which the radionuclide bolus has spread throughout the lung but has not yet reached the left ventricle. The distribution of the activity in that frame is taken as representative of the true background activity present during the left ventricular phase of the study. Ideally, it includes only activity in the pulmonary circulation and left atrium. Because the actual background activity is changing throughout the left ventricular phase as the radionuclide clears the lungs and left atrium, a correction for washout must be made. At the same time, the background activity is increasing in the myocardium itself owing to the coronary circulation, but this is a very small component compared with the amount of activity in the lungs or the ventricle.

The selection of the background frame is probably the most important operator intervention, with the exception of the drawing of the final ventricular regions of interest. As mentioned, overestimation of background results in a spuriously high ejection fraction. It is difficult to underestimate the background activity by much when using the lung-frame method. Because the counts preceding the lung phase are predominantly located in the right ventricle and many right ventricle pixels are common to the left ventricle in the anterior or shallow RAO views, selection of an early background frame typically results in assigning true left ventricular activity to the background, which results in oversubtraction. In that regard, the lung-frame background subtraction method becomes particularly problematic if there is poor separation between the right ventricular and left ventricular phases, as occurs with a delayed injection bolus, if there is right-sided pathology such as pulmonary hypertension or tricuspid insufficiency, or sometimes, inexplicably, in normal patients. If there is prolongation of right-side tracer transit, an accurate lung-frame background correction may be impossible. In that case, the ejection fraction may have to be estimated or calculated by a regression equation applied to the background uncorrected ejection fraction or calculated using an alternative background correction scheme.

Alternative approaches to background correction include a periventricular background region of interest, similar to that used in gated equilibrium studies, and subtraction of a constant background threshold from the entire left ventricular phase. Both of those approaches yield ejection fractions that correspond fairly well to those obtained at contrast angiography, although the lung-frame method has been shown to be statistically better in a comparison study.[24]

Representative Cycle

After the background correction has been performed, it becomes easier to redraw the ventricular regions of interest and, in particular, to identify the aortic valve plane on both the end-diastolic and end-systolic frames of the background-corrected representative cycle. These regions of interest are then used to generate a final representative cycle, from which all quantitative data are derived.

The LVEF is calculated from the end-diastolic and end-systolic counts after background correction as (ED − ES)/ED. The LVEF calculated by that approach has correlated closely with the LVEF measured during cardiac catheterization.[23, 24, 26] The accuracy of the first-pass LVEF is directly related to the statistical content of the data. The error of the measurement increases as the number of end-diastolic counts in the representative cycle decreases (Table 60–1). The percent error also increases as the LVEF decreases, because small changes in counts result in relatively large changes in low ejection fractions.[27]

Fortunately, as the LVEF decreases, counts within the left ventricle tend to be high because of the large volumes at end-diastole and end-systole. There is no absolute count rate limit below which first-pass data are guaranteed to be unacceptable, but the statistical

TABLE 60–1. PERCENT STATISTICAL ERROR IN CALCULATION OF EJECTION FRACTION

	Ejection Fraction						
ED Counts	***0.20***	***0.30***	***0.40***	***0.50***	***0.60***	***0.70***	***0.80***
500	30	24	17	13	10	8	6.5
2000	20	12	9	6	5	4	3
10000	9	5	4	3	2	1.5	1.5

Modified from Wackers, F. J. Th.: First-pass radionuclide angiocardiography. *In* Gerson, M. C. (ed.): Cardiac Nuclear Medicine. New York, McGraw-Hill, 1991, pp. 67–80, with permission.

error for measurement of an LVEF of 0.40 is almost 10 percent at an end-diastolic count rate of 2000 counts per frame, which means that the true LVEF could be anywhere from 0.36 to 0.44 ejection fraction units. Because the probability of survival after 2 years for a patient with stable coronary artery disease (CAD) is approximately 83 percent at an exercise LVEF of 0.36 but 93 percent at an LVEF of 0.44, it is of considerable clinical importance to reduce the statistical error of the measurement to as low a level as can reasonably be achieved. If the end-diastolic count rate were increased to 5000 counts per frame, the true LVEF in the same situation would range from 0.38 to 0.42, and the 2-year survival rate prediction would encompass a narrower range, from 85 to 90 percent.[28]

Variability in counts from study to study also affect the reproducibility of the measurement. When the same subjects were studied on two separate occasions and under similar hemodynamic conditions, the mean differences in ejection fraction measured by the processing scheme described were 0.04 and 0.03 at rest and at peak exercise, respectively.[29, 30] Interobserver variability was 2.0 percent at rest and 2.1 percent at peak exercise.[30]

Left Ventricular Volume

The volume of the ventricle may be calculated on a first-pass study by either geometric or count-proportional methods. The geometric technique is similar to the standard contrast angiographic approach and requires measurement of the area of the left ventricle at end-diastole and the length of the longest axis. The modified Sandler-Dodge equation can then be used to generate the end-diastolic volume. Because the left ventricular image is not as statistically reliable at end systole, the end-systolic volume is typically derived from the end-diastolic volume and the stroke volume, the latter being calculated as the product of the end-diastolic volume and the ejection fraction. Although reasonable correlations with contrast angiographic volumes have been obtained with this approach,[31] the geometric method is dependent on the accuracy of the edge detection scheme. Because the spatial resolution of the first-pass study is lower than that of other types of radionuclide imaging, geometric approaches are prone to error.

The count-proportional approach relies on the axiom that if the radioactivity is completely mixed in a chamber, the number of counts recorded from the chamber is directly proportional to its volume. The main problem with this approach is that the constant of proportionality differs for each patient because of differences in tissue attenuation, attenuation within the chamber, background activity, and the contribution of scattered activity.

Several investigators have proposed a count-proportional method that obviates the need to directly measure the constant of proportionality. First proposed by Nickel and colleagues[32] and modified by Massardo[33] and Levy[34] the method uses the ratio of the total counts recorded in the chamber to the peak count recorded in any single pixel within the chamber and has been applied to both equilibrium and first-pass data.[35] Application of the ratio between total counts and peak pixel counts eliminates the need to calculate or estimate attenuation because the attenuation would affect both the numerator and denominator, thereby canceling out. The area of a pixel for the acquisition system being used must also be known. The method has been rigorously validated with phantoms (both spherical and ellipsoidal balloons) and in clinical comparisons to contrast angiographic volumes. In 25 patients with contrast end-diastolic volumes ranging from 94 to 453 mL, the mean biplane contrast end-diastolic volume was calculated by the formula

$$V = 1.8\ (\text{Total/Peak} - 3.5)^{3/2}$$

where V= volume, Peak = peak pixel counts, and Total = observed counts in the entire LV phase. The angiographic volume obtained was 162±57, compared with 150±62 (*P* = NS) with FPRNA and a multicrystal camera. With a single-crystal camera and FPRNA, the radionuclide end-diastolic volume averaged 202±88 mL, compared with 210±92 mL (*P* = NS) for the biplane contrast study. Standard errors of the estimate using this technique compare favorably with methods that attempt to measure attenuation by blood sampling. For end-diastolic volume, the standard error of the estimate was 23 mL, or 14 percent of the average volume, and for end-systolic volume (calculated from stroke volume and LVEF), it was 16 mL, or 18 percent of the mean value.[35]

Normal values from our laboratory for ventricular volumes measured in the upright position by the count-proportional technique described are presented in Table 60–2. As one might expect, the end-diastolic volumes tend be be significantly lower in the upright compared with the supine position at rest, and they show a much greater increase during exercise than is typically seen during supine exercise.

Right Ventricular Function

The first-pass method is the technique of choice for the measurement of right ventricular ejection fraction (RVEF), but the acquisition technique requires some modification. When a bolus is rapidly injected into a vein close to the central circulation, it arrives in the right ventricle without much time for mixing and clears the ventricle quickly. Consequently, there are few beats available, and all of

TABLE 60–2. NORMAL VALUES FOR FIRST-PASS RADIONUCLIDE ANGIOGRAPHY WITH UPRIGHT ACQUISITION

	Heart Rate	**Ejection Fraction**	**End-Diastolic Volume Index (mL/m²)**	**End-Systolic Volume Index (mL/m²)**	**Cardiac Index (L/m²)**
Female					
Rest	76 ± 11	0.67 ± 0.04	61 ± 11	21 ± 4	3.0 ± 0.7
Exercise	168 ± 10	0.76 ± 0.04	88 ± 24	22 ± 6	11.0 ±3.2
Male					
Rest	75 ± 12	0.67 ± 0.06	60 ± 12	21 ± 6	2.0 ± 0.6
Exercise	163 ± 18	0.76 ± 0.06	83 ± 17	22 ± 7	9.9 ± 1.8

them have a rapidly changing concentration of the radionuclide. It is, therefore, helpful to delay the bolus injection if the evaluation of right ventricular function is the main indication for the study. Delay increases the number of right ventricular beats available for processing and provides a more stable radionuclide concentration during the right ventricular phase. It is also helpful to acquire the study in a 30-degree RAO view, because that view maximizes separation between the right atrium and the right ventricle.

Early attempts at measuring the RVEF with the first-pass technique yielded values that were frequently as low as those reported with the equilibrium technique.[36] This was primarily a result of the use of a single region of interest. Both atrial and pulmonary activity encroach on the end-diastolic right ventricular region of interest at end-systole, which spuriously lowers the RVEF. Use of separate end-diastolic and end-systolic regions of interest obviates that problem (Fig. 60–10). Various background correction schemes have been proposed for processing the right ventricular study.[36, 37] Most commonly, a periventricular region of interest with inclusion of right atrial activity has been used, but if separate end-diastolic and end-systolic regions of interest are used, there is no need for background correction. In fact, background correction may artificially increase the RVEF when separate regions of interest are used.

Although the RVEF is best measured with the first-pass technique, right ventricular regional wall motion is best evaluated with the higher-resolution gated equilibrium method. It is, therefore, beneficial to acquire both types of studies sequentially. A first-pass study should be acquired during the injection of technetium pertechnetate after pretreatment with stannous pyrophosphate, just as is done for a standard in vivo labeling procedure for a gated study. After the first-pass study has been acquired, a multiview gated study can be acquired.

Gated First-Pass Technique

Another approach to the measurement of RVEF is the so-called gated first-pass technique. In this case, the acquisition is set up as if a standard gated equilibrium study were to be performed. Instead of red blood cell labeling, however, a bolus of technetium is injected. The acquisition is started as soon as the bolus reaches the right ventricle, and it is stopped as soon as the majority of the bolus has cleared the right ventricle. This generates a gated study that includes the data from only those right ventricular beats that occurred while the camera was turned on. Although the resolution of the image is not as good as in a standard gated study, owing to the paucity of beats, the resolution is comparable to that of a standard right ventricular first-pass study, and the statistics are usually adequate for calculation of RVEF. The RVEF is systematically higher with this approach than that calculated by the standard gated equilibrium method in subjects with normal right ventricles and in those with valvular heart disease.[38] Morrison and colleagues showed that the linear correlation between gated first-pass RVEF and angiographic RVEF was significantly better than that obtained with standard gated equilibrium RVEF.[39]

Transit Times

The temporal separation of chambers in a first-pass study allows the calculation of the time required for the bolus to travel from one chamber to another or through a given chamber. That capability has not received much clinical application. However, the pulmonary blood volume may be calculated from the product of the pulmonary mean transit time and the cardiac output. Estimates of pulmonary blood volume have been shown to be of diagnostic value in detection of CAD.[40, 41] In addition, the lung uptake of thallium on exercise or in dipyridamole perfusion scans is of important prognostic value. It is conceivable, therefore, that pulmonary blood volume during exercise may also be of prognostic importance, although the hypothesis has never been tested.

To calculate the mean transit time through the lung, time-activity curves are generated from regions of interest over the left atrium and the pulmonary artery. The pulmonary transit time is then calculated as the left atrial mean transit time minus the pulmonary arterial mean transit time.

Motion Correction

There are two approaches to motion correction in first-pass studies. For lack of better terms, they may be referred to as internal and external approaches. The internal approach uses only the data available within the first-pass study itself, and the external approach requires application of a radioactive marker to the chest wall during study acquisition.

The assumption of the internal approach is that the ventricle must remain in the same *x-y* location throughout the acquisition. The *x-y* location of the center of the ventricle is then determined in each frame of the representative cycle with the use of a center-

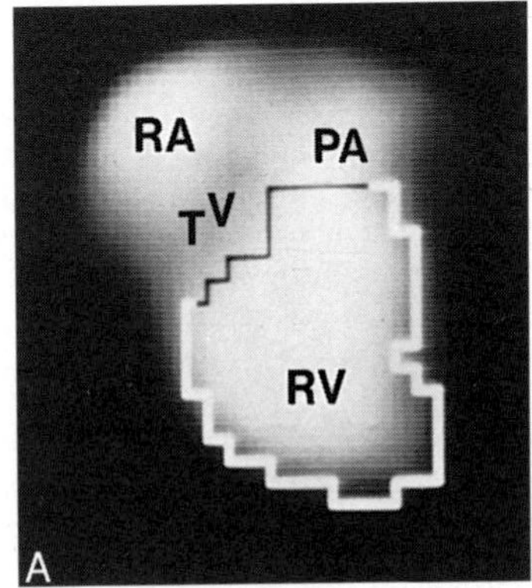

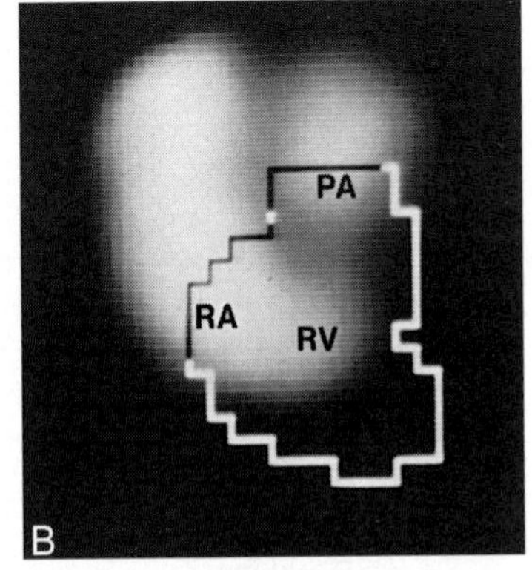

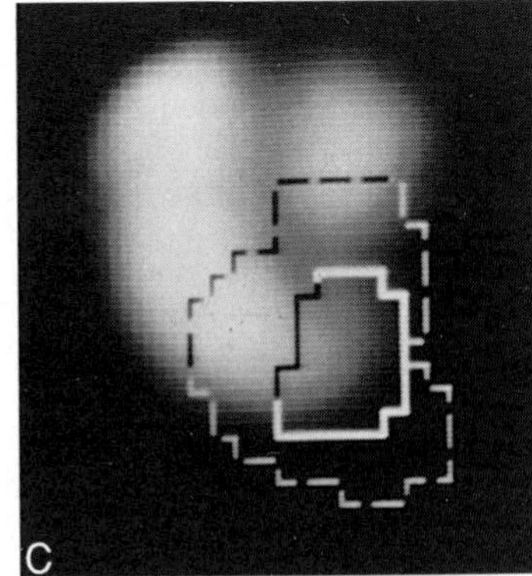

FIGURE 60–10. Right ventricular (RV) data processing is also best approached with the use of separate end-diastolic and end-systolic regions of interest (ROIs). *A*, The end-diastolic frame of a first-pass RV study acquired in a shallow right anterior oblique view, with an ROI drawn around the RV. *B*, The end-systolic frame, with the same end-diastolic ROI as in panel A. Because both the tricuspid and pulmonary valves move toward the RV body during systole, the activities of the both the right atrium (RA) and the pulmonary artery (PA) are contained within the end-diastolic ROI at end-systole. *C*, The end-diastolic ROI from panels *A* and *B*, with a separate end-systolic ROI drawn to exclude right atrial and pulmonary arterial activity. TV = tricuspid valve. (From Murphy, P., and Port, S.: Radionuclide evaluation of left ventricular function. *In* Sandler, M.P., Patton, J.A., Coleman, A.E., et al. [eds.]: Diagnostic Nuclear Medicine. Baltimore, Williams & Wilkins, 1996, with permission.)

of-mass algorithm. The average arithmetic x-y location of the center of mass is then considered to represent the correct location of the chamber, and each individual frame of the representative cycle is then re-registered to coincide with that location. This approach works fairly well for the magnitude of cardiac motion that is typically encountered during a bicycle exercise study, when the chest is forced against the collimator. During treadmill exercise, the chest and cardiac motion may be much more exaggerated, especially during the later stages of an exercise protocol. For treadmill motion correction, the external motion correction approach is recommended.

The external motion correction approach makes use of a chest wall marker that emits a gamma photon whose energy peak can be readily distinguished from the energy spectrum of technetium-99m. To date, both americium-241 and iodine-125 have been used for this purpose.[18, 19] A small, sealed radionuclide source is fixed to the anterior chest, usually over the sternum and slightly above the anticipated location of the left ventricle. The study is then set up for a dual-energy acquisition such that two first-pass data sets are acquired simultaneously. For the external approach to work properly, the marker must remain in the field of view throughout the study.

After acquisition, the location of the marker is determined in each frame of the study, and movement from one frame to the next is quantified. Each raw data frame of the technetium study is then shifted according to the magnitude and direction of motion calculated for the marker in that same frame. Data processing of the technetium study can then be performed as usual. Some degree of image distortion does occur as a result of this type of motion correction. The marker, which is akin to a point source, is tracked by use of a center-of-mass algorithm. Because the resolution of the first-pass study is not high, the point spread function is significant. It is therefore necessary to apply an arbitrary count threshold subtraction to the marker data in order to properly apply the algorithm for marker motion. After the technetium data are re-registered, some pixel values are changed because of an interpolation that must take place and some data are lost completely as the entire image is shifted. If the ventricle is too close to the edge of the field of view, that could result in loss of ventricular activity.

Overall, the external marker correction method works reasonably well (Fig. 60–11), and the LVEFs during treadmill exercise have been shown to be the same as the ejection fractions during bicycle exercise in the same subjects.[18, 19] However, we have found that the end-diastolic volumes obtained during marker-corrected treadmill exercise studies are significantly larger than the volumes obtained in the same subjects during bicycle exercise. We have also found it more difficult in certain cases to evaluate regional wall motion on the marker-corrected treadmill exercise studies.

FIGURE 60–11. See Color Plate 26.

DATA ANALYSIS AND INTERPRETATION

Tracer Transit

The normal sequential appearance of the radionuclide bolus in the superior vena cava, the right atrium, the right ventricle, the pulmonary circulation, the left side of the heart, and the aorta should be confirmed in every study. It is helpful to format the data into 1-second images in order to easily visualize the entire transit through the central circulation in 16 to 20 images (see Fig. 60–1). Occasionally, deviations from the normal sequence are encountered, suggesting a congenital or acquired anatomical abnormality (Fig. 60–12). From time to time, there are variations in the sequence of tracer transit that cannot easily be assessed with a display of serial static images; in these situations, it is particularly helpful to create a cinematic display of the raw data. The normal anatomical sequence of the bolus should be confirmed, and the duration of tracer transit through the right-heart and left-heart phases should be noted.

Tracer transit times vary with the heart rate, to some degree with the rhythm (e.g., atrial fibrillation may prolong transit), with the strength of contraction (e.g., severely depressed ejection fractions result in prolonged transit), and with the injection technique. In the presence of a good injection bolus, prolongation of tracer transit through the right-heart phase may occur because of pulmonary hypertension or tricuspid or pulmonary valve insufficiency. A left-to-right intracardiac shunt causes early reappearance of tracer in the right side of the heart, but the initial clearance may be normal. If tracer transit through the right-heart phase is normal, then prolongation of tracer transit through the left side of the heart suggests mitral or aortic insufficiency or a left-to-right shunt.

Because tracer transit varies with heart rate, ejection fraction,

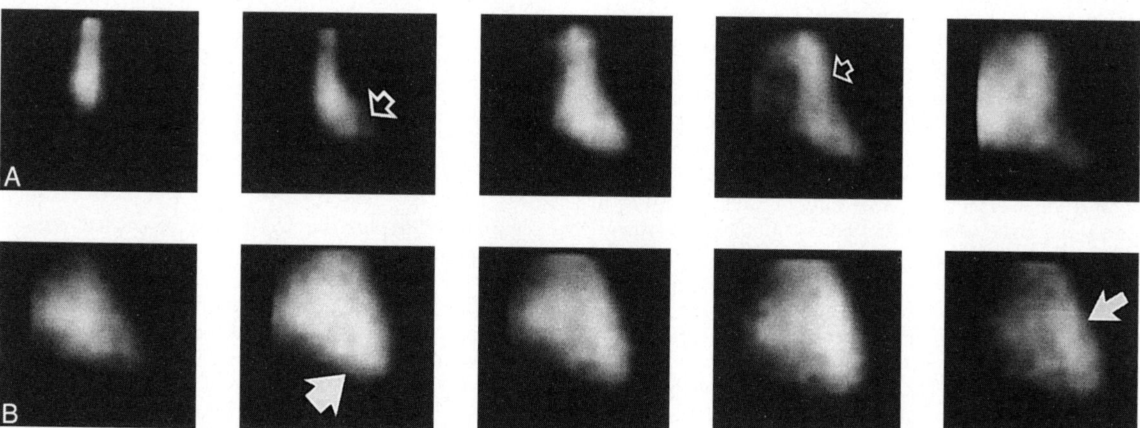

FIGURE 60–12. Although unusual, unsuspected deviations from normal tracer transit occasionally are encountered and may be diagnostically important. *A,* In this example, the bolus appears in a right-sided chamber whose shape is that of a left ventricle *(large open arrow)* and enters a pulmonary artery that is positioned more laterally than would be expected *(small open arrow)*. *B,* The left-sided ventricle has the typical appearance of a right ventricle *(large solid arrow)*, and the aorta is more medial than would be expected *(small solid arrow)*. These findings are diagnostic for corrected transposition of the great vessels. (From Gal, R., and Port, S.C.: Radionuclide angiography in congenitally corrected transposition of the great vessels in one adult. J. Nucl. Med. 28:116, 1987, with permission of the Society of Nuclear Medicine.)

rhythm, and injection technique, it is not a simple matter to detect mild prolongation of right- or left-heart tracer transit. There are no look-up tables to determine how many beats or how much time one can expect in the left side of the heart for any given combination of heart rate, ejection fraction, and bolus duration. Normally, there are 4 to 6 beats during the right-heart phase at rest and 2 to 4 beats during exercise. In the left side of the heart, those figures are 6 to 12 and 4 to 8 beats, respectively. If there are many more beats, then there must be some pathologic explanation; most typically, valvular insufficiency is responsible.

Cardiac Rhythm

If no ECG signal was recorded during the first-pass acquisition, then the interpreting physician must evaluate the time-activity curve to determine whether regular rhythm was present throughout the study. Atrial fibrillation, ventricular ectopy, or very premature supraventricular ectopy can alter the ejection fraction. One must be certain that the final representative cycle does not contain data from post-PVC or PVC beats unless a paucity of beats allows no alternative. In the latter situation, the clinician must be alerted to the fact that the reported ejection fraction and wall motion may be overestimated or underestimated, as the case may be. If ventricular bigeminy is present during the ventricular phase of the study, there is no way to accurately evaluate ventricular function, and one is obliged to report the results for the post-PVC beats.

Assessment of Systolic Function

The evaluation of systolic function begins with the inspection of the ventricular time-activity curve and the final ventricular region of interest. Proper beat selection should be confirmed, and the background frame should be checked. In an exercise study, the time-activity curve should also be inspected for evidence of cardiac motion. The final region of interest should be checked for accuracy and freedom from nonventricular activity.

Regional wall motion may be evaluated with the use of a cinematic display of the representative cycle, in which case abnormalities of regional wall motion should be characterized by the conventional terms hypokinesia, akinesia, and dyskinesia. The qualitative modifiers of mild, moderate, and severe should be used to further describe the severity of hypokinesia.

In the anterior view first-pass left ventricular study, the anterolateral, apical, and inferoseptal walls are defined by the perimeter of the image. In the 30-degree RAO view, the anterior, apical, and inferior walls are visible. In the LAO view, the septal, inferoapical, and lateral or true posterior walls may be evaluated. Semiquantitative assessment of regional wall motion with cinematic display of the representative cycle acquired in the RAO view has been compared with the results of contrast angiography in the same subjects.[13] The correlation between the anterior and apical walls was quite good. The weakest correlation was in the inferior wall, probably because of oversubtraction of inferior wall activity as a result of persistent right ventricular activity in the background frame. If the background activity is unavoidably high because of persistent right ventricular activity, it is better either to choose an alternative background approach (described in a previous section) or to analyze wall motion using the uncorrected representative cycle.

Because the first-pass study is typically acquired in only one view and resolution is somewhat limited, it may be difficult to separate regional wall motion abnormalities in contiguous or overlapping segments. A typical example of that shortcoming is the appearance of "anterior" hypokinesia on a study acquired in the anterior view in a patient whose actual dysfunction involves the circumflex territory. In that case, the three-dimensional effect of the posterior wall dysfunction is misinterpreted in two-dimensional analysis as a problem with the overlying anterior wall.

Visual assessment of regional function is obviously subjective. To improve interobserver variability, several parametric images may be generated to aid in the detection and characterization of regional dysfunction (Fig. 60–13). They can be as simple as a display of the superimposed end-diastolic and end-systolic perimeters after an edge-defining threshold has been applied to the data or as complex as a mean systolic transit time image.[42] Perhaps the most commonly used parametric image is the regional ejection fraction image, in which the ejection fraction of each pixel within the ventricular region of interest is calculated and color-coded. Based on reproducibility data, changes in regional ejection fraction of 0.25 have been considered as indicative of a true change in regional function. The amplitude image is similar, except that its output reflects the amplitude of the cosine function applied to each pixel after a Fourier transform has been performed. Phase images are typically used to characterize the timing of events during the cardiac cycle but may also help in detection of regional dysfunction because the latter is typically accompanied by altered timing as well as altered magnitude of contraction. Akinetic segments are easily detected in parametric images because the pixels of those segments will have a value of 0 (no change in counts) and be color-coded black. In dyskinetic regions, end-systolic counts may exceed end-diastolic counts. If end-diastolic counts are subtracted from end-systolic counts, only dyskinetic pixels will have positive values and show up on a color-coded image, the so-called paradox image.

FIGURE 60–13. See Color Plate 26.

In contrast angiography, regional wall motion has been quantified by calculation of regional shortening fractions applied to an arbitrary number of radii drawn from the center of the ventricle to the perimeter of the chamber at both end-diastole and end-systole.[43, 44] The same approach has been taken with gated equilibrium scintigraphy.[45] Because of the more limited spatial resolution of the first-pass study, that type of quantitation has not been applied to the first-pass ventriculogram.

Analysis of right ventricular systolic function is not as straightforward as that of the left ventricle because its geometry defies simple description and its contraction pattern is more complex. Furthermore, little clinical attention has been paid to right ventricular function, and no commonly accepted norms are available. Review of the cinematic display of the right ventricular representative cycle is perhaps the best way to evaluate regional right ventricular function, and application of the conventional terms, hypokinesia, akinesia, and dyskinesia is appropriate. The gated equilibrium study is better suited for description of regional right ventricular function because of its better spatial resolution.

Ejection Fraction

Normal values for the LVEF vary somewhat according to the exact type of processing used. At rest, an LVEF of 0.50 is usually accepted as the lower limit of normal for untrained individuals. Our most recent results (see Table 60–2), employing anterior view acquisitions, processing with dual regions of interest, and the latest generation of multicrystal gamma camera, showed that the resting LVEF was 0.66 ± 0.06 in a group of healthy male volunteers ($n = 33$) with an average age of 47. The lowest resting LVEF was 0.55. For healthy female volunteers ($n = 13$) with an average age of 44, the resting LVEF was 0.67 ± 0.04, and the lowest LVEF was 0.55. At peak exercise, the male subjects had an LVEF of 0.76 ± 0.04 with the lowest value being 0.64, whereas the female subjects had an average exercise LVEF of 0.76 ± 0.05 with the lowest value at 0.69. The exercise values represent those obtained during upright bicycle exercise and may not be applicable to either supine, semisupine, or treadmill exercise.

Left Ventricular Diastolic Function

The same analyses used for the evaluation of diastolic function with gated equilibrium imaging may be used for first-pass data (Fig. 60–14). The temporal resolution of a first-pass study acquired at 25 msec per frame is comparable to a 32 frames-per-cycle gated acquisition at a heart rate of 60 in which the frame time is 31 msec. The peak diastolic filling rate, time to peak filling rate, and filling fractions have been calculated.[46, 47] In two separate reports published within a year of each other, the normal peak diastolic filling rates were 3.13±0.85 in one[46] and 2.14±0.63 EDV/sec in the other.[47] Measurement of diastolic filling rates and intervals may vary with beat selection because of the changing radionuclide concentration throughout the ventricular phase of a first-pass study. Beats occurring early in the left ventricular phase tend to have higher peak filling rates than beats at the end of the left ventricular phase. It is, therefore, advisable to include only beats that closely surround the beat with the peak end-diastolic count rate, because those beats contain the best mixed concentration of radionuclide. If diastolic function is the primary reason for a radionuclide study, then it makes more sense to perform a gated study to ensure an adequate number of beats and to screen out ectopic beats. The clinical utility of the first-pass study in evaluation of diastole has been recently underscored by a study that used such data to distinguish between constrictive and restrictive disease,[48] two entities that are difficult to differentiate invasively (Fig. 60–15).

Assessment of Valvular Insufficiency

Prolongation of ventricular tracer transit, when not caused by a technical problem, is usually a result of valvular insufficiency. As indicated previously, prolonged tracer transit may be identified by an excessive number of beats during the ventricular phase. To quantify left-sided valvular insufficiency, it has been suggested that the pulmonary time-activity curve be used as a monoexponential input function to deconvolute the left ventricular time-activity curve. In that way, the contribution of regurgitation to the left ventricular curve can be isolated and quantified by standard curve analysis techniques. The correlation of that approach with results from invasive data has been favorable.[49] Tricuspid insufficiency has also been quantified by use of a curve analysis method.[50] Another approach is to calculate the total stroke output of the two ventricles, which would differ by a degree proportional to the amount of regurgitation.[51] If left-sided tracer transit is prolonged, the left ventricular image should be examined for the presence of a dilated left atrium (Fig. 60–16) or dilated aortic root, the former suggesting mitral and the latter aortic insufficiency.

Although radionuclide data may confidently be used to differentiate moderate to severe regurgitation from mild or no regurgitation, the ability to visualize the direction, width, and depth of penetration of regurgitant jets with Doppler echocardiography makes it the procedure of choice for the evaluation of valvular insufficiency.

Left-to-Right Shunts

The quantitation of left-to-right shunts with the use of radionuclides is an extension of classical indicator dilution theory. Any measurable, nondiffusible indicator injected into the central circulation has a finite circulation time and a typical monoexponential

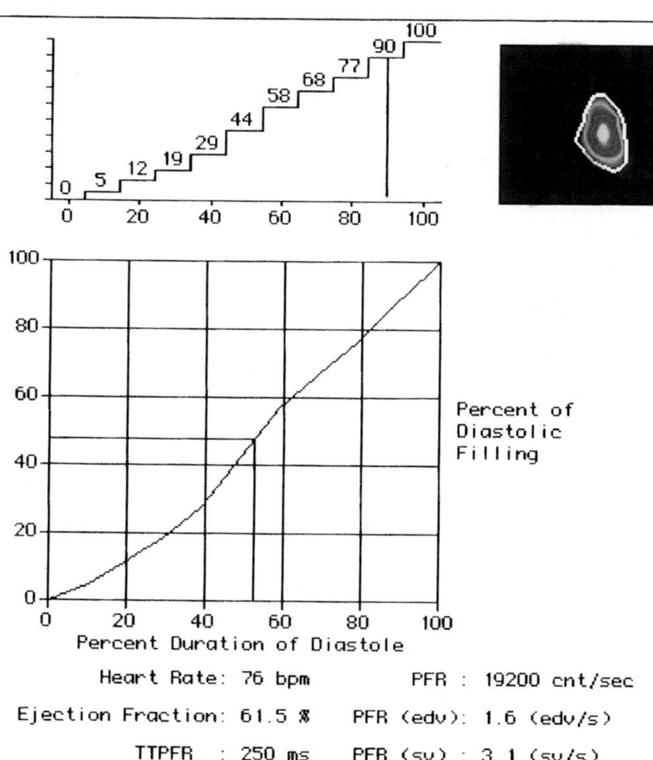

Counts at ES: 5633

Number of Frames: 20 (25 ms)

#	Slope	Cnts-ES	%dur	%filling
1	0	0	0.0	0.0
2	111	68	5.3	1.1
3	190	259	10.5	4.2
4	229	494	15.8	8.1
5	240	737	21.1	12.0
6	252	974	26.3	15.9
7	286	1219	31.6	19.9
8	352	1513	36.8	24.7
9	428	1900	42.1	31.0
10	480	2394	47.4	39.1
11	480	2922	52.6	47.7
12	429	3403	57.9	55.5
13	360	3797	63.2	61.9
14	314	4102	68.4	66.9
15	314	4376	73.7	71.4
16	354	4687	78.9	76.5
17	395	5077	84.2	82.8
18	374	5526	89.5	90.1
19	271	5932	94.7	96.8
20	101	6130	100.0	100.0

FIGURE 60–14. Diastolic function may be quantified with the same approach as that taken with gated equilibrium data. To minimize the effect of the changing radionuclide concentration during the ventricular phase, beats should be chosen symmetrically around the peak of the time-activity curve. The peak filling rate (PFR) is then calculated as the maximum rate of increase of counts during early diastolic filling and is typically expressed as end-diastolic volumes per second. The time to peak filling (TTPFR) is measured as the time in milliseconds from end-systole to the point at which the PFR occurs. In addition, the percent filling that has occurred at each frame of diastole may be expressed to generate variables such as first third or first half filling fractions. (edv = end-diastolic volume; esv = end-systolic volume; s, sec = seconds; %dur = percent of diastole.)

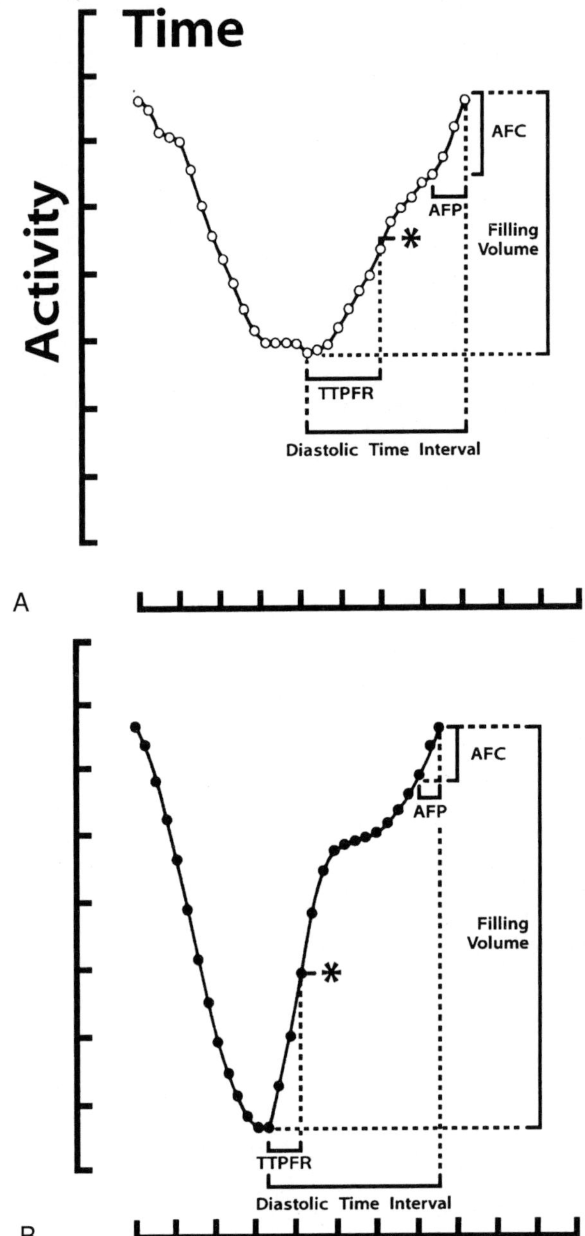

FIGURE 60–15. First-pass diastolic filling curves have recently been shown to be of value in differentiating restrictive myocardial disease *(A)* from constrictive pericardial disease *(B)*. Early diastolic filling tends to be delayed and reduced in restrictive disease but early and accelerated in constrictive disease. (AFC = atrial filling contribution; AFP = atrial filling period; TTPFR = time to peak filling rate.) (From Aroney, C.N., Ruddy, T.D., Dighero, H., et al.: Differentiation of restrictive cardiomyopathy from pericardial constriction: Assessment of diastolic function by radionuclide angiography. J. Am. Coll. Cardiol. 13:1010, 1989. Reprinted with permission from the American College of Cardiology.)

appearance and disappearance when sampled downstream from the injection site. In the catheterization laboratory, the traditional indicator was indocyanine green, which was sampled by drawing downstream blood through a densitometer.[52] In FPRNA, the indicator is technetium and the sampling is performed externally with the gamma camera. In the presence of a left-to-right shunt, the curve described by sampling the indicator downstream from the shunt is no longer monoexponential because of the early recirculation of the indicator through the shunt.

In FPRNA, the injection is performed as usual in a peripheral vein. The appearance in and clearance from the lungs is then recorded and graphed (Fig. 60–17). Standard curve analysis techniques such as exponential and gamma variate fitting are used to separate the observed curve into primary and shunt components. The areas of these two components are proportional to the systemic and shunt flows and allow calculation of the ratio of pulmonary to systemic flow or $\dot{Q}p:\dot{Q}s$ (Fig. 60–18). The $\dot{Q}p:\dot{Q}s$ is directly proportional to the magnitude of the shunt. With FPRNA, shunts with a $\dot{Q}p:\dot{Q}s$ of 1.2:1 can usually be detected. The early reports of results obtained with this technique showed excellent correlations with invasive oximetric data.[53, 54]

The pulmonary time-activity curves are usually generated from regions of interest over both the right and left lung. The right lung is more important, because it is spatially more separate from the left ventricle and aorta, whose cyclic changes in activity can contaminate the pulmonary curve analysis. The $\dot{Q}p:\dot{Q}s$ ratios calculated from the two lungs are rarely identical because of statistical fluctuations in the curves that influence the identification of the break point in the curve analysis. The raw pulmonary time-activity curves should be adequately smoothed to minimize the effect of the high-frequency statistical noise that can cause incorrect curve fitting.

The application of monoexponential curve analysis depends on the integrity of the bolus entering the pulmonary circulation. A delayed bolus or prolonged right-sided tracer transit (e.g., with tricuspid or pulmonary insufficiency) may preclude accurate quantitation of a shunt. The presence of a shunt, however, may almost always be confirmed visually. The sequential appearance of the radionuclide in the right atrium, right ventricle, pulmonary circulation, and left ventricle is obvious in a normal study, and the left ventricle is free of any right ventricular activity. If there is a significant intracardiac left-to-right shunt, the bolus initially transits the right heart normally, but on reaching the left side of the heart, it reappears in the right heart at the same time, preventing identification of a clear left ventricular phase (Fig. 60–19). Consequently, simple visual confirmation of a clearly identifiable left ventricle that is not contaminated by right ventricular activity excludes the presence of a significant left-to-right intracardiac shunt. With an extracardiac shunt (e.g., in patent ductus arteriosus), the right heart does not participate in the shunt, and the visual method cannot be used to exclude or confirm the presence of the shunt.

FIGURE 60–19. See Color Plate 27.

Attempts at quantitation of right-to-left shunts have been made with FPRNA. With placement of a region of interest over a systemic vessel that is uncontaminated by the pulmonary artery, early appearance of a radionuclide bolus in the systemic circulation after intravenous injection is consistent with a right-to-left shunt.[55] A more commonly used approach, however, is to inject radiolabeled macroaggregated albumin. The activity that bypasses the lung through the shunt and arrives in systemic organs is compared with the majority of activity that is trapped in the lung to arrive at a semiquantitative estimate of shunt magnitude.[56]

Cardiac Output by Curve Analysis

As mentioned previously, ventricular volumes may be measured both geometrically and by count-proportional techniques, and cardiac output may then be calculated as the product of the stroke volume and the heart rate. Those are the typical methods for measuring the cardiac output with FPRNA. However, there is another method that uses curve analysis to calculate the cardiac output directly from observed counts during the first pass and subsequently at "equilibrium." The area under the first-pass time activity-curve through the left ventricle is determined. Subsequently, the counts in the entire heart are recorded after equilibration. True equilibration never actually occurs, because the radionuclide is continuously withdrawn from the circulation by the kidneys.

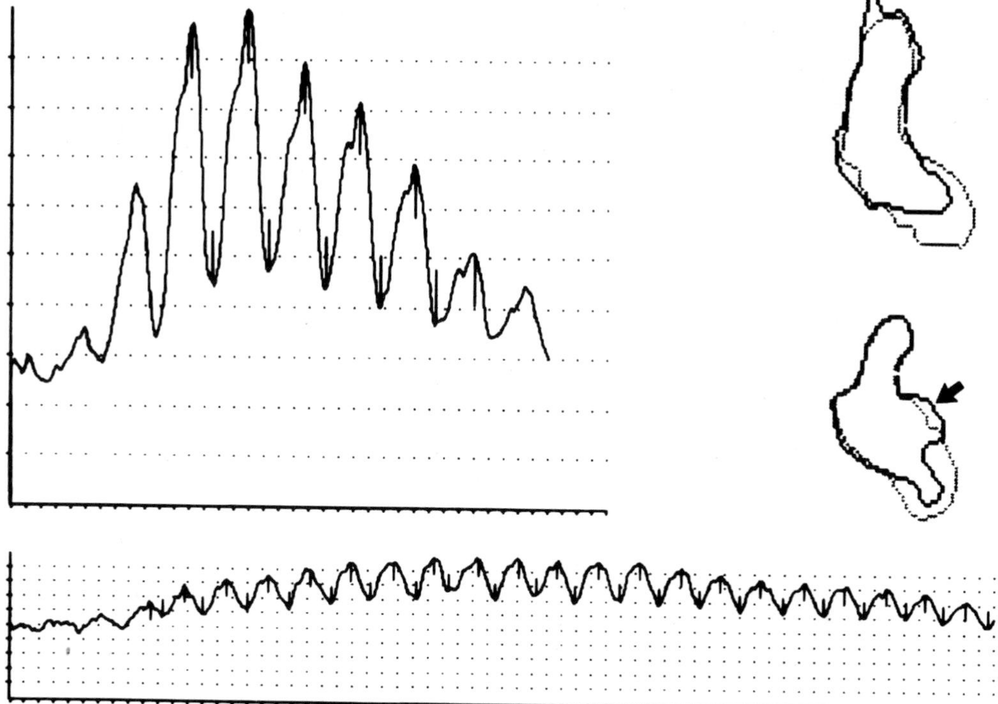

FIGURE 60–16. Prolongation of tracer transit is suggestive of valvular insufficiency. *Upper panel,* An example of normal tracer transit and a normal image. The time-activity curve *(lower panel)* shows markedly prolonged left ventricular tracer transit, and the image shows a very prominent left atrial appendage *(arrow),* suggesting moderate to severe mitral insufficiency.

CLINICAL APPLICATIONS OF FIRST-PASS RADIONUCLIDE ANGIOGRAPHY

FPRNA can theoretically be applied to any clinical situation in which the evaluation of ventricular function is important or in which the assessment of tracer transit is necessary (e.g., in quantitation of shunts). Practically, however, the technique is best applied to situations in which the unique characteristics of FPRNA make it superior to other modalities such as gated equilibrium imaging or echocardiography. FPRNA is not the procedure of choice for evaluation of ventricular function at rest. In that situation, the availability of enough acquisition time, the ability to acquire multiple views, and the superior spatial resolution of gated equilibrium imaging make it the procedure of choice. However, the extremely short acquisition time makes the first-pass method the technique of choice for the evaluation of ventricular function during exercise. The diagnostic and prognostic applications of imaging of ventricular function during exercise are, therefore, the main indications for first-pass studies.

Diagnosis of Coronary Artery Disease

Screening

In order for a test to be successfully used as a screening tool for a condition, several criteria must be met, only a few of which actually pertain to the test itself. First and foremost, the goal of the screening must be very focused. Many conditions exist in dichotomous states, that is, they are either present or not present. However, many conditions, of which CAD is a perfect example, exist in a wide range of severity. If the goal is to detect any CAD, regardless of severity, then perhaps ultrafast computed tomography scanning, with its ability to detect small amounts of calcium in arterial walls, is appropriate. If the goal is to detect only physiologically significant stenoses (which could be as mild as a 50 percent diameter stenosis), then some type of perfusion imaging that is very sensitive for small reductions in peak coronary blood flow would be more appropriate. In its current form, FPRNA cannot be advocated as a screening tool for the presence or absence of physiologically significant stenoses because its sensitivity and

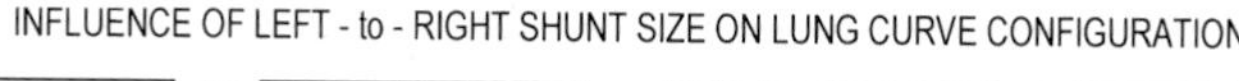

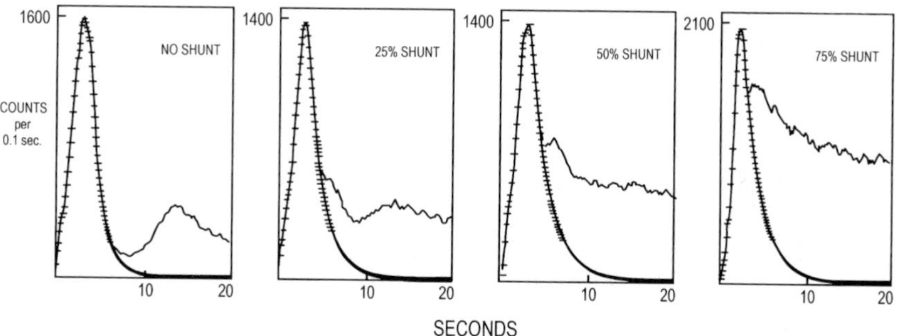

FIGURE 60–17. In the presence of a left-to-right shunt, the pulmonary time-activity curve shows an early recirculation peak, the magnitude of which varies directly with the size of the shunt. Early recirculation may be differentiated from normal recirculation by timing the primary and recirculation peaks. An early recirculation peak usually appears within 5 seconds of the primary peak, whereas a normal recirculation peak appears 10 to 20 seconds after the primary peak. (Courtesy of Robert H. Jones, M.D., Duke University Medical Center, Durham, NC.)

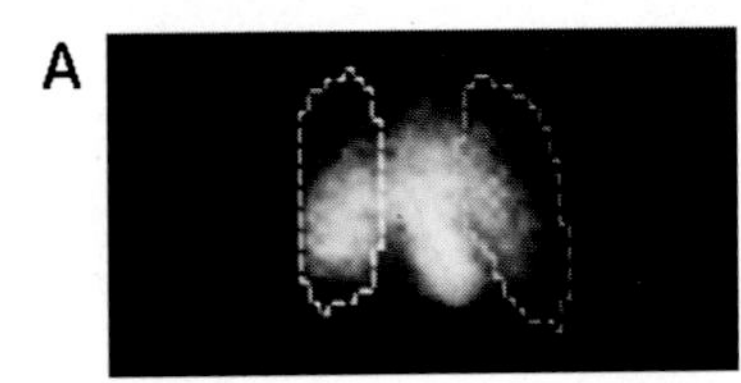

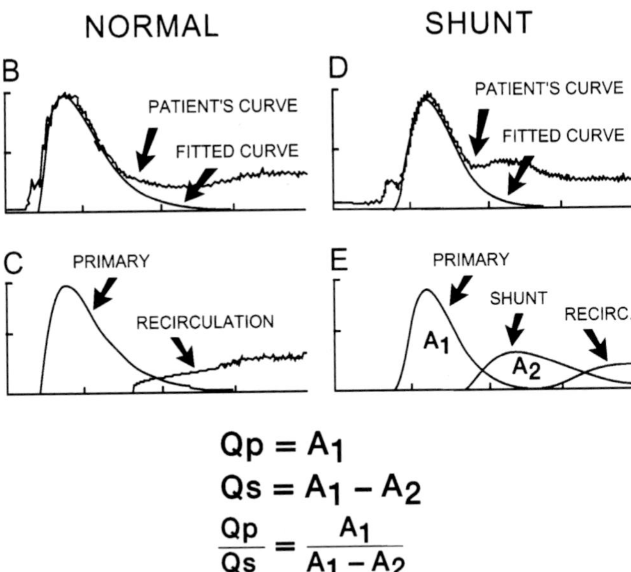

$$Qp = A_1$$
$$Qs = A_1 - A_2$$
$$\frac{Qp}{Qs} = \frac{A_1}{A_1 - A_2}$$

FIGURE 60–18. The left-to-right shunt calculation begins with the manual drawing of a pulmonary time-activity curve. *A,* The right lung is preferred because it is easier to avoid the beat-to-beat cyclic changes in activity from the neighboring ventricle that can influence the curve analysis. Examples of curves from a normal patient *(B and C)* are compared with curves from a patient with a left-to-right shunt *(D and E).* The patient's curve is fitted with an exponential or gamma variate fit to define the primary curve (A1), whose area represents pulmonary blood flow ($\dot{Q}p$). Curve A1 is then subtracted from the patient's data to leave the shunt component (A2), whose area represents the shunt flow. Systemic flow ($\dot{Q}s$) is the total pulmonary flow (A1) minus the shunt flow (A2), and $\dot{Q}p$:$\dot{Q}s$ is calculated purely in terms of the areas under the primary and shunt curves. (From Ports, S.: First-pass RNA. *In* Early, P.J., and Sodee, D.B. [eds.]: Principles and Practice of Nuclear Medicine. St. Louis, Mosby–Year Book, 1996, p. 381, with permission.)

specificity are inadequate for that purpose. If the goal is to detect only prognostically high-risk CAD, then either exercise ECG testing, myocardial perfusion imaging, exercise ventricular function imaging, or some combination of the three may be best.

After the goal has been established for the severity of disease to be detected, then one must establish the disease prevalence in the population to be screened, for that will greatly affect the predictive accuracy of the screening test. With a 5 percent disease prevalence, a test with a specificity of 90 percent and a sensitivity of 90 percent will incorrectly assign disease to 10 of 100 patients screened while correctly identifying 4.5 of 100 patients screened (positive predictive accuracy = 31 percent). Increase the disease prevalence to 25 percent, and the same test still incorrectly assigns disease to 10 of 100 but now correctly identifies 22.5 of 100 patients screened (positive predictive accuracy = 69 percent).

Because prognosis in stable CAD bears a quantitative relation to exercise LVEF, exercise first-pass ventricular function imaging could have a role in screening for prognostically high-risk CAD.[57–60] However, in one direct comparison, it did not perform significantly better than stress ECG for the detection of left main or severe three-vessel disease.[61]

Regional Wall Motion

Inadequate coronary perfusion for any given demand results in regional metabolic dysfunction, which, in turn, leads to regional mechanical dysfunction. If enough myocardium is rendered ischemic, there may be a compromise of global ventricular function (e.g., a drop in ejection fraction). Because radionuclide ventriculography can detect both regional and global ventricular dysfunction, it has been applied to the diagnosis of CAD. Typical changes in ventricular size and function during ischemia include a new or worsened regional wall motion abnormality, an increase in end-systolic volume, a decrease in ejection fraction, altered early diastolic filling, and a variable increase in end-diastolic volume (Fig. 60–20). However, all or none of those changes may occur, depending on the amount of myocardium involved.

FIGURE 60–20. See Color Plate 27.

The sensitivity of FPRNA for the detection of exercise-induced regional wall motion abnormalities in patients with known CAD has been reported to be as low as 53 percent.[62] In contrast, the specificity for detection of a new regional wall motion abnormality in the same study was more than 90 percent. The test appeared to perform more poorly in women than in men (Table 60–3), but the disease prevalence was much lower in the women than in the men. As one would expect, the sensitivity for detection of regional left ventricular dysfunction did increase as the disease became more extensive. Regional wall motion abnormalities were detected in 40 percent of patients with single-vessel CAD, 50 percent of those with two-vessel CAD, 60 percent of those with three-vessel CAD, and 65 percent of those with left main disease.

The low sensitivity of FPRNA for detection of exercise-induced regional wall motion abnormalities occurs for at least two important reasons. First, the exercise FPRNA is typically acquired in only one view, which precludes detection of disease in nonvisualized segments. Newer dual-headed detectors may permit biplane first-pass studies during exercise. Second, the spatial resolution of the first-pass technique is inadequate for detection of subtle changes in regional function. No large trials of sensitivity or specificity are available that take advantage of the newer generations of first-pass cameras, which have much better energy and spatial resolution than the cameras of the 1970s that were used to generate most of the existing data. As indicated previously, various parametric images that are more sensitive to three-dimensional count changes, and thereby potentially more sensitive than the standard visual assessment of the beating chamber, have been advocated to improve the sensitivity of the first-pass method;[42] however, such approaches have not been rigorously tested.

Ejection Fraction

The LVEF response to exercise has long been advocated as a criterion for the diagnosis of CAD. Early experience suggested that the LVEF would increase by at least 0.05 ejection fraction units during dynamic exercise in normal subjects. Failure to increase the LVEF by 0.05 became a diagnostic criterion with early claims of very high sensitivity.[63–66] Unfortunately, the early work in this area was skewed by the fact that the majority of subjects in the studies had extensive CAD, which would typically lead to global left ventricular dysfunction during exercise. If localized ischemia occurs that does not involve enough myocardium, there may be no changes in global left ventricular function, so LVEF alone would not have a high sensitivity for detection of a wide range of CAD extent and severity. In addition, after much more experience with radionuclide angiography, it has become clear that there are many possible reasons for failure of the LVEF to increase by 0.05 during exercise. Female patients seem to rely more on an increase in end-diastolic volume than on an increase in LVEF.[67, 68] Healthy older

TABLE 60–3. SENSITIVITY AND SPECIFICITY OF EXERCISE FIRST-PASS RADIONUCLIDE ANGIOGRAPHY FOR DETECTION OF CORONARY ARTERY DISEASE

	Men (n = 173)		Women (n = 56)		All	
Criterion	*Sens (%)*	*Spec (%)*	*Sens (%)*	*Spec (%)*	*Sens (%)*	*Spec (%)*
ΔEF less than 5%	82	73	78	46	81	60
Ex EF at least 6% less than predicted	85	81	50	71	79	76
Ex wall motion abnormality	56	96	38	88	53	92

Δ = Exercise minus rest; EF = left ventricular ejection fraction; Ex = exercise; Sens = sensitivity; Spec = specificity.
Adapted from Jones, R. H., McEwan, P., Newman, G. E., et al.: Accuracy of diagnosis of coronary artery disese by radionuclide measurement of left ventricular function during rest and exercise. Circulation 64:586, 1981, with permission.

subjects have been shown to have a blunted LVEF response to exercise.[69] Isometric exercise results in an acute drop in LVEF,[70] and the exact exercise protocol itself may influence the LVEF response.[71] Both the resting LVEF[72] and the change in end-diastolic volume during exercise[67] appear to influence the change in LVEF during exercise. The ejection fraction response may also be altered by hypertension or valvular heart disease.

Given all the factors that can affect the LVEF response to exercise, it is not surprising that the use of an LVEF criterion, whether it be failure to increase by 0.05, or failure to increase at all, or even a drop in LVEF, has a poor specificity for the diagnosis of CAD[40, 62] (see Table 60–3). In the largest study of the subject, the specificity of a failure to increase the LVEF by 0.05 was only 60 percent, and the sensitivity was 81 percent.[62] For that reason, some investigators have suggested the use of an equation to predict the LVEF response based on age, sex, change in end-diastolic volume, and other factors.[67] If the observed LVEF response is lower than that predicted by the model, CAD can diagnosed with an improved specificity of 76 percent, and sensitivity remains at 79 percent. Sensitivity is further increased by restriction of the analysis to those patients who achieve an adequate exercise end point. An alternative approach is to use an absolute exercise LVEF based on the lowest exercise LVEF of an age-matched, normal reference population. That value may vary from one laboratory to another because of differences in data processing, but an exercise LVEF of approximately 0.55 is reasonable.

Although ejection fraction criteria do not perform very well for the detection of all CAD, exercise LVEF does vary inversely with the extent and severity of coronary disease.[57] Therefore, it has been used to identify patients with a large ischemic burden—that is, those most likely to have multivessel or left main disease[58–60] and those most likely to benefit from revascularization.[73]

Pharmacologic Interventions

There is ample evidence to support the diagnostic use of myocardial perfusion imaging after pharmacologic coronary vasodilatation with dipyridamole[74, 75] and adenosine.[76] There is also evidence that myocardial perfusion imaging can be linked to catecholamine administration for the diagnosis of CAD.[77] There is less evidence that ventricular function imaging during pharmacologic stimulation is useful diagnostically. Some investigators have reported a high sensitivity for the detection of CAD by using transthoracic echocardiography during coronary vasodilatation[78, 79] or during dobutamine infusion.[80, 81] Gated equilibrium radionuclide angiography has been found to be modestly sensitive but quite specific for the diagnosis of CAD when performed after a dipyridamole infusion,[82] and it has recently been used with some success during dobutamine infusion as well.[83] We have tested the value of adding a first-pass acquisition to both dipyridamole and dobutamine myocardial perfusion imaging and have not found it to be incrementally useful. Our preliminary experience from a study comparing exercise to dobutamine first-pass left ventricular function suggests that the two types of stress produce very different results.

Combined Function-Perfusion Imaging

The combination of rest and exercise ventricular function imaging with rest and exercise tomographic myocardial perfusion imaging provides the most comprehensive noninvasive assessment of the patient with known or suspected CAD. Every important diagnostic and prognostic variable described noninvasively can be assessed or quantified. This approach has tremendous appeal and has rekindled interest in first-pass imaging.

Several attempts to perform both ventricular function and myocardial perfusion imaging during a single exercise test have been made in the past. The rationale was to improve the diagnostic sensitivity over that of either test alone and to add the well-recognized prognostic value of the exercise LVEF to the perfusion data. The early work used the simultaneous injection of short-lived radionuclides such as ^{195m}Au[84] and ^{191}Ir[85] along with ^{201}Tl. A first-pass study was acquired during exercise by imaging the gold or the iridium, and perfusion scanning then followed the decay of the short-lived isotope. More recently, the introduction of technetium-based myocardial perfusion imaging agents has made it possible to routinely acquire first-pass studies at peak exercise and subsequently to perform myocardial perfusion imaging of the same agent.[3–7] Preliminary evidence suggests that the diagnostic sensitivity is improved over that of perfusion imaging alone for the detection of ischemia[4] or of multivessel disease.[86] In a study of 86 patients with documented CAD, a stepwise analysis showed that the perfusion data contained two thirds of the diagnostic information and the first-pass exercise function data added an independent one third of the total diagnostic information.[4] More recently, it was shown that the addition of the first-pass wall motion analysis increased the detection of multivessel CAD from 64 percent to 83 percent.[86]

Because regional perfusion abnormalities, by definition, must be present before regional dysfunction can occur, one must question why functional imaging would improve the detection of multivessel disease. The answer is probably related to the fact that all single-photon perfusion imaging methods look at relative perfusion, comparing uptake in one segment to that of an adjacent segment. If perfusion is homogeneously reduced, as may occur in multivessel disease, it may be more difficult to appreciate all the abnormalities of perfusion. In contrast, ventricular dysfunction becomes progressively more extensive as the disease increases in extent. It would appear, then, that exercise ventricular function data do add diagnostically independent information to that contained in perfusion images.

From the standpoint of clinical practice and interpretation, we have found that the addition of functional imaging to perfusion imaging greatly enhances diagnostic confidence. An initial stress function-perfusion study allows us to be much more confident of our results, especially normal studies; as a result, fewer patients return for resting imaging, with consequent savings in time, radiation exposure, and cost. There are specific groups of patients in whom the exercise FPRNA may obviate the need for using imaging. One is the group of patients whose stress scans are equivocally abnormal. If exercise left ventricular function is unequivocally normal, such patients are diagnosed as being normal or as having prognostically insignificant CAD. The second group includes patients whose exercise perfusion scans are abnormal but whose exercise function is either so well preserved that further testing may not be necessary or so abnormal as to mandate catheterization.

In order to successfully implement the combined function-perfusion strategy, it is important to select the proper imaging sequence. We routinely perform the exercise study first and use 25-mCi injections to ensure a high-quality first-pass study. If a resting study is necessary, it must be performed on a separate day. We also use a dedicated multicrystal camera for the first-pass studies so that tomographic perfusion acquisitions are not interrupted. For studies that must be performed on the same day, a rest-stress sequence should be used so that the higher-dose study is the exercise study. The resting first-pass study, using 10 mCi, may be technically suboptimal in large patients, if there are few beats for analysis, or if a single-crystal gamma camera is used.

Preliminary comparisons of exercise LVEF to quantitative perfusion defect size suggest a linear correlation.[4] In general, subjects with small perfusion defects have exercise ejection fractions above 0.50, which would put them in a very favorable prognostic category, whereas subjects with large perfusion defect scores tend to have exercise LVEFs below 0.35, which would put them in an unfavorable prognostic category. Thus, for patients at the extremes of exercise perfusion defect sizes, the addition of functional data may not be helpful prognostically. However, for those patients with exercise perfusion defect scores in the intermediate range, the exercise LVEF can vary widely, suggesting that its prognostic role would be most important in that patient subset (Fig. 60–21).

Another important benefit of combined function-perfusion imaging is the enhanced diagnostic capability afforded the physician by the ability to interrogate diastole as well as systole. In Figure 60–22, the function-perfusion data from a patient with suspected coronary artery disease failed to confirm coronary disease but did demonstrate clear diastolic left ventricular dysfunction that had not been suspected clinically.

FIGURE 60–22. See Color Plate 28.

Perhaps the most important benefit of adding exercise function data to the perfusion data is the prognostic application of the exercise LVEF.

Prognosis in Stable Coronary Artery Disease

The prognosis of patients with stable CAD is directly related to the contractile state of the left ventricle. Large series of both medically and surgically treated patients have been followed for several years, and the data from different investigators confirm that the resting LVEF, measured either invasively or noninvasively, is a powerful predictor of subsequent outcome.[87, 88] Follow-up data are now available that address the prognostic roles of the resting LVEF, the exercise LVEF, and the change in LVEF from rest to exercise (ΔLVEF) in a cohort of patients with CAD followed during medical management after baseline catheterization. As noted in earlier work, the resting LVEF proved to be a powerful predictor of prognosis; however, the peak exercise LVEF proved to be even more powerful in predicting subsequent mortality.[28, 89] The ΔLVEF was of little prognostic significance if the exercise LVEF was included in a multivariable model. That finding has been confirmed by another group with the use of gated equilibrium data.[90] When the radionuclide data were compared with the clinical and catheterization-derived variables, it was shown that the combination of the radionuclide data and the clinical data contained as much or more prognostic information as that available from a catheterization (Table 60–4). Therefore, the noninvasive evaluation of patients with CAD, including a determination of exercise LVEF, may be used as a surrogate for cardiac catheterization for prediction of outcome.

TABLE 60–4. COMPARISON OF PROGNOSTIC INFORMATION FROM CLINICAL, RADIONUCLIDE, AND CATHETERIZATION VARIABLES

	Total Model Chi-Squared Test Values	
	CV Death	*CV Events*
Clinical	71	48
Catheterization	102	64
RNA	104	66
Clinical + RNA	120	78
Clinical + Catheterization	124	82
Clinical + Catheterization + RNA	138	93

CV = cardiovascular; RNA = radionuclide angiography.
From Lee, K. L., Pryor, D. B., Pieper, K. S., et al.: Prognostic value of radionuclide angiography in medically treated patients with coronary artery disease. Circulation 82:1705, 1990, with permission.

Figure 60–23 shows mortality and infarct-free survival plotted against the exercise LVEF. Patients with an exercise LVEF greater than 0.50 have an excellent long-term outlook. Mortality increases sharply after the exercise LVEF drops below 0.35. Other investigators, using gated equilibrium RNA, have suggested that there is prognostic information in the ΔLVEF. In a study of mildly symptomatic patients with three-vessel disease, those whose LVEF fell during exercise had more subsequent events than those whose LVEF increased during exercise.[91] All deaths in that study occurred in the subgroup with a drop in LVEF and 1-mm ST segment depression during exercise. The differences between study results

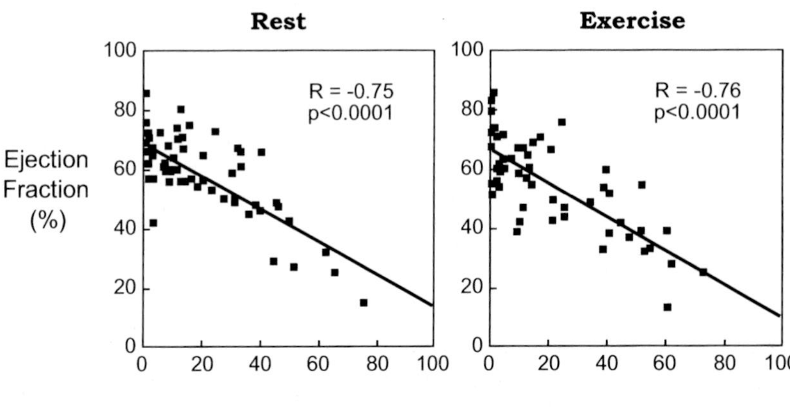

FIGURE 60–21. The ejection fraction does correlate linearly with the perfusion defect score acquired during the same exercise test, but there is a fairly wide scatter of ejection fractions for any given exercise perfusion defect score, especially for those in the intermediate range of severity. (From Borges-Neto, S., Coleman, R.E., Potts, J.M., et al.: Combined exercise radionuclide angiocardiography and single photon emission computed tomography perfusion studies for assessment of coronary disease. Semin. Nucl. Med. 21:223, 1991, reprinted with permission.)

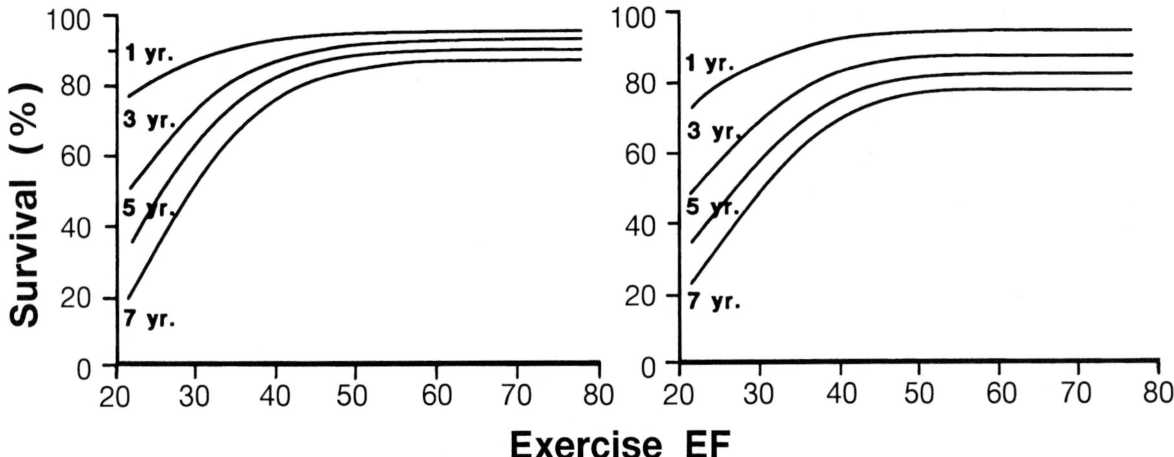

FIGURE 60–23. Total survival *(left)* and infarct-free survival *(right)* are plotted against the exercise ejection fraction. Prognosis is very stable for ejection fractions greater than 0.50. Survival drops sharply with exercise LVEFs below 0.35. (From Lee, K.L., Pryor, D.B., Pieper, K.S., et al.: Prognostic value of radionuclide angiography in medically treated patients with coronary artery disease. Circulation 82:1705, 1990, with permission.)

are certainly related, at least in part, to differences in the populations included. Although some controversy exists regarding which of the three variables (rest LVEF, exercise LVEF, or ΔLVEF) is most important in a particular population, there is certainly universal agreement that the LVEF can be used to stratify patients according to their likelihood of subsequent mortality. Although most of the data on prognosis and ejection fraction relate to patients with stable CAD, similar results have been demonstrated for patients soon after acute myocardial infarction.[92] There are also data to suggest that the same relation is true for predicting outcome in patients after surgical revascularization.

No prospective study has been performed that has examined the outcome of patients randomly assigned to treatment strategies based on the results of noninvasive testing. In a nonprospective, nonrandomized study of patients with normal resting left ventricular function, it was shown that those with the greatest fall in LVEF during exercise preoperatively showed the most benefit in terms of pain relief and longevity after bypass surgery.[73] Data such as these suggest that a prospective treatment trial based on pretreatment noninvasive descriptors would be appropriate.

Evaluation of Patients With Chronic Obstructive Pulmonary Disease

As with the left ventricle, the function of the right ventricle is related to the afterload presented to it, which in turn is related to the pulmonary arterial pressure or pulmonary vascular resistance. If pulmonary hypertension is present, RVEF may be decreased. Using first-pass data, RVEF has been shown to vary inversely with pulmonary pressure in patients with chronic obstructive pulmonary disease.[93] Patients with clinical cor pulmonale tend to have lower RVEF than those with chronic obstructive pulmonary disease without heart failure. In addition, an abnormal resting RVEF in the presence of chronic obstructive pulmonary disease may be predictive of the subsequent appearance of cor pulmonale.[94] Patients with chronic obstructive pulmonary disease and a normal resting RVEF may have an abnormal RVEF response to exercise.[95]

FIRST-PASS VERSUS EQUILIBRIUM RADIONUCLIDE ANGIOGRAPHY

The selection of first-pass or gated equilibrium radionuclide angiography should depend on the clinical question being asked. The gated equilibrium method provides higher spatial resolution and the ability to obtain multiple views or image multiple physiologic states. It requires prolonged acquisition times and is limited to the septal view for quantitative data. The first-pass study trades speed for spatial resolution and allows quantitation in multiple views. Some laboratories have little experience with FPRNA, and the local technical expertise must therefore be considered.

For most studies of left ventricular function at rest, the higher resolution, the ability to obtain multiple views, and the possibility of tomographic acquisitions make gated equilibrium imaging the procedure of choice. If right ventricular function is clinically important, a first-pass study may be performed in conjunction with a gated study in order to provide the best RVEF and high-resolution wall motion data. During exercise, the speed of the first-pass study is a major advantage and FPRNA becomes the procedure of choice. If there is a specific question about the presence or significance of a circumflex lesion, a gated exercise study may be preferable, because the septal LAO view on first-pass studies frequently suffers from left atrial–left ventricular overlap. The presence of baseline arrhythmias such as very irregular atrial fibrillation, frequent premature ventricular beats, or ventricular bigeminy is problematic for both methods, but the first-pass approach is more likely to produce an unacceptable result owing to the paucity of sinus beats during the ventricular phase of the study.

For the evaluation of congenital heart disease, especially in those cases in which a left-to-right shunt is suspected, the first-pass method or a combination of the two is preferable.

SUMMARY

Despite the proliferation of methods for imaging the heart, no technique surpasses the speed and simplicity of FPRNA for the evaluation of ventricular function during exercise. The technique therefore enjoys a unique role in the evaluation of coronary artery disease. The ability to combine first-pass imaging with tomographic perfusion imaging improves the diagnostic and prognostic capabilities of radionuclide exercise testing. This ability should increase the value of noninvasive testing and ultimately reduce the overall cost of the evaluation of the patient with known or suspected CAD.

References

1. Blumgart, H.L., and Weiss, S.: Studies on the velocity of blood flow: VII. The pulmonary circulation time in normal resting individuals. J. Clin. Invest. 4:399, 1927.
2. Mason, D.T., Ashburn, W.L., Harbert, J.C., et al.: Rapid sequential visualization

of the heart and great vessels in man using the wide-field Anger scintillation camera. Circulation 39:19, 1969.
3. Jones, R.H., Borges-Neto, S., and Potts, J.M.: Simultaneous measurement of myocardial perfusion and ventricular function during exercise from a single injection of technetium-99m sestamibi in coronary artery disease. Am. J. Cardiol. 66:68E, 1990.
4. Borges-Neto, S., Coleman, R.E., Potts, J.M., et al.: Combined exercise radionuclide angiocardiography and single photon emission computed tomography perfusion studies for assessment of coronary disease. Semin. Nucl. Med. 21:223, 1991.
5. Johnson, L.L., Rodney, R.A., Vaccarino, R.A., et al.: Left ventricular perfusion and performance from a single radiopharmaceutical and one camera. J. Nucl. Med. 33:1411, 1992.
6. Williams, K.A., Taillon, L.A., Draho, J.M., et al.: First-pass radionuclide angiographic studies of left ventricular function with technetium-99m-teboroxime, technetium-99m sestamibi and technetium-99m-DTPA. J. Nucl. Med. 34:394, 1993.
7. Takahashi, N., Tamaki, N., Tadamura, E., et al.: Combined assessment of regional perfusion and wall motion in patients with coronary artery disease with technetium-99m-tetrofosmin. J. Nucl. Cardiol. 1:29, 1994.
8. Treves, S., Cheng, C., Samuel, A., et al.: Iridium-191 angiocardiography for the detection and quantitation of left-to-right shunting. J. Nucl. Med. 21:1151, 1980.
9. Mena, I., Narahara, K.A., de Jong, R., et al.: Gold-195m, an ultra-short-lived generator-produced radionuclide: Clinical application in sequential first pass ventriculography. J. Nucl. Med. 24:139, 1983.
10. Adams, R., Lacy, J.L., Ball, M.E., et al.: The count rate performance of a multiwire gamma camera measured by a decaying source method with 9.3-minute tantalum-178. J. Nucl. Med. 31:1723, 1990.
11. Lacy, J.L., Layne, W.W., Guidry, G.W., et al.: Development and clinical performance of an automated, portable tungsten-178/tantalum-178 generator. J. Nucl. Med. 32:2158, 1991.
12. Verani, M.S., Lacy, J.L., Guidry, G.W., et al.: Quantification of left ventricular performance during transient coronary occlusion at various anatomic sites in humans: A study using tantalum-178 and a multiwire gamma camera. J. Am. Coll. Cardiol. 19:297, 1992.
13. Gal, R., Grenier, R.P., Carpenter, J., et al.: High count rate first-pass radionuclide angiography using a digital gamma camera. J. Nucl. Med. 27:198, 1986.
14. Nichols, K., DePuey, E.G., Gooneratne, N., et al.: First-pass ventricular ejection fraction using a single-crystal nuclear camera. J. Nucl. Med. 35:1292, 1994.
15. Bowyer, K.W., Konstantinow, G., Rerych, S.K., et al.: Optimum counting intervals in radionuclide cardiac studies. *In* Nuclear Cardiology: Selected Computer Aspects. Symposium Proceedings, New York, Society of Nuclear Medicine, 1978, p. 85.
16. Rerych, S.K., Scholz, P.M., Newman, G.E., et al.: Cardiac function at rest and during exercise in normals and in patients with coronary heart disease: Evaluation by radionuclide angiocardiography. Ann. Surg. 187:449, 1978.
17. Berger, H.I., Reduto, L.A., Johnstone, D.E., et al.: Global and regional left ventricular response to bicycle exercise in coronary artery disease. Am. J. Med. 66:13, 1979.
18. Potts, J.M., Borges-Neto, S., Smith, L.R., et al.: Comparison of bicycle and treadmill radionuclide angiocardiography. J. Nucl. Med. 32:1918, 1991.
19. Friedman, J.D., Berman, D.S., Kiat, H., et al.: Rest and treadmill exercise first-pass radionuclide ventriculography: Validation of left ventricular ejection fraction measurements. J. Nucl. Cardiol. 4:382, 1994.
20. Rerych, S.K., Scholz, P.M., Newman, G.E., et al.: Cardiac function at rest and during exercise in normals and in patients with coronary heart disease: Evaluation by radionuclide angiocardiography. Ann. Surg. 187:449, 1978.
21. Berger, H.I., Reduto, L.A., Johnstone, D.E., et al.: Global and regional left ventricular response to bicycle exercise in coronary artery disease. Am. J. Med. 66:13, 1979.
22. Jengo, M.A., Mena, I., Blaufuss, A., et al.: Evaluation of left ventricular function (ejection fraction and segmental wall motion) by single pass radioisotope aniography. Circulation 57:326, 1978.
23. Marshall, R.C., Berger, H.J., Costin, J.C., et al.: Assessment of cardiac performance with quantitative radionuclide angiocardiography. Circulation 56:820, 1977.
24. Gal, R., Grenier, R.P., Schmidt, D.H., et al.: Background correction in first-pass radionuclide angiography: Comparison of several approaches. J. Nucl. Med. 27:1480, 1986.
25. Scholz, P.M., Rerych, S.K., Moran, J.F., et al.: Quantitative radionuclide angiocardiography. Cathet. Cardiovasc. Diagn. 6:265, 1980.
26. Bodenheimer, M.M., Banka, V.S., Fooshee, C.M., et al.: Quantitative radionuclide angiography in the right anterior oblique view: Comparison with contrast ventriculography. Am. J. Cardiol. 41:718, 1978.
27. Wackers, F.J.Th.: First-pass radionuclide angiocardiography. *In* Gerson MC (ed.): Cardiac Nuclear Medicine. New York, McGraw-Hill, 1991, p. 67.
28. Pryor, D.B., Harrel, F.E., Lee, K.L., et al.: Prognostic indicators from radionuclide angiography in medically treated patients with coronary artery disease. Am. J. Cadiol. 53:18, 1984.
29. Marshall, R.C., Berger, H.J., Reduto, L.A., et al: Variability in sequential measures of left ventricular performance assessed with radionuclide angiocardiography. Am. J. Cardiol. 41:531, 1978.
30. Upton, M.T., Rerych, S.K., Newman, G.E., et al.: The reproducibility of radionuclide angiographic measurements of LV function in normal subjects at rest and during exercise. Circulation 62:126, 1980.
31. Anderson, P.A.W., Rerych, S.K., Moore, T.E., et al.: Accuracy of left ventricular end-diastolic dimension determinations obtained by radionuclide angiocardiography. J. Nucl. Med. 22:500, 1981.
32. Nickel, O., Schad, N., Andrews, E.J., et al.: Scintigraphic measurement of left ventricular volumes from the count-density distribution. J. Nucl. Med. 23:404, 1982.
33. Massardo, T., Gal, R.A., Grenier, R.P., et al.: Left ventricular volume calculations using a count based ratio method applied to multigated radionuclide angiography. J. Nucl. Med. 31:450, 1990.
34. Levy, W.C., Cerqueira, M.D., Matsuoka, D.T., et al.: Four radionuclide methods for left ventricular volume determination: Comparison of a manual and an automated technqiue. J. Nucl. Med. 33:763, 1992.
35. Gal, R., Grenier, R.P., Port, S.C., et al.: Left ventricular volume calculation using a count-based ratio method applied to first-pass radionuclide angiography. J. Nucl. Med. 33:2124, 1992.
36. Berger, H.J., Matthay, R.A., Loke, J., et al.: Assessment of cardiac performance with quantitative radionuclide angiocardiography: Right ventricular ejection fraction with reference to findings in chronic obstructive pulmonary disease. Am. J. Cardiol. 41:897, 1978.
37. Huang, P.J., Su, C.T., Lee, Y.T., et al.: Right ventricular ejection fraction: Validation of first-pass radionuclide studies by contrast angiography. Jpn. Heart J. 25:533, 1984.
38. Winzelberg, G.G., Boucher, C.A., Pohost, G.M., et al.: Right ventricular function in aortic and mitral valve disease. Chest 79:520, 1981.
39. Morrison, D.A., Turgeon, J., and Ouitt, T.: Right ventricular ejection fraction measurements: Contrast ventriculography versus gated blood pool and gated first-pass method. Am. J. Cardiol. 54:651, 1984.
40. Osbakken, M.D., Boucher, C.A., Okada, R.D., et al.: Spectrum of global left ventricular responses to supine exercise: Limitation in the use of ejection fraction in identifying patients with coronary artery disease. Am. J. Cardiol. 51:28, 1983.
41. Hanley, P.C., and Gibbons, R.J.: Value of radionuclide-determined changes in pulmonary blood volume for the detection of coronary artery disease. Chest 97:7, 1990.
42. Schad, N., Andrews, E.S., and Fleming, J.W.: Colour Atlas of First-Pass Functional Imaging of the Heart. Hingham, MTP Press Ltd., 1985.
43. Sheehan, F.H., Mathey, D.G., Schofer, J., et al.: Effect of interventions in salvaging left ventricular function in acute myocardial infarction: A study of intracoronary streptokinase. Am. J. Cardiol. 52:431, 1983.
44. Sheehan, F.H., Mathey, D.G., Schofer, J., et al.: Effect of interventions in salvaging left ventricular function in acute myocardial infarction: A study of intracoronary streptokinase. Am. J. Cardiol. 52:431, 1983.
45. Zaret, B.L., and Wackers, F.J.. Radionuclide methods for evaluating the results of thrombolytic therapy. Circulation 76:118, 1987.
46. Reduto, L.A., Wickemeyer, W.J., Young, J.B., et al.: Left ventricular diastolic performance at rest and during exercise in patients with coronary artery disease. Circulation 63:1228, 1981.
47. Polak, J.F., Kemper, A.J., Bianco, J.A., et al.: Resting early peak diastolic filling rate: A sensitive index of myocardial dysfunction in patients with coronary artery disease. J. Nucl. Med. 23:471, 1982.
48. Aroney, C.N., Ruddy, T.D., Dighero, H., et al.: Differentiation of restrictive cardiomyopathy from pericardial constriction: Assessment of diastolic function by radionuclide angiography. J. Am. Coll. Cardiol. 13:1007, 1989.
49. Philippe, L., Mena, I., Darcourt, J., et al.: Evaluation of valvular regurgitation by factor analysis of first-pass angiography. J. Nucl. Med. 29:159, 1988.
50. Kanishi, Y., Tatsuta, N., Hikasa, Y., et al.: Assessment of tricuspid regurgitation by analog computer analysis of dilution curves recorded by scintillation camera. Jpn. Circ. J. 46:1147, 1982.
51. Janowitz, W.R., and Fester, A.: Quantitation of left ventricular regurgitant fraction by first pass radionuclide angiocardiography. Am. J. Cardiol. 49:85, 1982.
52. Braunwald, E., Tannenbaum, H.L., and Morrow, A.G.: Localization of left-to right cardiac shunts by dye-dilution curves following injection into the left side of the heart and into the aorta. Am. J. Med. 24:203, 1958.
53. Maltz, D.L., and Treves, S.: Quantitative radionuclide angiocardiography: Determination of Qp:Qs in children. Circulation 47:1048, 1973.
54. Askenazi, J., Ahnberg, D.S., Korngold, E., et al.: Quantitative radionuclide angiocardiography: Detection and quantitation of left to right shunts. Am. J. Cardiol. 37:382, 1976.
55. Peter, C.A., Armstrong, B.E., and Jones, R.H.: Radionuclide quantitation of right-to-left intracardiac shunts in children. Circulation 64:572, 1981.
56. Dogan, A.S., Rezai, K., Kirchner, P.T., et al.: A scintigraphic sign for detection of right-to-left shunts. J. Nucl. Med. 34:1607, 1993.
57. DePace, N.L., Iskandrian, A.S., Hakki, A., et al.: Value of left ventricular ejection fraction during exercise in predicting the extent of coronary artery disease. J. Am. Coll. Cardiol. 1:1002, 1983.
58. Johnson, S.H., Bigelow, C., Lee, K.L., et al.: Prediction of death and myocardial infarction by radionuclide angiocardiography in patients with suspected coronary artery disease. Am. J. Cardiol. 67:919, 1991.
59. Weintraub, W.S., Schneider, R.M., Seelaus, P.A., et al.: Prospective evaluation of the severity of coronary artery disease with exercise radionuclide angiography and electrocardiography. Am. Heart J. 111:537, 1986.
60. Gibbons, R.J., Fyke, F.E., III, Clements, I.P., et al: Noninvasive identification of severe coronary artery disease using exercise radionuclide angiography. J. Am. Coll. Cardiol. 11:28, 1988.
61. Campos, C.T., Chu, H.W., D'Agostino, H.J., Jr., et al.: Comparison of rest and exercise radionuclide angiocardiography and exercise treadmill testing for diagnosis of anatomically extensive coronary artery disease. Circulation 67:1204, 1983.
62. Jones, R.H., McEwen, P., Newman, G.E., et al.: Accuracy of diagnosis of coronary artery disease by radionuclide measurement of left ventricular function during rest and exercise. Circulation 64:586, 1981.
63. Rerych, S.K., Scholz, P.M., Newman, G.E., et al.: Cardiac function at rest and

during exercise in normals and patients with coronary artery disease. Ann. Surg. 187:449, 1978.
64. Borer, J.S., Kent, K.M., Bacharach, S.L., et al.: Sensitivity, specificity and predictive accuracy of radionuclide cineangiography during exercise in patients with coronary artery disease. Circulation 60:572, 1979.
65. Berger, H., Reduto, L., Johnstone, D., et al.: Global and regional left ventricular response to bicycle exercise in coronary artery disease: Assessment by quantitative radionuclide angiocardiography. Am. J. Med. 66:13, 1979.
66. Jengo, J.A., Oren, V., Conant, R., et al.: Effects of maximal exercise stress on left ventricular function in patients with coronary artery disease using first pass radionuclide angiocardiography: A rapid noninvasive technique for determining ejection fraction and segmented wall motion. Circulation 59:60, 1979.
67. Gibbons, R.J., Lee, K.L., Cobb, F., et al.: Ejection fraction response to exercise in patients with chest pain and normal coronary arteriograms. Circulation 64:952, 1981.
68. Higginbotham, M.B., Morris, K.B., Coleman, R.E., et al.: Sex-related differences in the normal cardiac response to upright exercise. Circulation 70:357, 1984.
69. Port, S.C., Cobb, F.R., Coleman, E., et al.: Effect of age on the response of the left ventricular ejection fraction to exercise. N. Engl. J. Med. 303:1133, 1980.
70. Peter, C.A., and Jones, R.H.: Effects of isometric handgrip and dynamic exercise on left ventricular function. J. Nucl. Med. 21:1131, 1980.
71. Foster, C., Dymond, D.S., Anholm, J.D., et al.: Effect of exercise protocol on the left ventricular response to exercise. Am. J. Cardiol. 51:859, 1983.
72. Port, S.C., McEwan, P., Cobb, F.R., et al.: Influence of resting left ventricular function on the left ventricular response to exercise in patients with coronary artery disease. Circulation 63:856, 1981.
73. Jones, R.H., Floyd, R.D., Austin, E.H., et al.: The role of radionuclide angiocardiography in the preoperative prediction of pain relief and prolonged survival following coronary artery bypass grafting. Ann. Surg. 197:743, 1983.
74. Leppo, J., Boucher, C.A., Okada, R.D., et al.: Serial thallium-201, myocardial imaging after dipyridamole infusion:diagnostic utility in detecting coronary stenoses and relationship to reginal wall motion. Circulation 66:649, 1982.
75. Leppo, J.A.: Dipyridamole-thallium imaging: The lazy man's stress test. J. Nucl. Med. 30:281, 1989.
76. Verani, M.S., Mahmarian, J.J., Hixson, J.B., et al.: Diagnosis of coronary artery disease by controlled coronary vasodilation with adenosine and thallium-201 scintigraphy in patients unable to exercise. Circulation 82:80, 1990.
77. Pennell, D.J., Underwood, S.R., Swanton, R.H., et al.: Dobutamine thallium myocardial perfusion tomography. J. Am. Coll. Cardiol. 18:1471, 1991.
78. Picano, E., Lattanzi, F., Masini, M., et al.: High-dose dipyridamole echocardiography in effort angina pectoris. J. Am. Coll. Cardiol. 8:848, 1986.
79. Masini, M., Picano, E., Lattanzi, F., et al.: High dose dipyridamole-echocardiography test in women: Correlation with exercise-electrocardiography test and coronary arteriography. J. Am. Coll. Cardiol. 12:682, 1988.
80. Cohen, J.L., Greene, T.O., Ottenweller, J., et al.: Dobutamine digital echocardiography for detecting coronary artery disease. Am. J. Cardiol. 67:1311, 1991.
81. Baudhuin, T., Marwick, T., Melin, J., et al.: Diagnosis of coronary artery disease in elderly patients: Safety and efficacy of dobutamine echocardiography. Eur. Heart J. 14:799, 1993.
82. Cates, C.U., Kronenberg, M.W., Collins, H.W., et al.: Dipyridamole radionuclide ventriculography: A test with high specificity for severe coronary artery disease. J. Am. Coll. Cardiol. 13:841, 1989.
83. Bahl, V.K., Vasan, R.S., Malhotra, A., et al.: A comparison of dobutamine infusion and exercise during radionuclide ventriculography in the evaluation of coronary arterial disease. Int. J. Cardiol. 35:49, 1992.
84. Narahara, K.A., Mena, I., Maublaut, J.C., et al.: Simultaneous maximum exercise radionuclide angiography and thallium stress perfusion imaging. Am. J. Cardiol. 53:812, 1984.
85. Verani, M.S., Lacy, J.L., Ball, M.E., et al.: Simultaneous assessment of regional ventricular function and perfusion utilizing iridium-191m and thallium-201 during a single exercise test. Am. J. Cardiol. Imaging 2:206, 1988.
86. Palmas, W., Friedman, J.D., Kiat, H., et al.: Improved identification of multiple-vessel coronary artery disease by addition of exercise wall motion analysis to Tc-99m-sestamibi myocardial perfusion SPECT. (Abstract.) J. Nucl. Med. 34:1308, 1993.
87. Harris, P.J., Harrell, F.E., Jr., Lee, K.L., et al.: Nonfatal myocardial infarct in medically treated patients with coronary artery disease. Circulation 62:240, 1980.
88. Coronary Artery Surgery Study Principal Investigators: Coronary Artery Surgery Study (CASS): A randomized trial of coronary bypass surgery. Survival date. Circulation 68:989, 1983.
89. Lee, K.L., Pryor, D.B., Pieper, K.S., et al.: Prognostic value of radionuclide angiography in medically treated patients with coronary artery disease. Circulation 82:1705, 1990.
90. Iqbal, A., Gibbons, R.J., Zinmeister, A.R., et al.: Prognostic value of exercise radionuclide angiography in a population-based cohort of patients with known or suspected coronary artery disease. Am. J. Cardiol. 74:119, 1994.
91. Bonow, R.O., Kent, K.M., Rosing, D.R., et al.: Exercise-induced ischemia in mildly symptomatic patients with coronary artery disease and preseved left ventricular function: Identification of subgroups at risk of death during medical therapy. N. Engl. J. Med. 311:1339, 1984.
92. Morris, K.G., Palmeri, S.T., Califf, R.M., et al.: Value of radionuclide angiography for predicting specific cardiac events after acute myocardial infarction. Am. J. Cardiol. 55:318, 1985.
93. Brent, B.N., Mahler, D., Matthay, R.A., et al.: Noninvasive diagnosis of pulmonary arterial hypertension in chronic obstructive pulmonary disease: Right ventricular ejection fraction at rest. Am. J. Cardiol. 53:1349, 1984.
94. Berger, H.J., Matthay, R.A., Loke, J., et al.: Assessment of cardiac performance with quantitative radionuclide angiography: Right ventricular ejection fraction with reference to findings in chronic obstructive pulmonary disease. Am. J. Cardiol. 41:897, 1978.
95. Matthay, R.A., Berger, H.J., Davies, R.A., et al.: Right and left ventricular exercise performance in chronic obstructive pulmonary disease: Radionuclide assessment. Ann. Intern. Med. 93:234, 1980.

CHAPTER

61 Equilibrium Radionuclide Angiography

Raymond J. Gibbons, M.D.
Todd D. Miller, M.D.

TECHNICAL ASPECTS

Equilibrium radionuclide angiography, also known as radionuclide ventriculography or gated blood pool imaging, is a well-established, noninvasive technique for the assessment of ventricular function. Red blood cells are labeled with technetium-99m (^{99m}Tc), allowed to distribute uniformly throughout the blood volume, and then imaged with a standard single-crystal gamma camera.

This chapter reviews the technical aspects of equilibrium radionuclide angiography, the measurements that can be made with the use of this modality, and its application to a variety of clinical situations.

Red Blood Cell Labeling

The in vitro method[1, 2] of red blood cell labeling requires withdrawal of a small quantity (less than 10 mL) of blood from the patient. The blood is mixed with stannous citrate and gently agitated for approximately 5 minutes. After centrifugation, the red blood cells are mixed with ^{99m}Tc and incubated for 5 minutes, after which they are reinjected into the patient and allowed to distribute throughout the blood volume. This method is time-consuming and technically demanding. In contrast, the in vivo method,[3, 4] which is carried out completely within the patient, is rapid and technically simple. Several milligrams of stannous pyrophosphate are injected intravenously and allowed to circulate for approximately 30 minutes. During this time, the stannous ion binds to the red blood cells. A separate intravenous injection of 20 to 30 mCi of ^{99m}Tc-pertechnetate is then performed. The ^{99m}Tc will label red blood cells over the ensuing 5 minutes. Since ^{99m}Tc is injected separately as an intravenous bolus, first-pass measurements of right ventricular function can be performed during the same study. The major disadvantage of this method is that a significant portion of the injected radionuclide dose will distribute to the thyroid gland, the stomach, and the kidneys before binding to the red blood cells. The activity in noncardiac organs will therefore be considerable. The activity in the stomach may contribute significantly to the background counts within the cardiac image. In addition, this method has a reduced labeling efficiency in some patients, presumably because ^{99m}Tc has not remained within the blood pool long enough to permit satisfactory labeling.

The third method employed to label red blood cells is the modified in vivo method, which was first described by Callahan and associates.[5] This approach combines the speed of the in vivo method with the labeling efficiency of the in vitro method. The first step of the labeling procedure is an intravenous injection of stannous pyrophosphate identical to that performed in the in vivo method. Thirty minutes later, 30 to 50 mL of the patient's blood is withdrawn into a heparinized syringe through a three-way stopcock. ^{99m}Tc-pertechnetate, which is attached to the other port of the stopcock, is then injected into the syringe containing the patient's blood. The mixture is gently agitated for 5 minutes and then reinjected into the patient. Although this method is somewhat more time-consuming and technically demanding than the in vivo method, it does result in a uniformly high labeling efficiency and virtually eliminates the background activity in the stomach that occurs with in vivo labeling. Because rapid injection of the labeled red blood cells generally is not possible without significant red blood cell damage, first-pass studies of the right ventricle are not feasible with the use of this labeling method.

Once the red blood cells have been labeled by any of these methods, the major determinant of blood pool activity is the 6-hour half-life of ^{99m}Tc, as the biologic half-life of the labeled red blood cells is approximately 20 hours.[6] Depending on the body size of the patient, high-quality images are generally obtainable for at least 3 to 5 hours, permitting the assessment of ventricular function at multiple different levels of exercise, during different exercise protocols, and before and after drug interventions. Occasional difficulties with adequate labeling do occur. The majority are due to improper technique, including extravasation of the stannous pyrophosphate, improper preservation of the stannous pyrophosphate (which requires refrigeration), and injection of an inadequate quantity of ^{99m}Tc.

Rarely, technically suboptimal labeling can occur even with meticulous technique. Concurrent intravenous administration of heparin is recognized to reduce labeling efficiency.[7] Although multiple other drugs have been shown to interfere with labeling,[8, 9] usually through the formation of drug-antibody complexes, they do not usually prevent adequate clinical studies. In our experience, the modified in vivo labeling procedure will fail rarely (approximately once in every 1000 patients), usually because of the use of multiple drugs that are known to interfere with the labeling process.

Exercise Equipment and Techniques

In addition to the aforementioned standard single-crystal gamma camera, the performance of equilibrium radionuclide angiography requires an electrocardiographic monitoring device capable of generating a signal triggered by the R wave of the electrocardiogram as well as a computer system to acquire, organize, analyze, and display the data. Acquisition of the data occurs over many different cardiac cycles. The most common acquisition uses *frame mode*, in which counts recorded during the same time interval of successive cycles are added together to create an image of the great vessels and cardiac chambers. The R-wave trigger indicates the timing of each new cardiac cycle. The computer divides each cardiac cycle into a predetermined number of frames, ranging from 16 to 64. Each frame represents a predetermined time interval occurring at a specified time after the R wave. Data collected during the same frame of several hundred successive cardiac cycles are then added together (Fig. 61–1). The result is a sequence of 16 to 64 images, each representing a particular time interval in the cardiac cycle. These images may be displayed individually or in an endless-loop motion picture format for purposes of review and analysis. Less commonly used is *list mode* acquisition, in which all image data are recorded as a single list, along with frequent time markers and R-wave markers. The data are subsequently reformatted for image analysis. Although technically superior, this method is more time-consuming and requires more sophisticated computer hardware and software.

Multiple views of the heart at rest can be obtained from different angles to assess wall motion. The most commonly employed views for assessing the resting wall motion are an anterior view, a left anterior oblique view that is adjusted to visualize the interventricular septum optimally, and a steeper left anterior oblique or left lateral view.[10] Quantitative measurements are generally performed only on the "best septal" left anterior oblique view. Time constraints and the desire to perform quantitation studies generally restrict exercise studies to this view only. In selected patients who are able to exercise for a sufficiently long period, an anterior view may also be obtained at peak exercise. Occasionally, the additional information derived from an anterior view may justify a second exercise study.[11]

Exercise studies are performed with a bicycle ergometer. Before the introduction of exercise tables that could tilt to a semiupright

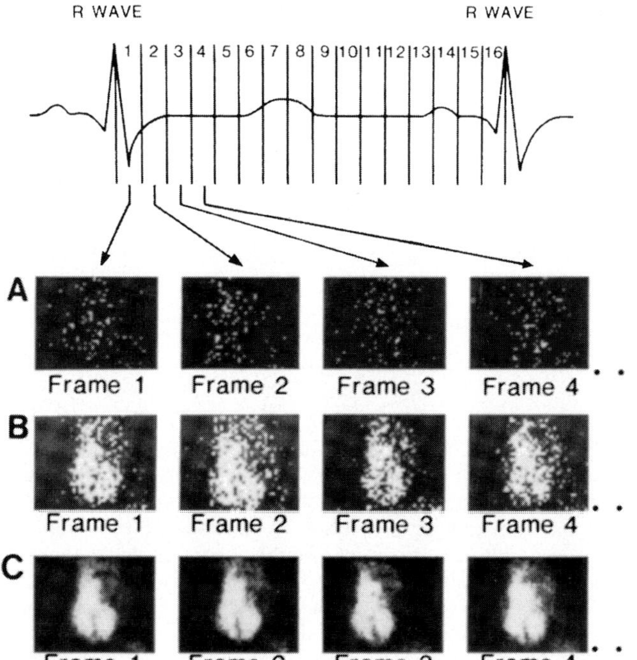

FIGURE 61–1. The cardiac cycle is divided into equal intervals (16 in this example). Counts recorded during each interval are stored in different computer frames. After a single cardiac cycle *(A)*, there are no recognizable images. After 20 cardiac cycles *(B)*, the images begin to be recognizable. After 400 cardiac cycles (300,000 counts per frame), image quality has improved considerably *(C)*. (From Parker, D.A., Thrall, J.H., Froelich, J.W., et al.: Radionuclide ventriculography: Methods. *In* Gerson, M.C. (ed.): Cardiac Nuclear Medicine. New York, McGraw-Hill, 1987, p. 68, with permission.)

position, supine bicycle exercise was most often employed as a means of minimizing patient motion during the radionuclide acquisitions. There are some clear physiologic differences between supine and semiupright exercise.[12–14] Patients who exercise in the supine position generally start with larger end-diastolic volumes, have less of an increase in heart rate and end-diastolic volume with exercise, and show a greater increase in systolic blood pressure with exercise. Although these differences are important for physiologic and drug intervention studies, they do not appear to have a major impact on the general clinical use of equilibrium radionuclide angiography for diagnostic and prognostic purposes.[15] Despite the lower exercise heart rates achieved in the supine position, electrocardiographic ST segment changes are somewhat more frequent with supine exercise, presumably because of greater ventricular wall tension.[16]

Exercise is performed in stages, each of which typically lasts for 3 minutes. During the first minute of each new exercise workload, the subject's heart rate and blood pressure increase to a nearly steady-state condition. The radionuclide acquisition is then performed during the last 2 minutes of the stage, when a reasonably steady hemodynamic state exists. There is a wide variation in the actual sequence of exercise bicycle workloads employed. Some evidence suggests that a sudden, severe workload will lead to spurious results.[17] With this exception, no clear evidence exists to support the use of one protocol rather than another. The most commonly employed protocols begin at workloads of 200 or 300 kg/m/min (37 to 50 watts) and increase in increments of 200 to 300 kg/m/min (37 to 50 watts).

One of the advantages of equilibrium radionuclide angiography is that multiple acquisitions can be obtained during exercise at different exercise workloads. One of the disadvantages of this modality is that the patient must be able to exercise for a minimum of 3 minutes to acquire any reasonable exercise data. Although cold pressor testing, psychologic stress, and dipyridamole and dobutamine infusions have been employed with equilibrium radionuclide angiography,[18–21] these techniques have not been as well validated as exercise. Since many successive cardiac cycles are added together to produce a composite image in equilibrium radionuclide angiography, the maintenance of a near steady state during exercise is critical. If the patient is not allowed sufficient time to reach a near steady state before the acquisition begins, considerable increases in heart rate and blood pressure may occur during the acquisition period, which may adversely affect the data. Similarly, reductions in bicycle workload during the 2-minute acquisition should be avoided, as the changes in hemodynamics that they create may lead to spurious results.[22]

Arrhythmias

Arrhythmias during exercise will clearly degrade the data. Sustained supraventricular or ventricular tachycardia is a clear cause for termination of an equilibrium radionuclide angiogram, since data from periods of different rhythm cannot be combined. Frequent premature ventricular contractions will lead to degradation of the data. If more than 10 percent of the cardiac cycles recorded are premature ventricular contractions, the data will be less accurate but usable.[23] If more than 20 percent of the cardiac cycles are premature ventricular contractions, it is generally advisable not to analyze or report the data. A change in the ventricular conduction pattern during the acquisition is also a cause for concern. Fixed left bundle branch block[24, 25] and rate-dependent left bundle branch block[26] have been clearly demonstrated to alter mechanical function. If left bundle branch block appears during an acquisition, the acquisition should either be aborted at that time or restarted so that it consists entirely of that conduction pattern.

The presence of atrial fibrillation will cause a wide variation in the RR interval in most patients. Although this variation will decrease somewhat during exercise, it will still influence the acquisition. The results, which represent an unusual "average" over many cardiac cycles of varying length, will provide a reasonable approximation of ventricular function but with less accuracy than an acquisition performed in sinus rhythm.

Two approaches are available to try to address the problem of arrhythmias during exercise. The first is pharmacologic. Intravenous lidocaine may be administered in an attempt to reduce the frequency of premature ventricular contractions. To the degree that this therapy is effective, it will improve the accuracy of the data. A second approach relies on computer processing. The most comprehensive computer method employed is that of list mode acquisition, which will permit the retrospective identification and elimination of all premature beats and other arrhythmias from the acquired data. This approach, however, is time-consuming and demanding from the standpoint of computer memory. As a result, it is fairly impractical for most busy clinical laboratories. More recent computer systems have enabled "on the fly" identification of premature beats during the acquisition, which has permitted their elimination from the data. However, these identification programs are not perfect, and the degree to which they correct the problem is not well documented.

Ambulatory Left Ventricular Function Monitoring

Practical methods are available for the continuous assessment of left ventricular function over a period of hours under a variety of physiologic and psychologic conditions. The most commonly used device (VEST, Capintec Inc., Ramsey, NJ) is worn on the chest as a plastic vest-like garment.[27] It consists of nonimaging radiation detectors positioned over the left ventricular blood pool and over the right lung (to monitor changes in pulmonary blood volume), electrocardiographic leads, and electronic instrumentation. Red blood cell labeling is performed by the conventional method using ^{99m}Tc, and a gamma camera is used to optimally position the detector over the left ventricle. Three major parameters are recorded simultaneously: the time-activity curve of the left ventricular blood pool, the background activity in the lungs, and electrocardiographic data. Many of the same parameters that can be measured by background-corrected equilibrium radionuclide angiography can be derived from the left ventricular time-activity curve.[27] These data can then be displayed over a period of several hours. The accuracy and reproducibility of these measurements obtained with the use of this device have been well validated.[28] Disadvantages of this particular device include its weight (nearly 3 kg) and the requirement of a gamma camera for positioning the radiation detector over the left ventricle. More recently, a miniature lightweight detector has been developed (Cardioscint, Oakfield Instruments Ltd., Oxford, UK) that can be positioned over the left ventricle without the use of a gamma camera; it can be held in place with only an elasticated harness.[29]

MEASUREMENTS FROM EQUILIBRIUM RADIONUCLIDE ANGIOGRAPHY

Left Ventricular Ejection Fraction

The parameters that can be measured by equilibrium radionuclide angiography are listed in Table 61–1. The most important measurement made from these studies is the left ventricular ejection fraction. The best-validated approach to the measurement of ejection fraction uses a semiautomated, operator-assisted method that identifies the border of the left ventricle throughout the cardiac cycle from the left anterior oblique view. The ejection fraction is computed from the formula:

$$\frac{\text{(end-diastolic counts} - \text{end-systolic counts)}}{\text{end-diastolic counts}}$$

where both end-diastolic and end-systolic counts are corrected for background. The region of interest employed to calculate background is usually placed along the left lateral edge of the end-systolic border. It is emphasized that this approach does not rely on any assumptions regarding the geometry of the left ventricle, which is a major strength of the technique. Although some investigators have employed a single, or fixed, region of interest method, in which the left ventricular border is identified only on the initial frame (which is assumed to represent end-diastole), the most commonly employed technique uses a variable region of interest in which the left ventricular border is outlined in every frame throughout the cardiac cycle. Multiple studies from different institutions have found that the left ventricular ejection fraction obtained in this fashion by equilibrium radionuclide angiography correlates well with that obtained by contract ventriculography over a wide range (Table 61–2).[30–35] The normal value for the resting left ventricular ejection fraction is generally considered to be greater than or equal to 0.5.[36] In addition, the technique has an acceptable intraobserver and interobserver variability, which is not

TABLE 61–1. MEASUREMENTS OBTAINED FROM EQUILIBRIUM RADIONUCLIDE ANGIOGRAPHY

- Left ventricle
  - Ejection fraction
  - Regional wall motion
  - Volumes
- Right ventricle
  - Ejection fraction
  - Regional wall motion
  - Volumes
- Phase analysis
- Left ventricular output
- Regurgitant fraction
- Pulmonary blood volume
- Diastolic filling measurements

TABLE 61–2. STUDIES COMPARING LEFT VENTRICULAR EJECTION FRACTION BY CONTRAST VENTRICULOGRAPHY AND RADIONUCLIDE ANGIOGRAPHY

Reference	No. of Subjects	r
Berman et al.[31]	27	0.93
Burow et al.[30]	17	0.93
Folland et al.[32]	30	0.84
Green et al.[33]	39	0.92
Pfisterer et al.[34]	24	0.92
Secker-Walker et al.[35]	16	0.87
Wackers et al.[38]	26	0.84

surprising, as most of the analysis is performed by computer with little modification by the operator.[37, 38] However, most of the validation studies were carried out with the use of a particular computer system and a particular generation of software. Other computer systems and software programs should not be assumed to yield identical results unless they have been similarly validated. It is therefore vital that every laboratory validate its own method and maintain a consistent technique thereafter. There are relatively little data assessing the intrinsic variability in ejection fraction over longer periods. In a group of 39 clinically stable patients who underwent two studies 6 weeks apart, one study reported that variation due to chance alone was unlikely to account for a 0.07 unit change in rest or a 0.10 unit change in the exercise ejection fraction.[39] The radionuclide angiographic measurement of ejection fraction may be more accurate than that obtained by other modalities, as it does not rely on any assumption regarding left ventricular geometry. The variation in attenuation with distance from the camera may occasionally lead to systematic errors, however, particularly in the presence of localized dyskinesia.[40]

Regional Wall Motion

Equilibrium radionuclide angiography also permits an accurate assessment of regional wall motion, which is usually judged visually from a video display of all the images throughout the cardiac cycle in an endless-loop motion picture format. As mentioned earlier, multiple different views of the heart are obtained at rest, whereas exercise studies are usually restricted to a single left anterior oblique view. Regional wall motion assessed by this technique has been demonstrated to correlate well with the subjective assessment of regional wall motion by contrast ventriculography.[41, 42] Furthermore, the interobserver variability of this technique is comparable with the interobserver variability of biplane contrast ventriculography (Fig. 61–2).[41] Right ventricular overlap makes the assessment of inferior wall motion on the anterior view difficult; for that reason, a steep left anterior oblique or left lateral view is required.[10] During exercise, the interobserver variability of the technique for regional wall motion is greater than that at rest as a result of the shorter imaging period and lower resolution images obtained during exercise. The assessment of regional wall motion change in the interventricular septum during exercise is generally more difficult than the assessment of the inferoapical or lateral walls.

Several different methods have been reported for the quantitative assessment of regional wall motion.[43–46] In each of these methods, the left ventricular end-diastolic frame in the left anterior oblique view is divided into several different regions. The change in counts during the cardiac cycle within each region is then employed to calculate a regional ejection fraction. Such measurements have been shown to correlate well with quantitative measurements on contrast ventriculography, although there is clearly an inherent difference between these two measurements. The count change measured by equilibrium radionuclide angiography represents a change in ventricular volume. It is, therefore, influ-

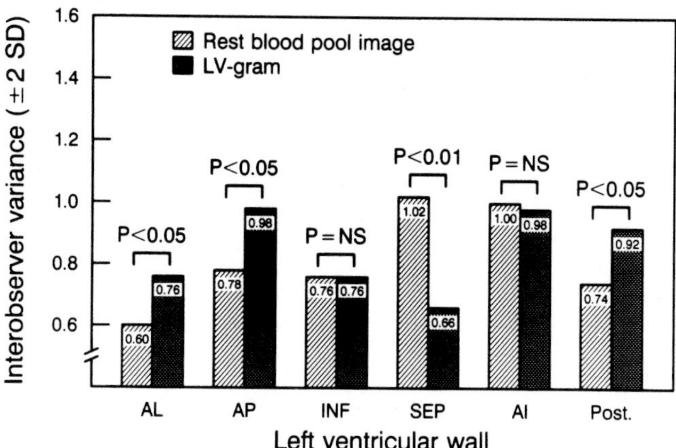

FIGURE 61–2. Left ventricular regional wall motion was judged on a five-point scale by equilibrium radionuclide angiography (rest blood pool image) and contrast ventriculography (LV-gram). The segments are anterolateral (AL), apical (AP), inferior (INF), septal (SEP), apical-inferior (AI), and posterior (Post.). The two modalities have a comparable interobserver variance. (From Okada, R., Kirshenbaum, H., Kushner, F., et al.: Observer variance in the qualitative evaluation of left ventricular wall motion and the quantitation of left ventricular ejection fraction using rest and exercise multi-gated blood pool imaging. Circulation 61:128, 1980, by permission of the American Heart Association, Inc.)

enced by the wall motion along surfaces that are tangential to the imaging plane. Conversely, contrast ventriculography measures wall motion in those segments that are perpendicular to the imaging plane. Two small studies have reported the application of quantitative regional ejection fractions to exercise studies and suggested that they are superior to the subjective assessment of wall motion.[43, 47] However, no quantitative method for the assessment of regional wall motion has achieved broad acceptance. Most clinical laboratories currently employ a subjective assessment of regional wall motion by one or more observers.

An alternative approach to the assessment of regional wall motion employs Fourier phase analysis of individual computer pixels.[48–52] Various phase parameters that are derived from the first Fourier harmonic will permit the detection of abnormal regional function. Although some reports have suggested that this technique is superior to the visual assessment of regional wall motion,[51] other studies have not found it to be as helpful,[49, 50] particularly in patients with abnormal wall motion at rest.[52] This technique has provided insights into a broad spectrum of ventricular conduction disturbances as well as ventricular arrhythmias.[48]

Left Ventricular Volumes

Left ventricular volumes also can be assessed by equilibrium radionuclide angiography. The first method described, which continues to be in common clinical use because of its simplicity, was a count-based method without any geometric assumptions.[53, 54] The formula used in this method is:

$$\text{Volume} = K \frac{\text{left ventricular activity}}{\text{number of cardiac cycles} \times \frac{\text{time}}{\text{frame}} \times \text{blood activity}}$$

where K is an attenuation correction factor.

The counts recorded from the ventricular region of interest in a particular frame are corrected for the time of acquisition for that frame and the activity of a blood sample of known volume (which can be determined in a well counter or by counting a sample placed directly on the camera face). The volume "units" determined by the equation are then related to volumes measured by contrast ventriculography. The constant K is determined from the resulting regression equation and represents an average attenuation correction. Ideally, every nuclear cardiology laboratory should develop its own regression equation and its own constant K to account for differences in equipment and technique. The particular volume measurements obtained by radionuclide angiography in this fashion have correlated well with those obtained from contrast ventriculography. The correlation coefficient reported by Dehmer and associates[54] was 0.98, with an average error of the estimate of 16 mL for end-diastolic volume and 15 mL for end-systolic volume (Fig. 61–3). However, since the constant represents an "average" attenuation correction, and since chest wall attenuation will clearly vary with body geometry, more substantial errors can be expected from this method in very thin and very obese patients. More substantial errors also can be expected in patients with very large ventricular volumes, as counts within the regions of the left ventricle that are farthest from the camera will be attenuated.

Despite these limitations, this methodology remains useful for making sequential measurements in the same patient, since attenuation can be assumed to be relatively constant unless body weight changes substantially. Thus, changes in ventricular volume between rest and different levels of exercise can be estimated with this method, as can changes in resting left ventricular volume over time in the same patient.[55–57] It has been demonstrated that the blood activity employed in the equation to measure left ventricular volume will change during exercise if labeling is performed by the in vivo method.[58] Although there have been conflicting studies using the modified in vivo method,[59, 60] blood activity probably also increases modestly using this technique. As a result, multiple blood samples must be obtained during exercise.

Many extensive efforts have been made to develop methods that calculate attenuation in individual patients to eliminate the problem of variable attenuation.[61–63] The actual distance from the gamma camera detector to the center of the left ventricle can be estimated in individual patients.[61] Even when this distance can be judged accurately, however, the actual attenuation coefficient may still vary from individual to individual. Thus, these more detailed methods, which clearly require additional time and effort compared with the simple count-based method, still will have some systematic error in the determination of absolute left ventricular volumes. In clinical situations in which the determination of absolute left ventricular volumes is of importance, these measurement techniques may be worthwhile. In general clinical practice, however, when relative volume changes are probably sufficient, the count-based volume method without attenuation correction provides important information with a modest amount of time and effort. Recently, count-based ratio methods that do not require attenuation correction or blood sampling have been developed.[64, 65] These methods are based

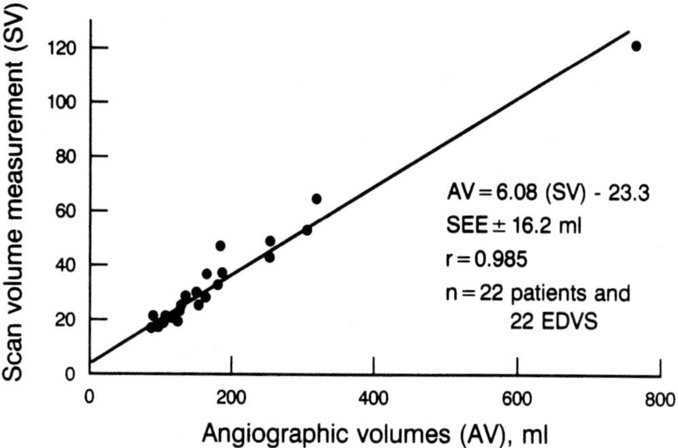

FIGURE 61–3. Left ventricular end-diastolic volumes (EDVS) measured by equilibrium radionuclide angiography (SV) and contrast ventriculography (AV). The results for end-systolic volume were comparable. (From Dehmer, G., Lewis, S., Hillis, L., et al.: Nongeometric determination of left ventricular volumes from equilibrium blood pool scans. Am. J. Cardiol. 45:293, 1980, with permission.)

on the count proportional volume theory, which states that the ratio of total counts–to–peak pixel counts in the left ventricle is a function of left ventricular volume. Measurement of left ventricular volume by these methods has been shown to be highly accurate when compared with contrast ventriculography.

Similar count-based techniques have been applied to the determination of right ventricular volume.[66] Unfortunately, it is difficult to validate these measurements, as there is no generally accepted ventriculographic "gold standard" for the measurement of right ventricular volume. The right ventricular stroke volume measured by a count-based method appears to agree closely with the stroke volume derived from thermodilution cardiac output measurements.[66] Thus, on the basis of this indirect validation, these measurements appear to be reasonably accurate.

Regurgitant Fraction

A variety of other measurements can be made from equilibrium radionuclide angiography. Although generally they are not employed on a routine clinical basis, they may be of great interest in particular clinical settings. One such measurement is the regurgitant fraction, a noninvasive determination of the severity of mitral or aortic regurgitation. Equilibrium radionuclide angiography is employed to calculate the stroke counts from the right ventricle and the left ventricle.[67–72] Generally, the stroke counts from the right ventricle are best measured from a left anterior oblique view that employs significant caudal-cranial angulation to minimize overlap between the right atrium and the right ventricle. Further processing of this image, including phase and amplitude images, may help delineate the tricuspid valve plane.[73] The ratio of left-to-right ventricular stroke counts or the difference between left ventricular and right ventricular stroke counts as a percentage of left ventricular stroke counts can be employed to estimate the severity of regurgitation. The ratio of stroke counts will be near unity in patients without evidence of left-sided regurgitation. This ratio will considerably exceed unity, and occasionally be as high as 5, in patients with mitral or aortic regurgitation. The stroke count ratio has been shown to agree well with the qualitative angiographic assessment of regurgitation. The regurgitant fraction that can be calculated from this ratio correlates well with the regurgitant fraction obtained from the difference of angiographic and Fick cardiac output measurements.[72] The major limitation of this approach is the presence of some right atrial and right ventricular overlap in most patients. As a result, there is a systematic error in this calculation, which can produce a regurgitant fraction as high as 20 percent and a stroke count ratio as high as 1.25 in normal patients without regurgitation. This systematic error reduces the ability of this parameter to detect minor degrees of regurgitation and causes an overestimation of the regurgitant fraction. For example, a calculated regurgitant fraction of 30 percent indicates, at most, mild left-sided regurgitation.

Right Ventricular Ejection Fraction

The right ventricular ejection fraction can be determined from equilibrium radionuclide angiography using a variety of methods.[74–76] One is similar to that employed for the determination of the left ventricular ejection fraction, in which a region of interest is drawn manually around the right ventricle in end-diastole and end-systole.[76] The major technical limitation of this technique is the determination of the tricuspid and pulmonic valve planes. Phase and amplitude images, as well as stroke volume images, can be employed to help locate these valve planes. As noted, however, right atrial and right ventricular overlap is unavoidable in many patients and is, in part, due to the motion of the tricuspid valve plane throughout the cardiac cycle, which is difficult to characterize on the left anterior oblique view. Despite these technical limitations, the right ventricular ejection fraction determined in this fashion agrees well with other methods and has acceptable interobserver and intraobserver variability.[74–76]

An alternative approach to the measurement of right ventricular ejection fraction is to acquire a gated, first-pass study during the initial injection of ^{99m}Tc. This technique, which uses the in vivo labeling method, allows visual determination of the motion of the tricuspid valve plane. The right ventricular ejection fraction determined by this method has been validated against contrast ventriculography[77] and ultrafast computed tomography.[78] The normal right ventricular ejection fraction is generally considered to be greater than or equal to 0.4.[36]

Pulmonary Blood Volume

It is also possible to measure changes in pulmonary blood volume during exercise with equilibrium radionuclide angiography.[79] This measurement has been demonstrated to be a valid noninvasive indicator of the changes that occur in pulmonary capillary wedge pressure with exercise.[80] Although the initial report describing this measurement suggested that it might be superior to the ejection fraction in detecting exercise-induced ischemia, work in our laboratory has shown that the change in pulmonary blood volume is not superior to ejection fraction and is more difficult to measure.[81]

Left Ventricular Output

Equilibrium radionuclide angiography also can estimate left ventricular output. This output is derived from the product of heart rate, ejection fraction, and end-diastolic volume. The methodology for the determination of ejection fraction and end-diastolic volume has already been described. The major source of error in the measurement of left ventricular output is the potential error in the measurement of end-diastolic volume due to variable attention. Left ventricular output determined in this fashion correlates surprisingly well ($r = 0.97$) with thermodilution measurements of cardiac output in patients without significant left-sided regurgitation.[82–84] Conversely, in the presence of aortic or mitral regurgitation, left ventricular output determined in this fashion will consistently exceed the Fick cardiac output. As a result, these outputs can be used to calculate a regurgitant fraction, which correlates with the severity of regurgitation assessed angiographically.[68]

Diastolic Parameters

All the measurements described thus far are derived from the systolic phase of the cardiac cycle. There has been increasing interest in the use of equilibrium radionuclide angiography to make diastolic measurements as well. Methodologic details are generally much more important for these measurements, as they are clearly more technically demanding. Higher temporal resolution is required, necessitating higher framing rates and longer acquisition times. Statistical fluctuations in counts within the ventricular region of interest impose a need for curve fitting, which can influence the results. The duration of diastole clearly depends on cardiac cycle length; minor variations in RR interval, therefore, will significantly influence diastolic filling parameters. Such variations in RR interval add greatly to the technical difficulty of performing diastolic measurements by equilibrium radionuclide angiography because of the difficulty of superimposing many different cardiac cycles of slightly different length. Atrial pacing will eliminate these variations and permit highly accurate measurements, but this step clearly complicates the procedure from a practical standpoint.

A variety of different methods has been used to make diastolic measurements by equilibrium radionuclide angiography.[85–94] List mode acquisition, the most accurate method, is the most technically demanding from the standpoint of time, computer software, and computer storage.[86, 87] With the use of this method, the cardiac cycle can be reconstructed in forward-backward fashion from the R wave. Cardiac cycles that are too long or too short can be eliminated from consideration. An alternative is to employ the same standard gating procedure that is used for systolic measurements but to increase the framing rate to 32 or 64 frames per cardiac cycle and increase the acquisition time to permit adequate counting statistics in each frame.[85, 91, 94] This method will avoid the technical demands of list mode acquisition, but its accuracy will be greatly affected by any variability in RR interval.[90] As a result, obtaining measurements in late diastole, including the atrial filling phase, will be virtually impossible. A third alternative, which is technically simple but permits late diastolic measurements, is alternate R-wave gating.[89] This method employs a simple filter that allows every other R-wave trigger signal to reach the computer. As a result, the cardiac "cycle" constructed by the computer actually consists of two successive cardiac cycles. This technically simple method permits measurements in both early diastole and late diastole, including the entire atrial filling phase. These measurements will still be affected, however, by variability in the RR interval.

A variety of different diastolic parameters has been measured, including the peak filling rate, the time-to-peak filling, the first one-third and first one-half filling fraction, and the atrial filling fraction.[95] These parameters generally contain a great deal of overlapping information. When one parameter is abnormal, all other parameters frequently will be abnormal as well. The exact significance of these parameters, and their relationship to left ventricular compliance, is a subject of ongoing research. One of the most useful applications of this technique has been in the identification of "diastolic dysfunction" in patients who present with left-sided heart failure but have a normal or near-normal left ventricular ejection fraction.[95] Perrone-Filardi and colleagues have suggested that among patients with coronary artery disease and preserved systolic function at rest, those with impaired diastolic filling have more functionally severe disease as manifested by a greater degree of exercise-induced ischemia.[96] Measurements of volume or rates of change in volume by equilibrium radionuclide angiography or any other technique are at best indirect indicators of left ventricular compliance in the absence of simultaneous pressure measurements. Simultaneous measurements of ventricular volume by radionuclide angiography and pressure by micromanometer have been reported.[97]

CLINICAL APPLICATIONS

Diagnosis of Chest Pain

Equilibrium radionuclide angiography is one of several different exercise modalities frequently employed to help establish the diagnosis of chest pain. The ultimate goal of clinical evaluation and noninvasive exercise testing is to establish the likelihood that an individual patient has significant coronary artery disease. To the statistician, this is what is known as the *post-test probability*. Ideally, one would like to separate all patients into two groups. In one group, no patient would have coronary artery disease, and in the other group, all the patients would have coronary artery disease. Such a separation, however, is not possible with our current testing modalities. One must be satisfied, therefore, with a characterization of a patient as "likely" or "unlikely" to have coronary artery disease.

The determination of the post-test probability requires a knowledge of the *pretest probability*, the performance characteristics of the test employed, and the test results.[98, 99] Detailed discussions of the proper application of Bayes theorem to such a determination have been published elsewhere.[100, 101] The pretest probability is simply the likelihood that a patient has coronary artery disease on the basis of clinical characteristics before any test is performed. Age, sex, and the patient's description of chest pain are the most important characteristics.[98] Published estimates of the pretest probability of disease on the basis of these three characteristics are shown in Tables 61–3 and 61–4. It is obvious that there is a wide range of pretest probability, ranging from 1 percent for a woman in her thirties with nonanginal chest pain to 94 percent for a man in his sixties with typical angina.

TABLE 61–3. PRETEST PROBABILITY OF CORONARY ARTERY DISEASE IN MEN

		Pretest Probability (%)	
Age (Years)	**Nonanginal Chest Pain**	***Atypical Angina***	***Typical Angina***
30–39	5	22	70
40–49	14	46	87
50–59	22	59	92
60–69	28	67	94

From Diamond, G.A., and Forrester, J.S.: Analysis of probability as an aid in the clinical diagnosis of coronary-artery disease. N. Engl. J. Med. 300:1350, 1979, with permission.

A number of other noninvasive characteristics are important in the determination of pretest probability. A detailed statistical analysis of 3627 patients from the Duke University Medical Center data bank[102] found that previous myocardial infarction by history or electrocardiogram, or both, as well as smoking, hyperlipidemia, ST-T wave changes on the resting electrocardiogram, and diabetes are all highly significant predictors ($P < .001$) of the presence of coronary artery disease in addition to age, sex, and a description of chest pain.

In addition to the pretest probability of disease, the ability of the test to distinguish normal from abnormal, that is, its performance characteristics, is important in determining post-test probability. The statistical parameters that have been most widely used to assess test performance are sensitivity and specificity. The sensitivity of the test is defined as the percentage of people *with disease* who have a positive test. The specificity of the test is the percentage of patients *without disease* who have a negative test.

Many different studies have compared equilibrium radionuclide angiography and first-pass radionuclide angiography with exercise thallium-201 (^{201}Tl) scintigraphy and exercise electrocardiographic testing for the diagnosis of coronary artery disease.[100, 101, 103–110] Equilibrium radionuclide angiography generally has been found to have a higher sensitivity and a lower specificity than exercise electrocardiographic testing. It is important to note, however, that these comparisons have often omitted patients whose treadmill tests were felt to be "inadequate" or "uninterpretable." If such treadmill tests were counted as negative, the difference in sensitivity between equilibrium radionuclide angiography and treadmill tests would widen considerably.

The exact specificity of equilibrium radionuclide angiography has been a subject of some controversy. The first large reported series described a specificity of 100 percent.[105] This, and similar early series, reported high values for specificity that were probably clinically unrealistic, since they were based on normal volunteers rather than on patients with chest pain. These normal volunteers generally were not representative of clinical patient populations with respect to age, sex, or exercise capacity. As a result, they tended to perform

TABLE 61–4. PRETEST PROBABILITY OF CORONARY ARTERY DISEASE IN WOMEN

		Pretest Probability (%)	
Age (Years)	**Nonanginal Chest Pain**	***Atypical Angina***	***Typical Angina***
30–39	1	4	26
40–49	3	13	55
50–59	8	32	79
60–69	19	54	91

From Diamond, G.A., and Forrester, J.S.: Analysis of probability as an aid in the clinical diagnosis of coronary-artery disease. N. Engl. J. Med. 300:1350, 1979, with permission.

better on these tests; they were "supernormals." Later series suggested that the specificity of radionuclide angiography was as low as 50 percent.[111] These estimates were probably falsely low, however, since the decision to send these patients to cardiac catheterization was influenced by the abnormal results of their radionuclide angiograms. As a result, there were many patients with normal radionuclide angiograms who did not undergo cardiac catheterization and therefore were not included in the calculation of specificity. This "post-test referral bias"[112] has resulted in declining estimates of specificity that are incorrectly low. The calculated level of specificity obviously will depend on the criteria required to label a test as abnormal, since a higher specificity can always be achieved by more stringent criteria at the cost of a lower sensitivity.[113] Various methods, such as "debiasing" algorithms, have been proposed to reduce the impact of pretest and post-test referral biases in an attempt to determine the true accuracy of different diagnostic testing modalities.[114]

The criteria employed to label an equilibrium radionuclide angiogram as abnormal have varied considerably among different reports. The earliest series used a combination of the peak exercise ejection fraction and the presence or absence of regional wall motion abnormalities.[105] Later workers tended to focus on the change in ejection fraction from rest to exercise and suggested that an increase in the ejection fraction of 0.05 from rest to exercise was necessary for a "normal" response.[103, 106, 108, 109] The change in ejection fraction from rest to exercise is clearly a complex response that is influenced by many physiologic and pathologic variables, including the rest ejection fraction, the gender of the patient, the change in end-diastolic volume index from rest to exercise, the rest pulse pressure, the presence of electrocardiographic changes with exercise, and the extent of coronary artery disease.[111, 115] Patients with higher resting ejection fractions tend to have a lesser increase in ejection fraction with exercise. Thus, a patient with a resting ejection fraction of 0.7 and an exercise fraction of 0.7 has a normal functional response to exercise, not an abnormal one as was once thought.[111, 116]

The peak exercise ejection fraction combines information about both prior ventricular damage (as reflected in the resting ejection fraction) and the presence of exercise-induced ischemia (as reflected in the change in ejection fraction). Thus, this parameter is an indicator of the "maximal performance" of the heart and is less subject to influence by resting conditions. A detailed analysis of 736 patients that compared the change in ejection fraction and the peak exercise ejection fraction for diagnostic purposes found that the latter was a better parameter for the detection of coronary artery disease.[117] Other series have confirmed the superiority of the peak exercise ejection fraction, not only for diagnosis[118, 119] but also for the identification of severe disease[120–122] and for prognosis.[123–126] Although this parameter is most appropriately considered as a continuous variable with a broad range rather than simply as normal or abnormal based on an arbitrary cutoff, a peak exercise ejection fraction of 0.5 to 0.6 has generally been used as a cutoff for diagnostic and prognostic purposes. For diagnostic purposes, Table 61–5 shows the actual values of sensitivity and normalcy rates for different cutoff values of peak exercise ejection fraction. A cutoff of 0.6 yields a sensitivity of 77 percent and a normalcy rate of 82 percent, which is clearly more sensitive than a treadmill exercise test but less specific.

The difference between men and women in the left ventricular response to exercise must be considered in the evaluation of both specificity and test criteria. The largest reported series of patients with chest pain and normal coronary arteriograms found that many patients had abnormal ejection fraction responses to exercise without evidence of other cardiovascular abnormality, and that such responses were clearly more common in women than in men.[111] Using equilibrium radionuclide angiography and upright exercise in a small series of normal volunteers, Higgenbotham and associates demonstrated that there was a clear gender difference in the response of the left ventricle to exercise.[127] The women in their series tended to have less increase in ejection fraction with exercise and a greater increase in end-diastolic volume index with exercise. Hanley and associates subsequently confirmed these findings in a much larger series of 259 patients with a low likelihood of coronary artery disease.[128] They identified a large number of gender differences in ejection fraction and end-diastolic volume index at rest and with exercise. More important, when the exercise response of the ejection fraction and end-diastolic volume index were plotted versus exercise intensity in metabolic equivalents, there was a clear gender difference in the slope of this response between men and women (Figs. 61–4 and 61–5). Women tended to have more left ventricular dilatation with exercise and less increase in ejection fraction than did men. This gender difference may be related to the long-standing observation that women tend to have smaller hearts than men, even after adjustment for body size.[129] This difference, which is not explained by differences in exercise capacity, clearly will affect the interpretation of the results of equilibrium radionuclide angiography in women.

The proper interpretation of the results of equilibrium radionuclide angiography requires careful consideration of all the information from the test, including the hemodynamics,[130] the symptoms,[117] and electrocardiographic changes during exercise.[117, 122, 131] The magnitude of myocardial oxygen demand achieved (as reflected in the exercise heart rate and blood pressure) and the presence or absence of symptomatic or electrocardiographic evidence of ischemia, or both, have been demonstrated to be complementary to radionuclide parameters for diagnostic and prognostic purposes. Thus, all the information from the test should be considered, and

TABLE 61–5. SENSITIVITY AND NORMALCY RATE FOR DIFFERENT VALUES OF PEAK EXERCISE EJECTION FRACTION

Peak Ejection Fraction	Sensitivity (%)	Normalcy Rate (%)
0.5	55	98
0.55	66	93
0.57	72	90
0.6	77	82
0.63	84	72
0.65	86	67

From Gibbons, R.J.: Rest and exercise radionuclide angiography for diagnosis in chronic ischemic heart disease. Circulation 84(Suppl. I):I–93, 1991. Reprinted with permission from the American Heart Association, Inc.

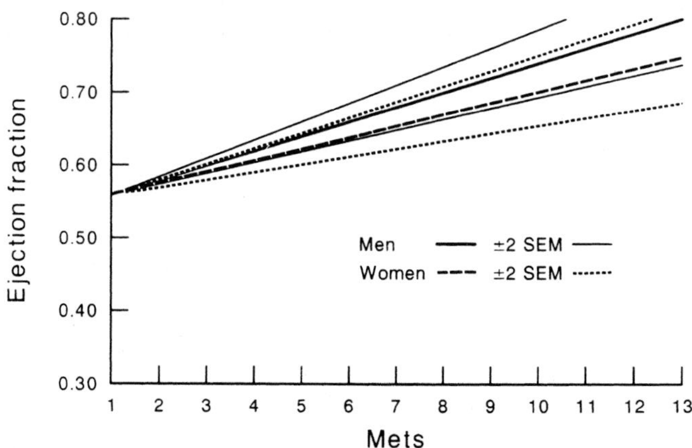

FIGURE 61–4. Relationship between ejection fraction and metabolic equivalents (Mets) of exercise for 192 men and 67 women with a low probability of coronary artery disease. Shown are the mean slopes ±2 standard errors of the mean (SEM). Men had greater increases in ejection fraction with exercise. (From Hanley, P., Gibbons, R., Zinsmeister, A., et al.: Sex-related differences in cardiac response to supine exercise assessed by radionuclide angiography. J. Am. Coll. Cardiol. 13:624, 1989. With permission of the American College of Cardiology.)

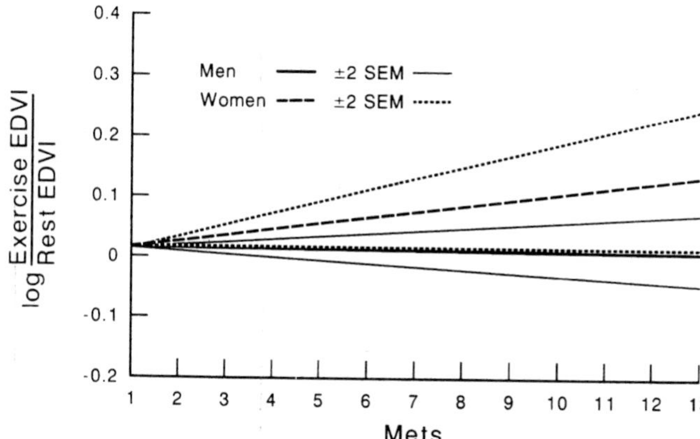

FIGURE 61–5. Relationship between end-diastolic volume index and metabolic equivalents (Mets) of exercise for 192 men and 67 women with a low probability of coronary artery disease. Shown are mean slopes ±2 SEM. Women have greater increases in end-diastolic volume index with exercise.(From Hanley, P., Gibbons, R., Zinsmeister, A., et al.: Sex-related differences in cardiac response to supine exercise assessed by radionuclide angiography. J. Am. Coll. Cardiol. 13:624, 1989. With permission of the American College of Cardiology.)

the results should be considered as a continuous variable rather than as a dichotomous one.

The choice of which exercise modality to employ in an individual patient is often dictated by the particular clinical circumstances and the particular expertise present in a given medical center. In addition to diagnostic information, equilibrium radionuclide angiography provides valuable additional information regarding ventricular function and prognosis. In the absence of left bundle branch block, frequent premature ventricular complexes, or other known exercise-induced arrhythmias, it is a valuable diagnostic tool, particularly in men. Little data exist comparing the accuracy of exercise radionuclide angiography to exercise perfusion imaging in the same patients. One unique clinical situation in which radionuclide angiography is superior to qualitative tomographic thallium imaging is for the detection of left circumflex coronary artery disease.[132]

Identification of Severe Coronary Artery Disease

Equilibrium radionuclide angiography may be employed noninvasively to identify patients who are likely to have severe anatomical coronary artery disease. The rationale for noninvasive screening of patients with chest pain and known or suspected coronary artery disease is based on two premises: (1) coronary artery bypass surgery is known to improve survival in certain patient subgroups and (2) coronary angiography is expensive, is not available in every community, and has a finite risk. Large randomized trials[133–135] have demonstrated that patients with significant left main coronary artery disease or three-vessel disease and abnormal resting left ventricular function have an improved survival when treated with initial surgical management rather than initial medical management. The impact of surgery on survival in patients with three-vessel disease and normal resting function is more controversial. The potential role of exercise radionuclide angiography in the identification of patients with three-vessel disease and normal left ventricular function who are most likely to benefit from coronary revascularization will be addressed in a later section.

Equilibrium radionuclide angiography can identify patient subsets likely to have left main or three-vessel coronary artery disease, or both. Initial studies using first-pass radionuclide angiography[120, 121] suggested that the exercise ejection fraction might be the most important variable in the identification of severe coronary artery disease. Subsequent studies using first-pass radionuclide angiography were generally promising but either failed to consider all the available data[136] or required the impractical calculation of multiple discriminant functions.[137]

TABLE 61–6. VARIABLES INDEPENDENTLY PREDICTIVE OF THE PRESENCE OF LEFT MAIN OR THREE-VESSEL CORONARY ARTERY DISEASE

Variable	*P*
Magnitude of ST segment depression	<0.0001
Exercise ejection fraction	<0.0001
Exercise heart rate × systolic blood pressure product	<0.0001
Patient gender	0.0001
Exercise end-systolic volume index	0.001
Exercise pressure/volume ratio/rest pressure/volume ratio	0.01
METS of exercise	0.02

Variables are listed in order of importance. METS = metabolic equivalents.

From Gibbons, R.J., Fyke, F., and Clements, I.: Noninvasive identification of severe coronary artery disease using exercise radionuclide angiography. J. Am. Coll. Cardiol. 11:28, 1988. With permission of the American College of Cardiology.

Our laboratory attempted to provide clinically useful noninvasive predictions of the likelihood of left main or three-vessel coronary artery disease using supine equilibrium radionuclide angiography.[122] The study group consisted of 681 patients who underwent equilibrium radionuclide angiography and coronary angiography within 6 months. Patients with significant valvular heart disease or previous coronary revascularization were excluded. Logistic regression analysis identified seven different variables that were independently predictive of the presence of left main or three-vessel coronary artery disease (Table 61–6). The first four variables were the most significant and provided most of the predictive power of the model. In order of importance, they were (1) the magnitude of ST segment depression with exercise, (2) the peak exercise ejection fraction, (3) the peak exercise heart rate–systolic blood pressure product, and (4) the gender of the patient. Patients could be separated into high-probability, intermediate-probability, and low-probability subgroups on the basis of their predicted likelihood of left main or three-vessel coronary artery disease (Table 61–7). Of the 216 patients predicted to be at low probability, 20 (9 percent) had left main or three-vessel coronary artery disease. In contrast, of the 258 patients predicted to have a high probability, 144 (56 percent) had left main or three-vessel coronary artery disease.[122]

These same four variables were employed to provide practical estimates of the risk of left main or three-vessel coronary artery disease using six simple graphs (Figs. 61–6 and 61–7). Each graph displays the probability of left main or three-vessel coronary artery disease as a function of exercise ejection fraction and exercise heart rate–systolic blood pressure product for a given degree of ST segment depression in a man or a woman. For example, a man with less than 1 mm of ST segment depression, an exercise ejection

TABLE 61–7. SEPARATION OF PATIENTS ACCORDING TO THE PROBABILITY OF LEFT MAIN OR THREE-VESSEL CORONARY ARTERY DISEASE

Group	Total Patients	Patients with Left Main or Three-Vessel Coronary Artery Disease	
		Number	%
Low probability	216	20	9
Intermediate probability	207	51	25
High probability	258	144	56
Total	681	215	32

From Gibbons, R.J., Fyke, F., and Clements, I.: Noninvasive identification of severe coronary artery disease using exercise radionuclide angiography. J. Am. Coll. Cardiol. 11:28, 1988. With permission of the American College of Cardiology.

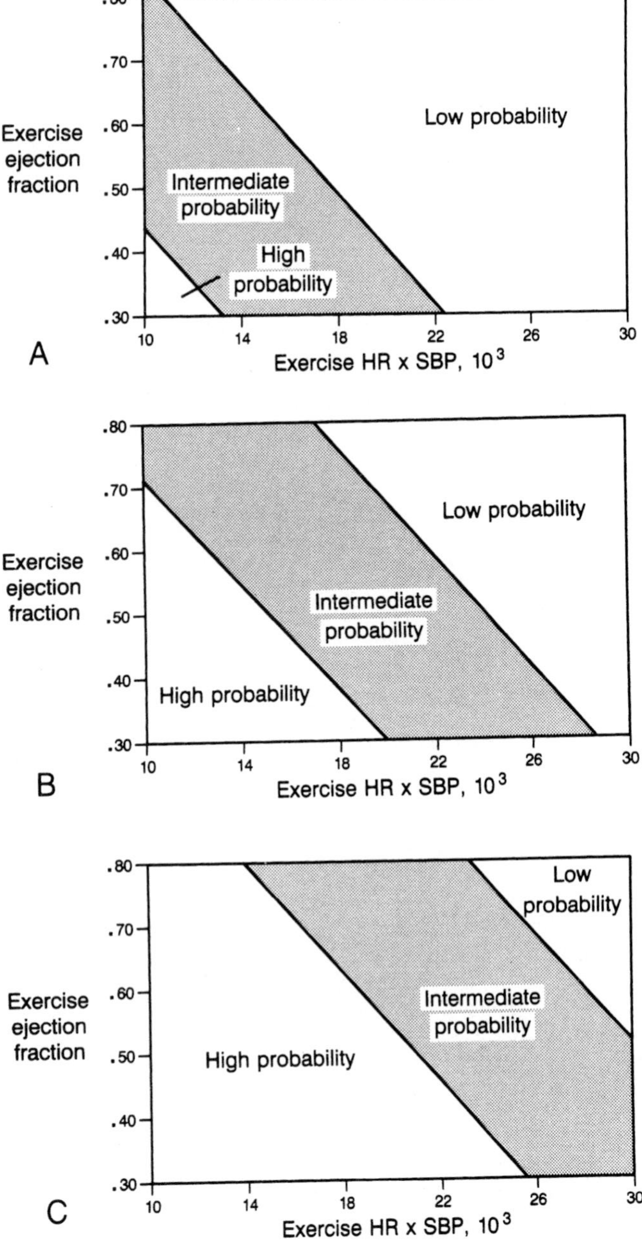

FIGURE 61–6. Estimated probability of left main or three-vessel coronary artery disease for women with less than 1-mm ST segment depression *(A)*, 1-mm ST segment depression *(B)*, and 2-mm ST segment depression *(C)*. Zones of different probability are shown. Exercise heart rate (HR) x systolic blood pressure (SBP) = exercise heart rate–systolic blood pressure product. (From Gibbons, R., Fyke, F., and Clements, I.: Noninvasive identification of severe coronary artery disease using exercise radionuclide angiography. J. Am. Coll. Cardiol. 11:28, 1988. With permission of the American College of Cardiology.)

fraction of 0.6, and an exercise heart rate–systolic blood pressure product of 20,000 would have a low probability of left main or three-vessel coronary artery disease (see Fig. 61–7). In contrast, a man with 1 mm of ST segment depression, an exercise ejection fraction of less than 0.6, and a heart rate–systolic blood pressure product of less than 18,000 would have a high probability of left main or three-vessel coronary artery disease (see Fig. 61–7). As indicated in Figure 61–7, for a given level of ST segment depression, exercise heart rate–systolic blood pressure product, and exercise ejection fraction, men generally have a greater probability of left main or three-vessel coronary artery disease.[122]

From the standpoint of clinical management, the prevalence of left main or three-vessel coronary artery disease in patients judged to be at low probability appears to be sufficiently low that the decision to proceed with coronary angiography should be based primarily on the severity of symptoms. Conversely, the prevalence of left main or three-vessel coronary artery disease in those patients judged to be at high probability exceeds 50 percent, and early coronary angiography appears to be warranted in this group. The management of those patients judged to be at intermediate probability remains a matter of clinical judgment. Thus, it appears that equilibrium radionuclide angiography can easily separate patients

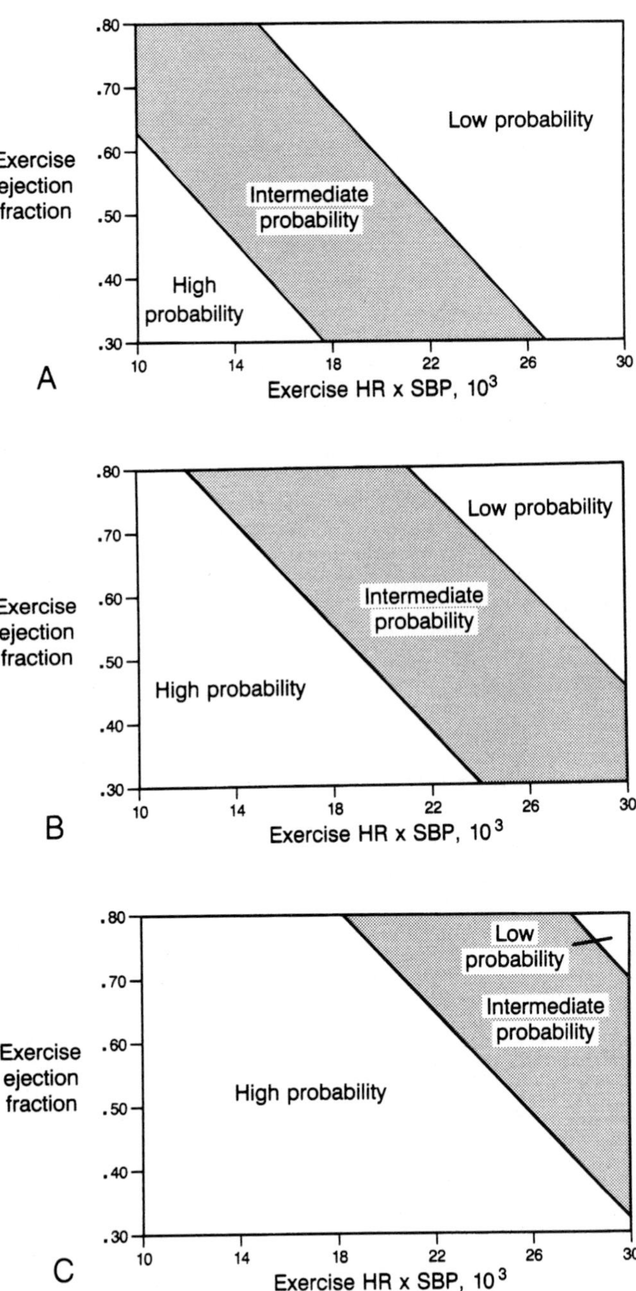

FIGURE 61–7. Estimated probability of left main or three-vessel coronary artery disease for men with less than 1-mm ST segment depression *(A)*, 1-mm ST segment depression *(B)*, and 2-mm ST segment depression *(C)*. Zones of different probability are shown. Exercise heart rate (HR) x systolic blood pressure (SBP) = exercise heart rate-systolic blood pressure product. (From Gibbons, R., Fyke, F., and Clements I.: Noninvasive identification of severe coronary artery disease using exercise radionuclide angiography. J. Am. Coll. Cardiol. 11:28, 1988. With permission of the American College of Cardiology.)

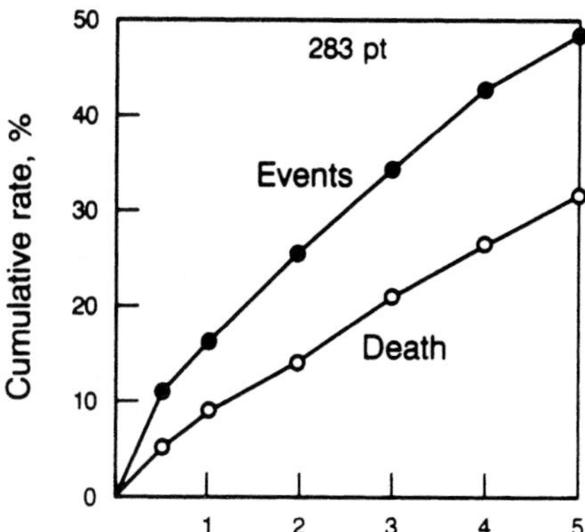

FIGURE 61-8. Five-year follow-up of 283 medically treated patients with three-vessel disease and moderate left ventricular dysfunction. Events consisted of death and nonfatal myocardial infarction. (From Harris, P., Lee, K., Harrell, F., et al.: Survival in medically treated coronary artery disease. Circulation 60:1259, 1979, by permission of the American Heart Association, Inc.)

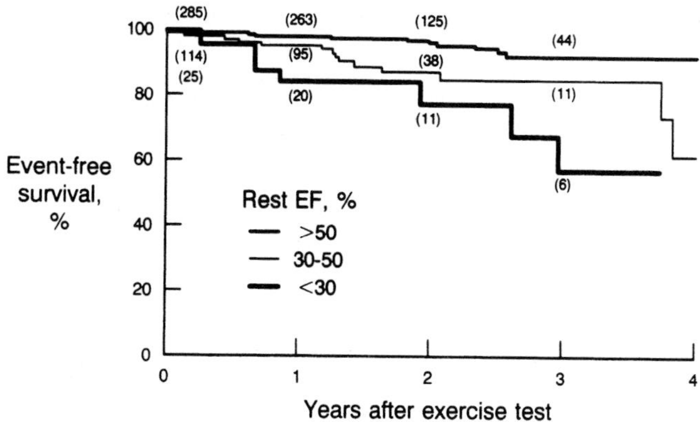

FIGURE 61-9. Event-free survival as a function of resting ejection fraction (EF) in 424 medically treated patients with known or suspected coronary artery disease. Events consisted of death, nonfatal myocardial infarction, and nonfatal out-of-hospital cardiac arrest. (From Taliercio, C.P., Clements, I.P., Zinsmeister, A.R., et al.: Prognostic value and limitations of exercise radionuclide angiography. Mayo Clin. Proc. 63:573, 1988, with permission.)

into low-probability, intermediate-probability, and high-probability groups using the four simple variables described.[122]

A subsequent study of 391 patients with normal resting electrocardiograms who were not taking digoxin showed that an exercise electrocardiographic model (which incorporated the variables gender, exercise heart rate, and magnitude of ST segment depression) was nearly as accurate as a radionuclide angiographic model (which incorporated the three variables in the electrocardiographic model and the variable exercise response of the pressure-to-volume ratio) for accurately characterizing patients as having or not having left main or three-vessel coronary artery disease, or both.[138] The electrocardiographic model correctly classified 60 percent of the population versus 63 percent for the radionuclide angiographic model. Thus, although radionuclide angiographic variables are clearly helpful in identifying patients with severe coronary artery disease in unselected patient populations, these variables add little additional value to the information that is available from clinical and standard exercise electrocardiographic variables *in patients with normal resting electrocardiograms.*

Prognostic Implications

The ultimate goal of the evaluation of patients with chest pain is to identify those who are most likely to benefit from subsequent coronary revascularization because they will have cardiac events if treated initially with medical therapy. Multiple large studies have demonstrated that both the number of diseased vessels and the state of resting left ventricular function are the most important determinants of subsequent patient outcome.[139–141] Even when these parameters are known, however, the subsequent outcome of an individual patient cannot be predicted with great certainty, a point that is obvious but often overlooked. For example, the cumulative event rate for nonfatal infarction and death in patients with three-vessel coronary artery disease and moderate left ventricular function is approximately 50 percent over 5 years of follow-up (Fig. 61–8).[142] If these data were used to predict whether or not an individual patient would need revascularization to prevent an event within the following 5 years, the likelihood that this prediction would be correct is only 50 percent.

At least part of this prognostic uncertainty can be attributed to widely recognized limitations of coronary angiography.[143, 144] It is now clear that the angiographic, or anatomical, assessment of the degree of coronary stenosis does not always correlate well with the physiologic significance of the stenosis. These limitations of angiography for the assessment of physiologic significance and the estimation of subsequent patient outcome have led to the evaluation of the potential complementary role of exercise testing modalities, including equilibrium radionuclide angiography.

Considered alone as a noninvasive prognostic tool, exercise radionuclide angiography is powerful.[123–126, 145] The initial published data, which employed first-pass radionuclide angiography, demonstrated that the exercise ejection fraction was the single most important variable for predicting subsequent cardiovascular death or nonfatal myocardial infarction.[123, 145] These findings have recently been confirmed in a larger series.[125] Exercise ejection fraction was the most powerful independent radionuclide angiographic variable for predicting both cardiovascular mortality and combined cardiovascular mortality or nonfatal myocardial infarction. The strength of the association between radionuclide angiographic variables and cardiovascular mortality was the same as that between catheterization variables and this end point. The radionuclide angiographic variables provided 84 percent of the prognostic information provided by the combination of clinical and catheterization variables.[125]

The prognostic value of equilibrium radionuclide angiography has also been demonstrated.[124] Using this technique, both the ejection fraction at rest (Fig. 61–9) and the ejection fraction with exercise (Fig. 61–10) can be employed to identify subsets of patients who are more likely to have cardiac events over the following 4 years. An exercise ejection fraction of less than 0.3 is associated with a cardiac event rate of almost 50 percent over the following 4 years.

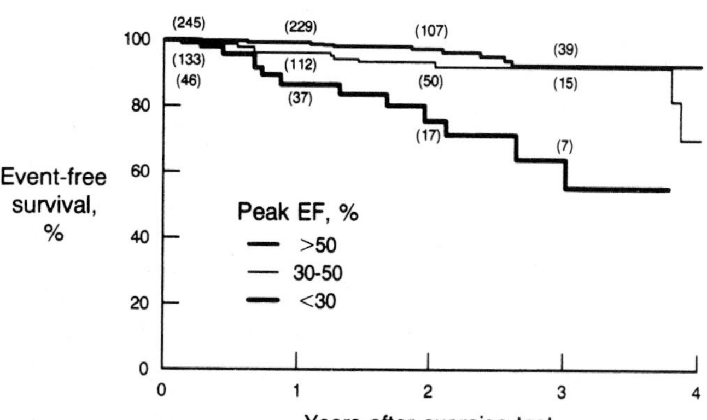

FIGURE 61-10. Event-free survival as a function of peak exercise ejection fraction (EF) in 424 medically treated patients with known or suspected coronary artery disease. Events are as defined for Figure 61–9. (From Taliercio, C.P., Clements, I.P., Zinsmeister, A.R., et al.: Prognostic value and limitations of exercise radionuclide angiography. Mayo Clin. Proc. 63:573, 1988, with permission.)

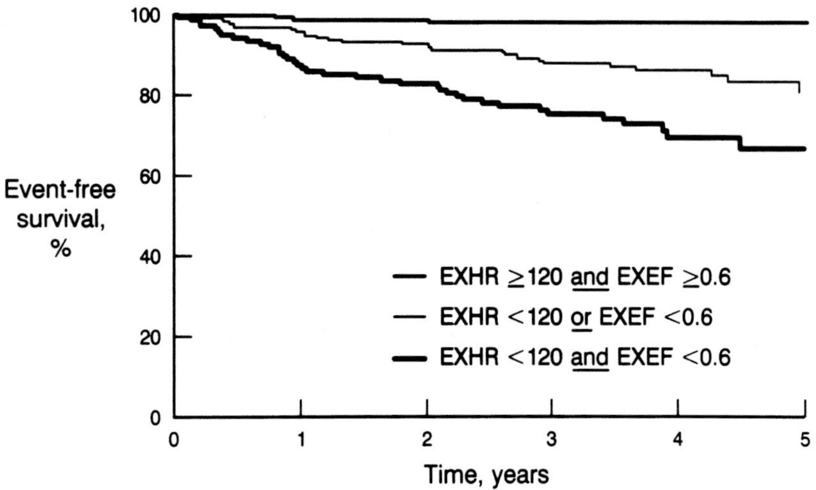

FIGURE 61–11. Event-free survival as a function of exercise ejection fraction (EF) and heart rate (HR) in 526 medically treated patients from a community-based population with known or suspected coronary artery disease. Events are defined as in Figure 61–9.

These findings, based on patients undergoing cardiac catheterization in tertiary referral centers, recently have been confirmed in a community population.[126] Among 536 residents of Olmsted County, Minnesota, who were followed for a median of 46 months, there were 71 cardiac events (26 deaths and 45 nonfatal myocardial infarctions). There were four independent predictors of outcome: (1) exercise ejection fraction, (2) exercise heart rate, (3) age, and (4) evidence of prior myocardial infarction (by history or electrocardiogram). Using the two most powerful variables (exercise ejection fraction and exercise heart rate), the patients could be divided into various prognostic groups (Fig. 61–11). One hundred fifty-seven patients in this community-based population (29 percent of the total group) had an exercise ejection fraction of less than 0.6 and an exercise heart rate of less than 120 beats per minute. This high-risk subgroup had a 4-year event-free survival rate of only 68 percent. These results clearly suggest that the noninvasive prognostic value of equilibrium radionuclide angiography applies to both tertiary care center patient populations and community populations.[126]

A more important issue is whether equilibrium exercise radionuclide angiography contributes prognostic information that is independent of the information (number of diseased vessels and resting ejection fraction) that can be obtained by cardiac catheterization. Does exercise radionuclide angiography add to our ability to predict outcome in an individual patient once his or her coronary anatomy and resting ejection fraction are known? This issue was rigorously examined in a large series of 571 patients with stable coronary disease followed for a median of 5.4 years.[125] A variety of clinical and catheterization variables were considered, including age, gender, indices of pain, myocardial damage, vascular disease, conduction defects, ejection fraction, number of diseased vessels, left main artery stenosis, proximal left anterior descending artery stenosis, and mitral insufficiency. After consideration of all these parameters, exercise radionuclide angiography provided significant additional prognostic information.

The impact of this information has been studied in specific patient subsets. Bonow and associates examined the outcome of medically treated, mildly symptomatic patients with three-vessel artery disease and normal or near-normal resting left ventricular function.[146] The presence of severe exercise-induced ischemia on equilibrium exercise radionuclide angiography identified a subset of patients who were at high risk for subsequent death (Fig. 61–12). The 18-month survival rate of the 19 patients with a decline in ejection fraction with exercise, ST segment depression, and a limited exercise capacity was less than 80 percent. In contrast, 24 patients with three-vessel coronary artery disease who did not have severe exercise-induced ischemia had a 4-year survival rate of 100 percent. This study clearly suggested that equilibrium radionuclide angiography provides prognostic information that is independent of the number of diseased vessels and resting left ventricular ejection fraction and that this modality could be used to identify patients with three-vessel artery disease and normal or near-normal resting function who were likely to benefit from coronary revascularization.

Taliercio and associates sought to confirm these findings in a group of 424 medically treated patients followed for a median of 21.7 months.[124] Univariate analysis demonstrated that multiple individual parameters were associated with subsequent cardiac death and nonfatal myocardial infarction, including both the exercise ejection fraction and the resting ejection fraction. As assessed by multivariate analysis, however, only three variables were independently associated with subsequent cardiac events: the number of diseased vessels, the resting ejection fraction, and patient age. Thus, exercise-induced ischemia did not contribute independent prognostic information in this study, even when a subgroup similar to that of Bonow and associates was analyzed (Fig. 61–13). The potential reasons for these apparently conflicting data have been well reviewed in detail elsewhere.[147]

Other studies have tended to confirm the independent prognostic value of exercise-induced ischemia assessed by equilibrium exercise radionuclide angiography. In a study of 53 mildly symptomatic patients with one-vessel or two-vessel coronary artery disease and abnormal resting left ventricular function (resting ejection

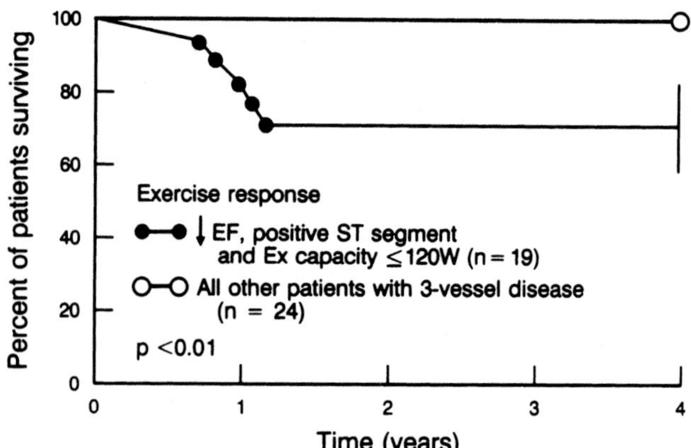

FIGURE 61–12. Survival in 43 patients from the National Institutes of Health with three-vessel disease and a resting ejection fraction of more than 0.4, as a function of the presence of a markedly abnormal exercise response. Patients with marked ischemia had a poor prognosis. (From Bonow, R., Kent, K., Rosing D., et al.: Exercise-induced ischemia in mildly symptomatic patients with coronary artery disease and preserved left ventricular function: Identification of subgroups at risk of death during medical therapy. N. Engl. J. Med. 311:1339, 1984, with permission.)

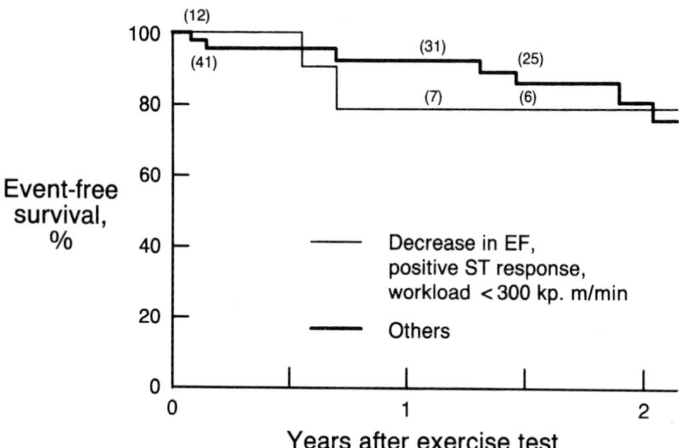

FIGURE 61–13. Event-free survival in 53 patients from the Mayo Clinic with three-vessel disease and an ejection fraction (EF) of more than 0.4 as a function of the presence of a markedly abnormal exercise response. There was no significant difference between the two groups. (From Taliercio, C.P., Clements, I.P., Zinsmeister, A.R., et al.: Prognostic value and limitations of exercise radionuclide angiography. Mayo Clin. Proc. 63:573, 1988, with permission.)

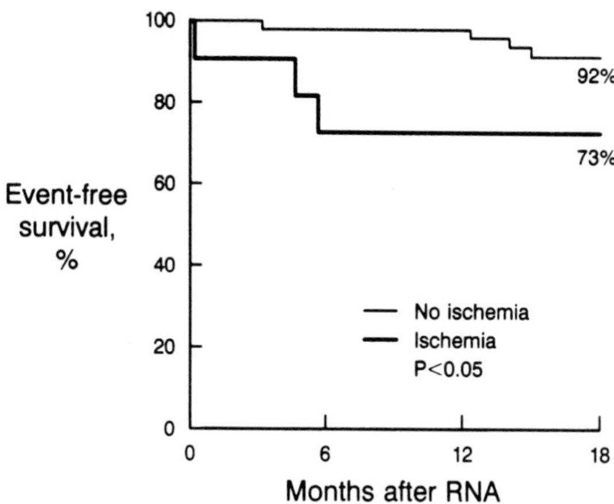

FIGURE 61–15. Event-free survival in 68 patients from the Mayo Clinic with one- or two-vessel disease and a resting ejection fraction of less than 0.5 as a function of the presence of a markedly abnormal exercise response. Patient outcome was significantly different in the two groups. (From Miller, T., Taliercio, C., Zinsmeister, A., et al.: Risk stratification of single- or double-vessel coronary artery disease and impaired left ventricular function using exercise radionuclide angiography. Am. J. Cardiol. 65:1317, 1990, with permission.)

fraction <0.4), Mazzotta and associates found that the exercise ejection fraction and the change in ejection fraction from rest to exercise were highly predictive of subsequent events (Fig. 61–14).[148] In the 17 patients with an exercise ejection fraction of less than 0.3, the 5-year survival rate was only 61 percent, compared with a 97 percent 5-year survival rate in the 36 patients with an exercise ejection fraction of greater than 0.3.

A study from our laboratory confirmed these findings in 68 patients with one-vessel or two-vessel coronary artery disease and a resting left ventricular ejection fraction of less than 0.5.[149] The presence of severe ischemia on equilibrium exercise radionuclide angiography, defined as a decrease in ejection fraction with exercise, a peak workload of less than or equal to 600 kg • m/min, and greater than or equal to 1 mm ST segment depression, was a significant ($P < .001$) predictor of subsequent patient outcome (Fig. 61–15). The 12 patients with ischemia had a 33 percent event rate within 1 year, compared with only 2 percent in the 56 patients without ischemia. Thus, both these studies confirmed the earlier findings of Bonow and colleagues, suggesting that equilibrium exercise radionuclide angiography provides prognostic information that is complementary to cardiac catheterization in predicting patient outcome.

Does exercise radionuclide angiography identify a high-risk subgroup of patients among low-risk populations? A study from our laboratory evaluated the outcome of 264 medically treated patients with normal resting left ventricular ejection fraction and one- or two-vessel coronary artery disease.[150] Fifty-six of these patients had severe exercise-induced ischemia (using the same three variables defined previously). During a median follow-up of 63 months, there were 12 cardiac deaths and 18 nonfatal myocardial infarctions. The 5-year event-free survival rate was equivalent for patients with (91 percent) and for those without (87 percent) severe exercise-induced ischemia (Fig. 61–16).

Similarly, in a study of 256 medically treated patients with normal resting electrocardiograms who were not taking digoxin, the event rate was low, and radionuclide angiography failed to augment the prognostic information provided by the exercise electrocardio-

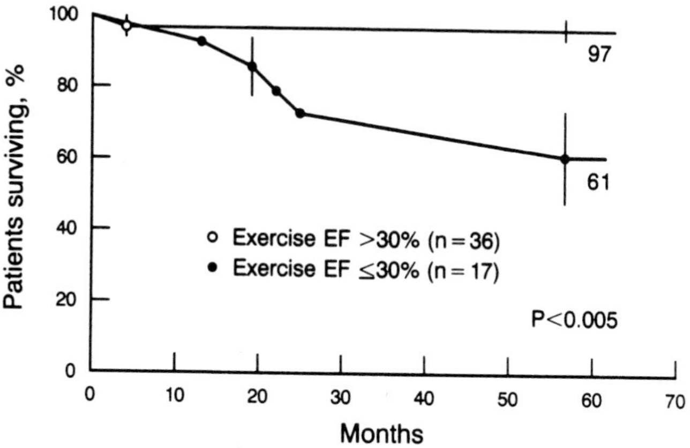

FIGURE 61–14. Survival in 53 patients from the National Institutes of Health with one- or two-vessel disease and a resting ejection fraction of less than 0.4. The exercise ejection fraction was highly predictive of survival. (From Mazzotta, G., Bonow, R., Pace, L., et al.: Relation between exertional ischemia and prognosis in mildly symptomatic patients with single or double-vessel coronary artery disease and left ventricular dysfunction at rest. J. Am. Coll. Cardiol. 13:567, 1989. With permission of the American College of Cardiology.)

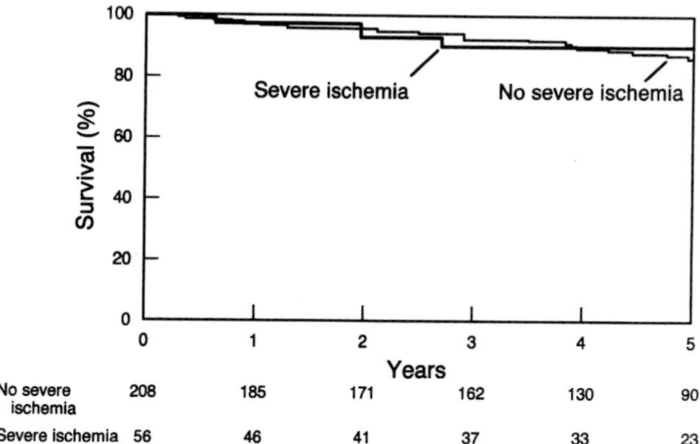

FIGURE 61–16. Survival free of cardiac death or nonfatal myocardial infarction in 264 patients from the Mayo Clinic with one- or two-vessel disease and an ejection fraction greater than or equal to 0.5 as a function of the presence of a markedly abnormal exercise test. Patient outcome was not significantly different between the two groups. (From Miller, T., Christian, T., Taliercio, C., et al.: Severe exercise-induced ischemia does not identify high-risk patients with normal left ventricular function and one- or two-vessel coronary artery disease. J. Am. Coll. Cardiol. 23:219, 1994. With permission of the American College of Cardiology.)

gram.[151] Finally, exercise radionuclide angiography cannot identify a high-risk subgroup among patients with normal or near-normal resting left ventricular function who do not have significant coronary artery disease. In a study of 79 patients with a resting left ventricular ejection fraction greater than or equal to 0.4 and no significant coronary artery disease who had a decrease in ejection fraction with exercise or a peak exercise ejection fraction less than 0.6, 4-year infarction-free survival was 97 percent.[152]

Thus, the available literature indicates that exercise radionuclide angiography can further refine risk stratification in anatomically defined high-risk patients with coronary artery disease but does not identify the few patients who have future events among low-risk patient groups.[153, 154]

Resting diastolic filling parameters have also been shown to refine risk stratification in patients with coronary artery disease and reduced resting left ventricular systolic function. Clements and colleagues reported that the variables peak filling rate and time-to-peak filling rate added independent prognostic information to resting left ventricular ejection fraction in a group of 93 patients with resting left ventricular ejection fractions of less than 0.5.[155] Survival free of cardiac death at 1 year was 73 percent in patients whose peak filling rate was below the median value and 98 percent in patients in whom this rate was above the median.

Functional Assessment and Patient Management

Equilibrium radionuclide angiography may also be used to guide patient management in patients with chronic angina. Most often this involves the assessment of the physiologic importance of anatomical coronary artery disease. For the reasons already outlined, such an assessment is often complementary to the information provided by coronary arteriography. Functional information is particularly important for clinical patient management when coronary arteriography has demonstrated arterial obstructions that are likely to be of borderline hemodynamic significance. The presence or absence of exercise-induced ischemia in such patients will help determine the physiologic significance of the lesion and greatly influence the management of the patient. In addition, there may be situations in which the symptomatology appears to be out of proportion to the coronary anatomy. Functional testing with equilibrium radionuclide angiography may help provide evidence that the patient's symptomatology is, in fact, due to myocardial ischemia. The ability of equilibrium radionuclide angiography to assess ventricular performance at multiple levels of exercise and thereby determine whether functional evidence of ischemia is present at low levels of exercise (and presumably low levels of myocardial oxygen demand) is particularly helpful in these circumstances.

Equilibrium radionuclide angiography may also be employed to assess the results of coronary revascularization. Such testing can be employed to provide objective confirmation of the relief of exercise-induced ischemia, to evaluate the physiologic importance of nonrevascularized lesions, to reassure the patient, and to provide a baseline for subsequent follow-up. Several studies have employed equilibrium radionuclide angiography to assess the impact of coronary artery bypass grafting on left ventricular function.[156–159] Many factors influence the result, including patient selection, coronary anatomy, perioperative infarction, graft patency, ventricular loading conditions, drug therapy, and the timing of the postoperative study. The findings in individual patients, therefore, may be highly variable. In groups of patients, the most consistent finding is an improvement in exercise left ventricular function, particularly in those patients who had the most exercise-induced ischemia preoperatively.[158] Recent evidence suggests that resting function may also improve postoperatively in selected patients.[160–162] Exercise radionuclide angiography performed after bypass surgery has also been shown to be useful for prognostic purposes. In a group of 192 patients studied an average of 26 months after bypass surgery and followed for an average of 8.7 years, Wallis and colleagues reported that the change in left ventricular ejection fraction between rest and exercise was the strongest independent predictor of both cardiac death and all cardiac events.[163] The risk of cardiac death increased more than twofold with each 10 percent decrement in change in the left ventricular ejection fraction with exercise.

Equilibrium radionuclide angiography early after successful percutaneous transluminal coronary angioplasty appears to predict the presence or absence of restenosis on coronary angiography months later. DePuey and colleagues found that severe degrees of restenosis were present in 43 percent of patients with positive radionuclide angiograms early after percutaneous transluminal coronary angioplasty.[164] In contrast, only 7 percent of those with a negative early radionuclide angiogram experienced severe late restenosis. O'Keefe and colleagues confirmed the ability of early radionuclide angiography to predict subsequent restenosis.[165] In those patients who had normal radionuclide angiograms within 1 month after percutaneous transluminal coronary angioplasty, no patient experienced late restenosis. In those patients with abnormal early radionuclide angiograms, the incidence of subsequent restenosis was 42 percent. Thus, early exercise radionuclide angiography identifies subgroups of patients who are at low risk and high risk for restenosis after percutaneous transluminal coronary angioplasty.

Myocardial Infarction

Equilibrium radionuclide angiography is useful for the evaluation of patients following acute myocardial infarction. Approximately one of four patients not treated with thrombolytic therapy who are discharged from the hospital following an acute myocardial infarction will suffer a recurrent infarction or die during the following year. The medical literature reports a great variety of different modalities to predict patient outcome following acute myocardial infarction. Two factors are consistently noted to relate to patient outcome: (1) the extent of myocardial damage and (2) the extent of exercise-induced ischemia.

The extent of myocardial damage clearly can be assessed by the resting ejection fraction. This measurement provides information that is complementary to clinical data and is predictive of the short-term prognosis.[166–169] In addition, the resting ejection fraction is an important determinant of survival during the following year. The Multicenter Post-infarction Research Group identified four independent predictors of survival following acute myocardial infarction in a large group of 799 patients.[170] One of these predictors was a resting ejection fraction of less than 0.4, a cutoff value selected for analysis before the study. A review of the data from that study clearly indicates, however, that 1-year cardiac mortality is inversely related to the ejection fraction in a continuous fashion (Fig. 61–17). Of note is the fact that the 1-year cardiac mortality approaches 50 percent in those patients with a resting ejection fraction of less than 0.20.

Regional wall motion from the resting radionuclide angiogram has been shown to contain prognostic information independent of the ejection fraction.[171] Weissler and associates demonstrated that a quantitative expression of the nonuniformity among all ventricular segments adds independent prognostic information to global ejection fraction.[171] At the present time, however, the ejection fraction is the variable most commonly used to assess the severity of myocardial damage and determine prognosis following a myocardial infarction.

Equilibrium radionuclide angiography is one of several noninvasive exercise testing modalities that have been employed prior to a patient's hospital discharge in an attempt to determine the presence and extent of exercise-induced ischemia. Corbett and colleagues examined the results of exercise radionuclide angiography in 117 patients with uncomplicated myocardial infarction, who were then followed for at least 6 months.[172, 173] The change in ejection fraction with submaximal exercise was the most useful parameter for predicting subsequent patient outcome. The ejection fraction failed to increase with exercise in 74 patients; of these individuals, 70 (95 percent) had events within 6 months. In contrast, of the 43 patients whose ejection fraction increased with exercise, only 4 (9 percent) had events. It should be noted, however, that congestive heart

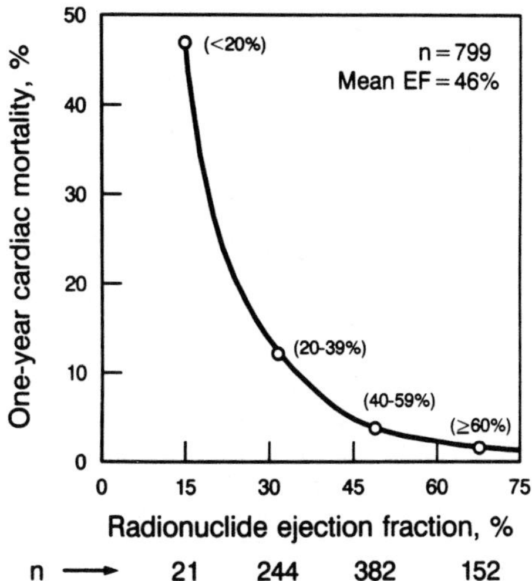

FIGURE 61–17. One-year cardiac mortality in 799 patients following acute myocardial infarction as a function of the resting ejection fraction (EF) on predischarge radionuclide angiography. n = number of patients in each category and the total population. (From Multicenter Post-infarction Research Group: Risk stratification and survival after myocardial infarction. N. Engl. J. Med. 309:331, 1983, with permission.)

failure, medically refractory angina, and limiting angina were all considered events in this analysis.

Dewhurst and Muir studied 100 consecutive patients who underwent exercise radionuclide angiography 1 month after infarction.[174] A resting ejection fraction of less than 0.35 identified a high-risk group with a very poor prognosis. In those patients with a resting ejection fraction of greater than 0.35, a decrease in ejection fraction of at least 0.05 with exercise identified patients who were at high risk for postinfarction angina. Their study is one of the few true "natural history" studies in the literature, as coronary revascularization was not undertaken in any of the patients.

Hung and associates compared the prognostic value of the treadmill exercise test, exercise ^{201}Tl scintigraphy, and equilibrium exercise radionuclide angiography in 117 men who received all three tests within 3 weeks after myocardial infarction.[175] They compared the ability of a large number of parameters from each of these modalities to predict the subsequent development of death, recurrent myocardial infarction, or ventricular fibrillation. The single best predictor of outcome was the change in ejection fraction at an exercise workload of 450 kg • m/min. The only other variable that provided additional prognostic information was the peak treadmill workload. Thus, on the basis of their study, equilibrium exercise radionuclide angiography appears to be the preferred technique for the assessment of prognosis following acute myocardial infarction. There is a clear variation in patient population across the various studies in the literature, however, suggesting the use of different selection criteria for testing.

It is particularly difficult to relate the previously published studies to current populations now that percutaneous transluminal coronary angioplasty, acute thrombolytic therapy, and early β-blockade are commonly used. In fact, one recent study demonstrated significant changes over time in multiple clinical and exercise parameters in those patients undergoing exercise radionuclide angiography early after myocardial infarction.[176] Recent studies have shown that patients treated with thrombolytic therapy who survive to hospital discharge have a much lower posthospital mortality rate compared with historical studies of conventionally treated patients.[177] Because these patients are a low-risk group, previously proven prognostic variables from the prethrombolytic era are less powerful for predicting outcome in these patients. Resting ejection fraction is still an important determinant of survival, but for a given level of left ventricular dysfunction, survival is better in patients treated with thrombolytic therapy compared with historical controls from the prethrombolytic era.[154, 178] Peak exercise ejection fraction is still a significant predictor of death and reinfarction,[179] but the event rate is low, at least partially because of a high rate of early revascularization. The applicability of previously published results to current patient populations, therefore, is in question.

Equilibrium radionuclide angiography is also frequently employed to assess the efficacy of acute intervention with thrombolytic therapy or percutaneous transluminal coronary angioplasty in patients with myocardial infarction. Such interventions are presumed to limit the extent of myocardial damage. The resting ejection fraction after infarction has been employed as an end point in many investigations of therapeutic efficacy.[176, 180–188] The Thrombolysis in Myocardial Infarction (TIMI) II study also evaluated the exercise ejection fraction as an end point.[189] Other studies have used the change in the resting ejection fraction measured during and after infarction as an end point to assess efficacy in an attempt to adjust for the variable amount of myocardium that is "at risk." The change in ejection fraction measured during and after infarction has generally demonstrated a more significant treatment effect than the ejection fraction measured after infarction only.[183, 184] It should be noted, however, that the resting ejection fraction measured during infarction is influenced by many factors other than the amount of hypoperfused myocardium, including preload, afterload, the duration of myocardial ischemia, and hyperkinesia in normal segments. These factors may contribute to the large spontaneous changes that occur in ejection fraction during the first 24 hours of acute myocardial infarction[190] and appear to persist at least until hospital discharge. In a study of patients treated with reperfusion therapy, there was no difference in mean ejection fraction measured at hospital discharge and at 6 weeks, but 34 percent of patients were found to have a significant change (≥8 ejection fraction points) between these two time points.[191] ^{99m}Tc-sestamibi is able to assess the amount of myocardium "at risk" in acute infarction without any delay in therapy. The change in myocardial perfusion determined by this radiopharmaceutical agent before and after therapy appears to be a superior measurement tool for the assessment of the efficacy of acute interventions.[192, 193]

LIMITATIONS OF RADIONUCLIDE ANGIOGRAPHY. Like any other sophisticated medical procedure, radionuclide angiography has both strengths and weaknesses. Although the limitations of this procedure have been mentioned previously, it is important to summarize and re-emphasize them here. First and foremost, the test must be performed carefully and correctly, with a great deal of attention to quality control. As with many other sophisticated procedures, exercise radionuclide angiography can be useful when performed and interpreted by experts, but it also can be misleading in the hands of unskilled practitioners. Second, the test requires approximately 2 minutes of a steady state during exercise for adequate exercise images. For a variety of cardiac and noncardiac reasons, many patients cannot sustain exercise for this amount of time. In other individuals who are able to exercise, left ventricular dysfunction may occur for only a brief period at the peak of exercise and will therefore be missed by this technology. Third, left ventricular response to exercise is a complex phenomenon dependent on gender, age, medications, exercise workload, ventricular loading, and exercise position. Fourth, the assessment of regional dysfunction by this technique is limited because of the nontomographic format and the usual use of only one projection during exercise. Fifth, significant arrhythmias, including atrial fibrillation, interfere with the gating required for accurate studies. Depending on their prevalence, arrhythmias will reduce the accuracy of the data or totally invalidate them. Finally, the previous validation studies mentioned throughout the chapter have often relied on comparison with coronary anatomy, as assessed by subjective estimates of percent diameter stenosis on coronary arteriography. The limitations of subjective assessment by coronary arteriography have now been well demonstrated.[143, 144] Such angiographic comparisons, however, are of importance primarily because of the demonstrated relationship of coronary anatomy to patient outcome. As previously mentioned, the prognostic significance of exercise radionuclide angiography is already well demonstrated.

Cardiomyopathy

Equilibrium radionuclide angiography is useful in the evaluation of patients with known or suspected congestive cardiomyopathies. Measurement of resting ejection fraction and resting left ventricular volume can provide objective documentation of left ventricular size and function. Those patients with a possible restrictive physiology may be identified. Radionuclide angiography may provide potential clues to the underlying cause. An early study suggested that a combination of radionuclide angiography and ^{201}Tl perfusion imaging could help identify patients with end-stage ischemic heart disease rather than a true cardiomyopathy,[194] although a more recent study concluded that these techniques cannot be used reliably to differentiate these two entities.[195]

The presence and importance of diastolic dysfunction in patients with hypertrophic cardiomyopathy and restrictive cardiomyopathy is now well established. Abnormalities of diastolic filling in such patients can be objectively documented by equilibrium radionuclide angiography.[95, 196, 197] The potential response to medical therapy, including calcium channel blockers, can be evaluated using diastolic filling measurements on equilibrium radionuclide angiography as an end point.[95, 197]

Radionuclide angiography can help guide the medical management and follow-up of patients with congestive cardiomyopathy as well. Since the clinical course of these patients is frequently variable, this modality may be employed as an objective means of assessing any temporal change in left ventricular size or function. The stability of equilibrium radionuclide angiography left ventricular volume measurements over time has been examined,[39, 55] and it has been determined that an end-diastolic volume index change of greater than 36 to 45 mL/m^2 is necessary to indicate a true change between two serial examinations. The response of the left ventricle to therapeutic interventions, including vasodilator therapy and abstention from alcohol, may be assessed objectively in this fashion.[198, 199] Such information clearly may be important in the clinical management of these patients.

Valvular Heart Disease

Equilibrium radionuclide angiography has little place at this time in the assessment of stenotic valvular lesions. Its principal role in valvular heart disease is in the assessment of left-sided regurgitant lesions, that is, mitral and aortic insufficiency, although it has been used to assess tricuspid insufficiency as well.[200]

In patients with mitral or aortic insufficiency, equilibrium radionuclide angiography may be employed to measure resting left ventricular size and resting left ventricular ejection fraction. As mentioned previously, the estimates of the volume of the left ventricle obtained by radionuclide angiography is this setting are subject to greater error than usual because of the attenuation of counts from the portions of the ventricle that are farthest away from the gamma camera. In addition, relatively few patients with very large hearts have been included in many of the previous studies validating methods for the assessment of volume. Despite these potential limitations with respect to absolute volumes, measurements of relative volume changes in the same patient remain highly accurate and therefore have been employed to assess the response to exercise[201–206] and the long-term response to medical therapy.[56]

Measurements of resting ejection fraction in patients with aortic insufficiency are highly accurate by equilibrium radionuclide angiography. Although the measurement of ejection fraction by contrast ventriculography may become difficult in the presence of severe left ventricular enlargement, the presence of such enlargement improves the accuracy of equilibrium radionuclide angiography by increasing the counts within the left ventricle and thereby reducing statistical fluctuation. In patients with mitral insufficiency, the increase in accuracy due to statistical considerations may be offset by the increasing degree of overlap between the left atrium and the left ventricle. This overlap can be reduced by increasing the caudal-cranial angulation of the gamma camera; in the presence of severe left atrial enlargement, it usually cannot be eliminated.

As described earlier, the magnitude of left-sided regurgitation can be quantified by using the regurgitant fraction and left ventricular output. Such measurements are useful when the magnitude of regurgitation is not evident from clinical examination. This is particularly true in cases of severe left ventricular enlargement with mitral regurgitation, when the magnitude of mitral regurgitation and the issue of whether it is a primary or secondary phenomenon often are not readily apparent from clinical examination.

Equilibrium radionuclide angiography potentially can make an important contribution to the timing of valve replacement in patients with severe left-sided regurgitation. This issue has been best studied in patients with aortic regurgitation. Despite substantial volume overload of the left ventricle, patients with aortic regurgitation may remain asymptomatic for many years. Once symptoms occur, the downhill course of patients treated medically is often rapid. Therefore, there is general agreement that patients with aortic insufficiency and significant symptoms should undergo aortic valve replacement.[207] The treatment of the asymptomatic or minimally symptomatic patient is a much more controversial issue. The long-term survival of patients who undergo aortic valve replacement for chronic aortic insufficiency is somewhat disappointing. Many of the late postoperative deaths in such patients have been related to chronic congestive heart failure.[208] The long-standing volume overload in these patients apparently has led to irreversible left ventricular dysfunction. Thus, there has been considerable interest in identifying such patients earlier in the natural history of disease so that aortic valve replacement can be undertaken before irreversible left ventricular dysfunction occurs. However, the benefit of performing early aortic valve replacement must be weighed against the risks of the surgery as well as the subsequent morbidity and mortality because of the presence of a prosthetic heart valve.

The issue of the timing of aortic valve replacement has been addressed in a series of published studies from Bonow and colleagues at the National Institutes of Health.[207–212] Preoperative left ventricular function, as assessed by the resting ejection fraction with equilibrium radionuclide angiography, is a major determinant of postoperative survival (Fig. 61–18). Survival at 5.5 years was 96

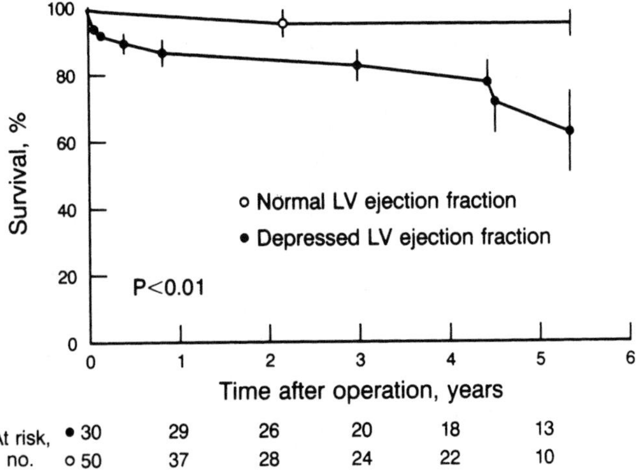

FIGURE 61-18. Survival of patients with aortic insufficiency after aortic valve replacement. Preoperative resting left ventricular (LV) ejection fraction is a determinant of postoperative survival. (From Bonow, R., Picone, A., McIntosh, C., et al.: Survival and functional results after valve replacement for aortic regurgitation from 1976 to 1983: Impact of preoperative left ventricular function. Circulation 72:1244, 1985, by permission of the American Heart Association, Inc.)

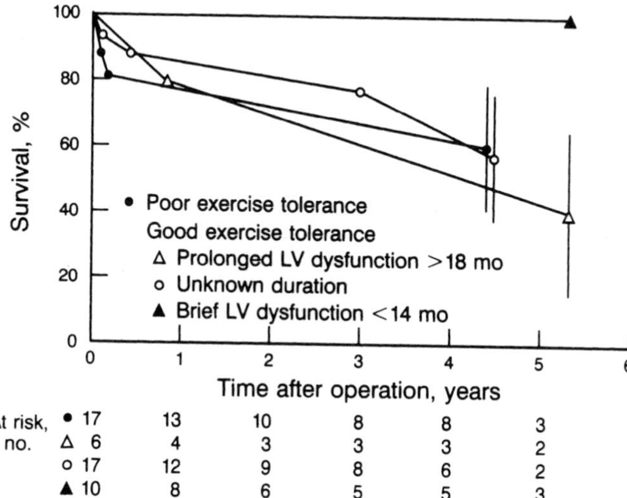

FIGURE 61–19. Postoperative survival of patients with aortic insufficiency and abnormal preoperative resting left ventricular (LV) ejection fraction. Exercise tolerance and the duration of left ventricular dysfunction are determinants of survival. (From Bonow, R., Picone, A., McIntosh, C., et al.: Survival and functional results after valve replacement for aortic regurgitation from 1976 to 1983: Impact of preoperative left ventricular function. Circulation 72:1244, 1985, by permission of the American Heart Association, Inc.)

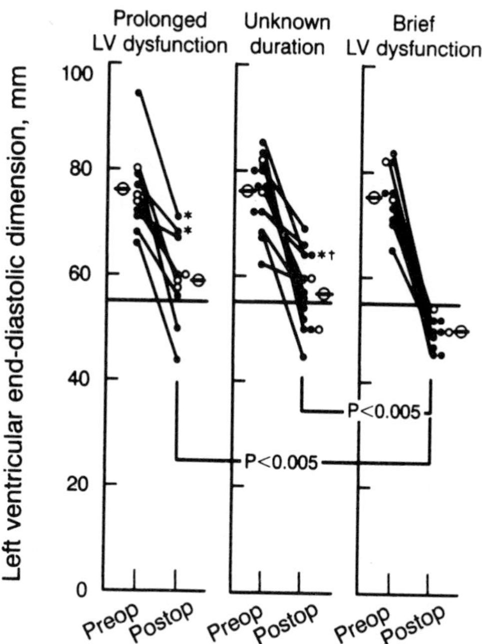

FIGURE 61–20. Change in echocardiographic left ventricular (LV) end-diastolic dimension from before (preop) to 6 months after (postop) aortic valve replacement. *Open symbols,* asymptomatic patients; *asterisks,* patients who subsequently died with symptoms of heart failure; *cross,* one patient who subsequently died with prosthetic valve dysfunction; *slashed circles,* mean values. The horizontal solid line at 55 mm indicates the upper limit of normal. (From Bonow, R., Rosing, D., Maron, B., et al.: Reversal of left ventricular dysfunction after aortic valve replacement for chronic aortic regurgitation: Influence of duration of preoperative left ventricular dysfunction. Circulation 70:570, 1984, by permission of the American Heart Association, Inc.)

percent in patients with a normal preoperative ejection fraction, compared with 63 percent in patients with an abnormal preoperative ejection fraction.[208] Further analysis demonstrated that the risk of postoperative death in patients with an abnormal preoperative ejection fraction depended on two other factors: preoperative exercise tolerance and the duration of resting left ventricular dysfunction. Postoperative survival was poor in patients with a poor exercise tolerance or resting left ventricular dysfunction either of unknown duration or known to have been present for greater than 18 months (Fig. 61–19). In contrast, postoperative survival was excellent in patients with a good exercise tolerance and an abnormal resting left ventricular ejection fraction of less than 14 months' duration (see Fig. 61–19). A more recent study examining the value of serial echocardiographic and radionuclide angiographic studies in these patients showed the rate of change in resting ejection fraction was an independent predictor of death or the development of symptoms necessitating operation.[212] These findings strongly suggest that patients with asymptomatic or minimally symptomatic aortic insufficiency should have their resting ejection fraction assessed by equilibrium radionuclide angiography at regular intervals. Surgery can be safely postponed until symptoms develop or until the resting ejection fraction becomes abnormal.

Bonow and associates have demonstrated that death is rare when this strategy is used in asymptomatic patients with aortic insufficiency and normal left ventricular function, and less than 4 percent of the patients require aortic valve replacement each year.[210] More important, when this strategy is followed, postoperative survival is excellent, and left ventricular size (Fig. 61–20) and resting function (Fig. 61–21) both improve postoperatively.[211]

Earlier studies had suggested that exercise-induced left ventricular dysfunction might be an early sign of impending irreversible left ventricular failure in patients with aortic insufficiency.[202] Exercise-induced changes in ejection fraction correlate with the end-systolic pressure-to-volume ratio[213] and with the resting systolic wall stress[214, 215] but not with left ventricular filling pressure.[216] Changes in regurgitant volume, end-diastolic volume, and stroke volume during exercise are variable, depending on when patients are studied during the natural history of the disease.[204, 205, 213] The ejection fraction response to exercise is clearly influenced by the marked changes in ventricular loading that occur in patients with aortic insufficiency. Patients with an increase in ejection fraction during exercise are unlikely to experience symptoms or left ventricular dysfunction during subsequent follow-up (Fig. 61–22).[210] In patients who have a decrease in ejection fraction with exercise, however, the magnitude of the decrease does not appear to predict

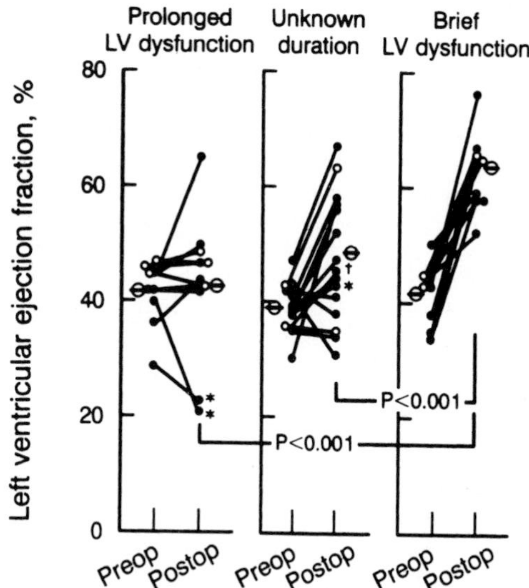

FIGURE 61–21. Change in radionuclide angiographic resting left ventricular (LV) ejection fraction from before to after aortic valve replacement. Symbols are as defined for Figure 61–19. (From Bonow, R., Rosing, D., Maron, B., et al.: Reversal of left ventricular dysfunction after aortic valve replacement for chronic aortic regurgitation: Influence of duration of preoperative left ventricular dysfunction. Circulation 70:570, 1984, by permission of the American Heart Association, Inc.)

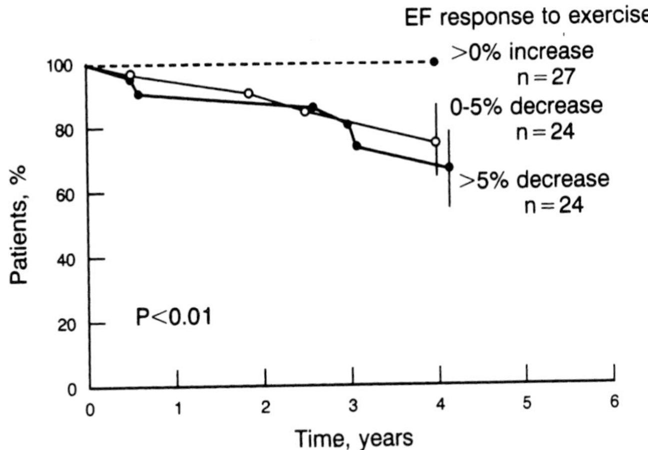

FIGURE 61–22. Influence of left ventricular ejection fraction (EF) response to exercise on the subsequent course of patients with asymptomatic aortic insufficiency. The onset of symptoms or the onset of resting left ventricular dysfunction was taken as an end point. (From Bonow, R., Rosing, D., and McIntosh, C.: The natural history of asymptomatic patients with aortic regurgitation and normal left ventricular function. Circulation 68:509, 1983, by permission of the American Heart Association, Inc.)

subsequent clinical course.[210] Thus, exercise radionuclide angiography can identify a subgroup of patients who are apparently in the earlier stage of the disease's natural history (and therefore unlikely to experience symptoms or resting left ventricular dysfunction over the following 4 years), but its routine use for follow-up purposes does not appear to be justified.

Radionuclide angiography also can assess the effects of aortic valve replacement on left ventricular size, left ventricular function, and exercise performance.[217] Such an assessment can be particularly important in postoperative patients with vague symptoms that may or may not be due to myocardial dysfunction, and it may identify patients who have suffered perioperative myocardial damage despite optimal preservation techniques. An early postoperative decrease in the resting ejection fraction may be seen in the presence of an altered loading condition, however, and does not necessarily imply a decline in ventricular contractility.[218] Measurements of left ventricular function at rest and with exercise generally improve and plateau at 2 to 3 years after surgery. In 21 patients who underwent serial radionuclide angiograms before and after aortic valve replacement, the mean resting ejection fraction improved from 0.45 preoperatively to 0.54 at postoperative year 1 to 2, and the mean exercise ejection fraction improved from 0.39 preoperatively to 0.60 at postoperative year 2 to 3.[219]

Published data regarding patients with severe mitral regurgitation are far fewer.[220, 221] The right ventricular ejection fraction is clearly important, as its resting value is correlated with exercise tolerance.[220] The resting right ventricular ejection fraction and resting left ventricular ejection fraction both predict survival in medically treated patients. Further studies are needed in this area.

Other Indications

Equilibrium radionuclide angiography may be employed in a wide variety of other clinical situations. A few of these miscellaneous indications will be briefly highlighted in this section.

Patients with a presenting complaint of dyspnea frequently may have known coexisting cardiac and pulmonary disease. The identification of the primary problem is often difficult on clinical grounds. Rest and exercise radionuclide angiography may provide an objective assessment of cardiac function to clarify the situation. The experience in our laboratory has been that cardiac dysfunction in such patients is often much greater than anticipated.

The potential cardiotoxic effects of antitumor drugs such as doxorubicin may be monitored by radionuclide angiography.[222, 223] Although one early study reported the use of exercise radionuclide angiography for this purpose, resting radionuclide angiography is usually sufficient. Serial measurements of the resting ejection fraction can provide evidence of impending cardiac dysfunction before there is any overt evidence of congestive failure. Discontinuation of the drug in these early stages can prevent irreversible cardiac dysfunction.

Finally, a wide variety of pathophysiologic and pharmacologic studies have employed rest and exercise radionuclide angiography as a measurement tool. This technique has been used to study several aspects of exercise physiology, including organ blood volume shifts with acute exercise[224] and the effects of exercise training in healthy individuals[225–227] and those with coronary heart disease.[228] The effects of drug intervention[229–232] on coronary artery disease have been well studied using this approach. Other studies have examined the effects of the aging process[85, 233] and cardiac performance after transplantation.[234, 235]

CONCLUSIONS

In the past 20 years, equilibrium radionuclide angiography has progressed from its first description as a research tool to a common clinical test that is widely used in the community. Although the technical aspects of this technique have changed little in recent years, our understanding of its proper use in clinical patient management continues to evolve.

References

1. Eckelman, W., Richards, P., Hauser, W., et al.: Technetium-labeled red blood cells. J. Nucl. Med. 12:22, 1971.
2. Smith, T., and Richards, P.: A simple kit for the preparation of Tc-99m-labeled red blood cells. J. Nucl. Med. 17:126, 1976.
3. Pavel, D., Zimmer, A., and Patterson, V.: In vivo labeling of red blood cells with ^{99m}Tc: A new approach to blood pool visualization. J. Nucl. Med 18:305, 1977.
4. Stokley, E., Parkey, R., Bonte, F., et al.: Gated blood pool imaging following Tc-99m stannous pyrophosphate imaging. Radiology 120:433, 1976.
5. Callahan, R., Froelich, J., McKusick, K., et al.: A modified method for the in vivo labeling of red blood cells with Tc-99m. Concise communication. J. Nucl. Med. 23:315, 1982.
6. Berger, H., and Zaret, B.: Nuclear cardiology. N. Engl. J. Med. 305:855, 1981.
7. Rao, S., Knobel, J., Collier, B., et al.: Effect of Sn(II) ion concentration and heparin on technetium-99m red blood cell labelling. J. Nucl. Med. 27:1202, 1986.
8. Hladik, W., Nigg, K., and Rhodes, B.: Drug induced changes in biologic distribution of radiopharmaceuticals. Semin. Nucl. Med. 12:184, 1982.
9. Lee, H., Wexler, J., Scarf, S., et al.: Pharmacologic alterations in Tc-99m binding by red blood cells. J. Nucl. Med. 24:397, 1983.
10. Kelly, M., Giles, R., Simon, T., et al.: Multigated equilibrium radionuclide angiocardiography: Improved detection of left ventricular wall motion abnormalities and aneurysms by the addition of the left lateral view. Radiology 139:167, 1981.
11. Berman, D., Maddahi, J., Garcia, E., et al.: Assessment of left and right ventricular function with multiple gated equilibrium cardiac blood pool imaging. *In* Berman, D., and Mason, D. (eds.): Clinical Nuclear Cardiology. New York, Grune & Stratton, 1981, p. 224.
12. Manyari, D., and Kostuk, W.: Left and right ventricular function at rest and during bicycle exercise in the supine and sitting positions in normal subjects and patients with coronary artery disease. Am. J. Cardiol. 51:36, 1983.
13. Poliner, L., Dehmer, G., Lewis, S., et al.: Left ventricular performance in normal subjects: A comparison of the responses to exercise in the upright and supine position. Circulation 62:528, 1980.
14. Stengart, R., Wexler, J., Slagle, S., et al.: Radionuclide ventriculographic responses to graded supine and upright exercise: Critical role of the Frank-Starling mechanism at submaximal exercise. Am. J. Cardiol. 53:1671, 1984.
15. Freeman, M., Berman, D., Staniloff, H., et al.: Comparison of upright and supine bicycle exercise in the detection and evaluation of extent of coronary artery disease by equilibrium radionuclide ventriculography. Am. Heart J. 102:182, 1981.
16. Currie, P., Kelly, M., and Pitt, A.: Comparison of supine and erect bicycle exercise electrocardiography in coronary heart disease: Accentuation of exercise-induced ischemic ST depression by supine posture. Am. J. Cardiol. 52:1167, 1983.
17. Foster, C., Dymond, D., Auholm, J., et al.: Effect of exercise protocol on the left ventricular response to exercise. Am. J. Cardiol. 51:859, 1983.
18. Coma-Canella, I., Martinez, M., Rodrigo, F., et al.: The dobutamine stress test with thallium-201 single-photon emission computed tomography and radionuclide angiography: Post-infarction study. J. Am. Coll. Cardiol. 22:399, 1993.
19. Harris, D., Taylor, D., Condon, B., et al.: Myocardial imaging with dipyridamole:

Comparison of the sensitivity and specificity of ^{201}Tl versus MUGA. Eur. J. Nucl. Med. 7:1, 1982.

20. Manyari, D., Nolewajka, A., Purves, P., et al.: Comparative value of the cold-pressor test and supine bicycle exercise to detect subjects with coronary artery disease using radionuclide ventriculography. Circulation 65:571, 1982.
21. Rozanski, A., Bairey, C., Krautz, D., et al.: Mental stress and the induction of silent ischemia in patients with coronary artery disease. N. Engl. J. Med. 318:1005, 1988.
22. Seaworth, J., Higginbotham, M., Coleman, R., et al.: Effect of partial decreases in exercise workload on radionuclide indices of ischemia. J. Am. Coll. Cardiol. 2:522, 1983.
23. Brash, H., Wraith, P., Hannan, W., et al.: The influence of ectopic heart beats in gated ventricular blood pool studies. J. Nucl. Med. 21:391, 1980.
24. Gibbons, R., and Essandoh, L.: Exercise radionuclide angiography in left bundle branch block. Dynamic Cardiovasc. Imaging 1:206, 1987.
25. Rowe, D., Depuey, E., Sonnemaker, R., et al.: Left ventricular performance during exercise in patients with left bundle branch block: Evaluation by gated radionuclide ventriculography. Am. Heart J. 105:66, 1983.
26. Bramlet, D., Mooris, K., Coleman, R., et al.: Effects of rate-dependent left bundle branch block on global and regional left ventricular function. Circulation 67:1059, 1983.
27. Ishibashi, M., Tamaki, N., Yasuda, T., et al.: Assessment of ventricular function with an ambulatory left ventricular function monitor. Circulation 83:II-166, 1991.
28. de Yang, L., Bairey, C., Berman, D., et al.: Accuracy and reproducibility of left ventricular ejection fraction measurements using an ambulatory radionuclide left ventricular function monitor. J. Nucl. Med. 32:796, 1991.
29. Broadhurst, P., Cashman, P., Crawley, J., et al.: Clinical validation of a miniature nuclear probe system for continuous on-line monitoring of cardiac function and ST-segment. J. Nucl. Med. 32:37, 1991.
30. Burow, R., Strauss, H., Singleton, R., et al.: Analysis of left ventricular function from multiple gated acquisition cardiac blood pool imaging: Comparison to contrast angiography. Circulation 56:1024, 1977.
31. Berman, D., Salel, A., Denardo, G., et al.: Clinical assessment of left ventricular regional contraction patterns and ejection fraction by high-resolution gated scintigraphy. J. Nucl. Med. 16:865, 1975.
32. Folland, E., Hamilton, G., Larson, S., et al.: The radionuclide ejection fraction: A comparison of three radionuclide techniques with contrast angiography. J. Nucl. Med. 18:1159, 1977.
33. Green, M., Brody, W., Douglas, M., et al.: Ejection fraction by count rate from gated images. J. Nucl. Med. 19:880, 1978.
34. Pfisterer, M., Ricci, D., Schuler, G., et al.: Validity of left-ventricular ejection fractions measured at rest and peak exercise by equilibrium radionuclide angiography using short acquisition times. J. Nucl. Med. 20:484, 1979.
35. Secker-Walker, R., Resnick, L., Kunz, H., et al.: Measurement of left ventricular ejection fraction. J. Nucl. Med. 14:798, 1973.
36. Zaret, B., and Wackers, F.: Nuclear cardiology (second of two parts). N. Engl. J. Med. 329:855, 1993.
37. Pfisterer, M., Battler, A., Swanson, S., et al.: Reproducibility of ejection fraction determinations by equilibrium radionuclide angiography in response to supine bicycle exercise: Concise communication. J. Nucl. Med. 20:491, 1979.
38. Wackers, F., Berger, H., Johnstone, D., et al.: Multiple gated cardiac blood pool imaging for left ventricular ejection fraction: Validation of the technique and assessment of variability. Am. J. Cardiol. 43:1159, 1979.
39. Mahmarian, J., Moye, L., Verani, M., et al.: Criteria for the accurate interpretation of changes in left ventricular ejection fraction and cardiac volumes as assessed by rest and exercise gated radionuclide angiography. J. Am. Coll. Cardiol. 18:112, 1991.
40. Schneider, R., Jaszczak, R., Coleman, R., et al.: Disproportionate effects of regional hypokinesis on radionuclide ejection fraction: Compensation using attenuation-corrected ventricular volumes. J. Nucl. Med. 25:747, 1984.
41. Okada, R., Kirshenbaum, H., Kushner, F., et al.: Observer variance in the qualitative evaluation of left ventricular wall motion and the quantitation of left ventricular ejection fraction using rest and exercise multigated blood pool imaging. Circulation 61:128, 1980.
42. Okada, R., Pohost, G., Nichols, A., et al.: Left ventricular regional wall motion assessment by multigated and end-diastolic, end-systolic gated radionuclide left ventriculography. Am. J. Cardiol. 45:1211, 1980.
43. Gibbons, R., Morris, K., Lee, K., et al.: Assessment of regional left ventricular function using gated radionuclide angiography. Am. J. Cardiol. 54:294, 1984.
44. Maddox, D., Wynne, J., Uren, R., et al.: Regional ejection fraction: A quantitative radionuclide index of regional left ventricular performance. Circulation 59:1001, 1979.
45. Papapietro, S., Yester, M., Logic, J., et al.: Method for quantitative analysis of regional left ventricular function with first pass and gated blood pool scintigraphy. Am. J. Cardiol. 47:618, 1981.
46. Steckley, R., Kronenberg, M., Born, M., et al.: Radionuclide ventriculography: Evaluation of automated and visual methods for regional wall motion analysis. Radiology 142:179, 1982.
47. Douglas, K., Links, J., Chen, D., et al.: Linear discriminant analysis of regional ejection fractions in the diagnosis of coronary artery disease. Eur. J. Nucl. Med. 12:602, 1987.
48. Botvinick, E., Dae, M., O'Connell, J., et al.: First Harmonic Fourier (Phase) Analysis of Blood Pool Scintigrams for the Analysis of Cardiac Contraction and Conduction. *In* Gerson, M. (ed.): Cardiac Nuclear Medicine. New York, McGraw-Hill, 1987.
49. Mancini, G., Peck, W., and Slutsky, R.: Analysis of phase-angle histograms from equilibrium radionuclide studies: Correlation with semi-quantitative grading of wall motion. Am. J. Cardiol. 55:535, 1985.
50. Norris, S., Slutsky, R., Gerber, K., et al.: Sensitivity and specificity of nuclear phase analysis versus ejection fraction in coronary artery disease. Am. J. Cardiol. 53:1547, 1984.
51. Ratib, O., Henze, E., Schon, M., et al.: Phase analysis of radionuclide ventriculograms for the detection of coronary artery disease. Am. Heart J. 104:1, 1982.
52. Schwaiger, M., Ratib, V., Henze, E., et al.: Limitations of quantitative phase analysis of radionuclide angiograms for detecting coronary artery disease in patients with impaired left ventricular function. Am. Heart J. 108:942, 1984.
53. Clements, I., Brown, M., and Smith, H.: Radionuclide measurement of left ventricular volume. Mayo Clin. Proc. 56:733, 1981.
54. Dehmer, G., Lewis, S., Hillis, L., et al.: Nongeometric determination of left ventricular volumes from equilibrium blood pool scans. Am. J. Cardiol. 45:293, 1980.
55. Brown, M., Vaqueiro, M., Clements, I., et al.: Stability of radionuclide left ventricular volume measurements. Nucl. Med. Commun. 9:117, 1988.
56. Greenberg, B., Massie, B., Bristow, J., et al.: Long-term vasodilator therapy of chronic aortic insufficiency. Circulation 78:98, 1988.
57. Warren, S., Royal, H., Markis, J., et al.: Time course of left ventricular dilation after myocardial infarction: Influence of infarct-related artery and success of coronary thrombolysis. J. Am. Coll. Cardiol. 11:21, 1988.
58. Konstam, M., Tumeh, S., Wynne, J., et al.: Effect of exercise on erythrocyte count and blood activity concentration after technetium-99m in vivo red blood cell labeling. Circulation 66:638, 1982.
59. Levy, W., Cerqueira, M., Veith, R., et al.: Factors influencing serial measurements of cardiac volumes by count-based methods: Effects of elevated catecholamines, position, and exercise on technetium-99m blood radioactivity concentration. J. Nucl. Med. 33:1324, 1992.
60. Vatterott, P., Gibbons, R., Hu, D., et al.: Assessment of left ventricular volume changes during exercise radionuclide angiography in coronary artery disease. Am. J. Cardiol. 61:912, 1988.
61. Links, J., Becker, L., Shindledecker, J., et al.: Measurements of absolute left ventricular volume from gated blood pool studies. Circulation 65:82, 1982.
62. Petru, M., Sorenson, S., Chandhuri, T., et al.: Attenuation correction of equilibrium radionuclide angiography for noninvasive quantitation of cardiac output and ventricular volumes. Am. Heart J. 107:1221, 1984.
63. Starling, M., Dell'Italia, L., Walsh, R., et al.: Accurate estimates of absolute left ventricular volumes from equilibrium radionuclide angiographic count data using a simple geometric attenuation correction. J. Am. Coll. Cardiol. 3:789, 1984.
64. Levy, W., Cerqueira, M., Matsuoka, D., et al.: Four radionuclide methods for left ventricular volume determination: Comparison of a manual and an automated technique. J. Nucl. Med. 34:763, 1992.
65. Massardo, T., Gal, R., Grenier, R., et al.: Left ventricular volume calculation using a count-based ratio method applied to multigated radionuclide angiography. J. Nucl. Med. 31:450, 1990.
66. Dehmer, G., Firth, B., Hillis, L., et al.: Nongeometric determination of right ventricular volumes from equilibrium blood pool scans. Am. J. Cardiol. 49:78, 1982.
67. Gobert, P., Kremer, R., Rigot, P., et al.: Value, sensitivity and specificity of stroke volume ratio in routine equilibrium gated scintigraphy. Eur. Heart J. 8:77, 1987.
68. Konstam, M., Wynne, J., Holman, B., et al.: Use of equilibrium (gated) radionuclide ventriculography to quantitate left ventricular output in patients with and without left-sided valvular regurgitation. Circulation 64:578, 1981.
69. Melchior, J., Chevigne, M., Righetti, A., et al.: Quantification of valvular regurgitation by cardiac blood pool scintigraphy: Correlation with catheterization. Eur. Heart J. 8:71, 1987.
70. Nicod, P., Corbett, J., Firth, B., et al.: Radionuclide techniques for valvular regurgitant index: Comparison in patients with normal and depressed ventricular function. J. Nucl. Med. 23:763, 1982.
71. Rigo, P., Alderson, P., Robertson, R., et al.: Measurement of aortic and mitral regurgitation by gated cardiac blood pool scans. Circulation 60:306, 1979.
72. Sorensen, S., O'Rourke, R., and Chaudhuri, T.: Noninvasive quantitation of valvular regurgitation by gated equilibrium radionuclide angiography. Circulation 62:1089, 1980.
73. Sciagra, R., Voth, E., Tebbe, U., et al.: Evaluation of three methods for quantifying valvular regurgitation using gated equilibrium radionuclide ventriculography. Eur. Heart J. 8:1109, 1987.
74. Holman, B., Wynne, J., Zielonka, J., et al.: A simplified technique for measuring right ventricular ejection fraction using the equilibrium radionuclide angiocardiogram and the slant-hole collimator. Radiology 138:429, 1981.
75. Korr, K., Gandsman, E., Winkler, M., et al.: Hemodynamic correlates of right ventricular ejection fraction measured with gated radionuclide angiography. Am. J. Cardiol. 49:71, 1982.
76. Maddahi, J., Berman, D., Matsuoka, D., et al.: A new technique for assessing right ventricular ejection fraction using rapid multiple-gated equilibrium cardiac blood pool scintigraphy. Circulation 60:581, 1979.
77. Morrison, D., Turgeon, J., and Ovitt, T.: Right ventricular ejection fraction measurement: Contrast ventriculography versus gated blood pool and gated first-pass radionuclide methods. Am. J. Cardiol. 54:651, 1984.
78. Rezai, K., Weiss, R., Stanford, W., et al.: Relative accuracy of three scintigraphic methods for determination of right ventricular ejection fraction: A correlative study with ultrafast computed tomography. J. Nucl. Med. 32:429, 1991.
79. Okada, R., Pohost, G., Kirshenbaum, H., et al.: Radionuclide-determined change in pulmonary blood volume with exercise: Improved sensitivity of multigated blood-pool scanning in detecting coronary artery disease. N. Engl. J. Med. 301:569, 1979.

80. Okada, R., Osbakken, M., Boucher, C., et al.: Pulmonary blood volume ratio response to exercise: A noninvasive determination of exercise-induced changes in pulmonary capillary wedge pressure. Circulation 65:126, 1982.
81. Hanley, P., and Gibbons, R.: The value of radionuclide determined changes in pulmonary blood volume for the detection of coronary artery disease. Chest 97:7, 1990.
82. Dehmer, G., Firth, B., Lewis, S., et al.: Direct measurement of cardiac output by gated equilibrium blood pool scintigraphy: Validation of scintigraphic volume measurements by a nongeometric technique. Am. J. Cardiol. 47:1061, 1981.
83. Melin, J., Wijns, W., Robert, A., et al.: Validation of radionuclide cardiac output measurements during exercise. J. Nucl. Med. 26:1386, 1985.
84. Sorensen, S., Ritchie, J., Caldwell, J., et al.: Serial exercise radionuclide angiography: Validation of count-derived changes in cardiac output and quantitation of maximal exercise ventricular volume change after nitroglycerin and propranolol in normal men. Circulation 61:600, 1980.
85. Arora, R., Machac, J., Goldman, M., et al.: Atrial kinetics and left ventricular diastolic filling in the healthy elderly. J. Am. Coll. Cardiol. 9:1255, 1987.
86. Bacharach, S., Green, M., Borer, J., et al.: Left ventricular peak ejection rate, filling rate, and ejection fraction-frame rate requirements at rest and exercise: Concise communication. J. Nucl. Med. 20:189, 1979.
87. Bonow, R., Bacharach, S., Green, M., et al.: Impaired left ventricular diastolic filling in patients with coronary artery disease: Assessment with radionuclide angiography. Circulation 64:315, 1981.
88. Bowman, L., Lee, F., Jaffe, C., et al.: Peak filling rate normalized to mitral stroke volume: A new Doppler echocardiographic filling index validated by radionuclide angiographic techniques. J. Am. Coll. Cardiol. 12:937, 1988.
89. Clements, I., Nelson, M., O'Connor, M., et al.: Diastolic measurements from alternate R-wave gating. Am. Heart J. 116:113, 1988.
90. Juni, J., and Chen, C.: Effects of gating modes on the analysis of left ventricular function in the presence of heart rate variation. J. Nucl. Med. 29:1272, 1988.
91. Miller, T., Grossman, S., Schechtman, K., et al.: Left ventricular diastolic filling and its association with age. Am. J. Cardiol. 58:531, 1986.
92. Miller, T., Fountos, A., Biello, D., et al.: Detection of coronary artery disease by analysis of ventricular filling. J. Nucl. Med. 28:837, 1987.
93. Mancini, G., Slutsky, R., Norris, L., et al.: Radionuclide analysis of peak filling rate, filling fraction, and time to peak filling rate: Response to supine bicycle exercise in normal subjects and patients with coronary disease. Am. J. Cardiol. 51:43, 1983.
94. Poliner, L., Farber, S., Glaeser, D., et al.: Alterations of diastolic filling rate during exercise radionuclide angiography: A highly sensitive technique for detection of coronary artery disease. Circulation 70:942, 1984.
95. Clements, I., Sinak, L., Gibbons, R., et al.: Determination of diastolic function by radionuclide ventriculography. Mayo Clin. Proc. 65:1007, 1990.
96. Perrone-Filardi, P., Bacharach, S., Dilsizian, V., et al.: Impaired left ventricular filling and regional diastolic asynchrony at rest in coronary artery disease and relation to exercise-induced myocardial ischemia. Am. J. Cardiol. 67:356, 1991.
97. Magorien, D., Shaffer, P., Bush, C., et al.: Assessment of left ventricular pressure-volume relations using gated radionuclide angiography, echocardiography and micromanometer pressure recordings: A new method for serial measurements of systolic and diastolic function in man. Circulation 67:844, 1983.
98. Diamond, G., and Forrester, J.: Analysis of probability as an aid in the clinical diagnosis of coronary-artery disease. N. Engl. J. Med. 300:1350, 1979.
99. Diamond, G., Forrester, J., Hirsch, M., et al.: Application of conditional probability analysis to the clinical diagnosis of coronary artery disease. J. Clin. Invest. 65:1210, 1980.
100. Gibbons, R.: Noninvasive exercise testing in cardiac disease. *In* Spittell, J. (ed.): Clinical Medicine. Philadelphia, Harper & Row, 1985.
101. Gibbons, R.: Nuclear cardiology. *In* Brandenburg, R., Fuster, V., Giuliani, E., et al. (eds.): Cardiology: Fundamentals and Practice. Chicago, Year Book Medical, 1987.
102. Pryor, D., Harrell, F., Jr., Lee, K., et al.: Estimating the likelihood of significant coronary artery disease. Am. J. Med. 75:771, 1983.
103. Berger, H., Reduto, L., Johnstone, D., et al.: Global and regional left ventricular response to bicycle exercise in coronary artery disease: Assessment by quantitative radionuclide angiocardiography. Am. J. Med. 66:13, 1979.
104. Bodenheimer, M., Banka, V., Fooshee, C., et al.: Comparative sensitivity of the exercise electrocardiogram, thallium imaging and stress radionuclide angiography to detect the presence and severity of coronary heart disease. Circulation 60:1270, 1979.
105. Borer, J., Kent, K., Bacharach, S., et al.: Sensitivity, specificity and predictive accuracy of radionuclide cineangiography during exercise in patients with coronary artery disease: Comparison with exercise electrocardiography. Circulation 60:572, 1979.
106. Caldwell, J., Hamilton, G., Sorensen, S., et al.: The detection of coronary artery disease with radionuclide techniques: A comparison of rest-exercise thallium imaging and ejection fraction response. Circulation 61:610, 1980.
107. Jengo, J., Oren, V., Conant, R., et al.: Effects of maximal exercise stress on left ventricular function in patients with coronary artery disease using first pass radionuclide angiocardiography: A rapid, noninvasive technique for determining ejection fraction and segmental wall motion. Circulation 59:60, 1979.
108. Jengo, J., Freman, R., Brizendine, M., et al.: Detection of coronary artery disease: Comparison of exercise stress radionuclide angiocardiography and thallium stress perfusion scanning. Am. J. Cardiol. 45:535, 1980.
109. Johnstone, D., Sands, M., Berger, H., et al.: Comparison of exercise radionuclide angiocardiography and thallium-201 myocardial perfusion imaging in coronary artery disease. Am. J. Cardiol. 45:1113, 1980.
110. Jones, R.H., McEwan, P., Newman, G., et al.: Accuracy of diagnosis of coronary artery disease by radionuclide measurement of left ventricular function during rest and exercise. Circulation 64:586, 1981.
111. Gibbons, R., Lee, K., Cobb, F., et al.: Ejection fraction response to exercise in patients with chest pain and normal coronary arteriograms. Circulation 64:952, 1981.
112. Rozanski, A., Diamond, G., Berman, D., et al.: The declining specificity of radionuclide ventriculography. N. Engl. J. Med. 309:518, 1983.
113. Metz, C.: Principles of ROC analysis. Semin. Nucl. Med. 8:283, 1978.
114. Rozanski, A.: Referral bias and the efficacy of radionuclide stress tests: Problems and solutions. (Editorial.) J. Nucl. Med 33:2074, 1992.
115. Gibbons, R., Lee, K., Cobb, F., et al.: Ejection fraction response to exercise in patients with chest pain, coronary artery disease, and normal resting ventricular function. Circulation 66:643, 1982.
116. Rozanski, A., Diamond, G., Jones, R., et al.: A format for integrating the interpretation of exercise ejection fraction and wall motion and its application in identifying equivocal response. J. Am. Coll. Cardiol. 5:2388, 1985.
117. Gibbons, R., Lee, K., Pryor, D., et al.: The use of radionuclide angiography in the diagnosis of coronary artery disease—a logistic regression analysis. Circulation 68:740, 1983.
118. Gibbons, R., Clements, I., Zinsmeister, A., et al.: Exercise response of the systolic pressure to end systolic volume ratio in patients with coronary artery disease. J. Am. Coll. Cardiol. 10:33, 1987.
119. Gibbons, R.: Rest and exercise radionuclide angiography for diagnosis in chronic ischemic heart disease. Circulation 84:I-93, 1991.
120. Depace, N., Iskandrian, A., Hakki, A., et al.: Value of left ventricular function during exercise in predicting the extent of coronary artery disease. J. Am. Coll. Cardiol. 1:1002, 1983.
121. Depace, N., Hakki, A., Weinreich, D., et al.: Noninvasive assessment of coronary artery disease. Am. J. Cardiol. 52:715, 1983.
122. Gibbons, R., Fyke, F., and Clements, I.: Noninvasive identification of severe coronary artery disease using exercise radionuclide angiography. J. Am. Coll. Cardiol. 11:28, 1988.
123. Pryor, D., Harrell, F., Lee, K., et al.: Prognostic indicators for radionuclide angiography in medically treated patients with coronary artery disease. Am. J. Cardiol. 53:18, 1984.
124. Taliercio, C., Clements, I., Zinsmeister, A., et al.: Prognostic value and limitations of exercise radionuclide angiography. Mayo Clin. Proc. 63:573, 1988.
125. Lee, K., Pryor, D., Pieper, K., et al.: Prognostic value of radionuclide angiography in medically treated patients with coronary artery disease. A comparison with clinical and catheterization variables. Circulation 82:1705, 1990.
126. Iqbal, A., Gibbons, R., Zinsmeister, A., et al.: Prognostic value of exercise radionuclide angiography in a population-based cohort of patients with known or suspected coronary artery disease. Am. J. Cardiol. 74:119, 1994.
127. Higgenbotham, M., Morris, K., Coleman, E., et al.: Sex-related differences in normal cardiac response to upright exercise. Circulation 70:357, 1984.
128. Hanley, P., Gibbons, R., Zinsmeister, A., et al.: Sex-related differences in cardiac response to supine exercise assessed by radionuclide angiography. J. Am. Coll. Cardiol. 13:624, 1989.
129. Smith, H.: The relation of the weight of the heart to the weight of the body and of the weight of the heart to age. Am. Heart J. 4:79, 1928.
130. Gibbons, R., Hu, D., Clements, I., et al.: Anatomic and functional significance of a hypotensive response during supine exercise radionuclide ventriculography. Am. J. Cardiol. 60:1, 1987.
131. Currie, P., Kelly, M., Harper, R., et al.: Incremental value of clinical assessment, supine exercise electrocardiography, and biplane exercise radionuclide ventriculography in the prediction of coronary artery disease in men with chest pain. Am. J. Cardiol. 52:927, 1983.
132. Dilsizian, V., Perrone-Filardi, P., Cannon, R., et al.: Comparison of exercise radionuclide angiography with thallium SPECT imaging for detection of significant narrowing of the left circumflex coronary artery. Am. J. Cardiol. 68:320, 1991.
133. CASS Principal Investigators and Associates: Coronary artery surgery study (CASS): A randomized trial of coronary artery bypass surgery: Survival data. Circulation 68:939, 1983.
134. European Coronary Study Group: Long-term results of prospective randomized study of coronary artery bypass surgery in stable angina pectoris. Lancet 2:1173, 1982.
135. Takaro, T., Hultgren, H., Lipton, M., et al.: VA Cooperative Randomized Study for coronary artery occlusive disease. II. Left main disease. Circulation 54:III-107, 1976.
136. Campos, C., Chu, H., D'Agostino, H., Jr., et al.: Comparison of rest and exercise radionuclide angiography and exercise treadmill testing for diagnosis of anatomically extensive coronary artery disease. Circulation 67:1204, 1983.
137. Weintraub, W., Schneider, R., Seelaus, P., et al.: Prospective evaluation of the severity of coronary artery disease with exercise radionuclide angiography and electrocardiography. Am. Heart J. 111:537, 1986.
138. Gibbons, R., Zinsmeister, A., Miller, T., et al.: Supine exercise electrocardiography compared with exercise radionuclide angiography in noninvasive identification of severe coronary artery disease. Ann. Intern. Med. 112:743, 1990.
139. Harris, P., Lee, K., Harrell, F., et al.: Survival in medically treated coronary artery disease. Circulation 60:1259, 1979.
140. Hammermeister, K., Derouen, T., and Dodge, H.: Variables predictive of survival in patients with coronary artery disease: Selection by univariate and multivariate analysis from the clinical, electrocardiographic, exercise, arteriographic and quantitative angiographic evaluations. Circulation 59:421, 1979.
141. Mock, M., Rengqvist, I., Fisher, L., et al.: Survival of medically treated patients in the Coronary Artery Surgery Study (CASS) registry. Circulation 66:562, 1982.

142. Harris, P., Lee, K., and Hurrell, F.: Outcome in medically treated coronary artery disease. Circulation 62:718, 1980.
143. Harrison, D., White, C., Hiratzka, L., et al.: The value of lesion cross-sectional area determined by quantitative coronary angiography in assessing the physiologic significance of proximal left anterior descending coronary arterial stenoses. Circulation 69:1111, 1984.
144. White, C., Wright, C., Doty, D., et al.: Does visual interpretation of the coronary arteriogram predict the physiologic importance of a coronary stenosis? N. Engl. J. Med. 310:819, 1984.
145. Iskandrian, A., Hakki, A.H., Schwartz, J.S., et al.: Prognostic implications of rest and exercise radionuclide ventriculography in patients with suspected or proven coronary heart disease. Int. J. Cardiol. 6:707, 1984.
146. Bonow, R., Kent, K., Rosing, D., et al.: Exercise-induced ischemia in mildly symptomatic patients with coronary artery disease and preserved left ventricular function: Identification of subgroups at risk of death during medical therapy. N. Engl. J. Med. 311:1339, 1984.
147. Bonow, R.: Prognostic implications of exercise radionuclide angiography in patients with coronary artery disease. Mayo Clin. Proc. 63:630, 1988.
148. Mazzotta, G., Bonow, R., Pace, L., et al.: Relation between exertional ischemia and prognosis in mildly symptomatic patients with single or double vessel coronary artery disease and left ventricular dysfunction at rest. J. Am. Coll. Cardiol. 13:567, 1989.
149. Miller, T., Taliercio, C., Zinsmeister, A., et al.: Risk stratification of patients with single or double vessel disease and impaired left ventricular function using exercise radionuclide angiography. Am. J. Cardiol. 65:1317, 1990.
150. Miller, T., Christian, T., Taliercio, C., et al.: Severe exercise-induced ischemia does not identify high risk patients with normal left ventricular function and one- or two-vessel coronary artery disease. J. Am. Coll. Cardiol. 23:219, 1994.
151. Simari, R., Miller, T., Zinsmeister, A., et al.: Capabilities of supine exercise electrocardiography versus exercise radionuclide angiography in predicting coronary events. Am. J. Cardiol. 67:573, 1991.
152. Miller, T., Taliercio, C., Zinsmeister, A., et al.: Prognosis in patients with an abnormal exercise radionuclide angiogram in the absence of significant coronary artery disease. J. Am. Coll. Cardiol. 12:637, 1988.
153. Bonow, R.: Radionuclide angiography for risk stratification of patients with coronary artery disease. Am. J. Cardiol. 72:735, 1993.
154. Bonow, R.: Prognostic assessment in coronary artery disease: Role of radionuclide angiography. J. Nucl. Cardiol. 1:280, 1994.
155. Clements, I., Brown, M., Zinsmeister, A., et al.: Influence of left ventricular diastolic filling on symptoms and survival in patients with decreased left ventricular systolic function. Am. J. Cardiol. 67:1245, 1991.
156. Freeman, M., Gray, R., Berman, D., et al.: Improvement in global and segmental left ventricular function after coronary bypass surgery. Circulation 64(Suppl. II):34, 1981.
157. Kent, K., Borer, J., Green, M., et al.: Effects of coronary artery bypass on global and regional left ventricular function during exercise. N. Engl. J. Med. 298:1434, 1978.
158. Kronenberg, M., Pederson, R., Harston, W., et al.: Left ventricular performance after coronary artery bypass surgery. Ann. Intern. Med. 99:305, 1983.
159. Lim, Y., Kalff, V., Kelly, M., et al.: Radionuclide angiographic assessment of global and segmental left ventricular function at rest and during exercise after coronary artery bypass graft surgery. Circulation 66:972, 1982.
160. Dilsizian, V., Bonow, R., Cannon, R., et al.: The effect of coronary artery bypass grafting on left ventricular systolic function at rest: Evidence for preoperative subclinical myocardial ischemia. Am. J. Cardiol. 61:1248, 1988.
161. Fernandes, V., Freedman, S., Allman, K., et al.: Detection of myocardial viability in stunned or hibernating myocardium by delayed emptying on radionuclide ventriculography. Am. J. Cardiol. 67:529, 1991.
162. Rozanski, A., Berman, D., Gray, R., et al.: Preoperative prediction of reversible myocardial asynergy by postexercise radionuclide ventriculography. N. Engl. J. Med. 307:212, 1982.
163. Wallis, J., Supine, P., and Borer, J.: Prognostic value of left ventricular ejection fraction response to exercise during long-term follow-up after coronary artery bypass graft surgery. Circulation 88:II-99, 1993.
164. Depuey, E., Leatherman, L., Leachman, R., et al.: Restenosis after transluminal coronary angioplasty detected with exercise gated radionuclide ventriculography. J. Am. Coll. Cardiol. 4:1103, 1984.
165. O'Keefe, J., Lapeyre, A., Holmes, D., et al.: Early radionuclide angiography identifies low risk patients for late restenosis after transluminal coronary angioplasty. Am. J. Cardiol. 61:51, 1988.
166. Nicod, P., Corbett, J., Sanford, C., et al.: Comparison of the influence of acute transmural and nontransmural myocardial infarction on ventricular function. Am. Heart J. 107:28, 1984.
167. Reduto, L., Berger, H., Cohen, L., et al.: Sequential radionuclide assessment of left and right ventricular performance after acute transmural myocardial infarction. Ann. Intern. Med. 89:441, 1978.
168. Sanford, C., Corbett, J., Nicod, P., et al.: Value of radionuclide ventriculography in the immediate characterization of patients with acute myocardial infarction. Am. J. Cardiol. 49:637, 1982.
169. Shah, P., Pichler, M., Berman, D., et al.: Left ventricular ejection fraction determined by radionuclide ventriculography in early states of first transmural myocardial infarction: Relation to short-term prognosis. Am. J. Cardiol. 45:542, 1980.
170. Multicenter Post-Infarction Research Group: Risk stratification and survival after myocardial infarction. N. Engl. J. Med. 309:331, 1983.
171. Weissler, A., Miller, B., Granger, C., et al.: Augmentation of mortality risk discriminating power of left ventricular ejection fraction by measures of nonuniformity in systolic emptying on radionuclide angiography. J. Am. Coll. Cardiol. 16:387, 1990.
172. Corbett, J., Nicod, P., and Huxley, R.: Left ventricular functional alterations at rest and during submaximal exercise in patients with recent myocardial infarction. Am. J. Med. 74:577, 1983.
173. Corbett, J., Nicod, P., Lewis, S., et al.: Prognostic value of submaximal exercise radionuclide ventriculography after myocardial infarction. Am. J. Cardiol. 52:82, 1983.
174. Dewhurst, N., and Muir, A.: Comparative prognostic value of radionuclide ventriculography at rest and during exercise in 100 patients after first myocardial infarction. Br. Heart J. 49:111, 1983.
175. Hung, J., Goris, M., Nash, E., et al.: Comparative value of maximal treadmill testing, exercise thallium myocardial perfusion scintigraphy and exercise radionuclide ventriculography for distinguishing high- and low-risk patients soon after acute myocardial infarction. Am. J. Cardiol. 53:1221, 1984.
176. Lavie, C., Gibbons, R., Zinsmeister, A., et al.: Interpreting results of exercise studies after acute myocardial infarction altered by thrombolytic therapy, coronary angioplasty or bypass. Am. J. Cardiol. 67:116, 1991.
177. Williams, D., Braunwald, E., Knutterud, G., et al.: One year results of the Thrombolysis in Myocardial Infarction investigation (TIMI) Phase II trial. Circulation 85:533, 1992.
178. Zaret, B., Wackers, J., Terrin, M., et al.: Does left ventricular ejection fraction following thrombolytic therapy have the same prognostic impact described in the prethrombolytic era? Results of the TIMI II Trial. J. Am. Coll. Cardiol. 17:214, 1991.
179. Zhu, W., Gibbons, R., Bailey, K., et al.: Predischarge exercise radionuclide angiography in predicting multivessel coronary artery disease and subsequent cardiac events after thrombolytic therapy for acute myocardial infarction. Am. J. Cardiol. 74:554, 1994.
180. Anderson, J., Marshall, H., Bray, B., et al.: A randomized trial of intracoronary streptokinase in the treatment of acute myocardial infarction. N. Engl. J. Med. 308:1312, 1983.
181. Khaja, F., Walton, J., Jr., Brymer, J., et al.: Intracoronary fibrinolytic therapy in acute myocardial infarction: Report of a prospective randomized trial. N. Engl. J. Med. 308:1305, 1983.
182. Leiboff, R., Katz, R., Wasserman, A., et al.: A randomized, angiographically controlled trial of intracoronary streptokinase in acute myocardial infarction. Am. J. Cardiol. 53:404, 1984.
183. O'Rourke, M., Baron, D., Keogh, A., et al.: Limitation of myocardial infarction by early infusion of recombinant tissue-type plasminogen activator. Circulation 77:1311, 1988.
184. Guerci, A., Gerstenbligh, G., Brinker, J., et al.: A randomized trial of intravenous tissue plasminogen activator for acute myocardial infarction with subsequent randomization to elective coronary angioplasty. N. Engl. J. Med. 317:1613, 1987.
185. Kennedy, J., Martin, G., Davis, K., et al.: The Western Washington Intravenous Streptokinase in Acute Myocardial Infarction Randomized Trial. Circulation 77:345, 1988.
186. Rentrop, K., Feit, F., Blanke, H., et al.: Effects of intracoronary streptokinase and intracoronary nitroglycerin infusion on coronary angiographic patterns and mortality in patients with acute myocardial infarction. N. Engl. J. Med. 311:1457, 1984.
187. Ritchie, J., Davis, K., Williams, D., et al.: Global and regional left ventricular function and tomographic radionuclide perfusion: The Western Washington Intracoronary Streptokinase in Myocardial Infarction Trial. Circulation 70:867, 1984.
188. Simoons, M., Serruys, P., van den Brand, M., et al.: Early thrombolysis in acute myocardial infarction: Limitation of infarct size and improved survival. J. Am. Coll. Cardiol. 7:717, 1986.
189. Zaret, B., Wackers, F., Terrin, M., et al.: Assessment of global and regional left ventricular performance at rest and during exercise after thrombolytic therapy for acute myocardial infarction: Results of the Thrombolysis in Myocardial Infarction (TIMI) II Study. Am. J. Cardiol. 69:1, 1992.
190. Wackers, F., Berger, H., Weinberg, M., et al.: Spontaneous changes in left ventricular function over the first 24 hours of acute myocardial infarction: Implications for evaluating early therapeutic interventions. Circulation 66:748, 1982.
191. Christian, T., Behrenbeck, T., Pellikka, P., et al.: Mismatch of left ventricular dysfunction and infarct size demonstrated by technetium-99m-isonitrile imaging after reperfusion therapy for acute myocardial infarction. J. Am. Coll. Cardiol. 16:1632, 1990.
192. Gibbons, R., Verani, M., Behrenbeck, T., et al.: Feasibility of tomographic technetium-99m-hexakis-2-methoxy-2-methylpropyl-isonitrile imaging for the assessment of myocardial area at risk and efficacy of thrombolytic therapy in acute myocardial infarction. Circulation 80:1277, 1989.
193. Gibbons, R., Holmes, D., Reeder, G., et al.: Immediate angioplasty compared with the administration of a thrombolytic agent followed by conservative treatment for myoardial infarction. N. Engl. J. Med. 328:685, 1993.
194. Bulkley, B., Hutchins, G., Bailey, I., et al.: Thallium-201 imaging and gated cardiac blood pool scans in patients with ischemic and idiopathic congestive cardiomyopathy: A clinical and pathologic study. Circulation 55:753, 1977.
195. Glamann, D., Lange, R., Corbett, J., et al.: Utility of various radionuclide techniques for distinguishing ischemic from nonischemic dilated cardiomyopathy. Arch. Intern. Med. 152:769, 1992.
196. Betocchi, S., Bonow, R., Bacharach, S., et al.: Isovolumic relaxation period in hypertrophic cardiomyopathy: Assessment by radionuclide angiography. J. Am. Coll. Cardiol. 7:74, 1986.
197. Bonow, R., Rosing, D., Bacharach, S., et al.: Effects of verapamil on left ventricu-

lar systolic function and diastolic filling in patients with hypertrophic cardiomyopathy. Circulation 64:787, 1981.
198. Hindman, M., Slosky, D., and Peter, R.: Rest and exercise hemodynamic effects of oral hydralazine in patients with coronary artery disease and left ventricular dysfunction. Circulation 61:751, 1980.
199. O'Connell, J., Robinson, J., Henkin, R., et al.: Immunosuppressive therapy in patients with congestive cardiomyopathy and myocardial uptake of gallium-67. Circulation 64:780, 1981.
200. Handler, B., Pavel, D., Peitras, R., et al.: Equilibrium radionuclide gated angiography in patients with tricuspid regurgitation. Am. J. Cardiol. 51:305, 1983.
201. Boucher, C., Kanarek, D., Okada, R., et al.: Exercise testing in aortic regurgitation: Comparison of radionuclide left ventricular ejection fraction with exercise performance at the anaerobic threshold and peak exercise. Am. J. Cardiol. 52:801, 1983.
202. Borer, J., Bacharach, S., Green, M., et al.: Exercise-induced left ventricular dysfunction in symptomatic and asymptomatic patients with aortic regurgitation: Assessment with radionuclide cineangiography. Am. J. Cardiol. 42:351, 1978.
203. Dehmer, G., Firth, B., and Hillis, L.: Alterations in left ventricular volumes and ejection fraction at rest and during exercise in patients with aortic regurgitation. Am. J. Cardiol. 48:17, 1981.
204. Huxley, R., Gaffney, F., Corbett, J., et al.: Early detection of left ventricular dysfunction in chronic aortic regurgitation as assessed by contrast angiography, echocardiography and rest and exercise scintigraphy. Am. J. Cardiol. 51:1542, 1983.
205. Johnson, L., Powers, E., Tzall, W., et al.: Left ventricular volume and ejection fraction response to exercise in aortic regurgitation. Am. J. Cardiol. 51:1379, 1983.
206. Steingart, R., Yee, C., Weinstein, L., et al.: Radionuclide ventriculographic study of adaptations to exercise in aortic regurgitation. Am. J. Cardiol. 51:488, 1983.
207. Bonow, R., Rosing, D., Kent, D., et al.: Timing of operation for chronic aortic regurgitation. Am. J. Cardiol. 50:325, 1982.
208. Bonow, R., Picone, A., McIntosh, C., et al.: Survival and functional results after valve replacement for aortic regurgitation from 1976 to 1983: Impact of preoperative left ventricular function. Circulation 72:1244, 1985.
209. Bonow, R., Borer, J., Rosing, D., et al.: Preoperative exercise capacity in symptomatic patients with aortic regurgitation as a predictor of postoperative left ventricular function and long-term prognosis. Circulation 62:1280, 1980.
210. Bonow, R., Rosing, D., and McIntosh, C.: The natural history of asymptomatic patients with aortic regurgitation and normal left ventricular function. Circulation 68:509, 1983.
211. Bonow, R., Rosing, D., Maron, B., et al.: Reversal of left ventricular dysfunction after aortic valve replacement for chronic aortic regurgitation: Influence of duration of preoperative left ventricular dysfunction. Circulation 70:570, 1984.
212. Bonow, R., Lakatos, E., Maron, B., et al.: Serial long-term assessment of the natural history of asymptomatic patients with chronic aortic regurgitation and normal left ventricular systolic function. Circulation 84:1625, 1991.
213. Schuler, G., von Olshausen, K., Schwarz, F., et al.: Noninvasive assessment of myocardial contractility in asymptomatic patients with severe aortic regurgitation and normal left ventricular ejection fraction at rest. Am. J. Cardiol. 50:45, 1982.
214. Goldman, M., Packer, M., Horowitz, S., et al.: Relation between exercise-induced changes in ejection fraction and systolic loading conditions at rest in aortic regurgitation. J. Am. Coll. Cardiol. 3:924, 1984.
215. Lewis, S., Riba, A., Berger, H., et al.: Radionuclide angiographic exercise left ventricular performance in chronic aortic regurgitation. Relationship to resting echographic ventricular dimensions and systolic wall stress index. Am. Heart J. 103:498, 1982.
216. Boucher, C., Wilson, R., Kanarek, D., et al.: Exercise testing in asymptomatic or minimally symptomatic aortic regurgitation: Relationship of left ventricular ejection fraction of left ventricular pressure during exercise. Circulation 67:1091, 1983.
217. Borer, J., Rosing, D., Kent, K., et al.: Left ventricular function at rest and during exercise after aortic valve replacement in patients with aortic regurgitation. Am. J. Cardiol. 44:1297, 1979.
218. Boucher, C., Bingham, J., Osbakken, M., et al.: Early changes in left ventricular size and function after correction of left ventricular volume overload. Am. J. Cardiol. 47:991, 1981.
219. Borer, J., Herrold, E., Hochreiter, C., et al.: Natural history of left ventricular performance at rest and during exercise after aortic valve replacement for aortic regurgitation. Circulation 84:III-133,1991.
220. Hochtreiter, C., Niles, N., Devereux, R., et al.: Mitral regurgitation: Relationship of noninvasive descriptors of right and left ventricular performance to clinical and hemodynamic findings and to prognosis in medically and surgically treated patients. Circulation 73:900, 1986.
221. Schuler, G., Peterson, K., Johnson, A., et al.: Temporal response of left ventricular performance to mitral valve surgery. Circulation 59:1218, 1979.
222. Alexander, J., Dainiak, N., Berger, H., et al.: Serial assessment of doxorubicin cardiotoxicity with quantitative radionuclide angiocardiography. N. Engl. J. Med. 300:278, 1979.
223. Gottdiener, J., Mathisen, D., Borer, J., et al.: Doxorubicin cardiotoxicity: Assessment of late left ventricular dysfunction by radionuclide cineangiography. Ann. Intern. Med. 94:430, 1981.
224. Flamm, S., Taki, J., Moore, R., et al.: Redistribution of regional and organ blood volume and effect on cardiac function in relation to upright exercise intensity in healthy human subjects. Circulation 81:1550, 1990.
225. Ehsani, A., Ogawa, T., Miller, T., et al.: Exercise training improves left ventricular systolic function in older men. Circulation 83:96, 1991.
226. Levy, W., Cerqueira, M., Abrass, I., et al.: Endurance exercise training augments diastolic filling at rest and during exercise in healthy young and older men. Circulation 88:116, 1993.
227. Spina, R., Ogawa, T., Miller, T., et al.: Effect of exercise training on left ventricular performance in older women free of cardiopulmonary disease. Am. J. Cardiol. 71:99, 1993.
228. Jensen, D., Atwood, J., Froelicher, V., et al.: Improvement in ventricular function during exercise studied with radionuclide ventriculography after cardiac rehabilitation. Am. J. Cardiol. 46:770, 1980.
229. Borer, J., Bacharach, S., Green, M., et al.: Effect of nitroglycerin on exercise-induced abnormalities of left ventricular regional function and ejection fraction in coronary artery disease. Assessment by radionuclide cineangiography in symptomatic and asymptomatic patients. Circulation 57:314, 1978.
230. Dehmer, G., Falkoff, M., Lewis, S., et al.: Effect of oral propranolol on rest and exercise left ventricular ejection fraction, volumes, and segmental wall motion in patients with angina pectoris. Assessment with equilibrium gated blood pool imaging. Br. Heart J. 45:656, 1981.
231. Ritchie, J., Sorensen, S., Kennedy, J., et al.: Radionuclide angiography: Noninvasive assessment of hemodynamic changes after administration of nitroglycerin. Am. J. Cardiol. 43:278, 1979.
232. Tan, A., Sadick, N., Kelly, D., et al.: Verapamil in stable effort angina: Effects on left ventricular function evaluated with exercise radionuclide ventriculography. Am. J. Cardiol. 49:425, 1982.
233. Bonow, R., Vitale, D., Bacharach, S., et al.: Effects of aging on asynchronous left ventricular regional function and global ventricular filling in normal human subjects. J. Am. Coll. Cardiol. 11:50, 1988.
234. Harmann, A., Maul, F.-D., Huth, A., et al.: Serial evaluation of left ventricular function by radionuclide ventriculography at rest and during exercise after orthotopic heart transplantation. Eur. J. Nucl. Med. 20:146, 1993.
235. Teo, K., Yusuf, S., Wittes, J., et al.: Preserved left ventricular function during supine exercise in patients after orthopic cardiac transplantation. Eur. Heart J. 13:321, 1992.

CHAPTER

62 Single-Photon Emitting Tracers for Imaging Myocardial Perfusion and Cell Membrane Integrity

Seth T. Dahlberg, M.D.
Jeffrey A. Leppo, M.D.

Myocardial blood flow can be assessed by imaging the regional deposition of radiolabeled perfusion agents. Localization of perfusion agents involves their extraction from myocardial capillaries and subsequent retention by cardiac myocytes.[1–5] Because intravascular tracers must traverse endothelial and sarcolemmal barriers by means of passive diffusion or active transport, myocardial extraction of these compounds generally falls as coronary flow increases. Also, when a perfusion agent is actively retained by energy-dependent processes, myocyte membrane disruption and cell death result in tissue loss or washout of tracer.[6–15] Therefore, the regional deposition of perfusion agents is affected by two factors: the level of coronary flow and cardiac myocyte viability. Optimal intepretation of clinical planar or tomographic perfusion images requires an understanding of how both coronary flow and cellular function affect the myocardial distribution of perfusion tracers.

MYOCARDIAL PERFUSION AGENTS

Radiolabeled perfusion tracers can be classified as cations or as neutral compounds.[16, 17] Because myocardial extraction of cations generally involves an active energy-dependent process, the cellular retention of these tracers typically reflects myocardial viability. Neutral compounds, on the other hand, can passively diffuse into cells and localize in lipid membranes, so their retention may be much less affected by membrane disruption or cell death. Table 62–1 summarizes the characteristics of several single-photon radiolabeled tracers that are either approved for clinical use or currently undergoing evaluation as myocardial perfusion agents. Radiation dosimetry includes both the effective dose and the critical organ dose.[18–22]

Early myocardial perfusion studies used the cation ^{43}K, which is actively concentrated within muscle cells.[23, 24] However, since the 1970s thallium-201 (^{201}Tl) has become the most widely used single-photon tracer for myocardial perfusion imaging.[25–30] Thallium-201 is a monovalent heavy-metal cation with a crystal radius similar to that of K^+ and Rb^+.[31] Whereas the cellular uptake of ^{201}Tl, like that of K^+, is caused in part by active transport by Na-K ATPase, ^{201}Tl has a higher extraction and more stable retention than K^+.[31–35] Despite the excellent physiologic properties of ^{201}Tl for imaging blood flow and assessing myocardial viability, its low-energy (68 to 80 keV) Hg x-rays and its relatively long 73-hour half-life have led to the development of technetium-99m (^{99m}Tc)-labeled perfusion agents.

Initial development of ^{99m}Tc-labeled cations focused on phosphine compounds, such as dimethylphosphinoethane, and isonitriles, such as t-butyl or carboxypropyl isonitrile.[36–42] However, problems such as poor myocardial retention, slow blood clearance, and high lung or liver uptake prevented their clinical use.[43] Further research resulted in the development of cations with favorable imaging properties, including the isonitrile sestamibi and the phosphine compounds tetrofosmin, furifosmin (also referred to as Q12), and ^{99m}Tc-N,N′ ethylene-bis(acetylacetone iminato)bis[tris(3-methoxy-l-propyl)-phosphine)] (also referred to as Q3).[21, 44–47] These compounds show moderate myocardial extraction, stable retention, and moderate liver uptake. Sestamibi is approved for clinical use, whereas the newer phosphine compounds are undergoing clinical evaluation at the present time.

One of the first neutral perfusion agents studied was xenon-133 (^{133}Xe).[48, 49] After the tracer was injected into a coronary artery, its clearance rates were used to assess regional blood flow. Technetium-99m teboroxime, a BATO (boronic acid adduct of technetium dioxime) compound with a high myocardial extraction and rapid clearance, is a neutral lipophilic perfusion agent currently available for clinical use.[50] Recent studies with teboroxime have also used regional clearance rates of the tracer to assess coronary stenoses, which is similar to the earlier work with ^{133}Xe.[51] Finally, ^{99m}TcN (NOET) is a neutral nitrido compound recently developed for perfusion imaging.[52, 53] The properties of this lipophilic compound, which can be modified by the addition of solubilizing cyclodextrins,[54] are currently being evaluated in basic and clinical studies.[55–57]

This work was supported in part by U.S. Public Health Service Grant HL34199 of the National Heart, Lung, and Blood Institute, Bethesda, MD, and performed during the tenure of a Clinician-Scientist Award from the American Heart Association (Seth T. Dahlberg, M.D.).

TABLE 62–1. SINGLE-PHOTON MYOCARDIAL PERFUSION AGENTS

	^{201}Tl	Sestamibi	Teboroxime	Tetrofosmin	Q12	NOET
Isotope	^{201}Tl	^{99m}Tc	^{99m}Tc	^{99m}Tc	^{99m}Tc	^{99m}Tc
Class	Metal	Isonitrile	BATO*	Diphosphine	Mixed ligand monophosphine	Nitrido
Emax*	0.73	0.39	0.89	0.24	0.26	NA
Enet* (5 min)	0.57	0.41	0.71	0.16	0.12	NA
Lipophilic	No	Yes	Yes	Yes	Yes	Yes
Charge	Cation	Cation	Neutral	Cation	Cation	Neutral
Cell uptake	Na-K ATPase	Mitochondria	Passive	Mitochondria	Unknown	Unknown
Myocardial clearance	Moderate	Slow	Rapid	Slow	Slow	Moderate
Redistribution	Yes	Minimal	Yes	No	No	Yes
Measure hyperemic flow	Good	Adequate	Excellent	Adequate	Adequate	Unknown
Effective dose (rem)	1.57/2 mCi	1.33/30 mCi	1.38/30 mCi	0.99/30 mCi	NA	NA
Critical organ dose (rad)	Kidney 3.89/2 mCi	Large bowel 8.44/30 mCi	Large bowel 2.79/30 mCi	Gall bladder 5.40/30 mCi	NA	NA

*Emax and Enet are maximum and net tracer extractions in isolated hearts; tetrofosmin data from isolated rat hearts; all others are from rabbit hearts.
BATO = boronic acid adduct of technetium dioxime; NA = not available; rem = radiation equivalent, man.

TRANSMEMBRANE KINETICS AND BLOOD-TISSUE EXCHANGE INDEPENDENT OF BLOOD FLOW

Measurement of cellular or tissue kinetics of perfusion agents is most accurate when the confounding effect of variable flow on tracer extraction is removed. This can be achieved by studying cardiac myocytes in culture or by measuring tracer blood-tissue exchange in isolated hearts maintained at constant flow.

When excess perfusion tracer is added to the culture medium of rat or chick cardiac myocytes, the cells concentrate the tracer to a level above that of the surrounding extracellular medium. The intracellular tracer concentration initially rises (reflecting predominant tracer influx) and then plateaus at a steady-state level, described as tracer net accumulation, when influx equals back diffusion. When cells are subsequently placed in a tracer-free medium, tracer efflux or washout occurs.[58] Table 62–2 summarizes cell culture data for several perfusion agents.

Teboroxime shows the most rapid influx (short T1/2) to a high intracellular accumulation, ^{201}Tl has a slightly slower influx, whereas the influx of sestamibi is much slower.[34, 59, 60] Therefore, the rate of cellular influx appears to correlate with in vivo myocardial extraction, in which teboroxime has the highest extraction, followed by ^{201}Tl and then sestamibi. The slow cellular efflux of sestamibi is consistent with its stable in vivo myocardial retention, whereas the faster efflux of ^{201}Tl also correlates with its myocardial washout.[59, 61–63] However, the relatively slow cellular efflux of teboroxime, at a rate comparable to that of ^{201}Tl,[59] contrasts with the rapid in vivo myocardial clearance of this tracer. Because the rate of teboroxime clearance is also similar to that of ^{201}Tl in many isolated heart studies,[64–66] noncardiac effects such as binding of teboroxime to blood components or changes in its chemical structure, may affect the compound's in vivo kinetics.[64, 67]

With the isolated perfused heart model, myocardial and capillary-tissue tracer kinetics can be studied at constant coronary flow in the absence of tracer recirculation. Whole-organ cardiac time activity curves can be measured with an external scintillation detector,[67–70] or coronary sinus blood can be collected for the determination of cardiac venous outflow dilution curves.[71–73] When diffusible tracers, such as ^{201}Tl and the ^{99m}Tc-labeled compounds, are coinjected into the coronary inflow together with an intravascular tracer, such as radiolabeled albumin, the multiple indicator-dilution technique can be used to measure the capillary permeability and myocardial kinetics of the perfusion agents.[3, 4, 74]

Figure 62–1 shows indicator-dilution data for ^{201}Tl and teboroxime. The venous outflow curves, referred to as h(t) curves, in Figure 62–1*A* are used to calculate instantaneous extraction, or E(t) (see Fig. 62–1*B*). The early maximum extraction (Emax at 50 seconds) (see Fig. 62–1*B*), which can be used to calculate the Crone-Renkin permeability-surface area product,[2, 4, 75, 76] is the best estimate of capillary-tissue permeability for the perfusion agents. The integral or net tissue tracer extraction, or Enet, (see Fig. 62–1*C*) can then be used to assess temporal changes in myocardial tracer retention or washout. Figure 62–2 shows net myocardial extraction of several perfusion agents for 1 hour after tracer injection. Both ^{201}Tl and teboroxime show gradual clearance, whereas sestamibi and tetrofosmin demonstrate avid myocardial retention. Isolated heart measurements of Emax and Enet (at 5 minutes) are included in Table 62–1.

TABLE 62–2. KINETICS OF PERFUSION AGENTS IN CULTURED MYOCYTES

	T1/2 (min)		Myocyte Net Accumulation*	Severe Cell Injury Reduces Accumulation	References
	Influx	*Efflux*			
Rat Cells					
^{201}Tl	5	5–6	0.88	Yes	35, 57, 59
$^{42}K^+$	12	12	NR	NR	34
MIBI	33–35	28–29	1.00	Yes	57, 59
Tebo	<2	13	3.77	Minimal	57, 59
NOET	18	>120	NR	Moderate	57
Chick Cells					
^{201}Tl	NR	NR	0.66	Yes	16, 83
MIBI	9.3	8–10	1.00	Yes	16, 60, 83
Tebo	NR	4†	3.77	Minimal	16

*Myocyte uptake is expressed in different units by various authors, so uptake is presented relative to sestamibi uptake.
NR = not reported; MIBI = sestamibi; Tebo = teboroxime.
†Efflux was biexponential; the larger rapidly clearing fraction had a 4-minute T1/2.

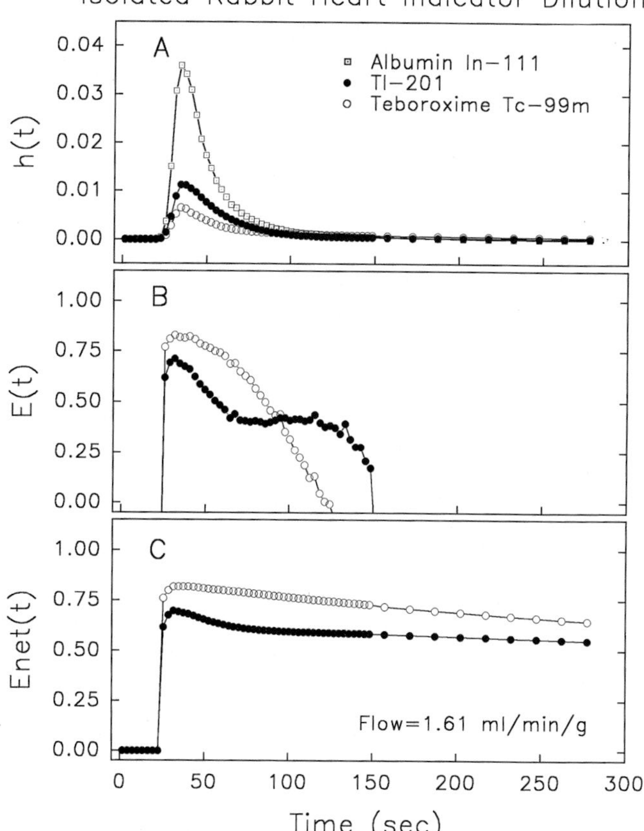

FIGURE 62–1. *A*, Coronary sinus venous dilution curves, h(t), from an isolated rabbit heart after bolus injection of the intravascular reference indium-111 albumin (Albumin In-111) and the diffusible tracers ^{201}Tl and teboroxime into the aortic inflow. *B*, Instantaneous extraction, E(t), of ^{201}Tl and teboroxime, showing higher early maximum extraction (Emax) of teboroxime. *C*, Net extraction, Enet(t), showing myocardial clearance of both tracers over 4.5-minute collection.

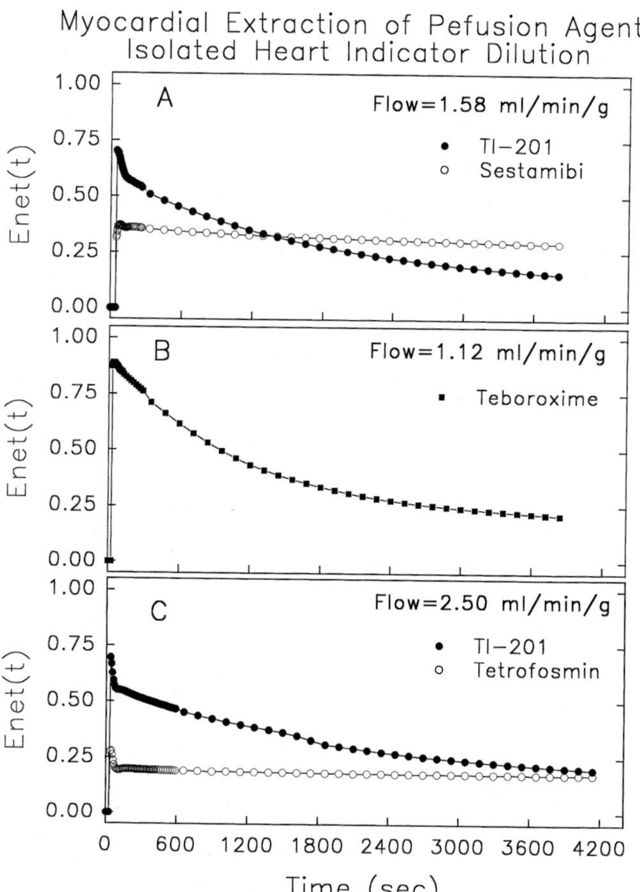

FIGURE 62–2. Net extraction, Enet(t), for myocardial perfusion agents measured for more than 1 hour in isolated hearts with multiple indicator-dilution method. *A and B*, Slow washout of ^{201}Tl and teboroxime that contrasts with stable retention of sestamibi in isolated rabbit hearts. *C*, Similar myocardial clearance of ^{201}Tl versus retention of tetrofosmin in an isolated rat heart.

A high myocardial extraction, reflecting rapid capillary-tissue exchange, suggests that regional tracer deposition can accurately image hyperemic coronary flow. Teboroxime and ^{201}Tl show the highest extractions, followed by more moderate extractions for sestamibi, tetrofosmin, and Q12.[64, 71, 72, 77, 78] These data demonstrate tracer kinetics for normal cardiac cells and myocardium. However, the retention of perfusion agents can also be significantly affected by metabolic insults or cellular injury.[7, 8, 14, 15, 79–82]

INTRACELLULAR BINDING MECHANISMS AND THE EFFECT OF CELLULAR INJURY

The mechanism of a perfusion agent's uptake and the effect of cell viability on its retention can be evaluated by studying cultured cardiac myocytes injured with metabolic inhibitors or toxins. Membrane disruption and cell death can be documented by the release of the cellular enzymes lactate dehydrogenase (LDH) or creatine kinase (CK) and correlated with loss of intracellular tracer.[58, 68, 83]

Cellular uptake of ^{201}Tl, which involves active transport of the ion by Na-K ATPase, is decreased 40 to 60 percent by ouabain, whereas sestamibi uptake remains unchanged or increases.[35, 60, 84] The loss of accumulated intracellular sestamibi after treatment of cells with the mitochondrial depolarizing agent carbonyl cyanide *m*-chlorophenylhydrazone (CCCP) has demonstrated the importance of an intact mitochondrial electrochemical gradient for cellular sestamibi retention.[62] Preliminary data also suggest that tetrofosmin actively accumulates in mitochondria.[85] Teboroxime uptake, on the other hand, is most likely a passive process, because cellular uptake of this tracer shows only a mild decrease after ouabain and no change with CCCP.[16, 84]

The importance of cell viability can be assessed by inhibiting glycolysis with iodoacetate and blocking mitochondrial respiration with rotenone or cyanide. Brief treatment with iodoacetate produces mild cell injury, whereas prolonged treatment, with the addition of rotenone or cyanide, causes irreversible injury manifested by lactate dehydrogenase release.[83, 84, 86]

Studies by Maublant and colleagues[84, 86] and Piwnica-Worms and associates[83] have shown that whereas intracellular ^{201}Tl uptake is reduced by mild cell injury, a reduction in sestamibi retention only occurs after severe irreversible damage. Cell injury may also affect tetrofosmin retention, because uncoupling of mitochondrial oxidative phosphorylation by dinitrophenol causes a marked reduction in mitochondrial tetrofosmin uptake.[85] Viability is probably less important for NOET retention, because cellular content of NOET was reduced only by 30 to 35 percent after iodoacetate-cyanide or osmotic cell lysis.[57] Teboroxime appears least affected by cell viability, because iodoacetate and cyanide only mildly reduce cell tracer uptake.[16] Even after osmotic lysis of cells, Maublant and colleagues[84] (Fig. 62–3) found no effect on teboroxime uptake, despite marked reductions in ^{201}Tl and sestamibi content.

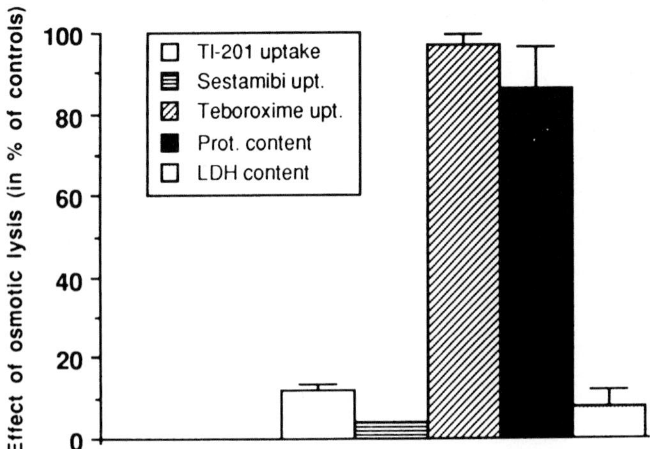

FIGURE 62–3. Effect of osmotic lysis of rat myocytes on cellular accumulation of ^{201}Tl, sestamibi, and teboroxime (after 20 minutes of incubation with tracer) and on protein (prot.) and LDH content. (From Maublant, J.C., Moins, N., Gachon, P., et al.: Uptake of technetium-99m-teboroxime in cultured myocardial cells: Comparison with thallium-201 and technetium-99m-sestamibi. J. Nucl. Med. 34:255–259, 1993, with permission.)

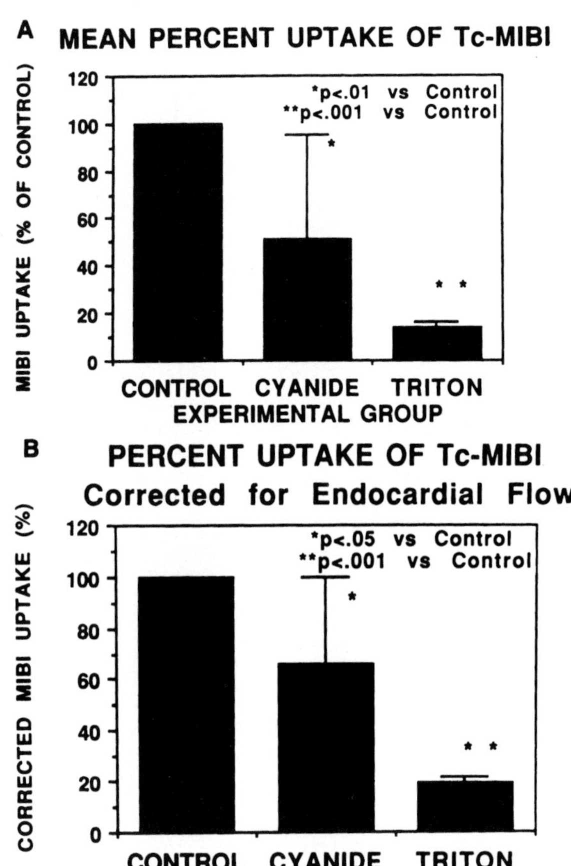

FIGURE 62–4. Peak sestamibi (MIBI) uptake by isolated rat hearts at control and after cyanide or Triton-X injury (*A*), as well as uptake corrected for changes in endocardial blood flow (*B*). Values are normalized to the control group uptake, which was assigned a value of 100 percent. (From Beanlands, R.S.B., Dawood, F., Wen, W.-H., et al.: Are the kinetics of technetium-99m methoxyisobutyl isonitrile affected by cell metabolism and viability? Circulation 82:1802–1814, 1990, with permission. © 1990, American Heart Association.)

Isolated heart studies by Meerdink and Leppo showed that whereas ^{201}Tl extraction was reduced after ouabain, sestamibi extraction increased.[87] Extraction of ^{201}Tl was also more sensitive than sestamibi to ischemic injury.[88] Beanlands and colleagues developed a model of cell injury by infusing cyanide or the detergent Triton-X into isolated rat hearts.[68] Reduced cardiac sestamibi uptake after cyanide injury or severe membrane disruption with Triton-X correlated with cell death as manifested by creatine kinase and lactate dehydrogenase release and the absence of vital staining with triphenyl tetrazolium (TTC) dye (Fig. 62–4). Preliminary data for Q12 and NOET suggest that the uptake of these tracers is not affected by moderate ischemic injury that does not cause cell disruption.[55, 89, 90] Infusion of Triton-X into isolated rat hearts, however, does cause loss of NOET.[55] Cell viability appears to have little effect on teboroxime retention by isolated hearts, because neither ischemia nor metabolic injury with cyanide or Triton-X affected the myocardial clearance of teboroxime.[66, 91] Therefore, basic data from cell culture and isolated heart models suggest that cardiac retention of the cations ^{201}Tl, sestamibi, and tetrofosmin requires cellular viabil-

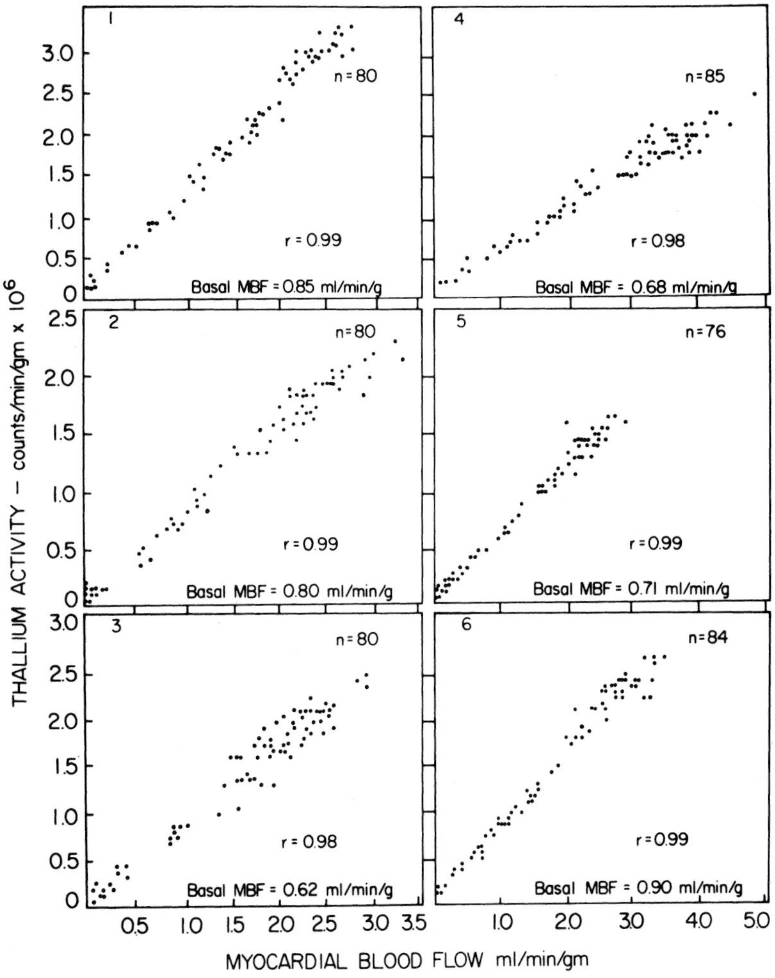

FIGURE 62–5. The relationship between ^{201}Tl activity and myocardial blood flow (MBF) in six dogs during exercise and ischemia; n = number of myocardial samples analyzed. (From Nielsen, A.P., Morris, K.G., Murdock R., et al.: Linear relationship between the distribution of thallium-201 and blood flow in ischemic and nonischemic myocardium during exercise. Circulation 61:797–801, 1980, with permission. © 1980, American Heart Association.)

ity, whereas uptake of teboroxime is nonspecific. Further studies of Q12 and NOET are warranted.

ANIMAL STUDIES OF MYOCARDIAL TRACER RETENTION AND CLEARANCE AS A FUNCTION OF BLOOD FLOW

Because a primary indication for perfusion agents involves their use as noninvasive markers of regional blood flow for the diagnosis of coronary disease and assessment of revascularization, it is important to know how accurately their deposition reflects flow.[92] To assess tracer uptake versus flow, a flow-limiting stenosis can be created in one coronary artery while hyperemic flow is produced in other territories with exercise or vasodilators.[93–98]

Nielsen and associates measured regional myocardial ^{201}Tl uptake versus microsphere blood flow in exercising dogs after placement of left circumflex stenoses.[98] Figure 62–5 shows nearly linear ^{201}Tl uptake over a wide range of coronary flow. The slight "roll off" or plateau in tracer uptake, which was also observed with dipyridamole,[99] is probably due to variable ^{201}Tl extraction or washout at high flow.[28, 94, 100–104]

The favorable flow characteristics of ^{201}Tl relate to its high myocardial extraction. Teboroxime has an even higher extraction of 90 percent and images hyperemic flow more accurately than ^{201}Tl.[96, 105, 106] However, as illustrated in Figure 62–6,[107] the uptake of rubidium (Rb), a cation tracer with a lower extraction, plateaus and underestimates flows higher than about 2.5 mL/min/g. Sestamibi also shows a plateau in tracer uptake at flows above 2.5 mL/min/g, whereas the phosphine compounds tetrofosmin and Q12 show a plateau in tracer uptake above flows of about 1 to 1.5 mL/min/g.[47, 108–110] Despite these differences, the different perfusion agents have generally shown comparable clinical accuracy for the detection of coronary disease.

The myocardial clearance or washout of a perfusion agent is determined not only by the intrinsic cellular retention of the compound but also by the level of coronary flow, the blood level of recirculating tracer, and myocardial viability.[95, 100, 111, 112] When ^{201}Tl is injected during a transient disparity in coronary perfusion, hypoperfused myocardium appears as a scan defect. Because the myocardial clearance rate of ^{201}Tl correlates with the level of coronary flow, differential washout results in apparent tracer "redistribution" over 3 to 4 hours, which can be detected by serial imaging.[101–103, 113] Teboroxime shows even faster myocardial washout. Using a canine model of coronary stenosis and adenosine hyperemia, Stewart and colleagues[114] showed that regional teboroxime clearance was faster in normally perfused myocardium (T1/2 = 6.3 minutes) than in the territory supplied by the stenotic artery (T1/2 = 11.2 minutes). This rapid differential washout, which can result in teboroxime redistribution within 5 to 10 minutes after intravenous injection, requires rapid imaging protocols for the accurate assessment of coronary flow.[96, 114–117] In contrast, sestamibi and the phosphine compounds tetrofosmin and Q12 show very slow myocardial clearance.[22, 46, 47, 118–120] Because of similar clearance rates from both ischemic and normally perfused territories, these compounds show minimal redistribution in most situations.

EFFECTS OF ISCHEMIA AND REPERFUSION

The delineation of reduced coronary flow and the separation of infarcted from viable ischemic myocardium make perfusion imaging useful for the study of acute and chronic ischemic syndromes. Retention of the cations ^{82}Rb and ^{201}Tl, as markers of membrane integrity during coronary occlusion and reperfusion, has correlated well with myocardial viability, as assessed by ^{18}F-labeled deoxyglucose (FDG) imaging or triphenyl tetrazolium staining.[111, 112, 121–124] Because sestamibi and tetrofosmin uptake require intact mitochondrial function, retention of these tracers is also a marker of myocardial viability. Infarct studies in canine models of occlusion-reperfusion have shown that injection of these tracers during coronary occlusion documents the total ischemic area "at risk." When these tracers are injected during reperfusion, the residual scan defect represents infarcted tissue, while improved uptake occurs in salvaged viable myocardium.[125–130]

Preliminary data for teboroxime suggest that when it is injected during reperfusion, its early distribution reflects primarily blood flow independent of myocardial viability.[131–133] Rapid serial imaging of this compound may permit early documentation of coronary artery patency during thrombolysis for acute myocardial infarction.[134] Little information is currently available regarding the effect of acute ischemia on the uptake of Q12 or NOET.

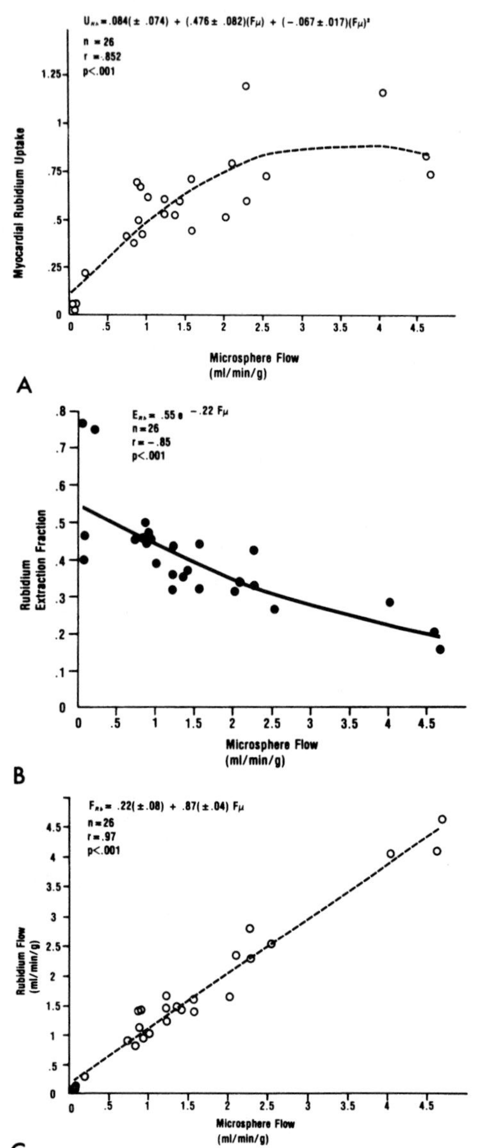

FIGURE 62–6. Relationship between myocardial rubidium uptake *(A)* and extraction fraction *(B)* versus microsphere-determined flow. Uptake (product of flow and extraction) is linearly related to flows up to 2.5 mL/min/g. Above this level of flow the fall in extraction results in a plateau in tracer uptake. After correction for variable extraction *(C)* rubidium and microsphere-determined flows are linearly related. (From Goldstein, R.A., Mullani, N.A., Marani, S.K., et al.: Myocardial perfusion with rubidium-82. II. Effects of metabolic and pharmacologic interventions. J. Nucl. Med. 24:907–915, 1983, with permission.)

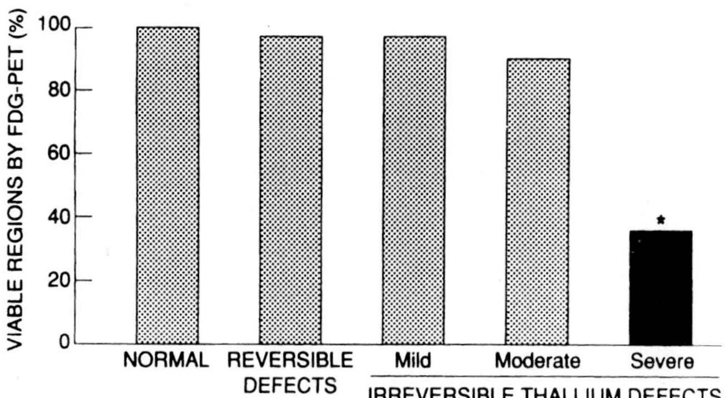

FIGURE 62–7. Percentage of myocardial regions showing evidence of preserved metabolic activity by ^{18}F-deoxyglucose (FDG) positron emission tomography (PET). The five groups were defined by the pattern of ^{201}Tl activity on stress-redistribution imaging. Most regions with normal ^{201}Tl uptake, reversible ^{201}Tl defects, and mild or moderate irreversible defects at redistribution imaging showed preserved FDG uptake. In contrast, most (64 percent) of the severe ^{201}Tl defects showed absent metabolic activity. All such severe defects that showed reversibility after ^{201}Tl reinjection showed preserved FDG uptake. (From Perrone-Filardi, P., Bacharach, S.L., Dilsizian, V., et al.: Regional left ventricular wall thickening: Relation to regional uptake of 18-fluorodeoxyglucose and 201-Tl in patients with chronic coronary artery disease and left ventricular dysfunction. Circulation 86:1125–1137, 1992, with permission. © 1992, American Heart Association.)

In a study of patients with chronic left ventricular dysfunction, Perrone-Filardi and colleagues[124] (Fig. 62–7) showed that most segments with preserved ^{201}Tl retention (>50 percent normal maximal activity) demonstrated viability by ^{18}F-deoxyglucose imaging even in the absence of ^{201}Tl redistribution. Although most segments with severe irreversible reductions in ^{201}Tl activity (<50 percent maximal activity) were not viable, use of the ^{201}Tl reinjection technique detected most of those segments with preserved ^{18}F-deoxyglucose metabolism.

FUTURE DIRECTIONS AND CONCLUSIONS

By detecting regional disparities in myocardial perfusion during physiologic or pharmacologic stress, all currently available perfusion agents permit the noninvasive diagnosis of coronary artery disease. Techniques that reduce imaging artifacts, such as photon scatter or variable attenuation, should increase diagnostic accuracy by improving the assessment of regional tracer distribution.[135–137] Dual-isotope studies, combining ^{201}Tl and sestamibi, are undergoing preliminary evaluation as a means of streamlining imaging protocols.[138, 139] New tracers such as ^{99m}Tc-nitroimidazole, a compound that is selectively retained within hypoxic cells, are being developed to specifically image ischemic myocardium.[140]

Myocardial perfusion agents can accurately delineate regions of reduced flow and can be used to determine infarct size or to document myocardial viability. As more radiolabeled perfusion agents with differing properties become available, the choice of the specific tracer for a given perfusion study will be based on which compound can answer the specific clinical question in the most cost-effective manner.

References

1. Marcus, M.L., and Harrison, D.G.: Physiologic basis for myocardial perfusion imaging. *In* Marcus, M.L., Skorton, D.J., Schelbert, H.R., et al. (eds.): Cardiac

Imaging: A Companion to Braunwald's Heart Disease. Philadelphia, W.B. Saunders, 1991, pp. 8–23.
2. Lassen, N.A., and Perl, W.: Tracer Kinetic Methods in Medical Physiology. New York, Raven Press, 1979.
3. Bassingthwaighte, J.B.: Physiology and theory of tracer washout techniques for the estimation of myocardial blood flow: Flow estimation from tracer washout. Prog. Cardiovasc. Dis. 20:165, 1977.
4. Bassingthwaighte, J.B., and Goresky, C.A.: Modeling in the analysis of solute and water exchange in the microvasculature. *In* Renkin, E.M., and Michel, C.C. (eds.): Handbook of Physiology. Sect. 2, The Cardiovascular System. Vol. IV. The Microcirculation. Bethesda, MD, American Physiological Society, 1984, pp. 549–626.
5. Bassingthwaighte, J.B., Raymond, G.M., and Chan, J.I.: Principles of tracer kinetics. *In* Zaret, B.L., and Beller, G.A. (eds.): Nuclear Cardiology: State of the Art and Future Directions. St. Louis, Mosby, 1993, pp. 3–23.
6. Leppo, J.A.: Overview: Clinical assessment of myocardial viability. Coron. Artery Dis. 4:481, 1993.
7. Dilsizian, V., and Bonow, R.O.: Current diagnostic techniques of assessing myocardial viability in patients with hibernating and stunned myocardium. Circulation 87:1, 1993.
8. Bonow, R.O., and Dilsizian, V.: Thallium-201 for assessment of myocardial viability. Semin. Nucl. Med. 21:230, 1991.
9. Lucas, J.R., Botvinick, E.H., and Dae, M.W.: Myocardial viability: Evidence provided by the analysis of left ventricular systolic function. Coron. Artery Dis. 4:485, 1993.
10. Gropler, R.J., and Bergmann, S.R.: Flow and metabolic determinants of myocardial viability by positron-emission tomography. Coron. Artery Dis. 4:495, 1993.
11. Tamaki, N.: Assessment of myocardial viability by use of multiple clinical parameters and effect on prognosis. Coron. Artery Dis. 4:521, 1993.
12. Hendel, R.C., and Bonow, R.O.: Disparity in coronary perfusion and regional wall motion: Effect on clinical assessment of viability. Coron. Artery Dis. 4:512, 1993.
13. Kuijper, A.F.M., van Eck-Smit, B.L.F., Bruschke, A.V.G., et al.: Flow and cellular function: Clinical assessment of myocardial viability by single-photon agents. Coron. Artery Dis. 4:505, 1993.
14. Bolli, R.: Mechanism of myocardial "stunning." Circulation 82:723, 1990.
15. Bolli, R.: Myocardial "stunning" in man. Circulation 86:1671, 1992.
16. Kronauge, J.F., Chiu, M.L., Cone, J.S., et al.: Comparison of neutral and cationic myocardial perfusion agents: Characteristics of accumulation in cultured cells. Nucl. Med. Biol. 19:141, 1992.
17. Dahlberg, S.T., and Leppo, J.A.: Physiologic properties of myocardial perfusion tracers. Cardiol. Clin. 12:169, 1994.
18. Johansson, L., Mattsson, S., Nosslin, B., et al.: Effective dose to the patient from radiopharmaceuticals calculated with the new ICRP tissue weighting factors. *In* Watson, E.E., and Schlafke-Stelson, A.T. (eds.): Fifth International Radiopharmaceutical Dosimetry Symposium, CONF-910529. Oak Ridge, TN, Oak Ridge Associated Universities, 1992, pp. 41–48.
19. Leide, S., Diemer, H., Ahlgren, L., et al.: In vivo distribution and dosimetry of Tc-99m MIBI in man. *In* Watson, E.E., and Schlafke-Stelson, A.T. (eds.): Fifth International Radiopharmaceutical Dosimetry Symposium, CONF-910529. Oak Ridge, TN, Oak Ridge Associated Universities, 1992, pp. 483–497.
20. Smith, T., Lahiri, A., Gemmell, H.G., et al.: Dosimetry of ^{99m}Tc-P53, a new myocardial perfusion imaging agent. *In* Watson, E.E., and Schlafke-Stelson, A.T. (eds.): Fifth International Radiopharmaceutical Dosimetry Symposium, CONF-910529. Oak Ridge, TN, Oak Ridge Associated Universities, 1992, pp. 467–481.
21. Higley, B., Smith, F.W., Smith, T., et al.: Technetium-99m-1,2-bis[bis(2-ethoxyethyl)phosphino]ethane: Human biodistribution, dosimetry and safety of a new myocardial perfusion imaging agent. J. Nucl. Med. 34:30, 1993.
22. Wackers, F.J.T., Berman, D.S., Maddahi, J., et al.: Technetium-99m hexakis 2-methoxyisobutyl isonitrile: Human biodistribution, dosimetry, safety, and preliminary comparison to thallium-201 for myocardial perfusion imaging. J. Nucl. Med. 30:301, 1989.
23. L'Abbate, A., Biagini, A., Michelassi, C., et al.: Myocardial kinetics of thallium and potassium in man. Circulation 60:776, 1979.
24. Zaret, B.L., Strauss, H.W., Martin, N.D., et al.: Noninvasive regional myocardial perfusion with radioactive potassium: Study of patients at rest, with exercise and during angina pectoris. N. Engl. J. Med. 288:809, 1973.
25. Lebowitz, E., Greene, M.V., Fairchild, R., et al.: Thallium-201 for medical use. I. J. Nucl. Med. 16:151, 1975.
26. Bradley-Moore, P.R., Lebowitz, E., Greene, M.W., et al.: Thallium-201 for medical use. II. Biologic behavior. J. Nucl. Med. 16:156, 1975.
27. Atkins, H.L., Budinger, T.F., Lebowitz, E., et al.: Thallium-201 for medical use. Part 3: Human distribution and physical imaging properties. J. Nucl. Med. 18:133, 1977.
28. Strauss, H.W., Harrison, K., Langan, J.K., et al.: Thallium-201 for myocardial imaging: Relation of thallium-201 to regional myocardial perfusion. Circulation 51:641, 1975.
29. Beller, G.A.: Myocardial perfusion imaging with thallium-201. *In* Marcus, M.L., Skorton, D.S., Schelbert, H.R., et al. (eds.): Cardiac Imaging: A Companion to Braunwald's Heart Disease. Philadelphia, W.B. Saunders, 1991, pp. 1047–1073.
30. Pohost, G.M., Alpert, N.M., Ingwall, J.S., et al.: Thallium redistribution: Mechanisms and clinical utility. Semin. Nucl. Med. 10:70, 1980.
31. Mullins, L.J., and Moore, R.D.: The movement of thallium ions in muscle. J. Gen. Physiol. 43:759, 1960.
32. Gehring, P.J., and Hammond, P.B.: The interrelationship between thallium and potassium in animals. J. Pharmacol. Exp. Ther. 155:187, 1967.
33. Gehring, P.J., and Hammond, P.B.: The uptake of thallium by rabbit erythrocytes. J. Pharmacol. Exp. Ther. 145:215, 1964.
34. McCall, D.: Cation exchange and glycoside binding in cultured rat heart cells. Am. J. Physiol. 236:C87, 1979.
35. McCall, D., Zimmer, L.J., and Katz, A.M.: Kinetics of thallium exchange in cultured rat myocardial cells. Circ. Res. 56:370, 1985.
36. Berman, D.S., Kiat, H., Leppo, J., et al.: Technetium-99m myocardial perfusion imaging agents. *In* Marcus, M.L., Skorton, D.J., Schelbert, H.R., et al. (eds.): Cardiac Imaging: A Companion to Braunwald's Heart Disease. Philadelphia, W.B. Saunders, 1991, pp. 1097–1109.
37. Gerson, M.C., Deutsch, E.A., Libson, K.F., et al.: Myocardial scintigraphy with ^{99m}Tc-tris-DMPE in man. Eur. J. Nucl. Med. 9:403, 1984.
38. Deutsch, E., Bushong, W., Glavan, K.A., et al.: Heart imaging with cationic complexes of technetium. Science 214:85, 1981.
39. Dudczak, R., Angelberger, P., Homan, R., et al.: Evaluation of ^{99m}Tc-dicholor bis(1,2-dimethylphosphino) ethane (^{99m}Tc-DMPE) for myocardial scintigraphy in man. Eur. J. Nucl. Med. 8:513, 1983.
40. Sia, I.B., Holman, B.L., McKusick, K., et al.: The utilization of Tc-99m-TBI as a myocardial perfusion agent in exercise studies: Comparison with Tl-201 thallous chloride and examination of its biodistribution in humans. Eur. J. Nucl. Med. 12:333, 1986.
41. Deutsch, E., Ketring, A.R., Libson, K., et al.: The Noah's Ark experiment: Species dependent biodistributions of cationic ^{99m}Tc complexes. Nucl. Med. Biol. 16:191, 1989.
42. Liu, X.-J., Wang, X., Liu, Y., et al.: Clinical evaluation of the ^{99m}Tc-CPI myocardial perfusion imaging. Eur. J. Nucl. Med. 15:277, 1989.
43. Gerundini, P., Savi, A., Gilardi, M.C., et al.: Evaluation in dogs and humans of three potential technetium-99m myocardial perfusion agents. J. Nucl. Med. 27:409, 1986.
44. Berman, D.S., Kiat, H., Van Train, K., et al.: Technetium 99m sestamibi in the assessment of chronic coronary artery disease. Semin. Nucl. Med. 21:190, 1991.
45. Kelly, J.D., Forster, A.M., Higley, B., et al.: Technetium-99m-tetrofosmin as a new radiopharmaceutical for myocardial perfusion imaging. J. Nucl. Med. 34:222, 1993.
46. Gerson, M.C., Lukes, J., Deutsch, E., et al.: Comparison of ^{99m}technetium-Q3 and thallium-201 for detection of coronary artery disease in humans. J. Nucl. Med. 35:580, 1994.
47. Gerson, M.C., Millard, R.W., Roszell, N.J., et al.: Kinetic properties of ^{99m}Tc-Q12 in canine myocardium. Circulation 89:1291, 1994.
48. Cannon, P.J., Weiss, M.B., and Sciacca, R.R.: Myocardial blood flow in coronary artery disease: Studies at rest and during stress with inert gas washout techniques. Prog. Cardiovasc. Dis. 20:95, 1977.
49. Cannon, P.J.: Radioisotopic studies of the regional myocardial circulation. Circulation 51:955, 1975.
50. Narra, R.K., Nunn, A.D., Kuczynski, B.L., et al.: A neutral technetium-99m complex for myocardial imaging. J. Nucl. Med. 30:1830, 1989.
51. Chua, T., Kiat, H., Germano, G., et al.: Technetium-99m teboroxime regional myocardial washout in subjects with and without coronary artery disease. Am. J. Cardiol. 72:728, 1993.
52. Pasqualini, R., Duatti, A., Bellande, E., et al.: Bis(dithiocarbamato) nitrido technetium-99m radiopharmaceuticals: A class of neutral myocardial imaging agents. J. Nucl. Med. 35:334, 1994.
53. Giganti, M., Cittanti, C., Colamussi, P., et al.: Biodistribution in man of bis[(*N*-ethyl, *N*-ethoxy) dithiocarbamate] nitrido technetium (V), a promising new tracer for myocardial perfusion imaging. J. Nucl. Med. 35:155P, 1994.
54. Bellande, E., Hoffschir, D., Comazzi, D., et al.: Interaction of the myocardial imaging agent TcN-NOET with cyclodextrins: Influence of the stability of the inclusion complex on the biological properties. J. Nucl. Med. 35:261P, 1994.
55. Johnson, G., III, Nguyen, K.N., and Okada, R.D.: Clearance of Tc-99m-NOET in normal, ischemic-reperfused and membrane-disrupted rat myocardium. Circulation 88:I-249, 1993.
56. Fagret, D., Marie, P.Y., Brunotte, F., et al.: Stress and delayed SPECT myocardial imaging with a new neutral technetium-99m nitrido dithiocarbamate complex (TcN-NOET): Comparison with thallium-201 SPECT imaging and coronary angiography. J. Nucl. Med. 35:114P, 1994.
57. Zhang, Z., Maublant, J.C., Ollier, M., et al.: Cellular uptake of Tc-99m-NOET, a potent myocardial blood flow imaging agent: Comparison with Tl-201, Tc-99m sestamibi and Tc-99m teboroxime. Circulation 86:I-708, 1992.
58. Piwnica-Worms, D., and Kronauge, J.F.: Transport mechanisms of SPECT perfusion tracers in cultured cells. *In* Zaret, B.L., and Beller, G.A. (eds.): Nuclear Cardiology: State of the Art and Future Directions. St. Louis, Mosby, 1993, pp. 25–34.
59. Maublant, J.C., Moins, N., and Gachon, P.: Uptake and release of two new Tc-99m–labeled myocardial blood flow imaging agents in cultured cardiac cells. Eur. J. Nucl. Med. 15:180, 1989.
60. Piwnica-Worms, D., Kronauge, J.F., Delmon, L., et al.: Effect of metabolic inhibition on technetium-99m-MIBI kinetics in cultured chick myocardial cells. J. Nucl. Med. 31:464, 1990.
61. Chiu, M.L., Kronauge, J.F., and Piwnica-Worms, D.: Effect of mitochondrial and plasma membrane potentials on accumulation of hexakis (2-methoxyisobutylisonitrile)technetium(I) in cultured mouse fibroblasts. J. Nucl. Med. 31:1646, 1990.
62. Piwnica-Worms, D., Kronauge, J.F., and Chiu, M.L.: Uptake and retention of hexakis (2-methoxyisobutyl isonitrile) technetium(I) in cultured chick myocardial cells: Mitochondrial and plasma membrane potential dependence. Circulation 82:1826, 1990.
63. Carvalho, P.A., Chiu, M.L., Kronauge, J.F., et al.: Subcellular distribution and analysis of technetium-99m-MIBI in isolated perfused rat hearts. J. Nucl. Med. 33:1516, 1992.
64. Dahlberg, S.T., Gilmore, M.P., and Leppo, J.A.: Interaction of technetium 99m-

labeled teboroxime with red blood cells reduces the compound's extraction and increases apparent cardiac washout. J. Nucl. Cardiol. 1:270, 1994.
65. Marshall, R.C., Leidholdt, E.M., Jr., Zhang, D.-Y., et al.: The effect of flow on technetium-99m-teboroxime (SQ30217) and thallium-201 extraction and retention in rabbit heart. J. Nucl. Med. 32:1979, 1991.
66. Stone, J.A., Dawood, F., Wen, W.-H., et al.: Is the myocardial uptake of teboroxime viability dependent? Circulation 86:I-707, 1992.
67. Rumsey, W.L., Rosenspire, K.C., and Nunn, A.D.: Myocardial extraction of teboroxime: Effects of teboroxime interaction with blood. J. Nucl. Med. 33:94, 1992.
68. Beanlands, R.S.B., Dawood, F., Wen, W.-H., et al.: Are the kinetics of technetium-99m methoxyisobutyl isonitrile affected by cell metabolism and viability? Circulation 82:1802, 1990.
69. Bergmann, S.R., Clark, R.E., and Sobel, B.E.: An improved isolated heart preparation for external assessment of myocardial metabolism. Am. J. Physiol. 236:H644, 1979.
70. Kampf, G., Muenze, R., Knop, G., et al.: Evaluation of potential heart affine compounds by use of the isolated perfused rat heart. Eur. J. Nucl. Med. 13:410, 1987.
71. Leppo, J.A., and Meerdink, D.J.: Comparison of the myocardial uptake of a technetium-labeled isonitrile analogue and thallium. Circ. Res. 65:632, 1989.
72. Marshall, R.C., Leidholdt, E.M., Jr., Zhang, D.-Y., et al.: Technetium-99m hexakis 2-methoxy-2-isobutyl isonitrile and thallium-201 extraction, washout and retention at varying coronary flow rates in rabbit heart. Circulation 82:998, 1990.
73. Dahlberg, S.T., Meerdink, D.J., Gilmore, M.P., et al.: Myocardial extraction of technetium-99m-[2-(1-methoxybutyl) isonitrile] in the isolated rabbit heart: A new myocardial perfusion agent with high extraction and stable retention. J. Nucl. Med. 34:927, 1993.
74. Bassingthwaighte, J.B., and Holloway, G.A.: Estimation of blood flow with radioactive tracers. Semin. Nucl. Med. 6:141, 1976.
75. Crone, C.: The permeability of capillaries in various organs as determined by use of the "indicator diffusion" method. Acta Physiol. Scand. 58:292, 1963.
76. Renkin, E.M.: Transport of potassium-42 from blood to tissue in isolated mammalian skeletal muscles. Am. J. Physiol. 197:1205, 1959.
77. Dahlberg, S.T., Gilmore, M.P., Flood, M., et al.: Extraction and washout of Tc-99m tetrofosmin in the isolated rat heart. J. Nucl. Med. 35:47P, 1994.
78. Meerdink, D.J., Dahlberg, S.T., Gilmore, M., et al.: Transcapillary exchange of Q12 and thallium-201 in isolated rabbit hearts. Circulation 88:I-249, 1993.
79. Porenta, G., Czernin, J., and Schelbert, H.R.: Assessment of myocardial viability with tracers of blood flow and metabolism of glucose. *In* Bergmann, S.R., and Sobel, B.E. (eds.): Positron Emission Tomography of the Heart. Mt. Kisco, NY, Futura Publishing, 1992, pp. 153–183.
80. Lerch, R.A., Bergmann, S.R., and Sobel, B.E.: Delineation of myocardial fatty acid metabolism with positron emission tomography. *In* Bergmann, S.R., and Sobel, B.E. (eds.): Positron Emission Tomography of the Heart. Mt. Kisco, NY, Futura Publishing, 1992, pp. 129–152.
81. Bergmann, S.R., and Sobel, B.E.: Quantification of regional myocardial oxidative utilization with positron emission tomography. *In* Bergmann, S.R., and Sobel, B.E. (eds.): Positron Emission Tomography of the Heart. Mt. Kisco, NY, Futura Publishing, 1992, pp. 209–229.
82. Kloster, G., Stöcklin, G., Smith, E.F., III, et al.: Omega-halo fatty acids: A probe for mitochondrial membrane integrity. Eur. J. Nucl. Med. 9:305, 1984.
83. Piwnica-Worms, D., Chiu, M.L., and Kronauge, J.F.: Divergent kinetics of ^{201}Tl and ^{99m}Tc-sestamibi in cultured chick ventricular myocytes during ATP depletion. Circulation 85:1531, 1992.
84. Maublant, J.C., Moins, N., Gachon, P., et al.: Uptake of technetium-99m-teboroxime in cultured myocardial cells: Comparison with thallium-201 and technetium-99m-sestamibi. J. Nucl. Med. 34:255, 1993.
85. Songadele, J.A., Younès, A., Maublant, J.C., et al.: Uptake of Tc-99m tetrofosmin in isolated mitochondria: Evidence for an active mechanism. J. Nucl. Med. 35:46P, 1994.
86. Maublant, J.C., Gachon, P., and Moins, N.: Hexakis (2-methoxy isobutylisonitrile) technetium-99m and thallium-201 chloride: Uptake and release in cultured myocardial cells. J. Nucl. Med. 29:48, 1988.
87. Meerdink, D.J., and Leppo, J.A.: Comparison of hypoxia and ouabain effects on the first-pass myocardial uptake kinetics of Tc-99m hexakis 2-methoxyisobutyl isonitrile and thallium-201. J. Nucl. Med. 30:1500, 1989.
88. Meerdink, D.J., and Leppo, J.A.: Myocardial transport of hexakis 2-methoxyisobutyl isonitrile and thallium before and after coronary reperfusion. Circ. Res. 66:1738, 1990.
89. Johnson, G., III, Nguyen, K.N., and Okada, R.D.: Myocardial Tc-99m Q-12 (TechneCard™) clearance is not affected by hypoxia or low flow in an isolated perfused rat heart model. Circulation 88:I-249, 1993.
90. Johnson, G., III, Nguyen, K.N., Alton, I.L., et al.: Myocardial Tc-99m Q-12 (TechneCard™) clearance is not affected by ischemia and reperfusion in an isolated perfused rat heart model. J. Am. Coll. Cardiol. 23:422A, 1994.
91. Beanlands, R.S.B., Palser, A., Masika, M., et al.: The effect of ischemic reperfusion flow on the myocardial kinetics of Tc-99m-teboroxime. J. Nucl. Med. 35:3P, 1994.
92. Gewirtz, H.: Present status and future directions for nuclear cardiology: Observations derived from intact animal models. *In* Zaret, B.L., and Beller, G.A. (eds.): Nuclear Cardiology: State of the Art and Future Directions. St. Louis, Mosby, 1993, pp. 53–61.
93. Gould, K.L.: Noninvasive assessment of coronary stenoses by myocardial perfusion imaging during pharmacologic coronary vasodilation. I. Physiologic basis and experimental validation. Am. J. Cardiol. 41:267, 1978.
94. Beller, G.A., Holzgrefe, H.H., and Watson, D.D.: Intrinsic washout rates of thallium-201 in normal and ischemic myocardium after dipyridamole-induced vasodilation. Circulation 71:378, 1985.
95. Okada, R.D., Leppo, J.A., Boucher, C.A., et al.: Myocardial kinetics of thallium-201 after dipyridamole infusion in normal canine myocardium and in myocardium distal to a stenosis. J. Clin. Invest. 69:199, 1982.
96. Gray, W.A., and Gewirtz, H.: Comparison of ^{99m}Tc-teboroxime with thallium for myocardial imaging in the presence of a coronary artery stenosis. Circulation 84:1796, 1991.
97. Caldwell, J.H., Martin, G.V., Link, J.M., et al.: Iodophenylpentadecanoic acid-myocardial blood flow relationship during maximal exercise with coronary occlusion. J. Nucl. Med. 30:99, 1990.
98. Nielsen, A.P., Morris, K.G., Murdock, R., et al.: Linear relationship between the distribution of thallium-201 and blood flow in ischemic and nonischemic myocardium during exercise. Circulation 61:797, 1980.
99. Mays, A.E., Jr., and Cobb, F.R.: Relationship between regional myocardial blood flow and thallium-201 distribution in the presence of coronary artery stenosis and dipyridamole-induced vasodilation. J. Clin. Invest. 73:1359, 1984.
100. Grunwald, A.M., Watson, D.D., Holzgrefe, H.H., Jr., et al.: Myocardial thallium-201 kinetics in normal and ischemic myocardium. Circulation 64:610, 1981.
101. Pohost, G.M., Okada, R.D., O'Keefe, D.D., et al.: Thallium redistribution in dogs with severe coronary artery stenosis of fixed caliber. Circ. Res. 48:439, 1981.
102. Beller, G.A., Watson, D.D., Ackell, P., and Pohost, G.M.: Time course of thallium-201 redistribution after transient myocardial ischemia. Circulation 61:791, 1980.
103. Pohost, G.M., Zir, L.M., Moore, R.H., et al.: Differentiation of transiently ischemic from infarcted myocardium by serial imaging after a single dose of thallium-201. Circulation 55:294, 1977.
104. Weich, H.F., Strauss, H.W., and Pitt, B.: The extraction of thallium-201 by the myocardium. Circulation 56:188, 1977.
105. Stewart, R.E., Schwaiger, M., Hutchins, G.D., et al.: Myocardial clearance kinetics of technetium-99m-SQ 30217: A marker of regional myocardial blood flow. J. Nucl. Med. 31:1183, 1990.
106. Beanlands, R., Muzik, O., Nguyen, N., et al.: The relationship between myocardial retention of technetium-99m teboroxime and myocardial blood flow. J. Am. Coll. Cardiol. 20:712, 1992.
107. Goldstein, R.A., Mullani, N.A., Marani, S.K., et al.: Myocardial perfusion with rubidium-82. II. Effects of metabolic and pharmacologic interventions. J. Nucl. Med. 24:907, 1983.
108. Glover, D.K., and Okada, R.D.: Myocardial kinetics of Tc-MIBI in canine myocardium after dipyridamole. Circulation 81:628, 1990.
109. Melon, P.G., Beanlands, R.S., DeGrado, T.R., et al.: Comparison of technetium-99m sestamibi and thallium-201 retention characteristics in canine myocardium. J. Am. Coll. Cardiol. 20:1277, 1992.
110. Sinusas, A.J., Shi, Q.-X., Saltzberg, M.T., et al.: Technetium-99m-tetrofosmin to assess myocardial blood flow: Experimental validation in an intact canine model of ischemia. J. Nucl. Med. 35:664, 1994.
111. Goldstein, R.A.: Kinetics of rubidium-82 after coronary occlusion and reperfusion: Assessment of patency and viability in open chested dogs. J. Clin. Invest. 75:1131, 1985.
112. Okada, R.D.: Kinetics of thallium-201 in reperfused canine myocardium after coronary artery occlusion. J. Am. Coll. Cardiol. 3:1245, 1984.
113. Leppo, J., Rosenkrantz, J., Rosenthal, R., et al.: Quantitative thallium-201 redistribution with a fixed coronary stenosis in dogs. Circulation 63:632, 1981.
114. Stewart, R.E., Heyl, B., O'Rourke, R.A., et al.: Demonstration of differential post-stenotic myocardial technetium-99m-teboroxime clearance kinetics after experimental ischemia and hyperemic stress. J. Nucl. Med. 32:2000, 1991.
115. Hendel, R.C., McSherry, B., Karimeddini, M., et al.: Diagnostic value of a new myocardial perfusion agent, teboroxime (SQ30217), utilizing a rapid planar imaging protocol: Preliminary results. J. Am. Coll. Cardiol. 16:855, 1990.
116. Dahlberg, S.T., Weinstein, H., Hendel, R.C., et al.: Planar myocardial perfusion imaging with technetium-99m-teboroxime: Comparison by vascular territory with thallium-201 and coronary angiography. J. Nucl. Med. 33:1783, 1992.
117. Weinstein, H., Dahlberg, S.T., McSherry, B.A., et al.: Rapid redistribution of teboroxime. Am. J. Cardiol. 71:848, 1993.
118. Taillefer, R., Primeau, M., Costi, P., et al.: Technetium-99m-sestamibi myocardial perfusion imaging in detection of coronary artery disease: Comparison between initial (1-hour) and delayed (3-hour) postexercise images. J. Nucl. Med. 32:1961, 1991.
119. Okada, R.D., Glover, D., Gaffney, T., et al.: Myocardial kinetics of technetium-99m-hexakis-2-methoxy-2-methylpropyl-isonitrile. Circulation 77:491, 1988.
120. Sridhara, B.S., Braat, S., Rigo, P., et al.: Comparison of myocardial perfusion imaging with technetium-99m tetrofosmin versus thallium-201 in coronary artery disease. Am. J. Cardiol. 72:1015, 1993.
121. Gould, K.L., Yoshida, K., Hess, M.J., et al.: Myocardial metabolism of fluorodeoxyglucose compared to cell membrane integrity for the potassium analogue rubidium-82 for assessing infarct size in man by PET. J. Nucl. Med. 32:1, 1991.
122. Sabia, P.J., Powers, E.R., Ragosta, M., et al.: Role of quantitative planar thallium-201 imaging for determining viability in patients with acute myocardial infarction and a totally occluded infarct-related artery. J. Nucl. Med. 34:728, 1993.
123. Ragosta, M., Beller, G.A., Watson, D.D., et al.: Quantitative planar rest-redistribution ^{201}Tl imaging in detection of myocardial viability and prediction of improvement in left ventricular function after coronary bypass surgery in patients with severely depressed left ventricular function. Circulation 87:1630, 1993.
124. Perrone-Filardi, P., Bacharach, S.L., Dilsizian, V., et al.: Regional left ventricular wall thickening: Relation to regional uptake of 18-fluorodeoxyglucose and 201-Tl in patients with chronic coronary artery disease and left ventricular dysfunction. Circulation 86:1125, 1992.

125. Verani, M.S., Jeroudi, M.O., Mahmarian, J.J., et al.: Quantification of myocardial infarction during coronary occlusion and myocardial salvage after reperfusion using cardiac imaging with technetium-99m hexakis 2-methoxyisobutyl isonitrile. J. Am. Coll. Cardiol. 12:1573, 1988.
126. Sinusas, A.J., Trautman, K.A., Bergin, J.D., et al.: Quantification of area at risk during coronary occlusion and degree of myocardial salvage after reperfusion with technetium-99m methoxyisobutyl nitrile. Circulation 82:1424, 1990.
127. Freeman, I., Grunwald, A.M., Hoory, S., et al.: Effect of coronary occlusion and myocardial viability on myocardial activity of technetium-99m-sestamibi. J. Nucl. Med. 32:292, 1991.
128. Beller, G.A., Glover, D.K., Edwards, N.C., et al.: ^{99m}Tc-sestamibi uptake and retention during myocardial ischemia and reperfusion. Circulation 87:2033, 1993.
129. Detre, K.M., Wright, E., Murphy, M.L., et al.: Observer agreement in evaluating coronary angiograms. Circulation 52:979, 1975.
130. Glover, D.K., Ruiz, M., Allen, T.R., et al.: Assessment of myocardial viability by Tc-99m tetrofosmin in a canine model of coronary occlusion and reperfusion. J. Am. Coll. Cardiol. 23:475A, 1994.
131. Heller, L.I., Villegas, B.J., Reinhardt, C.P., et al.: Teboroxime is a marker of blood flow following reperfusion of a myocardial infarction. J. Nucl. Med. 34:14P, 1993.
132. Chang, P.I., Shi, Q., Saltzberg, M.T., et al.: Myocardial distribution and clearance of Tc-99m-teboroxime during reperfusion after acute myocardial infarction. Circulation 86:I-707, 1992.
133. Chang, P.I., Shi, Q.-X., Maniawski, P., et al.: Tc-99m-teboroxime is a marker of reperfusion flow early after acute myocardial infarction. J. Am. Coll. Cardiol. 19:338A, 1992.
134. Grégoire, J., Pérez-Villa, F., and Théroux, P.: ^{99m}Tc-teboroxime scintigraphy for the early diagnosis of coronary reperfusion during thrombolytic therapy for acute myocardial infarction. J. Am. Coll. Cardiol. 23:475A, 1994.
135. Datz, F.L., Gullberg, G.T., Zeng, G.L., et al.: Application of convergent-beam collimation and simultaneous transmission emission tomography to single-photon emission computed tomography. Semin. Nucl. Med. 24:17, 1994.
136. King, M.A., Hademenos, G.J., and Glick, S.J.: A dual-photopeak window method for scatter correction. J. Nucl. Med. 33:605, 1992.
137. King, M.A., Luo, D.-S., Dahlberg, S.T., et al.: Transmission and emission SPECT imaging of attenuator and source distributions larger than the camera field of view. J. Nucl. Med. 35:92P, 1994.
138. Kiat, H., Germano, G., Friedman, J., et al.: Comparative feasibility of separate or simultaneous rest thallium-201/stress technetium-99m-sestamibi dual-isotope myocardial perfusion SPECT. J. Nucl. Med. 35:542, 1994.
139. Berman, D.S., Kiat, H., Van Train, K., et al.: Dual-isotope myocardial perfusion SPECT with rest thallium-201 and stress Tc-99m sestamibi. Cardiol. Clin. 12:261, 1994.
140. Kusuoka, H., Hashimoto, K., Fukuchi, K., et al.: Kinetics of a putative hypoxic tissue marker, technetium-99m-nitroimidazole (BMS181321), in normoxic, hypoxic, ischemic, and stunned myocardium. J. Nucl. Med. 35:1371, 1994.

CHAPTER

63 Myocardial Perfusion Imaging for the Detection and Evaluation of Coronary Artery Disease

Jamshid Maddahi, M.D.

In cardiology, myocardial perfusion scintigraphy has now become an established method of diagnosing and evaluating coronary artery disease (CAD). Since its introduction about 2 decades ago, myocardial perfusion scintigraphy has advanced significantly. The imaging technique has evolved from the conventional planar method to single-photon emission computed tomography (SPECT). Parallel with these developments, significant advances in the interpretation of test results have resulted from the development of objective, quantitative methods for analysis and display of myocardial perfusion images. In recent years, technetium-99m (^{99m}Tc)-labeled agents have become clinically available that offer improved imaging characteristics compared to those of conventional thallium-201 (^{201}Tl). The clinical applications have expanded from diagnosis to risk stratification of CAD and assessment of a variety of clinical conditions, such as myocardial infarction, reperfusion, and revascularization. This chapter provides an overview of the technical and clinical aspects of myocardial perfusion scintigraphy that uses single-photon radionuclides.

CLINICAL IMPLICATIONS OF MYOCARDIAL KINETICS OF THALLIUM-201 AND TECHNETIUM-99m LABELED AGENTS

Thallium-201

Thallium is a metallic element in group IIIA of the periodic table, with biologic properties similar but not identical to potassium. The ionic radii of these two elements are close to each another, and as with potassium, the distribution of the thallous ion following intravenous administration is primarily intracellular.[1–3] Transport of thallium across the cell membrane has been reported to occur partly via an ouabain inhibitable mechanism, presumed to be the sodium-potassium ATPase pump.[4]

After intravenous injection, the *initial distribution* of ^{201}Tl in the myocardium is related to regional blood flow[5, 6] and the extraction fraction (ability of the myocardium to extract the tracer from blood), which is 87 percent[7] at normal flow rates. At exceedingly low flow rates (less than 10 percent of baseline), ^{201}Tl uptake increases relative to blood flow because of an increase in myocardial extraction fraction. Conversely, at high flow rates (exceeding twice the control level), the myocardial extraction fraction for ^{201}Tl decreases, resulting in a "roll-off" of the relationship between myocardial uptake of ^{201}Tl and increasing flow.[8–10] Overall, the initial defects in myocardial ^{201}Tl images, whether injection is made at rest, during exercise, or after administration of a coronary vasodilator, are produced predominantly by regional deficits in myocardial blood flow distribution. In clinical situations, the additional role played by myocardial ischemia or drugs in producing image defects (by altering extraction fraction) is unclear but does not appear to be significant.

The distribution of ^{201}Tl in the myocardium is not static but changes as a function of time. This phenomenon is referred to as *redistribution.* Poshost and colleagues[5] demonstrated that after injection of ^{201}Tl in patients with exercise-induced ischemia but without infarction, delayed images revealed disappearance of the initial perfusion defects. Thallium-201 redistribution also has been observed after injection at rest in patients with severe fixed coronary stenosis without infarction.[11] This finding has been confirmed in experimental studies.[12, 13] The disappearance of initial exercise ^{201}Tl defects over time generally results from slower clearance of ^{201}Tl from the previously underperfused zones compared to that of the normal zones.[13, 14] The normal net myocardial clearance half-life of ^{201}Tl after intravenous injection is approximately 4 hours when injection is made during exercise[15] and is longer when injection is made at submaximal exercise heart rate[16, 17] or at rest.[18] Although changes in myocardial blood flow after intravenous administration of ^{201}Tl do not substantially alter myocardial ^{201}Tl clearance,[19, 20] the rate of disappearance of ^{201}Tl from the blood also affects myocardial clearance of ^{201}Tl,[18, 21] which in turn may influence the time course of ^{201}Tl defect reversibility. Budinger and colleagues[22] showed that rapid blood clearance of ^{201}Tl prevented perfusion defect reversibility in viable myocardial regions up to 24 hours after ^{201}Tl administration. Angello and colleagues[23] found that poststress glucose loading resulted in decreased blood ^{201}Tl concentration during the initial 2 hours after ^{201}Tl injection, causing a high frequency of nonreversible defects in regions that demonstrated reversibility at 4 hours when ^{201}Tl imaging was performed without glucose loading. Thus, fasting is recommended to patients on the day of and for the interval between sequential ^{201}Tl imaging.

Based on the change from exercise to the redistribution phase, ^{201}Tl defects may be categorized clinically as reversible, partially reversible, nonreversible, or as exhibiting reverse redistribution. The time period for redistribution may vary; complete redistribution may require 24 hours or more.[24, 25] This phenomenon of late redistribution has important implications with respect to differentiation of viable from nonviable myocardium. The following categorization of types of reversibility assumes that adequate time has been allowed for the ultimate redistribution pattern to be established. In *reversible defects,* the net myocardial washout rate of ^{201}Tl is slower in the defect region compared with that of normal areas, leading to equalization of the concentration of ^{201}Tl in normal and abnormal regions. This pattern indicates the presence of viable myocardium. In *partially reversible defects,* the concentrations of ^{201}Tl in the normal and defect regions become closer to each another during the redistribution phase but do not equalize. This pattern is believed to occur in myocardial regions that contain a mixture of nonviable and viable but ischemic myocardium. However, the redistribution process may be incomplete under such

Supported in part by a grant 1RO1-HL41628 from the National Institutes of Health, Bethesda, Maryland.

circumstances, with absence of nonviable myocardium. In *nonreversible defects,* the initial ratio of ^{201}Tl concentration between the abnormal and the normal regions is maintained over time because of similar net clearance rates for ^{201}Tl in the normal and abnormal zones. Nonreversible defects generally imply myocardial scar but may also be seen in myocardial regions with viable tissue. In defects that show *reverse redistribution,* the ratio of ^{201}Tl concentration between the defect and the normal region decreases over time because of faster than normal ^{201}Tl washout from the defect zone.[26] This pattern has been observed in the setting of nontransmural myocardial infarction, associated with a patent infarct-related coronary artery, and may result from higher than normal blood flow to the residual viable myocardium in the partially infarcted zone.[27]

Technetium-99m Labeled Agents

The imaging characteristics of ^{201}Tl are generally not considered to be optimal because its photon energy (68 to 80 keV) is not well suited to standard gamma cameras (which perform best at the 140-keV photon peak of ^{99m}Tc) and its 73-hour half-life limits the injected dose to 111 to 148 MBq (3 to 4 mCi), resulting in relatively low-count density of the images. This situation has encouraged the development and clinical testing of several ^{99m}Tc-labeled myocardial perfusion tracers. Two such agents, ^{99m}Tc-sestamibi and ^{99m}Tc-teboroxime, have been approved for clinical use.

Technetium-99m Sestamibi

Technetium-99m methoxyisobutyl isonitrile (^{99m}Tc-sestamibi) is a member of the ^{99m}Tc-isonitrile family that exhibited better biologic properties for clinical application[28–32] than other compounds in this family. ^{99m}Tc-sestamibi, like ^{201}Tl, is a positively charged particle, but its transport across the cell membrane is not dependent on ATP because of its high lipophilicity. Once inside the cells, it is predominantly (84 percent) bound irreversibly to cytosol proteins. The initial myocardial uptake of ^{99m}Tc-sestamibi is directly related to myocardial blood flow over a wide range of flow rates, with a roll-off in uptake occurring at high flow rates, similar to that observed with ^{201}Tl.[33–36] The peak extraction fraction of ^{99m}Tc-sestamibi is lower than that of ^{201}Tl,[34, 35] but myocardial retention is greater. ^{99m}Tc-sestamibi does not redistribute significantly,[35, 37] necessitating separate injections of the agent during exercise and at rest to assess reversibility of myocardial perfusion defects. Because of the short half-life (6 hours) of ^{99m}Tc and the prompt hepatobiliary and renal excretion of ^{99m}Tc, up to 1110 MBq (30 mCi) can be given as a single dose while keeping the similar radiation to the target organ (small intestine) at less than 50 mGy. The higher administration dose of ^{99m}Tc-sestamibi compared to that of ^{201}Tl results in a far greater count rate, allowing high-count density images to be recorded. The higher photon flux allows electrocardiographic gating of planar or tomographic images and the performance of first-pass studies.[38–41]

Because ^{99m}Tc-sestamibi does not significantly redistribute, two separate injections, one during stress and one at rest, are required. These two studies should be performed so that myocardial activity adequately decays from the first image, to minimize interference of the first with the second image. One protocol is to perform the rest and stress studies on two separate days. With this protocol, 814 to 1110 MBq (22 to 30 mCi) of ^{99m}Tc-sestamibi is injected, and imaging begins approximately 15 to 30 minutes after exercise and about 45 to 60 minutes after resting injection. Exercise and rest studies may be completed on the same day by injecting a lower dose of ^{99m}Tc-sestamibi (296 MBq or 8 mCi) during the first study, followed in a few hours by a higher dose (814 MBq or 22 mCi) injection during the second study. The time interval between injection and imaging is the same as in the 2-day protocol. This protocol was first introduced by Taillefer and co-workers,[42–44] who showed that using *rest-stress imaging sequence* and planar imaging ^{99m}Tc-sestamibi results had excellent agreement with the results of two separate-day ^{99m}Tc-sestamibi protocols as well as stress-redistribution ^{201}Tl studies for detecting perfusion defects and identifying their pattern of reversibility.[42] The rest-stress protocol appears more suitable than the stress-rest protocol for assessment of defect reversibility, because with the *stress-rest imaging sequence,* the residual activity of the stress injection causes an uneven background for the rest study, resulting in an underestimation of defect reversibility. Another drawback of the stress-rest protocol is that the quality of the exercise study, which is the most critical study, is reduced by injecting a lower dose and that gated imaging is suboptimal because of low count rate. An alternative rapid same-day protocol is *dual isotope imaging* with rest ^{201}Tl and stress ^{99m}Tc-sestamibi acquired separately, taking advantage of the different energies of these two single-photon agents.[45]

Technetium-99m Teboroxime

Technetium-99m teboroxime is another ^{99m}Tc-labeled myocardial perfusion agent that is approved by the FDA for clinical use.[46] It belongs to a class of neutral lipophilic complexes known as boronic acid adducts of technetium dioxime. In an isolated blood-perfused rabbit heart model, Leppo and Meerdink[47] showed that at a wide range of coronary flow rates (0.3 to 2.4), mean teboroxime extraction was higher than that of ^{201}Tl. The mean capillary flux for teboroxime was also higher than that for ^{201}Tl. In an experimental cell culture model, Maublant and associates[48] showed that ^{99m}Tc-teboroxime has the fastest uptake and greatest myocardial cell accumulation compared to those of both ^{201}Tl and ^{99m}Tc-sestamibi. They also showed that, in general, teboroxime is the least and ^{201}Tl is the most sensitive to metabolic inhibition at the cellular level. In open-chest dogs, Stewart and co-workers[49] demonstrated relatively high extraction of teboroxime after intracoronary injection and that myocardial washout of teboroxime appeared to be flow related and quite rapid. Studies in humans have shown that myocardial uptake of teboroxime is rapid, so myocardium is very well visualized within 2 minutes after injection.[50] Myocardial clearance of the agent is also rapid and biexponential. The effective half-life of the fast washout component is 5.2 minutes (representing two thirds of the original activity), and that of the slow component is 3.8 hours. These properties necessitate the completion of imaging within 10 to 15 minutes from the time of injection because almost one half of the myocardial clearance occurs during this time. To perform SPECT imaging with teboroxime, it is necessary for imaging to start 2 minutes after injection and be completed in about 13 minutes. Shortening of the time interval between injection and initiation of imaging may be facilitated by pharmacologic stress testing (with dipyridamole or adenosine). Shortening of SPECT acquisition could be achieved with continuous acquisition or three-headed cameras. In phase I and II clinical trials, teboroxime has been shown to be safe.[51]

METHODS OF STRESS TESTING

Treadmill Exercise

Treadmill exercise is by far the most common mode of stress testing used in conjunction with myocardial perfusion imaging. Even with the presence of moderate to severe (up to 80 percent) stenosis of an epicardial coronary artery, resting myocardial blood flow is maintained at the baseline level because of compensatory arteriolar coronary vasodilation. Therefore, in most patients with CAD, myocardial blood flow at rest is homogeneous; that is, it is equal in myocardial regions subtended by both normal and diseased coronary arteries. During exercise, myocardial oxygen demand increases because of increases in heart rate, myocardial contractility, and systemic blood pressure. This results in a 3- to 5-times increase in myocardial blood flow through vasodilation of normal coronary arteries. Blood flow through diseased coronary arteries, however, does not increase as much in response to exercise because vasodilatory reserve of stenosed coronary arteries is already exhausted. Thus, during exercise, myocardial blood flow becomes inhomogeneous, with relatively less flow to myocardial regions subtended by diseased coronary arteries. This results in the appearance of a relative perfusion defect when the myocardial perfusion tracer is injected during exercise. Detection of CAD and evaluation of the extent and severity of ischemia are enhanced when disparity in regional coronary flow between normal and diseased arteries is large. Because myocardial hyperemia is related to exercise heart rate, disparity in flow is accentuated when patients with CAD achieve a maximal heart rate response during exercise.[52] Therefore, it is recommended that patients not be under the influence of β-blocker and calcium-channel blocker medications when exercise myocardial perfusion imaging is being performed to evaluate the presence and extent of underlying CAD. The Bruce Protocol[53] is most commonly used for maximal stress testing, but low-level exercise, using protocols such as the Naughton Protocol,[54] may be employed in patients soon after myocardial infarction. Exercise at peak level is continued for about 60 seconds after injection of the myocardial perfusion tracer, so that maximal myocardial blood flow is maintained during the period of major myocardial uptake of the tracer. Assessment of ventricular function by first-pass imaging with ^{99m}Tc-labeled agents has traditionally required bicycle exercise to ensure lack of patient motion with respect to the collimator at peak exercise when images are acquired. With the use of a special algorithm for motion correction, first-pass ventricular function studies may be acquired during peak treadmill exercise.[55]

Pharmacologic Stress Testing

A significant proportion of patients are unable to exercise because of peripheral vascular, musculoskeletal, or neurologic diseases, or they cannot achieve an adequate exercise heart rate because of lack of motivation or poor physical condition or because they are taking β-blocker or calcium channel–blocking medications. In these patients, pharmacologic stress testing may be used effectively as a substitute for exercise in conjunction with myocardial perfusion imaging. Two of the three commonly used pharmacologic stress-testing agents, dipyridamole and adenosine, are coronary vasodilators that can increase myocardial blood flow 3 to 5 times the resting level in myocardial regions that are supplied by normal coronary arteries.[9, 56–58] Adenosine is a direct coronary vasodilator and activates the adenosine (A_2) receptors in the coronary arterial wall. This activation leads to an increase in adenosine cyclase and cyclic 3′, 5′-adenosine monophosphate levels, decreased transmembrane calcium uptake, and, ultimately, coronary vasodilation. Dipyridamole exerts its effect by raising endogenous adenosine blood levels through blocking of cell membrane transport and reuptake of endogenous adenosine. In myocardial regions that are supplied by diseased coronary arteries, the hyperemic response to these agents is attenuated. Not infrequently, after administration of coronary vasodilators, myocardial perfusion may actually decrease below the resting level in regions supplied by diseased coronary arteries, the result of a true "coronary steal."[59–65] Therefore, in patients with coronary artery disease, infusion of dipyridamole or adenosine induces a disparity in regional myocardial perfusion similar to that achieved with exercise testing. Because xanthines directly block the action of dipyridamole and adenosine, prior to pharmacologic vasodilation testing patients should avoid caffeine (coffee, tea, some soft drinks, and medications) for 24 hours and stop all xanthine-containing medications (e.g., aminophylline) for at least 36 hours. Contraindications to coronary vasodilator infusion include unstable angina, acute phase of myocardial infarction, critical aortic stenosis, and hypertrophic cardiomyopathy. Furthermore, these agents are contraindicated in patients with hypotension (systolic blood pressure < 90 mm Hg) because they lower systolic and diastolic blood pressures. Coronary vasodilators are also contraindicated in patients with asthma because they may exacerbate bronchospasm. Unlike exercise testing, however, coronary vasodilators can be used in patients with a high resting blood pressure. The third pharmacologic stress agent, dobutamine, is predominantly a β_1-agonist that increases heart rate, myocardial contractility, and systolic blood pressure. To meet the increased myocardial oxygen demand, normal coronary arteries dilate, whereas stenotic arteries do not dilate at all or dilate insufficiently. Thus, the coronary vasodilatory effect of dobutamine is similar to that of physiologic exercise and is unlike that of dipyridamole and adenosine, which are direct coronary vasodilators. In the study of Hays and co-workers,[66] dobutamine infusion increased heart rate and systolic blood pressure, while diastolic blood pressure decreased because of peripheral (β_2) vasodilator effect. Krivokapich and associates[67] showed that the increase in blood flow is significantly related to heart rate and suggested that increase in coronary flow seen with dobutamine is due to increased oxygen demand.

Pharmacologic Stress Testing With Dipyridamole

Dipyridamole is infused intravenously in a dose of 0.56 to 0.84 mg/kg over a 4-minute period. Three minutes after termination of infusion, at the time of maximal hyperemic effect,[9, 56, 57] ^{201}Tl is injected intravenously (Fig. 63–1A). Should severe ischemia develop, as evidenced by ST-segment depression or angina pectoris, the effects of dipyridamole may be reversed quickly, usually within 45 seconds, by intravenous administration of aminophylline (50 to 100 mg). Whenever possible, administration of aminophylline should be delayed until at least 1 minute after injection of the ^{201}Tl so that myocardial hyperemia is not abolished before substantial ^{201}Tl uptake by the myocardium has occurred. Several variations in this protocol have been proposed, including, the use of handgrip exercise (2 minutes after termination of dipyridamole infusion for a period of 3 to 4 minutes), the routine administration of aminophylline 1 to 2 minutes after ^{201}Tl injection, and low-level treadmill testing before ^{201}Tl injection, but the effect on the overall efficacy of dipyridamole ^{201}Tl scintigraphy for diagnosis of coronary disease is uncertain.

The side effects of dipyridamole infusion may be categorized into three groups.[68, 69] The first group of side effects is related to systemic vasodilation: dizziness, headache, hypotension, and flushing. The second group of side effects is related to the development of myocardial ischemia in the form of angina pectoris or ST-segment depression, or both. The third category of side effects relates to gastrointestinal effects in the form of nausea and an "uneasy feeling" in the abdomen. The combined major adverse

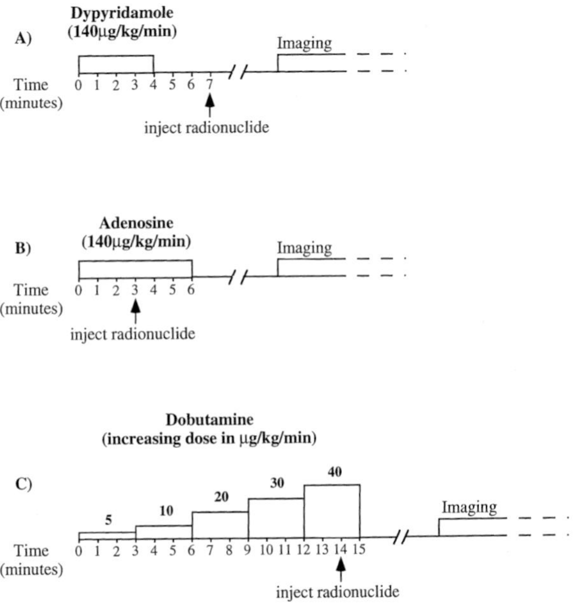

FIGURE 63–1. Protocols for pharmacologic stress testing with dipyridamole *(A)*, adenosine *(B)*, and dobutamine *(C)*.

events among 73,806 patients who were evaluated with dipyridamole ^{201}Tl testing[69] included cardiac death (0.95 per 10,000), nonfatal myocardial infarction (1.76 per 10,000), nonfatal sustained ventricular arrhythmias (0.81 per 10,000), transient cerebral ischemic attacks (1.22 per 10,000), and severe bronchospasms (1.22 per 10,000). It is generally believed that the risk of serious events is similar to that seen with exercise. Such risks may be diminished by careful screening of patients who are referred for dipyridamole stress testing and by proper attention to the aforementioned contraindications of dipyridamole testing. Physician monitoring of patients undergoing dipyridamole studies is clearly as important as it is in the case of exercise studies. Additionally, because the effects of dipyridamole can last longer than those of aminophylline, any patient requiring aminophylline to reverse side effects of dipyridamole should have physician monitoring for approximately 20 to 30 minutes after administration of aminophylline.

Pharmacologic Stress Testing With Adenosine

Adenosine is infused at the rate of 140 μg/kg per minute for 6 minutes. Adenosine has a very short half-life (several seconds) and reaches its peak effect within 1 to 2 minutes after start of infusion.[70, 71] The myocardial perfusion imaging agent is injected after 3 minutes of infusion (see Fig. 63–1*B*). After termination of infusion, the effects generally dissipate within 1 to 2 minutes (disappearance half-life of 37 seconds). Because of the short duration of effects after termination of infusion, aminophylline is rarely needed to terminate the side effects. Another advantage of the short half-life of adenosine is the feasibility of increasing or decreasing the dose, when necessary. The safety of adenosine pharmacologic stress testing has been evaluated in 5552 patients in the Phase III Multicenter Trial[72] and was recently updated in 9256 patients.[73] In general the side effects of adenosine are similar to those of dipyridamole but are more frequent. In addition, adenosine slows atrioventricular conduction, and different types of heart block may result from its infusion, such as first-degree (2.7 percent), second-degree (4 percent), or third-degree (0.7 percent) block.[73]

Pharmacologic Stress Testing With Dobutamine

Candidates for pharmacologic stress testing with dobutamine are patients who cannot undergo stress testing with dipyridamole or adenosine because of a history of asthma. The protocol for dobutamine infusion is shown in Figure 63–1*C*. Infusion begins with 5 μg/kg per minute for 3 minutes and is then increased to 10 μg/kg per minute for another 3 minutes and is increased every 3 minutes by 10 μg/kg per minute until a maximum of 40 μg/kg per minute is achieved. Myocardial perfusion tracer is injected 1 minute after the maximal tolerable dose, and infusion is continued for at least 1 or, preferably, 2 minutes after injection.

The most common adverse effects of dobutamine infusion are palpitations and chest pain. Less common adverse effects are headache, flushing, and dyspnea. The majority of these adverse effects are transient and last only a few minutes after cessation of infusion because of the 2-minute biologic half-life of dobutamine. More serious adverse effects of dobutamine infusion are the development of premature ventricular depolarizations and, occasionally, ventricular tachycardia (which is usually not sustained) or atrial fibrillation.[66] Therefore, patients with underlying cardiac arrhythmias must be observed closely for development of these side effects. The adverse effects of dobutamine may be neutralized by esmolol, which is a rapidly acting β-blocker.

IMAGING PROTOCOLS

Planar Imaging

Planar imaging has been widely used for the detection and evaluation of CAD. For planar imaging, a standard or a large field-of-view camera, equipped with 1/4- or 3/8-inch sodium iodide crystal thickness, is used. A medium-resolution (all-purpose) or a high-resolution, parallel-hole collimator is generally employed. The recommended energy windows are 20 percent, centered on the 69- to 83-KeV peak, and 10 percent, centered on the 167-KeV peak. Patients are imaged in three orientations: anterior, "best septal" left anterior oblique (LAO), and steep LAO or left lateral views. For the first two views, the patient lies supine on the imaging table, but for the steep LAO or left lateral view, the patient is positioned in the lateral decubitus position with the left side of the chest against the collimator. Imaging is begun 6 minutes after injection of ^{201}Tl and each image is acquired for a preset time of 10 minutes per view. The recommended acquisition matrix for planar imaging is 128 × 128 × 8 bits.

Single-Photon Emission Computed Tomography Imaging

Single-photon emission computed tomography allows separation of overlapping myocardial regions and provides a higher contrast resolution and, thus, overcomes the limitations of planar imaging. Since its introduction, SPECT imaging has been extensively evaluated for optimal image acquisition and processing. As with planar ^{201}Tl imaging, the SPECT technique is generally used in conjunction with stress. The patient is injected with 111 to 148 MBq (3 to 4 mCi) of ^{201}Tl at least 1 minute prior to termination of exercise or pharmacologic stress. For imaging, a large field-of-view camera specially designed to rotate around the patient is used. The most common protocol includes the use of an all-purpose, parallel-hole collimator and a 64 × 64 16 bit matrix. The patient lies on the imaging table in a supine position, and images are obtained over a semicircular 180-degree arc, extending from the 45-degree right anterior oblique to the 45-degree left posterior oblique (LPO) position, imaging 32 or 64 projections, each for 40 or 20 seconds, respectively. Single-photon emission computed tomography imaging in the prone position may be used to reduce the inferoseptal attenuation artifact.[74] Prone imaging, however, causes anterior wall attenuation artifact and is associated with reduced overall image count density because of photon attenuation by the imaging table. To diminish the frequency of the (upward creep) artifact, SPECT imaging does not begin until at least 10 minutes after injection of ^{201}Tl.[75] During this 10-minute waiting period, a single 5-minute anterior view planar image may be acquired to assess lung uptake of ^{201}Tl, transient ischemic dilation of the left ventricle, and the breast attenuation artifact. Because of the length of acquisition and the nature of the equipment, SPECT imaging is technically very demanding and requires more attention to quality control than does planar imaging. Important steps in quality control for SPECT acquisition are correction for nonuniformity and determination of the mechanical center of rotation. Because patient motion during SPECT imaging is a frequent cause of image artifacts, patients should be instructed to lie still during the entire acquisition, and projection images should be displayed at the end of acquisition in a cine-loop format to evaluate occurrence of patient motion.

IMAGE PROCESSING AND QUANTITATION

Thallium-201

Several methods have been developed and successfully applied clinically for objective, quantitative analysis of the initial myocardial count distribution and washout rate of ^{201}Tl on planar[14, 15, 76–84] and SPECT images.[52, 85–88] These quantitative approaches to ^{201}Tl image analysis have provided several advantages over qualitative (visual) analysis of images by (1) reducing interobserver and intraobserver variability; (2) aiding recognition of normal variant patterns, because image results are compared to a normal database; (3) providing a better estimate of the size and severity of perfusion defects;

and (4) assessing defect reversibility more accurately. It is important to note, however, that the results of quantitative analysis should be viewed as a "second expert opinion" and do not replace physician interpretation of the images.

Planar Imaging

There are several approaches to the quantitation of the initial myocardial distribution and washout of ^{201}Tl, but in general there are several steps involved. First, for each image, compensation for tissue cross-talk is achieved by performing *background subtraction*. The most commonly used method is bilinear interpolative background subtraction, described by Goris and co-workers[83] and modified by Watson and associates.[78] After background subtraction, image *smoothing* is done with the use of a standard algorithm for 9-point weighted averaging. Several methods may be employed for *myocardial sampling*,[15, 76–82, 84] but the most commonly used one is the circumferential count profile method.[14, 77, 81, 82, 84] With this method, the center of the left ventricle is assigned visually, and from this center 60 radii, spaced by 6 degrees, are generated toward the myocardium. Along each radius, the maximal count per pixel is automatically determined by the computer and is normalized to the maximal value observed in that view. The profile is then constructed by the computer from the values of the 60 samples, which are plotted clockwise. The redistribution images are processed with the use of the same approach. The *circumferential profiles* are then aligned by visually identifying the location of the scintigraphic apex on the stress and redistribution profiles. These profiles are subsequently plotted for both exercise and redistribution studies. The redistribution profiles are normalized to the maximal pixel value found on the stress images. In addition to initial and 4-hour redistribution profiles, percent washout circumferential profiles are calculated as a percent washout from the initial to the 4-hour redistribution time. The results thus obtained are then compared with results generated from a *normal database*.[14, 80, 81] The computer is programmed to identify any points of the profile that fall below normal limits.

Single-Photon Emission Computed Tomography

Single-photon emission computed tomography image processing involves several steps. Each of the projections is first corrected for nonuniformity with a 30-million count flood collected with the use of a cobalt-57 source. The mechanical center of rotation is determined from the projection data to align detector data with respect to the reconstruction matrix. Raw data are smoothed with a 9-point weighted averaging system. The filtered backprojection technique is used to reconstruct images. A Butterworth filter with a cutoff frequency of 0.2 cycles per pixel and order 5, which has the highest efficiency, is used for filtering of the images, prior to reconstruction.[86] However, with different camera-computer systems, different filters may be optimal. Images are reoriented into planes that are perpendicular to the long axis (short axis) and parallel to the long axis of the left ventricle (vertical and horizontal long axes). In all three planes, each tomographic slice is 1 pixel thick, representing thickness of approximately 6.2 mm. Several methods have been developed and are available for quantitation of relative myocardial count distribution on SPECT images.[52, 85–88] The technique described by Maddahi and associates[86] is briefly presented here to outline the various steps involved in quantitation and display of ^{201}Tl SPECT images. In contrast to planar image quantitation, assessment of myocardial percent washout of ^{201}Tl with the SPECT technique does not contribute to detection of disease in individual coronary arteries and is therefore not quantitated. Detection and localization of coronary disease by SPECT imaging relies on quantitative analysis of exercise images for the presence and location of perfusion defects. Myocardial ^{201}Tl activity of the apex is analyzed from the apical portion of the vertical long-axis slices, and the myocardial activity of the remaining portions of the left ventricle is analyzed from the short-axis slices. The choice of vertical long-axis slices for analysis of the apex is made, because the apex is subject to partial volume effect on the short-axis slices. For myocardial sampling, the center of the left ventricle and the radius of search on each slice are defined by the operator, and 60 equidistant radii (6 degrees apart) are then automatically generated. Along each radius, the computer searches and selects the maximal count value. The values are then normalized to the highest value found in each slice and are plotted for each angular location on the myocardial periphery, generating a circumferential count profile. For proper comparison of stress and redistribution images with the normal profiles and with one another, an anatomical landmark is defined at the inferior junction of the right and left ventricles on the short-axis cuts, to which the 102-degree angle is assigned. On the vertical long-axis cuts, the most apical point is used for alignment, and the 90-degree angle is assigned to it. As with planar imaging, development of a normal reference database is essential for objective analysis of results in patients. In males, normal myocardial count distribution on SPECT images is different from that in females, because of gender-related differences in soft-tissue attenuation patterns. Thus, for each gender, a different set of normal values is used. To develop normal reference circumferential profiles, mean circumferential profiles are generated for five left ventricular anatomical regions from pooled data of patients who had a low pre-^{201}Tl SPECT likelihood of CAD. From these mean normal circumferential profiles, lower limits of normal have been derived.

The most common format for display of myocardial counts with SPECT imaging is the "polar-map" or "bull's-eye" approach, in which the left ventricular myocardium is represented two-dimensionally, with the center of display corresponding to the apex and the periphery corresponding to the atrioventricular junction. Different portions of the left ventricular myocardium represent territories of various coronary arteries and their major branches. In a patient with a proximal left anterior descending (LAD) coronary stenosis, defects are noted in the anterior wall, the apex, the anteroseptal wall, and the anterolateral region (Fig. 63–2). In a patient with a distal LAD stenosis, the anteroseptal and anterolateral regions, representing the septal perforator and diagonal branch territories, are not involved, and the defect is limited to the distal anterior wall and apex (Fig. 63–3). In patients with disease in the diagonal branch of the LAD, perfusion defects are limited to the proximal and middle anterior-anterolateral left ventricular regions (Fig. 63–4). The territory of a nondominant left circumflex (LCX) coronary artery is represented by the proximal, middle, and distal anterolateral and inferolateral left ventricular regions (Fig. 63–5). The territory of a dominant LCX coronary artery includes the inferior and inferoseptal regions of the left ventricular myocardium, in addition to the territory of a nondominant LCX territory (Fig. 63–6). In a patient with disease in a dominant right coronary artery (RCA), the inferior and inferoseptal regions of the left ventricular myocardium are involved (Fig. 63–7).

FIGURE 63–2. See Color Plate 28.

Technetium-99m Sestamibi

Because the physical characteristics of ^{99m}Tc-sestamibi are different from those of ^{201}Tl, acquisition and processing parameters for ^{99m}Tc-sestamibi need to be specifically tailored to its physical and biologic characteristics. Comprehensive studies have addressed optimization of parameters, such as the type of collimator, acquisition matrix size, energy window setting, imaging time, and filtering. These studies have led to the development of a separate set of recommendations for planar and SPECT studies.[89, 90] As with ^{201}Tl, quantitative analysis is an important adjunct to the interpretation of ^{99m}Tc-sestamibi myocardial perfusion images, for the purpose of diagnosing and localizing coronary artery disease as well as the assessment of perfusion defect extent.

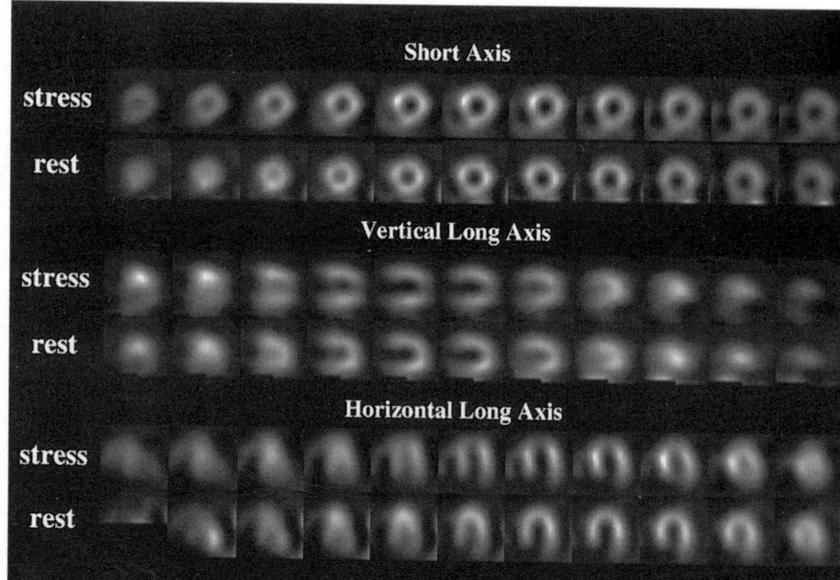

FIGURE 63–3. An example of a stress-rest myocardial perfusion SPECT study in a patient with 90 percent distal LAD stenosis. A reversible apical defect is noted on the vertical and horizontal long-axis slices.

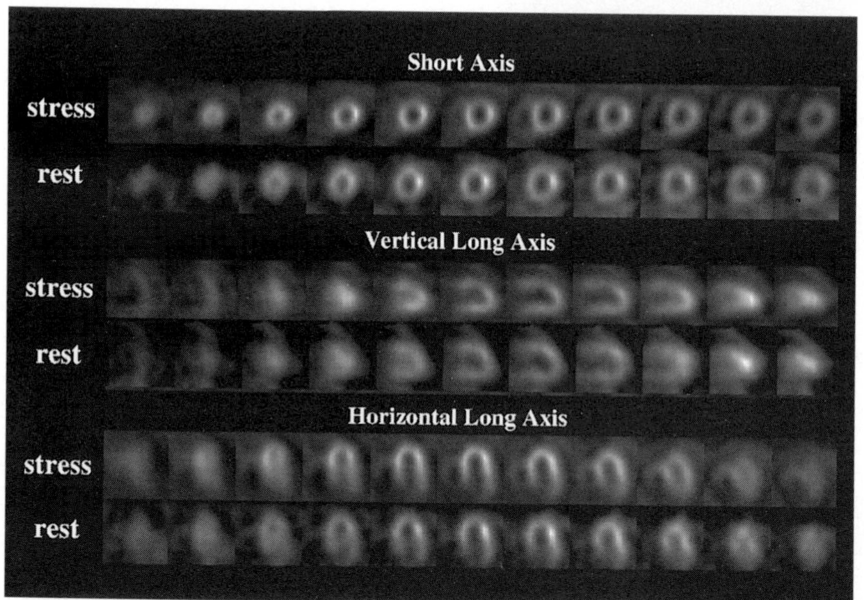

FIGURE 63–4. A stress-rest myocardial perfusion SPECT study in a patient with 80 percent proximal disease in the diagonal branch of the LAD. A reversible proximal and midanterior wall defect is present.

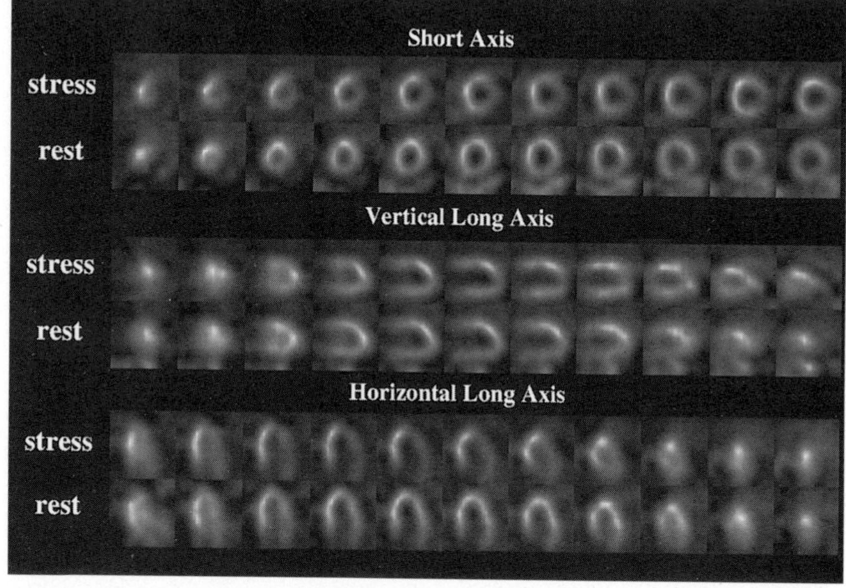

FIGURE 63–5. A stress-rest myocardial perfusion SPECT study in a patient with 85 percent proximal stenosis in a nondominant LCX coronary artery. A reversible lateral wall defect is noted.

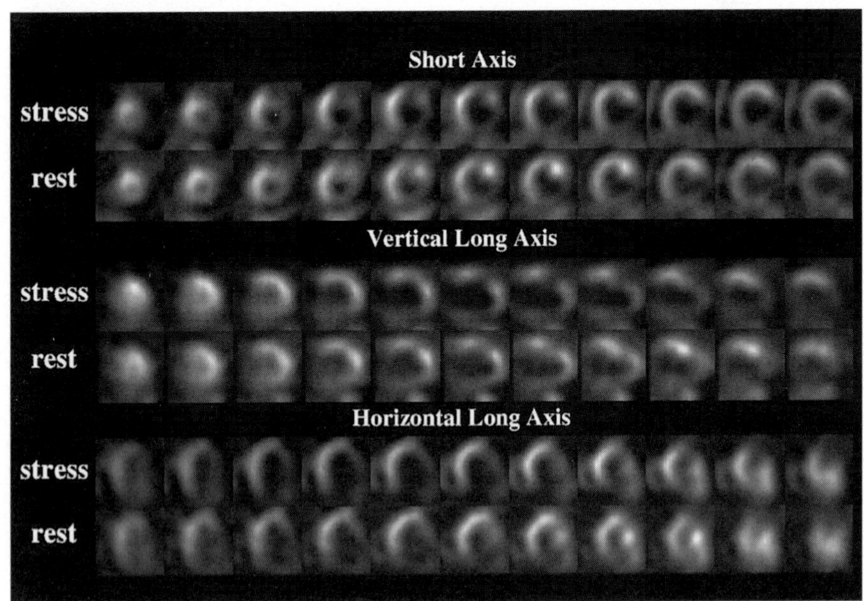

FIGURE 63–6. A stress-rest myocardial perfusion SPECT study in a patient with a severe disease in a proximal dominant LCX coronary artery. A nonreversible inferolateral and inferior wall defect is present.

Separate-Day Protocol Single-Photon Emission Computed Tomography

Several computerized algorithms are now available for objective analysis of separate-day protocol ^{99m}Tc-sestamibi SPECT images. A method that was reported by Kiat and colleagues[91] is based on an approach similar to that used for quantitation of ^{201}Tl SPECT studies, which incorporates a gender-specific ^{99m}Tc-sestamibi normal database. Another different technique for quantitation of ^{99m}Tc-sestamibi SPECT images has been reported by Kahn and colleagues,[92] with a similar diagnostic accuracy.

Same-Day Protocol Single-Photon Emission Computed Tomography

Since acquisition and processing parameters for the same-day ^{99m}Tc-sestamibi SPECT protocol are different from those of the separate-day protocol, new gender-specific quantitative normal databases are required for proper quantitative analysis of same-day rest-stress ^{99m}Tc-sestamibi SPECT images. Recently, a new, refined quantitative method for analysis of same-day ^{99m}Tc-sestamibi SPECT has been developed and validated.[93, 94] With this new method, maximal-count circumferential profiles are generated for all short-axis tomograms, including the base. A hybrid search algorithm is used to extract the three-dimensional tracer distribution by sampling perpendicular to the myocardial wall. The apical slices are sampled in a spherical manner, while the remainder of the myocardium is sampled with the use of a cylindrical search (Fig. 63–8).[90, 93] Maximal-count circumferential profiles are automatically generated from all short-axis slices with this two-part sampling scheme. The stress and rest profiles were normalized to the most normal wall of the entire patient's stress study prior to comparison to the normal limits. Several quantitative polar maps are then created from the profile data (see Fig. 63–8). Separate polar maps are generated for the rest and stress myocardial perfusion distributions and for the severity and reversibility of defects. Defect-extent polar maps for rest and stress are generated after the patients' profiles have been compared to gender-matched normal limits. For localization of CAD, the polar maps are divided into three territories (LAD, LCX, and RCA), according to the approach previously described for ^{201}Tl. In each of the three coronary vascular territories, the total percentage of circumferential profile points that fall below the normal limits is determined. Various criteria for perfu-

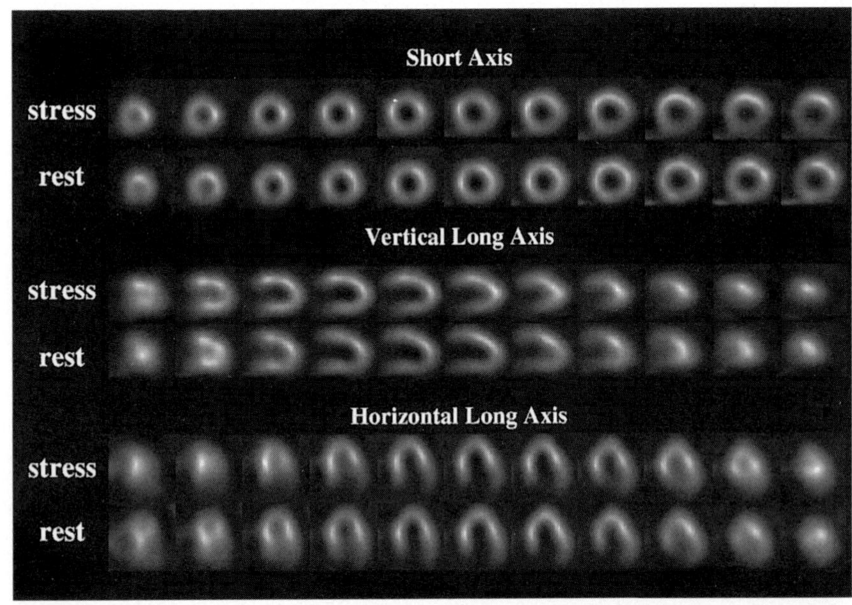

FIGURE 63–7. A stress-rest myocardial perfusion SPECT study in a patient with 75 percent stenosis in a proximal dominant RCA. A reversible proximal inferior wall defect is noted.

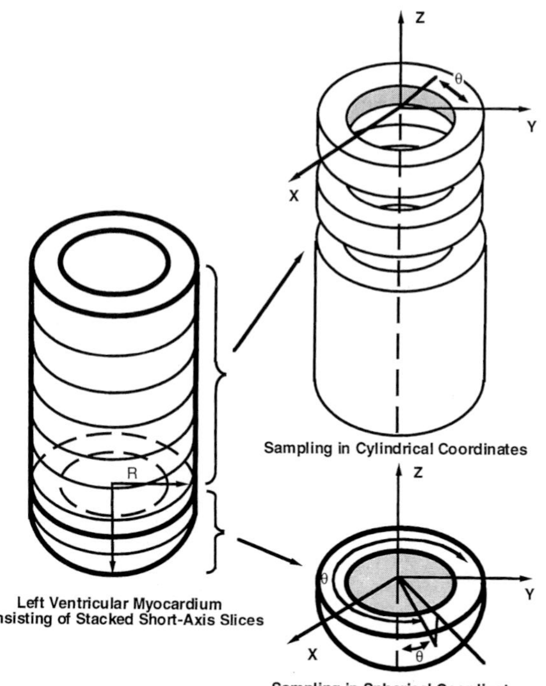

FIGURE 63–8. Method for quantitative analysis of ^{99m}Tc-sestamibi SPECT myocardial perfusion images. (From Garcia, E., Cook, C., Van Train, K., et al.: Technical aspects of myocardial SPECT imaging with technetium-99m sestamibi. Am. J. Cardiol. 66:23E, 1990, with permission.)

sion abnormality have been determined, based on the optimal true-positive versus false-positive tradeoff for identifying disease in each of the three coronary arteries, using receiver-operating characteristic curve analysis.

DIAGNOSTIC ACCURACY OF MYOCARDIAL PERFUSION IMAGING

As with other tests applied for the detection of CAD, the diagnostic accuracy of myocardial perfusion imaging is expressed by sensitivity and specificity. These indices depend on several technical factors, such as the imaging agent, planar versus tomographic imaging, qualitative (visual) versus quantitative analysis, and exercise versus pharmacologic stress testing. In addition, several characteristics of the patient population under study may affect sensitivity and specificity, such as presence or absence of myocardial infarction, threshold for defining significant CAD, referral bias, level of exercise, and the severity (percentage stenosis) and extent (number of diseased vessels) of CAD in the referred population.

Thallium-201 Imaging

Qualitative Analysis of Thallium-201 Images

By far, most of the literature available to date deals with the use of exercise redistribution ^{201}Tl imaging by planar acquisition and qualitative analysis. The combined reported sensitivity and specificity are shown in Table 63–1. The overall sensitivity and specificity of this technique in a total of 4678 patients reported in the literature[10, 14, 84, 95–139] are 82 and 88 percent, respectively. Differing reports from center to center are most likely the result of characteristics of the patient population under study. In an analysis of factors affecting sensitivity and specificity of exercise ^{201}Tl testing in 56 published reports, Detrano and colleagues[140] demonstrated that in patients without myocardial infarction, the sensitivity was 79 percent, lower than that of patients with prior myocardial infarction, which was 96 percent. The sensitivity of exercise ^{201}Tl testing is also affected by the threshold of percentage narrowing that is used for definition of angiographic disease, by how severe the stenoses are in a given population, and by the number of diseased coronary arteries. The effect of the latter can be derived from 11 published reports that specified the effect of extent of disease on test sensitiv-

TABLE 63–1. INDIVIDUAL AND COMBINED REPORTED SENSITIVITY AND SPECIFICITY OF EXERCISE-REDISTRIBUTION PLANAR THALLIUM-201 SCINTIGRAPHY BY QUALITATIVE ANALYSIS FOR DETECTION OF CORONARY ARTERY DISEASE

Year	Lead Author	Sensitivity No. of Patients	(%)	Specificity No. of Patients	(%)
1977	Ritchie[100]	58/76	(76)	23/25	(92)
	Bailey[101]	47/63	(75)	20/20	(100)
	Rosenblatt[102]	14/15	(93)	5/7	(71)
	Lenaers[95]	52/55	(95)	14/15	(93)
1978	Botvinick[103]	35/41	(85)	22/24	(92)
	Verani[104]	38/48	(79)	33/34	(97)
	Ritchie[105]	115/148	(78)	37/42	(88)
	Turner[106]	23/34	(68)	29/30	(97)
	Blood[107]	55/62	(89)	20/25	(80)
	Carillo[108]	34/39	(87)	16/16	(100)
	Hamilton[109]	82/107	(77)	28/30	(93)
1979	Vogel[84]	31/42	(74)	22/23	(96)
	Massie[96]	57/64	(89)	15/15	(100)
	McKillop[98]	43/47	(91)	31/34	(91)
	McCarthy[110]	81/95	(85)	26/33	(79)
	Caralis[111]	9/10	(90)	4/5	(80)
	Silber[112]	71/86	(83)	18/22	(82)
	Dash[97]	66/81	(81)	15/15	(100)
1980	Jengo[113]	39/42	(93)	15/16	(94)
	Rigo[99]	118/133	(89)	21/26	(81)
	Caldwell[114]	35/41	(85)	11/11	(100)
	Boucher[10]	141/162	(87)	44/64	(69)
	Iskandrian[115]	78/98	(80)	92/96	(96)
	Iskandrian[116]	75/91	(82)	28/30	(93)
	Schicha[117]	55/60	(92)	9/10	(90)
1981	Elkayam[118]	54/56	(96)	6/8	(75)
	Uhl[119]	28/41	(68)	142/150	(95)
	Guiney[120]	8/9	(89)	23/26	(88)
	Maddahi[14]	41/45	(91)	8/11	(73)
	Melin[121]	86/99	(87)	54/61	(89)
1982	Patterson[122]	42/50	(84)	26/46	(63)
	Faris[123]	69/87	(79)	20/20	(100)
	Kambara[124]	27/33	(82)	25/26	(96)
	Kambara[124]	56/67	(84)	39/40	(98)
1983	Brown[125]	67/81	(83)	39/58	(67)
	Cinotti[126]	52/69	(75)	24/27	(89)
	O'Keefe[127]	22/28	(79)	19/22	(86)
1984	Chaitman[128]	53/71	(75)	11/12	(92)
	Osbakken[129]	65/86	(76)	23/34	(68)
	Hung[130]	21/28	(75)	58/64	(91)
	Burke[131]	34/43	(79)	7/8	(88)
1985	Melin[132]	31/44	(70)	84/91	(92)
	Canhasi[133]	52/56	(93)	11/17	(65)
	Del Rio-Meraza[134]	50/57	(88)	19/23	(83)
	Hung[135]	94/117	(80)	47/54	(87)
	Rothendler[136]	26/42	(63)	13/18	(72)
	Weiner[137]	45/58	(78)	38/44	(86)
	Amor[138]	93/108	(86)	35/35	(100)
Overall		2568/3115	(82)	1369/1563	(88)

Modified from Maddahi, J., Rodrigues, E., Berman, D.S.: Assessment of myocardial perfusion by single-photon agents. *In* Pohost, G., and O'Rourke, R. (eds.): Principles and Practice of Cardiovascular Imaging. Boston, Little, Brown, & Co., copyright 1990; with permission.

TABLE 63–2. SENSITIVITY OF THALLIUM-201 SCINTIGRAPHY: INFLUENCE OF THE EXTENT OF DISEASED VESSELS

		Single Vessel		Double Vessel		Triple Vessel	
Year	Lead Author	*No. of Patients*	*(%)*	*No. of Patients*	*(%)*	*No. of Patients*	*(%)*
Qualitative Planar							
1977	Bailey[101]	20/28	(71)	13/20	(65)	14/15	(93)
	Lenaers[95]	12/13	(92)	16/17	(94)	24/25	(96)
1978	Botvinick[103]	6/8	(75)	16/18	(89)	13/15	(87)
	Verani[104]	11/14	(79)	15/18	(83)	12/16	(75)
1979	Massie[96]	11/15	(73)	13/15	(87)	33/34	(97)
	McKillop[98]	10/11	(91)	22/24	(92)	11/12	(92)
	McCarthy[110]	31/34	(78)	27/30	(90)	23/25	(92)
1980	Rigo[99]	46/56	(82)	33/35	(94)	39/42	(94)
1981	Elkayam[118]	9/10	(90)	17/18	(94)	28/28	(100)
	Uhl[119]	6/6	(100)	18/18	(100)	15/17	(88)
1984	Chaitman[128]	12/20	(60)	17/23	(74)	24/28	(86)
Total		193/247	(78)	244/275	(89)	303/328	(92)
		Single Vessel		**Double Vessel**		**Triple Vessel**	
		No. of Patients	*(%)*	*No. of Patients*	*(%)*	*No. of Patients*	*(%)*
Quantitative SPECT							
1988	DePasquale[87]	85/93	(91)	72/73	(99)	13/13	(100)
1989	Maddahi[86]	15/18	(83)	32/33	(97)	40/41	(98)
	Iskandrian[52]	45/70	(64)	93/107	(87)	86/95	(91)
1990	Van Train[153]	56/64	(88)	69/72	(96)	60/60	(100)
	Mahmarian[88]	119/142	(84)	60/66	(91)	13/13	(100)
1991	Nishimura[156]	26/32	(81)	20/22	(91)	15/16	(94)*
1993	Hacot[157]	28/31	(90)	17/18	(94)	8/8	(100)
Total		374/450	(83)	363/391	(93)	235/246	(96)

*Adenosine stress.

ity.* The mean sensitivity of the planar method increased from 78 percent for single-vessel disease to 89 percent for double-vessel disease and 92 percent for triple-vessel disease (Table 63–2).

Quantitative Analysis of Planar Images

The interobserver variability of qualitative analysis of ^{201}Tl images has been shown to range from 3 to 16 percent, and intraobserver variability from 4 to 11 percent.[96, 141–143] To overcome the subjectivity of interpretation inherent in qualitative visual analysis of ^{201}Tl images, several methods for semiquantitative analysis of planar ^{201}Tl images have been reported. The initial methods involved visual analysis of processed ^{201}Tl images.[123, 144, 145] However, subsequent quantitative techniques used objective criteria for detection of perfusion defects based on comparison of image data with results from a normal database.[14, 79, 82, 146, 147] Although quantitative analysis of ^{201}Tl scintigrams reduces inter- and intraobserver variability, its effect on the overall sensitivity and specificity of ^{201}Tl testing has not been major. This is well demonstrated by the results of reports comparing visual and quantitative analysis in the same patient population.[14] When the effect of quantitation of images on the sensitivity and specificity of ^{201}Tl testing is assessed by comparing mean literature results obtained in two different patient populations, there appears to be a trend toward increased sensitivity and decreased specificity. The mean sensitivity and specificity in the literature for quantitative planar ^{201}Tl imaging[14, 79, 146, 148] in a total of 800 patients are 89 and 68 percent, respectively (Table 63–3). The lower specificity and higher sensitivity, however, are most likely products of other confounding factors encountered in the comparison of results from two different patient populations. More specifically, it is likely that the increased referral bias (described below) encountered in more recent publications, which used quantitative analysis, explains the observed differences. In fact, normalcy rate (described below) has been used to represent nonbiased specificity of tests, and the mean literature[14, 148] normalcy rate for planar ^{201}Tl quantitative analysis has been 88 percent.

*See references 95, 96, 98, 99, 101, 103, 104, 110, 118, 119, and 128.

Effect of Referral Bias on Sensitivity and Specificity

The reported sensitivities and specificities of tests may be heavily distorted by selection bias. This bias results in an apparent increase in sensitivity and an apparent decrease in specificity. Rozanski and co-workers[149] demonstrated that the false-positive rate for radionuclide ventriculography increased substantially from 1978 to 1982. This observation was explained by two phenomena: *pretest selection bias* and *post-test referral bias.* The pretest selection bias was the result of increasing pretest likelihood of CAD in the population referred for testing. In other words, as the years went by and the

TABLE 63–3. SENSITIVITY AND SPECIFICITY OF QUANTITATIVE PLANAR THALLIUM-201 SCINTIGRAPHY

		Sensitivity		Specificity		Normalcy Rate	
Year	Lead Author	*No. of Patients*	*(%)*	*No. of Patients*	*(%)*	*No. of Patients*	*(%)*
1981	Maddahi[14]	42/45	(93)	9/11	(82)	11/11	(100)
1986	Van Train[148]	119/143	(83)	25/54	(46)	61/71	(86)
1986	Kaul[146]	253/281	(90)	34/44	(77)	—	—
1981	Berger[79]	100/110	(91)	27/30	(90)	—	—
Total		514/579	(89)	95/139	(68)	72/82	(88)

TABLE 63–4. SENSITIVITY AND SPECIFICITY OF THALLIUM-201 SINGLE-PHOTON EMISSION COMPUTED TOMOGRAPHY

Year	Lead Author	Sensitivity		Specificity		Normalcy Rate	
		No. of Patients	*(%)*	*No. of Patients*	*(%)*	*No. of Patients*	*(%)*
Qualitative Analysis							
1984	Tamaki[150]	76/82	(93)	20/22	(91)		
1988	DePasquale[87]	173/179	(97)	21/31	(68)		
1989	Fintel[151]	88/96	(92)	—	—		
1990	Mahmarian[88]	193/221	(87)	57/75	(76)		
1992	Quinones[152]	65/86	(76)	21/126	(81)		
Overall		595/664	(90)	110/154	(77)		
Quantitative Analysis							
1984	Tamaki[150]	80/82	(98)	20/22	(91)		
1988	DePasquale[87]	170/179	(95)	23/31	(74)		
	Tamaki[154]	46/48	(96)	3/3	(100)		
1989	Maddahi[86]	88/92	(96)	10/18	(56)	24/28	(86)
	Iskandrian[52]	224/272	(82)	36/58	(62)	123/131	(94)
1990	Van Train[153]	185/196	(94)	20/46	(43)	62/76	(82)
	Mahmarian[88]	192/221	(87)	65/75	(87)		
Overall		995/1090	(91)	177/253	(70)	209/235	(89)

test became established, sicker patients were referred for testing, such as those with left ventricular hypertrophy, multiple risk factors, and positive exercise ECG test. The sicker the population referred for testing, the more abnormalities may appear on the test, even though they do not have the disease in question. The second reason for an apparent increase in the false-positive rate of exercise radionuclide ventriculography in the study of Rozanski and colleagues was the post-test referral bias. In the early years of the technique, specificity of radionuclide ventriculography was determined by calculating the true-negative rate in patients who already had a normal coronary arteriogram and were subsequently referred for radionuclide ventriculography. Later on, however, clinical decisions were increasingly based on the results of radionuclide ventriculography, so that most patients referred for coronary angiography had already undergone radionuclide ventriculography and, in fact, had an abnormal test result to warrant cardiac catheterization. Detrano and colleagues[140] found a significant negative relationship between referral bias and test specificity. In their study, the effect on sensitivity was not significant. They showed that studies that attempted to reduce referral bias by not allowing the result of the exercise ^{201}Tl study to influence the decision to do a coronary angiogram had significantly higher specificities than those of studies that did not (84 versus 78 percent). Therefore, the actual specificity of exercise planar ^{201}Tl imaging may be higher than that reported by many investigators. In an attempt to determine a more representative specificity of ^{201}Tl testing, the authors introduced the use of the "normalcy rate," which is observed in patients with a low likelihood of angiographically significant CAD, based on analysis of age, sex, symptoms, and the results of exercise electrocardiography.[14, 148] This approach provides a proxy for specificity that can be used when the referral bias is operational, and it offers the advantage over healthy normal volunteers of studying a patient population that is closer in demographics to the patient population in question.

Qualitative and Quantitative Single-Photon Emission Computed Tomography Thallium-201 Imaging

Table 63–4 summarizes the results of the SPECT ^{201}Tl imaging technique. For the qualitative analysis, in a total of 818 patients reported,[87, 88, 150–152] the sensitivity and specificity were 90 and 77 percent, respectively. The literature results for the quantitative SPECT method are also shown in Table 63–4. In a total of 1578 patients reported,* the sensitivity, specificity, and normalcy rates have been 91, 70, and 89 percent, respectively. A trend is toward lower specificity noted for the SPECT method with a decrease in specificity from 91 to 43 percent from 1984 to 1990 and a decrease in sensitivity from 98 to 94 percent, during the same period of time. The decline of specificity with time is likely to be due, in part, to an increase in referral bias in the more recent studies. Although the true, unbiased specificity of the SPECT technique has not been determined, it may be implied from the normalcy rate of 89 percent in a total of 235 low-likelihood patients.[52, 86, 153] Therefore, it is likely that the true specificity of the SPECT technique is slightly lower than that of the planar imaging method, which may be due to the fact that SPECT imaging is technically more demanding and has many more sources of artifacts during acquisition and processing. In a total of 983 patients reported in the literature[155] that specified sensitivity with respect to the presence or absence of prior myocardial infarction, the overall sensitivity has been 90 percent, which is higher (99 percent) in the subgroup of 324 patients with prior myocardial infarction and is lower (85 percent) in the subgroup of 659 patients without prior myocardial infarction. In seven SPECT studies that specified the effect of extent of disease on test sensitivity,* the mean sensitivity of the SPECT method increased from 83 percent for single-vessel disease to 93 percent for double-vessel disease and 95 percent for triple-vessel disease (see Table 63–2). Sensitivity of SPECT ^{201}Tl imaging in patient without prior myocardial infarction has also been reported in relation to the extent of disease.[155] In this population of 135 patients, sensitivities for single-, double-, and triple-vessel coronary disease have been 75, 89, and 96 percent, respectively. The sensitivity of SPECT imaging in relation to the degree of underlying coronary narrowing has also been evaluated. In a total of 704 patients reported in the literature,[155] the sensitivity of ^{201}Tl SPECT for detecting moderate coronary stenoses (50 to 70 percent narrowing) has been 63 percent, and for those with severe coronary narrowing (70 to 100 percent) it has been 88 percent. Fintel and colleagues[151] compared the visual diagnostic performance of planar and tomographic imaging methods in 136 patients. In subgroup analysis, they found that ^{201}Tl tomography was superior in males and in patients with milder disease, such as those with no prior myocardial infarction or with single-vessel disease or in patients with 50 to 69 percent coronary stenosis.

Pharmacologic Versus Exercise Stress Testing

The mean literature sensitivity and specificity for dipyridamole ^{201}Tl scintigraphy in 18 published reports in a total of 1272 patients[143, 158–174] were 87 and 81 percent, respectively. These results

*See references 52, 86 to 88, 150, 153, and 154.

*See references 52, 86 to 88, 153, 156, and 157.

are similar to those noted with exercise ^{201}Tl scintigraphy. This observation has been confirmed by analysis of the results of five reports[143, 161–164] in which exercise and dipyridamole ^{201}Tl scintigraphy were compared in the same population totaling 207 patients. Dipyridamole and exercise ^{201}Tl sensitivities were 79 percent, and specificities were 95 and 92 percent, respectively. The overall sensitivity and specificity of dobutamine ^{201}Tl myocardial perfusion imaging for detection of coronary artery disease has been reported by Hays and associates[66] to be 86 and 90 percent, respectively. In the study of Pennell and colleagues,[175] dobutamine ^{201}Tl SPECT imaging in 50 patients had 97 percent sensitivity and 80 percent specificity. Dobutamine sestamibi imaging has been reported by Marwick and Forster to have sensitivities of 80 and 83 percent and specificities of 74 and 89 percent, respectively. Sensitivity of dobutamine perfusion imaging for detection of greater than 70 percent coronary stenosis has been reported to be 78 percent.[66]

Technetium-99m Sestamibi Imaging

Planar Imaging

Several investigators[32, 176–178] have compared 2-day stress-rest ^{99m}Tc-sestamibi studies with stress-redistribution ^{201}Tl studies for overall detection of CAD and detection of disease in individual coronary arteries. The combined results[139] demonstrate that ^{99m}Tc-sestamibi and ^{201}Tl had respective sensitivities of 84 and 90 percent and specificities of 83 and 67 percent for detection of CAD. Normalcy rates (true-negative rate in patients with a low likelihood of CAD) for the two agents were 94 and 88 percent, respectively. The differences between the two agents were not statistically significant. With respect to detection of disease in individual coronary arteries, the combined results of several groups[32, 176–178] showed similar sensitivities of 66 and 69 percent and specificities of 70 and 68 percent with ^{99m}Tc-sestamibi and ^{201}Tl, respectively.[139] In the North American Phase III Multicenter Clinical Trial,[179, 180] 22 centers from the United States and two centers from Canada participated in an open-label study designed to compare ^{99m}Tc-sestamibi with ^{201}Tl and coronary angiography. Of the 284 patients who had planar imaging, 73 had a low likelihood of CAD; 191 had angiographic CAD; and 20 had normal coronary arteriograms. There was a 92 percent agreement between the two agents for classifying patients as normal or abnormal. Of a total of 4622 segments, 4358 (94 percent) were concordantly detected as normal or abnormal by the two agents. The sensitivity, specificity, and normalcy rate for ^{99m}Tc-sestamibi were 85, 95, and 100 percent and for ^{201}Tl were 87, 55, and 100 percent. When sensitivity data were broken down according to the extent of CAD, the two agents were again comparable. Using planar imaging, the sensitivity for detecting one-vessel disease was 73 percent for ^{99m}Tc-sestamibi and 77 percent for ^{201}Tl. For detection two-vessel disease, the sensitivity was 87 percent for both agents. For three-vessel disease, the sensitivities for ^{99m}Tc-sestamibi and ^{201}Tl were 92 and 95 percent, respectively.

Single-Photon Emission Computed Tomography Imaging

Several investigators have compared ^{99m}Tc-sestamibi and ^{201}Tl SPECT imaging for overall detection of CAD and for detection of disease in individual coronary arteries. For detection of CAD,[92, 176, 181] the respective average sensitivities for ^{201}Tl and ^{99m}Tc-sestamibi were 83 and 90 percent; the respective average specificities were 80 and 93 percent, and the respective average normalcy rates were 77 and 100 percent.[139] The differences between ^{201}Tl and ^{99m}Tc-sestamibi were not statistically significant. For detecting CAD in individual vessels[92, 182] the two agents were again similar; the average sensitivity and specificity for ^{201}Tl were 70 and 75 percent and for ^{99m}Tc-sestamibi were 83 and 77 percent.[139] In the North American Phase III Multicenter Study,[179, 180] 2-day stress-rest ^{99m}Tc-sestamibi and stress-redistribution ^{201}Tl SPECT were compared in a total of 294 patients of whom 45 had normal coronary arteriograms, 170 had angiographically documented CAD, and 79 had less than a 5 percent likelihood of coronary disease based on Bayesian analysis of their age, sex, clinical symptoms, and the results of exercise electrocardiography.[86–88] The diagnostic accuracy of ^{99m}Tc-sestamibi and ^{201}Tl SPECT images for the identification of patients with coronary artery disease was evaluated in 215 patients who had coronary angiography. Among the 170 patients with coronary artery disease (≥50 percent luminal stenosis), the overall sensitivities of ^{99m}Tc-sestamibi and ^{201}Tl were 92 and 90 percent, respectively. The overall specificities, determined in the 45 patients who had normal coronary arteriograms, were 50 percent for ^{99m}Tc-sestamibi and 39 percent for ^{201}Tl. The observed low specificity with both agents is consistent with previously reported specificity for ^{201}Tl[52] and most likely is due to patient referral bias, in that patients with an abnormal perfusion study were predominantly referred to coronary angiography. Importantly, for both agents, the normalcy rates in the 79 patients with less than a 5 percent likelihood of coronary artery disease were significantly higher than those of their respective specificities. For ^{99m}Tc-sestamibi, the normalcy rate was 92 percent, and for ^{201}Tl it was 94 percent. Furthermore, sensitivity for detecting one-vessel disease was 90 percent for both agents. For detection of two-vessel disease, the sensitivity was 88 percent for ^{99m}Tc-sestamibi and 84 percent for ^{201}Tl. For three-vessel disease, the sensitivities for ^{99m}Tc-sestamibi and ^{201}Tl were 98 and 96 percent, respectively. Overall, the two agents again had comparable sensitivities according to the extent of CAD.

In a recent multicenter study,[94] the accuracy of an automated quantitative analysis of same-day rest-stress ^{99m}Tc-sestamibi SPECT images for detection and localization of CAD was reported in 161 patients from seven different clinical sites. The quantitative analysis method was associated with an overall sensitivity of 87 percent, a specificity of 36 percent, and a normalcy rate of 81 percent. Sensitivity for overall detection of CAD was similar in patients with and without myocardial infarction (MI) (90 and 89 percent, respectively). The sensitivities and specificities for identification of disease in individual coronary arteries were, respectively, 69 and 76 percent for LAD, 70 and 80 percent for LCX, and 77 and 85 percent for RCA (Fig. 63–9).

Technetium-99m Teboroxime Imaging

Results of phase I, II, and III clinical trials of ^{99m}Tc-teboroxime have suggested that this tracer yields image quality similar to that of ^{201}Tl, provided that the images are obtained very rapidly after injection. In 10 normal volunteers and 20 patients with coronary artery disease, ^{99m}Tc-teboroxime stress and rest studies were compared with ^{201}Tl stress redistribution studies that used planar imaging.[51] For the ^{99m}Tc-teboroxime studies, three-view planar im-

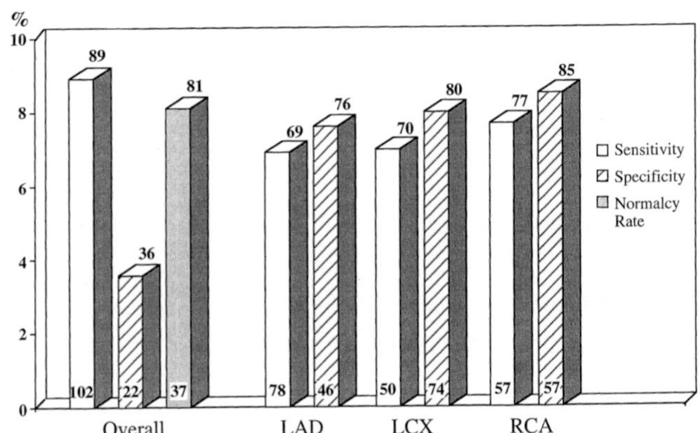

FIGURE 63–9. The diagnostic accuracy (sensitivity, specificity, and normalcy rate) for same-day rest-stress ^{99m}Tc-sestamibi imaging from a recent multicenter study. LAD = left anterior descending; LCX = left circumflex; RCA = right coronary artery. (From Van Train, K., Garcia, E., Maddahi, J., et al.: Multicenter trial validation for quantitative analysis of same-day rest-stress technetium-99m sestamibi myocardial tomograms. J. Nucl. Med. 35:609, 1994, with permission.)

aging was completed by approximately 16 minutes after injection. The ^{99m}Tc-teboroxime method detected abnormalities in 16 of the 20 patients with coronary artery disease (80 percent), which was not significantly different from the 17 of 20 (85 percent) detected by ^{201}Tl. Similarly, considering stenosis is greater than 70 percent as significant, no significant difference was noted between ^{99m}Tc-teboroxime and ^{201}Tl for identifying diseased coronary arteries, with 19 of 45 (42 percent) being detected by ^{99m}Tc-teboroxime and 21 of 45 (47 percent) being detected by ^{201}Tl. Both agents were found to be positive in 1 of 15 vessels without significant stenosis. It was reported that hepatic uptake of ^{99m}Tc-teboroxime obscured inferoapical segments in some views in 14 of the 20 CAD patients, but that this did not interfere with abnormal vessel identification. In a large multicenter trial,[183] 177 patients were studied with ^{99m}Tc-teboroxime imaging, using either planar or SPECT methods, and the results were compared to those with cardiac catheterization and/or ^{201}Tl imaging. In the angiographic correlations, the overall sensitivity for coronary artery disease was 84 percent, and specificity was 91 percent. Teboroxime imaging results agreed with ^{201}Tl interpretations in 91 percent of the cases. A preliminary report by Hendel and co-workers showed that rapid planar imaging techniques could be used with the patient in a seated position to collect complete diagnostic teboroxime studies within 5 minutes of injection.[184]

Unique Applications of Technetium-99m Labeled Agents

The high count rates and other physical and biologic properties of ^{99m}Tc-labeled agents has allowed development of several unique protocols.

Simultaneous Assessment of First-Pass Ventricular Function and Myocardial Perfusion

One of the most important advantages of ^{99m}Tc-sestamibi over ^{201}Tl is its ability to assess myocardial function and perfusion with a single injection.[38–41, 55, 185] Borges-Neto and co-workers[55] demonstrated the feasibility of treadmill exercise first-pass ^{99m}Tc-sestamibi procedures, followed by SPECT myocardial perfusion imaging. Rest and peak exercise first-pass measurements were obtained with a specially designed first-pass scintillation camera with a small detector head. The authors also showed that with respect to the assessment of left ventricular ejection fraction, there was no significant difference between same-day and separate (two)-day rest-exercise protocols. Because exercise left ventricular ejection fraction is a powerful prognostic indicator in CAD, its measurement may enhance the information obtained from the assessment of regional myocardial perfusion.

Gated Studies

Because of its high count rates, planar or SPECT ^{99m}Tc-sestamibi images may be acquired with cardiac gating to assess regional wall motion and wall thickening, in addition to myocardial perfusion. Wall motion and thickening may be objectively evaluated by analyzing regional count changes during the cardiac cycle.[186] Analysis of regional wall motion on gated planar or SPECT[187] studies may allow differentiation of viable and nonviable myocardial regions. Viable myocardial regions demonstrate regional wall motion in areas of reduced ^{99m}Tc-sestamibi activity, while nonviable myocardial regions show lack of motion in areas with perfusion defects. Analysis of diastolic ^{99m}Tc-sestamibi SPECT studies may, indeed, improve the ability to detect small perfusion defects and, thereby, improve the threshold for detection of myocardial perfusion abnormalities. In addition, review of gated ^{99m}Tc-sestamibi data should offer an additional quality-control method for identification of SPECT imaging artifacts (i.e., breast and diaphragmatic artifacts).

Attenuation and Scatter Correction

A major problem with ^{201}Tl and ^{99m}Tc-sestamibi SPECT studies is variable attenuation caused by varying distance of myocardial regions from the collimator and variable thickness of tissues interposed between the myocardium and the collimator. These attenuation patterns are frequently the source of false-positive studies. Various algorithms are being developed and validated through studies on phantom and experimental animals, which are aimed at correcting for attenuation and scatter.[188, 189] Attenuation correction is accomplished by first obtaining a transmission map, and this matrix is applied to the raw data prior to reconstruction using the first-order Chang correction method. This approach may ultimately add 10 minutes to the acquisition and another 10 minutes to the processing time. For scatter correction, myocardial images are obtained on two different photopeaks simultaneously, with the photopeak of 106 keV yielding a scatter image that is then used to correct the 140-keV "on-peak" study. Application of scatter and attenuation correction, as well as object size should make it feasible to obtain absolute measurement of regional myocardial counts. The author believes that incorporation of this technique will ultimately result in an improvement in the diagnostic accuracy for detection of CAD.

CLINICAL APPLICATIONS OF MYOCARDIAL PERFUSION IMAGING

Detection of Coronary Artery Disease in Asymptomatic and Symptomatic Patients

Asymptomatic Patients

A large percentage of patients with coronary events (sudden death or myocardial infarction) are totally asymptomatic. It is proposed that in such patients, CAD is silent and may be detected by use of noninvasive testing. The appropriateness of noninvasive testing in asymptomatic patients, however, should be viewed in light of Bayes' theorem. Bayes' theorem expresses the post-test likelihood of disease as a function of sensitivity and specificity of the test and the prevalence of disease in the population that is being tested. Stated differently, when the sensitivity and specificity of a test and the prevalence of disease in the population under study are known, one can calculate the likelihood of coronary disease being present on the basis of a normal or an abnormal test result. After an extensive literature search, Diamond and Forrester[190] have reported the prevalence of CAD, based on age, sex, and symptom classification. Literature reports of 28,948 patients were reviewed. For the prevalence of disease in symptomatic patients, the angiographic literature of 4952 patients was surveyed. With respect to symptoms, patients were classified into asymptomatic, nonanginal chest pain, atypical angina, and typical angina categories, using three major characteristics of chest pain (i.e., substernal location, provocation by exercise, and relief gained from rest or nitroglycerin within 10 minutes). For classification into the typical angina category, the patient is required to manifest all three characteristics. When any two of three characteristics of chest pain are present, the pain is classified as atypical angina. When any one of the characteristics is present, the pain is classified as nonanginal chest pain. Based on their results, the likelihood of CAD, prior to exercise ECG and nuclear imaging testing, may be determined based on the patient's age, sex, and symptoms, as shown in Figure 63–10. These results demonstrate that the prevalence of CAD in the asymptomatic population ranges from 0 to 20 percent and is, therefore, low.

The predictive accuracy of exercise ^{201}Tl myocardial perfusion imaging in 1000 asymptomatic patients (with approximately 10 percent prevalence of CAD) may be calculated, based on known sensitivity and specificity for exercise planar ^{201}Tl imaging (80 and 90 percent, respectively). Of the 100 patients with CAD, 80 percent (80 patients) had true-positive tests. Of the 900 patients without CAD, 10 percent (90 patients) had false-positive tests. Therefore, of a total of 170 positive tests in this population, only 80 showed results that were correctly positive, resulting in a positive predictive

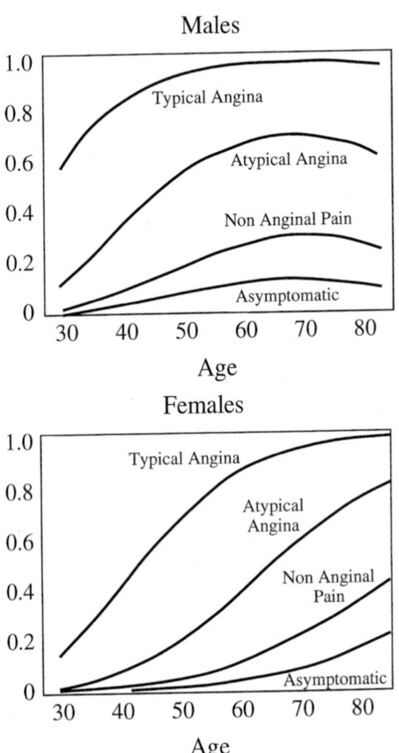

FIGURE 63–10. Relation between CAD prevalence and the patient's age, gender, and symptoms. (Based on data from Diamond, G., and Forrester, J.: Analysis of probability as an aid in the clinical diagnosis of coronary artery disease. N. Engl. J. Med. 300:1350, 1979.)

accuracy of only 47 percent. The post-test likelihood of CAD in asymptomatic patients with negative exercise ^{201}Tl testing, however, is very low (2 percent in the above example). This suggests that a positive exercise ^{201}Tl test in asymptomatic patients does not establish the presence of CAD, while a negative test effectively rules out the presence of CAD. These observations are also applicable to positive and negative exercise treadmill test results (sensitivity and specificity of approximately 70 percent) in asymptomatic patients. In these patients, the post-test likelihood of CAD after a positive exercise treadmill test is 20 percent, and the post-test likelihood of CAD after a negative treadmill test is 4.5 percent. It is of note, however, that when ^{201}Tl testing is applied to asymptomatic patients with positive exercise treadmill test results (20 percent likelihood of CAD), a positive ^{201}Tl test increases the CAD likelihood to 67 percent, and a negative ^{201}Tl test decreases the likelihood to less than 5 percent. Using the Bayesian analysis concept, therefore, it becomes apparent that only the subgroup of asymptomatic patients who have a low intermediate likelihood of CAD will benefit from exercise ^{201}Tl testing; that is, asymptomatic patients with a positive treadmill exercise test or asymptomatic patients with multiple risk factors increasing their likelihood of disease to a low intermediate range.

Several studies in the literature support this theoretical conclusion. Uhl and co-workers[191] demonstrated that of 130 asymptomatic U.S. Air Force pilots who were referred for cardiac catheterization because of a positive stress ECG or coronary risk factors, 22 (16 percent) had CAD. Of note, ^{201}Tl study was abnormal in all 22 who had CAD. In another study, Uhl and co-workers performed exercise ^{201}Tl imaging in 191 U.S. Air Force crew members who had an abnormal ST-segment response to exercise and underwent both exercise ^{201}Tl imaging and coronary angiography.[119] Of 135 patients with normal coronary arteries, 131 (91 percent) had normal ^{201}Tl studies. Of the 41 patients with CAD, 39 had abnormal exercise ^{201}Tl studies. Of the remaining 15 with insignificant coronary lesions, 10 had abnormal and 5 had normal exercise ^{201}Tl studies. In this population, the positive predictive accuracy of an abnormal ST-segment response to exercise was 21 percent, and exercise ^{201}Tl study increased the positive predictive accuracy to 91 percent. If both an abnormal ST-segment response and an abnormal ^{201}Tl study had been required before angiography was performed, 136 patients who were found to be free from significant CAD would not have undergone the risk of cardiac catheterization. On the other hand, five patients with insignificant disease and two patients with coronary narrowing of 50 percent or more would have gone undetected.

Symptomatic Patients

Bayes' theorem also helps define the appropriateness of stress ^{201}Tl testing for detection of CAD in symptomatic patients.[109, 190, 192, 193] Figure 63–11 demonstrates the post-test likelihood of CAD according to negative and positive ^{201}Tl test results in patients with differing pretest likelihood of CAD. A sensitivity of 85 percent and a specificity of 85 percent have been chosen for ^{201}Tl imaging. The center line, the line of identity, represents a test with sensitivity and specificity of 50 percent. At all points along the center line, the post-test likelihood is equal to the pretest likelihood; therefore, a test with these characteristics would have no diagnostic value. The degree to which the upper and lower curves representing abnormal and normal test results deviate from the line of identity can be viewed as a measure of the diagnostic value of the test; the greater the difference between the curves, the more valuable the test. It is evident that at the extremes of pretest likelihood or prevalence, the abnormal and normal test results have very little effect on post-test likelihood of CAD. However, in a patient with an intermediate likelihood of CAD (50 percent), a positive ^{201}Tl test increases the likelihood to more than 85 percent, and a negative test decreases the likelihood to less than 15 percent.

The application of the Bayesian analysis approach to proper utilization of nuclear cardiology procedures has also been demonstrated by several investigators. In a study of 135 women without prior myocardial infarction, Melin and co-workers[121] found that the use of ^{201}Tl scintigraphy in patients with an intermediate (10 to 90 percent) probability of CAD resulted in a marked increase in the proportion of patients with a high (>90 percent) or low (<10 percent) probability of CAD. They noted that this shift was appropriate, based on the angiographic findings, and they demonstrated that ^{201}Tl scintigraphy could be used to reduce unnecessary diagnostic catheterization without loss of diagnostic accuracy. In a separate study, Melin and co-workers[132] evaluated another 62 pa-

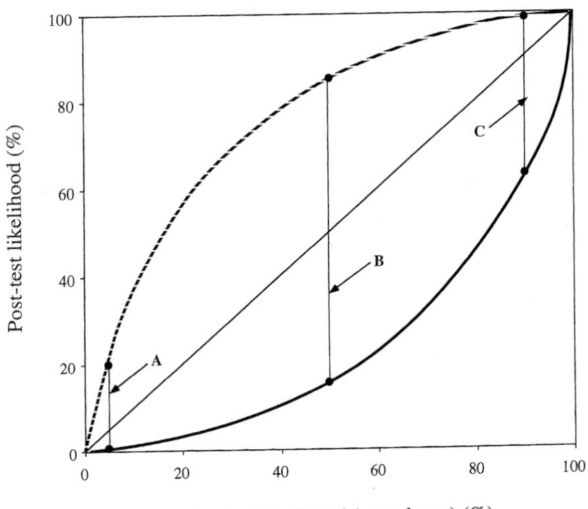

FIGURE 63–11. The effect of positive and negative exercise myocardial perfusion test results on the post-test likelihood of CAD in three patients with differing pretest likelihoods of CAD. A = low; B = intermediate; C = high.

tients with a low intermediate (average of 18 percent) pretest probability of disease. All six patients who had concordantly positive ECG and ^{201}Tl test had angiographically significant CAD. However, when the ^{201}Tl study failed to confirm the electrocardiographic results, the probability of CAD was low, with only 1 of 14 such patients angiographically documented as having CAD. Christopher and associates[194] also demonstrated the diagnostic usefulness of exercise radionuclide ventriculography, using a Bayesian approach. Among 250 patients undergoing exercise radionuclide ventriculography, post-test disease probability moved correctly downward in 85 percent of the 43 normal patients and upward in 72 percent of the 207 CAD patients. Failure to increase post-test probability in 28 percent of the CAD patients occurred most frequently in the groups of patients with anatomically mild CAD. None of the patients with left main CAD, and only 18 percent of the patients with triple-vessel disease, had a post-test probability less than their pre-test probability. Currie and colleagues[195] confirmed the diagnostic usefulness of exercise radionuclide ventriculography in patients with an intermediate probability of CAD. Examples of symptomatic patients with an intermediate pretest likelihood of CAD are those with (1) nonanginal chest pain and a positive or nondiagnostic exercise ECG; (2) atypical angina (unless ECG is markedly abnormal or is normal in a very young patient); and (3) atypical angina and a negative exercise ECG (especially in young females).

Detection of Disease in Individual Coronary Arteries

The coronary arteries and their branches supply different regions of the left ventricular myocardium. Based on the known anatomical relationship between coronary arteries and various myocardial regions and actual study of patients with single-vessel and multivessel CAD and with ^{201}Tl myocardial perfusion studies, general guidelines have been developed for assignment of various myocardial regions to specific coronary arteries. Therefore, it is possible to infer disease of a given coronary artery by noting the location of a perfusion defect on planar or tomographic myocardial images. Table 63–5 summarizes the sensitivity and specificity of the visually analyzed defects on planar ^{201}Tl imaging studies for identification of disease in the LAD, LCX, and RCA. As noted, the mean literature* sensitivities were 69, 37, and 65 percent, respectively, and the mean literature specificities were 94, 95, and 85 percent, respectively. The mean sensitivity and specificity for detection of disease in any coronary artery are 59 and 91 percent, respectively. It is of note that the sensitivity for detection of individual coronary stenosis is lower than the sensitivity of ^{201}Tl for detection of individual disease in patients with single-vessel disease and the sensitivity of overall detection of CAD. This relatively lower sensitivity of ^{201}Tl for detection of disease in individual coronary arteries may be explained by one or more of the following factors. First in patients with multivessel disease who have multiple adjacent areas of hypoperfusion, only the more hypoperfused regions may appear abnormal because of the relative nature of myocardial ^{201}Tl perfusion defect analysis. Second, it is possible that in patients with multivessel disease, exercise may be terminated because of development of limiting ischemia in one region before another region becomes ischemic. Third, the assignment of myocardial regions to coronary arteries is not perfect because of significant interindividual variability. Fourth, it is possible that coronary narrowings of 50 percent that are considered significant by angiography are not hemodynamically significant. Thus, myocardial regions subtended by these vessels do not become ischemic during exercise. Fifth, the role of collateral circulation in preventing ischemia in the distribution of a significant coronary region is variable and unpredictable. Sixth, the overlap of various myocardial regions that is inherent in the planar imaging technique may obscure small defects in a given coronary territory and thus lower the regional sensitivity. This factor may be particularly responsible for the lower sensitivity of ^{201}Tl testing for the detection of the circumflex CAD. The territory of the LCX coronary artery is observed in only one view represented by the posterolateral wall in the 45-degree LAO view with significant overlap of proximal and distal portions.

*See references 95, 96, 99, 118, 196, and 197.

Quantitative analysis of planar ^{201}Tl images has improved identification of disease in individual coronary arteries. As shown in Table 63–5, the mean literature[14, 148] sensitivities and specificities are, respectively, 77 and 74 percent for the LAD, 50 and 85 percent for the LCX, and 91 and 59 percent for the RCA. Overall, the sensitivity and specificity of the quantitatively analyzed planar images for identification of disease in any coronary artery are 74 and 73 percent, respectively. This improved sensitivity has been attributed to two factors. First, the slow regional washout rate of ^{201}Tl is used as an additional index of myocardial hypoperfusion. This index is spatially nonrelative and may demonstrate the presence of hypoperfusion in a relatively less hypoperfused myocardial region in patients with multivessel coronary disease and multiple adjacent regions of ischemia. Second, the use of background subtraction that is inherent in all quantitative methods may enhance ^{201}Tl perfusion defects that would otherwise be considered negative or equivocal by visual analysis of unsubtracted images. There have been reports of further improvement of sensitivity for the detection of disease in individual coronary arteries with the use of the SPECT technique. The mean literature[87, 150] sensitivities and specificities of the visually analyzed SPECT images (Table 63–5) are, respectively, 74 and 86 percent for the LAD, 57 and 94 percent for the LCX,

TABLE 63–5. SENSITIVITY AND SPECIFICITY OF THALLIUM-201 IMAGING FOR IDENTIFICATION OF DISEASE IN INDIVIDUAL CORONARY ARTERIES

	LAD		LCX		RCA		All Vessels	
	No. of Patients	*(%)*	*No. of Patients*	*(%)*	*No. of Patients*	*(%)*	*No. of Patients*	*(%)*
Qualitative Planar*								
Sensitivity	264/381	(69)	98/267	(37)	190/293	(65)	552/941	(59)
Specificity	60/64	(94)	23/97	(95)	82/98	(85)	234/258	(91)
Quantitative Planar[14, 148]								
Sensitivity	87/113	(77)	42/84	(50)	83/92	(91)	212/288	(74)
Specificity	51/69	(74)	83/98	(85)	54/91	(59)	188/258	(73)
Qualitative SPECT[87, 154, 261]								
Sensitivity	130/175	(74)	71/125	(57)	152/172	(88)	353/472	(75)
Specificity	145/169	(86)	206/219	(94)	143/172	(83)	494/560	(88)
Quantitative SPECT[86–88, 150, 153, 154]								
Sensitivity	422/530	(80)	264/367	(72)	438/528	(83)	1124/1419	(79)
Specificity	360/433	(83)	528/624	(85)	402/473	(85)	1290/1530	(84)

*See references 95, 96, 99, 118, 196, and 197.

88 and 83 percent for the RCA, with values of 75 and 88 percent for any coronary artery. The mean literature[86–88, 150, 153] sensitivities and specificities of the quantitatively analyzed SPECT ^{201}Tl images (Table 63–5) are, respectively, 80 and 83 percent for the LAD, 72 and 85 percent for the LCX, 83 and 85 percent for the RCA, and 79 and 84 percent for any coronary artery. By tomographic imaging, improved sensitivity is noted, particularly for detection of disease in the LCX coronary artery, as shown by pooled literature results and direct comparison of SPECT and planar quantitative imaging methods in the same patient population.[198] This improved sensitivity may be related to improved defect contrast and decreased overlap between myocardial regions that result from SPECT imaging.

Identification of Diagnostic Patients at Low Risk for Coronary Events

During the last decade, clinical application of myocardial perfusion imaging has evolved from diagnosis to risk stratification of CAD. The prognostic application of myocardial perfusion imaging plays an important role in patient management; the decision between using myocardial revascularization and medical therapy depends on the risk of coronary events with medical therapy versus the risk pertaining to myocardial revascularization procedure. In 1983, Brown and colleagues[125] demonstrated that among 61 patients with suspected CAD who had a negative exercise myocardial perfusion study, none died during an average of 46 months of follow-up, and three developed myocardial infarction during this period (0.85 percent event rate per year). These initial results were subsequently confirmed by several studies, summarized in Table 63–6. As noted, 2825 patients without myocardial infarction and with a normal ^{201}Tl exercise myocardial perfusion planar study have been reported in 13 separate publications. In these studies, the follow-up period has ranged from 12 to 56 months, with an average of 33.3 months. The weighted average incidence of cardiac death per year is 0.24 percent, ranging from 0 to 0.7 percent. Furthermore, the average incidence of developing myocardial infarction is 0.53 percent per year, ranging from 0 to 1.4 percent. These results suggest that a normal exercise myocardial perfusion study in patients without prior myocardial infarction is associated with a very low likelihood of coronary events during the subsequent year. The observed coronary event rates in this population are very similar to those of patients with normal coronary arteries, which suggests that further cardiac catheterization or intervention is not justified in these patients. An association between a normal stress myocardial perfusion study and a low coronary event rate has also been reported, in rather small groups of patients, using ^{201}Tl SPECT, ^{99m}Tc-sestamibi SPECT, atrial pacing planar ^{201}Tl stress testing, and dipyridamole stress planar ^{201}Tl imaging. An implication of excellent prognosis in patients with normal stress myocardial perfusion study is that the subgroup with coronary disease and normal perfusion studies also had good prognosis. The question as to whether normal ^{201}Tl studies would have the same benign predictive value for patients with angiographically significant CAD has been addressed in a recent study by Brown and Rowen.[199] These investigators demonstrated that of 75 patients with significant CAD who had normal exercise planar ^{201}Tl myocardial perfusion studies, 1 patient developed nonfatal myocardial infarction 28 months after the ^{201}Tl study, yielding an annual event rate of 7 percent per year. In comparison, 2 of the 101 patients with normal exercise planar ^{201}Tl studies who had either normal coronary arteries (14 patients) or a low likelihood of CAD developed hard events (nonfatal myocardial infarction at 28 months and cardiac death at 23 months), yielding an annual event rate of 1 percent per year. These results imply that a normal exercise ^{201}Tl myocardial perfusion study, even in the presence of significant CAD, carries a very benign prognosis with a very low rate of hard cardiac events.

TABLE 63–6. PROGNOSTIC VALUE OF A NORMAL THALLIUM-201 EXERCISE MYOCARDIAL PERFUSION PLANAR STUDY IN PATIENTS WITHOUT MYOCARDIAL INFARCTION

Lead Author	No. of Patients	Follow-Up (mos)	Myocardial Infarction (%/yr)	Death (%/yr)
Brown[125]	61	46	0.85	0.00
Pamelia[262]	345	34	0.61	0.51
Wackers[263]	95	22	1.15	0.00
Staniloff[264]	382	12	0.52	0.00
Gammage[265]	86	18	0.00	0.00
Heo[266]	519	27	0.34	0.17
Gill[267]	174	58	0.48	0.36
Koss[268]	309	36	0.43	0.11
Kaul[213]	39	64	0.48	0.00
Bairey[269]	144	12	1.40	0.70
Fleg[270]	352	56	0.61	0.30
Brown[271]	176	24	0.57	0.28
Oosterhuis[272]	143	24	1.40	0.35
Overall	2825	33.3	0.54	0.24

Identification of Extensive and High-Risk Coronary Artery Disease

An important goal of noninvasive methods currently used to assess patients with CAD is the correct identification of those with extensive coronary disease. Information regarding the extent of coronary disease may be derived from stress redistribution ^{201}Tl studies by assessing (1) the number of diseased vessels, as suggested by the number of coronary territories with perfusion defects or washout abnormalities; (2) diffuse slow washout rate of ^{201}Tl, as an index of extensive myocardial ischemia; (3) increased pulmonary capillary wedge pressure, as evidenced by increased lung uptake of ^{201}Tl; and (4) transient postexercise ischemic dilation of the left ventricle.

Identification of Left Main and Triple-Vessel Disease

Using the previously described schemes for assigning myocardial perfusion abnormalities to individual coronary arteries, it is possible to determine whether abnormalities involve the distribution of all three coronary arteries or of the left main coronary artery (combined territories of LAD and LCX). Several reports, however, have demonstrated that with this approach the sensitivity of conventional visual analysis of planar ^{201}Tl images for correct identification of extensive coronary disease is low.[97, 99, 197, 200, 201] This low sensitivity has been attributed to the limitation of relative perfusion defect analysis in revealing all hypoperfused myocardial regions in patients with multivessel coronary disease. The author observed that use of the combined criteria of exercise defect and abnormal regional washout of ^{201}Tl on planar images improved the sensitivity of visual ^{201}Tl analysis for correct identification of patients with left main and triple-vessel coronary disease (from 16 to 63 percent) without significant loss of specificity. Sixty-four percent of the patients who were misclassified by visual analysis as having less extensive disease were correctly classified as having extensive disease by virtue of quantitative analysis of regional myocardial ^{201}Tl washout. When the results of quantitative ^{201}Tl analysis were combined with those of blood pressure and electrocardiographic response to exercise,[200] the sensitivity and specificity for identification of patients with left main and triple main coronary disease were 86 and 76 percent, respectively, and the highest overall accuracy (82 percent) was obtained. When CAD is extensive and is of relatively uniform severity, regional myocardial hypoperfusion may be balanced during stress, precluding the development of spatially relative perfusion defects. The assessment of myocardial ^{201}Tl washout rate on planar ^{201}Tl images may provide diagnostic assistance in these cases.[202] Bateman and colleagues[203] demonstrated that with imaging studies, 13 (1 percent) had the pattern of diffuse slow ^{201}Tl washout rate in the absence of a regional perfusion defect. *Diffuse slow washout* was defined as the presence of washout abnormalities in the distribution of all three major coronary arteries but not uniformly in all. Of these 13 patients, 9 (69 percent) were found to have left main or triple-vessel coronary disease. In practice, it is important to keep in mind that the incidence of the diffuse ^{201}Tl slow washout pattern, indicating extensive disease, is low (approximately 1 percent). It should be noted that several factors, such as a low exercise heart rate, subcutaneous infiltration of the dose, arm vein uptake, low-count rate studies, inappropriate data acquisition, and imaging protocol deviations, may cause diffuse ^{201}Tl slow washout in the absence of coronary disease. With the SPECT imaging technique, sensitivity and specificity for correct identification of extensive disease, even without the use of regional washout rate of ^{201}Tl, is higher than the planar imaging method. The pooled literature results[52, 87, 88, 150] demonstrated that 69 percent of patients (291 of 423) with three-vessel CAD were correctly identified as such by the SPECT imaging method.

Size of Infarcted and Jeopardized Myocardium

The extent of myocardial ischemia may not be always inferred by the number of diseased coronary arteries because the size of myocardial ischemia is influenced by the size of the supplying coronary artery; the location, severity, and number of coronary narrowings; and the status of collateral blood flow. On stress myocardial perfusion studies, the magnitude of myocardial hypoperfusion may be expressed by the number of myocardial segments with a defect, the actual percentage of total left ventricular myocardium with perfusion defects, and the severity of hypoperfusion (reflecting the severity of underlying CAD). These defects can be further categorized to reflect infarcted myocardium (if they are nonreversible) or viable but jeopardized myocardium (if they are reversible). Several investigators have evaluated the relationship between the size of myocardial hypoperfusion and subsequent coronary events. Brown and co-workers[125] showed, by stepwise logistic regression analysis, that in 100 patients without prior myocardial infarction, potential predictors of cardiac death or myocardial infarction were the number of transient ^{201}Tl defects, the total number of ^{201}Tl defects, and the number of diseased vessels by angiography. Importantly, after the number of transient ^{201}Tl defects (which had the highest significant chi-square value) was included in the logistic regression model, no other predictor was found to be significant. In the study of Ladenheim and associates,[204] involving 1689 patients without prior myocardial infarction, stepwise logistic regression identified only 3 independent predictors of annual coronary events: the number of myocardial regions with reversible hyperperfusion, the magnitude of hypoperfusion, and achieved heart rate (Fig. 63–12).

Increased Pulmonary Uptake of Thallium-201

An increase in pulmonary ^{201}Tl activity may be noted on anterior view images in patients with CAD. Both experimental studies and clinical evidence suggest that this increased pulmonary ^{201}Tl activity is related to the development of left ventricular dysfunction with exercise.[10, 205, 206] To objectify assessment of pulmonary uptake of ^{201}Tl, two methods have been developed. In the method developed by Kushner and colleagues,[207] the degree of pulmonary ^{201}Tl activity is expressed as the quantitative fraction of the myocardial value. Another approach described by Levy and colleagues[208] quantifies the percentage of pulmonary ^{201}Tl washout from immediate postexercise to 4-hour redistribution anterior view images. With both techniques, abnormal values have been observed in patients with extensive coronary disease. In the study of Levy and colleagues,[208] abnormal pulmonary ^{201}Tl washout was related to both the anatomical extent and the functional severity of disease: It occurred with greater frequency in patients with multivessel coronary disease and in those with exercise-induced left ventricular dysfunction. It should be noted that increased pulmonary uptake of ^{201}Tl reflects increased pulmonary capillary wedge pressure, which may be caused by factors other than extensive and severe coronary disease, such as mitral valve regurgitation, mitral stenosis, decreased left ventricular compliance, and nonischemic cardiomyopathy with left ventricular dysfunction. Therefore, it is important to exercise caution in interpreting increased pulmonary uptake of ^{201}Tl as an index of extensive coronary disease when it occurs in isolation (without myocardial perfusion defects) or in patients with one or more of the aforementioned conditions.

Transient Ischemic Dilation of the Left Ventricle

The author's group[209] and others[210] have noted that some patients with CAD have a pattern of transient dilation of the left ventricle on the immediate poststress images, as compared with the 4-hour redistribution images. Because this dilation must be present for at least 10 to 15 minutes after exercise to be visualized on the postexercise anterior image, this pattern most likely represents severe and extensive CAD, causing transient ischemic dilation of the left ventricle after exercise. Transient dilation of the left ventricle was shown to have a sensitivity of 60 percent and a specificity of 95 percent for identifying patients with multivessel critical stenoses, and this phenomenon was more specific than other known markers of severe and extensive coronary disease, such as the presence of multiple perfusion defects or washout abnormalities, or both.[209] In routine practice, this phenomenon can be estimated by visual inspection of the immediate postinjection and 4-hour anterior views. This phenomenon may also be noted on SPECT images (Fig. 63–13). When transient dilation is observed, it should be interpreted as strong evidence of severe and extensive myocardial ischemia. The significance of transient dilation of the left ventricle after pharmacologic stress testing is similar to that of exercise testing.[211]

Incremental Prognostic Power of Thallium-201 Imaging

The incremental prognostic power of ^{201}Tl imaging, in comparison with other parameters, such as clinical variables, exercise treadmill results, and coronary angiography, has been extensively evaluated. Four of the reported studies have addressed the incremental value of exercise ^{201}Tl imaging over and above clinical, exercise ECG, and angiographic variables. As previously mentioned, in the study of Brown and co-workers,[125] multivariate regression analysis showed that the number of transient ^{201}Tl defects was a better predictor of future cardiac events than clinical, ECG, and angiographic data. Kaul and associates evaluated two large patient popu-

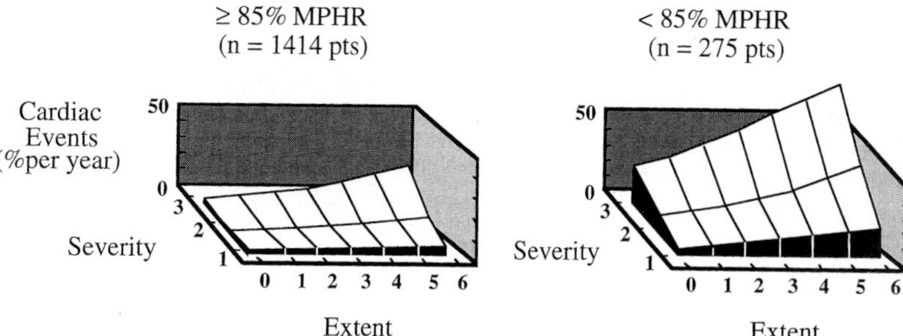

FIGURE 63–12. Relation between the extent and severity of exercise myocardial perfusion defects and subsequent coronary events, according to percent maximal predicted heart rate achieved during exercise. MPHR = maximum predicted heart rate. (From Ladenheim, M., Pollack, B., Rozanski, A., et al.: Extent and severity of myocardial hypoperfusion as predictors of prognosis in patients with suspected coronary artery disease. J. Am. Coll. Cardiol. 7:464, 1986, with permission.)

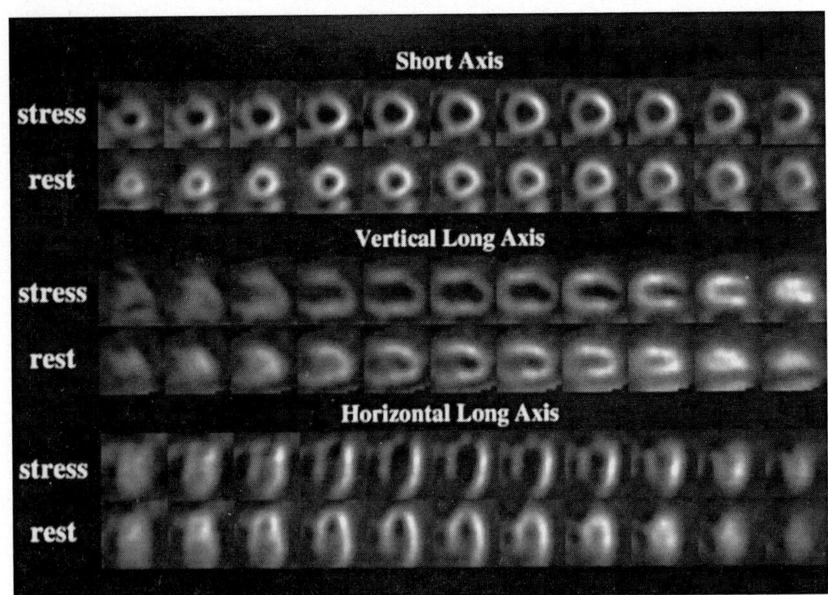

FIGURE 63–13. Transient postexercise dilation of the left ventricle, noted on SPECT images of a patient with a proximal subtotal occlusion of a large LAD coronary artery.

lations at two different institutions. In 293 patients who were studied at Massachusetts General Hospital,[212] Cox regression analysis showed that the quantitatively assessed lung-to-heart ratio of ^{201}Tl activity was the most important predictor of a future cardiac event. Other significant predictors were the number of diseased vessels, patient gender, and change in heart rate from rest to exercise. Although the number of diseased vessels was an important independent predictor of cardiac events, it did not add significantly to the overall ability of the exercise ^{201}Tl test to predict events. Furthermore, information obtained from ^{201}Tl imaging alone was marginally superior to that obtained from cardiac catheterization alone and significantly superior to that obtained from exercise testing alone in determining the occurrence of events. In addition, unlike the exercise ^{201}Tl test, which could predict the occurrence of all categories of events, catheterization data were not able to predict the occurrence of all categories of events, catheterization data were not able to predict the occurrence of nonfatal myocardial infarction. These data suggested that exercise ^{201}Tl imaging is superior to data from both exercise testing alone and cardiac catheterization data alone for predicting future events in patients with chronic CAD who have undergone both exercise ^{201}Tl imaging and catheterization for the evaluation of chest pain.

In a subsequent study, Kaul and colleagues[213] evaluated the prognostic utility of ^{201}Tl stress testing, compared to that of other parameters, in 382 patients from The University of Virginia who were followed up for a mean of 4.6 years. When all clinical, exercise, ^{201}Tl, and catheterization variables were analyzed by Cox regression analysis, the number of diseased vessels was the single most important predictor of future events, followed by the number of segments demonstrating redistribution on delayed ^{201}Tl images, except in the case of nonfatal myocardial infarction, for which redistribution was the most important predictor of future events. When CAD was defined as demonstrating 70 percent or greater luminal diameter narrowing, the number of diseased vessels significantly lost its power to predict events. In this study, when exercise ^{201}Tl stress test results were considered as a whole (in conjunction with a change in heart rate from rest to exercise, ST-segment depression on the ECG, and ventricular premature beats on exercise), they were as powerful as cardiac catheterization data. Of note, the combination of both catheterization and exercise ^{201}Tl data was superior to either alone in determining future events. In a more recent study by Pollack and associates from the same group of investigators,[214] the incremental prognostic value of data obtained in succession (clinical, exercise stress test, ^{201}Tl imaging, and coronary angiography) in patients with suspected CAD was evaluated. Thallium-201 imaging provided significant additional prognostic information compared with that provided by clinical and exercise stress test data. In a subgroup of patients in whom lung-to-heart ^{201}Tl ratio had been analyzed, coronary angiography did not provide additional prognostic information. In this subgroup of patients, the combination of clinical and exercise ^{201}Tl variables provided greater prognostic information than the combination of clinical and angiographic data. In the remaining subgroup of patients in whom the lung-to-heart ratio had not been analyzed, coronary angiography provided incremental prognostic information compared with clinical and exercise ^{201}Tl data alone.

Risk Stratification After Myocardial Infarction

In survivors of myocardial infarction, many high-risk clinical and laboratory variables have been identified. These variables include recurrent angina, left ventricular failure, shock, conduction abnormalities, malignant arrhythmia, and decreased left ventricular ejection fraction. In a subset of patients with uncomplicated myocardial infarction (asymptomatic and without evidence of severe left ventricular dysfunction), 1-year mortality ranges from 2 to 7.5 percent.[215] The aim of noninvasive testing prior to discharge of uncomplicated myocardial infarction patients, therefore, is the identification of those who are at relatively lower or higher risk for subsequent death or recurrent infarction on the basis of residual ischemic myocardium, either adjacent to or remote from the infarction. In 1983, Gibson and associates[216] compared the predictive value of predischarge of maximal exercise ^{201}Tl imaging with clinical, exercise treadmill, and coronary angiographic data. They demonstrated that the presence of reversible ^{201}Tl defects involving multiple vascular territories and increased lung uptake of ^{201}Tl were significant prognostic indicators in these patients. The combination of these ^{201}Tl variables had significantly greater sensitivity for predicting future cardiac events than that with exercise treadmill and coronary angiographic data.

With wide application of thrombolytic therapy in the acute phase of myocardial infarction, the role of myocardial perfusion imaging for risk stratification of patients after myocardial infarction has changed.[217] In patients treated with thrombolytic therapy, ^{201}Tl redistribution is still more prevalent than ST-segment depression (48 versus 14 percent), but the prevalence of inducible ischemia is less than that observed in the prethrombolytic era (59 percent for ^{201}Tl redistribution and 32 percent for ST-segment depression).[217] Therefore, although fewer ischemic responses are observed in patients who undergo reperfusion therapy, detection of ischemia is better achieved with exercise perfusion imaging than with exercise ECG alone. Another important prognostic variable in patients surviving uncomplicated acute myocardial infarction is presence of multivessel CAD. Haber and colleagues[218] demonstrated that the sensitivity of ST-segment depression, remote ^{201}Tl redistribution, and either of the two findings were 29, 35, and 58 percent, respectively. The respective specificities were 96, 87, and 78 percent for detection of multivessel CAD in patients with thrombolytic therapy for acute myocardial infarction. Table 63–7 summarizes the results of four studies[216, 219–221] that have assessed the usefulness of exercise ^{201}Tl myocardial perfusion imaging for risk stratification after myocardial infarction. In a total of 537 patients reported with exercise myocardial perfusion studies, the positive and negative predictive accuracies of myocardial perfusion imaging for prediction of future cardiac events have been 40 and 93 percent, respectively.

The availability of pharmacologic coronary vasodilation with dipyridamole and adenosine has provided a unique opportunity for early post–myocardial infarction risk stratification, using myocardial perfusion imaging. With pharmacologic vasodilation, maximal hyperemia may be achieved without the undesired effects of maximal exercise testing, such as increase of myocardial oxygen consumption, due to significant increase in heart rhythm blood pressure, and increase in intraventricular pressure and possible adverse effects on ventricular remodeling due to increase in systolic and mean blood pressure during exercise. Table 63–7 also summarizes studies that have employed pharmacologic coronary vasodilation for risk assessment after myocardial infarction.[222–226] A total of four studies are available that have used dipyridamole pharmacologic coronary vasodilation and ^{201}Tl imaging early after uncomplicated myocardial infarction in a total of 205 patients. The positive and negative predictive accuracies have been 30 and 94 percent, respectively.[222–225] Of note, in a recent study by Mahmarian and co-workers,[226] adenosine coronary vasodilation and ^{201}Tl imaging were used to predict cardiac death, myocardial infarction, unstable angina, and congestive heart failure in a total of 92 patients during 15 months of follow-up after uncomplicated myocardial infarction. The presence of reversible defect involving 5 percent of the left ventricle was 50 percent sensitive and 97 percent specific for predicting subsequent coronary events.

Evaluation of Patients With Resting Chest Pain and Unstable Angina

Unstable angina is a diagnostic challenge because of the low specificity of chest pain and ECG changes for its diagnosis. Uncertainty regarding diagnosis of unstable angina generally results in hospital admission for patients who present to the emergency room with resting chest pain, to avoid the serious consequences of inappropriate emergency room discharge of patients with true myocardial ischemia. One of the early applications of ^{201}Tl imaging has been differential diagnosis of resting chest pain. In 1978, Wackers and colleagues[227] injected ^{201}Tl at rest after episodes of chest pain and found reversible defects in 39 percent of patients with subsequent diagnosis of unstable angina. Reversible ^{201}Tl defects were associated with a more complicated subsequent clinical course. In 1981, Parodi and co-workers[228] showed transient reduction of regional myocardial perfusion during angina at rest with ST-segment depression or normalization of negative T waves in all patients who were injected during episodes of chest pain. Since ^{201}Tl readily redistributes after initial injection, it is logistically limited for such application because the time interval between injection and start of imaging in patients with unstable angina generally exceeds 15 minutes. Technetium-99m sestamibi is particularly suitable for evaluation of patients with unstable angina because of its minimal redistribution after resting injection. Bilodeau and associates[229] injected 45 patients with ^{99m}Tc-sestamibi during episodes of chest pain, followed by imaging in 1 to 6 hours. Of 26 patients with significant coronary stenosis, only 9 (35 percent) had diagnostic ECG changes, while 25 (96 percent) had a perfusion defect. The specificity of ^{99m}Tc-sestamibi was 88 percent, and the negative predictive value of a normal perfusion scan during pain was 94 percent.

Recently, Hilton and associates[230] evaluated 102 emergency room patients with typical angina during a normal or nondiagnostic ECG by injecting ^{99m}Tc-sestamibi during chest pain. All patients were followed for development of adverse cardiac events (cardiac death, nonfatal myocardial infarction, or coronary intervention) during subsequent hospital admission. Multivariate regression analysis identified an abnormal perfusion image as the only independent predictor of adverse cardiac events. Of 70 patients with a normal perfusion scan, only 1 had a cardiac event, compared with 15 patients with equivocal scans or 17 patients without normal scans with cardiac event rates of 13 and 71 percent, respectively. These investigators concluded that injection of ^{99m}Tc-sestamibi and subsequent imaging in the emergency department in patients with typical angina during a normal or nondiagnostic ECG is highly accurate in predicting cardiac events during subsequent admission. An implication of these data is that patients with a normal myocardial perfusion scan or small defects could be admitted to the observation unit, in contrast to those with large defects who would be

TABLE 63–7. COMPARISON OF EXERCISE VERSUS PHARMACOLOGIC CORONARY VASODILATORS FOR RISK ASSESSMENT AFTER MYOCARDIAL INFARCTION

Study	No. of Patients	Follow-Up (mos)	Events	Predictor	Positive Predictive Accuracy (%)	Negative Predictive Accuracy (%)
Exercise						
Wilson[221]	97	39	Death/MI/unstable angina	IZRD	42	77
Brown[220]	59	37	Death/MI/unstable angina	IZRD	28	100
Gibson[216]	140	15	Death/MI/unstable angina	RD	59	94
Gibson[219]	241	27	Death/MI	IZRD	31	97
Overall	537				40	93
Dipyridamole						
Gimple[224]	36	6	Death/MI/unstable angina	NIZRD	26 (42)	88
Younis[223]	68	12	Death/MI	RD	22	94
Leppo[222]	51	19	Death/MI	RD	33	94
Brown[225]	50	12	Death/MI/unstable angina	RD	45	100
Overall	205				30	94
Adenosine						
Mahmarian[226]	92	15	Death/MI/unstable angina/CHF	RD (5% LV)	50	97

IZ = infarct zone; MI = myocardial infarction; NIZ = noninfarct zone; RD = redistribution; LV = left ventricle.

Modified from Mahmarian, J.J., and Verani, M.S.: Myocardial perfusion imaging during pharmacologic stress testing. Cardiol. Clin. 12(2):223–245, 1994, with permission.

most appropriately admitted to an intensive care unit for monitoring. Brown[231] evaluated the prognostic value of exercise ^{201}Tl myocardial perfusion imaging in 52 consecutive patients with unstable angina who responded to medical treatment. Stress ^{201}Tl imaging was done within 1 week of discharge, and patients were followed up for an average of 39 months. Thallium-201 redistribution was the only significant predictor of cardiac death or nonfatal myocardial infarction. Furthermore, the number of myocardial segments with ^{201}Tl redistribution and a history of prior myocardial infarction were the only significant predictors of all cardiac events. Therefore, it appears that, similar to application of stress ^{201}Tl imaging in patients with stable coronary artery disease, in patients with unstable angina who respond to medical treatment, myocardial perfusion imaging is a powerful prognostic indicator of subsequent coronary events.

Risk Stratification of Patients Undergoing Noncardiac Surgery

Coronary artery disease is common among patients with peripheral vascular disease. Hertzer and co-workers[232] have shown that among 1000 consecutive patients with peripheral vascular disease who underwent coronary angiography, and had no clinical suspicion for CAD prior to angiography, 37 percent had one or more 70 percent coronary stenosis and 15 percent had CAD significant enough to warrant percutaneous transluminal coronary angioplasty or coronary artery bypass surgery. Mangano and associates[233] have demonstrated that approximately 50 percent of all deaths associated with elective noncardiac surgery in the United States are related to cardiac deaths. Thallium-201 myocardial perfusion imaging has been extensively investigated for its application to the identification of patients who are at high risk for developing cardiac complications during noncardiac surgery.

In 1985, Boucher and colleagues[234] applied pharmacologic stress testing in conjunction with ^{201}Tl myocardial perfusion planar scintigraphy to assess the perioperative risk of coronary events in 48 patients with peripheral vascular disease. They demonstrated that in 16 patients with reversible defects, 3 developed hard events (myocardial infarction or death), and 5 developed unstable angina perioperatively, while among 32 patients with normal or fixed defects, none had perioperative events. Subsequently, several investigators used the technique of dipyridamole stress ^{201}Tl planar imaging for risk stratification of patients prior to elective noncardiac surgery,[222, 235–244] and the results are summarized in Table 63–8. In a total of 2020 reported patients, 21 percent (194 of 905) of patients who had reversible defects developed perioperative cardiac events, in contrast to 2 percent (20 of 1115) of those who had normal studies or had fixed defects. These results suggest that lack of reversible defects of dipyridamole stress-redistribution of ^{201}Tl planar imaging defectively identifies a group of patients who are at very low risk for developing cardiac events during elective noncardiac surgery. However, the positive predictive accuracy is only 20 percent; that is, only 1 of 4 patients with reversible defects develop events. This low figure suggests that other factors influence the development of perioperative cardiac events in these patients.

NEWER TECHNETIUM-99m LABELED MYOCARDIAL PERFUSION IMAGING AGENTS UNDER INVESTIGATION

Recently, several second-generation ^{99m}Tc myocardial perfusion imaging agents have been evaluated for clinical use, including tetrofosmin, furifosmin (Q12), and Q3. An important clinical feature of these new agents is that they improve imaging convenience in the clinical setting by providing better target-to-background activity soon after injection of the tracer, as compared to ^{99m}Tc-sestamibi, and a longer duration of myocardial activity than that of ^{99m}Tc-teboroxime.

Technetium-99m Tetrofosmin

This agent is a diphosphine cation[245] with rapid myocardial uptake and fairly rapid clearance from background organs when injected during exercise, allowing the start of imaging at approximately 5 minutes after exercise.[246, 247] When tetrofosmin is injected at rest, however, clearance from background organs is not as fast, and optimal target-to-background ratio is reached at approximately 45 to 60 minutes after injection.[247, 248] In isolated perfused rabbit hearts, a linear relation between ^{99m}Tc-tetrofosmin myocardial uptake and coronary blood flow has been shown at flows up to 2.5 mL/min/g.[249] Experimental studies by Sinusas and associates[250] in an open-chest canine model demonstrated a high correlation between early myocardial ^{99m}Tc-tetrofosmin activity and macrosphere blood flow; however, relative ^{99m}Tc-tetrofosmin activity underestimated flow at high flow rates (>2.0 mL/min/g) and overestimated flow in low flow ranges (<0.2 mL/min/g). Technetium-99m tetrofosmin shows minimal myocardial washout in experimental studies[250] and in humans.[248, 251] The absorbed radiation dose from ^{99m}Tc-

TABLE 63–8. PREOPERATIVE RISK STRATIFICATION WITH DIPYRIDAMOLE

Study	No. of Patients	Follow-Up	Events	Positive Predictive Accuracy: No. of Patients	(%)	Negative Predictive Accuracy: No. of Patients	(%)
Brown[235]	231	30 days	Death/MI/UA	15/77	(19)	150/154	(97)
Levinson[236]	62	HD	Death/MI/UA	17/62	(27)	—	—
Lette[237]	355	HD	Death/MI	28/161	(17.5)	192/194	(99)
Coley[238]	100	HD	Death/MI/CHF/UA	8/36	(22)	63/64	(99)
Hendel[239]	327	HD	Death/MI	24/167	(14.4)	156/160	(99)
Camp[240]	40	HD	Death/MI/UA	6/9	(67)	31/31	(100)
Lane[241]	101	HD	Death/MI/UA/CH	10/71	(14)	29/30	(97)
Boucher[234]	48	HD	Death/MI/UA	8/16	(50)	32/32	(100)
Lette[237]	360	HD	Death/MI	28/60	(17.5)	198/200	(99)
Leppo[222]	89	HD	Death/MI	14/42	(33)	46/47	(98)
Eagle[242]	61	HD	Death/MI/UA/CHF	8/18	(44)	43/43	(100)
Sachs[243]	46	HD	Death/MI/UA	3/14	(21)	32/32	(96)
Eagle[244]	200	HD	Death/MI/UA/CHF	25/72	(35)	123/128	(96)
Total	2020			194/905	(21)	1095/1115	(98)

CHF = congestive heart failure; HD = hospital discharge; UA = unstable angina.
Modified from Mahmarian, J.J., and Verani, M.S.: Myocardial perfusion imaging during pharmacologic stress testing. Cardiol. Clin. 12(2):223–245, 1994, with permission.

tetrofosmin for various organs in humans is comparable to that of ^{201}Tl and ^{99m}Tc-sestamibi.[247]

As part of a phase II clinical study, same-day and 2-day planar imaging protocols were compared in 50 patients suspected of CAD.[252] Discrepancies between the two protocols for reversibility of defects were found in five patients, all in the inferior wall. In a recent phase III Multicenter International Trial, the sensitivity and specificity of planar exercise-rest ^{99m}Tc-tetrofosmin imaging was compared with those of planar ^{201}Tl imaging and coronary angiography in 252 patients suspected of having CAD and 58 subjects with a low likelihood of CAD.[253] A same-day exercise-rest imaging protocol was used, with the injection of 6 to 10 mCi ^{99m}Tc-tetrofosmin at peak exercise and 22 to 27 mCi at rest, after an interval of 2.5 to 4 hours. Generally, ^{99m}Tc-tetrofosmin images were of good quality and were easy to interpret. Concordance between ^{99m}Tc-tetrofosmin and ^{201}Tl images was 80.4 percent when patients were categorized as normal and abnormal. The concordance between the two agents was 59.4 percent when patients were categorized as having normal function, ischemia, infarction, or a mixture. In this multicenter study, sensitivities, normalcy rates, positive predictive accuracies, and negative predictive accuracies of ^{99m}Tc-tetrofosmin and ^{201}Tl planar imaging were comparable. The accuracy of ^{99m}Tc-tetrofosmin SPECT imaging was compared with that of ^{201}Tl SPECT in 25 patients in a recent study[254] that reported similar sensitivities, specificities, and defect reversibility between the two methods.

Technetium-99m Furifosmin (Q12)

Technetium-99m furifosmin belongs to a new class of nonreducible Tc(III) cationic complexes that was developed by Deutsche and colleagues.[255] The myocardial uptake of ^{99m}Tc-Q12 is linearly related to myocardial blood flow up to 2 ml/min/g flow rates, and myocardial extraction is reduced at higher flow rates.[256] Technetium-99m Q12 clears from the blood rapidly and does not exhibit myocardial washout or redistribution.[257] The initial human studies with ^{99m}Tc-Q12 suggest that this agent clears from the hepatobiliary system more rapidly than ^{99m}Tc-sestamibi, providing more favorable images early after resting injection of the agent.[258, 259]

Technetium-99m Q3

This agent, like Q12, belongs to the new class of nonreducible Tc(III) cationic complexes. In experimental studies, Gerson and associates have shown that myocardial activity of this tracer is linearly related to myocardial blood flow with minimal subsequent myocardial washout. Phase II clinical studies of ^{99m}Tc-Q3 were conducted by Gerson and colleagues in 17 patients.[260] A same-day rest-stress SPECT protocol was used, with the start of imaging 15 minutes after both rest and stress injection of the agent, and the entire study was completed in less than 2 hours. In this study, ^{99m}Tc-Q3 and ^{201}Tl SPECT images correlated highly for the presence and reversibility of perfusion defects.

Acknowledgments

I am grateful to Pooneh Hendi and Sepehr Rokhsar for their assistance in the literature search and to Diane Martin for preparation of the figures and Terri Meredith for typing of the manuscript.

References

1. Lebowitz, E., Greene, M., Fairchild, R., et al.: Tl-201 for medical use. J. Nucl. Med. 16:151, 1975.
2. Mullins, L., and Moore, R.: The movement of thallium ions in muscle. J. Gen. Physiol. 43:759, 1960.
3. Gehring, P., and Hammond, P.: The interrelationship between thallium and potassium in animals. J. Pharmacol. Exp. Ther. 155:187, 1967.
4. Zimmer, L., McCall, D., and D'Abbado, L.: Kinetics and characteristics of thallium exchange in cultured cells. Circulation 59:138, 1979.
5. Pohost, G., Zir, L., Moor, R., et al.: Differentiation of transiently ischemic from infarcted myocardium by serial imaging after a single dose of Tl-201. Circulation 55:294, 1977.
6. Nielsen, A., Morris, K., Murdock, R., et al.: Linear relationship between the distribution of Tl-201 and blood flow in ischemic and nonischemic myocardium during exercise. Circulation 61:797, 1980.
7. Weich, H., Strauss, H., and Pitt, B.: The extraction of Tl-201 by the myocardium. Circulation 56:188, 1977.
8. Strauss, H., and Pitt, B.: Noninvasive detection of subcritical coronary arterial narrowings with coronary vasodilator and myocardial perfusion imaging. Am. J. Cardiol. 39:403, 1977.
9. Gould, K.: Noninvasive assessment of coronary stenosis by myocardial perfusion imaging during pharmacologic coronary vasodilatation. Am. J. Cardiol. 41:267, 1978.
10. Boucher, C., Zir, L., Beller, G., et al.: Increased lung uptake of Tl-201 during exercise myocardial imaging: Clinical, hemodynamic and angiographic implications in patients with coronary artery disease. Am. J. Cardiol. 46:189, 1980.
11. Berger, B., Watson, D., Burwell, L., et al.: Redistribution of thallium at rest in patients with stable and unstable angina and the effect of coronary artery bypass surgery. Circulation 60:1114, 1979.
12. Pohost, G., O'Keefe, D., Gewirtz, H., et al.: Thallium redistribution in the presence of severe fixed coronary stenosis. J. Nucl. Med. 19:680, 1978.
13. Beller, G., and Pohost, G.: Mechanism for Tl-201 redistribution after transient myocardial ischemia. Circulation 56:141, 1977.
14. Maddahi, J., Garcia, E., Berman, D., et al.: Improved noninvasive assessment of coronary artery disease by quantitative analysis of regional stress myocardial distribution and washout of Tl-201. Circulation 164:924, 1981.
15. Garcia, E., Maddahi, J., Berman, D., et al.: Space/time quantitation of thallium-201 myocardial scintigraphy. J. Nucl. Med. 22:309, 1981.
16. Massie, B., Wisneski, J., Kramer, B., et al.: Comparison of myocardial thallium-201 clearance after maximal and submaximal exercise: Implications for diagnosis of coronary disease. (Concise communication.) J. Nucl. Med. 23:381, 1982.
17. Kaul, S., Chesler, D., Pohost, G., et al.: Influence of peak exercise heart rate on normal Tl-201 myocardial clearance. J. Nucl. Med. 27:26, 1986.
18. Maddahi, J., Van Train, K., Don Michael, T., et al.: Normal initial myocardial distribution and washout of Tl-201 at rest vs. exercise. Clin. Nucl. Med. 10:11, 1985.
19. Gewirtz, H., O'Keefe, D.D., Pohost, G.M., et al.: The effect of ischemia on thallium-201 clearance from the myocardium. Circulation 58:215, 1978.
20. Okada, R., and Pohost, G.: Effect of decreased blood flow and ischemia on myocardial thallium clearance. J. Am. Coll. Cardiol. 3:744, 1984.
21. Sklar, J., Kirch, D., Johnson, T., et al.: Slow late myocardial clearance of thallium: A characteristic phenomenon in coronary artery disease. Circulation 65:1504, 1982.
22. Budinger, T., Pohost, G., and Bichoff, P.: Tl-201 integral blood concentration over 2 hours explains persistent defects in patients with no evidence of MI by ECG. (Abstract.) Circulation 76:64, 1987.
23. Angello, D., Wilson, R., and Palac, R.: Effect of eating on Tl-201 myocardial redistribution after myocardial ischemia. Am. J. Cardiol. 60:528, 1987.
24. Gutman, J., Berman, D., Freeman, M., et al.: Time to completed redistribution of thallium-201 in exercise myocardial scintigraphy: Relationship to the degree of coronary artery stenosis. Am. Heart J. 106:989, 1983.
25. Kiat, H., Berman, D., Maddahi, J., et al.: Late reversibility of tomographic myocardial Tl-201 defects: An accurate marker of myocardial viability. J. Am. Coll. Cardiol. 12:1456, 1988.
26. Weiss, A., Maddahi, J., Lew, A., et al.: Reverse redistribution of Tl-201: A sign of nontransmural myocardial infarction with patency of the infarct-related coronary artery. J. Am. Coll. Cardiol. 7:61, 1986.
27. Maddahi, J., and Berman, D.: Reverse redistribution of thallium-201. J. Nucl. Med. 36:1019, 1995.
28. Williams, S., Mousa, S., Morgan, R., et al.: Pharmacology of Tc-99m isonitrile: Agents with favorable characteristics for heart imaging. (Abstract.) J. Nucl. Med. 27:877, 1986.
29. Sia, S., Holman, B., and McKusick, K.: The utilization of Tc-99m TBI as a myocardial perfusion agent in exercise studies: Comparison with Tl-201 thallous chloride and examination of its biodistribution in humans. Eur. J. Nucl. Med. 12:333, 1986.
30. Mousa, S., Williams, S., and Sands, H.: Characterization of in-vivo chemistry of cations in the heart. J. Nucl. Med. 28:1351, 1987.
31. McKusick, K., Holman, B., Jones, A., et al.: Comparison of three Tc-99m isonitriles for detection of ischemic heart disease in humans. J. Nucl. Med. 27:878, 1986.
32. Wackers, F., Berman, D., Maddahi, J., et al.: Technetium-99m hexakis 2-methoxy isobutyl isonitrile: Human biodistribution, dosimetry, safety, and preliminary comparison to thallium-201 for myocardial imaging (phase I and II studies). J. Nucl. Med. 30:301, 1989.
33. Mousa, S., Cooney, J., and Williams, S.: Regional myocardial distribution of RP-30 in animal models of myocardial ischemia and reperfusion. J. Nucl. Med. 28:620, 1987.
34. Marshall, R., Leidhodt, E., Barnett, C., et al.: Single-pass myocardial extraction and retention of a Tc-99m isonotrilevs Tl-201. Circulation 76:IV-218, 1987.
35. Okada, R., Glover, D., Gaffney, T., et al.: Myocardial kinetics of technetium-99m hexakis 2-methoxy e-methylpropyl isonitrile. Circulation 77:491, 1988.
36. Leppo, J., and Meerdink, D.: Comparison of the myocardial uptake of a technetium-labeled isonitrile analogue and thallium. Circ. Res. 64:632, 1989.
37. Stirner, H., Buell, U., Kleinhans, E., et al.: Myocardial kinetics of Tc-99m hexakis 2-methoxy isobutyl isonitrile (HMIBI) in patients with coronary heart disease: A comparative study versus Tl-201 with SPECT. Nucl. Med. Commun. 9:15, 1988.
38. Elliot, A., McKillop, J., Gillen, G., et al.: Simultaneous assessment of left ventric-

ular function and perfusion at rest and exercise using Tc-99m-RP-30A. Nucl. Med. Commun. 9:154, 1988.
39. Levy, R., Elstob, J., Wiseman, M., et al.: Myocardial perfusion and first pass ventriculography with technetium-99m MIBI in coronary artery disease. Nucl. Med. Commun. 9:155, 1988.
40. Sporn, V., Perez Balino, N., Holman, B., et al.: Simultaneous measurement of ventricular function and myocardial perfusion using the technetium-99m isonitriles. Clin. Nucl. Med. 13:77, 1988.
41. Baillet, G., Mena, I., Kuperus, J., et al.: Simultaneous Tc-99m MIBI angiography and myocardial perfusion imaging. J. Nucl. Med. 20:38, 1989.
42. Taillefer, R., La Flamme, L., Dupras, G., et al.: Myocardial perfusion imaging with Tc-99m methoxy-isobutyl-isonitrile (MIBI): Comparison of short and long time intervals between rest and stress injections. Preliminary results. Eur. J. Nucl. Med. 13:515, 1988.
43. Taillefer, R., Gagnon, A., La Flamme, L., et al.: Same-day injection of Tc-99m methoxy sidobutyl isonitrile (hexamibi) for myocardial tomographic imaging: Comparison between rest-stress and stress-rest injection sequences. Eur. J. Nucl. Med. 15:113, 1989.
44. Taillefer, R.: Technetium-99m sestamibi myocardial imaging: Same-day rest-stress studies and dipyridamole. Am. J. Cardiol. 66:80E, 1990.
45. Berman, D., Kiat, H., Friedman, J., et al.: Separate acquisition rest thallium-201/stress technetium-99m sestamibi dual-isotope myocardial perfusion SPECT: A clinical validation study. J. Am. Coll. Cardiol. 22:1455, 1993.
46. Rama, K., Nunn, A., Kuczynsk, B., et al.: A neutral technetium-99m complex for myocardial imaging. J. Nucl. Med. 30:1830, 1989.
47. Leppo, J., and Meerdink, D.: Comparative myocardial extraction of two technetium-labeled BATO derivatives (SQ30217, SQ32014) and thallium. J. Nucl. Med. 31:67, 1990.
48. Maublant, J., Moins, N., and Gachon, P.: Uptake and release of two new technetium-99m labeled myocardial blood flow imaging agents in cultured cardiac cells. Eur. J. Nucl. Med. 15:180, 1989.
49. Stewart, R., Hutchins, G., Brown, D., et al.: Myocardial retention and clearance of the flow tracer technetium-99m SQ30217 in canine heart. J. Nucl. Med. 30:860, 1989.
50. Narra, R., Feld, T., Wedeking, P., et al.: SQ30217, a technetium-99m labeled myocardial imaging agent which shows no interspecies difference in uptake. Nuklearmedizin 231 (Suppl.):489, 1987.
51. Seldin, D., Johnson, L., and Blood, D.: Myocardial perfusion imaging with technetium-99m SQ30217: Comparison with thallium-201 and coronary anatomy. J. Nucl. Med. 30:312, 1989.
52. Iskandrian, A., Heo, J., Kong, B., et al.: Effect of exercise level on the ability of thallium-201 tomographic imaging in detecting coronary artery disease: Analysis of 461 patients. J. Am. Coll. Cardiol. 14:1477, 1989.
53. Bruce, R.: Methods of exercise testing. Steptest, bicycle, treadmill, isometrics. Am. J. Cardiol. 33:715, 1974.
54. Naughton, J., and Haiden, R.: Methods of exercise testing. *In* Naughton, J., and Helerstein, H.K. (eds.): Exercise Testing and Exercise Training in Coronary Heart Disease. New York, Academic Press, 1973, pp. 79–91.
55. Borges-Neto, S., Coleman, R., and Jones, R.: Perfusion and function at rest and treadmill exercise using technetium-99m sestamibi: Comparison of one and two day protocols in normal volunteers. J. Nucl. Med. 31:1128, 1990.
56. Brown, B., Josephson, M., Peterson, R., et al.: Intravenous dipyridamole combined with isometric handgrip for near maximal acute increase in coronary flow in patients with coronary artery disease. Am. J. Cardiol. 48:1077, 1981.
57. Gould, K., Westcott, R., Albro, P., et al.: Noninvasive assessment of coronary stenoses by myocardial imaging during pharmacologic coronary vasodilation. II. Clinical methodology and feasibility. Am. J. Cardiol. 41:279, 1978.
58. Chan, S., Brunken, R., Czernin, J., et al.: Comparison of maximal myocardial blood flow during adenosine infusion with that of intravenous dipyridamole in normal men. J. Am. Coll. Cardiol. 20:979, 1992.
59. Hoffman, J.: Determinants and prediction of transmural myocardial perfusion. Circulation 58:381, 1978.
60. Becker, L.: Conditions for vasodilator-induced coronary steal in experimental myocardial ischemia. Circulation 57:1103, 1978.
61. Forman, R., Kirk, E., Downey, J., et al.: Nitroglycerine and heterogeneity of myocardial blood flow: Reduced subendocardial blood flow and ventricular contractile force. J. Clin. Invest. 52:905, 1973.
62. Flameng, W., Schaper, W., and Lewi, P.: Multiple experimental coronary occlusion without infarction. Effects of heart rate and vasodilatation. Am. Heart J. 85:767, 1973.
63. Flameng, W., Wusten, B., and Schaper, W.: On the distribution of myocardial blood flow. II. Effects of arterial stenosis and vasodilation. Basic Res. Cardiol. 69:435, 1974.
64. Flameng, W., Wusten, B., Winkler, B., et al.: Influence of perfusion pressure and heart rate on local myocardial flow in the collateralized heart with chronic coronary occlusion. Am. Heart J. 89:51, 1983.
65. Patterson, R., and Kirk, E.: Coronary steal mechanisms in dogs with one-vessel occlusion and other arteries normal. Circulation 67:1009, 1975.
66. Hays, J., Mahmarian, J., Cochran, A., et al.: Dobutamine thallium-201 tomography for evaluating patients with suspected coronary artery disease unable to undergo exercise or pharmacologic stress testing. J. Am. Coll. Cardiol. 21:1583, 1993.
67. Krivokapich, J., Huang, S-C, and Schelbert, H.: Assessment of the effects of dobutamine on myocardial blood flow and oxidative metabolism in normal human subjects using nitrogen-13 ammonia and carbon-11 acetate. Am. J. Cardiol. 71:1351, 1993.
68. Ranhosky, A., Kempthorne-Rawson, J., and Group TIDTIS.: The safety of intravenous dipyridamole thallium myocardial perfusion imaging. Circulation 81:1205, 1990.
69. Lette, J., Tatum, J., Fraser, S., et al.: Safety of dipyridamole testing in 73,806 patients: The Multicenter Dipyridamole Safety Study. J. Nucl. Cardiol. 2:3, 1995.
70. Belardinelli, L., Linden, J., and Berne, R.: The cardiac effects of adenosine. Prog. Cardiovasc. Dis. 32:73, 1989.
71. Rosen, J., Stenberg, R., Lopez, J., et al.: Coronary dilation with intravenous dipyridamole and adenosine: A comparative study. (Abstract.) Circulation 82:731, 1990.
72. Abreu, A., Mahmarian, J., and Nishimura, S.: Tolerance and safety of pharmacologic coronary vasodilation with adenosine in association with thallium-201 scintigraphy in patients with suspected coronary artery disease. J. Am. Coll. Cardiol. 18:730, 1991.
73. Cerqueira, M., Verani, M., Schwaiger, M., et al.: Safety profile of adenosine stress perfusion imaging: Results from the Adenoscan Multicenter Trial Registry. J. Am. Coll. Cardiol. 23:384, 1994.
74. Segall, G., and Davis, M.: Prone versus supine thallium myocardial SPECT: A method to decrease artifactual inferior wall defects. J. Nucl. Med. 30:548, 1989.
75. Friedman, J., Van Train, K., Maddahi, J., et al.: "Upward creep" of the heart: A frequent source of false-positive reversible defects during thallium-201 stress redistribution SPECT. J. Nucl. Med. 30:1718, 1989.
76. Meade, R., Bamrah, V., Horgan, J., et al.: Quantitative methods in the evaluation of Tl-201 myocardial perfusion images. J. Nucl. Med. 19:1175, 1978.
77. Burrow, R., Pond, M., Schafer, A., et al.: "Circumferential profiles": A new method for computer analysis of Tl-201 myocardial perfusion images. J. Nucl. Med. 20:771, 1979.
78. Watson, D., Campbell, N., Read, E., et al.: Spatial and temporal quantitation of planar thallium myocardial images. J. Nucl. Med. 22:577, 1981.
79. Berger, B., Watson, D., Taylor, G., et al.: Quantitative Tl-201 exercise scintigraphy for detection of coronary artery disease. J. Nucl. Med. 22:585, 1981.
80. Kaul, S., Chesler, D., Boucher, C., et al.: Quantitative aspects of myocardial perfusion imaging. Semin. Nucl. Med. 17:131, 1987.
81. Wackers, F., Bales, D., Fetterman, R., et al.: Non-uniform washout of Tl-201 (within normal range): Criterion for improved detection of single-vessel coronary artery disease. (Abstract.) Circulation 68:207, 1983.
82. Massie, B., Hollenberg, M., Wisneski, J., et al.: Scintigraphic quantitation of myocardial ischemia: A new approach. Circulation 68:747, 1983.
83. Goris, M., Daspir, S., McLaughlin, P., et al.: Interpolative background subtraction. J. Nucl. Med. 17:744, 1976.
84. Vogel, R., Kirch, D., LeFree, M., et al.: Tl-201 myocardial perfusion scintigraphy: Results of standard and multi-pinhole tomographic techniques. Am. J. Cardiol. 43:787, 1979.
85. Garcia, E., Maddahi, J., Berman, D., et al.: Quantification of rotational Tl-201 myocardial tomography. J. Nucl. Med. 26:17, 1985.
86. Maddahi, J., Van Train, K., Prigent, F., et al.: Quantitative single photon emission computerized thallium-201 tomography for detection and localization of coronary artery disease: Optimization and prospective validation of a new technique. J. Am. Coll. Cardiol. 14:1689, 1989.
87. DePasquale, E., Nody, A., DePuey, E., et al.: Quantitative rotational thallium-201 tomography for identifying and localizing coronary artery disease. Circulation 77:316, 1988.
88. Mahmarian, J., Boyce, T., Goldberg, R., et al.: Quantitative exercise thallium-201 single-photon emission computed tomography for the enhanced diagnosis of ischemic heart disease. J. Am. Coll. Cardiol. 15:318, 1990.
89. Smith, W., and Watson, D.: Technical aspects of myocardial planar imaging with technetium-99m sestamibi. Am. J. Cardiol. 66:16E, 1990.
90. Garcia, E., Cooke, C., Van Train, K., et al.: Technical aspects of myocardial SPECT imaging with technetium-99m sestamibi. Am. J. Cardiol. 66:23E, 1990.
91. Kiat, H., Van Train, K., Maddahi, J., et al.: Development and prospective application of quantitative two-day stress-rest Tc-99m methoxy isobutyl isonitrile SPECT for the diagnosis of coronary artery disease. Am. Heart J. 120:1255, 1990.
92. Kahn, J., McGhie, I., Akers, M., et al.: Quantitative rotational tomography with Tl-201 and Tc-99m 2-methoxy-isobutyl-isonitrile: A direct comparison in normal individuals and patients with coronary artery disease. Circulation 79:1282, 1989.
93. Van Train, K., Areeda, J., Garcia, E., et al.: Quantitative same-day-rest-stress technetium 99m sestamibi SPECT: Definition and validation and stress, normal limits and criteria for abnormality. J. Nucl. Med. 34:1494, 1993.
94. Van Train, K., Garcia, E., Maddahi, J., et al.: Multicenter trial validation for quantitative analysis of same-day rest-stress technetium-99m sestamibi myocardial tomograms. J. Nucl. Med. 35:609, 1994.
95. Lenaers, A., Block, P., Thiel, E., et al.: Segmental analysis of Tl-201 stress myocardial scintigraphy. J. Nucl. Med. 18:509, 1977.
96. Massie, B., Botvinick, E., and Brundage, B.: Correlation of Tl-201 scintigrams with coronary anatomy: Factors affecting region by region sensitivity. Am. J. Cardiol. 44:616, 1979.
97. Dash, H., Massie, B., Botvinick E., et al.: The noninvasive identification of left main and three-vessel coronary artery disease by myocardial stress perfusion scintigraphy and treadmill exercise electrocardiography. Circulation 60:276, 1979.
98. McKillop, H., Murray, R., Turner, J., et al.: Can the extent of coronary artery disease be predicted from Tl-201 myocardial images? J. Nucl. Med. 20:714, 1979.
99. Rigo, P., Bailey, I., Griffith, L., et al.: Value and limitation of segmental analysis of stress thallium myocardial imaging for localization of coronary artery disease. Circulation 61:973, 1980.
100. Ritchie, J., Trobaugh, G., Hamilton, G., et al.: Myocardial imaging with thallium at rest and during exercise: Comparison with coronary angiography and resting and stress electrocardiography. Circulation 56:66, 1977.
101. Bailey, I., Griffith, L., Rouleau, J., et al.: Thallium-201 myocardial perfusion

imaging at rest and during exercise: Comparative sensitivity to electrocardiography in coronary artery disease. Circulation 55:79, 1977.
102. Rosenblatt, A., Lowenstein, J., Kerth, W., et al.: Post exercise Tl-201 myocardial scanning: A clinical appraisal. Am. Heart J. 94:463, 1977.
103. Botvinick, E., Taradash, MR, Shames, D., et al.: Tl-201 myocardial perfusion scintigraphy for the clinical clarification of normal, abnormal and equivocal electrocardiographic stress tests. Am. J. Cardiol. 41:43, 1978.
104. Verani, M., Marcus, M., Razzak, M., et al.: Sensitivity and specificity of Tl-201 perfusion scintigrams under exercise in the diagnosis of coronary artery disease. J. Nucl. Med. 19:773, 1978.
105. Ritchie, J., Zaret, B., Strauss, H., et al.: Myocardial imaging with Tl-201: A multicenter study in patients with angina pectoris or acute myocardial infarction. Am. J. Cardiol. 42:345, 1978.
106. Turner, D., Battle, W., Deshmukh, H., et al.: The predictive value of myocardial perfusion scintigraphy after stress in patients without previous myocardial infarction. J. Nucl. Med. 19:249, 1978.
107. Blood, D., McCarthy, D., Sciacca, R., et al.: Comparison of single-dose and double-dose Tl-201 myocardial perfusion scintigraphy for the detection of coronary artery disease and prior myocardial infarction. Circulation 58:777, 1978.
108. Carrillo, A., Marks, D., Pickard, S., et al.: Correlation of exercise Tl-201 myocardial scan with coronary arteriograms and the maximum exercise test. Chest 73:321, 1978.
109. Hamilton, G., Trobaugh, G., Ritchie, J., et al.: Myocardial imaging with Tl-201: An analysis of clinical usefulness based on Bayes' theorem. Semin. Nucl. Med. 8:358, 1978.
110. McCarthy, D., Blood, D., Sciacca, R., et al.: Single dose myocardial perfusion imaging with Tl-201: Application in patients with nondiagnostic electrocardiographic stress tests. Am. J. Cardiol. 43:899, 1979.
111. Caralis, D., Bailey, L., Kennedy, H., et al.: Tl-201 myocardial imaging in evaluation of asymptomatic individuals with ischemic ST-segment depression on exercise electrocardiogram. Br. Heart J. 42:562, 1979.
112. Silber, S., Fleck, E., Klein, U., et al.: Wertigkeir der Tl-201 belastungselektrokardiographie bie patienten mit koronarer herzerkrankung ohne myokardinfarkt. Herz 4:359, 1979.
113. Jengo, J., Freeman, R., Brizendine, M., et al.: Detection of coronary artery disease: Comparison of exercise stress radionuclide angiocardiography and thallium stress perfusion scanning. Am. J. Cardiol. 45:535, 1980.
114. Caldwell, J., Ha, G., Sorenson, S., et al.: The detection of coronary artery disease with radionuclide techniques: A comparison of rest exercise thallium imaging and ejection fraction response. Circulation 61:610, 1980.
115. Iskandrian, A., Mintz, G., Croll, M., et al.: Exercise Tl-201 myocardial scintigraphy: Advantages and limitations. Cardiology 65:136, 1980.
116. Iskandrian, A., Segal, B., Haaz, W., et al.: Effects of coronary artery narrowing, collaterals, and left ventricular function on the pattern of myocardial perfusion. Cathet. Cardiovasc. Diagn. 6:159, 1980.
117. Schicha, H., Rentrop, P., Facorro, L., et al.: Results of quantitative myocardial scintigraphy with Tl-201 at rest and after maximum exercise—critical analysis of predictive value and clinical application. Z. Kardiol. 69:31, 1980.
118. Elkayam, U., Weinstein, M., Berman, D., et al.: Stress Tl-201 myocardia scintigraphy and exercise technetium ventriculography in the detection and location of chronic coronary artery disease: Comparison of sensitivity and specificity of these noninvasive tests alone and in combination. Am. Heart J. 101:657, 1981.
119. Uhl, G., Kay, T., and Hickman, J.: Computer-enhanced thallium scintigrams in asymptomatic men with abnormal exercise tests. Am. J. Cardiol. 48:1037, 1981.
120. Guiney, T., Pohost, G., McKusick, K., et al.: Differentiation of false from true positive ECG responses to exercise stress by Tl-201 perfusion imaging. Chest 80:4, 1981.
121. Melin, J., Piret, L., Vanbutsele, R., et al.: Diagnostic value of exercise electrocardiography and thallium myocardial scintigraphy in patients without previous myocardial infarction: A Bayesian approach. Circulation 63:1019, 1981.
122. Patterson, R., Horowitz, S., Eng, C., et al.: Can exercise electrocardiagraphy and Tl-201 myocardial imaging exclude the diagnosis of coronary artery disease? Bayesian analysis of the clinical limits of exclusion and indications for coronary angiography. Am. J. Cardiol. 49:1127, 1982.
123. Faris, J., Burt, R., Graham, M., et al.: Tl-201 myocardial scintigraphy: Improved sensitivity, specificity, and predictive accuracy by application of a statistical image analysis algorithm. Am. J. Cardiol. 49:733, 1982.
124. Kambara, H., Kawashita, K., Yoshida, A., et al.: Identification of patients with coronary artery disease using a scoring system of coronary risk factors, electrocardiography, and myocardial perfusion imaging (prospective and retrospective). Jpn. Circ. J. 46:235, 1982.
125. Brown, K., Boucher, C., Okada, R., et al.: Prognostic value of exercise thallium-201 imaging in patients presenting for evaluation of chest pain. J. Am. Coll. Cardiol. 1:994, 1983.
126. Cinotti, L., Meignan, M., Usdin, J., et al.: Diagnostic value of image processing in myocardial scintigraphy. J. Nucl. Med. 24:768, 1983.
127. O'Keefe, J., Edwards, A., Wiserman, J., et al.: Comparison of exercise electrocardiography, Tl-201 myocardial imaging, exercise-gated blood pool scan in patients with suspected coronary artery disease. Aust. NZ J. Med. 13:45, 1983.
128. Chaitman, B., Brevers, G., Dupras, G., et al.: Diagnostic impact of thallium scintigraphy and cardiac fluoroscopy when the exercise ECG is strongly positive. Am. Heart J. 108:260, 1984.
129. Osbakken, M., Okada, R., Boucher, C., et al.: Comparison of exercise perfusion and ventricular function imaging: An analysis of factors affecting the diagnostic accuracy of each technique. J. Am. Coll. Cardiol. 3:272, 1984.
130. Hung, J., Chaitman, B., Lam, J., et al.: Noninvasive diagnostic test for the evaluation of coronary artery disease in women: A multivariate comparison of cardiac fluoroscopy, exercise electrocardiography, and exercise thallium myocardial perfusion scintigraphy. J. Am. Coll. Cardiol. 4:8, 1984.
131. Burke, J., Morganroth, J., Soffer, J., et al.: The cardiokymography exercise test compared to the thallium-201 perfusion exercise test in the diagnosis of coronary artery disease. Am. Heart J. 107:718, 1984.
132. Melin, J., Wijns, W., Vanbutsele, R., et al.: Alternative diagnostic strategies for coronary artery disease in women: Demonstration of the usefulness and efficiency of probability analysis. Circulation 71:535, 1985.
133. Canhasi, B., Dae, M., Botvinick, E., et al.: Interaction of "supplementary" indicators of ischemia and stress electrocardiography in the diagnosis of multivessel coronary disease. J. Am. Coll. Cardiol. 6:581, 1985.
134. Del Rio-Meraza, A., Vilapando-Gutierrez, J., Nava-Lopez, G., et al.: Correlation between exercise electrocardiographic test, myocardial perfusion test with Tl-201, and contrast coronary arteriography in patients with ischyemic heart disease. Arch. Invest. Med. (Mex.) 16:175, 1985.
135. Hung, J., Chaitman, B., Lam, J., et al.: A logistic regression analysis of multiple noninvasive tests for the prediction of the presence and extent of coronary artery disease in men. Am. Heart J. 110:460, 1985.
136. Rothendler, J., Okada, R., Wilson, R., et al.: Effect of a delay in commencing imaging on the ability to detect transient thallium defects. J. Nucl. Med. 26:880, 1985.
137. Weiner, D.: Accuracy of cardiokymography during exercise resting: Results of a multicenter study. J. Am. Coll. Cardiol. 6:502, 1985.
138. Amor, M., Verdaguer, M., Karcher, G., et al.: Les examens isotopiques a l'effort dans l'isuffisance coronaire. Arch. Mal. Coeur. Vaiss 78:55, 1985.
139. Maddahi, J., Rodrigues, E., Berman, D., et al.: State-of-the-art myocardial perfusion imaging. Cardiol. Clin. 12:199, 1994.
140. Detrano, R., Janosi, A., Lyons, K., et al.: Factors affecting sensitivity and specificity of a diagnostic test: The exercise thallium scintigram. Am. J. Med. 84:699, 1988.
141. Atwood, J., Jensen, D., Froelicher, V., et al.: Agreement in human interpretation of analog thallium myocardial perfusion images. Circulation 64:601, 1981.
142. Okada, R., Boucher, C., Kirshenbaum, H., et al.: Improved diagnostic accuracy of Tl-201 stress test using multiple observers and criteria derived from interobserver analysis of variance. Am. J. Cardiol. 46:619, 1980.
143. Albro, P., Gould, K., Westcott, R., et al.: Noninvasive assessment of coronary stenoses by myocardial imaging during pharmacologic coronary vasodilatation. III Clinical trial. Am. J. Cardiol. 42:751, 1978.
144. Bodenheimer, M., Banka, V., Fooshee, C., et al.: Extent and severity of coronary heart disease: Determinations by thallous chloride Tl-201 myocardial perfusion scanning and comparison with stress electrocardiography. Arch. Intern. Med. 139:630, 1979.
145. Dunn, R., Kelly, D., Bailey, I., et al.: Serial exercise thallium myocardial perfusion scanning and exercise electrocardiography in the diagnosis of coronary artery disease. Aust. NZ J. Med. 9:547, 1979.
146. Kaul, S., Boucher, C., Newell, J., et al.: Determination of the quantitative thallium imaging variables that optimize detection of coronary artery disease. J. Am. Coll. Cardiol. 7:527, 1986.
147. Goris, M., Gordon, E., and Kim, O.: A stochastic interpretation of thallium myocardial perfusion scintigraphy. Invest. Radiol. 20:253, 1985.
148. Van Train, K., Berman, D., Garcia, E., et al.: Quantitative analysis of stress Tl-201 myocardial scintigrams: A multicenter trial. J. Nucl. Med. 27:17, 1986.
149. Rozanski, A., Diamond, G., Berman, D., et al.: The declining specificity of exercise radionuclide ventriculography. N. Engl. J. Med. 309:518, 1983.
150. Tamaki, N., Yonekura, Y., Mukai, T., et al.: Stress Tl-201 transaxial emission computed tomography: Quantitative vs qualitative analysis for evaluation of coronary artery disease. J. Am. Coll. Cardiol. 4:1213, 1984.
151. Fintel, D., Links, J., Brinker, J., et al.: Improved diagnostic performance of exercise Tl-201 single photon emission computed tomography over planar imaging in the diagnosis of coronary artery disease: A receiver operation characteristic analysis. J. Am. Coll. Cardiol. 13:600, 1989.
152. Quinones, M., Verani, M., Hiachin, R., et al.: Exercise echocardiography versus Tl-201 single-photon emission computed tomography in evaluation of coronary artery disease: Analysis of 292 patients. Circulation 85:1026, 1992.
153. Van Train, K., Maddahi, J., Berman, D., et al.: Quantitative analysis of tomographic stress thallium-201 myocardial scintigrams: A multicenter trial. J. Nucl. Med. 31:1168, 1990.
154. Tamaki, N., Yonekura, Y., Senda, M., et al.: Value and limitation of stress thallium-201 single photon emission computed tomography: Comparison with nitrogen-13 ammonia positron tomography. J. Nucl. Med. 29:1181, 1988.
155. Mahmarian, J., and Verani, M.: Exercise thallium-201 perfusion scintigraphy in the assessment of coronary artery disease. Am. J. Cardiol. 67:2D, 1991.
156. Nishimura, S., Mahmarian, J., Boyce, T., et al.: Quantitative thallium-201 single-photon emission computed tomography during maximal pharmacologic coronary vasodilation with adenosine for assessing coronary artery disease. J. Am. Coll. Cardiol. 18:736, 1991.
157. Hacot, J., Bojovic, M., Delonca, J., et al.: Comparison of planar imaging and single-photon emission computed tomography for the detection and localization of coronary artery disease. Int. J. Cardiac Imaging 9:113, 1993.
158. Leppo, J., Boucher, C., Okada, R., et al.: Serial thallium-201 myocardial imaging after dipyridamole infusion: Diagnostic utility in detecting coronary stenoses and relationship to regional wall motion. Circulation 66:649, 1982.
159. Taillefer, R., Lette, J., Phaneuf, D., et al.: Thallium-201 myocardial imaging during pharmacologic coronary vasodilation: Comparison of oral and intravenous administration of dipyridamole. J. Am. Coll. Cardiol. 8:76–83, 1986.
160. Ruddy, T., Dighero, H., Newell, J., et al.: Quantitative analysis of dipyridamole-

thallium images for the detection of coronary artery disease. J. Am. Coll. Cardiol. 10:142, 1987.
161. Timmis, A., Lutkin, J., Fenney, L., et al.: Comparison of dipyridamole and treadmill exercise for enhancing thallium-201 perfusion defects in patients with coronary artery disease. Eur. Heart J. 1:275, 1980.
162. Narita, M., Kurihara, T., and Usami, M., et al.: Noninvasive detection of coronary artery disease by myocardial imaging with thallium-201: The significance of pharmacologic interventions. Jpn. Circ. J. 45:127, 1981.
163. Machencourt, J., Denis, B., Wolf, J., et al.: Sensibilite et specificite respective de la scintigraphie myocardie realisee apres injection de thallium-201 au course de l'effort, apres injection de dipyridamole et au repos: Comparison chez 70 subjects coronarographies. Arch. Mal. Coeur. 74:147, 1981.
164. Wilde, P., Walke, P., Watt, I., et al.: Thallium myocardial imaging: Recent experience using a coronary vasodilator. Clin. Radiol. 33:43, 1982.
165. Ando, J., Yasuda, H., Kobayashi, T., et al.: Conditions for "coronary steal" caused by coronary vasodilator in man. Jpn. Heart J. 23:79, 1982.
166. Francisco, D., Collins, S., Go, R., et al.: Tomographic thallium-201 myocardial perfusion scintigrams after maximal coronary artery vasodilation with intravenous dipyridamole: Comparison of qualitative and quantitative approaches. Circulation 66:370, 1982.
167. Harris, D., Taylor, D., Condon, B., et al.: Myocardial imaging with dipyridamole: Comparison of the sensitivity and specificity of 201-Tl versus MUGA. Eur. J. Nucl. Med. 7:1, 1982.
168. Sochor, H., Pachiger, O., Ogris, E., et al.: Radionuclide imaging after coronary vasodilation: Myocardial scintigraphy with thallium-201 and radionuclide angiography after administration of dipyridamole. Eur. Heart 5:500, 1984.
169. Demangeat, J., and Wolff, F.: Redistribution of Tl-201 after myocardial scintigraphy with dipyridamole: Value in the detection of coronary stenosis and ventricular kinetic anomalies. Arch. Mal. Coeur 78:1902, 1985.
170. Laarman, G., Verzijlbergen, J., and Ascoop, C.: Ischemic ST-segment changes after dipyridamole infusion. Int. J. Cardiol. 14:384, 1987.
171. Lam, J., Chaitman, B., Glaenzer, M., et al.: Safety and diagnostic accuracy of dipyridamole-thallium imaging in the elderly. J. Am. Coll. Cardiol. 11:585, 1988.
172. Schmoliner, R., Dudczak, R., Kronik, G., et al.: Thallium-201 imaging after dipyridamole in patients with coronary multivessel disease. Cardiology 70:145, 1983.
173. Okada, R., Lim, Y., Rothendler, J., et al.: Split-dose thallium-201 dipyridamole imaging: A new technique for obtaining thallium images before and immediately after an intervention. J. Am. Coll. Cardiol. 1:1302, 1983.
174. Walker, P., James, M., Wilde, R., et al.: Dipyridamole combined with exercise for thallium-201 myocardial imaging. Br. Heart J. 55:321, 1986.
175. Pennell, D., Underwood, S., Swanton, R., et al.: Dobutamine thallium myocardial perfusion tomography. J. Am. Coll. Cardiol. 18:1471, 1991.
176. Kiat, H., Maddahi, J., Roy, L., et al.: Comparison of technetium-99m methoxy isobutyl isonitrile and thallium-201 for evaluation of coronary artery disease by planar and tomographic methods. Am. Heart J. 117:1, 1989.
177. Taillefer, R., Lambert, R., Dupras, G., et al.: Clinical comparison between thallium-201 and Tc-99m methoxy isobutyl isonitrile (hexamibi) myocardial perfusion imaging for detection of coronary artery disease. Eur. J. Nucl. Med. 15:280, 1989.
178. Maisey, M., Lowry, A., Bischof-Delaloye, A., et al.: European multi-centre comparison of thallium-201 and technetium-99m methoxisobutylisonitrile in ischemic heart disease. Eur. J. Nucl. Med. 16:869, 1990.
179. Maddahi, J., Kiat, H., Van Train, K., et al.: Myocardial perfusion imaging with technetium-99m sestamibi SPECT in the evaluation of coronary artery disease. Am. J. Cardiol. 66:55E, 1990.
180. Dupont. Data on File.
181. Iskandrian, A., Heo, J., Kong, B., et al.: Use of technetium-99m isonitrile (RP-30A) in assessing left ventricular perfusion and function at rest and during exercise in coronary artery disease, and comparison with coronary arteriography and exercise thallium-201 SPECT imaging. Am. J. Cardiol. 64:270, 1989.
182. Larock, M., Cantineau, R., Legrand, V., et al.: 99mTc-MIBI (RP-30) to define the extent of myocardial ischemia and evaluate ventricular function. Eur. J. Nucl. Med. 16:223, 1990.
183. Diagnostics: Squibb. Data on File.
184. Hendel, R., McSherry, B., Karimeddini, M., et al.: Diagnostic utility of a new Tc-99m myocardial imaging agent (SQ30217) utilizing a rapid imaging protocol. J. Nucl. Med. 70:730, 1989.
185. Friedman, J., Kiat, H., Beitendorf, J., et al.: Validation and preliminary application of simultaneous treadmill exercise ejection fraction and myocardial perfusion scintigraphy. Circulation 82:321, 1990.
186. Ziffer, J., La Pidus, A., Alazraki, N., et al.: Predictive value of systolic wall thickening for myocardial viability assessed by Tc-99m sestamibi using a count based algorithm. (Abstract.) J. Am. Coll. Cardiol. 17:251A, 1991.
187. Kahn, J., McGhei, I., Faber, T., et al.: Assessment of myocardial viability with technetium-99m-2-methoxy isobutylisonitrile (MIBI) and gated tomography in patients with coronary artery disease. (Abstract.) J. Am. Coll. Cardiol. 13:31A, 1989.
188. Maddahi, J., Prigent, F., Garcia, E., et al.: Validation of newly developed attenuation and scatter correction methods of quantitating myocardial perfusion by Tc-99 sestamibi SPECT. Circulation 82:64, 1990.
189. Cullom, S., Galt, J., Maddahi, J., et al.: Scatter and attenuation correction of SPECT Tc-99m sestamibi myocardial distributions: Experimental validation of the effect on uniformity and contrast. J. Nucl. Med. 32:1067, 1991.
190. Diamond, G., and Forrester, J.: Analysis of probability as an aid in the clinical diagnosis of coronary artery disease. N. Engl. J. Med. 300:1350, 1979.
191. Uhl, G., Kay, T., Hickman, J., et al.: Detection of coronary artery disease in asymptomatic aircrew members with thallium-201 scintigraphy. Aviat. Environ. Med. 51:1250, 1980.
192. Diamond, G., Forrester, J., Hirsch, M., et al.: Application of conditional probability analysis to the clinical diagnosis of coronary artery disease. J. Clin. Invest. 65:1210, 1980.
193. Dans, P., Weiner, J., Melin, J., et al.: Conditional probability in the diagnosis of coronary artery disease: A future tool for eliminating unnecessary testing. South. Med. J. 76:1118, 1983.
194. Christopher, T., Konstantinow, G., and Jones, R.: Incremental value of clinical assessment, supine exercise electrocardiography and biplane exercise radionuclide ventriculography in the prediction of coronary artery disease in men with chest pain. Am. J. Cardiol. 52:927, 1983.
195. Currie, P., Kelly, M., Harper, R., et al.: Incremental value of clinical assessment, supine exercise electrocardiography and biplane exercise radionuclide ventriculography in the prediction of coronary artery disease in men with chest pain. Am. J. Cardiol. 52:927, 1983.
196. McLaughlin, P., Martin, R., Doherty, P., et al.: Reproducibility of Tl-201 myocardial imaging. Circulation 55:497, 1977.
197. Rehn, T., Griffith, L., Aschuff, S., et al.: Exercise Tl-201 myocardial imaging in left main coronary artery disease: Sensitive but not specific. Am. J. Cardiol. 28:217, 1981.
198. Maddahi, J., Van Train, K., Wong, C., et al.: Comparison of Tl-201 SPECT and planar imaging for evaluation of coronary artery disease: Sensitive but not specific. J. Nucl. Med. 27:999, 1986.
199. Brown, K., and Rowen, M.: Prognostic value of a normal exercise myocardial perfusion imaging study in patients with angiographically significant coronary artery disease. Am. J. Cardiol. 71:865, 1993.
200. Maddahi, J., Abdulla, A., Garcia, E., et al.: Noninvasive identification of left main and triple-vessel coronary artery disease: Improved accuracy using quantitative analysis of regional myocardial stress distribution and washout of Tl-201. J. Am. Coll. Cardiol. 7:53, 1986.
201. Patterson, R., Horowitz, S., Eng, C., et al.: Can noninvasive exercise test criteria identify patients with left main or 3-vessel coronary disease after a first myocardial infarction? Am. J. Cardiol. 51:361, 1983.
202. Abdulla, A., Maddahi, J., Garcia, E., et al.: Slow regional clearance of myocardial Tl-201 in the absence of perfusion defect: Contribution to detection of individual coronary stenosis and mechanism for occurrence. Circulation 71:72, 1985.
203. Bateman, T., Maddahi, J., Gray, F., et al.: Diffuse slow washout of myocardial thallium-201: A new scintigraphic indicator of extensive coronary artery disease. J. Am. Coll. Cardiol. 4:55, 1984.
204. Ladenheim, M., Pollack, B., Rozanski, A., et al.: Extent and severity of myocardial hypoperfusion as predictors of prognosis in patients with suspected coronary artery disease. J. Am. Coll. Cardiol. 7:464, 1986.
205. Gibson, R., Watson, D., Carabello, B., et al.: Clinical implications of increased lung uptake of Tl-201 during exercise scintigraphy 2 weeks after myocardial infarction. Am. J. Cardiol. 49:1586, 1982.
206. Bingham, J., McKusick, K., Strauss, H., et al.: Influence of coronary artery disease on pulmonary uptake of Tl-201. Am. J. Cardiol. 46:821, 1980.
207. Kushner, F., Okada, R., Kirschenbaum, H., et al.: Lung Tl-201 uptake after stress testing in patients with coronary artery disease. Circulation 63:341, 1981.
208. Levy, R., Rozanski, A., Berman, D., et al.: Analysis of the degree of pulmonary thallium washout after exercise in patients with coronary artery disease. J. Am. Coll. Cardiol. 2:719, 1983.
209. Weiss, A., Berman, D., Lew, A., et al.: Transient ischemic dilation of the left ventricle on stress thallium-201 scintigraphy: A marker of severe and extensive coronary artery disease. J. Am. Coll. Cardiol. 9:752, 1987.
210. Stolzenberg, J.: Dilation of the left ventricular cavity on stress thallium scan as an indicator of ischemic disease. Clin. Nucl. Med. 5:289, 1980.
211. Chouraqui, P., Rodrigues, E., Berman, D., et al.: Significance of dipyridamole-induced transient dilation of the left ventricle during thallium-201 scintigraphy in suspected coronary artery disease. Am. J. Cardiol. 66:689, 1990.
212. Kaul, S., Finkelstein, D., Homma, S., et al.: Superiority of quantitative exercise thallium-201 variables in determining long-term prognosis in ambulatory patient with chest pain: A comparison with cardiac catheterization. J. Am. Coll. Cardiol. 12:25, 1988.
213. Kaul, S., Lilly, D., Gasho, J., et al.: Prognostic utility of the exercise thallium-201 test in ambulatory patients with chest pain: Comparison with cardiac catheterization. Circulation 77:745, 1988.
214. Pollack, S., Abbott, R., Boucher, C., et al.: Independent and incremental prognostic value of tests performed in hierarchial order to evaluate patients with suspected coronary artery disease. Circulation 85:237, 1992.
215. Epstein, S., Palmeri, S., and Patterson, E.: Evaluation of patients after acute myocardial infarction: Indications for cardiac catheterization and surgical intervention. N. Engl. J. Med. 307:1487, 1982.
216. Gibson, R., Watson, D., Craddock, G., et al.: Prediction of cardiac events after uncomplicated myocardial infarction: A prospective study comparing predischarge exercise thallium-201 scintigraphy and coronary angiography. Circulation 68:321, 1983.
217. Gimple, L., and Beller, G.: Assessing prognosis after acute myocardial infarction in the thrombolytic era. J. Nucl. Cardiol. 1:198, 1994.
218. Haber, H., Beller, G., Watson, D., et al.: Exercise thallium-201 scintigraphy after thrombolytic therapy with or without angioplasty for acute myocardial infarction. Am. J. Cardiol. 71:1257, 1993.
219. Gibson, R., Beller, G., Gheorghiade, M., et al.: The prevalence and clinical significance of residual myocardial ischemia 2 weeks after uncomplicated non-Q-wave myocardial infarction: A prospective natural history study. Circulation 73:1186, 1986.

220. Brown, K., Weiss, R., Clements, J., et al.: Usefulness of residual ischemic myocardium within prior infarct zone for identifying patients at high risk late after acute myocardial infarction. Am. J. Cardiol. 60:15, 1987.
221. Wilson, W., Gibson, R., Nygaard, T., et al.: Acute myocardial infarction associated with single-vessel coronary artery disease: An analysis of clinical outcome and the prognostic importance of vessel patency and residual ischemic myocardium. J. Am. Coll. Cardiol. 11:223, 1988.
222. Leppo, J., O'Brien, J., Rothendler, J., et al.: Dipyridamole-thallium-201 scintigraphy in the prediction of future cardiac events after acute myocardial infarction. N. Engl. J. Med. 310:1014, 1984.
223. Younis, L., Byers, S., Shaw, L., et al.: Prognostic value of intravenous dipyridamole thallium scintigraphy after an acute myocardial ischemic event. Am. J. Cardiol. 64:161, 1989.
224. Gimple, L., Hutter, A., Guiney, T., et al.: Prognostic utility of predischarge dipyridamole-thallium imaging compared to predischarge submaximal exercise thallium imaging after uncomplicated acute myocardial infarction. Am. J. Cardiol. 64:1243, 1989.
225. Brown, K., O'Meara, J., Chambers, C., et al.: Ability of dipyridamole-thallium-201 imaging one to four days after acute myocardial infarction to predict in-hospital and late recurrent myocardial ischemic events. Am. J. Cardiol. 65:160, 1990.
226. Mahmarian, J., Cochran, A., Marks, G., et al.: Models for predicting long-term outcome after acute myocardial infarction by quantitative adenosine tomography. J. Nucl. Med. 34:54P, 1993.
227. Wackers, F., Lie, K., Liem, K., et al.: Thallium-201 scintigraphy in unstable angina pectoris. Circulation 57:738, 1978.
228. Parodi, O., Uthurralt, N., Severi, S., et al.: Transient reduction of regional myocardial perfusion during angina at rest with ST segment depression or normalization of negative T waves. Circulation 63:1238, 1981.
229. Bilodeau, L., Theroux, P., Gregoire, J., et al.: Technetium-99m-sestamibi tomography in patients with spontaneous chest pain: Correlations with clinical, electrocardiographic, and angiographic findings. J. Am. Coll. Cardiol. 18:1684, 1991.
230. Hilton, T., Thompson, R., Williams, H., et al.: Technetium-99m sestamibi myocardial perfusion imaging in the emergency room evaluation of chest pain. J. Am. Coll. Cardiol. 23:1016, 1994.
231. Brown, K.: Prognostic value of thallium-201 myocardial perfusion imaging in patients with unstable angina who respond to medical treatment. J. Am. Coll. Cardiol. 17:1053, 1991.
232. Hertzer, N., Beren, B., Young, J., et al.: Coronary artery disease in peripheral vascular patients: A classification of 1000 coronary angiograms and results of surgical management. Ann. Surg. 199:223, 1984.
233. Mangano, D., Browner, W., Hollenberg, M., et al.: Association of perioperative myocardial ischemia with cardiac morbidity and mortality in men undergoing noncardiac surgery. The Study of Perioperative Ischemia Research Group. N. Engl. J. Med. 323:1781, 1990.
234. Boucher, C., Brewster, D., Darling, R., et al.: Determination of cardiac risk by dipyridamole-thallium imaging before peripheral vascular surgery. N. Engl. J. Med. 312:389, 1985.
235. Brown, K., and Rowen, M.: Extent of jeopardized viable myocardium determined by myocardial perfusion imaging best predicts perioperative cardiac events in patients undergoing noncardiac surgery. J. Am. Coll. Cardiol. 21:325, 1993.
236. Levinson, J., Boucher, C., Coley, C., et al.: Usefulness of semiquantitative analysis of dipyridamole thallium-201 redistribution for improving risk stratification before vascular surgery. Am. J. Cardiol. 66:406, 1990.
237. Lette, J., Waters, D., Bernier, H., et al.: Preoperative and long-term cardiac risk assessment: Predictive value of 23 clinical descriptors, 7 multivariate scoring systems, and quantitative dipyridamole imaging in 360 patients. Ann. Surg. 216:192, 1992.
238. Coley, C., Field, T., Abraham, S., et al.: Usefulness of dipyridamole-thallium scanning for preoperative evaluation of cardiac risk for nonvascular surgery. Am. J. Cardiol. 69:1280, 1992.
239. Hendel, R., Whitfield, S., Villegas, B., et al.: Prediction of late cardiac events by dipyridamole thallium imaging in patients undergoing elective vascular surgery. Am. J. Cardiol. 70:1243, 1992.
240. Camp, A., Garvin, P., Hoff, J., et al.: Prognostic value of intravenous dipyridamole thallium imaging in patients with diabetes mellitus considered for renal transplantation. Am. J. Cardiol. 65:1459, 1990.
241. Lane, S., Lewis, S., Pippin, J., et al.: Predictive value of quantitative dipyridamole-thallium scintigraphy in assessing cardiovascular risk after vascular surgery in diabetes mellitus. Am. J. Cardiol. 64:1275, 1989.
242. Eagle, K., Singer, D., Brewster, D., et al.: Dipyridamole-thallium scanning in patients undergoing vascular surgery: Optimizing preoperative evaluation of cardiac risk. JAMA 257:2185, 1987.
243. Sachs, R., Tellier, P., Larmignat, P., et al.: Assessment by dipyridamole-thallium-201 myocardial scintigraphy of coronary risk before peripheral vascular surgery. Surgery 103:584, 1988.
244. Eagle, K., Coley, C., Newell, J., et al.: Combining clinical and thallium data optimizes preoperative assessment of cardiac risk before major vascular surgery. Ann. Intern. Med. 110:859, 1989.
245. Kelly, J., Forster, A., Higley, B., et al.: Technetium-99m-tetrofosmin as a new radiopharmaceutical for myocardial perfusion imaging. J. Nucl. Med. 34:222, 1993.
246. Taillefer, R., Lambert, R., Essiambre, R., et al.: Comparison between thallium-201, technetium-99m sestamibi and technetium-99m teboroxime planar myocardial perfusion imaging in detection of coronary artery disease. J. Nucl. Med. 33:1091, 1992.
247. Higley, B., Smith, F., Smith, T., et al.: Technetium-99m-1,2-bis[bis(2-ethoxyethyl) phosphino]ethane: Human biodistribution, dosimetry and safety of a new myocardial perfusion imaging agent. J. Nucl. Med. 34:30, 1993.
248. Jain, D., Wackers, F., Mattera, J., et al.: Biokinetics of technetium-99m-tetrofosmin: Myocardial perfusion imaging agent: Implications for a one-day imaging protocol. J. Nucl. Med. 34:1254, 1993.
249. Dahlberg, S., Gilmore, M., and Leppo, J.: Effect of coronary blood flow on the "uptake" of tetrofosmin in the isolated rabbit heart. (Abstract.) J. Nucl. Med. 33:846, 1992.
250. Sinusas, A., Shi, Q., Saltzberg, M., et al.: Technetium-99m-tetrofosmin to assess myocardial blood flow: Experimental validation in an intact canine model of ischemia. J. Nucl. Med. 35:664, 1994.
251. Lahiri, A., Higley, B., Crawley, J., et al.: Novel functionalized diphosphine complexes of Tc-99m for myocardial imaging in man. J. Nucl. Med. 30:818, 1989.
252. Braat, S., Leclercq, B., Itti, R., et al.: Myocardial imaging with technetium-99m-tetrofosmin: Comparison of one-day and two-day protocols. J. Nucl. Med. 35:1581, 1994.
253. Zaret, B., Rigo, P., Wackers, F., et al.: Myocardial perfusion imaging with 99mTc tetrofosmin. Comparison to Tl-201 imaging and coronary angiography in a phase III multicenter trial. Circulation 91:313, 1995.
254. Tamaki, N., Takahashi, N., Kawamoto, M., et al.: Myocardial tomography using technetium-99m-tetrofosmin to evaluate coronary artery disease. J. Nucl. Med. 35:594, 1994.
255. Deutsche, E., Vanderheyden, J-L., Gerundini, P., et al.: Development of nonreducible technetium-99m(III) cations as myocardial perfusion imaging agents: Initial experience in humans. J. Nucl. Med. 28:1870, 1987.
256. De Rosch, M., Brodack, J., Grummon, G., et al.: Kit development for the Tc-99m myocardial imaging agent TechneCard. (Abstract.) J. Nucl. Med. 33:850, 1992.
257. Gerson, M., Millard, R., Roszelli, N., et al.: Kinetic properties of Tc-99m Q12 in dogs. Circulation 89:1291, 1994.
258. Rossetti, C., Best, T., Paganelli, G., et al.: Evaluation of a new nonreducible 99m-Tc(III) myocardial perfusion tracer: Biodistribution and initial clinical experience. (Abstract.) J. Nucl. Med. 34:223, 1990.
259. Rossetti, C., Vanoli, G., Paganelli, G., et al.: Evaluation in humans of a new tracer with optimized properties for myocardial perfusion imaging: [Tc-99m] Q12. (Abstract.) Eur. J. Nucl. Med. 18:540, 1991.
260. Gerson, M., Lukes, J., Deutsch, E., et al.: Comparison of technetium-99m-Q3 and Tl-201 for detection of coronary disease in man. J. Nucl. Med. 35:580, 1994.
261. Tartagni, F., Dondi, M., Limonetti, P., et al.: Dipyridamole technetium-99m-2-methoxy isobutyl isonitrile tomoscintigraphic imaging for identifying diseased coronary vessels: Comparison with thallium-201 stress-rest study. J. Nucl. Med. 32:369, 1991.
262. Pamelia, F., Gibson, R., Wason, D., et al.: Prognosis with chest pain and normal thallium-201 exercise scintigrams. Am. J. Cardiol. 55:920, 1985.
263. Wackers, F., Russo, D.J., Russo, D., et al.: Prognostic significance of normal quantitative planar thallium-201 stress scintigraphy in patients with chest pain. J. Am. Coll. Cardiol. 6:27, 1985.
264. Staniloff, H., Forrester, J., Berman, D., et al.: Prediction of death, myocardial infarction, worsening chest pain using thallium scintigraphy and exercise electrocardiography. J. Nucl. Med. 27:1842, 1986.
265. Gammage, M., Murray, D., Rafiqi, E., et al.: The clinical role of thallium-201 scintigraphy in the management and prognosis of coronary artery disease. Eur. Heart J. 7:412, 1986.
266. Heo, J., Thompson, W., and Iskandrian, A.: Prognostic implications of normal exercise thallium images. Am. J. Noninvas. Cardiol. 1:209, 1987.
267. Gill, J., Ruddy, T., Newell, J., et al.: Prognostic importance of thallium uptake by the lungs during exercise in coronary artery disease. N. Engl. J. Med. 317:1486, 1987.
268. Koss, J., Kobren, S., Grunwald, A., et al.: Role of exercise thallium-201 myocardial perfusion scintigraphy in predicting prognosis in suspected coronary artery disease. Am. J. Cardiol. 59:531, 1987.
269. Bairey, C., Rozanski, A., Maddahi, J., et al.: Exercise thallium-201 scintigraphy and prognosis in typical angina pectoris and negative exercise electrocardiography. Am. J. Cardiol. 64:282, 1989.
270. Fleg, J., Gerstenblith, G., Zonderman, A., et al.: Prevalence and prognostic significance of exercise induced silent myocardial ischemia detected by thallium scintigraphy and electrocardiography in asymptomatic volunteers. Circulation 81:428, 1990.
271. Brown, K., Altland, E., and Rowen, M.: Prognostic value of normal Tc-99m sestamibi myocardial perfusion imaging. J. Nucl. Med. 35:554, 1994.
272. Oosterhuis, W., Breeman, A., Niemeyer, M., et al.: Patients with a normal exercise thallium-201 myocardial scintigram: Always a good prognosis? Eur. J. Nucl. Med. 20:151, 1993.

CHAPTER

64 Myocardial Imaging for the Assessment of Myocardial Viability

George A. Beller, M.D.

INTRODUCTION

Myocardial systolic dysfunction characterized by absence of wall thickening can occur despite preservation of myocardial metabolism and cell membrane integrity. Severe regional dysfunction that leads to a depression of left ventricular ejection fraction (LVEF) can result from either myocardial necrosis, myocardial stunning, or hibernating myocardium. Assessment of left ventricular function alone, with techniques such as contrast ventriculography, echocardiography, radionuclide angiography, or magnetic resonance imaging, cannot distinguish among these three mechanisms of reduced contractile function. An accurate noninvasive determination of myocardial viability that can differentiate irreversible myocardial cellular injury from myocardial stunning or hibernation is critically important for clinical decision-making. It allows for the selection of patients with coronary artery disease (CAD) and resting left ventricular dysfunction who can most benefit from revascularization strategies. Results of clinical trials comparing the outcome of patients undergoing bypass operation with those being medically treated have demonstrated that patients with extensive multivessel CAD and depressed LVEF benefit most from revascularization, even if anginal symptoms are minimal or absent.[1] However, patients with extensive CAD and a profound depression in ejection fraction can experience improvement in function and amelioration of heart failure symptoms only if revascularization results in improvement in regional and global cardiac function. Only zones of asynergy that are viable but chronically hypoperfused should benefit from revascularization with improvement in function; areas of asynergy that reflect extensive necrosis should not be expected to improve with enhanced regional and global function. Many surgeons are reluctant to perform coronary bypass operation in patients with severe left ventricular dysfunction, particularly in the presence of associated comorbidities and less than optimum coronary angiographic findings for successful revascularization (e.g., small distal vessels, diffuse CAD). Demonstration of myocardial viability in asynergic regions in such patients would provide reassurance to the surgeon that a technically-successful revascularization procedure would have as its outcome improved global function, reduction in heart failure symptoms (if present), and enhanced survival with improved quality of life.

Detection of viability in noncontracting myocardium may be important in the decision-making process regarding the need for coronary angioplasty in patients with an acute myocardial infarction. Patients treated with thrombolytic therapy for acute infarction may have significant salvage of myocardium that is not apparent early after reperfusion on either contrast ventriculography, echocardiography, or radionuclide angiography. Demonstration of substantial viability in these reperfused but stunned regions could obviate the need for urgent referral for angiography and angioplasty because spontaneous recovery of function would be predicted. However, if resting or stress-induced ischemia were evident within or remote from the infarct zone in such patients by demonstration of reversible perfusion defects and substantial tracer uptake at rest, then an invasive strategy would be appropriate.

This chapter discusses the various radionuclide approaches to the assessment of myocardium viability that employ single-photon tracers and conventional planar or gamma camera imaging. The value of positron emission tomographic (PET) imaging of myocardial blood flow and metabolism for assessment of viability is discussed in detail in Chapter 71.

STUNNED AND HIBERNATING MYOCARDIUM

The term, "stunned myocardium," was first introduced by Braunwald and Kloner in 1982.[2] Myocardial stunning implies a reversible form of contractile dysfunction that occurs after restoration of coronary blood flow following a relatively brief period of transient myocardial ischemia (e.g., 15 minutes).[3] Return of function after myocardial stunning is usually slow, taking days to weeks. Stunning can also be seen after multiple transient flow diminutions, in which each period of flow cessation rarely exceeds 5 minutes.[4]

The precise pathophysiology of the stunning phenomenon is not completely comprehended. Proposed mechanisms include impairment of myocardial energy production,[5] impairment of transfer of energy into contraction of myocytes,[6, 7] ischemic damage to sympathetic nerves,[8] altered calcium sensitivity at the myofilament level,[9] intracellular calcium overload,[10, 11] microvascular dysfunction caused by obstruction of capillaries by neutrophils,[12] ischemic damage to the extracellular collagen matrix,[13] and detrimental effects of free radicals that result in myocardial membrane injury.[14] Certain clinical correlates of stunned myocardium include transient left ventricular dysfunction after thrombolytic therapy or direct angioplasty in acute myocardial infarction[15, 16]; repetitive episodes of coronary flow diminution in patients with unstable angina, possibly caused by coronary vasospasm or cyclic obstruction by intraluminal platelet or erythrocyte-rich thrombi[17, 18]; and occurrence immediately after exercise-induced myocardial ischemia.[19]

Several groups have shown gradual improvement in regional systolic function in the infarct zone in patients treated with either intracoronary or intravenous thrombolytic therapy.[16, 20] Touchstone and colleagues[21] from the University of Virginia evaluated regional systolic function by two-dimensional echocardiography in a group of patients with acute myocardial infarction who had received intravenous streptokinase on admission. Approximately 50 percent of the patients demonstrated an improvement in wall motion in the infarct zone at 10 days. Functional recovery was not evident at 1 to 3 days after admission.

The term "hibernating myocardium" refers to a state of persistently-impaired left ventricular function at rest caused by a chronic reduction in coronary blood flow.[22] By definition, hibernating myocardium implies that if coronary blood flow is enhanced, then ventricular function will improve. Edwards and colleagues[23] from the University of Virginia reported that in the presence of subendocardial hypoperfusion in open-chested dogs and preservation of subepicardial blood flow, transmural myocardial dysfunction can occur (Fig. 64–1). In this animal model, flow was reduced by approximately 50 percent in the distribution of the left anterior descending (LAD) coronary artery. With this flow reduction, epicardial blood flow remained normal, but endocardial blood flow was significantly reduced. Systolic dysfunction was observed in

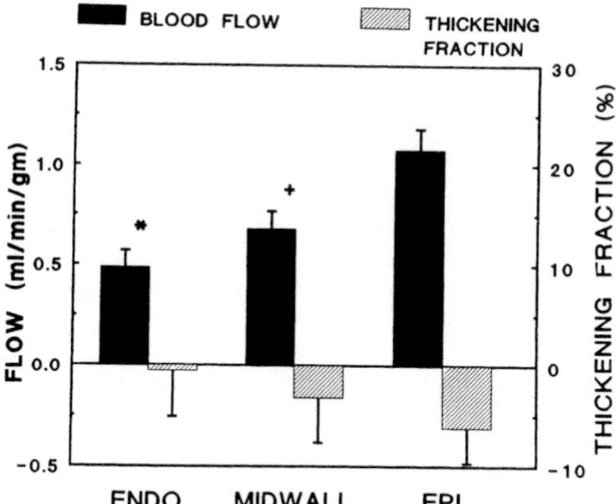

FIGURE 64–1. Transmural distribution of systolic wall thickening (means ± standard error of the mean) in subendocardium (ENDO), midwall, and subepicardium (EPI) in the perfusion zone of the left anterior descending coronary artery during partial stenosis of the vessel in a dog model. Thickening fraction *(crosshatched bars)* was not significantly different among the layers despite relative preservation of blood flow *(solid bar)* to the epicardium. *$P < .01$ versus midwall and EPI; †$P < .001$ versus EPI. (From Edwards, N.C., Sinusas, A.J., Bergin, J.D., et al.: Influence of subendocardial ischemia on transmural myocardial function. Am. J. Physiol. 262:H572, 1992, with permission.)

endocardial, midwall, and epicardial layers with equal severity, although hypoperfusion was confined to the subendocardium (see Fig. 64–1). Systolic thinning, reflecting severe asynergy, was seen in the epicardial layers in this canine model, yet subepicardial blood flow was not reduced. Severe subendocardial hypoperfusion may be a mechanism for hibernation characterized by transmural asynergy. Bolli and colleagues[24] suggest that hibernation may actually be the outcome of repeated episodes of myocardial stunning.

There are some clinical correlates of hibernating myocardium that deserve mention. Several groups have shown that regional and global function improve after revascularization in patients with chronic CAD and no prior evidence of myocardial infarction.[25–28] Topol and co-workers[27] found that improvement in segmental function after coronary bypass operation was greatest in segments that preoperatively exhibited the most severe dysfunction. Similarly, improvement in segmental function has been observed after angioplasty in patients with and without a recent myocardial infarction.[28–31] In one study,[28] wall motion did not improve at 4 days after balloon dilatation of a highly stenotic vessel but did show significant improvement by 5 months after the procedure. As with the stunned myocardial state, the noninvasive demonstration of viability in asynergic hibernating myocardial regions in patients with chronic CAD or after infarction would suggest that coronary revascularization would be of benefit in enhancing cardiac dynamics and improving markers of systolic ventricular performance (global LVEF). Patients who undergo revascularization of segments that are viable but chronically underperfused would have better enhancement of exercise tolerance and improvement in heart failure symptoms than patients who have primarily extensive myocardial scar that is revascularized.

THALLIUM-201 IMAGING FOR DETECTION OF MYOCARDIAL VIABILITY

Experimental Validation

The myocardial uptake and clearance kinetics of ^{201}Tl and other radionuclide tracers employed for assessment of myocardial perfusion and viability have been described by Dahlberg and Leppo in Chapter 62. Thallium-201 is a monovalent cation considered to be a potassium analog. After intravenous injection, the early myocardial distribution of ^{201}Tl is proportional to regional blood flow and the first-pass ^{201}Tl myocardial extraction fraction.[32–37] Under normal resting conditions, approximately 85 percent of an intracoronary dose of ^{201}Tl is extracted by the myocardial tissue on the first pass through the coronary circulation.[33] This avid extraction of ^{201}Tl by cardiac cells yields a high myocardial-to-background ratio of activity, which makes the tracer suitable for myocardial scintigraphy.

Perturbations such as acidosis, hypoxemia, and transient ischemia do not adversely affect the extraction of ^{201}Tl.[34, 38] The extraction of ^{201}Tl is unaltered in canine models of myocardial stunning. Moore and colleagues[39] from our group found that the initial myocardial extraction and subsequent intracellular clearance of ^{201}Tl were unaltered in stunned myocardium of dogs that underwent ten 5-minute periods of total LAD coronary occlusion, each separated by 10 minutes of reperfusion through a critical stenosis. This stunning protocol resulted in a reduction of systolic thickening in the distribution of the LAD to 0.4±2.4 percent in comparison with 32±2 percent thickening in the same region in sham-operated control animals. As shown in Figure 64–2, the first-pass extraction of ^{201}Tl was not significantly reduced despite severe systolic dysfunction in the stunned anterior wall. Both the extraction fraction and the intrinsic ^{201}Tl washout rate were not significantly different in the stunned animals compared with control animals. Sinusas and colleagues[40] also demonstrated preserved ^{201}Tl uptake in stunned myocardium in a model characterized by 15 minutes of total LAD occlusion followed by reperfusion through an entirely patent vessel.

Thallium-201 uptake has been evaluated in canine models of chronic sustained low flow intended to simulate "short-term

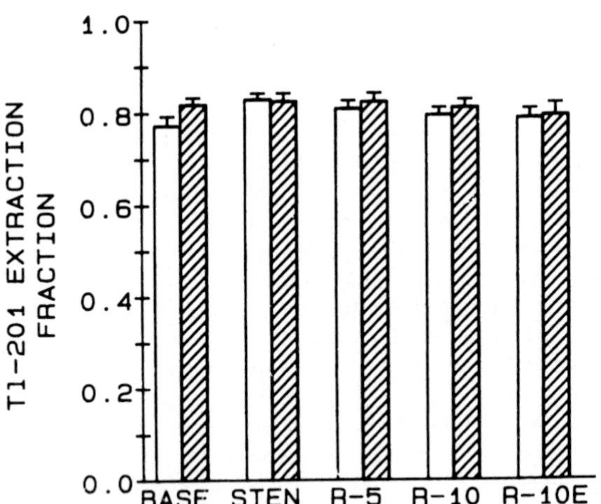

FIGURE 64–2. First-pass ^{201}Tl extraction fraction in stunned *(open bars)* and control *(crosshatched bar)* dogs that underwent ten 5-minute periods of left anterior descending coronary artery occlusions interspersed with 10-minute periods of reflow. BASE = baseline; STEN = stenosis; R-5 = end of fifth reperfusion; R-10 = end of tenth reperfusion; R-10E = 40 minutes after tenth reperfusion. Note that ^{201}Tl extraction fraction is preserved despite akinesis by R-5 which was produced by the stunning protocol (see text). (From Moore, C.A., Cannon, J., Watson, D.D., et al.: Thallium 201 kinetics in stunned myocardium characterized by severe postischemic systolic dysfunction. Circulation 81:1627, 1990, with permission.)

hibernation."[40, 41] If resting baseline flow is reduced by 40 to 50 percent, producing severe regional asynergy, myocardial ^{201}Tl uptake after intravenous injection is preserved. In fact, under such chronic low-flow conditions, ^{201}Tl is observed to demonstrate "rest redistribution."[42] This redistribution is characterized by an initially diminished myocardial uptake of ^{201}Tl with subsequent delayed accumulation or slow washout in the hypoperfused zone, coupled with more rapid ^{201}Tl washout from normally-perfused myocardium. This results in an initial resting ^{201}Tl defect with delayed defect resolution. In contrast, irreversibly damaged myocardial cells cannot concentrate ^{201}Tl intracellularly. Granato and associates[43] from our laboratory produced extensive myocardial necrosis with 3 hours of total LAD occlusion followed by reperfusion in anesthetized dogs. They showed that necrotic myocardium in the LAD risk zone did not take up ^{201}Tl administered after reflow. Goldhaber and co-workers,[44] in a cultured fetal mouse heart preparation, found that accumulation of ^{201}Tl in hearts subjected to an ischemia-like myocardial insult was related in a decreasing fashion to the loss of lactic dehydrogenase.

If myocardial necrosis is present, an initial defect is observed after ^{201}Tl injection, but no delayed ^{201}Tl redistribution can be detected in the region of irreversibly injured myocardial tissue.[42, 45] Regions that demonstrate a mixture of viable and irreversibly-injured myocardium show either partial redistribution or a mild persistent reduction in ^{201}Tl uptake between 1- and 4-hour images.[46] Taken together, this experimental work suggests that the intracellular transport of ^{201}Tl across the sarcolemmal membrane is not significantly impaired until irreversible myocardial cellular injury is present. Postischemic dysfunction causing stunning of the myocardium and chronic underperfusion causing hibernation do not markedly affect ^{201}Tl uptake as long as there is still some preserved microcirculatory flow (i.e., collaterals) to ensure adequate delivery of the radionuclide to the myocardial cell membrane for intracellular transport.

Exercise Scintigraphy and Assessment of Viability

Various approaches have been used to assess ischemia and viability by ^{201}Tl imaging in conjunction with exercise stress testing.[47] These approaches or protocols are summarized in Table 64–1. The basic protocol employed in most laboratories is characterized by imaging 5 minutes after administration of ^{201}Tl during stress to assess the initial distribution of the tracer, and repeat imaging 2.5 to 4 hours later to assess the presence and degree of redistribution or lack thereof.[35] To enhance detection of defect reversibility, some have advocated acquisition of images 24 hours after tracer injection or "reinjection" of a second dose of ^{201}Tl at rest after acquisition of the delayed redistribution images.

Early and 2.5- to 4-Hour Redistribution Imaging

Many clinicians desire to determine simultaneously the degree of jeopardized myocardium provoked under stress conditions and the extent of myocardial viability at rest in patients with CAD who undergo exercise ^{201}Tl scintigraphy. As mentioned, inducible ischemia is identified by the demonstration of reversible perfusion abnormalities from the stress to the resting states, whereas viability is determined by the degree of tracer uptake solely in the resting state or on redistribution images. An initial postexercise ^{201}Tl defect that demonstrates total redistribution on delayed images implies both ischemia and preserved viability.[46] The detection of redistribution on such serial images is enhanced by use of quantitative analysis of either serial planar images or serial single-photon emission computed tomographic (SPECT) images. The quantitative computer-assisted programs employed provide information concerning relative changes in ^{201}Tl activity in ischemic and normal areas. For planar imaging techniques, background must first be subtracted by means of an appropriate interpolative background subtraction algorithm.[48] Some defects that appear persistent on the basis of visual analysis of serial scans demonstrate redistribution when defect count ratios (i.e., the ratio of counts in the area of defect to counts in normal myocardium) are analyzed by quantitative scan analysis.

Approximately 30 to 40 percent of persistent ^{201}Tl defects represent myocardial viability rather than scar. Gibson and associates[46] evaluated 47 patients with CAD who underwent quantitative planar ^{201}Tl scintigraphy before and 4.3 weeks after coronary bypass operation. Ninety-three percent of defects in those patients who demonstrated preoperative total redistribution exhibited normal uptake and washout of ^{201}Tl on postoperative exercise scintigraphy (Fig. 64–3). Seventy-three percent of partial redistributing defects showed enhanced ^{201}Tl uptake and clearance after bypass operation. These investigators found that 45 percent of persistent defects seen on preoperative scans thought to represent scar demonstrated significant improvement in initial ^{201}Tl uptake on postoperative scintigraphic studies. The persistent defects that normalized postoperatively were often mild, demonstrating no more than 25 to 50 percent reduction in ^{201}Tl activity relative to normal region activity preoperatively. Fifty-seven percent of these mild defects demonstrating less than 50 percent reduction in regional counts normalized postoperatively, whereas only 3 of 14 severe persistent defects demonstrating more than 50 percent reduction in regional ^{201}Tl counts showed the same improvement after coronary bypass operation. Figure 64–4 shows that the percentage reduction in regional ^{201}Tl uptake preoperatively in those persistent defects that improved after operation was significantly lower than the percentage reduction in those persistent defects that did not improve. Other investigators also found that a substantial number of persistent ^{201}Tl

TABLE 64–1. APPROACHES TO ASSESSMENT OF MYOCARDIAL VIABILITY WITH MYOCARDIAL THALLIUM-201 PERFUSION IMAGING

1. Stress and 2.5- to 4.0-hour delayed redistribution imaging
2. Stress, 2.5- to 4.0-hour redistribution imaging, and repeat imaging at 18 to 24 hours
3. Stress, 2.5- to 4.0-hour redistribution imaging, and reinjection of a second ^{201}Tl dose at rest (either immediately after acquisition of redistribution images or on the next day)
4. Early and 4.0-hour delayed imaging solely in the resting state

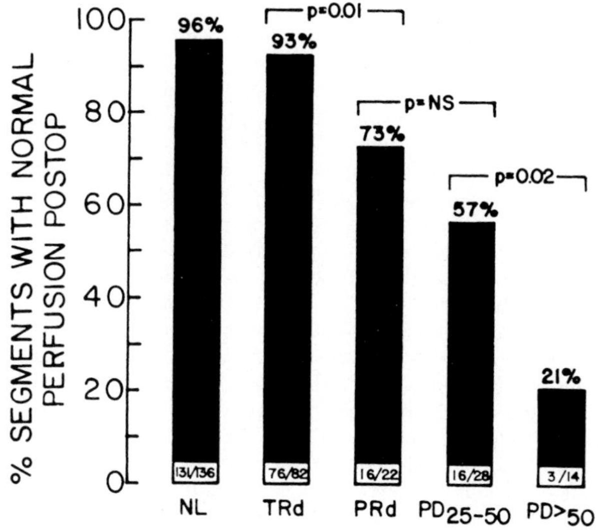

FIGURE 64–3. Relation between preoperative (PREOP) ^{201}Tl perfusion patterns on exercise scintigraphy and the percentage of segments with normal perfusion after coronary bypass operation (POSTOP) based on the type of preoperative segmental perfusion pattern. Data indicate that as preoperative perfusion abnormalities become progressively more severe *(abscissa)*, the probability of restoring ^{201}Tl uptake to normal postoperatively *(ordinate)* becomes progressively lower. NL = normal; TRd = total ^{201}Tl redistribution; PRd = partial ^{201}Tl redistribution; PD_{25-50} = mild persistent defect with 25 to 50 percent of normal uptake; PD $>_{50}$ = severe persistent defect with greater than 50 percent reduction in ^{201}Tl activity; NS = not significant. (From Gibson, R.S., Watson, D.D., Taylor, G.J., et al.: Prospective assessment of regional myocardial perfusion before and after coronary revascularization surgery by quantitative thallium-201 scintigraphy. J. Am. Coll. Cardiol. 1:810, 1983. With permission from the American College of Cardiology.)

defects seen on 3- to 4-hour delayed redistribution images normalize after revascularization.[49–52]

Yamamoto and colleagues[53] demonstrated that improvement in regional wall motion in infarct zones after angioplasty of the infarct-related vessel was more likely to occur if mean ^{201}Tl uptake on redistribution images was more than 50 percent of nonischemic uptake. In zones of greater than 50 percent uptake, mean regional ejection fraction appropriate to the infarct zone increased from 39 percent before angioplasty to 47 percent after angioplasty. In contrast, in zones demonstrating a reduction of more than 50 percent in regional ^{201}Tl activity, the preprocedure regional ejection fraction was 24 percent and did not change after balloon dilatation. Other evidence from the PET literature confirms the observation that some persistent ^{201}Tl defects on redistribution images represent viable but underperfused myocardium.[52] Brunken's study demonstrated enhanced ^{18}F-2,deoxyglucose (FDG) uptake in regions demonstrating a persistent reduction in ^{201}Tl activity from stress to redistribution images.

Late Redistribution Imaging

Redistribution imaging repeated at 18 to 24 hours after ^{201}Tl administration has been recommended to enhance the detection of viability in defects that do not demonstrate redistribution at 2.5 to 4 hours after tracer injection.[51, 54–56] The rationale for late redistribution imaging is that redistribution is an ongoing, kinetic process that depends on continued uptake of ^{201}Tl through recirculation in zones perfused by stenotic lesions and more rapid ^{201}Tl washout in normal myocardial zones.[57] Redistribution also requires some residual blood pool concentration, and that residual activity has been shown to persist for at least 24 hours after tracer injection.

Kiat and co-workers[54] reported that the presence or absence of late ^{201}Tl redistribution at 18 to 24 hours after tracer injection predicted the response to coronary revascularization. They demonstrated that 95 percent of scan segments that showed further relative ^{201}Tl uptake at 18 to 24 hours, compared with the uptake at 4 hours, improved after revascularization, whereas only 37 percent of scan segments that remained persistent at 18 to 24 hours showed similar improvement after either bypass operation or angioplasty.

In another study from the same group at the Cedars-Sinai Medical Center in Los Angeles,[55] the frequency of late redistribution was assessed prospectively in a cohort of 118 patients who underwent serial SPECT exercise ^{201}Tl scintigraphy. Fifty-three percent of patients in this study showed late redistribution in myocardial zones that correlated with persistent reduction in ^{201}Tl uptake on 4-hour redistribution images. Thirty-five percent of patients had late redistribution in two or more segments that appeared persistent on redistribution images. As shown in Figure 64–5, 27 percent of stress defects showed reversibility at 4 hours, and a further 16 percent showed reversibility between 4 and 24 hours.

The potential limitations of 24-hour redistribution imaging for enhancement of viability detection include suboptimal count statistics at 24 hours after ^{201}Tl injection, resulting in reduced image quality; the necessity to ask patients to return 24 hours later; and the inability to prospectively identify which patients may need to return for 24-hour imaging. Our experience has been that most defects that exhibit late redistribution at 24 hours do already demonstrate some evidence for redistribution on 2.5- to 4-hour images if quantitative scan analysis is employed.[58]

Reinjection Thallium-201 Imaging

Another approach to enhancing detection of defect reversibility involves the injection of a second dose of ^{201}Tl at rest, after acquisi-

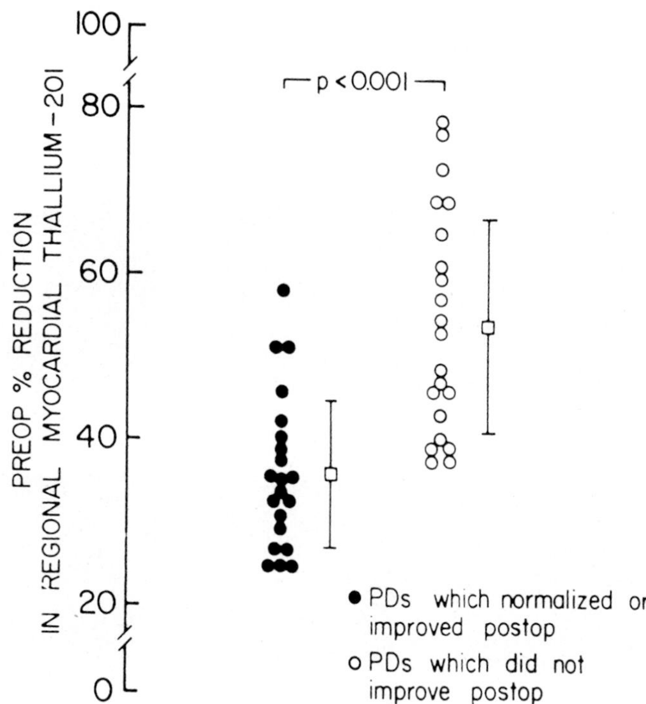

FIGURE 64–4. Percent reduction in regional ^{201}Tl uptake before operation (PREOP) for persistent defects (PDs) that normalized or improved *(solid circles)* compared with those that did not improve after coronary bypass operation *(open circles)*. The percent reduction in regional myocardial ^{201}Tl uptake was significantly less in those persistent defects that normalized or improved after operation. (From Gibson, R.S., Watson, D.D., Taylor, G.J., et al.: Prospective assessment of regional myocardial perfusion before and after coronary revascularization surgery by quantitative thallium-201 scintigraphy. J. Am. Coll. Cardiol. 1:811, 1983. With permission from the American College of Cardiology.)

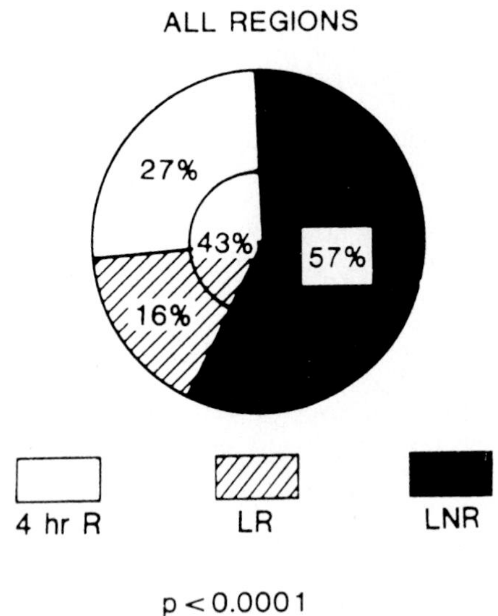

FIGURE 64–5. Comparative frequency of 4-hour reversibility (4 hr R) and late reversibility (LR) in 1047 segments with an initial stress perfusion defect. The *P* value compares the percentage of segments with reversibility at both 4-hour and 24-hour imaging (43%) with the percentage of segments with reversibility at 4-hour imaging alone (27%). LNR = late nonreversibility. (From Yang, L.D., Berman, D.S., Kiat, H., et al.: The frequency of late reversibility in SPECT thallium-201 stress-redistribution studies. J. Am. Coll. Cardiol. 15:337, 1990. With permission from the American College of Cardiology.)

tion of the 2.5- to 4-hour redistribution images, to optimize assessment of defect reversibility.[59–73] This is referred to as the ^{201}Tl "reinjection" technique. With this protocol, 50 percent of the original dose that was administered during stress is reinjected at rest. One of the first studies validating this technique, by Dilsizian and colleagues,[59] employed stress, redistribution, and reinjection SPECT ^{201}Tl scintigraphy in 100 patients with CAD. They found that 33 percent of abnormal segments (85 of 260) demonstrated persistent defects on 3- to 4-hour redistribution images. Approximately half of these demonstrated improved or were normal in ^{201}Tl uptake after reinjection of the second dose of ^{201}Tl. Figure 64–6 shows stress, redistribution, and reinjection tomographic images from a representative patient in this study. Note that ^{201}Tl uptake is enhanced in the anterior wall and septum after reinjection, compared with the redistribution images. These investigators demonstrated that 87 percent (13 of 15) of regions that exhibited enhanced ^{201}Tl uptake on preangioplasty reinjection images in a subgroup of 20 patients showed normal ^{201}Tl uptake and improved segmental wall motion after balloon dilatation. Regions demonstrating no enhanced ^{201}Tl uptake after reinjection preprocedures exhibited both abnormal ^{201}Tl uptake and persistently abnormal regional wall motion after the procedure. Similarly, Ohtani and associates[50] demonstrated that 47 percent (15 of 32) of persistent defects on 3-hour delayed images acquired in 20 patients demonstrated enhanced ^{201}Tl uptake after reinjection. The majority of these persistent defects demonstrated improved perfusion after revascularization as well as improved regional wall motion. Seventy-four percent of segments with preoperative redistribution exhibited improved function, and 71 percent of persistent defects at 3 hours that exhibited enhanced ^{201}Tl uptake after reinjection showed improvement in regional systolic function after revascularization.

Tamaki and co-workers[61] reported on a series of 60 patients with CAD who demonstrated improved ^{201}Tl uptake after reinjection of the tracer in 32 segments that had exhibited a persistent reduction in ^{201}Tl activity on SPECT redistribution images. In this study, 29 percent of patients with persistent defects and no evidence of redistribution in any segment on 3- to 4-hour delayed images showed enhanced ^{201}Tl uptake after reinjection. In this subset of patients, the reinjection protocol was the only way to demonstrate preserved viability.

Dilsizian and associates[62] investigated which persistent defects on redistribution ^{201}Tl imaging would most likely show enhanced

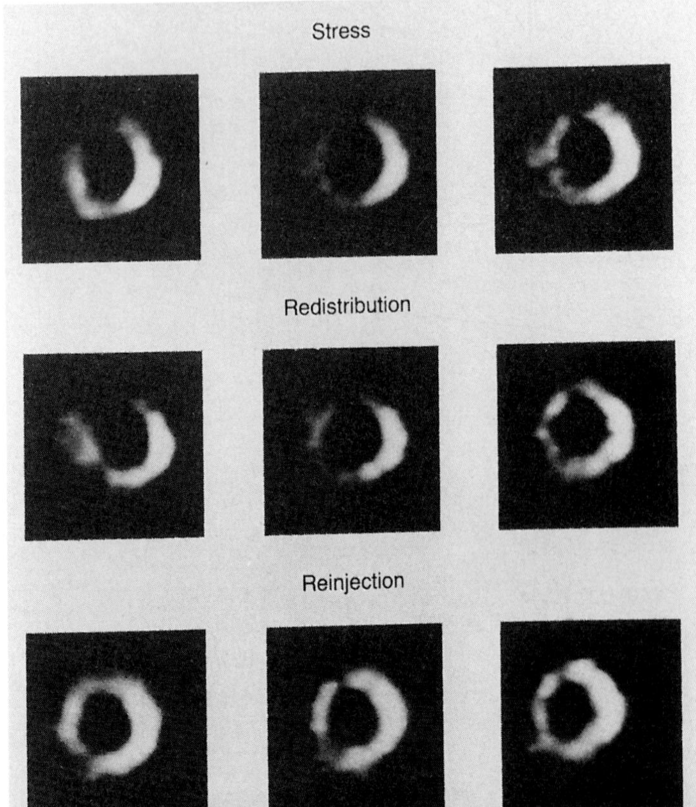

FIGURE 64–6. Stress, redistribution, and reinjection tomographic ^{201}Tl images demonstrating enhanced ^{201}Tl uptake in the anterior wall and septum after reinjection. (From Dilsizian, V., Rocco, T.P., Freedman, N.M., et al.: Enhanced detection of ischemic but viable myocardium by the reinjection of thallium after stress-redistribution imaging. N. Engl. J. Med. 323:143, 1990, with permission. Copyright 1990, Massachusetts Medical Society.)

^{201}Tl uptake after reinjection. Mild-to-moderate (51 to 85 percent of normal activity) persistent defects were more likely to show an increase in absolute ^{201}Tl activity after reinjection than the more severe persistent defects (i.e., those showing less than 50 percent of normal activity). These data are consistent with our findings,[46] in which mild persistent defects showing no more than 50 percent reduction in ^{201}Tl counts, relative to normal region counts, had the greatest likelihood of demonstrating improved ^{201}Tl uptake and systolic function after revascularization.

Some investigators have correlated findings on ^{201}Tl reinjection imaging with PET imaging in the same patients. Theoretically, ^{201}Tl uptake at redistribution or after reinjection should correlate well with preserved myocardial metabolism, because monovalent cation uptake is dependent on an intact sarcolemmal membrane and normal sodium pump activity. Bonow and colleagues[65] compared ^{201}Tl reinjection imaging to PET imaging with FDG in the same patients. FDG uptake was observed in 94 percent of defects on conventional postexercise imaging that corresponded to complete or partial ^{201}Tl redistribution. Fifty-one percent of the persistent defects demonstrated enhanced ^{201}Tl uptake after reinjection. The same percentage of these defects demonstrated preserved FDG uptake. Detection of myocardial viability in these persistent defects by the two techniques was concordant in 88 percent of segments. The authors concluded that ^{201}Tl reinjection provided the same predictive information with respect to viability as FDG imaging with PET in patients with CAD and regional left ventricular dysfunction. Mild persistent defects were shown to have a high prevalence of myocardial viability by FDG criteria. Mild defects on serial SPECT images were defined as 60 to 84 percent of peak activity, moderate defects as 50 to 59 percent of peak activity, and severe defects as less than 50 percent of peak activity. FDG uptake was seen in 91 percent of mild, 84 percent of moderate, and 51 percent of severe persistent defects. There was a greater percentage of FDG uptake in severe persistent defects that showed enhanced ^{201}Tl uptake with reinjection compared with those that did not. Therefore, the "absolute" level of ^{201}Tl activity in persistent defects can be used as an index to predict presence of viable myocardium.

Perrone-Filardi et al[66] compared magnetic resonance imaging (MRI) with ^{201}Tl and PET imaging in the same patients. They found that only regions with severe irreversible defects showed absence of thickening on gated MRI scanning (Fig. 64–7). In that study, the percentage of regions showing FDG uptake was similar

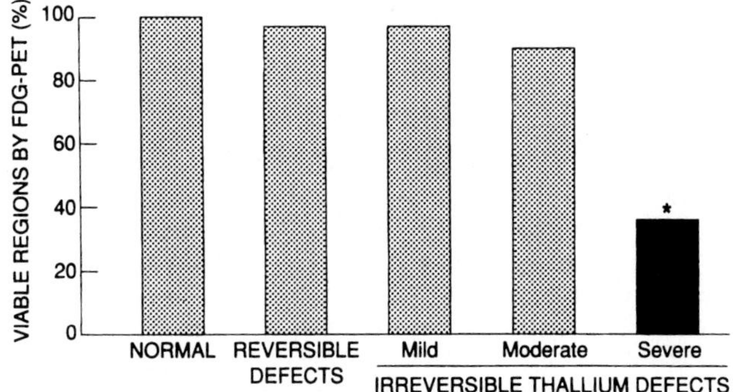

FIGURE 64–7. Percent of viable regions as determined by positron emission tomographic (PET) imaging of ^{18}F-2,deoxyglucose (FDG) uptake related to the type of ^{201}Tl single-photon emission computed tomographic (SPECT) defects on stress-redistribution imaging. The percent of regions showing presence of FDG uptake was similar among regions with normal ^{201}Tl uptake, reversible ^{201}Tl defects, and mild-or-moderate irreversible defects at redistribution imaging. Sixty-four percent of regions with severe ^{201}Tl defects showed absence of FDG uptake. *$P < .01$ compared with all other groups of regions. (From Perrone-Filardi, P., Bacharach, S.L., Dilsizian, V., et al.: Regional left ventricular wall thickening. Related to regional uptake of ^{18}fluorodeoxyglucose and ^{201}Tl in patients with chronic coronary artery disease and left ventricular dysfunction. Circulation 86:1133, 1992, with permission.)

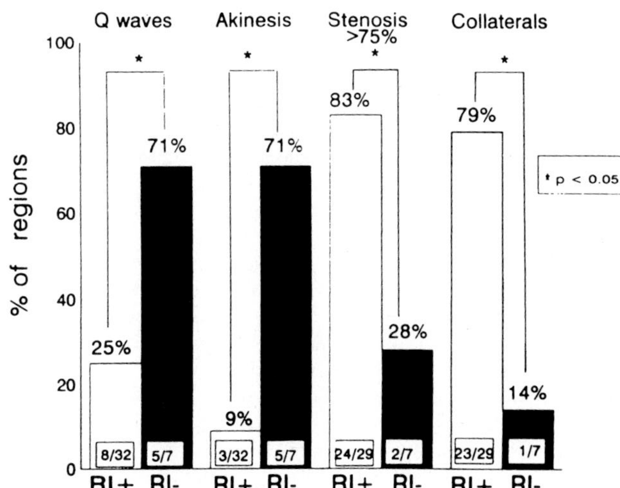

FIGURE 64–8. Frequency of Q waves, akinesis, stenoses greater than 75 percent, and presence of collateral circulation in regions of reverse redistribution with (RI+) and without (RI−) enhanced ^{201}Tl uptake after reinjection. (From Marin-Neto, J.A., Dilsizian, V., Arrighi, J.A., et al.: Thallium reinjection demonstrates viable myocardium in regions with reverse redistribution. Circulation 88:1741, 1993, with permission.)

in defects showing reversibility and mild-to-moderate irreversible defects.

Marin-Neto and associates[74] reported that 82 percent of defect regions showing reverse redistribution in 39 patients with stable chronic CAD showed enhanced ^{201}Tl activity after reinjection. Most of those regions showed either normal patterns of FDG uptake and flow or a mismatch pattern with enhanced FDG uptake relative to flow. Figure 64–8 shows the comparison of the frequency of Q waves, akinesis, and critically-stenosed arteries in regions of reverse redistribution with or without enhanced ^{201}Tl uptake after reinjection. The authors concluded that reverse redistribution in chronic CAD most often reflects viable myocardium.

Maublant and colleagues[75] compared 4-hour redistribution images with 4-hour reinjection images and images obtained at rest on a separate day in a group of patients with chronic stable CAD. They reported that the overall sensitivity for detection of coronary artery stenoses was significantly higher with reinjection at 4 hours ($P < .05$) or with a rest injection on a separate day ($P < .05$) than with redistribution imaging: 84 percent, 83 percent, and 70 percent, respectively. Among 11 patients who had no evidence of redistribution at 4 hours, 5 (45 percent) demonstrated ischemia with reinjection and 5 demonstrated ischemia when the separate rest study was compared with the stress study. The authors concluded that the 4-hour postexercise reinjection approach is as sensitive for detecting ischemia as a 2-day rest and exercise approach for detection of coronary artery stenoses.

Some variations have been proposed for the timing of reinjection after completion of the stress portion of an imaging protocol. Favaro and colleagies[73] studied 27 patients with ischemic heart disease who had at least one persistent defect on 3-hour redistribution images. One protocol involved reinjection of ^{201}Tl immediately after redistribution imaging, with imaging commencing 15 minutes later. In a "different-day" protocol, patients were reinjected 48 to 96 hours later and images were obtained at 30 and 180 minutes after reinjection. The uptake of ^{201}Tl in 111 irreversible segments at redistribution was enhanced in 35 percent with the protocol in which reinjection immediately followed acquisition of redistribution imaging, in 43 percent when reinjection images were acquired 30 minutes after a separate rest injection, and in 49 percent when imaging was acquired 180 minutes after reinjection on a different day. The authors concluded that perhaps the best technique to differentiate scarred from viable myocardium is the reinjection of a second dose of ^{201}Tl on a different day, followed by imaging 3 hours later. A 3-hour duration after a resting injection permits the process of "rest redistribution," which enhances the identification of underperfused but viable myocardium.[42]

The "reinjection" approach for assessment of viability is preferred by many to 24-hour delayed redistribution imaging to detect viable myocardium in defects that appear persistent on 4-hour redistribution images. In one study,[67] late 24-hour imaging after reinjection did not appear to detect further improvement in ^{201}Tl uptake, compared with images acquired 10 minutes after reinjection. Ninety-two percent of regions that demonstrated improved ^{201}Tl uptake on early reinjection images showed no further improvement on the 24-hour late study. The mean normalized ^{201}Tl activity in regions with enhanced tracer uptake after reinjection increased from 57 percent of normal on 4-hour redistribution images to 70 percent of normal after reinjection and 71 percent at 24 hours. In defects that remained persistent after reinjection, no enhanced activity was seen 24 hours later (57 percent at reinjection versus 58 percent at 24 hours). Of defects that remained irreversible after reinjection, all but one remained irreversible 24 hours later when imaging was repeated.

Kayden and co-workers[76] examined the issue of whether the reinjection protocol was superior to the stress-redistribution 24-hour delayed protocol for maximizing detection of reversibility. In their study, reinjection was performed immediately after acquisition of 24-hour redistribution images. These investigators found that slightly more than one-third of ^{201}Tl defects that remained irreversible on 24-hour redistribution images showed enhanced ^{201}Tl uptake after reinjection. Therefore, the reinjection technique was superior to late 24-hour imaging for detection of reversibility after a single dose of ^{201}Tl administered during stress.

Controversy still exists as to whether reinjection of a second dose of ^{201}Tl should be performed with each scintigraphic study in which a defect is noted on both the stress and redistribution images. It is difficult to "prospectively" identify those patients for whom reinjection will enhance detection of viability. In a preliminary study from our group, we compared redistribution images obtained 2.5 hours after ^{201}Tl administration with reinjection images.[77] We found only a slight improvement in ^{201}Tl uptake between redistribution and reinjection images when quantitative analysis of serial images was undertaken. Similarly, preliminary work in a canine model of coronary stenosis in which defects were produced by creation of a coronary stenosis and administration of a combination of dipyridamole and dobutamine, there was little improvement in defect magnitude between redistribution with reinjection images.[78] Nevertheless, many groups prefer to employ the reinjection technique when patients appear to have a persistent defect on both redistribution and initial stress images.

Serial Resting Thallium-201 Imaging for Assessment of Viability

Thallium-201 imaging can be undertaken entirely in the resting state for evaluation of resting myocardial perfusion and cellular viability. This approach should be undertaken in patients who have known CAD and exhibit a reduction in regional or global left ventricular dysfunction in order to determine whether coronary revascularization would have a high probability of improving cardiac function and perhaps symptoms of congestive heart failure.[79, 80] Berger and co-workers[81] studied 29 patients who had either severe stable angina (n = 15) or unstable angina (n = 14) and found that 76 percent of scan segments showing initial defects on early rest images showed delayed rest redistribution when images were repeated at 3 hours. Seventy-seven percent of segments showing rest redistribution exhibited improvement or normalization of ^{201}Tl uptake when rest imaging was repeated after coronary bypass operation. Improved wall motion on postoperative ventriculograms corresponded to scan segments showing improved ^{201}Tl uptake on postoperative resting ^{201}Tl scintigrams. Also in that study, 80 percent of patients who showed rest redistribution preoperatively showed at least a 5 percent increase in LVEF after revascularization. In contrast, only approximately one quarter of patients with preoperative persistent defects on serial rest imaging showed a comparable improvement.

A similar study was undertaken by Gewirtz and colleagues,[82] who found that most defects at rest that showed delayed rest redistribution correlated with normal or hypokinetic wall motion. In that study, 50 percent of akinetic segments had normal ^{201}Tl uptake or initial defects with delayed rest redistribution. No postoperative evaluation was undertaken, and mild and severe resting defects were not analyzed separately. Hakki and associates[83] reported that 50 percent of patients with an ejection fraction of less than 30 percent had preserved ^{201}Tl uptake at rest on serial ^{201}Tl scintigraphy. No postoperative assessment of left ventricular function or perfusion was undertaken.

Mori and associates[84] studied a group of patients with regional dysfunction and a prior myocardial infarction, all of whom underwent preoperative and postoperative radionuclide ventriculography and preoperative initial and delayed rest ^{201}Tl scintigraphy. They found that the majority of regions showing rest ^{201}Tl redistribution exhibited improved systolic function after revascularization. Conversely, most severe persistent defects did not show such an improvement. However, they found that some mild persistent defects did show improved wall motion after revascularization.

Our own group[85] performed rest ^{201}Tl scintigraphy and resting radionuclide ventriculography before and after bypass surgery in a group of 21 patients whose mean LVEF was 27 percent. Among severely-asynergic myocardial segments, 73 percent showed evidence for preserved viability, which was defined as either normal ^{201}Tl uptake, an initial resting defect with delayed redistribution at 3 hours, or a mild persistent defect with no more than 25 to 50 percent reduction in ^{201}Tl activity (Fig. 64–9). A significantly greater number of viable asynergic segments showed improved postoperative regional wall motion, compared with segments corresponding to severe persistent defects with greater than 50 percent reduction in ^{201}Tl activity. Patients who had more than seven viable asynergic segments preoperatively had a significant increase in LVEF at 8 weeks after coronary bypass operation, compared with patients with seven viable asynergic segments on preoperative rest ^{201}Tl scintigraphy (Fig. 64–10). In the 10 patients with more than seven viable asynergic segments (15-segment model), the mean LVEF increased from 29 ± 7 to 41 ± 11 percent (P = .002) after operation. In the 11 patients with seven viable asynergic segments, mean LVEF was 27 ± 5 percent before operation and 30 ± 8 percent after operation (P = NS). Figure 64–11 is an example of a resting single-photon emission computed tomographic (SPECT) ^{201}Tl study showing an initial resting defect that demonstrates delayed redistribution in the septum.

Altehoefer and colleagues[71] compared resting SPECT ^{201}Tl with PET imaging of FDG uptake for the assessment of myocardial viability in patients with chronic CAD. All 24 patients comprising this study cohort had a previous myocardial infarction. The mean LVEF was 45 percent. Segmental ^{201}Tl uptake on SPECT images and segmental normalized FDG uptake on PET images showed a close linear relation in the LAD territory (r = 0.79) and in the lateral wall (r = 0.77), whereas the correlation in the posterior myocardial region was lower (r = 0.52). On a segmental basis, concordancy was observed in 81 percent (439 of 541 segments). In myocardial segments with 50 percent or less ^{201}Tl reduction compared from normal, discordance was observed in 10 percent of segments in the LAD territory and lateral wall but in 44 percent of segments in the posterior myocardial zone.

Dilsizian and co-workers[86] reported a concordancy rate of 94 percent between rest and redistribution ^{201}Tl imaging and ^{201}Tl stress-redistribution-reinjection imaging for assessment of myocardial viability in 41 patients with chronic stable CAD. In that study, the criteria for viability by resting ^{201}Tl imaging was demonstration of defect reversibility or less than 50 percent defect magnitude relative to a normal region and a persistent resting defect. The "gold standard" for viability was defined by PET criteria. Finally,

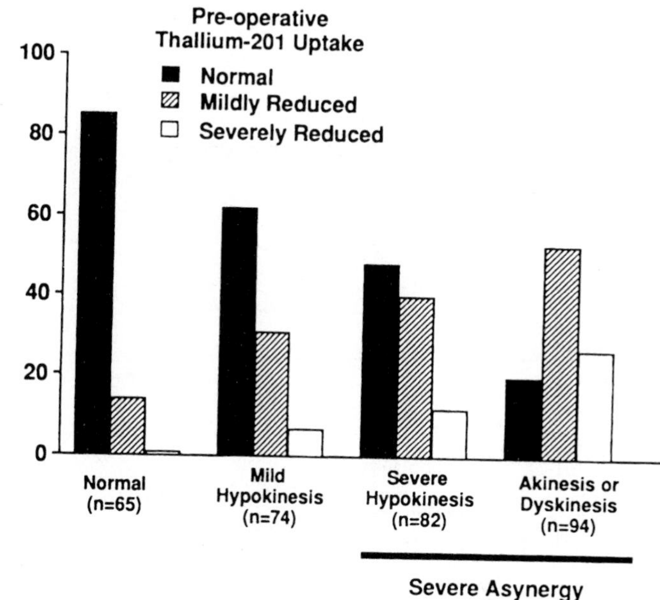

FIGURE 64–9. Relation between preoperative ^{201}Tl uptake patterns and regional wall motion by preoperative radionuclide ventriculography. In zones of severe asynergy (n = 176), the majority of segments demonstrate normal *(solid bar)* or mildly-reduced *(crosshatched bar)* ^{201}Tl uptake. (From Ragosta, M., Beller, G.A., Watson, D.D., et al.: Quantitative planar rest-redistribution ^{201}Tl imaging in detection of myocardial viability and prediction of improvement in left ventricular function after coronary bypass surgery in patients with severely depressed left ventricular function. Circulation 87:1634, 1993, with permission.)

Lomboy and associates[87] determined the utility of early rest-redistribution ^{201}Tl imaging for detection of myocardial viability after acute myocardial infarction. In that study, viability by ^{201}Tl criteria was defined as an initial resting defect showing redistribution or an initial mild resting defect, whether it showed redistribution or showed persistently-reduced ^{201}Tl uptake. Fifty percent of the patients were predicted to have viable myocardium in the infarct zone, and such patients were more likely to have a patent infarct-related artery, a higher initial ejection fraction, a higher infarct wall motion score, and fewer abnormal ^{201}Tl segments, compared with the patients who had nonviable myocardium in the infarct zone by ^{201}Tl criteria. On follow-up, ejection fraction improved from 57 ± 13 to 66 ± 10 percent ($P < .05$) in patients who were predicted to have viable myocardium in the infarct zone. In contrast, ejection fraction significantly fell from 53 ± 10 to 46 ± 8 percent ($P < .05$) in patients who had nonviable myocardium in the infarct zone. Figure 64–12 depicts the early and late LVEF values in both groups of patients in this study.

Patients who received streptokinase in the Western Washington Intravenous Thrombolytic Trial had significantly more ^{201}Tl uptake in the infarct zone than patients who received placebo.[88] Several

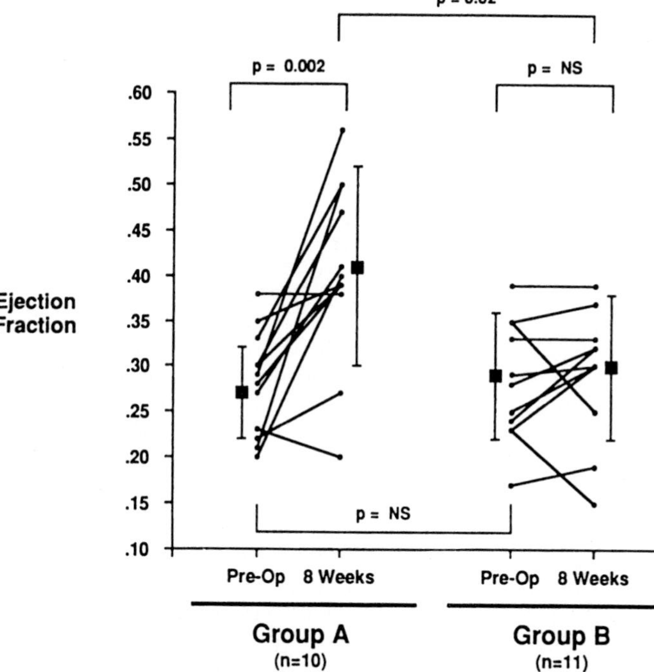

FIGURE 64–10. Left ventricular ejection fraction (LVEF) determined preoperatively (Pre-Op) and 8 weeks after coronary artery bypass graft operation in patients with seven *(group B)* or more than seven *(group A)* viable ^{201}Tl scan segments (15-segment model) before operation. LVEF significantly increased only in group A patients who demonstrated substantial preserved viability in asynergic myocardial scan segments. (From Ragosta, M., Beller, G.A., Watson, D.D., et al.: Quantitative planar rest-redistribution ^{201}Tl imaging in detection of myocardial viability and prediction of improvement in left ventricular function after coronary bypass surgery in patients with severely depressed left ventricular function. Circulation 87:1636, 1993, with permission.)

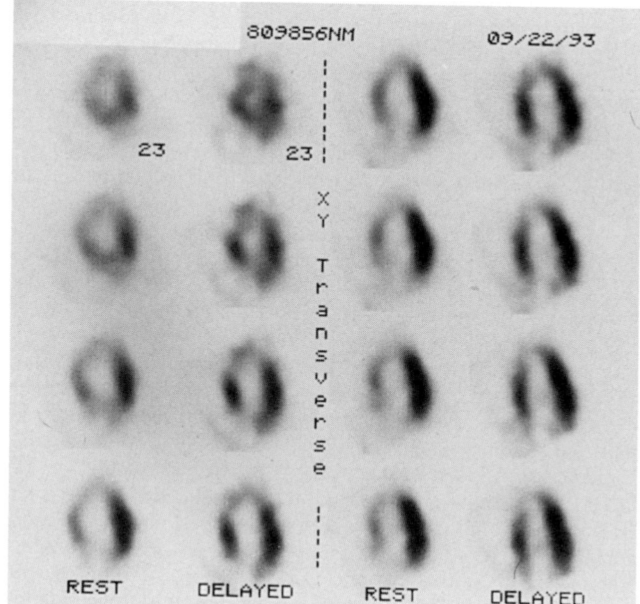

FIGURE 64–11. Rest and delayed rest redistribution horizontal long-axis single-photon emission computed tomographic (SPECT) ^{201}Tl images showing initial defects in the septum and apex that demonstrate delayed septal redistribution and a persistent reduction of ^{201}Tl activity in the apex.

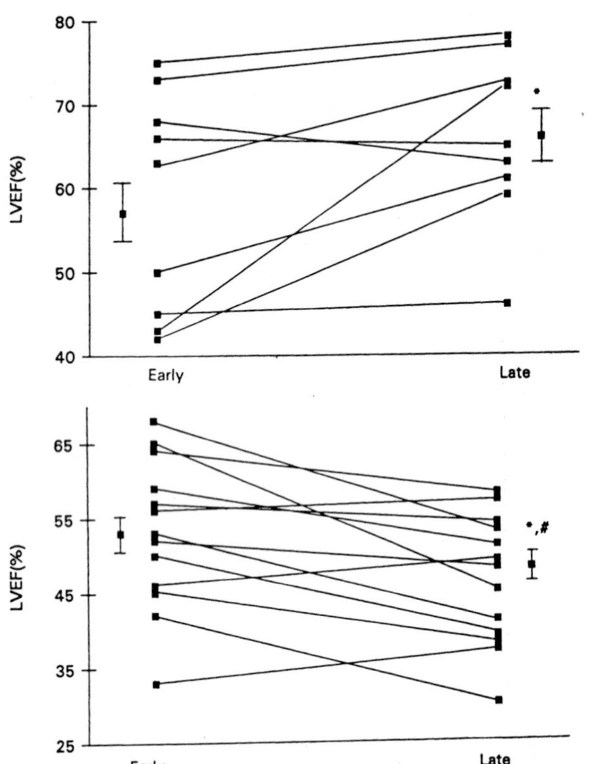

FIGURE 64–12. Early and late left ventricular ejection fraction (LVEF) in patients predicted to have viable myocardium by rest-redistribution ^{201}Tl imaging after myocardial infarction *(group 1, top)* and in patients predicted to have nonviable myocardium in the infarct zone *(group 2, bottom)*. Individual data and mean value ± standard error of the mean are presented. °$P < .01$, early versus late ejection fraction; †$P < .0001$, group 1 versus group 2. (From Lomboy, C.T., Schulman, D.S., Grill, H.P., et al.: Rest-redistribution thallium-201 scintigraphy to determine myocardial viability early after myocardial infarction. J. Am. Coll. Cardiol. 25:213, 1995. With permission from the American College of Cardiology.)

investigators administered ^{201}Tl intravenously before using a thrombolytic agent and obtained postthrombolysis images several hours later. These studies demonstrated that patients who exhibited successful thrombolysis had more ^{201}Tl redistribution and smaller final ^{201}Tl defects than patients who had persistently occluded infarct-related vessels.[89, 90] Patients who demonstrated redistribution 4 hours after thrombolytic therapy showed even further improvement in ^{201}Tl uptake when imaging was repeated several weeks later.[90] Resting ^{201}Tl scintigraphy is perhaps most useful when performed 48 hours or later after thrombolytic therapy to determine the success of reperfusion and to assess the degree of myocardial salvage.[91] If ^{201}Tl is administered too early after reflow, ^{201}Tl may be trapped in the infarct zone during the hyperemic phase that immediately follows reperfusion.[92] In that situation, the degree of ^{201}Tl uptake would overestimate the degree of myocardial salvage.

In summary, ^{201}Tl imaging performed solely in the resting state appears to have good positive and negative predictive value for predicting which asynergic myocardial segments will demonstrate improved regional systolic function after coronary revascularization. Segments corresponding to resting ^{201}Tl defects that show enhanced ^{201}Tl uptake on rest redistribution imaging exhibit the greatest amount of improvement in regional wall motion after revascularization, whereas segments corresponding to severe persistent ^{201}Tl defects (more than 50 percent reduction in ^{201}Tl uptake compared with normal) show the least improvement in systolic function after revascularization. Many mild persistent defects (more than 50 percent ^{201}Tl uptake compared with normal) also show substantial improvement in systolic function after revascularization. This implies that quantitation of regional ^{201}Tl activity is of paramount importance in differentiating between viable and nonviable asynergic myocardial regions.

Few studies have been undertaken to compare the value of quantitative resting SPECT ^{201}Tl scintigraphy with PET imaging of myocardial metabolism in situations in which the expertise in SPECT and PET is comparable. Such studies appear warranted in the era of cost-effective use of imaging technology. Perhaps, PET would be most valuable in patients with severe left ventricular dysfunction who have a potentially high postoperative morbidity and mortality and in whom SPECT ^{201}Tl results are equivocal. A cardiovascular surgeon may desire additional confirming data pertaining to the presence or absence of substantial viability in areas corresponding to left ventricular asynergy that are perfused by severely stenotic coronary arteries.

TECHNETIUM-99m LABELED RADIONUCLIDES FOR DETECTION OF MYOCARDIAL VIABILITY

The knowledge concerning uptake and clearance kinetics of the ^{99m}Tc-labeled myocardial perfusion agents that have emerged as alternatives to ^{201}Tl for the assessment of regional myocardial blood flow and myocardial cellular viability are reviewed in Chapter 62. Briefly, various ^{99m}Tc-labeled perfusion agents have been under investigation in recent years for determination of their efficacy in assessment of myocardial perfusion and viability.[79, 93–103] ^{99m}Tc-labeled radionuclides are superior to ^{201}Tl because of better physical characteristics. The 140-keV photon energy peak of ^{99m}Tc is optimal for imaging with a gamma camera and produces higher quality images than those produced by ^{201}Tl. The relatively short half-life of ^{99m}Tc (6 hours) permits administration of doses 10 to 15 times larger than those used for ^{201}Tl, yielding better image quality in a shorter time.

^{99m}Tc-Sestamibi

Experimental Validation

^{99m}Tc-sestamibi has been evaluated both in the experimental laboratory and in the clinical setting for its suitability as an agent for the evaluation of regional myocardial viability. Piwnica-Worms and his group[104–106] and Beanlands and associates[107] employed basic cellular preparations or isolated heart preparations to demonstrate that ^{99m}Tc-sestamibi is transported passively across plasma and mitochondrial membranes and at equilibrium is sequestered largely within mitochondria by the large negative transmembrane potential. If the mitochondrial membrane potential is depolarized, uptake of ^{99m}Tc-sestamibi is inhibited. Metabolic derangements simulating ischemia and hypoxia produced by these investigators resulted in diminished ^{99m}Tc-sestamibi uptake independent of flow. Our group has shown[108] that ^{99m}Tc-sestamibi retention was dependent on myocardial viability in intact dogs that were rendered severely ischemic. In dogs preloaded with ^{99m}Tc-sestamibi under normal conditions, a 3-hour period of LAD occlusion and 3 hours of reflow resulted in a loss of ^{99m}Tc-sestamibi in the endocardial zone of the ischemic region to 40±6 percent of nonischemic uptake (Fig. 64–13). Severe ischemia resulted in an efflux of ^{99m}Tc-sestamibi into the coronary venous effluent, presumably secondary to mitochondrial and sarcolemmal membrane injury. Further evidence that myocardial ^{99m}Tc-sestamibi uptake depends on cellular viability is that such uptake is not significantly affected by myocardial stunning or "short-term hibernation."[40] Despite severe systolic dysfunction, ^{99m}Tc-sestamibi uptake was preserved in myocardium that was stunned by a transient 15 minutes of LAD occlusion and total reflow.[40]

More recent studies from our group by Sansoy and colleagues[41] showed substantial ^{99m}Tc-sestamibi uptake (greater than 50 percent of normal) 2 hours after ^{99m}Tc-sestamibi injection in dogs with an approximate 50 percent reduction in regional blood flow. There

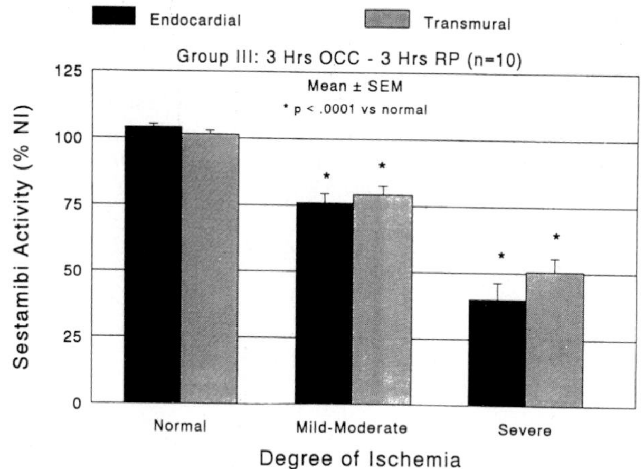

FIGURE 64–13. Bar graph of mean ^{99m}Tc-sestamibi values (percentage nonischemic [NI]) in dogs undergoing 3 hours of left anterior descending coronary artery occlusion (OCC) and 3 hours of reperfusion (RP). ^{99m}Tc sestamibi was administered at baseline conditions before OCC. Mild-to-moderate ischemia is defined as endocardial flow during OCC ranging between 0.3 and 0.8 mL/min/g; severe ischemia is defined as flow during OCC of less than 0.3 mL/min/g. Over time, there is a significant loss of ^{99m}Tc-sestamibi activity in the region of severe ischemia, which is worse in endocardial than epicardial layers. (From Beller, G.A., Glover, D.K., Edwards, N.C., et al.: ^{99m}Tc-sestamibi uptake and retention during myocardial ischemia and reperfusion. Circulation 87:2039, 1993, with permission.)

was a slight but significant amount of delayed ^{99m}Tc-sestamibi redistribution in this model, but greater ^{201}Tl redistribution than ^{99m}Tc-sestamibi redistribution was observed when both tracers were administered to the same animals. Nevertheless, ^{201}Tl uptake was only 5 percent greater, on the average, than ^{99m}Tc-sestamibi uptake in the region perfused by this severely-stenotic LAD. Some delayed ^{99m}Tc-sestamibi redistribution was also seen by Sinusas and associates[109] in dogs given ^{99m}Tc-sestamibi after a chronic reduction in LAD flow (Fig. 64–14). As seen in the previous study, the magnitude of redistribution was less than that observed with ^{201}Tl in the same animals. Glover and Okada[110] could not visually detect ^{99m}Tc-sestamibi redistribution in reperfused viable myocardium in a dog model but found evidence for delayed redistribution by gamma well counting after the animals were killed. Therefore, it can be concluded that, under conditions of sustained low flow, there is

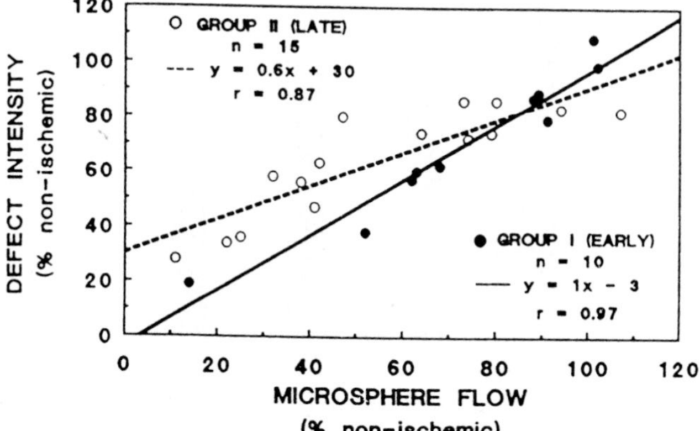

FIGURE 64–14. Scatterplot of quantitation of transmural defect intensity (percent nonischemic) from gamma camera images of ex vivo myocardial slices in dogs receiving ^{99m}Tc sestamibi during sustained low flow and sacrificed either 15 minutes *(group I)* or 2.5 hours *(group II)* after tracer injection. In group II dogs, ^{99m}Tc-sestamibi defect magnitude was less severe than the flow deficit, reflecting greater redistribution than occurred in the group I dogs. (From Sinusas, A.J., Bergin, J.D., Edwards, N.C., et al.: Redistribution of ^{99m}Tc-sestamibi and ^{201}Tl in the presence of a severe coronary artery stenosis. Circulation 89:2338, 1994, with permission.)

some redistribution of ^{99m}Tc-sestamibi, though to a lesser extent than seen for ^{201}Tl.

^{99m}Tc-sestamibi uptake in experimental models of myocardial infarction demonstrates that the defect area after reperfusion correlates well with histologic infarct size.[111, 112] Verani and colleagues[111] reported that perfusion defect size on SPECT ^{99m}Tc-sestamibi images in dogs undergoing 2 hours of coronary artery occlusion correlated well with pathologic infarct size. After 48 hours of reperfusion, scintigraphic defect size was markedly reduced and correlated with final infarct size in these animals. With reperfusion, myocardial uptake of ^{99m}Tc-sestamibi in the ischemic region correlated well with enhanced regional blood flow. Similar findings were reported by Sinusas and co-workers,[112] who measured ^{99m}Tc-sestamibi uptake before and after reperfusion in open-chested dogs undergoing 3 hours of LAD occlusion and 3 hours of reflow. If ^{99m}Tc-sestamibi was injected during occlusion, uptake of the radionuclide correlated well with the anatomic risk area as determined at postmortem examination.

In contrast, if ^{99m}Tc-sestamibi was injected after 90 minutes of reperfusion, uptake of the radionuclide correlated well with final histologically-determined infarct area ($r = 0.98$). In dogs injected with ^{99m}Tc-sestamibi after reperfusion, the myocardial uptake of the radionuclide did not correlate well with reperfusion flow. This was because a substantial increase in flow was observed after reperfusion despite severe irreversible myocardial injury. Flow was restored to 74 percent of nonischemic flow, whereas ^{99m}Tc-sestamibi activity was 25 percent of normal activity. This observation suggests that ^{99m}Tc-sestamibi does not behave solely like a radioactive microsphere in regional perfusion, but it requires viable myocytes for intracellular sequestration when administered after reperfusion. This is why myocardial uptake of the radionuclide during reflow correlated better with histologic infarct area than mere tracking of reperfusion flow.

Finally, it should be pointed out that the size of the ^{99m}Tc-sestamibi defect during ischemia and reperfusion is affected by alterations in left ventricular geometry.[113] Coronary occlusion produces regional systolic thinning, which can exaggerate perfusion defects on ^{99m}Tc-sestamibi images because of the partial volume effect.

Clinical Assessment of Viability With the Use of ^{99m}Tc-Sestamibi

As seen with animal experimental studies cited, some ^{99m}Tc-sestamibi redistribution can be observed either after exercise stress[114] or when imaging is performed solely in the resting state.[115] Dilsizian and colleagues[115] found that 38 percent of irreversible defects seen on rest-stress ^{99m}Tc-sestamibi SPECT images showed delayed redistribution when an additional 4-hour redistribution image was acquired.

^{99m}Tc-sestamibi imaging for detection of myocardial viability has been evaluated in various patient cohorts.[116–124] Cuocolo and associates[116] reported that ^{201}Tl reinjection imaging was superior to rest and stress ^{99m}Tc-sestamibi imaging for detection of defect reversibility. Marzullo and colleagues[117] reported that the sensitivity and specificity of ^{99m}Tc-sestamibi imaging for prediction of postrevascularization recovery of function by echocardiography were 83 percent and 71 percent, respectively. Viability was underestimated by ^{99m}Tc-sestamibi imaging in 25 percent of myocardial regions that were perfused by stenotic arteries but exhibited normal wall motion. In a subsequent study by this same group,[118] asynergic segments that improved after dobutamine administration had more ^{201}Tl uptake and a higher percentage of ^{99m}Tc-sestamibi uptake than segments that were unresponsive to dobutamine infusion. Compared with improved function after revascularization by echocardiography as the “gold standard” for viability, delayed ^{201}Tl images and dobutamine echocardiography had good sensitivity and specificity for detection of viable myocardium. ^{99m}Tc-sestamibi uptake was significantly less than early and delayed ^{201}Tl uptake in those segments that were perfused by stenotic vessels but showed normal systolic function.

Maurea and co-workers[119] found that resting ^{201}Tl uptake was higher than ^{99m}Tc-sestamibi uptake in segments supplied by a totally occluded artery; however, uptake of ^{201}Tl and ^{99m}Tc-sestamibi was comparable in segments supplied by arteries with 50 to 99 percent stenoses. In a subsequent study by the same researchers,[125] rest-redistribution ^{201}Tl and resting ^{99m}Tc-sestamibi images were compared in patients with chronic CAD and regional left ventricular dysfunction (mean LVEF 35 ± 9 percent). Regional left ventricular wall motion was assessed on gated ^{99m}Tc-sestamibi images, and both ^{201}Tl uptake and ^{99m}Tc-sestamibi uptake measurements were made quantitatively. ^{201}Tl and ^{99m}Tc-sestamibi uptake values were significantly higher in segments that demonstrated normal wall motion or hypokinetic wall motion, compared with akinetic and dyskinetic segments ($P < .05$). When ^{201}Tl and ^{99m}Tc-sestamibi uptake values were directly compared, no significant differences were seen in segments that showed normal wall motion or hypokinetic wall motion, whereas ^{99m}Tc-sestamibi uptake (67 ± 14 percent) was significantly lower ($P < .001$) than initial (72 ± 11 percent) and delayed ^{201}Tl uptake (73 ± 12 percent). These authors concluded that myocardial segments demonstrating severely impaired regional systolic function are better assessed by ^{201}Tl imaging than by ^{99m}Tc-sestamibi imaging. Figure 64–15 summarizes the data from this study. It should be pointed out that the difference in ^{99m}Tc-sestamibi uptake and ^{201}Tl uptake in segments with severe asynergy in that study was only 6 percent.

Rocco and associates[120] administered ^{99m}Tc-sestamibi at rest before and after revascularization operation in patients with chronic CAD. Preoperative ^{99m}Tc-sestamibi uptake correlated well with preoperative wall motion but seemed to underestimate extent of myocardial viability. That is, 61 percent of segments exhibiting severely-reduced tracer uptake preoperatively showed improved tracer uptake after operation. Dilsizian and co-workers[115] compared results of stress-redistribution-reinjection ^{201}Tl SPECT imaging with ^{99m}Tc-sestamibi imaging performed within an average of 5 days in a group of 54 patients. They reported that ^{99m}Tc-sestamibi imaging incorrectly identified 36 percent of scan segments as demonstrating irreversible defects and nonviability, compared with ^{201}Tl redistribution-reinjection imaging. PET imaging was used as the "gold standard" for viability in this study. Sawada and colleagues[121] compared resting SPECT ^{99m}Tc-sestamibi imaging results with PET imaging of FDG uptake. They reported that viability by PET criteria was evident in 50 percent of myocardial segments that demonstrated 40 percent or less uptake of ^{99m}Tc-sestamibi. In that study, most of the segments that underestimated viability by ^{99m}Tc-sestamibi were confined to inferior segments. This may be related to the known attenuation of ^{99m}Tc-sestamibi in midinferior and high posterior regions. PET imaging inherently corrects for attenuation by obtaining a transmission scan. Figure 64–16 shows ^{99m}Tc-sestamibi, ^{13}N-ammonia, and FDG polar maps from a patient in this study who demonstrated an inferior ^{99m}Tc-sestamibi defect and preserved FDG uptake.

FIGURE 64–16. See Color Plate 29.

More recently, Udelson and associates[122] compared rest-redistribution ^{201}Tl imaging with resting ^{99m}Tc-sestamibi imaging, employing quantitative SPECT techniques in a study population of 31 patients with chronic CAD, all of whom had a history of prior myocardial infarction. Figure 64–17 shows the results of quantitative analysis of rest ^{201}Tl activity, redistribution ^{201}Tl activity, and ^{99m}Tc-sestamibi activity in regions grouped according to the mean normalized resting ^{201}Tl activity. Segments judged to be normal or to demonstrate mild, moderate, or severe defects all showed ^{99m}Tc-sestamibi uptake that was comparable to the delayed resting ^{201}Tl uptake. For example, in 122 segments with a mild reduction in resting ^{201}Tl activity (65 to 79 percent of nonischemic activity), redistribution ^{201}Tl uptake was 74 ± 8 percent of peak, compared with ^{99m}Tc-sestamibi activity equal to 76 ± 10 percent of peak (P = NS). Similarly, in segments showing a moderately severe reduction in ^{201}Tl activity (50 to 64 percent of nonischemic activity), tracer uptake on redistribution ^{201}Tl imaging was 62 ± 9 percent of peak, which was comparable to the ^{99m}Tc-sestamibi activity of 60 ± 9 percent of peak nonischemic ^{99m}Tc-sestamibi activity. Concordancy in defect severity was observed in 87 percent of the 372 segments analyzed in this study. Seventy-five percent of segments with ^{201}Tl activity of 60 percent of peak activity demonstrated improved wall motion and thickening after revascularization. In comparison, 80 percent of segments with ^{99m}Tc-sestamibi regional activity of 60

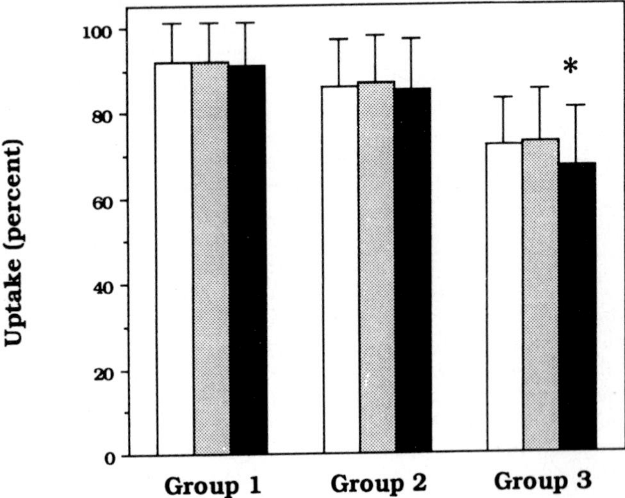

FIGURE 64–15. Initial *(open bars)* and delayed *(light bars)* ^{201}Tl and ^{99m}Tc-sestamibi *(dark bars)* regional uptake in myocardial segments with normal wall motion *(group 1)*, hypokinesia *(group 2)*, and akinesia or dyskinesia *(group 3)*. *P < .001 versus initial and delayed ^{201}Tl. (From Maurea, S., Cuocolo, A., Pace, L., et al.: Left ventricular dysfunction in coronary artery disease: Comparison between rest-redistribution thallium 201 and resting technetium 99m methoxyisobutyl isonitrile cardiac imaging. J. Nucl. Cardiol. 1:69, 1994, with permission.)

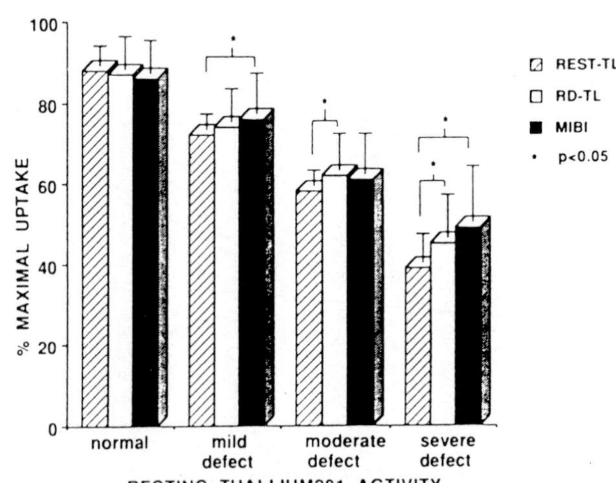

FIGURE 64–17. Resting ^{201}Tl activity represented as percent maximal uptake versus initial resting ^{201}Tl image *(crosshatched bar)*, delayed rest ^{201}Tl image at redistribution *(open bars)*, and ^{99m}Tc-sestamibi uptake *(solid bar)*. ^{99m}Tc-sestamibi uptake values are comparable to the delayed redistribution ^{201}Tl uptake in normal segments, segments with mild initial ^{201}Tl defects, those with moderate initial ^{201}Tl defects, and those with severe initial ^{201}Tl defects. (From Udelson, J.E., Coleman, P.S., Metherall, J., et al.: Predicting recovery of severe regional ventricular dysfunction: Comparison of resting scintigraphy with ^{201}Tl and ^{99m}Tc-sestamibi. Circulation 89:2554, 1994, with permission.)

percent demonstrated functional recovery. There was no difference between the two techniques in predicting enhanced function after revascularization.

Therefore, in comparison with the previous studies cited, quantitative analysis of regional activities of both ^{201}Tl and ^{99m}Tc-sestamibi after resting injection can distinguish between viable and nonviable myocardium. In addition, the two agents demonstrated comparable accuracy in predicting improvement in regional wall motion after revascularization. Preliminary data from our group[124] also demonstrate comparable ^{201}Tl and ^{99m}Tc-sestamibi uptake in zones of severe asynergy, as categorized by resting echocardiography. The patients in the study by Kauffman and colleagues[124] were comparable to those enrolled by Udelson and co-workers in the study described.

Assessment of Viability After Coronary Reperfusion

Because ^{99m}Tc-sestamibi demonstrates very little redistribution, separate injections of the tracer are required during stress and resting states. The separate injection technique can be employed for the assessment of the efficacy of myocardial salvage by thrombolytic therapy or direct angioplasty in patients with acute myocardial infarction. A dose of ^{99m}Tc-sestamibi is injected before thrombolytic therapy, and imaging is postponed for several hours after completion of the therapeutic intervention. The perfusion pattern visible at the time of subsequent imaging reflects the regional flow state at the time of injection, when the infarct vessel was presumably still occluded. The defect area and defect severity reflect the "area at risk." That is, a "snapshot" of the perfusion pattern before the intervention is demonstrated. A second injection of ^{99m}Tc-sestamibi is then administered 24 hours or later after the initial images are acquired in order to demonstrate improvement, or lack thereof, in regional flow and viability in the zone subtended by the infarct-related vessels.

Several clinical studies[126, 127] have been reported in which serial ^{99m}Tc-sestamibi imaging in patients with acute myocardial infarction who receive thrombolytic therapy was undertaken. Patients with a patent infarct vessel had a significantly greater decrease in defect size on the second set of images after thrombolytic therapy, compared with those patients with persistently-occluded vessels. A relative defect decrease of more than 30 percent predicted patency of the infarct-related vessel. Also, the final ^{99m}Tc-sestamibi defect size correlated well with the predischarge LVEF in these acute infarction patients.[126] The above observations may have clinical relevance because there are few reliable noninvasive techniques that can be employed to predict successful reperfusion after thrombolytic therapy. ^{99m}Tc-sestamibi imaging could be used as a tool in clinical trials aimed at evaluating the efficacy of new thrombolytic protocols or mechanical approaches to reperfusion in the setting of acute myocardial infarction.

Gated ^{99m}Tc-Sestamibi Imaging for Enhanced Detection of Viability

One advantage of ^{99m}Tc-sestamibi for assessment of viability is the capability to simultaneously assess regional myocardial perfusion and regional systolic wall thickening. This feature is applicable for the assessment of myocardial viability in patients with chronic CAD and in patients with a recent acute myocardial infarction. Myocardial scan segments that show preserved ^{99m}Tc-sestamibi uptake and preserved thickening are judged to represent viable myocardium. Segments that show persistently reduced uptake of ^{99m}Tc-sestamibi and no enhanced thickening from end-diastole to end-systole are judged to be nonviable. Figure 64–18 shows end-diastolic and end-systolic ^{99m}Tc-sestamibi SPECT tomograms in a patient with a myocardial perfusion abnormality. Increased systolic thickening can be appreciated in the zone underperfusion. Chua and colleagues[128] compared gated ^{99m}Tc-sestamibi SPECT images with echocardiography for the assessment of myocardial function. In that study, a high segmental score agreement existed between gated ^{99m}Tc-sestamibi SPECT and echocardiography for wall motion (91 percent, $\kappa = 0.68$) and thickening (90 percent, $\kappa = 0.62$). In 32 patients who had no prior myocardial infarction, excellent agreement for reversibility between stress gated ^{99m}Tc-sestamibi imaging and rest ^{201}Tl together with stress ^{99m}Tc-sestamibi imaging was observed ($r = 0.98$) employing the SPECT technique. Figure 64–19 correlates the number of reversible segments per patient by gated SPECT ^{99m}Tc-sestamibi imaging and stress ^{99m}Tc-sestamibi with rest ^{201}Tl dual imaging in patients with and without a prior infarction.

^{123}I-PHENYLPENTADECANOIC ACID FOR ASSESSMENT OF MYOCARDIAL VIABILITY

^{123}I-phenylpentadecanoic acid (IPPA) is a new metabolic agent that can be employed with SPECT imaging for the assessment of regional myocardial viability in patients with chronic CAD or patients with acute ischemic syndromes who have left ventricular dysfunction.[129–136] The initial uptake of IPPA is related to regional myocardial blood flow. After peak uptake, IPPA metabolism results in a biexponential myocardial clearance pattern with a rapid initial phase reflecting beta-oxidation and a slower second phase representing turnover of the remaining lipid pools. When myocardial ischemia causes a diminution in beta-oxidation of fatty acids, with a relative increase in the proportion of fatty acids in the slowly metabolizing intracardiac lipid pool, imaging demonstrates this alteration. That is, ischemia diminishes the myocardial washout rate of radiolabeled fatty acids when there is a reduction in the oxidative metabolism of fatty acids. Nonviable and irreversibly-injured myocardia demonstrate significantly reduced IPPA uptake after a resting injection, without much change in the activity in the defect region over time. With chronic underperfusion causing myocardial hibernation, IPPA uptake is initially decreased early after tracer administration, but over time there is relative "filling in" of the defect because of reduced beta-oxidation and clearance. The reduced washout in the underperfused zone, compared with more rapid washout from the normal zone, results in a defect pattern comparable to that of ^{201}Tl redistribution.

In clinical trials,[132] the assessment of viability in patients with left ventricular dysfunction by IPPA involves a serial SPECT imaging protocol wherein images are acquired 4, 12, 20, 28, and 36 minutes after tracer injection. Preliminary data from clinical studies have suggested that quantitative assessment of IPPA uptake and clearance on these serial images can assist differentiation between viable and nonviable myocardium and prediction of left ventricular function after revascularization.[130–135]

Murray and co-workers[133] reported a 92 percent sensitivity and 86 percent specificity for IPPA imaging for detection of viability. Myocardial biopsy findings at the time of revascularization were used as a pathologic criterion for viability. IPPA washout was 17.8 percent in biopsy-viable segments, compared with 21.2 percent in healthy volunteers and 13.4 percent in nonviable biopsy segments ($P < .001$ versus biopsy-viable segments). Hansen and co-workers[132] reported findings in which IPPA clearance slopes were predictive of improvement in left ventricular function after revascularization. Further studies are underway with a larger number of patients to compare the accuracy of IPPA imaging with other techniques such as ^{201}Tl imaging and PET imaging for the determination of myocardial viability in areas of left ventricular dysfunction.

SUMMARY

There is no doubt that the use of nuclear cardiology techniques for the assessment of myocardial viability can help predict outcome of coronary revascularization in the setting of severe left ventricular dysfunction. Zones of myocardial asynergy perfused by severely stenotic vessels that demonstrate substantial uptake of perfusion

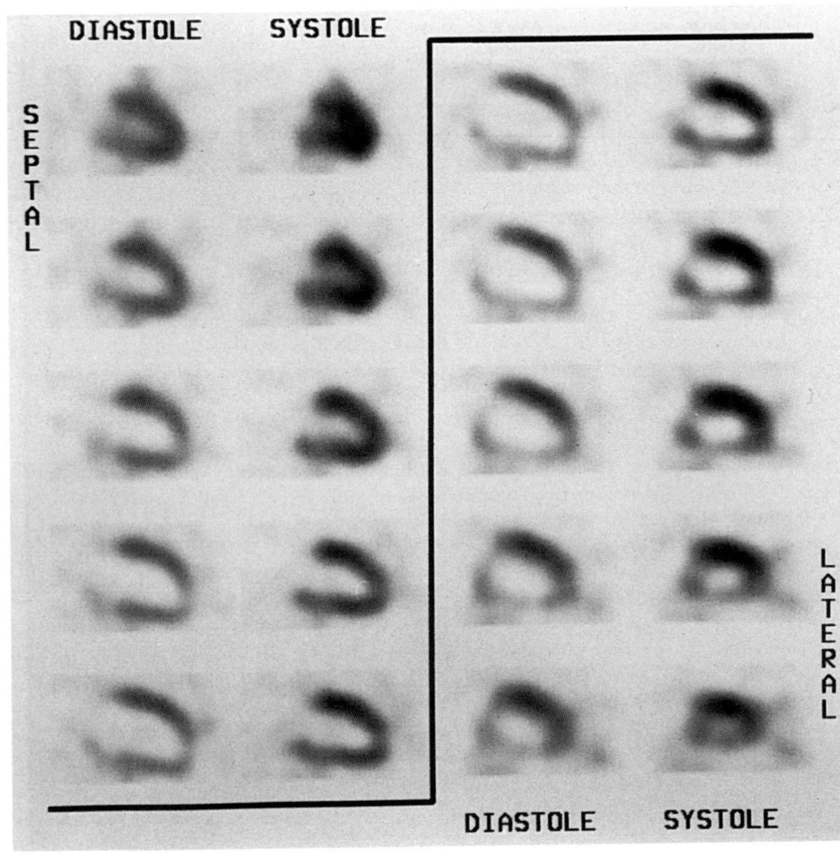

FIGURE 64–18. End-diastolic (DIASTOLE) and end-systolic (SYSTOLE) long-axis ^{99m}Tc-sestamibi gated tomograms demonstrating normal thickening of the anterior wall and diminished thickening of the inferior wall. The latter is most evident on the tomograms in the upper right corner, representing the midventricular region. The tomograms are oriented from the septal *(upper left)* to the lateral region *(lower right)*.

tracers such as ^{201}Tl, ^{99m}Tc-sestamibi, or some of the newer ^{99m}Tc-labeled agents can be expected to exhibit improved systolic function after successful revascularization. In contrast, zones of asynergy (particularly akinesis or dyskinesis) that demonstrate a severe reduction in tracer activity preoperatively are unlikely to demonstrate significant improvement in systolic function after either coronary angioplasty or bypass operation.

Several issues remain unresolved concerning the accuracy of these nuclear cardiology techniques for distinguishing between viable and nonviable myocardium and predicting improvement, or lack thereof, in regional and global function after coronary revascularization. First, studies in the literature are in conflict with respect to the accuracy of ^{99m}Tc-sestamibi imaging, compared with ^{201}Tl imaging, for the assessment of myocardial viability. Further studies in larger numbers of patients are warranted to determine whether gated resting ^{99m}Tc-sestamibi imaging provides information relevant to viability comparable to that obtained with rest-redistribution ^{201}Tl imaging.

A second issue relates to the magnitude of the superiority of PET imaging for the assessment of viability in comparison with the SPECT techniques. Studies in the literature to date would suggest that PET imaging of FDG or ^{11}C-acetate uptake remains the noninvasive "gold standard" for identifying myocardial viability in zones of myocardial asynergy in patients with chronic CAD. However, the magnitude of this superiority may be no more than 10 percent in accuracy compared with quantitative SPECT techniques. Further studies are warranted in a large number of patients to compare PET imaging with SPECT techniques for the assessment of viability where the definition of viability is significant improvement in global left ventricular function after revascularization. Such a study is warranted because of the greater expense of PET imaging compared with SPECT imaging. Cost-effectiveness is a criterion that has now emerged in comparison of different imaging modalities.

A third issue that remains to be resolved is the accuracy of low-dose dobutamine echocardiography for assessment of viability, compared with the nuclear cardiology techniques. The question is whether enhanced systolic thickening in response to dobutamine can provide comparable information with respect to predicting improvement in cardiac function after revascularization. Again, further clinical research appears warranted in this regard. Currently, dobutamine echocardiography lacks independent quantitative assessment of systolic thickening, and myocardial responsiveness is still assessed by visual inspection of digitized images.

Finally, there is the issue of whether the determination of viability adds supplementary diagnostic or prognostic information to assessment of clinical and ECG variables alone in selection of patients with chronic CAD and depressed left ventricular function who are candidates for coronary bypass operation. It is unknown whether mere assessment of coronary angiographic, contrast ventriculographic, and echocardiographic variables is sufficient to identify suitable candidates for myocardial revascularization who then may anticipate an enhanced life expectancy and an improved quality of life and functional capacity. It is uncertain whether all patients with depressed left ventricular function who have multivessel CAD benefit from revascularization as long as the anatomy is suitable for grafting. Larger studies in unselected patients with ischemic cardiomyopathy are warranted to test the hypothesis that patients with depressed LVEF and substantial areas of viable myocardium have a better outcome after operation with respect to survival, improvement in left ventricular function, improvement in heart failure symptoms, and enhanced quality of life, compared with patients who have a similar reduction in resting left ventricular function and a similar extent of angiographic CAD but who demonstrate a lesser extent of myocardial viability by the nuclear techniques before revascularization. The studies published to date with small numbers of patients are most encouraging in this regard.

Despite these unresolved issues, the radionuclide imaging approaches discussed in this chapter are currently helpful to physicians for differentiation of patients with severe left ventricular dysfunction resulting from hibernation or myocardial stunning from those with irreversible myocardial cellular injury. Further studies

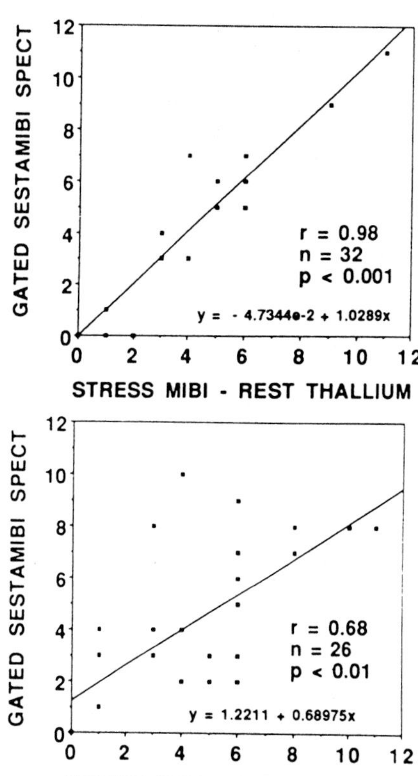

FIGURE 64–19. Correlation between the number of reversible segments per patient by stress gated ^{99m}Tc-sestamibi (MIBI) single-photon emission computed tomographic *(y axis)* and stress ^{99m}Tc-sestamibi together with rest ^{201}Tl *(x axis)* in patients without *(top)* and with *(bottom)* a previous infarction by history or electrocardiography. (From Chua, T., Kiat, H., Germano, G., Maurer, G., et al.: Gated technetium-99m sestamibi for simultaneous assessment of stress myocardial perfusion, postexercise regional ventricular function and myocardial viability: Correlation with echocardiography and rest thallium-201 scintigraphy. J. Am. Coll. Cardiol. 23:1111, 1994. With permission from the American College of Cardiology.)

will surely be undertaken to validate the use of these techniques for optimal selection of patients with CAD and left ventricular dysfunction for revascularization.

Acknowledgment

The author is grateful to Mr. Jerry Curtis for his superb editorial skills used in the preparation of this manuscript.

References

1. Alderman, E.L., Bourassa, M.G., Cohen, L.S., et al.: Ten-year follow-up of survival and myocardial infarction in the randomized Coronary Artery Surgery Study. Circulation 82:1629, 1990.
2. Braunwald, E., and Kloner, R.A.: The stunned myocardium: Prolonged, postischemic ventricular dysfunction. Circulation 66:1146, 1982.
3. Bolli, R., Zhu, W.X., Thornby, J.I., et al.: Time course and determinants of recovery of function after reversible ischemia in conscious dogs. Am. J. Physiol. 254:H102, 1988.
4. Nicklas, J.M., Becker, L.C., and Bulkley, B.H.: Effects of repeated brief coronary occlusion on regional left ventricular function and dimension in dogs. Am. J. Cardiol. 56:473, 1985.
5. Swain, J.L., Sabina, R.L., McHale, P.A., et al.: Prolonged myocardial nucleotide depletion after brief ischemia in the open-chest dog. Am. J. Physiol. 242:H818, 1982.
6. Greenfield, R.A., and Swain, J.L.: Disruption of myofibrillar energy use: Dual mechanisms that may contribute to postischemic dysfunction in stunned myocardium. Circ. Res. 60:283, 1987.
7. Stahl, L.D., Weiss, H.R., and Becker, L.C.: Myocardial oxygen consumption, oxygen supply/demand heterogeneity, and microvascular patency in regionally stunned myocardium. Circulation 77:865, 1988.
8. Ciuffo, A.A., Ouyang, P., Becker, L.C., et al.: Reduction of sympathetic inotropic response after ischemia in dogs. Contributor to stunned myocardium. J. Clin. Invest 75:1504, 1985.
9. Kusuoka, H., Porterfield, J.K., Weisman, H.F., et al.: Pathophysiology and pathogenesis of stunned myocardium. Depressed Ca^{2+} activation of contraction as a consequence of reperfusion-induced cellular calcium overload in ferret hearts. J. Clin. Invest. 79:950, 1987.
10. Zimmerman, A.N., and Hulsmann, W.C.: Paradoxical influence of calcium ions on the permeability of the cell membranes of the isolated rat heart. Nature 211:646, 1966.
11. Grinwald, P.M., and Brosnahan, C.: Sodium imbalance as a cause of calcium overload in post-hypoxic reoxygenation injury. J. Mol. Cell. Cardiol. 19:487, 1987.
12. Engler, R.L.: Free radical and granulocyte-mediated injury during myocardial ischemia and reperfusion. Am. J. Cardiol. 63:19E, 1989.
13. Zhao, M.J., Zhang, H., Robinson, T.F., et al.: Profound structural alterations of the extracellular collagen matrix in postischemic dysfunctional ("stunned") but viable myocardium. J. Am. Coll. Cardiol. 10:1322, 1987.
14. Bolli, R.: Oxygen-derived free radicals and postischemic myocardial dysfunction ("stunned myocardium"). J. Am. Coll. Cardiol. 12:239, 1988.
15. Topol, E.J., Weiss, J.L., Brinker, J.A., et al.: Regional wall motion improvement after coronary thrombolysis with recombinant tissue plasminogen activator: Importance of coronary angioplasty. J. Am. Coll. Cardiol. 6:426, 1985.
16. Anderson, J.L., Marshall, H.W., Bray, B.E., et al.: A randomized trial of intracoronary streptokinase in the treatment of acute myocardial infarction. N. Engl. J. Med. 308:1312, 1983.
17. de Feyter, P.J., Suryapranata, H., Serruys, P.W., et al: Effects of successful percutaneous transluminal coronary angioplasty on global and regional left ventricular function in unstable angina pectoris. Am. J. Cardiol. 60:993, 1987.
18. de Zwaan, C., Cheriex, E.C., Braat, S.H., et al.: Improvement of systolic and diastolic left ventricular wall motion by serial echocardiograms in selected patients treated for unstable angina. Am. Heart J. 121:789, 1991.
19. Armstrong, W.F.: Stress echocardiography for detection of coronary artery disease. Circulation 84(Suppl. I):I-43, 1991.
20. Stack, R.S., Phillips, H.R., Grierson, D.S., et al.: Functional improvement of jeopardized myocardium following intracoronary streptokinase infusion in acute myocardial infarction. J. Clin. Invest. 72:84, 1983.
21. Touchstone, D.A., Beller, G.A., Nygaard, T.W., et al.: Effects of successful intravenous reperfusion therapy on regional myocardial function and geometry in humans: A tomographic assessment using two-dimensional echocardiography. J. Am. Coll. Cardiol. 13:1506, 1989.
22. Rahimtoola, S.H.: The hibernating myocardium. Am. Heart J. 117:211, 1989.
23. Edwards, N.C., Sinusas, A.J., Bergin, J.D., et al.: Influence of subendocardial ischemia on transmural myocardial function. Am. J. Physiol. 262:H568, 1992.
24. Bolli, R.: Myocardial "stunning" in man. Circulation 86:1671, 1992.
25. Lewis, S.J., Sawada, S.G., Ryan, T., et al.: Segmental wall motion abnormalities in the absence of clinically documented myocardial infarction: Clinical significance and evidence of hibernating myocardium. Am. Heart J. 121:1088, 1991.
26. Brundage, B.H., Massie, B.M., and Botvinick, E.H.: Improved regional ventricular function after successful surgical revascularization. J. Am. Coll. Cardiol. 3:902, 1984.
27. Topol, E.J., Weiss, J.L., Guzman, P.A., et al.: Immediate improvement of dysfunctional myocardial segments after coronary revascularization: Detection by intraoperative transesophageal echocardiography. J. Am. Coll. Cardiol. 4:1123, 1984.
28. Nienaber, C.A., Brunken, R.C., Sherman, C.T., et al.: Metabolic and functional recovery of ischemic human myocardium after coronary angioplasty. J. Am. Coll. Cardiol. 18:966, 1991.
29. van den Berg, E.K. Jr., Popma, J.J., Dehmer, G.J., et al.: Reversible segmental left ventricular dysfunction after coronary angioplasty. Circulation 81:1210, 1990.
30. Linderer, T., Guhl, B., Spielberg, C., et al.: Effect on global and regional left ventricular functions by percutaneous transluminal coronary angioplasty in the chronic stage after myocardial infarction. Am. J. Cardiol. 69:997, 1992.
31. Montalescot, G., Faraggi, M., Drobinski, G., et al.: Myocardial viability in patients with Q wave myocardial infarction and no residual ischemia. Circulation 86:47, 1992.
32. Strauss, H.W., Harrison, K., Langan, J.K., et al.: Thallium-201 for myocardial imaging: Relation of thallium-201 to regional myocardial perfusion. Circulation 51:641, 1975.
33. Weich, H.F., Strauss, H.W., and Pitt, B.: The extraction of thallium-201 by the myocardium. Circulation 56:188, 1977.
34. Leppo, J.A.: Myocardial uptake of thallium and rubidium during alterations in perfusion and oxygenation in isolated rabbit hearts. J. Nucl. Med. 28:878, 1987.
35. Pohost, G.M., Zir, L.M., Moore, R.H., et al.: Differentiation of transiently ischemic from infarcted myocardium by serial imaging after a single dose of thallium-201. Circulation 55:294, 1977.
36. Mays, A.E. Jr., and Cobb, F.R.: Relationship between regional myocardial blood flow and thallium-201 distribution in the presence of coronary artery stenosis and dipyridamole-induced vasodilation. J. Clin. Invest. 73:1359, 1984.
37. Nielsen, A.P., Morris, K.G., Murdock, R., et al.: Linear relationship between the distribution of thallium-201 and blood flow in ischemic and nonischemic myocardium during exercise. Circulation 61:797, 1980.
38. Grunwald, A.M., Watson, D.D., Holzgrefe, H.H. Jr., et al.: Myocardial thallium-201 kinetics in normal and ischemic myocardium. Circulation 64:610, 1981.
39. Moore, C.A., Cannon, J., Watson, D.D., et al.: Thallium 201 kinetics in stunned myocardium characterized by severe postischemic systolic dysfunction. Circulation 81:1622, 1990.
40. Sinusas, A.J., Watson, D.D., Cannon, J.M. Jr., et al.: Effect of ischemia and postischemic dysfunction on myocardial uptake of technetium-99m-labeled methoxyisobutyl isonitrile and thallium-201. J. Am. Coll. Cardiol. 14:1785, 1989.
41. Sansoy, V., Glover, D.K., Watson, D.D., et al.: Comparison of thallium-201 rest redistribution with technetium-99m sestamibi uptake and functional response to dobutamine for assessment of myocardial viability. Circulation 99:994, 1995.

42. Pohost, G.M., Okada, R.D., O'Keefe, D.D., et al: Thallium redistribution in dogs with severe coronary artery stenosis of fixed caliber. Circ. Res. 48:439, 1981.
43. Granato, J.E., Watson, D.D., Flanagan, T.L., et al.: Myocardial thallium-201 kinetics and regional flow alterations with 3 hours of coronary occlusion and either rapid reperfusion through a totally patent vessel or slow reperfusion through a critical stenosis. J. Am. Coll. Cardiol. 9:109, 1987.
44. Goldhaber, S.Z., Newell, J.B., Alpert, N.M., et al.: Effects of ischemic-like insult on myocardial thallium-201 accumulation. Circulation 67:778, 1983.
45. Khaw, B.A., Strauss, H.W., Pohost, G.M., et al.: Relation of immediate and delayed thallium-201 distribution to localization of iodine-125 antimyosin antibody in acute experimental myocardial infarction. Am. J. Cardiol. 51:1428, 1983.
46. Gibson, R.S., Watson, D.D., Taylor, G.J., et al.: Prospective assessment of regional myocardial perfusion before and after coronary revascularization surgery by quantitative thallium-201 scintigraphy. J. Am. Coll. Cardiol. 1:804, 1983.
47. Wackers, F.J.: The maze of myocardial perfusion imaging protocols in 1994. J. Nucl. Cardiol. 1:180, 1994.
48. Berger, B.C., Watson, D.D., Taylor, G.J., et al.: Quantitative thallium-201 exercise scintigraphy for detection of coronary artery disease. J. Nucl. Med. 22:585, 1981.
49. Liu, P., Kiess, M.C., Okada, R.D., et al.: The persistent defect on exercise thallium imaging and its fate after myocardial revascularization: Does it represent scar or ischemia? Am. Heart J. 110:996, 1985.
50. Ohtani, H., Tamaki, N., Yonekura, Y., et al.: Value of thallium-201 reinjection after delayed SPECT imaging for predicting reversible ischemia after coronary artery bypass grafting. Am. J. Cardiol. 66:394, 1990.
51. Cloninger, K.G., DePuey, E.G., Garcia, E.V., et al.: Incomplete redistribution in delayed thallium-201 single photon emission computed tomographic (SPECT) images: An overestimation of myocardial scarring. J. Am. Coll. Cardiol. 12:955, 1988.
52. Brunken, R., Schwaiger, M., Grover-McKay, M., et al.: Positron emission tomography detects tissue metabolic activity in myocardial segments with persistent thallium perfusion defects. J. Am. Coll. Cardiol. 10:557, 1987.
53. Yamamoto, K., Asada, S., Masuyama, T., et al.: Myocardial hibernation in the infarcted region cannot be assessed from the presence of stress-induced ischemia: Usefulness of delayed image of exercise thallium-201 scintigraphy. Am. Heart J. 125:33, 1993.
54. Kiat, H., Berman, D.S., Maddahi, J., et al.: Late reversibility of tomographic myocardial thallium-201 defects: An accurate marker of myocardial viability. J. Am. Coll. Cardiol. 12:1456, 1988.
55. Yang, L.D., Berman, D.S., Kiat, H., et al.: The frequency of late reversibility in SPECT thallium-201 stress-redistribution studies. J. Am. Coll. Cardiol. 15:334, 1990.
56. Gutman, J., Berman, D.S., Freeman, M., et al.: Time to completed redistribution of thallium-201 in exercise myocardial scintigraphy: Relationship to the degree of coronary artery stenosis. Am. Heart J. 106:989, 1983.
57. Beller, G.A., Watson, D.D., Ackell, P., et al.: Time course of thallium-201 redistribution after transient myocardial ischemia. Circulation 61:791, 1980.
58. Watson, D.: Quantitative analysis of Tl-201 redistribution at 24 hours compared to 2 and 4 hours post-injection (Abstract). J. Nucl. Med. 31:763, 1990.
59. Dilsizian, V., Rocco, T.P., Freedman, N.M., et al.: Enhanced detection of ischemic but viable myocardium by the reinjection of thallium after stress-redistribution imaging. N. Engl. J. Med. 323:141, 1990.
60. Rocco, T.P., Dilsizian, V., McKusick, K.A., et al.: Comparison of thallium redistribution with rest "reinjection" imaging for the detection of viable myocardium. Am. J. Cardiol. 66:158, 1990.
61. Tamaki, N., Ohtani, H., Yamashita, K., et al.: Metabolic activity in the areas of new fill-in after thallium-201 reinjection: Comparison with positron emission tomography using fluorine-18-deoxyglucose. J. Nucl. Med. 32:673, 1991.
62. Dilsizian, V., Freedman, N.M., Bacharach, S.L., et al.: Regional thallium uptake in irreversible defects: Magnitude of change in thallium activity after reinjection distinguishes viable from nonviable myocardium. Circulation 85:627, 1992.
63. Kiat, H., Friedman, J.D., Wang, F.P., et al.: Frequency of late reversibility in stress-redistribution thallium-201 SPECT using an early reinjection protocol. Am. Heart J. 122:613, 1991.
64. Dilsizian, V., and Bonow, R.O.: Differential uptake and apparent ^{201}Tl washout after thallium reinjection: Options regarding early redistribution imaging before reinjection or late redistribution imaging after reinjection. Circulation 85:1032, 1992.
65. Bonow, R.O., Dilsizian, V., Cuocolo, A., et al.: Identification of viable myocardium in patients with chronic coronary artery disease and left ventricular dysfunction: Comparison of thallium scintigraphy with reinjection and PET imaging with ^{18}F-fluorodeoxyglucose. Circulation 83:26, 1991.
66. Perrone-Filardi, P., Bacharach, S.L., Dilsizian, V., et al.: Regional left ventricular wall thickening: Related to regional uptake of ^{18}fluorodeoxyglucose and ^{201}Tl in patients with chronic coronary artery disease and left ventricular dysfunction. Circulation 86:1125, 1992.
67. Dilsizian, V., Smeltzer, W.R., Freedman, N.M., et al.: Thallium reinjection after stress-redistribution imaging: Does 24-hour delayed imaging after reinjection enhance detection of viable myocardium? Circulation 83:1247, 1991.
68. Galli, M., and Marcassa, C.: Thallium-201 redistribution after early reinjection in patients with severe stress perfusion defects and ventricular dysfunction. Am. Heart J. 128:41, 1994.
69. Bartenstein, P., Schober, O., Hasfeld, M., et al.: Thallium-201 single photon emission tomography of myocardium: Additional information in rejection studies is dependent on collateral circulation. Eur. J. Nucl. Med. 19:790, 1992.
70. Cuocolo, A., Pace, L., Maurea, S., et al.: Enhanced thallium-201 uptake after reinjection: Relation to regional ventricular function, myocardial perfusion and coronary anatomy. J. Nucl. Biol. Med. 38:6, 1994.
71. Altehoefer, C., vom Dahl, J., Buell, U., et al.: Comparison of thallium-201 single-photon emission tomography after rest injection and fluorodeoxyglucose positron emission tomography for assessment of myocardial viability in patients with chronic coronary artery disease. Eur. J. Nucl. Med. 21:37, 1994.
72. Garcia, M.J., Neumann, D., Go, R.T., et al.: Comparison of persistent thallium perfusion defects by quantitative washout analysis with thallium reinjection in patients with coronary artery disease. Am. J. Cardiol. 74:977, 1994.
73. Favaro, L., Masini, F., Serra, W., et al.: Thallium 201 for detection of viable myocardium: Comparison of different reinjection protocols. J. Nucl. Cardiol. 1:515, 1994.
74. Marin-Neto, J.A., Dilsizian, V., Arrighi, J.A., et al.: Thallium reinjection demonstrates viable myocardium in regions with reverse redistribution. Circulation 88:1736, 1993.
75. Maublant, J.C., Lipiecki, J., Citron, B., et al.: Reinjection as an alternative to rest imaging for detection of exercise-induced ischemia with thallium-201 emission tomography. Am. Heart J. 125:330, 1993.
76. Kayden, D.S., Sigal, S., Soufer, R., et al.: Thallium-201 for assessment of myocardial viability: Quantitative comparison of 24-hour redistribution imaging with imaging after reinjection at rest. J. Am. Coll. Cardiol. 18:1480, 1991.
77. Watson, D.D., Smith, W., Vinson, E., et al.: Quantitative analysis of rest reinjection compared to redistribution (Abstract). J. Am. Coll. Cardiol. 19:129A, 1992.
78. Glover, D.K., Ruiz, M., Simanis, J.P., et al.: Tl-201 reinjection does not improve detection of defect reversibility compared with quantitative Tl-201 redistribution in a canine ischemia model (Abstract). Circulation 86:I-418, 1992.
79. Gimple, L.W., and Beller, G.A.: Myocardial viability: Assessment by cardiac scintigraphy. Cardiol. Clin. 12:317, 1994.
80. Iskandrian, A.S., Heo, J., and Stanberry, C.: When is myocardial viability an important clinical issue? J. Nucl. Med. 35(Suppl.):4S, 1994.
81. Berger, B.C., Watson, D.D., Burwell, L.R., et al.: Redistribution of thallium at rest in patients with stable and unstable angina and the effect of coronary artery bypass surgery. Circulation 60:1114, 1979.
82. Gewirtz, H., Beller, G.A., Strauss, H.W., et al.: Transient defects of resting thallium scans in patients with coronary artery disease. Circulation 59:707, 1979.
83. Hakki, A.H., Iskandrian, A.S., Kane, S.A., et al.: Thallium-201 myocardial scintigraphy and left ventricular function at rest in patients with rest angina pectoris. Am. Heart J. 108:326, 1984.
84. Mori, T., Minamiji, K., Kurogane, H., et al.: Rest-injected thallium-201 imaging for assessing viability of severe asynergic regions. J. Nucl. Med. 32:1718, 1991.
85. Ragosta, M., Beller, G.A., Watson, D.D., et al.: Quantitative planar rest-redistribution ^{201}Tl imaging in detection of myocardial viability and prediction of improvement in left ventricular function after coronary bypass surgery in patients with severely depressed left ventricular function. Circulation 87:1630, 1993.
86. Dilsizian, V., Perrone-Filardi, P., Arrighi, J.A., et al.: Concordance and discordance between rest-redistribution-reinjection thallium imaging for assessing viable myocardium: Comparison with metabolic activity by positron emission tomography. Circulation 88:941, 1993.
87. Lomboy, C.T., Schulman, D.S., Grill, H.P., et al.: Rest-redistribution thallium-201 scintigraphy to determine myocardial viability early after myocardial infarction. J. Am. Coll. Cardiol. 25:210, 1995.
88. Ritchie, J.L., Cerqueira, M., Maynard, C., et al.: Ventricular function and infarct size: The Western Washington Intravenous Streptokinase in Myocardial Infarction Trial. J. Am. Coll. Cardiol. 11:689, 1988.
89. Reduto, L.A., Freund, G.C., Gaeta, J.M., et al.: Coronary artery reperfusion in acute myocardial infarction: Beneficial effects of intracoronary streptokinase on left ventricular salvage and performance. Am. Heart J. 102:1168, 1981.
90. De Coster, P.M., Melin, J.A., Detry, J.M., et al.: Coronary artery reperfusion in acute myocardial infarction: Assessment by pre- and postintervention thallium-201 myocardial perfusion imaging. Am. J. Cardiol. 55:889, 1985.
91. Schwarz, F., Hofmann, M., Schuler, G., et al.: Thrombolysis in acute myocardial infarction: Effect of intravenous followed by intracoronary streptokinase application on estimates of infarct size. Am. J. Cardiol. 53:1505, 1984.
92. Granato, J.E., Watson, D.D., Flanagan, T.L., et al.: Myocardial thallium-201 kinetics during coronary occlusion and reperfusion: Influence of method of reflow and timing of thallium-201 administration. Circulation 73:150, 1986.
93. Berman, D.S., Kiat, H., Van Train, K., et al.: Technetium-99m sestamibi in the assessment of chronic coronary artery disease. Semin. Nucl. Med. 21:190, 1991.
94. Beller, G.A., and Watson, D.D.: Physiological basis of myocardial perfusion imaging with the technetium 99m agents. Semin. Nucl. Med. 21:173, 1991.
95. Sinusas, A.J., Beller, G.A., and Watson, D.D.: Cardiac imaging with technetium 99m-labeled isonitriles. J. Thorac. Imaging 5:20, 1990.
96. Leppo, J.A., DePuey, E.G., and Johnson, L.L.: A review of cardiac imaging with sestamibi and teboroxime. J. Nucl. Med. 32:2012, 1991.
97. Liu, P.: New technetium 99m imaging agents: Promising windows for myocardial perfusion and viability. Am. J. Card. Imaging 6:28, 1992.
98. Beller, G.A., and Sinusas, A.J.: Experimental studies of the physiologic properties of technetium-99m isonitriles. Am. J. Cardiol. 66:5E, 1990.
99. Maddahi, J., Kiat, H., Friedman, J.D., et al.: Technetium-99m-sestamibi myocardial perfusion imaging for evaluation of coronary artery disease. *In* Zaret, B.L., Beller, G.A. (eds.): Nuclear Cardiology: State of the Art and Future Directions. St. Louis, C.V. Mosby, 1993.
100. Berman, D.S., Kiat, H.S, Van Train, K.F., et al.: Myocardial perfusion imaging with technetium-99m-sestamibi: Comparative analysis of available imaging protocols. J. Nucl. Med. 35:681, 1994.
101. Hendel, R.C.: Single-photon perfusion imaging for the assessment of myocardial viability. J. Nucl. Med. 35(Suppl.):23S, 1994.

102. Bonow, R.O., and Dilsizian, V.: Thallium-201 and technetium-99m-sestamibi for assessing viable myocardium. J. Nucl. Med. 33:815, 1992.
103. Iskandrian, A.S., Heo, J., and Nguyen, T.: Current and emerging scintigraphic methods to assess myocardial viability and their critical importance. Am. J. Card. Imaging 6:16 (with editorial comments, 26), 1992.
104. Piwnica-Worms, D., Kronauge, J.F., and Chiu, M.L.: Uptake and retention of hexakis (2-methoxyisobutyl isonitrile) technetium(I) in cultured chick myocardial cells: Mitochondrial and plasma membrane potential dependence. Circulation 82:1826, 1990.
105. Piwnica-Worms, D., Chiu, M.L., and Kronauge, J.F.: Divergent kinetics of ^{201}Tl and ^{99m}Tc-sestamibi in cultured chick ventricular myocytes during ATP depletion. Circulation 85:1531, 1992.
106. Carvalho, P.A., Chiu, M.L., Kronauge, M., et al.: Subcellular distribution and analysis of technetium-99m-MIBI in isolated perfused rat hearts. J. Nucl. Med. 33:1516, 1992.
107. Beanlands, R.S., Dawood, F., Wen, W.H., et al.: Are the kinetics of technetium-99m methoxyisobutyl isonitrile affected by cell metabolism and viability? Circulation 82:1802, 1990.
108. Beller, G.A., Glover, D.K., Edwards, N.C., et al.: ^{99m}Tc-sestamibi uptake and retention during myocardial ischemia and reperfusion. Circulation 87:2033, 1993.
109. Sinusas, A.J., Bergin, J.D., Edwards, N.C., et al.: Redistribution of ^{99m}Tc-sestamibi and ^{201}Tl in the presence of a severe coronary artery stenosis. Circulation 89:2332, 1994.
110. Glover, D.K., and Okada, R.D.: Myocardial technetium 99m sestamibi kinetics after reperfusion in a canine model. Am. Heart J. 125:657, 1993.
111. Verani, M.S., Jeroudi, M.O., Mahmarian, J.J., et al.: Quantification of myocardial infarction during coronary occlusion and myocardial salvage after reperfusion using cardiac imaging with technetium-99m hexakis 2-methoxyisobutyl isonitrile. J. Am. Coll. Cardiol. 12:1573, 1988.
112. Sinusas, A.J., Trautman, K.A., Bergin, J.D., et al.: Quantification of area at risk during coronary occlusion and degree of myocardial salvage after reperfusion with technetium-99m methoxyisobutyl isonitrile. Circulation 82:1424, 1990.
113. Sinusas, A.J., Shi, Q., Vitols, P.J., et al.: Impact of regional ventricular function, geometry, and dobutamine stress on quantitative ^{99m}Tc-sestamibi defect size. Circulation 88:2224, 1993.
114. Taillefer, R., Primeau, M., Costi, P., et al.: Technetium-99m-sestamibi myocardial perfusion imaging in detection of coronary artery disease: Comparison between initial (1-hour) and delayed (3-hour) postexercise images. J. Nucl. Med. 32:1961, 1991.
115. Dilsizian, V., Arrighi, J., Diodati, J.G., et al.: Myocardial viability in patients with chronic coronary artery disease: Comparison of ^{99m}Tc-sestamibi with thallium reinjection and [^{18}F]-fluorodeoxyglucose. Circulation 89:578, 1994.
116. Cuocolo, A., Pace, L., Ricciardelli, B., et al.: Identification of viable myocardium in patients with chronic coronary artery disease: Comparison of thallium-201 scintigraphy with reinjection and technetium-99m-methoxyisobutyl isonitrile. J. Nucl. Med. 33:505, 1992.
117. Marzullo, P., Sambuceti, G., and Parodi, O.: The role of sestamibi scintigraphy in the radioisotopic assessment of myocardial viability. J. Nucl. Med. 33:1925, 1992.
118. Marzullo, P., Parodi, O., Reisenhofer, B., et al.: Value of rest thallium-201/technetium-99m sestamibi scans and dobutamine echocardiography for detecting myocardial viability. Am. J. Cardiol. 71:166, 1993.
119. Maurea, S., Cuocolo, A., Pace, L., et al.: Rest-injected thallium-201 resistribution and resting technetium-99m methoxyisobutylisonitrile uptake in coronary artery disease: Relation to the severity of coronary artery stenosis. Eur. J. Nucl. Med. 20:502, 1993.
120. Rocco, T.P., Dilsizian, V., Strauss, H.W., et al.: Technetium-99m isonitrile myocardial uptake at rest: Relation to clinical markers of potential viability. J. Am. Coll. Cardiol. 14:1678, 1989.
121. Sawada, S.G., Allman, K.C., Muzik, O., et al.: Positron emission tomography detects evidence of viability in rest technetium-99m sestamibi defects. J. Am. Coll. Cardiol. 23:92, 1994.
122. Udelson, J.E., Coleman, P.S., Metherall, J., et al.: Predicting recovery of severe regional ventricular dysfunction: Comparison of resting scintigraphy with ^{201}Tl and ^{99m}Tc-sestamibi. Circulation 89:2552, 1994.
123. Sinusas, A.J., Beller, G.A., Smith, W.H., et al.: Quantitative planar imaging with technetium-99m methoxy-isobutyl isonitrile: Comparison of uptake patterns with thallium-201. J. Nucl. Med. 30:1456, 1989.
124. Kauffman, G.J., Boyne, T.S., Watson, D.D., et al.: Comparison of resting ^{201}Tl imaging and resting ^{99m}Tc-sestamibi imaging to assessment of myocardial viability in patients with coronary artery disease and severe left ventricular dysfunction. J. Am. Coll. Cardiol. (in press).
125. Maurea, S., Cuocolo, A., Pace, L., et al.: Left ventricular dysfunction in coronary artery disease: Comparison between rest-redistribution thallium 201 and resting technetium 99m methoxyisobutyl isonitrile cardiac imaging. J. Nucl. Cardiol. 1:65, 1994.
126. Wackers, F.J., Gibbons, R.J., Verani, M.S., et al.: Serial quantitative planar technetium-99m isonitrile imaging in acute myocardial infarction: Efficacy for noninvasive assessment of thrombolytic therapy. J. Am. Coll. Cardiol. 14:861, 1989.
127. Gibbons, R.J., Verani, M.S., Behrenbeck, T., et al.: Feasibility of tomographic ^{99m}Tc-hexakis-2-methoxy-2-methylpropyl-isonitrile imaging for the assessment of myocardial area at risk and the effect of treatment in acute myocardial infarction. Circulation 80:1277, 1989.
128. Chua, T., Kiat, H., Germano, G., et al.: Gated technetium-99m sestamibi for simultaneous assessment of stress myocardial perfusion, postexercise regional ventricular function and myocardial viability: Correlation with echocardiography and rest thallium-201 scintigraphy. J. Am. Coll. Cardiol. 23:1107, 1994.
129. Reske, S.N.: Experimental and clinical experience with iodine 123-labeled iodophenylpentadecanoic acid in cardiology. J. Nucl. Cardiol. 1(Suppl.):S58, 1994.
130. Corbett, J.: Clinical experience with iodine-123-iodophenylpentadecanoic acid. J. Nucl. Med. 35(Suppl.):32S, 1994.
131. Hansen, C.L.: Preliminary report of an ongoing phase I/II dose range, safety and efficacy study of iodine-123-phenylpentadecanoic acid for the identification of viable myocardium. J. Nucl. Med. 35(Suppl.):38S, 1994.
132. Hansen, C.L., Heo, J., and Iskandrian, A.S.: Prediction of improvement of left ventricular function after coronary revascularization from alterations in myocardial metabolic activity detected with I-123 phenylpentadecanoic acid dynamic SPECT imaging (Abstract). J. Am. Coll. Cardiol. February 1994; 344A.
133. Murray, G.L., Schad, N.C., Magill, H.L., et al.: Myocardial viability assessment with dynamic low-dose iodine-123-iodophenylpentadecanoic acid metabolic imaging: Comparison with myocardial biopsy and reinjection SPECT thallium after myocardial infarction. J. Nucl. Med. 35(Suppl.):43S, 1994.
134. Powers, J., Cave, V., Wasserleben, V., et al.: Mechanisms and implications of redistribution during dynamic rest SPECT I-123 IPPA imaging. J. Am. Coll. Cardiol. February 1994; 423A.
135. Tamaki, N., and Kawamoto, M.: The use of iodinated free fatty acids for assessing fatty acid metabolism. J. Nucl. Cardiol. 1(Suppl.):S72, 1994.
136. Kuikka, J.T., Mussalo, H., Hietakorpi, S., et al.: Evaluation of myocardial viability with technetium-99m hexakis-2-methoxyisobutyl isonitrile and iodine-123 phenylpentadecanoic acid and single photon emission tomography. Eur. J. Nucl. Med. 19:882, 1992.

CHAPTER

65 Imaging Acute Myocardial Necrosis (Monoclonal Antibodies and Technetium-99m Pyrophosphate)

Lynne L. Johnson, M.D.

The standard tests in general clinical use to diagnose myocardial infarction (MI), the electrocardiogram (ECG) and cardiac enzymes, have a fairly high sensitivity and specificity for including or excluding recent myocardial necrosis. However, in some patients the diagnosis remains in question, and additional tests are needed to plan future care. Assessment of left ventricular function and myocardial perfusion imaging have major limitations in excluding or confirming the diagnosis of acute MI.

Analysis of global and regional left ventricular function to diagnose and assess the extent of MI is limited by the recognized discordance between the extent and severity of wall motion abnormalities and the extent of myocardial viability and scar. Regional or global left ventricular function may be reversibly depressed in patients with ischemic heart disease because of stunning, hibernation, or both. Function may be down-regulated as a consequence of reduced energy production to adjust to limited resting blood flow in the process described as "hibernation."[1] In stunning, brief episodes of myocardial ischemia can lead to reversible reduction in myocardial contractility. Myocardial stunning can develop in patients who have repeated episodes of angina or "silent ischemia," as well as in patients after acute MI.[2] Myocardial stunning resolves with time after the ischemic insult, and hibernating myocardium improves function with revascularization. In addition to hibernation or stunning, regional left ventricular dysfunction not related to the acute ischemic event may be due to remote MI or to coexisting myocardial disease consequent to hypertensive heart disease, postviral myocarditis, or idiopathic dilated cardiomyopathy. These situations confound the ability to use wall motion analysis to diagnose or localize regions of recent myocardial necrosis.

The detection and localization of myocardial perfusion defects with thallium- or technetium-based myocardial perfusion scans also have limited accuracy in confirming or excluding the diagnosis of recent myocardial necrosis. Regions of remote myocardial scar are indistinguishable from regions of recent myocardial necrosis or acute ischemia on perfusion scans. Reduction in left ventricular contraction secondary to ischemic myocardial stunning can, in itself, lead to reduction in regional uptake of a perfusion tracer.[3] In addition, nontransmural necrosis can reduce the sensitivity of perfusion tracers in diagnosing recent myocardial necrosis, because on nongated images, uptake of a perfusion tracer in the epicardium may hide mild hypoperfusion to the subendocardium.

For all the reasons described, a noninvasive imaging modality to diagnose and localize recent myocardial necrosis continues to have a niche in diagnostic medicine, despite the advent of new therapies and imaging modalities. This chapter describes the use of radiolabeled tracers taken up into myocardium that is recently infarcted; these tracers are therefore categorized as "hot spot" imaging agents. Two classes of infarct-avid radiotracers will be discussed: technetium-99m (^{99m}Tc) pyrophosphate and monoclonal antibodies directed against cardiac myosin. At the time of the writing of this chapter, antimyosin antibodies were not available in the United States but were available in a number of European countries.

TECHNETIUM-99M PYROPHOSPHATE

Mechanism of Uptake

Technetium-99m pyrophosphate binds to calcium and has been used primarily for bone scans. Twenty years ago it was observed that some patients undergoing bone scanning showed cardiac uptake of ^{99m}Tc-pyrophosphate and had a clinical history of recent MI.[4] It was also observed a number of years ago by several groups of investigators that in severely ischemic and infarcted myocardium, calcium localizes within the mitochondria and that mitochondrial calcium is incorporated within a crystalline structure similar to that of hydroxyapatite.[5–7] Buja and colleagues[8] performed a number of experiments to localize the sites of pyrophosphate uptake in ischemic and infarcted myocardium. In in vitro experiments, they found that pyrophosphate binds to hydroxyapatite and amorphous calcium phosphate. On electromyography (EMG), they found that mitochondria of necrotic myocytes exhibit electron-dense calcific deposits and less dense amorphous matrix densities that resemble hydroxyapatite and are thought to be binding sites for pyrophosphate.[8] Other radiotracers are known to bind to hydroxyapatite, including ^{99m}Tc-diphosphonate.[9, 10] In an experimental study in dogs that compared infarct uptake of ^{99m}Tc-pyrophoshate and ^{99m}Tc-diphosphonate, ^{99m}Tc-pyrophosphate provided slightly better infarct to normal myocardial count ratios and slightly less favorable (for MI imaging) bone content.[9] Both agents provided diagnostic images.

To enable pyrophosphate to bind to intracellular myocardial calcium, the radiotracer must be delivered to the tissue that is acutely ischemic, infarcted, or both. If the infarct-related artery is occluded (nonreperfused) and there are sparse collaterals to the ischemic region, radiotracer delivery to the central infarct zone will be impaired. Likewise, in late reperfused infarctions, blood flow to the central infarct zone is impaired because of the effects of cell swelling on limiting nutrient flow at the microvascular level.[11] Because pyrophosphate requires some flow for delivery to the necrotic tissue and because calcium flux across the sarcolemma is increased in myocytes with severe but reversible ischemic injury, pyrophosphate uptake is greatest at the infarct borders, where blood flow is only moderately reduced.[12] This phenomenon explains the observation of a "doughnut" pattern of tracer uptake observed in patients with large anterior infarctions. It also explains why pyrophosphate uptake, when used to map out the infarction, overestimates the extent of necrosis.

The mechanism of pyrophosphate binding also helps explain the window of scan positivity. It takes a period of time, following initiation of ischemia, before changes in calcium flux produce accumulations of intracellular calcium sufficient to result in positive pyrophosphate scans. In general, it takes 24 to 48 hours from the onset of symptoms until pyrophosphate scans are positive, with a range of time from 12 to 72 hours. Because of these pharmacokinetics, pyrophosphate cannot be used to confirm or exclude the presence of recent necrosis in patients coming through the emergency room with chest pain. The window for scan positivity for pyrophosphate is 2 to 14 days, although some patients have persistently positive scans for months after their infarction. Persistently positive scans correlate with large anterior infarctions and aneurysm formation.

Radiotracer Preparation and Imaging Parameters

A dose of approximately 25 mCi of ^{99m}Tc is added to a vial of commercially available stannous pyrophosphate. The radiotracer is administered intravenously and should not be injected through an intravenous line used to infuse heparin, because in vivo breakdown of the radiolabel will occur, resulting in poor scan quality. Technetium-99m pyrophosphate clears from the blood pool relatively rapidly, with a clearance half-life (T1/2) of about 15 minutes. To allow for blood pool clearance, imaging is delayed for about 2.5 hours after injection. Because blood pool clearance is further prolonged in patients with renal impairment, the time from injection to imaging should be prolonged to 4 hours in patients with renal failure.

Planar imaging is sufficient in the majority of patients. Three to four planar scans are acquired, using a 15 percent window centered over the 140-keV photopeak of ^{99m}Tc and a general all-purpose (low-energy, high-resolution) collimator or a high-resolution collimator, in a 128 × 128 matrix, for a total count level of 500,000 counts in the anterior image. Intensity of tracer uptake on the planar scans is scored with reference to sternal uptake of tracer (0 = no cardiac uptake; 1+ = faint or equivocal cardiac uptake; 2+ = tracer uptake in the myocardial region less intense than sternal uptake but greater than background; 3+ = tracer uptake in myocardial region less intense than sternal uptake but greater than background; and 4+ = myocardial uptake more intense than sternal uptake) (Fig. 65–1).

Rib and sternal uptake of pyrophosphate, as well as persistent blood pool activity, can interfere with visualization of small or faint regions of cardiac uptake of tracer. Because of its greater contrast resolution, tomographic imaging may help resolve some of these defects. A suggested approach to pyrophosphate imaging is to perform the planar imaging and interpret the scans before allowing the patient to leave the department. When the planar scans are clearly positive or clearly negative and the clinical probability of a positive scan is low, the test is finished and the patient can leave the department. When the planar scans are equivocal and the clinical probability is moderate to high, tomographic imaging should be performed. Even with the use of tomography, small regions of tracer uptake in the heart may not be resolved. Corbett and co-workers developed a technique of simultaneously labeling the blood pool and, with color tables and scan overlays, subtracting blood pool activity to reveal small regions of focal pyrophosphate uptake.[13]

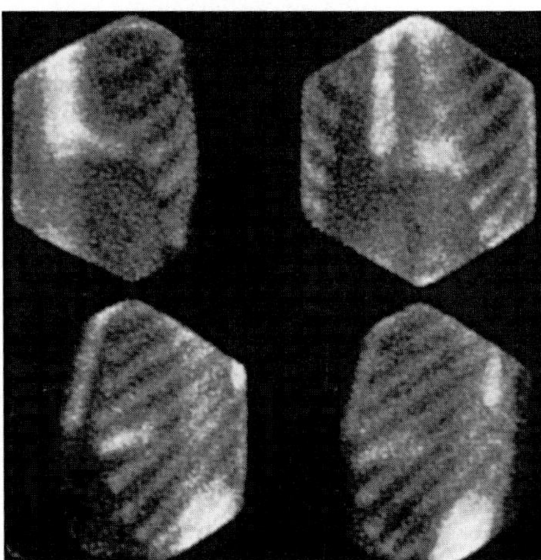

FIGURE 65–1. Four planar ^{99m}Tc-pyrophosphate scans in the anterior, shallow, steep left anterior oblique, and left lateral projections. There is grade 3 intensity of tracer uptake (equal to sternal uptake) in the inferoposterior wall of the left ventricle in a patient with recent inferior wall infarction. (Courtesy of Dr. James R. Corbett, University of Michigan Hospital, Ann Arbor.)

A suggested protocol for tomographic imaging of pyrophosphate includes the following. For a single-detector camera, use a 64 × 64 matrix with a 180-degree orbit, 60 stops (3-degree increments, 15 to 20 seconds per stop). For multidetector cameras the imaging time can be decreased and continuous acquisition performed. For processing, a Butterworth filter can be used, with cutoff frequencies selected according to image statistics. Transaxial slices are interpreted, or oblique reconstruction performed. The axes selected for oblique reconstruction of the left ventricle must be estimated in the absence of tracer uptake, which delineates the heart borders.

ANTIMYOSIN ANTIBODIES

Antibody Development

Several years after the observation was made that pyrophosphate is taken up into necrotic myocardium, Khaw and co-workers began developing radiolabeled antibodies that can be used as infarct-avid radiotracers.[14] They observed that heavy-chain myosin is a highly insoluble protein, making it a good target antigen for antibody imaging because the antigen remains at the site where the antibody must bind to localize the infarction. Because heavy-chain myosin constitutes about 10 percent of the myocyte contents, it is an antigen that provides an abundance of antibody binding sites. In a series of experiments Khaw and co-workers demonstrated that antimyosin uptake is highly specific for myocyte necrosis.[15, 16] For the antibody to gain access to bind to the antigen, the sarcolemmal membrane must be disrupted, a process that signals irreversible cell injury and subsequent cell death. This specificity for binding to irreversibly injured myocytes is distinct from that of ^{99m}Tc-pyrophosphate, which is also taken up into severely but reversibly ischemic myocardium. In an animal experiment directly comparing the uptake of the two tracers, Beller and co-workers found that ^{99m}Tc-pyrophosphate uptake was greatest at the infarct borders, where blood flow was only moderately reduced, whereas uptake of antimyosin correlated inversely with blood flow levels measured by microspheres.[12]

The first antimyosin antibody used experimentally was a murine whole immunoglobulin G (IgG) antibody directed against canine myocardium and labeled with iodine-125 or iodine-133.[12] Over the next several years the antibody underwent a series of modifications. With the use of hybridoma technology and human heavy-chain myosin as the antigen, murine monoclonal antibodies directed against human heavy-chain myosin were developed. To decrease antigenicity and hasten blood pool clearance, the whole antibody was cleaved by papain digestion to produce Fab fragments.[18] These fragments were labeled via diethylenetriamine pentaacetic acid to ^{99m}Tc, but because of apparent breakdown of the radiotracer and antibody complex in the blood due to transchelation of ^{99m}Tc to transferrin, the antibody fragments were then labeled via diethylenetriamine pentaacetic acid to indium-111 (^{111}In) in citrate buffer at pH 5.5.[19] The citrate buffer prevents the ^{111}In from forming a colloid, thereby minimizing damage to the protein during preparation.

Because ^{111}In is cyclotron produced, it is not readily available and is relatively expensive. The two photopeaks of ^{111}In (167 and 247 keV, respectively) are relatively high, requiring use of a medium-energy collimator for imaging. In addition the biologic T1/2 of ^{111}In is relatively long, limiting the administered dose to about 2 mCi. Because ^{99m}Tc is generator produced, widely available, and less costly, further work has recently been performed to produce technetium-labeled monoclonal antibody fragments that do not break down in vivo and have more rapid blood pool clearances.

There are three approaches to improving the labeling of ^{99m}Tc to antibody fragments: development of novel chelators, direct labeling of ^{99m}Tc to the antibody fragments via the native cysteine residues, and conjugating a preformed ^{99m}Tc complexes to the antibody protein. A novel bifunctional chelator (RP-1) was developed to attach to the sulfhydryls of the C-terminus region of the antibody Fab′ fragments via an ester linkage.[20, 21] This linkage facilitates breakdown of the antibody complex in the kidneys, which hastens renal clearance of antibody and blood pool clearance. The direct method of antibody labeling has been pursued by a Canadian group. They developed a mixture of monoclonal murine Fab′ and $F(ab')_2$ fragments directed against heavy-chain human cardiac myosin that they labeled with ^{99m}Tc by reducing both the protein sulfhydryl groups and the technetium, allowing the two to bind.[22]

Other antibody modifications have been pursued to improve image quality and dosimetry and to hasten blood pool clearance to allow earlier imaging. To decrease the nonspecific organ uptake of radiolabeled antibody fragments, Torchilin and co-workers and Khaw and colleagues developed a polylysine antimyosin.[23, 24] All cell membranes possess a global negative charge that contributes to nonselective binding of the positively charged antibody fragments. By modifying the antibody by means of negatively charged, low-molecular polylysine, the nonspecific interaction of the antibody with other organs, especially the liver, is decreased. The linking of polyvalent cations such as ^{111}In to protein polymers requires chelating agents to bind to the polymer. Chelator groups can be substituted on the polymer, increasing the ratio of the number of moles of ^{111}In to moles of Fab, thereby increasing the specific activity of the antibody complex and diminishing the administered dose of ^{111}In.

The antibody modification that most successfully speeds blood pool clearance to allow earliest imaging is the sFv fragment of antimyosin antibody.[25] This fragment contains only the antigenic binding sites. Because of its small size, it is cleared from the blood pool much more rapidly than the Fab fragment. In an animal infarct model, imaging of a ^{99m}Tc-labeled sFv antimyosin fragment was possible as early as 1 hour after injection. Because this antibody fragment is a fusion protein produced in *Escherichia coli*, at present it is too costly to manufacture for clinical use.

The ^{111}In-labeled Fab fragment of antimyosin is the radiolabeled antibody used in clinical trials in the United States and is available clinically in some European countries; therefore, the clinical and imaging parameters discussed below will apply to ^{111}In antimyosin.

Radiotracer Preparation and Imaging Parameters

Two mCi of ^{111}In is added to a vial containing 50 mg of antibody in citrate buffer, and following incubation, chromatography is performed to assess the protein binding. The radiolabeled antibody is injected intravenously at the bedside. Because of the relatively slow blood pool clearance (T1/2 = about 6 hours), imaging must be delayed for 24 to 48 hours after injection. In 13 to 20 percent of patients the blood pool activity at 24 hours is still too great to show discrete myocardial uptake. Three to four planar images are acquired, with the use of two 15 percent windows centered over the 171- and 247-keV photopeaks of ^{111}In, using a medium energy collimator and a 128 × 128 matrix for approximately 10 minutes per image. Significant extracardiac uptake of ^{111}In antimyosin occurs in the liver and kidneys. A scheme for scoring the intensity of radiotracer uptake in the heart by comparing the count intensity to a reference organ uptake, which is similar to the method described for ^{99m}Tc-pyrophosphate, can be performed for antimyosin. Intensity of cardiac uptake is compared to hepatic tracer uptake (0 = negative; 1+ = equivocal; 2+ = greater than background but less than liver; and 3+ = equal to liver uptake). A strategy for clinical imaging similar to that described for ^{99m}Tc-pyrophosphate is as follows. Planar imaging is performed at 24 hours after injection, and, when clearly positive, the test is completed; however, when the scans are equivocal or when there is too much residual blood pool activity, the patient must return at 48 hours for repeat imaging (Fig. 65–2). If the planar scans are clearly negative, the test is completed, but when equivocal, tomography should be performed. The imaging protocol recommended for a single-detector camera and medium-energy collimator is 32 projections at 60 seconds per projection. The use of filters must be optimized for each camera.

DIAGNOSTIC ACCURACIES OF INFARCT-AVID IMAGING

The diagnostic accuracy of infarct-avid imaging is limited by the physiologic parameters of the infarction that may affect tracer

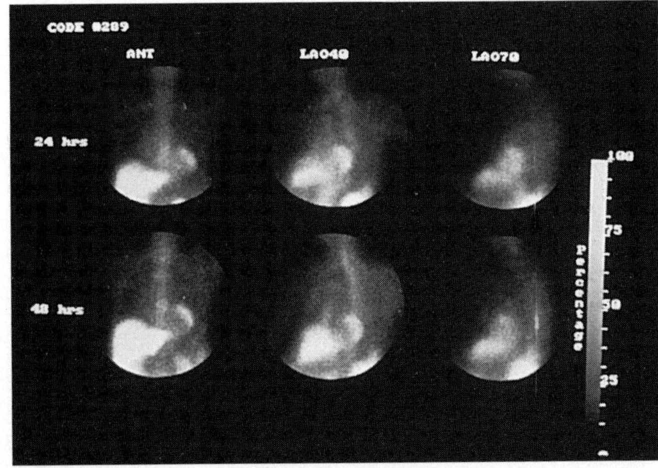

FIGURE 65–2. Planar ^{111}In antimyosin antibody (AMA) scans performed at 24 hours *(top row)* and 48 hours *(bottom row)* following tracer injection. In this patient, blood pool activity cleared well by 24 hours, allowing clear visualization of focal uptake in the lateral wall of the left ventricle.

delivery or imaging, such as status of the infarct vessel, presence or absence of collaterals, infarct size, and location. In a dog infarct model, intensity of antimyosin uptake on planar scans was found to be greater in infarctions reperfused following 2 hours of occlusion than in infarctions reperfused following 6 hours of balloon occlusion (close to no reflow), despite the larger sizes of infarctions reperfused after 6 hours of occlusion (Fig. 65–3).[26] In a more recent nonimaging experimental study, it was found that ^{111}In antimyosin activity in infarct zones increases with increasing ischemic injury, as measured by triphenyl tetrazolium chloride (TTC) for both early reperfused and nonreperfused infarctions, but that this relationship is attenuated in the nonreperfused infarctions.[27] The difference in ratios of indium activity to TTC grade between reperfused and nonreperfused infarctions was abolished when the indium activity was corrected for residual blood flow. These observations made in experimental studies have correlated well with what has been observed clinically, using infarct-avid tracers. Uptake of ^{111}In antimyosin is more intense in reperfused infarctions. Equivocal scans or false-negative scans correlate with both posterior infarct location and total occlusion of the infarct-related vessel and absent collaterals.[28]

The diagnostic accuracy of ^{99m}Tc-pyrophosphate in diagnosing acute MI was addresed in a study that comprised 52 patients who underwent ^{99m}Tc-pyrophosphate imaging and subsequently died and underwent necropsy.[29] Predictive indices for the recognition of microscopic or gross MI by the radionuclide imaging technique were evaluated. The sensitivity was 80 percent, the specificity was 100 percent, the predictive value of a positive scan was 100 percent, and for a negative scan it was 72 percent. These results compare fairly well with what one would expect from the known limitations of the technique to detect small areas of necrosis due to interference with overlying rib uptake, residual blood pool activity, and limited resolution of the camera.

The safety and diagnostic accuracy of planar antimyosin imaging was evaluated in a large multicenter trial in which 497 patients were enrolled in the United States and Europe.[30] The "gold standard" for myocardial necrosis used in this clinical trial was the ECG and enzyme measurements. For this reason, patients with uninterpretable ECGs, such as left bundle branch block, or late presenters were excluded from enrollment. The overall sensitivity for detecting myocardial necrosis was 89 percent, with 94 percent sensitivity for detection of Q wave infarctions and 82 percent for non-Q infarctions. Specificity was 95 percent, as assessed from patients admitted to the hospital with chest pain subsequently determined not to be cardiac in origin. These sensitivity and specificity values are similar to those reported in two smaller published trials. In general, "false-positive" scans occurred in patients with myocarditis. Most of the false-negative scans occurred in patients with inferoposterior infarctions and patients with total occlusion of the infarct vessel and absent collaterals.

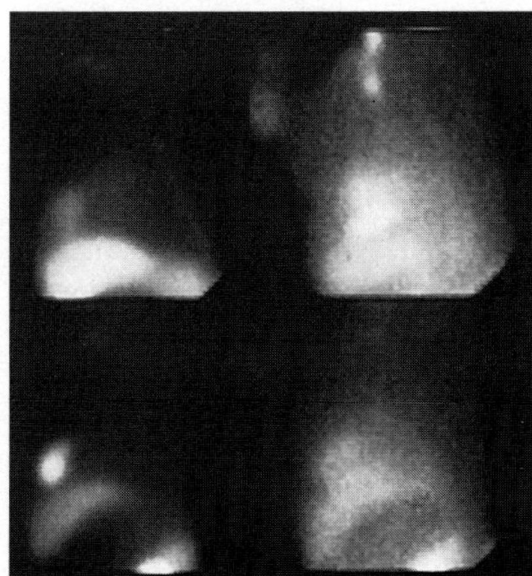

FIGURE 65–3. Simultaneously acquired dual-isotope (^{111}In antimyosin antibody [AMA] and ^{201}Tl) left lateral planar images acquired in a 6-hour balloon occlusion left anterior descending artery (LAD) infarction (late reflow) *(top)* and 2-hour balloon occlusion LAD infarction (early reflow) *(bottom)*. ^{111}In AMA scans are on the left, and ^{201}Tl scans on the right. Note the more intense ^{111}In uptake in relationship to hepatic uptake in the early reperfused infarction.

The diagnostic accuracy of antimyosin images is also affected by the incidence of late-scan positivity. In the clinical trials described previously, only patients with acute infarctions and onset of chest pain within 48 hours of antibody injection were reported. A subsequent study of 182 patients who were given injections at intervals after the acute infarction revealed that antimyosin scans can remain positive for up to 6 months after infarction in a fairly high percentage of patients: 65 percent positive at 2 to 4 months, 62 percent at 4 to 6 months, 51 percent at 6 to 8 months, 46 percent at 8 to 10 months, and 29 percent at 10 to 12 months. These data, which have not been published in manuscript form to date, are supported by data from several smaller published studies.[31, 32] The presumed mechanism for late positivity is the existence of residual strands of myosin embedded in the infarction that present binding sites for the ^{111}In-labeled antibody. This fairly high prevalence of late positive antimyosin scans decreases specificity of the technique in identifying patients with acute necrosis, because a prior infarction within one year may take up radiolabeled antibody. The clinical history for each patient undergoing antimyosin scanning must be considered when one interprets scans.

The safety of Fab antimyosin antibodies was also investigated in the large multicenter trial. There were no acute allergic reactions to antibody injection and no episodes of serum sickness. Human antimouse antibody titers were measured before and after antibody injection, and the results did not show any significant rise in titers following a single antibody injection. Rises in titer have not been detected after multiple injections of antibody into patients who were enrolled in the late positivity study, nor were they detected in patients with myocarditis, cardiomyopathy, or cardiac transplant rejection who received multiple injections.[33, 34]

Antimyosin scans can be positive in patients with unstable angina. The degree of ischemic injury to the heart muscle represents a continuum of damage related to the length of vessel occlusion, ranging from unstable angina with transient thrombus and/or local vasospasm to non–Q wave infarctions (which are usually reperfused infarctions) to Q wave infarctions that are frequently late reperfused or nonperfused infarctions. It is not surprising, therefore, that in the large multicenter clinical trial, 37 percent of patients who received the diagnosis of unstable angina from review of the clinical and laboratory data had positive antimyosin scans. In these cases, transient reductions in flow were sufficient to result in myocardial necrosis that could not be detected by determinations of the MB isoenzyme of creatine kinase (CK-MB).

In addition to MI, myocyte necrosis is the hallmark of acute myocarditis, the early stages of cardiomyopathy, and cardiac transplant rejection. A number of studies have been performed that evaluated the clinical efficacy of antimyosin in these conditions.[35–39] Patients with acute myocarditis, new onset of left ventricular failure thought to be due to myocarditis, or new onset of left ventricular failure thought to be due to myocarditis or cardiomyopathy show varying degrees of diffuse myocardial uptake of ^{111}In antimyosin. The degree of myocardial uptake is expressed in relation to lung uptake of the radiotracer as the heart-to-lung ratio. In patients with a diffuse myocardial process, care must be taken to ensure that blood pool activity has cleared before one attempts to interpret antimyosin uptake. Positive scans in patients with new onset of left ventricular dysfunction identify patients who show spontaneous improvement in left ventricular function over time as the scan changes from positive to negative, implying that an inflammatory or a reversible process was operative.[36, 39] Using heart-to-lung ratios to quantitate diffuse antimyosin uptake in patients after cardiac transplantation, Carrio and co-workers found an overall correlation with the histopathologic rejection score made from the endomyocardial biopsy samples, but there was a wide range in the intensity of antimyosin uptake within each rejection score classification.[33] This group of investigators found the ratio of 2.0 to be a cutoff separating patients who went on to have further rejection-related complications from those who did not.[37]

CLINICAL INDICATIONS FOR INFARCT-AVID SCANNING

As discussed in the introductory paragraphs, clinical tests routinely performed in patients admitted with chest pain, such as the ECG and cardiac enzymes, are sufficient to establish or rule out MI in the majority of patients. However, in some patients the diagnosis will still be in doubt, including patients with equivocal enzymes and nonspecific ECG abnormalities, patients with left bundle branch block, and late presenters. The late presenter is the patient who comes to the hospital at least 1 week after onset of symptoms with an infarct pattern of indeterminant age on the ECG, too late after the acute event for the enzymes to be elevated. For further management it is important to establish the diagnosis of recent infarction; therefore, in these patients, performing an infarct-avid scan is clinically indicated.

DUAL-ISOTOPE IMAGING

Based on the premise that the combined uptake patterns of an infarct-avid tracer such as ^{111}In antimyosin and a flow or viability agent such as thallium-201 (^{201}Tl) can provide information on location and extent of infarction, as well as location and extent of viable myocardium at further ischemic risk, simultaneous imaging of ^{111}In antimyosin and ^{201}Tl was investigated, first in an animal model and then in a clinical trial. The physical properties of ^{201}Tl and ^{111}In make them uniquely suited for simultaneous imaging. Their half-lives are similar, making the injected doses almost equivalent, and their photopeaks are well separated. An animal experiment was performed in which half the animals underwent balloon occlusion of a coronary artery followed by reflow at 2 hours and half underwent balloon occlusion followed by reflow at 6 hours, a situation approximating a no-reflow state.[26] Following balloon deflation, the animals were injected with ^{111}In antimyosin and, 24 hours later, were injected with ^{201}Tl and underwent simultaneous dual-isotope planar and tomographic imaging using the high (247-keV) photopeak of ^{111}In and the 70-keV photopeak of ^{201}Tl. In the late reflow group, the pattern of uptake of the two tracers fit together like pieces in a puzzle. The early reflow infarcts were smaller, showed more intense tracer uptake, and showed a greater degree of overlap with ^{201}Tl uptake than did the 6-hour reperfused infarcts. A more recent experimental study using ^{99m}Tc-sestamibi as the perfusion agent and ^{111}In antimyosin documented overlap of the two tracers in myocardial segments of infarctions demonstrated to be nontransmural on histopathology.[40] Animal infarct models cannot reproduce variables encountered in patients, such as multivessel disease and presence or absence of collaterals.

To investigate the hypothesis that the pattern of uptake of ^{111}In antimyosin and ^{201}Tl on simultaneously obtained tomograms can map out regions of recent necrosis, viable nonjeopardized myocardium, and jeopardized viable myocardium, 87 patients underwent simultaneous dual-isotope imaging at Columbia-Presbyterian Medical center. This study comprised 81 patients with myocardial necrosis confirmed by CK-MB fractions and 6 with unstable angina. There were 54 men and 33 women, with a mean age of 59 ± 12 years. Sixty-one patients had Q wave infarctions (anterior in 27, inferoposterior in 34), 17 had non-Q infarctions, and 3 had infarctions that could not be localized by ECG. Only 10 of these patients received thrombolytic therapy.[41, 42]

Radiotracer Preparation and Imaging Parameters

Indium-111 antimyosin was prepared as described previously and injected at the bedside within 48 hours of the onset of chest pain. Forty-eight hours later each patient was brought to the nuclear cardiology laboratory, was given an injection of 2.2 mCi of ^{201}Tl, and underwent simultaneous dual-isotope tomographic imaging. A 15 percent window was set over the 247-keV photopeak of ^{111}In and a 20 percent window was set over the 70-keV photopeak of ^{201}Tl. A medium-energy collimator was used on a single-detector camera, with a 180-degree circular orbit, a 64 × 64 matrix, and 32 projections at 60 seconds per projection. A Metz prefilter was used with ramp backprojection. The two simultaneously acquired studies were split apart, and the ^{201}Tl study was reconstructed first. The angles used to produce the obliquely reconstructed short-axis and vertical long-axis slices for the ^{201}Tl study were duplicated for reconstructing the ^{111}In antimyosin data. When cardiac uptake was present, the slices were scaled to the hottest pixel in the heart.

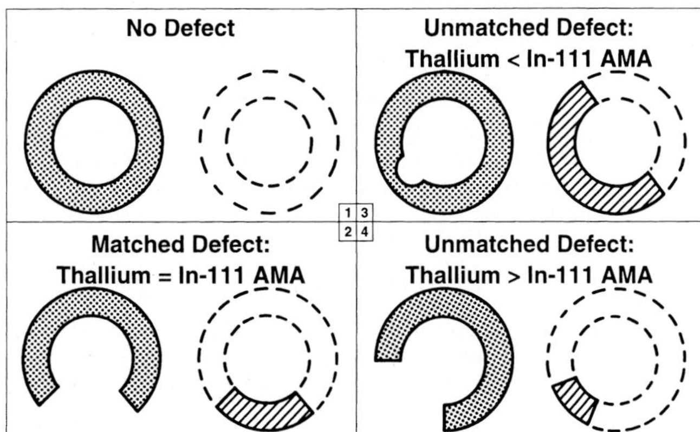

FIGURE 65–4. Scheme for classifying patterns of uptake of ^{111}In antimyosin antibody (AMA) and ^{201}Tl on simultaneously acquired dual-isotope tomography.

Scan Interpretation

Corresponding short-axis, vertical long-axis, and horizontal long-axis slices from both the ^{201}Tl and the ^{111}In antimyosin tomograms were lined up next to each other on a color display monitor for qualitative interpretation. Patterns of the relative uptake of the two tracers were classified as matches, mismatches, or overlap (Fig. 65–4). Thallium defects corresponding in extent and location to antimyosin uptake were classified as "matches." Thallium-201 defects seen in vascular territories without antimyosin uptake or thallium defects more extensive than antimyosin uptake were classified as "mismatches." Both thallium and antimyosin uptake occurring in the same myocardial segment were classified as "overlap." Not uncommonly, one patient had several patterns of uptake of the two tracers in different vascular territories, for instance, a matching pattern in the left anterior descending territory and another unmatched thallium defect in the right coronary artery territory, or both match and overlap of the two tracers in the same vascular territory. Because of the small number of scans showing overlap alone and because the overlap pattern denotes nontransmural necrosis, all scans showing a mismatch, an overlap, or both were classified as mismatches, and all scans showing a single matching pattern of uptake of the two tracers were classified matches.

The 87 patients described earlier were followed for 6 weeks after their MIs to evaluate the dual-isotope scan patterns as predictors of ischemic end points defined as recurrent angina, recurrent MI, death, or evidence for ischemia on the 6-week symptom-limited stress test. During the period of follow-up, 39 patients developed further ischemic end points. A total of 38 of these 39 patients had dual-isotope scan patterns interpreted as mismatches, yielding a sensitivity of 97 percent in detecting patients with further ischemic end points in the first 6 weeks after infarction (Fig. 65–5). Of the 48 patients who were event free for up to 6 weeks, the dual-isotope

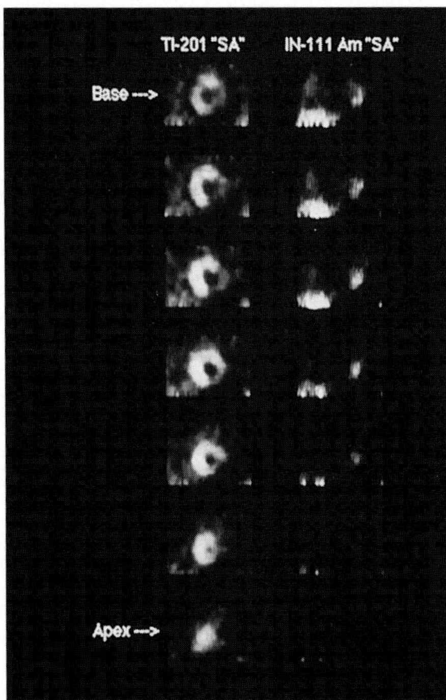

FIGURE 65–5. Side-by-side display of simultaneously acquired ^{201}Tl short-axis tomographic slices on the left and ^{111}In antimyosin antibody (AMA) short-axis slices on the right from a patient admitted with an acute lateral wall MI who received thrombolytic therapy with clinical evidence for reperfusion. The inferolateral thallium defect is more extensive than the region of ^{111}In AMA uptake (mismatch in infarct territory). The patient subsequently developed recurrent chest pain and was brought to the catheterization laboratory, where angiography revealed single-vessel disease with a patent but highly stenotic infarct vessel (left circumflex coronary artery).

scan patterns were almost evenly divided between matches and mismatches, yielding a specificity of only 56 percent. Sources of false-positive ischemic scan patterns include old infarctions and perfusion defects due to myocardial stunning; sources of false-negative ischemic antimyosin scan patterns include poor tracer delivery to the area of infarction. It is interesting to note that nine of the patients in this "false-negative" category who underwent coronary angiography had large anterior infarctions with areas of moderate to intense antimyosin uptake in part but not all of the risk region as delineated by the thallium defect extent and totally occluded left anterior descending coronary artery. It is tempting to hypothesize that the dual-isotope scan patterns were able to identify patients with residual myocardium at risk in the infarct vessel territory who are candidates for rescue angioplasty.

DIAGNOSIS OF RIGHT VENTRICULAR INFARCTION

Right ventricular infarction occurs in about 45 percent of patients with acute occlusion of the right coronary artery (inferior-wall MIs). Because the right ventricular muscle mass is less than the left ventricular mass, right ventricular infarctions are small in comparison. In addition, the right ventricle is resilient to ischemic insults, even in the absence of reperfusion, and right ventricular function returns to normal over time in most patients. Making the diagnosis of infarction of the right ventricle in the setting of acute inferior-wall MI becomes clinically important when a patient is admitted with acute infarction and hypotension. The differential diagnosis includes hypovolemia, cardiogenic shock, and right ventricular infarction. Because the treatments of these conditions differ, making the correct diagnosis is important. Since the advent of routine placement of pulmonary artery catheters in patients with acute MIs and the performance of bedside echocardiography, relying on nuclear imaging modalities to make the diagnosis of right ventricular infarction is not necessary. The following discussion will serve to inform the reader about the patterns of uptake of infarct-avid tracers in the right ventricle, so that these patterns can be recognized and commented on during the interpretation of infarct-avid scans performed on patients with recent MIs.

Studies evaluating the efficacy of ^{99m}Tc-pyrophosphate in identifying right ventricular necrosis were performed 15 years ago. The low muscle mass of the right ventricle, combined with sternal uptake of pyrophosphate, makes it difficult to identify pyrophosphate uptake localized to the right ventricle. Despite these difficulties, several groups of investigators were able to diagnose right ventricular infarctions on planar pyrophosphate scans, reporting an incidence of 33 to 37 percent among patients with acute inferior-wall infarctions and demonstrating a correlation between right ventricular uptake of pyrophosphate and reduced right ventricular ejection fraction.[43, 44]

It is even more difficult to see tracer uptake localized to the right ventricle on planar antimyosin scans. In addition to the limitations intrinsic in imaging right ventricular necrosis, the higher energy and longer T1/2 of ^{111}In limit the injected dose and reduce scan quality. Although sternal uptake of ^{111}In antimyosin does not usually interfere with identifying right ventricular uptake, hepatic uptake of ^{111}In antimyosin may cause difficulties in seeing small discrete areas of uptake in the region of the right ventricle on planar scans. Tomographic imaging improves contrast over planar imaging, and when a perfusion tracer such as ^{201}Tl is injected and simultaneous dual-isotope imaging is performed, thallium uptake affords landmarks that help localize small areas of ^{111}In antimyosin to the territory of the right ventricle. A subgroup analysis was performed on 30 of 87 patients with acute inferoposterior Q wave infarctions who underwent simultaneous dual-isotope imaging at Columbia-Presbyterian Medical Center.[45] Uptake of ^{111}In antimyosin anterior and to the right of the septum was seen in 14 of 30 (47 percent) patients. Although the numbers studied are small, the incidence is higher than that reported from planar pyrophosphate scans and more closely approximates reported autopsy data. Three patterns of tracer uptake in the right ventricle were identified (Fig. 65–6). Either antimyosin uptake appeared as a "crescent"-shaped pattern of uptake on the short-axis slices, corresponding anatomically to the free wall of the right ventricle, or it appeared as focal uptake, either in the free wall of the right ventricle on short-axis slices or localized to the apex of the right ventricle, best seen on vertical long-axis slices taken to the right of the septum.

INFARCT SIZING

Several methods have been developed to quantitate the muscle mass infarcted from tomographic scans, using either perfusion tracers or infarct-avid tracers. A simple and accurate method of measuring infarct size would be helpful clinically, because prognosis is related to infarct size, and most of the available clinical parameters, such as CK-MB and ejection fraction, have limitations in assessing infarct size. The levels of cardiac enzymes measured in the blood depend on blood flow to the infarction and enzyme washout from the infarct zone, in addition to infarct size. The reported methods of measuring infarct size using radionuclides include applying a threshold technique to size the defect on either ^{201}Tl or ^{99m}Tc-sestamibi scans, applying a count-based method to quantitate count reduction on ^{201}Tl tomograms, and applying a threshold technique to size the uptake of either ^{99m}Tc-pyrophosphate or ^{111}In antimyosin.[46–52] There are theoretical drawbacks to all these approaches. Perfusion defect size, determined with a threshold method, would include old scar, hibernating, or stunned myocardium, in addition to acutely infarcted myocardium. Thallium redistribution and quantitation of thallium uptake may help identify

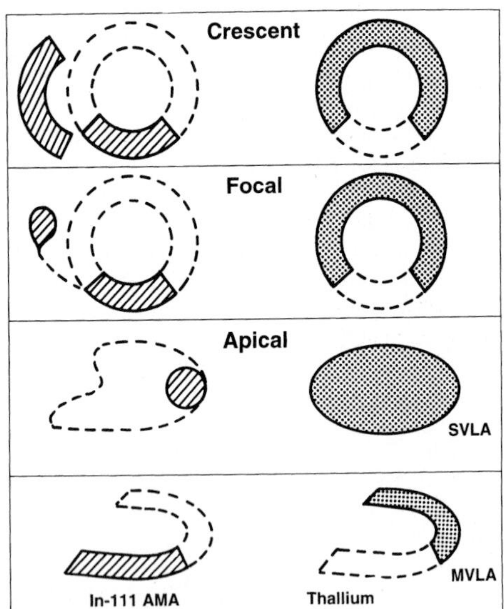

FIGURE 65–6. Schematic description of patterns of uptake of ^{111}In antimyosin antibody (In-111 AMA) in the right ventricle in patients with acute inferior wall infarctions and right ventricle involvement. The top two rows show crescent and focal patterns of uptake of ^{111}In AMA in the free wall of the right ventricle *(striped)* and thallium uptake *(dashes)*. The bottom two rows show focal uptake of ^{111}In AMA (In-111 AMA) confined to the apex of the RV seen on the VLA slices taken to the right of the septum. SVLA = septal vertical long axis; MVLA = midvertical long axis. (From Antunes, M. L., Johnson, L. L., Seldin, D. W., et al.: Diagnosis of right ventricular acute myocardial infarction by dual-isotope thallium-201 and indium-111 antimyosin SPECT imaging. Am. J. Cardiol. 70:426, 1992, with permission.)

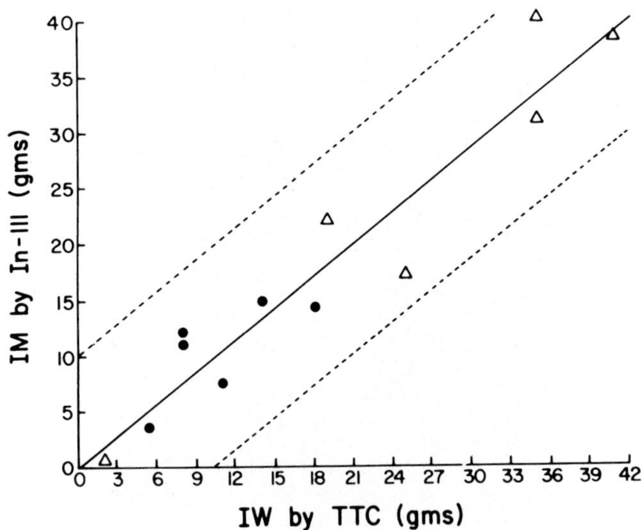

FIGURE 65–7. Correlation between infarct mass (IM) calculated from the ^{111}In AMA (In-111 AMA) tomographic slices using a threshold technique and infarct weight (IW) calculated from the triphenyl tetrazolium chloride (TTC) infarct size and left ventricle weight. (Johnson, L. L., Lerrick, K. S., Coromilas, J., et al.: Measurement of infarct size and percentage myocardium infarcted in a dog preparation with single photon emission computed tomography, thallium-201 and indium-111 monoclonal antimyosin. Fab. Circulation 76:181, 1987, with permission.)

viable myocardium in the early postinfarction period but may not help separate non-Q infarction from hibernation or stunning. Sizing infarctions from uptake of infarct-avid tracers also has limitations. With the limited resolution of gamma cameras, subendocardial infarctions cannot be distinguished from transmural infarctions. In the thrombolytic therapy era, non-Q infarctions are becoming more prevalent. Applying a threshold to either ^{99m}Tc-pyrophosphate or ^{111}In antimyosin uptake on tomograms performed in patients with nontransmural infarctions leads to overestimation of the mass of left ventricular muscle infarcted.

In the experimental study mentioned earlier in this chapter, the accuracy of a threshold method applied to antimyosin uptake to measure infarct size was evaluated.[26] The animals underwent simultaneous dual-isotope tomographic imaging, and the extent of antimyosin uptake was sized with a threshold technique and was expressed in grams and as a percentage of the entire left ventricular mass (assessed from the ^{201}Tl uptake). It was observed that the intensity of antimyosin uptake was greater in the early reperfused infarctions than in the late (no-reflow) reperfused infarctions. To investigate whether a single threshold value could be applied to infarctions with varying intensity of tracer uptake, phantom experiments were performed with the use of different-sized balls filled with different concentrations of ^{111}In placed in baths with varying concentrations of ^{111}In activity. These experiments demonstrated that the ^{111}In-filled objects of varying count intensity can be accurately sized by applying a single threshold when background activity is subtracted before the threshold is applied. From the raw tomographic data acquired in the dog experiments, background subtraction was performed, and the threshold value determined in the first few experiments was applied to the regions of ^{111}In antimyosin uptake. There was an excellent correlation between infarct size calculated from the reconstructed tomographic slices and infarct size determined by TTC (Fig. 65–7). It must be noted, however, that the early reperfused infarcts were small and showed intense uptake of ^{111}In antimyosin. A subsequent experimental study demonstrated overlap of a perfusion tracer and an infarct-avid tracer in nontransmural infarctions.[40] Any attempt to size nontransmural infarctions in grams or as a percentage of the left ventricular mass leads to an overestimation of infarct size.

A similar method of sizing infarctions by applying a threshold value to ^{111}In antimyosin uptake was used in patients with Q wave infarctions, who underwent simultaneous dual-isotope acquisitions and were found to have matched patterns of ^{201}Tl and ^{111}In antimyosin on the tomographic slices.[52] The following method was used to size the infarctions. Hepatic activity was masked out. Myocardial ^{111}In antimyosin activity was normalized to the short-axis slice with maximum myocardial activity. Background activity was subtracted by the operator by increasing the lower level cutoff percentage until extracardiac activity disappeared. The pixel value corresponding to this percentage was uniformly subtracted from all slices. For

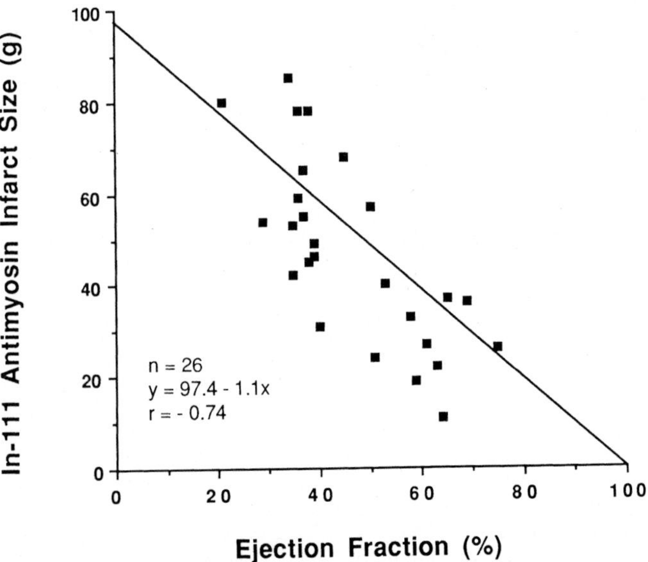

FIGURE 65–8. Statistically significant inverse correlation between infarct size in grams calculated from the ^{111}In AMA tomographic slices, using a threshold technique and left ventricular ejection fraction.

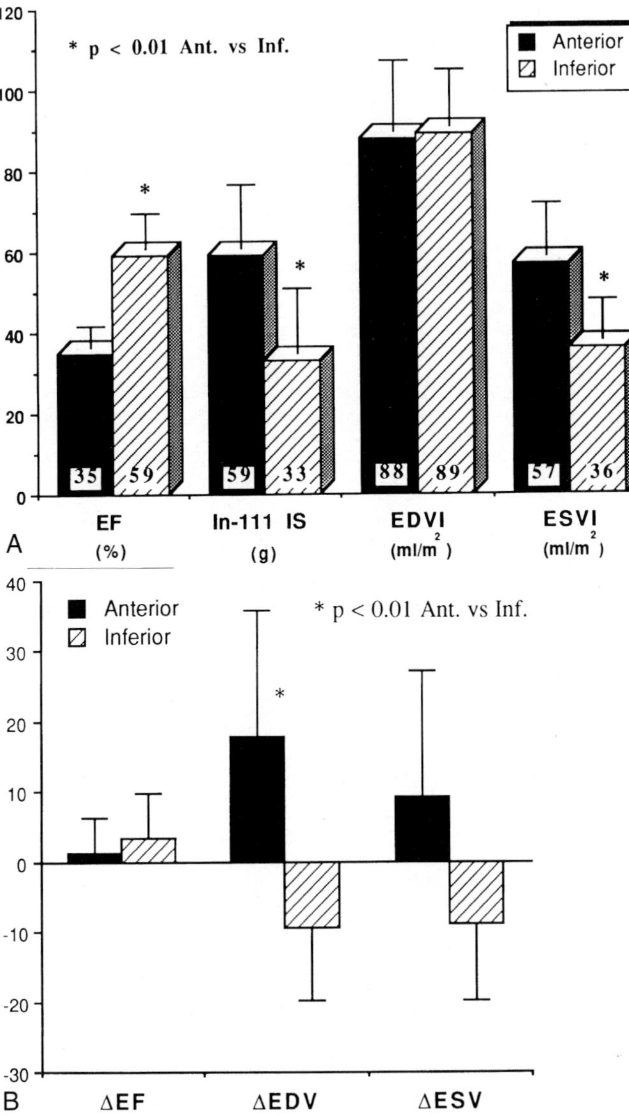

FIGURE 65–9. *A, Bars* representing left ventricular ejection fraction, infarct size (IS) calculated from ^{111}In AMA uptake and end-diastolic volume index (EDVI) and end-systolic volume index (EDVI) from predischarge gated blood pool scans in patients with anterior and inferior infarctions. *B,* Late follow-up demonstrated remodeling of the hearts with anterior infarctions. (From Antunes, M.L., Tresgallo, M.E., Seldin, D.W., et al.: Effect of infarct size measured from antimyosin single-photon computed tomographic scans on left ventricular remodeling. J. Am. Coll. Cardiol. 18:1267, 1991. With permission from the American College of Cardiology.)

these patient studies, the threshold value applied to find the infarct borders was determined from a torso phantom experiment. This threshold value was applied to the tomographic slices that had undergone liver masking and background subtraction, and the number of voxel elements in each slice was determined. All voxel elements from slices with antimyosin uptake were summed to obtain the infarct volume, which was then multiplied by the specific gravity of heart muscle to obtain infarct mass. Infarct size ranged from 11 to 87 g and was higher in anterior (60 ± 20 g) than inferior (34 ± 21 g) than infarctions. There was an excellent inverse correlation between infarct size in grams and left ventricular ejection fraction measured from the predischarge gated blood pool scan (Fig. 65–8).

A similar method applying a threshold level to determine the borders and measure infarct size was reported for ^{99m}Tc-pyrophosphate.[50] In this method, ^{99m}Tc was labeled both to the infarct via pyrophosphate and to the blood pool. Thresholds were applied to both the infarct and the blood pool, and the blood pool was subtracted to delineate the endocardial border. Infarct size determined by this technique ranged from 2.5 to 81.2 g and correlated with CK-MB values.

Clinical follow-up in both of the antimyosin and ^{99m}Tc-pyrophosphate studies showed that patients with large infarctions (above 60 g in the antimyosin study and above 40 g in the pyrophosphate study) had increased event rates relating to large infarctions, such as left ventricular failure, malignant arrhythmias, and death. In addition to providing data to help determine prognosis after infarction, sizing infarctions may also help predict remodeling. A study measuring infarctions from ^{111}In antimyosin uptake showed that at hospital discharge the end-diastolic volumes in patients with large anterior wall infarctions were not significantly greater than those in patients with smaller inferior wall infarctions, although end-systolic volumes were higher in the large infarct group. The patients with larger infarctions and higher end-systolic volumes underwent cardiac remodeling over the ensuing year, which was demonstrated by significant increases in their end-diastolic volumes (Fig. 65–9).

SUMMARY

Because the ECG and cardiac enzymes are sufficiently accurate to confirm or exclude the diagnosis of acute MI in the majority of patients who are admitted to the hospital with chest pain to rule out MI, infarct-avid scanning is not performed frequently in most nuclear medicine departments. However, there does exist a subset of patients in whom the results of routine clinical tests are equivocal and the diagnosis remains in question after performance of the routine tests. In these patients, the results of infarct-avid imaging with either ^{99m}Tc-pyrophosphate or ^{111}In antimyosin may aid in establishing a diagnosis and in patient management. The more interesting and potentially more widely applicable use of infarct-avid imaging, is its combination with perfusion or viability tracers such as ^{201}Tl to identify myocardium at further ischemic risk after infarction.

References

1. Braunwald, E., and Rutherford, J.D.: Reversible ischemic left ventricular dysfunction: Evidence for the "hibernating myocardium." J. Am. Coll. Cardiol. 8:1467, 1986.
2. Vanoverschelde, J.L.J., Wijns, W., Depré, C., et al.: Mechanisms of chronic regional postischemic dysfunction in humans: New insights from the study of noninfarcted collateral-dependent myocardium. Circulation 87:1513, 1993.
3. Sinusas, A.J., Qing, X.S., Vitols, P.J., et al.: Impact of regional ventricular function, geometry, and dobutamine stress on quantitative ^{99m}Tc-sestamibi defect size. Circulation 88:2224, 1993.
4. Parkey, R.W., Bonte, F.J., Meyer, S.L., et al.: A new method for radionuclide imaging of acute myocardial infarction in humans. Circulation 50:540, 1974.
5. D'Agostino, A.N., and Chiga, M.: Mitochondrial mineralization in human myocardium. Am. J. Clin. Pathol. 53:820, 1970.
6. Shen, A.C., and Jennings, R.B.: Kinetics of calcium accumulation in acute myocardial ischemic injury. Am. J. Pathol. 67:441, 1972.
7. Shen, A.C., and Jennings, R.B.: Myocardial calcium and magnesium in acute ischemic injury. Am. J. Pathol. 67:417, 1972.
8. Buja, M., Tofe, A., Kulkarni, P.V., et al.: Sites and mechanisms of localization of technetium-99 phosphorus radiopharmaceuticals in acute myocardial infarcts and other tissues. J. Clin. Invest. 60:724, 1977.
9. Bonte, F.J., Parkey, R.W., Graham, K.D., et al.: Distribution of several agents useful in imaging myocardial infarction. J. Nucl. Med. 16:132, 1975.
10. Zweiman, F.G., Holman, B.L., O'Keefe, A., et al.: Selective uptake of Tc-99m complexes and Ga-67 in acutely infarcted myocardium. J. Nucl. Med. 16:975, 1975.
11. Kloner, R.A., Ganote, C.E., and Jennings, R.B.: The "no-reflow" phenomenon after temporary coronary occlusion in the dog. J. Clin. Invest. 54:1496, 1974.
12. Beller, G.A., Chow, B.A., Haber, E., et al.: Localization of radiolabeled cardiac myosin-specific antibody in myocardial infarcts—comparison with technetium-99m stannous pyrophosphate. Circulation 55:74, 1977.
13. Corbett, J.R., Lewis, M., Willerson, J.T., et al.: Technetium-99m pyrophosphate imaging in patients with acute myocardial infarction: Comparison of planar images with single photon tomography with and without blood pool overlay. Circulation 69:1120, 1984.
14. Khaw, B.A., Beller, G.A., Haber, E., et al.: Localization of cardiac myosin-specific antibody in myocardial infarction. J. Clin. Invest. 58:439, 1976.

15. Khaw, B.A., Fallon, J.T., Beller, G.A., et al.: Specificity of localization of myosin-specific antibody fragments in experimental myocardial infarction, histologic, histochemical, autoradiographic and scintigraphic studies. Circulation 60:1527, 1979.
16. Khaw, B.A., Scott, J., Fallon, J.T., et al.: Myocardial injury: Quantification by cell sorting initiated with antimyosin fluorescent spheres. Science 217:1050, 1982.
17. Khaw, B.A., Beller, G.A., and Haber, E.: Experimental myocardial infarct imaging following intravenous administration of iodine-131 labeled antibody $F(ab)_2$ fragments specific for cardiac myosin. Circulation 57:743, 1978.
18. Khaw, B.A., Gold, H.K., Yasuda, T., et al.: Scintigraphic quantification of myocardial necrosis in patients after intravenous injection of myosin-specific antibody. Circulation 74:501, 1986.
19. Khaw, B., Yasuda, T., Gold, H.K., et al.: Acute myocardial infarct imaging with indium-111–labeled monoclonal Fab. J. Nucl. Med. 28:1671, 1987.
20. Weber, R.W., Boutin, R.H., Nedelman, M.A., et al.: Enhanced kidney clearance with an ester-linked ^{99m}Tc-radiolabeled antibody Fab′-chelator conjugate. Bioconjugate Chem. 2:431, 1990.
21. Senior, R., Bhattacharya, S., Manspeaker, P., et al.: ^{99m}Tc-antimyosin antibody imaging for the detection of acute myocardial infarction in human beings. Am. Heart J. 126:536, 1993.
22. Rhodes, B.A., Zamora, P.O., Newell, K.D., et al.: Technetium-99m labeling of murine monoclonal antibody fragments. J. Nucl. Med. 27:685, 1986.
23. Torchilin, V.P., Klibanov, A.L., Nossiff, N.D., et al.: Monoclonal antibody modification with chelate-linked high-molecular-weight polymers: Major increases in polyvalent cation binding without loss of antigen binding. Hybridoma 6:229, 1987.
24. Khaw, B.A., Torchilin, V.P., Klibanov, A.L., et al.: Modification of monoclonal antimyosin antibody: Enhanced specificity of localization and scintigraphic visualization in acute experimental myocardial infarction. J. Mol. Cell. Cardiol. 21(Suppl. 1):31, 1989.
25. Nedelman, M.A., Shealy, D.F., Boulin, R., et al.: Rapid infarct imaging with a technetium-99m–labeled antimyosin recombinant single-chain Fv: Evaluation in a canine model of acute myocardial infarction. J. Nucl. Med. 34:234, 1993.
26. Johnson, L.L., Lerrick, K.S., Coromilas, J., et al.: Measurement of infarct size and percentage myocardium infarcted in a dog preparation with single photon emission computed tomography, thallium-201 and indium-111 monoclonal antimyosin Fab. Circulation 76:181, 1987.
27. Vaghaiwalla, F., Buxton, D.B., Araujo, L.I., et al.: Blood flow–dependent uptake of indium-111 monoclonal antimyosin antibody in canine acute myocardial infarction. J. Am. Coll. Cardiol. 21:233, 1993.
28. Johnson, L.L., Seldin, D.W., Becker, L.C., et al.: Antimyosin imaging in acute transmural myocardial infarctions: Results of a multicenter clinical trial. J. Am. Coll. Cardiol. 13:27, 1989.
29. Poliner, L.R., Buja, L.M., Parkey, R.W., et al.: Clinicopathologic findings in 52 patients studied by technetium-99m stannous pyrophosphate myocardial scintigraphy. Circulation 59:257, 1979.
30. Berger, H., Lahiri, A., Leppo, J., et al.: Antimyosin imaging in patients with ischemic chest pain: Initial results of phase III multicenter trial (Abstract). J. Nucl. Med. 29:805, 1988.
31. Matsumori, A., Yamada, T., Tamaki, N., et al.: Persistent uptake of indium-111-antimyosin monoclonal antibody in patients with myocardial infarction. Am. Heart J. 120:1026, 1990.
32. Tamaki, N., Yamada, T., Matsumori, A., et al.: Indium-111 antimyosin antibody imaging for detecting different stages of myocardial infarction: Comparison with technetium-99m pyrophosphate imaging. J. Nucl. Med. 31:136, 1990.
33. Ballester-Rhodes, M., Carrio-Gasset, I., Abadal-Berini, L., et al.: Patterns of evolution of myocyte damage after human heart transplantation detected by indium-111 monoclonal antimyosin. Am. J. Cardiol. 62:623, 1988.
34. Obrador, D., Ballester, M., Carrio, I., et al.: Presence, evolving changes, and prognostic implications of myocardial damage detected in idiopathic and alcoholic dilated cardiomyopathy by In-111 monoclonal antimyosin antibodies. Circulation 89:2054, 1994.
35. Carrio, I., Berna, L., Ballester, M., et al.: Indium-111 antimyosin scintigraphy to assess myocardial damage in patients with suspected myocarditis and cardiac rejection. J. Nucl. Med. 29:1893, 1988.
36. Dec, G.W., Placios, I., Yasuda, T., et al.: Antimyosin antibody cardiac imaging: Its role in the diagnosis of myocarditis. J. Am. Coll. Cardiol. 16:97, 1990.
37. Ballester, M., Obrador, D., Carrio, I., et al.: Indium-111 monoclonal antimyosin antibody studies after the first year of heart transplantation. Circulation 82:2100, 1990.
38. Ballester, M., Obrador, D., Carrio, I., et al.: Early postoperative reduction of monoclonal antimyosin antibody uptake is associated with absent rejection-related complications after heart transplantation. Circulation 85:61, 1992.
39. Obrador, D., Ballester, M., Carrio, I., et al.: Presence, evolving changes, and prognostic implications of myocardial damage detected in idiopathic and alcoholic dilated cardiomyopathy by In-111 monoclonal antimyosin antibodies. Circulation 89:2054, 1994.
40. Morguet, A.J., Munz, D.L., Klein, H.H., et al.: Myocardial distribution of indium-111 antimyosin Fab and technetium-99m sestamibi in experimental non-transmural infarction. J. Nucl. Med. 33:223, 1992.
41. Johnson, L.L., Seldin, D.W., Keller, A.M., et al.: Dual-isotope thallium and indium antimyosin SPECT imaging to identify acute infarct patients at further ischemic risk. Circulation 81:37, 1990.
42. Johnson, L.L.: Dual-isotope thallium-201 and indium-111 antimyosin antibody tomographic imaging to identify viable myocardium at further ischemic risk after myocardial infarction. J. Nucl. Biol. Med. 36:91, 1992.
43. Wackers, F.J. T., Lie, K.I., Sokole, E.B., et al.: Prevalence of right ventricular involvement in inferior wall infarction assessed with myocardial imaging with thallium-201 and technetium-99m pyrophosphate. Am. J. Cardiol. 43:358, 1978.
44. Sharpe, D.V., Botvinick, E.H., Shames, D.M., et al.: The noninvasive diagnosis or right ventricular infarction. Circulation 57:483, 1978.
45. Antunes, M.L., Johnson, L.L., Seldin, D.W., et al.: Diagnosis of right ventricular acute myocardial infarction by dual-isotope thallium-201 and indium-111 antimyosin SPECT imaging. Am. J. Cardiol. 70:426, 1992.
46. Holman, M.L., Moore, S.C., Shulkin, P.M., et al.: Quantitation of perfused myocardial mass through thallium-201 and emission computed tomography. Invest. Radiol. 4:322, 1983.
47. Prigent, F., Maddahi, J., Garcia, E.V., et al.: Comparative methods for quantifying myocardial infarct size by thallium-201 SPECT. J. Nucl. Med. 28:325, 1987.
48. Christian, T.F., Clements, I.P., and Gibbrons, R.J.: Noninvasive identification of myocardium at risk in patients with acute myocardial infarctions and nondiagnostic electrocardiograms with technetium-99m sestamibi. Circulation 83:1615, 1992.
49. Holman, B.L., Goldhaber, S.Z., Kirsch, L., et al.: Measurement of infarct size using single photon emission computed tomography and technetium-99m pyrophosphate: A description of the method and comparison with patient prognosis. Am. J. Cardiol. 50:503, 1982.
50. Corbett, J.R., Lewis, S.E., Wolfe, C.L., et al.: Measurement of myocardial infarct size by technetium pyrophosphate single photon tomography. Am. J. Cardiol. 54:1231, 1984.
51. Jansen, D.E., Corbett, J., Wolfe, C.L., et al.: Quantification of myocardial infarction: A comparison of single-photon emission computed tomography with pyrophosphate to serial plasma MB-creatine kinase measurement. Circulation 72:327, 1985.
52. Antunes, M.L., Seldin, D.W., Wall, R.M., et al.: Measurement of acute Q-wave myocardial infarct size with single photon emission computed tomography imaging of indium-111 antimyosin. Am. J. Cardiol. 63:777, 1989.

CHAPTER

66 Metabolic Imaging With Single-Photon Emitting Tracers

Johannes Czernin, M.D.
Heinz Sochor, M.D.
Heinrich R. Schelbert, M.D.

Insertion of radioactive isotopes into physiologically active compounds offers the exciting prospect of noninvasive evaluation and quantification of local organ function with radionuclide imaging techniques. These prospects have largely materialized for positron-emitting isotopes of elements such as carbon, nitrogen, and fluorine and for positron emission tomography but remain limited with single-photon emitting isotopes. This is because only a small number of radioisotopes are suitable for imaging with conventional nuclear medicine instrumentation. Furthermore, labeling of physiologic substrates with, for example, technetium-99m or iodine-123 so dramatically alters their biologic properties that, in most cases, the resulting radiopharmaceuticals no longer behave like their natural, unlabeled parents. Radioiodination of free fatty acids thus far has been the only exception for which studies of myocardial metabolism appear feasible. This chapter reviews briefly the historical development of myocardial imaging with radioiodinated fatty acids, then describes the behavior of these radiotracers in the myocardium and how it relates to myocardial fatty acid metabolism, and concludes with a review of clinical observations with this radionuclide imaging technique in ischemic heart disease, cardiomyopathy, and left ventricular hypertrophy.

HISTORICAL PERSPECTIVE

Myocardium avidly extracts long-chain free fatty acids. Steady-state extraction fractions in human myocardium average 45 percent for oleic acid and 32 percent for palmitic acid.[1] If labeled with radioactive markers, these long-chain fatty acids therefore appear attractive for myocardial scintigraphy because they can serve as vehicles for transport of radioisotopes into myocardium. Evans and co-workers[2] in 1965 were first to demonstrate this possibility. They radioiodinated the double carbon bond of oleic acid and obtained myocardial scintigrams of adequate diagnostic quality. Limited imaging capabilities at that time, the high radiation burden associated with the iodine-131, and the altered biologic behavior of the radioiodinated fatty acid, caused by the radioiodination of the carbon double bond, prevented widespread acceptance of this compound for myocardial imaging.

In order to preserve the structural integrity of long-chain fatty acids and, consequently, their biologic behavior, Robinson and Lee[3,4] replaced the methyl group in the terminal (or omega) position with a radioactive iodine atom. The same group of investigators demonstrated that adequate myocardial images could be obtained with this newly synthesized iodinated fatty acid analog.[5,6] The biexponential clearance of the radioisotope from myocardium suggested further the possibility that metabolic information could be derived noninvasively with these tracers. Comparative studies with ^{14}C- and ^{11}C-labeled palmitate subsequently demonstrated the correspondence of the biexponential clearance pattern of iodinated fatty acid analogs to the known metabolic fate of free fatty acid in myocardium. Serial imaging and construction of regional tissue time-activity curves offered the possibility of noninvasive exploration of regional myocardial fatty acid metabolism.

Limitations, however, remained. Rapid clearance of tracer from the myocardium, together with liberation of free iodine and high radioiodine blood levels, required complicated and error-sensitive corrections. To obviate the need for such corrections, Machulla and associates[7,8] introduced a new radioiodinated aromatic fatty acid analog. Stabilization of radioiodide on a terminal phenyl ring prevented rapid deiodination. Myocardial uptake and subsequent clearance generally corresponded to those of the iodine-for-methyl group straight-chain fatty acid analogs and to those of ^{11}C-palmitate. In contrast to earlier fatty acid analogs, the radioiodine was released from the myocardium in the form of benzoic acid and subsequently cleared from blood by the kidney in the form of hippuric acid. The rapid clearance of this tracer from the myocardium continued to present limitations, especially because newly introduced tomographic imaging techniques required longer myocardial residence times in order to record adequate tomographic images. This prompted the search for tracers that would be retained in or clear more slowly from myocardium.

The notion that branched-chain fatty acids were less susceptible to β-oxidation led to the synthesis of numerous iodinated fatty acids with methyl branches.[9–14] Other approaches included insertion of elements such as tellurium into the central position of the long-chain fatty acid, which resulted in isosteric fatty acid analogs.[15] These two groups of fatty acid analogs have remained in a developmental stage, and their metabolic fate in myocardium is understood only incompletely.[16] Numerous iodinated fatty acid analogs are important, but a detailed description of their merits and limitations is beyond the scope of this chapter. The following review therefore focuses on those iodinated fatty acid analogs that have been tested more extensively and have been employed in humans.

TRACER TISSUE KINETICS OF IODINATED FATTY ACID ANALOGS

General Considerations

The myocardial tissue kinetics of ^{11}C-labeled palmitate serve as a yardstick for determining the quality and type of metabolic information that is available through iodinated fatty acid analogs. As detailed in Chapter 69, this tracer most closely approximates the uptake and subsequent metabolic fate of free fatty acids in myocardium. Injected intravenously, the tracer rapidly accumulates in myocardium and subsequently clears from it in a biexponential fashion (Fig. 66–1). The biexponential clearance curve implies distribution of tracer between two functional pools, from which it clears at different rates. These two functional pools have been shown to correspond to oxidation of free fatty acid (the rapid

Dr. Schelbert is affiliated with the Laboratory of Structural Biology and Molecular Medicine, operated for the U.S. Department of Energy by the University of California under Contract #DE-AC03-76-SF00012. This work was supported in part by the Director of the Office of Energy Research, Office of Health and Environmental Research, Washington, D.C., by Research Grants #HL 29845 and #HL 33177, the National Institutes of Health, Bethesda, M.D., and by an Investigative Group Award by the Greater Los Angeles Affiliate of the American Heart Association, Los Angeles, CA.

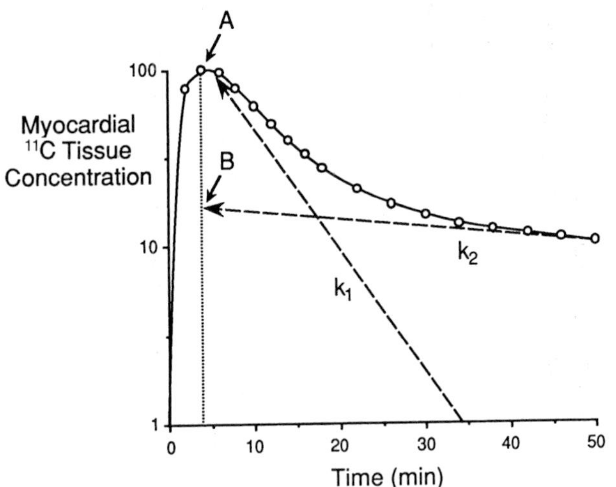

FIGURE 66–1. Schematic representation of the myocardial uptake and subsequent clearance of ^{11}C-palmitate. The tissue time-activity curves are obtained from serially acquired positron emission tomographic images of intravenous injection of ^{11}C-palmitate. Note the rapid accumulation of activity in myocardium; peak activity concentrations are reached within 4 to 5 minutes. Least square fitting of the subsequent clearance of tracer from myocardium indicates two distinct clearance phases, defined by slopes k_1 and k_2 and their intercepts. The relative sizes as an index of the fractional distribution of fatty acid in myocardium are estimated by extrapolation of the slow clearance-curve component to the time of peak activity, A. The activity concentration, B, is an estimate of the fraction of tracer incorporated into the slow turnover functional pool. Its relative size is estimated by the ratio of B to A. The relative size of the rapid clearance phase is the difference between A and B, divided by A. The clearance rate constants (slopes of the two phases) can be converted into clearance half-times and are expressed in minutes.

clearance curve component) and storage of fatty acid in the endogenous lipid pool (the slow clearance phase). The latter pool includes diglycerides, triglycerides, and phospholipids.

After crossing the capillary and cellular membranes, free fatty acid becomes esterified by an energy-requiring reaction to acyl coenzyme A (acyl-CoA), as shown in Figure 66–2). The reaction is largely unidirectional and represents effective sequestration of free fatty acid into myocardium. The metabolism of acyl-CoA can follow several paths thereafter. It can be synthesized to glycerides of phospholipids (the slow functional pool) or transported by the carnitine shuttle to the inner mitochondrial membrane, where β-oxidation metabolizes the acyl-CoA to two carbon units, which then enter the tricarboxylic acid cycle for oxidation to carbon dioxide and water (see Fig. 66–2), for details see Chapter 4. Transport into mitochondria, β-oxidation, tricarboxolic acid cycle oxidation, and release of end products from myocardium correspond to the rapid clearance phase on the tissue time-activity curve and represent a rapid-turnover, functional pool. The relative size of the rapid phase corresponds to the fraction of fatty acid that is immediately oxidized (see Fig. 66–1), and its slope is related to the transmembranous transport, oxidation of fatty acid, and release of metabolic end products. The relative size of the slow clearance phase is related to the fraction of fatty acid that is incorporated into the endogenous lipid pool and its slope to its turnover rate.

Physiologic interventions alter the clearance curve in a predictable manner (see Chapter 69 for details). These alterations are important for understanding the tissue clearance kinetics of iodinated fatty acid analogs. Higher cardiac workload and, thus, higher oxygen consumption increase the relative size and slope of the rapid clearance phase as a reflection of increased fatty acid oxidation. Conversely, ischemia reduces the relative size and clearance rate of the rapid phase as a reflection of impaired fatty acid oxidation. The relative size of the slow clearance phase increases as an expression of increased incorporation of radiolabeled compound into the endogenous lipid pool. Changes in myocardial substrate utilization affect the shape of the clearance curve in a similar fashion. The preferential oxidation of fatty acid in the fasted state, when plasma fatty acid levels are high and glucose and insulin levels are low, is reflected on the time-activity curve by high tracer uptake, a large relative size, and a steep slope of the rapid clearance phase. Increases in plasma glucose and insulin levels in the postprandial state shift substrate oxidation from free fatty acid to glucose or lactate. The time-activity curve mirrors this change by a decrease in the relative size and slope of the rapid clearance curve component, together with an increase in the relative size of the slow clearance phase.

The various iodinated fatty acid analogs participate in the overall fatty acid metabolism and its responses to physiologic intervention to different extents. They therefore provide different degrees of information on myocardial fatty acid metabolism. As listed in Table 66–1, iodinated fatty acid analogs are grouped into iodine-for-methyl group analogs, aromatic fatty acid analogs, branched-chain fatty acid analogs, and isosteric fatty acid analogs.

Iodine-for-Methyl Group Fatty Acid Analogs

In this group of fatty acid analogs, the radioactive iodine replaces a methyl group in the terminal (or omega) position of the long-chain fatty acid[3, 4] (Fig. 66–3). The two most commonly used fatty acid analogs in this group are 16-^{123}I-iodohexadecanoic acid (IHDA) and 17-^{123}I-iodoheptadecanoic acid (IHPA). They differ in chain length by one carbon but exhibit comparable tracer properties, and they are therefore reviewed together.

Administered intravenously, both IHDA and IHPA accumulate rapidly in the myocardium. Poe and associates[5, 6] reported first-pass extraction fractions as high as 80 percent after intracoronary injection in dogs. In both animal experimental studies and clinical investigations, the radiotracer was found to clear from myocardium in a biexponential manner.[7, 17, 18] Correlative studies in rabbit myo-

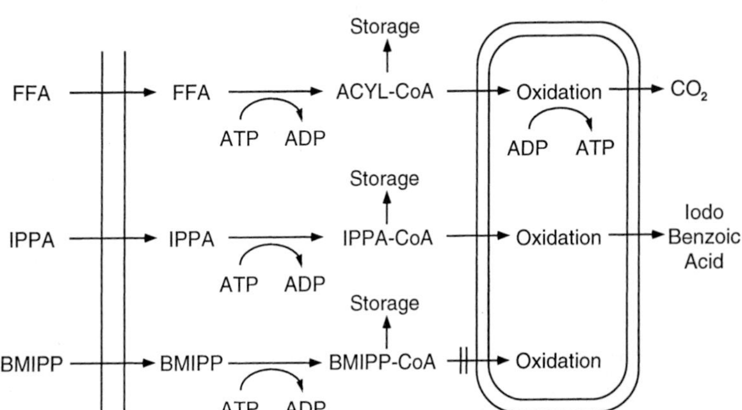

FIGURE 66–2. Schematic representation of metabolic fate of free fatty acid (FFA) and iodinated analogs in myocardium. ADP = adenosine diphosphate; ATP = adenosine triphosphate; CoA = coenzyme A; IPPA = 15-para-iodophenyl pentadecanoic acid (IPPA); BMIPP = 15-(para-iodophenyl)-3-R, S-methyl pentadecanoic acid.

cardium with ^{14}C-labeled palmitate demonstrated comparable clearance characteristics and provided additional support for the utility of these two iodinated fatty acid analogs as tracers of fatty acid metabolism.[7, 19–21] Further, studies in six patients revealed similar clearance characteristics for ^{11}C-palmitate and IHDA in human myocardium.[22] For ^{11}C-palmitate, clearance half-times averaged 6.0 ± 1.1 minutes for the early phase and 157 ± 103 minutes for the slow phase. The corresponding values for IHDA were 9 ± 3 and 43 ± 26 minutes. Discrepancies between the tracer results were attributed by the authors to differences in heart rate and blood pressure products between studies that affected myocardial oxygen consumption.

Consistent with the change in myocardial fatty acid oxidation, the relative size and slope of the clearance curve component of IHDA was found to be decreased in ischemic myocardium.[23, 24] Global ischemia in isolated rabbit hearts was associated with monoexponential rather than biexponential IHDA clearance, with mean clearance half-times of 60.5 minutes.[20] A small fraction of the total tissue activity cleared rapidly from myocardium, with an average half-time of 3.8 minutes. The loss of the rapid clearance phase was thought to reflect the impairment of fatty acid oxidation. The residual slow clearance may have been related to some extent to residual fatty acid oxidation or to release of nonmetabolized tracer after hydrolysis of labeled triglycerides. The initial, rapid loss of a small fraction of activity, on the other hand, may have resulted from back-diffusion of nonmetabolized iodinated fatty acid or from enhanced diffusibility because of a possible increase in the mitochondrial surface area and, consequently, a higher permeability surface product. Either possibility remains unconfirmed, because the chemical species containing the radiotracer in the myocardial effluent was not determined.

Infusion of glucose and insulin in patients altered the clearance curve in a fashion similar to that of ^{11}C-palmitate (Fig. 66–4). The decrease in the relative size and slope of the rapid clearance phase reflected the known shift in oxidative metabolism from fatty acid to glucose.[19, 25] The observed changes in the clearance curve in response to physiologic interventions therefore confirmed the utility of this fatty acid analog for the noninvasive evaluation of regional myocardial fatty acid metabolism. There were, however, inconsistencies. The failure of the clearance slope to increase with exercise[24] and the accelerated clearance rates in infarcted human myocardium[26] raised questions as to what extent or how accurately the slope of this rapid clearance phase reflected the rate of fatty acid oxidation.

In addition to the fractional distribution of radiotracer in myocardium, subsequent studies elucidated several factors that determine the slope of the rapid clearance curve component. Tissue assays of myocardium from isolated heart preparations and from dogs demonstrated that the radioiodine label was in fact incorporated into triglycerides and phospholipids[20, 27–29] (Fig. 66–5). They also revealed high intracellular concentrations of free iodine early after

TABLE 66–1. IODINATED FATTY ACID ANALOGS FOR EVALUATION OF MYOCARDIAL FATTY ACID METABOLISM

Iodine-for-methyl group analogs
17-[*p*-^{123}I]-heptadecanoic acid (IHPA)
16-[*p*-^{123}I]-hexadecanoic acid (IHDA)
Aromatic fatty acid analogs
15-(*p*-[^{123}I]-iodophenyl)-pentadecanoic acid (IPPA)
Branched-chain fatty acid analogs
14-(*p*-[^{123}I]-iodophenyl)-β methyltetradecanoic acid (BMTDA)
15-(*p*-[^{123}I]-iodophenyl)-3,3-dimethyl pentadecanoic acid (DMIPP)
15-(*p*-[^{123}I]-iodophenyl)-3-methylpentadecanoic acid (BMIPP)
Isosteric analogs
17-[*p*-^{123}I]-iodo-9-tellura heptadecanoic acid
15-(*p*-[^{123}I]-iodophenyl)-6-tellura pentadecanoic acid

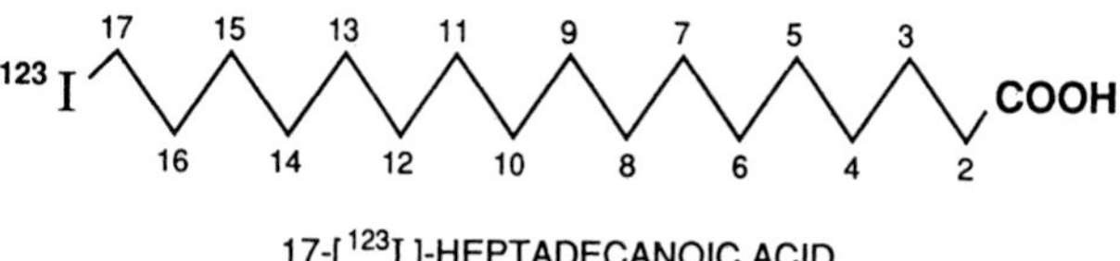

17-[^{123}I]-HEPTADECANOIC ACID

15-(p-[^{123}I]-IODOPHENYL)PENTADECANOIC ACID

15-(p-[^{123}I]-IODOPHENYL)-3,3-DIMETHYLPENTADECANOIC ACID

FIGURE 66–3. Schematic representation of examples of three different types of radioiodinated fatty acid analogs (see text).

tracer administration. Ischemia caused a predicted change in the fractional distribution of tracer. The decline of the ratio of free to lipid-bound radioiodine appeared to reflect the reduced oxidation as well as the augmented deposition of fatty acid in the endogenous lipid pool.[28] Nevertheless, free iodine still represented 41 to 84 percent of the total tissue activity at 5 and 120 minutes. These observations raised two questions: was there nonspecific deiodination, and was the transfer of free iodine from mitochondria into cytosol and across the cellular membrane into blood the rate-limiting step for clearance of radiotracer from myocardium?

Observations in isolated hearts implicated oxidation rather than a nonspecific process as the primary mechanism for the rapid liberation and accumulation of free iodine in the cell.[30] Depending on the length of the carbon chain, the radiotracer resides after β-oxidation in either acetic acid or propionic acid and is subsequently released as halide ion.[21] These observations, together with findings in normal and ischemic myocardium of dogs, suggested that transmembranous exchange of iodine rather than rates of oxidation primarily account for the rate of tracer clearance from myocardium.[29–31] "Prelabeling" of isolated perfused rabbit hearts with free iodine led to similar conclusions.[20] Tissue clearance half-times of free iodine from myocardium averaged 14 ± 2.1 minutes and thus were similar to those observed after IHDA labeling. More recent observations in canine myocardium further supported this possibility.[32] Comparative studies of IHDA and ^{14}C-labeled palmitate failed to demonstrate a direct relation between changes in the clearance rates of IHDA and of ^{14}C-palmitate in response to changes in myocardial oxygen consumption. In fact, the slope of the early clearance phase of IHDA declined with higher oxygen consumption. The authors concluded that the fractional distribution of tracer between the rapid and slow clearance phases or the ratio of the relative sizes better reflected changes in fatty acid oxidation rather than the slope of the rapid clearance phase.

In summary, high first-pass extraction fractions indicate that the initial uptake of IHDA and IHPA in the myocardium largely depends on blood flow. Although the shape of the biexponential clearance curve generally corresponds to the fractional distribution of fatty acid between oxidation and incorporation into the endogenous lipid pool, clearance rates of tracer from the myocardium may not accurately reflect rates of fatty acid oxidation, because transfer of iodine across the mitochondrial or cellular membranes is the rate-limiting step. On the other hand, the fractional distribution of

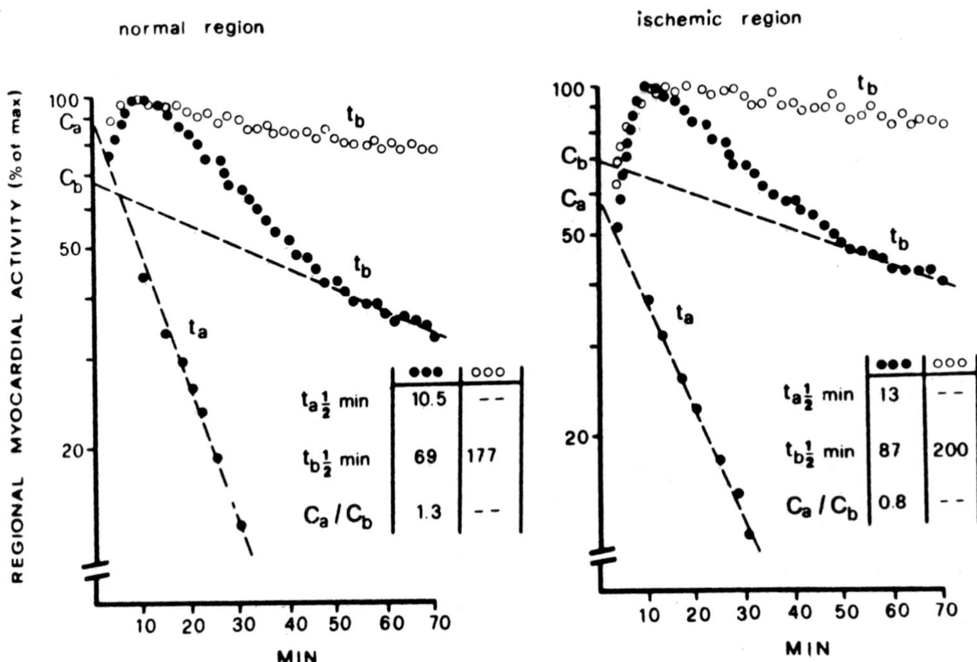

FIGURE 66–4. Uptake and clearance of 16-(p-^{123}I)-hexadecanoic acid (IHDA) in normal (*left*) and ischemic (*right*) myocardium in a patient with coronary artery disease studied in the fasted state and again after glucose and insulin infusion. In the fasted state, iodine activity clears biexponentially from both myocardial regions. The relative size and slope of the rapid clearance phase are lower in ischemic than in normal myocardium. Glucose and insulin infusion abolishes the rapid clearance curve component, consistent with a shift from fatty acid to glucose oxidation. The terms t_a and t_b are the clearance half-times for the rapid and the slow clearance curve components, and C_a and C_b are their relative sizes. (From Dudczak, K., Kletter, K., and Frischauf, H.: The use of I-123 heptadecanoic acid (HDA) as a metabolic tracer: Preliminary report. Eur. J. Nucl. Med. 9:81, 1984, with permission.)

tracer in myocardium, as reflected by the relative sizes of the two clearance curve components, can provide information on myocardial fatty acid metabolism.

Aromatic Fatty Acid Analogs

Machulla and colleagues[7, 8] proposed 15-para-iodophenyl pentadecanoic acid (IPPA) as an alternate and potentially useful tracer of myocardial fatty acid metabolism. As illustrated in Figure 66–3, the radioiodine is stabilized on the terminal phenyl ring of the straight-chain fatty acid. The compound undergoes β-oxidation with release of radioiodine from myocardium in the form of benzoic acid, which the liver metabolizes to glucuronic and hippuric acid (see Fig. 66–2). Both substances clear from blood through the kidney.[33] Initial investigations in rabbits and in patients with coronary artery disease or cardiomyopathy established the utility of this new compound for myocardial imaging and for the evaluation of regional myocardial fatty acid metabolism.[17] The biodistribution of this new agent and its subcellular distribution in myocardium have been determined. Within 5 minutes of intravenous administration, its uptake in myocardium averaged 4.4 percent of the total injected dose, compared with only 2.7 percent of coinjected ^{14}C-labeled palmitate.[33] IPPA subsequently cleared biexponentially from myocardium. Fractional distributions and clearance rates were similar to those of radiolabeled palmitate, although myocardial IPPA concentrations remained higher than those of ^{14}C-labeled palmitate.

Other studies[34] have demonstrated the anticipated effects of dietary interventions on the myocardial uptake and fractional distribution of IPPA. Higher incorporation of tracer into triglycerides and phospholipids in the postprandial state (70 to 80 percent in triglycerides and 6 to 15 percent in phospholipids) than in the fasted state (40 to 57 percent in triglycerides and 17 to 28 percent in phospholipids) suggested that preferential fatty acid utilization results in enhanced β-oxidation of IPPA and reduced incorporation into the endogenous lipid pool.

Additional studies by the same investigators confirmed the similarity of the fractional distributions of the radioiodine label of IPPA and of radiolabeled oleic acid and palmitic acid in rat myocardium.[35] In isolated rat heart experiments, the rate of release of iodobenzoic acid as a metabolite of IPPA was found to correlate closely to the rate of release of ^{14}C-labeled carbon dioxide as the oxidative end product of coinjected ^{14}C-labeled palmitate.[35] Isoproterenol-mediated increases and lactate-induced decreases in fatty acid oxidation in these studies were associated with comparable changes in rates of ^{14}C-labeled carbon dioxide and iodobenzoic acid release. DeGrado and associates[36] inhibited pharmacologically in isolated working rat hearts the carnitine palmitoyl transferase I and observed a suppression of oxidation of IPPA of almost 70 percent, compared with a reduction of about 90 percent in ^{14}C-palmitate oxidation. These changes were correctly identified by a decline of the relative size of the rapid clearance curve component. In summary, considerable experimental evidence supports the utility of IPPA as a tracer of myocardial fatty acid metabolism.

The orthoisomer of IPPA, which has been found to be retained in the myocardium, may be useful as a myocardial perfusion agent, and the paraisomer, which is metabolized by β-oxidation, could serve as an indicator of myocardial fatty acid metabolism. Dual-isotope imaging with these agents could provide information on perfusion and metabolism. However, species-related differences in tracer kinetics have been reported recently by Dormehl and colleagues,[37] who demonstrated in baboons a similar degree of β-oxidation for both isomers. This finding is in contrast to previous studies in rats, which failed to demonstrate prolonged retention of ortho-IPPA in the left ventricular myocardium.[38] Because of these differences in tracer kinetics between species, Dormehl and group recommended caution for the interpretation of the kinetics of radioiodinated fatty acids in humans.

Most studies indicate higher myocardial uptake of IPPA, compared with ^{11}C-labeled palmitate. Altered binding of IPPA to albumin and differences in transmembranous exchange or in metabolic handling may serve as possible explanations.[39] Regional myocardial clearance rates and changes in the biexponential clearance curve after substrate intervention or during ischemia appear to accurately identify directional changes in myocardial fatty acid oxidation and storage in the endogenous lipid pool.

The rapid accumulation of IPPA in myocardium and its subsequent biexponential clearance pattern has been demonstrated in humans. By means of high temporal sampling and serial gamma camera imaging, myocardial activity concentrations were shown to reach a plateau phase within 5 to 10 minutes after injection; this phase lasted from 8 to 18 minutes and was followed by biexponential clearance of tracer from myocardium[40] (Fig. 66–6). Tissue clearance half-times, as determined by Dudczak and co-workers[17] by monoexponential curve fitting, were found to average 43.8 ± 6.2 minutes in normal myocardium (Table 66–2).

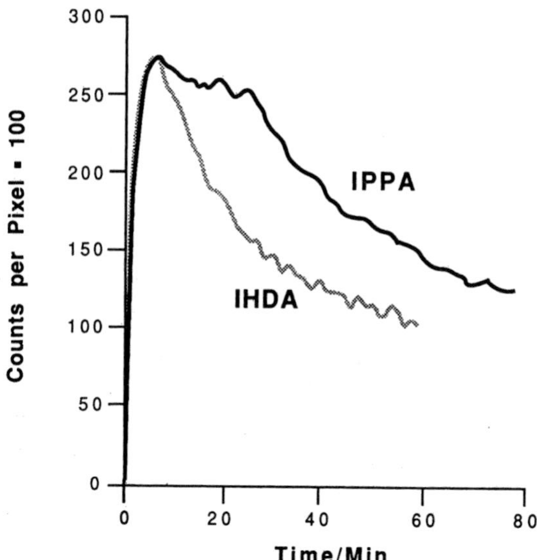

FIGURE 66–6. Myocardial uptake and clearance of 16-(*p*-^{123}I)-hexadecanoic acid (IHDA) and 15-(*p*-[^{123}I]-iodophenyl)-pentadecanoic acid (IPPA) in normal human myocardium after intravenous tracer injection and serial planar gamma camera imaging. The two time-activity curves were normalized to the same maximum activity. Note the plateau phase for IPPA that is not present for IHDA. (Adapted from Vyska, K., Machulla, H., and Stremmel, W. Regional myocardial free fatty acid extraction in normal and ischemic myocardium. Circulation 78:1218, 1988, with permission of the American Heart Association Inc.)

Branched-Chain Fatty Acid Analogs

The search for iodinated fatty acid analogs with longer myocardial retention times prompted the development of this class of compounds. As discussed by Otto and colleagues,[41] methyl branching of the fatty acid chain is thought to protect these compounds against β-oxidation. Provided they retain some of the physiologic properties critical for the initial transmembranous exchange and for effective sequestration into myocardium, these modified fatty acid analogs should be retained in myocardium for longer periods. They therefore would be more suitable for the lower temporal sampling capabilities of single-photon emission computed tomography (SPECT). Based on findings with several newly synthesized fatty acid analogs, Otto and group concluded that branching of the fatty acid chain significantly lowered the heart-to-blood ratios relative to straight-chain analogs but resulted in constant myocardial activity concentrations.[41] The degree of branching and the length of the chain determined the myocardial uptake of these tracers.

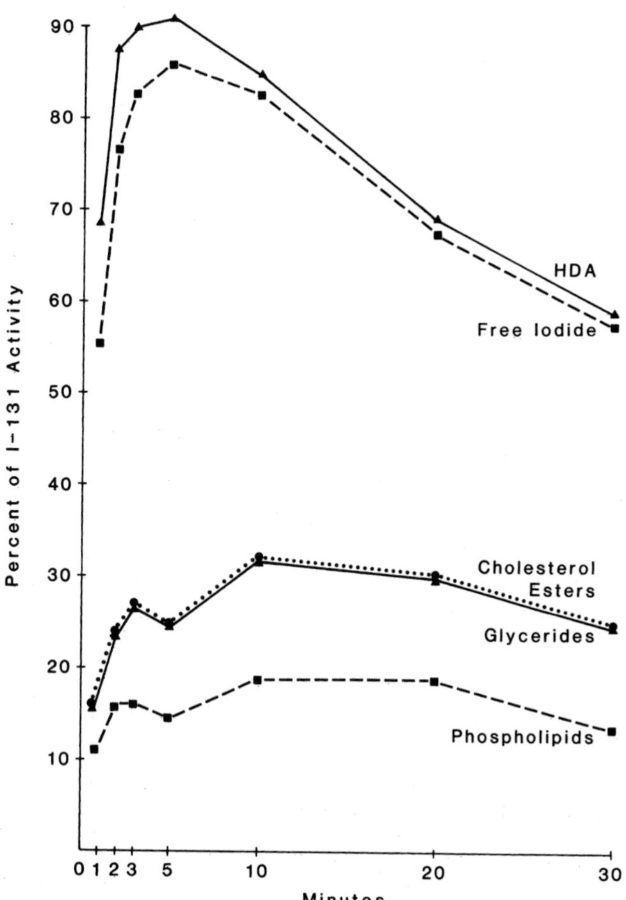

FIGURE 66–5. Fractional distribution of the radiotracer 16-(*p*^{123}I)-hexadecanoic acid (IHDA) in myocardium and its changes over time, as determined from serial myocardial biopsies and tissue assays in normal canine myocardium after intravenous administration of IHDA. Note the large fraction of free iodine in myocardium. (Adapted from Visser, F., van Eenige, M., and Westera, G.: Metabolic fate of radioiodinated heptadecanoic acid in the normal canine heart. Circulation 72:5651, 1985. Reproduced from Schelbert H.: Current status and prospects of new radionuclides and radiopharmaceuticals for cardiovascular nuclear medicine. Semin. Nucl. Med. 17:145, 1987, with permission.)

An example of this class of compounds is β-methyl-heptadecanoic acid, which contains a methyl group in the 2-carbon (or β-carbon) position of the straight-chain fatty acid. Labeled with iodine or ^{11}C and examined in isolated, arterially perfused hearts or in intact animals,[13, 42, 43] the compound rapidly accumulates in myocardium but clears from it only slowly. The agent has been employed in several experimental animal studies for delineation of regional differences in myocardial fatty acid uptake.[44, 45] Images obtained with this type of fatty acid analog in normal volunteers and in patients with cardiac disease were of excellent diagnostic quality.[14]

More information on the biologic properties of this type of iodinated fatty acid analog is available for two other side-branch aromatic fatty acids, 15-(*p*-iodophenyl)-3-R, S-methyl pentadecanoic acid (BMIPP) (see Fig. 66–2) and 15-(*p*-iodophenyl)-3,3-dimethyl pentadecanoic acid (DMIPP).[9, 10, 46–48] As illustrated in Figure 66–3, either one (BMIPP) or two (DMIPP) methyl side branches are attached to the 3-carbon of the straight-chain fatty acid with a terminal, radioiodinated phenyl ring. Comparative studies in fasted rat myocardium revealed distinct differences between these two compounds and the earlier-described IPPA.[49] All three compounds rapidly accumulated in myocardium. At 5 minutes, an average of about 4 percent of the total injected dose resided in 1 g of myocardium (or about 2 percent in the whole heart). As

TABLE 66–2. CLEARANCE HALF-TIMES OF IODINATED FATTY ACID ANALOGS IN NORMAL AND DISEASED MYOCARDIUM

Study	Number	Clearance Half-Times (min)			Radioiodinated Fatty Acid Analog
		Normal Myocard.	*Infarcted Myocard.*	*Ischemic Myocard.*	
Normal Volunteers					
Freundlieb et al. 1980	10	25.5±5.0	—	—	
Poe et al. 1977		>25	—	—	
Stoddart et al. 1987	9	18.8±3.3	—	—	IHDA
Van der Wall et al. 1981	6	27.5±3.0	—	—	IHDA
Hock et al. 1983	6	24.7±2.5	—	—	IHDA
		24.7±2.0*	—	—	IHDA
Coronary Artery Disease					
Freundlieb et al. 1980	10			31.8±19.6	IHDA
Van der Wall et al. 1981	25	34.0±8.4	18.5±2.5	46.7±7.1*	
		34.8±7.7	16.8±3.5	29.1±4.7	IHPA
Stoddart et al. 1987	10			35.5±41.5	IHDA
Dudczak et al. 1983	40	20.8±4.0	15.5±7.8	54.5±9.6	IPPA
Kennedy et al. 1986	18	43.8±6.2	66.1±15.1	Prolonged‡	IPPA
Cardiomyopathy					
Dudczak et al. 1983	10	68.3±29.6	—	—	IPPA
Rabinovich et al. 1985	16	15.0–105†	—	—	IHDA
Ugolini et al. 1988	19	accelerated	—	—	IPPA
Hock et al. 1983	20	15.1–116.2†	—	—	IHPA

*Studied after exercise.
†Range of regional clearance values.
‡No absolute values available.
IHDA = 16-[p-^{123}I]-hexadecanoic acid; IHPA = 17-[p-^{123}I]-heptadecanoic acid; IPPA = 15-(p-[^{123}I]-iodophenyl)-pentadecanoic acid; Myocard. = myocardium.

expected, IPPA cleared most rapidly from myocardium. Over the 2-hour observation period, myocardial activity concentrations declined by more than 50 percent. Myocardial concentrations of BMIPP declined more slowly (by only 25 percent) over the same observation period. In contrast, DMIPP exhibited virtually no clearance. These differences in clearance kinetics were associated with differences in the ratio of heart to blood activity. At 30 minutes after administration, the ratio was highest for DMIPP at 12:1, compared with ratios of 2:1 or less for BMIPP and IPPA.

The fractional distribution of the radiotracers between the functional and structural compartments in myocardium similarly differed among the three compounds.[50] Thirty minutes after injection in fasted rats, 65 to 80 percent of the total radioactivity resided in the triglyceride fraction for all three compounds. The fraction of total tissue activity contained in free fatty acid, however, markedly differed among the three compounds early after injection (at 5 minutes). It ranged from 10 to 15 percent for IPPA, was about 20 percent for BMIPP, and was more than 60 percent for DMIPP. Competition of oxidation with lipid incorporation for activated free fatty acid probably accounts for these differences. For example, if oxidation is reduced or impaired, as appears to be true for DMIPP, more tracer is available for esterification to triglycerides. Moreover, 34 and 38 percent of the total activity for DMIPP was associated at 30 minutes with the mitochondrial and microsomal fractions, respectively, compared with only 18 percent and 15 percent for IPPA. The same studies further indicated that DMIPP cleared most rapidly from blood, which largely accounted for the high ratio of myocardium to blood activity.

In summary, experimental data support the notion of a protective effect of the side branch against β-oxidation (see Fig. 66–2). However, the clearance of radioactivity from myocardium observed for some of these compounds implies some degree of metabolic degradation. Whether this occurs by β-oxidation, α-oxidation, or other metabolic pathways or whether it can be explained, at least in part, by hydrolysis of triglycerides and backdiffusion of nonmetabolized tracer remains uncertain at present. Branched-chain fatty acid analogs with virtually complete trapping may prove useful for noninvasive measurements of total fatty acid utilization, although some uncertainty remains as to whether these analogs trace only the uptake of that fraction of fatty acid that is subsequently incorporated into the endogenous lipid pool. Although this class of compounds is unlikely to provide comprehensive information on fatty acid metabolism, they offer an opportunity for quantitative measurement of total myocardial fatty acid utilization. The virtually unidirectional transport, together with the high myocardium-to-blood activity ratios, permits design of relatively simply tracer kinetic models for the external quantification of myocardial fatty acid utilization, analogous to the ^{18}F-2-fluoro-2-deoxyglucose method described in Chapter 69.

Isosteric Fatty Acid Analogs

Other attempts to protect fatty acid analogs against degradation by β-oxidation resulted in the development of isosteric fatty acid analogs. The inclusion of a tellurium atom at a central position within the fatty acid chain has been one modification.[51] Several animal experimental studies have conclusively demonstrated that these isosteric fatty acid analogs continue to be avidly extracted by myocardium but are then, as postulated, retained in the myocardium.[15, 51] Although the initial distribution of these tracers in the myocardium depends on regional myocardial blood flow, there is little information on their subsequent metabolic fate.[12]

Comparison of Fatty Acid Analogs

Fatty acid analogs are avidly extracted by myocardium independent of their structural differences. Their initial uptake in myocardium depends largely on blood flow but may be modified by dietary interventions or by regional myocardial ischemia. Both iodine-for-methyl group (IHDA and IHPA) and aromatic (IPPA) fatty acid analogs clear biexponentially from myocardium. Myocardial tissue clearance half-times for IPPA are moderately longer than those for IHDA and IHPA (see Table 66–2). For both groups of fatty acid analogs, the shape of the biexponential clearance curve reflects the fractional distribution of tracer between oxidation and storage of free fatty acid. Mitochondrial membranes apparently exert a significant barrier effect to the egress of liberated free iodide. Therefore, the slope of the early clearance phase of IHDA and IHPA may not reflect accurately the changes in the rate of β-oxidation of free fatty acid. This does not pertain to the rate for clearance of IPPA, during which the radiotracer is released from myocardium in the form of benzoic acid.

It appears that the fractional distribution of IHDA and IHPA, as reflected by the ratio of the relative sizes of the two clearance phases, offers more accurate information on fatty acid metabolism than does determination of individual clearance rates. The higher blood pool and background activity for IHDA and IHPA (compared with the aromatic fatty acid analog IPPA) degrade image quality and necessitate complex corrections for determination of regional myocardial tissue clearance rates. Furthermore, the longer myocardial residence time of IPPA renders this compound more suitable for tomographic radionuclide imaging. In terms of image quality, branched-chain fatty acids like BMIPP and isosteric fatty acid analogs appear to be superior. They are metabolically trapped in myocardium; blood pool and background activities are low. The metabolic information provided by the latter compounds is, however, limited and pertains largely to the initial uptake by and metabolic sequestration of fatty acid into myocardium.

TECHNICAL ASPECTS OF IODINATED FATTY ACID IMAGING

The metabolic information derived noninvasively by imaging of the myocardial uptake and subsequent clearance of radioiodinated fatty acid analogs depends on several factors.

Type of Fatty Acid Analog

The particular type of fatty acid analog employed largely determines the specific information that can be obtained. Tracers that are virtually trapped in myocardium provide information mostly on regional myocardial fatty acid utilization and, because of their high first-pass extraction fraction, on regional myocardial blood flow. In contrast, radiotracers that subsequently clear from myocardium offer information on fatty acid oxidation as well as on storage of fatty acid in the endogenous lipid pool. The relative sizes of the two clearance curve components correspond to the fractional distribution of tracer between oxidation and storage of free fatty acid, whereas their slopes or clearance half-times can provide information on rates of fatty acid oxidation and of turnover of the endogenous lipid pool.

Image Acquisition

The duration of image acquisition is an equally important factor.[52, 53] Because clearance half-times differ significantly between the various iodinated fatty acid analogs, acquisition times must be sufficiently long to adequately delineate the biexponential clearance pattern. Short image acquisition times offer information on the initial uptake and the initial clearance of tracer from the myocardium but do not provide information on fatty acid metabolism. Dudczak and colleagues[18] pointed out the need for sufficiently long acquisition times, as long as 70 minutes. Adequately high temporal sampling rates are readily available with planar imaging[54] yet are limited with SPECT imaging. Several investigators rely on acquisition of an initial uptake image and a subsequent "redistribution" image[55]; others acquire serial SPECT images—for example, every 8 minutes for a total acquisition time of 40 minutes.[56]

Dietary Conditions

The dietary state must be standardized or at least monitored. As with ^{11}C-palmitate, the relative size and slope of the early clearance curve component, as the reflection of fatty acid oxidation, depend on substrate availability and, consequently, on substrate utilization. In the postprandial state, when glucose and insulin plasma levels are high, the myocardium preferentially oxidizes glucose, and less free fatty acid is oxidized. Therefore, both the size and slope of the rapid clearance curve component are likely to be low, as implied by the findings after infusion of glucose and lactate.[18, 57]

Background Activity

Correction of myocardial uptake for background activity is also important. The need for such correction depends on the type of fatty acid analog. It applies especially to iodine-for-methyl group analogs, which produce high concentrations of free iodide in blood. Freundlieb and associates have devised a special correction technique.[58] After acquisition of IHDA images, a separate dose of ^{123}I-sodium iodide is injected intravenously. The resulting step-increase in activity concentrations, determined from a region of interest assigned to myocardium, indicates the magnitude of contamination of myocardial uptake by background activity and serves as a measure for the correction of myocardial activity. Because of an additional injection of radioactive iodine and an increase in cost as well as radiation burden to the patient, this approach has not been widely accepted. No such corrections have been developed for or are employed with the aromatic fatty acid analog IPPA.

Planar Versus Tomographic Imaging

Another important technical aspect is the mode of image acquisition. Early investigations employed only planar imaging. Studies with limited-angle tomography (e.g., the seven-pinhole collimator), have now been replaced by SPECT imaging. Emergence of iodinated fatty acid analogs such as IPPA that have long myocardial residence times has favored the latter approach. The images are of high diagnostic quality with good contrast resolution. Adequate delineation of temporal changes in myocardial tissue activity concentrations, such as that caused by intravenous administration of radio-iodine for iodine-for-methyl group fatty acid analog, appears possible at present only with conventional planar imaging. However, the rate of temporal sampling depends on the type of fatty acid analog employed. With IPPA, Hansen and associates were able to detect regional abnormalities in tracer tissue clearance rates from only two SPECT image sets acquired for 20 minutes each at an interval of 40 minutes.[55] With the same approach, the investigators succeeded in detecting with a high degree of sensitivity regional impairments of fatty acid metabolism after exercise in patients with coronary artery disease. Recently, Iskandrian and associates[56] used higher sampling rates with SPECT for myocardial IPPA imaging. These investigators recorded 8-minute SPECT images for a total of 40 minutes (Fig. 66–7). Therefore, depending on the type of fatty acid analog employed, low temporal sampling may not necessarily limit the detection of metabolic abnormalities. Generally, the superior image quality achievable with SPECT has favored the use of iodinated fatty acid tracers with slower myocardial clearance rates.

FIGURE 66–7. See Color Plate 29.

CLINICAL EXPERIENCE WITH IODINATED FATTY ACID ANALOGS

The promise of iodinated fatty acid analogs for the evaluation of regional myocardial blood flow and, more importantly, for the evaluation of fatty acid metabolism has prompted clinical investigations in patients with acute and chronic coronary artery disease and with cardiomyopathies. The utility of fatty acid analogs also has been explored for delineating responses to therapeutic interventions such as coronary thrombolysis, coronary angioplasty, and coronary artery bypass grafting.

Myocardial Infarction

Animal Experimental Observations

The initial uptake of iodinated fatty acid analogs in infarcted myocardium is reduced in direct proportion to regional myocardial blood flow. This is expected because of the high first-pass extraction of iodinated fatty acid and the flow-dependent tracer net extraction. However, discrepancies between blood flow and uptake of iodinated fatty acid can occur and have been observed in both experimental animal studies and clinical investigations. Miller and co-workers explored the issue in a coronary occlusion-reperfusion dog model in which the utility of BMIPP for identification of viability in reperfused myocardium was examined.[59] As mentioned, this agent does not undergo β-oxidation and therefore traces primarily myocardial fatty acid uptake. In these experiments, coronary occlusions were maintained for either 15 minutes ($n = 5$) or 60 minutes ($n = 5$) and were followed by reperfusion for 3 hours. Myocardial blood flow was measured with microspheres, and segmental systolic function was measured with ultrasonomicrometry. Myocardial tissue samples were submitted to staining by triphenyl tetrazolium chloride (TTC) and then examined by electron microscopy. An additional group of dogs underwent a 60-minute occlusion of the left anterior descending coronary artery, followed by 3 hours of reperfusion. However, the distal portion of the artery remained occluded in these dogs in order to create an anteroapical perfusion defect that could be visualized on SPECT imaging. In this latter group of dogs, dual imaging with thallium-201 and BMIPP was performed.

Iodinated fatty acid activity concentrations were 37 percent higher in TTC-staining than in TTC-nonstaining tissue samples but occlusion blood flows and contractile function were similarly depressed during occlusion. After 3 hours of reperfusion, TTC-nonstaining segments remained akinetic, whereas TTC-staining zones had partially recovered systolic function. Furthermore, regional BMIPP activity concentrations in TTC-staining myocardium significantly exceeded those of myocardial blood flow. Electron microscopy demonstrated ultrastructural changes in these segments that were consistent with reversible injury. In the third group of dogs, SPECT imaging disclosed that uptake of the fatty acid analog exceeded the uptake of thallium-201. The discordant uptakes of tracers of blood flow and of fatty acid metabolism noninvasively identified myocardial segments as viable or ischemically stunned. Because methyl-branch fatty acid analogs do not undergo β-oxidation, their metabolic fate in myocardium is relatively limited. Most of the tracer is incorporated into the triglyceride pool, from which it may be released by lipoprotein lipase-mediated hydrolysis and back-diffusion of tracer into blood. Incorporation of the tracer into the triglyceride pool most likely accounts for tracer retention in postischemic myocardium. Branched-chain fatty acid analogs may therefore prove useful for delineation of adenosine triphosphate–dependent esterification of free fatty acid and fatty acid storage in the endogenous triglyceride pool as an indicator of myocardial viability. These studies further compared the initial uptake of the fatty acid analog to blood flow, as assessed either by microspheres or with thallium-201. If the delivery and initial extraction of the fatty acid tracer depend on myocardial blood flow, these disparities between regional myocardial blood flow and retention of the fatty acid analog may represent an abnormality in the initial metabolic sequestration process and, thus, in regional fatty acid metabolism.

Clinical Observations

Early investigations with IHDA and IHPA and serial planar scintigraphic imaging demonstrated the possibility of accurate localization of acute or recent myocardial infarctions and determination of their extent.[26] Severity and extent of segmental reductions in uptake of myocardial iodinated fatty acid correlated with defects on thallium-201 scintigraphy (Fig. 66–8) or with the electrocardiographic infarct location. Although ischemia had been expected to prolong the tissue clearance rates of iodinated fatty acid significantly, investigations in 30 patients studied within 1 week of onset of acute symptoms demonstrated accelerated clearance rates in recently infarcted myocardium.[26] The rates averaged 18.5 ± 2.5 minutes and were 46 percent shorter than the clearance half-times in presumably normal myocardium (34.0 ± 8.4 minutes) (see Table 66–2). Stoddart and colleagues more recently confirmed these unexpected findings in a group of 20 patients restudied within 1 week of acute myocardial infarction.[60] Clearance half-times in myocardial infarcted regions averaged 15.5 ± 7.5 minutes, compared with 20.8 ± 4.0 minutes in noninfarcted myocardium (see Table 66–2). Several mechanisms for the shortened rather than prolonged clearance half-times in acutely infarcted myocardium have been proposed. They range from possible contamination of myocardial uptake by blood pool activity to increased contractile work by noninfarcted myocardium in the epicardial layer of the left ventricular wall.[26] Studies in isolated hearts suggest another possibility. An increase in the mitochondrial surface associated with severe but reversible ischemia may facilitate the rate of exchange of free iodide across the mitochondrial membrane.[20, 27]

In the study by Stoddart and colleagues in patients early after infarction, global left ventricular function was found to have improved at 6 months' follow-up in patients with prolonged clearance half-times in infarcted myocardium, whereas shortened tissue clearance half-times in the infarcted region were associated with a decline of left ventricular function.[60] Although the small number of observations precludes definitive conclusions, differences in clearance half-times may be related to the severity of the ischemic injury and thus may be of prognostic significance.

Other investigators observed consistently prolonged regional tissue clearance rates in patients with remote myocardial infarction with both IHDA[61] and IPPA.[17] Uptake of IPPA in infarcted regions was reduced by 38 percent, and regional tissue clearance half-times were markedly prolonged. They averaged 66.5 ± 15.1 minutes, compared with 43.6 ± 6.2 minutes in myocardium supplied by normal coronary arteries. Fridrich and co-workers reported similar clearance half-times for IHDA for infarcted and normal myocardial segments (29.8 ± 6.2 versus 25.8 ± 4.2 minutes, respectively).[61] However, there was a considerable overlap of tissue clearance half-times between infarcted myocardium and myocardium supplied by stenosed but patent coronary arteries. Nevertheless, the difference in clearance half-times for IPPA between ischemic and infarcted areas was statistically significant (54.4 ± 9.6 minutes versus 66.5 ± 15.1 minutes; $P < .025$). Tracer clearance rates in both types of myocardial regions were significantly slower than those in myocardium supplied by normal coronary arteries or by the least severely stenosed coronary artery. There was a statistically significant positive correlation between clearance half-times of IPPA and the degree of impairment in regional contractile function.[17]

Rösler and colleagues examined 28 patients with limited-angle tomography and IHDA within 10 days of acute myocardial infarction and again at 6 months.[62] Two different infarct patterns were observed: pattern 1 was associated with low uptake and accelerated washout, and pattern 2 was associated with reduced tracer uptake but delayed clearance. Pattern 1 was attributed to scar tissue and pattern 2 to viable but ischemically injured myocardium. For both patterns, the extent and severity of the defect size declined with time, but infarct size remained significantly larger in areas with accelerated washout during the initial study. However, left ventricular performance, as assessed by radionuclide ventriculography, did not correlate with these different patterns, which were further unrelated to the clinical outcome of patients. It therefore remains unclear to what extent the impairment of fatty acid oxidation, as evidenced by regional clearance rates, may be directly related to the severity of the ischemic injury, as evidenced by the severity of wall motion abnormality. It is also possible that reduced

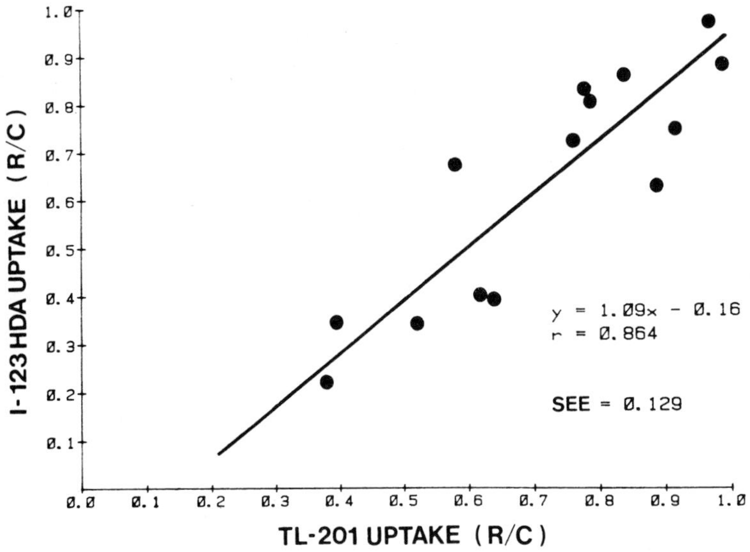

FIGURE 66–8. Comparison of the relative concentrations of 16-[*p*-^{123}I]-hexadecanoic acid (IHDA) and thallium-201 in patients with acute myocardial infarction after coronary thrombolysis. Values for both tracers are given as relative reductions in activity concentrations in the infarcted or risk myocardium (R) and in normal myocardium (C).

energy demand in dysfunctional myocardium could have resulted in a proportionate reduction in fatty acid oxidation. Both explanations also may pertain to findings by Vyska and colleagues.[63] In three patients examined before and after an acute myocardial infarction, the location and extent of postinfarction thallium-201 defects corresponded to regions of delayed IPPA clearance before infarction. The investigators suggested that delayed clearance may have identified myocardium at risk, but no information was provided on pre-existing wall motion abnormalities or the severity of coronary artery disease.

Clinical observations in patients after coronary thrombolysis also disclosed differences between myocardial blood flow and the initial myocardial uptake of iodinated fatty acid analogs. For example, Pachinger and colleagues observed, in patients who had undergone thrombolysis, segmental defects in myocardial iodinated fatty acid analog uptake that were larger and more severe than the perfusion defects seen on thallium-201 scintigrams.[64] Follow-up studies of such defects in a subset of patients indicated that reperfused myocardium with this blood flow metabolism discrepancy recovered more often than myocardium in which blood flow and fatty acid uptake were concordantly reduced. In agreement with this observation is a report by Franken and associates,[65] who studied 22 patients within 4 to 10 days after an acute myocardial infarction and thrombolytic therapy. These authors found a "mismatch" between blood flow and BMIPP distribution, with less severely reduced uptake of the latter in segments that had maintained contractile reserve, by low-dose dobutamine echocardiography. In contrast, segments without adequate response to inotropic stimulation with dobutamine were characterized by concordant reductions in blood flow and fatty acid uptake. Similar discrepancies between uptakes of ^{201}Tl and of BMIPP in 4 of 6 patients after acute myocardial infarction were reported by Saito and co-workers.[66]

Tamaki and colleagues[67] examined 28 patients with acute or chronic myocardial infarction with BMIPP and ^{201}Tl. They reported discordant tracer uptake in 69 percent of patients with recent myocardial infarction (within 4 weeks) but in only 47 percent of patients with a chronic myocardial infarction (more than 4 weeks). Again, a "mismatch" between regional myocardial blood flow and fatty acid uptake, with more severely reduced fatty acid uptake, suggested myocardial viability. More recently, Kawamoto and coworkers[68] compared regional BMIPP and ^{201}Tl uptake to regional glucose metabolic activity as assessed with positron emission tomography and F-18 deoxyglucose in 22 patients with recent myocardial infarctions. Uptake of BMIPP was reduced more severely than that of ^{201}Tl in 27 of 75 hypoperfused segments, whereas the remaining 48 segments exhibited concordant reductions in tracer uptake. Eighty-one percent of the discordant segments but only 2 percent (1 of 48) of the concordant segments revealed redistribution on late ^{201}Tl imaging. Thirty-three hypoperfused segments in 10 patients were also studied with F-18 deoxyglucose and positron emission tomography. Glucose metabolic activity was maintained in 7 (88 percent) of 8 discordant but in only 5 (20 percent) of 25 concordant segments, suggesting that dual-isotope imaging of myocardial blood flow with ^{201}Tl and fatty acid uptake with BMIPP may be useful for identification of ischemically injured but viable myocardium.

These studies suggest an uncoupling of fatty acid uptake from blood flow in acutely injured but potentially viable myocardium. Myocardial SPECT imaging with fatty acid analogs in combination with tracers of myocardial blood flow may develop into a useful clinical tool for the assessment of myocardial viability in patients with recent myocardial infarction. However, the significance of these findings needs to be verified in larger patient cohorts and by careful evaluation of wall motion abnormalities and their changes over time.

Chronic Coronary Artery Disease

Effects on Regional Uptake and Clearance

Initial studies after exercise in patients with chronic coronary artery disease failed to demonstrate the anticipated prolongation of regional clearance half-times of fatty acid analogs in myocardial regions supplied by stenosed coronary arteries. The fact that IHDA was injected after exercise, after the double product and thus fatty acid oxidation most probably had returned to normal, presumably accounted for the failure to demonstrate metabolic abnormalities. Planar imaging with IPPA also established the relation between reduced IPPA uptake and clearance rates in the presence of significant coronary artery disease (Fig. 66–9).

Kennedy and colleagues employed SPECT to determine whether exercise-induced ischemia in 18 patients with coronary artery disease resulted in identifiable segmental reductions in myocardial IPPA uptake and clearance rates.[69] The radioiodinated fatty acid analog was injected 1 minute before the end of exercise, and SPECT images were recorded at 9 and at 40 minutes after tracer injection. Normal values were established in a group of 15 normal volunteers studies in an identical fashion. Overall, early and delayed IPPA imaging detected the presence of coronary artery disease with a sensitivity of 89 percent and a specificity of 67 percent if a limit of one standard deviation from the mean, as determined in the normal volunteers, was employed as the upper limit of normal. Use of a limit of two standard deviations lowered the sensitivity to 72 percent but raised the specificity to 100 percent. Abnormal

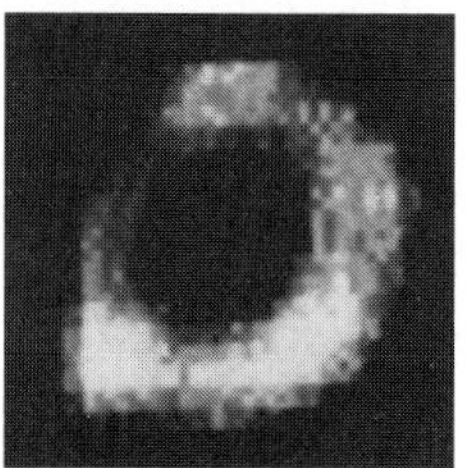

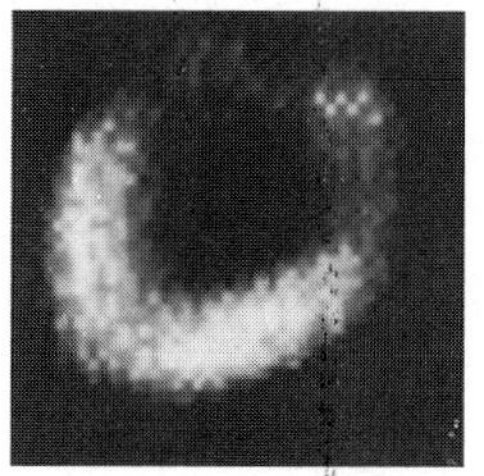

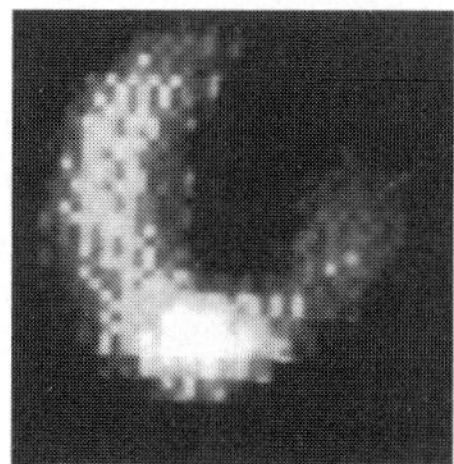

FIGURE 66–9. Serial planar myocardial scintigrams recorded after intravenous injection of 15-(*p*-[^{123}I]-iodophenyl)-pentadecanoic acid (IPPA) at rest in a patient with a 70 percent diameter stenosis of the left anterior descending coronary artery. Note the initially decreased tracer uptake in the interventricular septum, which subsequently resolves on the late images. As seen on the 80-minute image, tracer is retained in the interventricular septum but has cleared from myocardium (lateral wall) that is supplied by normal coronary arteries. (From Dudczak, R., Kletter, K., Angelberger, P., et al: Imaging with I-123–labeled fatty acids. *In* Biersack, H.J., and Cox, P.H. [eds.]: Radioisotope Studies in Cardiology. Hingham, MA, Kluwer Academic Publishers [Martin Nijhoff Publishers], 1985, pp. 295–317, with permission.)

IPPA uptake or washout patterns were observed in 26 of a total of 27 noninfarcted regions. Increased tracer uptake in myocardial regions supplied by significantly stenosed coronary arteries was seen on the early images; differential clearance rates most likely accounted for this observation. Although the tracer rapidly cleared from normal myocardium, it was retained in postischemic segments. The even more prominent relative increase in segmental tracer uptake, as demonstrated in some of the patients on the late images, appears to support this explanation.

With the use of the same study protocol in 33 patients with stable symptomatic coronary artery disease and with at least one coronary artery with an arteriographically determined stenosis equal to or greater than 70 percent diameter, segmental abnormalities in tracer uptake or clearance, or both, were found in 27 patients (82 percent) if the aforementioned limit of two standard deviations was used. A subgroup of 25 patients underwent treadmill exercise testing with both IPPA and ^{201}Tl. Workloads were comparable for the two exercise studies. The ^{201}Tl images were abnormal in 18 (or 72 percent) and the IPPA images in 21 (or 84 percent) of the 25 patients. Although IPPA tended to detect coronary artery disease with a greater sensitivity than ^{201}Tl imaging, this difference failed to reach statistical significance. More recently, Kaiser and colleagues[70] evaluated the use of ortho-IPPA and reported a lower sensitivity of 76 percent for detection of disease in 41 patients with coronary artery disease.

Reske and associates studied 41 patients with coronary artery disease and 10 normal volunteers after maximal bicycle exercise[39] (Fig. 66–10). The investigators observed that 65 and 89 percent, respectively, of myocardial segments supplied by coronary arteries that had luminal narrowing of either 50 to 75 percent or greater than 75 percent exhibited reduced uptake on early imaging (acquired 5 to 7 minutes after injection) or increased retention (i.e., delayed washout) at the time of late imaging, or both. Segmental metabolic abnormalities persisted for significantly longer time periods than exercise-induced chest pain or ECG abnormalities. In normal subjects, uptake and clearance of the iodinated fatty acid analog were homogeneous, but patients with coronary artery disease revealed retention of tracer in ischemic zones and persistent defects in infarcted territories. In a semiquantitative analysis for three tomographic planes, the investigators found a correlation between severity of stenosis and extent of the uptake abnormality. The results derived from these studies in patients with exercise-induced ischemia by SPECT and IPPA imaging are comparable to those achieved with ^{11}C-palmitate and positron emission tomography in experimental animals with segmentally reduced ^{11}C-palmitate uptake and washout and enhanced ^{18}F-2-fluoro-2-deoxyglucose uptake in ischemic segments (see Chapter 71).

Vyska and colleagues examined the myocardial extraction of IPPA in 18 normal volunteers and in patients with coronary artery disease at rest and after exercise.[63] A subgroup of patients were studied after interventional revascularization. In 15 of the 20 patients, exercise-induced defects of fatty acid uptake were larger than those seen on the ^{201}Tl images, suggesting that acute, stress-induced ischemia had reduced the extraction fraction of IPPA. After angioplasty, stress scintigraphy revealed an improvement in segmental uptake of ^{201}Tl and IPPA, although the extraction fraction of IPPA remained depressed in 7 of 10 patients. Stoddart and colleagues studied eight patients with chronic coronary artery disease before and after coronary angioplasty.[71] Clearance half-times for IHDA averaged 35.7 ± 41.2 minutes in poststenotic segments and tended to be longer than in regions supplied by normal coronary arteries, which had an average clearance half-time of 18.8 ± 3.4 minutes (see Table 66–2). The researchers failed to demonstrate a significant change in tracer half-times after successful angioplasty.

In summary, exercise stress in patients with chronic coronary artery disease is frequently associated with segmental reductions in myocardial uptake and prolonged myocardial clearance half-times of iodinated fatty acid analogs. Segmentally reduced tracer uptake is largely a function of the reduced blood flow but may be modified by an ischemia-related effect on metabolic trapping of fatty acid in myocardium. The longer clearance half-times are likely to reflect abnormal rates of fatty acid oxidation and increased incorporation into the endogenous lipid pool. Lastly, iodinated fatty acid analogs appear to allow detection of coronary artery disease with a sensitivity and specificity comparable to those of myocardial perfusion scintigraphy.

Assessment of Myocardial Viability

Although numerous studies have interpreted disparities between blood flow and iodinated fatty acid uptake as evidence of "myocardial viability," only two investigations tested this hypothesis by correlating the findings on iodinated fatty acid images to the outcome after revascularization in regional contractile function. Both studies employed IPPA. Murray and colleagues[54] determined the initial tracer kinetics from rapid, serially acquired planar images for 25 minutes. Based on findings in 17 healthy volunteers with an average tracer washout rate of 21 ± 5 percent during the initial 25 minutes, myocardium was defined as viable if the initial washout was equal to or greater than 16 percent. Compared with interoperatively obtained biopsy samples, there was a 91 percent agreement between the degree of fibrosis and the tracer clearance rate. Myocardium was defined histologically as "nonviable" if more than 50 percent of the biopsy sample demonstrated fibrosis. More important, the regional IPPA clearance rates were 75 percent accurate (12 of 16 segments) in predicting that wall motion would improve after revascularization and 67 percent accurate (4 out of 6 segments) in predicting that it would not. Furthermore, in the patients

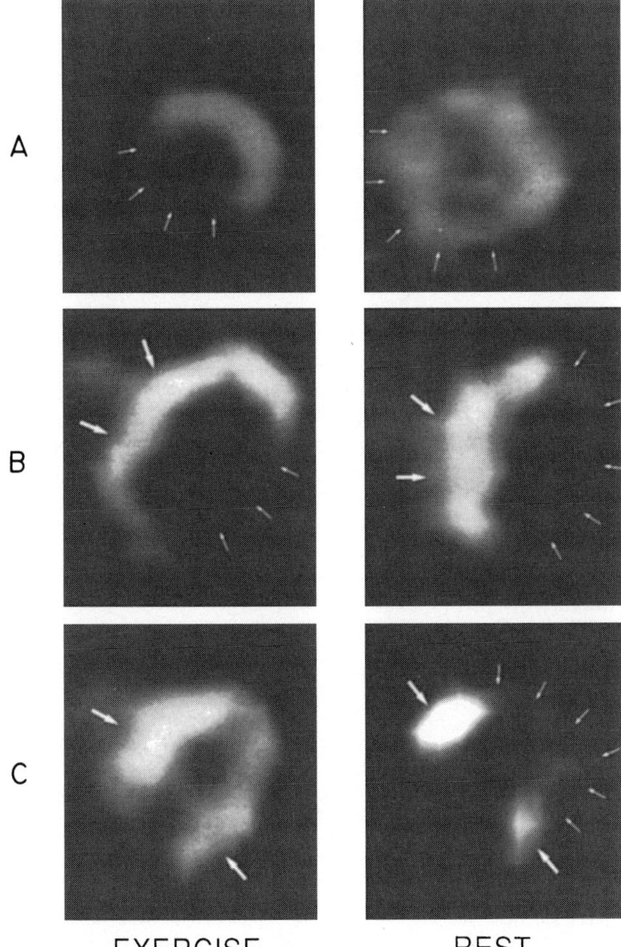

FIGURE 66–10. Single-photon emission computed tomographic images of the initial myocardial uptake of 15-(*p*-[^{123}I]-iodophenyl)-pentadecanoic acid (IPPA) in three patients (*A*, *B*, and *C*) early (5 minutes, *left*) and late (35 minutes) after exercise. Panel *A* represents a short-axis cut through the middle left ventricle and indicates reduced uptake of IPPA in the interventricular septum and the inferior wall on the early postexercise images, with increased tracer retention on the late images. Angiography in this patient revealed a 95 percent diameter stenosis of the left anterior descending coronary artery. Panel *B* shows long-axis cuts in a patient with a prior myocardial infarction, complete occlusion of the left circumflex coronary artery, and a high-grade stenosis of the left anterior descending coronary artery after bypass grafting. The early postexercise image reveals a large defect in the posterolateral wall, with normal uptake in the interventricular septum and the anterior wall. The late image indicates increased retention of tracer in the interventricular septum. Panel *C* shows horizontal long-axis cuts in a patient with a complete occlusion of the right coronary artery and a 70 percent diameter stenosis of the left circumflex coronary artery. The early image reveals relatively homogeneous uptake of IPPA, whereas the late image indicates increased retention of tracer in the lateral wall. (From Reske, S., Koischwitz, D., and Reichmann, K.: Cardiac metabolism of 15(*p*-I-123)phenylpentadecanoic acid after intracoronary tracer application. Eur. J. Radiol. 4:144, 1984, with permission.)

with viable myocardium, the left ventricular ejection fraction increased from 28 ± 7 to 43 ± 14 percent ($P < .001$) after surgery. The results of a more recent study, performed also with IPPA but employing serial SPECT image acquisition for 40 minutes, similarly indicated a potentially useful role of iodinated fatty acid analogs for the assessment of myocardial viability.[56] This study in 21 patients reported an 89 percent agreement between rest ^{201}Tl redistribution and IPPA redistribution findings. Regional and global left ventricular function was reevaluated after revascularization in 14 patients. IPPA demonstrated "viability" in 16 (89 percent) of 18 segments with a postrevascularization improvement in wall motion but also in 18 (47 percent) of 38 segments without such improvement. Patients with an improvement in global left ventricular function exhibited a significantly greater number of "viable" segments than those without a revascularization improvement.

Kawamoto and co-workers[72] compared the tracer kinetics of BMIPP to those of ^{11}C-palmitate in 10 patients, 6 with chronic coronary artery disease and 4 with hypertrophic cardiomyopathy, and found a significant correlation between BMIPP and early ^{11}C-palmitate uptake. In contrast, BMIPP uptake was unrelated to the early clearance component of ^{11}C-palmitate as a marker of β-oxidation. Thus, BMIPP uptake probably reflects myocardial blood flow and fatty acid extraction but not β-oxidation.

In summary, iodinated fatty acid analogs can be used to evaluate myocardial blood flow and viability in patients with chronic coronary artery disease. However, larger patient populations need to be studied prospectively with IPPA or BMIPP to determine the clinical role of these tracers of blood flow and fatty acid metabolism.

Cardiomyopathy

Several clinical investigations have explored the utility of iodinated fatty acid analogs for identification of metabolic abnormalities in dilated cardiomyopathies.

Idiopathic Dilated Cardiomyopathy

With the use of IHPA, Höck and group studied 20 patients with congestive cardiomyopathy of varying origin after a 3-minute, low-level stress test.[73] In addition to heterogeneous uptake of tracer in myocardium, clearance half-times were markedly prolonged (see Table 66–2). In a subgroup of seven patients with normal left ventricular ejection fractions and normal wall motion but abnormally increased pulmonary wedge pressures during exercise, myocardial clearance half-times averaged 26.8 ± 6.7 minutes and did not differ from those of normal volunteers. In contrast, the remaining 13 patients with reduced left ventricular ejection fractions had clearance half-times that were markedly prolonged, averaging 42 ± 13.1 minutes. Values derived from six normal volunteers averaged 21.7 ± 2 minutes after stress and 24 ± 5 minutes at rest. Furthermore, the regional clearance half-times significantly varied between the interventricular septum and the inferior and posterolateral walls. This variability was greater than that observed in normal volunteers. Although an elevated pulmonary wedge pressure alone would appear to be a tenuous indicator of impending dilated cardiomyopathy, the investigators argued that a correlation existed between the severity of disease and the impairment of myocardial fatty acid metabolism.

Other investigations with IPPA[17] revealed a similar heterogeneity in myocardial tracer uptake and prolonged clearance half-times (see Table 66–2). They averaged 69.3 ± 29.6 minutes in the 10 study patients and were significantly longer than those in normal and ischemic myocardium of patients with coronary artery disease (43.8 ± 6.2 minutes and 54.4 ± 9.6 minutes, respectively). Both uptake and clearance of IPPA were normal in four patients. In the remaining six patients, there were regional abnormalities in uptake and clearance rates, although there was no close correlation between uptake and clearance abnormalities.

The utility of IHDA as a metabolic probe for cardiomyopathy was examined in 16 patients with different types of cardiomyopathies.[35] These included idiopathic dilated cardiomyopathy in four patients and myotonic dystrophy in another four patients. The remaining patients had Duchenne muscular dystrophy, complex congenital heart disease, hypertrophic heart disease, and other types of disease. Mean clearance half-times for the patient group were similar to those observed for normal controls (32.7 ± 7.0 versus 33.0 ± 7.0). This finding is not surprising in view of the heterogeneous patient population. Only two patients revealed prolonged clearance half-times. One of these patients suffered from carnitine deficiency, which can be associated with cardiomyopathy.

With the use of IPPA and SPECT imaging, Ugolini and colleagues[74] demonstrated highly heterogeneous myocardial uptake but, in contrast to other reports, they observed shortened clearance half-times. The degree of heterogeneity of the initial myocardial IPPA uptake was related to the clinical status as classified by the New York Heart Association. Yet there was no significant relation between the initial uptake and left ventricular ejection fractions as determined by radionuclide ventriculography. The researchers postulated that increased catecholamine levels in their patients may have enhanced rates of β-oxidation and therefore accelerated the myocardial clearance of IPPA. They argued further that the degree of heterogeneity in tracer uptake potentially could provide prognostic information.

In summary, the observed heterogeneous uptake of iodinated fatty acid analogs is consistent with that as observed with ^{11}C-palmitate and positron emission tomography (see Chapter 69). However, myocardial clearance rates varied between studies, possibly because of heterogeneous patient populations or inadequate standardization of study conditions. The reports also failed to demonstrate convincingly a significant correlation between tracer uptake or clearance half-times and left ventricular function that could be of predictive value. Finally, the mechanisms that accounted for the delay of tracer tissue clearance, as observed in the majority of these studies, remain unexplained.

Hypertrophic Cardiomyopathy

More recently, BMIPP has emerged as a potentially useful tracer to identify abnormalities in fatty acid metabolism in patients with cardiomyopathy. Early animal experimental studies had demonstrated reductions in BMIPP uptake relative to blood flow in cardiomyopathic hamsters.[75] Consequently, Shimonagata and colleagues[76] examined possible discrepancies between myocardial blood flow and free fatty acid metabolism in patients with hypertrophic cardiomyopathy. These investigators reported a reduction in BMIPP uptake relative to ^{201}Tl uptake in 40 percent of all segments, suggesting an impairment in fatty acid metabolism in these patients. Furthermore, Hase and associates[77] correlated regional wall motion by two-dimensional echocardiography with fatty acid metabolism by BMIPP in 15 patients with coronary artery disease, left ventricular hypertrophy, or hypertrophic cardiomyopathy (Fig. 66–11). In this study, the incidence of disagreement between ^{201}Tl and BMIPP uptake scores was significantly higher in patients with cardiomyopathy than in those with coronary artery disease or hypertension.

FIGURE 66–11. See Color Plate 30.

Similar observations were made by Taki and associates in 13 of 17 patients with hypertrophic cardiomyopathy and regions with lower BMIPP than ^{201}Tl uptake.[78] In addition to differences between fatty acid uptake and blood flow by ^{201}Tl abnormalities in tracer retention and washout were reported by Torizuka and colleagues in almost 50 percent of 55 patients with hypertrophic cardiomyopathy.[79] However, both tracer washout and fill-in were observed in these patients. In contrast, no such changes were noted in 88 percent of 91 patients with ischemic heart disease.

Overall, these findings suggest an abnormality in fatty acid esterification in patients with hypertrophic cardiomyopathy. However, the clinical relevance of metabolic imaging with iodinated fatty acids in patients with cardiomyopathy and its potential clinical role have not been defined.

SUMMARY AND CONCLUSIONS

Animal experimental studies and clinical investigations with a variety of radioiodinated fatty acid analogs have demonstrated the possibility of noninvasively deriving metabolic information with single-photon and tomographic imaging. The extent of metabolic information obtained with these tracers depends on their specific properties and ranges from myocardial uptake of exogenous fatty acid to incorporation of fatty acid into the endogenous lipid pool and β-oxidation of free fatty acid. At present, the fractional distribution of tracer in myocardium, rather than its rate of clearance from myocardium, appears to be an indicator of fatty acid metabolism. Observations in patients with coronary artery disease have demonstrated the known impairment of oxidation of fatty acid and increased incorporation into the endogenous lipid pool as consequences of myocardial ischemia. Findings in patients with cardiomyopathy have been less conclusive and warrant further studies. Quantification of exogenous fatty acid utilization may ultimately become possible with some of the described fatty acid analogs and an appropriate tracer kinetic model. Although this class of metabolic tracers has remained underutilized, possibly because of the limited availability, cost, and complexities of tracer synthesis, it nevertheless appears to offer the potential of identifying viable myocardium as well as gaining novel insights into the pathophysiology of cardiovascular disease.

Acknowledgments

The authors thank Wendy Wilson and Mary Lee Griswold for preparing the illustrations for this chapter and Eileen Rosenfeld for her secretarial assistance in preparing this manuscript.

References

1. Rothlin, M.E, and Bing, R.J.: Extraction and release of individual free fatty acids by the heart and fat depots. J. Clin. Invest. 40:1380, 1961.
2. Evans, J.R., Gunton, R.W., Baker, R.G., et al.: Use of radioiodinated fatty acid for photoscans of the heart. Circ. Res. 16:1, 1965.
3. Robinson, G.D.: Rapid synthesis of high specific activity biologically active ^{18}F-fluoroaliphatic analog compounds. J. Nucl. Med. 14:446, 1973.
4. Robinson, G.D., and Lee, A.W.: Radioiodinated fatty acids for heart imaging: Iodine monochloride addition compared with iodine replacement labeling. J. Nucl. Med. 16:17, 1975.
5. Poe, N.D., Robinson, G.D., Jr., Graham, L.S., et al.: Experimental basis for myocardial imaging with ^{123}I-labeled hexadecanoic acid. J. Nucl. Med. 17:1077, 1976.
6. Poe, N.D., Robinson, G.D., Jr., Zielinski, F.W., et al.: Myocardial imaging with ^{123}I-hexadecanoic acid. Radiology 124:419, 1977.
7. Machulla, H.J., Stöcklin, G., Kupfernagel, C.H., et al.: Comparative evaluation of fatty acids with C-11, Cl-34m, Br-77, I-23, for metabolic studies of the myocardium: Concise communication. J. Nucl. Med. 19:298, 1978.
8. Machulla, H., Marsmann, M., and Dutschka, K.: Biochemical concept and synthesis of a radioiodinated phenylfatty acid for in vivo metabolic studies of the myocardium. Eur. J. Nucl. Med. 5:171, 1980.
9. Goodman, M., Kirsch, G., and Knapp, F.: Synthesis of radioiodinated ω-(*p*-iodophenyl)-substituted methyl-branched long-chain fatty acids. J. Lab. Comp. Radiopharm. 19:1316, 1982.
10. Goodman, M., Knapp, F., Elmaleh, D., et al.: Synthesis and evaluation of radioiodinated terminal *p*-iodophenyl-substituted alpha- and beta-methyl-branched fatty acids. J. Med. Chem. 25:390, 1984.
11. Kirsch, G., Goodman, M., and Knapp, F.: Orano-tellurium compounds of biological interest: Unique properties of the *N*-chlorosuccinimide oxidation product of 9-telluraheptadecanoic acid. Organometallics 2:357, 1983.
12. Knapp, F., Ambrose, K., and Callahan, A.: Effects of chain length and tellurium position on the myocardial uptake of Te-123m fatty acids. J. Nucl. Med. 22:988, 1981.
13. Livni, E., Elmaleh, D.R., Levy, S., et al.: Beta-methyl-[1-^{11}C]heptadecanoic acid: A new metabolic tracer for positron emission tomography. J. Nucl. Med. 23:169, 1982.
14. Livni, E., Elmaleh, D., and Barlai-Kovach, M.: Radioiodinated beta-methyl phenyl fatty acids as potential tracers for myocardial imaging and metabolism. Eur. Heart J. 6:(Suppl. B):85, 1985.
15. Goodman, M., and Knapp, F.: Synthesis of 15-(*p*-iodo-phenyl)-6-tellurapentadecanoic acid: A new myocardial imaging agent. J. Org. Chem. 47:3004, 1982.
16. Bianco, J., Pape, L., and Alpert, J.: Accumulation of radioiodinated 15-(*p*-iodophenyl)-6-tellurapentadecanoic acid in ischemic myocardium during acute coronary occlusion and reperfusion. J. Am. Coll. Cardiol. 4:80, 1984.
17. Dudczak, R., Schmoliner, R., and Kletter, K.: Clinical evaluation of I-123-labeled *p*-phenyl pentadecanoic acid (*p*-IPPA) for myocardial scintigraphy. J. Nucl. Med. Allied Sci. 27:267, 1983.
18. Dudczak, K., Kletter, K., and Frischauf, H.: The use of I-123 heptadecanoic acid (HDA) as metabolic tracer: Preliminary report. Eur. J. Nucl. Med. 9:81, 1984.
19. Dudczak, K., Kletter, K., and Frischauf, H.: Myocardial turnover rates of I-123 heptadecanoic acid (HD). Radioakt. Isotope Klin. Forsch. 15:685, 1982.
20. Kloster, G., Stöcklin, G., Smith, E., et al.: Omega-halofatty acids: A probe for

mitochondrial membrane integrity: In vitro investigations in normal and ischaemic myocardium. Eur. J. Nucl. Med. 9:305, 1984.

21. Knust, E.J., Kupfernagel, C.H., and Stocklin, G.: Long chain F-18 fatty acids for the study of regional metabolism in heart and liver: Odd-even effects of metabolism in mice. J. Nucl. Med. 20:1170, 1979.
22. Notohamiprodjo, G., Schmid, A., and Spohr, G.: Comparison of ^{11}C-palmitic acid (CPA) and ^{123}I-heptadecanoic acid (IHA) turnover in human heart. J. Nucl. Med. 26:P88, 1985.
23. van der Wall, E., Heidendal, G., and den Hollander, W.: I-123–labeled hexadecanoic acid in comparison with thallium-201 for myocardial imaging in coronary heart disease: A preliminary study. Eur. J. Nucl. Med. 5:401, 1980.
24. van der Wall, E., Heidendal, G., and Hollander, W.: Metabolic myocardial imaging with I-123–labeled heptadecanoic acid in patients with angina pectoris. Eur. J. Nucl. Med. 6:391, 1981.
25. Dudczak, R., Homan, R., and Zanganeh, A.: Myocardial metabolic studies in patients with cardiomyopathy. J. Nucl. Med. 24:P20, 1983.
26. van der Wall, E., Hollander, W., and Heidendal, G.: Dynamic myocardial scintigraphy with I-123–labeled free fatty acids in patients with myocardial infarction. Eur. J. Nucl. Med. 6:383, 1981.
27. Kloster, G., and Stoecklin, G.: Determination of the rate-determining step in halofatty acid turnover in the heart. Radioakt. Isotope Klin. Forsch. 15:235, 1982.
28. Visser, F., van Eenige, M., and Westera, G.: Metabolic fate of radioiodinated heptadecanoic acid in the normal canine heart. Circulation 72:565, 1985.
29. Visser, F., Westera, G., and van Eenige, M.: The myocardial elimination rate of radioiodinated heptadecanoic acid. Eur. J. Nucl. Med. 10:118, 1985.
30. Cuchet, P., Demaison, L., and Bontemps, L.: Do iodinated fatty acids undergo a nonspecific deiodination in the myocardium? Eur. J. Nucl. Med. 10:505, 1985.
31. Visser, F., van Eenige, M., Duwel, C., et al.: Radioiodinated free fatty acids: Can we measure myocardial metabolism? Eur. J. Nucl. Med. 12:S20, 1986.
32. Schön, H., Senekowitsch, R., and Berg, D.: Measurement of myocardial fatty acid metabolism: Kinetics of iodine-123–heptadecanoic acid in normal dog hearts. J. Nucl. Med. 27:1449, 1986.
33. Reske, S., Sauer, W., Machulla, H., et al.: 15(p-[^{123}I]iodophenyl)pentadecanoic acid as a tracer of lipid metabolism: Comparison with [I-^{14}C]palmitic acid in murine tissues. J. Nucl. Med. 25:1335, 1984.
34. Reske, S., Machulla, H., and Winkler, C.: Metabolic turnover of p-I-123 phenylpentadecanoic acid in the hearts of rats. J. Nucl. Med. 23:P10, 1982.
35. Rabinovitch, M., Kalff, V., and Allen, R.: Omega-^{123}I-hexadecanoic acid metabolic probe of cardiomyopathy. Eur. J. Nucl. Med. 10:222, 1985.
36. DeGrado, T., Holden, J., and Ng, C.: Quantitative analysis of myocardial kinetics of 15-p-[iodine-125] iodophenylpentadecanoic acid. J. Nucl. Med. 30:1211, 1989.
37. Dormehl, I., Feinendegen, L., Hugo, N., et al.: Comparative myocardial imaging in the baboon with ^{123}I-labelled ortho and para isomers of 15-(iodophenyl)pentadecanoic acid (IPPA). Nucl. Med. Commun. 14:998, 1993.
38. Kaiser, K.P., Geuting, B., Grobmann, K., et al.: Tracer kinetics of 15-(ortho-$^{123/131}$I-phenyl)-pentadecanoic acid (oPPA) and 15-(para-$^{123/131}$I-phenyl)-pentadecanoic acid (pPPA) in animals and man. J. Nucl. Med. 31:1608, 1990.
39. Reske, S., Koischwitz, D., and Reichmann, K.: Cardiac metabolism of 15(p-I-123)phenylpentadecanoic acid after intracoronary tracer application. Eur. J. Radiol. 4:144, 1984.
40. Vyska, K., Machulla, H., and Stremmel, W.: Regional myocardial free fatty acid extraction in normal and ischemic myocardium. Circulation 78:1218, 1987.
41. Otto, C., Brown, L., and Scott, A.: Radioiodinated branched-chain fatty acids: Substrates for beta oxidation? Concise communication. J. Nucl. Med. 25:75, 1985.
42. Elmaleh, D., Livni, E., and Levy, S.: Comparison of ^{11}C- and ^{14}C-labeled fatty acids and their beta-methyl analogs. Int. J. Nucl. Med. 10:81, 1983.
43. Jones, G., Livni, E., and Strauss, H.: Synthesis and biologic evaluation of 1-[^{11}C]-3,3-dimethylheptadecanoic acid. J. Nucl. Med. 29:68, 1988.
44. Yamamoto, K., Som, P., and Brill, A.: Dual tracer autoradiographic study of β-methyl-(1-^{14}C) heptadecanoic acid and 15-p(^{131}I)-iodophenyl-β-methyl-pentadecanoic acid in normotensive and hypertensive rats. J. Nucl. Med. 27:1178, 1986.
45. Yonekura, Y., Brill, A., and Som, P.: Regional myocardial substrate uptake in hypertensive rats: A quantitative autoradiographic measurement. Science 227:1494, 1985.
46. Goodman, M., Knapp, F., Elmaleh, D., et al.: New myocardial imaging agents: Synthesis of 15(p-iodo-phenyl)-3-(R,S)-methyl-pentadecanoic acid by decomposition of a 3,3-(1,5-pentanedyl) triazene precursor. J. Org. Chem. 49:2322, 1984.
47. Knapp, F., Goodman, M., Kirsch, G., et al.: Radioiodinated 15-(p-iodophenyl)-3-3-dimethylpentadecanoic acid (DMIPP): A new agent to evaluate regional myocardial fatty acid uptake. J. Nucl. Med. 26:123, 1985.
48. Knapp, F., Ambrose, K., and Goodman, M.: New radioiodinated methyl-branched fatty acids for cardiac studies. Eur. J. Nucl. Med. 12:S39, 1986.
49. Knapp, F., Goodman, M., Callahan, A., et al.: Radioiodinated 15-(p-iodophenyl)-3,3-dimethylpentadecanoic acid: A useful new agent to evaluate myocardial fatty acid uptake. J. Nucl. Med. 27:521, 1986.
50. Ambrose, K., Owen, B., Goodman, M., et al.: Evaluation of the metabolism in rat hearts of two new radioiodinated 3-methyl-branched fatty acid myocardial imaging agents. Eur. J. Nucl. Med. 12:486, 1987.
51. Goodman, M., Knapp, F., and Callahan, A.: Synthesis and biological evaluation of 17-[^{131}]-iodo-9-telluraheptadecanoic acid, a potential imaging agent. J. Med. Chem. 25:613, 1982.
52. von Eenige, M., Visser, F., and Duwel, C.: Analysis of myocardial time-activity curves of ^{123}I-heptadecanoic acid: II. The acquisition time. Nuklearmedizin 26:248, 1987.
53. von Eenige, M., Visser, F., and Duwel, C.: Analysis of myocardial time-activity curves of ^{123}I-heptadecanoic acid: I. Curve fitting. Nuklearmedizin 26:241, 1987.
54. Murray, G., Schad, N., Ladd, W., et al.: Metabolic cardiac imaging in severe coronary disease: Assessment of viability with iodine-123–iodophenylpentadecanoic acid and multicrystal gamma camera, and correlation with biopsy. J. Nucl. Med. 33:1269, 1992.
55. Hansen, C., Corbett, J., and Pippin, J.: Iodine-123 phenylpentadecanoic acid and single-photon emission computed tomography in identifying heart disease: Comparison with thallium-201 myocardial tomography. J. Am. Coll. Cardiol. 12:78, 1988.
56. Iskandrian, A., Powers, J., Cave, V., et al.: Assessment of myocardial viability by dynamic tomographic iodine-123 iodophenylpentadecanoic acid imaging: Comparison with rest-redistribution thallium-201 imaging. J. Nucl. Cardiol. 2:101, 1995.
57. Dudczak, R., Schmoliner, R., and Angelberger, P.: Structurally modified fatty acids: Clinical potential as tracers of metabolism. Eur. J. Nucl. Med. 12:S45, 1986.
58. Freundlieb, C., Höck, A., and Vyska, K.: Myocardial imaging and metabolic studies with (17-^{123}I) iodoheptadecanoic acid. J. Nucl. Med. 21:1043, 1980.
59. Miller, D., Gill, J., and Elmaleh, D.: Fatty acid analogue accumulation: A marker of myocyte viability in ischemic-reperfused myocardium. Circulation 63:681, 1988.
60. Stoddart, P., Papouchado, M., and Wilde, P.: Prognostic value of 123-iodo-heptadecanoic acid imaging in patients with acute myocardial infarction. Eur. J. Nucl. Med. 12:525, 1987.
61. Fridrich, L., Pichler, M., and Gassner, A.: Tracer elimination in I-123 heptadecanoic acid: Half-life, component ratio and washout profiles in patients with cardiac disease. Eur. Heart J. 6(Suppl. B):61, 1985.
62. Rösler, H., Noelpp, U., and Toth, T.: On the prognostic potential of the sequential ^{123}I-HDA tomoscintigram after the first MI. Eur. Heart J. 6:(Suppl. B):49, 1985.
63. Vyska, K., Machulla, H., and Stremmel, W.: Regional myocardial free fatty acid extraction in normal and ischemic myocardium. Circulation 78:1218, 1988.
64. Pachinger, O., Sochor, H., Probst, P., et al.: Selective thrombolysis in acute myocardial infarction: Evaluation of functional result by metabolic studies and perfusion imaging. Acta Med. Austriaca 9:65, 1982.
65. Franken, P., De Geeter, F., Dendale, P., et al.: Abnormal free fatty acid uptake in subacute myocardial infarction after coronary thrombolysis: Correlation with wall motion and inotropic reserve. J. Nucl. Med. 35:1758, 1994.
66. Saito, S., Yasuda, T., Gold, H., et al.: Differentiation of regional myocardial perfusion and fatty acid uptake in zones of myocardial injury. Nucl. Med. Commun. 12:663, 1991.
67. Tamaki, N., Kawamoti, M., Yonekura, Y., et al.: Regional metabolic abnormality in relation to perfusion and wall motion in patients with myocardial infarction: Assessment with emission tomography using an iodinated branch chain fatty acid analog. J. Nucl. Med. 33:659, 1992.
68. Kawamoto, M., Tamaki, N., Yonekura, Y., et al.: Combined study with I-123 fatty acid and thallium-201 to assess ischemic myocardium: Comparison with thallium redistribution and glucose metabolism. Ann. Nucl. Med. 8:47, 1994.
69. Kennedy, P., Corbett, J., and Kulkarni, P.: Iodine I-123 phenylpentadecanoic acid myocardial scintigraphy: Usefulness in identifying myocardial ischemia. Circulation 74:1007, 1986.
70. Kaiser, K., Grossmann, K., Geuting, B., et al.: Semiquantitative analysis of SPECT with the iodinated fatty acid 15-(ortho-^{123}I-phenyl)-pentadecanoic acid. Nucl. Med. Commun. 12:927, 1991.
71. Stoddart, P., Papouchado, M., Vann Jones, J., et al.: Assessment of percutaneous transluminal coronary angioplasty with ^{123}iododo-heptadecanoic acid. Eur. J. Nucl. Med. 12:605, 1987.
72. Kawamoto, M., Tamaki, N., Yonekura, Y., et al.: Significance of myocardial uptake of iodine-123–labeled beta-methyl iodophenyl pentadecanoic acid: Comparison with kinetics of C-11–labeled palmitate in positron emission tomography. J. Nucl. Cardiol. 1:522, 1994.
73. Höck, A., Freundlieb, D., and Vyska, K.: Myocardial imaging and metabolic studies with (17-^{123}I) iodoheptadecanoic acid in patients with congestive cardiomyopathy. J. Nucl. Med. 24:22, 1983.
74. Ugolini, V., Hansen, C., and Kulkarni, P.: Abnormal myocardial fatty acid metabolism in dilated cardiomyopathy detected by iodine-123 phenyl pentadecanoic acid and tomographic imaging. Am. J. Cardiol. 62:923, 1988.
75. Nishimura, T., and Sago, M.: Comparison of myocardial thallium and beta-methyl-iodo-phenyl pentadecanoic acid (BMIPP) distribution in cardiomyopathy hamsters. J. Nucl. Med. 30:80, 1989.
76. Shimonagata, T., Nishimura, T., Uehara, T., et al.: Discrepancies between myocardial perfusion and free fatty acid metabolism in patients with hypertrophic cardiomyopathy. Nucl. Med. Commun. 14:1005, 1993.
77. Hase, M., Nakata, T., Yonekura, S., et al.: Correlation of regional wall motion and fatty acid metabolism in coronary artery disease, hypertension and hypetrophic cardiomyopathy: Assessment by dual-isotope SPECT with thallium-201 and iodine-123 beta-methyl fatty acid analog. Kaku Igaku 30:529, 1993.
78. Taki, J., Nakajima, K., Bunko, H., et al.: ^{123}I-labeled BMIPP fatty acid myocardial scintigraphy in patients with hypertrophic cardiomyopathy: SPECT comparison with stress ^{201}Tl. Nucl. Med. Commun. 14:181, 1993.
79. Torizuka, K., Yonekura, Y., Nishimura, T., et al.: Phase 2 study of beta-methyl-p-(^{123}I)-iodophenyl-pentadecanoic acid metabolism. Kaku Igaku 29:305, 1992.

CHAPTER

67 Thrombosis Imaging With Indium-111–Labeled Platelets

John R. Stratton, M.D.

The central role of platelets in cardiovascular diseases has become increasingly apparent. Several lines of evidence indicate that platelets contribute to the genesis of the atherosclerotic lesion, in part by the production and release of growth factors that promote smooth muscle cell hyperplasia. In addition, intra-arterial platelet-fibrin thrombus formation is the final common pathway leading to most of the complications that ensue after an atherosclerotic lesion forms, including acute myocardial infarction, unstable angina, stroke, transient cerebral ischemia, and sudden cardiac death. Another important pathophysiologic function of platelets is the platelet thrombus formation that uniformly occurs after implantation of intravascular prosthetic materials, which are increasingly used for the construction of arterial and venous substitutes, heart valves, vascular catheters, and artificial hearts. With virtually all these prosthetic materials, thrombotic and embolic complications caused by platelet thrombus formation are an important long-term side effect. The importance of platelets in causing cardiovascular events is also indicated by the success of platelet-inhibitory therapy in reducing mortality or morbidity in a variety of vascular disease states.

Given the great importance of intravascular platelet-fibrin thrombosis in causing cardiovascular diseases, a noninvasive, in vivo method of diagnosing the presence and extent of intravascular thrombi would be of great clinical value. Thrombosis imaging by radionuclide techniques involves the injection of a tracer that accumulates preferentially in areas of thrombosis. Multiple approaches to thrombosis imaging are being explored, including the labeling of monoclonal antibodies directed against platelets or fibrin and the labeling of other compounds, such as tissue plasminogen activator (t-PA) or annexin V, that also localize in areas of thrombosis. To date, however, most thrombosis imaging in humans has used platelets labeled with indium-111. Thrombosis imaging with ^{111}In-labeled platelets has shown promise as a technique for studying localized thrombosis as well as for the assessment of therapies in a wide variety of human disease states. The main advantages of ^{111}In-labeled platelet imaging over previously used techniques for the detection of thrombosis are that it is noninvasive, it can be performed in humans, it can be done serially to assess the effects of time or therapy, and it provides semiquantitative, organ-specific information. In addition to defining the presence and location of localized thrombosis, platelet imaging also provides kinetic information regarding thrombus activity, unlike anatomical methods such as angiography or ultrasonography.

Indium-111–labeled platelet imaging has proved particularly useful as a research tool in animal studies, because an accurate measurement of the magnitude of platelet thrombus formation can be made either by external, in vivo imaging or by ex vivo counting of resected specimens. This chapter focuses on a discussion of platelet imaging findings in humans. In addition to the cardiovascular disorders reviewed in this chapter, platelet imaging has been used in humans to assess platelet survival and the sites of platelet destruction in thrombocytopenic syndromes and has been used to aid in the diagnosis of organ rejection. A review of ^{111}In platelet labeling, imaging, and quantitative techniques appears first, followed by a discussion of findings in patients with intracardiac thrombi, arterial thrombi, venous thrombi, and intravascular prosthetic materials.

LABELING, DOSIMETRY, IMAGING, AND QUANTITATIVE METHODS

Platelet-Labeling Techniques

During ^{111}In decay, the two gamma rays that are emitted, at 171 and 245 keV, are responsible for 87 percent of the energy released. Both of these gamma rays can be detected readily by conventional gamma cameras. The 2.8-day half-life of ^{111}In corresponds reasonably closely to the half-life of normal circulating platelets (approximately 4 days) and therefore allows the assessment of the dynamics of platelet deposition over several days. Since Thakur and associates[1] originally described the preparation of ^{111}In-oxine–labeled platelets in 1976, numerous additional methods of platelet labeling have been described.[2–25] The techniques vary widely with regard to the blood volume used, the chelate (e.g., oxine, tropolone, acetylacetone, mercaptopyridine-*N*-oxide), the centrifugal forces, the medium in which platelets are labeled (e.g., acid citrate dextrose, saline solution, plasma, Tyrode buffer), the labeling efficiency, the duration of the procedure, and the injected dose of radioactivity. Techniques also vary as to whether the platelets are labeled in an open test tube, with the use of a laminar flow hood to minimize airborne contamination, or in a closed blood bag system, which effectively eliminates the possibility of airborne contamination.

Several steps are common to all labeling techniques. All procedures require the separation of platelets from other blood cells and plasma. Whole blood is drawn into an anticoagulant mixture, and platelet-rich plasma is separated by a "soft" (640 to 2000 *g*) centrifugation to yield platelet-rich plasma. A platelet pellet is then formed, washed, and resuspended in plasma or another physiologic medium, such as Ringer citrate dextrose or a modified Tyrode solution. Indium complexed to oxine or another chelate is then added, and the platelets are incubated for up to 30 minutes. Indium alone will not penetrate the platelet membrane because it is not lipid soluble. The labeled platelets are then typically recentrifuged, washed, and finally resuspended in autologous platelet-poor plasma. The injected dose ranges between 100 and 500 μCi in human studies. Depending on the technique, labeling requires 30 minutes to 3.5 hours. Contamination with other cells (e.g., leukocytes, erythrocytes) has been estimated to be less than 5 percent by Dewanjee and colleagues.[3]

After the ^{111}In complex is inside the cell, the oxine or other ligand is probably displaced, with subsequent, almost irreversible binding of the ^{111}In to intracellular components such as cytoplasmic proteins, organelles, and the cell membrane. More than 70 percent of the ^{111}In is located in the platelet cytosol,[4, 5] and the remainder is distributed between the alpha and dense granules and the platelet membrane. The mechanism of labeling probably involves an exchange reaction between the oxine carrier and subcellular cytosol platelet components that chelate ^{111}In more strongly than oxine.[5–9] In addition, minimal release of the ^{111}In tracer from human platelets occurs during incubation in vitro at 37° C.[1, 5, 6, 8, 10] Because of the long life span of labeled platelets and their relatively small mass, the estimated radiation dose to an individual platelet incubated with 1 mCi of ^{111}In is 129 Gy.[11] As the ^{111}In-labeled platelets disintegrate in vivo, the major portion circulates in the blood and is sequestered by the reticuloendothelial system.

The lipophilic technetium-99m–hexamethylpropyleneamine-oxime (HMPAO) complex can be used for labeling autologous platelets with ^{99m}Tc as well, and several authors have described preliminary studies with this ^{99m}Tc compound.[12–19] With these methods, the tracer is continuously lost from the platelets, which leads to renal excretion of the tracer and to significant kidney and bladder activity.

Function of Labeled Platelets: Aggregation, Recovery, Survival

Platelets can be relatively easily damaged during the labeling process by improper centrifugation, by the use of normal saline solution, and by the use of improper anticoagulant or pH. Damaged platelets may have reduced survival or aggregability and may not participate in thrombosis.[20] Although platelets clearly undergo some mechanical, chemical, and radiation-induced trauma as a result of the labeling procedure, multiple lines of evidence suggest that minimal permanent damage is inflicted with careful labeling methodology, because platelets largely retain their normal function. Several studies have demonstrated almost normal aggregation patterns of labeled platelets with several labeling techniques.[1, 4, 6, 7, 9, 21–25] Additionally, Thakur and associates reported no marked change in the ultrastructure of labeled platelets with their labeling methods.[9, 26] No differences in survival or recovery have been reported in studies comparing platelet labeling with plasma versus saline solution[25] or in studies comparing two different chelates, oxine and tropolone.[3, 27]

The author and others have noted that, after injection into humans, typically less than 5 to 10 percent of the ^{111}In present in whole blood is "free" circulating ^{111}In unattached to cells, confirming that ^{111}In remains complexed to platelets in vivo. In addition, Peters and colleagues[28] and Kotze and group[29] have demonstrated that there is minimal elution of ^{111}In once it is taken up by reticuloendothelial cells after platelet senescence. Because of the minimal redistribution of ^{111}In over time, it is well suited for quantifying sites of platelet destruction. Total-body ^{111}In activity remains at almost 100 percent after isotope injection, indicating minimal loss in the urine or feces.[21, 30, 31]

Studies of platelet recovery and platelet survival in humans offer more convincing evidence that ^{111}In-labeled platelets retain normal function after injection. Trauma during the labeling procedure would be expected to decrease recovery and survival, because damaged cells would be removed from the circulation rapidly. With the use of a variety of platelet-labeling techniques, platelet recovery rates with ^{111}In-labeled platelets have ranged between 52 and 72 percent,[6, 7, 21, 31–33] which is similar to that found with autologous chromium-51–labeled platelets (59 ± 4 percent). Platelet survival time is also a measure of the viability of labeled platelets; however, Peters considers survival time alone to be a doubtful marker of viability, because survival time can be normal even if the platelets fail to function normally.[34] Nevertheless, several laboratories have demonstrated that ^{111}In- and ^{51}Cr-labeled platelet survival times are similar in normal subjects and in patients with reduced survival times.[3, 35–38] In the author's laboratory, in 13 normal subjects the autologous platelet survival time with the use of ^{111}In was 7.7 ± 1.5 days, versus 7.6 ± 1.2 days with ^{51}Cr; in 14 patients with a variety of thrombocytopenic disorders, survival time was also similar with ^{111}In and with ^{51}Cr (3.9 ± 2.4 and 3.9 ± 1.9 days, respectively). Heaton reviewed other available data comparing ^{111}In and ^{51}Cr platelet labeling and concluded that there was little difference in vivo in terms of either survival time or recovery rate.[35] Dewanjee and associates noted similar platelet survival times with ^{111}In-oxine–labeled, ^{111}In-tropolone–labeled, and ^{51}Cr-labeled platelets; they found no difference between the two indium markers in terms of isotope distribution.[3] In 1988, the International Committee for Standardization in Hematology recommended a specific method of labeling for studies performed to calculate platelet survival time.[39]

Additional evidence that labeled platelets retain viability is the demonstration of labeled platelet uptake in areas of active thrombosis. In summary, although there is clear evidence that improper labeling techniques can adversely affect function of labeled platelets, multiple in vitro and in vivo tests suggest that labeled platelets can retain viability despite labeling trauma.

Radiation Dosimetry in Humans

Based on human studies in which platelets were labeled with ^{111}In by a variety of methods, the Medical Internal Radiation Dose Committee of the Society of Nuclear Medicine recently published dose estimates for radioindium-labeled autologous platelets in humans. For ^{111}In-labeled platelets injected, the estimated spleen dose is 8.0 mGy/MBq, the red marrow dose is 0.29 mGy/MBq, the liver dose is 0.56 mGy/MBq, the male gonad dose is 0.12 mGy/MBq, the ovarian dose is 0.12 mGy/MBq, the blood dose is 0.14 mGy/MBq, and the dose to the remainder of the body is 0.004 mGy/MBq.[40] Prior estimates in individual studies were similar.[31, 41–43]

Because of the splenic dose, although it is within acceptable limits, the author does not perform more than one study in young normal subjects, and he limits the total injected dose to 0.33 mCi. In subjects with vascular diseases, the author limits the total injected dose to 1 mCi per year. The author does not study women of childbearing potential.

Imaging Techniques

Imaging of labeled platelets can be performed with either conventional planar techniques or single-photon emission computed tomography. Owing to the relatively low count rates, simultaneous collection of both 171- and 245-keV photopeaks of ^{111}In is desirable. The author uses a medium-energy parallel-hole collimator and 15 to 20 percent energy windows. The low count rates obtained from most vascular structures necessitate relatively long imaging times (15 to 30 minutes per view).

Owing to the platelet life span of approximately 8 days in the circulation, there is substantial blood pool background for several days after injection. Therefore, serial imaging over a period of 4 to 5 days is usually necessary to differentiate areas of increased uptake caused by thrombosis from circulating blood pool activity. Areas of active thrombosis become more apparent on later images because of continued accumulation of labeled platelets over time and a reduction in the circulating background blood pool as senescent platelets are removed from the circulation. Extended imaging clearly improves lesion detection; in one study of patients with left ventricular thrombi, only one half of the images were positive at 24 hours after injection, compared with images obtained at 48 or 72 hours.[44] Static and whole-body scanning techniques have been reviewed,[45] as have dual-isotope imaging methods.[46] Despite the low count rates, tomographic imaging of labeled platelets is feasible (Fig. 67–1) and probably improves thrombus detection as well as allowing improved quantification of platelet uptake.[47, 48]

For planar images of the thorax and heart, the author typically obtains 300,000 counts per view. For lower abdominal images that exclude the liver and spleen, the author obtains 150,000 counts per view. For single-photon emission computed tomographic imaging of labeled platelets, the patient is positioned lying supine, and 64 sequential images of 30 seconds each are obtained at 2.8-degree angular intervals over the 180 degrees centered on the region of interest.[47, 49] Tomographic reconstruction is performed in a transaxial projection at increments of 0.6 cm with the use of filtered backprojection techniques without attenuation correction.

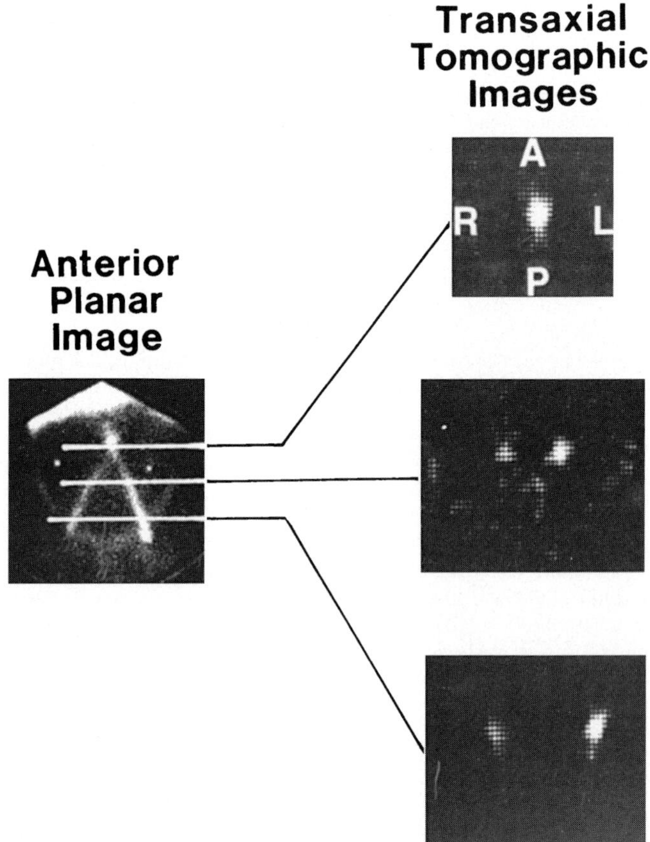

FIGURE 67–1. Single-photon emission tomographic images of indium-111 platelet deposition on a Dacron aortic bifurcation graft. The transaxial tomographic images are 1.8 cm thick. The approximate level from which each tomographic image was obtained is depicted on a standard anterior planar image of the same patient, on the left. Activity in the upper left of the planar image is caused by the liver; the two localized white spots are anatomical markers used for patient positioning. The orientation of the tomographic images is in standard x-ray computed tomographic format. A = anterior; P = posterior; R = patient's right; L = patient's left. (From Stratton, J.R., and Ritchie, J.L.: Reduction of indium-111 platelet deposition on Dacron vascular grafts in humans by aspirin plus dipyridamole. Circulation 73:326, 1986, with permission of the American Heart Association.)

Image Quantitation Techniques

The in vivo quantification of ^{111}In-labeled platelet images in humans has not been standardized, and many approaches have been described. Experimental studies have demonstrated that small areas of deposition, as well as relatively large changes induced by drugs, cannot adequately be assessed by simple visual analysis of the images.[50] To quantify thrombus activity, localized platelet activity in a region has been compared with a noninvolved area in the same image, with simultaneously collected whole-blood activity or with injected ^{111}In dose.

Although no quantitative methods have been validated in human studies, several techniques have been assessed in animal models. For measurement of platelet uptake in large organs like the liver and spleen, a geometric mean method has been developed by van Reenen and Heyns and their colleagues,[51, 52] in which activity in an organ is expressed as a percentage of whole-body activity. In studies in baboons, the values obtained in vivo correlated closely with in vitro values. This method is relatively simple and practical, but whether it will offer similar results for smaller regions of platelet uptake remains to be determined. Other authors have described methods to correct ^{111}In activity for attenuation.[45, 53] Mortelmans and associates[54] compared quantitative methods in patients with vascular grafts with either a nonimaging detector alone or a gamma camera. They concluded that the gamma camera method, with background subtraction and indexing of the graft activity to whole blood, was the preferable method. Hanson and colleagues have described methods of quantitation that emphasize various kinetic measurements of platelet uptake, including the residence time of the deposited platelets, the rate of deposition per day, the maximum radioactivity present in the region of interest (expressed as a percentage of total-body activity), and the time to maximal deposition.[55, 56]

A background subtraction technique has been developed by Powers and associates, Mathias and Welch, and Allen and colleagues[46, 57, 58] in which autologous red blood cells are labeled with ^{99m}Tc and estimated ^{111}In counts contributed by the blood radioactivity are subtracted from an ^{111}In image. This technique attempts to compensate for the fact that circulating platelet activity may obscure the detection of platelets incorporated into a thrombus. The results of this dual-isotope technique of quantification correlate closely with in vitro well-counting results in animals with prosthetic grafts ($r = 0.94$) and in animals with arterial thrombi.[57, 58] However, one report compared the blood pool subtraction technique of quantification with a simpler indium excess ratio that related counts in the region of interest to a reference region in dogs with vascular prostheses.[59] The blood pool subtraction method had a very poor correlation to the actual gamma activity of excised grafts, but the indium excess ratio, which did not require the injection of a second radioisotope, had a much better correlation with the in vitro results.[59] In addition, Powers did not find that the blood pool subtraction technique improved the detection of localized platelet deposition compared with simple visual analysis alone in 28 patients.[60] Similarly, Machac and colleagues found that blood pool subtraction techniques did not improve the visual detection of abnormal uptake of ^{111}In-labeled platelets compared with standard visual analysis in subjects with a variety of thrombi,[61] and blood pool subtraction was associated with a decreased specificity. The superiority of blood pool subtraction techniques to simpler methods therefore has not been established.

Other in vivo approaches to quantification with the use of planar images have been described by Dewanjee and colleagues,[62, 63] Goldman and colleagues,[64] Pumphrey and colleagues,[65] and Stratton and colleagues[66] but without in vitro validation. In addition, the author and colleagues have described methods for quantifying platelet uptake on tomographic images.[47, 48] The findings suggest that the quantification of platelet uptake on grafts is improved by tomographic imaging compared with standard planar imaging, because tomographic quantification was able to detect more subtle changes.[47] Further studies that develop and validate accurate methods of quantifying platelet uptake are needed.

Nonspecific binding of ^{111}In to the object being studied may lead to overestimation of the degree of platelet deposition. For example, in a flow chamber model that used human arteries, Garrett and colleagues estimated that approximately 23 percent of ^{111}In activity was not platelet associated.[67]

CARDIAC THROMBI

Coronary Artery Thrombi

Because of the great importance of coronary artery thrombi in causing acute myocardial infarction, unstable angina, and sudden cardiac death, a noninvasive method of detection would be of immense clinical importance. Such a technique would allow the assessment of the efficacy of thrombolytic therapy. To date, the only clinically valid method for determining clot lysis in an individual patient has been invasive contrast angiography; a noninvasive substitute would be very helpful. In animal models of coronary artery thrombosis, labeled platelets have detected thrombi with either unprocessed images[68] or a blood pool subtraction technique.[69] However, old (more than 24 hours) or small (11 to 17.5 g) thrombi were not detectable externally.

In humans, the evidence that coronary artery thrombi can be externally imaged has been less convincing (Table 67–1). Although Fox and colleagues described the possible detection of coronary thrombi in nine patients by a blood pool subtraction technique, no patient had independent confirmation of thrombus, and only one thrombus was visualized on an unprocessed image.[70] Their encouraging findings have not been replicated. In 27 survivors of sudden cardiac death, Stratton and colleagues detected no coronary artery thrombi.[71] In the setting of acute infarction, platelet uptake on left ventricular thrombi or platelet accumulation in reperfused infarcted areas has been documented[72, 73]; uptake in these areas may be confused with uptake on a coronary artery thrombus, further restricting the ability to diagnose coronary artery thrombi.

Clinical and experimental studies suggest that platelet mechanisms contribute to angioplasty failure as well as to coronary artery vein bypass graft failure. Although platelet accumulation has been demonstrated at coronary angioplasty sites in animal models, preliminary reports in humans have noted no detectable deposition.[20, 74] Similarly, although animal studies have demonstrated that in vivo imaging of deposition in recently implanted vein grafts is possible,[63, 75] platelet uptake in 10 patients with recent saphenous vein bypass grafts was not detectable.[3] Attempts to image platelet deposition in the coronary arteries or in vein bypass grafts in humans after infarction, angioplasty, or coronary bypass grafting have been disappointing. Some contributory factors include the poor intrinsic spatial resolution of gamma imaging systems, attenuation effects, the relatively low injected isotope dose, surrounding background activity, cardiac motion, and the small amounts of deposition that occur in the coronary vasculature.

TABLE 67–1. STUDIES OF CARDIAC THROMBI IN HUMANS

	Reference Numbers
Coronary artery thrombi	70, 71
Left ventricular thrombi	44, 61, 78, 80–87, 89–91, 93, 94, 107, 218–226
Atrial thrombi	95–99, 219, 223
Bacterial endocarditis	61, 62, 219
Percutaneous transluminal coronary angioplasty	20, 74
Coronary artery bypass grafts	62
Prosthetic heart valves	62, 77, 161, 184

Valvular Thrombi and Vegetations

Platelet imaging has detected uptake in experimental models of endocarditis,[76] but detection of platelet thrombus in humans with endocarditis has not been possible.[62]

Although Dewanjee and colleagues were able to detect platelet deposition in experimental animal models of prosthetic valve placement,[3] detection of platelet thrombus in humans with endocarditis or with prosthetic heart valves was not possible in their laboratory.[62] Acar and associates[77] studied 41 patients with 45 prosthetic valves (37 mechanical and 8 tissue valves). All patients had suspected valve thrombosis as a result of prior thromboembolic events. All 10 patients who went on to surgery or autopsy had thrombus present; platelet imaging was positive in 8 of 10, suggesting a sensitivity of 80 percent. Of the subjects who did not have surgery or autopsy validation, platelet imaging was positive in 16 of 31. The overall proportion of positive findings did not appear to be influenced by the presence or absence of heparin, oral anticoagulants, or antiplatelet drugs. These findings have not yet been confirmed in another laboratory.

Left Ventricular Thrombi

Although the detection of small intracardiac thrombi is not possible, larger thrombi, such as left atrial or left ventricular thrombi, can be imaged with the use of labeled platelets. Left ventricular thrombi occur in approximately one third of patients with either transmural anterior myocardial infarction or idiopathic congestive cardiomyopathy, and left atrial thrombi occur in approximately 10 percent of patients with atrial fibrillation. Left ventricular and left atrial thrombi are of clinical importance because they lead to embolic events. Overall, it is estimated that left ventricular or left atrial thrombi account for approximately 10 percent of all acute stroke syndromes, and other cardiac thrombotic conditions (e.g., prosthetic valves, endocarditis) account for an additional 5 percent. The detection of intracardiac thrombi can be of clinical importance because it allows the identification of patients at risk for embolism and may permit the selection of optimal drug therapy.

Indium-111–labeled platelet imaging can detect left ventricular thrombi in humans.[44, 78–90] Imaging is said to be positive for left ventricular thrombi if one or more discrete areas of intracardiac activity are present on at least two views. Obtaining late images in multiple views is essential for accurate thrombus detection and localization.[44, 84] Of 10 patients with left ventricular thrombi that Stratton and colleagues initially studied, no images were positive at 2 hours after platelet injection, only five were positive at 24 hours, but all were positive at 48 or 72 hours after injection (Fig. 67–2).[44] Similarly, Ezekowitz and associates found that the sensitivity of platelet imaging at 3 to 4 days was twofold to threefold greater than at 1 to 2 days after platelet injection.[84]

In surgically excised specimens, the ratio of left ventricular thrombus to whole-blood radioactivity counts has ranged from 10:1 to 355:1 in patients with positive platelet imaging results and from 0.03:1 to 16:1 in patients with negative imaging findings.[44, 82]

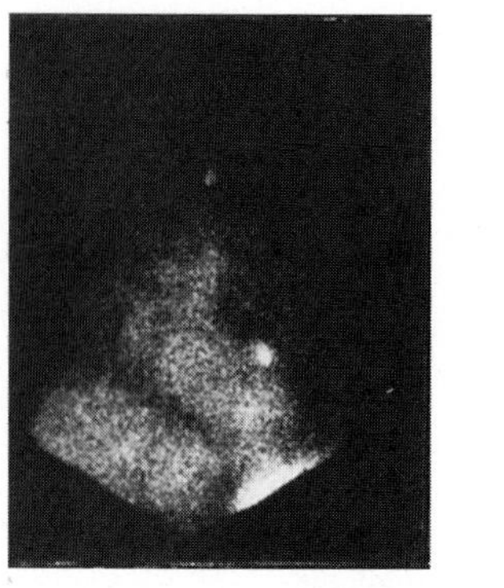

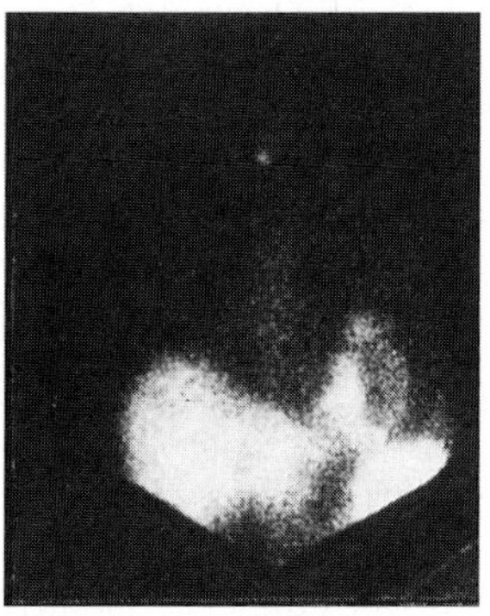

FIGURE 67–2. Left ventricular thrombus. Indium-111 platelet images in the anterior view obtained at 24 and 96 hours after labeled platelet injection (300,000 counts per view). On the later image, platelet uptake within thrombus was more apparent. Improved lesion detection at later imaging times is the result of continued accretion of labeled platelets onto the thrombus and a reduction in circulating background blood pool activity. The liver is at the lower left and the spleen at the lower right in both images.

Ezekowitz and associates have determined the sensitivity of platelet imaging to range from 65 to 71 percent and the specificity to be 99 to 100 percent.[81, 82, 84] Among 47 patients with remote anterior infarction (2 to 36 months, mean = 10 months) with left ventricular thrombi who were not receiving antithrombotic drugs, 68 percent had positive ^{111}In-labeled platelet images and 32 percent were negative.[91] In other words, only two thirds of left ventricular thrombi have externally detectable platelet uptake by platelet imaging. However, the risk of a false-positive study is very low. It is possible that tomographic imaging can improve the sensitivity. The failure to detect some thrombi probably relates to decreased thrombus activity over time or to small thrombus size.

In an experimental animal study of left ventricular thrombi, Seabold and colleagues noted that the apparent sensitivity of platelet imaging for the detection of a left ventricular thrombus decreased over time after thrombus formation; among recently formed thrombi, 75 percent (9 of 12) were detected by platelet imaging, but among 1-week-old thrombi, only 57 percent (4 of 7) were detected.[92] In a cross-sectional study, Bellotti and associates noted that the hematologic activity of recent thrombi (less than 1 month) was significantly greater than that of older thrombi (2 to 14 months).[93] However, despite the apparent decrease in activity over time, all thrombi continued to be externally detectable.

Embolic Risk Stratification With Platelet Imaging

Platelet imaging findings appear to predict the subsequent risk of embolization. To determine whether a positive ^{111}In-labeled platelet image for a left ventricular thrombus, which indicates ongoing thrombogenic activity, is associated with an increased risk of systemic embolization, Stratton and colleagues compared the embolic rate in patients with positive imaging findings to the rate in patients with negative imaging findings during a mean follow-up period of 31 ± 24 months. The groups were similar with respect to all clinical features, including antithrombotic therapy, the prevalence of anterior infarction, the prevalence of aneurysm formation, and the time since infarction. During follow-up, embolic events occurred in 12 percent (4 of 33) of patients with platelet images that were positive for left ventricular thrombi, compared with only 2 percent (1 of 65) of patients with negative images (P = .02).[86] By actuarial methods at 5 years of follow-up, only 71 percent of patients with positive imaging results were embolus-free, compared with 98 percent of patients with negative results.

These data also suggest that platelet imaging offers additional predictive value to two-dimensional echocardiography in the prediction of embolic events. Among 53 patients who had evidence of a left ventricular thrombus by echocardiography, 29 had a positive result on platelet imaging. Among patients with both positive echocardiographic and positive platelet imaging results, embolic events occurred in 23 percent (7 of 30), compared with 4 percent (1 of 28) in patients with a positive echocardiogram but negative findings on platelet imaging (P = .03) (Fig. 67–3). These data strongly suggest that a positive finding on platelet imaging predicts an increased embolic risk, even among patients with echocardiographically documented left ventricular thrombi. Platelet imaging stratifies patients into those with a high risk of subsequent embolization and those with a low risk of embolization. Thrombosis imaging therefore may be useful to assess the risk of thromboembolic complications in patients with left ventricular thrombi.

Antithrombotic Drug Effects on Left Ventricular Thrombi

The effects of antithrombotic drugs on left ventricular thrombi have been assessed in several studies. In a randomized trial of patients with acute myocardial infarction, Funke-Kupper and colleagues found no effect of low-dose aspirin (100 mg daily) in preventing the development of left ventricular thrombi or in reducing the activity of established thrombi as studied by platelet imaging.[94] Similarly, in uncontrolled series, aspirin in various doses (300 to 2400 mg daily) did not prevent platelet uptake onto the left ventricular thrombus surface in five patients,[81] nor did subcutaneous heparin.[83, 90]

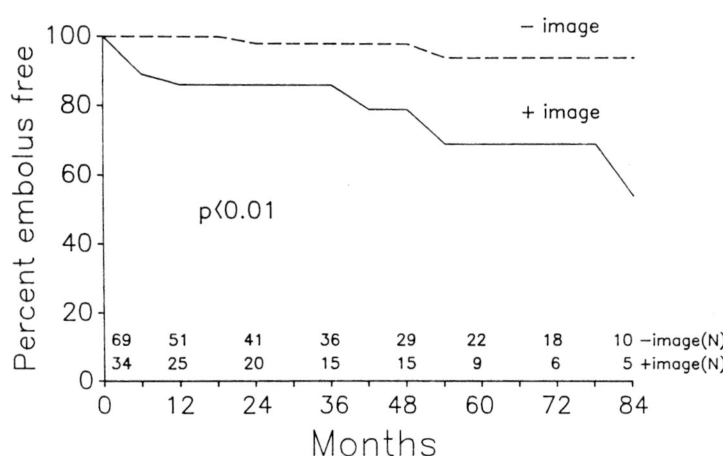

FIGURE 67–3. The probability of remaining free from embolus, for patients with a left ventricular thrombus documented by echocardiography, was less in patients who had positive findings on platelet scan than in those with negative platelet imaging findings. Among patients with both positive echocardiography and positive platelet imaging results, 23 percent had embolic events during a mean follow-up period of 38 months, compared with only 4 percent of subjects who had positive results on echocardiography but negative platelet imaging findings. (From Stratton, J.R., and Ritchie, J.L.: Indium-111 platelet imaging of left ventricular thrombi: Predictive value for systemic emboli. Circulation 81:1186, 1990, with permission of the American Heart Association.)

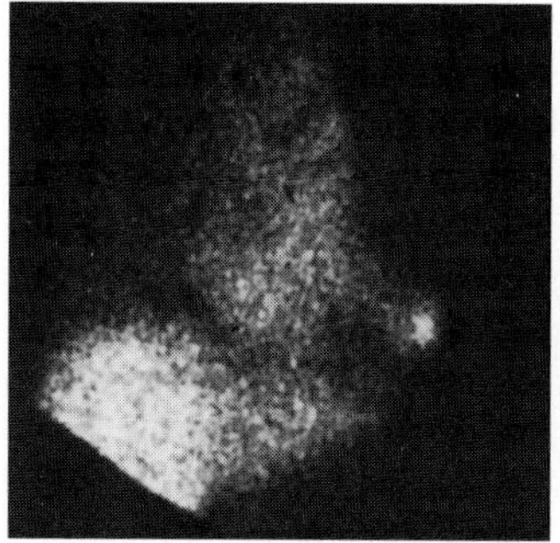
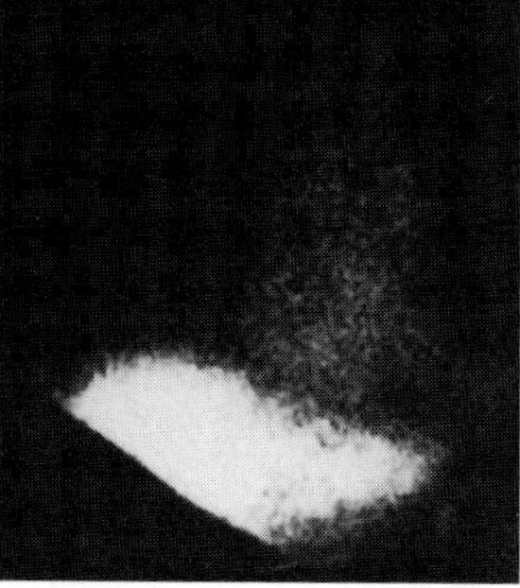

FIGURE 67–4. Anterior 72-hour images obtained from a patient with a left ventricular thrombus at baseline while receiving no therapy *(left panel)* and then while receiving warfarin *(right panel)*. During warfarin therapy, platelet deposition ceased. (From Stratton, J.R., and Ritchie, J.L.: The effects of antithrombotic drugs in patients with left ventricular thrombi: Assessment with indium-111 platelet imaging and two-dimensional echocardiography. Circulation 69:565, 1984, with permission of the American Heart Association.)

In patients with chronic left ventricular thrombi (i.e., longer than 3 months after myocardial infarction), the author assessed the effects of 2 to 3 weeks of therapy with sulfinpyrazone (200 mg q.i.d.), aspirin (325 mg t.i.d.) plus dipyridamole (75 mg t.i.d.), or full-dose warfarin. To establish the reproducibility of platelet imaging findings, five subjects with thrombi were serially restudied on no medications; all studies remained positive.[85] Among seven patients treated with sulfinpyrazone, five had evidence of decreased platelet deposition by platelet imaging (three became negative, two equivocal). Among six patients treated with aspirin plus dipyridamole, three had decreased deposition (one became negative, three equivocal). Among four warfarin-treated patients, three became negative and one was unchanged (Fig. 67–4). Despite evidence of reduced or absent platelet uptake in many patients during drug therapy, thrombus resolution by echocardiography was seen only in one of the patients who had received warfarin; the remaining studies showed no change or only a small decrease in estimated thrombus size. Bellotti and colleagues had similar findings with other platelet-inhibitory agents, ticlopidine and indobufen.[91] Among 32 patients with platelet imaging results that were initially positive for left ventricular thrombi, reduced deposition was seen in 63 percent of those treated with ticlopidine, 42 percent of those treated with indobufen, and only 11 percent of control subjects. By echocardiography, none of the 32 subjects had complete resolution of the thrombus, and only 1 of the patients treated with ticlopidine had an apparent reduction in thrombus size.

These results suggest that platelet-active agents or warfarin diminishes left ventricular thrombus activity in some patients. Furthermore, the results suggest that platelet imaging may be superior to echocardiography as an early indicator of drug effect.

Atrial Thrombi

There are only limited data regarding the ability of ^{111}In-labeled platelet imaging to detect left atrial thrombi.[65, 78, 95, 96] Yamada and associates reported findings compatible with left atrial thrombi in 7 of 28 patients with mitral valve disease.[96] Only 12 patients had operative or autopsy confirmation of the findings; platelet imaging detected four of five proven thrombi and was negative in all seven patients without thrombi. In case reports, platelet imaging has detected uptake onto a left atrial myxoma,[97] onto a right atrial tumor thrombus,[98] and onto a right atrial thrombus associated with pericardial constriction.[99]

The role of platelet imaging in the detection and management of patients with suspected intracardiac thrombi remains unclear. For left ventricular thrombi, the sensitivity of platelet imaging is approximately 71 percent and the specificity is almost 100 percent; false-negative studies can occur in patients receiving antithrombotic drugs or in patients with very small or inactive thrombi. In general, echocardiography is preferable as a diagnostic test for left ventricular thrombi because it is relatively quick, involves no radiation exposure, is widely available, and has a sensitivity of 80 to 90 percent and a specificity of 90 to 95 percent. However, platelet imaging may have a role in identification of left ventricular thrombi in patients who have technically poor or equivocal echocardiograms. In addition, because thrombosis imaging appears to stratify embolic risk even in patients who have thrombi detected by echocardiography, platelet imaging or some other form of thrombosis imaging may help in making decisions regarding long-term anticoagulation.

For left atrial thrombi, additional data are needed, but the preliminary results suggest that platelet imaging may have a reasonably high accuracy. Transthoracic echocardiography, in contrast, has a very poor sensitivity (50 percent or lower) for left atrial thrombi. In a recent study in experimental animals, platelet imaging detected 100 percent (17 of 17) of recently formed left atrial appendage thrombi, but two-dimensional echocardiography detected only 18 percent (3 of 17). However, platelet imaging had a low sensitivity for chronic thrombi present for 4 to 8 days before platelet injection.[100]

ARTERIAL THROMBI

Platelet imaging has been used to assess platelet accumulation at sites of atherosclerosis or arterial injury and to evaluate pharmacologic and other interventions. In humans, studies have evaluated carotid artery platelet deposition in patients with cerebral ischemia, platelet uptake in carotid arteries after endarterectomy, platelet uptake after injury or peripheral angioplasty, and platelet uptake in aneurysms or atherosclerotic plaques (Table 67–2). Experimental studies have demonstrated that maximal platelet accumulation occurs very early after an arterial injury.[50, 101, 102]

Carotid Artery Disease

Atherosclerosis of the internal carotid artery, with associated platelet-fibrin thrombus formation, is one mechanism that leads to stroke and transient ischemic attacks. Other nonplatelet mechanisms, such as intracranial lesions or intraplaque hemorrhage, are also potential causes of ischemic cerebral vascular disease.[41] Several groups have attempted to determine whether platelet deposition in the region of the carotid artery is externally detectable in patients with known or suspected cerebral vascular disease.[60, 103–111] In an early report, labeled platelet uptake was detected in 61 percent of 33 atherosclerotic carotid arteries with the use of unblinded

TABLE 67–2. STUDIES OF ARTERIAL AND VENOUS DISEASES IN HUMANS

	Reference Numbers
Carotid artery disease	31, 60, 103–106, 108–110, 112–114, 117, 118, 227–234
Cause of stroke	95, 107, 111, 117, 235, 236
Carotid endarterectomy	119–121, 237
Endothelial or arterial injury	103, 128, 132
Percutaneous peripheral angioplasty or thrombolysis	125, 128, 130–132, 134, 231
Arterial aneurysms, thrombosis	56, 122–124, 126, 238–243
Intracranial aneurysm, sagittal sinus thrombosis	115, 116, 244
Homocystinuria	245
Atherosclerotic plaques	104, 136, 137, 185, 246, 247
Deep venous thrombosis	138, 139, 144–149, 151, 152, 154, 159, 248–251
Pulmonary emboli	144, 151, 155–159, 185

interpretation; however, lesion detection dropped to 36 percent with blinded interpretation.[103] The largest series are summarized in Table 67–3.

Powers and colleagues studied 100 patients, 54 with clinically suspected carotid artery disease and 46 with a variety of other syndromes, including seizures, syncope, and migraine.[109] The frequency of positive imaging results was not different between patients with carotid artery symptoms and patients without carotid artery symptoms. Moreover, among patients with clinically symptomatic carotid artery disease, images of the asymptomatic carotid artery were as likely to be abnormal as those of the symptomatic carotid artery. Platelet deposition was detected in 14 percent of angiographically normal sites and in 43 percent of stenotic or ulcerative sites detected angiographically. There was no correlation between platelet imaging findings and the subsequent risk of stroke or frequency of symptoms. Kessler and colleagues found that symptomatic carotid arteries were associated with positive imaging results in 44 percent of cases, but 22 percent of asymptomatic carotid arteries were also associated with positive platelet images.[108] However, the correlation between angiographic and imaging findings was poor, with 63 percent of angiographically normal or near-normal arteries demonstrating abnormal scans and only 47 percent of angiographically abnormal arteries demonstrating abnormal scans. In a subsequent study of 68 patients with the diagnosis of a carotid source of stroke, 57 percent of the presumed affected carotid arteries demonstrated positive scans; however, 29 percent of the asymptomatic carotid arteries also were found to be positive on platelet imaging, and 17 percent of carotid arteries in subjects with a noncarotid cause of stroke were also positive in the carotid area.[112]

Goldman and group found a modest increase in positive imaging results in symptomatic versus asymptomatic arteries (64 and 40 percent, respectively) and in arteriographically abnormal versus arteriographically normal regions (60 and 38 percent, respectively).[105] On 11 resected specimens, uptake of ^{111}In-labeled platelets was present but relatively minor.

Minar and colleagues had the most negative findings.[113] Among 60 subjects with presumed carotid symptoms, only 12 percent of vessels on the symptomatic side were positive by platelet imaging, which was not different from the result of 10 percent positive or equivocal on the asymptomatic side. In their study, only 2 percent of carotid arteries in patients without carotid symptoms were positive, in contrast to some of the previously described studies. They concluded that platelet imaging had no value in the clinical evaluation of carotid artery disease.

Isaka and colleagues noted that the blood pool subtraction technique appeared to improve the specificity of the analysis compared with visual techniques.[106] By visual analysis, 31 percent of normal arteries had evidence of abnormal platelet uptake, but only 6 percent of normal arteries had semiquantitative evidence of abnormal deposition by blood pool subtraction. Isaka and associates studied the efficacy of aspirin (325 mg b.i.d.) or ticlopidine (100 mg t.i.d.) in 12 subjects with symptomatic carotid artery disease and positive platelet imaging findings.[114] Aspirin reduced platelet uptake in the affected carotid arteries, but there was no significant change after ticlopidine. Additional studies in patients with neurologic syndromes have demonstrated platelet uptake in patients with giant intracranial aneurysms[115] and in a patient with a superior sagittal sinus thrombosis.[116]

Two case reports have presented patients in whom arterioarterial emboli, documented by platelet imaging, were implicated as the cause of stroke.[117, 118]

In summary, the correlation between platelet imaging findings and clinical symptoms and arteriographic findings in patients with suspected carotid artery disease has been poor. In addition, Powers and associates noted no prognostic value of a positive scan result in this patient population in regard to subsequent risk of stroke or transient ischemic attack.[109] The high rate of positive results obtained in angiographically normal vessels in several studies suggests a high rate of false-positivity. In addition, observer disagreement in two of the studies was high at 20 percent[106] and 24 percent.[105]

Other Causes of Stroke

Approximately 10 to 15 percent of all stroke syndromes result from a cardiac embolic source. In 27 patients with cerebral ischemic syndromes possibly from a cardiac cause (16 with stroke

TABLE 67–3. PLATELET IMAGING IN PATIENTS WITH CAROTID DISEASE

			Findings on Symptomatic vs. Asymptomatic Carotid % and Proportion of Positive Findings on Platelet Scans			Correlation With Arteriography % Positive Platelet Scans	
Author	**Patients**	**Analysis Method**	Symptomatic Carotid	Asymptomatic Carotid	Number of Patients	Abnormal Artery	Normal Artery
Kessler[108]	62 With cerebral ischemia (52 with carotid symptoms)	Visual	44% (23/52)	22% (13/60)	64	47% (21/45)	63% (12/19)
Kessler[112]	68 With carotid cause of stroke	Visual	57% (39/68)	29% (20/68)			
	53 With noncarotid stroke	Visual	17% (9/53)	17% (9/53)			
Minar[113]	60 With carotid symptoms	Visual	12% positive or equivocal (7/60)	10% positive or equivocal (6/60)		"Not different"	"Not different"
	63 Controls	Visual	NA	2% positive or equivocal (2/126)			
Isaka[106]	37 Patients (25 with carotid symptoms)	a) Blinded visual			25	65% positive or equivocal (22/34)	31% positive or equivocal (5/16)
		b) Semiquantitative			25	56% (19/34)	6% (1/16)
Powers[109]	100 Patients (54 with carotid symptoms)	Visual	"Not different"	"Not different"	64 (4 sites each)	43% (32/75)	14% (20/155)
Goldman[105]	25 With carotid symptoms	Visual	64% (16/25)	40% (10/25)	18	60% (16/23)	38% (5/13)

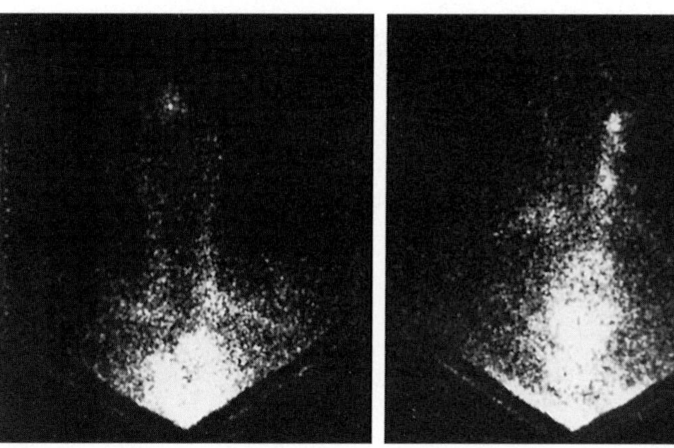

FIGURE 67–5. Anterior indium-111 platelet images of the head and neck of a young normal control subject on the left and of a patient with a recent left carotid endarterectomy on the right. In the patient imaged after endarterectomy, localized platelet accumulation was apparent at the endarterectomy site. Labeled platelets were injected 30 minutes after operation, and images were obtained 48 hours later. (From Stratton, J.R., Zierler, R.E., and Kazmers, A.: Platelet deposition at carotid endarterectomy sites in humans. Stroke 18:725, 1987, with permission of the American Heart Association.)

and 11 with transient ischemic attack), Kessler and colleagues obtained platelet imaging of the heart within 10 days of the onset of the stroke syndrome.[95, 107] Associated cardiac diseases were prior myocardial infarction (n = 8), atrial fibrillation (n = 10), cardiomegaly (n = 6), coronary artery disease (n = 7), and rheumatic heart disease (n = 3). Among the 27 patients, 13 had platelet images that were interpreted as positive for an intracardiac source; 9 had evidence of a left ventricular thrombus, 3 of a left atrial thrombus, and 1 of an aortic valve thrombus. The data suggest that platelet imaging may have some role in detection of embolic sources in patients with clinically suspected embolic strokes, but further confirmation is needed. The high rate of positive findings in this study is not concordant with the very low yield of transthoracic and even transesophageal echocardiography in most studies.

Carotid Endarterectomy

Endarterectomy involves the removal of atherosclerotic plaque, with substantial exposure of underlying media and adventitia. The complications of carotid endarterectomy include early thrombotic occlusion (approximately 2 percent of vessels) and late recurrent high-grade stenosis (9 to 18 percent of vessels). Both of these complications may be related to platelet mechanisms.

In an animal study, Lusby and colleagues demonstrated labeled platelet accumulation at recent endarterectomy sites; deposition decreased by 2 to 3 weeks after surgery owing to re-endothelialization.[119] Among 17 patients who had platelet injection within 1 hour after endarterectomy, 16 had externally detectable deposition.[119]

In a study in the author's laboratory, we injected labeled platelets less than 30 minutes after carotid endarterectomy and obtained images 24 to 96 hours later[120] (Fig. 67–5). Semiquantitative analysis was performed by means of an index that compared activity in the operated side with that in the unoperated side. Patients with recent endarterectomy had a mean deposition index of 1.7 ± 0.5, compared with a similarly determined ratio of 1.1 ± 0.1 in normal subjects without surgery (Fig. 67–6). In addition, to determine the amount of uptake caused by surgical dissection in the absence of endarterectomy, the author studied a surgical control group composed of six patients with noncarotid surgery. Among the surgical controls, the deposition index ratio was only 1.2 ± 0.1. Twelve patients had follow-up studies 0.5 to 24 months after endarterectomy. The deposition index decreased at follow-up in all subjects to a mean of 1.0 ± 0.1, documenting reduced platelet deposition over time, compatible with re-endothelialization of the endarterectomized surface (Fig. 67–7).

To determine whether aspirin (330 mg t.i.d.) plus dipyridamole (75 mg t.i.d.) reduces platelet uptake at endarterectomy sites, Findlay and co-workers conducted a randomized double-blind trial in 22 patients.[121] Treated patients had a significant reduction in labeled platelet accumulation measured at approximately 48 hours

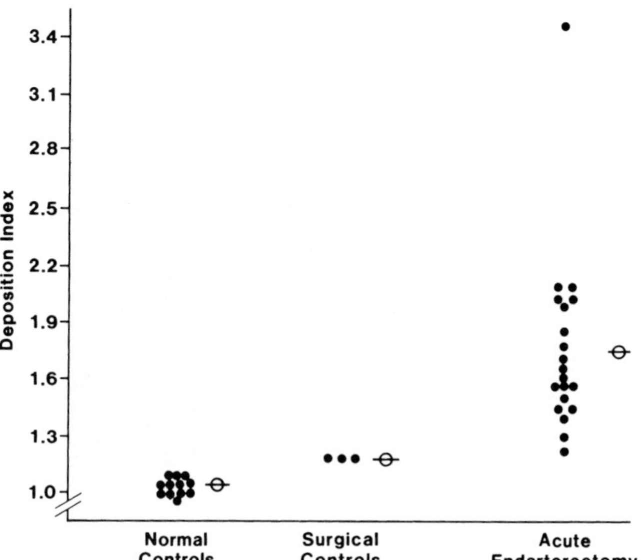

FIGURE 67–6. The deposition index in patients with a recent carotid endarterectomy was greater than in either normal control subjects or surgical control subjects ($P \leq .05$). Only one subject with a recent endarterectomy overlapped with either control group. (From Stratton, J.R., Zierler, R.E., and Kazmers, A.: Platelet deposition at carotid endarterectomy sites in humans. Stroke 18:724, 1987, with permission of the American Heart Association.)

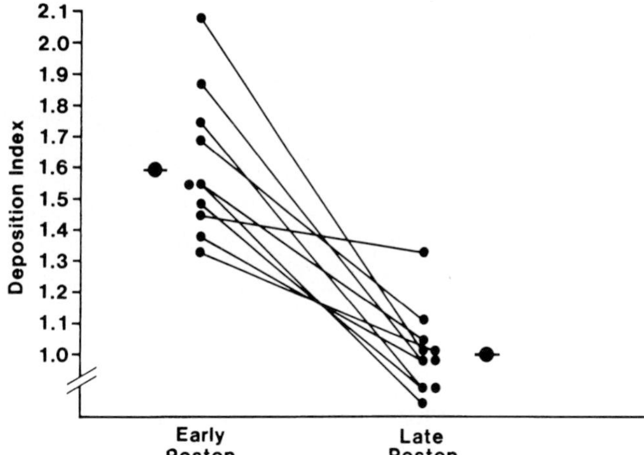

FIGURE 67–7. The deposition index decreased in all subjects who had both acute and follow-up studies. (From Stratton, J.R., Zierler, R.E., and Kazmers, A.: Platelet deposition at carotid endarterectomy sites in humans. Stroke 18:725, 1987, with permission of the American Heart Association.)

after carotid endarterectomy. Meek and colleagues had similar findings and also noted that closure of the arteriotomy with a patch was associated with greater platelet deposition than simple direct closure with no patch.[237]

These data indicate that the arterial injury of carotid endarterectomy results in predictable early platelet deposition, which decreases later and which may be reduced by pretreatment with platelet-inhibitory agents.

Arterial Aneurysms and Arterial Injury

Large-vessel aneurysms are frequently associated with mural thrombus. Ritchie, Stratton, and colleagues studied 18 unoperated patients with either abdominal aortic aneurysms (n = 17) or bilateral femoral artery aneurysms (n = 1).[122] By visual analysis, 12 studies were definitely positive, 2 equivocal, and 4 negative (Fig. 67–8). In two resected specimens, the portion of thrombus in contact with flowing blood had 3.4 and 6.0 times more ^{111}In activity per gram than the outer section of thrombus in contact with the arterial wall. Heyns and colleagues studied the kinetics of accumulation of platelets in abdominal aortic aneurysm thrombi.[123] Shortly after the injection of labeled platelets, 1.5 ± 1.1 percent of whole-body activity was in the aneurysm thrombus, which increased to 4.7 ± 3.6 percent at 132 hours. These quantitative data confirm the visual impression that greater platelet uptake occurs at later imaging times. In a subsequent study, Hanson and associates found that aortic aneurysms accounted for a maximum of 3.3 percent of whole-body ^{111}In activity, that the mean residence time of deposited radioactivity in aneurysms was 1.4 days, and that the rate of labeled platelet accumulation was 5 percent of radioactivity per day.[56]

Asymptomatic aortic aneurysms are not uncommon. Among 860 patients imaged for other reasons, Sinzinger and co-workers detected 21 asymptomatic aneurysms as a result of the presence of localized platelet uptake in the aneurysm thrombus.[124] Infusions of prostacyclin (PGI_2; 95 ng/kg per minute) caused a reduction in platelet uptake in four patients. Arterial injury from puncture causes detectable platelet deposition, as noted by several investigators.[31, 104, 125] In addition, a femoral artery embolus has been detected.

The "blue toe syndrome" is caused by microembolization from atheromatous or aneurysmal lesions, usually in the abdominal aorta. In one study, platelet scanning was positive in 14 of 26 patients examined.[126] In another study, platelet imaging revealed a source in 8 of 20 patients with the syndrome, and all 8 positive studies were true positives.[127] Among the patients having operation, platelet imaging was falsely negative in 5, who had thrombus found at surgery. The authors concluded that the lack of sensitivity of the technique limited its value as a screening tool for microembolic disease.

Peripheral Angioplasty

In contrast to the negative findings with coronary angioplasty, several investigators have noted detectable uptake at the sites of peripheral percutaneous transluminal angioplasty. Pope and associates detected uptake in 73 percent (11 of 15) of patients undergoing peripheral angioplasty, despite the fact that all subjects received either heparin, warfarin, streptokinase, or platelet-inhibitory drugs.[128] Among 15 subjects who underwent injection of labeled platelets before neodymium-yttrium-aluminum-garnet (Nd:YAG) laser–assisted balloon angioplasty, the 2 subjects who had restenosis at 3 to 6 months had markedly increased uptake 24 and 48 hours after the procedure.[129] In another study, the postangioplasty ^{111}In uptake radioactivity ratio tended to be higher in vessels that ultimately had restenosis than in those that did not have restenosis (3.1 ± 0.6 versus 1.9 ± 0.3).[130] However, in the largest study, involving 92 subjects, the platelet uptake ratio was *lower* in the subjects who went on to have restenosis compared with subjects who did not develop restenosis.[131]

Kadir and colleagues reported uptake in three subjects despite treatment with aspirin,[132] and Minar and colleagues[131] noted no difference in uptake between subjects receiving high-dose and those receiving low-dose aspirin. In contrast, Cunningham and coworkers detected deposition at 0 of 11 sites in patients pretreated with aspirin versus 6 of 8 sites in patients not pretreated with aspirin.[133] One study found no difference in uptake of labeled platelets in patients randomly assigned to infusions of streptokinase or t-PA after angioplasty.[134] Two studies in which platelet imaging was done early after angioplasty found that higher platelet deposition appeared to be associated with early thrombosis of the angioplasty site.[129, 134]

Peripheral Atherosclerosis

Peripheral atherosclerotic plaques are occasionally associated with platelet deposition. Powers and colleagues found evidence of

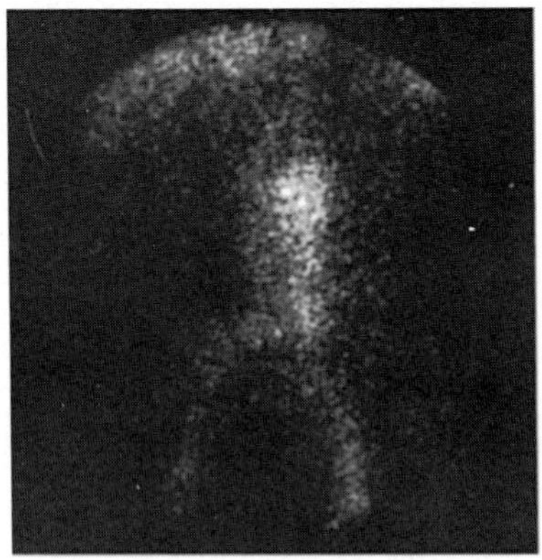

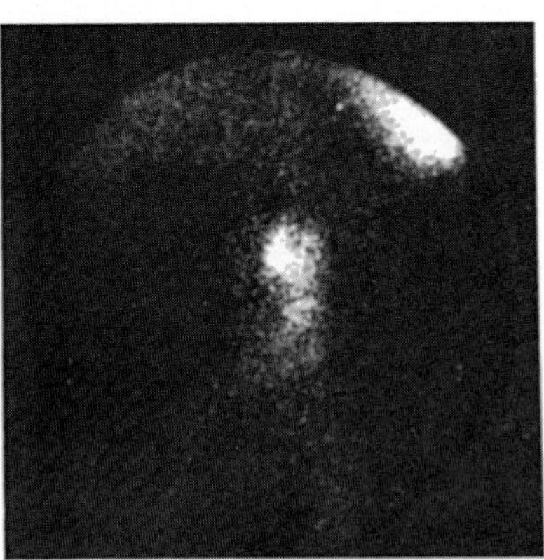

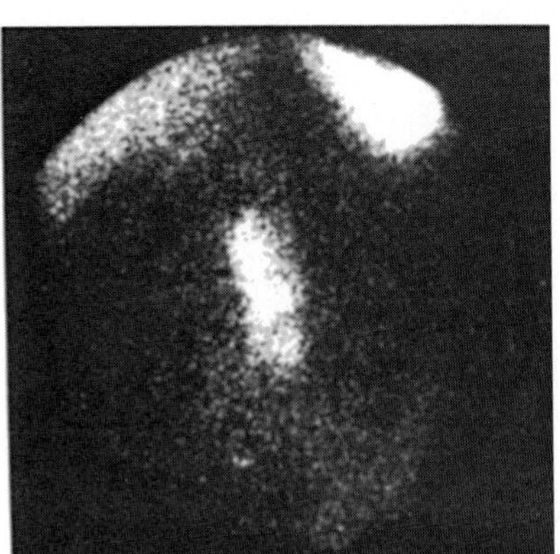

FIGURE 67–8. Serial anterior abdominal views of a patient with a 6-cm abdominal aortic aneurysm that contained a thrombus at surgery. Over time, platelet deposition in the aneurysm increased relative to the background blood pool in the iliac and femoral arteries. The liver edge is at the upper left, the spleen edge at the upper right, and the aortic bifurcation in the lower midsection of each image. (From Ritchie, J.L., Stratton, J.R., Thiele, B., et al.: Indium-111 platelet imaging for detection of platelet deposition in abdominal aneurysms and prosthetic arterial grafts. Am. J. Cardiol. 47:884, 1981, with permission of the American Journal of Cardiology.)

platelet deposition in the abdominal aortas of macaques with diet-induced atherosclerosis with the use of blood pool subtraction techniques, but not with unprocessed, visually interpreted images.[135] At autopsy, however, the extent of apparent deposition did not correlate with the severity of atherosclerosis. Animal studies suggest that only relatively large de-endothelialized areas can be imaged and small lesions cannot.[136]

Among 36 patients with angiographically proved femoral artery stenosis, 61 percent had abnormally high platelet uptake in the diseased leg, compared with the contralateral leg, documenting increased platelet uptake in atherosclerotic vessels. Patients who had ulceration or recent thrombus subsequently noted at surgery had particularly high uptake ratios.[137]

VENOUS THROMBOSIS AND PULMONARY EMBOLISM

In animal models of venous thrombosis, labeled platelets have detected uptake over a several-day period in both the calf and the proximal leg,[138, 139] and ^{111}In-labeled platelet imaging has offered radioactivity count ratios superior to those obtained with iodine-125 (^{125}I) fibrinogen.[140] The age of the thrombus at the time of platelet injection critically influences the ability to image thrombus[138–143]; older thrombi are either undetectable or take longer to visualize. In addition, antithrombotic agents can inhibit labeled platelet uptake and lead to negative images. For example, heparin in high doses blocks platelet incorporation, as does PGI_2.[138, 139]

Platelet imaging, in contrast to some other techniques, may be capable of detecting venous thrombi at all sites, including the calf, thigh, and pelvis (see Table 67–2). In studies in humans, the sensitivity of ^{111}In-labeled platelet imaging for the detection of deep venous thrombosis has varied widely, with reported sensitivities of between 38 and 100 percent.[144–149] Specificity has ranged from 67 to 100 percent. In a study of 31 patients, only two of whom were receiving heparin, the sensitivity of platelet imaging was 100 percent and the specificity was 89 percent.[148] The sensitivity of platelet imaging appears to drop dramatically if patients are receiving heparin. In a study by Ezekowitz and colleagues of patients with deep venous thrombosis documented by prior venography, platelet imaging was positive in 80 percent (4 of 5) of patients not receiving heparin but in only 33 percent (5 of 15) of patients receiving heparin at the time of platelet imaging.[145, 150] Imaging at least 24 hours after the injection of labeled platelets appears to improve the sensitivity. In one study of nonheparinized subjects at 120 minutes after injection, the sensitivity was only 36 to 48 percent, although the specificity was high.[149] In another study, the sensitivity improved from 69 percent at 4 hours to 100 percent at 24 hours after platelet injection.[148]

Platelet imaging has been used to monitor patients who are at high risk for development of deep venous thrombosis, usually because of recent surgery.[144, 151–154] Clarke-Pearson and co-workers noted positive images (deep vein thrombi or pulmonary emboli) in 30 percent of patients after abdominal or pelvic surgery.[144] Winter and associates noted positive images for deep venous thrombi in 64 percent of 64 patients with femur fractures[153] and in 45 percent of 29 patients with respiratory failure.[154]

Platelet imaging appears to offer little promise in the diagnosis of pulmonary emboli. Although acute pulmonary emboli have been detected by platelet imaging in animal models, older thrombi (more than 24 hours) could not be detected. In addition, heparin blocked the ability to detect pulmonary emboli platelet uptake.[136] Although isolated case reports[155–158] have noted pulmonary emboli in humans, platelet imaging failed to detect platelet uptake in 11 of 12 heparinized patients with pulmonary emboli.[159] Clarke-Pearson and colleagues detected five asymptomatic pulmonary emboli among 146 patients studied with platelet imaging after abdominal or pelvic surgery.[144]

To summarize, platelet imaging has demonstrated some promise in the noninvasive diagnosis of deep venous thrombosis, and in particular it may be capable of detecting calf, thigh, and pelvic thrombi. The detection of pulmonary emboli, in contrast, does not appear to be routinely possible. The sensitivity of platelet imaging for the detection of deep venous thrombosis appears to be adversely affected by concomitant heparin therapy and by early imaging times. It is possible that platelet imaging may prove useful in the serial monitoring of patients at high risk for the development of deep venous thrombosis. However, other thrombosis imaging techniques, possibly using antifibrin antibodies or peptides, may be able to detect thrombi at earlier imaging times and potentially may be less influenced by heparin therapy.

PROSTHETIC MATERIALS

Intravascular prosthetic materials are increasingly used as arterial and venous substitutes, vascular catheters, membrane oxygenators, heart valves, and ventricular assist devices and even as totally artificial hearts (Table 67–4). Owing to improved materials and improved fabrication techniques, mechanical failure of prosthetic devices is now extremely rare. The most common current complications of prosthetic materials are thromboembolic events. There is now abundant evidence that platelet mechanisms play a dominant role in the thrombotic and embolic events caused by intravascular prosthetic materials. Despite improved materials, all currently used prosthetic devices are thrombogenic when placed in humans (Fig. 67–9). Two strategies have been used to reduce thromboembolic complications: the construction of new, less thrombogenic materials and the development of improved, safe antithrombotic drug regimens. Testing of either new materials or new drug regimens before widespread clinical use is necessary. However, the assessment of thrombogenicity of prosthetic materials in the past has been limited by the lack of suitable methods. Platelet imaging has been widely used in animal studies to measure platelet uptake in vivo or in vitro after death.[160] Platelet imaging also has been increasingly used in human studies to quantitatively evaluate new materials and new drug regimens.

Natural History of Platelet Deposition on Prosthetic Arterial Grafts

Deposition of ^{111}In-labeled platelets is detectable in virtually all recently implanted large-caliber prosthetic arterial grafts in humans by both visual and quantitative analysis.[55, 56, 64, 65, 102, 122, 160–165] In contrast, autologous vein grafts typically do not have visually detectable platelet accumulation.[64]

After implantation, as grafts mature they become less thrombogenic and have less associated platelet deposition.[162, 163, 165–167] Among 24 patients studied at 1 to 2 weeks and again at 6 to 9 months after implantation of Dacron bifurcation grafts, the graft thrombogenicity index decreased from 0.16 ± 0.02 to 0.08 ± 0.01 ($\pm$SEM).[162] Similarly, Stratton and colleagues noted a reduction in a graft-to-blood ratio from 4.4 ± 2.1 ($\pm$SD) at 1 to 2 weeks after

TABLE 67–4. STUDIES OF PROSTHETIC GRAFT MATERIALS IN HUMANS

	Reference Numbers
Acutely placed grafts	64, 65, 122, 161, 162, 165, 168, 169
"Chronic" grafts (>1 month)	54–56, 66, 102, 162–165, 170, 184
Endothelial cell seeding	167, 172, 176, 177, 179
Comparison of different graft materials	64, 66, 162, 166, 168, 171, 182, 252
Drug effects on graft platelet deposition	47, 48, 65, 168, 182, 186, 189–191, 241
Cardiopulmonary bypass	183

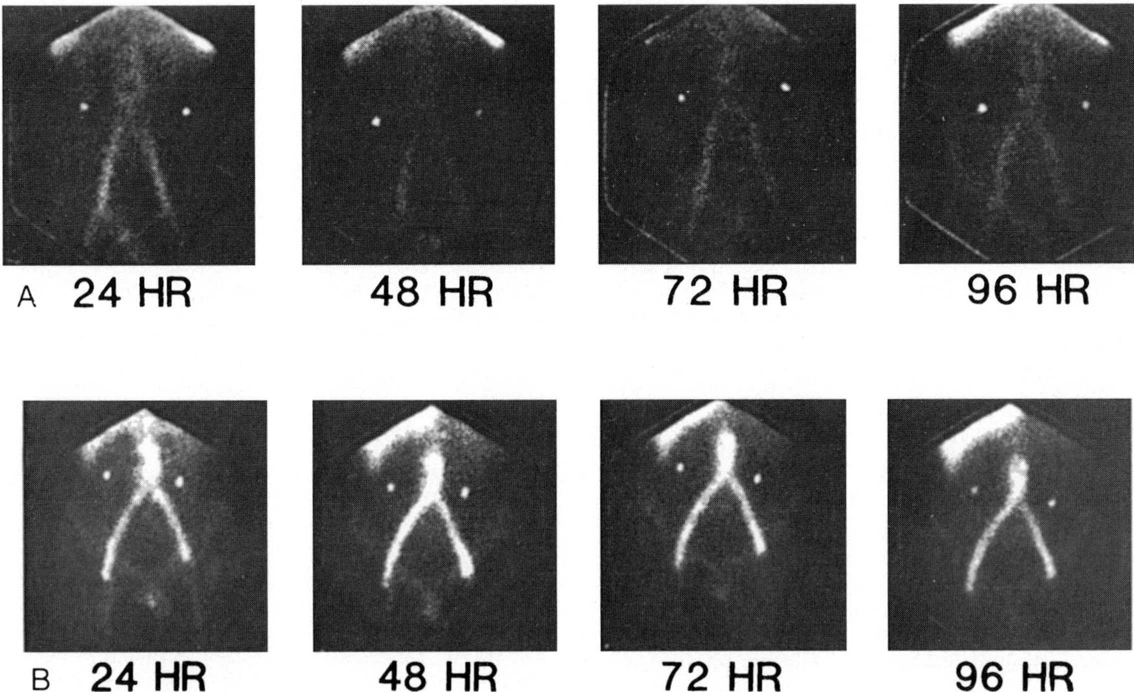

FIGURE 67–9. *A*, Serial anterior abdominal images in a young normal subject show only faint circulating platelet activity present in the aortofemoral vessels (150,000 counts). The two white spots are anatomical markers that are placed 8 cm to each side of the umbilicus to aid in patient positioning. *B*, Anterior abdominal images (150,000 counts) of a 13-month-old Dacron aortic graft demonstrate diffuse uptake throughout the graft. (From Stratton, J.R., Thiele, B.L., and Ritchie, J.L.: Platelet deposition on Dacron aortic bifurcation grafts in man: Quantitation with indium-111 platelet imaging. Circulation 66:1289 and 1291, 1982, with permission of the American Heart Association.)

operation to 3.0 ± 1.8 at 31 weeks ($P = .02$) in patients with Dacron bifurcation grafts. There was no further decrease at 55 weeks (2.8 ± 2.0).[165] Goldman and colleagues also found a significant reduction in platelet deposition over time, with the mean thrombogenicity index decreasing from 0.21 at 1 week to 0.08 at 6 to 12 months after Dacron graft implantation.[102] Similarly, in patients with woven Dacron grafts, the deposition index decreased from 0.19 to 0.06 over the first 6 to 9 months after graft implantation.[162] Isaka and group noted a significant negative correlation between their semiquantitative estimate of graft platelet accumulation and graft age ($r = -0.76$).[163] In summary, multiple studies have reached a similar conclusion: in humans, platelet uptake onto prosthetic grafts significantly decreases with time after implantation in the absence of therapy.

Platelet imaging done early after operation may predict ultimate graft patency in patients with prosthetic femoral popliteal bypass grafts. The mean thrombogenicity index 1 week after surgery in 21 femoropopliteal grafts that eventually occluded within 1 year was 0.19 ± 0.02 ($\pm$SEM), compared with 0.07 ± 0.01 in 36 grafts that remained patent ($P < .001$).[168] If grafts with a thrombogenicity index below the median at 1 week after implantation were compared with those with a higher thrombogenicity index, there was a marked difference in the patency rate at 1 year by life table methods. Among patients with a low index, the patency rate at 1 year was 90 percent, compared with a patency rate of only 39 percent in those with a higher thrombogenicity index.[168] In another study of 18 grafts, of the 9 that had little uptake, all remained patent at a mean of 24 months of follow-up; in contrast, all 9 of the grafts with early marked uptake went on to occlude.[169] These two studies indicate that early platelet imaging of grafts may be useful in prediction of long-term patency.

Substantial data document that platelet deposition continues after implantation, albeit at a lesser rate. Several studies have reported both visual and quantitative evidence that Dacron grafts have ongoing deposition for indefinite periods up to 10 years after implantation (Fig. 67–10).[66, 102, 162–166, 170] In a study of patients with chronically implanted Dacron grafts (9 months to 10 years), 12 of 15 subjects had visually positive evidence of platelet deposition (see Fig. 67–9*B*). In contrast, among 12 normal subjects, all had visually negative studies[66] (see Fig. 67–9*A*). The quantitative results more convincingly demonstrate that continued platelet accumulation occurs (Fig. 67–11). In the case of the normal subjects, the

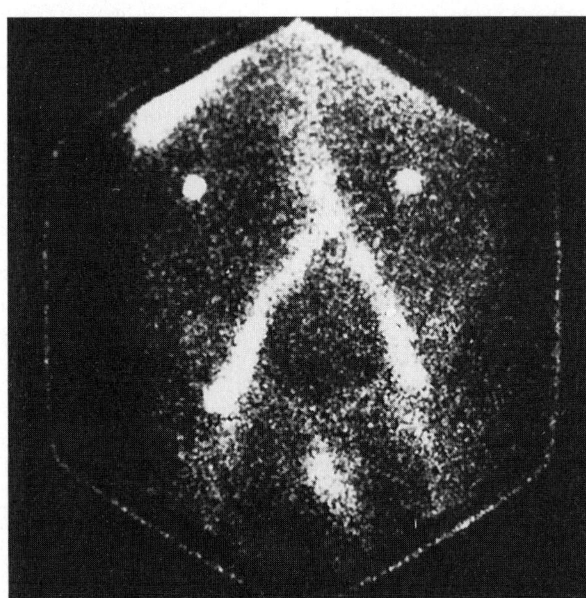

FIGURE 67–10. Diffuse platelet accumulation was present in this 10-year-old Dacron bifurcation graft (48 hours, 150,000 count image). Deposition appears to continue for indefinite periods after placement of Dacron grafts in humans.

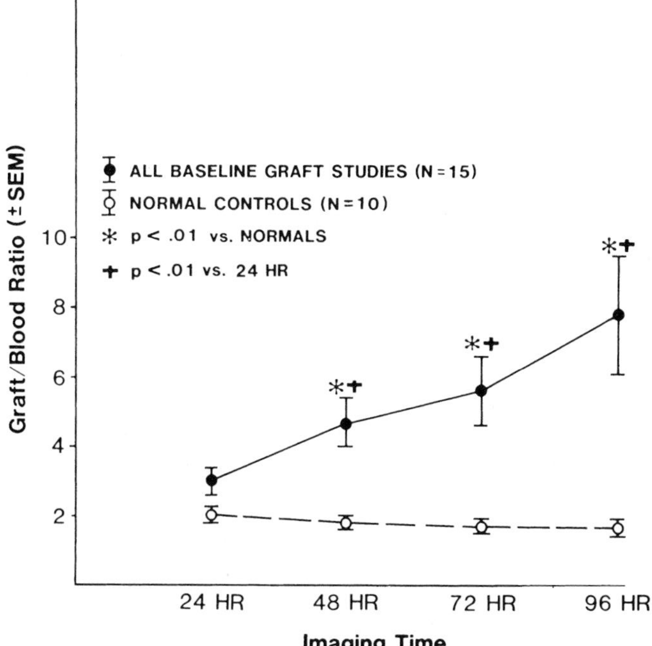

FIGURE 67–11. The graft-to-blood ratio obtained in 15 patients with grafts that were in place for longer than 9 months and in 10 normal controls without grafts. In normal subjects, the ratio represents the aortofemoral blood pool versus whole blood. Patients with grafts had a higher ratio at all imaging times than did normal subjects. Patients with grafts had an increasing ratio over time, in contrast to normal subjects, who exhibited no change. By quantitative analysis, later imaging times (72 or 96 hours) better differentiated patients with grafts from normal subjects. (From Stratton, J.R., Thiele, B.L., and Ritchie, J.L.: Platelet deposition on Dacron aortic bifurcation grafts in man: Quantitation with indium-111 platelet imaging. Circulation 66:1291, 1982, with permission of the American Heart Association.)

graft-to-blood ratio was unchanged at serial imaging times between 24 and 96 hours after platelet injection (2.0±0.7, 1.8±0.6, 1.7±0.8, and 1.7±0.9, respectively). In contrast, among 15 patients with chronically implanted prosthetic grafts, there was a significant serial increase in the graft-to-blood ratio over time after platelet injection (from 3.0±1.6 at 24 hours to 7.8±5.0 at 96 hours).[66] Most subjects with chronically implanted grafts have evidence of diffuse deposition. However, some also have relatively irregular foci of deposition.[66, 163]

Evaluation of Different Graft Materials

There are limited data in humans comparing the thrombogenicity of different types of graft materials. Recently implanted Dacron and polytetrafluoroethylene (PTFE) femoropopliteal grafts have significantly higher thrombogenicity indices than autologous vein grafts (0.25, 0.16, and 0.03, respectively). The autologous vein grafts are less thrombogenic than either type of prosthetic material.[64, 168] In a randomized trial, Goldman and colleagues found no difference in platelet deposition between woven Dacron grafts (USCI, DeBakey) and more porous, double-velour, knitted Dacron grafts (Microvel, Meadox Medical) in 24 patients studied at 1 week and at 6 to 9 months.[162] Similarly, they noted no qualitative or quantitative difference in platelet accumulation between knitted DeBakey Dacron (n = 6) and knitted Sauvage double-velour Dacron grafts (n = 8).[66] In a uniquely designed study, 20 patients who received aortobifemoral grafts had one limb constructed of knitted Dacron and the other limb constructed of woven Dacron. Patients were then studied at a single time, which varied from 1 week to 42 months after implantation. Platelet accumulation was almost identical in the two graft limbs, documenting no significant difference in thrombogenicity between knitted and woven Dacron arterial grafts.[166]

In baboon models, larger graft pore size causes improved endothelial coverage of the graft flow surface.[171] To evaluate this effect in humans, 10 above-knee femoropopliteal grafts composed of equal lengths of 60-μm and 30-μm PTFE were placed in eight patients. These grafts were reinforced (wrapped) for human use. Because biopsy of the grafts was not possible, endothelialization was assessed noninvasively by ^{111}In-labeled platelet imaging 1 week and 3 months after surgery. There was no difference in indium uptake between the 60-μm and 30-μm graft segments at either time.[171]

Platelet imaging has been extensively used to evaluate the effects of endothelial cell seeding of prosthetic graft surfaces.[167, 172–180] Endothelial cell seeding has been pursued because of the assumption that the presence of a normally functioning endothelial layer in contact with circulating blood reduces the thrombogenic potential of prosthetic materials. Fasol and colleagues found no difference in patients receiving seeded versus nonseeded PTFE grafts, but only 17 subjects were studied at 1 year.[179] In studies by Ortenwall and colleagues, each subject received both an unseeded and a seeded graft segment. These human trials demonstrated reduced uptake of ^{111}In-labeled platelets on Dacron-seeded versus unseeded grafts at 1, 4, and 12 months after implantation and reduced platelet deposition in seeded versus unseeded PTFE grafts at 1 and 6 months.[167, 176, 177]

The influence of collagen and albumin presealants on knitted Dacron aortoiliac grafts compared with standard Dacron grafts was assessed in a randomized trial of 36 subjects.[181] At 5 days and at 2 months after implantation, there were no differences between the three graft types, suggesting that sealing of Dacron grafts with collagen or albumin does not reduce early graft thrombogenicity. Small numbers of patients with vascular access grafts,[182] cardiopulmonary bypass grafts,[183] mechanical heart valves,[62] extracardiac valved conduits that incorporate xenograft valves,[184] and indwelling catheters[185] have also been assessed in regard to platelet uptake onto differing prosthetic surfaces.

Drug Effects on Platelet Deposition on Grafts

The combination of aspirin plus dipyridamole has been most extensively studied in patients with both acute and chronically implanted grafts. In eight subjects with recently implanted Dacron aortofemoral grafts, the combination of aspirin (325 mg t.i.d.) plus dipyridamole (100 mg q.i.d. preoperatively and 75 mg t.i.d. postoperatively) decreased platelet uptake in all portions of the graft, compared with eight untreated control patients.[65] In contrast, the same regimen had no apparent effect in five patients with PTFE femoropopliteal grafts compared with controls. In a randomized trial involving 47 patients with recently implanted Dacron, PTFE, or vein grafts, aspirin plus dipyridamole treatment decreased the deposition index in recently implanted Dacron grafts from 0.25±0.09 to 0.16±0.05 ($P < .05$) and in PTFE grafts from 0.16±0.03 to 0.05±0.01 ($P < .05$); but in vein grafts no detectable reduction in deposition was induced by drug therapy.[186] The reduction in early platelet deposition was associated with an improved patency rate in drug-treated patients at 1 year (67 percent), compared with placebo-treated controls (36 percent, $P < .05$).[168] In patients with older Dacron bifurcation grafts (10 to 121 months), short-term therapy with aspirin (325 mg t.i.d.) plus dipyridamole (75 mg t.i.d.) also reduced platelet accumulation (Fig. 67–12).[48] The mean drug-induced decrease in the tomographically obtained graft-to-blood ratio was 13±4 percent, and the decrease in planar imaging graft-to-blood ratio was 12±4 percent. A study by Lane and colleagues found a 9 percent reduction in thrombogenicity index with aspirin plus dipyridamole in similar patients with chronic grafts; this reduction was not statistically significant.[187]

PGI_2 also reduces platelet deposition in both recently implanted and chronically implanted grafts in humans.[188] The magnitude of the reduction was greater among patients with more recently implanted grafts, compared with patients with chronically implanted

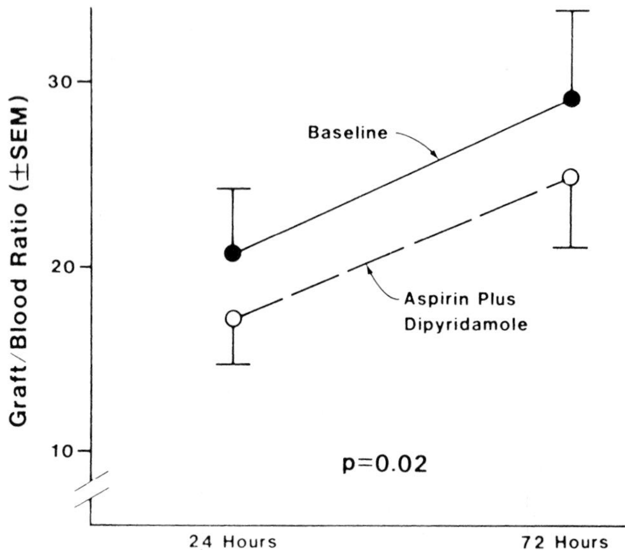

FIGURE 67–12. The effects of aspirin plus dipyridamole on the tomographic graft-to-blood ratio are summarized here. The graft-to-blood ratio was significantly reduced by aspirin plus dipyridamole compared with control testing ($P = .02$). (From Stratton, J.R., and Ritchie, J.L.: Reduction of indium-111 platelet deposition on Dacron vascular grafts in humans by aspirin plus dipyridamole. Circulation 73:327, 1986, with permission of the American Heart Association.)

grafts. Some evidence suggests that the PGI_2 effect persists after discontinuation of the infusion. A new thromboxane A_2-receptor antagonist, Bay u3405, substantially reduced uptake of ^{111}In-labeled platelets on Dacron aortic grafts in 12 subjects, even though mean platelet survival was not altered.[189] The thrombogenicity index was reduced by 26 percent with the drug, compared with placebo. Another trial, which used a different thromboxane A_2-receptor blocking drug, AH23848, also found a significant 40 percent reduction in platelet uptake on mature Dacron aortobifemoral grafts measured by the thrombogenicity index[187]; in contrast, the combination of aspirin and dipyridamole caused only a 9 percent reduction, which was not statistically significant.

In general, results of drug therapy in patients with chronically implanted grafts have been much less impressive than in patients with recently implanted prostheses. Stratton and co-workers have assessed the effects of three agents in patients with chronically implanted grafts (more than 9 months). In randomized, placebo-controlled crossover studies, the experimental agents suloctidil (200 mg t.i.d.) and ticlopidine (250 mg b.i.d.) failed to cause a significant reduction in platelet uptake onto the surface of chronic grafts.[47, 190] Similarly, sulfinpyrazone (200 mg q.i.d.) also failed to reduce platelet uptake on chronic grafts.[191]

To summarize, platelet deposition on prosthetic arterial grafts has been present on all materials studied in humans. Deposition is greatest soon after implantation. Despite a reduction in deposition over the first few months after implantation, detectable deposition appears to remain present indefinitely in most, if not all, patients. Deposition is decreased on both recently and chronically implanted grafts by aspirin plus dipyridamole, and by prostacyclin and thromboxane A_2-receptor antagonists. On chronically implanted grafts, suloctidil, ticlopidine, and sulfinpyrazone have failed to reduce deposition. Deposition is clearly less on autologous vein grafts, compared with either PTFE or Dacron grafts. The magnitude of platelet uptake detected early on prosthetic materials appears to predict ultimate graft patency.

ALTERNATIVE IMAGING METHODS IN HUMANS

Although ^{111}In-labeled platelets have been the predominant form of thrombus imaging used in humans to date, other methods have been described in recent years. Because thrombi are formed of platelets, fibrin, and other blood elements, it is rational to attempt to image thrombi using agents that have a high specificity for one or more of these elements. Several other radiolabeled materials have been tested in animal models for their ability to bind to and permit scintigraphic detection of thrombi. These have included labeled fibrinogen, monoclonal antibodies directed against platelets or fibrinogen or other thrombus components, fibrin fragment E_1, thrombospondin, plasminogen activators, annexin V, and radiolabeled peptides that bind with certain receptors.[192–194]

Because fibrin, unlike fibrinogen, is present only in areas of active thrombosis, antifibrin imaging has appeared promising in animal models of venous and arterial thrombosis.[195–199] More recently, human studies suggest antifibrin antibody imaging can detect *venous* thrombi with the use of a variety of monoclonal antibodies or antibody fragments.[12, 197, 200–206] In human studies of deep venous thrombosis, labeled antifibrin antibodies (or fragments) appeared promising, with sensitivities of 81 to 97 percent and specificities of 84 to 100 percent compared to contrast venography.[200, 203–206]

The author investigated the ability of ^{99m}Tc-labeled monoclonal T2G1s antifibrin Fab′ to detect *arterial thrombi* in humans and compared ^{111}In-labeled platelet imaging results to those with ^{99m}Tc-labeled monoclonal T2G1s antifibrin Fab′. Compared with venous thrombi, which are composed predominantly of fibrin and red blood cells, arterial thrombi, at least acute arterial thrombi, contain more platelets with less fibrin and fewer red cells.[207] With ^{99m}Tc-labeled T2G1s antifibrin Fab′, results in humans with large-vessel arterial thrombi were disappointing and clearly inferior to the results achieved with ^{111}In-labeled platelet imaging (Fig. 67–13).[49]

FIGURE 67-13. See Color Plate 30.

Eighteen subjects with chronic arterial thrombi were studied with planar and tomographic imaging of ^{99m}Tc-labeled T2G1s monoclonal antifibrin antibody fragment and ^{111}In-labeled platelets. Images were visually graded by two observers as 0, 1, 2, or 3 (i.e., no, faint, moderate, or marked) uptake, and quantitative analysis of tomographic images was done in 13 subjects. On visual analysis of tomographic images, 61 percent (11 of 18) of antifibrin studies were graded 1.0 or greater, compared with 100 percent (17 of 17) of platelet studies ($P < .01$) (Fig. 67–14). Planar imaging results were similar. The tomographic target-background ratio was also higher with platelets than with antifibrin antibody (2.5 ± 1.4 versus 1.8 ± 1.0, $P < .05$). In the large-vessel chronic arterial thrombi studied, ^{99m}Tc-labeled monoclonal T2G1s antifibrin Fab′ imaging

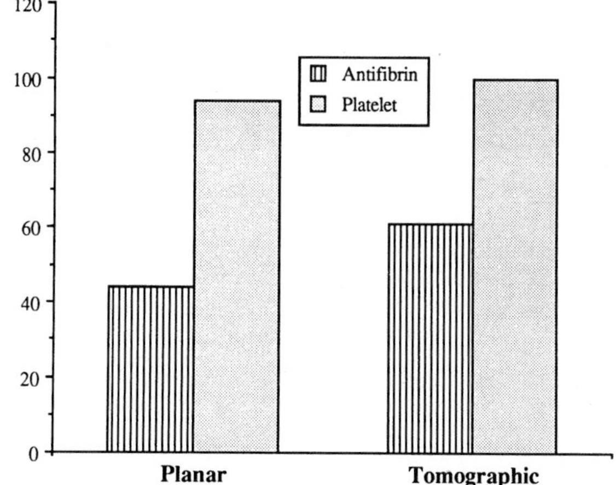

FIGURE 67–14. The percentage of patient studies graded visually as 1.0 or greater (faint or greater uptake) was higher for both planar and tomographic platelet imaging than for antifibrin imaging (both $P < .01$).

was positive in significantly fewer subjects than platelet imaging, which was positive in all subjects.

Very encouraging early results have been reported in animal and human studies with the use of the synthetic peptide P280, which is a 26–amino acid dimer that binds with high affinity to the GPIIb/IIIa receptor expressed on activated platelets. In preliminary canine studies of venous thrombi, ^{99m}Tc-labeled P280 accumulated in fresh thrombi with thrombus-to-background ratios using region-of-interest analysis of 2.3 at 4 hours after injection.[253, 254] In preliminary human studies in nine subjects, ^{99m}Tc-labeled P280 detected deep venous thrombi in eight of nine cases within 1 hour after injection.[255] In addition, uptake compatible with pulmonary emboli was detectable in two subjects. Blood clearance was rapid, with less than 5 percent of the injected dose circulating 1 hour after injection. The in vivo thrombus-to-background ratios obtained from region-of-interest analysis averaged 1.6 to 1.8 at 1 to 4 hours after injection and dropped to 1.4 at 24 hours in the human studies. These early findings need further verification.

Another approach has been the use of fragment E_1, which is a 60-kilodalton fragment of human fibrin that binds to fibrin dimers and polymers but not to fibrinogen or fibrin monomer.[192, 208–211] In preliminary human studies, the agent has appeared promising for the detection of venous thrombi, as might be predicted from its binding properties.[209] To the author's knowledge, this agent has not been tested in human arterial thrombi. Based on the disappointing findings with antifibrin antibodies, fragment E_1, which also binds to fibrin, may have limited value in detection of arterial thrombi.

Other approaches that have been tested in animal models but not in humans include the use of antibodies to an antigen that is expressed only on activated platelets, the alpha-granule protein GMP-140, also known as PADGEM protein.[212, 213] Palabrica used an iodine-123–labeled anti-PADGEM antibody in an ex vivo graft model and achieved approximately sixfold higher thrombus-to-blood ratios with the specific antibody than with a nonspecific control.[213] Uptake on venous thrombi was less, with thrombus-to-blood ratios of 3:1. With a ^{99m}Tc-labeled anti-PADGEM antibody, Miller and colleagues found in vivo imaging ratios of injured to uninjured artery of only 1.3:1 to 1.6:1 after angioplasty in a rabbit model.[212]

Another approach has been to label t-PA, which also binds to fibrin.[214–216] With the use of inactive labeled t-PA, Ord and associates[215] found thrombus-to-blood ratios ranging from 3:1 to 18:1 if thrombi were formed 10 to 60 minutes before t-PA infusion, and even higher if t-PA was present when the thrombi were formed; however, uptake of control proteins was not reported. More recently, DeBruyn and colleagues described the detection of pulmonary emboli in nine dogs using inactivated ^{99m}Tc-labeled t-PA.[256]

Yet another approach that has shown promise in animal studies is the use of annexin V.[193, 194] Annexin V is a human phospholipid-binding protein that binds to the phosphatidylserine that becomes exposed on the extracellular face of the plasma membrane of activated platelets in vitro. Because activated platelets are concentrated at sites of thrombosis, the author sought to determine the potential of this agent for imaging intracardiac thrombi in swine. It was hoped that by selective targeting of active platelets, higher ratios between thrombi and background blood could be obtained. Annexin V has a higher affinity for the thrombus than fibrin-targeted or t-PA–targeted approaches, and it is selective, binding to activated but not to quiescent platelets. In initial nonimaging experiments, the selectivity of intravenous ^{125}I-labeled human annexin V for left atrial thrombus uptake was assessed. The mean thrombus-to-blood ratio was 13.4 ± 4.8 for the entire thrombus. Subsequently, the author and associates labeled annexin V with ^{99m}Tc. In 12 experiments, planar or tomographic images were positive or equivocal in all animals with left atrial thrombi, and negative in all 12 control animals. By tomographic imaging, the mean thrombus-to-blood ratio at 2 hours in animals with a thrombus was 3.90 ± 1.12, compared with a comparable ratio of 0.84 ± 0.10 in closed-chest and 1.01 ± 0.23 in open-chest control subjects ($P <$ .001). By well counting of resected specimens, the mean left atrial thrombus-to-blood ratio was 14.2 ± 10.6 for the entire thrombus; the peak thrombus-to-blood ratio in any section was 26.2 ± 14.9. In contrast, the corresponding uptake ratio for a control protein, ovalbumin, was 1.0 ± 0.2, documenting the thrombus specificity of labeled annexin V.

Multiple factors influence thrombus composition. Probably two of the most important are thrombus location and thrombus age. Thrombi that form in the arterial circulation, where shear forces are higher, tend to be richer in platelets and have less fibrin than thrombi in the venous system.[207, 217] In addition, thrombi have a life cycle. Several studies have suggested that arterial thrombi have reduced uptake of ^{111}In-labeled platelets over time.[92, 93, 100, 165] Thrombi can be identified by agents that are incorporated into the thrombus while it is forming, such as labeled platelets, or by agents that target an element found in thrombi but not in surrounding blood, such as annexin V. Based on these considerations and the other factors that determine thrombus composition, it is likely that no single thrombosis imaging approach will offer success for all types of thrombi.

SUMMARY AND CONCLUSIONS

The ability of ^{111}In-labeled platelet imaging to localize noninvasively and define platelet kinetics during life already has offered a new window for examination of the pathophysiologic role of platelets in a broad range of diseases. Thrombosis imaging with labeled platelets has proved to be a very useful research tool in experimental animal studies and is increasingly used to study a variety of diseases in humans. To date, platelet imaging as a method of thrombosis detection has several constraints that have limited its clinical utility. Current labeling and imaging techniques are time consuming and costly, and rapid diagnosis is not possible because delayed imaging is usually necessary. The resolution of platelet imaging has been limited to some extent by the relatively high circulating blood pool activity that occurs and in part by the inherent limitations of all gamma imaging techniques.[110] Small arterial thrombi that have great clinical importance, such as coronary artery thrombi, cannot routinely be detected with ^{111}In-labeled platelet imaging in humans. The lack of simple, validated methods for quantification of platelet uptake in humans is also a limitation, because quantitative analysis is necessary to detect small changes in platelet accumulation induced by drugs or by time.

To realize the full potential of thrombosis imaging, both improvements in imaging techniques and improved thrombosis tracers are needed. The development of positron emitters for thrombosis imaging may improve spatial resolution and quantification, but positron production and imaging facilities are unlikely to be widely available because of their cost. It is more likely that superior methods of thrombosis detection will be found that employ gamma-emitting isotopes tagged to tracers that localize in areas of ongoing thrombosis. Improved thrombosis imaging may be possible with labeling of compounds, such as t-PA, annexin V, peptides, or antifibrin or antiplatelet monoclonal antibodies, that are incorporated into thrombus. To be clinically useful, new approaches need to offer thrombus-to-background ratios that exceed those achieved with ^{111}In-labeled platelets at earlier times after injection. With future improvements, it is likely that thrombosis imaging will play an increasingly important role in detecting localized thrombosis and assessing the effects of therapy in humans.

References

1. Thakur, M.L., Welch, M.J., Joist, J.H., et al.: Indium-111–labeled platelets: Studies on preparation and evaluation of in vitro and in vivo functions. Thromb. Res. 9:345, 1976.
2. Sinzinger, H., Virgolini, I., and Vinazzer, H.: Autologous platelet-labeling in thrombocytopenia. Thromb. Res. 60:223, 1990.
3. Dewanjee, M.K., Wahner, H.W., Dunn, W.L., et al.: Comparison of three platelet markers for measurement of platelet survival time in healthy volunteers. Mayo Clin. Proc. 61:327, 1986.

4. Hudson, E.M., Ramsey, R.B., and Evatt, B.L.: Subcellular localization of indium-111 in indium-111–labeled platelets. J. Lab. Clin. Med. 97:577, 1981.
5. Joist, J.H., Baker, R.K., and Welch, M.J.: Methodologic and basic aspects of indium-111 platelets. Semin. Thromb. Hemost. 9:86, 1983.
6. Heaton, W.A., Davis, H.H., Welch, M.J., et al.: Indium-111: A new radionuclide label for studying human platelet kinetics. Br. J. Haematol. 42:613, 1979.
7. Hawker, R.J., Hawker, L.M., and Wilkinson, A.R.: Indium (^{111}In)-labelled human platelets: Optimal method. Clin. Sci. 58:243, 1980.
8. Joist, J.H., Baker, R.K., Thakur, M.L., et al.: Indium-111–labeled human platelets: Uptake and loss of label and in vitro function of labeled platelets. J. Lab. Clin. Med. 92:829, 1978.
9. Thakur, M.L., Walsh, L., Malech, H.L., et al.: Indium-111–labeled human platelets: Improved method, efficacy, and evaluation. J. Nucl. Med. 22:381, 1981.
10. Schmidt, K.G., and Rasmussen, J.W.: Labelling of human and rabbit platelets with ^{111}In-oxine complex. Scand. J. Haematol. 23:97, 1979.
11. Bassano, D.A., and McAfee, J.G.: Cellular radiation doses of labeled neutrophils and labeled platelets. J. Nucl. Med. 20:255, 1979.
12. Vorne, M.S., Honkanen, T.T., Lantto, T.J., et al.: Thrombus imaging with ^{99m}Tc-HMPAO–labeled platelets and ^{111}In-labeled monoclonal antifibrin antibodies. Acta Radiol. 34:59, 1993.
13. Dewanjee, M.K., Robinson, R.P., Hellman, R.L., et al.: Technetium-99m–labeled platelets: Comparison of labeling with a new lipid-soluble Sn(II)-mercaptopyridine-*N*-oxide and ^{99m}Tc-HMPAO. Int. J. Rad. Appl. Instrum. [B] 18:461, 1991.
14. Sundrehagen, E., Urdal, P., Heggli, D.E., et al.: Radiolabelling of platelets with technetium-99m. Thromb. Res. 57:737, 1990.
15. Hardeman, M.R.: Thrombocytes labelled with ^{99m}Tc-HMPAO: In vitro studies and preliminary clinical experience. Prog. Clin. Biol. Res. 355:49, 1990.
16. Becker, W., Borst, U., Krahe, T., et al.: ^{99m}Tc-HMPAO–labelled human platelets: In vitro and in vivo results. Eur. J. Nucl. Med. 15:296, 1989.
17. Vorne, M., Honkanen, T., Karppinen, K., et al.: Radiolabelling of human platelets with ^{99m}Tc-HMPAO. Eur. J. Haematol. 42:487, 1989.
18. Becker, W., Börner, W., and Borst, U.: ^{99m}Tc-hexamethylpropyleneamineoxime (HMPAO) as a platelet label: Evaluation of labelling parameters and first in vivo results. Nucl. Med. Commun. 9:831, 1988.
19. Honkanen, T., Jauhola, S., Karppinen, K., et al.: Venous thrombosis: A controlled study on the performance of scintigraphy with ^{99m}Tc-HMPAO–labelled platelets versus venography. Nucl. Med. Commun. 13:88, 1992.
20. Thakur, M.L.: A look at radiolabeled blood cells. Int. J. Rad. Appl. Instrum. [B] 13:147, 1986.
21. Heyns, A.D., Lotter, M.G., Badenhorst, P.N., et al.: Kinetics, distribution and sites of destruction of ^{111}In-labelled human platelets. Br. J. Haematol. 44:269, 1980.
22. Mathias, C.J., and Welch, M.J.: Radiolabeling of platelets. Semin. Nucl. Med. 14:118, 1984.
23. Schmidt, K.G., Rasmussen, J.W., and Arendrup, H.: Function ex vivo of ^{111}In-labelled human platelets: Simultaneous aggregation of labelled and unlabelled platelets induced by collagen. Scand. J. Haematol. 29:51, 1982.
24. Schmidt, K.G., Rasmussen, J.W., and Lorentzen, M.: Function and morphology of ^{111}In-labelled platelets: In vitro, in vivo and ex vivo studies. Haemostasis 11:193, 1982.
25. Isaka, Y., Kimura, K., Matsumoto, M., et al.: Functional alterations of human platelets following indium-111 labelling using different incubation media and labelling agents. Eur. J. Nucl. Med. 18:326, 1991.
26. Thakur, M.L., and Sedar, A.W.: Ultrastructure of human platelets following indium-111 labeling in plasma. Nucl. Med. Commun. 8:69, 1987.
27. Kotze, H.F., Heyns, A.D., Lotter, M.G., et al.: Comparison of oxine and tropolone methods for labeling human platelets with indium-111. J. Nucl. Med. 32:62, 1991.
28. Peters, A.M., Klonizakis, I., Lavender, J.P., et al.: Elution of ^{111}In from reticuloendothelial cells. J. Clin. Pathol. 35:507, 1982.
29. Kotze, H.F., Lotter, M.G., Heyns, A.D., et al.: ^{111}In-labelled baboon platelets: The influence of in vivo redistribution and contaminating ^{114m}In on the radiation dose. Int. J. Rad. Appl. Instrum. [B] 14:593, 1987.
30. Goodwin, D.A.: Cell labeling with oxine chelates of radioactive metal ions: Techniques and clinical implications. (Editorial.) J. Nucl. Med. 19:557, 1978.
31. Goodwin, D.A., Bushberg, J.T., Doherty, P.W., et al.: Indium-111–labeled autologous platelets for location of vascular thrombi in humans. J. Nucl. Med. 19:626, 1978.
32. Klonizakis, I., Peters, A.M., Fitzpatrick, M.L., et al.: Radionuclide distribution following injection of ^{111}In-labelled platelets. Br. J. Haematol. 46:595, 1980.
33. Stratton, J.R., Ballem, P.J., Gernsheimer, T., et al.: Platelet destruction in autoimmune thrombocytopenic purpura: Kinetics and clearance of indium-111–labeled autologous platelets. J. Nucl. Med. 30:629, 1989.
34. Peters, A.M.: Should platelets be labelled in plasma or saline? Consider the clinical indication. (Editorial; Comment.) Eur. J. Nucl. Med. 18:305, 1991.
35. Heaton, W.A.L.: Indium-111 (^{111}In) and chromium-51 (^{51}Cr) labeling of platelets: Are they comparable? Transfusion 26:16, 1986.
36. Peters, A.M., and Lavender, J.P.: Platelet kinetics with indium-111 platelets: Comparison with chromium-51 platelets. Semin. Thromb. Hemost. 9:100, 1983.
37. Schmidt, K.G., Rasmussen, J.W., Rasmusen, A.D., et al.: Comparative studies of the in vivo kinetics of simultaneously injected ^{111}In- and ^{51}Cr-labeled human platelets. Scand. J. Haematol. 30:465, 1983.
38. Wadenvik, H., and Kutti, J.: The in vivo kinetics of ^{111}In- and ^{51}Cr-labelled platelets: A comparative study using both stored and fresh platelets. Br. J. Haematol. 78:523, 1991.
39. International Committee for Standardization in Hematology: Recommended method for indium-111 platelet survival studies. J. Nucl. Med. 29:564, 1988.
40. Robertson, J.S., Ezekowitz, M.D., Dewanjee, M.K., et al.: MIRD dose estimate no. 15: Radiation absorbed dose estimates for radioindium-labeled autologous platelets. J. Nucl. Med. 33:777, 1992.
41. Robertson, J.S., Dewanjee, M.K., Brown, M.L., et al.: Distribution and dosimetry of ^{111}In-labeled platelets. Radiology 140:169, 1981.
42. Scheffel, U., Tsan, M.F., Mitchell, T.G., et al.: Human platelets labeled with In-111 8-hydroxyquinoline: Kinetics, distribution, and estimates of radiation dose. J. Nucl. Med. 23:149, 1982.
43. van Reenen, O.R., Lotter, M.G., Minnaar, P.C., et al.: Radiation dose from human platelets labelled with indium-111. Br. J. Radiol. 53:790, 1980.
44. Stratton, J.R., Ritchie, J.L., Hamilton, G.W., et al.: Left ventricular thrombi: In vivo detection by indium-111 platelet imaging and two dimensional echocardiography. Am. J. Cardiol. 47:874, 1981.
45. Badenhorst, P.N., and Pieters, H.: Methodology of platelet imaging. *In* Heyns, A., Badenhorst, P., and Lotter, M. (eds.): Platelet Kinetics and Imaging. Vol. 1. Boca Raton, CRC Press, 1985, pp. 160–168.
46. Mathias, C.J., and Welch, M.J.: Dual isotope scintigraphy for the detection of platelet deposition. *In* Heyns, A., Badenhorst, P., and Lotter, M. (eds.): Platelet Kinetics and Imaging. Vol. 1. Boca Raton, CRC Press, 1985, pp. 89-106.
47. Stratton, J.R., and Ritchie, J.L.: Effect of suloctidil on tomographically quantitated platelet accumulation in Dacron aortic grafts. Am. J. Cardiol. 58:152, 1986.
48. Stratton, J.R., and Ritchie, J.L.: Reduction of indium-111 platelet deposition on Dacron vascular grafts in humans by aspirin plus dipyridamole. Circulation 73:325, 1986.
49. Stratton, J.R., Cerqueira, M.D., and Kohler, T.: Imaging arterial thrombosis in humans: Comparison of technetium-99m–labeled monoclonal antifibrin antibodies and indium-111–labeled platelets. J. Nucl. Med. 35:1731, 1994.
50. Wu, K.K., Chen, Y.C., Fordham, E., et al.: Differential effects of two doses of aspirin on platelet-vessel wall interaction in vivo. J. Clin. Invest. 68:382, 1981.
51. Heyns, A.D., Lotter, M.G., Kotzë, H.F., et al.: Quantification of in vivo distribution of platelets labeled with indium-111 oxine. (Letter.) J. Nucl. Med. 23:943, 1982.
52. van Reenen, P.C., Lotter, M.G., Heyns, A.D., et al.: Quantification of the distribution of ^{111}In-labelled platelets in organs. Eur. J. Nucl. Med. 7:80, 1982.
53. van Rensburg, A.J., Lotter, M.G., Heyns, A.D., et al.: An evaluation of four methods of ^{111}In planar image quantification. Med. Phys. 15:853, 1988.
54. Mortelmans, L., Verbruggen, A., DeBakker, C., et al.: Comparison of quantification methods of ^{111}In-labelled platelet deposition in peripheral bypass grafts. Nuklearmedizin 26:87, 1987.
55. Kotze, H.F., Heyns, A.D., Nel, C.J., et al.: The influence of platelet-graft interaction on platelet survival in patients with aortobifemoral Dacron grafts. S. Afr. Med. J. 81:27, 1992.
56. Hanson, S.R., Kotze, H.F., Pieters, H., et al.: Analysis of indium-111 platelet kinetics and imaging in patients with aortic grafts and abdominal aortic aneurysms. Arteriosclerosis 10:1037, 1990.
57. Allen, B.T., Mathias, C.J., Sicard, G.A., et al.: Platelet deposition on vascular grafts: The accuracy of in vivo quantification and the signficance of in vivo platelet reactivity. Ann. Surg. 203:318, 1986.
58. Powers, W.J., Hopkins, K.T., and Welch, M.J.: Validation of the dual radiotracer method for quantitative ^{111}In platelet scintigraphy. Thromb. Res. 34:135, 1984.
59. Wakefield, T.W., Lindblad, B., Graham, L.M., et al.: Nuclide imaging of vascular graft-platelet interactions: Comparison of indium excess and technetium subtraction techniques. J. Surg. Res. 40:388, 1986.
60. Powers, W.J.: Indium-111 platelet scintigraphy: Carotid atherosclerosis and stroke. J. Nucl. Med. 25:626, 1984.
61. Machac, J., Vallabhajosula, S., Goldman, M.E., et al.: Value of blood-pool subtraction in cardiac indium-111–labeled platelet imaging. J. Nucl. Med. 30:1445, 1989.
62. Dewanjee, M.K.: Cardiac and vascular imaging with labeled platelets and leukocytes. Semin. Nucl. Med. 14:154, 1984.
63. Dewanjee, M.K., Tago, M., Josa, M., et al.: Quantification of platelet retention in aortocoronary femoral vein bypass graft in dogs treated with dipyridamole and aspirin. Circulation 69:350, 1984.
64. Goldman, M., Norcott, H.C., Hawker, R.J., et al.: Femoropopliteal bypass grafts: An isotope technique allowing in vivo comparison of thrombogenicity. Br. J. Surg. 69:380, 1982.
65. Pumphrey, C.W., Chesebro, J.H., Dewanjee, M.K., et al.: In vivo quantitation of platelet deposition on human peripheral arterial bypass grafts using indium-111–labelled platelets: Effect of dipyridamole and aspirin. Am. J. Cardiol. 51:796, 1983.
66. Stratton, J.R., Thiele, B.L., and Ritchie, J.L.: Platelet deposition on Dacron aortic bifurcation grafts in man: Quantitation with indium-111 platelet imaging. Circulation 66:1287, 1982.
67. Garrett, K.O., Bentz, M.L., Macpherson, T., et al.: Quantitation of platelet deposition on human arteries: Assessment of the disparity between results obtained with indium-111 (^{111}In) labelling versus scanning electron microscopy. Thromb. Res. 71:495, 1993.
68. Riba, A.L., Thakur, M.L., Gottschalk, A., et al.: Imaging experimental coronary artery thrombosis with indium-111 platelets. Circulation 60:767, 1979.
69. Bergmann, S.R., Lerch, R.A., Mathias, C.J., et al.: Noninvasive detection of coronary thrombi with indium-111 platelets: Concise communication. J. Nucl. Med. 24:130, 1983.
70. Fox, K.A., Bergmann, S.R., Mathias, C.J., et al.: Scintigraphic detection of coronary artery thrombi in patients with acute myocardial infarction. J. Am. Coll. Cardiol. 4:975, 1984.
71. Stratton, J.R., Ritchie, J.L., and Werner, J.A.: Indium-111 platelet imaging for the detection of intracardiac thrombi in survivors of sudden cardiac death. (Abstract.) Clin. Res. 28:68A, 1980.

72. Laws, K.H., Clanton, J.A., and Starnes, V.A.: Kinetics and imaging of indium-111–labelled autologous platelets in experimental myocardial infarction. Circulation 67:110, 1983.
73. Romson, J.L., Hook, B.G., Rigot, V.H., et al.: The effect of ibuprofen on accumulation of indium-111–labeled platelets and leukocytes in experimental myocardial infarction. Circulation 66:1002, 1982.
74. Callahan, R.J., Bunting, R.W., and Block, P.C.: Evaluation of platelet deposition at the site of coronary angioplasty using indium-111–labeled platelets. (Abstract.) J. Nucl. Med. 24:P60, 1983.
75. Fuster, V., Dewanjee, M.K., Kaye, M.P., et al.: Noninvasive radioisotopic technique for detection of platelet deposition in coronary artery bypass grafts in dogs and its reduction with platelet inhibitors. Circulation 60:1508, 1979.
76. Riba, A.L., Thakur, M.L., Gottschalk, A., et al.: Imaging experimental infective endocarditis with indium-111–labeled blood cellular components. Circulation 59:336, 1979.
77. Acar, J., Vahanian, A., Dorent, R., et al.: Detection of prosthetic valve thrombosis using indium-111 platelet imaging. Eur. Heart J. 11:389, 1990.
78. Benichou, M., Bernard, P.J., Sarrat, P., et al.: Detection of intracardiac thrombi by scintigraphy with indium-111–labeled platelets: Correlation with 2-dimensional echography and cardiac scanning. Arch. Mal. Coeur Vaiss. 77:1054, 1984.
79. Benichou, M., Camilleri, J.F., Bernard, P.J., et al.: Development of left intraventricular thrombi: Monitoring by two-dimensional echocardiography and scintigraphy with indium-111–labelled platelets. Arch. Mal. Coeur Vaiss. 81:1317, 1988.
80. Ezekowitz, M.D., Leonard, J.C., Smith, E.O., et al.: Identification of left ventricular thrombi in man using indium-111–labeled autologous platelets: A preliminary report. Circulation 63:803, 1981.
81. Ezekowitz, M.D., Cox, A.C., Smith, E.O., et al.: Failure of aspirin to prevent incorporation of indium-111–labelled platelets into cardiac thrombi in man. Lancet 2:440, 1981.
82. Ezekowitz, M.D., Wilson, D.A., Smith, E.O., et al.: Comparison of indium-111 platelet scintigraphy and two-dimensional echocardiography in the diagnosis of left ventricular thrombi. N. Engl. J. Med. 306:1509, 1982.
83. Ezekowitz, M.D., Kellerman, D.J., Smith, E.O., et al.: Detection of active left ventricular thrombosis during acute myocardial infarction using indium-111 platelet scintigraphy. Chest 86:35, 1984.
84. Ezekowitz, M.D., Burrow, R.D., Heath, P.W., et al.: Diagnostic accuracy of indium-111 platelet scintigraphy in identifying left ventricular thrombi. Am J Cardiol 51:1712, 1983.
85. Stratton, J.R., and Ritchie, J.L.: The effects of antithrombotic drugs in patients with left ventricular thrombi: Assessment with indium-111 platelet imaging and two-dimensional echocardiography. Circulation 69:561, 1984.
86. Stratton, J.R., and Ritchie, J.L.: Indium-111 platelet imaging of left ventricular thrombi: Predictive value for systemic emboli. Circulation 81:1182, 1990.
87. Verheugt, F.W., Lindenfeld, J., Kirch, D.L., et al.: Left ventricular platelet deposition after acute myocardial infarction: An attempt at quantification using blood pool subtracted indium-111 platelet scintigraphy. Br. Heart J. 52:490, 1984.
88. Vandenberg, B.F., Seabold, J.E., Schroder, E., et al.: Noninvasive imaging of left ventricular thrombi: Two dimensional echocardiography and indium-111 platelet scintigraphy. Am. J. Card. Imaging 1:289, 1987.
89. Ezekowitz, M.D.: Imaging techniques for identifying left ventricular thrombi. Am. J. Card. Imaging 8:81, 1994.
90. Salehi, N.F., Chan, W.C., McHutchinson, J., et al.: Early detection of left ventricular mural thrombi after acute Q wave myocardial infarction using ^{111}In-oxine–labelled autologous platelets. Nucl. Med. Commun. 11:857, 1990.
91. Bellotti, P., Claudiani, F., Chiarella, F., et al.: Left ventricular thrombi: Changes in size and in platelet deposition during treatment with indobufen and ticlopidine. Cardiology 77:272, 1990.
92. Seabold, J.E., Schroder, E., Conrad, G.R., et al.: Indium-111 platelet scintigraphy and two-dimensional echocardiography for detection of left ventricular thrombus: Influence of clot size and age. J. Am. Coll. Cardiol. 9:1057, 1988.
93. Bellotti, P., Claudiani, F., Chiarella, F., et al.: Activity of left ventricular thrombi of different ages: Assessment with indium-oxine platelet imaging and cross-sectional echocardiography. Eur. Heart J. 8:855, 1987.
94. Funke-Kupper, A.J., Verheugt, F.W., Peels, C.H., et al.: Effect of low dose acetylsalicylic acid on the frequency and hematologic activity of left ventricular thrombus in anterior wall acute myocardial infarction. Am. J. Cardiol. 63:917, 1989.
95. Kessler, C., Henningsen, H., and Reuther, R.: Der Nachweis intrakardialer Thromben mit der ^{111}In-Plattchenszintigraphie. Nervenarzt 56:311, 1985.
96. Yamada, M., Hoki, N., Ishikawa, K., et al.: Detection of left atrial thrombi in man using indium-111–labelled autologous platelets. Br. Heart J. 51:298, 1984.
97. Ezekowitz, M.D., Kellerman, D.J., Smith, E.O., et al.: Left atrial mass: Diagnostic value of transesophageal 2-dimensional echocardiography and indium-111 platelet scintigraphy. Am. J. Cardiol. 51:1563, 1983.
98. Takeda, T., Ishikawa, N., Sakakibara, Y., et al.: A giant tumor thrombus in the right atrium clearly detected by ^{111}In-oxine–labeled platelet scintigraphy. Eur. J. Nucl. Med. 11:49, 1985.
99. Nishimura, T., Misawa, T., Park, Y.D., et al.: Visualization of right atrial thrombus associated with constrictive pericarditis by indium-111 oxine platelet imaging. J. Nucl. Med. 28:1344, 1987.
100. Vandenberg, B.F., Seabold, J.E., Conrad, G.R., et al.: Indium-111 platelet scintigraphy and two-dimensional echocardiography for the detection of left atrial appendage thrombi: Studies in a new canine model. Circulation 78:1040, 1988.
101. Finklestein, S., Miller, A., Callahan, R.J., et al.: Imaging of acute arterial injury with ^{111}In-labeled platelets: A comparison with scanning electron micrographs. Radiology 145:155, 1982.
102. Goldman, M., Norcott, H.C., Hawker, R.J., et al.: Platelet accumulation on mature Dacron grafts in man. Br. J. Surg. 69:S38, 1982.
103. Davis, H.H., Siegel, B.A., Sherman, L.A., et al.: Scintigraphic detection of carotid atherosclerosis with indium-111–labeled autologous platelets. Circulation 61:982, 1980.
104. Davis, H.H., Heaton, W.A., Siegel, B.A., et al.: Scintigraphic detection of atherosclerotic lesions and venous thrombi in man by indium-111–labelled autologous platelets. Lancet 1:1185, 1978.
105. Goldman, M., Leung, J.O., Aukland, A., et al.: Indium-111 platelet imaging, Doppler spectral analysis and angiography compared in patients with transient cerebral ischaemia. Stroke 14:752, 1983.
106. Isaka, Y., Kimura, K., Yoneda, S., et al.: Platelet accumulation in carotid atherosclerotic lesions: Semiquantitative analysis with indium-111 platelets and technetium-99m human serum albumin. J. Nucl. Med. 25:556, 1984.
107. Kessler, C., Henningsen, H., Reuther, R., et al.: Identification of intracardiac thrombi in stroke patients with indium-111 platelet scintigraphy. Stroke 18:63, 1987.
108. Kessler, C., Reuther, R., Berentelg, J., et al.: The clinical use of platelet scintigraphy with ^{111}In-oxine. J. Neurol. 229:255, 1983.
109. Powers, W.J., Siegel, B.A., Davis, H.H., et al.: Indium-111 platelet scintigraphy in cerebrovascular disease. Neurology 32:938, 1982.
110. Powers, W.J., and Siegel, B.A.: Thrombus imaging with indium-111 platelets. Semin. Thromb. Hemost. 9:115, 1983.
111. Pramsohler, B., Lupattelli, G., Scholz, H., et al.: Platelet scintigraphy and survival in juvenile stroke patients. Prog. Clin. Biol. Res. 355:71, 1990.
112. Kessler, C.: Carotid ^{111}In–platelet scintigraphy and correlation to stroke pathogenesis. Prog. Clin. Biol. Res. 355:63, 1990.
113. Minar, E., Ehringer, H., Dudczak, R., et al.: Indium-111–labeled platelet scintigraphy in carotid atherosclerosis. Stroke 20:27, 1989.
114. Isaka, Y., Kimura, K., Etani, H., et al.: Effect of aspirin and ticlopidine on platelet deposition in carotid atherosclerosis: Assessment by indium-111 platelet scintigraphy. Stroke 17:1215, 1986.
115. Sutherland, G.R., King, M.E., Peerless, S.J., et al.: Platelet interaction within giant intracranial aneurysms. J. Neurosurg. 56:53, 1982.
116. Bridgers, S.L., Strauss, E., Smith, E.O., et al.: Demonstration of superior sagittal sinus thrombosis by indium-111 platelet scintigraphy. Arch. Neurol. 43:1079, 1986.
117. Kessler, C.M.: Intracerebral platelet accumulation as evidence for embolization of carotid origin. Clin. Nucl. Med. 17:728, 1992.
118. Nakagawa, H., Isaka, Y., Nakajima, S., et al.: Multiple cerebral infarcts caused by emboli from carotid atheroma: A case confirmed by indium-111 platelet scintigraphy. Neurol. Med. Chir. (Tokyo) 31:159, 1991.
119. Lusby, R.J., Ferrell, L.D., Englestad, B.L., et al.: Vessel wall and indium-111–labelled platelet response to carotid endarterectomy. Surgery 93:424, 1983.
120. Stratton, J.R., Zierler, R.E., and Kazmers, A.: Platelet deposition at carotid endarterectomy sites in humans. Stroke 18:722, 1987.
121. Findlay, J.M., Lougheed, W.M., Gentili, F., et al.: Effect of perioperative platelet inhibition on postcarotid endarterectomy mural thrombus formation: Results of a prospective randomized controlled trial using aspirin and dipyridamole in humans. J. Neurosurg. 63:693, 1985.
122. Ritchie, J.L., Stratton, J.R., Thiele, B., et al.: Indium-111 platelet imaging for detection of platelet deposition in abdominal aneurysms and prosthetic arterial grafts. Am. J. Cardiol. 47:882, 1981.
123. Heyns, A.D., Lotter, M.G., Badenhorst, P.N., et al.: Kinetics and fate of indium-111-oxine-labeled platelets in patients with aortic aneurysms. Arch. Surg. 117:1170, 1982.
124. Sinzinger, H., O'Grady, J., Fitscha, P., et al.: Detection of aneurysms by gamma-camera imaging after injection of autologous labelled platelets. Lancet 2:1365, 1984.
125. O'Connor, M.K., Brennan, S.S., and Shanik, D.G.: Indium-111–labeled platelet deposition following transfemoral angiography. Radiology 158:191, 1986.
126. Comerford, J.A., Broe, P.J., Wilson, I.A., et al.: Digital ischaemia and palpable pedal pulses. Br. J. Surg. 74:493, 1987.
127. Comerfold, J., Dowsett, G., Kennedy, J., et al.: Indium-111 labelled platelet scanning in the diagnosis of microembolic disease: A prospective study. Ir. J. Med. Sci. 155:121, 1986.
128. Pope, C.F., Ezekowitz, M.D., Smith, E.O., et al.: Detection of platelet deposition at the site of peripheral balloon angioplasty using indium-111 platelet scintigraphy. Am. J. Cardiol. 55:495, 1985.
129. Mohan, S.R., Hawker, R.J., Wolinski, A.P., et al.: Detection of arterial thrombosis after laser angioplasty by platelet scintigraphy. Eur. J. Nucl. Med. 16:865, 1990.
130. Poskitt, K.R., Harwood, A., Scott, D.J., et al.: Failure of peripheral arterial balloon angioplasty: Does platelet deposition play a role? Eur. J. Vasc. Surg. 5:541, 1991.
131. Minar, E., Ehringer, H., Ahmadi, R., et al.: Platelet deposition at angioplasty sites and its relation to restenosis in human iliac and femoropopliteal arteries. Radiology 170:767, 1989.
132. Kadir, S., Hill, Z.R., and Tsan, M.F.: Evaluation of arterial injury due to balloon angioplasty by ^{111}In-labelled platelets. Nuklearmedizin 22:324, 1983.
133. Cunningham, D.A., Kumar, B., Siegel, B.A., et al.: Aspirin inhibition of platelet deposition at angioplasty sites: Demonstration by platelet scintigraphy. Radiology 151:487, 1984.
134. Berridge, D.C., Frier, M., Wastie, M., et al.: ^{111}In platelet deposition following peripheral arterial thrombolysis. Nucl. Med. Commun. 11:565, 1990.
135. Powers, W.J., Mathias, C.J., Welch, M.J., et al.: Scintigraphic detection of platelet deposition in atherosclerotic macaques: A new technique for investigation of anti-thrombotic drugs. Thromb. Res. 25:137, 1982.

136. Sinzinger, H., and Virgolini, I.: Nuclear medicine and atherosclerosis. Eur. J. Nucl. Med. 17:160, 1990.
137. Sinzinger, H., and Fitscha, P.: Scintigraphic detection of femoral artery atherosclerosis with indium-111–labeled autologous platelets. Vasa 13:350, 1984.
138. Moser, K.M., and Fedullo, P.F.: Imaging of venous thromboemboli with labeled platelets. Semin. Nucl. Med. 14:188, 1984.
139. Moser, K.M., and Fedullo, P.F.: Imaging of venous thromboemboli with ^{111}In-labeled platelets. *In* Heyns, A.D., Badenhorst, P.N., and Lotter, M.G. (eds.): Platelet Kinetics and Imaging. Vol. 2. Boca Raton, CRC Press, 1985, pp. 57–70.
140. Knight, L.C., Primeau, J.L., Siegel, B.A., et al.: Comparison of ^{111}In-labeled platelets and iodinated fibrinogen for the detection of deep vein thrombosis. J. Nucl. Med. 19:891, 1978.
141. Dormehl, I.C., Jacobs, D.J., duPlessis, M., et al.: Evaluation of the diagnostic efficacy of autologous ^{111}In-labelled platelets as a scanning agent for deep vein thrombosis in the chacma baboon. Eur. J. Nucl. Med. 10:432, 1985.
142. Dormehl, I.C., Jacobs, D.J., Pretorius, J.P., et al.: Baboon *(Papio ursinus)* model to study deep vein thrombosis using ^{111}In-labeled autologous platelets. J. Med. Primatol. 16:27, 1987.
143. Grossman, Z.D., Rosebrough, S.F., McAfee, J.G., et al.: Imaging fresh venous thrombi in the dog with I-131 and In-111–labeled fibrin-specific monoclonal antibody and F(ab′)2 fragments. Radiographics 7:913, 1987.
144. Clarke-Pearson, D.L., Coleman, R.E., Siegel, R., et al.: Indium-111 platelet imaging for the detection of deep venous thrombosis and pulmonary embolism in patients without symptoms after surgery. Surgery 98:98, 1985.
145. Ezekowitz, M.D., Pope, C.F., Sostman, H.D., et al.: Indium-111 platelet scintigraphy for the diagnosis of acute venous thrombosis. Circulation 73:668, 1986.
146. Fenech, A., Hussey, J.K., Smith, F.W., et al.: Diagnosis of deep vein thrombosis using autologous indium-111–labelled platelets. B.M.J. 282:1020, 1981.
147. Grimley, R.P., Rafiqi, E., Hawker, R.J., et al.: Imaging of ^{111}In-labelled platelets: A new method for the diagnosis of deep vein thrombosis. Br. J. Surg. 68:714, 1981.
148. Seabold, J.E., Conrad, G.R., Ponto, J.A., et al.: Deep venous thrombophlebitis: Detection with 4-hour versus 24-hour platelet scintigraphy. Radiology 165:355, 1987.
149. Farlow, D.C., Ezekowitz, M.D., Rao, S.R., et al.: Early image acquisition after administration of indium-111 platelets in clinically suspected deep venous thrombosis. Am. J. Cardiol. 64:363, 1989.
150. Ezekowitz, M.D., Migliaccio, F., Farlow, D., et al.: Comparison of platelet scintigraphy, impedance plethysmography gray scale and color flow duplex ultrasound and venography for the diagnosis of venous thrombosis. Prog. Clin. Biol. Res. 355:23, 1990.
151. Hansberry, K.L., Thompson, I.J., Bauman, J., et al.: A prospective comparison of thromboembolic stockings, external sequential pneumatic compression stockings and heparin sodium/dihydroergotamine mesylate for the prevention of thromboembolic complications in urological surgery. J. Urol. 145:1205, 1991.
152. Siegel, R.S., Rae, J.L., Ryan, N.L., et al.: The use of indium-111–labeled platelet scanning for the detection of asymptomatic deep venous thrombosis in a high risk population. Orthopedics 12:1439, 1989.
153. Winter, J.H., Fenech, A., Bennett, B., et al.: Preoperative antithrombin III activities and lipoprotein concentrations as predictors of venous thrombosis in patients with fracture of neck of femur. J. Clin. Pathol. 36:570, 1983.
154. Winter, J.H., Buckler, P.W., Bautista, A.P., et al.: Frequency of venous thrombosis in patients with an exacerbation of chronic obstructive lung disease. Thorax 38:605, 1983.
155. Ezekowitz, M.D., Eichner, E.R., Scatterday, R., et al.: Diagnosis of a persistent pulmonary embolus by indium-111 platelet scintigraphy with angiographic and tissue confirmation. Am. J. Med. 72:839, 1982.
156. Sostman, H.D., Neumann, R.D., Loke, J., et al.: Detection of pulmonary embolism in man with ^{111}In-labeled autologous platelets. AJR 138:945, 1982.
157. Poskitt, K.R., Payne, M.N., Lane, I.F., et al.: Radiolabeled platelets in detecting the source of recurrent pulmonary emboli: A case report. Angiology 38:62, 1987.
158. Uchida, Y., Minoshima, S., Anzai, Y., et al.: A case of pulmonary embolism diagnosed by ^{111}In-labeled platelet scintigraphy. Kaku Igaku 27:869, 1990.
159. Davis, H.H., Siegel, B.A., Sherman, L.A., et al.: Scintigraphy with ^{111}In-labeled autologous platelets in venous thromboembolism. Radiology 136:203, 1980.
160. Stratton, J.R.: Platelet kinetics and imaging of prosthetic materials. *In* Heyns, A.D., Badenhorst, P.N., and Lotter, M.G. (eds.): Platelet Kinetics and Imaging. Vol. 2. Boca Raton, CRC Press, 1985, pp. 21–44.
161. Agarwal, K.C., Wahner, H.W., Dewanjee, M.K., et al.: Imaging of platelets in right-sided extracardiac conduits in humans. J. Nucl. Med. 23:342, 1982.
162. Goldman, M., McCollum, C.N., Hawker, R.J., et al.: Dacron arterial grafts: The influence of porosity, velour, and maturity on thrombogenicity. Surgery 92:947, 1982.
163. Isaka, Y., Kimura, K., Etani, H., et al.: Imaging platelet deposition on Dacron bifurcation grafts in man: Quantification by a dual-tracer method using ^{111}In-labeled platelets and ^{99m}Tc-labeled human serum albumin. Eur. J. Nucl. Med. 11:386, 1986.
164. Kotze, H.F., Pieters, H., Heyns, A.D., et al.: Quantification of the thrombogenicity of Dacron aortic prostheses. S. Afr. J. Surg. 24:65, 1986.
165. Stratton, J.R., Thiele, B.L., and Ritchie, J.L.: Natural history of platelet deposition on Dacron aortic bifurcation grafts in the first year after implantation. Am. J. Cardiol. 52:371, 1983.
166. Robicsek, F., Duncan, G.D., Anderson, C.E., et al.: Indium-111–labeled platelet deposition in woven and knitted Dacron bifurcated aortic grafts with the same patient as a clinical model. J. Vasc. Surg. 5:833, 1987.
167. Ortenwall, P., Wadenvik, H., Kutti, J., et al.: Endothelial cell seeding reduces thrombogenicity of Dacron grafts in humans. J. Vasc. Surg. 11:403, 1990.
168. Goldman, M., Hall, C., Dykes, J., et al.: Does ^{111}indium-platelet deposition predict patency in prosthetic arterial grafts? Br. J. Surg. 70:635, 1983.
169. Zwas, S.T., Walden, R., Elkanovitz, R., et al.: Simplified assessment of arterial graft patency using indium-labelled–platelet scintigraphy. Nucl. Med. Commun. 8:727, 1987.
170. Yui, T., Uchida, T., Matsuda, S., et al.: Detection of platelet consumption in aortic graft with ^{111}In-labeled platelets. Eur. J. Nucl. Med. 7:77, 1982.
171. Kohler, T.R., Stratton, J.R., Kirkman, T.R., et al.: Conventional versus high-porosity polytetrafluoroethylene grafts: Clinical evaluation. Surgery 112:901, 1992.
172. Zilla, P., Fasol, R., Deutsch, M., et al.: Endothelial cell seeding of polytetrafluoroethylene vascular grafts in humans: A preliminary report. J. Vasc. Surg. 6:535, 1987.
173. Sicard, G.A., Allen, B.T., Long, J.A., et al.: Prostaglandin production and platelet reactivity of small-diameter grafts. J. Vasc. Surg. 1:774, 1984.
174. Seeger, J.M., and Klingman, N.: Improved in vivo endothelialization of prosthetic grafts by surface modification with fibronectin. J. Vasc. Surg. 8:476, 1988.
175. Seeger, J.M., and Klingman, N.: Improved endothelial cell seeding with cultured cells and fibronectin-coated grafts. J. Surg. Res. 38:641, 1985.
176. Ortenwall, P., Wadenvik, H., and Risberg, B.: Reduced platelet deposition on seeded versus unseeded segments of expanded polytetrafluoroethylene grafts: Clinical observations after a 6-month follow-up. J. Vasc. Surg. 10:374, 1989.
177. Ortenwall, P., Wadenvik, H., Kutti, J., et al.: Reduction in deposition of indium-111–labeled platelets after autologous endothelial cell seeding of Dacron aortic bifurcation grafts in humans: A preliminary report. J. Vasc. Surg. 6:17, 1987.
178. Koveker, G.B., Graham, L.M., Burkel, W.E., et al.: Extracellular matrix preparation of expanded polytetrafluoroethylene grafts seeded with endothelial cells: Influence on early platelet deposition, cellular growth, and luminal prostacyclin release. Surgery 109:313, 1991.
179. Fasol, R., Zilla, P., Deutsch, M., et al.: Human endothelial cell seeding: Evaluation of its effectiveness by platelet parameters after one year. J. Vasc. Surg. 9:432, 1989.
180. Allen, B.T., Long, J.A., Clark, R.E., et al.: Influence of endothelial cell seeding on platelet deposition and patency in small-diameter Dacron arterial grafts. J. Vasc. Surg. 1:224, 1984.
181. Bearn, P.E., McCollum, C.N., and Greenhalgh, R.M.: The influence of collagen and albumin presealants on knitted Dacron grafts. Eur. J. Vasc. Surg. 7:271, 1993.
182. Ritchie, J.L., Lindner, A., Hamilton, G.W., et al.: ^{111}In-oxine platelet imaging in hemodialysis patients: Detection of platelet deposition at vascular access sites. Nephron 31:333, 1982.
183. Hope, A.F., Heyns, A.D., Lotter, M.G., et al.: Kinetics and sites of sequestration of indium-111–labeled human platelets during cardiopulmonary bypass. J. Thorac. Cardiovasc. Surg. 81:880, 1981.
184. Kawata, H., Matsuda, H., Isaka, Y., et al.: Imaging analysis of platelet deposition on the extracardiac valved conduit in humans. ASAIO Trans. 35:190, 1989.
185. Schmidt, K.G., and Rasmussen, J.W.: Scintigraphic visualization of haemostatic and thromboembolic processes using ^{111}In-labelled platelets. Acta Med. Scand. 215:173, 1984.
186. Goldman, M.D., Simpson, D., Hawker, R.J., et al.: Aspirin and dipyridamole reduce platelet deposition on prosthetic femoro-popliteal grafts in man. Ann. Surg. 198:713, 1983.
187. Lane, I.F., Lumley, P., Michael, M.F., et al.: A specific thromboxane receptor blocking drug, AH23848, reduces platelet deposition on vascular grafts in man. Thromb. Haemost. 64:369, 1990.
188. Sinzinger, H., O'Grady, J., Fitscha, P., et al.: Effect of epoprostenol on platelet deposition on synthetic arterial grafts. Lancet 2:1212, 1984.
189. Pieters, H., Roodt, J.P., Badenhorst, P.N., et al.: Antithrombotic activity of Bay u3405, a thromboxane A_2-antagonist, in patients with Dacron aortic grafts: A random controlled clinical trial. Thromb. Haemost. 70:903, 1993.
190. Stratton, J.R., and Ritchie, J.L.: Failure of ticlopidine to inhibit deposition of indium-111–labeled platelets on Dacron prosthetic surfaces in humans. Circulation 69:677, 1984.
191. Stratton, J.R., and Ritchie, J.L.: The effect of sulfinpyrazone on platelet deposition on Dacron vascular grafts in man. Am. Heart J. 109:453, 1985.
192. Knight, L.C.: Scintigraphic methods for detecting vascular thrombus. J. Nucl. Med. 34:554, 1993.
193. Tait, J.F., Cerqueira, M.D., Dewhurst, T.A., et al.: Evaluation of annexin V as a platelet-directed thrombus targeting agent. Thromb. Res. 75:491, 1994.
194. Stratton, J.R., Dewhurst, T.A., Kasina, S., et al.: Selective uptake of radiolabeled annexin V on acute porcine left atrial thrombi. Circulation 1995 (in press).
195. Cerqueira, M.D., Stratton, J.R., Vracko, R., et al.: Noninvasive arterial thrombus imaging with ^{99m}Tc monoclonal antifibrin antibody. Circulation 85:298, 1992.
196. Rosebrough, S.F., Kudryk, B., Grossman, Z.D., et al.: Radioimmunoimaging of venous thrombi using iodine-131 monoclonal antibody. Radiology 156:515, 1985.
197. Knight, L.C., Maurer, A.H., Ammar, I.A., et al.: Technetium-99m antifibrin Fab′ fragments for imaging venous thrombi: Evaluation in a canine model. Radiology 173:163, 1989.
198. Rosebrough, S.F., Grossman, Z.D., McAfee, J.G., et al.: Aged venous thrombi: Radioimmunoimaging with fibrin-specific monoclonal antibody. Radiology 162:575, 1987.
199. Wasser, M.N., Koppert, P.W., Arndt, J.W., et al.: An antifibrin monoclonal antibody useful in immunoscintigraphic detection of thrombi. Blood 74:708, 1989.
200. DeFaucal, P., Peltier, P., Planchon, B., et al.: Evaluation of indium-111–labeled antifibrin monoclonal antibody for the diagnosis of venous thrombotic disease. J. Nucl. Med. 32:785, 1991.
201. Wasser, M.N., Pauwels, E.K., and Nieuwenhuizen, W.: Thrombus detection using

a ^{99m}Tc-labeled antifibrin monoclonal antibody (MoAb): Experiments in vitro and in animals. Thromb. Res. Suppl. 10:91, 1990.
202. Koblik, P.D., DeNardo, G.L., and Berger, H.J.: Current status of immunoscintigraphy in the detection of thrombosis and thromboembolism. Semin. Nucl. Med. 19:221, 1989.
203. Alavi, A., Palevsky, H.I., Gupta, N., et al.: Radiolabeled antifibrin antibody in the detection of venous thrombosis: Preliminary results. Radiology 175:79, 1990.
204. Aronen, H.: Diagnosis of deep venous thrombosis of the leg using immunoscintigraphy with indium-111–labelled monoclonal antifibrin antibody fragments. Acta Radiol. 30:159, 1989.
205. Jung, M., Kletter, K., Dudczak, R., et al.: Deep vein thrombosis: Scintigraphic diagnosis with indium-111–labeled monoclonal antifibrin antibodies. Radiology 173:469, 1989.
206. Lusiani, L., Zanco, P., Visona, A., et al.: Immunoscintigraphic detection of venous thrombosis of the lower extremities by means of human antifibrin monoclonal antibodies labeled with indium-111. Angiology 40:671, 1989.
207. Cadroy, Y., and Hanson, S.R.: Effects of red blood cell concentration on hemostasis and thrombus formation in a primate model. Blood 75:2185, 1990.
208. Knight, L.C.: Imaging thrombi with radiolabelled fragment E1. Nucl. Med. Commun. 9:849, 1988.
209. Knight, L.C., Maurer, A.H., Robbins, P.S., et al.: Fragment E1 labeled with I-123 in the detection of venous thrombosis. Radiology 156:509, 1985.
210. Knight, L.C., Abrams, M.J., Schwartz, D.A., et al.: Preparation and preliminary evaluation of technetium-99m–labeled fragment E1 for thrombus imaging. J. Nucl. Med. 33:710, 1992.
211. Knight, L., Olexa, S., Malmud, L., et al.: Specific uptake of radioiodinated fragment E1 by venous thrombi in pigs. J. Clin. Invest. 72:2007, 1983.
212. Miller, D.D., Boulet, A.J., Tio, F.O., et al.: In vivo technetium-99m S12 antibody imaging of platelet alpha-granules in rabbit endothelial neointimal proliferation after angioplasty. Circulation 83:224, 1991.
213. Palabrica, T.M., Furie, B.C., Konstam, M.A., et al.: Thrombus imaging in a primate model with antibodies specific for an external membrane protein of activated platelets. Proc. Natl. Acad. Sci. U.S.A. 86:1036, 1989.
214. Hnatowich, D.J., Virzi, F., Doherty, P.W., et al.: Characterization of indium-111–labeled recombinant tissue plasminogen activator for the imaging of thrombi. Eur. J. Nucl. Med. 13:467, 1987.
215. Ord, J.M., Hasapes, J., Daugherty, A., et al.: Imaging of thrombi with tissue-type plasminogen activator rendered enzymatically inactive and conjugated to a residualizing label. Circulation 85:288, 1992.
216. Uehara, A., Isaka, Y., Etani, H., et al.: Binding of ^{131}I-labeled tissue-type plasminogen activator on de-endothelialized lesions in rabbits. Nuklearmedizin 26:224, 1987.
217. Harker, L., and Hanson, S.: Experimental arterial thromboembolism in baboons: Mechanism, quantitation, and pharmacologic investigation. J. Clin. Invest. 64:559, 1979.
218. Claudiani, F., Bellotti, P., Strada, P., et al.: Semiquantitative imaging of left ventricular thrombi with ^{111}In-oxine–labelled platelets. J. Nucl. Med. Allied Sci. 31:287, 1987.
219. Kimura, M., Ojima, K., Tsuda, T., et al.: Indium-111-oxine–labeled platelet scintigraphy for detection of intracardiac and intravascular thrombi. J. Cardiogr. 13:499, 1983.
220. Stratton, J.R., and Resnick, A.D.: Increased embolic risk in patients with left ventricular thrombi. Circulation 75:1004, 1987.
221. Stratton, J.R.: Common causes of cardiac emboli: Left ventricular thrombi and atrial fibrillation. West. J. Med. 151:172, 1989.
222. Stratton, J.R.: Chronic left ventricular thrombi: Embolic potential and therapy. G. Ital. Cardiol. 24:269, 1994.
223. Benichou, M., Camilleri, J.F., Bernard, P.J., et al.: Comparison of two-dimensional echocardiography with scanography and indium-111 platelet scintigraphy in detection of intracardiac thrombi. Acta Cardiol. 43:93, 1988.
224. Funke-Kupper, A.J., Verheugt, F.W., Jaarsma, W., et al.: Detection of ventricular thrombosis in acute myocardial infarction: Value of indium-111 platelet scintigraphy in relation to two-dimensional echocardiography and clinical course. Eur. J. Nucl. Med. 12:337, 1986.
225. Ikeoka, K., Todo, Y., Konishiike, A., et al.: Scintigraphic detection of thrombi using indium-111–labeled autologous platelets. J. Cardiogr. 15:67, 1985.
226. Tsuda, T., Kubota, M., Iwakubo, A., et al.: Availability of ^{111}In-labeled platelet scintigraphy in patients with postinfarction left ventricular aneurysm. Ann. Nucl. Med. 3:15, 1989.
227. Branchereau, A., Bernard, P.J., Ciosi, G., et al.: Indium-111 platelet scintigraphy in carotid disease. Ann. Vasc. Surg. 2:215, 1988.
228. Henningsen, H., Kessler, C., Bihl, H., et al.: Detection of carotid thrombi with indium-111 platelet scintigraphy. Acta Radiol. Suppl. 369:14, 1986.
229. Isaka, Y., Handa, N., Imaizumi, M., et al.: Effect of TRK-100, a stable orally active prostacyclin analogue, on platelet function and plaque size in atherothrombotic strokes. Thromb. Haemost. 65:344, 1991.
230. Isaka, Y., Kimura, K., Uehara, A., et al.: Platelet aggregability and in vivo platelet deposition in patients with ischemic cerebrovascular disease: Evaluation by indium-111–platelet scintigraphy. Thromb. Res. 56:739, 1989.
231. Kachel, R., Endert, G., Reiss-Zimmermann, U., et al.: ^{111}In-thrombocyte scintigraphy and percutaneous transluminal dilatation (angioplasty) of supra-aortic vascular stenoses: A new method for deciding therapy and for follow-up control. Rofo Fortschr. Geb. Rontgenstr. Nuklearmed. 145:336, 1986.
232. Kessler, C., Reuther, R., and Rösch, M.: Dual isotope carotid scintigraphy in patients with amaurosis fugax attacks. Eur. Arch. Psychiatry Neurol. Sci. 234:106, 1984.
233. Kessler, C., Hipp, M., Langkau, G., et al.: Platelet scintigraphy findings in carotid thrombosis following whiplash trauma of the cervical spine. Nervenarzt 58:428, 1987.
234. Sinzinger, H., Silberbauer, K., Fitscha, P., et al.: Value of the detection of arteriosclerotic lesions with labeled autologous thrombocytes. Acta Med. Austriaca 9:181, 1982.
235. Joubert, J., Pilloy, W.J., vanReenen., O.R., et al.: Use of indium-111–labelled platelets in black stroke patients: A pilot study. S. Afr. Med. J. 77:246, 1990.
236. Allard-Latour, G., Schlama, S., Aubran, M., et al.: Contribution of complementary examinations in the diagnosis and treatment of emboligenic cardiopathies: Retrospective study apropos of 46 cases. Arch. Mal. Coeur Vaiss. 78:1249, 1985.
237. Meek, A.C., Chidlow, A., Lane, I.F., et al.: Platelet kinetics following carotid endarterectomy: The effect of aspirin and patch angioplasty. Eur. J. Vasc. Surg. 2:99, 1988.
238. Serradimigni, A., Bernard, P.J., B'enichou, M., et al.: Detection of arterial thrombi using blood platelets labeled with indium-111. Arch. Mal. Coeur Vaiss. 79:1766, 1986.
239. Etani, H., Kimura, K., Isaka, Y., et al.: Platelet accumulation in abdominal aortic aneurysms and the effect of antiplatelet drugs: Assessment by indium platelet scintigraphy. Kaku Igaku 29:651, 1992.
240. Mukaiyama, H., Shionoya, S., Ikezawa, T., et al.: Abdominal aortic aneurysm complicated with chronic disseminated intravascular coagulopathy: A case of surgical treatment. J. Vasc. Surg. 6:600, 1987.
241. Fitscha, P., Kaliman, J., and Sinzinger, H.: Is gamma-camera imaging of platelet deposition useful to assess the effectiveness of prostacyclin treatment? Biomed. Biochim. Acta 43:S403, 1984.
242. Forstrom, L., Thorpe, P., Weir, E.K., et al.: Detection of an abdominal aneurysm by indium-111 platelet imaging. Clin. Nucl. Med. 10:683, 1985.
243. Fenech, A., Hussey, J.K., Smith, F.W., et al.: Diagnosis of aortic aneurysm using autologous platelets labelled with indium-111. B.M.J. 282:1020, 1981.
244. Maruyama, M., Asai, T., Kuriyama, Y., et al.: Positive platelet scintigram of a vertebral aneurysm presenting thromboembolic transient ischemic attacks. Stroke 20:687, 1989.
245. Hill-Zobel, R.L., Pyeritz, R.E., Scheffel, U., et al.: Kinetics and distribution of ^{111}In-labeled platelets in patients with homocystinuria. N. Engl. J. Med. 307:781, 1982.
246. Sinzinger, H., Virgolini, I., and Fitscha, P.: Platelet kinetics in patients with atherosclerosis. Thromb. Res. 57:507, 1990.
247. Sinzinger, H., O'Grady, J., and Fitscha, P.: Platelet deposition on human atherosclerotic lesions is decreased by low-dose aspirin in combination with dipyridamole. J. Int. Med. Res. 16:39, 1988.
248. Fenech, A., Dendy, P.P., Hussey, J.K., et al.: Indium-111–labelled platelets in diagnosis of leg-vein thrombosis: Preliminary findings. B.M.J. 280:1571, 1980.
249. Grice, G.D., Smith, R.B., Robinson, P.H., et al.: Primary popliteal venous aneurysm with recurrent pulmonary emboli. J. Vasc. Surg. 12:316, 1990.
250. Clarke-Pearson, D.L., Coleman, R.E., Petry, N., et al.: Postoperative pelvic vein thrombosis and pulmonary embolism detected by indium-111–labeled platelet imaging: A case report. Am. J. Obstet. Gynecol. 149:796, 1984.
251. Winter, J.H., Fenech, A., Mackie, M., et al.: Treatment of venous thrombosis in antithrombin III deficient patients with concentrates of antithrombin III. Clin. Lab. Haematol. 4:101, 1982.
252. Wakefield, T.W., Shulkin, B.L., Fellows, E.P., et al.: Platelet reactivity in human aortic grafts: A prospective, randomized midterm study of platelet adherence and release products in Dacron and polytetrafluoroethylene conduits. J. Vasc. Surg. 9:234, 1989.
253. Knight, L., Lister-James, J., Dean, R.T., et al.: Evaluation of Tc-99m-labeled cyclic peptides for thrombus imaging. (Abstract.) J. Nucl. Med. 34(Suppl.):17P, 1993.
254. Knight, L.C., Radcliffe, R., Maurer, A.H., et al.: Thrombus imaging with technetium-99m synthetic peptides based upon the binding domain of a monoclonal antibody to activated platelets. J. Nucl. Med. 35:282, 1994.
255. Muto, P., Lastoria, S., Varrella, P., et al.: Detecting deep venous thrombosis with technetium-99m labeled synthetic peptide P280. J. Nucl. Med 36:1384, 1995.
256. DeBruyn, V.H., Bergmann, S.R., Keyt, B.A., et al.: Visualization of thrombi in pulmonary arteries with radiolabeled, enzymatically inactivated tissue-type plasminogen activator. Circulation 92:1320, 1995.

CHAPTER

68 Imaging the Cardiac Autonomic Nervous System

Gary D. Hutchins, Ph.D.
Douglas P. Zipes, M.D.

The autonomic nervous system helps regulate the chronotropic, dromotropic, and inotropic responses necessary to maintain normal cardiovascular performance under extremely diverse physiologic conditions. Disruption of the excitatory and inhibitory balance of the autonomic system may be responsible, at least in part, for decreased performance and rhythm disturbances in a variety of cardiac disorders, including coronary artery disease, hypertrophy, cardiomyopathy, and electrophysiologic disturbances in apparently normal hearts. With the development of radiopharmaceuticals selectively targeted to measure specific neuronal processes, powerful new scintigraphic approaches have been established to investigate noninvasively the role of the autonomic nervous system in normal physiology and its failure in disease. Radiopharmaceuticals have been developed for use with conventional nuclear medicine imaging systems (planar and single-photon emission computed tomography [SPECT]) as well as for positron emission tomography (PET). This chapter describes the validation and application of radiopharmaceuticals to probe the function of the autonomic nervous system with conventional nuclear imaging systems. A detailed presentation of PET imaging applications is described in Chapter 73 and summarized in reference 1.

AUTONOMIC NERVOUS SYSTEM PRINCIPLES

The autonomic nervous system regulates chronotropic, dromotropic, and inotropic responses of the heart through two main subdivisions: the sympathetic and the parasympathetic nervous systems.[2] The sympathetic system provides excitatory stimulation and increases the heart rate, shortens the conduction time of several fiber types, and increases the force of ventricular contraction.[3] In contrast, the parasympathetic system tends to exert the opposite effects. Each of these systems affects control through the synthesis, storage, and release of neurotransmitters that interact with receptor sites on cardiomyocytes and neurons. The primary neurotransmitter of the sympathetic system is norepinephrine, and in the parasympathetic system it is acetylcholine.[4] The sympathetic nerve fibers travel along the arterial vasculature on the heart surface and penetrate into the ventricular myocardium, analogous to the coronary artery distribution.[5] High concentrations of norepinephrine are observed throughout the human heart, suggesting a high density of innervation with a small innervation gradient, extending from the base to the apex of the left ventricle (Fig. 68–1).[5]

Parasympathetic innervation, as assessed by the levels of choline acetyltransferase,[6] is highest in the atria, followed by the atrioventricular node.[7] Parasympathetic innervation appears to be relatively sparse within the ventricles of the heart. In contrast with the patterns of sympathetic nerve fiber distribution in the ventricles, the parasympathetic fibers enter the ventricles at the epicardial surface with the sympathetic fibers but quickly penetrate the myocardium and appear to be distributed along the endocardial surfaces of the ventricles (see Fig. 68–1).[8]

The processes of neurotransmitter synthesis, release, and interaction in the autonomic nervous system are diagrammed in Figure 68–2. Norepinephrine is synthesized from tyrosine in the presynaptic nerve terminals of the sympathetic system by a series of chemical reactions.[9, 10] Each neuron of the sympathetic system has approximately 12 μg of norepinephrine contained in 25,000 vesicles.[11] On nerve stimulation, a small number of the vesicles exocytose and release their contents into the synapse between the presynaptic terminal and the postsynaptic cardiomyocytes. The potential fate of the released norepinephrine is threefold. First, it can bind to pre- or postsynaptic adrenergic receptors on the surface of neurons or cardiomyocytes, producing an inhibitory or a stimulatory effect. Second, it can be rapidly returned to the presynaptic nerve terminal by the uptake-1 transport system, in which its action is terminated by conversion to 3,4-hydroxymandelic acid by monoamine oxidase (MAO) or vesicular storage. Third, it can diffuse into the vascular space of the heart and be removed from the myocardium by blood flow, in which it is converted to normetanephrine by catechol-*O*-methyltransferase.[12] Only small amounts of norepinephrine bind to receptor sites or spill over into the venous blood.

Approximately 75 percent of the norepinephrine released is rapidly returned to the presynaptic nerve terminal via the reuptake mechanism and stored for rerelease. In a manner analogous to the function of the sympathetic neurons, parasympathetic neurons synthesize acetylcholine from choline and store the product in vesicles for release via nerve stimulation. After release, however, acetylcholine has a very short period of action because of the high levels of acetylcholinesterase in the heart, which rapidly inactivate the neurotransmitter through hydrolysis.[13]

The primary function of the autonomic nervous system, the regulation of heart rate and contractility, is mediated to a large extent by postsynaptic β-receptors located on effector cells. Two specific types of β-receptor have been classified, based on the action produced through stimulation.[13] They are β_1-receptors, responsible for mediation of cardiac stimulation and lipolysis, and β_2-receptors, responsible for mediation of vascular and bronchial smooth muscle relaxation.[14] Most of the β-receptors found in the heart are of the β_1 subtype.[15–17] The β_1-receptors are predominantly located in close proximity to adrenergic synapses, whereas β_2-receptors tend to be located in a position remote from the synapses.[18] As a consequence, β_1-receptors appear to respond primarily to synaptically released norepinephrine, and β_2-receptors to circulating catecholamines (primarily, epinephrine).

Adrenergic neurons also express a variety of presynaptic receptors. The primary role of these receptors is the regulation of the rate of release of norepinephrine into the synaptic cleft.[13] External control of norepinephrine release, by the parasympathetic nervous system, occurs when acetylcholine interacts with adrenergic presynaptic muscarinic receptors. Feedback control occurs when released norepinephrine interacts with either presynaptic α_2 (inhibitory) receptors or β (stimulatory) receptors of the adrenergic neuron.

SCINTIGRAPHIC ASSESSMENT OF SYMPATHETIC INNERVATION

Ideally, noninvasive imaging methods would permit investigation of both presynaptic and postsynaptic processes throughout the autonomic nervous system. With an appropriate combination of tracer probes, one would expect that a complete picture of the mechanisms responsible for life-threatening dysfunction in cardiac disorders could be discerned. Unfortunately, radiopharmaceuticals suitable for routine imaging of each component of the autonomic system have not been developed and validated. At the present time, the majority of scintigraphic studies performed with conventional nuclear imaging systems have examined the distribution and function of the presynaptic nerve terminals of the sympathetic nervous system. A very small number of studies were devoted to the measurement of postsynaptic receptor distributions. In the sections that follow, specific emphasis is placed on the description of the validation and application of scintigraphic methods for the study of the presynaptic sympathetic nervous system.

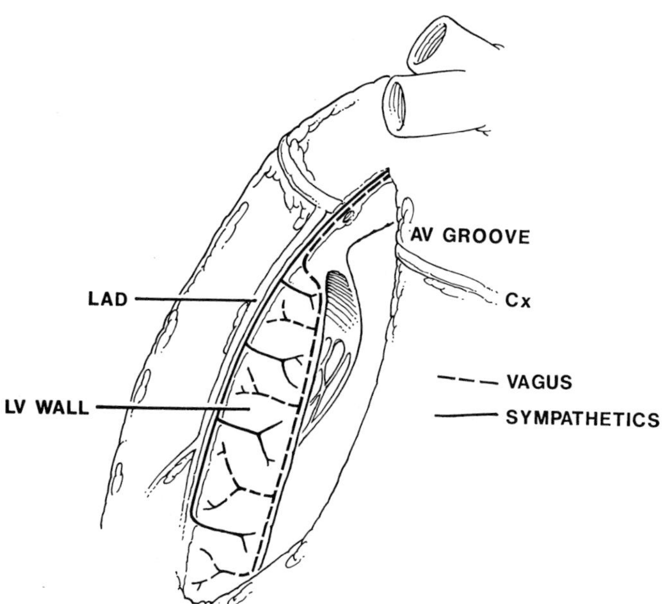

FIGURE 68–1. Patterns of autonomic innervation in the left ventricle. Sagittal view of the left ventricle wall showing the pathways of the afferent and efferent sympathetic and vagal nerve fibers. The sympathetic nerves tend to travel along the epicardial surface of the heart, and the vagal nerves travel along the endocardial surface.

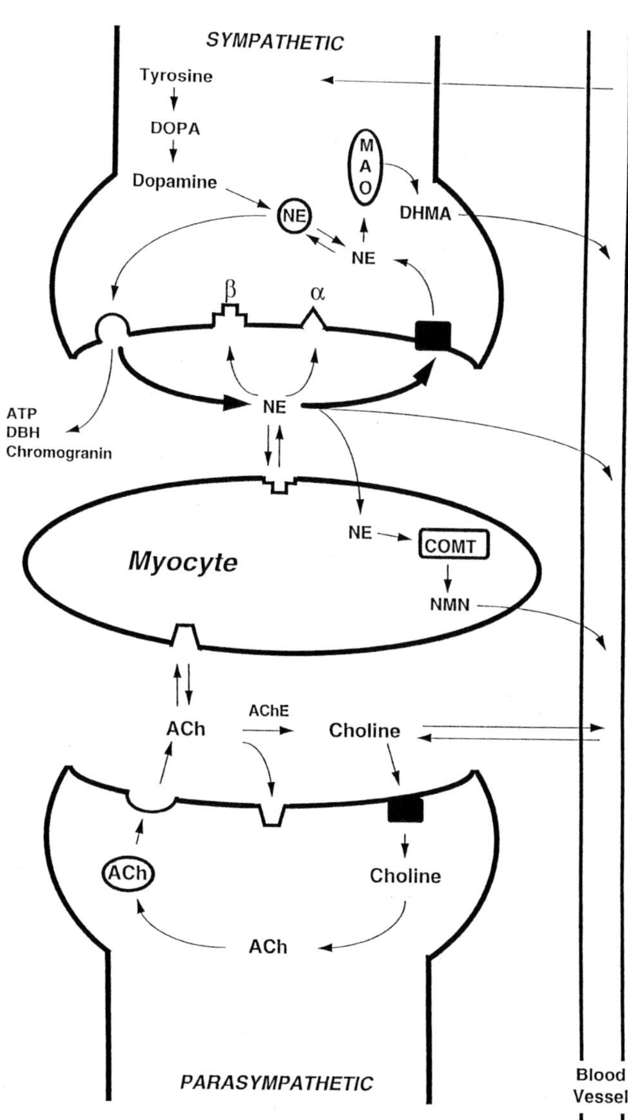

FIGURE 68–2. Autonomic nervous system. The mechanisms involved in the biosynthesis, release, receptor binding, reuptake, and metabolism of the two primary neurotransmitters of the autonomic nervous system are shown. Norepinephrine is derived from tyrosine in sympathetic nerve terminals, and acetylcholine is generated from choline in parasympathetic terminals. Control of cardiac chronotropic, dromotropic, and inotropic responses is produced by neurotransmitter interactions on effector cells (myocytes). Presynaptic receptors provide feedback control of the neurotransmitter release rates. All the processes diagrammed in the figure are potential targets for radiopharmaceutical-based imaging studies. NE = norepinephrine; MAO = monoamine oxidase; COMT = catechol-*O*-methyltransferase; ACh = acetylcholine; AChE = acetylcholinesterase; NMN = normetanephrine; DHMA = 3,4-dihydroxymandelic acid; DBH = dopamine-β-hydroxylase.

Radiolabeled Tracers

Studies designed to evaluate the autonomic nervous system of the heart with scintigraphic imaging techniques have been based on radiolabeled analogs of the "false neurotransmitter" guanethidine. In the early 1960s, bretylium and guanethidine were shown to interfere selectively with adrenergic neuron function.[19] These observations, and the development by medicinal chemists of related compounds with even higher potencies for interaction in the adrenergic system, stimulated the development of radioiodinated forms of substituted aralkyl guanidines for human imaging studies.[20–22] These compounds share the same mechanisms as those used for the uptake, storage, and release of the endogenous neurotransmitter norepinephrine. As implied by the categorization of false neurotransmitters, these compounds have a greatly diminished ability to stimulate postsynaptic excitation through receptor interactions. The guanethidine analog used for the scintigraphic evaluation of sympathetic innervation is metaiodobenzylguanidine (MIBG) with radioiodine incorporated into the phenyl ring.[22] A comparison of the chemical structures of norepinephrine, guanethidine, and MIBG is shown in Figure 68–3.

Imaging studies of adrenergic β-receptors have been limited by the availability of radiopharmaceuticals with specific localization on β-receptors in the heart. Radiolabeled forms of both pindolol[23] and iodocyanopindolol[24] have been studied. However, these compounds have limited applications as imaging agents because of high levels of nonspecific binding (pindolol) or significant pulmonary uptake (iodocyanopindolol) impairing the interpretation of cardiac tracer uptake. Studies of both β- and muscarinic receptor systems with PET-based radiopharmaceuticals have been much more successful (see Chapter 73).

Experimental Validation Studies

Numerous experimental studies have been performed to validate the capability of MIBG to map the distribution and function of presynaptic adrenergic neurons. These studies include (1) comparison of MIBG biodistribution with endogenous catecholamine levels, (2) selective pharmacologic blocking of cellular and vesicular uptake transport mechanisms, (3) pharmacologic and experimental sympathectomies, (4) MIBG turnover rates as a function of sympathetic system activity or tone, (5) correlation of MIBG uptake with myocardial electrophysiology, and (6) MIBG studies in experimental disease models. Collectively, these studies provide convincing evidence for the highly specific accumulation and storage of MIBG by the same mechanisms responsible for the storage of endogenous catecholamines. A summary of the important observations in each of these categories is provided below.

Metaiodobenzylguanidine Biodistribution

Initial studies of the biodistribution of iodobenzylguanidine compounds were performed by Wieland and colleagues[21] in the early 1980s by measuring tracer uptake at a series of time points after the intravenous injection of iodine-125 (^{125}I)–labeled MIBG in three species (rats, dogs, and primates). These initial studies demonstrated striking similarity between the uptake of MIBG in the heart and the endogenous distribution of norepinephrine.

Careful distribution studies in rat hearts by Matsunari and associates[25] demonstrate significant regional variation in MIBG uptake, with doses of 0.45 and 0.30 percent kg dose per g accumulating in the right and left ventricles, respectively. Within the left ventricle, uptake in the endocardial wall (0.32 percent kg dose per g) was greater than in the epicardial wall (0.25 percent kg dose per g). These observations are consistent with the known distribution of adrenergic neurons in the left ventricle of the mammalian heart.[5]

Glowniak and co-workers[26] demonstrated that MIBG is specific for the norepinephrine transporter by studying uptake in cell lines that were transfected with DNA encoding the human norepinephrine transporter. A ninefold increase in MIBG uptake was observed in transfected cell lines, compared with that of cells that did not express this system. Cells transfected with other transporter systems did not show enhanced accumulation of MIBG.

Shiga and colleagues[27] examined the distribution and clearance of MIBG in normal subjects ($n = 12$). Single-photon emission computed tomography images were obtained both early and late after the administration of MIBG, and the regional accumulation, expressed as the ratio of heart-to-mediastinum uptake, was measured in the anterior, septal, inferior, and lateral walls. With the exception of the inferior wall, the uptake of MIBG was uniform in both the immediate and the late images. The results of this study, as well as results from other studies in control subjects, are summarized in Table 68–1. Regional clearance rates for the four walls of the left ventricle were also calculated (see Table 68–1). The regional clearance rate was significantly higher in the inferior and lateral walls than in the anterior or septal regions. In a related study of the distribution of MIBG uptake in humans, Gill and associates[28] examined young subjects with supraventricular tachycardia and older control subjects. Results similar to the observations made by Shiga and colleagues were obtained (see Table 68–1).[27] Figure 68–4 shows an example of the uniformity of ^{123}I-labeled MIBG and thallium-201 (^{201}Tl) uptake in a normal subject.

The biodistribution data and studies of cellular uptake transport systems reviewed here support the hypothesis of neuronal accumulation of MIBG. However, these data alone do not demonstrate the relationship between the fate of MIBG in the neuron and endogenous catecholamines, nor do they provide evidence of this relationship in dysfunctional sympathetic nerves.

Pharmacologic Inhibition of Cellular and Vesicular Transport Mechanisms

Studies of the extraction fraction of MIBG in the heart of pigs have helped clarify the mechanisms responsible for the accumulation of MIBG in myocardium.[29] The extraction fraction of MIBG in the normal heart averaged 0.79. Following pharmacologic vasodilation that increased myocardial blood flow by a factor of 1.46, the extraction fraction dropped to 87 percent of the control value. Administration of agents that should inhibit neuronal uptake of MIBG, namely, cocaine and imipramine, produced either no change or a small increase in extraction fraction (7 percent), respectively.[29] These studies indicate that the initial extraction of MIBG into the heart is governed primarily by diffusion of the tracer into the extravascular space and probably is not regulated by neuronally mediated processes. However, once the MIBG has entered the extravascular space of the myocardial tissue, it diffuses back out into the vascular space and is removed from the tissue by blood flow, diffuses across cell membranes and enters the cytoplasm, or is transported by a carrier system into the cellular cytoplasm. Therefore, the fate of MIBG appears to be similar to that of norepinephrine. Unlike norepinephrine, MIBG is not a substrate for catechol-*O*-methyltransferase or MAO and, therefore, is not

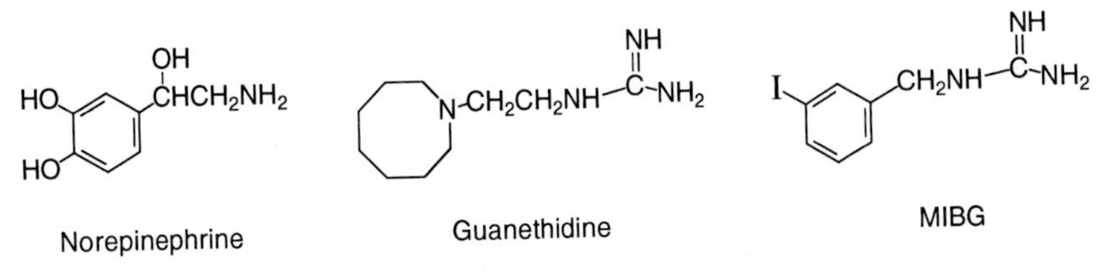

FIGURE 68–3. Chemical structures. The chemical structure for the endogenous catecholamine norepinephrine is compared to the structure of the "false transmitters" guanethidine and MIBG. The site for radioiodination of MIBG on the phenyl ring is indicated in the chemical structure.

TABLE 68–1. MYOCARDIAL MIBG DISTRIBUTION

Region	MIBG Uptake (Delayed Images)				% Washout
	Lerch et al.[88*]	*Gohl et al.*[84*]	*Gill et al.*[28†]	*Shiga et al.*[27‡]	*Shiga et al.*[27]
Anterior	88.8 ± 6.1	86.1 ± 4.2	100 ± 12.3	100 ± 0	25.1 ± 4.6
Septal	79.4 ± 6.1	81.6 ± 11.5	79.7 ± 16.2	96.8 ± 9.6	22.5 ± 8.2
Inferior	80.5 ± 2.6	86.1 ± 6.7	90.6 ± 15.8	79.4 ± 8.3	29.7 ± 8.3
Lateral	83.5 ± 5.5	84.1 ± 6.4	81.5 ± 36.4	99.1 ± 7.9	29.3 ± 3.4
Basal	80.9 ± 6.1	83.7 ± 8.2	88.5 ± 21.0	100 ± 0	26.5 ± 5.9
Mid	87.3 ± 4.9	87.7 ± 5.8	88.7 ± 21.0	103.9 ± 4.5	27.0 ± 4.6
Apical	76.2 ± 5.2	72.2 ± 12.9	88.0 ± 19.6	96.8 ± 15.2	28.3 ± 6.2

*Average polar map segments.
†Regional count data normalized by anterior wall uptake.
‡Heart-to-mediastinum ratios normalized to anterior wall.

metabolized appreciably in the heart.[30] After pretreatment with the uptake-1 inhibitor desmethylimipramine, a significant reduction in MIBG uptake in rat heart that qualitatively corresponded with the level of ^{3}H-norepinephrine uptake in the same animals was observed.[31] However, the reduction in ^{3}H-norepinephrine levels was significantly greater than the MIBG reduction after treatment with desmethylimipramine (94 versus 50 percent). These differences may indicate that a non-negligible amount of MIBG enters the presynaptic neuron by diffusion.

Pretreatment of cells expressing the human norepinephrine transporter with desipramine, mazinol, or elevated norepinephrine concentrations produced a 94, 97, and 87 percent inhibition of MIBG uptake, respectively.[26] It has also been shown that elevated levels of circulating catecholamines partially inhibit MIBG uptake in human subjects.[32] These studies provide additional evidence for the accumulation of MIBG within adrenergic neurons of the heart.

The intraneuronal fate of MIBG has been examined by blocking vesicular uptake with reserpine and measuring changes in the level of accumulated MIBG. Wieland and co-workers[30] showed that administration of 1 mg/kg of reserpine with an intramuscular injection in dogs 4 hours prior to MIBG administration produced a 30 percent reduction in uptake at 2 hours after tracer injection. In a similar study, a reduction of MIBG uptake in rat hearts after administration of reserpine to approximately 37 percent of control levels was observed.[25] In this study, a reduction in the differential endocardial-epicardial uptake relative to normal hearts was observed. These pharmacologic blocking studies provide further evidence for specific neuronal localization of MIBG via the transport

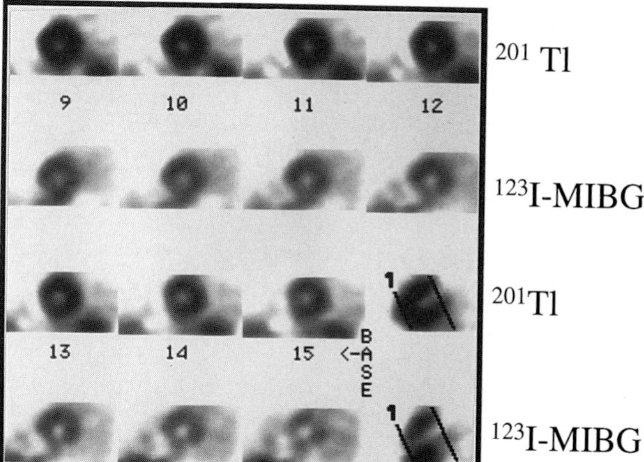

FIGURE 68–4. ^{123}I-MIBG and ^{201}Tl in the normal human heart. The images represent long-axis views of the left ventricle. Images were acquired 4 hours after injection of ^{123}I-MIBG. Uniformity of uptake reflects the relatively homogeneous distribution of presynaptic nerve terminals throughout the left ventricle.

mechanisms that accumulate and store endogenous catecholamines. However, it is also clear that the neuronal fate of MIBG and norepinephrine in myocardial tissue is not identical. Further study is necessary to determine whether these differences are caused by the relative affinities of MIBG and norepinephrine for metabolic enzymes and transport carrier sites, differences in hydrophilicity and lipophilicity, or a combination of these factors.

Pharmacologic and Experimental Sympathectomies

Three approaches have been adopted to produce sympathetically denervated myocardial tissue to study the specificity of MIBG uptake. These approaches include (1) 6-hydroxydopamine administration to chemically degenerate sympathetic nerves, (2) phenol application to the epicardial surface of the heart to destroy sympathetic fibers, and (3) transection of sympathetic nerve fibers proximal to the heart by cardiac transplantation or selective cutting of the stellate ganglia to produce global or regional denervation, respectively. Chemical denervation studies that used 6-hydroxydopamine (100 mg/kg) have been performed in rats by Sisson and colleagues.[31] They observed globally decreased uptake of ^{3}H-norepinephrine (12 percent of control) and ^{125}I-MIBG (31 percent of control) after denervation. The endogenous norepinephrine concentration in these same animals fell to 9 percent of the control concentration. Dae and associates[33] performed MIBG studies in dogs 1 week after the administration of 6-hydroxydopamine, 50 mg/kg. Early (5-minute) and late (3-hour) images showed good myocardial localization in all dogs studied at baseline. However, the studies performed after 6-hydroxydopamine MIBG administration showed good early uptake but failed to show any myocardial MIBG localization at 3 hours. The endogenous norepinephrine concentration in these dogs fell to 6 percent of the control animal concentrations.

Dae and co-workers[34] performed another series of studies in which regional denervation was created by the application of phenol or via removal of the left or right stellate ganglion. Imaging studies in normal hearts showed uniform perfusion (measured with ^{201}Tl) and uniform uptake of MIBG. Left and right stellectomies produced MIBG uptake defects, in the presence of normal ^{201}Tl uptake, in the posterior and anterior left ventricles, respectively. Hearts treated with phenol showed a broad area of reduced MIBG uptake that extended beyond the territory of phenol application. All hearts showed normal ^{201}Tl uptake in the regions of decreased MIBG uptake. Significant reductions in endogenous norepinephrine concentration in the areas of MIBG defects confirmed neuronal dysfunction or denervation.

Metaiodobenzylguanidine Turnover Rates Versus Sympathetic Activity or Tone

The presynaptic nerve terminals of the autonomic nervous system regulate both the uptake and the release of endogenous catecholamines. An ideal tracer of the adrenergic system, therefore, could provide information about the integrity and distribution of the nervous system as well as about stimulation rate, or "tone," of the system. Sisson and colleagues[31] have examined the washout rate of MIBG in animals, using both pharmacologic manipulation and physiologic stimulation of sympathetic tone. In each of these studies, MIBG was administered to the animal and allowed to accumulate for 2 hours. In one group of rats, the sympathomimetic drug, phenylpropanolamine, was administered at 2 hours after MIBG injection (4 doses of 50 mg/kg given every 15 minutes). The concentrations of MIBG and ^{3}H-labeled norepinephrine fell to 47 and 63 percent of the control values, respectively. In this same study, the washout rate of MIBG from the heart was compared in fed (food being known to simulate sympathetic activity) and fasted rats. The halftime for the washout of MIBG was significantly shorter in the fed rats (6 hours) than in the fasted rats (10.3 hours). These results are consistent with similar studies based on norepinephrine loss in fed ($T\frac{1}{2}$ = 12.8 hours) and fasted ($T\frac{1}{2}$ = 23.6 hours) rats.

The sympathetic tone of the heart can also be regulated through the administration of α_2-adrenergic receptor agonist and antagonists. Sisson and colleagues[35] performed a series of studies in rats and dogs to examine the washout of both ^{3}H-labeled norepinephrine and MIBG under control conditions, after stimulation of the adrenergic system with the α_2-receptor antagonist yohimbine, and following inhibition of the adrenergic system with the α_2-receptor agonist, clonidine. The rate of loss of MIBG was greater than that of ^{3}H-labeled norepinephrine under control conditions, was nearly identical with increased sympathetic tone, and was greater for MIBG (with both washout rates approaching zero) with inhibition of sympathetic activity. These results were reproduced in humans in a subsequent study.[36]

The results of these studies provide important evidence for the capability to assess the rate of stimulation in the adrenergic system of the heart on the basis of MIBG washout rates. Coupling the information provided by washout of the tracer (sympathetic tone) with evaluation of sympathetic system integrity or distribution based on MIBG uptake, an overall assessment of the presynaptic function of the sympathetic nervous system can be made.

Correlation of Metaiodobenzylguanidine Uptake With Cardiac Electrophysiology

It is clear that the studies described previously demonstrate the ability of MIBG imaging to measure disruption of presynaptic uptake of catecholamines as well as infer the rate of sympathetic tone in regions of the heart with normal uptake. However, those studies do not provide any information about the functional implications in regions of the heart that do not accumulate MIBG.

Several studies have been performed to address this issue. Minardo and associates[37] performed MIBG and ^{201}Tl scintigraphy after epicardial phenol application or transmural myocardial infarction produced by latex injection into the coronary arteries. The defects observed in the scintigraphic images were compared with the electrophysiologic responses obtained during sympathetic stimulation or after norepinephrine infusion. In both the phenol and the infarct models, regions of MIBG defects with normal ^{201}Tl uptake were observed. With ansae subclavia stimulation, the effective refractory period shortening in the regions of the apical MIBG defects was less than that in the basal regions with normal MIBG uptake. However, after the infusion of norepinephrine, the effective refractory period shortened more at the denervated apex than at the base, demonstrating both viable myocardium capable of responding to the sympathetic stimulation in the apex and a supersensitivity phenomenon, presumably caused by the lack of normal sympathetic stimulation. In another set of dogs in Minardo and associates' study, normalization of sympathetic function occurred after approximately 14 weeks. However, the supersensitivity to norepinephrine in the apex persisted.

Mori and colleagues[38] also studied the functional implication of MIBG uptake defects in dogs generated by phenol application, by measuring contractile response with ultrasonic crystals during stellate stimulation, tyramine infusion, and isoproterenol infusion. In studies performed 1 to 2 hours after phenol application, MIBG uptake and tissue norepinephrine levels were normal. Contractile response, however, was diminished. Animals studied 3 to 7 days after the application of phenol showed decreased MIBG uptake, which corresponded with decreased endogenous norepinephrine concentrations. Neither stellate ganglion stimulation nor intracoronary tyramine infusion produced any augmentation in contractile function. However, these regions maintained a response to β-receptor stimulation by isoproterenol.

In a more recent study, Newman and associates[39] examined the correlation between electrophysiology and MIBG uptake in dogs with experimentally produced infarction. In this study, the area of the MIBG defect always exceeded the ^{201}Tl perfusion defect produced by coronary artery occlusion followed by ligation. During constant ventricular pacing in these animals, stellate ganglion stimulation significantly shortened the epicardial monophasic action potential duration at 50 percent repolarization in innervated areas, compared with that of areas demonstrating MIBG defects.

Metaiodobenzylguanidine Studies in Experimental Disease Models

Studies of MIBG uptake in myocardial infarction, in addition to those studies previously discussed, have focused on the relationship between the size of the MIBG defect relative to ^{201}Tl perfusion defects and recovery of sympathetic function in peri-infarct zones. Sisson and co-workers[40] created myocardial infarcts in 12 dogs and compared the size of MIBG and ^{201}Tl defects on scintigraphic images. The MIBG defects were regularly larger than the defects observed on the ^{201}Tl images and were consistent with endogenous norepinephrine concentrations in ex vivo measurements.

Barber and associates[41] first demonstrated that transmural myocardial infarction sympathetically denervated noninfarcted, otherwise normal myocardium. They used studies of functional response to sympathetic neural stimulation, myocardial norepinephrine concentrations, and tissue histofluorescence to identify denervation. Minardo and colleagues[37] were the first to image these denervated regions with MIBG. Nishimura and associates[42] studied acute myocardial infarction with ^{201}Tl and MIBG in dogs. In studies performed at 6 hours, 1 week, 4 weeks, and 6 weeks following infarction, the MIBG-^{201}Tl uptake defect size ratios were 1.0 ± 0.04, 2.48 ± 0.15, 1.88 ± 0.14, and 1.61 ± 0.12, respectively. In this study, the norepinephrine content in all regions of the heart fell during the first week after infarction. By week 6, the control areas of the heart returned to normal norepinephrine levels, the norepinephrine content in peri-infarct zones significantly increased, and no improvement was observed in the infarct zones. Consistent with the observations of Minardo and co-workers,[37] these results suggest either the recovery of function or the reinnervation of previously dysfunctional sympathetic systems.

Inoue and Zipes[43] showed that a nontransmural infarction spared the sympathetic fibers because they were localized in the subepicardium. In another study with dogs, Dae and colleagues[44] produced both transmural and nontransmural infarcts and compared MIBG and ^{201}Tl image patterns with tissue norepinephrine content and histofluorescence microscopic findings in biopsy samples. Transmural infarction produced MIBG uptake defects adjacent and distal to the ^{201}Tl defects. Denervation in these regions was confirmed by reduction in norepinephrine content and the absence of nerve fluorescence. With nontransmural infarcts, the areas of the ^{201}Tl defect and MIBG defect were matched, with minimal apparent sympathetic involvement outside of the infarct area. As with the transmural infarcts, norepinephrine content and nerve fluorescence studies demonstrated denervation in the regions showing reduced MIBG uptake.

Miyazaki and Zipes[45] demonstrated that short periods of coronary occlusion preconditioned the myocardium to withstand the effects of prolonged total occlusion, with preservation of sympathetic and vagal neural function. Nohara and colleagues[46] produced stunned myocardium in dogs with short periods of ischemia and imaged the uptake of MIBG. With up to 40 minutes of ischemia, MIBG uptake remained normal, which was consistent with the previously described observation of Dae and associates.[44] MIBG uptake decreased in this study as the tissue progressed from ischemic to the development of infarction. MIBG uptake also showed a linear relationship with wall motion.

Dysfunction of the sympathetic nervous system in cardiomyopathy has also been studied, using MIBG in animal models. Wakasugi and co-workers[47, 48] performed studies on rats to monitor the induction of cardiomyopathy as a result of doxorubicin (Adriamycin) administration. Animals were treated with 2 mg/kg doxorubicin once per week for up to 9 weeks. The studies in mice showed normal uptake in the myocardium during the first 2 weeks of treatment, with a progressive decline in MIBG uptake during the period between 4 and 8 weeks of treatment. After 8 weeks of treatment, the MIBG uptake was 18 and 14 percent of control values in the right and left ventricles, respectively. Histopathologic studies showed some correlation between regions of myocyte damage and sympathetic denervation. However, sympathetic denervation was observed in regions of apparently normal myocytes. Studies of left ventricular ejection fraction in the same animals with gated blood pool imaging did not show a decline until 7 weeks of therapy, followed by a very rapid decline in function over the final 2 weeks of the study. These results suggest that sympathetic denervation due to administration of doxorubicin precedes functional changes in the heart.

Finally, recent data show that direct-current shocks delivered to the epicardium of the heart can cause sympathetic dysfunction for 3 hours or more.[49] Preliminary studies in humans (unpublished) suggest that a similar event can occur in patients with implantable defibrillators.

Summary

The studies of MIBG uptake in animals and control human subjects reviewed in this section demonstrate the close relationship that exists between the kinetics of MIBG in the heart and function of the sympathetic nervous system. The accumulation of MIBG is highly correlated with the functional status of presynaptic sympathetic neurons and, in many cases, failure to accumulate MIBG represents sympathetic denervation. In addition, regions with minimal MIBG accumulation demonstrated electrophysiologic abnormalities and impaired contractility in response to sympathetic stimulation. Based on the studies described previously, it is also evident that the rate of MIBG washout in normal tissue corresponds with the level of sympathetic activity in the heart, suggesting that MIBG may be useful for measuring the functional status as well as the distribution of adrenergic neurons. However, because denervation and functional impairment are presumably both characterized by increased MIBG washout rates, differentiating partial denervation and dysfunction in cardiac disorders remains a significant challenge. Nonetheless, these studies provide an important framework, demonstrating the validity of MIBG imaging in human cardiac disorders.

Clinical Studies

In many reports, MIBG imaging in human subjects parallels the animal studies just presented. Studies have been performed in patients with both regional and global denervation resulting from a heterogeneous group of cardiac disorders. In these studies, good correspondence between electrophysiologic abnormalities and regional MIBG accumulation defects has been observed. In this section, we present an overview of the characteristics of MIBG uptake and washout in a variety of cardiac conditions that lead to apparent sympathetic denervation.

Coronary Artery Disease and Myocardial Infarction

Studies of MIBG uptake in myocardial infarction have focused primarily on the relationship between the size of the MIBG and perfusion defects. In the acute stage after infarction, numerous studies have confirmed the initial observations of Stanton and colleagues[50] demonstrating defects in MIBG uptake that exceed the volume of the perfusion defect imaged with ^{201}Tl or technetium-99m (^{99m}Tc) sestamibi.[51–67] It is apparent in these studies that the abnormality in adrenergic function is more extensive with anterior wall infarction than in other regions of the heart. Figure 68–5 shows an example of the mismatch between MIBG and ^{201}Tl uptake in a patient studied in the authors' laboratory. In a subset of the studies examining patients in the chronic stage after myocardial infarction, evidence of recovery or reinnervation of the sympathetic system is evident. In paired MIBG-^{201}Tl SPECT studies performed between 1 week and 8 months after myocardial infarction, five of six patients demonstrated partial sympathetic reinnervation. The reinnervation occurred within 2 months in four patients and within 6 months in one patient. Interestingly, the time frame of this reinnervation is consistent with the heightened risk of lethal arrhythmias during the initial 6 months after myocardial infarction.[60] In a similar study, Nishimura and associates[61] observed recovery of sympathetic catecholamine uptake in 7 of 14 patients studied at 86 days, on the average, after myocardial infarction. The remaining subjects in this study showed no improvement in the MIBG defect. In another related study by Guertner and co-workers,[63] MIBG and sestamibi imaging studies performed in 16 patients with coronary artery disease before and after percutaneous transluminal angioplasty showed reinnervation in five subjects 3 to 4 months after therapy.

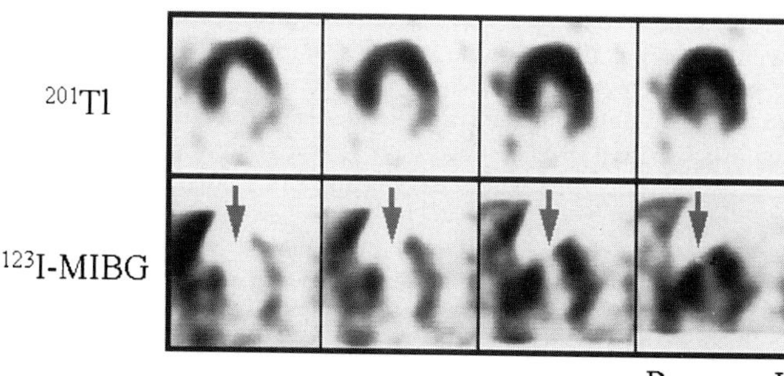

FIGURE 68–5. ^{123}I-MIBG and ^{201}Tl uptake after myocardial infarction. The images represent long-axis views of the left ventricle. Images were acquired at 4 hours after injection of ^{123}I-MIBG. A mismatch between ^{123}I-MIBG and ^{201}Tl uptake in the anterior wall of the left ventricle is readily apparent. The greater extent of the MIBG defect reflects sympathetic system dysfunction or denervation.

In a small number of studies, some evidence is provided to suggest that the regions of MIBG defect in peri-infarct zones with apparent preservation of perfusion are ischemically compromised regions of tissue. In a study by Terada and colleagues,[65] it was observed that exercise-induced perfusion defects in the areas of MIBG-perfusion mismatch at rest created a matched defect. However, this phenomenon is not observed in all subjects undergoing exercise. Based on the presented data, taken collectively, one may hypothesize that there exists an ischemic threshold for the production of irreversible damage for sympathetic neurons that is different from that for cardiomyocytes. This observation suggests that the regions of MIBG defect that extend beyond the perfusion defect or infarct are at least partially related to ischemic episodes in the tissue. Consistent with this suggestion is the observation of MIBG defects with normal ^{201}Tl uptake in patients with stunned myocardium.[68] This hypothesis is further supported by paired imaging studies of MIBG uptake and perfusion that demonstrate recovery of regional tissue perfusion and contractile function with persistent MIBG defects after successful therapy. Further quantitative studies are required to adequately test this hypothesis.

Heart Failure Studies

Over the past several years, a number of studies evaluating the function of the sympathetic nervous system in heart failure due to various causes have been investigated. These studies include patients with ischemic and idiopathic cardiomyopathy, left and right ventricular hypertrophy, diabetic neuropathy, and chemotherapeutic cardiotoxicity. Across this heterogeneous population of subjects, a consistent pattern of relatively normal or slightly reduced MIBG uptake was observed with a significantly increased rate of tracer washout from the myocardium. In addition, areas of MIBG defects with preserved perfusion were frequently observed.

In studies of subjects with dilated cardiomyopathy by Yamakado and colleagues[69] and Morozumi and associates,[70] initial MIBG uptake and washout rate were compared with those of control subjects. In Yamakado and colleagues' studies, the percentage decrease of myocardial MIBG at 3 hours was 46.9 ± 13.8 percent in 8 patients versus 18 ± 7.7 percent in control subjects. During the early phase of the study (15 to 45 minutes), the differences between the patient and the control washout rates were even greater (21.2 ± 7.5 percent in patients versus 5.3 ± 4.0 percent in control subjects). In these studies, the initial uptake of MIBG, as well as ^{201}Tl uptake and washout, showed no significant differences between the groups. Morozumi and co-workers examined the uptake and washout of MIBG in six patients with dilated cardiomyopathy and one patient with doxorubicin-induced cardiomyopathy. Consistent with the results of Yamakado and colleagues' studies, an enhanced washout rate was observed in the patients (58 ± 13 percent over 3 hours), compared to that in control subjects (33 percent over 3 hours [n = 2]). However, Morozumi and associates' study also demonstrated a reduction in the initial uptake (at 15 minutes after injection) of MIBG, relative to that of control subjects. Schofer and colleagues[71] also demonstrated a good correlation between MIBG uptake and myocardial norepinephrine concentration in patients with idiopathic dilated cardiomyopathy.

In an interesting study by Merlet and colleagues,[72] the prognostic value of MIBG imaging in patients suffering from either ischemic (n = 24) or idiopathic (n = 66) cardiomyopathy was compared with that of other noninvasive cardiac imaging indices. Analysis of these data showed that MIBG uptake was a better predictor of both survival and life duration than radionuclide left ventricular ejection fraction, x-ray cardiothoracic ratio, and echographic M-mode data. These results suggest that MIBG uptake may provide valuable information in the assessment of patients for cardiac transplantation. In a related study, Maeno and colleagues[73] performed MIBG and ^{201}Tl imaging studies in 17 patients with idiopathic dilated cardiomyopathy. Eleven patients had ventricular tachycardia, and six did not. Imaging studies performed at 15 minutes and 5 hours after injection showed a greater number of MIBG-^{201}Tl mismatches in the ventricular tachycardia group. These results are consistent with the observation of increased incidence of electrophysiologic distrubances in patients with large MIBG defects after myocardial infarction and suggest that regional sympathetic denervation is a possible factor in provoking ventricular tachycardia.[5]

Studies of MIBG uptake in hypertrophic cardiomyopathy have examined the uptake and washout of tracer with respect to the degree of wall thickness and electrophysiologic changes. Nakajima and associates[74] classified 29 hypertrophic cardiomyopathy patients into one of three categories: (1) those with wall thickness less than 16 mm, (2) those with wall thickness from 16 to 20 mm, and (3) those with wall thickness greater than 20 mm. The uptakes of both MIBG and ^{201}Tl were increased in the patients with more hypertrophic septa compared with those of control subjects. This increase in uptake could be explained by increased myocardial perfusion and/or reduction in the partial volume effect due to wall thickness. A consistent decrease in MIBG accumulation at 3 hours, corrected for flow, was observed as the myocardial wall became more hypertrophic. The perfusion-corrected uptake values were 0.69 ± 0.20, 0.50 ± 0.10, and 0.39 ± 0.23 for groups 1, 2, and 3, respectively. In addition, the regional MIBG clearance rate in the septum was significantly higher in group 3 than in group 1 (13 versus 1.5 percent per hour).

Shimizu and co-workers[75] studied 22 patients with hypertrophic cardiomyopathy and classified subjects according to serial electrophysiologic changes. Group A consisted of 15 patients with an increase in or appearance of a negative T wave, and group B consisted of 7 patients with a conduction disturbance or a decrease or disappearance of the negative T wave. An increase in the appearance of MIBG uptake defects was observed in group B relative to that of group A. In these studies, the areas of decreased activity or defects corresponded with the hypertrophied portion of the left ventricular wall. The MIBG defects were attributed to increased tracer washout rate, rather than to impaired uptake. The MIBG clearance rate was significantly higher in group B (0.25 ± 0.17) than in group A (0.10 ± 0.15) (expressed as early uptake minus late uptake divided by early uptake). A recent study in patients with left ventricular hypertrophy secondary to valvular stenosis demonstrated lower initial myocardial MIBG uptake and enhanced washout, compared to those of control subjects.

In a pair of studies in diabetic patients, the uptake and washout of MIBG and ^{201}Tl showed characteristics similar to those of patients in the cardiomyopathy and hypertrophy studies just discussed. Mantysaari and colleagues observed a decrease in initial uptakes of MIBG in patients with and without autonomic neuropathy, compared to those of control subjects.[76] Six hours after MIBG administration, the autonomic neuropathy group showed a larger reduction in tracer accumulation than the diabetic patients without neuropathy, when compared with that of control subjects. ^{201}Tl imaging appeared normal in these subjects. Katono and associates[77] examined the regional distribution of MIBG uptake in patients with or without diabetic neuropathy. In all subjects studied with neuropathy, MIBG defects were observed in the apical and inferior walls of the left ventricle. In addition, rapid clearance was observed in the apical and inferior regions of the heart in two of six cases without neuropathy. Again, no anatomical or perfusion defects were detected in these subjects.

The mechanisms responsible for the reduction in MIBG uptake in heart failure subjects were evaluated by Rabinovitch and co-workers.[78] They performed serial MIBG imaging in 33 volunteers, 10 orthotopic cardiac transplant patients, and 26 subjects with chronic mechanical overload of the left ventricle. The volunteer and transplant patient data were used to develop a mathematical model describing specific and nonspecific uptake of MIBG. Application of this compartmental model to analyze the chronic mechanical overload subjects suggests that the accelerated myocardial egress of tracer is due to a specific impairment in vesicular storage, rather than to a more rapid turnover of an intact vesicular pool.

Cardiac Transplantation

A small number of studies examining MIBG uptake in cardiac transplant subjects have been used to help assess the level of nonspecific accumulation of MIBG in the heart. Transection of the cardiac nerves in the process of removing a human heart produces global denervation of the sympathetic nervous system. MIBG imaging studies performed within a short period of time after a cardiac transplant show a dramatic reduction in tracer accumulation in the presence of normal perfusion. Dae and colleagues[33] performed imaging studies a mean of 4.3 months after transplantation and showed no uptake in either initial (5-minute) or delayed (3-hour) MIBG images. Studies performed in subjects approximately 6 months after transplantation by Gill and associates[28] also demonstrated a dramatic reduction in the myocardial uptake of MIBG.

In studies performed at later times after transplantation (1 to 1.5 years, on the average), results similar to those of the early transplant subjects were observed,[78, 79] namely, a marked reduction in initial uptake of MIBG, followed by a rapid washout of the tracer from the heart. In a study by Rabinovitch and co-workers,[78] the average accumulation of MIBG at 30 minutes after injection was only 21 percent of control values and fell to 9 percent by 2 hours. In another study of patients examined at approximately the same period of time after transplantation, the myocardial uptake of MIBG was approximately 13 percent that of control at 1 hour after injection and remained at the same fraction of control up to 4 hours after injection.[79]

In a more recent study, Dae and colleagues[80] have observed apparent reinnervation in 4 of 10 transplant patients studied for a mean of 13 months after surgery. Consistent with a recent PET study using ^{11}C-hydroxyephedrine, the pattern of reinnervation in these subjects appears confined to the anterior and basal segments of the heart.[81] However, this apparent reinnervation was observed only in patients with transplants performed more than 2 years before the PET imaging study.

Cardiotoxicity

Two reports of sympathetic system disruption measured with MIBG scintigraphy as a result of chemotherapy-induced cardiotoxicity in humans have been published.[82, 83] Morozumi and colleagues[82] described the enhanced washout of MIBG over 4 hours in a subject being treated with doxorubicin for breast cancer. At the time of the imaging study, the left ventricular ejection fraction in this subject was 22 percent. The initial uptake of MIBG and ^{201}Tl distributions were normal. In a more recent report, six patients with doxorubicin-related cardiotoxicity were studied with MIBG.[83] The washout rate of MIBG in this study appeared inversely related to the patients' ejection fraction. In four patients with severely decreased left ventricular ejection fractions, the 4-hour washout rate varied from 43 to 56 percent. Two patients with moderate cardiotoxicity had washout rates of 37 and 35 percent, respectively.

Electrophysiologic Abnormalities

Studies of the correlation between electrophysiologic disturbances of the heart and patterns of sympathetic innervation have been performed in a heterogeneous population of patients. To date, these studies include subjects with long QT syndrome, ventricular tachycardia in structurally normal hearts, cardiomyopathy, left ventricular hypertrophy, valvular disease, right ventricular disease, and myocardial infarction. In patients from families with long QT syndrome, MIBG studies revealed regional disruption of sympathetic system function.[84, 85] In a study by Gohl and associates,[84] the MIBG defects were observed primarily in the inferior and inferior septal regions of the left ventricle. In contrast to these observations, Muller and co-workers[85] observed MIBG uptake defects preferentially in the anterior and lateral walls of the left ventricle near the apex. In this study, MIBG uptake at 2 hours was reduced relative to that of controls (1.43 ± 0.13 versus 1.66 ± 0.15). The halftime values of MIBG washout from the left ventricle were significantly reduced in the long QT syndrome (6.4 ± 1.5 hours), compared to those of controls (16.7 ± 15.3 hours).

Apparent regional denervation is also observed in MIBG studies in subjects with structurally normal hearts.[86, 87] In a study by Gill and colleagues,[86] subjects studied with ventricular tachycardia, both related to and independent of exercise, had a high proportion of asymmetrical MIBG scans. In 75 percent of the patients with exercise-induced ventricular tachycardia, defects in MIBG uptake were observed in the septal wall of the left ventricle, except for one subject, who had a posterior wall defect. Similar defects were also observed in 28.6 percent of the patients with non–exercise-induced ventricular tachycardia.

Mitrani and associates[87] performed MIBG and ^{201}Tl imaging studies in 18 patients with ventricular tachycardia and compared the results with those of 12 control subjects with cardiomyopathy or structurally normal hearts and no evidence of ventricular tachycardia. Regional MIBG defects with normal ^{201}Tl uptake were observed in 67 percent of the patients with ventricular tachycardia. However, only 1 of 12 subjects (8.35 percent) without ventricular tachycardia had evidence of sympathetic dysfunction in the MIBG studies. In the nine patients with structurally normal hearts with ventricular tachycardia examined in this study, five had regional cardiac sympathetic denervation.

The influence of arrhythmogenic disease of the right ventricle on the innervation patterns in the left ventricle was examined in studies by Lerch and colleagues[88] and Wichter and associates.[89] In the study by Lerch and colleagues,[88] 25 patients with arrhythmogenic right ventricular disease of unknown origin were imaged with MIBG, and the results were compared to those of 7 control subjects. Regional reductions in MIBG uptake were observed in 22 of these subjects. The abnormal areas were located predominantly in posterior and posteroseptal segments of the heart. Thallium-201 studies were normal in 16 patients. The remaining nine patients showed areas of slight hypoperfusion correlated with the reduced MIBG uptake. In the study by Wichter and co-workers,[89] 48 patients with arrhythmogenic right ventricular cardiomyopathy were imaged with MIBG, and the results were compared with those of nine patients with idopathic ventricular tachycardia and seven control subjects without known cardiac disease. Regional MIBG defects were observed in the left ventricle in 40 (83 percent) of the arrhythmogenic right ventricular cardiomyopathy patients. In 38 of these 40 patients, the MIBG defect was located in the basal posteroseptal left ventricle, with involvement in the adjacent lateral wall in 10 subjects, the anterior wall in 2 subjects, and the apex in 12 patients. These studies nicely demonstrate that arrhythmogenic right ventricular disease can produce regional disruption of adrenergic function in the left ventricle. This regional disruption may also be responsible for the frequent incidence of ventricular arrhythmias in exercise or after catecholamine exposure.

Summary

When one compares the results obtained in the heterogeneous population of patients described above, some consistent observations become apparent. Subjects who present with MIBG defects in viable myocardial territories, as determined by perfusion, have a higher propensity for electrophysiologic disturbances than patients with matched MIBG-perfusion defects. It also becomes apparent that when larger regions of sympathetic denervation are observed, the likelihood of electrophysiologic dysfunction is greater. Unfortunately, the information provided by MIBG scintigraphy enables the assessment of only one component of the autonomic nervous system. To obtain a clear picture of the relationship between the distribution and volume of sympathetic denervation and electrophysiologic abnormalities, a more complete assessment of sympathovagal interactions and dysfunction must be available. Although the results obtained with MIBG imaging in cardiac disorders are exciting, it is clear that significant challenges remain before the relevance of information obtained from these studies can be accurately associated with the underlying pathophysiology.

CLINICAL INDICATIONS

It is clear from the discussion presented in this chapter that the information obtained from MIBG imaging provides a noninvasive evaluation of sympathetic nervous system function in clinical disorders observed in patients. The studies on the prognostic value of MIBG imaging and its usefulness as an indicator of survival and life duration by Merlet and colleagues[72] suggest that this technique may play a role in the management and selection of patients for cardiac transplantation. In addition, the small number of studies on cardiotoxicity suggest that MIBG may be an important indicator of cardiac damage caused by chemotherapy. In general, however, the clinical use of MIBG imaging techniques requires an enhanced understanding of the relevance of observed defects to development of cardiac arrhythmias and to the underlying remodeling of the heart that has occurred as a result of disease.[90] In the future, as myocardial remodeling becomes better understood and therapeutic methods for correcting these defects are developed, MIBG may play a very important role in defining the extent and nature of remodeling, as well as the effectiveness of therapeutic approaches.

FUTURE DIRECTIONS

The most important challenge at the present time for the noninvasive evaluation of the autonomic nervous system of the heart is the development of methods of examining vagal innervation. Radiopharmaceuticals developed to image the presynaptic nerve terminals of the parasympathetic system, coupled with imaging of the sympathetic system distribution and function, are expected to provide insight into the pathophysiology of the heart in disease, particularly regarding the development of arrhythmias and sudden cardiac death, and remodeling patterns that have a high likelihood of developing life-threatening events. In addition, the development of improved SPECT instrumentation capable of accurately measuring the kinetics of radiopharmaceuticals will enhance our understanding of the relationship between tracer behavior and function of the autonomic nervous system. With these continued developments, scintigraphic imaging will play an important role in future investigations of autonomic nervous system function and potentially aid the clinical management and therapy of patients with cardiac disorders.

References

1. Schwaiger, M., Hutchins, G., Allman, K., et al.: Neurocardiology: Is there a future for imaging? *In* Zaret, B., and Beller, G. (eds.): Nuclear Cardiology: State of the Art and Future Directions. St. Louis, Mosby Year Book, 1993.
2. Rossi, L.: Neuroanatomopathology of the cardiovascular system. *In* Kulbertus, H., and Franck, G. (eds.): Neurocardiology. Mt. Kisco, NY, Futura Publishing, 1988.
3. Levy, M.: Sympathetic-parasympathetic interactions in the heart. *In* Kulbertus, H., and Franck, G. (eds.): Neurocardiology. Mt. Kisco, NY, Futura Publishing, 1988.
4. Randall, W., and Ardell, J.: Functional anatomy of the cardiac efferent innervation. *In* Kulbertus, H., and Franck, G. (eds.): Neurocardiology. Mt. Kisco, NY, Futura Publishing, 1988.
5. Zipes, D.: Autonomic modulation and cardiac arrhythmias. *In* Zipes, D., and Jalife, J. (eds.): Cardiac Electrophysiology from Cell to Bedside. Philadelphia, W.B. Saunders, 1994.
6. Schmid, P., Greif, B., Lund, D., et al.: Regional choline acetyltransferase activity in the guinea pig heart. Circ. Res. 42:657, 1978.
7. Stanley, R., Conatser, J., and Dettbarn, W.D.: Acetylcholine, choline acetyltransferase and cholinesterases in the rat heart. Biochem. Pharmacol. 27:2409, 1987.
8. Takahashi, N., Barber, M., and Zipes, D.: Efferent vagal innervation of canine ventricle. Am. Physiol. Soc. 246:H89, 1985.
9. Goldstein, D., Chang, P., Eisenhofer, G., et al.: Positron emission tomographic imaging of cardiac sympathetic innervation and function. Circulation 81(5):1606, 1990.
10. Perth, W.: The nature of splenic sympathin. J. Physiol. 108:491, 1949.
11. Crout, J.: The uptake and release of ^{3}H-epinephrine by the guinea pig heart in vivo. Naunyn Schmiedebergs Arch. Pharmacol. 248:85, 1964.
12. Landsberg, L., and Young, J.: Catecholamines and the adrenal medulla. *In* Wilson, J., and Foster, D. (eds.): Williams' Textbook of Endocrinology. Philadelphia, W.B. Saunders, 1985.
13. Braunwald, E., Sonnenblick, E., and Ross, J.: Mechanisms of cardiac contraction and relaxation. *In* Braunwald, E. (ed.): Heart Disease: A Textbook of Cardiovascular Medicine. Philadelphia, W.B. Saunders, 1988.
14. Lands, A., Arnold, A., McAuliff, J., et al.: Differentiation of receptor systems activated by sympathomimetic amines. Nature 214:597, 1967.
15. Lefkowitz, R., Stadel, J., and Caron, M.: Adenylate cyclase-coupled beta-adrenergic receptors: Structure and mechanisms of activation and desensitization. Annu. Rev. Biochem. 52:159, 1983.
16. Watanabe, A.: Recent advances in knowledge about beta-adrenergic receptors: Application to clinical cardiology. J. Am. Coll. Cardiol. 1:82, 1983.
17. Homey, C., and Graham, R.: Molecular characterization of adrenergic receptors. Circ. Res. 56:635, 1985.
18. Willfart, B., Tummermans, P.B.M.W.M., and van Zwieten, P.A.: Extrasynaptic location of alpha-2 and non-innervated beta-2 adrenoceptors in the vascular system in the pithed normotensive rat. J. Pharmacol. Exp. Ther. 221:762, 1982.
19. Nickerson, M., and Collier, B.: Drugs inhibiting adrenergic nerves and structures innervated by them. *In* Goodman, L.S., and Gilman, A. (eds.): The Pharmacological Basis of Therapeutics. 5th ed. New York, Macmillan, 1975.
20. Short, J.H., and Darby, T.D.: Sympathetic nervous system blocking agents. III. Derivatives of benzylguanidine. J. Med. Chem. 10:833, 1967.
21. Wieland, D.M., Swanson, D.P., Brown, L.E., et al.: Imaging the adrenal medulla with a I-131-labeled antiadrenergic agent. J. Nucl. Med. 20:155, 1979.
22. Wieland, D.M., Wu, J.-L., Brown, L.E., et al.: Radiochemistry and radiopharmaceuticals: Radiolabeled adrenergic neuron-blocking agents: Adrenomedullary imaging with [^{131}I]iodobenzylguanidine. J. Nucl. Med. 21(4):349, 1980.
23. Hughes, B., Marshall, D.R., Sobel, B.E., et al.: Characterization of beta-adrenoreceptors in vivo with iodine-131 pindolol and gamma scintigraphy. J. Nucl. Med. 27:660, 1986.
24. Sisson, J., Wieland, D., Johnson, J., et al.: Portrayal of cardiac beta receptors in living animals. J. Am. Coll. Cardiol. 13:64A, 1989.
25. Matsunari, I., Bunko, H., Taki, J., et al.: Regional uptake of iodine-125-metaiodobenzylguanidine in the rat heart. Eur. J. Nucl. Med. 20(11):1104, 1993.
26. Glowniak, J.V., Kilty, J.E., Amara, S.G., et al.: Evaluation of metaiodobenzylguanidine uptake by the norepinephrine, dopamine and serotonin transporters. J. Nucl. Med. 34(7):1140, 1993.
27. Shiga, K., Sugihara, H., Inoue, T., et al.: The distribution and kinetics of ^{123}I-MIBG in normal human hearts. Jpn. J. Nucl. Med. 30(11):1359, 1993.
28. Gill, J.S., Hunter, G.J., Gane, G., et al.: Heterogeneity of the human myocardial sympathetic innervation: In vivo demonstration by iodine 123-labeled metaiodobenzylguanidine scintigraphy. Am. Heart J. 126(2):390, 1993.
29. Glowniak, J.V., Wilson, R.A., Joyce, M.E., et al.: Evaluation of metaiodobenzylguanidine heart and lung extraction fraction by first-pass analysis in pigs. J. Nucl. Med. 33(5):716, 1992.
30. Wieland, D.M., Brown, L.E., Rogers, W.L., et al.: Myocardial imaging with a radioiodinated norepinephrine storage analog. J. Nucl. Med. 22:22, 1981.
31. Sisson, J., Wieland, D., Sherman, P., et al.: Metaiodobenzylguanidine as an index of the adrenergic nervous system integrity and function. J. Nucl. Med. 28(10):1620, 1987.
32. Wafelman, A.R., Hoefnagel, C.A., Maes, R.A., et al.: Radioiodinated metaiodobenzylguanidine: A review of its biodistribution and pharmacokinetics, drug interactions, cytotoxicity and dosimetry. Eur. J. Nucl. Med. 21:545, 1994.
33. Dae, M.W., De Marco, T., Botvinick, E., et al.: Scintigraphic assessment of MIBG uptake in globally denervated human and canine hearts—implications for clinical studies. J. Nucl. Med. 33(8):1444, 1992.
34. Dae, M., O'Connell, J., Botvinick, E., et al.: Scintigraphic assessment of regional cardiac adrenergic innervation. Circulation 79(3):634, 1989.
35. Sisson, J.C., Bolgos, G., and Johnson, J.: Measuring acute changes in adrenergic nerve activity of the heart in the living animal. Am. Heart J. 121:1119, 1991.
36. Sisson, J.C., Shapiro, B., Meyers, L., et al.: Metaiodobenzylguanidine to map scintigraphically the adrenergic nervous system in man. J. Nucl. Med. 28(10):1625, 1987.
37. Minardo, J., Tuli, M., Mock, B., et al.: Scintigraphic and electrophysiological evidence of canine myocardial sympathetic denervation and reinnervation produced by myocardial infarction or phenol application. Circulation 78(4):1008, 1988.
38. Mori, H., Pisarri, T., Aldea, G., et al.: Usefulness and limitations of regional cardiac sympathectomy by phenol. Am. J. Physiol. 257:H1523, 1989.
39. Newman, D., Munoz, L., Chin, M., et al.: Effects of canine myocardial infarction on sympathetic efferent neuronal function: Scintigraphic and electrophysiologic correlates. Am. Heart J. 126(5):1106, 1993.
40. Sisson, J.C., Johnson, J., Bolgos, G., et al.: Portrayal of adrenergic denervation in the presence of myocardial infarction: A feasibility study. Am. J. Physiol. Imaging 5(4):151, 1990.
41. Barber, M., Mueller, T., Henry, D., et al.: Transmural myocardial infarction in the dog produces sympathectomy in noninfarcted myocardium. Circulation 67:787, 1983.
42. Nishimura, T., Oka, H., Sago, M., et al.: Serial assessment of denervated but viable myocardium following acute myocardial infarction in dogs using iodine-123 metaiodobenzylguanidine and thallium-201 chloride myocardial single photon emission tomography. Eur. J. Nucl. Med. 19(1):25, 1992.
43. Inoue, H., and Zipes, D.: Time course of denervation of efferent sympathetic and vagal nerves after occlusion of the coronary artery in the canine heart. Circ. Res. 62:1111, 1988.
44. Dae, M.W., Herre, J.M., O'Connell, J.W., et al.: Scintigraphic assessment of sympathetic innervation after transmural versus nontransmural myocardial infarction (see Comments). J. Am. Coll. Cardiol. 17(6):1416, 1991.
45. Miyazaki, T., and Zipes, D.: Protection against autonomic denervation following acute myocardial infarction by preconditioning ischemia. Circ. Res. 64:437, 1989.
46. Nohara, R., Kambara, H., Okkuda, K., et al.: Effects of cardiac sympathetic nervous system on the stunned myocardium: Experimental study with ^{123}I-metaiodobenzylguanidine. Jpn. Circ. J. (Engl. edition) 55(9):893, 1991.
47. Wakasugi, S., Wada, A., Hasegawa, Y., et al.: Detection of abnormal cardiac adrenergic neuron activity in adriamycin-induced cardiomyopathy with iodine-125-metaiodobenzylguanidine (see Comments). J. Nucl. Med. 33(2):208, 1992.
48. Wakasugi, S., Fischman, A.J., Babich, J.W., et al.: Metaiodobenzylguanidine: Evaluation of its potential as a tracer for monitoring doxorubicin cardiomyopathy. J. Nucl. Med. 34(8):1283, 1993.
49. Ito, M., Pride, H., and Zipes, D.: Defibrillating shocks delivered to the heart impair efferent sympathetic responsiveness. Circulation 88:2661, 1993.
50. Stanton, M.S., Tuli, M.M., Radtke, N.L., et al.: Regional sympathetic denervation after myocardial infarction in humans detected noninvasively using I-123-metaiodobenzylguanidine. J. Am. Coll. Cardiol. 14(6):1519, 1989.
51. Nishimura, T., Uehara, T., Oka, H., et al.: Serial assessment of denervated but viable myocardium following acute myocardial infarction by using ^{123}I-MIBG and ^{201}Tl-Cl myocardial SPECT (in Japanese). Kaku Igaku 27(7):709, 1990.
52. Nishimura, T., Uehara, T., Hayashida, K., et al.: Newly developed myocardial imaging by using single photon emission computed tomography (SPECT). Jpn. Circ. J. (Engl. edition) 54(3):328, 1990.
53. Satoh, K., Katoh, K., Murata, H., et al.: Assessment of ischemic damage of the cardiac sympathetic nerve function by semiquantitative analysis of ^{123}I-MIBG (metaiodobenzylguanidine)-SPECT—comparison with ^{201}Tl-Cl-SPECT (in Japanese). Kaku Igaku 27(8):821, 1990.
54. Morozumi, T., Ishida, Y., Tani, A., et al.: Myocardial adrenergic derangement due to myocardial ischemia: Decreased myocardial uptake of I-123 metaiodobenzylguanidine after PTCA in a patient with effort angina (in Japanese). Kaku Igaku 27(7):735, 1990.
55. McGhie, A.I., Corbett, J.R., Akers, M.S., et al.: Regional cardiac adrenergic function using I-123 meta-iodobenzylguanidine tomographic imaging after acute myocardial infarction. Am. J. Cardiol. 67(4):236, 1991.
56. Hirosawa, K., Tanaka, T., Hisada, K., et al.: Clinical evaluation of ^{123}I-MIBG for assessment of the sympathetic nervous system in the heart (multi-center clinical trial) (in Japanese). Kaku Igaku 28(5):461, 1991.
57. Tanaka, T., Aizawa, T., Kato, K., et al.: Interesting PYP, ^{201}Tl, MIBG, AM and

BMIPP myocardial SPECT images in a patient under successful reperfusion therapy (in Japanese). Kokyu To Junkan 40(6):609, 1992.
58. Tahara, Y., Taya, M., Nishimura, T., et al.: Assessment of denervated but viable myocardium in patients with myocardial infarction—by myocardial imaging with ^{201}Tl and ^{123}I-MIBG (in Japanese). Kokyu To Junkan 39(8):795, 1991.
59. Wharton, J.M., Friedman, I.M., Greenfield, R.A., et al.: Quantitative perfusion and sympathetic nerve defect size after myocardial infarction in humans. J. Am. Coll. Cardiol. 19(3):264A, 1992.
60. Mitrani, R., Burt, R.W., Klein, L.S., et al.: Regional cardiac sympathetic denervation and reinnervation following myocardial infarction in humans. (Abstract.) Circulation 86:I-247, 1992.
61. Nishimura, T., Uehara, T., Shimonagata, T., et al.: Assessment of myocardial viability by using newly developed myocardial SPECT imaging. Jpn. Circ. J. (Engl. edition) 56(6):603, 1992.
62. Tanaka, T., Aizawa, T., Katou, K., Ogasawara, K., et al.: Interesting PYP, Tl-201, MIBG and AM myocardial SPECT images in a patient under successful reperfusion therapy (in Japanese). Kaku Igaku 28(9):1099, 1991.
63. Guertner, C., Klepzig, H., Maul, F.D., et al.: Noradrenaline depletion in patients with coronary artery disease before and after percutaneous transluminal coronary angioplasty with iodine-123 metaiodobenzylguanidine and single-photon emission tomography. Eur. J. Nucl. Med. 20(9):776, 1993.
64. Spinnler, M.T., Lombardi, F., Moretti, C., et al.: Evidence of functional alterations in sympathetic activity after myocardial infarction. Eur. Heart J. 14(10):1334, 1993.
65. Terada, K., Sugihara, H., Taniguchi, Y., et al.: A case of acute coronary syndrome followed by ^{201}Tl, ^{123}I-BMIPP and ^{123}I-MIBG myocardial imagings before and after PTCA (in Japanese). Kaku Igaku 30(12):1459, 1993.
66. Lekakis, J., Antoniou, A., Vassilopoulos, N., et al.: I-123 metaiodobenzylguanidine–thallium-201 mismatch following myocardial infarction. Clin. Cardiol. 17(1):21, 1994.
67. Tanaka, T., Aizawa, T., Kato, K., et al.: Study of sympathetic nervous function under effort induced ischemia in patients with angina pectoris with I-123 metaiodobenzylguanidine (MIBG) myocardial SPECT images (in Japanese). Kaku Igaku 27(2):143, 1990.
68. Katoh, K., Nishimura, S., Nakanishi, S., et al.: Stunned myocardium and sympathetic denervation—clinical assessment using MIBG scintigraphy. Jpn. Circ. J. (Engl. edition) 55(9):919, 1991.
69. Yamakado, K., Takeda, K., Kitano, T., et al.: Serial change of iodine-123 metaiodobenzylguanidine (MIBG) myocardial concentration in patients with dilated cardiomyopathy. Eur. J. Nucl. Med. 19(4):265, 1992.
70. Morozumi, T., Ishida, Y., Tani, A., et al.: Clinical significance of I-123 MIBG myocardial scintigraphy for evaluating the severity of congestive heart failure (in Japanese). Kaku Igaku 28(3):271, 1991.
71. Schofer, J., Spielmann, R., Schuchert, A., et al.: Iodine-123 metaiodobenzylguanidine scintigraphy: A noninvasive method to demonstrate myocardial adrenergic nervous system disintegrity in patients with idiopathic dilated cardiomyopathy. J. Am. Coll. Cardiol. 12(5):1252, 1988.
72. Merlet, P., Valette, H., Dubois-Rande, J.-L., et al.: Prognostic value of cardiac metaiodobenzylguanidine imaging in patients with heart failure (see Comments). J. Nucl. Med. 33(4):471, 1992.
73. Maeno, M., Ishida, Y., Shimonagata, T., et al.: The significance of ^{201}Tl/^{123}I MIBG (metaiodobenzylguanidine) mismatched myocardial regions for predicting ventricular tachycardia in patients with idiopathic dilated cardiomyopathy (in Japanese). Kaku Igaku 30(10):1221, 1993.
74. Nakajima, K., Bunko, H., Taki, J., et al.: Quantitative analysis of ^{123}I-metaiodobenzylguanidine (MIBG) uptake in hypertrophic cardiomyopathy. Am. Heart J. 119(6):1329, 1990.
75. Shimizu, M., Sugihara, N., Kita, Y., et al.: Long-term course and cardiac sympathetic nerve activity in patients with hypertrophic cardiomyopathy. Br. Heart J. 67(2):155, 1992.
76. Mantysaari, M., Kuikka, J., Mustonen, J., et al.: Noninvasive detection of cardiac sympathetic nervous dysfunction in diabetic patients using [^{123}I]metaiodobenzylguanidine. Diabetes 41(9):1069, 1992.
77. Katono, E., Owada, K., Takeda, H., et al.: Usefulness of myocardial imaging by ^{123}I-MIBG in assessment of diabetic neuropathy (in Japanese). Kaku Igaku 30(10):1235, 1993.
78. Rabinovitch, M.A., Rose, C.P., Schwab, A.J., et al.: A method of dynamic analysis of iodine-123-metaiodobenzylguanidine scintigrams in cardiac mechanical overload hypertrophy and failure. J. Nucl. Med. 34(4):589, 1993.
79. Fagret, D., Wolf, J., Vanzetto, G., et al.: Myocardial uptake of metaiodobenzylguanidine in patients with left ventricular hypertrophy secondary to valvular aortic stenosis (see Comments). J. Nucl. Med. 34(1):57, 1993.
80. Dae, M.W., De Marco, T., Bovinick, E.H., et al.: MIBG uptake at one year post cardiac transplant—evidence for partial reinnervation in man. (Abstract.) J. Nucl. Med. 33:896, 1992.
81. Schwaiger, M., Hutchins, G., Kalff, V., et al.: Evidence for regional catecholamine uptake and storage sites in the transplanted human heart by positron emission tomography. J. Clin. Invest. 87:1681, 1991.
82. Morozumi, T., Ishida, Y., Tani, A., et al.: Gallium-67 myocardial imaging for the detection of adriamycin cardiomyopathy (in Japanese). Kaku Igaku 27(5):477, 1990.
83. Valdes Olmos, R., ten Bokkel Huinink, W., Greve, J., et al.: I-123 MIBG and serial radionuclide angiocardiography in doxorubicin-related cardiotoxicity. Clin. Nucl. Med. 17(3):163, 1992.
84. Gohl, K., Feistel, H., Weikl, A., et al.: Congenital myocardial sympathetic dysinnervation (CMSD)—a structural defect of idiopathic long QT syndrome. PACE Pacing Clin. Electrophysiol. 14:1544, 1991.
85. Muller, K.D., Jakob, H., Neuzner, J., et al.: ^{123}I-metaiodobenzylguanidine scintigraphy in the detection of irregular regional sympathetic innervation in long QT syndrome. Eur. Heart J. 14(3):316, 1993.
86. Gill, J.S., Hunter, G.J., Gane, J., et al.: Asymmetry of cardiac [^{123}I] metaiodobenzylguanidine scans in patients with ventricular tachycardia and a "clinically normal" heart. Br. Heart J. 69(1):6, 1993.
87. Mitrani, R.D., Klein, L.S., Miles, W.M., et al.: Regional cardiac sympathetic denervation in patients with ventricular tachycardia in the absence of coronary artery disease. J. Am. Coll. Cardiol. 22(5):1344, 1993.
88. Lerch, H., Bartenstein, P., Wichter, T., et al.: Sympathetic innervation of the left ventricle is impaired in arrhythmogenic right ventricular disease. Eur. J. Nucl. Med. 20(3):207, 1993.
89. Wichter, T., Hindricks, G., Lerch, H., et al.: Regional myocardial sympathetic dysinnervation in arrhythmogenic right ventricular cardiomyopathy. An analysis using ^{123}I-meta-iodobenzylguanidine scintigraphy. Circulation 89(2):667, 1994.
90. Zipes, D.P.: Sympathetic stimulation and arrhythmias. (Editorial.) N. Engl. J. Med. 325:656, 1991.

PART 8

POSITRON EMISSION TOMOGRAPHY

CHAPTER 69

Principles of Positron Emission Tomography

Heinrich R. Schelbert, M.D.

Positron emission tomography offers several unique advantages over conventional scintigraphic approaches for the noninvasive study of the human heart. The number of positron-emitting tracers available for exploring specific aspects of myocardial tissue function is virtually unlimited. The concentrations of these tracers in blood and in myocardium and their changes over time can be quantified noninvasively by static or by rapid serial imaging. The combination of the quantitative imaging capabilities with positron-emitting tracers of myocardial tissue function permits the application of tracer kinetic principles in vivo and, consequently, the noninvasive quantification of blood flow and substrate fluxes in human myocardium. With these capabilities, positron emission tomography offers the opportunity to examine and characterize directly in human myocardium biologic processes that previously had been defined in animal experiments only. Such opportunities should provide new insights into the physiology of the normal and diseased human heart and result in a more accurate definition and characterization of human myocardial disease.

This chapter describes the major components of positron emission tomography for the noninvasive study of myocardial tissue function. It examines currently used tracers as probes for various aspects of myocardial tissue function, describes methodologic aspects of positron emission tomography, reviews concepts of tracer compartment modeling, and finally describes how these various

Dr. Schelbert is affliated with The Laboratory of Biomedical and Environmental Sciences, operated for the U.S. Department of Energy by the University of California under Contract #DE-AC03-76-SF00012. This work was supported in part by the Director of the Office of Energy Research, Office of Health and Environmental Research, Washington, D.C., by Research Grants #HL 29845 and #HL 33177, National Institutes of Health, Bethesda, M.D., and by an Investigative Group Award by the Greater Los Angeles Affiliate of the American Heart Association, Los Angeles, CA.

components are combined for the quantitative assessment of regional myocardial tissue function.

POSITRON-EMITTING TRACERS FOR CARDIAC STUDIES

General Considerations

The tracers employed most commonly with positron emission tomography are labeled with positron-emitting isotopes of elements that are abundantly present in nature (Table 69–1). These radioisotopes are inserted into organic compounds without altering their structural and biologic properties. For example, despite insertion of a radioactive carbon-11 (^{11}C) atom, radiolabeled palmitate or acetate continue to behave like natural myocardial fuel substrates and are metabolized by myocardium in a fashion identical to that of their unlabeled "parents." Other positron-emitting isotopes—for example, nitrogen-13 (^{13}N) and oxygen-15 (^{15}O)—can similarly be inserted into numerous other organic substances. The availability of isotopes such as ^{11}C, ^{13}N, and ^{15}O, thus accounts for the large number of potentially useful tracers for positron emission tomography.[1] Only the rapid physical decay limits their number because it necessitates synthesis of tracer compounds within one or two physical half-lives and thus within usually less than 1 hour. Automated synthesis methods for routine production of high specific activity tracers have become available for several radiopharmaceuticals.

Generally, positron-emitting substances must meet several criteria to be suitable for positron emission tomography. First, they must clear from blood into the myocardium and be retained there at high concentrations for time periods long enough to permit external imaging. Second, their specific activity must be high so that they do not exert a mass effect and perturb the very process to be studied. Third, the externally measured signal—that is, the concentrations of radioactivity in tissues and their changes over time—must closely and predictably correspond to the physiologic process to be examined. The last requirement is especially important because images of myocardial tracer uptake provide information only on the activity concentrations of the radiolabel and do not yield information on the chemical species to which it is bound. Therefore, careful delineation of the relationships between the externally measured signal, the metabolic fate of the label, and the process under study is essential.

The labeled compounds currently used with positron emission tomography can be generally classified into tracers of blood flow, those of metabolism, and those of presynaptic and postsynaptic neuron activities.

TABLE 69–1. POSITRON-EMITTING ISOTOPES FOR CARDIAC STUDIES

Isotope	Physical Half-Life	Parent Isotope	Physical Half-Life
Cyclotron Produced			
Carbon-11	20.4 min	—	—
Fluorine-18	109.7 min	—	—
Nitrogen-13	9.96 min	—	—
Oxygen-15	2.07 min	—	—
Rubidium-81	4.58 hr	—	—
Potassium-38	7.60 min	—	—
Technetium-94m	53 min	—	—
Generator Produced			
Rubidium-82	1.26 min	Strontium-82	25 d
Gallium-68	68.1 min	Germanium-68	288 d
Copper-62	9.73 min	Zinc-62	9.2 hr

d = days.

TABLE 69–2. TRACERS OF MYOCARDIAL BLOOD FLOW AND THEIR MYOCARDIAL EXTRACTION PROPERTIES

Agent	Physical Half-Time	Flow-Extraction Relationship
^{11}C or ^{68}Ga-albumin microspheres	20.4 min	
^{15}O-water	2.07 min	$E = 0.96 \pm 0.05$
^{82}R	1.26 min	$E = 1 - 0.73e^{-0.59/F}$
^{13}N-ammonia	10.0 min	$E = 1 - 0.607e^{-1.25/F}$
^{64}Cu-PTSM	9.7 min	$E = 1 - 0.89e^{-0.45/F}$
^{94m}Tc-sestamibi	53 min	$E = 1 - 0.74e^{-0.30/F}$
^{94m}Tc-teboroxime	53 min	Not reported
^{11}C-alcohol	20.4 min	Not reported

E = first-pass extraction or retention fraction; F = myocardial blood flow.

Data for ^{15}O-water were obtained from Bergmann et al. (1984) in canine myocardium,[27] those for ^{82}Rb from Glatting et al. (1995),[41] those for ^{13}N-ammonia from Schelbert et al. (1981) in canine myocardium,[18] those for PTSM from Beanlands et al. (1992) in human myocardium,[59] and those for sestamibi from Marshall et al. (1990) in isolated rabbit hearts.[57] The relationship between blood flow and the first-pass extraction is described by a modified Renkin-Crone model (see text).

Tracers of Myocardial Blood Flow

General Principles

The tracers of blood flow are categorized generally into (1) particulate, and (2) diffusable, extractable tracers (Table 69–2). The ideal tracer of blood flow accumulates in or clears from myocardium in linear proportion to myocardial blood flow. The relationship between uptake and clearance of the tracer and blood flow should be constant and should be unaffected by blood flow itself, by the physiologic and pathophysiologic changes of the myocardial tissue state, and by myocardial metabolism. As discussed later, not all tracers of blood flow fully meet these requirements.

Tracers of blood flow share several common features. The concentration of a tracer in myocardium (Q_t) at time t after injection depends on several factors and can be described by the following:

$$Q_t = E \cdot F \int_0^t C_a(t)dt \qquad (1)$$

where E is the first-pass unidirectional extraction or (in some instances more appropriately) retention fraction of tracer, F is myocardial blood flow, and C_a is the concentration of radiotracer in arterial blood. In a given heart, the arterial input function and its integral to time t are the same for all myocardial regions. Therefore, regional differences in myocardial tracer concentration depend only on E and regional blood flow. If the extraction fraction E were 1, then regional differences in tracer concentrations would depend solely on blood flow and would be related linearly to regional differences in blood flow.

The first-pass unidirectional extraction fraction E is the fraction of tracer that exchanges across the capillary membrane during a single transit of a tracer bolus through the coronary circulation. For most diffusible tracers, E is less than 1 and declines further as blood flow increases. This phenomenon occurs because higher flow velocities in the capillaries reduce the time for exchange of tracer across the capillary membrane. Assuming a model of rigid cylindrical tubes, Renkin[2] and Crone[3] described this relationship by the following:

$$E = 1 - e^{-PS/F} \qquad (2)$$

where P is the capillary permeability ($cm \cdot min^{-1}$) and S the exchangeable surface area ($cm^2 \cdot g^{-2}$). The product of P and S (the permeability surface area product) is unique to each tracer. The term PS/F is defined as the extraction coefficient and reflects the competitive rates between extraction in tissue and clearance by blood.

Experimentally measured first-pass extraction fractions do not conform fully to the relationship described by equation 2. Measured values at higher flow exceed the values predicted by the equation, implying that the PS product is not constant but increases with flow. Recruitment of capillaries may account for a flow-dependent increase in the PS product,[4, 5] which can be accommodated in the flow extraction fraction relationship by modifying the original Renkin-Crone equation to

$$E = 1 - e^{-(a+b/F)/F} \tag{3}$$

where a and b are derived from the best fit of the experimentally obtained data. The term (a+b/F) represents the flow-dependent PS product. The single-capillary transit extraction fraction must be distinguished from the steady-state extraction fraction, E_s, which, as described by equation 4, is defined as the ratio of the difference between tracer concentrations in arterial (C_a) and coronary sinus blood (C_s) over the concentration of tracer in arterial blood (C_a):

$$E_s = \frac{C_a - C_{cs}}{C_a} \tag{4}$$

E_s reflects the bidirectional or forward and reverse transmembranous transport of tracer and is therefore usually lower than the first-pass unidirectional extraction fraction.

The first-pass extraction fraction, E, should be distinguished further from the first-pass retention fraction, R, or the fraction of tracer that is effectively retained in myocardium after a transit of a tracer bolus through the coronary circulation. As illustrated in Figure 69–1, E and R may differ significantly. After tracer exchanges across the capillary membrane and enters the interstitial space, further transport of it across the sarcolemmal membranes and trapping of it in cytosol competes with backdiffusion of tracer into the blood. The rate of backdiffusion may depend on blood flow. At higher flows, a greater fraction of tracer returns from the extravascular space into the blood and results in lower retention fractions.

Last, different mechanisms account for exchange of tracer across the capillary and sarcolemmal membranes. Tracers can exchange across membranes via passive diffusion along a concentration gradient. Energy independent but saturable transport mechanisms may

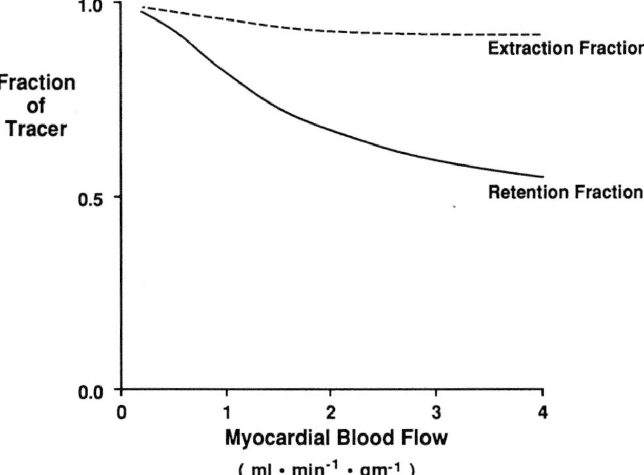

FIGURE 69–1. First-pass extraction and retention fractions of ^{13}N-ammonia and myocardial blood flow. The extraction fraction denotes the fraction of tracer that exchanges across the capillary and sarcolemmal membranes during a single capillary transit of tracer, whereas the retention fraction is metabolically retained in myocardium. Metabolic trapping competes with flow-dependent backdiffusion of tracer, this competition accounting for the progressive decline in retention fractions with increasing blood flow.

facilitate the exchange. Glucose transporters serve as an example of such facilitated transmembranous exchange. Conversely, tracers may be transported actively through energy-requiring processes against concentration gradients across the sarcolemmal membranes. The latter mechanism accounts, for example, for the transmembranous exchange of radioactive potassium or its analogs and its retention in myocardium.

Positron-Labeled Albumin Microspheres

Microspheres meet most closely the requirements of an ideal tracer of blood flow. Because their size exceeds the diameter of the myocardial capillaries, they are mechanically trapped in myocardium. Nearly 100 percent of microspheres are retained during a single capillary transit. Therefore, their first-pass extraction fraction is 1 and is independent of flow and changes in tissue state or in myocardial metabolism. For positron emission tomography, biodegradable human serum albumin microspheres, 15 to 20 μm in diameter, are labeled with either gallium-68 (^{68}Ga)[6] or with ^{11}C.[7] Whereas ^{68}Ga is generator produced and thus does not require an on-site cyclotron, the gallium-chelate complex is susceptible to disruption by plasma constituents, as demonstrated in animal experiments.[8] Therefore, the ^{11}C label is preferable because of its more stable covalent binding to microspheres. Once the tracers are trapped in myocardium, tissue activity concentrations have been found to remain constant for both tracers for at least 60 minutes.[8, 9] The amount of tracer retained in myocardium is a function of its first-pass extraction fraction and of blood flow. Because the first-pass extraction fraction is 1, the net uptake of microspheres in myocardium as the product of E and F is related linearly to blood flow (Fig. 69–2).

Positron-labeled microspheres have been successfully employed for qualitative and quantitative evaluations of regional myocardial blood flow.[8–10] Quantification is based on equation 1, in which blood flow is calculated from the microsphere concentrations in the myocardium, Q_t, and the integral of the arterial input function. With positron emission tomography, Q_t can be determined directly from the cross-sectional images, instead of by in vitro counting of postmortem obtained tissue samples. The arterial input function is obtained by withdrawal of arterial blood. In dogs, in vivo estimates of blood flow by this approach correlated closely with simultaneous blood flow measurements by the standard microsphere technique using in vitro counting of tissue samples.[8, 11] In humans with retrograde delivery of ^{11}C-labeled microspheres into the left ventricular cavity, the approach predicted average blood flows of 0.8 ± 0.3 mL $\cdot$ min^{-1} $\cdot$ g^{-1} in presumably normal myocardium.[10] In previously infarcted myocardial regions, blood flows ranged from 0 to 0.4 mL $\cdot$ min^{-1} $\cdot$ g^{-1}.

Although most accurate, the microsphere approach for measurements of blood flow in humans has been largely abandoned in favor of techniques with diffusible extractable tracers that do not require delivery of tracer into the left ventricular cavity but can be conveniently administered intravenously or by inhalation.

^{13}N-Ammonia

First proposed by Hunter and Monahan[12] and Harper and coworkers,[13] the use of ^{13}N-ammonia as a tracer of blood flow was subsequently demonstrated in animals[14, 15] and in clinical investigations.[16] In blood, ^{13}N-ammonia (NH_3) exists primarily in its ionic species, the ammonium ion (NH_4^+). In red blood cells, the ammonium ion can substitute for K^+ on the sodium-potassium transmembranous exchange system.[17] Thus, it may be actively transported into myocardium. Another route of exchange that most likely predominates is that in which the lipid soluble ^{13}N-ammonia passively diffuses across the capillary and sarcolemmal membranes, because its first-pass extraction fraction exceeds that of potassium ions.[18, 19] If the tracer leaves the vascular space in the form of ammonia, it then must be rapidly replenished by conversion of NH_4^+ to NH_3. Equilibrium between both species is achieved within about 19 μsec,[5] which is fast enough to permit almost

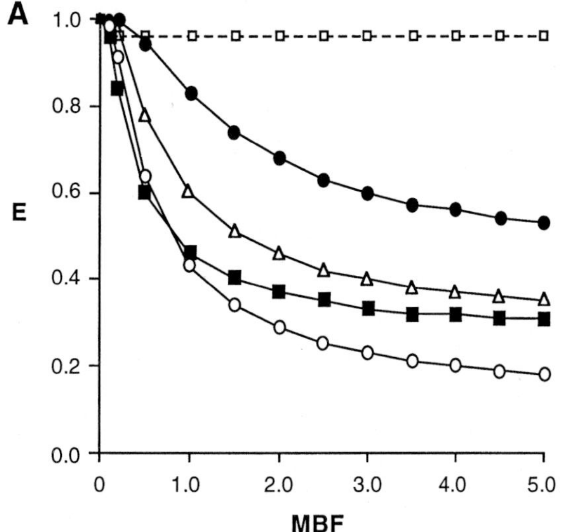

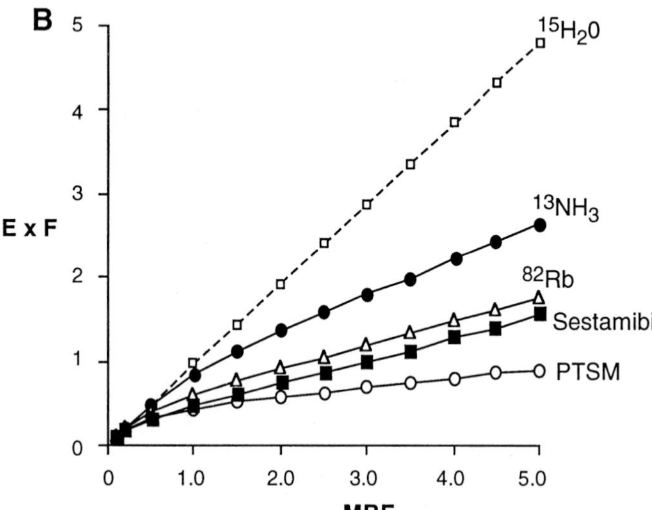

FIGURE 69–2. First-pass extraction fraction *(A)* and net extraction *(B)* of flow tracers in myocardium as a function of blood flow. The data for ^{13}N-ammonia were taken from the study by Schelbert and colleagues (1981),[18] those for rubidium-82 (Rb^{82}) from the study by Glatting and associates (1995),[41] those for Cu-62 PTSM from Beanlands and co-workers (1992),[59] and those for Tc-94m sestamibi from Marshall and colleagues (1990).[57] The first-pass extraction fraction is the fraction of tracer that exchanges across the capillary membrane during a single pass through the coronary circulation, whereas the net extraction is the product of the first-pass extraction fraction and blood flow. Note the progressive decreases in the first-pass extraction fraction for diffusible tracers and the nonlinear changes in the myocardial net extraction in response to myocardial blood flow.

complete extraction of ^{13}N-ammonia during a 2- to 3-second transit through the coronary circulation.

Several metabolic routes are available to the cell for fixation of ^{13}N-ammonia. Foremost are the α-ketoglutarate-glutamate acid and the glutamate-glutamine reactions. The latter reaction appears to be the predominant one, because inhibition of glutamine synthetase with L-methionine sulfoximine abolishes the retention of tracer in myocardium.[18, 20, 21] Because of a large intracellular pool of glutamine and its slow turnover rate, the ^{13}N label clears only slowly from myocardium (clearance half-times range from 100 to 400 minutes in canine myocardium).[18] Therefore, for the duration of the study time, ^{13}N-ammonia becomes effectively trapped in myocardium.

Residue function measurements in canine myocardium have demonstrated that as much as 95 to 100 percent of tracer initially exchanges across the capillary membrane (see Fig. 69–1).[18] Metabolic fixation competes with backdiffusion of tracer into the vascular space. Because backdiffusion depends on blood flow, the fraction of tracer that is ultimately retained in myocardium declines with higher flows. This relationship, as shown in Figure 69–1, can be described by the following:

$$E = 1 - 0.607e^{-1.25/F} \quad (5)$$

where E is the first-pass retention fraction, and F is blood flow. Equation 5 predicts for a flow of 1 $mL \cdot min^{-1} \cdot g^{-1}$ a first-pass retention fraction of 0.83, which however declines progressively with increasing flow and averages 0.60 at flows of 3 $mL \cdot min^{-1} \cdot g^{-1}$. The net extraction of ^{13}N-ammonia as the product of first-pass retention fraction and flow and its relationship to blood flow are shown in Figure 69–2 and compared with net extractions of other diffusible tracers. The nonlinear relationship describes an initial steep rise of the net extractions in response to blood flow. Further increases in the higher flow range, however, are associated with successively smaller increments in net extraction and thus tracer tissue concentrations.

Although tracer is trapped metabolically in myocardium, changes in cardiac work and in inotropic state, as well as in myocardial metabolism, do not significantly perturb the observed relationship between tracer tissue concentrations and blood flow.[18] Only unphysiologically low plasma pH levels and acute myocardial ischemia reduced moderately but significantly the retention fraction of ^{13}N-ammonia, without however invalidating its utility as a flow tracer.

Nitrogen-13 ammonia is now widely employed for the evaluation of regional myocardial blood flow with positron emission tomography in humans.[22–25] Typically, 370 to 740 MBq (10 to 20 mCi) of ^{13}N-ammonia are injected intravenously. Imaging commences 4 to 7 minutes later, to allow for sufficient clearance of tracer from the blood (about 5 percent of peak activity). Whereas uptake of ^{13}N-ammonia is usually low in lung tissue, it may be high and degrade image quality in patients with severely depressed left ventricular function or with pulmonary disease and in smokers. Because the tracer clears more rapidly from the lungs than from myocardium, longer time intervals between tracer injection and imaging may improve the myocardium-to-background signal ratios.

^{15}O-Water

This agent meets most closely the criteria of an ideal tracer of blood flow. It is virtually freely diffusible, and its first-pass extraction fraction approaches unity, is independent of blood flow, and does not vary with changes in metabolic state.[20, 26, 27]

Water labeled with the short-lived positron-emitting ^{15}O (physical half-life of 75 seconds) readily diffuses across the capillary and sarcolemmal membranes. Based on residue function measurements in dogs, the first-pass extraction fraction approaches unity at flows of 1.0 $mL \cdot min^{-1} \cdot g^{-1}$ and remains constant despite increases in blood flow. The high first-pass extraction fraction substantiates the notion that the capillary and sarcolemmal membranes exert only little if any resistance to the exchange of labeled water. The concentration of ^{15}O-water in myocardium relative to blood flow depends further on the volume of distribution of water in both myocardium and blood.[4, 27] This relation, frequently defined as the tissue-to-blood partition coefficient, represents the ratio of the tracer concentrations in myocardium to those in blood at equilibrium and depends on the water content in myocardium and in blood. The latter strictly represents the plasma water content and is therefore a function of the hematocrit.

The advantages of ^{15}O-labeled water are offset partly by physical and physiologic properties. The rapid physical decay of radioactivity results in low-count and, at times, diagnostically unsatisfactory images. Furthermore, the tracer also distributes into tissue adjacent to myocardium, for example, arterial blood and lungs. Although this activity can be removed by blood pool imaging and image subtraction, it further reduces image count statistics. This subtraction is accomplished by labeling of red blood cells with ^{15}O-labeled carbon monoxide.[27] Inhaled during a single breath, ^{15}O-carbon monoxide firmly binds to hemoglobin by forming ^{15}O-carboxyhemoglobin. The carbon monoxide blood pool images are normalized to and then subtracted from the ^{15}O-water images.

Oxygen-15 water can be administered as either a short or a distributed single intravenous bolus[27–29] or by continuous inhalation of ^{15}O-labeled carbon monoxide. Carbonic anhydrase rapidly converts CO_2 to H_2O. Depending on the performance characteristics of the positron emission tomograph, doses of 18 MBq/kg or 555 MBq (15 mCi) of ^{15}O-water[28, 30] are administered intravenously and imaging commences either immediately[28] or after 2 to 3 minutes. After ^{15}O has physically decayed, the blood pool is labeled with a single-breath inhalation of ^{15}O-carbon monoxide, imaged and subtracted from the ^{15}O-water images. For the continuous tracer-delivery approach, the subject inhales ^{15}O-carbon dioxide for about 3 to 4 minutes or until labeled water has equilibrated with blood and myocardium.[31] Serial images are recorded throughout the inhalation phase and for several minutes thereafter. The blood pools are then labeled with ^{15}O-carbon monoxide and subtracted from the equilibrium water images. A more recently described modification utilizes differential clearance rates of tracer from blood and myocardium to correct for blood pool activity and thus eliminates the need for an additional blood pool scan.[32]

The water-perfusible tissue index represents a more recent extension of the ^{15}O-water approach. As described later in this chapter, the index indicates the fraction of extravascular myocardial tissue that is able to rapidly exchange water.[33] In theory, this fraction should approach unity in normal myocardium because water can freely exchange into all normal tissue cells.

^{82}Rb

This cation substitutes for potassium on the sodium-potassium–dependent transmembranous ion exchange system and is actively transported across the sarcolemmal membranes into the cell. As demonstrated by residue function measurements in arterially perfused isolated hearts, rubidium-82 (^{82}Rb) ions rapidly exchange across the capillary membranes.[34] Active transport across the sarcolemmal membrane then competes with backdiffusion of tracer from the interstitial to the vascular space. Because the rate of backdiffusion is a function of blood flow, first-pass retention fractions decline in a nonlinear fashion with increasing myocardial blood flows (see Fig. 69–2). In isolated arterially perfused rabbit myocardium, retention fractions were related to blood flow by 0.84/(F + 0.84).[34] Comparable relationships have been observed in canine myocardium with the use of either external scintillation detectors[35–37] or dynamic imaging with positron emission tomography.[38, 39] Budinger and colleagues[40] report a value of 0.9 min^{-1} for the PS product in canine myocardium. Based on the Renkin-Crone equation,[2, 3] this value predicts an ^{82}Rb rest extraction fraction of 0.59 at a flow of 1 $mL \cdot min^{-1} \cdot g^{-1}$. More recently, Glatting and colleagues reported a PS product of 0.82 ± 0.09 for human myocardium.[41] The extraction and flow data from the same study can be entered into equation 3 to derive a flow-extraction relationship with a variable flow-dependent PS product (see Table 69–2).

Theoretically, the energy-requiring active transport of tracer into the cell potentially renders myocardial tracer uptake susceptible to metabolic alterations. However, Goldstein and associates[36] failed to demonstrate significant effects of hyperglycemia, insulin, digoxin, and propranolol on the first-pass extraction fraction. Increased plasma pH levels similarly remained without effect on the extraction fraction, whereas acidosis reduced it. The authors attributed the latter effect to hyperkalemia and competition of potassium for uptake of ^{82}Rb.[36] The first-pass extraction fraction in acutely ischemic and postischemic myocardium did not significantly deviate from the flow extraction fraction relationship.[42] However, ^{82}Rb subsequently leaked from irreversibly injured (non–triphenyltetrazolium chloride [TTC]-staining) myocardium but was retained or continued to accumulate in only reversibly injured (TTC-staining) myocardium. Thus, differences in regional tracer clearance kinetics may prove useful for distinguishing between reversible and irreversible ischemic injury.[43] On the other hand, studies by Wilson and co-workers[44] suggested that the tracer first-pass extraction fraction may already be significantly reduced in postischemic though viable myocardium.

One major advantage of ^{82}Rb is its availability through a generator infusion system.[45, 46] Strontium-82 is the parent isotope, has a 23-day physical half-life, and permits the use of a generator system for about 4 to 5 weeks. Furthermore, the short 78-second physical half-life of ^{82}Rb affords studies of blood flow during short time intervals, for example, 8 to 10 minutes. Largely automated infusion systems are now available. They are push-button operated and deliver a preselected dose of activity at a preselected rate of infusion.[45] Typically, 1480 to 2220 MBq (40 to 60 mCi) is administered intravenously and 60 to 90 seconds is allowed for clearance of tracer from blood before imaging begins.[47–50] Myocardial ^{82}Rb images are generally of good diagnostic quality. However, rapid radioactivity decay and increased photon attenuation, particularly in obese patients, may result in low-count and diagnostically suboptimal images.

Other Tracers of Blood Flow

Other agents such as ^{11}C-labeled alcohols (e.g., butanol and ^{11}C-labeled antipyrine) have been proposed as alternative tracers of blood flow but still remain unexplored.[51–53] Potassium-38 similarly has been employed as a cationic tracer of blood flow.[54]

More recently, a lipophilic copper (II) complex of derivatives of pyruvaldehyde-bis-(thiosemicarbazone), referred to as PTSM, labeled with a positron-emitting isotope of copper has been proposed as a potentially useful tracer of flow. In tumors, these complexes diffuse across the cell membrane and are reduced by sulfhydryl groups, with liberation of copper, which binds nonspecifically to intracellular macromolecules.[55] If the same redox process does, in fact, occur in myocardium, it explains the retention of radioactive copper (Cu), as observed by Green and colleagues[55] in hearts of rats, monkeys, and gerbils. Of the total administered dose of Cu-labeled PTSM, 4.0 percent and 2.2 percent were retained in the hearts of monkeys and of rats, respectively. In isolated arterially perfused rabbit hearts, the first-pass extraction fraction of Cu-labeled PTSM averaged 0.45 ± 0.07 at flows of 1.5 $mL \cdot min^{-1} \cdot g^{-1}$ (ref. 56) and, as demonstrated by Marshall and co-workers,[57] declined with flow. Hypoxia and ischemia failed to significantly alter the extraction fraction of Cu-PTSM. Importantly, the radiolabel becomes fixed in myocardium, as evidenced by clearance half-times greater than 3600 minutes,[58] whereas it rapidly clears from blood, as demonstrated in preliminary dog studies. Myocardial blood flow images recorded with positron emission tomography were of good diagnostic quality and reflected accurately the regional distribution of blood flow, as confirmed by the close correlation between tracer and microsphere concentrations in myocardial tissue samples by in vitro counting.[58]

Images in humans have been of equally good quality.[59] Myocardial clearance half-times averaged 105 ± 49 minutes at rest and 101 ± 65 minutes after adenosine administration. The myocardial retention as an index of the net uptake was 0.41 ± 0.10 at rest and increased to 0.79 ± 0.24 (arbitrary units) during adenosine-induced hyperemia. Therefore, the compound appears particularly attractive as a tracer of myocardial blood flow with positron emission tomography because it can be labeled with generator-produced positron-emitting isotopes of copper, for example, ^{62}Cu and ^{64}Cu.[55, 60] Thus, its use does not require an on-site cyclotron; the half-life of the parent isotope of the zinc-62/copper-62 generator amounts to 9.2 hours, so one generator system could be used clinically for 1 to 2 days.

Initial reports also indicate the feasibility of labeling technetium-based myocardial blood flow–imaging agents used with single-photon emission computed tomography with the positron-emitting isotope technetium-94m (^{94m}Tc). This isotope is produced with the cyclotron by irradiation of a natural molybdenum foil target and then is separated by electrolytic dissociation in HCl and H_2O_2 solution and solvent extraction in methyl-ethylketone.[61, 62] With its physical half-life of 53 minutes, the positron-emitting ^{94m}Tc, like its single photon–emitting counterpart, can be labeled to isonitriles or borons used for myocardial blood flow imaging with single-photon emission tomography. In fact, Stone and colleagues[63] recently presented myocardial blood flow images of good diagnostic quality obtained in humans after intravenous administration of ^{94m}Tc methoxyisobutyl isonitrile (sestamibi); similarly, teboroxime again labeled with ^{94m}Tc yielded myocardial flow images of diagnostic quality.[62] Figure 69–2 depicts the first-pass extraction fractions of ^{94m}Tc-sestamibi, their flow dependency, and the net extraction as a function of myocardial blood flow. Despite lower first-pass extraction fractions and net uptakes, ^{94m}Tc-sestamibi accurately depicted flow defects, as noted on ^{13}N-ammonia images.[63]

Choice of Flow Tracer

The three major tracers of blood flow, ^{13}N-ammonia, ^{82}Rb, and ^{15}O-water, yield comparable diagnostic information on regional myocardial blood flow. The specific advantages of one tracer are often offset by its limitations and drawbacks. For example, ^{15}O-water is theoretically the most ideal tracer of flow. On the other hand, its use is technically demanding and requires additional image manipulation, for example, acquisition of a blood pool image and subtraction from the ^{15}O-water image. The resulting low-count statistics may degrade the image quality. In contrast, imaging of regional myocardial blood flow is more convenient with ^{13}N-ammonia because the tracer is fixed in myocardium; the longer physical half-life of ^{13}N allows a more flexible acquisition schedule. Furthermore, longer acquisition times yield images of higher count densities. Yet, lower and flow-dependent first-pass extraction fractions render the tracer less than perfect. Also, the reduced retention of ^{13}N-ammonia in the posterolateral wall of the left ventricle may give rise to artifacts and must be considered during image interpretation.[64, 65] Production of both ^{15}O-water and ^{13}N-ammonia depends on an on-site cyclotron. Therefore, blood flow studies with either tracer need to be coordinated with cyclotron production. In contrast, ^{82}Rb is available through a generator-infusion system that largely facilitates the logistics of blood flow imaging. Furthermore, studies can be repeated at short time intervals, and their timing can be closely coordinated with responses to interventions, rather than with the cyclotron production schedule. These significant practical advantages must be weighed against the cost and the short physical half-life of ^{82}Rb. About 50 percent of the activity is lost to physical decay during the interval from tracer injection to the beginning of image acquisition alone. Further decay during image acquisition may result in low count and diagnostically inadequate marginal image quality. Additionally, newer tracers of blood flow, such as the Cu-labeled PTSM or the ^{94m}Tc-labeled sestamibi offer potential alternatives for evaluating myocardial blood flow at imaging laboratories without an on-site cyclotron. Therefore, the preference for a given tracer depends often on practical and economic considerations such as the availability of an ^{82}Rb generator system, multiorgan use of a given tracer, and sharing of the same cyclotron-produced batch of tracer between studies performed simultaneously on two or more tomographs.

Tracers of Myocardial Metabolism

Several positron-emitting tracers are currently employed for the evaluation and quantification of regional myocardial metabolism (Table 69–3). Because free fatty acid has long been considered the heart's preferred fuel substrate, early efforts focused on the evaluation and testing of ^{11}C-labeled palmitate as a tracer of myocardial fatty acid metabolism. However, depending on substrate availability or circulating levels of substrates, often as a function of the dietary state or dependent on physical activity, a greater share in myocardial substrate metabolism may fall to other substrates, for example, glucose. Furthermore, utilization of glucose can assume a predominant role under certain conditions, for example, ischemia and hypoxia. For the evaluation and quantification of exogenous glucose utilization, fluorine-18 (^{18}F) 2-deoxyglucose is available. Both tracers, ^{11}C-palmitate and ^{18}F-2-deoxyglucose, fall short, however, of providing sufficient information on overall oxidative metabolism as the sum of all oxidative processes, which has now become possible with ^{11}C-acetate.

TABLE 69–3. TRACERS FOR CARDIAC EVALUATION BY POSITRON EMISSION TOMOGRAPHY

Tracer	Target
Substrate Metabolism	
^{11}C-palmitate	Free fatty acid metabolism
^{18}F-2-fluoro-2-deoxyglucose	Exogenous glucose utilization
^{11}C-acetate	TCA cycle activity; peak of oxidative metabolism
^{15}O-oxygen	Oxygen extraction, myocardial oxygen consumption
^{11}C- or ^{13}N-amino acids	Amino acid metabolism; protein synthesis
Tracers of Cardiac Innervation	
^{11}C-hydroxyephedrine	Norepinephrine uptake-1
^{11}C-epinephrine	
^{11}C-CGP-12177	β-Receptor density and affinity
^{11}C-MQNB	Cholinergic muscarinic receptors
Other Tracers	
^{18}F-misonidazole	Hypoxic or ischemic tissue
^{11}C-PK-11195	Peripheral benzodiazepine receptors
^{15}O or ^{11}C-carbon monoxide	Blood pool

CGP-12177 and PK-11195 are the catalog numbers of industrial research compounds.
PTSM = pyruvaldehyde-bis-(N_4-methylthiosemicarbazone); MQNB = methiodide salt of quinuclinidyl benzylate.

^{11}C-Palmitate

Uptake and subsequent turnover of this tracer in myocardium provide information on regional myocardial fatty acid metabolism. This information is derived from regional tissue time-activity curves constructed from serially acquired cross-sectional images. Image acquisition commences at the time of intravenous bolus injection of tracer and continues for about 40 to 60 minutes. Images recorded early after tracer injection depict the initial bolus transit through the central circulation, followed by tracer accumulation in myocardium and clearance from blood (Fig. 69–3).[66] The late images depict the decrease in myocardial activity concentrations over time.

After assigning regions of interest to the left ventricular myocardium, tissue time-activity curves are constructed and reveal a characteristic biexponential clearance pattern (Fig. 69–4). The clearance curve morphology corresponds to the metabolic fate of ^{11}C-palmitate in the myocardium and thus provides information on myocardial fatty acid metabolism. The biexponential clearance implies that the tracer enters at least two metabolic pools of different sizes and different turnover rates. Quantitative parameters of the tissue activity curves can be obtained by biexponential least-square-fitting routines and extrapolation of the slow clearance phase to the time of myocardial peak activity. Both the rapid and the slow clearance-curve components are then defined by their slopes and relative sizes.

The ^{11}C label is attached to palmitate in the one position of the 16-carbon fatty acid chain (1-^{11}C-palmitate). It is suspended in 6 percent albumin and, after intravenous administration into blood, continues to be reversibly bound to albumin. Because of first-pass extraction fractions of about 0.67 at flows of 1 $mL \cdot min^{-1} \cdot g^{-1}$ (as observed in dog experiments),[67, 68] the initial uptake and regional distribution of tracer in the myocardium are determined largely by regional myocardial blood flow. Transmembranous exchange occurs presumably via passive diffusion across a concentration gradient,

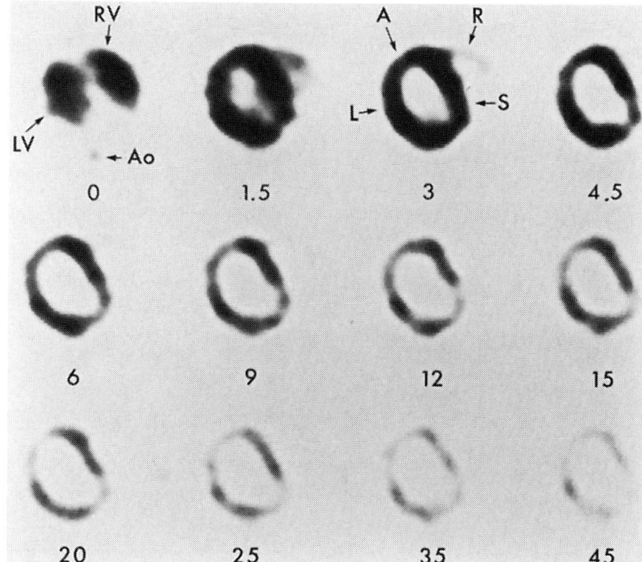

FIGURE 69–3. Serially acquired cross-sectional images following intravenous ^{11}C-palmitate administration. The images are recorded for a 45-minute period beginning at the time of tracer injection. The numbers under each frame indicate the time of acquisition after tracer injection (in minutes). RV and LV = right and left ventricle; Ao = aorta; A = anterior; L = lateral; S = septum; R = right ventricular myocardium. The first image reveals most of the activity in the right and left ventricular blood pool. After clearance of ^{11}C activity from blood, myocardium is optimally visualized at 3 minutes. The decline in intensity of myocardial activity indicates clearance of ^{11}C activity from myocardium.

although other mechanisms, including a facilitated transport system, have been proposed.[69] As depicted schematically in Figure 69–5, the radiotracer becomes esterified in cytosol to ^{11}C-acyl-CoA. The thiokinase-mediated and energy-dependent reaction is largely unidirectional and is therefore thought of as the effective step of tracer sequestration into myocardium.[70] Esterification of tracer competes, however, with backdiffusion of nonmetabolized ^{11}C-palmitate into the vascular space. Once activated to acyl-CoA, the metabolic fate of ^{11}C-palmitate branches thereafter. A fraction of esterified tracer moves via the carnitine shuttle to the inner mitochondrial membrane, where β-oxidation cleaves off the long carbon chain two carbon fragments, which enter the tricarboxylic acid (TCA) cycle and are completely oxidized to carbon dioxide and water. Another fraction of acyl-CoA becomes further esterified and is deposited as triglycerides and phospholipids in the endogenous lipid pool.

A large amount of animal experimental data supports the notion that the rapid clearance curve component reflects oxidation of ^{11}C-palmitate and thus corresponds to fatty acid oxidation. Its slope and relative size correlate with cardiac work and oxygen consumption[35, 68, 71–73] as well as with production and release of ^{11}C-carbon dioxide as the oxidative end product of ^{11}C-palmitate. Further, the clearance-curve morphology appropriately changes in response to physiologic interventions and thus correctly tracks known changes in fatty acid metabolism. For example, increases in plasma glucose and lactate levels associated with a decline in plasma free fatty acid levels induce changes in myocardial substrate selection and oxidation (Fig. 69–6). The resultant decrease in fatty acid oxidation in favor of an increase in carbohydrate oxidation is associated with a proportionate decline in the relative size and slope of the rapid clearance-curve component.[74–77] Changes in the clearance-curve morphology in response to inhibition of specific steps in the fatty acid metabolic pathway have further substantiated the nature of the rapid clearance-curve component. For example, impairment of fatty acid oxidation by inhibiting the transfer of acyl-CoA units into mitochondria with 2-tetradecylglycidic acid, an inhibitor of the carnitine acyltransferase I, resulted in a marked decline or even a disappearance of the rapid clearance component and cessation of release of ^{11}C-carbon dioxide.[77] The known impairment of fatty acid oxidation and disproportionate increase in fatty acid deposition in the endogenous lipid pool during ischemia or hypoxia are reflected on the clearance curve by a decline in the slope and relative size of the early clearance-curve component[67, 72, 73, 78, 79] and are associated with a proportionate decrease in the release of ^{11}C-carbon dioxide, as demonstrated in isolated arterially perfused rat hearts and in dog experiments.[67, 68, 78, 80]

Biochemical assays of myocardial tissue samples at various times after intracoronary bolus injection of tracer have confirmed that the slow tissue-clearance phase corresponds to incorporation of the ^{11}C label into the endogenous lipid pool.[80] In control hearts in dogs, about 75 percent of the initially extracted tracer was oxidized to ^{11}C-carbon dioxide and 10 percent diffused back into the vascular space in nonmetabolized form (Fig. 69–7*A*). The remainder of the ^{11}C label was retained in tissue in the form of diglycerides, triglycerides, and phospholipids and corresponded to the slow clearance phase on the tissue time-activity curve. Water-soluble ^{11}C-containing metabolites, for example, carbon dioxide, acyl-CoA, and acetyl CoA, were found to account for most of the activity cleared from myocardium in the form of ^{11}C-carbon dioxide. As predicted, ischemia dramatically altered the distribution of the radiolabel between metabolic pools (see Fig. 69–7*B*). Consistent with an impairment of oxidation of fatty acid, a significantly smaller fraction of label was released as ^{11}C-carbon dioxide, and backdiffusion of nonmetabolized ^{11}C-palmitate markedly increased. The fraction present in the aqueous pools declined, while the fractions of label in the diglyceride, triglyceride, and phospholipid pools markedly increased.

Together with the earlier established relationship to functional and metabolic indices, the results of the biochemical tissue assays

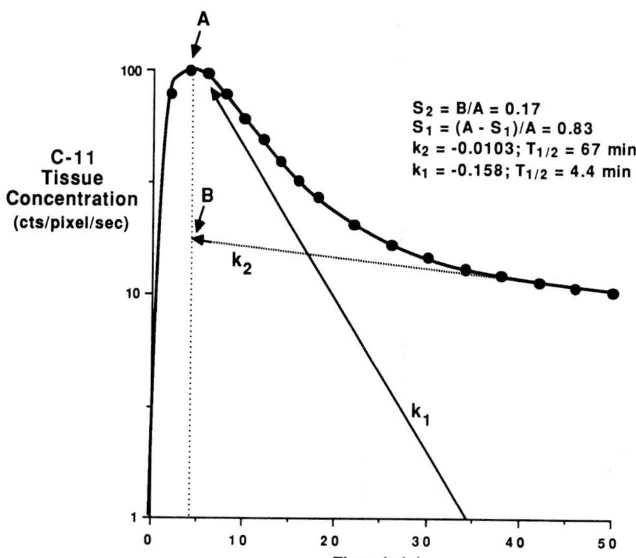

FIGURE 69–4. Myocardial tissue time-activity curves of ^{11}C-palmitate obtained from serially acquired cross-sectional images after intravenous tracer injection. Note the initial rapid increase in myocardial ^{11}C activity concentrations. Maximal activity, A, occurs at 4 minutes, followed by biexponential clearance of ^{11}C activity from myocardium. The slopes of the two clearance phases k_1 and k_2 are determined by biexponential least-square-fitting routines. Extrapolation of the slope k_2 to the time of peak activity (A) permits determination of the relative size (S_2) of the slow clearance phase by dividing B by A. The relative size of the rapid clearance phase is obtained from the difference between A and B divided by A. T½ is the tissue clearance half-time expressed in minutes. In this example, 83 percent of the tracer enters the rapid clearance phase, the remainder enters the slow clearance phase. The two clearance phases correspond to different metabolic fates of the radiolabel in form of deposition in the endogenous lipid pool and immediate oxidation and release as ^{11}C-carbon dioxide (as depicted schematically in Figure 69–5).

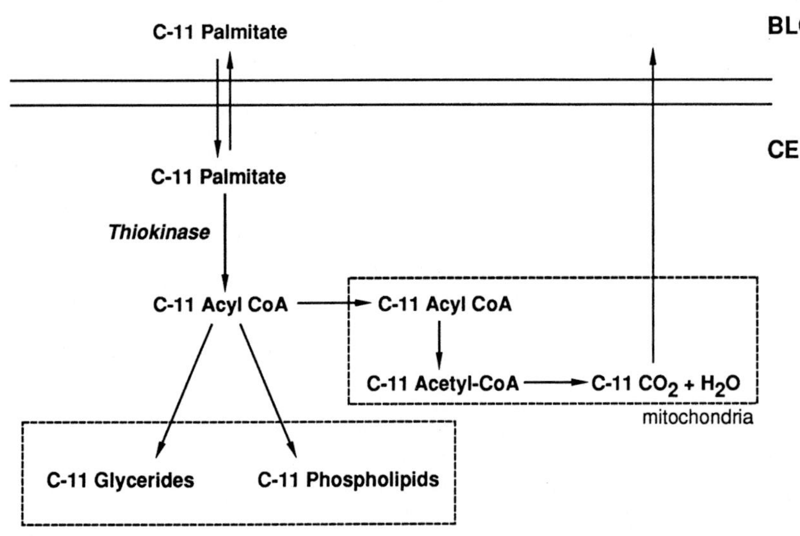

FIGURE 69–5. The metabolic fate of ^11^C-palmitate in the myocardium. (See text.) The two boxes indicate the two major pathways of the ^11^C label, oxidation of ^11^C-palmitate to ^11^C-carbon dioxide and deposition of the ^11^C label in the endogenous lipid pool, as reflected on the biexponential clearance curve as shown in Figure 69–4.

are important for adequate interpretation of the tissue time-activity curves. They confirm that the late slow clearance-curve component corresponds to incorporation of ^{11}C label into the endogenous lipid pool. The early clearance-curve component reflects oxidation of ^{11}C-palmitate and the rate of release of metabolic end products from myocardium. The results further point out limitations of the slope of the early clearance-curve component as an index of fatty acid oxidation. First, the slope of the clearance-curve component may be contaminated by increased backdiffusion of nonmetabolized ^{11}C-palmitate. Recent observations have suggested that the rate of backdiffusion exceeds the rate of release of ^{11}C-carbon dioxide from myocardium.[77] Second, the rate of tissue activity clearance depends not only on substrate flux through the oxidative pathways but also on the volume of distribution of metabolites. For example, the increase in the fraction of label present in the aqueous phase, reflecting ^{11}C bound to carbon dioxide, acyl-CoA, and acetyl CoA, may delay the tissue tracer clearance rate and thus cause an underestimation of the true flux rate through oxidative pathways.

For studies in humans, 555 to 740 MBq (15 to 20 mCi) of ^{11}C-palmitate is injected intravenously. Myocardial uptake of ^{11}C-palmitate and its relative distribution can be evaluated from a single image, recorded after tracer clearance from blood in about

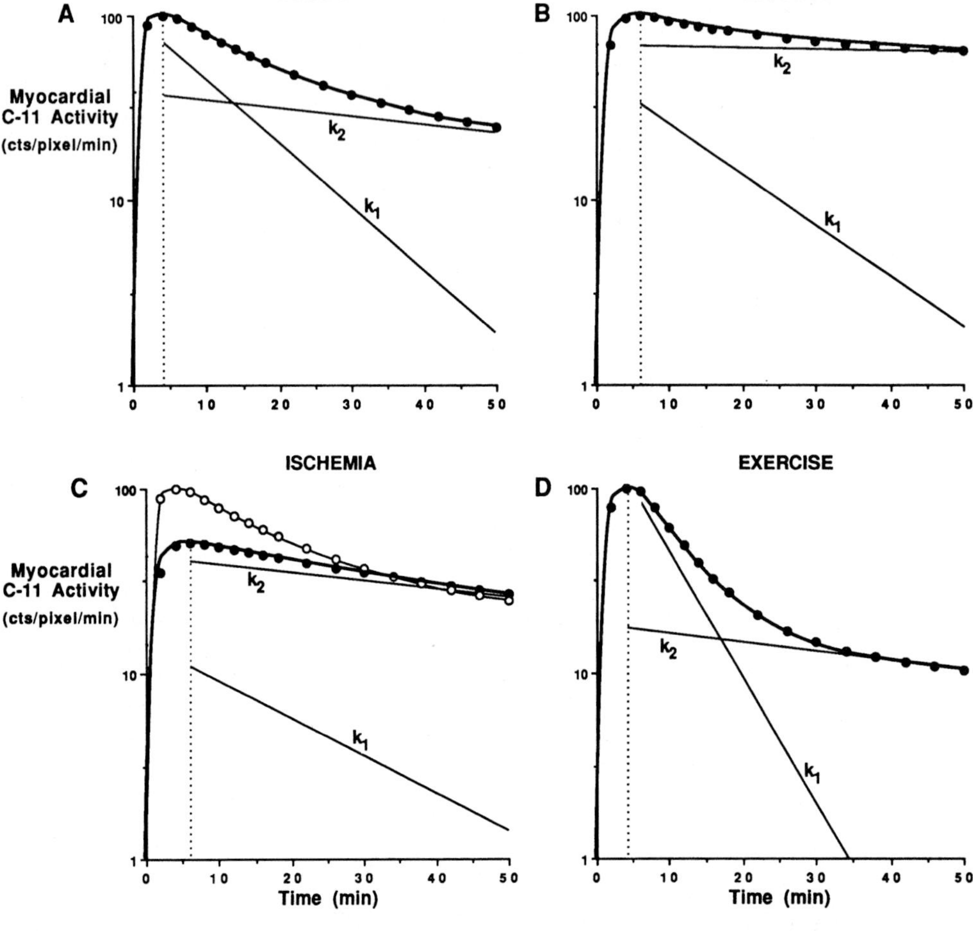

FIGURE 69–6. The effects of substrate availability, cardiac work, and ischemia on the clearance-curve morphology of ^{11}C-palmitate. *A,* In the fasted state, when plasma fatty acid levels are high and glucose levels are low, myocardium meets its energy requirements by oxidizing predominantly free fatty acid. The relative size and slope of the rapid clearance phase are high. *B,* An increase in glucose concentrations in plasma associated with a decline in free fatty acid levels after a carbohydrate-rich meal results in a shift in myocardial substrate selection from free fatty acid to glucose, which is reflected on the tissue clearance curve by a decrease in the relative size and slope of the rapid clearance-curve phase, indicating a decrease in the rate of fatty acid oxidation. *C,* Regional myocardial ischemia results in a regional impairment of fatty acid oxidation, which the regional time activity curve *(solid circles)* mirrors by a corresponding decline in regional ^{11}C-palmitate uptake and a decrease in both the relative size and slope of the rapid clearance-curve component. The time-activity curve derived from ischemic myocardium is compared with that in normal myocardium *(open circles). D,* The increase in myocardial oxygen consumption in response to exercise and increased cardiac work is reflected by an increase in the relative size and slope of the rapid clearance-curve component, reflecting augmented fatty acid oxidation.

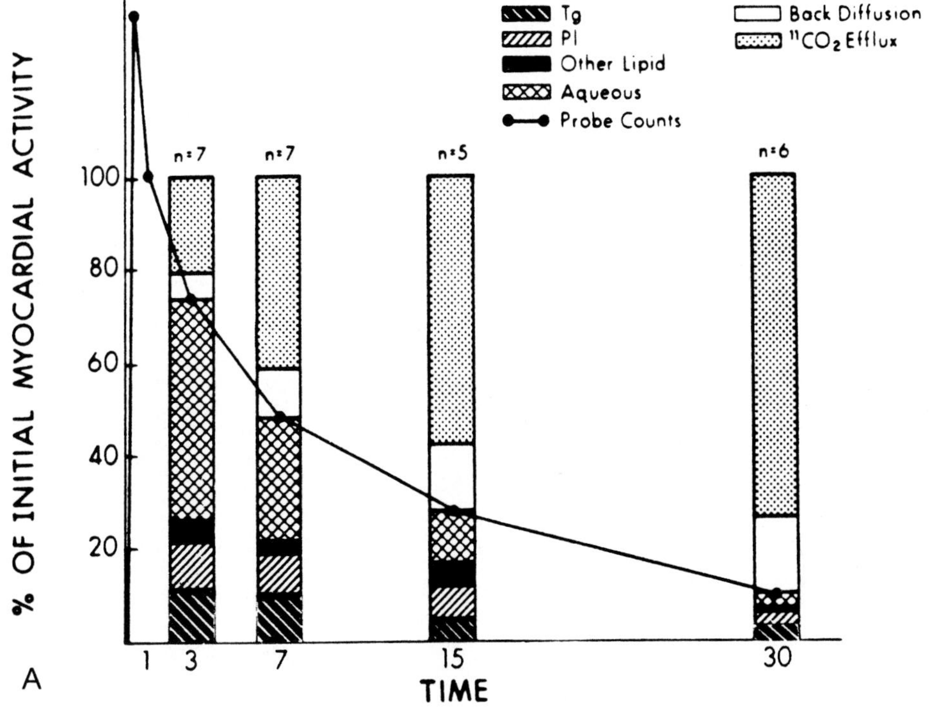

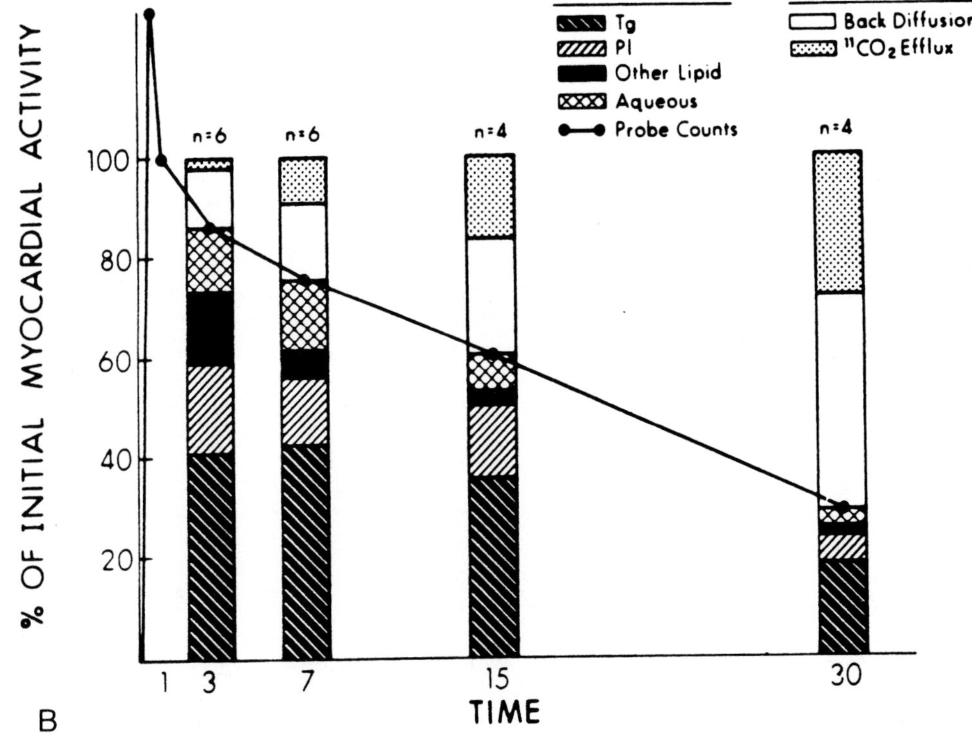

FIGURE 69–7. The metabolic fate of ^{11}C-palmitate in myocardium and coronary sinus effluent following intracoronary bolus administration of ^{11}C-palmitate in open-chest dog experiments at control *(A)* and low-flow ischemia *(B)*. The solid lines depict the tissue residue function and represent the average percentage of initially extracted tracer at each biopsy time point. The values above the curve at each time point indicate the cumulative contributions of ^{11}C-carbon dioxide and ^{11}C-palmitate efflux to tracer clearance from myocardium. The values below the curves depict the fractional distribution of the radiolabel between various pools of fatty acid metabolites in myocardium as determined by tissue assays. As shown in *B,* ischemia causes an increase in the efflux of nonmetabolized ^{11}C-palmitate and a disproportionate increase in the fraction of ^{11}C label deposited in tissue as triglycerides (Tg) and phospholipids (Pl). (From Rosamond, T. L., Abendschein, D. R., Sobel, B. E., et al.: Metabolite fate of radiolabeled palmitate in ischemic canine myocardium: Implications for positron emission tomography. J. Nucl. Med. 28:1322–1329, 1987, with permission of The Society of Nuclear Medicine.)

5 to 8 minutes following tracer administration.[81–83] As mentioned earlier, the initial distribution of tracer in myocardium is largely a function of regional blood flow. Nevertheless, these images of the initial uptake contain some metabolic information because retention or effective trapping of tracer in myocardium requires energy-dependent esterification of tracer to ^{11}C-acyl-CoA. More complete evaluation of myocardial fatty acid metabolism requires serial imaging that commences at the time of tracer administration and continues for about 40 to 60 minutes.[74–76] Regional myocardial tissue time-activity curves are then obtained from regions of interest assigned to the left ventricular myocardium on the serial cross-sectional images. Because of the dependence of fatty acid metabolism, and thus of the tissue clearance kinetics of ^{11}C-palmitate, on myocardial substrate selection, standardization of study conditions, including overnight fasting or determination of plasma substrate levels, is critical for adequate interpretation of the time-activity curves.

Although a tracer compartmental model for the quantification of regional myocardial fatty acid metabolism has been proposed for ^{11}C-palmitate, this model needs further refinement and validation.[84] Therefore, assessment of myocardial fatty acid metabolism with ^{11}C-palmitate remains qualitative or semiquantitative at present. Regional myocardial tissue time-activity curves are analyzed by biexponential least-square-fitting routines for determination of the relative sizes and slopes of the rapid and slow clearance-curve components. Alternatively, the slope of the early clearance-curve component is derived by monoexponential least square fitting.

Tissue time-activity curves characteristic for different dietary states, exercise, and ischemia are depicted in Figure 69–6. Under conditions of preferential fatty acid utilization, for example, after an overnight fast, the major fraction of tracer enters the rapid turnover pool and is rapidly oxidized, as indicated by the large relative size and steep slope of the rapid clearance-curve component. Under conditions of low plasma levels of fatty acids and high plasma levels of glucose, disproportionately more glucose is oxidized, a phenomenon reflected on the tissue time-activity curves by the decrease in both relative size and slope of the same clearance-curve component. Impairment of fatty acid oxidation during ischemia causes a similar decline in both curve parameters but occurs characteristically in a well-defined myocardial region and strikingly differs from the normal appearance of the clearance curve in normally perfused myocardial regions.

^{18}F-2-Fluoro-2-Deoxyglucose

Among several potentially useful tracers, the glucose analog ^{18}F-2-fluoro-2-deoxyglucose has emerged as the tracer of myocardial glucose metabolism of choice. It traces only one step—but a well-defined and representative one—the initial metabolism of exogenous glucose and is amenable to tracer kinetic modeling and thus more suitable for quantification of glucose metabolic rates with positron emission tomography.[85, 86] In contrast, glucose labeled with ^{11}C, which is also available,[73] participates in the entire metabolic fate of glucose. Distribution of the ^{11}C label into numerous metabolic pools and loss of label during the transit of metabolic intermediates through the glycolytic and final oxidative pathway of glucose put considerable limitations on the adequate interpretation of the externally recorded tissue time-activity curve as well as on tracer kinetic modeling.

As shown schematically in Figure 69–8, ^{18}F-2-fluoro-2-deoxyglucose exchanges across the capillary and sarcolemmal membranes in proportion to glucose. In cytosol, it competes with glucose for hexokinase and is phosphorylated to ^{18}F-2-fluoro-2-deoxyglucose-6-phosphate.[86] Unlike natural glucose-6-phosphate, the phosphorylated glucose analog is a poor substrate for glycogen synthesis, glycolysis, and the fructose-phosphate shunt. It is also relatively impermeable to the sarcolemmal membrane. Because the activity of phosphatase, the enzyme that reverses the initial phosphorylation of glucose, is low in normal myocardium, transport of tracer into the cell is largely unidirectional. The tracer is sequestered into the myocardium by the hexokinase reaction in proportion to glucose, so that images of the myocardial ^{18}F tissue concentrations reflect the relative distribution of exogenous glucose utilization in myocardium.

Following intravenous administration (about 185 to 370 MBq or 5 to 10 mCi in humans), ^{18}F-2-fluoro-2-deoxyglucose rapidly exchanges across the capillary and cellular membranes. Concentrations of ^{18}F initially rise rapidly in the myocardium. Backdiffusion of tracer then competes with phosphorylation and effective sequestration of tracer into myocardium. The rate of rise of myocardial ^{18}F activity concentrations progressively declines and may finally reach a plateau. This leveling-off occurs at about 50 to 60 minutes after tracer injection, when tracer concentrations in arterial blood have declined and a relative equilibrium state between phosphorylated tracer, tracer in tissue, and tracer in arterial blood has been attained. At that time, more than 80 percent of the ^{18}F label in myocardium is contained as ^{18}F-2-fluoro-2-deoxyglucose-6-phosphate.[87] In normal myocardium, the rate of effective sequestration of ^{18}F-2-deoxyglucose (e.g., transmembranous transport and phosphorylation minus loss due to backdiffusion of tracer) relative to phosphorylation of glucose has been found to be relatively constant.[88] Studies in in vitro experimental systems have suggested that this constancy is also maintained during abnormal states, for example, hypoxia and ischemia.[89, 90] However, further studies are needed to more definitively determine this relationship over a wide range of physiologic and pathophysiologic conditions.

Because ^{18}F-2-fluoro-2-deoxyglucose traces only the initial metabolic steps of exogenous glucose in myocardium, the compound provides only limited information on the metabolic fate of glucose beyond the major branch point between glycolysis and glycogen formation. The tracer does not indicate the fraction of glucose that

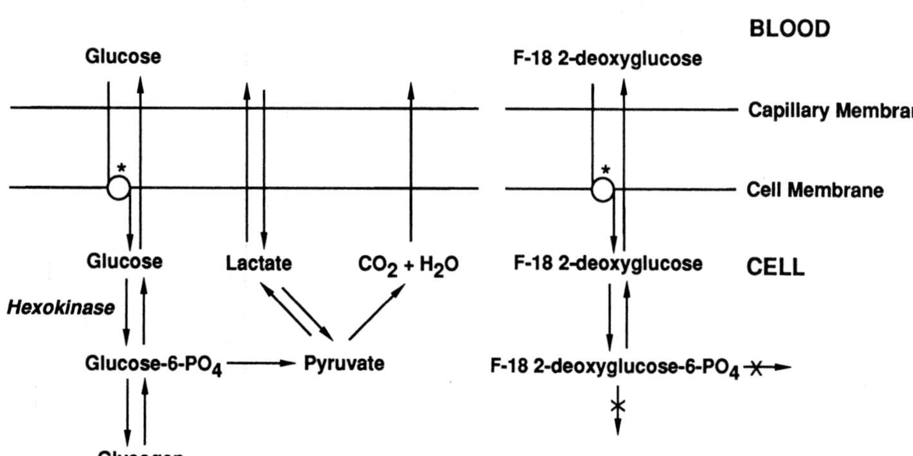

FIGURE 69–8. A comparison of the transmembranous exchange in the initial metabolic steps of glucose and of ^{18}F-2-fluoro-2-deoxyglucose in myocardium (asterisks denote facilitated transport across the sarcolemmal membrane). (See text.)

is subsequently synthesized to glycogen or the fraction that is directly catabolized through glycolysis. The contribution of endogenous glucose to the overall glycolytic flux also remains unknown. However, when the tracer is employed under strict steady-state conditions when rates of exogenous glucose utilization can be assumed to be at equilibrium with rates of glycogen formation and breakdown through glycolysis, some inferences in overall glycolytic flux should be possible. Furthermore, under extreme conditions, for example, during ischemia, when glycogen stores are depleted, the rate of exogenous glucose utilization determined with this tracer should approach the rate of glycolytic flux.

The qualitative evaluation of the relative distribution of myocardial glucose utilization requires acquisition of a single set of cross-sectional images at about 30 to 50 minutes after tracer injection or at the time of the plateau phase. On these images, regional activity concentrations represent relative rates of regional glucose utilization. If exogenous glucose utilization is to be quantified, acquisition of serial images commences at the time of tracer injection and continues for about 60 minutes. As described later, regions of interest can then be assigned to myocardium and arterial blood, and rates of glucose utilization derived from the tissue time-activity curves.

^{11}C-Acetate

This tracer permits the evaluation of flux through the TCA cycle and, because of its close linkage to oxidative phosphorylation, of myocardial oxygen consumption.

Myocardium avidly extracts acetate. First-pass extraction fractions of ^{11}C-acetate in canine myocardium average 63 percent at flows of 1 mL · min^{-} · g^{-1} and are inversely related to blood flow.[91] In cytosol, the tracer is activated to acetyl-CoA, which is oxidized in mitochondria by the TCA cycle to ^{11}C-carbon dioxide and water. Following intravenous bolus injection, ^{11}C-acetate rapidly clears from blood into myocardium. Serial images reveal subsequent clearance of ^{11}C activity from the myocardium. Regional time-activity curves, as shown in Figure 69–9, demonstrate a biexponential clearance pattern, which implies distribution of tracer between at least two metabolic pools of largely different sizes and turnover rates. The rapid clearance phase, however, corresponds closely to release of ^{11}C-carbon dioxide from myocardium and thus to the rate of oxidation of ^{11}C-acetate to ^{11}C-carbon dioxide in the TCA cycle and its release from the myocardium. In both in vitro experimental systems and in intact dogs, the rate of efflux of carbon dioxide correlated closely and linearly with the externally measured rate of ^{11}C activity clearance from myocardium or with consumption of oxygen.[91–97] Furthermore, the clearance rate is independent of blood flow and thus appears to depend almost exclusively on the rate of oxygen consumption and flux through the TCA cycle. Although nonmetabolized ^{11}C-acetate clears together with ^{11}C-carbon dioxide from myocardium, it represents only about 5 to 10 percent of the total activity released. This fraction remains relatively constant, even during markedly abnormal states, such as ischemia, hypoxia, postischemia state, and hyperemia, so that the tissue clearance slope of ^{11}C activity reliably and accurately reflects the rate of oxidative turnover of ^{11}C-acetate and, consequently, of oxidative metabolism.[91]

Tissue activity clearance curves of ^{11}C-acetate are analyzed by biexponential or monoexponential least-square-fitting routines (Fig. 69–9).[91, 96] On biexponential fitting, the relative size and slope of the slow clearance phase have been found to remain relatively constant over a wide range of oxygen consumption. In contrast, the slope of the rapid clearance-curve component correlates linearly in intact dogs with the rate of oxygen consumption,[91, 94, 96] and in normal human volunteers with the heart rate–blood pressure product as an index of cardiac work and oxygen consumption (Fig. 69–10).[98, 99]

Because the slow clearance phase is not always adequately visualized on the tissue time-activity curves, especially when tissue clearance rates are slow, for example, at rest, biexponential clearance-curve fitting often proves to be difficult or impossible. Slopes are then obtained by least square fitting of only the early monoexponential portion of the clearance curve (see Fig. 69–9). These monoexponential slopes are less sensitive to fitting errors because of low count rates and thus statistical noise toward the end of the clearance curve. Slopes by monoexponential fitting correlate well with oxygen consumption in dogs and with the heart rate–blood pressure product in humans.[96, 98]

Early investigations in normal volunteers demonstrated a homogeneously distributed clearance of ^{11}C-acetate in the normal left ventricular myocardium, implying a homogeneously distributed myocardial oxygen consumption.[91, 100] The determination of regional clearance rates in these studies was based on analysis of one or more sets of serial transaxial images. Yet, after reorientation of the transaxially acquired images into short-axis cross sections and, further, display of the three-dimensional distribution of functional processes in the form of two-dimensional polar maps, clearance rates of ^{11}C-acetate from the normal left ventricular myocardium have been reported to be heterogeneous. For example, these studies noted regional variations in the myocardial clearance rate of about 5 to 9 percent; clearance rates were higher in the septum than in the lateral wall. Although this difference was small, it achieved statistical significance.[101, 102] Also, clearance rates were highest in the most basal portions of the left ventricular myocardium and declined progressively from the base to the middle-left ventricle and to the apex. While methodologic reasons, including regional differences in the degree of spillover of activity from the blood pool into the myocardium, may account in part for such regional variations, they may also be physiologic as a consequence of regional differences in wall tension and shortening, such as that demonstrated with ultrafast computed tomography or gated magnetic resonance imaging.[103, 104] Consistent with these variations may also be the heterogeneity of myocardial blood flow, as observed in nonhuman primates and in dogs.[105, 106]

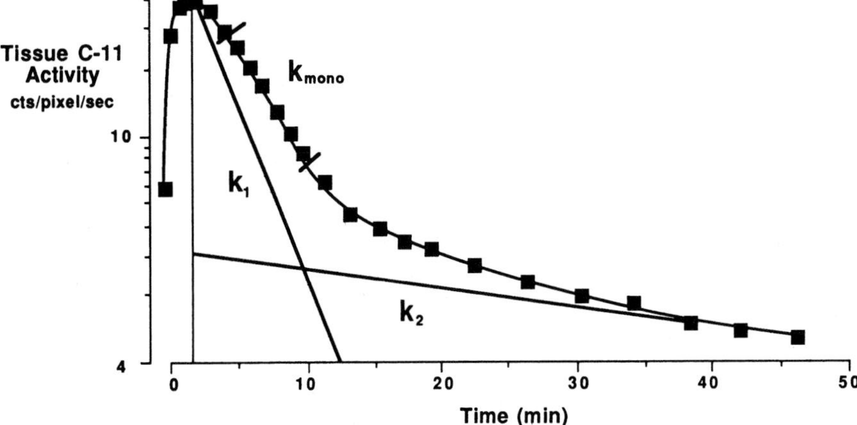

FIGURE 69–9. Myocardial ^{11}C-acetate tissue time-activity curve. Note the biexponential clearance of tracer from myocardium. The slopes of the two clearance phases are obtained by biexponential least square fitting and are denoted as k_1 and k_2. Monoexponential fitting of the early portion of the clearance phase yields the slope k_{mono}.

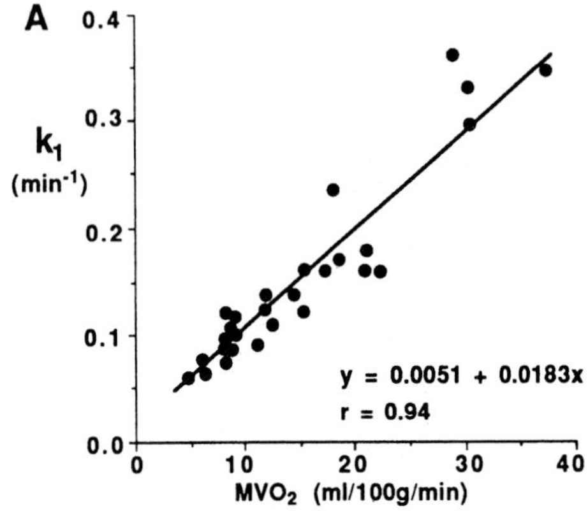

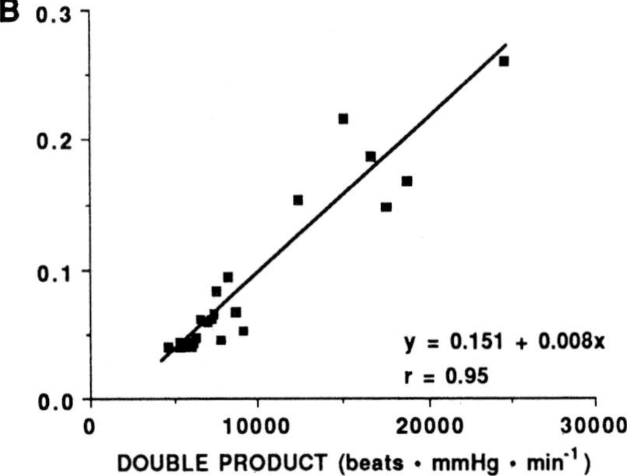

FIGURE 69–10. The relationship between the slope of the rapid clearance phase, k_1, of ^{11}C-acetate by serial positron emission tomography and myocardial oxygen consumption in dogs *(A)* and the heart rate–blood pressure product in normal human volunteers *(B)*. (Adapted from Buxton, D. B., Nienaber, C. A., Luxen, A., et al.: Noninvasive quantitation of regional myocardial oxygen consumption in vivo with [1-^{11}C]acetate and dynamic positron emission tomography. Circulation 79:134–142, 1989; and Armbrecht, J. J., Buxton, D. B., Brunken, R. C., et al.: Regional myocardial oxygen consumption determined noninvasively in humans with [1-^{11}C] acetate and dynamic positron tomography. Circulation 80:863, 1989, by permission of the American Heart Association, Inc.)

Both uptake and clearance rates of ^{11}C-acetate change with regional abnormalities in blood flow and metabolism. In ischemic myocardial regions, the initial uptake of ^{11}C-acetate decreases in proportion to myocardium blood flow. High tracer first-pass extraction fractions, as observed in canine myocardium,[91] account for the flow dependence of the initial tracer uptake. Regional clearance rates are reduced in proportion to regional reductions in oxidative metabolism.[91] For example, Selwyn and associates[107] observed a 30 percent reduction in regional clearance rates in acutely ischemic myocardium relative to normal myocardium in patients with severe coronary artery disease during supine bicycle exercise. Similarly, recently infarcted myocardial regions revealed delayed clearance of ^{11}C-acetate as an expression of regionally reduced oxidative metabolism. Gropler and colleagues[108] noted that the severity of the delay distinguished a reversibly ischemic from an irreversibly ischemic insult to the myocardium. Czernin and co-workers[109] showed that the reduction in oxidative metabolism, as demonstrated with ^{11}C-acetate in recently infarcted myocardial regions, correlated with reductions in blood flow, although in a biphasic rather than a linear fashion. The authors attributed this biphasic correlation to compensatory mechanisms, for example, an increase in the oxygen extraction. Once this compensatory mechanism was exhausted, oxidative metabolism declined precipitously with further decreases in blood flow.

Changes in plasma substrate concentrations and, thus, in myocardial substrate selection affect myocardial tissue clearance rates of ^{11}C-acetate only little. Shifts in substrate selection from predominantly fatty acid to glucose in experimental dogs resulted in a small but statistically significant increase in clearance rates for the same amount of oxygen consumption.[96] Differences in the proportions of oxygen consumption utilized in TCA oxidation of fatty acid versus glucose may account for this effect. For example, for glucose and lactate, 67 percent of overall myocardial oxygen consumption occurs via the TCA cycle, compared with 70 percent for palmitate and 72 percent for oleate. Nevertheless, this effect is only small and is likely to remain undetected on tissue clearance curves obtained in vivo with positron emission tomography in humans.[26, 98]

The average values of myocardial clearance rates of ^{11}C-acetate in normal volunteers are listed in Table 69–4.[98, 100, 101, 110, 111] Generally, the tissue clearance rates were obtained in these studies by monoexponential fitting of the early portion of the myocardial clearance time-activity curve. Recent studies have suggested that oxidative metabolism can be estimated also in the thin-walled myocardium of the right ventricle.[112] Clearance rates in nine normal volunteers indicated that oxidative metabolism in the right ventricular myocardium was 42 ± 10 percent lower than that in the interventricular septum. This difference is comparable to that observed with invasive techniques. In the same study, clearance rates in the right ventricular myocardium in patients with aortic valve disease but normal right ventricular pressures averaged 0.037 ± 0.007 minute^{-1}, compared with 0.065 ± 0.11 minute^{-1} in the interventricular septum.

More recent investigations in isolated, arterially perfused rabbit hearts have validated biochemically a six-compartment tracer kinetic model for ^{11}C-acetate.[113] These studies demonstrated that release of the tracer label from the myocardium occurs during the second turn through the TCA cycle. Further, in myocardial tissue, the major fraction of the ^{11}C label resides in the glutamate pool. Subsequent studies examined the feasibility of using such tracer compartment model in vivo. Investigations in acute dog experiments indicated that a simplified and, consequently, less error-sensitive model adequately described the experimental data and provided estimates of myocardial oxygen consumption in absolute units rather than rate constants.[114] The validity of this tracer compartment model is currently being tested in humans.

Evaluation of Myocardial Substrate Metabolism

Both ^{18}F-2-deoxyglucose and ^{11}C-palmitate afford the evaluation of well-defined aspects of myocardial substrate metabolism, whereas ^{11}C-acetate traces the overall myocardial oxidative metabolism of myocardium. Information obtainable with ^{18}F-2-deoxyglucose is confined to the initial steps of exogenous glucose utilization, whereas ^{11}C-palmitate traces the entire metabolic pathway of fatty acid, including deposition of fatty acid in the endogenous lipid pool and oxidation of fatty acid. The latter includes both β-oxidation and final oxidation of the two-carbon fragments via the TCA cycle. The information obtained with these two tracers therefore depends largely on the specific state of substrate selection and further on substrate availability and plasma substrate levels. In the fasted state, when plasma fatty acid levels are high and glucose insulin levels are low, and when myocardium preferentially utilizes fatty acid, little if any ^{18}F-2-deoxyglucose accumulates in the myocardium (Fig. 69–11). Conversely, on the tissue clearance curves of ^{11}C-palmitate, the relative size of the rapid clearance curve component will be large, and its clearance slope steep. Changes in substrate levels, such as a postprandial increase in glucose and decline in fatty acid levels, dramatically alter the clearance kinetics of ^{11}C-palmitate and the myocardial uptake of ^{18}F-2-deoxyglucose (see Figs. 69–6 and 69–11). The latter increases in response to augmented myocardial usage of exogenous glucose, while the slope and relative size of the rapid ^{11}C-palmitate clearance-curve component decline, consistent with lesser oxidation of fatty acid in favor of glucose. The effects of substrate availability and of resultant changes in myocardial substrate selection on the uptake and turnover of tracers in myocardium emphasize the need for standardization of study conditions and for monitoring of plasma substrate

TABLE 69–4. NORMAL VALUES FOR MYOCARDIAL OXIDATIVE METABOLISM BY ^{11}C-ACETATE

Study	Condition	n	RPP	k (min^{-1})
Armbrecht et al. (1989)[98]	Rest (fast)	7	6516±1553	0.048±0.004
	Rest (post-glucose)	9	6496±1154	0.052±0.009
	Supine exercise	6	17,198±4121	0.121±0.025
Henes et al. (1989)[100]	Rest	7	7328±1445	0.054±0.014
	Dobutamine	7	17,493±3582	0.198±0.043
Kotzerke et al. (1990)[101]	Rest	5	6420±826	0.057±0.009
vom Dahl et al. (1993)[110]	Rest	9	6592±891	0.053±0.006
Krivokapich et al. (1993)[111]	Rest	4	7017±974	0.050±0.010
	Dobutamine	11	20,960±3997	0.180±0.020

n = number of normal volunteers included in each study; RPP = rate pressure product (mm Hg · beats · min^{-1}); k = clearance rate of ^{11}C-acetate from myocardium.

levels. Changes in tracer tissue kinetics in response to alterations in substrate availability can also be used advantageously to elicit abnormal and normal responses.[75] Last, the combined use of metabolic tracers, for example, ^{11}C-palmitate and ^{11}C-acetate, permits the assessment of the contribution of free fatty acid or of glucose to overall oxidative metabolism[95] or, under conditions of ischemia, an assessment of anaerobic versus oxidative glucose metabolism.

FIGURE 69–11. See Color Plate 31.

Amino Acids Labeled With ^{13}N or ^{11}C

The usefulness of positron-emitting amino acids for the study of myocardial amino acid metabolism and rates of protein synthesis remains largely unexplored. As demonstrated in canine myocardium, the clearance-curve morphology of these agents depends on the specific label. When labeled with ^{11}C, the activity clears from myocardium in three phases, compared with only two phases when amino acids are labeled with ^{13}N. The rapid clearance phase is thought to represent a pool of amino acids that communicates with the vascular space by backdiffusion, with a slow turnover pool presumably reflecting labeled precursors for protein synthesis as well as with a third, oxidative pool, presumably representing oxidation via the TCA cycle and release of ^{11}C-carbon dioxide into blood.[89, 115–119]

Low first-pass retention fractions and, consequently, low myocardial uptake of labeled amino acids in canine myocardium are most likely species related because amino acids, for example, ^{13}N-glutamate, avidly accumulate in human myocardium.[118, 120–123] Comparisons to ^{13}N-ammonia uptake suggest that the distribution of ^{13}N-glutamate in human myocardium depends largely on regional myocardial blood flow.[118, 124] Nevertheless, Zimmerman and colleagues[125] reported relative or absolute increases in ^{13}N-glutamate uptake in acutely ischemic human myocardium and suggested the potential utility of ^{13}N-glutamate for exploring and delineating ischemia-related abnormalities in amino acid metabolism. Labeled amino acids further offer the possibility of measuring rates of myocardial protein synthesis.[126, 127]

Tracers of Cardiac Innervation and Receptors

Several positron-emitting tracers are available for the study of myocardial adrenergic neuron densities and of β-adrenergic and cholinergic muscarinic receptors. The properties of ^{11}C-labeled β-receptor antagonists and especially of the ^{11}C-labeled experimental drug CGP-12177 as probes for myocardial β-receptors as well as of ^{11}C-labeled MQNB (methiodide salt of quinuclinidyl benzylate) for the study of myocardial cholinergic muscarinic receptors are described in detail in Chapter 73.

Several other tracers of myocardial adrenergic neuron density have recently become available. Fluorine-18–labeled metaraminol, a norepinephrine analog, accumulates in myocardium in proportion to regional catecholamine concentrations.[128] The agent traces recapture and uptake of circulating norepinephrine by adrenergic nerve endings and is thought to accumulate in storage granules.[129] Because ^{18}F-metaraminol can be synthesized in only low specific activity, pharmacologic doses of tracer are required for imaging. Therefore, another agent, ^{11}C-hydroxyephedrine, has been developed and used to study regional myocardial adrenergic density and function in normal subjects and in patients with a variety of cardiovascular disorders. More recent additions have been the development of ^{11}C-labeled epinephrine[130] and ^{18}F-labeled dopamine.[131] Both agents should prove useful for gaining mechanistic insights into abnormalities of adrenergic function. The properties and findings of these tracers are reviewed in detail in Chapter 73.

Other Tracers for Cardiac Positron Emission Tomography

Several other tracers potentially useful for studies of myocardial tissue function with positron emission tomography have recently been described.

^{81}Rb

The 4.6-hour physical half-life of this cation offers the possibility of studying the equilibrium distribution of cations between blood and myocardium, rather than only the initial, flow-dependent uptake of the short-lived ^{82}Rb in myocardium. When imaged several hours after intravenous administration and after ^{81}Rb has equilibrated between blood and myocardium, tracer activity concentrations in myocardium probably reflect the potassium pool.[132, 133] The regional size of this pool and its variations in disease may prove useful as a reference to which metabolic measurements can be related. Equilibrium ^{81}Rb images have also been found useful for assessing partial volume–related, "artifactual" underestimation of regional true tracer tissue concentrations in abnormally contracting myocardial regions.[132]

Membrane Function

A peripheral type of benzodiazepine receptor antagonist, referred to as PK-11195 and labeled with ^{11}C, has been reported to specifically bind to peripheral-type benzodiazepine receptors in canine and human myocardium.[134] The agent is of potential interest for cardiac studies because the authors postulated a possible relationship between peripheral-type benzodiazepine receptors and calcium channels in the heart.

^{18}F-Misonidazole

Among currently emerging tracer compounds, ^{18}F-misonidazole is perhaps the most attractive one because it specifically labels ischemic or hypoxic myocardium. Based on investigations in tumors, the agent appears to diffuse across sarcolemmal membranes. Nitro reduction then results in formation of the RNO_2 radical anion, which, in the presence of oxygen, is oxidized to superoxide and noncharged misonidazole, which diffuses back into blood. If oxygen is absent, the RNO_2 radical is reduced to nitroso compounds and, further, to hydroxylamines and other amines that covalently bind to intracellular macromolecules, with effective trapping of radiolabel in hypoxic or ischemic cells.[135–138] Initial studies in isolated perfused rabbit hearts and in dogs have confirmed the usefulness of ^{18}F-misonidazole as a marker of hypoxic or ischemic myocardium. Isolated perfused hearts retained during hypoxia or low-flow ischemia 40 to 50 percent of the total administered tracer activity, compared with only 16 to 18 percent tracer retention in normal or postischemic hearts.[139] In dog experiments, 1.5 ± 0.8 percent of the tracer was extracted by normal myocardium, compared with 34 ± 24 percent in ischemic myocardium 75 minutes after coronary ligation.[140] The magnitude of tracer retention depends on the time after coronary occlusion. It declines to 12 ± 3 percent at 150 minutes and to only 3 ± 2 percent at 24 hours after coronary ligation. Thus, as ischemia proceeds to necrosis, progressively less tracer accumulates in ischemically injured myocardium, suggesting that the tracer specifically binds to ischemic rather than necrotic tissue. Imaging studies in dog experiments after coronary ligation have demonstrated segmentally enhanced tracer uptake in hypoperfused myocardial regions.[140, 141]

IMAGING WITH POSITRON EMISSION TOMOGRAPHY

General Principles

The quantitative imaging capability as a feature unique to positron emission tomography enables noninvasive measurements of regional tracer tissue concentrations. Cross-sectional images acquired with positron emission tomography represent quantitatively regional tracer tissue concentrations. The images are therefore comparable to autoradiographs but are acquired in vivo. The quantitative imaging capability derives from two technical aspects of positron emission tomography: (1) a relatively uniform or depth-independent spatial resolution and (2) appropriate correction for photon attenuation. Both are related to physical decay characteristics specific for positrons. Chapter 59 describes the technical aspects of positron emission tomographs in detail. Key features, such as the high spatial resolution, the high temporal sampling capability, and contrast resolution, account for the superior image quality relative to that available with single-photon emission computed tomography.

Image Acquisition

The relatively limited, 10- to 16-cm-long axial field of view of current tomographs mandates careful patient positioning. Some laboratories rely on a supine chest radiograph and demarcate the upper and lower limits of the cardiac silhouette on the patient's chest. Other laboratories record a rectilinear or two-dimensional transmission scan that resembles a low-spatial-resolution chest tomograph. Cursors on the computer display are moved to the cardiac silhouette and define the upper and lower imaging planes and thus the available axial field of view. They control the tomographs' bed position and automatically move the patient into the predefined position.

The imaging procedure itself begins with acquisition of cross-sectional transmission images with the use of a ring source or a rotating rod of positron-emitting isotope inserted into the imaging gantry. The transmission images measure the photon attenuation and are used for correction of the emission images. Acquisition times typically range from 10 to 20 minutes. The positron-emitting tracer is then injected intravenously, and sequential or static images are acquired. Static images display the relative distribution of functional processes throughout the left ventricular myocardium and are acquired after accumulation of radiotracer in myocardium and clearance from blood (Fig. 69–12). Therefore, the time interval between tracer injection and image acquisition depends on the type of tracer and may range from 5 to 50 minutes. If regional functional processes are to be determined quantitatively, serial images are recorded (Fig. 69–13). Image acquisition commences at the time of tracer administration and continues, depending on the type of tracer, for 10 to 60 minutes. For short-lived tracers, for example, ^{82}Rb or ^{13}N-ammonia, acquisition of an image set is typically completed within 10 to 15 minutes, whereas definition of the tissue clearance-curve morphology of, for example, ^{11}C-palmitate or ^{11}C-acetate requires acquisition periods of 40 to 50 minutes.

Rapid acquisition of serial images, also referred to as dynamic imaging, visualizes, as seen in Figure 69–13, the transit of the tracer bolus through the central circulation as well as its subsequent accumulation and clearance in myocardium. From these dynamically acquired images, the arterial input function of tracer and the myocardial tissue response can be determined (Fig. 69–14).

Image acquisition can also be synchronized with the patient's electrocardiogram (Fig. 69–15). As many as 16 to 32 frames per cardiac cycle can be collected and permit, as described later, the evaluation of regional myocardial wall motion or wall thickening.[8, 142, 143] Gated image acquisition has also been employed for minimizing motion artifacts and for improving the accuracy with which regional myocardial tracer concentrations can be determined from the cross-sectional images.[8, 144]

Identical patient positioning during transmission and emission image acquisition is critical because positional changes are likely to cause inadequate correction for photon attenuation and, consequently, to introduce image artifacts.[145] Therefore, most tomographs are equipped with low-power neon laser beams, which facilitate patient positioning as well as permit the monitoring of constancy of patient positioning during image acquisition. Other efforts to minimize changes in patient positioning include measurements of photon attenuation after tracer injection, for example, with rotating sources of positron-emitting tracers, as recently proposed,[146, 147] so that emission and transmission images are recorded in close temporal proximity. An alternative approach entails acquisition of a transmission scan for only a short time period. On these images or on post-tracer injection images, as described earlier, the boundaries of the chest and its organs are defined to determine the spatial distribution of various tissues, for example, chest wall, lungs, and mediastinum. Fixed attenuation coefficients for each tissue type are then employed for correction of photon attenuation.[148]

A set of 15 contiguous cross-sectional images obtained with a multislice tomograph in a normal volunteer is shown in Figure 69–12. These images depict the distribution of tracer within the left and right ventricular myocardium. The anterior and posterior papillary muscles are visualized clearly. The sets of transaxially acquired images are then reoriented into short- and long-axis cuts of the left ventricle (Fig. 69–16). The image reorientation also reduces the partial volume–related variability of apparent regional tracer concentrations due to regional differences in myocardial wall thickness and the angle between myocardium and image plane. Also, the activity profiles derived from contiguous short-axis cuts can be displayed in the form of "polar maps," as employed routinely with single-photon emission computed tomography (Fig. 69–17).[149] "Surface displays" are an alternative means of presenting the three-dimensional distribution of tracer throughout the left ventricular myocardium (Fig. 69–18).[150]

FIGURES 69–17 and 69–18. See Color Plate 31.

Surface displays or polar maps can provide estimates of the size and extent of regional abnormalities in blood flow or metabolism. For example, in dog experiments, Sun and co-workers[151] corrected for the geometric distortion inherent to polar maps by weighting

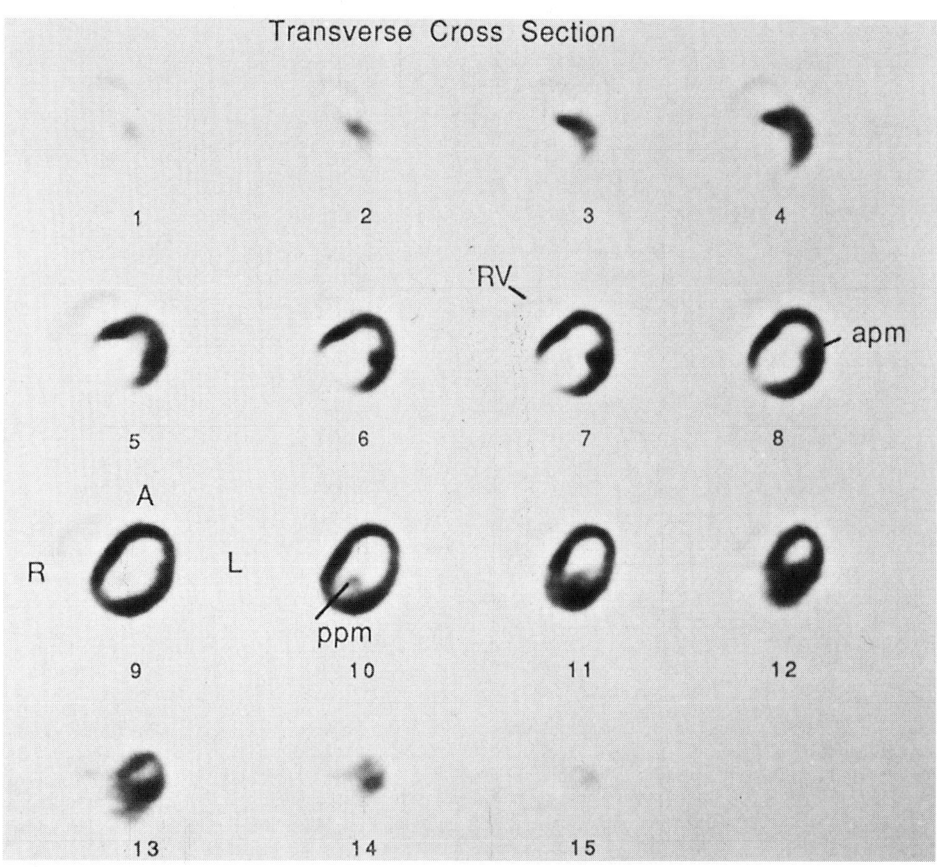

FIGURE 69–12. Contiguous cross-sectional images of the distribution of a positron-emitting tracer in the myocardium of a normal volunteer. The images were acquired with a state-of-the-art multislice positron emission tomograph after intravenous administration of ^{18}F-2-fluoro-2-deoxyglucose and are viewed from the subject's feet. The images begin at the base of the heart (levels 2 to 4) and proceed to the middle (levels 7 to 9) and diaphragmatic (levels 11 to 14) portions of the left ventricle. A = anterior; L = lateral; S = septum; R = right ventricular myocardium; APM and PPM = anterior and posterior papillary muscles; B = base; and AP = apex of the left ventricle.

the contribution of each short-axis slide or concentric ring on the polar map to the total left ventricular mass and compared the regional ^{13}N-ammonia concentrations with a database of normal. Regions with tracer concentrations of less than 1.5 standard deviations below the mean were defined as flow defects. The noninvasively estimated extent of blood flow defects correlated well with that derived independently by microspheres (Fig. 69–19). The approach further offered estimates of the average severity of such flow defects. Additionally, by determining the wall thickness of each short-axis slice and its thickness, measures of the total left ventricular mass can be obtained. For example, the noninvasive estimates in five dogs averaged 101.7 ± 23.7 g, which was similar to the average postmortem weight of the left ventricle of 100.9 ± 24.8 g.

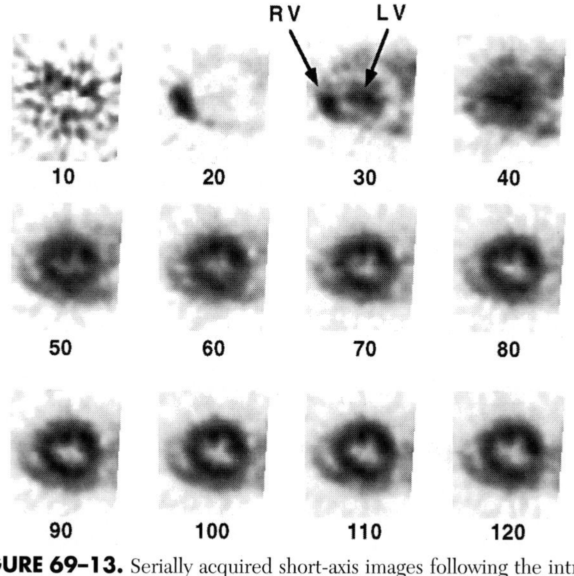

FIGURE 69–13. Serially acquired short-axis images following the intravenous bolus injection of ^{13}N-ammonia. Note the visualization of the right and left ventricular blood pools on the initial images. ^{13}N-ammonia subsequently clears from blood into the myocardium. From these serial images, the arterial input function and the myocardial tissue response can be directly obtained by assigning regions of interest to the center of the left ventricular blood pool as well as the left ventricular myocardium.

Assessment of Global and Regional Left Ventricular Function

Acquisition of electrocardiogram-gated images of the left ventricular blood pool or myocardium permits the assessment of global

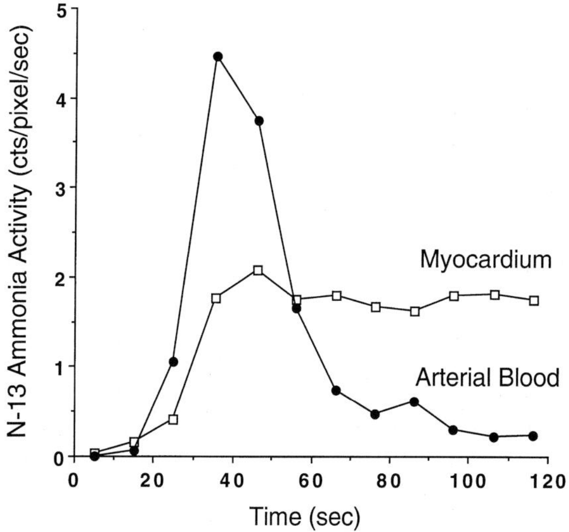

FIGURE 69–14. The arterial ^{13}N-ammonia input function and the myocardial tissue response for ^{13}N-ammonia in a dog study derived by assigning regions of interest to the images shown in Figure 69–13.

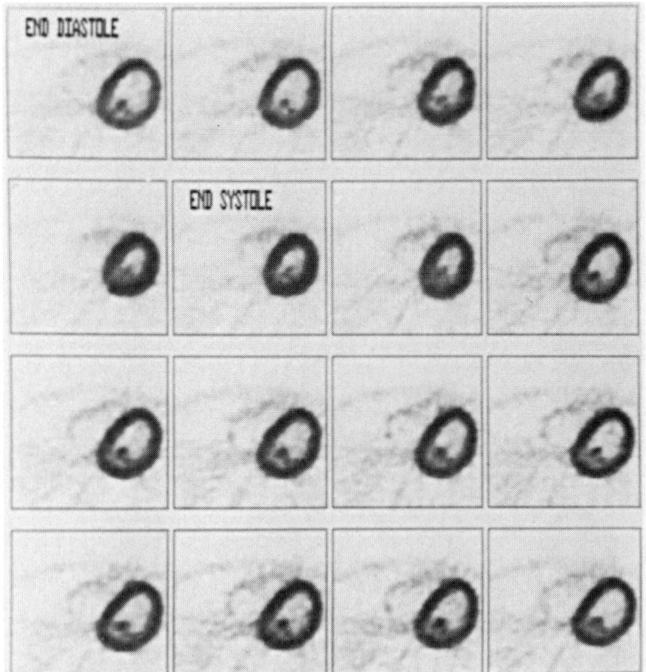

FIGURE 69–15. Multiple gated myocardial images acquired with positron emission tomography. The image plane was positioned through the middle left ventricle and the RR interval divided into 16 frames, each of 50 msec's duration. The sequence of images is presented from left to right and proceeds from end-diastole to end-systole and back to end-diastole. Note the corresponding changes in left ventricular size and myocardial wall thickness between diastole and systole. (From Schelbert, H. R., and Schwaiger, M.: PET studies of the heart. *In* Phelps, M., Mazziotta, J., and Schelbert, J. [eds.]: Positron Emission Tomography and Autoradiography: Principles and Applications for the Brain and Heart. New York, Raven Press, 1986, pp. 581–661, with permission.)

and regional left ventricular function. Gated blood pool imaging performed after in vivo red blood cell labeling via inhalation of minute tracer quantities of ^{15}O- or ^{11}C-carbon monoxide, similar to the conventional equilibrium radionuclide angiography, offers estimates of the end-diastolic and end-systolic volumes and thus of the left ventricular ejection fraction. Regional wall motion can be evaluated on cine-like displays of surface-rendered blood pool images; regional or segmental systolic wall motion can also be determined quantitatively and can be depicted in the form of two-dimensional polar maps.[152] In 16 chronic coronary artery disease patients, Miller and colleagues[152] demonstrated a close and linear correlation between left ventricular ejection fractions determined from gated ^{15}O-carbon monoxide positron emission tomography images and plasma ^{99m}Tc-labeled red blood cell images. Further, regional wall motion abnormalities were equally well detected by visual inspection of gated positron emission tomography and of planar equilibrium blood pool images. Changes in left ventricular cavity dimensions from diastole to systole can be determined from gated positron emission tomography images of the myocardium, compared with two-dimensional echocardiography or gated magnetic resonance imaging.[144] Last, consistent with the partial volume effect, an increase in myocardial thickness from diastole to systole is associated with a proportional increase in observed (rather than true) myocardial activity concentrations. As initially demonstrated in open-chest dog experiments, the increase in the observed tracer activity concentration correlates well with the percent systolic wall thickening as determined with echocardiography.[8] Yamashita and co-workers[153] reported a good agreement between abnormal regional wall thickening by gated positron emission tomography and abnormal systolic wall motion on contrast ventriculography in 16 coronary artery disease patients. The same investigators[154] subsequently demonstrated a significant correlation between segmental reductions and resting myocardial blood flow by ^{13}N-ammonia and systolic wall thickening as determined from gated myocardial ^{13}N-ammonia images. Thus, it is possible to explore the interrelationships between regional contractile function and blood flow or, alternatively, metabolism from the same gated myocardial images on positron emission tomography.

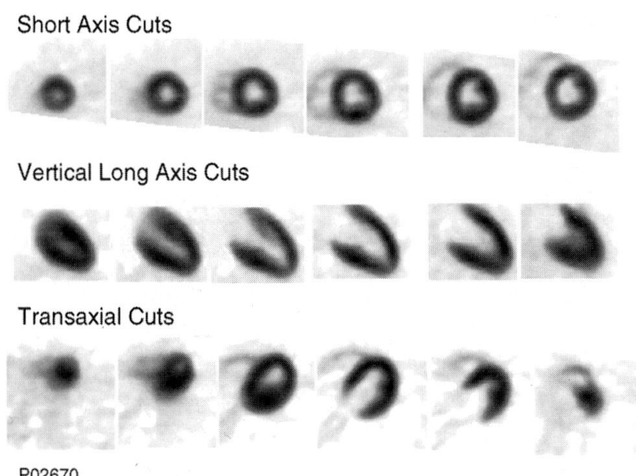

FIGURE 69–16. Reoriented transaxial images into short-axis and horizontal and vertical long-axis cuts in a normal volunteer. This reorientation results in images that are related to the orientation of the left ventricular myocardium.

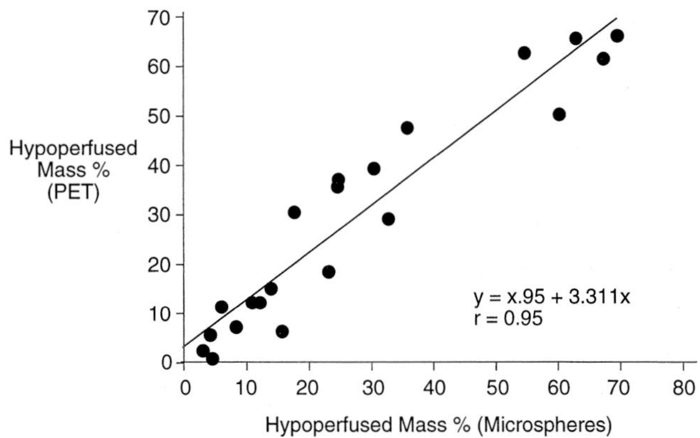

FIGURE 69–19. Determination of the extent of blood flow defects based on polar mapping. The figure shows the excellent correlation between the noninvasively measured extent of ^{13}N-ammonia defects following experimental coronary occlusions in dog experiments. The extent of flow abnormalities was determined independently by microspheres and in vitro counting of the myocardial tissue samples. Note the excellent linear correlation between both measurements, indicating that the size of blood flow defects can, in fact, be determined accurately in vivo with positron emission tomography from polar maps.

Determination of True Tissue Tracer Concentrations

Positional changes between transmission and emission images and low-count statistics can result in erroneous or inaccurate measurements of regional tracer concentrations. Additional errors can result from (1) partial volume effect and (2) activity spillover.

Partial Volume Effect

Regional tracer concentrations as seen on or determined quantitatively from the cross-sectional images depend on the size of the object or, in the case of the heart, on the regional myocardial wall thickness. As demonstrated in phantom experiments, apparent

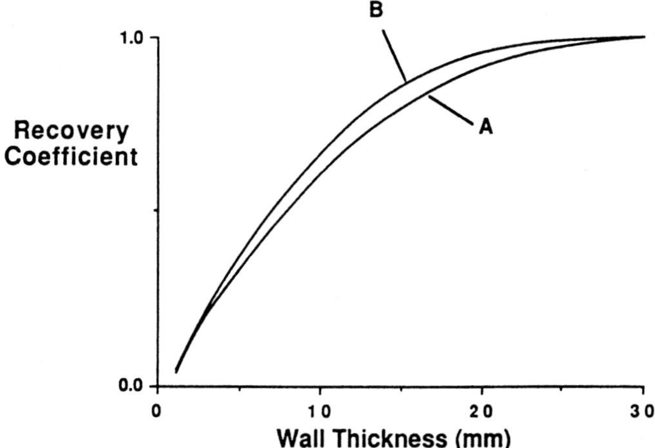

FIGURE 69–20. Partial volume effect and underestimation of true tracer tissue concentrations as a function of myocardial wall thickness and the tomograph's performance characteristics. The recovery coefficient as the ratio of observed–to–true tracer tissue concentrations increases with myocardial wall thickness (in millimeters). Curve A was obtained from bar phantom images reconstructed with an effective spatial resolution of 13.7 mm full-width half-maximum (FWHM) and curve B with an effective spatial resolution of 11.9 mm FWHM.

tissue concentrations equal true tissue concentrations only when the regional myocardial wall thickness is at least twice the spatial resolution of the imaging device.[155, 156] Observed tracer tissue concentrations, however, decrease nonlinearly with decreasing object size or regional myocardial wall thickness (Fig. 69–20).[8, 156] Loss of systolic thickening alone, for example, during ischemia, as demonstrated in dogs,[157] can result in an apparent further reduction in regional tracer activity on ungated images because of a decline in the average myocardial wall thickness.

Corrections for the partial volume–related underestimation of true tracer tissue concentrations are possible when the regional wall thickness is known.[156] From the relationship between recovered and true tissue activity concentrations and the object size, a recovery coefficient, RF, is derived. The recovery coefficient is a nonlinear function of the regional wall thickness. When the wall thickness is known, the true tracer tissue concentration (C_m) is calculated by the following:

$$C_m = \frac{C_{mo}}{RF} (\text{cts} \cdot \text{min}^{-1} \cdot \text{g}^{-1}) \qquad (6)$$

where C_{mo} is the observed tracer tissue concentration as derived from a region of interest. Myocardial wall thickness can be determined with echocardiography[8] or, as proposed more recently, directly from the positron emission tomographic images.[144] The magnitude of the partial volume effect and, thus, the recovery coefficient vary with the performance characteristics of the tomograph and should be determined for each instrument.

Activity Spillover

This effect results from the imperfect spatial resolution of the imaging device and misplaces activity between adjacent structures or organs. For example, if the regional myocardial tracer concentration is determined from a region of interest assigned to the left ventricular myocardium, the observed activity will be contaminated by spillover of activity from the left ventricular blood pool, as well as by activity in the vascular space of the left ventricular myocardium itself. Correction for activity spillover is especially important for dynamically acquired images when there is a time when tracer concentrations are high in blood but low in myocardium and, conversely, after tracer clearance from blood into myocardium, when activity is high in myocardium but low in blood. Thus, early after tracer injection, activity predominantly spills from blood into myocardium, whereas late after injection, the spillover direction reverses (Fig. 69–21). The degree of activity spillover is defined as spillover fraction, as the ratio of activity measured in a region of interest outside but adjacent to the structure to the activity recorded directly from the same structure. The spillover fraction is then applied to observed tissue concentrations to remove or correct for contamination by "misplaced" activity.

The magnitude of the spillover depends on the proximity of the organ or measurement regions of interest and the performance characteristics of the tomograph. For an intrinsic resolution of 5 to 6 mm, the spillover fraction from the blood pool into myocardium was found to amount to as much as 40 percent after blood pool labeling with ^{15}O-carbon monoxide in dogs.[158] Spillover of activity from blood into myocardium is caused only in part by instrument-related misplacement of activity, for it also includes activity in the vascular space of the myocardium. The myocardial blood volume amounts to about 10 percent of the myocardial volume but may vary considerably, for example, during hyperemia. Therefore, accu-

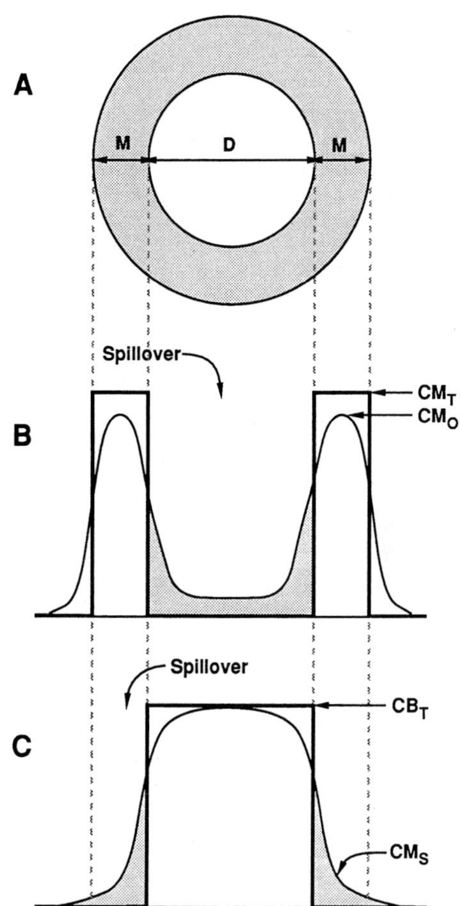

FIGURE 69–21. Partial volume and activity spillover. *A*, Schematic drawings of a cross section through the left ventricle with cavity diameter D and myocardial wall thickness M. *B*, Activity profile through the left ventricular cross section at a time when concentrations are high in myocardium and low in arterial blood and *C*, at a time when myocardial concentrations are low or negligible and are high in arterial blood. The bold lines in *B* and *C* reflect the true and the fine lines the observed tissue activity profiles. Because myocardial wall thickness M is less than twice the spatial resolution of the tomograph, the observed tracer tissue concentration (CM_O) is less than the true tracer tissue concentration (CM_T). CM_O can be corrected for by the recovery coefficient if M is known. In arterial blood, the observed tissue concentrations approximate the true blood activity concentration (CB_T) because the diameter of the blood pool is more than twice the spatial resolution. Misplacement of activity from myocardium to blood is shown in *B* and from blood into myocardium in *C*. The spillover fraction can be determined from the blood pool image from the ratio of activity in myocardium due to spillover (CM_S) and CB_T.

rate determinations of regional tracer concentrations in myocardium as well as in arterial blood require corrections for activity spillover. Such corrections are possible and are based on the performance characteristics of the tomograph as well as the dimensions of the left ventricular cavity in myocardium.[159–161]

Quantification of Tissue Activity Concentrations

Circumferential profile analysis approaches are employed to determine relative tracer concentrations throughout the left ventricular myocardium.[22, 24, 25, 162] Radii, originating from the center of the left ventricular blood pool at 6-degree intervals, search for the maximal, or average, activity of the myocardium and plot relative regional tracer concentrations as a function of the angle along the circumference. Individual patient profiles are compared with standard profiles derived from normal volunteers to define the extent and magnitude of segmental increases or reductions in tracer uptake.

Quantification of regional tissue concentrations from dynamically recorded images is facilitated by semiautomated analysis routines.[162] They define the inner and outer borders of the left ventricular myocardium and divide the myocardium into sectorial regions of interest. Together with an additional region of interest assigned to the left ventricular blood pool, this matrix is then copied to all serial images and regional tissue tracer concentrations, and their changes over time are determined in counts per second per pixel. They are then corrected for physical decay, partial volume effect, and activity spillover and are used for construction of time-activity curves for arterial blood and regional myocardium. Measurements of the arterial input function and of myocardial tracer activity concentrations determined in this manner have been validated and were found to correlate well with in vivo counting of tissue samples.[8, 163] High count rates at the time of the transit of the bolus activity through the central circulation can exceed count-rate capabilities of positron emission tomographs and result in losses in counts because of deadtime. Excessive peak activities and thus significant deadtime losses can be avoided with the use of a more distributed bolus input function, achieved by spreading out the tracer injection over a longer time period (e.g., 30 seconds) and by lowering tracer activities (e.g., 15 mCi) when the arterial input function is to be determined quantitatively by dynamic imaging. Correction routines for deadtime losses have also been developed[8, 164] and are implemented in commercially available positron emission tomographs.

In instances in which the arterial input function cannot be obtained directly from the serially acquired images, activity concentrations in arterial blood can be counted in vitro and then can be related to the noninvasively derived activity concentrations in, for example, myocardium. In vitro measurements are normalized to in vivo measurements of tissue concentrations by calibrating the cross-sectional images.[8] A small sample of the tracer is diluted in water and imaged in a cylindrical phantom 20 cm in diameter. An aliquot of the radioactive solution in the phantom is then submitted to well counting. A calibration factor K is determined by the following:

$$K = \frac{\text{in vitro counts } (g^{-1} \cdot \text{sec}^{-1})}{\text{in vivo counts } (mL^{-1} \cdot \text{sec}^{-1})} \cdot S \tag{7}$$

where the imaged volume in mL is a function of the number of picture or volume elements (pixels or voxels) in the region of interest and at S, the specific gravity ($mL \cdot g^{-1}$). The factor K converts in vivo derived activity concentrations into activity concentrations per gram of tissue per time and thus effectively calibrates the tomograph against in vitro measurements of tissue activity concentrations.

TRACER KINETIC MODELS AND APPLICATIONS

In vivo quantification of concentrations of positron-emitting tracers in blood and in myocardium and determination of their changes over time provide the basis for the in vivo application of tracer kinetic principles. Such models describe the time-dependent distribution of radiolabel between various functional (rather than anatomical) pools or compartments in tissue and the rate of exchange of radiolabel between such pools. They relate the tracer tissue kinetics and thus the externally measured signal to the process to be studied and form the basis for an operational equation that serves to derive quantitative estimates of rates of blood flow, biochemical reactions, or mass fluxes through metabolic pathways from externally measured tracer tissue concentrations.

The myocardial tissue response to a tracer input function largely determines the general configuration of a tracer compartmental model. The tissue response depends on the type of tracer as well as on its distribution in arterial blood.[4] As seen in *A* of Figure 69–22, a distributed tracer bolus input function with slow tracer clearance from blood results in slow but continuous tracer accumulation in myocardial tissue. The continued rise in tracer tissue concentrations during the observation period implies that the tracer becomes effectively trapped in myocardium. The tracer compartment model describes the exchange of tracer between blood and tissue accordingly. There is forward and reverse transport between the blood and the tissue compartments but unidirectional exchange from the tissue to, for example, a third and metabolic compartment. For the same tracer and the same process, the tissue response markedly changes when the tracer input function is shortened. The tissue concentrations rise rapidly and subsequently reach a plateau. An equilibrium state between tracer present in the three compartments has been attained. Analysis of the tissue response alone would indicate a change in the process examined with the tracer. However, because the tracer compartment model relates the tissue response to the tracer input function, it adjusts for differences in the tissue response to different input functions. The same distribution of the tracer input function, however, for a different tracer results in an entirely different tissue response. As shown in Figure 69–22*C*, myocardial activity concentrations rapidly rise but subsequently decline again. After initially being transported into myocardium, the tracer label must therefore be released again from the myocardium into blood in either nonmetabolized form or bound to metabolites.

The myocardial clearance-curve morphology offers additional information for tracer kinetic modeling. For example, monoexponential clearance of activity from myocardium implies distribution of tracer in a single functional pool and clearance from it. In contrast, a biexponential clearance pattern indicates that the tracer label distributes in tissue between at least two functional pools of different sizes and turnover rates. These differences must be large enough to be reflected clearly on the time-activity curves. When the pools are of similar size and turnover rate, the clearance rates are similar for different pools and are difficult to distinguish by examination of the clearance curves. Often, such "similar" pools are, for purposes of tracer kinetic modeling, lumped into one functional pool.

The error sensitivity of estimates predicted by tracer kinetic models increases with the number of functional pools.[4] Therefore, model approaches attempt to reduce the number of compartments while maintaining an acceptable degree of accuracy of predicted measurements. It is recognized that metabolism of tracer compounds results in transfer of the radiolabel to numerous metabolites that may distribute between numerous metabolic pools. Some of these pools may be small and therefore contribute little to the overall tracer tissue kinetics. These pools are then lumped together with other, more dominant pools.

Careful characterization of the metabolic fate of the radiolabel in tissue through biochemical assays is essential for the formulating as well as testing of tracer kinetic models. An initial model configuration must be examined for its accuracy in predicting the distribution of the radiolabel between various pools and how well estimates of functional processes correlate with actual independent measurements. Adjustments are then made, followed by retesting, until

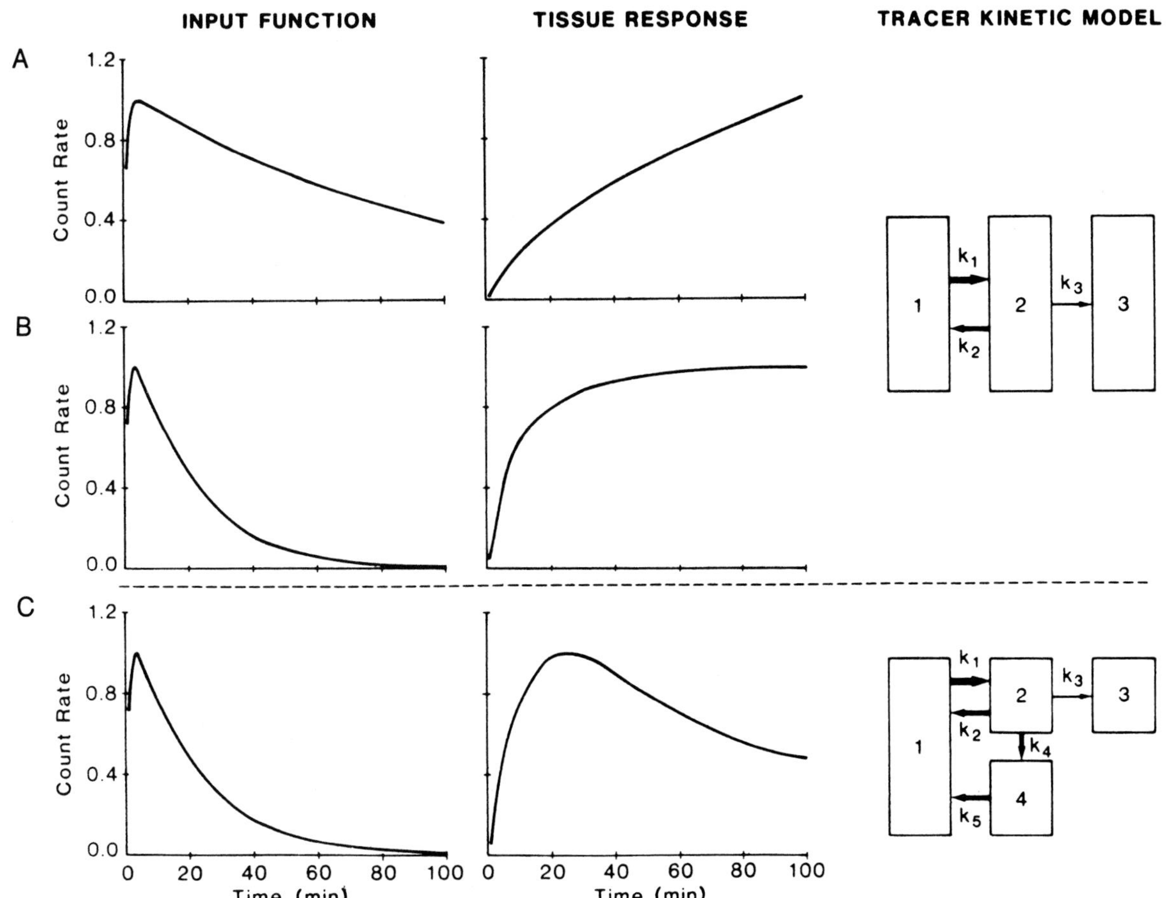

FIGURE 69–22. Dependence of the tissue response on changes in the distribution of the arterial tracer input function and on the specific tracer itself. Panels *A* and *B* compare, for the same tracer, the effects of changes in the tracer input function on the tissue response; panels *B* and *C* compare the tracer-specific differences in the tissue response to an identical distribution of the tracer input function. The rate of the functional process under study is the same in *A* and *B*. In response to the distributed arterial input function as seen in *A*, the tissue concentrations increase over the entire study period. Tracer exchanges from compartment 1 (blood) to compartment 2 (tissue). Effective sequestration of tracer from compartment 2 into compartment 3 (metabolic pool) competes with reversed transport of tracer from compartment 2 to compartment 1. The rates of exchange of tracer between the three compartments are identical in the example shown in *B*; however, the arterial input function is shorter. An initial rapid increase in tissue concentrations is followed by a plateau when tracer concentrations in blood have decreased and an equilibrium state is attained. Tracer kinetic models account for the effects of variations in the arterial input function on the tissue response, which, if it were measured alone, would erroneously indicate a change in the functional process. *C* depicts the same arterial input function as in *B*; however, for a different tracer. Tissue concentrations rapidly rise but subsequently decline, indicating exchange of tracer from blood into tissue (compartments 1 and 2), return of tracer into compartment 1, and unidirectional sequestration into compartment 3 and movement of tracer into compartment 4 with release of radiolabel bound to metabolites from myocardium into blood (compartment 1). (From Phelps, M. E., Mazziotta, J. M., and Huang, S. C.: Study of cerebral function with positron computed tomography. J. Cereb. Blood Flow Metab. 2:113–162, 1982, with permission.)

model estimates approximate actual measurements over a wide range of altered conditions.

An important requirement for the application of tracer kinetic models is that conditions be in equilibrium at the time of the study. Unstable study conditions may alter relative pool sizes and rate constants for tracer exchange and thus degrade the accuracy or even invalidate estimates of functional processes. Furthermore, the assumptions inherent to a model configuration must be valid over a wide range of physiologic and pathophysiologic conditions.

NONINVASIVE MEASUREMENT OF FUNCTIONAL PROCESSES

The noninvasive quantification of functional processes, such as quantification of regional myocardial blood flow and myocardial rates of substrate metabolism, takes advantage of the quantitative imaging capability of positron emission tomography and of the availability of positron-emitting substances that trace a specific process in a well-defined manner and applies tracer kinetic principles in vivo. Because adequate tracer kinetic models have not been developed or validated for all currently employed tracers, evaluation of some functional processes, for example, fatty acid and oxidative metabolism, remains at present only qualitative or semiquantitative.

Evaluation and Quantification of Regional Myocardial Blood Flow

Initial attempts to derive quantitative indices of regional myocardial blood flow relied on either the "fractionation principle" or normalized the myocardial tracer uptake to the arterial input function, which resulted in a quantitative index of blood flow.

The Fractionation Principle

As described by Sapirstein,[165] this principle implies that tracer distributes and is retained in an organ in proportion to the fractional cardiac output it receives. Applied to positron emission tomography, this relationship can be described by the following:

$$\frac{A_R}{A_T} = \frac{Q_F}{CO} \tag{8}$$

where A_R is the activity concentration in a myocardial region of interest, A_T the total activity administered, Q_F the fraction of flow to the myocardial region of interest, and CO cardiac output. The fractional flow Q_F is then determined by rearranging equation 6 to

$$Q_F = \frac{A_R}{A_T} \cdot CO = \frac{(ct \cdot min^{-1} \cdot g^{-1})}{(ct \cdot min^{-1})} \cdot (mL \cdot min^{-1}) = \frac{mL}{g \cdot min} \tag{9}$$

Changes in regional myocardial blood flow induced by an intervention are then calculated by the following:

$$\frac{Q_F \text{ intervention}}{Q_F \text{ control}} = \frac{A_R \text{ intervention}}{A_R \text{ control}} \times \frac{A_T \text{ control}}{A_T \text{ intervention}} \times \frac{CO \text{ control}}{CO \text{ intervention}} \tag{10}$$

Assuming that cardiac output remains unchanged from control to intervention and only flow to the region of interest increases and that the same amount of activity (A_T) is administered at control and during the intervention, the change in blood flow to the region of interest is then estimated by the following:

$$\frac{Q_F \text{ intervention}}{Q_F \text{ control}} = \frac{A_R \text{ intervention}}{A_R \text{ control}} \tag{11}$$

Changes in regional myocardial blood flow induced pharmacologically with intravenous dipyridamole estimated by this approach indicated, however, an only 50 to 100 percent increase in regional myocardial blood flow, which is strikingly less than the previously reported four- to fivefold increase in normal volunteers.[23, 42] Several factors account for this underestimation. First, myocardial concentrations of diffusible tracers do not increase linearly increase with blood flow. As predicted by the Renkin-Crone equation (equation 2) and as shown in Figure 69–2, the myocardial net extraction for ^{13}N-ammonia increases by only 220 percent for a fivefold increase in myocardial blood flow from a control value of 0.9 $mL \cdot min^{-1} \cdot g^{-1}$. Second, the cardiac output is assumed to be constant. However, changes in heart rate and arterial blood pressure during dipyridamole infusion indicate a systemic effect of this agent and thus a change in cardiac output. For example, if cardiac output increases by 50 percent and blood flow to the myocardial region of interest by 400 percent, then the fractional flow to the region of interest will increase only 3.3 instead of 5.0 times. If the increases in both myocardial blood flow and cardiac output were constant for all patients, then fixed values for correction of the flow-dependent decline of the first-pass extraction fraction and the change in cardiac output could be used and the actual increase in myocardial blood flow could be predicted more accurately.

Net Extraction of Tracers

An alternative approach for deriving a quantitative index of myocardial blood flow has been the normalization of the myocardial tracer uptake to the measured arterial input function. As seen in equation 1, the net myocardial tracer uptake is defined as the product of extraction fraction and blood flow and can be calculated from the myocardial tracer concentration Q_t divided by the integral of the arterial input function to that time. Measurements of tracer net extractions have been performed with both ^{13}N-ammonia and ^{82}Rb with the use of either an equilibrium or a tracer bolus approach.

In dog experiments, net extractions of ^{13}N-ammonia were estimated from the myocardial ^{13}N tissue activity concentrations and the arterial input function initially determined by constant withdrawal of arterial blood[166] or, more recently, with dynamic imaging and noninvasive measurements of arterial tracer concentrations.[163, 167] Net extractions at control and changes in response to increases in myocardial blood flow correlated well with the noninvasively determined relationship between first-pass extraction fractions and blood flow and thus provide a noninvasive though quantitative index of regional myocardial blood flow.

As expected, this index, as well as its increase during exercise, underestimates true blood flows and its changes for several reasons: (1) the first-pass extraction fraction is less than 1; (2) it declines with increasing flow; and (3) the arterial input function is artifactually high because of contamination by ^{13}N activity bound to amino acids rather than to ammonia and by spillover of activity from the myocardium into the blood pool. In dogs, as much as 75 percent of the total ^{13}N activity in arterial blood is bound to amino acids 1 minute after intravenous administration of ^{13}N-ammonia.[168] In humans, the ^{13}N label similarly transfers from ammonia to amino acids, although at a slower rate. About 6 percent of the ^{13}N activity in arterial blood was found to be bound to amino acids at 2 minutes after tracer injection.[169] To avoid this contamination as well as the effects of tracer recirculation, Bellina and colleagues[170] extrapolated the "end" of the initial bolus transit, and thus of the arterial input function, by fitting exponentially the early downslope. They derived the net extraction from the quotient of the tracer activity concentration in the myocardium at 2 minutes and the integral of the extrapolated tracer input function. Because the tracer net uptake underestimates the true myocardial blood flow, these investigators then corrected the net uptake at 2 minutes by the first-pass extraction fractions as derived in their study from the correlation between in vitro microsphere–measured blood flow and the ^{13}N-ammonia myocardial net extraction. The resulting estimates of blood flow correlated linearly with those by microspheres over a range from about 0.2 to about 5 $mL \cdot min^{-1} \cdot g^{-1}$.

While this approach yields estimates of myocardial blood flow in humans that are consistent with those derived by other techniques,[171, 172] it is potentially susceptible to errors because flow estimates depend on a single time point, which may be subject to statistical noise especially in low-count situations. Tracer compartment models usually overcome such shortcomings.

Use of Tracer Compartment Models

Different from the more qualitative or semiquantitative indices of blood flow, tracer kinetic models, used in conjunction with quantitative imaging, yield direct estimates of regional myocardial blood flow in milliliters of blood per minute per gram of myocardium. Such models have been developed or are already in use for several tracers of blood flow, for example, ^{13}N-ammonia and ^{15}O-labeled water.

^{13}N-Ammonia

Measurements of myocardial blood flow with this tracer employ model configurations that describe best the kinetics of the tracer and the myocardium. There are two configurations for ^{13}N-ammonia, one with three compartments[173, 174] and the other with only two.[168, 175] The first (three-compartment) configuration approximates more the anatomical pools of the tracer (vascular, extravascular, and metabolic pools), whereas the second (two-compartment) approach lumps the freely diffusible tracer in the intravascular and extravascular spaces into one functional compartment. First-pass extraction fractions of ^{13}N-ammonia approaching unity support the latter configuration, as they imply the absence of a true barrier effect on the transmembranous exchange of the freely diffusible

^{13}N-ammonia. Both model approaches do not differ in principle; in the three-compartment approach, the tracer mass flux rate from compartment 1 to compartment 2 (K_1) represents the blood flow rate and thus acknowledges the absence of a true barrier effect of the capillary wall or between the two compartments.

Because of this similarity, the following discussion focuses mainly on the two-compartment model, as first used by Krivokapich and associates[175] and subsequently validated by Kuhle and co-workers.[168] As mentioned earlier, the model contains one compartment, which represents the freely diffusible ^{13}N-ammonia in the myocardium and lumps the intravascular and extravascular spaces into one functional pool (Fig. 69–23). The second compartment represents the metabolically trapped ^{13}N label in the myocardium, mainly in the forms of glutamate and mostly glutamine. The rate constant K_1 describes the rate of the glutaminase reaction, e.g., the incorporation of the labeled amino group into glutamic acid to form ^{13}N activity in the myocardium, averaging 273 minutes, and because the model is applied to only the first 2 minutes of time activity data, the trapping of the ^{13}N label in the myocardium is considered "unidirectional," so loss of label during such time from the myocardium is negligible.

Measurements of myocardial blood flow with this approach are obtained with an intravenous 30-second bolus injection of ^{13}N-ammonia (555 to 740 MBq or 15 to 20 mCi) and acquisition of ten 12-second dynamic images, followed by two frames of 30 seconds each, one frame of 60 seconds, and one frame of 900 seconds. The latter static image of the myocardial ^{13}N activity concentrations reflects the relative distribution of myocardial blood flow. The transaxially acquired image sets are then reoriented into short-axis images. Sectorial regions of interest are assigned to the left ventricular myocardium, and a small circular region of interest to the center of the left ventricular blood pool. To diminish the negative effects of patient motion, the regions of interest are assigned to the first of the serially acquired images that adequately visualizes the left ventricular myocardium. The regions of interest are then copied to the first 2-minute image data; limitation of the analysis to this initial portion only diminishes the effects of contamination by ^{13}N-ammonia metabolites. The time-activity curves are then corrected for physical decay of ^{13}N as well as the partial volume effects. One model-based approach, as recently described by Porenta and colleagues,[144] derives estimates of regional myocardial thickness from the static ^{13}N-ammonia images. Such estimates of regional myocardial wall thickness in humans correlate well with estimates by echocardiography or by gated magnetic resonance imaging. Other, more recently proposed algorithms correct for patient motion and account for partial volume effects as well as for activity spillover.[176] When compared for independent noninvasive measurements of myocardial blood flow with the microsphere technique,[11] the noninvasive ^{13}N-ammonia positron emission tomography approach appropriately and adequately tracked regional myocardial blood flow.[168] The noninvasive flow estimates correlated linearly with independently measured blood flows (Fig. 69–24). The error bars in Figure 69–24 indicate the variability of regional flow measurements in a given dog experiment, presumably, and as described later, as a function of the spatial- and method-related flow heterogeneity. Additional animal experimental studies have confirmed the validity of the ^{13}N-ammonia blood flow approach.[174, 177] Essential to the measurement approach is the relationship of flow to the first-pass extraction fraction, as established in canine myocardium.[18] Thus, this relationship may not necessarily apply fully to human myocardium. On the other hand, the close correlation of blood flows as determined by the ^{13}N-ammonia and by the ^{15}O-water approach in human myocardium[178] argues against such species-related effect.

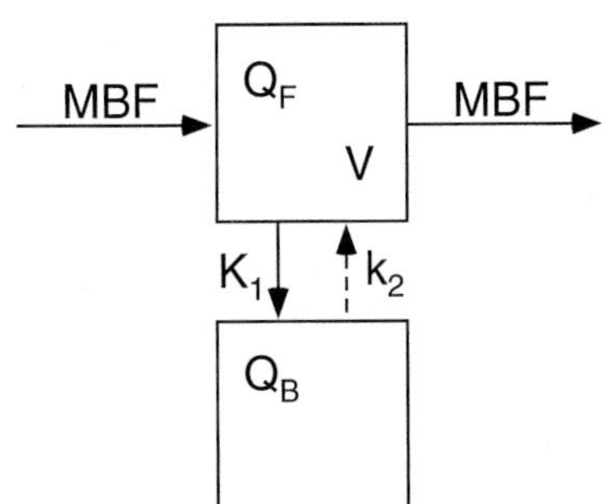

FIGURE 69–23. Two-compartment tracer kinetic model for measurements of myocardial blood flow. Compartment 1 reflects a functional pool of freely exchangeable ^{13}N-ammonia. It combines the activity in the vascular and extravascular spaces. Compartment 2 reflects the ^{13}N activity that has been trapped metabolically. The sum of activity in both compartments at any time after tracer injection reflects the total activity present in the myocardial tissue.

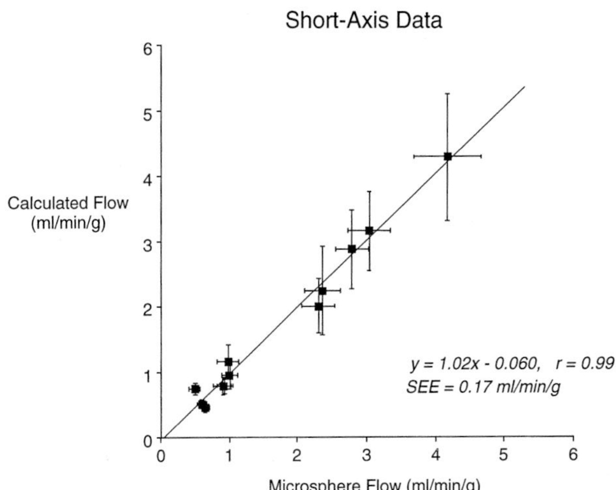

FIGURE 69–24. Validation of the noninvasive approach for the measurement of regional myocardial blood flow with ^{13}N-ammonia in canine myocardium. Note the close correlation of the noninvasive estimates of myocardial blood flow and the independent measurements with the standard microsphere technique. The correlation includes 12 dog experiments. The arrow bars indicate the standard deviation of regional flow measurements and are an index of the total flow heterogeneity as a function of the spatial-, temporal-, and method-related heterogeneity.

Estimates of myocardial blood flow with ^{13}N-ammonia range in normal humans at rest from 0.4 to 1.5 mL · min^{-1} · g^{-1}.[171, 173, 175, 179] During exercise or during intravenous dobutamine stimulation, blood flow increases in proportion to cardiac work, as defined by the product of heart rate and systolic blood pressure (RPP product). As shown in Figure 69–25 and discussed in detail in Chapter 70, myocardial blood flow correlates with cardiac work as a determinant of oxygen demand. Uncoupling of myocardial blood flow from oxygen demand by dipyridamole or adenosine produces three- to fivefold increases in myocardial blood flow. Last, to be of use in examining changes in myocardial blood flow in response to pharmacologic or therapeutic interventions, flow measurements must be reproducible. As shown by Czernin and colleagues[180] in normal volunteers, average flow values for initial and repeat measurement at rest were virtually identical (0.62 ± 0.14 versus 0.66 ± 0.15 mL · min^{-1} · g^{-1}). The random difference amounted to 15.8 ± 15.8 percent. Hyperemic blood flows were similarly reproducible. The initial measurements averaged 2.01 ± 0.39 mL · min^{-1} · g^{-1}, and the repeat measurements 2.03 ± 0.31 mL · min^{-1} · g^{-1}. Again, the random difference averaged 11.8 ± 9.4 percent. Importantly, repeat flow measurements performed on different days were as reproducible as those performed during the same study session with the study participants remaining in the tomograph between studies.

^{15}O-Water

Measurements of myocardial blood flow with ^{15}O-labeled water are based largely on a single tracer compartmental model (Fig.

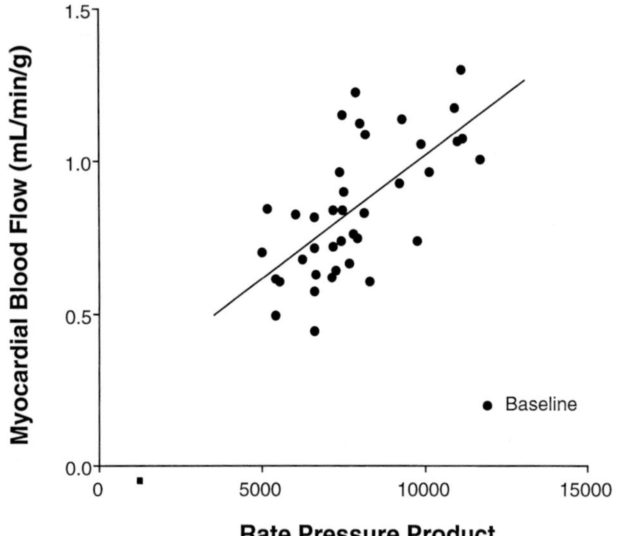

FIGURE 69–25. Myocardial blood flow as a function of cardiac work. The figure compares measurements of myocardial blood flow by the ^{13}N-ammonia approach with the rate-pressure product as an index of cardiac work. Note the close correlation between both estimates.

69–26). The model lumps the concentrations of tracer in tissue and blood into a single compartment and assumes that the tracer immediately and completely equilibrates between plasma and tissue. Differences in tracer concentrations between blood and tissue are then a function of the respective distribution volumes, which depend in blood on the hematocrit and in tissue on its water content.[20] Application of this model to ^{15}O-water assumes (1) that the tracer freely exchanges across the capillary membrane and instantaneously achieves equilibrium, and (2) that the partition coefficient between plasma and myocardium is constant. First-pass extraction fractions of 0.95 or more, as observed by Bergmann and co-workers[27] and described earlier, are in support of the first assumption that the capillary and sarcolemmal membranes exert a negligible barrier effect. According to equation 1, the tracer concentration in myocardium, Q, at time t is equal to the product of the integral of the arterial tracer concentrations to time t and blood flow corrected for the flow-dependent first-pass extraction fraction, E. The latter is assumed to be 1. By rearranging equation 1, myocardial blood flow, F, is then obtained by the following:

$$F = \frac{Q_t}{\int_0^t C_a(t)dt \cdot \lambda} \qquad (12)$$

where 1 is the partition coefficient and represents the ratio of distribution volumes of water in myocardium and in blood. The volume of distribution in myocardium is assumed to equal the myocardial water content (0.7 g H_2O/g muscle). In blood, the volume of distribution corresponds to the plasma water content and depends on the hematocrit.

Single intravenous bolus injections of ^{15}O-water and continuous ^{15}O-labeled carbon dioxide administration techniques have been employed. In experimental animals, estimates of blood flow after single bolus tracer injections correlated with independent measurements by the microsphere technique.[20, 31] Employed in human myocardium and incorporating correction techniques for partial volume and activity spillover into the operational equation, Iida and colleagues[28] recently reported values of 0.95 ± 0.09 mL · min^{-1} · g^{-1} in myocardium of normal subjects and significant reductions of regional flow in patients with severe coronary artery disease with and without prior myocardial infarction. Bergmann and associates[20] further developed a parameter estimation procedure that corrects for partial volume effect, activity spillover, and cardiac motion. Inclusion of these parameters in the operational equation of the flow model in experimental animals resulted in noninvasively obtained flow values that closely and linearly correlated with independent microsphere measurements over a range of 0.3 to 5.0 mL · min^{-1} · g^{-1}. Importantly, the slope of the regression line between noninvasive and invasive flow measurements approached unity (1.096; r = 0.95). Used in 11 normal human volunteers at rest, the approach yielded flow values that were uniform throughout the left ventricular myocardium and averaged, similar to those reported by Iida and co-workers,[28] 0.90 ± 0.22 mL · min^{-1} · g^{-1}. Intravenous dipyridamole in the same normal volunteers raised myocardial blood flow 4.35 times to 3.55 ± 1.15 mL · min^{-1} · g^{-1}. Again, in 11 normal volunteers, Araujo and colleagues[31] used the ^{15}O-carbon dioxide inhalation approach and derived estimates of myocardial blood flow at rest of 0.84 ± 0.09 mL · min^{-1} · g^{-1} and for dipyridamole-induced hyperemia of 3.52 ± 1.12 mL · min^{-1} · g^{-1}. Thus, both approaches yielded nearly identical values. While this approach has been validated against microsphere measurements in dog experiments, two investigations in normal volunteers and patients support the validity of the approach in human myocardium. Shelton and colleagues[181] reported in nine patients with chest pain but angiographically normal coronary arteries nearly identical average values for the myocardial flow reserve (3.5 ± 0.9) and for the coronary flow velocity reserve (3.5 ± 1.2) as assessed with intracoronary flow velocity probes. Similar to the highly significant correlation between both measurements, Merlet and colleagues[182] observed in another study a tight linear correlation between coronary flow velocity reserve and myocardial flow reserve in normal volunteers and patients with idiopathic dilated cardiomyopathy. Despite the potential shortcomings of intracoronary flow velocity measurements, both studies nevertheless support the accuracy with which pharmacologically induced changes in myocardial blood flow can be measured. Although the reproducibility of the ^{15}O-water approach has not been tested yet, a recent multicenter trial in 53 patients in seven different institutions with different imaging equipment reported comparable values for different laboratories.[183] This then would allow pooling of blood flow data from multiple institutions, as has already been done in an earlier investigation that examined the effects of coronary stenosis on hyperemic blood flows.[184]

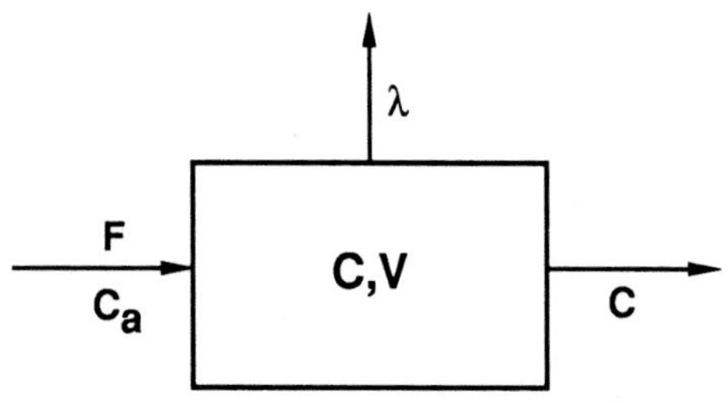

FIGURE 69–26. One-compartment model for ^{15}O-water. F = blood flow; C_a = tracer concentration in arterial blood; C = tracer concentration; V = volume of distribution in tissue; λ = physical decay constant of ^{15}O. (See text.)

Perfusible Tissue Fraction

Iida and colleagues[28] explored novel strategies for solving the partial volume effect. One evolving concept was that of the "tissue fraction," or the fraction of tissue in a given region of interest. What evolved from this concept was the "perfusible tissue fraction."[33] The term describes the fraction of the myocardium that exchanges water rapidly. It is derived by subtraction of blood pool images, obtained with ^{15}O-labeled carbon monoxide from the transmission images, which yields the extravascular myocardial tissue volume. The portion of this volume that on imaging with ^{15}O-water exchanges water rapidly is then referred to as the "water perfusible tissue fraction." Theoretically, this fraction should be at unity in normal myocardium, as all myocytes should be capable of rapid water exchanges. Yet, in infarcted myocardial regions, the perfusible tissue fraction should decline in proportion to the fraction of necrotic or scar tissue if, as postulated, these tissues do not freely and rapidly exchange water.[185, 186] Indeed, Iida and colleagues (personal communication) reported an inverse correlation between the perfusible tissue index and the extent of tissue fibrosis as determined morphometically in dog experiments.

The approach offers two obvious advantages: (1) a measure of the amount of fibrosis in a given myocardial region, and (2) the fraction of viable myocardium to which functional processes can be related. Findings both in early postinfarction patients and in patients with coronary artery disease imply that the perfusible tissue index does, in fact, provide a measure of the extent necrosis or fibrosis, or both,[185, 186] which at the same time contains prognostic information regarding the long-term outcome in regional contractile function. When more than 30 percent of a given myocardial segment no longer exchanges water rapidly, contractile function is found to be impaired irreversibly. Second, most approaches to the measurement of blood flow yield average transmural values. Accordingly, Yamamoto and co-workers[185] reported 64 ± 14 percent reductions in total transmural flow in previously infarcted regions in patients with chronic coronary artery disease. Yet, when blood flow was related to only the "viable portion" in a given infarcted segment, this reduction in regional flow in viable myocardium amounted to only 28 ± 38 percent.

Despite these encouraging results, the water-perfusible tissue index is not without shortcomings. One relates to the low count and, thus, statistically noisy images that diminish the certainty with which regional processes can be determined. Second, corrections for spillover of activity from the blood pool into the myocardium, especially in the interventricular septum, which is affected by activity originating from both the left and the right ventricular cavities, remain unsatisfactory. Last, separation of the activity in the anterior wall of the left ventricle from that in the anterior chest wall remains incomplete. All three limitations may adversely affect estimates of blood flow and of the perfusible tissue fraction and thus diminish the confidence in individual regional measurements.

Other Tracers

Early investigations by Mullani, Gould, and Goldstein and their co-workers[36, 187] focused on the development of quantitative approaches to the measurement of regional myocardial blood flow with ^{82}Rb. A two-compartment model, similar to that established for ^{13}N-ammonia, had been developed and tested with time-activity curves derived with β-probes attached to the left ventricular myocardium in open-chest dog experiments. In these studies, the proposed tracer compartment model did, in fact, fit the experimental data and predicted estimates of blood flow that were indeed consistent with those obtained independently with the microsphere technique. Use of the ultra-short-lived ^{82}Rb for quantitative blood flow studies is, however, challenging. The 75-second physical half-life requires high-activity doses to recover adequate counts from the myocardium after tracer clearance from blood. This requirement, on the other hand, necessitates the intravenous bolus injection of 40 to 60 mCi of ^{82}Rb; the activity during the initial bolus transit through the central circulation is therefore rather high and exceeds the count capability of most current positron emission tomographs. This limitation precludes the noninvasive derivation of the arterial input function. Nevertheless, Herrero and colleagues[188, 189] succeeded in testing in vivo in intact dogs a mathematical model that yielded with ^{82}Rb estimates of blood flow that correlated with those determined simultaneously with microspheres. Overall, the noninvasive ^{82}Rb approach underestimated true blood flows by about 10 percent and, further, yielded less reliable estimates in acutely ischemic myocardium.

Lastly, Herrero and co-investigators[190] demonstrated the possibility of estimating regional myocardial blood flow with ^{62}Cu-labeled PTSM both in experimental animals and in humans. With the use of a two-compartment tracer kinetic model and correcting for contamination of the arterial input function by tracer bound to red blood cells, the noninvasively derived estimates of myocardial blood flow correlated linearly with those obtained with the microsphere technique. In five normal volunteers, the approach yielded an average flow value of 1.05 ± 0.36 mL · min^{-1} · g^{-1}, which is similar to that derived from any simultaneous measurements with ^{15}O-water.

Choice of Flow Measurement Techniques

At present, the choice of flow measurement techniques is between the ^{13}N-ammonia and the ^{15}O-water approaches. Both techniques appear to yield comparable results. Yet, the issue of which technique is superior has been intensely and at times heatedly debated. Undoubtedly, ^{15}O-water meets more closely the requirements of an ideal flow tracer. It is metabolically inert, its first-pass extraction fraction is 1 and does not vary with flow. In contrast, ^{13}N-ammonia has a high though less than complete first-pass extraction fraction that declines with increasing flows. Further, its metabolic trapping mechanism may be susceptible to metabolic derangements. The latter may account for the reduced trapping of ^{13}N-ammonia in the posterolateral wall of the normal human left ventricle. While still unexplained, the reduced trapping may, in fact, be related to regional alterations in metabolism, as also evidenced by the enhanced ^{18}F-deoxyglucose uptake in the same region.[191, 192] Given these differences in the basic physiologic properties, it would seem that the issue must be decided primarily on practical terms. The main criteria are the image quality and the accuracy and statistical confidence with which regional blood flows can be quantified.

IMAGE QUALITY. Because ^{15}O-water freely diffuses across capillary and cellular membranes, it distributes into the water spaces of myocardium but also of blood and adjacent tissues which results in a low target to background ratio. The need for blood pool substraction with ^{15}O-carbon monoxide in addition to the rapid loss of tracer from myocardium and its short physical half-life may result in low count, statistically noisy images. Misalignments between the water and the blood pool images are additional sources of error. Nitrogen-13 ammonia, in contrast, becomes effectively trapped in myocardium, though in nonlinear proportion to blood flow, and rapidly clears from blood. The resulting higher target to background ratios together with the longer physical half-life and, consequently, longer imaging times permit acquisition of high count density images with high target to background ratios. Thus, ^{13}N-ammonia offers images of higher diagnostic quality. On the other hand, the longer physical half-life of ^{13}N precludes rapid serial studies as they are possible with only the 2.5 minute short-lived ^{15}O-water.

ACCURACY OF REGIONAL MEASUREMENTS OR OBSERVED HETEROGENEITY. The observed heterogeneity of blood flow serves as another criterion for determining how well regional myocardial blood flow can be assessed with either technique. It is important to emphasize that myocardial blood flow, per se, is spatially and temporally heterogeneous. Such heterogeneity has been demonstrated with radiolabeled microspheres in awake baboons[105] and awake dogs.[106] The coefficient of variation of flow or the relative dispersion (RD) as a measure of this heterogeneity was found to average 0.28 ± 0.07 in the baboons. The observed relative dispersion ($RD_{observed}$) is a function of the following:

$$RD^2_{observed} = RD^2_{temporal} + RD^2_{spatial} + RD^2_{method} \qquad (13)$$

that is, a function of the temporal- ($RD_{temporal}$), spatial- ($RD_{spatial}$), and method-related (RD_{method}) heterogeneity.[105] Of interest is that the values in awake dogs were lower (0.21 ± 0.02) than those in baboons. Much of this difference can be attributed to the sample sizes from which the RD is determined. The findings in the baboons were based on myocardial tissue samples of only 0.17 g, compared with 1.08 g tissue samples in dogs. The relative dispersion values in different studies can be related to each other by the square root of the ratio of the sample sizes or masses.[193]

These invasive studies in animal experiments provide a framework for evaluating heterogeneities in blood flow values observed with the noninvasive positron emission tomography approaches in human myocardium and for comparing method-related relative dispersions. Coefficients of variations reported for blood flow estimates in normal volunteers with the ^{15}O-water approach averaged 0.15 for an average sample size of about 10 g[31] and 0.35 for a sample volume of about 3.9 g[20], compared with an average value of 0.18 for a sample volume of 4.2 g for the ^{13}N-ammonia technique.[194] In the earlier discussion, the sample sizes were estimated from the slice thicknesses and the region-of-interest sizes as described in each of the three reports and are only approximations. If adjusted to an average sample size of 4 cm^3, the observed relative dispersions would amount to 0.24 and 0.35 for the two ^{15}O-water studies and to about 0.18 for the ^{13}N-ammonia approach. If one assumes the same values for spatial and temporal heterogeneities in the three studies in normal volunteers, then the above calculations suggest a somewhat lesser method-related heterogeneity for the ^{13}N-ammonia approach.

From the aforementioned considerations, one can see that either approach offers advantages but also has shortcomings. Thus, the choice of a specific measurement approach often seems to depend on laboratory specific conditions. Such conditions may include availability of a given tracer, ease of radiotracer synthesis, proximity of the cyclotron and of radiochemistry to the scanner, instrument performance, other research activities and type of studies performed in the same laboratory, and associated needs for a given tracer.

Measurements of Myocardial Glucose Metabolism

Quantification of regional rates of glucose utilization in millimoles of glucose per minute per gram of myocardium takes advantage of the unidirectional transport of labeled 2-deoxyglucose and a three-compartment tracer kinetic model proposed initially by Sokoloff and colleagues[195] for autoradiographic measurements of regional cerebral glucose metabolism in cats. Labeling of the glucose analog with the positron emitter ^{18}F with substitution of the methyl group by fluorine in the 2 position permitted the application of the deoxyglucose tracer compartmental model to the in vivo study of regional glucose metabolism in human brain and heart.[88, 196–198]

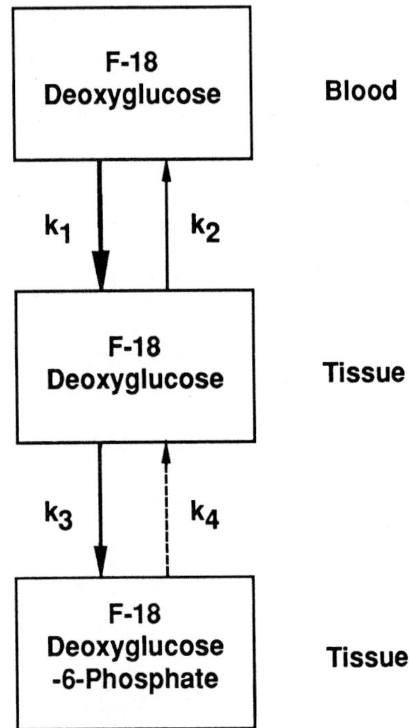

FIGURE 69–27. Three-compartment model for ^{18}F-2-fluoro-2-deoxyglucose (see text).

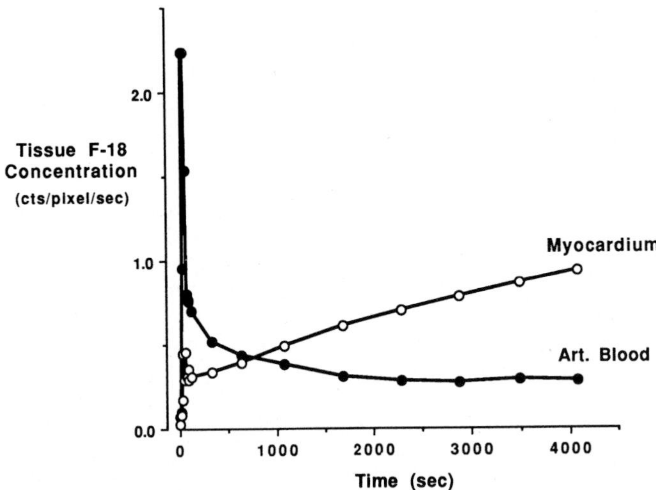

FIGURE 69–28. Fluorine-18 activity concentrations in arterial blood and myocardium following intravenous injection of ^{18}F-2-fluoro-2-deoxyglucose in a normal volunteer. The time-activity curves were derived from serially acquired cross-sectional positron emission tomography images.

A three-compartment model describes the tissue kinetics of ^{18}F-2-fluoro-2-deoxyglucose. As seen in Figure 69–27, compartment 1 represents tracer concentrations in blood, compartment 2 the tracer concentration in tissue, and compartment 3 the concentration of the phosphorylated compound ^{18}F-2-deoxyglucose-6-phosphate in myocardium. The linear rate constants k_1 and k_2 describe the forward and reverse transport of tracer between blood and tissue (transmembranous exchange), k_3 the hexokinase-mediated rate of phosphorylation, and k_4 the rate of phosphatase-mediated dephosphorylation. Although the activity of phosphatase is very low in myocardium, modifications of Sokoloff's initial tracer kinetic model now accommodate dephosphorylation rates.[197–199]

The model relates the myocardial metabolic rate of exogenous glucose utilization (MMRGlc) to the measured rate constants for ^{18}F-deoxyglucose by the following:

$$\text{MMRGlc} = \frac{C_p}{LC} \cdot \frac{k_1 k_3}{k_2 + k_3} (\mu\text{mol} \cdot \text{min}^{-1} \cdot \text{g}^{-1}) \quad (14)$$

where $k_1 \cdot k_3/k_2 + k_3$ (also referred to as K) reflects the rate of effective metabolic sequestration or clearance of ^{18}F-2-fluoro-2-deoxyglucose from plasma into myocardium. The term C_p is the concentration of glucose in plasma. The lumped constant LC adjusts for differences in transport and phosphorylation rates between glucose and ^{18}F-2-deoxyglucose as both compete for the same transport sites and are competitive substrates for hexokinase.

For measurements of rates of myocardial utilization of exogenous glucose, ^{18}F-deoxyglucose is administered intravenously. Serial images are acquired for 60 to 90 minutes, and regional myocardial tissue time-activity curves obtained. Least square fitting of the time activity curves (see Fig. 69–28) with the operational equation yields the individual rate constants k_1 to k_4, which are then entered together with the arterial plasma glucose concentrations into equation 14. For the lumped constant, LC, a fixed value of 0.67 is used, as determined in canine myocardium.[88] Estimates of glucose utilization by this approach were found to correlate in dog experiments with glucose consumption rates, as determined by the Fick principle (Fig. 69–29),[88] and predicted in normal human subjects glucose utilization rates that were similar to those reported previously in the literature.[135, 200]

More recent developments promise to simplify data analysis and facilitate the use of the approach in humans. As proposed by Patlak and co-workers,[201, 202] and as shown in Figure 69–30, the rate of glucose consumption can also be estimated graphically.[36] Tracer concentrations at time t in myocardium (A_m) over tracer concentra-

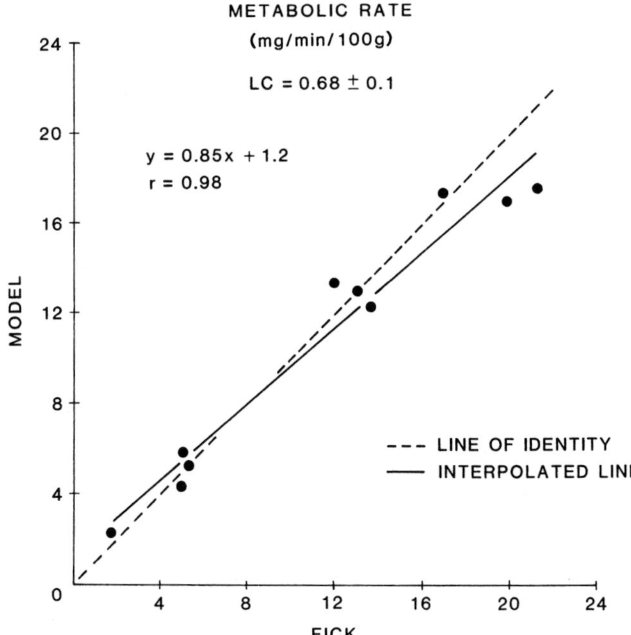

FIGURE 69–29. Comparison of noninvasively obtained estimates of regional myocardial exogenous glucose utilization rates with the ^{18}F-2-deoxyglucose positron emission tomography approach and simultaneous invasive measurements by the Fick method in dog experiments. (From Ratib, O., Phelps, M. E., Huang, S. C., et al.: Positron tomography with deoxyglucose for estimating local myocardial glucose metabolism. J. Nucl. Med. 23:577–586, with permission of The Society of Nuclear Medicine.)

tions in plasma are plotted against the integral of the arterial tracer input function divided by the arterial tracer concentration at time t. The slope corresponds to $k_1 \cdot k_3/k_2 + k_3$ and thus indicates the fraction of ^{18}F-2-deoxyglucose in plasma that is phosphorylated and metabolically sequestered into myocardium. The approach as described by Gambhir and colleagues[199] includes corrections for bidirectional spillover of activity between myocardium and blood and provides for k_4 or phosphatase activity. The graphical analysis approach provided in six normal volunteers estimates of glucose metabolism that were in close agreement with those obtained by the traditional derivation of individual rate constants by least square fitting of the time-activity curve. The graphical approach offers several advantages: It is computationally fast, corrects for activity spillover, and can be performed from only three tissue time points. In addition to reducing sampling requirements (only three myocardial images are required), the approach also appears suitable for development of parametric images with pixel-by-pixel display of regional glucose utilization rates.[203]

The myocardial uptake of ^{18}F-deoxyglucose and, consequently, glucose utilization rates depend on the concentrations of circulating plasma substrate and hormone (e.g., insulin, norepinephrine) levels. Early investigations in animals and subsequently in humans had pointed out this dependence of ^{18}F-deoxyglucose uptake and MMRGlc on plasma fatty acid, glucose, and lactate levels.[85, 88, 204, 205] Investigations in normal human volunteers has also emphasized the poor diagnostic quality of myocardial ^{18}F-deoxyglucose uptake images when studies were performed in the fasted rather than in the glucose-loaded state.[204, 205]

More recent investigations explored more systematically this dependence on circulating substrate levels and on the dietary state. Table 69–5 summarizes the glucose-utilization rates as reported for different dietary conditions or after manipulation of substrate plasma levels.[110, 205–207] These noninvasively derived estimates of MMRGlc in human myocardium are indeed comparable to those obtained with invasive study techniques and the Fick principle. At the same time, the observed interindividual variability has prompted the development of techniques to standardize the dietary state or circulating plasma glucose and insulin levels. One approach is the oral administration of 50 to 100 g of glucose about 1 hour prior to the administration of ^{18}F-deoxyglucose.[90] In normal volunteers, this results in a prompt increase in circulating plasma glucose concentrations, which, in turn, stimulates secretion of insulin. For example, one study reports an increase in insulin levels from 8 ± 3 mU · mL^{-1} under fasted conditions to 42 ± 18 mU · mL^{-1} after oral glucose loading. Another approach entails the hyperinsulinemic-euglycemic clamp.[208] A continuous infusion of insulin (its rate being adjusted to the body weight and tritrated to achieve plasma glucose levels in the range of 80 to 95 mg%), combined in some laboratories with an infusion of 20 percent dextrose in water, is preceded by a loading dose of regular insulin. Depending on the specific protocol used in a given laboratory, the clamp results in glucose utilization rates of 0.44 ± 0.12 µmol · min^{-1} · g^{-1} [110] or, in another study, of 0.74 ± 0.029 mmol · min^{-1} · g^{-1}.[206] The higher values in the latter study presumably result from the additional infusion of 20 percent dextrose in water. It is also of interest that the hyperinsulinemic-euglycemic clamp in the latter study resulted in MMRGlcs that were similar to those calculated after oral glucose administration (30 g). Both standardization approaches yield comparable interindividual variabilities, as expressed by coefficients of variation (e.g., 26.3 percent for the clamp, and 22.5 percent for oral glucose-loading studies). Unlike the glucose-loading approach, the hyperinsulinemic clamp resulted in approximately a 50 percent higher K value, the rate constant for transmembranous exchange and the hexokinase reaction that indicates significantly greater phosphorylation of glucose to glucose-6-phosphate. This increase, in turn, caused more clearance of ^{18}F activity from blood and, consequently, higher myocardial–to–blood pool (background) activity ratios.

Similar values for glucose metabolic rates were observed[205] after oral glucose loading (see Table 69–5). This study examined quantitatively the effects of glucose loading and of different time periods of fasting on the rate of exogenous glucose utilization by myocardium in 16 normal volunteers. Glucose administration resulted in a 2.9-fold increase in the MMRGlc from that in the fasted state. Further, the study demonstrated comparable MMRGlcs for different periods of fasting, for example, for 6 ± 2 hours and 16 ± 2 hours.

The hyperinsulinemic-euglycemic clamp has also proved useful for enhancing the image quality in diabetic patients and for stimulating myocardial glucose utilization.[209] As an alternative means of enhancing myocardial glucose utilization and, thus, ^{18}F-deoxyglucose uptake, oral administration of nicotinic acid derivatives may prove useful. For example, niacin lowers circulating free fatty acid

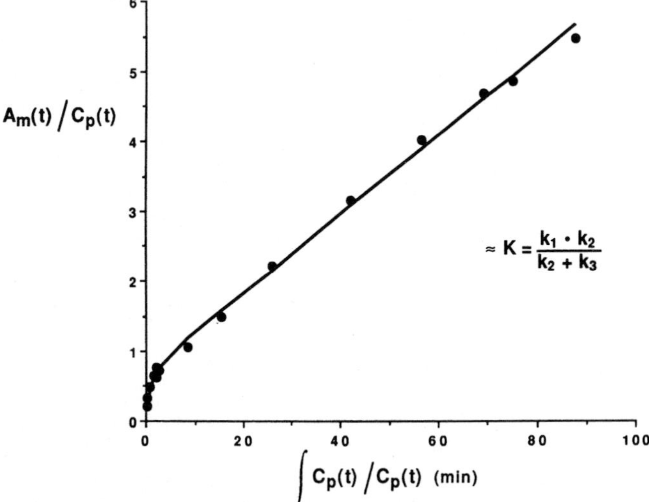

FIGURE 69–30. Patlak graphic analysis for the noninvasive quantification of myocardial rates of exogenous glucose utilization. A_m = activity concentrations in myocardium; C_p = tracer concentration in arterial blood. The slope of the plot corresponds to K or $k_1 \times k_3/k_2 + k_3$.

TABLE 69–5. MYOCARDIAL GLUCOSE UTILIZATION RATES IN NORMAL HUMAN MYOCARDIUM

Study	n	Plasma FFA (mEq · L^{-1})	Glucose mg%	Insulin µL · mL^{-1}	MMRGlc µmol · min^{-1} · g^{-1}
Fasting					
Choi et al.[205]	18	0.30±0.25	87±6	8±3	0.24±0.17
Ohtake et al.[209]	17	1.07±0.46	90±9	4±1	0.13±0.09
Oral Glucose Loading					
Choi et al.[205]	18	0.19±0.14	154±32	42±18	0.69±0.11
Knuuti et al.[206]	8	N/A	151±14	45±8	0.69±0.03
Ohtake et al.[209]	17	0.31±0.20	126±15	45±19	0.52±0.05
Euglycemic-Hyperinsulinemic Clamp					
Knuuti et al.[206]	8	N/A	92±4	104±71	0.74±0.03
vom Dahl et al.[110]	9°	0.12±0.04	85±7	75±14	0.44±0.12
Ohtake et al.[209]	17	0.34±0.17	98±17	90±41	0.54±0.11

n = number of normal volunteers; FFA = free fatty acid concentrations; MMRGlc = rate of myocardial glucose metabolic utilization; N/A = not reported.

levels; this diminishes the inhibitory effects of fatty acids on glycolysis and pyruvate oxidation and thus accelerates glucose utilization. Stone and colleagues[61] recently reported that oral administration of niacin (250 mg in 100 to 150 mL of water) in five normal volunteers after an overnight fast significantly lowered plasma free fatty acid levels and, in turn, produced a two- to threefold increase in myocardial glucose utilization rates as determined with ^{18}F-2 deoxyglucose. Similarly, Knuuti and associates[210] observed in 12 patients that lipid lowering with the nicotinic acid derivative acipimox was as effective as that with the hyperinsulinemic-euglycemic clamp in standardizing MMRGlc.

While initial investigations with ^{18}F-deoxyglucose reported homogeneous myocardial ^{18}F-deoxyglucose uptake and MMRGlcs,[211] Gropler and co-workers[191] drew attention to a marked heterogeneity. In nine healthy volunteers, these investigators reported approximately a 20 percent higher ^{18}F-deoxyglucose uptake in the lateral and posterolateral wall than in the septum and the anterior wall of the left ventricle ($P < .03$). This heterogeneity was most prominent in the fasted state but was also noted after oral glucose loading, when it no longer reached statistical significance. These findings were based on the analysis of transaxial images of the heart. Subsequent measurements based on short-axis cuts of the left ventricular myocardium and polar maps confirmed these observations. Regional differences in myocardial oxygen consumption, in wall motion, or in wall thickness do not explain the observed heterogeneity. Measurements of MMRGlc from short-axis cross sections and after corrections for regional partial volume effects indicated further that the observed heterogeneity does not depend on the preferential substrate selection of the myocardium. For example, Choi and colleagues[205] noted a difference in MMRGlc between the posterolateral and the anterior wall of 0.13 mmol · min^{-1} · g^{-1} in the fasted and of 0.18 mmol · min^{-1} · g^{-1} in the glucose-loaded state. Both values did not differ significantly, although, in relative terms, this difference was significantly lower in the glucose-loaded (24 percent) than in the fasted state (32 percent).

Although the ^{18}F-2-deoxyglucose approach has been successfully employed for noninvasive quantification of regional myocardial glucose utilization rates, several issues remain unresolved at present. Foremost is the use of a fixed value for the LC. Although this value has been found relatively constant over a wide range of normal and abnormal conditions in isolated arterially perfused rat hearts[89, 90] and in dogs,[88] other investigations in the isolated working rat-heart preparations suggest that the LC may be affected by glucose and insulin concentrations in the perfusate. In one study, addition of physiologic concentrations of insulin to the glucose-containing perfusate increased the LC,[212] while in another study markedly higher concentrations of insulin were noted to lower the LC.[213] Again, fasting and feeding as well as postischemia failed to significantly alter LC in isolated rat hearts.[214] Last, perturbation of the steady-state condition in the isolated arterially perfused rat heart, as recently reported by Hariharan and associates,[215] again affected the LC and thus re-emphasized one of the fundamental conditions of tracer kinetic principles, that is, the presence of steady-state conditions during measurements.

SUMMARY AND FUTURE DEVELOPMENTS

Recent logistical and technical developments promise a greater role for positron-emitting tracers in general nuclear medicine. It is now clear that myocardial ^{18}F-deoxyglucose uptake can be imaged with conventional and widely available though modified single-photon emission computed tomography equipment.[216–218] An ever-increasing geographic density of medical cyclotrons and radiopharmaceutical delivery systems and, thus, a greater availability of positron-emitting tracers offer the opportunity for a far greater clinical utilization of positron-emitting tracers of metabolism. This then would expand the scope of diagnostic possibilities in the more conventional setting of the nuclear medicine laboratory.

At the same time, "traditional" positron emission tomography will probably maintain its course. Initial developments have demonstrated the possibility of quantifying regional functional processes in myocardium. They advantageously combined the unique quantitative imaging capability of positron emission tomography with use of physiologically active positron-emitting tracers of myocardial tissue function. At present, most advanced are the quantification of regional myocardial blood flow and glucose metabolism. Other tracers have permitted the qualitative evaluation of additional aspects of tissue function, for example, fatty acid metabolism and overall oxidative metabolism. Appropriate tracer kinetic models await development and validation before these functions can be quantified. Furthermore, the emergence and characterization of new tracers will expand the scope with which myocardial tissue function can be characterized noninvasively in human myocardium. These new approaches, together with the ones already developed, should permit more accurate and complete definition of the human heart's normal and abnormal physiology.

Acknowledgments

The author thanks Diane Martin and Melissa Sheldon for preparing the illustrations and Eileen Rosenfeld for her skillful assistance in preparing this manuscript.

References

1. Fowler, J. S., and Wolf, A. P.: Positron emitter–labeled compounds: Priorities and problems. *In* Phelps, M., Mazziotta, J., and Schelbert, H. (eds.): Positron Emission Tomography and Autoradiography: Principles and Applications for the Brain and Heart. Vol. 9. New York, Raven Press, 1986, p. 391.

2. Renkin, E. M.: Transport of potassium-42 from blood tissue in isolated mammalian skeletal muscles. Am. J. Physiol. 197:1205, 1959.
3. Crone, C.: Permeability of capillaries in various organs as determined by use of the indicator diffusion method. Acta Physiol. Scand. 58:292, 1963.
4. Huang, S. C., and Phelps, M. E.: Principles of tracer kinetic modeling in positron emission tomography and autoradiography. *In* Phelps, M., Mazziotta, J., and Schelbert, H. (eds.): Positron Emission Tomography and Autoradiography: Principles and Applications for the Brain and Heart. Vol. 9. New York, Raven Press, 1986, p. 287.
5. Phelps, M., Huang, S., Hoffman, E., et al.: Cerebral extraction of N-13 ammonia: Its dependence on cerebral blood flow and capillary permeability surface area product. Stroke 12:607, 1981.
6. Hnatowich, D. J.: Labeling of human albumin microspheres with Ga-68. J. Nucl. Med. 17:57, 1976.
7. Turton, D. R., Brady, F., Pike, V. W., et al.: Preparation of human serum [methyl-^{11}C] methylalbumin microspheres and human serum [methyl-11] methylalbumin for clinical use. Int. J. Appl. Radiat. Isot. 35:337, 1984.
8. Wisenberg, G., Schelbert, H. R., Hoffman, E. J., et al.: In vivo quantitation of regional myocardial blood flow by positron emission computed tomography. Circulation 63:1248, 1981.
9. Wilson, R. A., Shea, M. J., De Landsheere, C. H., et al.: Validation of quantitation of regional myocardial blood flow in vivo with ^{11}C-labeled human albumin microspheres and positron emission tomography. Circulation 70:717, 1984.
10. Selwyn, A. P., Shea, M. J., Foale, R., et al.: Regional myocardial and organ blood flow after myocardial infarction: Application of the microsphere principle in man. Circulation 73:433, 1986.
11. Heymann, M. A., Payne, B. D., Hoffman, J. I. E., et al.: Blood flow measurements with radionuclide-labeled particles. Prog. Cardiovasc. Dis. 20:55, 1977.
12. Hunter, W., and Monahan, W. G.: A new physiologic radiotracer for nuclear medicine. J. Nucl. Med. 12:368, 1971.
13. Harper, P. V., Lathrop, K. A., Krizek, H., et al.: Clinical feasibility of myocardial imaging with $^{13}NH_3$. J. Nucl. Med. 13:278, 1972.
14. Phelps, M. E., Hoffman, E. J., Coleman, R. E., et al.: Tomographic images of blood pool and perfusion in brain and heart. J. Nucl. Med. 17:603, 1976.
15. Schelbert, H. R., Phelps, M. E., Hoffman, E. J., et al.: Regional myocardial perfusion assessed with N-13 labeled ammonia and positron emission computerized axial tomography. Am. J. Cardiol. 43:209, 1979.
16. Walsh, W. F., Harper, P. V., Resnekov, L., et al.: Noninvasive evaluation of regional myocardial perfusion in 112 patients using a mobile scintillation camera and intravenous nitrogen-13 labeled ammonia. Circulation 54:226, 1976.
17. Post, R. L., and Jolly, P. C.: The linkage of sodium, potassium and ammonium active transport across the human erythrocyte membrane. Biochim. Biophys. Acta. 25:118, 1957.
18. Schelbert, H. R., Phelps, M. E., Huang, S. C., et al.: N-13 ammonia as an indicator of myocardial blood flow. Circulation 63:1259, 1981.
19. Poe, N. D.: Comparative myocardial uptake and clearance characteristics of potassium and cesium. J. Nucl. Med. 13:557, 1972.
20. Bergmann, S. R., Herrero, P., Markham, J., et al.: Noninvasive quantitation of myocardial blood flow in human subjects with oxygen-15–labeled water and positron emission tomography. J. Am. Coll. Cardiol. 14:639, 1989.
21. Krivokapich, J., Barrio, J. R., Phelps, M. E., et al.: Kinetic characterization of $^{13}NH_3$ and ^{13}N-glutamine metabolism in rabbit heart. Am. J. Physiol. 246:H267, 1983.
22. Brunken, R., Schwaiger, M., Grover-McKay, M., et al.: Positron emission tomography detects tissue metabolic activity in myocardial segments with persistent thallium perfusion defects. J. Am. Coll. Cardiol. 10:557, 1987.
23. Schelbert, H. R., Wisenberg, G., Phelps, M. E., et al.: Noninvasive assessment of coronary stenoses by myocardial imaging during pharmacologic coronary vasodilation. VI. Detection of coronary artery disease in man with intravenous N-13 ammonia and positron computed tomography. Am. J. Cardiol. 49:1197, 1982.
24. Tamaki, N., Yonekura, Y., Senda, M., et al.: Value and limitation of stress thallium-201 single photon emission computed tomography: Comparison with nitrogen-13 ammonia positron tomography. J. Nucl. Med. 29:1181, 1988.
25. Tillisch, J., Brunken, R., Marshall, R., et al.: Reversibility of cardiac wall motion abnormalities predicted by positron tomography. N. Engl. J. Med. 314:884, 1986.
26. Walsh, M. N., Brown, M. A., Henes, C. G., et al.: Estimation of regional myocardial oxidative metabolism by positron emission tomography with carbon-22–acetate in patients. Circulation 78:II-599, 1988.
27. Bergmann, S. R., Fox, K. A. A., Rand, A. L., et al.: Quantification of regional myocardial blood flow in vivo with $H_2{}^{15}O$. Circulation 70:724, 1984.
28. Iida, H., Kanno, I., Takahashi, A., et al.: Measurement of absolute myocardial blood flow with $H_2{}^{15}O$ and dynamic positron-emission tomography: Strategy for quantification in relation to the partial-volume effect. Circulation 78:104, 1988.
29. Knabb, R. M., Fox, K. A. A., Sobel, B. E., et al.: Characterization of the functional significance of subcritical coronary stenoses with $H_2{}^{15}O$ and positron-emission tomography. Circulation 71:1271, 1985.
30. Walsh, M. N., Bergmann, S. R., Steele, R. L., et al.: Delineation of impaired regional myocardial perfusion by positron emission tomography with $H_2{}^{15}O$. Circulation 78:612, 1988.
31. Araujo, L., Lammertsma, A., Rhodes, C., et al.: Noninvasive quantification of regional myocardial blood flow in coronary artery disease with oxygen-15–labeled carbon dioxide inhalation and positron emission tomography. Circulation 83:875, 1991.
32. Lammertsma, A. A., DeSilva, R., Araujo, L. I., et al.: Measurement of regional myocardial blood flow using $C^{15}O_2$ and positron emission tomography: Comparison of tracer models. Clin. Physics Physiol. Meas. 13:1, 1992.
33. Iida, H., Rhodes, C., de Silva, R., et al.: Myocardial tissue fraction: Correction for partial volume effects and measure of tissue viability. J. Nucl. Med. 32:2169, 1991.
34. Huang, S. C., Williams, B. A., Krivokapich, J., et al.: Rabbit myocardial ^{82}Rb kinetics and a compartmental model for blood flow estimation. Am. J. Physiol. 256:H1156, 1989.
35. Goldstein, R. A., Klein, M. S., Welch, M. J., et al.: External assessment of myocardial metabolism with C-11 palmitate in vivo. J. Nucl. Med. 21:342, 1980.
36. Goldstein, R. A., Mullani, N. A., Marani, S. K., et al.: Perfusion imaging with rubidium-82: II. Effects of pharmacologic interventions on flow and extraction. J. Nucl. Med. 24:907, 1983.
37. Mullani, N. A., Goldstein, R. A., Gould, K. L., et al.: Perfusion imaging with rubidium-82: I. Measurement of extraction and flow with external detectors. J. Nucl. Med. 24:898, 1983.
38. Bergmann, S., Shelton, M., Weinheimer, C., et al.: Accuracy of quantitative estimates of myocardial blood flow with rubidium-82 and positron emission tomography. J. Nucl. Med. 30:807, 1989.
39. Grover-McKay, M., Huang, S. C., Hoffman, E. J., et al.: Noninvasive quantification of myocardial blood flow in dogs with rubidium-82 and PET. J. Nucl. Med. 27:976, 1986.
40. Budinger, T. F., Yano, Y., Moyer, B., et al.: Myocardial extraction of Rb-82 vs. flow determined by positron emission tomography. J. Nucl. Med. 68:III-81, 1983.
41. Glatting, G., Bergmann, K., Stollfub, J., et al.: Myocardial Rb extraction fraction: Determination in humans. J. Am. Coll. Cardiol. 25:364, 1995.
42. Goldstein, R. A.: Kinetics of rubidium-82 after coronary occlusion and reperfusion: Assessment of patency and viability in open-chested dogs. J. Clin. Invest. 75:1131, 1985.
43. Gould, L., Yoshida, K., Hess, M., et al.: Myocardial metabolism of fluorodeoxyglucose compared to cell membrane integrity for the potassium analogue rubidium-82 for assessing infarct size in many by PET. J. Nucl. Med. 32:1, 1991.
44. Wilson, R. A., Shea, M., De Landsheere, C., et al.: Rubidium-82 myocardial uptake and extraction after transient ischemia: PET characteristics. J. Comput. Assist. Tomogr. 11:60, 1987.
45. Gennaro, G. P., Neirinckx, R. D., Bergner, B., et al.: A radionuclide generator and infusion system for pharmaceutical quality Rb-82. *In* Knapp, F. F., Jr., and Butler, T. A. (eds.): American Chemical Society Series #241, Radionuclide Generators: New Systems for Nuclear Medicine Applications, 1984, p. 135.
46. Grant, P. M., Erdal, B. R., and O'Brien, H. A.: A ^{82}Sr-^{82}Rb isotope generator for use in nuclear medicine. J. Nucl. Med. 16:300, 1975.
47. Go, R., Marwich, T., MacIntyre, W., et al.: Initial results of comparative rubidium-82 and thallium-201 myocardial perfusion imaging in diagnosis of CAD. J. Nucl. Med. 30:759, 1989.
48. Goldstein, R. A., Mullani, N. A., Wong, W. H., et al.: Positron imaging of myocardial infarction with rubidium-82. J. Nucl. Med. 27:1824, 1986.
49. Goldstein, R. A., Kirkeeide, R. L., Smalling, R. W., et al.: Changes in myocardial perfusion reserve after PTCA: Noninvasive assessment with positron tomography. J. Nucl. Med. 28:1262, 1987.
50. Kalus, M. E., Stewart, R. E., Gacioch, G. M., et al.: Comparison of Rb-82 PET and Tl-201 SPECT for the detection of regional coronary artery disease. J. Nucl. Med. 30:829, 1989.
51. Hack, S. N., Eichling, J. O., Bergmann, S. R., et al.: External quantification of myocardial perfusion by exponential infusion of positron-emitting radionuclides. J. Clin. Invest. 66:918, 1980.
52. Ducan, C. C., Shiue, C. Y., Wolf, A. P., et al.: ^{18}F-4-fluoroantipyrene for the measurement of cerebral blood flow. J. Cereb. Blood Flow Metabol. Suppl. 1:S78, 1981.
53. Tewson, T. J., and Welch, M.: Preparation and preliminary biodistribution of no carrier added ^{18}F-fluoroethanol. J. Nucl. Med. 21:559, 1980.
54. Melon, P., Brihaye, C., Degueldre, C., et al.: Myocardial kinetics of potassium-38 in humans and comparison with copper-62-PTSM. J. Nucl. Med. 35:1116, 1994.
55. Green, M. A., Klippenstein, D. L., and Tennison, J. R.: Copper(II)-bis-(thiosemicarbazone) complexes as potential tracers for evaluation of cerebral and myocardial blood flow with PET. J. Nucl. Med. 29:1549, 1988.
56. Shelton, M. E., Green, M. A., Mathias, C. J., et al.: Microsphere-like retention in isolated hearts of copper-PTSM: A potential generator-produced tracer for measuring blood flow with PET. J. Nucl. Med. 30:768, 1989.
57. Marshall, R., Leidholdt, E. J., Zhang, D., et al.: Technetium-99m hexakis 2-methoxy-2-isobutyl isonitrile and thallium-201 extraction, washout, and retention at varying coronary flow rates in rabbit heart. Circulation 82:998, 1990.
58. Shelton, M., Green, M., Mathias, C., et al.: Measurement of regional blood flow using copper-PTSM and positron emission tomography (PET). J. Nucl. Med. 30:807, 1989.
59. Beanlands, R. S., Muzik, O., Mintun, M., et al.: The kinetics of copper-62-PTSM in the normal human heart. J. Nucl. Med. 33:684, 1992.
60. Robinson, J. G. D.: Generator systems for positron emitters. *In* Reivich, M., and Alair, A. (eds.): Positron Emission Tomography. New York, A. R. Liss, 1985, p. 81.
61. Stone, C., Holden, J., Stanley, W., et al.: Effect of nicotinic acid on exogenous myocardial glucose utilization. J. Nucl. Med. 36:996, 1995.
62. Nickles, R., Nunn, A., Stone, C., et al.: Technetium-94m-teboroxime: Synthesis, dosimetry and initial PET imaging studies. J. Nucl. Med. 34:1058, 1993.
63. Stone, C., Christian, B., Nickles, R., et al.: Technetium 94m-labeled methoxyisobutyl isonitrile: Dosimetry and resting cardiac imaging with positron emission tomography. J. Nucl. Cardiol. 1:425, 1994.
64. Porenta, G., Kuhle, W., Czernin, J., et al.: Semiquantitative assessment of myocardial viability and perfusion utilizing polar map displays of cardiac PET images. J. Nucl. Med. 33:1623, 1992.
65. Beanlands, R., Muzik, O., Hutchins, G., et al.: Heterogeneity of regional nitrogen-13–labeled ammonia tracer distribution in the normal human heart: Compar-

ison with rubidium-82 and copper-62–labeled PTSM. J. Nucl. Cardiol. 1:225, 1994.
66. Hoffman, E. J., Phelps, M. E., Weiss, E. S., et al.: Transaxial tomographic imaging of canine myocardium with ^{11}C-palmitic acid. J. Nucl. Med. 18:57, 1977.
67. Schön, H. R., Schelbert, H. R., Najafi, A., et al.: C-11 labeled palmitic acid for the noninvasive evaluation of regional myocardial fatty acid metabolism with positron computed tomography. II. Kinetics of C-11 palmitic acid in acutely ischemic myocardium. Am. Heart J. 103:548, 1982.
68. Schön, H. R., Schelbert, H. R., Najafi, A., et al.: C-11 labeled palmitic acid for the noninvasive evaluation of regional myocardial fatty acid metabolism with positron computed tomography. I. Kinetics of C-11 palmitic acid in normal myocardium. Am. Heart J. 103:532, 1982.
69. Little, S. E., van der Vusse, G. J., Moffett, T. C., et al.: Myocardial transcapillary transport of palmitate. J. Nucl. Med. 27:966, 1986.
70. Rose, C. P., and Goresky, C. A.: Constraints on the uptake of labeled palmitate by the heart: The barriers at the capillary and sarcolemmal surfaces and the control of intracellular sequestration. Circ. Res. 41:534, 1977.
71. Klein, M. S., Goldstein, R. A., Welch, M. J., et al.: External assessment of myocardial metabolism with ^{11}C-palmitate in rabbit hearts. Am. J. Physiol. 237:H51, 1979.
72. Lerch, R. A., Ambos, H. D., Bergmann, S. R., et al.: Kinetics of positron emitters in vivo characterization by a beta-probe. Am. J. Physiol. 11:H62, 1982.
73. Weiss, E. S., Hoffman, E. J., Phelps, M. E., et al.: External detection and visualization of myocardial ischemia with ^{11}C-substrates in vitro and in vivo. Circ. Res. 39:24, 1976.
74. Schelbert, H. R., Henze, E., Schön, H. R., et al.: C-11 palmitate for the noninvasive evaluation of regional myocardial fatty acid metabolism with positron computed tomography. III. In vivo demonstration of the effects of substrate availability on myocardial metabolism. Am. Heart J. 105:492, 1983.
75. Schelbert, H. R., Henze, E., Sochor, H., et al.: Effects of substrate availability on myocardial C-11 palmitate kinetics by positron emission tomography in normal subjects and patients with ventricular dysfunction. Am. Heart J. 111:1055, 1986.
76. Schelbert, H. R., Henze, E., Schön, H. R., et al.: C-11 palmitic acid for the noninvasive evaluation of regional myocardial fatty acid metabolism with positron computed tomography. IV. In vivo demonstration of impaired fatty acid oxidation in acute myocardial ischemia. Am. Heart J. 106:736, 1983.
77. Wyns, W., Schwaiger, M., Huang, S. C., et al.: Effects of inhibition of fatty acid oxidation on myocardial kinetics of C-11 labeled palmitate. Circ. Res. 65:1787, 1989.
78. Fox, K. A. A., Abendschein, D. R., Ambos, H. D., et al.: Efflux of metabolized and nonmetabolized fatty acid from canine myocardium: Implications for quantifying myocardial metabolism tomographically. Circ. Res. 57:232, 1985.
79. Lerch, R. A., Bergmann, S. A., Ambos, H. D., et al.: Effect of flow-independent reduction of metabolism on regional myocardial clearance of ^{11}C-palmitate. Circulation 65:731, 1982.
80. Rosamond, T. L., Abendschein, D. R., Sobel, B. E., et al.: Metabolic fate of radiolabeled palmitate in ischemic canine myocardium: Implications for positron emission tomography. J. Nucl. Med. 28:1322, 1987.
81. Sobel, B. E., Weiss, E. S., Welch, M. J., et al.: Detection of remote myocardial infarction in patients with positron emission tomography and intravenous ^{11}C-palmitate. Circulation 55:853, 1977.
82. Ter-Pogossian, M. M., Klein, M. S., Markham, J., et al.: Regional assessment of myocardial metabolic integrity in vivo by positron-emission tomography with ^{11}C-labeled palmitate. Circulation 61:242, 1980.
83. Weiss, E. S., Ahmed, S. A., Welch, M. J., et al.: Quantification of infarction in cross sections of canine myocardium in vivo with positron emission transaxial tomography and ^{11}C-palmitate. Circulation 55:66, 1977.
84. Huang, S., Schwaiger, M., Selin, C., et al.: Tracer kinetic model of C-11 palmitate (CPA) for estimating regional free fatty acid (FFA) utilization in myocardium. J. Nucl. Med. 24:P12, 1983.
85. Phelps, M. E., Hoffman, E. J., Selin, C. E., et al.: Investigation of [^{18}F]2-fluoro-2-deoxyglucose for the measure of myocardial glucose metabolism. J. Nucl. Med. 19:1311, 1978.
86. Schelbert, H. R., and Schwaiger, M.: PET studies of the heart. *In* Phelps, M., Mazziotta, J., Schelbert, H., (eds.): Positron Emission Tomography and Autoradiography: Principles and Applications for the Brain and Heart. Vol. 12. New York, Raven Press, 1986, p. 581.
87. Krivokapich, J., Huang, S. C., Phelps, M. E., et al.: Estimation of rabbit myocardial metabolic rate for glucose using fluorodeoxyglucose. Am. J. Physiol. 243:H884, 1982.
88. Ratib, O., Phelps, M. E., Huang, S. C., et al.: Positron tomography with deoxyglucose for estimating local myocardial glucose metabolism. J. Nucl. Med. 23:577, 1982.
89. Keen, R. E., Krivokapich, J., Phelps, M. E., et al.: Nitrogen-13 flux from L-[^{13}N]glutamate in the isolated rabbit heart: Effect of substrates and transaminase inhibition. Biochim. Biophys. Acta 884:531, 1986.
90. Marshall, R. C., Huang, S. C., Nash, W. W., et al.: Investigation of the 18-fluorodeoxyglucose tracer kinetic model to accurately measure the myocardial metabolic rate for glucose during ischemia: Preliminary notes. J. Nucl. Med. 24:1060, 1983.
91. Armbrecht, J. J., Buxton, D. B., and Schelbert, H. R.: Validation of [1-^{11}C] acetate as a tracer for noninvasive assessment of oxidative metabolism with positron emission tomography in normal, ischemic, post-ischemic and hyperemic canine myocardium. Circulation 81:1594, 1991.
92. Budinger, T. F., Yano, Y., Derenzo, S. E., et al.: Infarction sizing and myocardial perfusion measurements using rubidium-82 and positron emission tomography. Am. J. Cardiol. 45:39, 1980.
93. Brown, M., Marshall, D. R., Burton, B. S., et al.: Delineation of myocardial oxygen utilization with carbon-11–labeled acetate. Circulation 76:687, 1987.
94. Brown, M. A., Myears, D. W., and Bergmann, S. R.: Noninvasive assessment of canine myocardial oxidative metabolism with ^{11}C-acetate and positron emission tomography. J. Am. Coll. Cardiol. 12:1054, 1988.
95. Buxton, D. B., Schwaiger, M., Nguyen, A., et al.: Radiolabeled acetate as a tracer of myocardial tricarboxylic acid cycle flux. Circ. Res. 63:628, 1988.
96. Buxton, D. B., Nienaber, C. A., Luxen, A., et al.: Noninvasive quantitation of regional myocardial oxygen consumption in vivo with [1-^{11}C] acetate and dynamic positron emission tomography. Circulation 79:134, 1989.
97. Brown, M. A., Myears, D. W., and Bergmann, S. R.: Validity of estimates of myocardial oxidative metabolism with carbon-11 acetate and positron emission tomography despite altered patterns of substrate utilization. J. Nucl. Med. 30:187, 1989.
98. Armbrecht, J. J., Buxton, D. B., Brunken, R. C., et al.: Regional myocardial oxygen consumption determined noninvasively in humans with [1-^{11}C] acetate and dynamic positron tomography. Circulation 80:863, 1989.
99. Henes, C., Bergmann, S., Walsh, M., et al.: Noninvasive quantification of myocardial metabolic reserve by positron emission tomography (PET) with C-11 acetate and dobutamine. Circulation 80:II-312, 1989.
100. Henes, C. G., Bergmann, S. R., Walsh, M. N., et al.: Assessment of myocardial oxidative metabolic reserve with positron emission tomography and carbon-11 acetate. J. Nucl. Med. 30:1489, 1989.
101. Kotzerke, J., Hicks, R., Wolfe, E., et al.: Three-dimensional assessment of myocardial oxidative metabolism: A new approach for regional determination of PET-derived carbon-11-acetate kinetics. J. Nucl. Med. 31:1876, 1990.
102. Hicks, R., Herman, W., Kalff, V., et al.: Quantitative evaluation of regional substrate metabolism in the human heart by positron emission tomography. J. Am. Coll. Cardiol. 18:101, 1991.
103. Feiring, A., and Rumberger, J.: Ultrafast computed tomography analysis of regional radius-to-wall thickness ratios in normal and volume-overloaded human left ventricle. Circulation 85:1423, 1992.
104. Pflugfelder, P., Sechtem, U., White, R., et al.: Quantification of regional myocardial function by rapid cine MR imaging. AJR 150:523, 1988.
105. King, R., Bassingthwaighte, J., Hales, J., et al.: Stability of heterogeneity of myocardial blood flow in normal awake baboons. Circ. Res. 57:285, 1985.
106. Marcus, M., Kerber, R., Erhardt, J., et al.: Spatial and temporal heterogeneity of left ventricular perfusion in awake dogs. Am. Heart J. 94:748, 1977.
107. Selwyn, A. P., Allan, R. M., Pike, V., et al.: Positive labeling of ischemic myocardium: A new approach to patients with coronary disease. Am. J. Cardiol. 47:81, 1981.
108. Gropler, R. J., Geltman, E. M., Sampathkumaran, K., et al.: Comparison of carbon-11-acetate with fluorine-18-fluorodeoxyglucose for delineating viable myocardium by positron emission tomography. J. Am. Coll. Cardiol. 22:1587, 1993.
109. Czernin, J., Porenta, G., Brunken, R., et al.: Regional blood flow, oxidative metabolism, and glucose utilization in patients with recent myocardial infarction. Circulation 88:884, 1993.
110. vom Dahl, J., Herman, W., Hicks, R., et al.: Myocardial glucose uptake in patients with insulin-dependent diabetes mellitus assessed quantitatively by dynamic positron emission tomography. Circulation 88:395, 1993.
111. Krivokapich, J., Huang, S. -C., and Schelbert, H.: Assessment of the effects of dobutamine on myocardial blood flow and oxidative metabolism in normal human subjects using nitrogen-13 ammonia and carbon-11 acetate. Am. J. Cardiol. 71:1351, 1993.
112. Hicks, R., Kalff, V., Savas, V., et al.: Assessment of right ventricular oxidative metabolism by positron emission tomography with C-11 acetate in aortic valve disease. Am. J. Cardiol. 67:753, 1991.
113. Ng, C., Huang, S. -C., Schelbert, H., et al.: Validation of a model for [1-^{11}C] acetate as a tracer of cardiac oxidative metabolism. Am. J. Physiol. 266:H1304, 1994.
114. Sun, K., Cyhen, K., Huang, S., et al.: A workable compartmental model for simultaneous measurement of myocardial blood flow and oxygen consumption using C-11 acetate. J. Nucl. Med. 34:4, 1993.
115. Barrio, J. R., Egbert, J. E., Henze, E., et al.: L-[4-^{11}C]aspartic acid: Enzymatic synthesis, myocardial uptake and metabolism. J. Med. Chem. 25:93, 1982.
116. Barrio, J. R., Baumgartner, F. J., Henze, E., et al.: Synthesis and myocardial kinetics of N-13 and C-11 labeled branched chain L-amino acids. J. Nucl. Med. 24:937, 1983.
117. Baumgartner, F. J., Barrio, J. R., Henze, E., et al.: ^{13}N-labeled L-amino acids for in vivo assessment of local myocardial metabolism. J. Med. Chem. 24:764, 1981.
118. Krivokapich, J., Huang, S., Hoffman, E., et al.: N-13 glutamate as a tracer of blood flow at rest and with exercise in human myocardium. Circulation 76:IV-4, 1987.
119. Ropchan, J. R., and Barrio, J. R.: Enzymatic synthesis of [1-^{11}C]pyruvic acid, L-[1-^{11}C] lactic acid and L-[1-^{11}C]alanine. J. Nucl. Med. 25:887, 1984.
120. Gelbard, A. S., Clarke, L. P., McDonald, J. M., et al.: Enzymatic synthesis and organ distribution studies with ^{13}N-labeled L-glutamine and L-glutamic acid. Radiology 116:127, 1975.
121. Gelbard, A. S., McDonald, J. M., Reiman, R. E., et al.: Species differences in myocardial localization of N-13 labeled amino acids. J. Nucl. Med. 16:529, 1975.
122. Gelbard, A. S., Benua, R. S., Reiman, R. E., et al.: Imaging of the human heart after administration of L-[N-13]glutamate. J. Nucl. Med. 21:988, 1980.
123. Knapp, W. H., Helus, F., Ostertag, H., et al.: Uptake and turnover of L-(^{13}N)-

glutamate in the normal human heart and patients with coronary artery disease. Eur. J. Nucl. Med. 7:211, 1982.
124. Rigo, P., Beckers, J., De Landsheere, C., et al.: N-13 glutamate as a myocardial imaging agent in man. J. Nucl. Med. 27:891, 1986.
125. Zimmerman, R., Tillmanns, H., Knapp, W. H., et al.: Regional myocardial nitrogen-13 glutamate uptake in patients with coronary artery disease: Inverse poststress relation to thallium-201 uptake in ischemia. J. Am. Coll. Cardiol. 11:549, 1988.
126. Ishiwata, K., Vaalburg, W., Elsinga, P. H., et al.: Comparison of L-[1-^{11}C]methionine and L-methyl-[^{11}C]methionine for measuring in vivo protein synthesis rates with PET. J. Nucl. Med. 29:1419, 1988.
127. Ishiwata, K., Vaalburg, W., Elsinga, P. H., et al.: Metabolic studies with L-[1-^{14}C]tyrosine for the investigation of a kinetic model to measure protein synthesis rates with PET. J. Nucl. Med. 29:524, 1988.
128. Wieland, D., Rosenspire, K., Hutchins, G., et al.: Validation of 6-[^{18}F]fluorometaraminol (FMR) for positron tomography. Circulation 78:II-598, 1988.
129. Hutchins, G., Schwaiger, M., Haka, M., et al.: Compartmental analysis of the behavior of catecholamine analogs in myocardial tissue. J. Nucl. Med. 30:735, 1989.
130. Chakraborty, P., Gildersleeve, D., Jewett, D., et al.: High-yield synthesis of high specific activity R-(−)-[^{11}C]epinephrine for routine PET studies in humans. Nucl. Med. Biol. 20:939, 1993.
131. Goldstein, D., Eisenhofer, G., Dunn, B., et al.: Positron emission tomographic imaging of cardiac sympathetic innervation using 6-[^{18}F]fluorodopamine: Initial findings in humans. J. Am. Coll. Cardiol. 22:1961, 1993.
132. Shea, M. J., Wilson, R. A., de Landsheere, C. M., et al.: A new and independent measure of the volume of viable myocardium: The effects of transient ischemia. J. Am. Coll. Cardiol. 3:475, 1984.
133. Shea, M. J., Wilson, R. A., Delandsheere, C. M., et al.: Use of short- and long-lived rubidium tracers for the study of transient ischemia. J. Nucl. Med. 28:989, 1987.
134. Charbonneau, P., Syrota, A., Crouzel, C., et al.: Peripheral-type benzodiazepine receptors in the living heart characterized by positron emission tomography. Circulation 73:476, 1986.
135. Grierson, J. R., Link, J. M., Mathis, C. A., et al.: A radiosynthesis of fluorine-18 fluoromisonidazole. J. Nucl. Med. 30:343, 1989.
136. Martin, G., Caldwell, J., McGrath, P., et al.: Positron tomographic imaging of the hypoxic cell marker F-18 fluoromisonidazole in ischemic myocardium. Circulation 78:II-598, 1988.
137. Rasey, J. S., Grunbaum, Z., Magee, S., et al.: Characterization of radiolabeled fluoromisonidazole as a probe for hypoxic cells. Radiat. Res. 111:292, 1987.
138. Woods, S. D., Rasey, J. S., Graham, M. M., et al.: A model for fluoromisonidazole retention as a function of local PO_2: In vitro calibration for interpretation of PET images. J. Nucl. Med. 30:735, 1989.
139. Shelton, M. E., Dence, C. S., Hwang, D. R., et al.: Myocardial kinetics of fluorine-18 misonidazole: A marker of hypoxic myocardium. J. Nucl. Med. 30:351, 1989.
140. Shelton, M., Dence, C., Hwang, D. -R., et al.: Enhanced extraction of [F-18]fluoromisonidazole by jeopardized myocardium assessed with PET. J. Nucl. Med. 30:730, 1989.
141. Martin, G. V., Caldwell, J. H., Graham, M. M., et al.: Noninvasive detection of hypoxic myocardium using fluorine-18-fluoromisonidazole and positron emission tomography. J. Nucl. Med. 33:2202, 1992.
142. Hoffman, E. J., Phelps, M. E., Huang, S. C., et al.: Dynamic, gated, and high-resolution imaging with the ECAT III. I. E. E. E. Trans. Nucl. Sci. 33:452, 1986.
143. Hoffman, E. J., Phelps, M. E., Wisenberg, G., et al.: Electrocardiographic gating in positron emission computed tomography. J. Comput. Assist. Tomogr. 3:731, 1979.
144. Porenta, G., Kuhle, W., Sinha, S., et al.: Parameter estimation of cardiac geometry by ECG-gated PET imaging: Validation using magnetic resonance imaging and echocardiography. J. Nucl. Med. 36:1123, 1995.
145. Bacharach, S., and Buvat, I.: Attenuation correction in cardiac positron emission tomography and single-photon emission computed tomography. J. Nucl. Cardiol. 2:246, 1995.
146. Carson, R. E., Daube-Witherspoon, M. E., Jacobs, G. I., et al.: Validation of postinjection transmission measurements for PET. J. Nucl. Med. 30:825, 1989.
147. Ranger, N. T., Thompson, C. J., and Evans, A. C.: The application of a masked orbiting transmission source for attenuation correction in PET. J. Nucl. Med. 30:1056, 1989.
148. Huang, S. C., Carson, R. E., Phelps, M. E., et al.: A boundary method for attenuation in positron emission computed tomography. J. Nucl. Med. 22:627, 1981.
149. Hicks, K., Ganti, G., Mullani, N., et al.: Automated quantitation of three-dimensional cardiac positron emission tomography for routine clinical use. J. Nucl. Med. 30:1787, 1989.
150. Laubenbacher, C., Rothley, J., Sitomer, J., et al.: An automated analysis program for the evaluation of cardiac PET studies: Initial results in the detection and localization of coronary artery disease using nitrogen-13 ammonia. J. Nucl. Med. 34:968, 1993.
151. Sun, K., De Groof, M., Yi, J., et al.: Quantification of the extent and severity of perfusion defects in canine myocardium by PET polar mapping. J. Nucl. Med. 35:2031, 1994.
152. Miller, T., Wallis, J., Landy, B., et al.: Measurement of global and regional left ventricular function by cardiac PET. J. Nucl. Med. 35:999, 1994.
153. Yamashita, K., Tamaki, N., Yonekura, Y., et al.: Quantitative analysis of regional wall motion by gated myocardial positron emission tomography: Validation and comparison with left ventriculography. J. Nucl. Med. 30:1775, 1989.
154. Yamashita, K., Tamaki, N., Yonekura, Y., et al.: Regional wall thickening of left ventricle evaluated by gated positron emission tomography in relation to myocardial perfusion and glucose metabolism. J. Nucl. Med. 32:679, 1991.
155. Hoffman, E., and Phelps, M.: Positron emission tomography: Principles and quantitation. *In* Phelps, M., Mazziotta, J., and Schelbert, H. (eds.): Positron Emission Tomography and Autoradiography: Principles and Applications for the Brain and Heart. New York, Raven Press, 1986, p. 237.
156. Hoffman, E. J., Huang, S. C., and Phelps, M. E.: Quantitation in positron emission computed tomography. J. Comput. Assist. Tomogr. 3:299, 1979.
157. Parodi, P., Schelbert, H. R., Schwaiger, M., et al.: Cardiac emission computed tomography: Underestimation of regional tracer concentrations due to wall motion abnormalities. J. Comput. Assist. Tomogr. 8:1083, 1984.
158. Nienaber, C., Ratib, O., Bidaut, L., et al.: Simultaneous measurement of regional myocardial metabolism and function by multi-gated positron emission tomography (PET). J. Am. Coll. Cardiol. 11:38, 1988.
159. Henze, E., Huang, S. C., Ratib, O., et al.: Measurements of regional tissue and blood pool radiotracer concentrations from serial tomographic images of the heart. J. Nucl. Med. 24:987, 1983.
160. Huang, S. C., Schwaiger, M., Carson, R. E., et al.: Quantitative measurement of myocardial blood flow with oxygen-15 water and positron computed tomography: An assessment of potential and problems. J. Nucl. Med. 26:616, 1985.
161. Huang, S., Grover, M., Hoffman, E., et al.: Use of temporal information for spillover correction in dynamic PET studies of the heart. J. Nucl. Med. 27:980, 1986.
162. Ratib, O., Bidaut, L., Nienaber, C., et al.: Semiautomatic software for quantitative analysis of cardiac positron tomography studies. Proc. Soc. Photo-Optical Instrumentation Engineers 914:412, 1988.
163. Weinberg, I. N., Huang, S. C., Hoffman, E. J., et al.: Validation of PET-acquired functions for cardiac studies. J. Nucl. Med. 29:241, 1988.
164. Germano, G., and Hoffman, E. J.: Investigation of count rate capability and deadtime for a high-resolution PET system. J. Comput. Assist. Tomogr. 12:836, 1988.
165. Sapirstein, L. A.: Regional blood flow by fractional distribution of indicators. Am. J. Physiol. 193:161, 1958.
166. Shah, A., Schelbert, H. R., Schwaiger, M., et al.: Measurement of regional myocardial blood flow with N-13 ammonia and positron emission tomography in intact dogs. J. Am. Coll. Cardiol. 5:92, 1985.
167. Nienaber, C., Ratib, O., Weinberg, I., et al.: Noninvasive quantification of regional myocardial blood flow with N-13 ammonia and dynamic positron tomography. J. Am. Coll. Cardiol. 11:10, 1988.
168. Kuhle, W., Porenta, G., Huang, S. -C., et al.: Quantification of regional myocardial blood flow using ^{13}N-ammonia and reoriented dynamic positron emission tomographic imaging. Circulation 86:1004, 1992.
169. Rosenspire, K., Schwaiger, M., Mangner, T., et al.: Metabolic fate of N-13 ammonia in human blood: Implications for quantification of myocardial blood flow by PET. J. Nucl. Med. 29:783, 1988.
170. Bellina, C., Parodi, O., Camici, P., et al.: Simultaneous in vitro and in vivo validation of nitrogen-13 ammonia for the assessment of regional myocardial blood flow. J. Nucl. Med. 31:1335, 1990.
171. Camici, P., Chiriatti, G., Oorenzoni, R., et al.: Coronary vasodilation is impaired in both hypertrophied and nonhypertrophied myocardium of patients with hypertrophic cardiomyopathy: A study with nitrogen-13 ammonia and positron emission tomography. J. Am. Coll. Cardiol. 17:879, 1991.
172. Sambuceti, G., Parodi, O., Marzullo, P., et al.: Regional myocardial blood flow in stable angina pectoris associated with isolated significant narrowing of either the left anterior descending or left circumflex coronary artery. Am. J. Cardiol. 72:990, 1993.
173. Hutchins, G., Schwaiger, M., Rosenspire, K., et al.: Noninvasive quantification of regional blood flow in the human heart using N-13 ammonia and dynamic positron emission tomographic imaging. J. Am. Coll. Cardiol. 15:1032, 1990.
174. Muzik, O., Beanlands, R. S. B., Hutchins, G. D., et al.: Validation of nitrogen-13 ammonia tracer kinetic model for quantification of myocardial blood flow using PET. J. Nucl. Med. 34:83, 1993.
175. Krivokapich, J., Smith, G. T., Huang, S. C., et al.: N-13 ammonia myocardial imaging at rest and with exercise in normal volunteers: Quantification of absolute myocardial perfusion with dynamic positron emission tomography. Circulation 80:1328, 1989.
176. Muzik, O., Beanlands, R., Wolfe, E., et al.: Automated region definition for cardiac nitrogen-13 ammonia PET imaging. J. Nucl. Med. 34:336, 1993.
177. Bol, A., Melin, J. A., Vanoverschelde, J. -L., et al.: Direct comparison of [^{13}N]ammonia and [^{15}O]water estimates of perfusion with quantification of regional myocardial blood flow by microspheres. Circulation 87:512, 1993.
178. Nitzsche, E., Choi, Y., Czernin, J., et al.: Comparison of O-15 water and N-13 ammonia PET measurements of myocardial blood flow in humans. Circulation 88:I-274, 1993.
179. Czernin, J., Barnard, J., Sun, K., et al.: Beneficial effect of cardiovascular conditioning on myocardial blood flow and coronary vasodilator capacity. Circulation 88:I-51, 1993.
180. Czernin, J., Kim, A., Dominquez, V., et al.: How reproducible are measurements of myocardial blood flow by N-13 ammonia and PET? J. Nucl. Med. 35:24, 1994.
181. Shelton, M. E., Senneff, M. J., Ludbrook, P. A., et al.: Concordance of nutritive myocardial perfusion reserve and flow velocity reserve in conductance vessels in patients with chest pain with angiographically normal coronary arteries. J. Nucl. Med. 34:717, 1993.
182. Merlet, P., Mazoyer, B., Hittinger, L., et al.: Assessment of coronary reserve in man: Comparison between positron emission tomography with oxygen-15–labeled water and intracoronary Doppler technique. J. Nucl. Med. 34:1899, 1993.

183. Iida, H., and Tamaki, N.: Quantitative assessment of regional myocardial blood flow using O-15 water and PET: A multi-center project by 7 independent institutes in Japan. J. Nucl. Med. 36:78, 1995.
184. Uren, N., Melin, J., De Bruyne, B., et al.: Maximal myocardial flow as a function of stenosis severity in man. Circulation 88:1, 1993.
185. Yamamoto, Y., De Silva, R., Rhodes, C., et al.: A new strategy for the assessment of viable myocardium and regional myocardial blood flow using ^{15}O-water and dynamic positron emission tomography. Circulation 86:167, 1992.
186. de Silva, R., Yamamoto, Y., Rhodes, C. G., et al.: Preoperative prediction of the outcome of coronary revascularization using positron emission tomography. Circulation 86:1738, 1992.
187. Mullani, N. A., and Gould, K. L.: First-pass regional blood flow measurement with external detectors. J. Nucl. Med. 24:577, 1983.
188. Herrero, P., Markham, J., Shelton, M., et al.: Noninvasive quantification of regional myocardial perfusion with rubidium-82 and positron emission tomography. Circulation 82:1377, 1990.
189. Herrero, P., Markham, J., Shelton, M., et al.: Implementation and evaluation of a two-compartment model for quantification of myocardial perfusion with rubidium-82 and positron emission tomography. Circ. Res. 70:496, 1992.
190. Herrero, P., Markham, J., Weinheimer, C. J., et al.: Quantification of regional myocardial perfusion with generator-produced ^{62}Cu-PTSM and positron emission tomography. Circulation 87:173, 1993.
191. Gropler, R., Siegel, B., Lee, K., et al.: Nonuniformity in myocardial accumulation of fluorine-18-fluorodeoxyglucose in normal fasted humans. J. Nucl. Med. 31:1749, 1990.
192. Choi, Y., Huang, S., Hawkins, R., et al.: A refined method for quantification of myocardial oxygen consumption rate using mean transit time with carbon-11-acetate and dynamic PET. J. Nucl. Med. 34:2038, 1993.
193. Papoulis, A.: Probability, Random Variables and Stochastic Processes. New York, McGraw-Hill, 1965, p. 245.
194. Chan, S., Brunken, R., Czernin, J., et al.: Comparison of maximal myocardial blood flow during adenosine infusion with that of intravenous dipyridamole in normal men. J. Am. Coll. Cardiol. 20:979, 1992.
195. Sokoloff, L., Reivich, M., Kennedy, C., et al.: The [^{14}C]-deoxyglucose method for the measurement of local cerebral glucose utilization: Theory, procedure and normal values in the conscious and anesthetized albino rat. J. Neurochem. 28:897, 1977.
196. Gallagher, B. M., Ansari, A., Atkins, H., et al.: Radiopharmaceuticals XXVII. 18F-labeled 2-deoxy-2-fluoro-D-glucose as a radiopharmaceutical for measuring regional myocardial glucose metabolism in vivo: Tissue distribution and imaging studies in animals. J. Nucl. Med. 18:990, 1977.
197. Huang, S. C., Phelps, M. E., Hoffman, E. J., et al.: Non-invasive determination of local cerebral metabolic rate of glucose in man. Am. J. Physiol. 238:E69, 1980.
198. Phelps, M. E., Huang, S. C., Hoffman, E. J., et al.: Tomographic measurement of local cerebral glucose metabolic rate in humans with (F-18) 2-fluoro-2-deoxy-D-glucose: Validation of method. Ann. Neurol. 6:371, 1979.
199. Gambhir, S. S., Schwaiger, M., Huang, S. C., et al.: Simple noninvasive quantification method for measuring myocardial glucose utilization in humans employing positron emission tomography and fluorine-18-deoxyglucose. J. Nucl. Med. 30:359, 1989.
200. Schwaiger, M., Huang, S., Krivokapich, J., et al.: Myocardial glucose utilization measured noninvasively in man by positron tomography. J. Am. Coll. Cardiol. 1:688, 1983.
201. Patlak, C. S., Blasberg, R. G., and Fenstermacher, J. D.: Graphical evaluation of blood-to-brain transfer constants from multiple-time uptake data. J. Cereb. Blood Flow Metab. 3:1, 1983.
202. Patlak, C. S., and Blasberg, R. G.: Graphical evaluation of blood-to-brain transfer constants from multiple-time uptake data. J. Cereb. Blood Flow Metab. 5:584, 1985.
203. Choi, Y., Hawkins, R., Huang, S., et al.: Parametric images of myocardial metabolic rate of glucose generated from dynamic cardiac PET and 2-[^{18}F]fluoro-2-deoxy-D-glucose studies. J. Nucl. Med. 32:733, 1991.
204. Berry, J., Baker, J., Pieper, K., et al.: The effect of metabolic milieu on cardiac PET imaging using fluorine-18-deoxyglucose and nitrogen-13-ammonia in normal volunteers. J. Nucl. Med. 32:1518, 1991.
205. Choi, Y., Brunken, R. C., Hawkins, R. A., et al.: Factors affecting myocardial 2-[F-18]fluoro-2-deoxy-D-glucose uptake in positron emission tomography studies of normal humans. Eur. J. Nucl. Med. 20:308, 1993.
206. Knuuti, M., Nuutila, P., Ruotsalainen, U., et al.: Euglycemic hyperinsulinemic clamp and oral glucose load in stimulating myocardial glucose utilization during positron emission tomography. J. Nucl. Med. 33:1255, 1992.
207. Hicks, R., von Dahl, J., Lee, K., et al.: Insulin-glucose clamp for standardization of metabolic conditions during F-18-fluoro-deoxyglucose PET imaging. J. Am. Coll. Cardiol. 17:381, 1991.
208. DeFronzo, R., Tobin, J., and Andres, R.: Glucose clamp technique: A method for quantifying insulin secretion and resistance. Am. J. Physiol. 237:E214, 1979.
209. Ohtake, T., Yokoyama, I., Watanabe, T., et al.: Myocardial glucose metabolism in noninsulin-dependent diabetes mellitus patients evaluated by FDG-PET. J. Nucl. Med. 36:456, 1995.
210. Knuuti, M., Yki-Järvinen, H., Voipio-Pulkki, L., et al.: Enhancement of myocardial [fluorine-18] fluorodeoxyglucose uptake by a nicotinic acid derivative. J. Nucl. Med. 35:989, 1994.
211. Marshall, R. C., Tillisch, J. H., Phelps, M. E., et al.: Identification and differentiation of resting myocardial ischemia and infarction in man with positron computed tomography ^{18}F-labeled fluorodeoxyglucose and N-13 ammonia. Circulation 67:766, 1983.
212. Russell, R., Mrus, J., Mommessin, J., et al.: Compartmentation of hexokinase in rat heart: A critical factor for tracer kinetic analysis of myocardial glucose metabolism. J. Clin. Invest. 90:1972, 1992.
213. Ng, C. K., Holden, J. E., DeGrado, T. R., et al.: Sensitivity of myocardial fluorodeoxyglucose lumped constant to glucose and insulin. Am. J. Physiol. 260:H593, 1991.
214. Schneider, C., Nguyen, V., and Taegtmeyer, H.: Feeding and fasting determine postischemic glucose utilization in isolated working rat hearts. Am. J. Physiol. 260:H542, 1991.
215. Hariharan, R., Bray, M., Ganim, R., et al.: Fundamental limitations of [^{18}F]2-deoxy-2-fluoro-D-glucose for assessing myocardial glucose uptake. Circulation 91:2435, 1995.
216. Bax, J., Visser, F., van Lingen, A., et al.: Feasibility of assessing regional myocardial uptake of ^{18}F-fluorodeoxyglucose using single photon emission computed tomography. Eur. Heart J. 14:1675, 1993.
217. Burt, R., Perkins, O., Oppenheim, B., et al.: Direct comparison of fluorine-18-FDG SPECT, fluorine-18-FDG PET and rest thallium-201 SPECT for detection of myocardial viability. J. Nucl. Med. 36:176, 1995.
218. Martin, W., Delbeke, D., Patton, J., et al.: FDG-SPECT: Correlation with FDG-PET. J. Nucl. Med. 36:988, 1995.
219. Phelps, M. E., Mazziotta, J. C., and Huang, S. C.: Study of cerebral function with positron computed tomography. J. Cereb. Blood Flow Metabol. 2:113, 1982.

CHAPTER

70 Evaluation of Myocardial Blood Flow in Cardiac Disease

Heinrich R. Schelbert, M.D.
Linda L. Demer, M.D.

Imaging and, more recently, measurements of myocardial blood flow with positron emission tomography (PET) have been used for exploring cardiovascular physiology and are now gaining recognition as useful clinical tools. Several studies, including more than 1000 patients with suspected coronary artery disease, that used PET for the noninvasive assessment of myocardial blood flow have been reported in the scientific literature. Myocardial blood flow imaging with PET appears well suited for the evaluation of coronary artery disease, for it provides information complementary to that obtained with invasive coronary arteriography—not directly substituting for it. Arteriographic imaging identifies the location and anatomical severity of epicardial coronary artery stenoses. However, the physiologic significance of such lesions may be difficult to assess from angiographic data alone; blood flow abnormalities may occur in the absence of arteriographically evident stenoses. Noninvasive PET imaging complements arteriography by revealing the effects of the stenosis on the blood supply that reaches the myocardium. For example, PET blood flow images are useful for identifying physiologic abnormalities of perfusion in the absence of arteriographic abnormalities and for assessing the significance of known stenoses in terms of absolute or relative perfusion or perfusion reserve and the amount of heart wall involved. Conventional noninvasive methods, such as planar imaging and, more recently, single-photon emission computed tomography (SPECT) with thallium-201 (^{201}Tl) or technetium-99m (^{99m}Tc) labeled compounds, provide conceptually similar information, but they are theoretically less accurate, owing to the dependence of tracer attenuation and resolution on the distance of the tracer from the detectors and the lower signal-to-noise ratio.

The three primary clinical applications of PET perfusion imaging

Dr. Schelbert is affiliated with The Laboratory of Structural Biology and Molecular Medicine, operated for the U.S. Department of Energy by the University of California under Contract #DE-AC03-76-SF00012. This work was supported in part by the Director of the Office of Energy Research, Office of Health and Environmental Research, Washington, D.C., by Research Grants #HL 29845 and #HL 33177, the National Institutes of Health, Bethesda, M.D., and by an Investigative Group Award by the Greater Los Angeles Affiliate of the American Heart Association, Los Angeles, CA.

are qualitative detection of coronary artery disease with potentially greater accuracy than that of conventional noninvasive methods, assessment of responses to medical and surgical interventions designed to augment myocardial blood flow, and quantitative measurements of myocardial blood flow in milliliters of blood per minute per gram of myocardium. The first application has undergone the most extensive clinical evaluation, revealing high sensitivity and specificity. In progress is research that compares directly PET with SPECT imaging to assess the relative diagnostic accuracies of both approaches. Last, the usefulness of quantitative measurements of myocardial blood flow with PET is currently being explored. Such measurements begin to offer novel insights into the coronary circulation, its regulation, and its changes in disease in the human heart.

TECHNICAL ASPECTS

Evaluation of Regional Myocardial Blood Flow

Tracers of Myocardial Blood Flow

The most widely used positron-emitting tracers of myocardial blood flow are nitrogen-13 (^{13}N) ammonia, rubidium-82 (^{82}Rb) and oxygen-15 (^{15}O) water. Rubidium-82 (RbCl) is available through a generator; a specially designed infusion system permits the intravenous administration of tracer at preselected infusion rates, volumes, and radioactivity doses. The short physical half-life of ^{82}Rb, only 75 seconds, permits repeated measurements at short time intervals yet requires relatively high doses of activity (1850 to 2220 MBq or 50 to 60 mCi per intravenous administration) to obtain images of adequate count densities. In contrast, the longer physical half-time of ^{13}N-ammonia (10 minutes) yields statistically adequate images at lower activity doses (e.g., 370 to 740 MBq or 10 to 20 mCi) yet requires longer time intervals between repeat studies (40 to 50 minutes). Unlike ^{82}Rb and ^{13}N-ammonia, which selectively accumulate in the myocardium, the cyclotron-produced ^{15}O-water distributes into the water spaces of both the myocardium and the blood. Therefore, adequate visualization of the myocardium itself requires subtraction of blood pool activity, accomplished with ^{15}O-water or carbon-11 (^{11}C) labeled carbon monoxide. Together with the already short physical half-life of ^{15}O (2.1 minutes), this subtraction lowers the count density of the myocardial blood flow images further, so they are frequently of suboptimal diagnostic quality. Thus, ^{15}O-water is best suited for serial measurements of myocardial blood flow.

Physical or Pharmacologic Stress

Myocardial blood flow can be evaluated and measured with PET at rest, during physical exercise, or during pharmacologically induced hyperemia. For physical stress, patients undergo supine bicycle exercise while positioned in the tomograph.[1–3] Most laboratories, however, employ pharmacologic agents to induce stress, including dipyridamole, adenosine, and, more recently, dobutamine, because the patient remains in the same position, which minimizes misalignments between transmission and emission images (see later, and Chapter 69). Typically, patients fast for 4 to 8 hours before stress testing, because of potential side effects such as nausea and vomiting. Further, for studies with either adenosine or dipyridamole, patients are required to refrain from consumption of caffeine or theophylline for at least 8 hours or, preferentially, for 24 hours because these agents interfere with the vasodilatory effect of dipyridamole or adenosine.[4] Table 70–1 summarizes the key features of several stress agents, and Table 70–2 the induced hyperemic blood flows. Typically, and as seen in Figure 70–1, myocardial blood flow is evaluated first at rest and then again during stress. The stress should be maintained for at least 90 to 120 seconds after tracer administration to allow sufficient time for trapping and retention of the tracer in the myocardium. Both ^{13}N-ammonia and ^{82}Rb accumulate in the myocardium in proportion to myocardial blood flow, so images of their activity concentrations represent the relative distribution of blood flow in the myocardium.

Quantitative Aspects of Pharmacologic Stress Testing

The ability of PET to measure myocardial blood flow in absolute units ($mL \cdot min^{-1} \cdot g^{-1}$) has been used to quantitate flow responses to pharmacologic vasodilation. As demonstrated with either the ^{15}O-water or the ^{13}N-ammonia approach, intravenous dipyridamole (0.56 mg/kg over 4 minutes) produces a three- to fivefold increase in myocardial blood flow.[5–9] The ratio of hyperemic to rest blood flows represents the "myocardial flow reserve." Most quantitative studies demonstrate a considerable interpatient variability in hyperemic blood flows and, consequently, in the myocardial flow reserves. For example, in a group of 20 normal volunteers studied by Chan and co-workers,[8] myocardial flow reserves ranged from 1.5 to 5.8 (average 4.0). As the ratio of hyperemic to resting blood flows, the myocardial flow reserve depends on both measures.

RESTING MYOCARDIAL BLOOD FLOW. Reported values for resting blood flow vary between studies but also between individuals. Some of the variability appears to be related to method. Most of it, however, results from interindividual differences in myocardial oxygen demand and thus cardiac work. Several investigations have demonstrated a highly significant correlation between

TABLE 70–1. PHARMACOLOGIC STRESS AGENTS

Agent and Dosage	Mechanism of Action	Tracer Injection	Treatment and Adverse Reaction
Dipyridamole IV 0.142 $mg \cdot min^{-1} \cdot kg^{-1}$ BW for 4 min	Raises adenosine levels by inhibiting adenosine deaminase; adenosine causes smooth muscle relaxation	2 to 4 minutes after end of infusion, when hyperemic response is maximum	Aminophylline IV (75 to 125 mg)
Adenosine IV 140 $\mu g \cdot min^{-1} \cdot kg^{-1}$ BW	Direct vascular smooth muscle relaxant via A_2 receptors; increases myocardial blood flow independent of cardiac work, as does dipyridamole	Infuse IV at constant rate for 6 minutes; inject tracer at 4 minutes	Discontinue infusion (biologic half-time in about 10 seconds); if necessary, aminophylline IV.
Dobutamine IV 5 to 50 $\mu g \cdot min^{-1} \cdot kg^{-1}$ BW	Synthetic sympathomimetic amine with stimulation of predominantly β_1-receptors but also β_2- and α-receptors; increases blood flow in proportion to cardiac work	Infused at 5-µg incremental doses until systolic blood pressure or heart rate increases; maintain for 3 to 4 minutes while the flow tracer is administered; continue at least for another minute.	About 2 minutes biologic half-time in plasma; discontinue infusion; antiarrhythmics if indicated

BW = body weight; IV = intravenously.

TABLE 70–2. REST AND HYPEREMIC BLOOD FLOWS AND MYOCARDIAL FLOW RESERVES IN NORMAL PATIENTS AND THOSE WITH CARDIAC DISEASE

	MBF Rest ($mL \cdot min^{-1} \cdot g^{-1}$)	MBF Hyper ($mL \cdot min^{-1} \cdot g^{-1}$)	MFR	MBF Rest ($mL \cdot min^{-1} \cdot g^{-1}$)	MBF Hyper ($mL \cdot min^{-1} \cdot g^{-1}$)	MFR
Pharmacologic Stress	*Adenosine*			*Dipyridamole*		
(Chan et al. 1992)[8]	1.1±0.2	4.4±0.9	4.3±1.6	1.1±0.2	4.3±1.3	4.0±1.3
Pharmacologic Plus Physical Stress	*Adenosine*			*Adenosine and supine exercise*		
(Müller et al. 1994)[2]	0.53±0.07	2.61±0.38	5.0±0.9	0.53±0.07	2.21±0.31	4.3±1.0°
Effect of Age	*<50 years of age*			*>50 years of age*		
(Czernin et al. 1993)[9]	0.76±0.17	3.0±0.76	4.1±0.9	0.92±0.25°	2.66±0.58	3.0±0.7[.001]
Normal Regions in CAD						
(Di Carli et al. 1995)[66]	*10 age-matched controls (64±13 y)*			*18 patients (66±8 y)*		
	0.90±0.02	2.30±0.50	2.6±0.7	0.90±0.20	2.30±0.60	2.4±0.4
(Uren et al. 1993)[11]	*15 controls (21 to 55 y, mean 34 y)*			*10 patients (47 to 76 yrs, mean 60 y)*		
	0.92±0.13	3.67±0.94	4.1±1.0	1.06±0.19°	2.89±0.93°	2.7±0.9†
(Sambuceti et al. 1993)[69]	*14 controls (49±7 y)*			*30 patients (56±10 y)*		
	1.03±0.25	3.66±0.92	3.6±0.9	0.77±0.19†	1.76±0.68†	2.3±0.8†
Hypercholesteremia	*11 low-risk males (48±9 y)*			*16 hypercholesteremic males (49±1 y)*		
(Dayanikli et al. 1994)[73]	0.66±0.08	2.64±0.39	4.3±0.5	0.76±0.18	2.17±0.56°	2.9±0.9‡
CV Conditioning	*Before*			*After 6 weeks of conditioning*		
(Czernin et al. 1995)[15]	0.78±0.18	2.06±0.35	2.8±1.1	0.69±0.14°	2.25±0.40†	3.4±0.9†
Syndrome X	*No control group*			*45 patients (52±8 y)*		
(Camici et al. 1992)[96]	—	—	—	1.04±0.22	2.52±0.96	2.5±0.9
(Rosen et al. 1994)[97]	*20 controls (51±15 yrs)*			*20 patients (54±8 y)*		
	1.00±0.22	3.00±081	3.1±1.1	1.05±0.25	2.73±0.81	2.7±0.8
Hypertrophic CMP	*12 controls (51±8 y)*			*23 patients (48±15 y), hypertrophied septum*		
(Camici et al. 1991)[110]	1.04±0.25	2.99±1.06	N/A	1.14±0.43	1.63±0.58‡	N/A
Transplant Rejection	*Acute rejection (10 transplant recipients)*			*After immunosuppressive treatment*		
(Chan et al. 1994)[106]	1.70±0.20	2.50±0.90	1.5±0.5	1.20±0.30‡	3.90±1.10†	3.4±1.0‡

CAD = coronary artery disease; CV = cardiovascular; CMP = cardiomyopathy; MBF = myocardial blood flow; MFR = myocardial flow reserve; N/A = not applicable. Comparisons are made with either a normal control group or within the same group to values prior to the intervention. *P* values for statistically significant differences to the control or preintervention studies: ° = $P<.05$; † = $P<.01$; ‡ = $P<.001$ versus control of comparison group or measurements.

the rate-pressure product as an index of cardiac work and myocardial blood flow (Fig. 70–2) and therefore normalize blood flow to the rate-pressure product.[8–11] The correlation between blood flow and the rate-pressure product is consistent with that obtained previously through highly invasive means.[12] Increases in cardiac work in response to supine bicycle exercise[3] or intravenous dobutamine[13] produce proportional increases in myocardial blood flow, as measured with the ^{13}N-ammonia PET technique.

HYPEREMIC MYOCARDIAL BLOOD FLOW. The level of hyperemia achieved during pharmacologic vasodilation depends on many factors, among which are the effectiveness of the vasodilator stimulus, the coronary driving pressure and heart rate, extravascular resistive forces, and the intactness of the large epicardial vessels or the microcirculation, or both. The standard dose schedule for dipyridamole (0.56 mg/kg of body weight infused over a 4-minute period) typically produces a three- to fivefold increase in myocardial blood flow in normal volunteers.[5–8] Higher amounts of dipyridamole (0.8 mg/kg for 4 minutes) failed to produce further in-

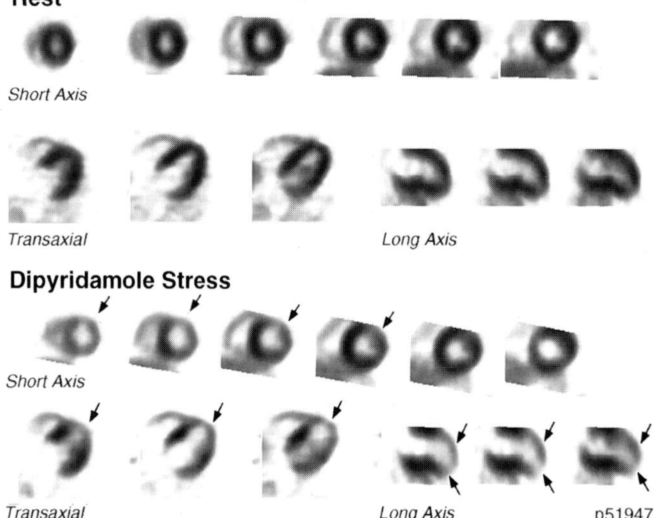

FIGURE 70–1. Myocardial blood flow images obtained at rest and after intravenous administration of dipyridamole in a patient with coronary artery disease. The transaxially acquired images have been resliced into short-axis and vertical long-axis images. In addition, selected transaxially acquired images are shown. Note the homogeneous myocardial ^{13}N-ammonia concentrations in the images obtained at rest. However, after dipyridamole administration, a reduction in ^{13}N-ammonia uptake and thus in myocardial blood flow is noted in the anterior wall, as seen on the short-axis and the vertical long-axis images.

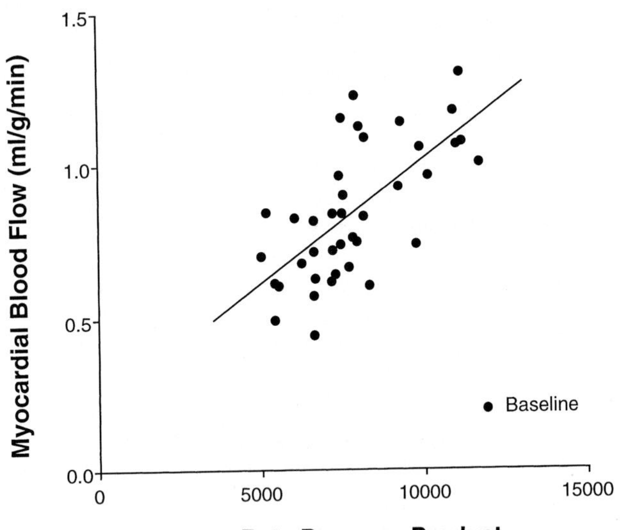

FIGURE 70–2. Correlation between myocardial blood flow and cardiac work at rest. Myocardial blood flow was measured with intravenous ^{13}N-ammonia, and cardiac work is expressed by the product of systolic blood pressure and heart rate (rate-pressure product). Note the linear correlation between the two parameters. (From Czernin, J., Müller, P., Chan, S., et al.: Influence of age and hemodynamics on myocardial blood flow and flow reserve. Circulation 88:62, 1993, with permission of the American Heart Association, Inc.)

creases in normal volunteers (2.13 ± 0.28 mL · min^{-1} · g^{-1} for standard versus 2.08 ± 0.20mL · min^{-1} · g^{-1} for high-dose dipyridamole). In, addition, higher doses did not reduce the variability of the hyperemic flow responses.[14]

In normal volunteers, the level of hyperemic blood flow appears to be independent of the heart rate. Increases in coronary driving pressure as a determinant of the hyperemic flow produced by bicycle exercise (mean arterial blood pressure rose from 125 ± 17 to 186 ± 24 mm Hg)[2] or by isometric handgrip (systolic arterial blood pressure rose from 123 ± 8 to 147 ± 10 mm Hg)[15] during pharmacologic vasodilation lowered, rather than raised, hyperemic blood flows (from 2.13 ± 0.28 mL · min^{-1} · g^{-1} without to 1.87 ± 0.32 mL · min^{-1} · g^{-1} with handgrip and from 2.61 ± 0.38 during adenosine infusion alone to 2.21 ± 0.31 mL · min^{-1} · g^{-1} during adenosine infusion plus supine bicycle exercise; see Table 70–2). This decline—rather than the expected increase—was ascribed to higher extravascular resistive forces resulting from increased end-diastolic pressures and myocardial contractility.

Another intriguing finding from quantitative blood flow measurements with PET is an age-dependent decline in the myocardial flow reserve.[9, 16] One study ascribed this decline to a decrease in the vasodilator capacity,[16] whereas a second study in 40 normal volunteers ranging in age from 19 to 86 years demonstrated an age-dependent progressive increase in resting blood flow as a result of an increase in the rate-pressure product as the primary cause of the age-dependent fall in the myocardial flow reserve (Fig. 70–3).[9] Of note, the same study observed a modestly lower vasodilator capacity in normal volunteers older than 50 years of age compared with younger ones. This age-dependent decline in the myocardial flow reserve must be considered when absolute flow responses are evaluated in disease states (see Table 70–2). If patient findings are compared with those from a group of young volunteers, then differences may result not from disease but rather from normal, age-related changes.

Selection of Stress Agent

Dipyridamole

The coronary vasodilator effects of dipyridamole are thought to be mediated through an inhibition of adenosine deaminase and, consequently, an increase in adenosine level. Stimulation of the A_2 receptors on the coronary smooth muscle cells causes vasodilation and therefore a marked decline in coronary resistance, which profoundly increases coronary and, in turn, myocardial blood flow (see Table 70–1). Measurements of myocardial blood flow with ^{13}N-ammonia or ^{15}O-water and PET have demonstrated a normal, three- to fivefold increase in myocardial blood flow (see Table 70–2). Dipyridamole lowers also the peripheral vascular resistance, which accounts for some of its side effects and produces an increase in cardiac output.[17] In the maximally dilated coronary artery, coronary and, in turn, myocardial blood flow depend on the coronary driving pressure. To relate these measurements and thereby to account for possible differences in hyperemic flows, some laboratories calculate a "myocardial flow resistance index" as the quotient of mean arterial blood pressure and myocardial blood flow.

Dipyridamole is infused intravenously at a rate of 0.142 mg · kg^{-1}

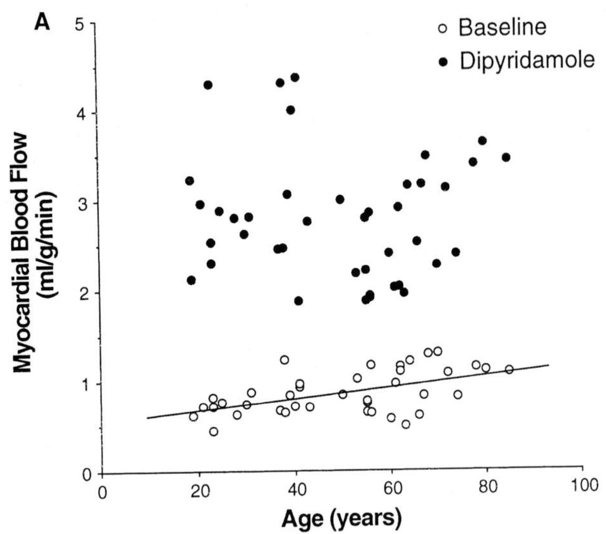

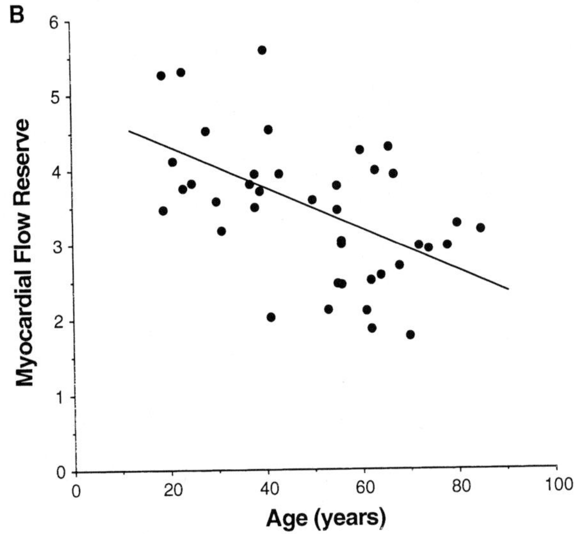

FIGURE 70–3. The age dependence of myocardial blood flow (*A*) and myocardial flow reserve (*B*). Measurements at rest and during dipyridamole-induced hyperemia were obtained in 40 normal volunteers with a low likelihood of coronary artery disease. As shown in (*A*), there was no significant trend in hyperemic blood flow, yet there was a progressive increase in the resting myocardial blood flow. Myocardial flow reserve, calculated from the ratio of hyperemic blood flow to rest blood flow, accordingly declined progressively with age, as shown in (*B*). (From Czernin, J., Müller, P., Chan, S., et al.: Influence of age and hemodynamics on myocardial blood flow and flow reserve. Circulation 88:62, 1993, with permission of the American Heart Association, Inc.)

body weight for 4 minutes. The maximum flow response occurs between 2 and 4 minutes after the end of the 4-minute infusion of the agent.[17] Although higher doses of dipyridamole have been proposed as a means to achieve higher and more consistent levels of hyperemic blood flows, measurements in normal volunteers have failed to confirm these claims.[14] Intravenous aminophylline promptly abolishes the effects of dipyridamole. Dosages vary between laboratories; most inject initially doses from 75 to 125 mg of aminophylline followed by a second, similar dose if the side effects are not promptly relieved. Further, some investigators routinely administer aminophylline, and others use aminophylline only if patients experience side effects.[18, 19] Table 70–3 summarizes the incidence of major and minor adverse reactions.

Adenosine

Adenosine serves as an alternative agent for inducing coronary vasodilation. It was thought to produce greater flow increases than dipyridamole, but comparative flow measurements with PET did not confirm this claim.[8] Adenosine infused intravenously at a rate of 140 $\mu g \cdot min^{-1} \cdot g^{-1}$ produces hyperemic blood flows that are comparable to those achieved with standard doses of intravenous dipyridamole. In a given individual, the responses to dipyridamole and adenosine may vary considerably.[8] Usually, adenosine is infused intravenously at a constant rate for a total of 6 minutes. The flow tracer is administered at 4 minutes so that 2 minutes of hyperemia remain for trapping of the tracer in the myocardium. Side effects,[20] as listed in Table 70–3, can rapidly be abolished by discontinuing the adenosine infusion because the agent has a biological half-life in plasma of less than 15 to 20 seconds.

Dobutamine

Dobutamine increases myocardial contractility and thus myocardial oxygen demand, which in turn raises myocardial blood flow. In contrast to dipyridamole or adenosine, which increase myocardial blood flow independent of cardiac work, changes in blood flow induced by dobutamine stimulation remain coupled to changes in myocardial oxygen consumption and myocardial work. Infusion rates of dobutamine range from 5 to 40 $\mu g \cdot min^{-1} \cdot kg^{-1}$; in most instances, infusion rates at the lower end of the spectrum are sufficient to induce flow defects and ischemia.[13] Normally, dobutamine infusion begins with doses of 5 or 10 $\mu g \cdot min^{-1} \cdot g^{-1}$. If no significant rise in systolic blood pressure occurs, the rate of infusion is progressively increased by 5 $\mu g \cdot min^{-1} \cdot kg^{-1}$ every 3 minutes. Most common side effects[21] include ventricular arrhythmias (see Table 70–3).

Cold Pressor Testing

This test has also been employed in the evaluation of coronary artery disease. Typically, the patient places a hand in a slush of ice water while heart rate and blood pressure are measured repeatedly. The flow tracer is usually administered at 30 seconds, and the hand remains immersed in the ice water for another 60 seconds to allow for tracer accumulation in the myocardium. Characteristically, the test causes a prompt increase in heart rate and blood pressure and thus in cardiac work; the effects are thought to be mediated by adrenergic neuronal stimulation. As demonstrated by highly invasive measurements, the procedure produces in coronary artery disease patients a constriction of the large epicardial coronary arteries,[22] possibly because of an α-mediated smooth muscle constriction unopposed by an α-receptor mediated endothelial-dependent vasodilatory effect. In coronary artery disease, endothelial dysfunction may be associated with an absence or attenuation of this endothelial-dependent vasodilator effect. Zeiher and coworkers[23] described a statistically significant correlation between the responses to intracoronary acetylcholine and those to cold pressor testing. Although such a correlation may imply that cold pressor testing does in fact evaluate endothelial function, given the complexity of this test, the authors refer more cautiously to this test as a means to evaluate "coronary vasomotion."

To summarize, dipyridamole and adenosine cause comparable increases in myocardial blood flow, although individual responses may vary considerably. Higher dipyridamole doses and exercise supplementation to raise coronary driving pressure do not augment further hyperemic blood flows but rather cause a modest decline. Last, the myocardial blood flow reserve depends on resting blood flow as a function of baseline cardiac work; flow reserves progressively decline with age, so flow reserve measurements in patients need to be compared with those of age-matched controls.

TABLE 70–3. MAJOR AND MINOR SIDE EFFECTS OF PHARMACOLOGIC STRESS TESTING

Symptoms	Dipyridamole	Adenosine	Dobutamine
Major Adverse Events			
Cardiac death	0.95 per 10,000*	0	0
Nonfatal MI	1.76 per 10,000*	1.08 per 10,000	0
Bronchospasm	1.22 per 10,000*	0.1%	0
Hypertension	1.5%	1.8%	1.4%
Hypotension	4.6%	Not reported	Not reported
Minor Side Effects			
Headaches	12.2%	14.2%	14.0%
Flushing	3.4%	36.5%	14.0%
Dyspnea	2.6%	35.2%	14.0%
Chest pain	19.7%	34.5%	31.0%
GI discomfort/nausea	4.6%	14.6%	9.0%
Lightheadedness/dizziness	11.8%	8.5%	4.0%
AV block	Not reported	7.6%*	0.7%
ST-T changes	7.5%	5.7%	50.0%
Arrhythmias	5.2%‡	3.3%	53.8%†

MI = myocardial infarction; GI = gastrointestinal; AV = atrial ventricular.

Data for dipyridamole were taken from Ranhosky et al.[18] and Lette et al.[19*] The report by Lette et al. describes a multicenter study that included 73,806 patients with dipyridamole. The data on adenosine were taken from the report by Cerqueira et al.,[20] who surveyed in a multicenter trial a total of 9256 consecutive patients studied with intravenous adenosine at a dose of 140 μg/kg body weight/min. Last, the data on dobutamine were taken from the report by Hays et al.[21] on 144 patients.

*This number includes all types of AV blocks, including a 2.8% incidence of first degree, 4.1% incidence of second degree, and of only 0.8% incidence of third degree AV blocks.

†Arrhythmias as listed here included unifocal or multifocal premature ventricular complexes, couplets, and nonsustained ventricular tachycardia (in 2.8%); 74.3% of all patients were studied with a maximum dose of 40 μg/kg/min.

‡Arrhythmias here represented mostly ventricular extrasystoles.

Stress Testing and Patient Monitoring

Vital signs and a 12-lead electrocardiogram (ECG) are obtained before imaging. The heart rate and rhythm should be monitored continuously throughout the study. Vital sign measurements are repeated every 2 minutes after the start of the dipyridamole, adenosine, or dobutamine infusion, and the ECG is repeated every 5 minutes for a total of 30 minutes, or longer if necessary, for resolution of any ST changes that develop. Vials of aminophylline (125 mg injectable) and a fully equipped resuscitation cart are kept in the imaging room.

Image Acquisition and Analysis

Images of the distribution of myocardial blood flow are obtained for 5 to 8 minutes for ^{82}Rb or 15 to 20 minutes for ^{13}N-ammonia. After isotope decay, 10 minutes after administration of the first dose of ^{82}Rb or 40 minutes after ^{13}N-ammonia, the pharmacologic stress study is performed. If blood flow is to be quantified, serial image acquisition commences with the intravenous tracer administration. For details see Chapter 69.

Image Display

Images of the distribution of the flow tracer in the myocardium at rest and during stress are acquired and displayed initially in the form of contiguous transaxial images. The transaxial image sets are typically reoriented into short-axis and long-axis cuts (see Fig. 70–1). Further processing allows the generation of polar maps, which display the three-dimensional distribution of the activity concentrations throughout the myocardium in the form of two-dimensional maps (Fig. 70–4). At the center of the polar map is the apical short-axis slice, with concentric rings of sequentially more superior short-axis slices. That is, the breadloaf slices are organized concentrically. The method introduces distortions by stretching the most superior slices to fit around the more apical slices. As a result, the area of the polar map is not proportional to the area of the myocardium that it represents. However, the contribution of each slice (or ring) to the total area of the polar map can be weighted appropriately so that accurate estimates of regional blood flow defect sizes can be obtained.[24] Software also has been developed for three-dimensional reconstruction and for display of the ratio of myocardial tracer uptake during stress and at rest.[25] Other displays have been proposed. One resembles a modified Mercator-type map similar to that employed by cartographers; it seeks to achieve a geometrically less distorted display of the tracer activity concentrations in the myocardium.[26] Finally, three-dimensional displays recently described[25] almost completely eliminate any geometric distortion and could, if applied routinely, reflect most accurately the location, extent, and severity of coronary artery disease.

FIGURE 70–4. See Color Plate 32.

Image Analysis

The relative distribution of flow tracer activity in the myocardium may be assessed subjectively or by quantitative criteria. Subjective interpretation is based on recognition of defects, similar to the conventional interpretation of scintigraphic images. A defect on an image obtained at rest usually represents myocardial infarction or ischemia, but it also may be caused by normal anatomical thinning, such as at the apex. The key finding is a defect that appears only on the hyperemic (vasodilator stress or exercise) image, which is evidence of a coronary artery stenosis of sufficient severity to reduce coronary flow reserve (see Figs. 70–1 and 70–4). Modern approaches of objective image and data interpretation include the use of databases of normal subjects, semiquantitative estimates of changes in regional myocardial blood flow from rest to stress, and quantitative estimates of regional myocardial blood flow in milliliters per minute per gram of myocardium.

COMPARISON TO DATABASES OF NORMAL SUBJECTS. In this approach, the patient's polar map is compared to a database established in normal volunteers for both resting and hyperemia studies. Regional reductions in tracer uptake exceeding two standard deviations below the mean or below a region-specific threshold are defined as regional flow defects; in order to reduce the effects of statistical noise, the geographic extent of such reductions must also exceed a predefined threshold to be considered as true flow defects.[8, 24, 27, 28] Region-specific thresholds have been established with the use of receiver operating curves[25, 29] and may differ among various positron-emitting tracers of blood flow. For the determination of stress-induced flow defects, "difference polar maps" (obtained by subtraction of the stress from the rest images) have been proposed but remain investigational.[25]

ESTIMATES OF MYOCARDIAL FLOW RESERVE. This approach seeks to quantify the dipyridamole-induced increase in regional myocardial blood flow. It employs "calibrated" myocardial activity images in which regional counts are normalized to the total administered activity.[30] The ratio of the normalized counts of the hyperemic images to those of the resting images serve as an estimate of the myocardial flow reserve. Although intriguing because of its simplicity, the approach is based on several assumptions that entail a consistent four- to fivefold increase in myocardial blood flow in response to dipyridamole and a constant dipyridamole-produced change in cardiac output and its fractional distribution to the myocardium. Accordingly, the myocardial flow reserve in a given region of the myocardium is defined as the ratio of flow at maximal vasodilation to resting perfusion of the same region. This ratio is closely related to stenosis flow reserve and coronary flow reserve (Fig. 70–5). Although the approach, referred to as the "uptake index ratio," enhances the accuracy of detection of coronary artery disease, the underlying assumptions do not hold under all conditions. The approach adjusts for the nonlinear tracer uptake in response to higher flows; however, as mentioned, the flow responses to pharmacologic vasodilations may vary considerably.[9]

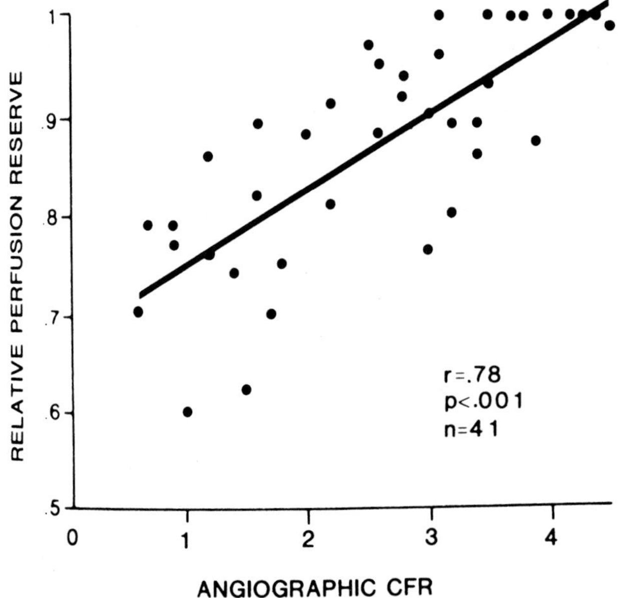

FIGURE 70–5. The relation of relative myocardial perfusion reserve and stenosis flow reserve derived from quantitative coronary arteriography. (From Goldstein, R., Kirkeeide, R., Demer, L., et al.: Relation between geometric dimensions of coronary artery stenoses and myocardial perfusion reserve in man. J. Clin. Invest. 79:1473, 1987, with permission of the American Society of Clinical Investigation.)

Also, it assumes a 50% increase in cardiac output, although the increase may be much more variable. Thus, use of a fixed correction factor may be practical but at times incorrect.

NONINVASIVE MEASUREMENTS OF MYOCARDIAL BLOOD FLOW. Regional myocardial blood flow can now be quantified noninvasively with either ^{15}O-water or ^{13}N-ammonia and dynamic PET imaging.[3, 5–7, 31, 32] Also, regional myocardial blood flow can be displayed in the form of a parametric image in which color codes correspond to discrete values of milliliters of blood flow per minute per gram of myocardium.[33] Measurements of regional myocardial blood flow appear to enhance the accuracy of determining the hemodynamic significance of coronary stenoses and to allow responses to interventions or treatment to be monitored. Such measurements may also prove useful for uncovering alterations in coronary vasomotion in early preclinical coronary artery disease and in cardiac diseases with normal coronary arteries.

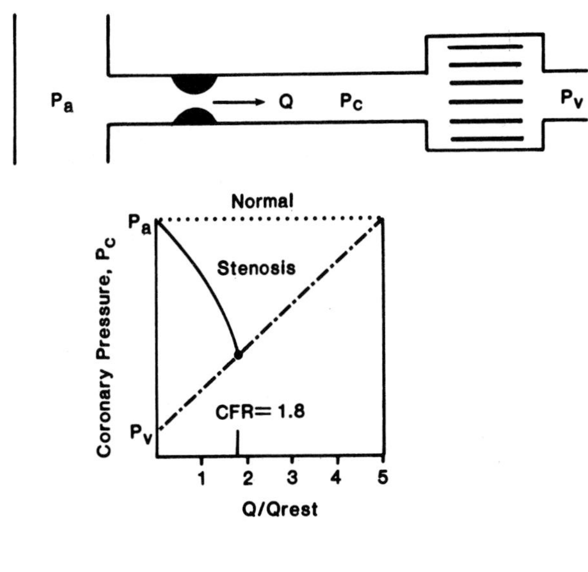

$$Pc = Pa - \left[A(Q/Qrest) + B\,(Q/Qrest)^2\right]$$

Stenosis Pressure Drop

FIGURE 70–6. The correlation of distal coronary perfusion pressure with coronary flow reserve. For a constant absolute diameter and length, the measurement of coronary flow reserve under conditions of maximal coronary vasodilation predicts the distal perfusion pressure as well as the percent diameter narrowing. (From Gould, K., Mullani, N., and Kirkeeide, R. L.: Coronary circulation. *In* Phelps, M. E., Mazziotta, J. C., and Schelbert, H. R. (eds.): PET and Autoradiography: Principles and Applications for the Brain and Heart. New York, Raven Press, 1986, p. 133, with permission.)

DETECTION OF CORONARY ARTERY DISEASE

Diagnosis of coronary artery disease is one of the primary clinical applications of PET blood flow imaging. Theoretically, it promises to be more accurate for the detection of coronary disease than exercise ECG testing and planar or even SPECT imaging. The basis for improved accuracy is that PET provides quantitative attenuation correction, has a higher spatial resolution than SPECT, which is rather homogeneous, and has a higher contrast resolution than SPECT.

Standards for Comparison

Subjective Versus Quantitative Arteriography

Conventionally, results of myocardial blood flow imaging have been tested against visually assessed coronary stenosis severity in terms of percent diameter reduction estimated from coronary arteriograms. This subjective method is no longer considered acceptable for research purposes because of the high interobserver variability.[34–36] Percent diameter narrowing is also not meaningful in the presence of diffuse disease or after percutaneous transluminal coronary angioplasty because there is no appropriate reference diameter.[37, 38] A more objective approach to assessment of stenosis severity is measurement of absolute stenosis diameter and cross-sectional area by quantitative arteriography.[39]

Percent Narrowing Versus Stenosis Flow Reserve

One method of assessing stenosis severity is measurement of its dimensions and calculation of its pressure-flow relation. This method allows comparison of anatomical stenosis severity from patient to patient independent of hemodynamic factors. The pressure-flow relation may be more conveniently described in terms of "stenosis flow reserve." It is the expected flow reserve of an artery with the given stenosis dimensions under standard hemodynamic conditions. Stenosis flow reserve may be determined from computed quantitative arteriography. Coronary perfusion pressure distal to each stenosis may be calculated as a function of flow.[40, 41]

Under conditions of maximal coronary arteriolar vasodilation, the pressure-flow relation is represented by a straight line. Stenosis flow reserve is identified as the flow at maximal coronary vasodilation, relative to resting flow, under standardized hemodynamic conditions. Graphically, this may be represented by the intersection of the two lines representing the pressure-flow relation at maximal vasodilation with the pressure-flow relation of the stenosis (Fig. 70–6). Predicted stenosis flow reserve correlates with direct, electromagnetic flow measurements in animals with artificial stenosis (r = .91).[40] Similarly, measurements of the coronary flow reserve in humans based on direct invasive transtenotic pressure measurements during maximum coronary vasodilation demonstrated a highly significant correlation between the invasively measured fractional flow reserve (described later) and myocardial flow reserve as determined quantitatively with ^{15}O-water and PET.[42]

Stenosis Flow Reserve Versus Coronary Flow Reserve

Anatomy alone does not predict the full physiologic consequence of coronary stenoses. Accordingly, physiologic measures of stenosis severity have been developed to incorporate effects of other factors. As described originally, "coronary flow reserve" referred to the ratio of maximal to resting flow in the proximal portion of the coronary artery. Flow velocities are measured with intracoronary Doppler flow probes; the coronary cross-sectional areas are determined by intracoronary ultrasound or by quantitative coronary angiography. "Coronary flow reserve" is then calculated from the product of flow velocity and the coronary cross-sectional areas as the ratio of hyperemic to rest coronary blood flow.

Coronary flow is determined at rest and after injection of intracoronary papaverine or during adenosine infusion. Directly measured coronary flow reserve of the same stenosis may be different in different patients or in the same patient at different times, depending on the moment-to-moment hemodynamic conditions.

Coronary flow reserve depends on the coronary driving pressure, the total resistance of the system, the strength of the hyperemic stimulus and the coronary venous tone. Two stenoses of exactly the same geometry (and thus the same stenosis flow reserve) may have entirely different values of coronary flow reserve in different patients, or even in the same patient at different times under different hemodynamic conditions. In contrast, stenosis flow reserve is independent of hemodynamic conditions, by definition. It indicates the conductance of the stenosis itself, as if the arterial segment were excised and studied ex vivo under controlled conditions.

The difference between stenosis flow reserve and coronary flow reserve is best described by analogy to the difference between the automobile mileage estimated by the automobile manufacturer and the actual automobile mileage. The former is obtained under standardized conditions, the same for all makes, for purposes of comparing one car model to another on a uniform scale, allowing objective comparison. Actual mileage depends on the individual driving conditions, such as load and velocity. Two cars of exactly the same make and nominal mileage may have entirely different values of actual mileage with different drivers or even with the same driver at different times under different load conditions. The two measures are likely to differ, but each is useful for its own purpose.

In analogy, stenosis flow reserve is obtained under standardized conditions, the same for all arteries, for purposes of comparing one artery to another on a uniform scale. Stenosis flow reserve differs from the actual coronary flow reserve, depending on hemodynamic conditions. The two measures are likely to differ, but each is useful for its own purpose. Even coronary flow reserve may not be directly comparable to a flow defect severity, because it is measured at the time of cardiac catheterization rather than at the time of PET imaging, and hemodynamic conditions may change. Thus, neither stenosis flow reserve nor coronary flow reserve provides the value of flow reserve at the time of the PET study; the choice is between stenosis flow reserve, based on standardized hemodynamic conditions, or coronary flow reserve, based on hemodynamic conditions at the time of cardiac catheterization, when anxiety or sedative effect may alter hemodynamics.

Coronary Flow Reserve Versus Myocardial Flow Reserve

Even directly measured coronary flow reserve does not always reflect the ultimate physiologic significance of a stenosis, which is its effect on myocardial blood flow. A large artery with the same coronary flow reserve as a small artery may have a more profound effect on blood flow. Arteries with the same coronary flow reserve may have different values of perfusion reserve in the presence of collaterals.

Accuracy of Detection of Coronary Artery Disease

The practical limit of detection of a flow reserve impairment by PET was estimated first with labeled microspheres, which are virtually 100 percent extracted, and by direct gamma camera imaging of the ex vivo cross-sectional myocardial slices.[43] The least amount of coronary narrowing detected using this method with submaximal coronary vasodilation in animals was 40 to 50 percent diameter narrowing. These "ex vivo data" were subsequently found to be consistent with findings in chronically instrumented dogs. Coronary stenoses of different degrees of the left circumflex coronary artery were produced with inflatable cuffs, and images of myocardial blood flow before and after intravenous infusion of dipyridamole were obtained with ^{13}N-ammonia and PET. Defects were identified subjectively during vasodilation with circumflex coronary artery narrowing of as little as 47 percent diameter by quantitative arteriography.[44]

Sensitivity and Specificity of Detecting Coronary Artery Disease

Sensitivity and specificity have been remarkably high in patient studies (Table 70–4). An initial study with ^{13}N-ammonia PET imaging at rest and with dipyridamole stress demonstrated a 97 percent sensitivity and 100 percent specificity for patients with arteriographically documented coronary artery disease and for 13 healthy subjects.[45] Overall, 52 of 58 stenotic vessels were identified correctly. However, in this study, coronary artery disease was defined visually as a 50 percent or greater narrowing by coronary arteriography. Similarly, high sensitivity and specificity have been found despite inclusion of patients without angina. In 50 patients studied with ^{82}Rb or ^{13}N-ammonia at rest and again with dipyridamole and hand-grip stress, images were 98 percent sensitive and 100 percent specific for coronary artery disease defined by quantitative arteriographic criteria for stenosis flow reserve.[46] When this study group was expanded to 193 patients, accuracy was minimally reduced.[47, 48] PET perfusion imaging was performed with dipyridamole stress and compared with stenosis flow reserve derived from quantitative arteriographic measurements. The authors defined a stenosis flow reserve of less than 3 as a critical stenosis and a reserve between 3 and 4 as a mild stenosis. PET was 94 percent sensitive in detecting critical coronary stenoses and 49 percent sensitive in detecting mild coronary stenoses. Other investigators have criticized this classification of coronary stenosis. However, other studies resort to even less well defined and validated indices of what constitutes a critical stenosis. Some studies simply rely on visual assessment of coronary stenosis; others use quantitative arteriography but employ only a given threshold of percent diameter or cross-sectional narrowing.

Sensitivity and specificity remain high for exercise instead of pharmacologic stress. Tamaki and colleagues found 95 percent sensitivity and 98 percent specificity for rest and exercise PET imaging with ^{13}N-ammonia in 25 patients, and 98 percent sensitivity in a group of 48 patients with known coronary artery disease.[1, 49] Specificity was not assessed because only 3 normal patients were studied. These results were based on subjective assessment of arteriographic percent diameter narrowing, with coronary disease defined as one or more stenoses of greater than 50 percent diameter narrowing.

Including these early clinical investigations, a total of 1083 patients studied with PET for the detection of coronary artery disease have been reported on in the peer-reviewed literature.[49–53] As summarized in Table 70–4, the sensitivities range from 82 to 97 percent, the specificities from 78 to 100 percent, and the diagnostic accuracies from 85 to 98 percent. Almost all studies relied on pharmacologic stress. Demer and co-workers[47] employed in their study either ^{82}Rb or ^{13}N-ammonia and concluded that both tracers were equally accurate in the identification of coronary artery disease.

Oxygen-15 water has also been found useful for imaging relative blood flow defects in coronary artery disease. Walsh and colleagues recently showed the feasibility of identifying relative flow defects

TABLE 70–4. SENSITIVITY AND SPECIFICITY OF POSITRON-EMISSION TOMOGRAPHY (PET) BLOOD FLOW IMAGING FOR THE DETECTION OF CORONARY ARTERY DISEASE

Investigation	No. of Patients	Stenosis	Tracer	Stress	Sensitivity	Specificity	Accuracy
Schelbert et al., 1982[45]	45	>50%	NH_3	DIP	97	100	98
Demer et al., 1989[47]	193	SFR<3	NH_3, Rb	DIP	94	95	94
Yonekura et al., 1987[49]	50	≥50%	NH_3	EX	93	100	94
Stewart et al., 1991[50]	81	≥50%	Rb	DIP	84	88	85
Go et al., 1990[51]	202	≥50%	Rb	DIP	93	78	90
Williams et al., 1994[52]	287	≥67%	Rb	DIP	87	88	88
Simone et al., 1992[53]	225	≥67%	Rb	DIP	82	91	89

The table represents a total of 1083 patients studied. Stenosis = degree of diameter narrowing considered hemodynamically significant; NH_3 = ^{13}N-ammonia; ^{82}Rb = rubidium-82; DIP and EX = dipyridamole and supine bicycle exercise used as stress; SFR = stenosis flow reserve as derived by quantitative arteriography.

using ^{15}O-water with dipyridamole stress in 33 patients.[54] Uniformity was significantly greater for the nine normal subjects than for the patients with coronary artery disease. However, the ^{15}O-water cardiac images were of lower diagnostic quality than the ^{13}N-ammonia or ^{82}Rb images because of low signal-to-noise ratios, so the main advantage of ^{15}O-water is its utility for measurements of blood flow.

Confidence Limits

Because the sensitivity and specificity values such as those shown in Table 70–4 are merely statistical estimates of the true sensitivity and specificity for a larger population, descriptions for comparison to other imaging methods in terms of sensitivity should include confidence intervals to indicate the accuracy of the estimate. The accuracy of the estimate depends on the population sizes and consistency. Confidence intervals indicate the accuracy of an estimate as a function of probability. For example, applying standard statistical tables[55] to data from Schelbert and associates,[45] the lower limit of the 95 percent confidence interval for sensitivity is 84 percent, and the lower limit for specificity is 75 percent. For Gould and colleagues,[46] the corresponding lower limits of the 95 percent confidence intervals are 77 percent and 66 percent, respectively. The overlap of these wide confidence intervals with the sensitivity and specificity values reported for planar thallium imaging, and even for ECG exercise testing, indicates the need for larger study populations. In the one large study, coronary artery disease severity was described in terms of three rather than two levels of severity to reduce the effects of binary classification, as described later.

Limitations of Sensitivity and Specificity Analysis

Most reports of the diagnostic accuracy of PET and SPECT or of planar blood flow imaging of the heart are based on sensitivity and specificity analysis.[45, 46, 56–60] Unfortunately, reported sensitivity and specificity values of tests are not comparable if they are based on different patient populations, different criteria for coronary artery disease, different criteria for positive flow defects, or different imaging methods.

First, threshold values that yield optimal sensitivity and specificity for one imaging method may yield suboptimal values for another test with a different threshold for detection. For example, a hypothetic test with perfect sensitivity and specificity using a cutoff value of 40 percent diameter narrowing will have falsely low specificity if the cutoff value is defined as 50 percent, particularly if the study population includes many patients with stenosis severity between 40 and 50 percent.

In addition, binary (positive or negative) classification of imaging and arteriographic results does not reflect the continuous nature of coronary artery disease severity. In the past, arteriographic results have been classified by the arbitrary cutoff values of 50, 70, or 75 percent diameter narrowing. Defining a 45 percent stenosis as normal and a 50 percent stenosis as abnormal has questionable meaning. Blood flow imaging results also have been classified into a binary scale as normal or abnormal despite a continuous spectrum of defect severity in terms of both defect intensity and size. However, criteria for differentiating positive from borderline defects are even more subjective than arteriographic percent diameter narrowing.

A third limitation of sensitivity and specificity analysis is the dependence on distribution of disease severity in the study population.[61] A sample population with a high frequency of mild disease, near the cutoff points, tends to have lower sensitivity and specificity for the same amount of scatter. Sensitivity and specificity determined for one population may not apply to a different population, as in symptomatic and asymptomatic patients. Use of a continuous variable has been proposed to overcome these limitations.[61] Regional myocardial blood flow at rest and during pharmacologic vasodilation has been measured with PET with continuous scales over the entire range of disease severity, using direct correlation analysis and quantitative coronary arteriography.[62]

Localization of Coronary Artery Disease

To assess the accuracy of PET imaging in identifying the specific coronary arteries with significant stenoses, it is necessary to assign each myocardial region to a particular artery (Fig. 70–7; see Fig. 70–4). However, anatomical variations in the coronary tree, such as right- and left-dominant systems and overlap of perfusion beds, limit any algorithm for matching each stenosis to a corresponding defect. With this limitation, most studies have shown a fairly strong relation between the region supplied by a narrowed coronary artery and the location of the PET defect, assuming standard anatomy. With acknowledgment of these limitations, polar map approaches have been developed and have been found useful for localization of coronary stenoses.[25, 29] These approaches also serve to define the amount of myocardium affected by a particular coronary stenosis as a fraction of the entire left ventricular myocardium or of a particular coronary territory.[24] It is also possible to derive an index of the severity of the flow defect[28] by determining the average reduction of tracer activity below the threshold. Indices of both the geographic extent and the severity of flow defects may prove useful for assessment of the amount myocardium at risk and for characterization or quantification of responses to physiologic or pharmacologic interventions or to medical and interventional treatment.

Stenosis Severity and Vasodilator Capacity

As pointed out by Gould,[26] if pharmacologic vasodilation reduces maximally the peripheral resistance in the coronary circulatory system, then the major resistance in a coronary vessel moves to the site of the coronary stenosis. Therefore, the stenosis severity should be correlated with the resistance to blood flow and, thus, the degree of the attenuation of blood flow during pharmacologic vasodilation. Early, semiquantitative studies with PET did in fact demonstrate such a relation (Fig. 70–8).[63] The degree of attenuation was estimated in this study by the ratio of tracer concentration in the stenosis-dependent myocardium to that in myocardium supplied by normal coronary arteries. As seen in Figure 70–9, the curvilinear correlation between angiographic estimates of stenosis flow reserves and the relative attenuation of hyperemic blood flow resembles the correlation originally described by Gould and co-workers.[64]

More recent investigations took advantage of the capability of PET to measure myocardial blood flow in absolute terms. One investigation by Uren and co-workers[10] combined flow values obtained with the ^{15}O-water approach in patients from different PET laboratories with different imaging equipment. In a total of 35 coronary artery disease patients and 21 normal subjects, this study reported the anticipated nonlinear correlation between stenosis severity, from less than 40 to greater than 80 percent diameter narrowing, and the decline in hyperemic blood flow and in flow reserve, together with a curvilinear increase in "minimal" coronary resistance (as estimated during dipyridamole administration). Another study with ^{13}N-ammonia blood flow measurements in 13

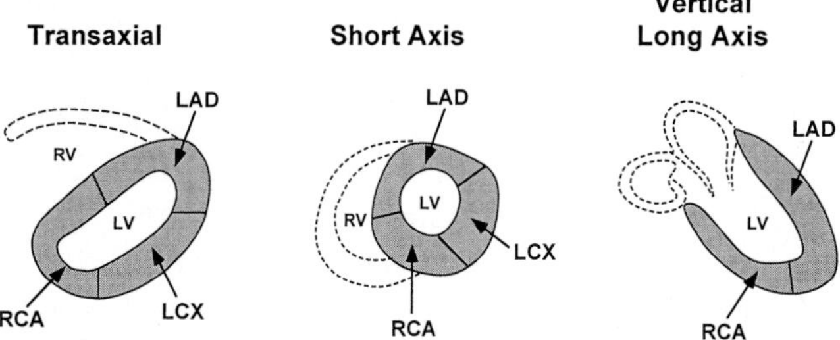

FIGURE 70–7. Schematic representation of the coronary artery territories relative to the left ventricular myocardium. LAD = left anterior descending artery; LCX = left circumflex coronary artery; RCA = right coronary artery.

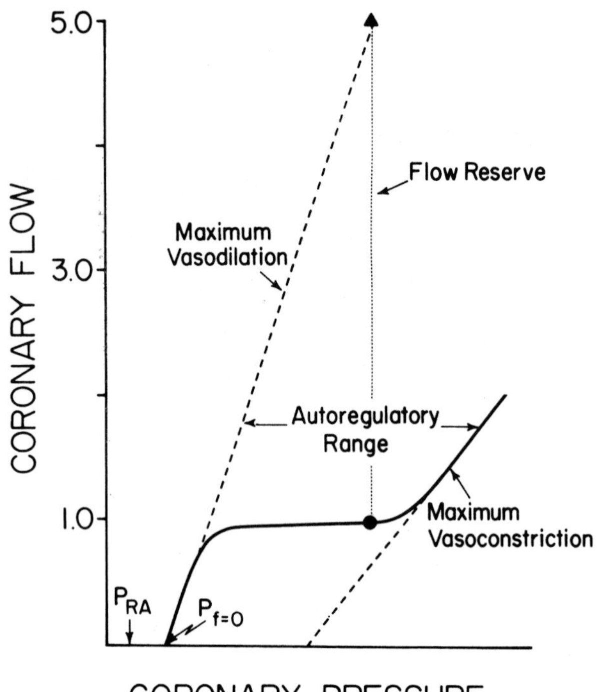

FIGURE 70–8. The steady-state relation between coronary flow and coronary arterial pressure in the left ventricle. The solid line depicts the normal relation. At a constant level of myocardial metabolic demand, coronary flow is maintained constant over a wide range of coronary pressure, between the bounds of maximal coronary vasodilation and constriction *(dashed lines)*. (From Klocke, F.: Measurements of coronary flow reserve: Defining pathophysiology versus making decisions about patient care. Circulation 76:1183, 1987. With permission from the American Heart Association, Inc.)

coronary artery disease patients similarly demonstrated reduced hyperemic blood flows and flow reserves in myocardium subtended by diseased coronary arteries.[65] A third study by Di Carli and coworkers[66] compared the percent cross-sectional area narrowing by quantitative angiography with the myocardial flow reserve calculated from ^{13}N-ammonia PET measurements of blood flow at rest and after standard-dose dipyridamole infusion. Hyperemic flows and flow reserve were determined in the territories of 41 non–infarct-related coronary arteries of 18 patients and compared with findings in 10 age-matched normal volunteers. The stenosis severity in this study ranged from 30 to 86 percent cross-sectional area reduction. Complete coronary occlusions and territories supplied by collaterals were excluded from analysis. Figure 70–10 depicts the nonlinear correlations between regional myocardial flow reserves and the stenosis severity. Hyperemic blood flows and flow reserves in vascular territories supplied by vessels without flow-limiting stenoses were virtually identical to those observed in the age-matched group of healthy normal volunteers.

Several aspects of these studies deserve comment. First, despite statistically significant correlations between stenosis severity and flow reserves, there is considerable scatter of the data about the regression line. To some extent, method-related limitations may account for this scatter. This is especially the case for ^{15}O-water studies for two reasons: (1) the higher coefficient of variation[67] and, consequently, a lesser degree of accuracy of regional flow measurements, and (2) combination of the study data from two different laboratories with different imaging equipment in the study by Uren and co-workers.[10] On the other hand, Iida and associates[68] recently demonstrated a rather good agreement of flow measurements performed at different institutions with different instruments so this issue may be of less concern. Further, effects of

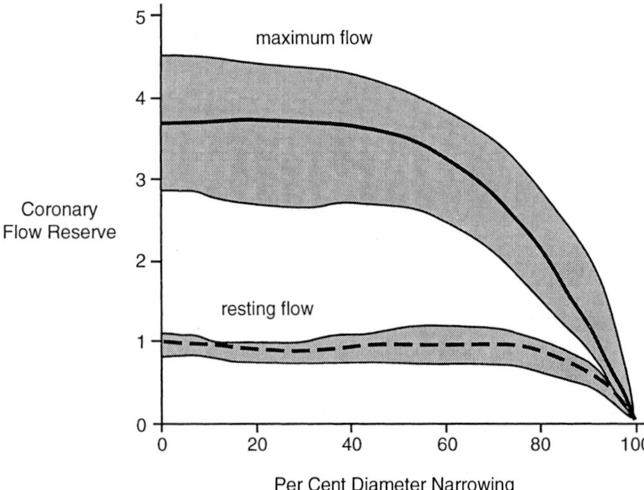

FIGURE 70–9. The relation between coronary artery diameter narrowing and coronary blood flows at rest and during hyperemia, as observed in dog experiments. (From Gould, K. L., Lipscomb, K., and Hamilton, G. W.: Physiologic basis for assessing critical coronary stenosis: Instantaneous flow response and regional distribution during coronary hyperemia as measures of coronary flow reserve. Am. J. Cardiol. 33:87, 1974, with permission.)

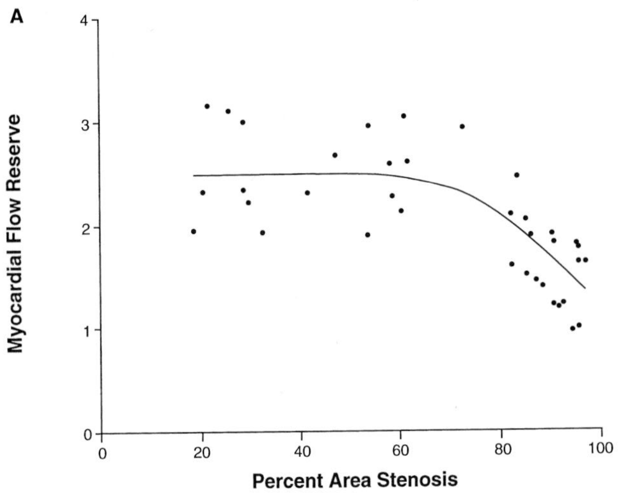

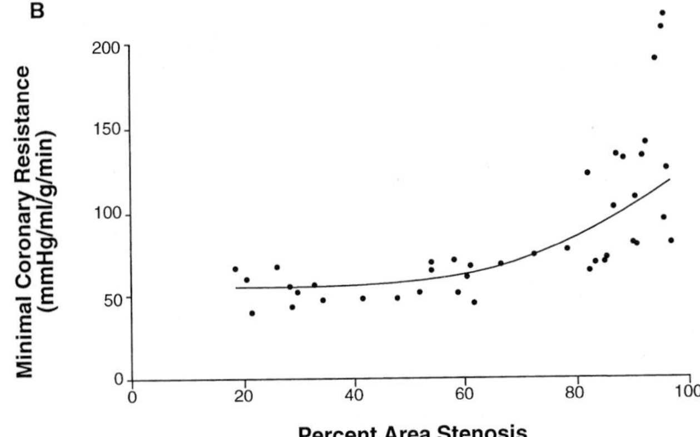

FIGURE 70–10. The effects of coronary stenosis on myocardial flow reserve *(A)* and the minimal coronary resistance *(B)* in human myocardium. Note the curvilinear correlation between the percent reduction in cross-sectional area, as determined by quantitative angiography, and the myocardial flow reserve as assessed through measurements of myocardial blood flows at rest and during dipyridamole hyperemia with ^{13}N-ammonia PET. (From Di Carli, M., Czernin, J., Hoh, C., et al.: Relation among stenosis severity, myocardial blood flow, and flow reserve in patients with coronary artery disease. Circulation 91:1944, 1995, with permission of the American Heart Association, Inc.)

collateral blood flow, especially in patients with complete coronary occlusions, may have contributed to the data scatter. In addition, the known variability of the flow responses to dipyridamole may have contributed further to the scatter of the data. Last, angiography characterizes primarily the anatomical features of a coronary lesion; likely discrepancies between "structure" and function may add further to the data scatter. At the same time, this raises the question as to whether the flow measurements define more accurately than angiography the degree of stenosis severity.

Findings in Preclinical or Non–Flow-Limiting Coronary Artery Disease

The possibility of demonstrating noninvasively through measurements of myocardial blood flow the presence of preclinical or non–flow-limiting coronary artery disease is currently being explored. Observations to date have been disappointing and, at the same time, encouraging. Di Carli and co-workers[66] demonstrated, in mildly diseased or angiographically normal vessels of patients with flow-limiting disease of other vessels, hyperemic blood flow and flow reserve values that were similar to values observed in age-matched healthy volunteers. The comparison with age-matched controls is important given the earlier-described age-dependent decline in myocardial flow reserve.[9, 16] Uren and co-workers[11] did in fact report an attenuated hyperemic flow response in normal territories of patients with single-vessel coronary artery disease, compared with a group of younger normal volunteers. Although the authors concluded that the vasodilator response in vessels without angiographic coronary artery disease was attenuated, they nevertheless entertained the possibility that their conclusions may indeed have been predicated by the comparison of their findings to a group of significantly younger normal controls. In contrast, Sambuceti and co-workers[69] noted a marked reduction in hyperemic flows and flow reserve in normal territories of patients with single-vessel disease. Hyperemic flows averaged 1.76 ± 0.68 $mL \cdot min^{-1} \cdot g^{-1}$ in patients, compared with 3.66 ± 0.92 $mL \cdot min^{-1} \cdot g^{-1}$ in normal volunteers. Because both groups were of similar ages, age dependency does not explain these findings.

Other studies again support the possibility of detecting preclinical or even very early stages of coronary artery disease. For example, observations with cold pressor testing indicated an attenuated flow response in normal territories of a small group of patients with coronary artery disease.[70] Cold pressor testing had been used in this study as a means to test endothelial function. Although the blunted flow response to cold pressor testing in normal territories is intriguing, these observations are based on a very small patient group and await further confirmation.

If in fact coronary artery disease begins at the endothelial level,[71] then the demonstration of endothelial dysfunction or, alternatively, associated abnormalities in coronary vasomotion may provide the earliest evidence of coronary artery disease. Recent observations in transplant vasculopathy may support such a possibility. Although not strictly comparable to the findings in regular coronary artery disease, these studies reported an attenuated or even absent flow response to cold pressor testing in patients with angiographically normal coronary arteries but with intimal thickening as determined by intracoronary ultrasound.[72] The same studies reported a highly significant inverse correlation between smooth muscle–mediated vasodilation, as tested with intravenous dipyridamole, and the maximal intimal thickening by intracoronary ultrasound. Furthermore, the minimal coronary resistance during dipyridamole administration correlated directly with the coronary resistance during cold pressor testing (coronary resistance was estimated from the ratio of the mean arterial blood pressure over myocardial blood flow). What these studies indicate is that quantitative flow measurements may uncover abnormal coronary vasomotion in angiographically normal vessels. Furthermore, these abnormalities may correlate with structural abnormalities as detected only invasively by intracoronary ultrasound.

Again, it remains uncertain to what extent transplant vasculopathy represents native coronary artery disease and whether findings in this model can be extrapolated to the more common "coronary artery disease." In hypercholesteremic patients without clinical evidence of coronary artery disease, dipyridamole-induced hyperemic blood flows and, especially, myocardial flow reserve were significantly attenuated when compared with an age matched control group.[73] Hyperemic blood flows averaged 2.18 ± 0.56 $mL \cdot min^{-1} \cdot g^{-1}$, compared with 2.64 ± 0.39 $mL \cdot min^{-1} \cdot g^{-1}$ in normal subjects; myocardial flow reserve was reduced to 2.93 ± 0.87, compared with 4.28 ± 0.5 ($P < .001$) in the normal control group (Fig. 70–11). In addition, the authors noted a statistically significant inverse correlation between the myocardial flow reserve and the ratio of total cholesterol to high-density lipoprotein cholesterol. It is possible that the elevated levels of total and low-density lipoprotein cholesterol impaired the normal endothelial function[74] and, via mechanoreceptors, a flow-mediated, endothelium-dependent augmentation of hyperemic blood flow.

Given the normal variability in flow responses to pharmacologic vasodilation, it remains unclear how specific such flow measurements can be for the detection of latent coronary artery disease. On the other hand, if such disease can be detected through a combination of flow measurements during several pharmacologic and physiologic interventions or in conjunction with other clinical parameters, given the high reproducibility of blood flow measurements with PET,[75] such interventions may indeed become useful for monitoring the progression of coronary artery disease or, conversely, responses to dietary and lifestyle changes.

Detection of Coronary Artery Disease by Positron Emission Tomography and by Single-Photon Emission Computed Tomography

Given its higher spatial and contrast resolution, PET would be expected to detect the presence of coronary artery disease more accurately than SPECT. Also, the appropriate correction for measured photon attenuation would diminish or eliminate artifacts frequently encountered by SPECT and render PET more specific. In fact, a survey of the literature supports these notions. Figure 70–12 depicts the sensitivity and specificity for several studies with ^{201}Tl SPECT, as described in Chapter 63, and for ^{13}N-ammonia or ^{82}Rb PET, as already summarized in this chapter and in Table 70–4. Both approaches offer comparable sensitivities, but SPECT appears to be less specific than PET. Such lower specificity is not surprising, because image artifacts occur more frequently with SPECT than with PET. In SPECT, such artifacts frequently arise from inhomogeneous photon attenuation, a limitation that PET overcomes by correction of the emission images with measured photon attenuation.

The higher spatial and contrast resolution of PET implies that it may have the ability to uncover the presence of less severe coronary artery disease. Some studies support this point. Two studies, one with PET and the other with ^{201}Tl SPECT,[60, 62] characterized stenosis severity by quantitative angiography in exactly the same manner and used "stenosis flow reserve" as a measure of stenosis severity. A comparison between the studies indicates a 94 percent sensitivity for PET and a 72 percent sensitivity for ^{201}Tl SPECT for detection of critical coronary stenoses, as defined by a stenosis flow reserve of 3 or less. Importantly, PET detected almost half (49 percent) but ^{201}Tl SPECT none of the intermediate coronary stenoses, as defined angiographically by a stenosis flow reserve between 3 and 4.

More compelling, however, are comparisons of both imaging modalities in the same patients. Such comparisons have been performed in a total of 331 patients in three separate clinical trials.[50, 51, 76] As shown in Table 70–5, Tamaki and collaborators[76] found comparable diagnostic accuracies with ^{201}Tl SPECT and ^{13}N-ammonia PET. Patients in this study underwent physical stress testing (either supine or upright), whereas patients in the other two investigations were submitted to pharmacologic stress alone or to pharma-

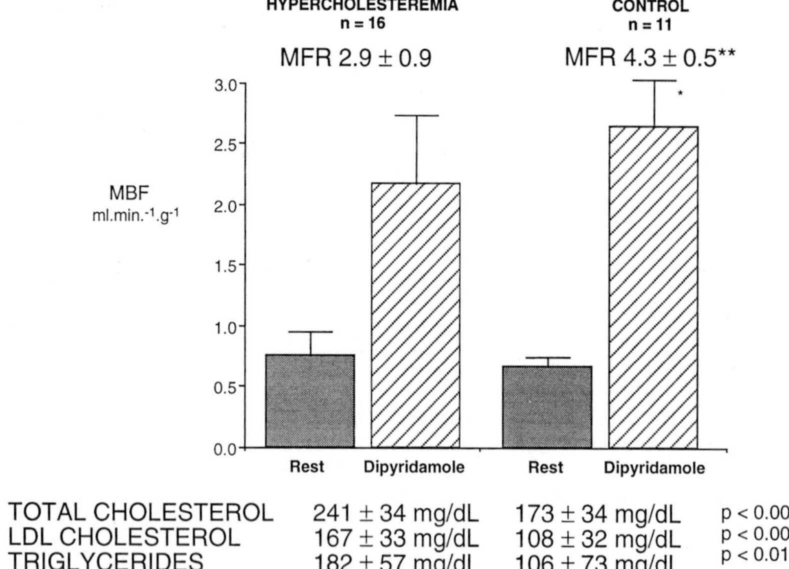

*p < 0.05 and p < 0.01 hypercholesteremia vs. control group

FIGURE 70–11. Myocardial blood flows at rest and during adenosine-induced hyperemia in hypercholesteremic patients. At rest, blood flows in the hypercholesteremic group *(left)* were similar to those in an age-matched control group with normal plasma lipid profiles. However, the hyperemic blood flows are significantly attenuated, resulting in a markedly lower myocardial flow reserve in hypercholesteremic patients. (From Dayanikli, F., Grambow, D., Muzik, O., et al.: Early detection of abnormal coronary flow reserve in asymptomatic men at high risk for coronary artery disease using positron emission tomography. Circulation 90:808, 1994, with permission of the American Heart Association, Inc.)

cologic stress on PET and to physical or pharmacologic stress on SPECT. Those studies also reached somewhat different conclusions. Go and colleagues[51] reported a higher sensitivity for PET and SPECT but comparable specificities. Stewart and co-workers,[50] however, found comparable sensitivities but a markedly higher specificity for PET than for SPECT. In spite of this discrepancy, both studies demonstrated significantly higher diagnostic accuracies for PET than for SPECT.

The reasons for these interstudy differences remain unclear. The Tamaki study[76] employed first-generation PET equipment with a more coarse spatial resolution. Further, potential shortcomings related to photon attenuation may have been minimized by the leaner body habitus of his patients (Tamaki, personal communication, 1994). More difficult to explain is the higher sensitivity for PET in the Go study.[51] In this study, both ^{82}Rb and ^{201}Tl were administered consecutively during the same pharmacologic stress intervention. It has been argued that, at the time of the ^{201}Tl administration (about 6 minutes later than the ^{82}Rb administration), the level of the dipyridamole-induced hyperemia had already declined. However, according to Brown and co-workers,[17] who described a decay half-time of 33 minutes for the hyperemic effect of dipyridamole, such interval decline would amount to only about 10 to 12 percent of the peak flow rate and should have had only a modest effect on stenosis detection. Conversely, the higher specificity in the Stewart study[50] would be expected, because PET does correct for photon attenuation and thus reduces the fraction of falsely positive studies.

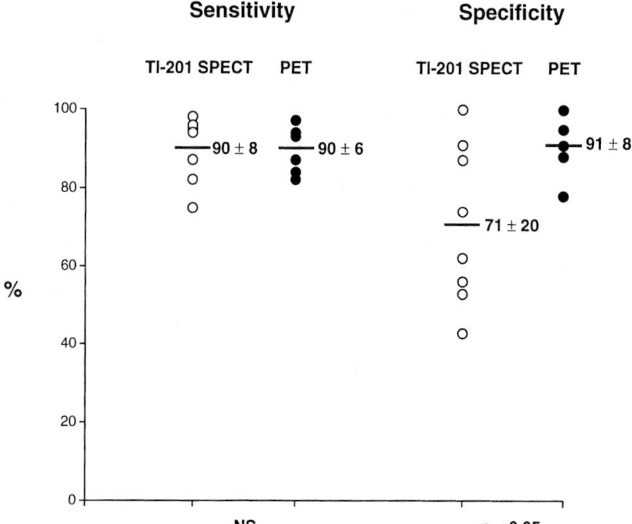

FIGURE 70–12. Summary of the sensitivities and specificities for the detection of coronary artery disease by SPECT and by PET. (See text.)

Limitations

In general, sensitivity and specificity of perfusion imaging for coronary artery disease depend on four factors: the patient population studied (i.e., the pretest probability), the standard of comparison used to define presence and absence of coronary artery disease, the subjective or objective criteria for defining positive and negative scans, and the adequacy of the vasodilator stimulus.

Unfortunately, there is no ideal "gold standard" for assessing accuracy of perfusion imaging in the identification of coronary artery disease severity. Myocardial flow reserve may not correspond to stenosis flow reserve in the presence of altered physiologic conditions, such as very high or very low perfusion pressure, marked bradycardia or tachycardia, collateral vessels, increased resting flow, ventricular hypertrophy, abnormal venous pressure, or inadequate vasodilatory stimulus.[77] Perfusion reserve may not correspond to directly measured coronary flow reserve in the presence of collateral vessels or if hemodynamic conditions change between the time of catheterization and the time of PET imaging.

Coronary Collaterals

Coronary collateral vessels are thought to be associated with a "coronary collateral steal," defined as an absolute decrease in blood flow in collateral-dependent myocardium after coronary arteriolar vasodilation. The conditions underlying the occurrence of a collateral steal remain controversial, although the following mechanism has been proposed. With dilation of distal coronary arteriolar beds (e.g., by dipyridamole or adenosine) flow increases in the supply artery, causing pressure to fall at the origin of the collaterals. As a result, collateral perfusion pressure falls (Fig. 70–13). Because the collateral channels appear to lack normal vasoregulation, collateral flow depends primarily on this driving pressure at the arteriolar level of the supply artery. To the extent that collaterals supply a

TABLE 70–5. COMPARISON OF SINGLE-PHOTON EMISSION COMPUTED TOMOGRAPHY (SPECT) AND POSITRON EMISSION TOMOGRAPHY (PET) FOR THE DETECTION OF CORONARY ARTERY DISEASE

			Sensitivity		Specificity		Accuracy	
Investigation	**No. of Patients**	**Stenosis**	**PET**	**SPECT**	**PET**	**SPECT**	**PET**	**SPECT**
Tamaki et al., 1988[76]	48	≥50%	98%	96%	N/A	N/A	N/A	N/A
Go et al., 1990[51]	202	≥50%	93%	76%*	78%	80%	90%	77%*
Stewart et al., 1991[50]	81	≥50%	84%	84%	88%	53%†	85%	79%†

Tamaki et al. submitted patients to supine bicycle exercise; Go et al. used near-simultaneous injections of rubidium-82 and thallium-201 during dipyridamole-induced hyperemia. Stewart et al. employed dipyridamole stress for all PET studies but only for 53 percent of the SPECT thallium-201 studies; the remaining patients underwent exercise treadmill stress for thallium-201 SPECT.

*$P < .001$; †$P < .05$ for the difference between PET and SPECT; stenosis = percent diameter narrowing.

portion or all of resting perfusion to a given region, a corresponding degree of steal occurs in that bed with coronary arteriolar dilation. According to simulation analysis, the greater the collateral conductance, the greater the decrease in collateral blood flow with vasodilation. Hence, collateral steal may be recognized as a myocardial flow reserve of less than 1; that is, blood flow after vasodilation is less than at baseline. The lower the myocardial flow reserve, the greater the functional collateral conductance.

Using a semiquantitative analysis approach, Demer and co-workers[78] did in fact demonstrate such decrease. With the use of intravenous ^{82}Rb or ^{13}N-ammonia and normalization of the regional tracer activity concentrations to the injected amount of activity, tracer concentrations in collateral-dependent myocardium were found to decline after administration of intravenous dipyridamole. Regional tracer concentrations decreased in 25 of the 28 patients with arteriographic collaterals, compared with a similar decrease in only 4 of 25 control patients with coronary artery disease but without angiographic collaterals. Although the authors ascribe this decline in activity concentrations to a "coronary steal," measurements of myocardial blood flow in absolute units with ^{13}N-ammonia and PET in other patients failed to confirm such decline. Rather, blood flow in the collateral-dependent anterior wall of 26 patients with

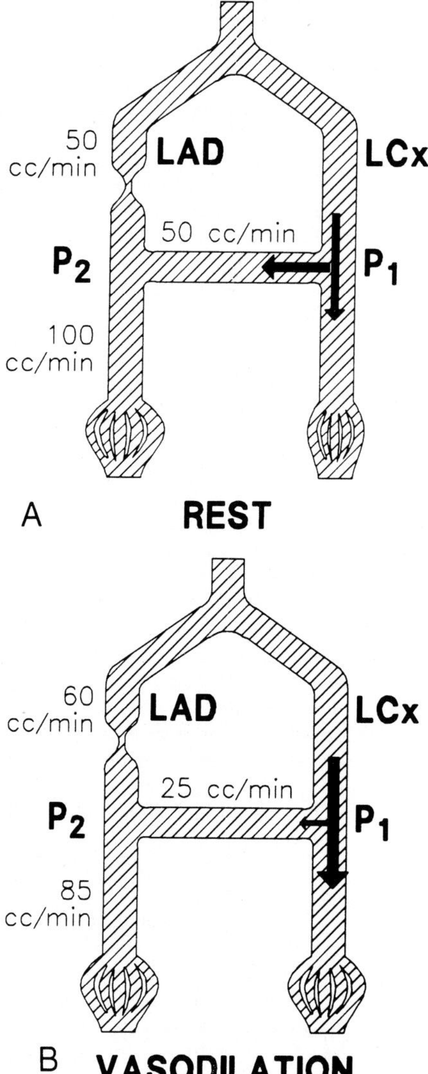

FIGURE 70–13. A hydraulic model illustrating possible mechanism of coronary steal. For this example, the left circumflex (LCX) is the supply artery, with the vascular distribution of the left anterior descending (LAD) artery being supplied by collaterals from the LCx coronary artery. P_1 is the perfusion pressure at the origin of the collaterals from distal circumflex branches. P_2 is the perfusion pressure of the vascular distribution of the LAD, which is severely stenotic. In *A*, the recipient bed vasodilates to maintain normal resting perfusion, thus expending its flow reserve. In *B*, with pharmacologic vasodilation, collateral driving pressure falls as LCx flow increases. (From Demer, L. L., Gould, K. L., and Kirkeeide, R.: Assessing stenosis severity: Coronary flow reserve, collateral function, quantitative coronary arteriography, positron imaging, and digital subtraction angiography: A review and analysis. Prog. Cardiovasc. Dis. 30:312, 1988, with permission.)

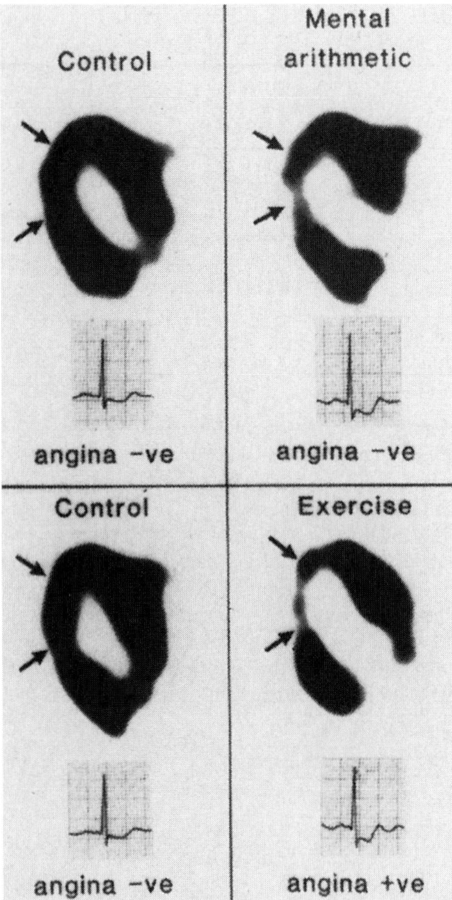

FIGURE 70–14. Changes in regional myocardial uptake of ^{82}Rb with silent ST-segment depression induced by mental stress: anterior and free wall ischemia. (From Deanfield, J. E., Kensett, M., Wilson, R. A., et al.: Silent myocardial ischemia due to mental stress. Lancet 2:1003, 1984, with permission.)

complete occlusions of the proximal left anterior descending coronary artery increased after administration of dipyridamole.[79, 80] The authors described considerable interindividual variations in the flow response but noted that in collateral-dependent myocardium with normally preserved systolic wall motion, blood flow increased by an average of 205 percent (from 0.78 ± 0.05 to 2.38 ± 0.54 mL · min^{-1} · g^{-1}), compared with a mean increase of only 27 percent (from 0.88 ± 0.17 to 1.12 ± 0.44 mL · min^{-1} · g^{-1}) in collateral-dependent myocardium with impaired systolic wall motion. Similarly, McFalls and co-workers[80] observed an increase rather than a decrease in blood flow after administration of dipyridamole in collateral-dependent myocardium of only 5 patients, using the ^{15}O-water technique with dynamic PET imaging. Dipyridamole induced a 90 percent increase in blood flow (range 0 to 201 percent) in collateral-dependent myocardium, compared with an average increase of 210 percent in remote myocardium in the same patients.

The reasons for these disparate observations remain unclear. To some extent, they may result from the differences in measurement technique, with the semiquantitative approach underestimating true regional myocardial blood flow. However, it must be remembered that PET measures only transmural blood flows. Although a subendocardial steal may indeed have occurred in some of the patients studied by Vanoverschelde and McFalls and co-workers,[79, 80] such decline may have been offset by an increase in flow in the more epicardial layers of the myocardium so that the sum of the subendocardial and subepicardial changes amounted to a net increase in blood flow.

Detection of Transient and Silent Ischemia

Transient changes in perfusion occurring during spontaneous coronary spasm, smoking, or mental stress cannot be detected by conventional perfusion imaging owing to the long physical half-life of ^{201}Tl. Selwyn and colleagues[81–83] have demonstrated the usefulness of PET blood flow imaging with ^{82}Rb for recognizing the causes of short-term variations in myocardial blood flow.

Mental Stress

Deanfield and colleagues first documented PET flow defects occurring during episodes of silent ST-segment depression induced by mental stress.[84] Abnormal regional ^{82}Rb uptake and ST-segment depression developed in patients undergoing a mental arithmetic test consisting of serial subtraction of sevens from 100 (Fig. 70–14). In 12 of 16 patients with chronic stable angina and exercise-induced PET defects, PET defects occurred with mental stress in the same regions as the exercise-related defects. Only half of these patients had ST-segment changes on ECG, and two thirds had no associated chest discomfort.

Smoking

Relative perfusion defects and absolute reduction in tracer uptake have been documented during smoking (Fig. 70–15) in patients with coronary artery disease.[85] Abnormal regional uptake of ^{82}Rb was found in 6 of 13 chronic smokers with typical stable angina (Fig. 70–16). Patients with smoking-induced flow defects also had exercise-induced defects. The degree of heterogeneity of blood flow images, which indicates the presence of relative flow defects, doubled with smoking and tripled with exercise. Regional uptake decreased approximately 30 percent with smoking, without concomitant angina. The mechanism of smoking's effect on myocardial blood flow is not known. However, because absolute reduction in perfusion tracer uptake occurred at lower levels of oxygen consumption than those required for exercise-induced defects, the supply side is implicated, suggesting effects of smoking on neurohumoral, prostaglandin, platelet, or vasomotor function, or all of these.

Measurements of myocardial blood flow in a group of young smokers without clinical evidence of coronary artery disease suggest an effect of smoking at the level of the vasomotor function.[86] Acute cigarette smoking increased diastolic blood pressure and heart rate; the rate-pressure product increased by about 22 percent and was associated with a proportional increase in the resting myocardial blood flow of about 25 percent. During maximum vasodilation,

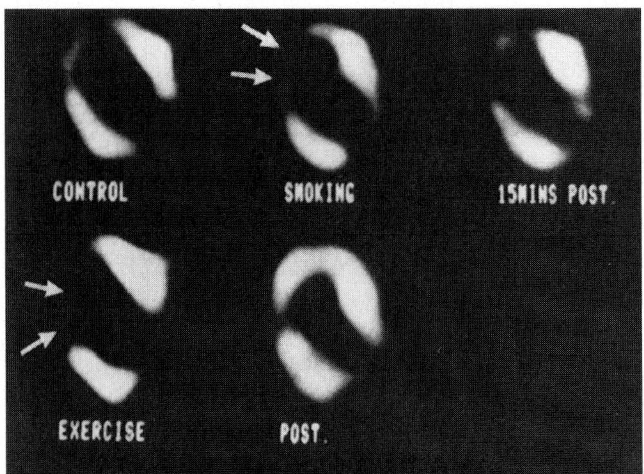

FIGURE 70–15. Tomograms from a patient showing changes in regional uptake of ^{82}Rb with smoking and exercise. (From Deanfield, J. E., Shea, M. J., Wilson, R. A., et al.: Direct effects of smoking on the heart: Silent ischemic disturbances of coronary flow. Am. J. Cardiol. 57:1007, 1986, with permission.)

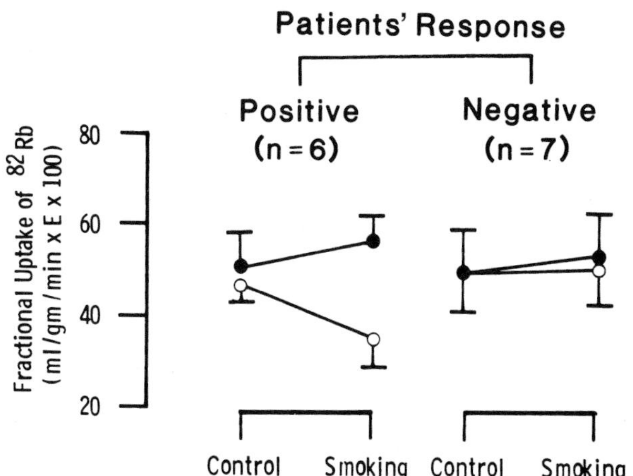

FIGURE 70–16. The effects of smoking on regional myocardial uptake of ^{82}Rb in 13 patients. Six patients showed a positive response with abnormal inhomogeneity and an absolute reduction in ^{82}Rb uptake in an affected segment, which was always the same segment that developed abnormal uptake after exercise. (From Deanfield, J. E., Shea, M. J., Wilson, R. A., et al.: Direct effects of smoking on the heart: Silent ischemic disturbances of coronary flow. Am. J. Cardiol. 57:1007, 1986, with permission.)

acute smoking reduced myocardial blood flow from 2.23 ± 0.35 to 1.98 ± 0.32 mL · min^{-1} · g^{-1} and increased myocardial flow resistance by 13 percent. This increase in resistance may have been related to an α-adrenergically–mediated vasoconstrictor effect of nicotine. As an additional observation of this study, resting and hyperemic blood flow in this group of young smokers with only a 6 ± 3 pack-year history of smoking did not differ from those of an age-matched group of nonsmokers, implying that chronic smoking in these young volunteers had not altered significantly the resting or hyperemic myocardial blood flows.

Daily Activities

PET also has been used to evaluate the importance of ST-segment changes seen on ambulatory ECG monitoring. Deanfield and associates documented temporary impairment of segmental myocardial perfusion coinciding with ST-segment depression on ECG in 30 patients with coronary artery disease.[87, 88] Transient, segmental reductions of uptake were present in 97 percent of 63 episodes of ST-segment depression with angina and in all 30 episodes of asymptomatic ST-segment depression at rest and with mental or exercise stress. Perfusion normalized simultaneously with resolution of ECG changes (Fig. 70–17). The duration of such defects associated with transient ischemic ECG changes is shortened by nitrates.

These findings imply that ischemic episodes are more common than previously suspected and that daily activities, such as mental stress and smoking, may be more common triggers of silent ischemia than is physical exertion.

Potential for Screening of Asymptomatic Patients

It is now recognized that angina pectoris is an insensitive marker for transient myocardial ischemia. If dipyridamole-PET imaging is found to have sufficient accuracy, it may ultimately permit screening of high-risk asymptomatic individuals. Asymptomatic coronary artery disease is now appreciated as a significant problem. In the Framingham study population, more than 25 percent of all infarctions were discovered only by routine ECG testing, and the prognosis for these "unrecognized" infarctions was found to be as serious as that for "recognized" infarctions.[89] In a Finnish study population, 67 percent of coronary heart disease deaths in men aged 40 to 59 years occurred in patients who were without a history of symptoms.[90] Asymptomatic coronary artery disease is found in up to 13 percent of patients undergoing preoperative cardiac catheterization for valvular heart disease.

If it is sufficiently severe, asymptomatic coronary artery disease also may be detected by ^{201}Tl SPECT imaging. The two features of PET that render it potentially more suitable for screening are its potential for higher specificity and sensitivity of detection and its potential for early detection of coronary stenoses, as mild as a 47 percent reduction in diameter.[44]

It is essential to recognize that the specificity for a test depends on the study population, that is, the pretest probability of disease. More false-positive results are expected in an asymptomatic population. Even a small likelihood of false-positive tests may result in large numbers of unnecessary invasive procedures when a large population is studied. For this reason, PET accuracy must be established in asymptomatic patients as well as symptomatic patients, and patient selection for clinical applications must be performed with this statistical problem in mind. At present, it is difficult to measure the accuracy of PET perfusion imaging in a large group of asymptomatic individuals without known coronary artery disease or myocardial infarction, because the standard for comparison, coronary arteriography, is rarely warranted in such patients.

Responses to Therapy

Interventional Revascularization

Using a semiquantitative analysis approach, Goldstein and co-workers[63] were first to demonstrate a postangioplasty improvement in regional myocardial flow reserve. This approach largely relied on regional tracer activity concentrations and their postangioplasty changes relative to activity concentrations in normal myocardium. The investigators demonstrated a linear correlation between the change in angiographic stenosis severity and the improvement in relative regional myocardial blood flow. Subsequent studies measured regional myocardial blood flow in absolute units. For example, Walsh and co-workers[91] demonstrated a normalization of the vasodilator response to intravenous dipyridamole 7.5 months after coronary angioplasty, compared with a markedly blunted prean-

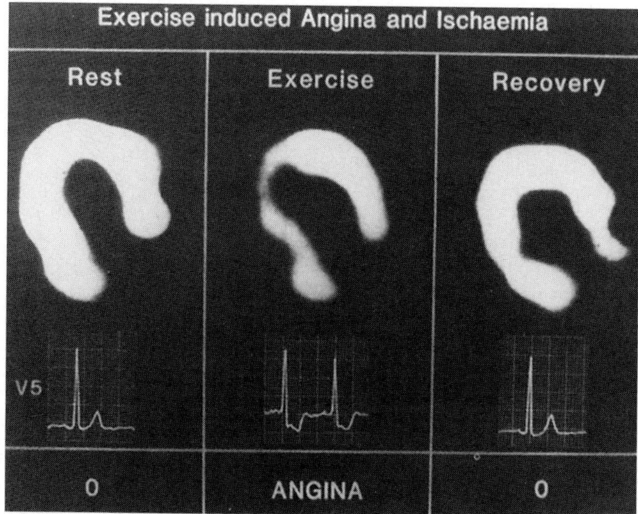

FIGURE 70–17. Tomograms through the midportion of the left ventricle, recorded in a patient with chronic stable angina and three-vessel coronary artery disease. Under control conditions, the regional myocardial perfusion to the anterior wall of the left ventricle is normal. During exercise, there is a marked decrease in the regional uptake of ^{82}Rb, suggesting a decrease in myocardial perfusion. Simultaneous recordings of a 12-lead electrocardiogram demonstrate isoelectric ST segments during control conditions and ST-segment depression during exercise. (From Nabel, E. G., Rocco, M. B., and Selwyn, A. P.: Characteristics and significance of ischemia detected by ambulatory electrocardiographic monitoring. Circulation 75:V–74, 1987, by permission of the American Heart Association, Inc.)

gioplasty response. More recent investigations in a relatively small patient population by Uren and co-workers[11] confirmed this earlier observation. Importantly, however, these investigators explored the vasodilator capacity in 9 patients at 7 days and again at 3 months after angioplasty. Initially, hyperemic blood flows in the territory of the culprit vessel failed to increase (2.28 ± 0.73, compared with 2.11 ± 0.80 mL · min^{-1} · g^{-1} before angioplasty). At 3 months, however, hyperemic flows had increased to 2.77 ± 0.74 mL · min^{-1} · g^{-1} and differed no longer from those in control myocardium (Fig. 70–18). Taken together, the studies indicate a normalization of myocardial flow reserve after successful angioplasty. Yet, the vasodilator capacity recovers slowly, possibly because of an altered resistive function downstream of a hemodynamically significant coronary stenosis.

Changes in Diet and Lifestyle

Several investigators have demonstrated beneficial effects of changes in lifestyle, regular exercise, and cholesterol-lowering diet on the progression of coronary artery disease. In fact, Gould,[92] in a passionate plea, advocated strict dietary and lifestyle changes as an important alternative to conventional mechanical revascularization with either coronary angiography or coronary arterial bypass grafting; according to Gould, the response to these changes should be monitored noninvasively by imaging the relative distribution of myocardial blood flow with PET. The same author presented data to support the cost-effectiveness of this approach. An earlier study by the same author and his collaborators supported to the validity of this approach and showed that associated improvements in regional blood flow could be demonstrated by PET imaging (Fig. 70–19). More recently, Czernin and co-workers[15] provided quantitative data for the beneficial effects of short-term cardiovascular conditioning on resting myocardial blood flow and myocardial flow reserve. Most notably, resting myocardial blood flow declined after a 6-week course of daily exercise and dietary changes associated with a decline in total and low-density lipoprotein cholesterol and in triglycerides. Resting blood flow declined in proportion to the decrease in the resting rate-pressure product and, thus, in cardiac work. This alone resulted in an improvement in the myocardial flow reserve. Also, hyperemic blood flow in response to standard-dose intravenous dipyridamole increased modestly, reflecting an augmented vasodilator capacity. These changes were most prominent in patients with coronary artery disease or hypertension. Because these changes occurred within 6 to 7 weeks after the cardiovascular conditioning program began, they most likely represented beneficial effects at the level of the coronary resistance vessels. Such short-term changes may indeed play a protective role in coronary artery disease, increasing the pressure gradients across a coronary stenosis and thereby augmenting distal, nutrient myocardial blood flow.

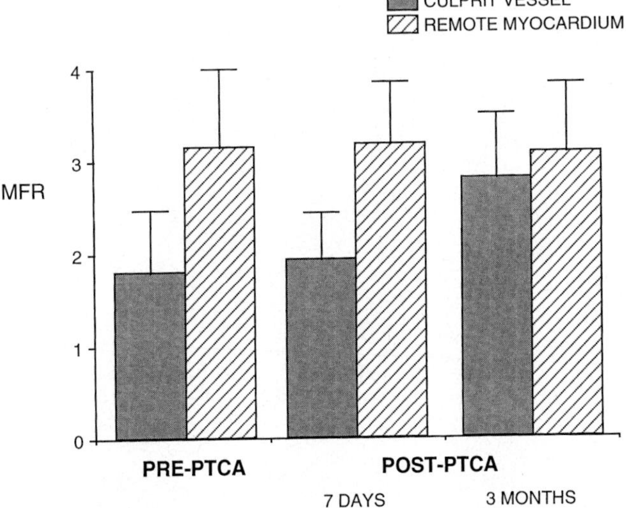

FIGURE 70–18. Recovery of myocardial flow reserve (MFR) after angioplasty. MFR was determined by measurements of myocardial blood flow at rest and during dipyridamole-induced hyperemia with the ^{15}O-water–positron emission tomography approach in seven patients submitted to coronary angioplasty (PTCA). As seen in the figure, the MFR in the culprit vessel was markedly attenuated before angioplasty. This attenuation existed when the patients were re-evaluated 7 days after successful angioplasty, but it was no longer noted when MFR was evaluated 3 months after angioplasty. (From Uren, N., Marraccini, P., Gistri, R., et al.: Altered coronary vasodilator reserve and metabolism in myocardium subtended by normal arteries in patients with coronary artery disease. J. Am. Coll. Cardiol. 22:650, 1993, with permission.)

FIGURE 70–19. See Color Plate 32.

SYNDROME X

Patients afflicted by this syndrome typically exhibit exertional chest pain or ischemic ST-segment changes on treadmill exercise testing yet have normal coronary arteries on angiography. Abnormalities of the coronary microcirculation or of coronary vasomotion are possible mechanisms, but no single underlying mechanism has been identified, and because of its unknown origin, this syndrome has been designated by an "X." It is also possible that this syndrome X does not result from one specific abnormality but rather represents a variety of abnormal states.

Because of its unknown cause, the syndrome has been targeted for exploration by several PET investigations, with measurements of blood flow at rest and during pharmacologic vasodilation. For example, Geltman and colleagues[94] measured resting and hyperemic blood flows with the ^{15}O-water technique in 17 syndrome X patients. Compared with a group of 16 normal volunteers, there were no significant differences in resting and hyperemic blood flows or in myocardial flow reserve. However, the individual flow responses to dipyridamole varied greatly in the syndrome X group. Eight of 9 patients had a flow reserve of less than 2.5 as the lower limit of the normal control group. These 8 patients revealed a significantly higher resting blood flow and lower hyperemic blood flows than the remaining 9 patients with a normal flow reserve or the normal control group. A later investigation from the same laboratory in 9 syndrome X patients revealed normal resting and hyperemic blood flows and a normal flow reserve.[95] The same group of patients had been studied with intracoronary Doppler flow velocity probes; both intracoronary papaverine and adenosine raised flow velocities 3.5 times, which was similar to the flow reserve of 3.5 ± 1.0 measured by PET. Like these investigators, Camici and co-workers,[96] using the ^{13}N-ammonia PET approach in 45 patients, and Rosen and colleagues,[97] using the ^{15}O-water approach in 29 patients, observed normal myocardial blood flow at rest and during pharmacologic vasodilation (see Table 70–2). The patients in Camici's study also underwent atrial pacing. The flow increases during pacing correlated significantly with the flow reserve during dipyridamole. Further, about one third of the patients had "blunted" flow reserve, without, however, a statistically significant increase in the occurrence of ST-segment depression during treadmill exercise relative to the normal flow responders. Finally, Galassi and co-investigators[98] observed in 13 syndrome X patients a somewhat more heterogeneous distribution of blood flow at rest and during dipyridamole-induced hyperemia than in a normal control group.

The flow measurements at rest and during pharmacologically induced hyperemia, as performed with PET, thus far have failed to uncover a uniform mechanism or even observation in patients with syndrome X. One reason may be that this particular patient population is very heterogeneous. Secondly, the pharmacologic stress targets primarily vascular smooth muscle function, and if the primary lesion resides at a different site of the coronary vessel or in myocytes, then other, more selective interventions would be needed to uncover the underlying mechanism.

MYOCARDIAL BLOOD FLOW IN CARDIAC TRANSPLANT RECIPIENTS

Intracoronary Doppler flow velocity probes permit the measurement of coronary flow velocity at baseline and after intracoronary administration of papaverine, adenosine, or acetylcholine. Such measurements have offered estimates of the coronary flow reserve and vasodilator capacity in cardiac transplants. These invasive studies in transplantation patients demonstrated a preserved coronary vasodilator capacity, provided rejection, left ventricular hypertrophy, and regional wall motion abnormalities were absent.[99, 100] Even mild to moderate diffuse atherosclerosis, as evidenced on coronary angiography, did not appear to diminish the maximal coronary vasodilator capacity.[99] Furthermore, the peak vasodilator capacity was found to remain normal for as long as 3 to 4 years after cardiac transplantation, after which a modest but statistically significant decline was observed.[101] Acute transplant rejection lowered the coronary flow velocity reserve (again, defined as the ratio of hyperemic to baseline coronary flow velocities); the reserve, however, appeared to normalize after successful immunosuppressive treatment of the acute rejection episode.[102]

Although these invasive studies offered initial insights into the coronary circulatory function of cardiac transplants, they suffered from several shortcomings. First, the measurements yielded only flow velocity ratios; from such ratios it is not possible to define whether abnormalities are caused by increased flow velocities at rest, diminished flow velocities during pharmacologic vasodilation, or both. Second, the information obtained with this approach is only regional because measurements are typically obtained in only one coronary artery and thus offer information on only one vascular territory. Third, these measurements yield only flow velocities but not true coronary blood flows or estimates of true myocardial blood flow. In contrast, measurements of myocardial blood flow with either ^{15}O-water or ^{13}N-ammonia and dynamic PET offer information on myocardial blood flow at rest or during hyperemia in absolute terms, examine blood flow in the entire myocardium rather than within only one vascular territory, and, importantly, are noninvasive.

In order to elucidate possible mechanisms accounting for the reduced maximal exercise capacity of cardiac transplant recipients, Krivokapich and co-workers[103] studied 12 transplant recipients without angiographic evidence of accelerated atherosclerosis and without rejection. Myocardial blood flow was measured with ^{13}N-ammonia and PET at rest and again during supine bicycle exercise. When compared with a group of 10 normal volunteers, blood flow at rest in the transplant recipients tended to be higher (1.05 ± 0.39 versus 0.83 ± 0.46 mL · min^{-1} · g^{-1}), but this difference was statistically insignificant. Despite markedly higher plasma levels of lactate during exercise in transplant recipients, both study groups achieved similar rate-pressure products and similar levels of myocardial blood flow during supine bicycle exercise (1.56 ± 0.171 mL · min^{-1} · g^{-1} in transplants versus 1.70 ± 0.60 mL · min^{-1} · g^{-1} in normal hearts). Further, myocardial blood flow during exercise increased in proportion to cardiac work; in fact, blood flows at exercise in the transplantation group were found to be appropriate for the level of cardiac work, as evidenced by a comparison with the normal control group. Senneff and collaborators[104] subsequently explored the vasodilator capacity in 35 nonrejecting transplant recipients 7 to 84 months (mean 31 months) after transplantation. Myocardial blood flow at rest was significantly higher than that in a group of normal volunteers (1.63 ± 0.51 versus 1.17 ± 0.33; $P < .001$). This increase was independent of prior rejection episodes but corresponded to the elevated rate-pressure product, most likely as a consequence of nephrotoxic effects of the immunosuppressive regimen. Both groups, normal subjects and transplant recipients, achieved comparable peak flows during administration of standard-dose dipyridamole (3.49 ± 1.70 mL · min^{-1} · g^{-1} in transplant patients versus 3.60 ± 1.5 mL · min^{-1} · g^{-1} in normal subjects), implying that the vasodilator capacity was indeed preserved although the myocardial flow reserve was markedly diminished (2.3 ± 1.1 mL · min^{-1} · g^{-1}, versus 3.3 ± 1.5 mL · min^{-1} · g^{-1} in normal subjects) because of the elevated resting blood flows. In a somewhat smaller group of only 14 transplant recipients, Rechavia and co-investigators[105] reached similar conclusions. Myocardial blood flow at rest and during dipyridamole-induced hyperemia was distributed homogeneously throughout the left ventricular myocardium. Resting myocardial blood flow, measured as in the Senneff study[104] with ^{15}O-water, was elevated at rest but in proportion to the increased rate-pressure product, whereas dipyridamole-induced hyperemic blood flows were similar to those in normal volunteers.

As shown by Chan and co-workers[106] in 16 transplant recipients, mild to moderate transplant rejection altered the normal relation between cardiac work, as estimated from the rate-pressure product, and myocardial blood flow at rest. In the 10 rejecting transplant recipients, myocardial blood flow averaged 1.7 ± 0.2 mL · min^{-1} · g^{-1} as compared to 0.9 ± 0.2 mL · min^{-1} · g^{-1} in 6 nonrejecting transplant patients (see Table 70–2). Myocardial blood flow, in relation to the rate-pressure product at rest, demonstrated a disproportionate, "inflammatory-like" increase (1.63 ± 0.20 versus 0.99 ± 0.40 MBF/RPP $\times$ 10^4; $P < .05$); conversely, intravenous dipyridamole (0.56 mg · kg^{-1}) induced markedly lower hyperemic flows in rejecting than in nonrejecting transplant recipients (2.45 ± 0.91 versus 3.88 ± 0.64 mL · min^{-1} · g^{-1}; $P < .01$). Successful immunosuppressive treatment restored the vasodilator reserve to dipyridamole (3.86 ± 1.08 mL · min^{-1} · g^{-1} versus 3.88 ± 0.64 mL · min^{-1} · g^{-1} in nonrejecting transplant recipients) and lowered both resting cardiac work and resting myocardial blood flow. However, both remained modestly higher than in nonrejecting counterparts so that myocardial flow reserve did not return to normal values (3.41 ± 0.95, versus 4.46 ± 0.74 in nonrejecting transplants $P < .05$). The somewhat higher resting myocardial blood flows corresponded, on average, to the higher rate-pressure products. The latter most likely reflected the consequences of the known nephrotoxicity of immunosuppressive treatment, which were more prominent in the rejecting transplant group because they were studied at an average of 22 ± 11 weeks after transplantation, compared with only 8 ± 5 weeks for the nonrejecting transplant patients.

In 43 heart transplant recipients studied from 3 months to more than 4 years after allografting, resting myocardial blood flow, as assessed with ^{13}N-ammonia and PET, was found to decline as a function of time.[107] Repeat measurements at 1-year intervals in 35 patients revealed a significant 9 ± 5 percent decline in resting myocardial blood flow (from 0.65 ± 0.18 to 0.54 ± 0.16 mL · min^{-1} · g^{-1}; $P < .001$). Although resting blood flow remained homogeneous and coronary angiography failed to reveal flow-limiting coronary stenosis, the decline in the resting blood flow data were significantly more pronounced in the 10 patients with irregular coronary artery surfaces and diffuse concentric narrowing on angiography (thought to reflect transplant vasculopathy), compared with the same measurements in those with smooth surfaces and vessels of normal diameter (14.4 ± 4 versus 5 ± 1 percent decrease in resting blood flow; $P < .02$).

More recent studies have demonstrated alterations in the vasodilator capacity and coronary vasomotion in transplant recipients with angiographically normal coronary arteries but evidence of intimal thickening as measured with intravascular ultrasound.[72] In these studies, published in only preliminary form, hyperemic blood flows (induced by dipyridamole) and myocardial flow reserve correlated inversely with the maximal intimal thickening in the left anterior descending coronary artery. Furthermore, the myocardial flow reserve correlated directly with the myocardial flow response to cold pressor testing as a means for exploring coronary vasomotion (as already described). This highly significant correlation may imply that the mechanism accounting for the diminished vasodilator capacity and abnormal coronary vasomotion in transplant vasculopathy resides at the same location. Further, because most of the 32 patients had normal coronary arteriograms, myocardial blood flow was homogeneous at rest and during dipyridamole stress testing. The transplant vasculopathy would have remained undetected except for the noninvasive measurement of intimal thickening or, conversely, through noninvasive means by measurements of myocardial blood flow at rest and during physiologic and pharmacologic interventions. What remains uncertain at present is to what extent the morphologic alterations as observed with intravascular ultrasound resemble changes in the more common setting of coronary artery disease. If transplant vasculopathy represents a model of coronary artery disease, then these observations may point toward the possibility of detecting early and angiographically silent coronary artery disease.

MYOCARDIAL BLOOD FLOW IN CARDIOMYOPATHIES

Idiopathic Dilated Cardiomyopathy

Findings in relation to myocardial blood flow and vasodilator reserve in idiopathic dilated cardiomyopathy have remained controversial. Fung and co-workers[108] reported normal values for myocardial blood flow at rest and during pharmacologic vasodilation and, thus, a normally preserved vasodilatory capacity in 7 patients with idiopathic cardiomyopathy and an average left ventricular ejection fraction of 30 ± 9 percent. In contrast, Merlet and colleagues[109] determined myocardial blood flow with the ^{15}O-water technique in 6 patients with idiopathic dilated cardiomyopathy and an average left ventricular ejection fraction of only 22 ± 7 percent. Myocardial blood flow averaged 0.73 ± 0.41 $mL \cdot min^{-1} \cdot g^{-1}$ at rest and increased to $1.68 \pm 1.08 mL \cdot min^{-1} \cdot g^{-1}$ after intravenous dipyridamole. The resulting myocardial flow reserve averaged 2.3 ± 0.5, which was similar to the coronary flow velocity reserve of 2.37 ± 0.53 determined with intracoronary Doppler flow velocity probes positioned in the left anterior descending coronary artery. Hyperemic blood flow, myocardial flow reserve, and coronary flow velocity reserve were all significantly lower than in a group of 6 age-matched normal volunteers (hyperemic blood flows averaged 3.50 ± 0.82, myocardial flow reserve 3.99 ± 0.67, and flow velocity reserve 4.13 ± 77 $mL \cdot min^{-1} \cdot g^{-1}$).

Hypertrophic Cardiomyopathy

In 23 patients with hypertrophic cardiomyopathies, Camici and collaborators[110] measured myocardial blood flow at rest and during dipyridamole-induced hyperemia. At rest, myocardial blood flow was modestly higher in the hypertrophied interventricular septum than in the lateral wall (1.14 ± 0.43 versus 0.90 ± 0.35 $mL \cdot min^{-1} \cdot g^{-1}$; $P < .05$), although no such difference existed in 12 control subjects (see Table 70–2). Furthermore, the blood flows at rest in the hypertrophy patients were within the normal range. Intravenous dipyridamole evoked a markedly attenuated response in the hypertrophic cardiomyopathy patients. On average, myocardial blood flow rose by 188 percent in normal volunteers but by only 43 percent in the hypertrophied septum of the patients. The impairment of the vasodilator response extended also to the free wall, where blood flow increased by only 63 percent. Furthermore, the dipyridamole-induced decline in coronary resistance was markedly less in hypertrophic cardiomyopathy patients who had chest pain than in those without chest pain.

Although pharmacologic vasodilation appears to appropriately reflect changes in vasodilator capacity, blood flow responses to physiologic interventions (e.g., physical exercise) may be influenced by additional factors. For example, as shown by Müller and coinvestigators,[2] superimposition of physical exercise and pharmacologic vasodilation diminished hyperemic blood flows. Cigarette smoking similarly lowered hypertrophic blood flows.[86] Thus, α-adrenergically mediated vasoconstriction and extravascular resistive forces may increase the total coronary resistance. Both factors may explain the observations by Nienaber and colleague[111] in hypertrophic cardiomyopathy. In a very small group of patients, supine bicycle exercise failed to increase myocardial blood flow, possibly because of an excessive increase in the extravascular resistive forces. This suggests that pharmacologic assessments and characterization of the coronary vasodilator capacity and of coronary vasomotion may offer only limited insights into coronary circulatory responses during physiologic activities.

SUMMARY

Technical aspects of PET imaging continue to improve. PET perfusion imaging is now entering the stage of routine clinical application. Quantitative assessment of tracer uptake is readily available, and the ability to measure absolute regional myocardial perfusion is imminent. Enormous clinical benefit may be derived from appropriate applications of PET for noninvasive, quantitative characterization of blood supply to the heart.

Acknowledgments

The authors thank Diane Martin and Melissa Sheldon for preparing the illustrations and are grateful to Eileen Rosenfeld for her skillful assistance in preparing this manuscript.

References

1. Tamaki, N., Yonekura, Y., Senda, M., et al.: Myocardial positron computed tomography with ^{13}N-ammonia at rest and during exercise. Eur. J. Nucl. Med. 11:246, 1985.
2. Müller, P., Czernin, J., Choi, Y., et al.: Effect of exercise supplementation during adenosine infusion on hyperemic blood flow and flow reserve. Am. Heart J. 128:52, 1994.
3. Krivokapich, J., Smith, G., Huang, S., et al.: Nitrogen-13 ammonia myocardial imaging at rest and with exercise in normal volunteers: Quantification of absolute myocardial perfusion with dynamic positron emission tomography. Circulation 80:1328, 1989.
4. Böttcher, M., Czernin, J., Sun, K., et al.: Effect of caffeine on myocardial blood flow at rest and during pharmacologic vasodilation. J. Nucl. Med. 36:2016, 1995.
5. Bergmann, S., Herrero, P., Markham, J., et al.: Noninvasive quantitation of myocardial blood flow in human subjects with oxygen-15–labeled water and positron emission tomography. J. Am. Coll. Cardiol. 14:639, 1989.
6. Araujo, L., Lammertsma, A., Rhoses, C., et al.: Noninvasive quantification of regional myocardial blood flow in coronary artery disease with oxygen-15–labeled carbon dioxide inhalation and positron emission tomography. Circulation 83:875, 1991.
7. Hutchins, G., Schwaiger, M., Rosenspire, K., et al.: Noninvasive quantification of regional blood flow in the human heart using ^{13}N-ammonia and dynamic positron emission tomographic imaging. J. Am. Coll. Cardiol. 15:1032, 1990.
8. Chan, S., Brunken, R., Czernin, J., et al.: Comparison of maximal myocardial blood flow during adenosine infusion with that of intravenous dipyridamole in normal men. J. Am. Coll. Cardiol. 20:979, 1992.
9. Czernin, J., Müller, P., Chan, S., et al.: Influence of age and hemodynamics on myocardial blood flow and flow reserve. Circulation 88:62, 1993.
10. Uren, N., Melin, J., De Bruyne, B., et al.: Relation between myocardial blood flow and the severity of coronary-artery stenosis. N. Engl. J. Med. 330:1782, 1994.
11. Uren, N., Marraccini, P., Gistri, R., et al.: Altered coronary vasodilator reserve and metabolism in myocardium subtended by normal arteries in patients with coronary artery disease. J. Am. Coll. Cardiol. 22:650, 1993.
12. Holmberg, S., Serzysko, W., and Varnauskas, E.: Coronary circulation during heavy exercise in control subjects and patients with coronary heart disease. Acta Med. Scand. 190:465, 1971.
13. Krivokapich, J., Huang, S.-C., and Schelbert, H.: Assessment of the effects of dobutamine on myocardial blood flow and oxidative metabolism in normal human subjects using nitrogen-13 ammonia and carbon-11 acetate. Am. J. Cardiol. 71:1351, 1993.
14. Czernin, J., Auerbach, M., Sun, K., et al.: Effects of modified pharmacologic stress approaches on hyperemic myocardial blood flow. J. Nucl. Med. 36:575, 1995.
15. Czernin, J., Barnard, J., Sun, K., et al.: Effect of short-term cardiovascular

conditioning and low-fat diet on myocardial blood flow and flow reserve. Circulation 92:197, 1995.
16. Senneff, M., Geltman, E., Bergmann, S., et al.: Noninvasive delineation of the effects of moderate aging on myocardial perfusion. J. Nucl. Med. 32:2037, 1991.
17. Brown, B., Josephson, M., Peterson, R., et al.: Intravenous dipyridamole combined with isometric handgrip for near maximal acute increase in coronary flow in patients with coronary artery disease. Am. J. Cardiol. 48:1077, 1981.
18. Ranhosky, A., and Kempthorne, R. J.: The safety of intravenous dipyridamole thallium myocardial perfusion imaging. Intravenous Dipyridamole Thallium-Imaging Study Group. Circulation 81:1205, 1990.
19. Lette, J., Tatum, J., Fraser, S., et al.: Safety of dipyridamole testing in 73,806 patients: The Multicenter Dipyridamole Safety Study. J. Nucl. Cardiol. 2:3, 1995.
20. Cerqueira, M., Verani, M., Schwaiger, M., et al.: Safety profile of adenosine stress perfusion imaging: Results from the Adenoscan Multicenter Trial Registry. J. Am. Coll. Cardiol. 23:384, 1994.
21. Hays, J., Mahmarian, J., Cochran, A., et al.: Dobutamine thallium-201 tomography for evaluating patients with suspected coronary artery disease unable to undergo exercise or vasodilator pharmacologic stress testing. J. Am. Coll. Cardiol. 21:1583, 1993.
22. Nabel, E., Ganz, P., Gordon, J., et al.: Dilation of normal and constriction of atherosclerotic coronary arteries caused by the cold pressor test. Circulation 77:43, 1988.
23. Zeiher, A., Drexler, H., Wollschlaäger, H., et al.: Endothelial dysfunction of the coronary microvasculature is associated with impaired coronary blood flow regulation in patients with early atherosclerosis. Circulation 84:1984, 1991.
24. Sun, K., De Groof, M., Yi, J., et al.: Quantification of the extent and severity of perfusion defects in canine myocardium by PET polar mapping. J. Nucl. Med. 35:2031, 1994.
25. Laubenbacher, C., Rothley, J., Sitomer, J., et al.: An automated analysis program for the evaluation of cardiac PET studies: Initial results in the detection and localization of coronary artery disease using nitrogen-13–ammonia. J. Nucl. Med. 34:968, 1993.
26. Gould, K.: Coronary Artery Stenosis. New York, Elseiver, 1990.
27. Hicks, R., Molina, E., Wolfe, E., Jr., et al.: Quantitative analysis of ^{82}Rb-PET images for the detection of coronary artery disease. J. Am. Coll. Cardiol. 15:171, 1990.
28. Porenta, G., Kuhle, W., Czernin, J., et al.: Semiquantitative assessment of myocardial viability and perfusion utilizing polar map displays of cardiac PET images. J. Nucl. Med. 33:1623, 1992.
29. Khanna, S., DeGroof, M., Maddahi, J., et al.: Quantitative analysis of adenosine stress ^{13}N-ammonia myocardial perfusion PET images: Definition of normal limits and criteria for detection and localization of coronary artery disease. J. Nucl. Med. 33:825, 1992.
30. Hicks, K., Ganti, G., Mullain, N., et al.: Automated quantitation of three-dimensional cardiac positron emission tomography for routine clinical use. J. Nucl. Med. 30:1787, 1989.
31. Kuhle, W., Porenta, G., Huang, S.-C., et al.: Quantification of regional myocardial blood flow using ^{13}N-ammonia and reoriented dynamic positron emission tomographic imaging. Circulation 86:1004, 1992.
32. Muzik, O., Beanlands, R., Hutchins, G., et al.: Validation of nitrogen-13–ammonia tracer kinetic model for quantification of myocardial blood flow using PET. J. Nucl. Med. 34:83, 1993.
33. Choi, Y., Huang, S.-C., Hawkins, R., et al.: A simplified method for quantification of myocardial blood flow using ^{13}N-ammonia and dynamic PET. J. Nucl. Med. 34:488, 1993.
34. Marcus, M., Skorton, D., Johnson, M., et al.: Visual estimates of percent diameter coronary stenosis: "A battered gold standard." J. Am. Coll. Cardiol. 11:882, 1988.
35. White, C., Wright, C., Doty, D., et al.: Does visual interpretation of the coronary arteriogram predict the physiologic importance of a coronary stenosis. N. Engl. J. Med. 310:819, 1984.
36. Zir, L., Miller, S., Dinsmore, R., et al.: Interobserver variability in coronary angiography. Circulation 53:627, 1976.
37. Beatt, K., Luijten, H., DeFeyter, P., et al.: Change in diameter of coronary artery segments adjacent to stenosis after percutaneous transluminal coronary angioplasty: Failure of percent diameter stenosis measurement to reflect morphologic changes induced by balloon dilation. J. Am. Coll. Cardiol. 12:315, 1988.
38. Marcus, M., Armstrong, M., Heistad, D., et al.: Comparison of three methods of evaluating coronary obstructive lesions: Postmortem arteriography, pathologic examination and measurement of regional myocardial perfusion during maximal vasodilation. Am. J. Cardiol. 49:1699, 1982.
39. Brown, B., Bolson, E., Frimer, M., et al.: Quantitative coronary arteriography: Estimation of dimensions, hemodynamic resistance and atheroma mass of coronary artery lesions using the arteriogram and digital computation. Circulation 55:329, 1977.
40. Kirkeeide, R., Gould, K., and Parsel, L.: Assessment of coronary stenoses by myocardial perfusion imaging during pharmacologic coronary vasodilation: VII. Validation of coronary flow reserve as a single integrated functional measure of stenosis severity reflecting all its geometric dimensions. J. Am. Coll. Cardiol. 7:103, 1986.
41. Mates, R., Gupta, R., Bell, A., et al.: Fluid dynamics of coronary artery stenosis. Circ. Res. 42:152, 1978.
42. De Bruyne, B., Baudhuin, T., Melin, J., et al.: Coronary flow reserve calculated from pressure measurements in humans: Validation with positron emission tomography. Circulation 89:1013, 1994.
43. Gould, K.: Assessment of coronary stenoses with myocardial perfusion imaging during pharmacologic vasodilation: IV. Limits of detection of stenosis with idealized experimental cross-sectional myocardial imaging. J. Am. Coll. Cardiol. 42:761, 1978.
44. Gould, K., Schelbert, H., Phelps, M., et al.: Noninvasive assessment of coronary stenoses with myocardial perfusion imaging during pharmacologic coronary vasodilation: V. Detection of 47 percent diameter coronary stenosis with intravenous ^{13}N-ammonia and emission-computed tomography in intact dogs. Am. J. Cardiol. 43:200, 1979.
45. Schelbert, H., Wisenberg, G., Phelps, M., et al.: Non-invasive assessment of coronary stenoses by myocardial imaging during pharmacologic coronary vasodilation: VI. Detection of coronary artery disease in man with intravenous $^{13}NH_3$ and positron computed tomography. Am. J. Cardiol. 49:1197, 1982.
46. Gould, K., Goldstein, R., Mullani, N., et al.: Noninvasive assessment of coronary stenoses by myocardial perfusion imaging during pharmacologic coronary vasodilation: VIII. Clinical feasibility of positron cardiac imaging without cyclotron using generator-produced rubidium-82. J. Am. Coll. Cardiol. 7:775, 1986.
47. Demer, L., Gould, K., Goldstein, R., et al.: Diagnosis of coronary artery disease by positron emission tomography: Comparison to quantitative arteriography in 193 patients. Circulation 79:825, 1989.
48. Demer, L., Gould, K., Goldstein, R., et al.: Diagnosis of coronary artery disease by positron imaging: Large-scale clinical trial. J. Am. Coll. Cardiol. 11:11, 1988.
49. Yonekura, Y., Tamaki, N., Senda, M., et al.: Detection of coronary artery disease with ^{13}N-ammonia and high-resolution positron emission computed tomography. Am. Heart J. 113:645, 1987.
50. Stewart, R., Schwaiger, M., Molina, E., et al.: Comparison of rubidium-82 positron emission tomography and thallium-201 SPECT imaging for detection of coronary artery disease. Am. J. Cardiol. 67:1303, 1991.
51. Go, R., Marwick, T., MacIntyre, W., et al.: A prospective comparison of rubidium-82 PET and thallium-201 SPECT myocardial perfusion imaging utilizing a single dipyridamole stress in the diagnosis of coronary artery disease. J. Nucl. Med. 31:1899, 1990.
52. Williams, B., Millani, N., Jansen, D., et al.: A retrospective study of the diagnostic accuracy of a community hospital–based PET center for the detection of coronary artery disease using rubidium-82. J. Nucl. Med. 35:1586, 1994.
53. Simone, G., Mullani, N., Page, D., et al.: Utilization statistics and diagnostic accuracy of a nonhospital-based positron emission tomography center for the detection of coronary artery disease using rubidium-82. Am. J. Physiol. Imaging 7:203, 1992.
54. Walsh, M., Bergmann, S., Baird, T., et al.: Improved myocardial perfusion after angioplasty delineated by positron emission tomography and $H_2{}^{15}O$. Circulation 76:IV–401, 1987.
55. Diem, K. (ed.): Documenta Geigy: Scientific Tables. Summit, NJ, Geigy Pharmaceuticals, 1962.
56. DePasquale, E., Nody, A., DePuey, E., et al.: Quantitative rotational thallium-201 tomography for identifying and localizing coronary artery disease. Circulation 77:316, 1988.
57. Hamilton, G., Trobaugh, G., Ritchie, J., et al.: Myocardial imaging with intravenously injected thallium-201 in patients with suspected coronary artery disease: Analysis of technique and correlation with electrocardiographic coronary anatomic and ventriculographic findings. Am. J. Cardiol. 39:347, 1977.
58. Ritchie, J., Zaret, B., Strauss, H., et al.: Myocardial imaging with thallium-201: A multicenter study in patients with angina pectoris or acute myocardial infarction. Am. J. Cardiol. 42:345, 1978.
59. Van Train, K., Berman, D., Garcia, E., et al.: Quantitative analysis of stress thallium-201 myocardial scintigrams: A multicenter trial. J. Nucl. Med. 27:17, 1986.
60. Zijlstra, F., Fioretti, P., Reiber, J., et al.: Which cineangiographically assessed anatomic variable correlates best with functional measurements of stenosis severity? A comparison of quantitative analysis of the coronary cineangiogram with measured coronary flow reserve and exercise/redistribution thallium-201 scintigraphy. J. Am. Coll. Cardiol. 12:686, 1988.
61. Hlatky, M., Mark, D., Harrell, F., et al.: Rethinking sensitivity and specificity. Am. J. Cardiol. 59:1195, 1987.
62. Demer, L. L., Gould, K. L., Goldstein, R. A., et al.: Assessment of coronary artery disease severity by positron emission tomography: Comparison with quantitative arteriography in 193 patients. Circulation 79:825, 1989.
63. Goldstein, R., Kirkeeide, R., Demer, L., et al.: Relation between geometric dimensions of coronary artery stenoses and myocardial perfusion reserve in man. J. Clin. Invest. 79:1473, 1987.
64. Gould, K. L., Lipscomb, K., and Hamilton, G. W.: Physiologic basis for assessing critical coronary stenosis: Instantaneous flow response and regional distribution during coronary hyperemia as measures of coronary flow reserve. Am. J. Cardiol. 33:87, 1974.
65. Beanlands, R., Muzik, O., Sutor, R., et al.: Noninvasive determination of regional perfusion reserve in coronary artery disease using ^{13}N-ammonia PET. J. Nucl. Med. 33:826, 1992.
66. Di Carli, M., Czernin, J., Hoh., C., et al.: Relation among stenosis severity, myocardial blood flow, and flow reserve in patients with coronary artery disease. Circulation 91:1944, 1995.
67. Schelbert, H.: Consideration of measurements of myocardial blood flow with positron emission tomography. Invest. Radiol. 28:S47, 1993.
68. Iida, H., and Tamaki, N.: Quantitative assessment of regional myocardial blood flow using ^{15}O-water and PET: A multi-center project by seven independent institutes in Japan. J. Nucl. Med. 36:78, 1995.
69. Sambuceti, G., Parodi, O., Marcassa, C., et al.: Alteration in regulation of myocardial blood flow in one-vessel coronary artery disease determined by positron emission tomography. Am. J. Cardiol. 72:538, 1993.
70. Grambow, D., Dayanikli, F., Muzik, O., et al.: Assessment of endothelial function

with PET cold pressure test in patients with various degrees of coronary atherosclerosis. J. Nucl. Med. 34:P36, 1993.

71. Fuster, V., Badimon, L., Badimon, J., et al.: The pathogenesis of coronary artery disease and the acute coronary syndromes. N. Engl. J. Med. 326:242, 1992.
72. Kofoed, K., Czernin, J., Kobashigawa, J., et al.: Coronary vasomotion and vasodilatory capacity are impaired after heart transplantation. J. Nucl. Med. 36:3, 1995.
73. Dayanikli, F., Grambow, D., Muzik, O., et al.: Early detection of abnormal coronary flow reserve in asymptomatic men at high risk for coronary artery disease using positron emission tomography. Circulation 90:808, 1994.
74. Flavahan, N.: Atherosclerosis or lipoprotein-induced endothelial dysfunction. Circulation 85:1927, 1992.
75. Czernin, J., Kim, A., Dominquez, V., et al.: How reproducible are measurements of myocardial blood flow by ^{13}N-ammonia and PET? J. Nucl. Med. 35:24, 1994.
76. Tamaki, N., Yonekura, Y., Senda, M., et al.: Value and limitation of stress thallium-201 single photon emission computed tomography: Comparison with nitrogen-13 ammonia positron tomography. J. Nucl. Med. 29:1181, 1988.
77. Klocke, F.: Measurements of coronary flow reserve: Defining pathophysiology versus making decisions about patient care. Circulation 76:1183, 1987.
78. Demer, L., Gould, K., Goldstein, R., et al.: Noninvasive assessment of coronary collaterals in man by PET perfusion imaging. J. Nucl. Med. 31:259, 1990.
79. Vanoverschelde, J., Wijns, W., Depre, C., et al.: Mechanisms of chronic regional postischemic dysfunction in humans: New insights from the study of noninfarcted collateral-dependent myocardium. Circulation 87:1513, 1993.
80. McFalls, E., Araujo, L., Lammertsma, A., et al.: Vasodilator reserve in collateral-dependent myocardium as measured by positron emission tomography. Eur. Heart J. 14:336, 1993.
81. Chierchia, S., Lazzari, M., Freedman, B., et al.: Impairment of myocardial perfusion and function during painless myocardial ischemia. J. Am. Coll. Cardiol. 1:924, 1983.
82. Selwyn, A., Shea, M., Deanfield, J., et al.: The character of transient myocardial ischemia: Clinical studies and progress using positron emission tomography. Int. J. Card. Imaging 1:61, 1985.
83. Selwyn, A., Shea, M., Deanfield, J., et al.: Clinical problems in coronary disease are caused by wide variety of ischemic episodes that affect patients out of hospital. Am. J. Med. 79:12, 1985.
84. Deanfield, J., Kensett, M., Wilson, R., et al.: Silent myocardial ischemia due to mental stress. Lancet 2:1001, 1984.
85. Deanfield, J., Shea, M., Wilson, R., et al.: Direct effects of smoking on the heart: Silent ischemic disturbances of coronary flow. Am. J. Cardiol. 57:1005, 1986.
86. Czernin, J., Sun, K., Brunken, R., et al.: Effect of acute and long-term smoking on myocardial blood flow and flow reserve. Circulation 91:2891, 1995.
87. Deanfield, J., Shea, M., Ribiero, P., et al.: Transient ST segment depression as a marker of myocardial ischemia during daily life. Am. J. Cardiol. 54:1195, 1984.
88. Nabel, E., Rocco, M., and Selwyn, A.: Characteristics and significance of ischemia detected by ambulatory electrocardiographic monitoring. Circulation 75:V–74, 1987.
89. Kannel, W., and Abbott, R.: Incidence of unrecognized myocardial infarction: An update on the Framingham study. N. Engl. J. Med. 311:1144, 1984.
90. Reuanen, M., Aromaa, A., Pyorala, K., et al.: The Social Insurance Institution's coronary heart disease study: Baseline data and 5-year mortality experience. Acta Med. Scand. 673:67, 1983.
91. Walsh, M., Geltman, E., Steele, R., et al.: Augmented myocardial perfusion reserve after coronary angioplasty quantified by positron emission tomography with $H_2{}^{15}O$. J. Am. Coll. Cardiol. 15:119, 1990.
92. Gould, K.: Reversal of coronary atherosclerosis: Clinical promise as the basis for noninvasive management of coronary artery disease. Circulation 90:1558, 1994.
93. Gould, K., Martucci, J., Goldberg, D., et al.: Short-term cholesterol lowering decreases size and severity of perfusion abnormalities by positron emission tomography after dipyridamole in patients with coronary artery disease: A potential noninvasive marker of healing coronary endothelium. Circulation 89:1530, 1994.
94. Geltman, E., Henes, C., Senneff, M., et al.: Increased myocardial perfusion at rest and diminished perfusion reserve in patients with angina and angiographically normal coronary arteries. J. Am. Coll. Cardiol. 16:586, 1990.
95. Shelton, M., Senneff, M., Ludbrook, P., et al.: Concordance of nutritive myocardial perfusion reserve and flow velocity reserve in conductance vessels in patients with chest pain with angiographically normal coronary arteries. J. Nucl. Med. 34:717, 1993.
96. Camici, P., Gistri, R., Lorenzoni, R., et al.: Coronary reserve and exercise ECG in patients with chest pain and normal coronary angiograms. Circulation 86:179, 1992.
97. Rosen, S., Uren, N., Kaski, J., et al.: Coronary vasodilator reserve, pain perception, and sex in patients with syndrome X. Circulation 90:50, 1994.
98. Galassi, A., Crea, F., Araujo, L., et al.: Comparison of regional myocardial blood flow in syndrome X and one-vessel coronary artery disease. Am. J. Cardiol. 72:134, 1993.
99. McGinn, A. L., Wilson, R. F., Olivari, M. T., et al.: Coronary vasodilator reserve after human orthotopic cardiac transplantation. Circulation 78:1200, 1988.
100. Nitenberg, A., Tavolaro, O., Loisance, D., et al.: Maximal coronary vasodilator capacity of orthotopic heart transplants in patients with and without rejection. Am. J. Cardiol. 64:513, 1989.
101. Treasure, C. B., Vita, J. A., Ganz, P., et al.: Loss of the coronary microvascular response to acetylcholine in cardiac transplant patients. Circulation 86:1156, 1992.
102. Nitenberg, A., Tavolaro, O., Benvenuti, C., et al.: Recovery of a normal coronary vascular reserve after rejection therapy in acute human cardiac allograft rejection. Circulation 81:1312, 1990.
103. Krivokapich, J., Stevenson, L., Kobashigawa, J., et al.: Quantification of absolute myocardial perfusion at rest and during exercise with positron emission tomography after human cardiac transplantation. J. Am. Coll. Cardiol. 18:512, 1991.
104. Senneff, M. J., Hartman, J., Sobel, B. E., et al.: Persistence of coronary vasodilator responsivity after cardiac transplantation. Am. J. Cardiol. 71:333, 1993.
105. Rechavia, E., Araujo, L., De Silva, R., et al.: Dipyridamole vasodilator response after human orthotopic heart transplantation: Quantification by oxygen-15–labeled water and positron emission tomography. J. Am. Coll. Cardiol. 19:100, 1992.
106. Chan, S., Kobashigawa, J., Stevenson, L., et al.: Myocardial blood flow at rest and during pharmacological vasodilation in cardiac transplants during and after successful treatment of rejection. Circulation 90:204, 1994.
107. Zhao, X.-M., Delbeke, D., Sandler, M., et al.: Nitrogen-13–ammonia and PET to detect allograft coronary artery disease after heart transplantation: Comparison with coronary angiography. J. Nucl. Med. 36:982, 1995.
108. Fung, C., Czernin, J., Müller, P., et al.: Noninvasive demonstration of normal myocardial perfusion reserve in patients with dilated idiopathic cardiopathy. J. Am. Coll. Cardiol. 19:120, 1992.
109. Merlet, P., Mazoyer, B., Hittinger, L., et al.: Assessment of coronary reserve in man: Comparison between positron emission tomography with oxygen-15–labeled water and intracoronary Doppler technique. J. Nucl. Med. 34:1899, 1993.
110. Camici, P., Chiriatti, G., Oorenzoni, R., et al.: Coronary vasodilation is impaired in both hypertrophied and nonhypertrophied myocardium of patients with hypertrophic cardiomyopathy: A study with nitrogen-13 ammonia and positron emission tomography. J. Am. Coll. Cardiol. 17:879, 1991.
111. Nienaber, C., Gambhir, S., Mody, F., et al.: Regional myocardial blood flow and glucose utilization in symptomatic patients with hypertrophic cardiomyopathy. Circulation 87:1580, 1993.

CHAPTER

71 Evaluation of Myocardial Substrate Metabolism in Ischemic Heart Disease

Richard C. Brunken, M.D.
Heinrich R. Schelbert, M.D.

GENERAL CONSIDERATIONS

Cardiac myocytes metabolize a wide variety of substrates via compartmentalized biochemical pathways.[1] The energy liberated by oxidative substrate metabolism sustains life and provides the "fuel" that powers the contractile proteins of the cardiac cell. Myocardial viability and function thus depend on the ability of the coronary circulation to maintain a steady supply of energy-rich substrates and molecular oxygen commensurate with tissue needs. Inhibitory by-products of cellular biochemical reactions such as lactate and hydrogen ion must also be removed to maintain substrate flux through the metabolic pathways used to generate vital cellular energy. If myocardial blood flow is diminished or disrupted, cellular metabolism, function, and viability are jeopardized.

Transient or sustained reductions in myocardial blood flow relative to regional work occur in a variety of clinical settings in patients with coronary artery disease, and all are associated with impaired myocardial function. In myocardial stunning, a transient reduction in blood flow temporarily impairs regional wall motion. Although regional wall motion eventually returns to baseline, recovery of function is delayed relative to restoration of blood flow.[2, 3] Myocardial hibernation is the term used to describe the impairment in contractile function associated with a sustained chronic blood flow reduction.[4–6] When myocardial blood flow is restored,

Dr. Schelbert is affiliated with the laboratory of Structural Biology and Molecular Medicine operated for the U.S. Department of Energy, Washington, D.C. by the University of California under Contract No. DE-AC03-76-SF00012. This work was supported in part by the Director of the Office of Energy Research, Office of Health and Environmental Research, Washington, D.C., by Grants No. HL 29845 and No. HL 33177 from the National Institutes of Health, Bethesda, MD, and by an Investigative Group Award from the Greater Los Angeles Affilate of the American Heart Association, Los Angeles, CA.

function improves or normalizes, indicating that hibernating tissue retains clinically important viability. Myocardial infarction results when a blood flow reduction is severe enough or prolonged enough to inhibit basic cellular life functions, for example, maintenance of cell membrane integrity. Myocytes die and are eventually replaced by fibrous scar, resulting in an irreversible loss of myocardial function. Although regional alterations in blood flow and ventricular dysfunction can be observed in each of these conditions, optimal medical treatment can differ substantially for each situation. As such, the physician must reliably distinguish among these entities to provide the best quality of clinical care to the patient.

By employing specific radiotracers of compartmentalized cellular metabolic pathways, positron emission tomography can be used in the clinical setting to evaluate and quantify the fundamental biochemical processes sustaining cellular life and function. This provides clinically useful information about the state of the myocardium beyond that provided by the assessment of either regional perfusion or function alone. The metabolic tissue characterization provided by positron emission tomography reliably predicts recovery from an ischemic insult and distinguishes viable but functionally compromised tissue from the fibrosis of completed infarction. Accumulating clinical studies further indicate that maintained metabolism in hypoperfused myocardium identifies the patient with coronary artery disease who is at risk for future adverse cardiac events. Accurate characterization of regional myocardial metabolism is therefore increasingly important for the clinical management of patients with coronary artery disease who have left ventricular dysfunction.

Although it is possible to image relative myocardial glucose metabolism using fluorine-18 (^{18}F) 2-fluoro-2-deoxyglucose and gamma cameras equipped with specifically designed collimators,[7, 8] single-photon emission tomographic (SPECT) imaging remains subject to attenuation artifact even for the higher energy radionuclides and has spatial and temporal resolutions that are poorer than those of positron emission tomography. Furthermore, direct assessment of myocardial oxidative substrate metabolism is not feasible with current SPECT imaging agents. Therefore, physicians will likely continue to rely on metabolic imaging with positron emission tomography to assist in the clinical management of their patients.

This chapter focuses on metabolic imaging with positron emission tomography in ischemic heart disease. It describes how metabolic imaging is used for disease characterization and illustrates how this information contributes to the clinical management. The chapter begins with a description of the metabolic disturbances that characterize acute myocardial ischemia and explains how these disturbances are identified with positron emission tomography. It then reviews the disturbances in tissue metabolism observed in acute myocardial infarction and stunning and proceeds to a summary of the biochemical abnormalities characteristic of chronic coronary artery disease and myocardial hibernation. In each section, a brief summary of the observations in animal experimental studies precedes the description of the metabolic findings in human ischemic heart disease. The relative clinical merits of metabolic imaging for the assessment of myocardial viability are then compared with those of routinely performed tests. Finally, the chapter describes how metabolic imaging can identify patients with coronary artery disease and left ventricular dysfunction who are at risk for future adverse cardiac events, thereby permitting intervention to reduce the likelihood of an unfortunate outcome.

MYOCARDIAL METABOLIC RESPONSES TO ACUTE ISCHEMIA

The severity and the anatomical extent of the metabolic disturbances resulting from acute ischemia reflect both the magnitude of the blood flow reduction and the duration of the ischemic insult.[9] In addition, the rapidity with which the blood flow reduction occurs may also influence the cellular response to the ischemic event.[10] Under normoxic conditions, the heart preferentially metabolizes free fatty acids; their oxidation accounts for about 60 to 70 percent of total myocardial oxygen consumption in the fasting state.[11] Ischemia limits cellular oxygen availability and interferes with mitochondrial respiration and substrate oxidation.[12, 13] Ischemia depresses mitochondrial β-oxidation of fatty acids and reduces the uptake, cytosolic activation, and transmitochondrial transport of fatty acids.[12] Because oxygen deprivation impairs fatty acid metabolism at several points in the biochemical pathway, acute ischemia could affect the tissue kinetics of a labeled fatty acid such as carbon-11 palmitate (^{11}C-palmitate) to a greater degree than those of C-11 acetate, a tracer of oxidative flux through the tricarboxylic acid cycle. ^{11}C-palmitate imaging may therefore prove more sensitive for detecting the metabolic perturbations resulting from acute ischemia than ^{11}C-acetate imaging, even though the kinetics of the labeled fatty acid quantitatively reflect changes in oxidative substrate flux less directly than those of ^{11}C-acetate. For example, Heyndrickx and associates[14] noted in stunned canine myocardium a 31 percent decrease in the rate of initial clearance of ^{11}C-palmitate as compared with only a 24 percent reduction in the rate of ^{11}C-acetate clearance.

Inhibition of mitochondrial oxidative substrate metabolism in acute myocardial ischemia is accompanied by enhanced glycogenolysis and anaerobic glycolysis.[9, 12] Early experimental studies demonstrated that exogenous glucose use is accelerated in acutely ischemic myocardium.[13, 15] In patients with coronary artery disease, atrial pacing to the point of lactate production is associated with an increase in myocardial glucose extraction,[16] and intravenous infusion of low-dose glucose during atrial pacing lengthens the time to the onset of angina and reduces the severity of associated electrocardiographic ST-segment changes.[17] These observations confirm that acutely ischemic human myocardium also exhibits an increase in exogenous glucose use, providing the rationale for the use of ^{18}F-2-fluoro-2-deoxyglucose, a radiolabeled tracer of exogenous glucose use, for identifying and characterizing acutely ischemic human myocardium with positron emission tomography.

Evaluation of Fatty Acid Metabolism With Carbon-11 Palmitate

Observations in isolated arterially perfused hearts and in situ in acute and chronic animal experiments serve as an underpinning for the use of ^{11}C-palmitate in human myocardial ischemia. Serial positron emission tomographic imaging during the acute ischemia in experimental animals demonstrates segmentally decreased uptake of ^{11}C-palmitate as a function of reduced blood flow and lower extraction fractions as well as a prolongation of the half-time of the rapid tissue clearance phase.[18–20] The findings indicate a decrease in the relative amount of fatty acid entering oxidative metabolic pathways and an impaired metabolism of substrate that does enter aerobic pathways. Furthermore, the relative proportion of labeled fatty acid entering the endogenous lipid pool increases.[21] The abnormalities in oxidative substrate metabolism identified with positron emission tomography and ^{11}C-palmitate occur in tissue without ultrastructural evidence of irreversible cellular damage, indicating the sensitivity of this imaging technique for detecting cellular dysfunction in acute ischemia.[22] Finally, the increase in the fraction of ^{11}C-palmitate that diffuses back from myocardium in nonmetabolized form may limit the accuracy of the clearance half-time as a quantitative index of fatty acid oxidation.[19, 23]

To assess the effects of acute ischemia on oxidative substrate metabolism in human myocardium, Grover-McKay and colleagues[24] employed serial positron emission tomographic imaging with ^{11}C-palmitate in 10 patients with exertional angina and significant (>70 percent) coronary stenoses. Relative myocardial blood flow was first evaluated at rest with ^{13}N-ammonia. Serial imaging with ^{11}C-palmitate was then performed at rest (control) and again during atrial pacing at heart rates 10 percent less than those provoking angina. Segmental wall motion was assessed with two-dimensional echocardiography at rest and during atrial pacing.

Atrial pacing increased the mean heart rate of the subjects from 65 ± 12 beats per minute to 102 ± 15 beats per minute but had no significant effect on mean systolic or diastolic pressures. Plasma levels of fatty acids, triglycerides, lactate, and pyruvate did not differ significantly between the control and pacing studies, whereas there was a slight but statistically significant decrease in plasma glucose levels (99 ± 22 versus 92 ± 16 mg/dL). Increases in the myocardial workload therefore resulted primarily from increases in the heart rate. The resting ^{13}N-ammonia images revealed homogeneous myocardial blood flow in eight patients, whereas two individuals with prior myocardial infarction had resting perfusion defects in the clinical infarct zone. Both patients had regional akinesis or dyskinesis at rest and corresponding Q waves on their electrocardiograms. With atrial pacing, five patients acquired new regional akinesis or severe hypokinesis, three patients experienced new hypokinesis that was mild, and two patients had no apparent change in regional function. Visual analysis of the resting metabolic studies in the eight patients without prior myocardial infarction revealed homogeneous myocardial uptake and washout of ^{11}C-palmitate. In the two patients with previous infarction, visual defects were apparent on both the early and late ^{11}C-palmitate images, which corresponded to the defects noted on the ^{13}N-ammonia perfusion studies. Half-times of the initial rapid phase of myocardial ^{11}C-palmitate clearance were similar in both normal myocardium and myocardium at risk, signifying that fatty acid oxidation was not impaired in the resting state (Fig. 71–1). The fraction of ^{11}C-palmitate activity retained in myocardium and, conversely, the fraction of ^{11}C-palmitate oxidized were virtually identical in normal myocardium and myocardium at risk.

With atrial pacing, the mean half-time of the rapid clearance phase decreased in both normal myocardium and myocardium at risk, consistent with an increase in myocardial oxygen consumption and fatty acid oxidation as a result of the increased cardiac workload.[25] Half-times in myocardium at risk, however, were significantly longer than those in reference myocardium (15.6 ± 4.0 minutes versus 13.4 ± 2.5 minutes, $P < .01$), indicating an impaired oxidative metabolic reserve in the regions supplied by the vessels with significant coronary stenoses (see Fig. 71–1). The fraction of ^{11}C-palmitate activity retained in myocardium at the end of the initial rapid phase during pacing was significantly greater in the risk zones when compared with reference myocardium (41.8 ± 10.9 percent versus 36.4 ± 9.0 percent, $P < .002$) implying that the flux of ^{11}C-palmitate through oxidative pathways during pacing-induced ischemia was not commensurate with tissue demands as determined by measurements in normal myocardium. For both the control and atrial pacing studies, tracer uptake in risk myocardium relative to remote myocardium remained unchanged (97.3 ± 14.3 percent at rest versus 97.9 ± 14.1 percent during pacing, P = NS).

When the alterations in ^{11}C-palmitate kinetics were correlated with changes in regional function, the five patients with new akinesis or severe hypokinesis in the risk zones during atrial pacing also had a significant change in the percent difference in ^{11}C-palmitate clearance half-times between risk myocardium and reference myocardium (−5.8 ± 13.2 percent at control versus 26.1 ± 30.6 percent during pacing, $P = .01$). In contrast, the percent difference in ^{11}C-palmitate clearance half-times between risk and reference myocardium in the five individuals with only mild hypokinesis or no change in function with pacing did not differ significantly between the resting and pacing studies (−10.1 ± 18.2 percent versus 8.2 ± 11.2 percent, P = NS). Thus, the regions with the most pronounced functional deterioration during the stress of atrial pacing also had the greatest impairment in myocardial oxidative reserve. Conversely, in regions without apparent stress-induced wall motion abnormalities, the changes in ^{11}C-palmitate tissue kinetics tended to be attenuated, although not significantly when compared with control myocardium. This suggests that the ability to maintain systolic function in human myocardium may be coupled to the oxidative metabolic capacity of the tissue. Alternatively, normal regional function might have been maintained by a shift in local tissue metabolism to preferential use of glucose, a more oxygen-efficient substrate. However, further studies would be required to confirm these possibilities.

Evaluation of Oxidative Metabolism With Carbon-11 Acetate

The validity of ^{11}C-acetate as a tracer of oxidative metabolism and its alterations in myocardial ischemia have been documented in experimental animals.[26–30] These investigations have demonstrated that the myocardial clearance of radiolabeled acetate parallels regional oxygen consumption during acute myocardial ischemia. Because ^{11}C-acetate is a "pure" tracer of tricarboxylic acid cycle flux, variations in plasma substrate levels affect its clearance from myocardium only slightly.[27, 28] Although backdiffusion of ^{11}C label from ischemic myocardium does occur with ^{11}C-acetate, the relative amount of backdiffusion is small and does not seriously affect the quantitative determinations of regional myocardial oxygen consumption made with this tracer.

Although early clinical metabolic studies initially focused on the assessment of fatty acid metabolism in human myocardium with ^{11}C-palmitate, the effects of substrate availability on its tissue kinetics and the observed increase in backdiffusion of tracer into the vascular space in myocardial ischemia as demonstrated previously prompted new investigations into the use of ^{11}C-acetate as a more direct tracer of myocardial oxidative metabolism.

Selwyn and colleagues[31] assessed monoexponential ^{11}C-acetate clearance constants (k_{mono}) in five patients with coronary artery disease and angina undergoing treadmill exercise. ^{11}C-acetate was administered intravenously 1 to 2 minutes before the appearance of ischemic electrocardiographic changes. Although myocardial uptake of ^{11}C-acetate was homogeneous on images obtained at 3 minutes, abnormal retention of activity was noted in ischemic regions on images obtained at 12 minutes. Accordingly, ischemic regions were positively labeled on the delayed ^{11}C-acetate images. Compared with normal regions, clearance half-times were significantly longer (10.1 minutes versus 7.7 minutes, $P < .01$) and clearance constants were significantly less (0.069 versus 0.09, $P < .01$) in ischemic regions. This initial report demonstrated that serial positron emission tomographic imaging with ^{11}C-acetate could identify impaired myocardial oxidative metabolism in patients with angina at a workload insufficient to produce electrocardiographic signs of myocardial ischemia.

Similar findings were noted by these investigators[32] in five patients with coronary artery disease undergoing supine bicycle exercise. Serial ^{11}C-acetate images were obtained at rest and during exercise. In normal myocardium, clearance constants averaged 0.065 ± 0.01 min^{-1} at rest and increased to 0.102 ± 0.009 min^{-1} with exercise, commensurate with an increase in regional myocardial oxygen consumption due to the increase in cardiac workload. In contrast, regions with stress-induced ischemia had clearance constants that remained depressed at 0.065 ± 0.011 min^{-1}, indicating an impaired oxidative metabolic reserve in these areas.

Evaluation of Glucose Metabolism With Fluorine-18 2-Fluoro-2-Deoxyglucose

Early observations in acute animal experiments gave the impetus for exploring the utility of ^{18}F-2-fluoro-2-deoxyglucose for demonstrating noninvasively metabolic responses to acute myocardial ischemia. Schelbert and collaborators[33] produced acute myocardial ischemia in canine myocardium by rapid atrial pacing after partially constricting the left anterior descending coronary artery. The acutely ischemic myocardium demonstrated reduced ^{13}N-ammonia uptake but enhanced ^{18}F-2-fluoro-2-deoxyglucose accumulation that correlated with a regional increase in glucose uptake as verified by the Fick principle and that was readily appreciated on positron emission tomographic images. This resulted in a visual "mismatch"

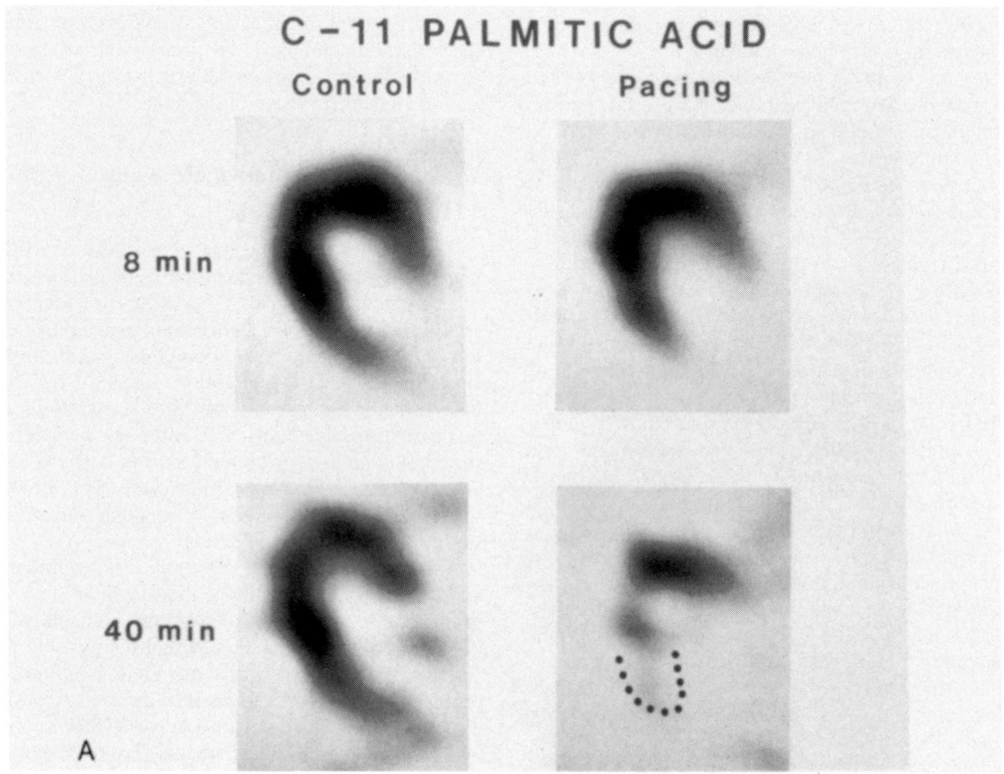

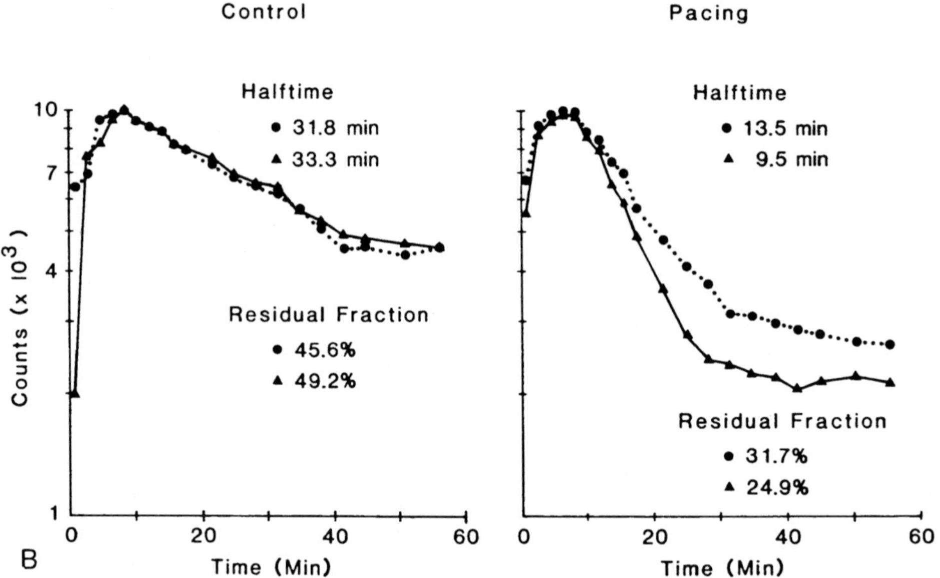

FIGURE 71-1. *Panel A,* Representative cross-sectional images of myocardial ^{11}C-palmitate activity in a patient with a proximal 90 percent stenosis of the left anterior descending coronary artery. The control images obtained in the resting state 8 and 40 minutes after the administration of the radiolabeled fatty acid are depicted in the column on the left, whereas images obtained at the corresponding time intervals during atrial pacing are displayed in the column on the right. Homogeneous uptake of the radiolabeled fatty acid is noted on the 8-minute images obtained both at control and during pacing. In the control resting state, there is uniform clearance of the labeled fatty acid from all myocardial regions, as indicated by a homogeneous distribution of the radiolabel on the delayed image at 40 minutes. In contrast, during atrial pacing there is rapid clearance of ^{11}C activity from the normally perfused lateral wall *(dotted region)* and an impairment in clearance of ^{11}C activity from the vascular territory of the anterior descending artery. *Panel B,* Representative myocardial ^{11}C time activity curves from the same patient at control and with atrial pacing. During the resting control study, uptake and clearance of ^{11}C activity in both the normal *(triangles)* and the anteroseptal regions *(circles)* are virtually identical. With atrial pacing, the ^{11}C clearance half-time is longer and the residual fraction is greater in the anteroseptal region, indicating impairment of free fatty acid oxidation during stress-induced myocardial ischemia and a relative increase in the amount of ^{11}C label entering the endogenous lipid pool. (From Grover-McKay, M., Schelbert, H. R., Schwaiger, M., et al.: Identification of impaired metabolic reserve by atrial pacing in patients with significant coronary artery disease. Circulation 74:281, 1986. With permission of the American Heart Association.)

between the ^{13}N-ammonia perfusion defect and the uptake of ^{18}F-2-fluoro-2-deoxyglucose on the metabolic images. Thus, acute myocardial ischemia is associated with augmented uptake of glucose relative to blood flow, and this metabolic disturbance can readily be identified with positron emission tomography and ^{18}F-2-fluoro-2-deoxyglucose.

Camici and coinvestigators[34] applied this newly found concept to humans to examine the effects of acute exercise-induced ischemia on myocardial glucose use in 12 patients with stable coronary artery disease. They compared the findings in the patients to those of 10 normal volunteers. Five of the 12 patients had evidence of prior transmural myocardial infarction, and 2 of the patients had poor R-wave progression in the anterior precordial leads on electrocardiography. None of the subjects had clinical histories of infarction in the 3 months prior to study.

Regional myocardial blood flow and glucose metabolism were examined at rest with rubidium-82 and ^{18}F-2-fluoro-2-deoxyglucose in six patients and five volunteers. Eight patients (including two with ^{18}F-2-fluoro-2-deoxyglucose studies at rest) and five volunteers had ^{82}Rb studies at rest, during supine bicycle exercise, and immediately following exercise. Glucose metabolism in these eight patients was evaluated after heart rate, blood pressure, and the electrocardiogram had returned to baseline and after the exercise-induced perfusion defect had resolved. Blood flow and glucose use were both evaluated semiquantitatively by measuring the fractional uptakes of ^{82}Rb and ^{18}F-2-fluoro-2-deoxyglucose. The latter was calculated by dividing myocardial ^{18}F activity concentrations at time t by the integral of the arterial ^{18}F-2-fluoro-2-deoxyglucose plasma concentration to time t.

At rest, myocardial fractional uptakes of ^{82}Rb were similar in the patients and the normal controls (0.44 ± 0.06 versus 0.47 ± 0.07). When segments were classified according to exercise performance as ischemic or nonischemic, the fractional uptake of ^{82}Rb at rest was similar in both the ischemic and nonischemic segments (0.41 ± 0.04 versus 0.45 ± 0.04, P = NS). During supine bicycle exercise, all patients experienced chest pain and ST-segment depression. At peak exercise, the average myocardial uptake of ^{82}Rb in the patients was lower than that in the normal subjects (0.52 ± 0.08 versus 0.65 ± 0.09, $P < .005$). ^{82}Rb uptake increased significantly with exercise in the nonischemic segments (0.45 ± 0.04 versus 0.63 ± 0.07) but not in the ischemic segments (0.41 ± 0.04 versus 0.39 ± 0.04, P = NS). In five patients, regional ^{82}Rb uptake actually decreased with exercise in myocardium supplied by diseased coronary arteries. Following exercise, fractional uptake of ^{82}Rb in the ischemic segments persisted unchanged (0.42 ± 0.08, P = NS versus either baseline or exercise values) whereas uptake in the nonischemic segments returned to baseline levels (0.51 ± 0.09, $P < .02$ as compared with exercise, P = NS as compared with initial resting values).

The fractional uptake of ^{18}F-2-fluoro-2-deoxyglucose at rest in the patients with coronary artery disease did not differ from that in the normal subjects (0.11 ± 0.03 versus 0.07 ± 0.04, P = NS). Following exercise, uptake of ^{18}F-2-fluoro-2-deoxyglucose in the nonischemic segments was similar to that in normal subjects (0.33 ± 0.18 versus 0.35 ± 0.21) yet was augmented in ischemic segments (0.47 ± 0.18, $P < .05$) relative to nonischemic regions (Fig. 71–2). Moreover, when compared with regional ^{82}Rb uptake after exercise, uptake of ^{18}F-2-fluoro-2-deoxyglucose per unit of fractional ^{82}Rb uptake in ischemic myocardium was 1.7 times higher than in normal segments, indicating that exogenous glucose use after exercise was augmented relative to flow in the segments with stress-induced perfusion defects. Despite return of blood flow to resting levels, glucose metabolic imaging identified an abnormal postischemic state, suggesting delayed cellular recovery from the acute ischemic insult, which may have represented the metabolic expression of "stunned myocardium."

To determine if myocardial segments with stress-induced perfusion defects exhibit augmented use of glucose remote from the episodes of exercise-induced ischemia, Yonekura and coinvestigators[35] performed resting and stress ^{13}N-ammonia perfusion studies

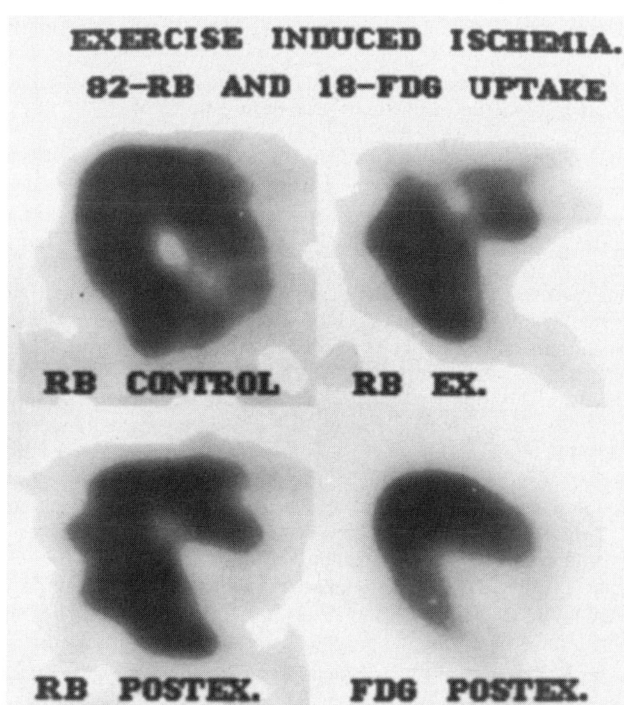

FIGURE 71–2. Representative ^{82}Rb *(RB)* perfusion and ^{18}F-2-fluoro-2-deoxyglucose (FDG) metabolic positron emission tomographic images in a patient with an 80 percent stenosis of the left anterior descending coronary artery. At rest *(RB CONTROL)*, perfusion is homogeneous throughout all ventricular regions. With exercise *(RB EX.)*, a stress-induced perfusion defect is identified in the anteroseptal region of the ventricle. On the postexercise perfusion image *(RB POSTEX.)* obtained 6 minutes after termination of exercise, perfusion has normalized in the anteroseptal region. However, the glucose metabolic image *(FDG POSTEX.)* obtained 60 minutes later reveals prominent uptake of the glucose analog in the anteroseptal region (1.55 times higher than in the lateral wall). The study with ^{18}F-2-fluoro-2-deoxyglucose thus demonstrates a persistently abnormal metabolic state in myocardium perfused by the diseased anterior descending artery despite the return of regional blood flow to normal levels. (From Camici, P., Araujo, L. I., Spinks, T., et al.: Increased uptake of ^{18}F-fluorodeoxyglucose in postischemic myocardium of patients with exercise-induced angina. Circulation 74:81, 1986. With permission of the American Heart Association.)

and separate (within 1 week) ^{18}F-2-fluoro-2-deoxyglucose glucose metabolic studies in 26 patients with angiographically confirmed coronary artery disease. Six patients had single-vessel disease, 12 patients had double-vessel disease, and 6 patients had triple-vessel disease as defined by a luminal diameter narrowing of 75 percent or greater on coronary angiography. Two patients with stenoses of less than 75 percent were considered to have significant lesions because of clinically documented myocardial infarctions in the corresponding vascular territories.

The resting ^{13}N-ammonia studies revealed flow defects in 26 (52 percent) of the vascular territories supplied by significantly stenosed coronary arteries. In 20 of these 26 territories, the electrocardiogram indicated evidence of antecedent infarction. The other six regions were perfused by vessels with 90 to 100 percent stenoses. In the two regions perfused by vessels with mild stenoses and electrocardiographic evidence of prior infarction, no resting perfusion abnormalities were identified. Stress imaging was performed using supine bicycle exercise. On the stress ^{13}N-ammonia images, there was no change in the perfusion defects in 13 (50 percent) regions with resting abnormalities, whereas relative perfusion had deteriorated further in the other 13 regions. In addition, 13 regions with normal resting perfusion exhibited stress-induced perfusion defects, including the two regions perfused by vessels with mild stenoses and electrocardiographic evidence of prior infarction and one region perfused by a circumflex artery with a 50 percent stenosis.

Evaluation of regional myocardial glucose metabolism at rest revealed augmented exogenous glucose use in 12 of the 13 (92.3 percent) regions with resting flow defects that became more severe with exercise (Fig. 71–3); six of the 13 (46.2 percent) regions with only stress-induced perfusion defects also exhibited augmented exogenous glucose use. Thus, a significant proportion of myocardial regions with stress-induced defects or with stress-induced deterioration of a resting perfusion exhibit abnormally increased exogenous glucose use at rest. The identification of regionally abnormal glucose metabolism at times remote from acute ischemic events in myocardium at risk suggests a persistently abnormal tissue metabolic state despite apparently normal resting blood flow. This observation would be consistent with the concept that repetitive stunning might presage or eventually result in a state of myocardial hibernation.[36] Of interest also was the observation that 4 of the 13 (31 percent) regions with resting perfusion defects and no change in perfusion defect with exercise also exhibited augmented uptake of ^{18}F-2-fluoro-2-deoxyglucose. This observation indicates that a fixed perfusion defect is not synonymous with the absence of metabolic tissue viability (see section on metabolic activity as a clinical indicator of tissue viability).

FIGURE 71–3. See Color Plate 33.

The relationship between stress-induced perfusion abnormalities and resting glucose metabolism was also examined by Fudo and coworkers[37] in 22 patients with prior anterior infarction. The mean interval from clinical infarction to positron emission tomography was 20 weeks (range of 5 to 80 weeks). Of 21 patients with coronary arteriography, 8 had single-vessel disease, 5 had double-vessel disease, 5 had triple-vessel disease, and 2 had less than 75 percent diameter stenosis of the anterior descending coronary arteries.

Perfusion defects were identified on resting ^{13}N-ammonia perfusion images that corresponded to the site of clinical infarction in 19 (86 percent) of the patients. Three patients with non–Q-wave infarctions did not have a resting perfusion abnormality. With supine bicycle exercise, 16 of the 22 (73 percent) patients exhibited peripheral expansion of a resting perfusion defect. Six of these 16 patients exhibited augmented uptake of ^{18}F-2-fluoro-2-deoxyglucose in the peripheral zones on remote (within 1 week) metabolic imaging with positron emission tomography (Fig. 71–4), indicating that an altered myocardial metabolic state can be detected with positron emission tomography and ^{18}F-2-fluoro-2-deoxyglucose in the border zone in these patients with stress-induced expansion of their resting perfusion defects.

Of interest relative to these observations are the beneficial effects of low-dose intravenous glucose infusions on the pacing-induced anginal threshold in patients with coronary artery disease.[17] During atrial pacing, the administration of glucose significantly prolonged the time to the onset of angina (140 ± 24 versus 110 ± 24 seconds, $P < .05$) and decreased the extent of ST-segment depression (0.9 ± 0.2 versus 1.8 ± 0.3 mm, $P < .01$). With glucose infusion, myocardial uptake of glucose increased by 100 percent, whereas free fatty acid uptake fell by 50 percent. In addition, intravenous infusion of glucose prevented efflux of citrate from the myocardium during pacing, suggesting a glycogen-sparing effect. Thus, it is possible that the enhanced uptake of ^{18}F-2-fluoro-2-deoxyglucose in postischemic myocardium might denote cellular replenishment of glycogen stores depleted during exercise-induced ischemia.

Araujo and associates[38] examined regional myocardial perfusion and glucose metabolism in patients with unstable angina. The study population consisted of 6 normal volunteers, 7 patients with chronic stable angina, and 22 patients with unstable angina. The diagnosis of unstable angina was based on a clinical history of a crescendo anginal pattern and the presence of electrocardiographic ST-segment depression during chest pain. None of the individuals studied had evidence of recent infarction by serial plasma enzyme levels or serial electrocardiography. Patients with stable angina were studied after all medications were discontinued for 48 hours. Patients with unstable angina were admitted to the coronary care unit and were treated with aspirin and, if necessary, sublingual nitrates. Twenty-four hour Holter monitoring was performed immediately before positron emission tomography. Fractional myocardial uptake of ^{82}Rb was calculated as described previously, whereas an index of myocardial glucose use was obtained employing a modified Patlak graphic approach.[39]

None of the patients with stable angina had chest pain or ST-segment depression in the 24 hours prior to positron emission tomography. Of the 22 patients with unstable angina, 8 had chest pain with ST-segment depression, whereas 6 had chest pain without ST-segment depression in the 24 hours prior to study. Five of these individuals had an episode of chest pain or ST-segment depression within 2 hours of positron emission tomography.

The positron emission tomographic images revealed similar mean fractional myocardial uptakes of ^{82}Rb for unstable angina patients (0.45 ± 0.07), normal volunteers (0.43 ± 0.09), and stable angina patients (0.44 ± 0.06). In contrast, mean rates of myocardial glucose use were significantly higher in the patients with unstable angina (0.084 ± 0.047 μmol/mL per minute) than in normals (0.012 ± 0.008 μmol/mL per minute, $P < .001$) or in patients with stable angina (0.023 ± 0.32 μmol/mL per minute, $P < .01$). The elevation in glucose use in the patients with unstable angina was diffuse rather than segmental. The mean myocardial glucose use rate for patients with stable angina did not differ significantly from the mean rate for normals.

In order to assess differences in dietary state and plasma substrate availability as possible explanations for their findings, the investigators measured plasma substrate levels and assessed rates of glucose use in skeletal muscle. Rates of glucose use in chest wall skeletal muscle were similar in the patients with unstable angina, in individuals with stable angina, and in the normal volunteers. Plasma glucose and insulin levels were similar in all three groups, indicating that differences in dietary state were unlikely to account for the observed differences in myocardial ^{18}F-2-fluoro-2-deoxyglucose uptake. Patients with chest pain or ST-segment depression within 2 hours of positron emission tomography had myocardial glucose use rates that were similar to the patients without chest pain or ST-segment depression immediately prior to imaging (0.085 ± 0.05 versus 0.078 ± 0.06 μmol/mL per minute, P = NS), implying that there was no association between clinically identified episodes of myocardial ischemia and the metabolic findings on positron emission tomography.

Although the authors of this report postulated that the increased rates of myocardial glucose use observed in the patients with unstable angina might have reflected a prolonged metabolic derangement occurring as a result of multiple transient episodes of ischemia, it is unclear why a global increase in glucose myocardial use rates would be anticipated in patients with unstable angina, particularly in individuals with single-vessel disease. Because discrete regions of resting hypoperfusion were not identified on the ^{82}Rb perfusion images, the authors were unable to distinguish myocardium at risk from normal myocardium. Thus, further studies of the metabolic abnormalities in individuals with unstable angina appear to be warranted, particularly in patients in whom a clearly defined risk zone can reliably be identified.

Synopsis of Metabolic Findings in Acute Myocardial Ischemia

As predicted by animal experimental studies, both overall oxidative metabolism and fatty acid metabolism per se are depressed during acute ischemic episodes in human myocardium. Both effects can be readily demonstrated as prolongation of the myocardial clearance rates of ^{11}C-acetate and ^{11}C-palmitate, respectively, in

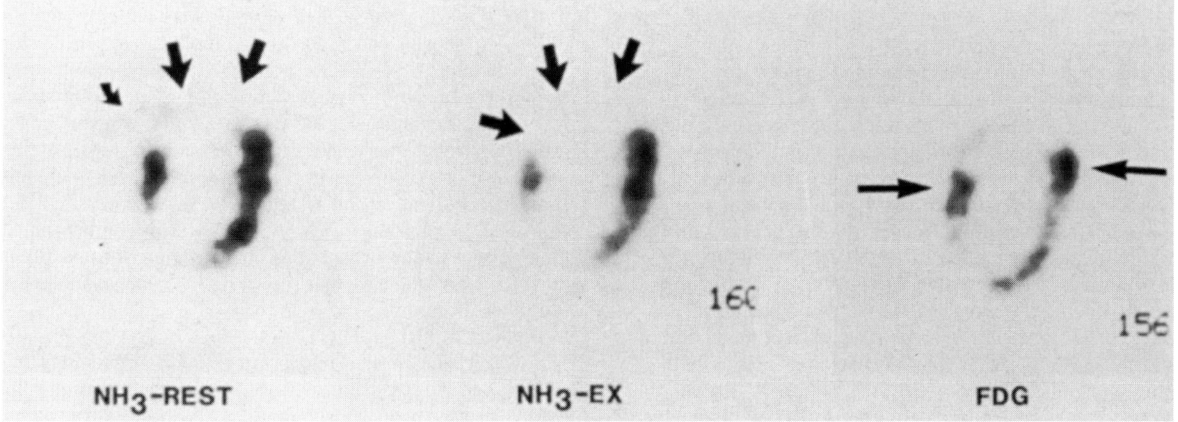

FIGURE 71–4. Rest *(NH_3-REST)* and stress *(NH_3-EX)* ^{13}N-ammonia perfusion and ^{18}F-2-fluoro-2-deoxyglucose (FDG) metabolic images from a 63-year-old man with a history of prior anterior infarction. The resting ^{13}N-ammonia study demonstrates a perfusion defect involving the anteroseptal and anterolateral regions of the ventricle *(thick arrows)*. With exercise, there is peripheral expansion of the resting perfusion defect *(thick arrows)*. On the glucose metabolic study performed on a different day, there is enhanced uptake of ^{18}F-2-fluoro 2-deoxyglucose in the peripheral zones of perfusion defect expansion *(thin arrows)*, indicating an abnormal postischemic metabolic state in the myocardium adjacent to the area of infarction. (From Fudo, T., Kambara, H., Hashimoto, T., et al.: F-18 deoxyglucose and stress N-13 ammonia positron emission tomography in anterior wall healed myocardial infarction. Am. J. Cardiol. 61:1191, 1988, with permission.)

acutely ischemic human myocardium. Studies with ^{11}C-palmitate also demonstrate increased retention of ^{11}C activity in acutely ischemic myocardium, suggesting that a disproportionately greater fraction of the labeled fatty acid is deposited in the endogenous lipid pool. The disturbances in fatty acid metabolism in acutely ischemic myocardium detected on positron emission tomography can occur in tissue without ultrastructural evidence of irreversible cellular damage, indicating the sensitivity of this imaging technique for detecting cellular dysfunction. Under conditions of impaired tissue oxygen delivery, myocardial consumption of exogenous glucose increases. This is identified on positron emission tomographic imaging by augmented uptake of the glucose analog ^{18}F-2-fluoro-2-deoxyglucose in hypoperfused myocardial regions, resulting in a "mismatch" between perfusion and exogenous glucose use on the images.

Additional clinical studies indicate that there is an increase in segmental glucose consumption as identified by a relative or absolute increase in ^{18}F-2-fluoro-2-deoxyglucose uptake. An unexpected finding in these studies, however, was that increased glucose use may persist for some time after a single discrete ischemic event. This increase in glucose use may in fact represent a metabolic correlate to mechanical "stunning." From the available investigations, however, it is uncertain how long such an abnormal metabolic state may persist. Although the observed increase in glucose use in normally perfused myocardial regions at rest suggests that such an abnormal metabolic state may exist for prolonged periods, the fact that the abnormal glucose uptake frequently occurs in regions with stress-induced perfusion defects raises the possibility that repeated episodes of acute ischemia alternating with "reperfusion" may result in a persistently abnormal metabolic state, which may presage progression to myocardial hibernation.

ACUTE MYOCARDIAL INFARCTION AND REPERFUSION

Acute myocardial infarction is a complex pathophysiologic process. It typically begins as an interruption of myocardial blood flow, which results in temporally and spatially inhomogeneous ischemia and cellular death.[40, 41] A disruption of blood flow of sufficient severity and duration to cause cellular necrosis in one area of a vascular territory might also "stun" or produce transient myocardial mechanical dysfunction in adjacent tissue. In stunned tissue, myocardial blood flow is sufficient (either through collateral vessels or through "recanalization" of the occluded vessel) to maintain viability and prevent cellular death.[42] It is also possible that persistence or restoration of some degree of blood flow results in a state of myocardial "hibernation."

Because early coronary angiography in patients with acute myocardial infarction often reveals an occluded infarct artery,[43] treatment of these individuals seeks to achieve timely restoration of antegrade perfusion to the zone of clinical infarction to limit myocardial infarct size.[44] As such, assessment of the adequacy of reperfusion, whether occurring spontaneously[45] or as a result of the administration of thrombolytic agents[46] or mechanical intervention,[47] and determination of salvage of endangered myocardium in the clinical infarct zone are assuming increasingly important roles in clinical cardiology. Because it is difficult with routine tests to distinguish ischemically compromised tissue from that with irreversible injury early in the course of an infarction, the clinician may be unable to identify the patient with viable but jeopardized myocardium that could be salvaged by early intervention. Laboratory and clinical research efforts therefore have been directed at assessing the utility of metabolic imaging with positron emission tomography for identifying viable, and therefore potentially salvageable, tissue early in the course of an acute ischemic injury.

General Considerations

As the importance of early restoration of antegrade perfusion for salvage of viable but jeopardized tissue in patients with acute infarction was recognized, clinical investigators began to use the noninvasive metabolic tissue characterization afforded by positron emission tomography to better understand and therefore more definitively treat acute human myocardial ischemic injury. As noted, experimental studies have suggested that viable but ischemically compromised tissue resorts to anaerobic glycolysis to sustain production of high-energy phosphate and thus to maintain cellular viability. Hence, most of the clinical studies of patients with acute myocardial infarction have focused on regional glucose metabolism in the clinical infarct zone. However, increasing interest in "purer" tracers of oxidative metabolism such as ^{11}C-acetate, whose tissue kinetics are more directly related to regional oxygen consumption, have also prompted in-depth studies of the clinical utility of the assessment of oxidative substrate metabolism in patients with acute ischemic injury.

Observations made with positron emission tomography in experimental animals serve as an underpinning of investigations in humans. Moreover, animal experimental findings aid in explaining and understanding unexpected findings in patients during or after the acute phase of a myocardial infarction. These animal experimental studies have also confirmed the dynamic nature of an acute ischemic event, its progression to necrosis, or its recovery as a result of reperfusion. These studies have characterized the interplay among blood flow, oxidative metabolism, glucose use, and anaerobic glycolysis, and contractile function. Early postreperfusion uptake of ^{11}C-palmitate has been found to predict the long-term outcome of ischemically injured, although reperfused, myocardium better than measures of regional myocardial blood flow.[48, 49] Oxidation of fatty acid as evidenced by the clearance pattern of ^{11}C-palmitate from reperfused myocardium recovers slowly and, possibly, in concert with an improvement in regional contractile function.[48–51] Overall oxidative metabolism as defined with ^{11}C-acetate remains depressed early after reperfusion.[52, 53] Inotropic stimulation of stunned myocardium largely restores contractile function associated with a near normalization of regional blood flow and oxidative metabolism.[53] If oxidative metabolism remains depressed for some time after reperfusion, glucose use may increase regionally[52] presumably because of an augmentation of anaerobic glycolysis.[54] This augmentation as demonstrated with ^{18}F-2-fluoro-2-deoxyglucose depends on the severity of the ischemic insult as well as on the time of the reperfusion period.[50, 55] Although absent early after restoration of blood flow, it appears to be most prominent after several days and may disappear as contractile function returns to normal.[50]

Multitracer approaches may allow a more complete characterization of the severity of the postischemic injury. For example, technetium-99m (Sn) pyrophosphate is retained most avidly in marginally reperfused myocardium.[56] In contrast, ^{18}F-2-fluoro-2-deoxyglucose accumulates best in myocardium with appreciable (more than 30 percent of control) to full restoration of blood flow.[56] The early postinjection uptake of thallium-201 (^{201}Tl) in reperfused myocardium parallels myocardial blood flow.[56] Finally, other observations indicate that ^{201}Tl redistribution and preserved glucose metabolic activity are both accurate indicators of viability in reperfused canine myocardium.[57]

Clinical Investigations

Metabolic Characterization of Acutely Infarcted Human Myocardium

In the initial study of myocardial glucose metabolism in patients with recent ischemic myocardial injury, Marshall and coinvestigators[58] employed positron emission tomography with ^{13}N-ammonia and ^{18}F-2-fluoro-2-deoxyglucose to assess relative myocardial perfusion and glucose metabolism in 15 patients in the subacute phase of myocardial infarction. Four electrocardiographically defined infarct regions were studied: anterior, septal, lateral, and inferoposterior. The study population included nine patients with postinfarction angina and six patients without postinfarction angina. The mean interval from the onset of chest pain to positron emission tomography was similar in both groups (2.2 ± 3.0 versus 3.7 ± 3.9 weeks, respectively, P = NS). Eleven patients had Q-wave infarctions involving 13 electrocardiographic infarct regions, whereas four individuals had non-Q wave infarctions. In addition, two individuals had histories of remote Q-wave infarctions. Thus, there were clinical histories of 19 infarctions (17 recent, 2 remote) in the patients studied.

On positron emission tomography, concordant decreases in myocardial perfusion and glucose use were noted on circumferential count profile analysis in 14 ventricular regions in 11 patients, consistent with completed infarction (Fig. 71–5). In contrast, myocardial uptake of ^{18}F-2-fluoro-2-deoxyglucose was preserved relative to that of ^{13}N-ammonia in 11 regions in 10 patients (see Fig. 71–5), indicating accelerated glucose metabolism relative to blood flow and providing evidence for residual tissue metabolic viability. Of the 11 regions exhibiting the metabolism-perfusion mismatch of myocardial ischemia, 5 were in the vascular territory of the infarct artery, whereas three regions of ischemia were noted in the territories of remote coronary arteries. In one patient with left bundle branch block and lateral ischemia, it was not possible to correlate the metabolic findings with an electrocardiographic infarct region. One patient had ischemia both in the region of the acute infarction and in a remote vascular bed. Right ventricular ischemia was identified in two patients.

Eight of the 10 patients with the metabolism-perfusion mismatch of myocardial ischemia had postinfarction angina at rest, whereas only one of the five patients without positron emission tomographic evidence of myocardial ischemia had postinfarction angina ($0.05 < P < .10$). In five patients with transient electrocardiographic ST-T changes and chest pain, the regions of ischemia identified with positron emission tomography correlated with the electrocardiographic regions demonstrating the ST-T changes. Thirteen of the patients had coronary angiography. In these, the metabolism-perfusion mismatch pattern of myocardial ischemia was associated with more extensive coronary disease (2.9 ± 0.4 versus 1.5 ± 0.6 coronary artery lesions, $P < .02$). Postmortem examination in two patients who died 10 days and 4 weeks, respectively, after imaging confirmed the presence of significant amounts of viable tissue in the myocardial regions exhibiting the positron emission tomographic pattern of myocardial ischemia. Thus, these seminal findings indicated that glucose metabolic imaging could identify viable tissue in some hypoperfused infarct regions in patients in the subacute stage of myocardial infarction and implied that positron emission tomography could prove useful for identifying viable tissue early in patients with acute infarction.

Schwaiger and coinvestigators[59] subsequently assessed relative myocardial perfusion and exogenous glucose metabolism within 72 hours of the onset of chest pain in 13 patients presenting with acute myocardial infarction. Regional function was determined with two-dimensional echocardiography on the day of imaging and at 6.0 ± 4.6 weeks. All patients revealed electrocardiographic or serum enzymatic evidence of acute myocardial infarction, or both. Q waves evolved on the electrocardiogram in 12 of the 13 individuals, whereas 1 patient had left bundle branch block. The electrocardiographic site of the infarction was anterior in 10 patients, inferior in 1 patient, posteroinferior in 1 patient, and undeterminable in the patient with left bundle branch block. In two patients, there was electrocardiographic evidence of old inferior infarction. Peak serum levels of creatine kinase were 1384 ± 1640 U/L (normal = 20 to 120 U/L) and peak serum levels of the creatine kinase-MB isoenzyme were 39.9 ± 43.9 U/L (normal < 4 U/L). None of the patients underwent thrombolytic therapy or angioplasty.

Positron emission tomography was performed 54 ± 12 hours after the onset of chest pain. In the 13 patients, ^{13}N-ammonia imaging identified 32 segments with diminished resting blood flow. In these hypoperfused segments, relative ^{13}N-ammonia activity was 46 ± 13.9 percent of maximal myocardial ^{13}N-ammonia activity. Regional myocardial perfusion was reduced in the anterior and apical segments in the 10 patients with electrocardiographic anterior infarctions, whereas in the single patient with an acute inferior infarction, hypoperfusion was noted in the inferior and apical segments. The patient with a posteroinferior infarction exhibited a perfusion defect involving the inferior, apical, and lateral segments. In one of the two individuals with chronic inferior infarction, a perfusion defect was identified in the inferior wall.

On metabolic imaging with ^{18}F-2-fluoro-2-deoxyglucose, there were concordant decreases in exogenous glucose use in 16 (50 percent) of the hypoperfused regions, indicating an absence of metabolic tissue viability. In contrast, preserved glucose metabolism was identified in the remaining 16 (50 percent) hypoperfused segments, indicating residual tissue metabolic viability. Of the 13 patients, 9 (69.2 percent) had residual tissue glucose metabolism

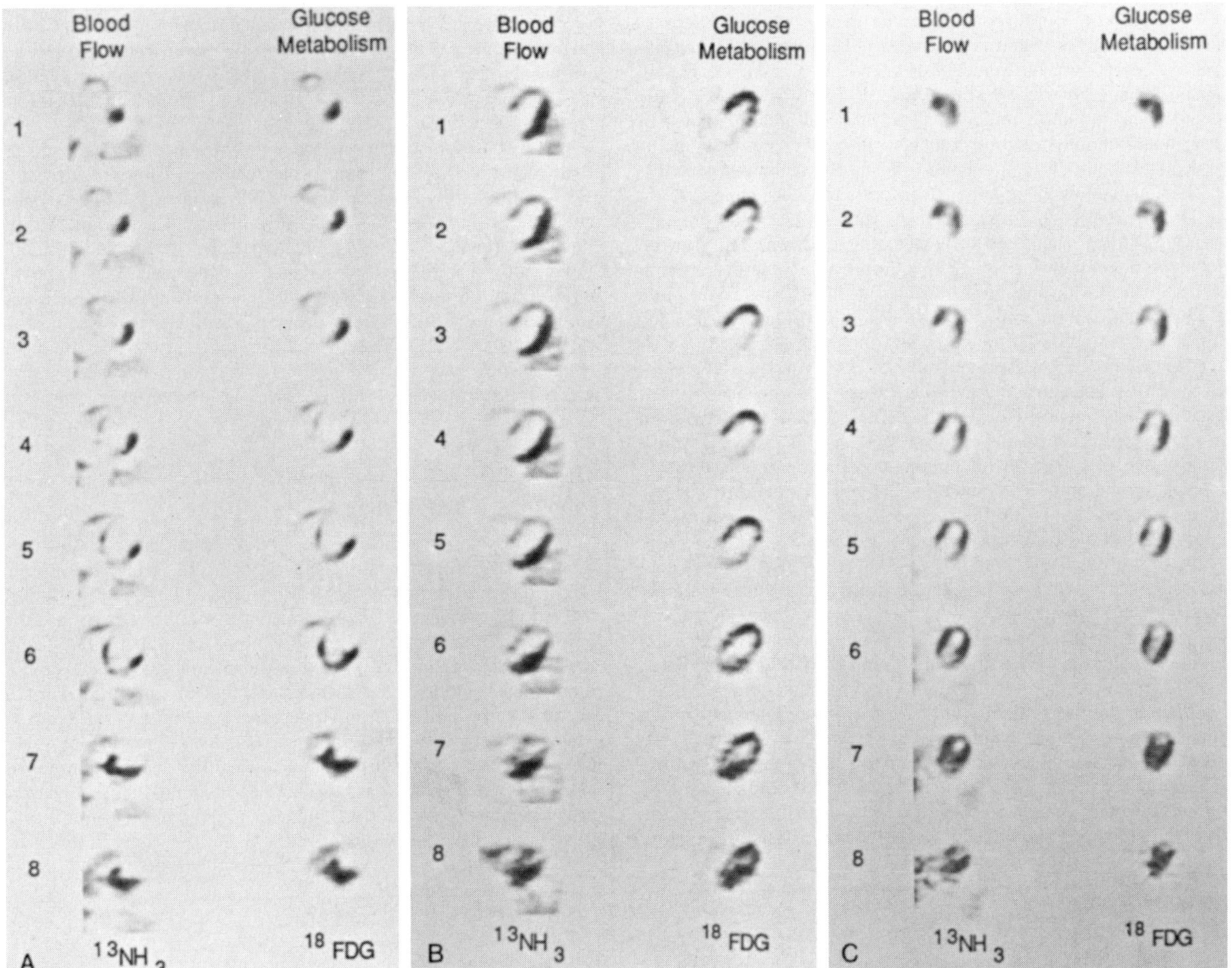

FIGURE 71–5. Representative ^{13}N-ammonia perfusion (*$^{13}NH_3$*) and ^{18}F-2-fluoro-2-deoxyglucose metabolic (*^{18}FDG*) images in three different patients with acute myocardial infarction. *Panel A,* Images from the study of a 52-year-old man with an uncomplicated acute anterolateral myocardial infarction. Matching defects in perfusion and glucose metabolism are noted in the anteroseptal and anteroapical regions of the ventricle, indicating completed infarction. *Panel B,* Representative images from a 76-year-old man with an acute anteroseptal infarction. On the ^{13}N-ammonia images, a large perfusion defect is identified in the anteroseptal and anteroapical region of the ventricle. On the metabolic images, there is prominent uptake of the labeled glucose tracer, indicating metabolic viability in the hypoperfused infarct tissue. *Panel C,* Perfusion and glucose metabolic images from the study of a 71-year-old woman with an acute uncomplicated anteroseptal myocardial infarction. Only modest reductions in perfusion and glucose use are noted in the anteroapical region, indicating substantial residual myocardial viability in the clinical infarct zone.

in hypoperfused ventricular segments, whereas concordant reductions in perfusion and glucose metabolism indicative of completed infarction were observed in 4 patients (30.8 percent). Each of the five patients who had postinfarction angina had preservation of glucose metabolism in the hypoperfused infarct zone. In the segments with residual tissue metabolic viability as identified with ^{18}F-2-fluoro-2-deoxyglucose, relative ^{13}N-ammonia activity was not significantly different from that in the segments with a loss of metabolic viability (48.2 ± 15.9 percent versus 46.0 ± 7.4 percent of maximal myocardial ^{13}N-ammonia activity, P = NS), indicating that assessment of myocardial perfusion alone could not have discriminated between the segments with and those without residual tissue metabolic viability on imaging with ^{18}F-2-fluoro-2-deoxyglucose.

Changes in contractile function were assessed by two independent observers who graded segmental wall motion in each of five myocardial segments according to the following scoring system: −1 = dyskinesia, 0 = akinesia, 1 = severe hypokinesia, 2 = mild hypokinesia, and 3 = normal function. On the day of positron emission tomography, there was no significant difference between the mean segmental wall motion score in segments with and those without preserved uptake of ^{18}F-2-fluoro-2-deoxyglucose (0.34 ± 0.84 versus 0.67 ± 0.83, P = NS), indicating that assessment of segmental wall motion could not have discriminated between segments with and those without metabolic evidence of viability. Mean left ventricular ejection fraction in patients with preserved glucose metabolism in the hypoperfused segments (44.4 ± 14.9 percent) did not significantly differ from that for the patients with the concordant reductions in flow and glucose metabolism (38.5 ± 4.4 percent, P = NS).

On follow-up assessment of segmental function in 12 patients at 6.0 ± 4.6 weeks, segments with a concordant reduction in perfusion and glucose metabolism exhibited no significant improvement in wall motion score (0.69 ± 0.99 versus 0.67 ± 0.83, P = NS) and the mean left ventricular ejection fraction also did not change (38.8 ± 6 percent versus 38.5 ± 4.4 percent, P = NS). In contrast, the mean wall motion score improved significantly in the hypoperfused segments with metabolic activity on the early ^{18}F-2-fluoro-2-deoxyglucose images (1.12±1.4 versus 0.34±0.84, $P < .01$). Of the 16 hypoperfused segments with preserved ^{18}F-2-fluoro-2-deoxyglucose uptake, 8 showed improvement in segmental wall motion of at least one grade, whereas function remained unchanged in 6 segments and deteriorated in 2 segments. As a result, the mean left ventricular ejection fraction for these nine patients did not change significantly at 6 weeks (46.7±12.9 percent versus 44.4±14.9 percent, P = NS). Thus, segments with matching perfusion and glucose metabolic defects uniformly failed to improve in function. In contrast, segments with perfusion-metabolism mismatches had a more variable functional outcome, with a substantial proportion showing improved function on follow-up echocardiography.

A case report by Brunken and colleagues[60] illustrates the clinical utility of metabolic imaging for identifying viable but jeopardized tissue in acute myocardial infarction. Both fatty acid metabolism and exogenous glucose use were assessed in a 71-year-old woman admitted with an acute anteroseptal myocardial infarction. Positron emission tomography with ^{13}N-ammonia and ^{18}F-2-fluoro-2-deoxyglucose was performed on the second hospital day and revealed a prominent mismatch between regional perfusion and glucose use in the anteroseptal region of the ventricle (Fig. 71–6), suggesting residual tissue viability in the clinical infarct zone. On subsequent study with ^{11}C-palmitate, serial positron emission tomographic images demonstrated impaired tissue clearance of ^{11}C activity in the hypoperfused infarct zone, indicating impaired fatty acid oxidation in the myocardial region with preserved exogenous glucose use.

Although the patient did not have postinfarction angina, the positron emission tomographic metabolic studies suggested the presence of a substantial amount of residual viable tissue in the clinical infarct region. The patient was referred for angiography and underwent angioplasty of a long 80 percent stenosis of the anterior descending artery. Unfortunately, the patient sustained a second infarction in the same vascular distribution 3 days after the angioplasty (felt clinically to have been caused by plaque dissection with acute occlusion of the vessel), convincingly demonstrating that a significant amount of viable tissue had resided in the clinical infarct zone following the initial ischemic insult.

Observations made in the prethrombolytic era thus indicated that positron emission tomography with ^{18}F-2-fluoro-2-deoxyglucose could identify viable but compromised myocardium early after an acute myocardial infarction. Hypoperfused segments without metabolic tissue viability on imaging with positron emission tomography and ^{18}F-2-fluoro-2-deoxyglucose rarely exhibited improved wall motion on delayed assessment of segmental function. In contrast, segments with diminished blood flow but evidence of residual metabolic activity as evidenced by the uptake of ^{18}F-2-fluoro-2-deoxyglucose had a variable functional outcome if intervention was not performed to salvage ischemically compromised tissue (Fig. 71–7).

Electrocardiographic Changes and Metabolic Abnormalities

To assess the significance of electrocardiographic ST-segment depression remote from the site of an acute ischemic injury, or "reciprocal" ST-segment depression, Billadello and coworkers[61] studied 20 patients with acute myocardial infarction using positron emission tomography and ^{11}C-palmitate. In the 20 patients, there were 7 anterior and 13 inferior electrocardiographically defined infarctions. Significant ST-segment depression was defined by 0.1 mV or greater depression in at least two precordial (V_1 through V_6) or two inferior (II, III, aVF) leads. Total ST-segment depression was defined as the sum of the ST-segment depression in the anterior or inferior leads. Electrocardiograms were recorded 3.4±3.3 hours and positron emission tomography was performed 9±7 hours after the onset of chest pain. The mean interval be-

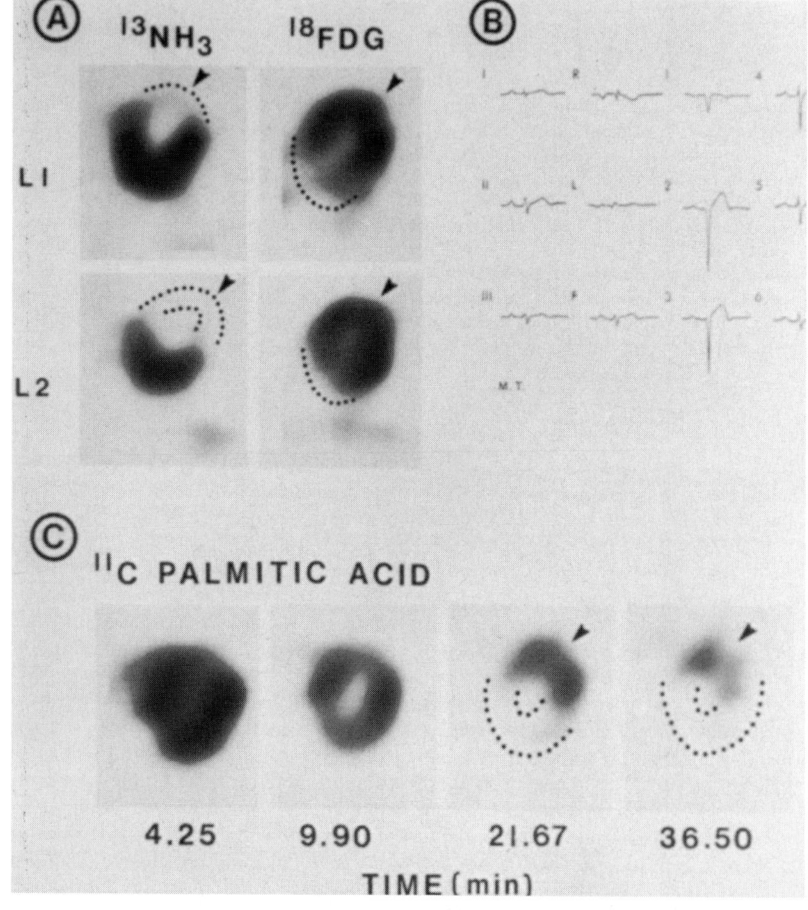

FIGURE 71–6. *Panel A,* Representative cross-sectional ^{13}N-ammonia (*$^{13}NH_3$*) perfusion and ^{18}F-2-fluoro-2-deoxyglucose (*^{18}FDG*) metabolic images from the study of a 71-year-old woman with a recent anteroseptal myocardial infarction. The images demonstrate an extensive mismatch between perfusion and glucose use in the clinical infarct zone, indicating residual tissue viability. *Panel B,* The patient's 12-lead electrocardiogram at the time of positron emission tomography. Q waves are present in V_1 and V_2 and there is a loss of R wave in the other anterior precordial leads. *Panel C,* Serial ^{11}C-palmitate images from the same patient. The ^{11}C-palmitate study demonstrates impaired uptake and delayed clearance of ^{11}C activity in the zone of clinical infarction, indicating impaired fatty acid oxidation. (From Brunken, R. C., Schwaiger, M., and Schelbert, H. R.: PET detection of residual, viable tissue in acute MI. Appl. Radiol. 14:82, 1985, with permission.)

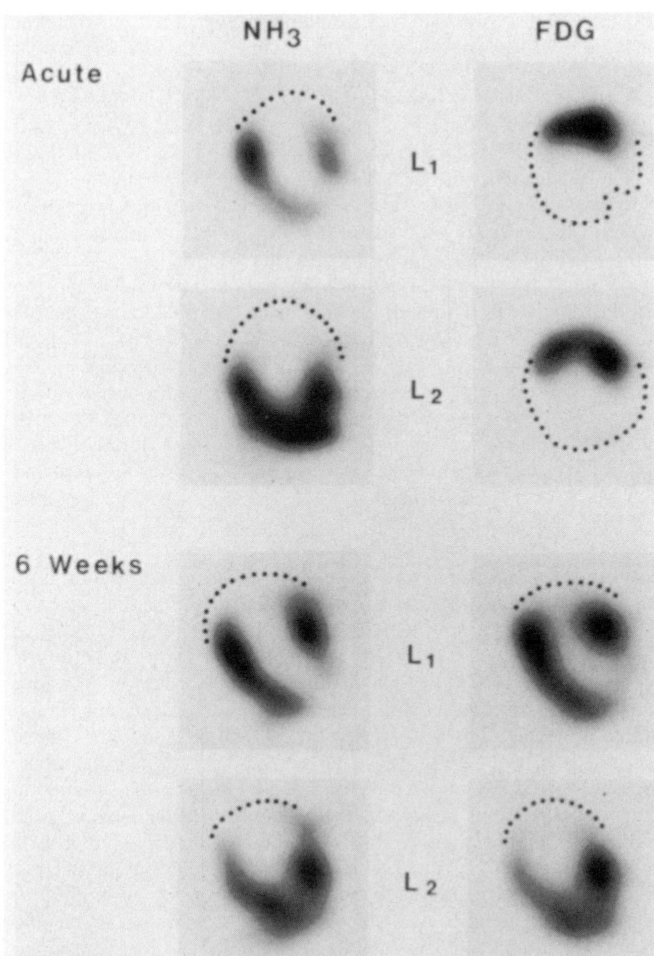

FIGURE 71–7. *Acute Study:* Representative cross-sectional ^{13}N-ammonia *(NH_3)* perfusion and ^{18}F-2-fluoro-2-deoxyglucose *(FDG)* metabolic images obtained 48 hours after the onset of chest pain in a 71-year-old man with an acute anterior myocardial infarction. Coronary angiography revealed an 80 percent stenosis of the anterior descending coronary artery and 50 percent stenosis of the circumflex artery. On the ^{13}N-ammonia perfusion images, there is an extensive anteroapical perfusion defect. The glucose metabolic study, performed in the fasting state, reveals enhanced uptake of the radiolabeled glucose analog in the zone of clinical infarction. *Study at 6 Weeks:* Corresponding images obtained in the same patient 6 weeks after the patient's clinical myocardial infarction. In contrast to the initial study, there are concordant perfusion and glucose metabolic defects in the anteroapical region of the ventricle, consistent with completed myocardial infarction. In this patient, positron emission tomography early after infarction demonstrated evidence of residual metabolic viability in the clinical infarct zone. On the study at 6 weeks, however, the patient's infarct was complete. This suggests that interventional restoration of blood flow early after infarction might have salvaged viable but endangered myocardium in the clinical infarct region. (From Schwaiger, M., Brunken, R., Grover-McKay, M., et al.: Regional myocardial metabolism in patients with acute myocardial infarction assessed by positron emission tomography. J. Am. Coll. Cardiol. 8:800, 1986, with permission.)

tween electrocardiography and positron emission tomography was 3 ± 3.2 hours. Imaging was repeated prior to hospital discharge at 14 ± 7 days. The patients were not treated with thrombolytic agents.

Of the seven patients with anterior infarction, none had reciprocal ST-segment depression in the inferior leads. Each had defects in ^{11}C-palmitate uptake limited to the septum and anterior and apical regions of the ventricle on the initial imaging studies, and there were no new defects identified on delayed imaging at 14 ± 7 days. Each of the individuals with anterior infarction had angiographic evidence of significant (>50 percent reduction in luminal diameter) stenoses in the left anterior descending artery. Significant stenoses were also noted in the right coronary artery in one patient and in the circumflex artery in three patients. The mean left ventricular ejection fraction in this group was 45 ± 9 percent. Assessment of regional function revealed wall motion abnormalities limited to the anterior wall, septum, and apex.

Of the 13 patients with electrocardiographic inferior infarctions, nine (69 percent) had ST depression in the anterior precordial leads. In each of the nine patients, positron emission tomography with ^{11}C-palmitate revealed decreased accumulation of tracer in the inferior, posterior, apical, and posterolateral segments. In addition, accumulation of ^{11}C-palmitate in the septal and anterior regions was reduced in three patients, corresponding to the anterior reciprocal ST-segment changes noted on electrocardiography. At the time of hospital discharge, two of the three patients with the anterior ^{11}C-palmitate defects showed improvement but not normalization of tracer uptake in the anterior and septal segments. This was observed despite normalization of the electrocardiographic anterior ST-segment changes. In the third patient, there was no change in the diminished accumulation of ^{11}C-palmitate in the anterior wall on delayed positron emission tomography. The three patients with the anterior ^{11}C-palmitate defects each had multivessel coronary artery disease on coronary angiography. Of the six patients with reciprocal anterior ST-segment depression and normal ^{11}C-palmitate accumulation in the anterior and septal segments, two had stenoses of the right coronary artery only, one had stenoses of both the right and left anterior descending arteries, and two had severe three-vessel coronary artery disease. The remaining patient did not undergo cardiac catheterization. The three patients with abnormal uptake of ^{11}C-palmitate had impaired wall motion in the anterior region, whereas the six patients with reciprocal ST changes and normal ^{11}C-palmitate uptake had no anterior wall motion abnormalities. The mean left ventricular ejection fraction for these nine patients was 51 ± 12 percent.

Of the four individuals with an acute inferior infarction without ST-segment depression, none had regional wall motion abnormalities in the anterior or septal regions of the ventricle. The mean left ventricular ejection fraction was 58 ± 17 percent. Uptake of ^{11}C-palmitate was reduced in the inferoposterior region in each patient. In one individual with a nonhemodynamically significant (<50 percent) stenosis in the anterior descending artery, there was a small anterior region with decreased accumulation of ^{11}C-palmitate. In this latter individual, the diminished accumulation of ^{11}C-palmitate in the anterior region was no longer present at the time of hospital discharge, suggesting a transient depression of oxidative metabolism in this area of the ventricle.

Both the total inferior ST-segment elevation (0.48 ± 0.35 versus 0.07 ± 0.19 mV, $P < .05$) and peak plasma creatine kinase-MB levels (354 ± 134 versus 80 ± 34 IU/L, $P < .05$) in the patients with inferior infarction and reciprocal anterior ST-segment changes were significantly larger than in the patients with inferior infarctions without reciprocal ST-segment changes. In addition, the mean extent of metabolic compromise, the size of the defect on the ^{11}C-palmitate images, was larger (58 ± 13 versus 33 ± 10 positron emission tomographic gram equivalents, $P < .02$). Thus, in this study, positron emission tomography with ^{11}C-palmitate identified "ischemia at a distance" in one third of the patients with inferior infarctions and reciprocal anterior ST-segment changes, and this ischemia was associated with impairment in regional wall motion.

Relationship Between Metabolic Findings and Coronary Anatomy

Schwaiger and coinvestigators[62] explored the relationship between coronary artery anatomy and the metabolic findings in patients with acute myocardial infarction. Positron emission tomography with ^{13}N-ammonia and ^{18}F-2-fluoro-2-deoxyglucose was performed 5.1 days (range of 2 to 14 days) after the onset of chest pain in 15 patients with acute myocardial infarction. The physiologic and metabolic information derived from the imaging studies was then correlated with the anatomical information derived from coronary angiography.

Ten patients had anterior infarctions and five had inferior infarctions. Plasma creatine kinase-MB levels averaged 63.9±38.1 U/L (normal < 4 U/L). The mean interval between positron emission tomography and coronary angiography was 4.4±6.7 days. Segmental function was assessed in each of five ventricular segments within 24 hours of positron emission tomography in 14 patients using two-dimensional echocardiography (12 patients) or radionuclide ventriculography (2 patients).

Imaging with ^{13}N-ammonia identified 37 hypoperfused left ventricular segments. In 20 (54.1 percent) of the segments, the decrease in relative perfusion was paralleled by a concordant decrease in exogenous glucose use on metabolic imaging with ^{18}F-2-fluoro-2-deoxyglucose, consistent with completed infarction. In contrast, 17 (45 percent) of the hypoperfused segments exhibited preserved uptake of ^{18}F-2-fluoro-2-deoxyglucose, consistent with metabolic tissue viability. On assessment of regional function, segments with preserved ^{18}F-2-fluoro-2-deoxyglucose uptake had wall motion scores that were as poor as those of the segments with matching perfusion and metabolic defects (0.79±0.76 versus 0.52±0.82, P = NS), signifying that assessment of function could not discriminate between segments with and those without tissue metabolic viability.

On coronary angiography at 8.4±7.5 days, the infarct-related artery was occluded in eight patients and patent in seven patients. When segmental function was compared with coronary angiographic classification, segments in the distribution of patent arteries had wall motion scores as poor as those in the distribution of occluded arteries (0.68±0.91 versus 0.60±0.84, P = NS). Sixteen of the 20 (80 percent) infarct segments distal to an occluded artery exhibited matching defects on metabolic imaging, indicating completed infarction. Although significant collateral flow was noted on coronary angiography in seven of these segments, only two (28.6 percent) had preserved uptake of ^{18}F-2-fluoro-2-deoxyglucose, implying that the presence of visible collateral vessels on coronary angiography exerted no significant beneficial effect on tissue viability. The absence of such effect, however, may have also been related to the relatively small sample size. In contrast, 13 of the 17 (75.5 percent) hypoperfused infarct segments in the territory of a patent artery exhibited residual metabolic activity (χ^2 = 11.9, P < .001).

Thus, this investigation in patients with acute myocardial infarction suggests a positive association between the presence of antegrade flow in the infarct artery and residual tissue metabolic activity. These observations are consistent with the hypothesis that anaerobic metabolism can be supported in acutely ischemic myocardium if some degree of residual blood flow exists for removal of inhibitory metabolites such as hydrogen ion and lactate. This study also illustrates how metabolic imaging with positron emission tomography can provide new and clinically useful insights into the pathophysiology of acute human myocardial ischemia. For example, neither assessment of segmental wall motion nor determination of the presence or absence of visible coronary collaterals on coronary angiography would have allowed discrimination between segments with and those without residual metabolic viability in these individuals.

Effects of Coronary Thrombolysis and Revascularization

The observations described previously in patients with acute myocardial infarction are consistent with previous clinicopathologic studies[63–67] demonstrating that myocardial infarction is a heterogeneous process. Reimer and Jennings[41] have suggested that a "wavefront" of myocardial necrosis spreads from the subendocardial to the epicardial layer of the myocardium in acute infarction and that the duration of coronary occlusion is related to the ultimate extent of myocardial necrosis. As such, early restoration of myocardial blood flow has the potential to prevent irreversible injury of the outer portion of the myocardial wall. Ultimate recovery of contractile function, therefore, would be inversely related to the amount of myocardial wall sustaining irreversible injury relative to the amount of stunned myocardium in the vascular territory at risk. Thus, limitation of infarct size by early restoration of blood flow to the zone of ischemic injury would be clinically desirable.

A case report illustrates this concept.[68] A 64-year-old man with an acute anterior infarction was treated within 3 hours of the onset of chest pain with intravenous streptokinase. The patient's chest pain resolved, and there were several brief episodes of ventricular tachycardia, indicating successful reperfusion of the infarct-related artery. Coronary angiography on the first hospital day revealed a 60 percent stenosis of the left anterior descending artery, and the patient was treated medically. The peak creatine kinase plasma level was 1142 U/L (normal 40 to 180 U/L), whereas the peak plasma creatine kinase-MB level was 71.5 EU/L (normal < 3.5 EU/L). The initial electrocardiogram revealed a loss of anterior R waves, ST-segment elevation in V_1 through V_5, and small Q waves in V_2 and V_3. On serial tracings, a Q-wave infarction did not evolve, but at 2 weeks, the patient had persistent ST-segment elevation and T-wave inversion in V_2 through V_6 (Fig. 71–8). Echocardiography revealed severe anterior and apical hypokinesis with a global left ventricular ejection fraction of 40 percent.

On infarct-avid scintigraphy with ^{111}In-antimyosin antibody fragments, prominent tracer uptake was noted in the septal, anterior, and apical regions of the ventricle, indicating acute myocardial necrosis (see Fig. 71–8). Positron emission tomography with ^{13}N-ammonia and ^{18}F-2-fluoro-2-deoxyglucose, performed on the fifth hospital day, revealed perfusion defects in the anterior, apical, and superior septal regions of the ventricle, which generally corresponded with the focal areas of uptake of ^{111}In-antimyosin uptake (see Fig. 71–8). Metabolic imaging revealed a concordant reduction in tracer activity in the apical region (consistent with irreversible tissue injury) but preserved tracer uptake in the hypoperfused septal and anterior segments (indicating myocardial viability). Thus, the ^{111}In-antimyosin and glucose metabolic studies identified an admixture of necrotic and viable myocardium in the septal and anterior segments and a completed infarction at the ventricular apex.

The patient was discharged on medical therapy and did well over the ensuing 2 months. A second positron emission tomographic study revealed improved perfusion in the septal and anterior regions and a persistent apical defect (see Fig. 71–8). On the metabolic images, exogenous glucose use had normalized in the septal and anterior segments, whereas the defect in the apical segment persisted. On stress echocardiography at 6 months, the patient's resting electrocardiogram was essentially normal (see Fig. 71–8). With exercise to a heart rate of 153 beats per minute and a blood pressure of 180/80 mm Hg, there were no ST-segment changes to suggest exercise-induced ischemia. On the baseline echocardiogram, the apex was akinetic to dyskinetic and there was normal function in the remaining ventricular segments. The resting left ventricular ejection fraction was 58 percent and it increased to 88 percent with exercise.

This case study illustrates the utility of glucose metabolic imaging for early myocardial tissue characterization in patients with acute infarction. Despite identification of cellular necrosis with ^{111}In-antimyosin, positron emission tomography with ^{13}N-ammonia and ^{18}F-2-fluoro-2-deoxyglucose indicated that substantial amounts of viable tissue persisted in the clinical infarct region, suggesting that thrombolysis had prevented transmural extension of the patient's infarction. Perhaps more importantly, early identification of tissue glucose metabolic activity predicted the delayed recovery of wall motion in the stunned myocardium in the septal and anterior segments.

In order to examine the relationships among recovery of myocardial blood flow, oxidative metabolism, and regional function following thrombolytic therapy for acute infarction, Henes and coworkers[69] performed positron emission tomography with oxygen-15 water and ^{11}C-acetate in eight patients with acute myocardial infarction treated with tissue-type plasminogen activator (t-PA). Seven of the eight patients had infarct-related artery patency con-

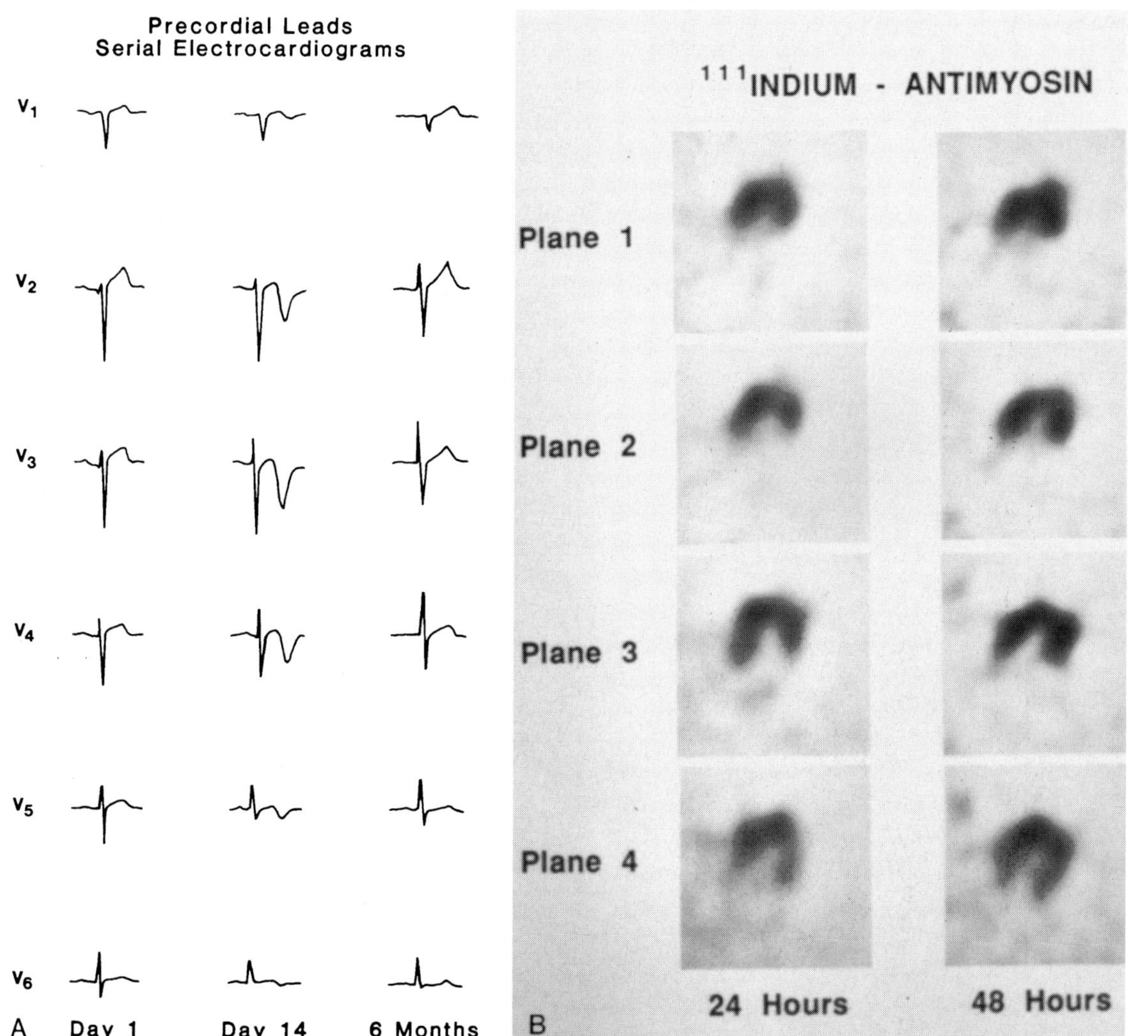

FIGURE 71–8. *Panel A,* Serial precordial electrocardiographic tracings obtained from a 64-year-old man with an acute anterior myocardial infarction who was treated with streptokinase. The initial set of tracings, obtained on the day of admission, demonstrate ST-segment elevation in leads V_1 through V_5. On the second set of tracings, obtained 2 weeks following the onset of chest pain, there is persistent ST-segment elevation and T-wave inversion in leads V_2 through V_6. By 6 months, there is relatively normal R-wave progression and only minor ST-T changes. Associated with the acute episode of chest pain was an elevation in the creatine kinase-MB level to 71.5 EU/L (normal = 0.0 to 3.5 EU/L). In light of the serial changes in enzymes, the clinical diagnosis of acute non-Q wave anterior myocardial infarction was established. *Panel B,* Representative single-photon emission tomographic ^{111}In-antimyosin images obtained 24 and 48 hours following the onset of chest pain in the patient whose electrocardiographic tracings are displayed in *Panel A.* In this display, the left ventricle points to the upper right-hand corner of the images. There is prominent uptake of the labeled antimyosin in the septum and anteroapical region of the ventricle, indicating an acute anteroseptal and anteroapical myocardial infarction.

Illustration continued on following page

firmed by angiography. Absolute myocardial blood flows were determined from the dynamic ^{15}O-water study, whereas ^{11}C-acetate clearance constants were derived from monoexponentially fitting myocardial ^{11}C time activity curves. Changes in segmental wall motion were identified on two-dimensional echocardiography.

Positron emission tomographic imaging was performed 18±6 hours, 45±5 hours and 8.6±7 days after t-PA administration. Absolute myocardial blood flow in the region of clinical infarction averaged 1.16±0.60 mL · g^{-1} · min^{-1} on the early postthrombolytic study and did not differ significantly at 45 hours (1.00±0.34 mL · g^{-1} · min^{-1} or at 9 days (1.26±0.25 mL · g^{-1} · min^{-1}). Blood flows were comparable in reperfused and remote normal myocardium at each time point.

In contrast, regional myocardial oxygen consumption in reperfused myocardium was significantly reduced relative to that in normal myocardium on each of the three imaging studies. As estimated from the monoexponential tissue clearance rate constants for ^{11}C-acetate, myocardial oxygen consumption averaged only 45±25 percent of that in reference myocardium on the initial study, 59±16 percent of normal at 45 hours, and 68±17 percent on day 9 ($P < .01$ relative to normal for all three times). ^{11}C-acetate clearance constants in reperfused myocardium were significantly improved relative to the early postthrombolytic study only at 9 days, indicating that recovery of oxidative substrate metabolism was delayed relative to restoration of blood flow. Improved wall motion was noted in six patients and tended to parallel recovery of oxidative substrate metabolism.

In order to test the hypothesis that positron emission tomographic imaging would identify differences in regional oxidative metabolism in acutely infarcted, hypoperfused myocardium with and without preserved glucose metabolism, Vanoverschelde and colleagues[70] performed dynamic positron emission tomographic im-

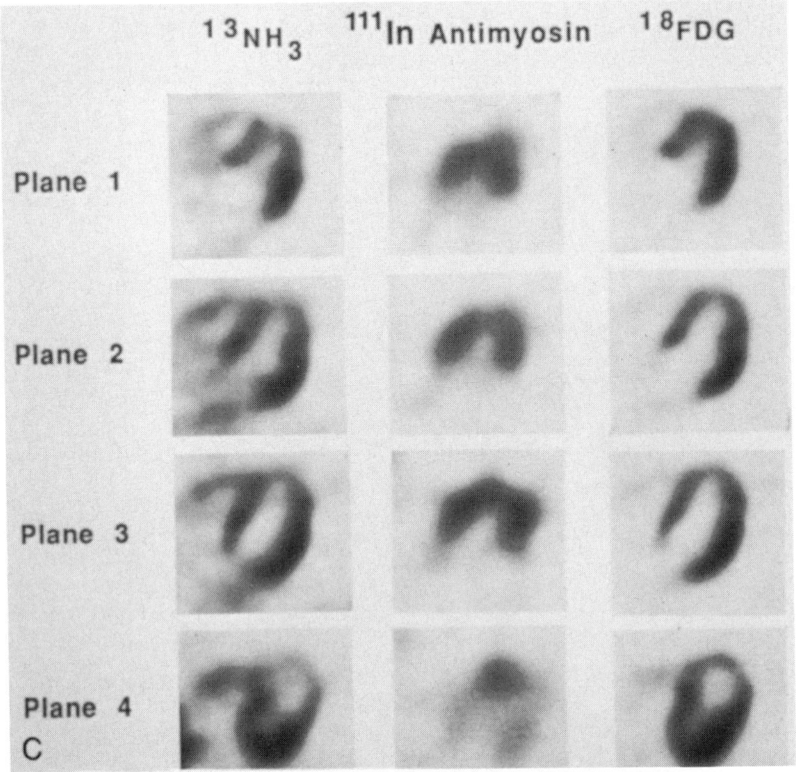

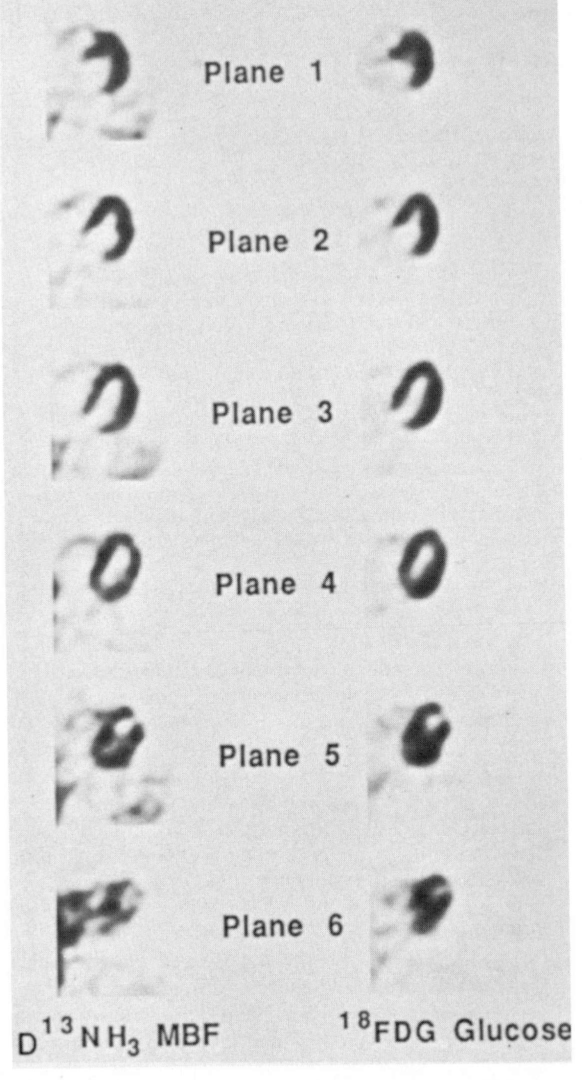

FIGURE 71–8 *Continued Panel C,* Corresponding ^{13}N-ammonia (*$^{13}NH_3$*) perfusion and ^{18}F-2-fluoro-2-deoxyglucose (*^{18}FDG*) metabolic images in the patient whose ^{111}In-antimyosin study is displayed in *Panel B.* On the ^{13}N-ammonia perfusion images defects present in the anteroseptal and anteroapical region correspond to the areas with ^{111}In-antimyosin. In the more superior aspect of the heart, glucose use is well preserved on the ^{18}F-2-fluoro-2-deoxyglucose metabolic images, indicating residual tissue viability. There is a small apical area that exhibits a concordant reduction in ^{18}F-2-fluoro-2-deoxyglucose uptake, consistent with completed infarction. *Panel D,* Repeat positron emission tomographic study in the same patient 8 weeks later. Concordant decreases in perfusion and glucose metabolism are noted in a small apical area of the ventricle, indicating completed infarction. Perfusion and glucose metabolism are essentially normal in the anterior segment and the interventricular septum. The resting left ventricular ejection fraction increased from 40 to 58 percent and segmental function in the septal and anterior segments improved from dyskinesia to normal. The apical segment remained akinetic to dyskinetic. Thus, positron emission tomography identified a large area of stunned myocardium that was successfully salvaged by thrombolytic therapy and correctly predicted the observed improvement in segmental wall motion. (From Brunken, R. C., and Schelbert, H. R.: Acute myocardial infarction: A case for metabolic imaging. Leading Edge Cardiol. 3:1, 1989, with permission.)

aging in 15 patients with reperfused anterior myocardial infarction using ^{13}N-ammonia, ^{11}C-acetate, and ^{18}F-2-fluoro-2-deoxyglucose. The patient population was composed of individuals admitted for a first acute anterior myocardial infarction who were treated either with thrombolytic therapy or intravenous heparin. The average time interval from the onset of chest pain to the beginning of thrombolytic therapy was 207 ± 183 minutes, and peak serum levels of creatine kinase averaged 2393 ± 1249 IU/L (normal is 40 to 160 IU/L).

Anterior Q waves developed on the electrocardiograms of each of the patients, and patency of the infarct-related artery was confirmed in each individual by angiography (mean residual diameter stenosis = 80 ± 11 percent). Seven individuals had anterior dyskinesis, seven patients had anterior akinesis, and one patient had mild anterior hypokinesis. The left ventricular ejection fraction ranged from 29 to 70 percent and averaged 52 ± 11 percent. Twelve of the 15 patients had stress and 4-hour redistribution planar thallium imaging. Nine of the 12 patients had persistent anterior ^{201}Tl defects, whereas 3 had transient anterior ^{201}Tl defects.

Eight of the 15 patients had concordant reductions in both flow and glucose metabolism on circumferential profile analysis. Five individuals had perfusion-metabolism mismatches throughout the infarct area, whereas two patients exhibited perfusion-metabolism mismatches at the periphery of the infarction. Twenty-four myocardial segments had mismatches, whereas 38 segments had matching defects. Segments with perfusion-metabolism mismatches had wall motion scores that were as poor as the segments with matching perfusion and glucose metabolic defects.

Relative ^{13}N-ammonia activity averaged 60 ± 10 percent in segments with perfusion-metabolism mismatches and 61 ± 14 percent in segments with matching defects (P = NS). Thus, assessment of relative myocardial perfusion alone would not have distinguished between hypoperfused segments with and those without preserved glucose metabolic activity. Absolute myocardial blood flows were 0.80 ± 0.14 $mL \cdot g^{-1} \cdot min^{-1}$ and 0.87 ± 0.18 $mL \cdot g^{-1} \cdot min^{-1}$ in remote normal myocardium of the patients with matches and mismatches, respectively. Myocardial segments with perfusion-metabolism mismatches had higher blood flows than the segments with matching defects (0.54 ± 0.13 $mL \cdot g^{-1} \cdot min^{-1}$ versus 0.45 ± 0.08 $mL \cdot g^{-1} \cdot min^{-1}$, $P < .01$). However, there was considerable overlap in the absolute blood flow measurements in the two groups.

Relative ^{18}F-2-fluoro-2-deoxyglucose concentrations in mismatched segments were 108 ± 26 percent, whereas those in the segments with matching defects averaged 60 ± 15 percent. As anticipated, ratios of absolute rates of glucose consumption in hypoperfused regions relative to normal myocardial areas were higher in the segments with perfusion-metabolism mismatches than in the hypoperfused segments with matching metabolic defects (0.23 ± 0.36 versus 0.59 ± 0.19).

Rates of ^{11}C-acetate clearance in the myocardial segments with perfusion-metabolism mismatches were significantly higher than those in the segments with matching perfusion and glucose metabolic defects (0.035 ± 0.014 min^{-1} versus 0.023 ± 0.009 min^{-1}, $P < .01$). A strong linear relationship was noted between absolute myocardial blood flow measurements and ^{11}C-acetate clearance constants. Thus, the differences in ^{11}C-acetate clearance constants in the segments with and those without perfusion-metabolism mismatches paralleled the differences in absolute myocardial blood flow measurements, irrespective of the presence or absence of a perfusion-metabolism mismatch.

Gropler and coworkers[71] sought to determine the importance of oxidative substrate metabolism for the recovery of regional function after revascularization in patients with acute myocardial infarction. They performed positron emission tomographic imaging with ^{15}O-water, ^{11}C-acetate, and ^{18}F-2-fluoro-2-deoxyglucose in 11 patients with acute myocardial infarction approximately 6 days following the acute event. The findings on positron emission tomography were then correlated with changes in regional function observed on echocardiography following coronary revascularization (eight percutaneous transluminal coronary angioplasty, three coronary artery bypass surgery). Dysfunctional but viable myocardium was distinguished from nonviable myocardium by postoperative improvement in regional function following revascularization. Repeat positron emission tomography was performed in nine individuals at 3.3 months (range of 1.5 to 10 months) following revascularization.

Sixty-two segments were examined in the 11 patients. On comparison of segmental wall motion before and after coronary revascularization, 33 segments were considered normal, 19 were classified dysfunctional but viable, and 10 had no improvement in function and were considered nonviable. Before coronary revascularization, segmental wall motion scores were comparable in the viable and nonviable dysfunctional segments, and both were significantly poorer than those in normal segments. Relative myocardial perfusion averaged 70.2 ± 21 percent of peak normal in hypoperfused, viable segments and 57.8 ± 19.6 percent in the nonviable segments ($P < .02$ versus normal segments; P = NS for viable versus nonviable).

^{11}C-acetate clearance constants (k_1), as indicators of regional oxidative metabolism, averaged 0.065 ± 0.02 min^{-1} in normal segments, 0.048 ± 0.018 min^{-1} in viable segments, and 0.029 ± 0.007 min^{-1} in nonviable segments. Ratios of relative regional glucose use to relative myocardial blood flow were variable but were significantly higher in viable segments (1.32 ± 0.67) than in normal segments (0.98 ± 0.15; $P < .02$). Although the ratios in viable myocardium also tended to be higher than those in nonviable myocardium (1.08 ± 0.58), this difference did not achieve statistical significance. Following revascularization, perfusion, oxidative metabolism, and glucose use to blood flow ratios in the viable segments no longer differed from those in normal segments. Although these parameters also improved in nonviable myocardium, they remained significantly depressed relative to normal values. The authors concluded that assessment of regional oxidative metabolism with positron emission tomography can facilitate identification of viable myocardium in patients with acute myocardial infarction and assist in identifying individuals likely to benefit from coronary revascularization.

Kalff and colleagues[72] demonstrated a direct effect of β-blockade on regional myocardial oxygen consumption. Dynamic positron emission tomography with ^{11}C-acetate was performed in 31 patients with acute myocardial infarction who were treated either with acute angioplasty or thrombolytic therapy. Twenty-four patients were imaged within 4 days and seven patients were studied within 8 days of the acute event. Eighteen individuals had anterior infarctions, and 13 had either inferior or lateral infarctions. Rates of ^{11}C-acetate clearance in the patients were compared with those obtained from the study of six healthy male volunteers.

On the 2- to 4-minute ^{11}C-acetate positron emission tomographic images, the area of clinical infarction was defined by a reduction in the initial uptake of the radiolabeled tracer. The initial myocardial uptake of ^{11}C-acetate reflects relative regional myocardial blood flow,[73, 74] and therefore the images obtained early following its intravenous administration can be used to assess relative myocardial perfusion. Regions of interest were defined over clinical infarct regions as well as in normal reference myocardium.

Rate constants for the clearance of ^{11}C-acetate averaged 0.051 ± 0.006 min^{-1} in normal volunteers and were substantially higher than those in the regions of anterior infarction (0.025 ± 0.010 min^{-1}) or inferior and lateral infarctions (0.034 ± 0.010 min^{-1}; $P < .008$ for both). Rate constants for regions of anterior myocardial infarction were significantly lower ($P < .04$) than those of inferior or lateral infarctions. Interestingly, washout rate constants of remote myocardium in patients with anterior infarction (0.60 ± 0.017 min^{-1}) and inferior and lateral infarcts (0.065 ± 0.011 min^{-1}) were slightly but significantly higher ($P < .04$) than those in the normal volunteers. This may reflect differences in regional myocardial workload. For both remote and infarct-related ^{11}C-acetate clearance constants, there was a significant linear relationship between rate-pressure product as a clinical index of myocardial oxygen consumption and k_{mono}.

The authors performed a multivariate regression analysis to examine the factors related to the observed regional ^{11}C-acetate clearance constants. Variables that were included in the statistical model included rate-pressure product; use of β-blockers; use of other medications, such as nitrates, angiotensin-converting enzyme inhibitors, digoxin, calcium channel blockers; and the left ventricular ejection fraction. Rate-pressure product was related to rates of ^{11}C-acetate clearance in infarct regions (P = .005), whereas both rate-pressure product and β-blockade were correlated to ^{11}C-acetate clearance constants in remote myocardium (P = .025 for rate-pressure product; P = .02 for β-blockade). Thus, β-blockade had no significant effect on myocardial oxygen consumption within the zone of clinical infarction, but separately and independently of rate-pressure product resulted in a reduction in ^{11}C-acetate clearance constants in remote tissue.

The authors also examined the effect of other clinical variables on the observed ^{11}C-acetate clearance constants. On stepwise multiple regression analysis, the time from the onset of symptoms to opening of the infarct artery and location of infarct were significantly related to ^{11}C-acetate kinetics in the infarct territory. The authors concluded that an analysis of ^{11}C-acetate kinetics from dynamic positron emission tomographic imaging in patients with acute infarction can assist in determining the degree and extent of infarct-related injury. In addition, the authors considered that the technique may prove helpful in assessing the efficacy of pharmacologic treatment of acute myocardial infarction by providing objective measurements of regional oxygen consumption. These measurements could be used to optimize clinical management to reduce myocardial damage and enhance tissue recovery. Further clinical studies appear to be warranted.

Czernin and associates[75] correlated regional myocardial perfusion, oxidative metabolism, and glucose consumption in 22 patients with recent myocardial infarction. Fourteen patients had Q-wave infarctions, whereas six individuals had non-Q wave infarctions. Two patients had left bundle branch block, precluding the diagnosis of either Q-wave or non–Q-wave infarction. The peak creatine phosphokinase and creatine kinase-MB levels averaged 1357 ± 865 and 74 ± 66 U/L, respectively. Eight patients were treated with thrombolytic therapy within 8 hours, whereas direct angioplasty was performed in two patients within 8 hours of the onset of chest pain.

Positron emission tomography was performed 86 ± 38 hours (range 21 to 170 hours) following the onset of chest pain. Sixteen of the patients had imaging with ^{13}N-ammonia, ^{11}C-acetate, and ^{18}F-2-fluoro-2-deoxyglucose, whereas six patients had imaging with ^{13}N-ammonia and ^{18}F-2-fluoro-2-deoxyglucose only. Segmental wall motion was assessed with two-dimensional echocardiography on the day of the study. Regional wall motion was graded on a four-point scale, where 3 = normal, 2 = mild hypokinesis, 1 = severe hypokinesis, and 0 = akinesis-dyskinesis. An echocardiographic wall motion score was derived by dividing the sum of all echocardiographic scores for each of seven anatomical segments by the number of projections on which the segment was visualized.

In the 22 patients, flow and metabolism were assessed in 154 anatomical segments. Of the 51 hypoperfused segments, 29 exhibited concordant reductions in perfusion and glucose metabolism, whereas 22 exhibited perfusion-metabolism mismatches. The severity of the regional wall motion abnormalities in the clinical infarct zones ranged from mild hypokinesis to akinesis, and wall motion scores in the segments with perfusion-metabolism mismatches were as poor as those in segments with matching perfusion and metabolic defects.

In normal segments, resting myocardial blood flows averaged 0.83 ± 0.2 mL · g^{-1} · min^{-1}. In myocardial segments with perfusion-metabolism mismatches, mean blood flows were 0.57 ± 0.2 mL · g^{-1} · min^{-1}, significantly higher than those observed in segments with matching perfusion and metabolic defects, 0.32 ± 0.12 mL · g^{-1} · min^{-1} (P < .05). The relative flow reduction in the areas of perfusion-metabolism mismatches averaged 65 ± 20 percent, as compared to 42 ± 18 percent in areas with matching perfusion and metabolic defects (P < .05). There was, however, considerable overlap in both the absolute and relative myocardial blood flow values in the segments with matched and the segments with mismatched defects.

Rates of ^{11}C-acetate clearance were determined in 76 normal segments, 17 segments with perfusion-metabolism mismatches, and 9 segments with matching defects (16 patients). In normal myocardium, ^{11}C-acetate clearance rates averaged 0.063 ± 0.012 min^{-1}, significantly higher than in segments with either matching defects, 0.037 ± 0.010 min^{-1}, or segments with perfusion-metabolism mismatches, 0.055 ± 0.010 min^{-1} (P < .05 for all pairwise comparisons). Relative reductions in ^{11}C-acetate clearance constants were 84 ± 15 percent in segments with perfusion-metabolism mismatches and 52 ± 19 percent in segments with matching defects (P < .05 for all pairwise comparisons).

Rates of exogenous glucose use averaged 0.57 ± 0.28 μmol · g^{-1} · min^{-1} in 93 normal segments, significantly higher than the 0.41 ± 0.20 μmol · g^{-1} · min^{-1} noted in the 22 segments with perfusion-metabolism mismatches and the 0.20 ± 0.10 μmol · g^{-1} · min^{-1} noted in the segments with the concordant perfusion and metabolic defects (P < .05 for all pairwise comparisons). Relative ^{18}F-2-fluoro-2-deoxyglucose concentrations averaged 35 ± 15 percent in the segments with perfusion-metabolism matches and 100 ± 16 percent in segments with mismatches. Thus relative to blood flow, glucose consumption was strikingly increased in the myocardial segments with perfusion-metabolism mismatches. Myocardial blood flows and rates of ^{11}C-acetate clearance in normal myocardium were correlated linearly with the rate-pressure product as an index of cardiac work.

No correlation was noted between absolute myocardial blood flows and rates of glucose consumption, likely reflecting differences in dietary and hormonal state as well as regional cardiac workload. When glucose metabolic rates and absolute myocardial blood flows were normalized to values in reference myocardium, reductions in relative glucose use paralleled those in blood flow in the segments with the matching perfusion and metabolic defects. As anticipated, relative rates of glucose use exceeded relative blood flows in the segments with perfusion-metabolism mismatches (Fig. 71–9).

In contrast, ^{11}C-acetate clearance constants, as indices of myocardial substrate oxidative metabolism, were correlated significantly with absolute myocardial blood flows. As illustrated in Figure 71–10, the relationship between k_{mono} and absolute myocardial blood flows was actually best described by a piecewise linear function with an inflection point at myocardial blood flow of 0.56 mL · g^{-1} · min^{-1} (Fig. 71–10). For absolute blood flows less than this value, the relationship was given as k_{mono} = 0.065 · myocardial blood flow + 0.017. For blood flows exceeding 0.56 mL · g^{-1} · min^{-1} the observed regression equation was k_{mono} = 0.03 · absolute myocardial blood flow + 0.037. Similar findings were noted when relative ^{11}C clearance constants and relative myocardial blood flows were plotted. The difference in the observed slopes at about 0.56 mL · g^{-1} · min^{-1} might reflect a critical threshold at which increases in oxygen extraction can no longer compensate for reductions in myocardial blood flow and oxygen delivery. Rates of oxygen consumption then fall more precipitously with more pronounced reductions in myocardial blood flow.

The findings are consistent with previously reported animal experimental observations.[76] Of interest was the observation that 17 (80 percent) of the 21 segments with greater than 30 percent reductions in k_{mono}, 17 (80 percent) had matching perfusion and glucose metabolic defects, whereas 13 of 14 (93 percent) segments with reductions in k_{mono} of less than 25 percent exhibited perfusion-metabolism mismatches. Thus, the data suggest that both a compensatory increase in oxygen extraction and glucose consumption are employed by hypoperfused myocardium to compensate for the impaired oxygen delivery in acute ischemic injury.

Synopsis of Findings in Acute Myocardial Infarction and Reperfusion

Myocardial infarction is a tissue injury characterized by both spatial and temporal inhomogeneity. Transient ventricular dysfunction caused by stunning of adjacent viable myocardium may render early estimation of the actual extent of tissue necrosis difficult. However, it is at this point, early in the course of an acute infarction, that therapy to restore blood flow is most successful in salvaging jeopardized myocardium and thereby limiting infarct size.

In animal models of acute ischemic injury, assessment of myocardial metabolism with positron emission tomography predicts eventual recovery of regional function more successfully than assessment of myocardial perfusion alone, primarily by providing a better estimate of the amount of stunned myocardium relative to that which has undergone necrosis. Tissue that has been stunned by an acute reduction in blood flow exhibits impaired oxidative substrate metabolism and an enhanced uptake of exogenous glucose. Because of the impaired supply of molecular oxygen, stunned myocardium may rely more on anaerobic glycolytic pathways to sustain cellular viability. Because cellular glycogen stores are rapidly depleted during ischemia, accelerated extraction of glucose from the vascular space is an important means of maintaining substrate for the glycolytic processes operant in stunned myocardium. This augmented glycolytic flux is manifested on positron emission tomography by an enhanced uptake of ^{18}F-2-fluoro-2-deoxyglucose relative to substrate delivery (blood flow). Following restoration of blood flow by thrombolysis, recovery of segmental function in stunned myocardium seems to parallel recovery of the altered metabolic state.

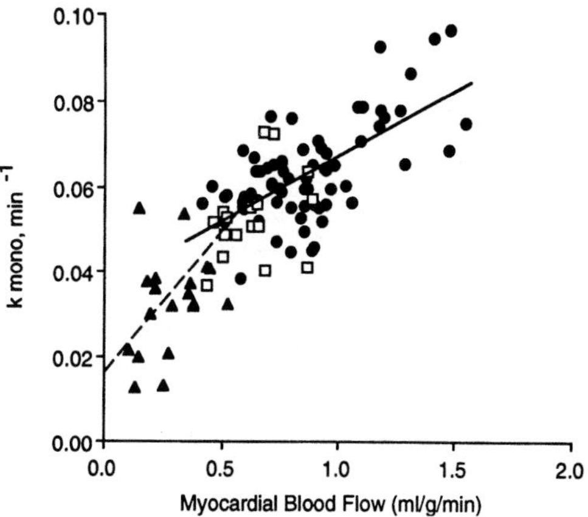

FIGURE 71–10. Relationship between k_{mono} measurements and absolute myocardial blood flows in patients with acute myocardial infarction. The data are best fit using a piecewise linear fit, with the best discrimination between the two pieces of the curve if an absolute blood flow value of 0.56 $mL \cdot g^{-1} \cdot min^{-1}$ is chosen as the break point. (From Czernin, J., Porenta, G., and Brunken, R., et al: Regional blood flow, oxidative metabolism and glucose utilization in patients with recent myocardial infarction. Circulation 88:891, 1993. With permission of the American Heart Association.)

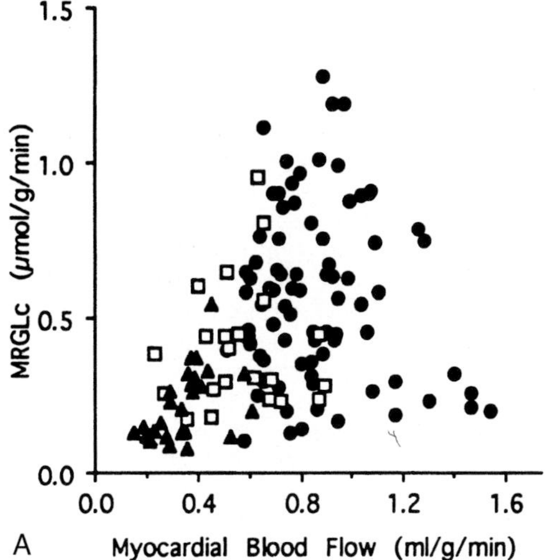

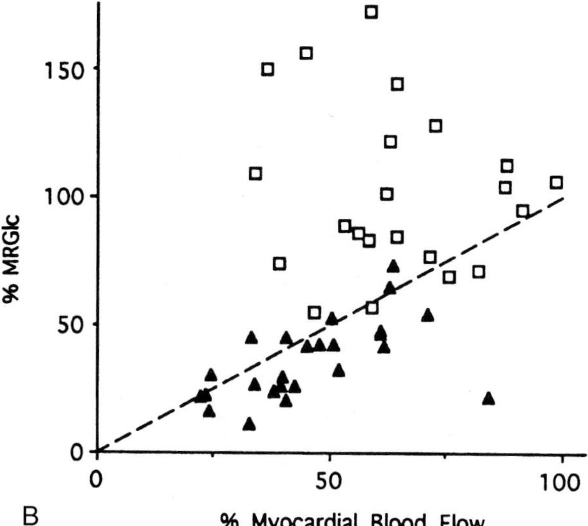

FIGURE 71–9. *Panel A,* Relationship between absolute rates of myocardial glucose consumption, in $\mu mol \cdot min^{-1} \cdot g^{-1}$ and absolute myocardial blood flows in $mL \cdot g^{-1} \cdot min^{-1}$ in patients with an acute myocardial infarction. *Panel B,* Relationship between normalized rates of glucose consumption and normalized blood flows. The black circles represent normal myocardium, the open boxes represent segments with perfusion-metabolism mismatches, and the black triangles represent segments with matching perfusion and metabolic defects. In the segments with perfusion-metabolism mismatches, normalized rates of glucose consumption exceed normalized blood flows, indicating an increase in glucose extraction. (From Czernin, J., Porenta, G., Brunken, R., et al.: Regional blood flow, oxidative metabolism and glucose utilization in patients with recent myocardial infarction. Circulation 88:891, 1993. With permission of the American Heart Association.)

Clinical studies of patients with acute myocardial infarction using positron emission tomography have demonstrated that myocardial infarction is an inhomogeneous process in humans as well as in the laboratory animal. Metabolic imaging reveals impairment of fatty acid and oxidative metabolism in the clinical infarct zone. Oxidative substrate flux in myocardium remote from the infarct region may actually be increased, perhaps as a result of the compensatory increase in regional myocardial work.

On metabolic imaging, a lack of residual tissue glucose metabolism or a markedly reduced rate of oxidative substrate metabolism in the hypoperfused infarct zone often presages a persistent depression in regional wall motion, suggesting completed infarction. In contrast, the presence of residual glucose metabolism or relatively maintained levels of oxidative substrate metabolism in the zone of infarction is associated with a more variable functional outcome, suggesting viable myocardium. Correlative studies with coronary angiography suggest that angiographically visible collateral vessels might not consistently exert a beneficial effect on myocardial metabolic viability in the clinical infarct region. Residual antegrade blood flow through the infarct vessel does appear to exert a favorable effect on regional metabolic viability, however, and several reports suggest that thrombolytic therapy or mechanical intervention to open the infarct-related artery affects the metabolic integrity and functional recovery of the affected region beneficially.

ASSESSMENT OF TISSUE VIABILITY IN CHRONIC CORONARY ARTERY DISEASE

Early patient studies employing positron emission tomography with ^{18}F-2-fluoro-2-deoxyglucose clearly indicated that residual tissue glucose metabolism could be identified in hypoperfused human myocardium. However, the clinical implications of these observations were uncertain. Although laboratory investigations indicated that exogenous glucose use was accelerated both in acutely ischemic tissue and in reperfused myocardium and that the metabolic findings correlated with the histologic presence of significant amounts of viable myocytes, it was unclear whether these observations could be extrapolated to patients with ischemic heart disease and, further, whether they would affect patient care. In particular, it was unknown whether identification of tissue glucose metabolism in hypoperfused ventricular regions in individual subjects would indeed indicate that clinically significant amounts of viable tissue were present. Thus, clinical studies were undertaken to determine if metabolic imaging with positron emission tomography could reliably identify viable tissue in patients with ischemic heart disease and, further, to determine how the metabolic assessment of myocardial viability would translate into improvement in regional and global ventricular function if coronary blood flow were restored.

Effect of Revascularization on Hypoperfused, Metabolically Active Tissue

To test the hypothesis that the presence of glucose metabolism in hypoperfused or dysfunctional myocardium, or both, represents clinically important tissue viability, Tillisch and coinvestigators[77] studied patients with resting wall motion abnormalities prior to elective coronary bypass surgery. The findings on positron emission tomography with ^{13}N-ammonia and ^{18}F-2-fluoro-2-deoxyglucose prior to revascularization were compared with postoperative changes in segmental function. Because scar tissue is both avascular and metabolically inert, asynergic myocardial segments with concordant reductions in perfusion and glucose metabolism were not expected to improve in function following revascularization. In contrast, segments with metabolically active tissue (either the metabolism-perfusion mismatch of myocardial ischemia or segments with a relatively normal perfusion and metabolic pattern) were predicted to exhibit improved function once blood flow had been restored.

The study population consisted of 17 patients referred for coronary artery bypass surgery who had resting regional wall motion abnormalities identified on either contrast left ventriculography (4 patients) or radionuclide angiography (13 patients). Indications for coronary revascularization included double- or triple-vessel coronary artery disease with an ejection fraction less than 40 percent in 11 patients, persistent angina or a positive stress test at a low workload after myocardial infarction in 5 patients, and angina refractory to medical therapy in 1 patient. Sixteen of the 17 patients had histories of antecedent myocardial infarction. Two patients had positron emission tomography within 2 weeks of an acute myocardial infarction, whereas the remaining 15 were studied 8 weeks (range of 6 to 14 weeks) after myocardial infarction. Segmental wall motion abnormalities were graded on a scale of 0 (normal) to 4 (dyskinesis) in seven myocardial segments. Following coronary artery bypass surgery, follow-up wall motion studies were performed within 3 weeks in 2 patients, at 6 to 10 weeks in 2 patients, and at 12 to 18 weeks in the remaining 13 patients.

Prior to coronary artery bypass surgery, 73 segments with resting wall motion abnormalities were identified in the 17 patients. After revascularization, improvement in the mean segmental score of at least one grade occurred in 9 of 21 (43 percent) mildly hypokinetic, 21 of 37 (57 percent) severely hypokinetic, and 6 of 14 (43 percent) akinetic segments. The only dyskinetic segment also exhibited improved function. There was no correlation between the severity of a wall motion abnormality prior to surgery and the extent of functional improvement on the postoperative studies. Of the segments with normal function before operation, two septal segments exhibited deterioration in function on the postoperative wall motion studies.

Of the 73 segments with abnormal resting wall motion, 67 were adequately revascularized. Of 46 segments with preserved glucose metabolism, 41 were successfully revascularized. Of these 41 segments, 22 of 25 (88 percent) regions considered normal by circumferential profiles and 13 of 16 (81 percent) with the metabolism-perfusion mismatch of myocardial ischemia had improved wall motion postoperatively (Table 71–1). The mean segmental wall motion score in these segments improved significantly on the delayed study (2.0 ± 0.08 versus 0.6 ± 0.6, $P < .05$). Furthermore, in the 11 patients with preserved glucose metabolism in three or more asynergic segments, the mean left ventricular ejection fraction increased significantly from 30 ± 11 percent to 45 ± 14 percent following coronary revascularization (Table 71–2). This suggests that the patients with the largest amounts of jeopardized tissue derived the greatest benefit from revascularization, as determined by improvement in global left ventricular function. Three of the six segments with preserved glucose metabolism that did not exhibit improved function after revascularization were septal segments, in which determination of wall motion is complicated by the mechanical effects of the bypass operation itself.[78]

TABLE 71–1. POSITRON EMISSION TOMOGRAPHIC METABOLIC IMAGING FOR RECOVERY OF LEFT VENTRICULAR FUNCTION AFTER REVASCULARIZATION

			Segments With Improved Wall Motion		
No. of Patients	Number of Segments	Procedure	*With ^{18}F-2-Fluoro-2-Deoxyglucose Uptake*	*No ^{18}F-2-Fluoro-2-Deoxyglucose Uptake*	Reference
17	67	CABG	35/41 (85%)	2/26 (8%)	Tillisch et al.[77]
22	46	CABG	18/23 (78%)*	5/23 (22%)	Tamaki et al.[79]
11	56	CABG	40/50 (80%)*	0/6 (0%)	Tamaki et al.[80]
16	85	PTCA, CABG	25/37 (68%)*	10/48 (21%)	Marwick et al.[81]
14	54	CABG	37/39 (95%)*	3/15 (20%)	Lucignani et al.[82]
21	23	CABG	16/19 (84%)	1/4 (25%)	Carrel et al.[83]
34	116	CABG, PTCA	38/73 (52%)	8/43 (19%)	Gropler et al.[84, 85]
48	90	PTCA, CABG	23/87 (85%)	10/63 (16%)	Knuuti et al.[86]
37	110	PTCA, CABG	24/59 (41%)†	7/51 (14%)†	vom Dahl et al.[87]
43	130	CABG, PTCA	45/59 (76%)*	6/71 (8%)	Tamaki et al.[88]
12‡	12	PTCA, CABG	12/12 (100%)	—	Vanoverschelde et al.[89]
20‡	20	CABG	8/12 (67%)	2/8 (25%)	Maes et al.[90]
Totals 295	809		321/451 (71%)	54/358 (15%)	

*Metabolic imaging performed in the fasting state.
†Segments with moderate hypokinesis or worse function.
‡Histopathologic correlation performed.
CABG = coronary artery bypass graft; PTCA = percutaneous transluminal coronary angioplasty.

TABLE 71–2. EFFECT OF REVASCULARIZATION AND LEFT VENTRICULAR EJECTION FRACTION

		Extensive Mismatch Region				Small or No Mismatch Region			
Reference	No. of Patients	*n*	*Pre-Left Ventricular Ejection Fraction*	*Post-Left Ventricular Ejection Fraction*	*P*	*n*	*Pre-Left Ventricular Ejection Fraction*	*Post-Left Ventricular Ejection Fraction*	*P*
Tillisch et al.[77]	17	11	30±11	45±14	<.05	6	30±11	31±12	NS
Marwick et al.[81]	24	9	37±11	40±9	NS	15	38±13	38±13	NS
Carrel et al.[83]	21	21	34±14	52±11	<.01	—	—	—	—
Lucignani et al.[82]	14	13	38±5	48±4	<.001	—	—	—	—
Depré et al.[91]	23	°	43±18	52±15	<.001		35±9	23±8	NS

°Values not given; n = number of patients with and without mismatches.

The results in the segments with concordant reductions in perfusion and glucose metabolism were strikingly different. Of the 27 segments with concordant reductions in perfusion and glucose metabolism, 26 were adequately revascularized. Of these 26 segments, 24 (92 percent) had no improvement or further deterioration in wall motion following revascularization. In addition, the mean segmental wall motion score did not improve in these segments (2.4±0.5 versus 2.6±0.04, P = NS), implying that there was little functional benefit derived by revascularizing these myocardial regions. Thus, this study indicated that metabolic imaging with positron emission tomography and ^{18}F-2-fluoro-2-deoxyglucose had an 85 percent positive predictive accuracy and a 92 percent negative predictive accuracy for identifying segments with functional improvement following coronary revascularization. Although the study was limited by the heterogeneity in the intervals from revascularization to postoperative determination of segmental function and by use of only a semiqualitative method to assess the anatomical extent of reversibly compromised tissue, this study was the first to indicate the utility of metabolic imaging for identifying viable but functionally compromised tissue that will benefit from restoration of blood flow (see Table 71–1).

The Tillisch study noted three distinct patterns of blood flow metabolism in myocardial regions with impaired wall motion (Fig. 71–11).

PATTERN A. Both blood flow and metabolism were normal in this pattern. Eighty-eight percent of such segments had improved contractile function after revascularization. Thus, this pattern presumably represented stunned or "repetitively stunned" myocardium.

PATTERN B. In this pattern, blood flow was reduced yet glucose use was preserved or even elevated. Eighty-one percent of such segments had improved contractile function after revascularization. This pattern presumably represented "hibernating myocardium" or, depending on the severity of flow reduction, in nontransmural infarction coexisting with "hibernating" or "stunned myocardium." This pattern is referred to as perfusion-metabolism mismatch.

PATTERN C. Both perfusion and glucose use were concordantly reduced in pattern C. Ninety-two percent of such patterns failed to have improved contractile function after revascularization. This pattern is referred to as blood flow–metabolism match. The varying degrees of reduced blood flow and metabolic activity most likely represent various degrees of tissue necrosis or scar formation coexisting with normal myocardium.

FIGURE 71–11. See Color Plate 34.

Tamaki and coworkers[79] confirmed the findings of Tillisch and colleagues in 22 consecutive patients who were examined with ^{13}N-ammonia and ^{18}F-2-fluoro-2-deoxyglucose and positron emission tomography within the 4 weeks prior to coronary artery bypass grafting. Segmental wall motion by equilibrium radionuclide ventriculography was abnormal in 46 segments in 20 of the 22 patients. Positron emission tomography prior to surgery revealed concordantly reduced blood flow and glucose metabolism in 23 of the 46 segments with abnormal wall motion, whereas both blood flow and glucose uptake were normal in four segments and blood flow decreased but glucose uptake increased in 19 segments. Thus, abnormal wall motion was considered to be associated with ischemic but viable myocardium in 23 segments, whereas the remaining 23 segments were considered infarcted. When re-examined 5 to 7 weeks after surgery, wall motion had improved in 18 (78 percent) of the 23 segments with metabolic evidence of viability, but in only 5 (22 percent) of the other 23 segments with evidence of scar tissue on preoperative imaging (see Table 71–1). In this study, therefore, the positive predictive accuracy of metabolic imaging for predicting improvement in segmental function following revascularization was 78 percent and the negative predictive accuracy was 78 percent.

Although generally comparable to the findings of Tillisch and colleagues,[77] Tamaki and coworkers[79] reported a lower negative predictive accuracy of the blood flow–metabolism match. The value of only 78 percent as compared with 92 percent by Tillisch and coinvestigators[77] may have resulted from two methodologic differences. First, Tamaki and colleagues[79] examined all patients in the fasting state, in which low plasma insulin and glucose levels and high free fatty acid levels suppressed ^{18}F-2-fluoro-2-deoxyglucose uptake in normal myocardium and in which only ischemic but viable myocardium characteristically exhibits tracer uptake. In contrast, Tillisch and associates[77] examined patients after glucose loading, resulting in ^{18}F-2-fluoro-2-deoxyglucose uptake in both ischemic and normal myocardium. Thus, the approach of Tamaki and coworkers detected even subtle increases in uptake of ^{18}F-2-fluoro-2-deoxyglucose, possibly caused by only small amounts of viable myocardium, which, if revascularized, may not have resulted in an improvement of segmental wall motion. Second, only visual inspection was employed for Tamaki and colleagues' metabolic image analysis, whereas Tillisch and coworkers submitted both the ^{13}N-ammonia perfusion and the ^{18}F-2-fluoro-2-deoxyglucose images to circumferential profile analysis of regional myocardial tracer activity concentrations. Viable myocardial regions were identified only if the difference between blood flow and glucose used exceeded 2 SD of a normal control population. It is therefore likely that Tamaki and colleagues' approach is more sensitive for detecting myocardial viability, whereas the approach used by Tillisch and associates is more specific for identifying myocardium in which contractile function will improve if blood flow is restored.

In a subsequent study, Tamaki and coinvestigators[80] correlated changes in regional wall motion following coronary revascularization in 11 coronary artery disease patients with the findings on ^{201}Tl reinjection scintigraphy and on positron emission tomography with ^{18}F-2-fluoro-2-deoxyglucose (see Table 71–1). In the 11 patients, the authors identified 56 segments with preoperative wall motion abnormalities. Improved segmental function was noted in 40 segments, whereas the other 16 segments had no change or further deterioration in function. Forty (80 percent) of the 50 segments with preserved uptake of ^{18}F-2-fluoro-2-deoxyglucose on positron emission tomography had improved function, whereas none of the

6 segments without metabolic activity exhibited improved wall motion following revascularization. The positive and negative predictive accuracies of metabolic imaging for predicting improvement in segmental wall motion were therefore 80 and 100 percent, respectively. In contrast, 11 of 17 (65 percent) segments with "fill-in" and two of eight (25 percent) segments without "fill-in" on ^{201}Tl reinjection had improved function following revascularization, for positive and negative predictive accuracies of 65 and 75 percent, respectively. In this study, one quarter of the segments with persistent ^{201}Tl defects following reinjection exhibited preserved tissue metabolic viability on positron emission tomographic imaging with ^{18}F-2-fluoro-2-deoxyglucose, and both of the segments with persistent ^{201}Tl defects with improved function following revascularization had perfusion-metabolism mismatches on positron emission tomography.

Marwick and colleagues[81] examined the influence of coronary revascularization on both segmental function and perfusion and metabolism. Sixteen patients with previous myocardial infarction were studied using digitized two-dimensional echocardiography, rest and dipyridamole ^{82}Rb perfusion and postexercise ^{18}F-2-fluoro-2-deoxyglucose metabolic imaging before and 4.9±2.6 months following coronary revascularization (coronary angioplasty in nine patients and coronary artery bypass in seven patients). Segments were considered to harbor hibernating myocardium if the echocardiographic wall motion score improved by one or more grades following revascularization.

Of 85 segments with fixed perfusion defects and resting wall motion abnormalities on the preoperative studies, 35 (41 percent) had improved function following revascularization and were classified as hibernating, whereas 50 (59 percent) failed to improve and were considered scarred. Relative myocardial perfusion improved significantly in the hibernating segments (57±11 to 69±13 percent, P = .001) but was unchanged in the nonhibernating segments (55±13 to 58±13 percent, P = NS). On metabolic imaging with ^{18}F-2-fluoro-2-deoxyglucose, 25 (71 percent) of the 35 hibernating segments were considered viable, whereas 38 (76 percent) of the 50 nonhibernating segments were considered nonviable. The positive and negative predictive accuracies for poststress metabolic imaging for predicting functional improvement following revascularization were therefore 68 and 79 percent, respectively (see Table 71–1). The relatively low positive predictive accuracy may reflect the fact that metabolic imaging was performed in the fasting state and also the fact that these were poststress metabolic studies. If lactate levels increased with exercise, this would favor myocardial use of this substrate over glucose.

On the postoperative positron emission tomographic studies, relative ^{18}F-2-fluoro-2-deoxyglucose metabolic activity returned to the normal range in 25 of the 35 hibernating segments. In the 10 segments (four patients) with persistently elevated ^{18}F-2-fluoro-2-deoxyglucose, regional perfusion and function did not differ from the segments in which ^{18}F-2-fluoro-2-deoxyglucose activity had normalized. However, these 10 segments were characterized by more severe perfusion and metabolic abnormalities on the preoperative studies, suggesting that full cellular reversibility of ischemic damage might not have been achievable with revascularization. Conversely, a more pronounced temporal delay in recovery of function in these areas may have produced similar findings, as function was assessed relatively early following restoration of blood flow.

Using an imaging protocol incorporating SPECT perfusion imaging and positron emission tomographic metabolic imaging, Lucignani and coworkers[82] studied 14 patients with coronary artery disease prior to elective coronary artery bypass surgery. Myocardial perfusion and glucose metabolism were assessed on ^{99m}Tc-sestamibi SPECT and ^{18}F-2-fluoro-2-deoxyglucose positron emission tomographic images, respectively, in 70 segments. Of these 70 segments, 54 (77 percent) had abnormal function and 53 (76 percent) had abnormal perfusion prior to revascularization. Segmental wall motion improved in 37 (95 percent) of the 39 segments with preserved ^{18}F-2-fluoro-2-deoxyglucose uptake and remained unchanged in 12 (80 percent) of the 15 segments without ^{18}F-2-fluoro-2-deoxyglucose uptake. The overall positive and negative predictive accuracies for this dual imaging technique were therefore 95 and 80 percent, respectively (see Table 71–1). The mean left ventricular ejection fraction increased from 38±4.9 to 47.9±4.1 percent following coronary artery bypass surgery. The authors concluded that SPECT imaging with ^{99m}Tc-sestamibi and positron emission tomographic imaging with ^{18}F-2-fluoro-2-deoxyglucose is a reliable means of identifying hibernating myocardium in patients with coronary artery disease and left ventricular dysfunction prior to coronary artery bypass surgery.

Carrel and colleagues[83] performed positron emission tomographic imaging with ^{82}Rb and ^{18}F-2-fluoro-2-deoxyglucose in 23 patients with advanced coronary artery disease prior to bypass surgery. Rest and stress two-dimensional echocardiography and coronary angiography were performed before and after revascularization. In 21 patients with patent coronary bypass grafts, revascularization resulted in a significant improvement in both the resting left ventricular ejection fraction (34±14 to 52±11 percent, $P < .01$) and the exercise left ventricular ejection fraction (31±14 to 58±13 percent, $P < .01$). Of the 19 segments with perfusion-metabolism mismatches, 16 (84 percent) had improved function postoperatively, including 4 of 7 akinetic segments and 2 of 5 dyskinetic segments (see Table 71–1). Of the four segments with concordant perfusion and metabolic defects, only one (25 percent) had improved function after coronary revascularization.

Gropler and colleagues[84] sought to ascertain the importance of maintained oxidative substrate metabolism for predicting improvement in segmental function in chronic coronary artery disease patients. Positron emission tomography with ^{15}O-water, ^{11}C-acetate, and ^{18}F-2-fluoro-2-deoxyglucose was performed prior to coronary revascularization in 16 patients with chronic coronary artery disease. Eleven of the patients had clinical histories of prior myocardial infarction. Dysfunctional but viable myocardium was distinguished from nonviable myocardium by postoperative improvement in segmental function when assessed 3.1±2.2 months following revascularization.

Of the 95 segments examined, 42 were normal, 24 were dysfunctional but viable, and 29 were considered nonviable. Preoperatively, neither the severity of the resting wall motion abnormality nor the level of relative myocardial perfusion distinguished viable from nonviable dysfunctional segments (relative blood flow in viable segments = 69.2±22.5 percent versus 63.9±25.4 percent for nonviable). Rates of ^{11}C clearance (k_1 values) in viable segments were significantly higher than in the nonviable segments (0.061±0.014 min^{-1} versus 0.042±0.013 min^{-1}, $P < .003$) and did not differ significantly from values in the normal segments (0.064±0.015 min^{-1}). Relative rates of glucose use when normalized to relative myocardial perfusion averaged 1.24±0.41 in viable segments, 19 percent higher than in normal segments (1.04±0.24, $P < .01$). The corresponding ratios for the nonviable segments (1.33±0.85) did not differ statistically from those of the normal or viable segments. Of the 24 segments with enhanced uptake of ^{18}F-2-fluoro-2-deoxyglucose relative to perfusion, 19 (79 percent) were viable; of the 29 segments with matching ^{18}F-2-fluoro-2-deoxyglucose and perfusion defects, 24 (83 percent) were nonviable.

Eleven patients underwent positron emission tomographic imaging following revascularization. Both relative perfusion and ratios of glucose use to perfusion improved significantly in the viable segments. In contrast, nonviable myocardium exhibited persistent defects in perfusion, oxidative metabolism, and glucose metabolism. Thus, this study confirmed the accuracy of positron emission tomography with ^{18}F-2-fluoro-2-deoxyglucose for identifying reversibly dysfunctional myocardium in patients with chronic coronary artery disease. Although the authors also surmised that assessment of regional myocardial oxygen consumption with dynamic ^{11}C-acetate imaging can also identify patients likely to benefit from coronary revascularization, a specific or relative "threshold" for k_1 values was not established in this report.

In a subsequent report,[85] the same investigators sought to compare the relative clinical utilities of ^{11}C-acetate clearance rates and preserved glucose metabolism on imaging with ^{18}F-2-fluoro-2-deoxyglucose for identifying reversibly dysfunctional myocardium in patients with chronic coronary artery disease. The study population consisted of the 16 patients previously reported[84] and 18 additional patients studied with ^{11}C-acetate and ^{18}F-2-fluoro-2-deoxyglucose. Regional myocardial perfusion was assessed in the latter individuals using the initial ^{11}C-acetate images. ^{11}C-acetate clearance constants were deemed indicative of viable myocardium if they were within 2 SD of the mean normal segmental values observed in 10 healthy volunteers. For the normal volunteers, ^{11}C-acetate clearance constants ranged from 0.052 ± 0.007 min^{-1} in the apex to 0.057 ± 0.006 min^{-1} in the inferior wall. On the ^{18}F-2-fluoro-2-deoxyglucose studies, viable myocardium was considered present if segmental values were within 2 SD of the normal mean, and perfusion-metabolism mismatches were considered present if relative ^{18}F-2-fluoro-2-deoxyglucose values normalized for blood flow exceeded mean normal segmental value by greater than 2 SD. Dysfunctional but viable myocardium was again distinguished from nonviable myocardium by postoperative improvement in segmental function, as assessed approximately 2 months after coronary revascularization.

Regional function was examined in the 34 patients in 116 segments. Seventy segments exhibited no improvement in function following revascularization and were considered nonviable, whereas 46 segments improved functionally and were classified viable. Of the 60 segments considered viable on the ^{11}C-acetate studies, 40 (67 percent) exhibited improved wall motion after restoration of blood flow, whereas 50 (89 percent) of the 56 segments considered nonviable had no improvement on the postrevascularization wall motion studies. Thus, metabolic imaging with ^{11}C-acetate had a 67 percent positive and an 89 percent negative predictive accuracy when all segments were considered for identifying reversibly dysfunctional myocardial segments prior to revascularization. The authors also examined the data in segments with akinesis and dyskinesis. Of 26 severely dysfunctional segments considered viable on the ^{11}C-acetate studies, 22 (85 percent) had improved function after revascularization. Of 31 segments considered nonviable, 27 (87 percent) had no change or deterioration in function after intervention. Thus, in these severely dysfunctional segments, the positive and negative predictive accuracies for metabolic imaging with ^{11}C-acetate were 85 and 87 percent, respectively.

On the ^{18}F-2-fluoro-2-deoxyglucose metabolic studies, segments were considered viable if relative metabolic tracer concentrations were within 2 SD of the normal mean or if ratios of the relative ^{18}F-2-fluoro-2-deoxyglucose activity to relative perfusion exceeded 2 SD from the mean. Importantly, relative ^{18}F-2-fluoro-2-deoxyglucose concentrations were calculated by normalizing to peak ^{18}F concentrations rather than to ^{18}F activity in normally perfused myocardium. The authors reported that 38 (52 percent) of the 73 segments considered viable on the ^{18}F-2-fluoro-2-deoxyglucose studies exhibited improved function after revascularization, whereas 35 (81 percent) of the 43 segments considered nonviable did not have improved wall motion following intervention ($P < .01$ for both positive and negative predictive accuracies versus ^{11}C-acetate). Of the 31 severely dysfunctional segments with criteria for viability on the ^{18}F-2-fluoro-2-deoxyglucose studies, 21 (72 percent) had improved function after coronary revascularization, whereas 23 (82 percent) of the segments considered nonviable had no change or deterioration in function following intervention. For the severely dysfunctional segments, the positive and negative predictive accuracies for the ^{11}C-acetate and the ^{18}F-2-fluoro-2-deoxyglucose studies were not statistically different. When all segments were considered, analysis of receiver operating characteristic curves indicated that ^{11}C-acetate clearance constants were more robust for predicting functional recovery than estimates of glucose metabolism. The authors concluded that quantification of oxidative substrate metabolism by positron emission tomography and ^{11}C-acetate can accurately predict functional recovery of dysfunctional myocardial segments following coronary revascularization.

This study raises the question of which metabolic tracer is the best to use to identify clinically important viability in dysfunctional myocardial segments. First, although the observed negative predictive accuracy for ^{18}F-2-fluoro-2-deoxyglucose is generally comparable to other studies, the observed positive predictive accuracy is substantially lower than in most other clinical investigations in which glucose loading was performed prior to imaging. Although the reasons for this are unclear, it may relate in part to the manner in which ^{18}F-2-fluoro-2-deoxyglucose concentrations were normalized on the circumferential profile analysis. These investigators normalized ^{18}F activities in myocardial defect areas to the highest ^{18}F concentrations on the metabolic study. Because ^{18}F concentrations in abnormal myocardium can sometimes exceed those in normal myocardium, many imaging centers instead normalize ^{18}F activity to that in the best perfused area of the heart. In this way, interpatient variations in dietary and hormonal state are minimized.

Second, ^{11}C-acetate clearance constants were considered normal or abnormal based on the segmental values obtained in normal volunteers. Because absolute ^{11}C-acetate clearance constants reflect myocardial oxygen consumption, increases or decreases in myocardial workload (rate-pressure product) in the normal subjects would also increase or decrease the observed k_1 values. In addition, rate-pressure products may be higher in patients with coronary artery disease because of a tendency to higher heart rates and blood pressures. Comparison of absolute patient k_1 values to those in a normal database therefore assumes relatively comparable rate-pressure products in the patients and the normals used to generate the reference database. Finally, exponential curve-fitting is a time-consuming process, and the practicality of using rate constants derived from ^{11}C time-activity in the clinical environment has yet to be established. Further studies comparing the relative efficacy of metabolic imaging with ^{11}C-acetate and ^{18}F-2-fluoro-2-deoxyglucose for identifying clinically important myocardial viability would appear to be indicated.

Knuuti and coworkers[86] examined the utility of relative tissue concentrations of ^{18}F-2-fluoro-2-deoxyglucose for identifying reversibly dysfunctional myocardium in 48 patients with prior myocardial infarction. In addition to positron emission tomography with ^{18}F-2-fluoro-2-deoxyglucose, resting perfusion was also assessed in 43 patients using SPECT (^{201}Tl in 25 patients, ^{99m}Tc-sestamibi in 18 patients). On circumferential profile analysis, ^{18}F-2-fluoro-2-deoxyglucose concentrations were normalized to those in the myocardial segment with the highest tracer uptake on the perfusion images or (in the five patients without perfusion images) to myocardial areas that were without infarction and supplied by a normal coronary artery.

In the 48 patients, there were 90 segments with preoperative wall motion abnormalities that were successfully revascularized. Of these 90 segments, 27 had improved function following revascularization, whereas 63 had no improvement or deterioration in function. Initially, relative ^{18}F-2-fluoro-2-deoxyglucose tracer concentrations that were less than the mean normal values minus 2 SD were considered to represent nonviable myocardium, whereas values above this threshold were considered to represent viable myocardium. Using this criterion, 27 (54 percent) of 50 segments viable on the ^{18}F-2-fluoro-2-deoxyglucose studies had improved function after revascularization, whereas none of the 40 segments without metabolic criteria for viability improved. However, the authors suggested that the mean -2 SD might not be the optimal threshold to distinguish viable from nonviable myocardium. On closer inspection of their data, they found that a relative ^{18}F-2-fluoro-2-deoxyglucose concentration of 85 to 90 percent of peak normal values provided a positive predictive accuracy of 85 percent and a negative predictive accuracy of 84 percent, respectively (see Table 71–1) for improvement in segmental function following revascularization. This study illustrates the importance of appropriate normalization of ^{18}F-2-fluoro-2-deoxyglucose to healthy reference myocardium. In addition, variations in local practice may necessitate a sensitivity-specificity analysis such as that performed by these authors in order for the clinical imaging center to optimize the diagnostic performance of ^{18}F-2-fluoro-2-deoxyglucose metabolic imaging in that location for identifying myocardial viability.

vom Dahl and colleagues[87] analyzed the positron emission tomographic findings in 37 patients with advanced coronary artery disease undergoing elective coronary artery bypass surgery. The goal of the study was to correlate changes in segmental function following revascularization with the severity of the preoperative resting wall motion abnormality as well as with the findings on the ^{13}N-ammonia and ^{18}F-2-fluoro-2-deoxyglucose images. Each of the 37 patients had multivessel coronary artery disease. Global and segmental left ventricular function was assessed before and 13±13 weeks after revascularization using gated radionuclide ventriculography. Segmental wall motion was scored visually according to the following scale: 1 = normal, 2 = mild hypokinesis, 3 = severe hypokinesis, 4 = akinesis, and 5 = dyskinesis. Improvement in segmental function was defined by an improvement in wall motion score of one or more grades.

On the positron emission tomographic images, relative segmental tracer accumulation was scored visually according to the following scale: 1 = normal, 2 = slight reduction, 3 = severe reduction, 4 = tracer uptake comparable to background activity. The authors considered that segments with a normal perfusion score were viable and that segments with perfusion and metabolic scores greater than 2 were nonviable. In addition, segments with a metabolic score less than or equal to 2 and with a perfusion score minus the metabolic score less than 1 were deemed "viable without mismatch." Segments with an ^{18}F-2-fluoro-2-deoxyglucose score less than or equal to 2 and with a difference in perfusion and metabolic scores of 1 or greater were said to be "viable with mismatch." Thus, segments that appeared normal or had "incomplete" matching defects of modest severity or perfusion-metabolism mismatches were considered viable and therefore anticipated to derive functional improvement from coronary revascularization.

In the 37 patients, the authors identified 191 segments with resting wall motion abnormalities. Fifty of the segments were considered normal on positron emission tomography, 43 were classified as viable without mismatch, 36 were considered viable with mismatch, and 62 were considered nonviable. Mean wall motion scores improved significantly for the normal segments (1.54±0.66 versus 1.37±0.54, $P < .05$) and for the segments with perfusion-metabolism mismatches (2.24±1.09 versus 1.87±0.98, $P < .01$). In contrast, no significant change in mean wall motion scores was noted in either the segments classified as viable without mismatch (1.97±1.04 versus 1.92±0.95, P = NS) or in the nonviable segments (2.87±1.08 versus 2.82±1.06, P = NS).

Overall, the absence of viability on the ^{13}N-ammonia and ^{18}F-2-fluoro-2-deoxyglucose images had a high negative predictive accuracy of 86 percent for improvement in segmental function. However, the positive predictive accuracy for the presence of viability as defined by the authors was quite variable, ranging from 21 to 86 percent, depending on the severity of the associated wall motion abnormality and the scintigraphic pattern. The authors presented data for 110 segments with wall motion scores greater than or equal to 2 according to the pattern identified on positron emission tomography. Segments that were viable without mismatch had positive predictive accuracies ranging from 21 to 31 percent, with the best predictive accuracy noted in the segments that were akinetic or dyskinetic. Thus, segments exhibiting the pattern of an incomplete matching defect were not likely to derive functional improvement from restoration of blood flow, suggesting completed nontransmural myocardial infarction.

For segments appearing normal on positron emission tomography, positive predictive accuracies ranged from 53 to 75 percent, again increasing as the severity of the associated wall motion abnormality increased. For segments with perfusion-metabolism mismatches, positive predictive accuracies ranged from 48 percent for segments with mild hypokinesis to 86 percent for segments with akinesis or dyskinesis exclusive of the apex. Thus for all three categories of viability, the positive predictive accuracy of metabolic imaging with ^{18}F-2-fluoro-2-deoxyglucose progressively increased with increasing severity of associated wall motion abnormality. Conversely, the negative predictive accuracy for absence of viability on the ^{18}F-2-fluoro-2-deoxyglucose images was 100 percent for segments that were akinetic or dyskinetic.

The investigators also correlated the image findings with changes in global left ventricular function. Patients with an improvement in left ventricular ejection fraction of greater than 5 percent had significantly more viable segments (80±18 versus 60±16 percent, $P < .01$) than those with a smaller improvement in left ventricular ejection fraction. Seven patients with perfusion-metabolism mismatches in greater than 50 percent of revascularized segments had an average improvement in left ventricular ejection fraction of 7±7 percent, whereas 13 patients without perfusion-metabolism mismatches in revascularized segments had an average increase in left ventricular ejection fraction of 1±6 percent ($P < .05$). The 12 patients with an ejection fraction of less than or equal to 30 percent had a mean ejection fraction of 23±6 percent, which increased to 28±7 percent after surgery. In contrast, the 25 patients with baseline ejection fractions greater than 30 percent had essentially no increase in ejection fraction following revascularization, 39±7 percent versus 40±8 percent ($P < .05$ for change in ejection fraction versus patients with baseline ejection fractions ≤ 30 percent). The authors concluded that the predictive value of positron emission tomography with ^{18}F-2-fluoro-2-deoxyglucose for identifying viable myocardium that will benefit from revascularization is highest in left ventricular regions with severe dysfunction and perfusion-metabolism mismatches and, further, that all clinical information should be used for optimal selection of patients with advanced coronary artery disease and impaired ventricular function for revascularization.

This investigation illustrates the very real physiologic differences between hypoperfused ventricular regions with matching reductions in glucose metabolism and hypoperfused ventricular regions with glucose metabolism increased relative to blood flow. In the situation in which blood flow and metabolism are reduced in parallel, one might envision a situation in which subendocardial fibrosis coexists with essentially normal (adequately perfused) tissue in the middle and epicardial layers. Segmental dysfunction in this scenario reflects primarily the inability of the normal myocardium to compensate for the loss of contractility in the subendocardium. Transmural function would be unlikely to benefit further from revascularization of the affected segment, since the subendocardial scar will continue to dominate transmural function. The distinction among "normal," "viable without mismatch," and "nonviable" on positron emission tomography will then merely relate to the severity of the observed reductions in defect tracer activity on the positron emission tomographic images. Particularly for visual image analysis, it may be difficult to gauge the severity of the observed perfusion and metabolic defects accurately. Even with a circumferential profile technique, proper normalization of counts to peak tracer concentrations is essential to make the distinction between viable and nonviable myocardium. A major lesson from this study, therefore, is that "viable without mismatch" segments are almost as unlikely to exhibit functional improvement following revascularization as segments considered nonviable, probably because of the presence of considerable amounts of subendocardial scar.

The segment with a perfusion-metabolism mismatch represents a different pathophysiologic state. In this situation, viable tissue is "distressed" because the oxygen supply is inadequate for its needs. As a result, it compensates by increasing its consumption of exogenous glucose and by shutting down all noncritical energy-requiring functions. In this situation, it is possible to envision substantial amounts of viable myocardium that are dysfunctional because of compensatory down-regulation of contractile function and in which the accelerated consumption of exogenous glucose can be readily identified on positron emission tomography as a perfusion-metabolism mismatch. In this example, restoration of blood flow will be expected to be of benefit because the wall motion abnormality primarily results from dysfunction of viable tissue. Thus, the finding that perfusion-metabolism mismatches had the highest positive predictive accuracy for functional improvement is not surprising. It is also not surprising that the positive predictive accuracy for segments with relatively preserved function and perfusion-metabolism mismatches was lower than that for segments with more profound wall motion abnormalities. Since assessment of wall motion was performed using visual analysis only, it may have been more difficult to identify accurately further functional improvement in a segment in which baseline function was only marginally impaired. For the segments with pronounced dysfunction, the observed positive and negative predictive accuracies of 86 and 100 percent, respectively, agree reasonably well with the values of 85 and 92 percent initially reported by Tillisch and colleagues.[77] Thus, the study of vom Dahl and coworkers does not negate the previously reported observations indicating a high positive and negative predictive accuracy for identifying viable myocardium with positron emission tomography and metabolic imaging with ^{18}F-2-fluoro-2-deoxyglucose.

In a subsequent study, Tamaki and colleagues[88] correlated the findings on rest and stress ^{13}N-ammonia perfusion images and ^{18}F-2-fluoro-2-deoxyglucose metabolic images with changes in ventricular function following coronary revascularization (see section on comparison to other diagnostic tests for determination of tissue viability, perfusion defect severity for additional discussion of this article). They studied 43 patients with chronic myocardial infarction (mean left ventricular ejection fraction = 41 percent) with rest and stress ^{13}N-ammonia perfusion imaging along with metabolic imaging with ^{18}F-2-fluoro-2-deoxyglucose in the fasting state. Three observers visually scored regional wall abnormalities on pre- and postoperative (4 to 8 weeks after surgery) biplane contrast ventriculograms using a five-point scoring system. Function was considered to have improved if regional scores improved by one or more grades.

In the 43 patients, there were 130 asynergic segments identified on the preoperative ventriculograms. Function improved in 51 of the segments following revascularization, whereas no change in function was noted in 79 segments. On positron emission tomography, glucose metabolism was preserved in 59 of the 130 asynergic regions. Forty-five (76 percent) of the regions exhibited improved function following revascularization, whereas only 6 (8 percent) of the 71 regions without metabolic activity had improved wall motion. The positive and negative predictive accuracies of metabolic imaging with ^{18}F-2-fluoro-2-deoxyglucose were therefore 76 and 92 percent, respectively (see Table 71–1), comparable to the values previously reported by these investigators.

In addition to the preceding studies, Vanoverschelde, Maes, and Depré and their colleagues[89–91] have correlated the findings on positron emission tomography prior to coronary revascularization with changes in segmental wall motion and histopathologic studies of affected myocardium. These investigations are discussed in detail in the section on histopathologic correlation in human myocardium. To date, the validity of positron emission tomography with ^{18}F-2-fluoro-2-deoxyglucose for identifying reversibly dysfunctional myocardial segments has been examined in 295 coronary artery disease patients in more than 800 myocardial segments (see Table 71–1). These clinical studies have involved 10 major medical centers in Europe, the United States, and Japan. In the accumulated experience, the absence of ^{18}F-2-fluoro-2-deoxyglucose activity in hypoperfused myocardial segments has an 85 percent negative predictive value for identifying irreversible tissue injury. The aggregated positive predictive value, 71 percent, is somewhat less than that of initial reports, primarily because of inclusion of studies performed in the fasting or postexercise state, or both, in which visual (as opposed to circumferential profile) analysis of the positron emission tomographic images was performed. Thus, aggregate experience indicates that positron emission tomographic imaging with ^{18}F-2-fluoro-2-deoxyglucose is an accurate means of identifying reversibly dysfunctional myocardium in patients with chronic coronary artery disease.

Histopathologic Correlation in Human Myocardium

Macroscopic Correlations

Several investigators have directly correlated the results of positron emission tomography with histopathologic findings in diseased human myocardium. Berry and coinvestigators[92] imaged the myocardial ^{13}N-ammonia and ^{18}F-2-fluoro-2-deoxyglucose uptake in nine patients with an average ejection fraction of 13 percent prior to cardiac transplantation. The image findings were then correlated with the histopathologic findings in the hearts removed at the time of transplantation. Four patients had chronic myocardial infarction with ischemic cardiomyopathy, whereas five individuals had nonischemic cardiomyopathy. The time interval between imaging and cardiac transplantation ranged from 7 to 87 days.

After removal, the hearts were fixed for 2 days in a formalin solution. A midventricular transaxial slice from each explanted heart was selected to correspond to a well-visualized imaging level on positron emission tomography. The slice was divided into eight or nine sectors and stained with hematoxylin and eosin and Masson trichrome stains. Using a circumferential profile technique, the percent of viable tissue was determined by planimetry in each 10-degree myocardial sector. The profiles generated from the excised myocardial slices were then compared with ^{13}N and ^{18}F circumferential profiles derived from the positron emission tomographic images (Fig. 71–12). Histologic myocardial infarction was defined as a dense confluent area of fibrosis with an associated loss of normal myocardial architecture.

In the patients with ischemic cardiomyopathy, circumferential profile analysis revealed a close correlation between the percent of viable myocardium determined histologically and relative ^{13}N and ^{18}F count densities on the positron emission tomographic images (Figs. 71–13 and 71–14; see Figs. 71–3 and 71–4). Relative tracer concentrations paralleled the percent of viable myocardium in most myocardial sectors. In one patient, there were two small areas with transmural myocardial infarction in which modest ^{13}N and ^{18}F counts were noted on the positron emission tomographic images. The authors attributed this activity to partial volume effects and the inability of positron emission tomography to resolve count differences in small anatomical regions. For the ^{13}N-ammonia perfusion images, correlation coefficients relating relative ^{13}N counts to the percent of viable myocardium ranged from 0.60 to 0.84. In three patients with technically adequate ^{18}F-2-fluoro-2-deoxyglucose images, the correlation coefficients ranged from 0.73 to 0.88. The authors concluded that areas of matching perfusion and metabolic defects on positron emission tomographic images correspond closely in extent and severity to the amount of irreversible tissue damage identified pathologically in ischemic human cardiomyopathy.

FIGURE 71–13. See Color Plate 35.

Similarly, there was a close correlation between the left ventricular mass and infarct size by histologic and histochemical studies of explanted hearts from transplant recipients and ^{13}N-ammonia and ^{18}F-2-fluoro-2-deoxyglucose images acquired prior to explantation of the recipients' hearts.[93] Tomographically derived measurements of the absolute total ventricular mass were correlated linearly in 11 hearts with gravimetric masses (r = .93; SEE = 61.5 g) although positron emission tomography systematically overestimated the true mass, presumably as a consequence of partial volume averaging and cardiac motion artifacts. Moreover, estimates of both absolute infarct mass and percent infarcted myocardium by external imaging were correlated linearly to the actual infarct mass and the actual percentage of infarcted myocardium (r = .93; $P < .01$ for both).

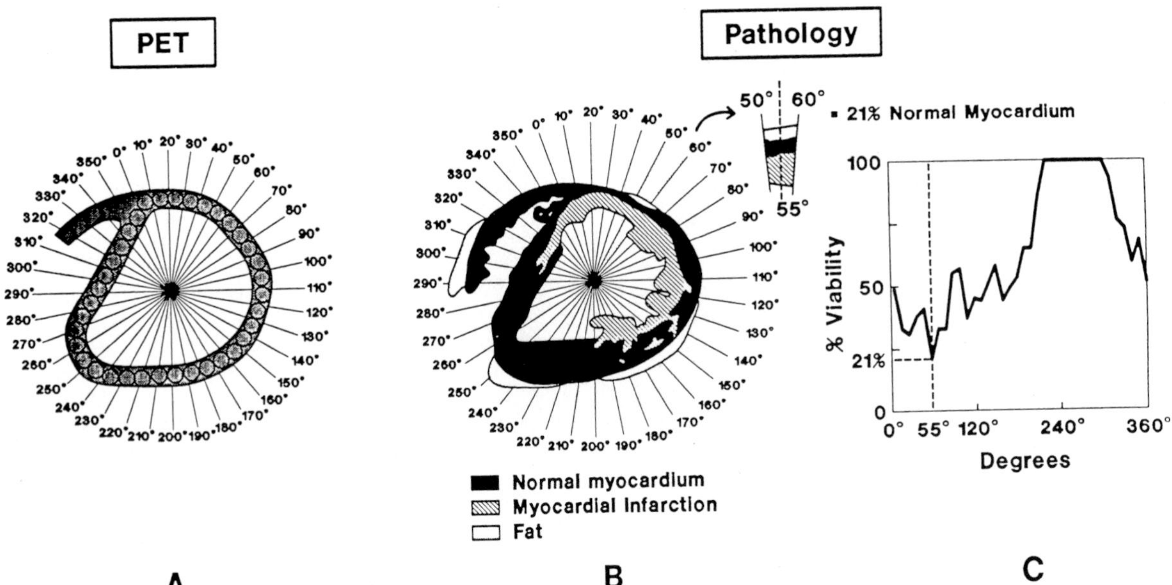

FIGURE 71–12. Circumferential profile method used by Berry and colleagues to relate ^{13}N-ammonia perfusion and ^{18}F-2-fluoro-2-deoxyglucose positron emission tomography *(PET)* images to the histopathologic findings noted in human hearts explanted at the time of cardiac transplantation. On a midventricular transaxial slice, the percent of viable tissue was determined by planimetry of each of 36 10-degree sectors. Using the insertion of the right ventricle as the starting point for the analysis, histopathologic profiles displaying the relative amount of viable myocardium were generated and compared with relative ^{13}N and ^{18}F tracer concentrations. A representative positron emission tomographic image and corresponding tissue slice are displayed in *Panels* A and *B*, respectively, illustrating the assignment of the 10-degree sectors used for the circumferential profile analysis. For the sector between 50 and 60 degrees, planimetric measurements reveal that 21 percent of the myocardial wall is viable. *Panel C* depicts the circumferential profile of the relative amount of viable myocardium as a function of the angle about the tissue slice. (From Berry, J. J., Hoffman, J. M., Steenbergen, C., et al.: Human pathologic correlation with PET in ischemic and nonischemic cardiomyopathy. J. Nucl. Med. 34:41, 1993, with permission).

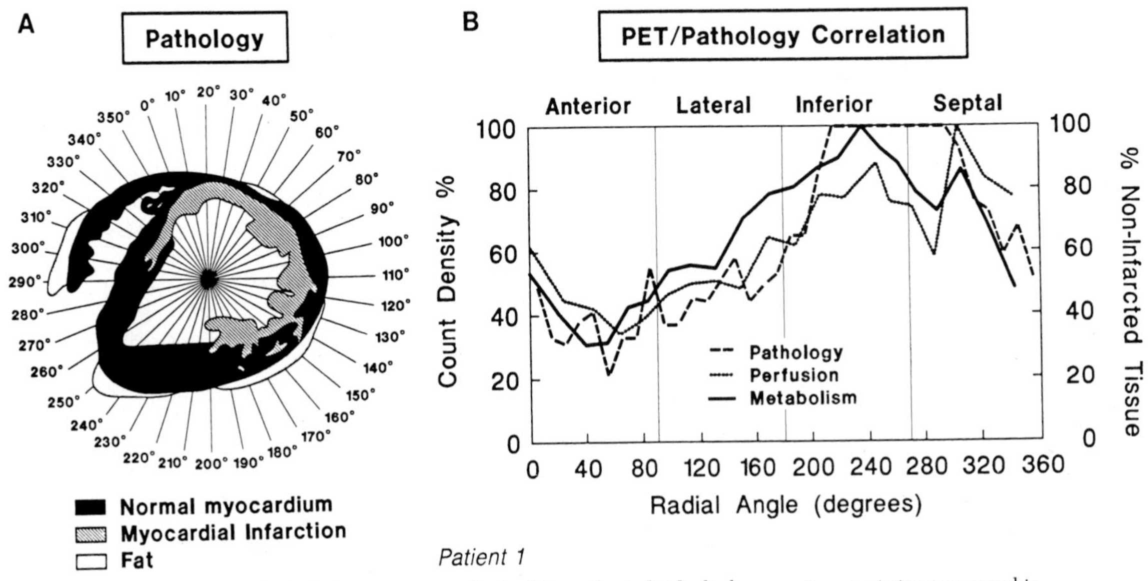

FIGURE 71–14. Pathologic specimen obtained from the individual whose positron emission tomographic images are shown in Figure 71–12. *Panel* A depicts the extensive anteroseptal, anterior, and anterolateral nontransmural myocardial infarction in this individual. *Panel B,* The circumferential profiles derived from the histopathologic specimen and the positron emission tomogrpahic images are seen. Relative ^{13}N-ammonia *(Perfusion)* and ^{18}F-2-fluoro-2-deoxyglucose *(Metabolism)* counts correlate well with the relative amount of viable tissue *(Pathology)*. (From Berry, J. J., Hoffman, J. M., Steenbergen, C., et al.: Human pathologic correlation with PET in ischemic and nonischemic cardiomyopathy. J. Nucl. Med. 34:43, 1993, with permission).

Histologic and Ultrastructural Changes

Several studies have correlated regional ^{13}N-ammonia and ^{18}F-2-fluoro-2-deoxyglucose findings on positron emission tomography with morphometric measurements and histologic and ultrastructural and histochemical findings (Fig. 71–15) in biopsy samples removed at the time of surgical revascularization.[89–91] Similar to findings by Flameng and colleagues,[94] Vanoverschelde and coworkers[89] noted various degrees of tissue fibrosis and, on electromicroscopy, abnormal cells characterized by a severe reduction in contractile filaments, extensive glycogen accumulation, a reduction in the sarcoplasmic reticulum, and the presence of numerous although small mitochondria (Fig. 71–16). The biopsy samples removed from collateral-dependent myocardium of the anterior wall with normal or near-normal wall motion exhibited less fibrosis and abnormal cells than biopsy samples removed from collateral-dependent myocardium in the anterior wall with reduced contractile function. Although these authors entertained the possibility that the augmented glycogen deposition in such cells might account for the enhanced ^{18}F-2-fluoro-2-deoxyglucose uptake, Maes and colleagues[90] disputed such a notion because of their failure to demonstrate a significant correlation between the fraction of such "dedifferentiated cells" and the relative ^{18}F-2-fluoro-2-deoxyglucose uptake. Nevertheless, these authors noted that the percentage of fibrosis (35 ± 25 percent) was significantly greater in "match" segments without a postrevascularization improvement in contractile function as compared with the percentage of fibrotic tissue of only 11 ± 6 percent in mismatch segments with improved contractile function after successful revascularization (Fig. 71–17). Interestingly, the fraction of dedifferentiated cells was almost identical in both types of segments (24 ± 15 percent versus 25 ± 13 percent; P = NS). Furthermore, the relative reductions in blood flow correlated significantly and linearly with the degree of tissue fibrosis in "match segments" but not in "mismatch segments."

More recent observations by Depré and colleagues[91] are generally in agreement with those described in the two earlier investigations with the exception of a statistically significant correlation between the transmural fraction of altered (dedifferentiated) myocytes and the relative ^{18}F-2-fluoro-2-deoxyglucose concentrations. The authors imply a relationship between the enhanced glucose use and the accumulation of glycogen in such altered cells. Nevertheless, this possibility remains as speculative as the arguments against an augmentation in a compartmentalized glycolysis.[95] As another intriguing possibility, the authors invoke a re-expression of the glucose transporter GLUT-1, which predominates in neonatal myocytes and is insulin-independent. Ischemia might cause the re-expression of GLUT-1.[96] Such enhanced expression of the insulin-independent GLUT-1 transporter could also be consistent with findings in chronic coronary artery disease patients in whom changes in glucose use rates as determined by quantitative measurements with ^{18}F-2-fluoro-2-deoxyglucose were significantly attenuated in response to changes in circulating glucose and, in particular, insulin levels.[97]

Further, interpatient variations in the fractional distribution of fibrosis, normal, dedifferentiated myocytes, and perhaps ultrastructurally normal yet compromised cells in myocardial regions with blood flow metabolism mismatches are likely to be of clinical importance. The fraction of tissue fibrosis is likely to determine the magnitude of a postrevascularization improvement in contractile function. Similarly, if dedifferentiated cells can "redifferentiate" and reconstitute their contractile machinery in a meaningful manner, one might expect a prolonged period of recovery of regional wall motion. Conversely, if the ultrastructural damage is small, function is likely to recover fully and rapidly.

Pathophysiologic Considerations

Different mechanisms are likely to account for the various patterns of blood flow and metabolism in dysfunctional myocardial

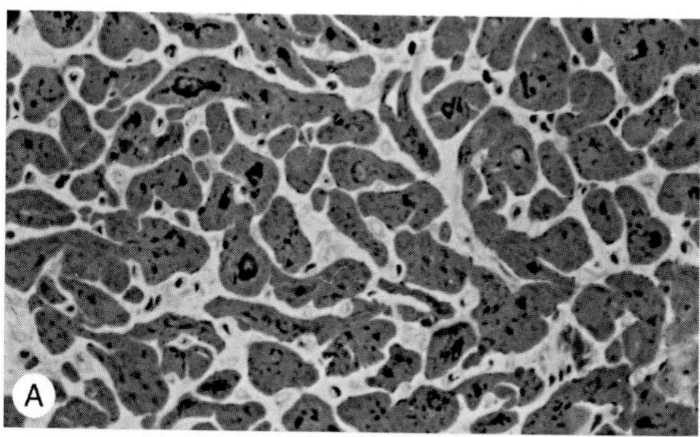

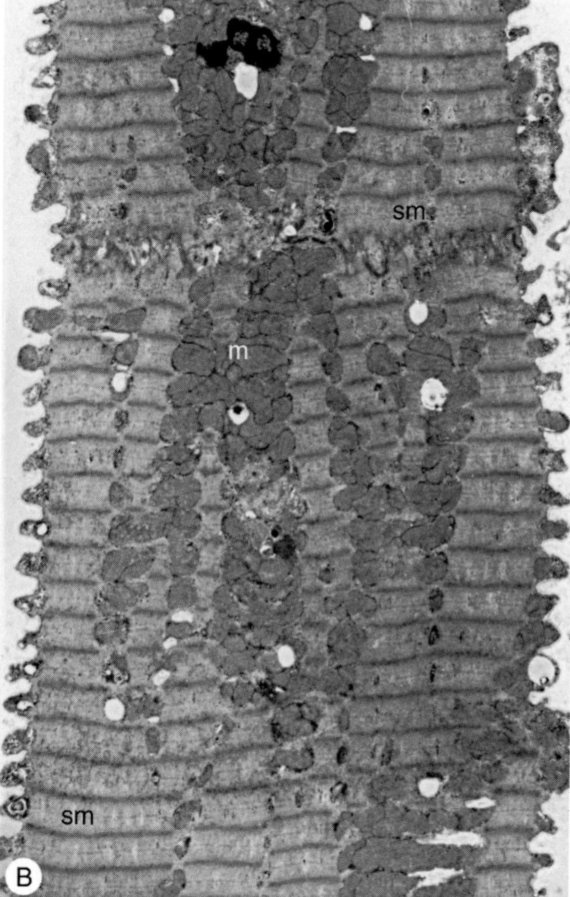

FIGURE 71–15. Light *(Panel A)* and electron microscopic *(Panel B)* images from a patient with coronary artery disease, normal regional wall motion, and normal ^{13}N-ammonia perfusion and ^{18}F-2-fluoro-2-deoxyglucose metabolic positron emission tomographic images. On the light micrograph of the periodic acid–Schiff (PAS)-stained tissue, a normal amount of glycogen is present. On the electron micrograph, the cellular cytoplasm is filled with rows of sarcomeres *(sm)* and normal-sized mitochondria *(m)*. (From Maes, A., Flameng, W., Nuyts, J., et al.: Histologic alterations in chronically hypoperfused myocardium. Correlation with PET findings. Circulation 90:740, 1994. With permission of the American Heart Association.)

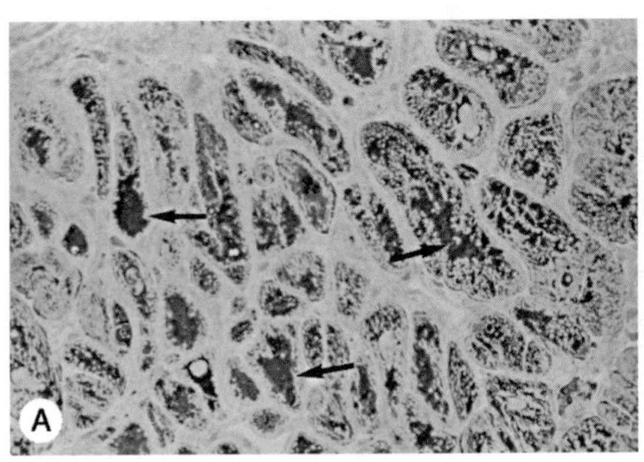

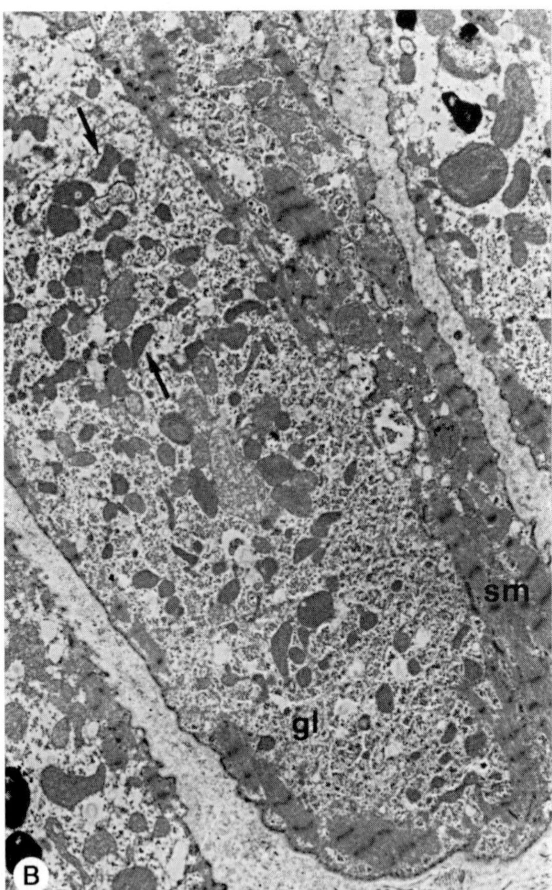

FIGURE 71–16. Light *(Panel A)* and electron microscopic *(Panel B)* images from a patient with anterior wall hypokinesis and a perfusion-metabolism mismatch on positron emission tomography. The arrows in *Panel A* depict accumulation of glycogen in this PAS-stained specimen. On the electron micrograph, sarcomeres are absent from the center of the cell and are identified only at the periphery *(sm)*. Cytosolic accumulation of glycogen is noted *(gl)* and small mitochondria are present *(arrows)*. The regional ejection fraction increased from 46 to 55 percent following coronary revascularization. (From Maes, A., Flameng, W., Nuyts, J., et al.: Histologic alterations in chronically hypoperfused myocardium. Correlation with PET findings. Circulation 90:741, 1994. With permission of the American Heart Association.)

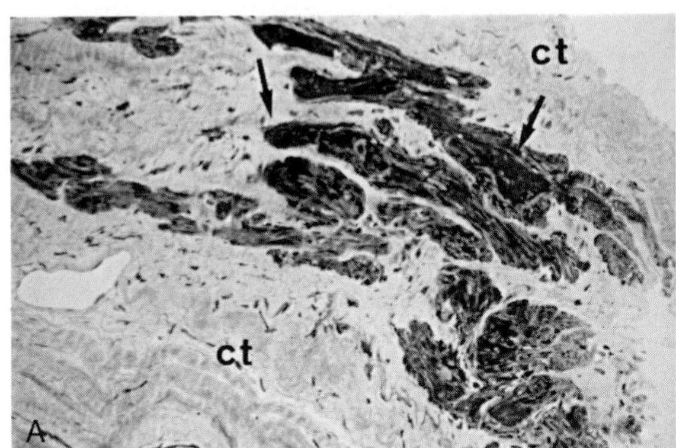

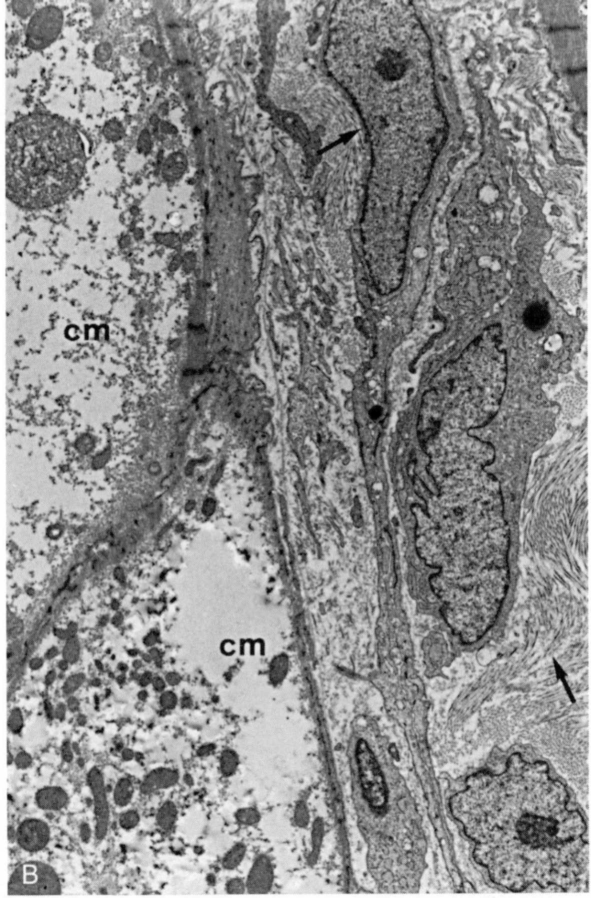

FIGURE 71–17. Light *(Panel A)* and electron microscopic *(Panel B)* images from a patient with coronary artery disease, anterior wall hypokinesis, and matching perfusion and metabolic defects on positron emission tomographic imaging. Exuberant amounts of fibrosis are noted on the light micrograph, along with glycogen-accumulating cells *(arrows)* on this PAS-stained specimen. On the electron micrograph, abundant collagen is noted *(arrows)* next to the cardiomyocytes *(CM)*. Following revascularization, the regional ejection fraction decreased from 23 to 17 percent. (From Maes, A., Flameng, W., Nuyts, J., et al.: Histologic alterations in chronically hypoperfused myocardium. Correlation with PET findings. Circulation 90:742, 1994. With permission of the American Heart Association.)

segments. Pattern A, that is, normal blood flow and glucose metabolism, might indeed be consistent with stunned myocardium. In the study by Nienaber and coworkers,[98] blood flow rapidly normalized after successful angioplasty, whereas ^{18}F-2-fluoro-2-deoxyglucose uptake remained elevated slightly and wall motion remained impaired initially. Such "stunning" might differ from "repetitive stunning" as demonstrated by Vanoverschelde and colleagues.[89] In collateral-dependent myocardium with near-normal blood flow yet slightly enhanced glucose use, wall motion was impaired in those patients with a markedly reduced myocardial flow reserve but not in patients with a normal flow reserve. Thus, one might argue that repeated increases in demand cannot be met by an appropriate increase in flow, thereby causing repetitive ischemic or stunning episodes alternating with episodes of recovery and stunned myocardium.

Although acknowledging the variability in the degree of tissue injury, segments with reduced blood flow but preserved or even enhanced glucose use might indeed represent the metabolic correlate of "myocardial hibernation." Glucose in this case is used as a more oxygen-efficient substrate. Contractile function is downregulated to match the reduced supply. Indeed, such segments may lose their flow reserve as demonstrated with pharmacologic stress.[99] Inotropic stimulation of such segments enhances contractile function yet produces an only marginal, although statistically significant, increase in blood flow.[100] At the same time, regional glucose use markedly and disproportionately increases, perhaps as an expression of an even greater reliance on the oxygen-efficient glucose or, alternatively, as an expression of acute ischemia superimposed on hibernation.

Lastly, pattern C with a concordant reduction in both flow and glucose use most probably represents scar tissue. The different degrees of reduction to flow and metabolism may reflect the fractional distributions of coexisting scar tissue with normal myocytes.

Recovery of Functional Capacity After Revascularization

Although physicians may be concerned primarily with the beneficial effects of coronary revascularization on segmental and global left ventricular function in individuals with coronary artery disease, patients tend to be more interested in whether an intervention will provide relief of cardiac symptoms. Marwick and coinvestigators[101] sought to determine the relationship between the amount of myocardium exhibiting postexercise uptake of ^{18}F-2-fluoro-2-deoxyglucose and changes in left ventricular function and exercise capacity following coronary revascularization. In 23 patients with previous Q-wave myocardial infarction, echocardiography and symptom-limited treadmill exercise testing were performed before and 22 ± 14 weeks after coronary revascularization. Five patients (22 percent) were in New York Heart Association Functional class III, 11 (48 percent) were in class II, and the remaining seven individuals were in class I. The results were correlated with resting and dipyridamole ^{82}Rb perfusion and postexercise ^{18}F-2-fluoro-2-deoxyglucose metabolic images prior to revascularization. Metabolic imaging was performed in the fasting state after antianginal medications were discontinued for 24 hours. The uptake of both ^{82}Rb and ^{18}F-2-fluoro-2-deoxyglucose was assessed visually in each of seven anatomical segments. In the 23 patients, the authors identified 73 segments with persistent ^{82}Rb perfusion defects and resting wall motion abnormalities. Increased uptake of ^{18}F-2-fluoro-2-deoxyglucose was noted on the postexercise metabolic images in 30 segments (26 segments with wall motion abnormalities, 4 segments with normal function) in 19 patients. The average resting ^{82}Rb concentration in the segments with increased ^{18}F-2-fluoro-2-deoxyglucose uptake did not differ from that in the 47 segments without increased uptake of the metabolic tracer (60 ± 8 percent versus 55 ± 11 percent, P = NS), meaning that resting perfusion did not discriminate between these two tissue types.

Following revascularization, wall motion improved in 19 (73 percent) of the 26 dysfunctional segments with increased ^{18}F-2-fluoro-2-deoxyglucose uptake and failed to improve in 35 (74 percent) of the 47 dysfunctional segments without enhanced uptake of the metabolic tracer. In nine patients, two or more segments had increased ^{18}F-2-fluoro-2-deoxyglucose uptake and these individuals demonstrated a significant postoperative improvement in achieved rate-pressure product (20 ± 4 to $26 \pm 4 \cdot 10^3$, $P < .02$) and percent of maximal predicted heart rate (84 ± 10 to 93 ± 6 percent, $P = .04$). In contrast, no significant improvement in these exercise parameters was noted in the patients with one or no segments with enhanced ^{18}F-2-fluoro-2-deoxyglucose uptake. Five of the 9 patients with two or more segments with ^{18}F-2-fluoro-2-deoxyglucose uptake had an improvement of one or more functional classes, whereas improvement in functional class was noted in only 3 of the other 14 patients. The authors concluded that analysis of postexercise ^{18}F-2-fluoro-2-deoxyglucose uptake is useful for predicting improvement in regional systolic function and exercise capacity following revascularization in chronic coronary artery disease patients.

In a study of patients with more profound left ventricular dysfunction, Di Carli and associates[102] correlated the findings on preoperative positron emission tomographic imaging with improvement in functional status following coronary artery bypass grafting. The study population consisted of 36 individuals with ischemic cardiomyopathy (mean left ventricular ejection fraction = 27 ± 7 percent) referred for coronary bypass surgery. Twenty-eight patients had a history of prior infarction and nine had prior coronary bypass surgery. Prior to surgery, all the patients had symptoms of congestive heart failure and 13 patients also had angina. Thirty-two patients were in class III and four were in class IV heart failure.

The patients' functional status was assessed before and 25 ± 14 months after coronary revascularization using the Specific Activity Scale.[103] Using a standard interview, the Specific Activity Scale approximates the metabolic costs of a variety of personal care, housework, occupational, and recreational activities. The Specific Activity Scale has a higher agreement with exercise treadmill performance than do the classifications of the New York Heart Association and the Canadian Cardiovascular Society. In a subset of 15 patients, these authors noted a highly significant linear relationship between treadmill exercise capacity and that approximated by the Specific Activity Scale (Specific Activity Scale metabolic equivalents = 0.5 · treadmill metabolic equivalents + 2.3, r = .73, SEE = 1.02, $P = .002$).

Positron emission tomography was performed prior to coronary artery bypass surgery using ^{13}N-ammonia and ^{18}F-2-fluoro-2-deoxyglucose. The images were analyzed using a polar mapping technique that quantifies both the extent and severity of perfusion defects and perfusion-metabolism mismatches.[104, 105] The perfusion defect size and severity averaged 63 ± 13 percent and 33 ± 12 percent, respectively, for the population as a whole. The average extent of matching perfusion and metabolic defects was 41 ± 23 percent, indicating extensive myocardial scarring. Significant areas of perfusion-metabolism mismatches were also noted, however, averaging 23 ± 22 percent of the left ventricle.

On univariate analysis relating perfusion defect extent and severity, extent and severity of perfusion-metabolism mismatches, left ventricular size, left ventricular ejection fraction, and age to changes in heart failure symptoms, only variables relating to the extent, severity, and location of perfusion-metabolism mismatches were found to be significantly related to the percent improvement in functional capacity following revascularization. Age was of borderline significance ($P = .08$). On a subsequent stepwise multivariate analysis, only the total extent of a perfusion-metabolism mismatch (F = 40.2, $P = .0001$) and patient age (F = 4.1, $P = .05$) were independent predictors of the change in the functional state after coronary revascularization. Perhaps most importantly, the percent improvement in functional capacity was linearly related to the extent of the postrevascularization perfusion-metabolism mismatch (percent improvement = 2.04 · percent of left ventricle with perfusion-metabolism mismatch + 24.27, r = 0.87, SEE = 10.8,

$P < .001$). Thus improvement in functional capacity was directly related to the amount of left ventricular myocardium exhibiting a perfusion-metabolism mismatch on preoperative positron emission tomographic imaging. A perfusion-metabolism mismatch involving 18 percent or more of the left ventricle had a positive predictive accuracy of 76 percent and a negative predictive accuracy of 78 percent for predicting an improvement in functional class of at least one grade. Thus, the studies of Marwick and coworkers[101] and Di Carli and colleagues[102] indicate that the patients with compromised ventricular function who benefit most from coronary revascularization are the ones with the largest perfusion-metabolism mismatches on preoperative metabolic imaging with ^{18}F-2-fluoro-2-deoxyglucose.

Relationships Among Recovery of Blood Flow, Metabolism, and Function After Revascularization

In animal models of stunned myocardium, restoration of blood flow precedes recovery of both myocardial function and metabolism.[50, 52] To assess both the temporal and quantitative relationships among recovery of myocardial perfusion, glucose metabolism, and segmental function following restoration of blood flow to ischemic human myocardium, Nienaber and coinvestigators[98] studied patients with ischemic heart disease and resting segmental wall motion abnormalities who were undergoing percutaneous transluminal coronary angioplasty. Positron emission tomography with ^{13}N-ammonia and ^{18}F-2-fluoro-2-deoxyglucose and two-dimensional echocardiography were performed just before and within 72 hours of successful coronary angioplasty in 12 patients with resting wall motion abnormalities involving 13 vascular territories. Late echocardiograms (10 patients) and positron emission tomography studies (8 patients) were obtained 2 to 3 months after coronary angioplasty. Segmental function was assessed with two-dimensional echocardiography.

Quantitative indices of abnormal wall motion were derived by multiplying visually assessed segmental wall motion scores by the percent of myocardium with abnormal function. Quantitative indices of abnormal perfusion were derived from the ^{13}N-ammonia circumferential count profiles by multiplying the percent of visualized myocardium with abnormal perfusion by the severity of the deviation from laboratory normal values. In a similar fashion, quantitative indices of myocardial ischemia were calculated by multiplying the percent of visualized myocardium with an elevated ^{13}N-^{18}F count difference by the severity of deviation from normal values. Changes in coronary lesion geometry following angioplasty were assessed with quantitative coronary angiography.

Coronary angioplasty improved coronary stenosis dimensions as determined by a significant decrease in the percent of area stenosis from 84.8±14.6 percent to 55.1±23.6 percent ($P < .001$) on quantitative coronary angiography. This was associated with a significant improvement in the mean ^{13}N-ammonia perfusion defect score (Fig. 71–18) on the early postangioplasty images (115.9±166.3 versus 31.2±50.5, $P < .002$). However, despite the early improvement in resting myocardial perfusion, the mean echocardiographic wall motion score index did not improve significantly (111±76 versus 81±72, P = NS), indicating the persistence of myocardial dysfunction despite improvement in blood flow.

Although there was improvement in the ^{13}N-ammonia perfusion–^{18}F-2-fluoro-2-deoxyglucose metabolism mismatch score (159±175 versus 65±117, $P < .01$) performed early after angioplasty, rates of myocardial glucose use obtained in eight of the patients revealed that ratios of values in myocardium at risk relative to normal myocardium did not change significantly from the pre- to the early postangioplasty studies (1.7±0.8 versus 1.3±0.4, P = NS). This suggests that the early improvement in the perfusion-metabolism mismatch score resulted primarily from an improvement of perfusion.

Two months following angioplasty, no further improvement in mean perfusion score was noted (31.2±50.5 versus 24.2±19.2, P = NS). However, there was further improvement in the perfusion-metabolism mismatch score (65±117 to 26±29, P = NS). Because rates of glucose use in myocardium at risk had normalized relative to reference myocardium, the late improvement in the perfusion-metabolism mismatch score resulted primarily from a normalization of metabolism. A significant improvement in mean wall motion score was noted on the delayed studies at 2 months (43±46, $P < .005$ as compared with before angioplasty). The quantitative extent of recovery of segmental function was linearly related to the preangioplasty mismatch score (change in wall motion score = 0.29 · preangioplasty mismatch score + 22.5, SEE = 27.9, r = .87, $P < .001$). Improvement in segmental function correlated only weakly with the preangioplasty perfusion score (r = .72) and depended on a single data point, indicating that the tissue characterization afforded by concurrent perfusion and metabolic imaging rather than perfusion imaging alone predicted the ultimate degree of improvement in segmental function following restoration of blood flow.

Thus, full recovery of left ventricular function may be delayed following relief of chronic myocardial ischemia in humans. Improvement in tissue metabolism appears to be paralleled by recovery of segmental function. Although there is a significant improvement in myocardial perfusion early after interventional restoration of blood flow, metabolic imaging with ^{18}F-2-fluoro-2-deoxyglucose identifies the persistence of an abnormal metabolic state. As demonstrated in animal experiments, this metabolic state is characterized by an accelerated rate of exogenous glucose use, which may reflect a period of cellular repair necessary for return of full contractile function. Alternatively, it is also possible that the early persistence of enhanced regional glucose use reflects slow normalization of a chronic metabolic adaptive process to a persistent reduction in blood flow.[106] For example, in the 22 patients studied by Tamaki and colleagues,[79] repeat positron emission tomography at 5 to 7 weeks after coronary artery bypass surgery demonstrated persistently elevated myocardial uptake of ^{18}F-2-fluoro-2-deoxyglucose in 6 of the 19 (32 percent) segments with abnormal wall motion and enhanced glucose use prior to revascularization. Three of the six segments (50 percent) with persisting uptake of ^{18}F-2-fluoro-2-deoxyglucose failed to exhibit an improvement in wall motion. In contrast, wall motion invariably improved in the segments with normalized ^{18}F-2-fluoro-2-deoxyglucose uptake. These data suggest that recovery of function in chronically ischemic human myocardium following restoration of blood flow may not be fully achieved until the abnormalities in tissue glucose metabolism have resolved.

The relationship between the severity of ischemic human myocardial dysfunction and the time course of recovery of left ventricular function after restoration of blood flow has not been well defined. However, the case report of Luu and coworkers[107] dramatically illustrates that recovery of left ventricular function may be prolonged following coronary artery revascularization. Their patient, a 45-year-old man with ischemic cardiomyopathy (New York Heart Association class IV), had an ejection fraction of 16 percent. Although tomographic ^{201}Tl imaging revealed extensive persistent perfusion defects, metabolic imaging with positron emission tomography uncovered significant viability in virtually all myocardial segments (Fig. 71–19). Based on the scintigraphic findings, the patient was referred for coronary revascularization rather than cardiac transplantation. The patient's postoperative course was complicated by marked left ventricular failure requiring the use of an intra-aortic balloon pump and the administration of vasopressors. Eventually, the patient's condition stabilized and he was discharged on medical therapy with little improvement in left ventricular function (Table 71–3). Over the ensuing 3 months, the patient was admitted to the hospital on two separate occasions for treatment of congestive heart failure despite improvement on follow-up positron emission tomography (see Fig. 71–19). On medical therapy, the patient's symptoms gradually improved to functional class II and he returned to work. On serial noninvasive testing, it was clear that left ventricular function had slowly improved over the 12 months after bypass

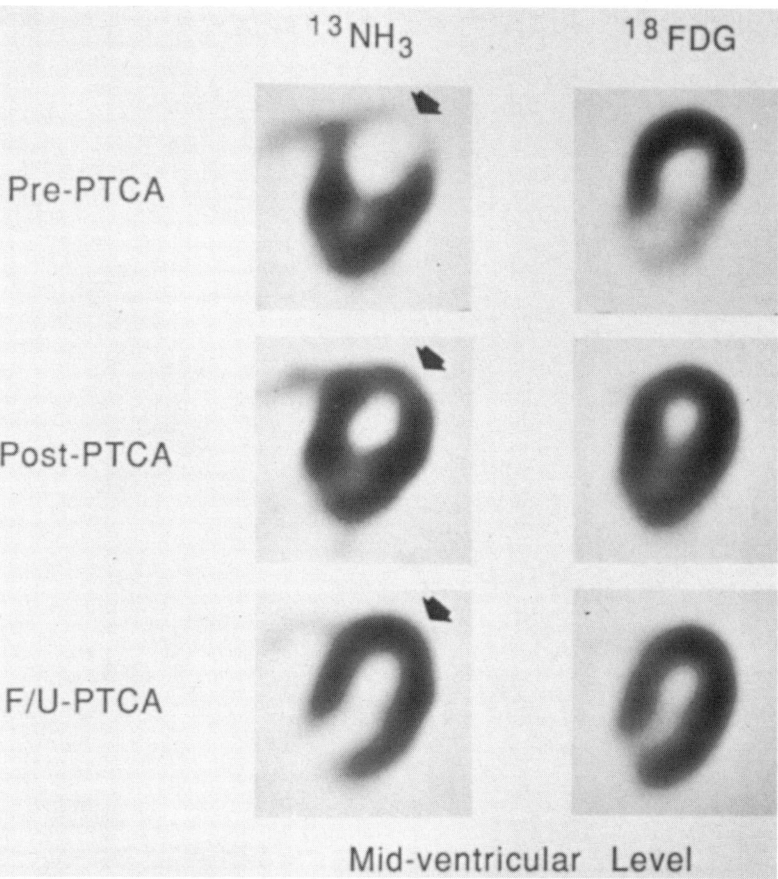

FIGURE 71–18. Sequential ^{13}N-ammonia perfusion (*$^{13}NH_3$*) and ^{18}F-2-fluoro-2-deoxyglucose (*^{18}FDG*) metabolic images in a patient just before *(Pre-PTCA)*, early after *(Post-PTCA)*, and 2 months *(F/U-PTCA)* following angioplasty of a proximal anterior left anterior descending coronary artery stenosis. The pre-PTCA positron emission tomographic study demonstrates an extensive metabolism perfusion mismatch in the anteroseptal and anteroapical regions of the ventricle. Early after successful angioplasty of the left anterior descending coronary lesion, there is considerable improvement in myocardial perfusion *(arrow)*. However, glucose use remains enhanced relative to blood flow in the territory of the anterior descending coronary artery. By 2 months, both perfusion and glucose metabolism have normalized, indicating full recovery of tissue metabolism following successful restoration of blood flow by angioplasty of the culprit coronary lesion.

surgery, indicating that the beneficial effects of restoration of blood flow to the chronically ischemic myocardium in this patient were not fully achieved for a considerable time. This case study would suggest that recovery of contractile function after revascularization may require a significant amount of time. Consequently, beneficial effects of revascularization may be underestimated if assessment of function is performed too soon after restoration of blood flow.

Synopsis of Metabolic Activity As an Indicator of Viability

Identification of residual glucose metabolism in hypoperfused ventricular segments with positron emission tomography and ^{18}F-2-fluoro-2-deoxyglucose in patients with ischemic heart disease is a reliable marker of clinically important myocardial viability. This has been documented by the improvement in regional contractile function in metabolically active myocardial segments following interventional restoration of blood flow. Ultimately, the observed improvement in global left ventricular ejection fraction as well as in the functional capacity of the patient is related to the anatomical extent and severity of the prerevascularization mismatch between perfusion and glucose metabolism on the preoperative positron emission tomographic images. Those individuals with the most extensive perfusion-metabolism mismatches will benefit most from revascularization. Clinical studies also suggest that the recovery of both myocardial function and metabolism may be delayed following restoration of blood flow, perhaps indicating that a period of cellular repair is necessary before full contractile function can be achieved.

In patients with end-stage ischemic cardiomyopathy with discrete, completed myocardial infarctions, relative tracer concentrations on positron emission tomographic images generally parallel the amount of viable myocardial tissue and can be used to derive accurate estimates of infarct size. In coronary artery disease patients with left ventricular dysfunction and perfusion-metabolism mismatches, relatively high numbers of viable but abnormal myocytes can be identified in affected myocardial regions. These abnormal myocytes are characterized histologically by sarcomere depletion, particularly in the perinuclear region, and also by an increase in cellular glycogen content. In addition to direct histologic evidence for cellular viability of the abnormal cardiac myocytes in these studies, indirect clinical evidence of viability was also provided by recovery of function following successful coronary revascularization in these patients. Thus, the disturbances in myocardial metabolism identified noninvasively with positron emission tomography have associated histologic abnormalities that indicate viable but functionally impaired tissue.

COMPARISON WITH OTHER DIAGNOSTIC TESTS FOR TISSUE VIABILITY

Although the identification of preserved tissue glucose metabolism in initial clinical studies indicated the presence of ischemically compromised but viable myocardium in patients with coronary artery disease, it remained uncertain whether this approach provided information unobtainable with routine clinical tests. Accordingly, clinical studies were performed in patients with chronic ischemic heart disease to compare the tissue characterization afforded by metabolic imaging with positron emission tomography with that derived from routine clinical tests.

Electrocardiography

Q Waves

Although pathologic Q waves on the resting electrocardiogram have been attributed to "transmural" myocardial infarction,[108] care-

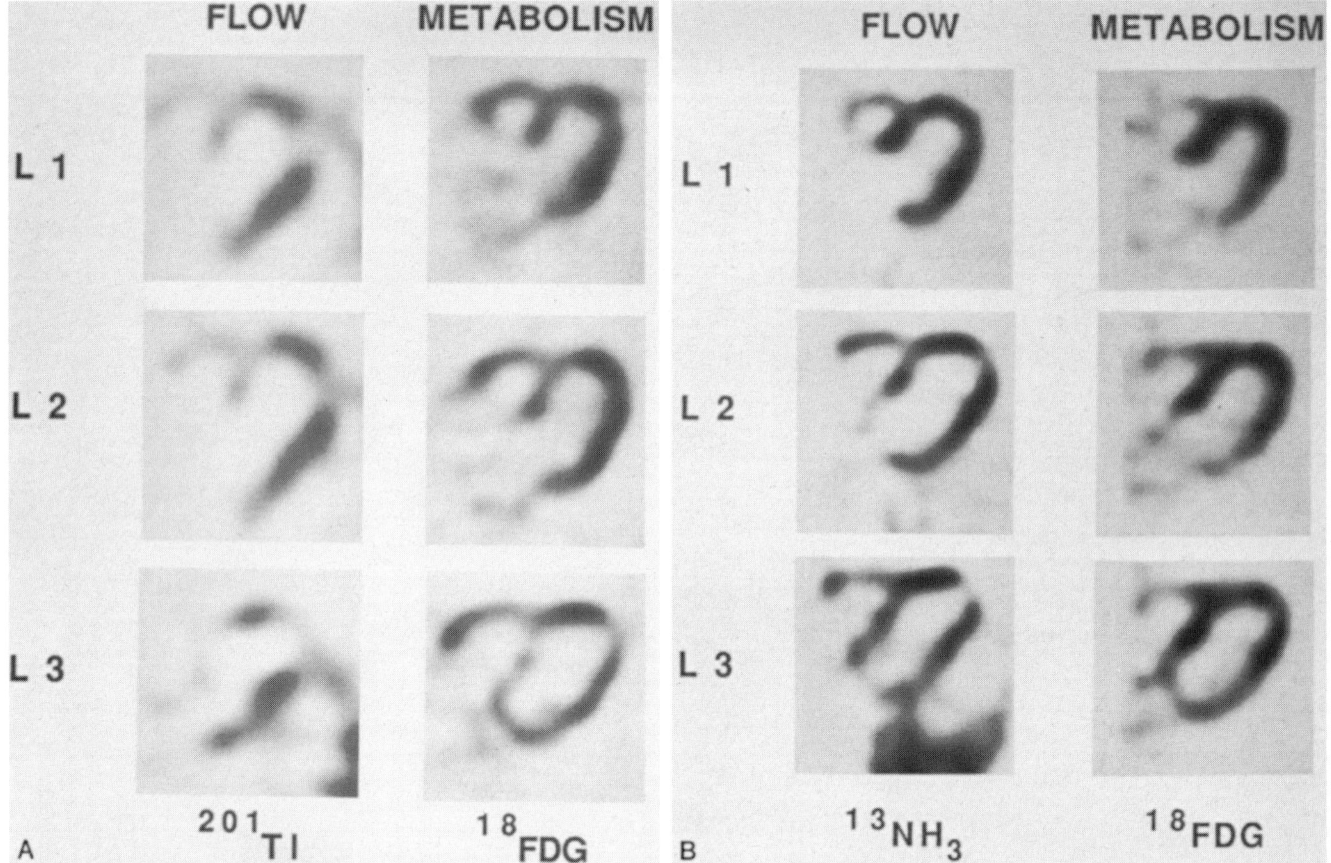

FIGURE 71–19. *Panel A,* Representative cross-sectional SPECT 24-hour redistribution ^{201}Tl images (^{201}*Tl*) and the corresponding ^{18}F-2-fluoro-2-deoxyglucose (^{18}*FDG*) metabolic images from the studies of a 45-year-old man with ischemic cardiomyopathy. On the ^{201}Tl images, extensive perfusion defects are identified in the anterolateral, septal, inferior, and inferolateral regions of the ventricle. In contrast, glucose metabolism is well preserved in the same ventricular regions, indicating residual myocardial viability. *Panel B,* Representative cross-sectional ^{13}N-ammonia ($^{13}NH_3$) perfusion and ^{18}F-2-fluoro-2-deoxyglucose (^{18}*FDG*) metabolic images in the same patient 2 months after coronary bypass surgery. Myocardial perfusion has markedly improved in the septal, inferior, inferolateral, and anteroapical regions of the ventricle. Although the resting left ventricular ejection fraction had increased from 16 to 26 percent at this time, ultimate recovery of ventricular function was not achieved until a full year after coronary bypass surgery (see Table 71–3). (From Luu, M., Stevenson, L. W., Brunken, R. C., et al.: Delayed recovery of revascularized myocardium after referral for cardiac transplantation. Am. Heart J. 119(Part I):668, 1990, with permission.)

ful clinicopathologic studies have shown that Q waves do not reliably distinguish transmural from subendocardial infarction.[64–67] Both Durer and colleagues[109] and Savage and associates[66] have reported that even small subendocardial infarctions may be associated with significant Q waves. In addition, chronic anterior Q waves

TABLE 71–3. LEFT VENTRICULAR FUNCTION FOLLOWING CORONARY ARTERY BYPASS GRAFTING IN A PATIENT WITH ISCHEMIC CARDIOMYOPATHY

Date	Echocardiography End-Diastolic Dimension (mm)	Left Ventricular Ejection Fraction (Radionuclide Ventriculography)	
		Rest	*Exercise*
Preoperatively	66	16%	15%
1 month	68	26%	24%
6 months	52	33%	34%
12 months	52	40%	47%

From Luu, M., Stevenson, L., Brunken, R., et al: Delayed recovery of revascularized myocardium after referral for cardiac transplantation. Am. Heart J. 119(Part I):668, 1990, with permission.

have disappeared and associated regional ventricular dysfunction has improved following coronary revascularization,[110, 111] indicating that electrocardiographic Q waves and regional wall motion abnormalities are not always indicative of transmural scar formation.

Brunken and coinvestigators[112] examined regional myocardial perfusion and glucose metabolism in 20 patients with 31 chronic electrocardiographic Q-wave infarctions. All patients had clinical histories of one or more antecedent myocardial infarctions. The mean interval from the most recent clinical infarction to positron emission tomography was 20.6 months. Of the 20 patients, 10 (50 percent) had a history of congestive heart failure and the mean left ventricular ejection fraction was depressed at 35.1 ± 12.1 percent. The mean interval between electrocardiography and positron emission tomography was 15.4 ± 20.1 days.

There were 31 Q-wave regions in the 20 patients: 11 septal, 7 anterior, 3 lateral, and 10 inferior. Only 10 of the 31 Q-wave infarct regions (32 percent) exhibited the concordant reductions in perfusion and glucose metabolism indicative of completed infarction (Fig. 71–20). Six of the Q-wave regions (20 percent) had the metabolism-perfusion mismatch of myocardial ischemia (Fig. 71–21). In 15 of the Q-wave infarct regions, regional tracer concentrations were within 2 SD of established normal limits and therefore were considered normal (Fig. 71–22). Thus, positron emission tomography revealed metabolic evidence of tissue viability in 21 of 31 (68 percent) Q wave-infarct regions.

Because previous investigations have shown an inexact relationship between the anatomical site of abnormal electrical activity and the surface electrocardiographic leads displaying Q waves,[113] a second analysis of the data was performed to avoid inadvertent bias in favor of positron emission tomography. In this analysis, Q-wave regions were reassigned to maximize the agreement between the positron emission tomographic and the electrocardiographic "infarct regions." Even when this second analysis of the data was performed, the majority of myocardial Q-wave infarct regions, 15 of 28 Q-wave regions (54 percent), exhibited evidence of metabolic activity. There were no characteristic ST-segment or T-wave changes that distinguished regions with metabolic criteria for ischemia from regions with criteria for completed infarction. T-wave inversion and ST-segment elevation and depression were noted with equal frequency in both groups. Thus, this report indicated

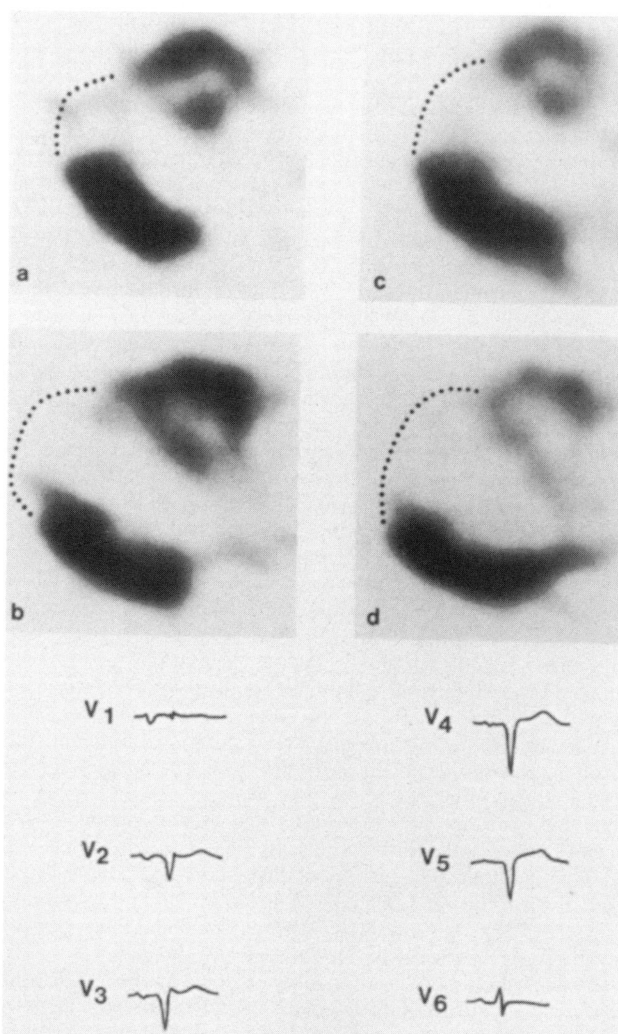

FIGURE 71–20. Representative ^{13}N-ammonia perfusion images *(Panels A and B)* and ^{18}F-2-fluoro-2-deoxyglucose metabolic images *(Panels C and D)* and the precordial electrocardiogram in a 68-year-old man with a history of myocardial infarction 5 months prior to study. On the electrocardiogram, deep Q waves are noted in V_1 through V_5 in agreement with the concordant decreases in perfusion and glucose metabolism identified in the anteroapical and septal regions of the ventricle. The electrocardiogram and positron emission tomography both indicate completed myocardial infarction. (From Brunken, R., Tillisch, J., Schwaiger, M., et al.: Regional perfusion, glucose metabolism and wall motion in patients with chronic electrocardiographic Q-wave infarctions: Evidence for persistence of viable tissue in some infarct regions by positron emission tomography. Circulation 73:951, 1986. With permission of the American Heart Association.)

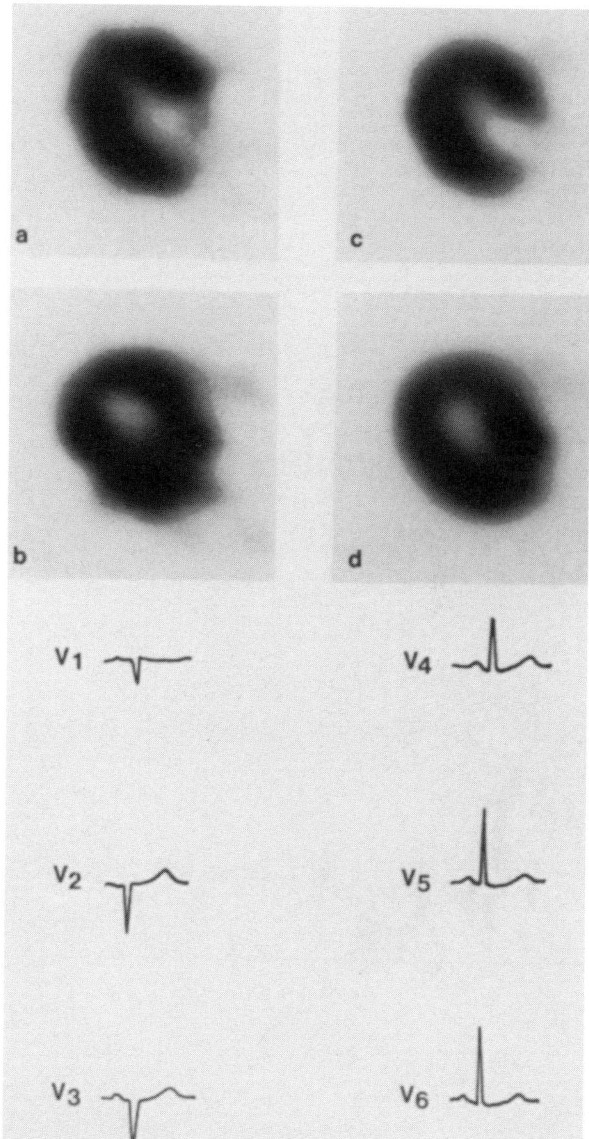

FIGURE 71–21. Precordial electrocardiogram and representative ^{13}N-ammonia perfusion images *(Panels A and B)* and ^{18}F-2-fluoro-2-deoxyglucose metabolic images *(Panels C and D)* in a 59-year-old man who sustained an anterior myocardial infarction 1 year prior to study. On the electrocardiogram, pathologic Q waves are noted in V_1 through V_4. On the ^{13}N-ammonia perfusion images, defects are identified in the anterior and septal regions of the ventricle. In contrast, exogenous glucose use is well preserved in these hypoperfused ventricular regions, indicating the metabolism-perfusion mismatch of myocardial ischemia. (From Brunken, R., Tillisch, J., Schwaiger, M., et al.: Regional perfusion, glucose metabolism and wall motion in patients with chronic electrocardiographic Q-wave infarctions: Evidence for persistence of viable tissue in some infarct regions by positron emission tomography. Circulation 73:951, 1986. With permission of the American Heart Association.)

that tissue viability could be identified with ^{18}F-2-fluoro-2-deoxyglucose and positron emission tomography in a significant proportion (54 percent) of electrocardiographic Q-wave infarct regions and that neither ST-segment nor T-wave changes were helpful in distinguishing hypoperfused regions with metabolic viability from regions with completed infarction.

Confirmation that glucose metabolic viability can be identified with metabolic imaging in regions with chronic myocardial infarction was provided in a subsequent report by Fudo and colleagues[37] who studied 22 patients with chronic anterior myocardial

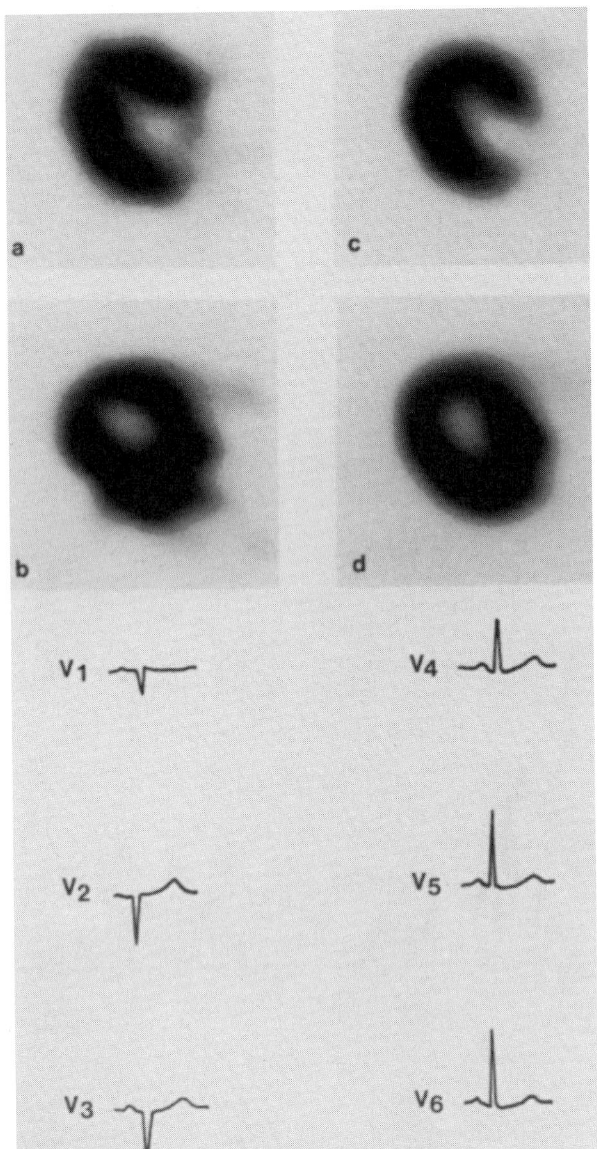

FIGURE 71–22. Representative ^{13}N-ammonia perfusion images *(Panels A and B)* and ^{18}F-2-fluoro-2-deoxyglucose metabolic images *(Panels C and D)* and precordial electrocardiogram of a 45-year-old woman with a well-documented anterior myocardial infarction 3 years prior to study. Although the electrocardiogram demonstrates pathologic Q waves in V_1 through V_3, regional perfusion and exogenous glucose use are within normal laboratory limits, indicating substantial tissue viability in the region with the electrocardiographic Q-wave infarction. (From Brunken, R., Tillisch, J., Schwaiger, M., et al.: Regional perfusion, glucose metabolism and wall motion in patients with chronic electrocardiographic Q-wave infarctions: Evidence for persistence of viable tissue in some infarct regions by positron emission tomography. Circulation 73:951, 1986. With permission of the American Heart Association.)

infarctions using resting and stress ^{13}N-ammonia perfusion and remote (within 1 week) ^{18}F-2-fluoro-2-deoxyglucose metabolic imaging. The mean interval from anterior myocardial infarction to the positron emission tomographic study was 20 weeks. Although the myocardial infarctions were diagnosed by "electrocardiographic and enzymatic criteria," their report did not indicate the number of the patients with Q waves on the electrocardiogram.

When studied with positron emission tomography, 19 of the 22 patients (86 percent) had resting ^{13}N-ammonia perfusion defects in the anterior wall. With exercise, 16 of the patients exhibited peripheral expansion of their resting perfusion defects, and 6 of these individuals had augmented uptake of ^{18}F-2-fluoro-2-deoxyglucose in these zones of peripheral perfusion defect expansion (see previous discussion). More importantly, 12 of the patients (54.5 percent) had diffuse uptake of ^{18}F-2-fluoro-2-deoxyglucose in the hypoperfused anterior regions, whereas an additional 2 patients (9.1 percent) without resting perfusion defects had elevated uptake of ^{18}F-2-fluoro-2-deoxyglucose in the electrocardiographic infarct region.

Hashimoto and coworkers[114] compared ^{13}N-ammonia and ^{18}F-2-fluoro-2-deoxyglucose images in 11 patients with chronic non-Q wave infarctions with those obtained in 11 patients with chronic Q-wave infarctions. The population consisted of 22 patients with documented anterior or lateral wall infarctions. Electrocardiographic Q-wave infarction was defined by the presence of Q waves greater than or equal to 30 msec in duration in at least two adjacent electrocardiographic leads. Non-Q wave myocardial infarction was defined by a history of precordial chest pain of greater than 30 minutes' duration and elevation of creatine kinase-MB levels on serial studies along with significant evolution of ST-segment or T-wave changes, or both, on serial electrocardiograms. The mean interval from the most recent clinical infarction to positron emission tomography was 3.3 ± 2.6 months in patients with the non-Q wave infarctions and 5.8 ± 6.7 months in patients with the Q-wave infarctions (P = NS).

On the ^{13}N-ammonia images, only 5 (45 percent) of the 11 patients with non-Q wave infarctions had resting perfusion defects. With exercise, 8 (73 percent) demonstrated a perfusion defect. In contrast, all 11 patients with Q-wave myocardial infarction had perfusion defects on both the resting and stress studies. Of the 15 patients who had coronary angiography and resting perfusion defects, all had significant stenoses (greater than or equal to 90 percent) in the infarct-related artery. Four of the 6 patients without a resting perfusion defect had coronary stenoses of less than or equal to 50 percent in the infarct vessel. One patient with a 90 percent stenosis did not exhibit a perfusion defect either at rest or with exercise, and this was attributed to the patient's use of a β-blocker.

Of the 11 patients with Q-wave myocardial infarction, 4 (36 percent) exhibited enhanced uptake of ^{18}F-2-fluoro-2-deoxyglucose in the hypoperfused infarct region. In contrast, 10 (91 percent) of the 11 patients with non-Q wave infarction had increased uptake of the labeled glucose tracer in the clinical infarct region ($P <$ .01). Thus, although this study suggests that myocardial metabolic viability is observed more frequently in individuals with non-Q wave infarction than in those with Q-wave infarctions, it also confirms that a significant proportion (36 percent) of patients with chronic Q-wave infarction will exhibit residual metabolic tissue viability.

Although electrocardiographic Q waves are most frequently observed in the setting of coronary artery disease, other coronary arterial disease processes may also lead to myocardial ischemia and infarction. Coronary arterial lesions are identified in about 20 percent of patients with Kawasaki disease,[115] and some patients with Kawasaki disease experience myocardial infarction.[116] Typically, the diagnosis of myocardial infarction is made by the new appearance of abnormal Q waves on the electrocardiogram, and these Q waves may disappear over the subsequent course of the illness.

The clinical utility of positron emission tomography for assessing the myocardial effects of the coronary arterial lesions was illustrated in 14 pediatric patients, aged 3 to 14 years, with Kawasaki disease and coronary arterial stenoses confirmed by selective coronary angiography.[117] The time interval from the onset of the disease to positron emission tomographic imaging ranged from 6 to 163 months (mean of 67 months). The images were compared with serial electrocardiograms that had been obtained monthly from the clinical onset of the disease process. Each of the individuals studied demonstrated either persistent or transient abnormal Q waves on serial electrocardiograms.

Positron emission tomography was performed in the fasting state using ^{13}N-ammonia and ^{18}F-2-fluoro-2-deoxyglucose. Myocardial segments were classified into four categories: normal perfusion and normal ^{18}F-2-fluoro-2-deoxyglucose uptake; hypoperfused with no increase in ^{18}F-2-fluoro-2-deoxyglucose uptake; hypoperfused with increased ^{18}F-2-fluoro-2-deoxyglucose uptake; and normal perfusion with increased ^{18}F-2-fluoro-2-deoxyglucose uptake.

Positron emission tomography revealed abnormalities in six of seven myocardial segments with persistent electrocardiographic Q waves. In three of these segments, ^{18}F-2-fluoro-2-deoxyglucose uptake was augmented relative to perfusion consistent with myocardial hibernation. In three myocardial segments, matching reductions in perfusion and glucose metabolism were observed, suggesting myocardial scar. In the final segment with persistent Q waves, both perfusion and glucose metabolism appeared normal. Thus, 57 percent (4 of 7) of myocardial Q wave regions exhibited evidence of tissue viability on positron emission tomography. In six myocardial segments with transient electrocardiographic Q waves, only two exhibited matching reductions in perfusion and glucose metabolism consistent with scar formation. Normal perfusion with augmented uptake of ^{18}F-2-fluoro-2-deoxyglucose was noted in three segments, whereas perfusion and glucose metabolism appeared normal in the final segment. Thus, 67 percent (4 of 6) of myocardial electrocardiographic Q wave regions appeared viable on positron emission tomography. Interestingly, the severity of the associated wall motion abnormalities did not reliably distinguish between the scintigraphic patterns observed in the myocardial electrocardiographic Q-wave regions. Thus, analysis of regional wall motion would have failed to discriminate between myocardial areas with scar formation and those with viable tissue.

The chronicity of the presence of the persistent Q waves on the electrocardiogram differed significantly between the myocardial segments with metabolically active tissue and those without. The mean duration of the abnormal Q waves in the myocardial regions with metabolically active tissue was 18.5 ± 17.1 months, which was significantly shorter than the duration of the persistence of the abnormal Q waves in the patients with matching metabolic and perfusion defects, 92.4 ± 26.8 months ($P < .01$). Thus, in the myocardial Q-wave regions with persistent electrocadiographic abnormalities, the longer the persistence of the electrocardiographic Q wave, the greater the likelihood of myocardial scar on positron emission tomographic imaging. The authors concluded that in patients with Kawasaki disease, the new appearance of abnormal Q waves is a reliable clue to the presence of ischemic myocardial injury and that a high proportion of transient Q waves are associated with metabolically active myocardium. The disappearance of abnormal Q waves did not necessarily imply the normalization of regional myocardial perfusion, metabolism, or function, however, and thus were not a reliable indicator of the presence or absence of jeopardized myocardium.

These clinical investigations are consistent with previous histologic studies demonstrating that myocardial infarction is an inhomogeneous process. In some patients, an infarction may be nearly transmural in extent, whereas in other patients, there may be only small amounts of subendocardial fibrosis. As noted previously, electrocardiographic Q waves reflect only abnormal electrical activation of the myocardium and they do not establish a cause nor imply irreversibility of the underlying process (Fig. 71–23). Thus, glucose metabolic imaging provides an additional means of tissue characterization in patients with previous myocardial infarction. Also, the presence of chronic Q waves on the electrocardiogram does not preclude the existence of substantial amounts of viable tissue in the clinical infarct zone.

ST-Segment Elevation

Prior clinical studies have indicated that exercise-induced ST-segment elevation in electrocardiographic leads with a pathologic Q wave is a marker for poor left ventricular function and an adverse prognosis.[118] Exercise-induced ST-segment elevation has been noted in about 30 percent of patients with anterior myocardial infarctions and 15 percent of patients with inferior infarctions when studied within 2 weeks of the acute event.[119] The prevalence of exercise-induced ST-segment elevation decreases in frequency over the 6 weeks following the acute event.

Margonato and colleagues[120] studied 34 patients with prior Q-wave infarction (anterior in 21 and inferior in 13) using resting SPECT perfusion imaging with ^{99m}Tc-sestamibi, positron emission tomography with ^{18}F-2-fluoro-2-deoxyglucose, and coronary angiography. The average time interval between the clinical infarction and the positron emission tomographic metabolic study was 72 ± 108 days in 18 patients with ST-segment elevation and 516 ± 545 days in 16 patients without exercise-induced ST-segment elevation. Each patient underwent maximal treadmill exercise following an overnight fast. Exercise-induced ST-segment elevation was defined by an elevation greater than 1 mm above the baseline ST-segment level, 8 msec after the J-point in more than one lead with abnormal Q waves. Resting myocardial perfusion was assessed with SPECT on the day after the positron emission tomographic metabolic study. Positron emission tomography was performed in the fasting state to enhance the detection of viable myocardium by suppressing uptake of the radiolabeled tracer in normal tissue. In each of six myocardial segments, hypoperfused tissue was considered viable when ^{18}F-2-fluoro-2-deoxyglucose uptake divided by the activity within the ventricular cavity exceeded the 95 percent confidence interval determined by the study of five normal, fasting subjects.

Of the 18 patients with exercise-induced ST-segment elevation, 14 had an anterior infarction and 4 had an inferior myocardial infarction. In the 16 individuals without exercise-induced ST-segment elevation, there were seven anterior infarctions and nine inferior infarctions. Eight individuals with exercise-induced ST-segment elevation had been treated with thrombolytic therapy, whereas seven in the remaining group were treated with thrombolytic therapy. The achieved rate-pressure product at exercise and the total exercise time for both groups were similar. Six (33 percent) of the patients with exercise-induced ST-segment elevation reported anginal symptoms, whereas only one (6 percent) reported anginal symptoms ($P = .05$). Each of the 34 patients had a resting perfusion defect that agreed with the site of previous clinical infarction. On contrast left ventriculography, each of the 34 patients had abnormal wall motion in the areas corresponding to the electrocardiographic Q waves. The severity of the associated wall motion abnormality was significantly more pronounced in the individuals with ST-segment elevation than in the individuals without. Furthermore, 14 of the individuals with exercise-induced ST-segment elevation had occluded infarct-related vessels, whereas 8 of the individuals without ST-segment elevation had occluded infarct vessels. All patients with exercise-induced ST-segment elevation also exhibited enhanced uptake of ^{18}F-2-fluoro-2-deoxyglucose in the zone of clinical infarction. In contrast, only 9 (56 percent) of the 16 individuals without exercise-induced ST-segment elevation displayed enhanced metabolic activity. The sensitivity, specificity, and positive predictive accuracy of exercise-induced ST-segment elevation for detecting residual tissue viability were 67, 100, and 74 percent, respectively. When only anterior myocardial infarctions were considered, sensitivity, specificity, and positive predictive accuracy were 82, 100, and 86 percent, respectively. The authors concluded that the presence of exercise-induced ST-segment elevation in electrocardiographic leads with Q-wave infarctions is highly specific for the detection of residual viability within the zone of clinical infarction.

Several factors should be considered in interpreting the results of this investigation. The first factor is the temporal disparity between the time of clinical infarction and enrollment in the study. As noted, exercise-induced ST-segment elevation and preserved glucose metabolism within the zone of clinical infarction are both relatively common findings early after the acute event. For both findings, the relative frequency of observation of these markers declines as time progresses from the acute ischemic injury. Thus the differences in relative prevalence of preserved metabolic viability in the two patient groups may, in part, be influenced by the difference in time from clinical infarction to study in these individuals. Second, preserved metabolic viability was noted in 56 percent of the clinical infarct zones in which ST-segment elevation was not

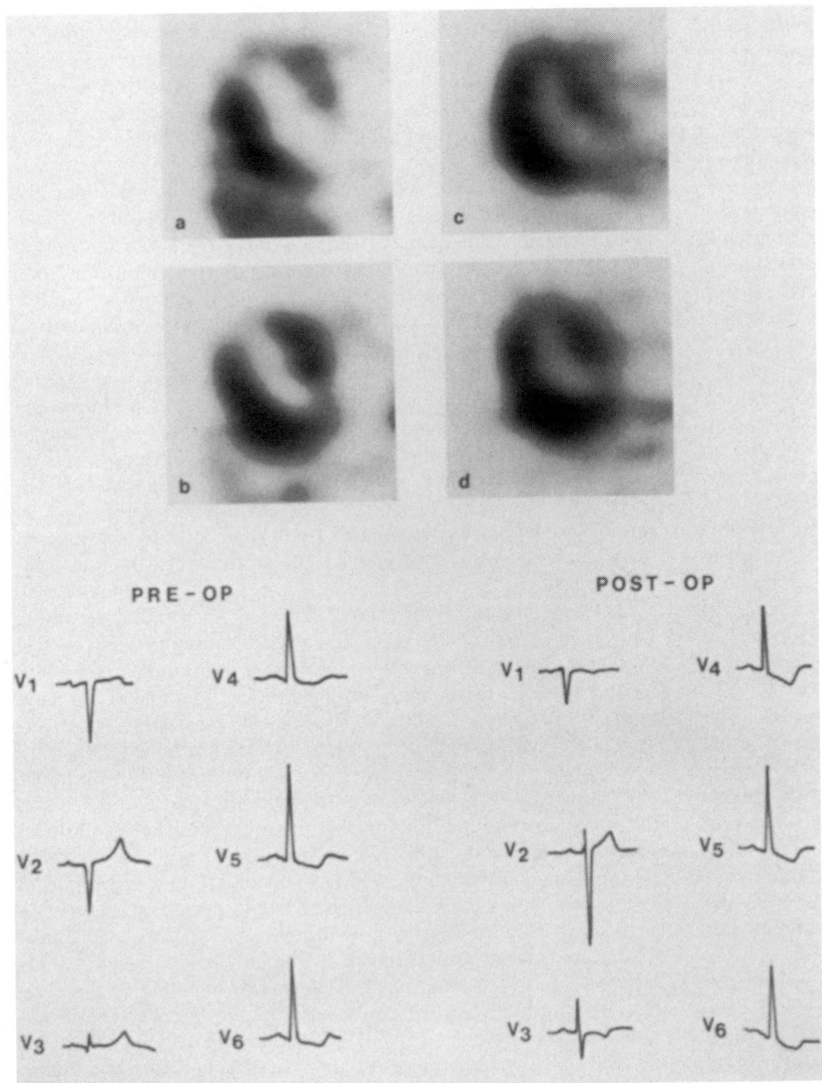

FIGURE 71–23. Precordial electrocardiograms obtained before *(PRE-OP)* and after *(POST-OP)* coronary bypass surgery along with representative preoperative ^{13}N-ammonia perfusion images *(Panels A and B)* and ^{18}F-2-fluoro-2-deoxyglucose metabolic images *(Panels C and D)* in a 73-year-old woman with a history of two remote myocardial infarctions and recurrent angina. The ^{13}N-ammonia perfusion images demonstrate an anteroapical perfusion defect. On the metabolic images there is preserved glucose metabolism in the hypoperfused region, indicating myocardial viability. On the preoperative electrocardiogram, pathologic Q waves are noted in leads V_1 through V_3. Following coronary bypass surgery, the anterior Q waves are replaced by normal-appearing R waves. Along with the electrocardiographic changes, the patient's left ventricular ejection fraction increased from 25 to 45 percent following coronary revascularization, and there was improvement in wall motion in the anteroapical region of the ventricle from akinesis to severe hypokinesis. (From Brunken, R., Tillisch, J., Schwaiger, M., et al.: Regional perfusion, glucose metabolism and wall motion in patients with chronic electrocardiographic Q-wave infarctions: Evidence for persistence of viable tissue in some infarct regions by positron emission tomography. Circulation 73:951, 1986. With permission of the American Heart Association.)

identified. The absence of this electrocardiographic finding does not reliably discriminate between patients with and those without myocardial metabolic viability in the zone of clinical infarction. As noted by the authors, further prospective studies to examine the relationship between the identification of residual myocardial metabolic activity and exercise-induced ST-segment elevation in patients with prior myocardial infarction appear to be warranted.

Regional Myocardial Wall Motion and Thickening

Although assessment of segmental wall motion has been used to infer the presence or absence of viable myocardium in patients with ischemic heart disease, previous histopathologic studies have indicated that the severity of a resting wall motion abnormality is not always related to the extent of myocardial fibrosis.[94, 121] To determine if analysis of regional wall motion might assist in distinguishing regions with and without metabolic activity, Brunken and coworkers[112] also assessed segmental wall motion in Q-wave and non-Q wave regions considered normal, ischemic, and infarcted on positron emission tomography (see previous discussion). Resting left ventricular wall motion abnormalities were assessed with gated radionuclide ventriculography in 14 patients, with two-dimensional echocardiography in 4 patients, and with contrast left ventriculography in 2 patients. The mean interval from the wall motion study to positron emission tomography was 20.5 ± 21.9 days. Regional wall motion was graded according to the following scale: normal = 0, mild hypokinesis = 1, severe hypokinesis = 2, akinesis = 3, and dyskinesis = 4. Three independent observers graded segmental wall motion, and their scores were averaged to give a mean regional wall motion score.

Regions with electrocardiographic Q waves that were considered normal on positron emission tomography had a mean wall motion score of 1.27 ± 0.85, whereas ischemic regions had a score of 2.17 ± 0.81, and infarcted regions had a score of 2.69 ± 0.59. The score for normal regions was significantly better than the score for ischemic regions ($P < .025$) or for infarcted regions ($P < .0005$). Perhaps more importantly, there was no significant difference between the scores for ischemic and infarcted regions, indicating that assessment of wall motion failed to distinguish between hypoperfused regions with and those without metabolic evidence of tissue viability.

Analysis of wall motion in 52 non–Q wave regions yielded similar findings. Normal regions had a mean wall motion score of 1.02 ± 0.71, ischemic regions had a mean score of 1.82 ± 0.88 ($P <$ .05 versus normal), and infarcted regions had a score of 2.00 ± 0.71 ($P < .01$ versus normal, P = NS versus ischemic regions). Thus, the findings in this study indicate that the assessment of regional wall motion cannot successfully discriminate between hypoperfused regions with and those without metabolic viability as determined on metabolic imaging with positron emission tomography.

Fudo and colleagues[37] also correlated the results of metabolic imaging with regional wall motion (see previous discussion) in their study of patients with chronic anterior myocardial infarctions. They grouped their patients according to regional function in the anterior wall. Group I consisted of eight patients with dyskinesis; in group II there were seven patients with anterior akinesis and in group III there were seven patients with anterior hypokinesis. Of the eight patients in group I, 3 (37.5 percent) exhibited diffuse uptake of ^{18}F-2-fluoro-2-deoxyglucose in the anterior dyskinetic region. Of the seven patients in group II, 3 (42.9 percent) exhibited uptake of the glucose metabolic tracer in the akinetic zone of infarction. In contrast, six of seven (85.7 percent) patients in group III had diffuse uptake of ^{18}F-2-fluoro-2-deoxyglucose in the hypokinetic anterior regions. Thus, although the results of this study indicate that the myocardial regions with chronic infarction and less severe impairment in wall motion have a better probability of exhibiting metabolic viability, a significant proportion of dyskinetic (37.5 percent) and akinetic (42.9 percent) clinical infarct regions manifest metabolic evidence of viability. The results also suggest that reliance on the severity of a regional wall motion abnormality alone may seriously underestimate the extent of tissue viability in patients with ischemic heart disease.

Using a more sophisticated means of assessing ventricular function, Perone-Filardi and colleagues[122] performed positron emission tomography with ^{15}O-water and ^{18}F-2-fluoro-2-deoxyglucose in 25 patients with chronic coronary artery disease and correlated these findings with measurements of regional end-diastolic wall thicknesses and systolic wall thickening obtained from spin-echo gated nuclear magnetic resonance imaging (MRI).

Of 355 regions evaluated, 89 were akinetic or dyskinetic (mean systolic wall thickening = -1.2 ± 1.8 mm), 95 were hypokinetic (mean systolic wall thickening = 1.3 ± 0.5 mm), and 171 had normal systolic function (mean systolic thickening = 4.2 ± 1.7 mm). Importantly, absolute myocardial blood flows did not distinguish among these three groups of regions (0.87 ± 0.34 versus 0.84 ± 0.34 versus 0.90 ± 0.34 mL $\cdot$ g^{-1} $\cdot$ min^{-1}, respectively). Although mean relative ^{18}F-2-fluoro-2-deoxyglucose activity was significantly lower in the akinetic-dyskinetic and hypokinetic regions than in normal regions, there was a large degree of overlap among the three groups. Relative ^{18}F-2-fluoro-2-deoxyglucose activities did not correlate well with either end-diastolic wall thickness or systolic wall thickening.

Of the 89 regions with akinesia-dyskinesia, 66 (74 percent) had preserved metabolic activity (defined as a relative tracer concentration greater than 50 percent of a normal reference region), and regional systolic thickening did not distinguish between regions with and without metabolic activity (-1.1 ± 1.7 versus -1.1 ± 1.9 mm, P = NS). Regions with preserved metabolic activity had greater end-diastolic wall thicknesses (11 ± 4 versus 7 ± 3 mm, $P < .001$) and greater regional blood flows (0.90 ± 0.34 versus 0.67 ± 0.34 mL $\cdot$ g^{-1} $\cdot$ min^{-1}, $P < .05$) than akinetic-dyskinetic regions without metabolic activity. An end-diastolic thickness of 8 mm provided the best discrimination between akinetic and dyskinetic regions, yet metabolic activity was present in 14 of 31 (45 percent) regions with end-diastolic wall thicknesses less than 8 mm. Of the 95 regions with hypokinesia, 87 (92 percent) exhibited metabolic activity. The relative ^{18}F-2-fluoro-2-deoxyglucose concentrations in regions less than 8 mm thick at end-diastole did not differ from those with end-diastolic thicknesses greater than 8 mm. These investigators concluded that measures of regional left ventricular anatomy and systolic function are of limited value in distinguishing nonviable from viable dysfunctional myocardium in patients with chronic coronary artery disease.

The metabolic observations made in these studies are consistent with previous clinicopathologic investigations indicating that myocardial infarction is a heterogeneous process and that the extent of myocardial fibrosis in patients with ischemic heart disease may vary considerably among individuals. For example, in the autopsy study of Idecker and colleagues,[123] the measured percentage of fibrosis in hypokinetic segments ranged from 0 to 60 percent, from 0 to 85 percent in akinetic segments, and from 5 to 85 percent in dyskinetic segments. In addition, these authors also reported that some segments with normal wall motion displayed as much as 40 percent fibrosis on histologic examination. Comparable findings were reported by Stinson and Billingham,[124] who correlated the results of transmural apical biopsy specimens obtained at the time of coronary bypass surgery with regional function. Normal or only mild to moderate fibrosis was found in 81 percent (17 of 21) of hypokinetic regions, 47 percent (9 of 19) of akinetic regions, and 21 percent (3 of 14) of dyskinetic regions.

Further indirect evidence for the frequent presence of viable tissue in asynergic ventricular regions comes from the functional outcome after revascularization. In individuals with stable angina, improvement or normalization of resting wall motion abnormalities occurs in 34 to 66 percent of segments following successful coronary bypass grafting,[125–127] including 29 percent of segments with previous infarction.[126] In addition, both Cohen and colleagues[128] and Melchior and coworkers[129] have reported that 83 and 65 percent, respectively, of patients with chronic ischemic left ventricular dysfunction will have improvement in regional function following angioplasty of the culprit vessel. Thus, assessment of segmental wall motion is not a reliable indicator of myocardial viability. The tissue characterization afforded by metabolic imaging with positron emission tomography is helpful in distinguishing asynergic regions with extensive fibrosis from regions with viable but ischemically compromised tissue.

Thallium-201 Scintigraphy

^{201}Tl redistribution scintigraphy has played an important clinical role in assessing myocardial viability in patients with coronary artery disease.[130] Initially, ^{201}Tl defects that persisted on 3- or 4-hour redistribution images were attributed to completed infarction, whereas fill-in of defects was associated with ischemic but viable tissue.[131] Several early clinical observations, however, suggested that ^{201}Tl redistribution imaging at 4 hours underestimates the extent of myocardial viability in some patients. For example, Liu and colleagues[132] reported that 12 of 16 (75 percent) myocardial segments with persistent defects on stress ^{201}Tl scintigraphy prior to angioplasty normalized on ^{201}Tl imaging after interventional restoration of blood flow. Further, Gibson and coworkers[133] noted that 19 of 42 (45 percent) myocardial segments with persistent defects on preoperative stress and redistribution ^{201}Tl scintigraphy had normal tracer uptake and normal washout kinetics after coronary revascularization. Thus, these early reports indicated that some myocardial segments with fixed defects on ^{201}Tl scintigraphy might indeed harbor viable tissue.

Stress-Resting Redistribution Scintigraphy

In order to determine if myocardial metabolic viability could be identified in segments with persistent ^{201}Tl defects, Brunken and coinvestigators[134] studied 12 consecutive patients with fixed defects on stress and 4-hour redistribution planar scintigraphy. Ten of the patients had a history of 14 prior myocardial infarctions. The mean left ventricular ejection fraction was depressed at 32.1 ± 14.7 percent.

Of the 51 segmental ^{201}Tl defects identified by three independent observers, 36 were fixed, 11 were partially reversible, and 4 were completely reversible. Of the 36 segments with a fixed ^{201}Tl defect, only 15 (42 percent) exhibited the concordant defects in perfusion and glucose metabolism indicative of myocardial infarction on positron emission tomography (Table 71–4). In contrast, the metabolism-perfusion mismatch of myocardial ischemia was present in 9 segments (25 percent), whereas 12 segments (33 percent) were normal on study with positron emission tomography. Thus, the majority of myocardial segments with a fixed ^{201}Tl defect (58 percent) exhibited evidence of myocardial metabolic viability on study with positron emission tomography (see Table 71–4).

Of the 11 segments with a partially reversible ^{201}Tl defect, 4 (36 percent) exhibited the concordant decreases in perfusion and glucose metabolism indicative of myocardial infarction. Four of the segments (36 percent) had a metabolism-perfusion mismatch, whereas three segments (27 percent) were normal on positron

TABLE 71–4. POSITRON EMISSION TOMOGRAPHY VERSUS THALLIUM-201 FOR MYOCARDIAL VIABILITY

			Segmental Defects With Positron Emission Tomographic Metabolic Viability					
Thallium-201	**Images**	**Number of Studies**	***Fixed***	***Partial Thallium-201 Redistribution***	***Complete Thallium-201 Redistribution***	***Reinjection* +**	***Reinjection* −**	**Reference**
Planar	4-hr RD	12	21/36 (58%)	7/11 (67%)	4/4 (100%)			Brunken et al.[134]
SPECT	3-hr RD	28	15/39 (38%)		21/22 (95%)			Tamaki et al.[135]
SPECT	3-hr RD	28	56/136 (41%)		52/77 (68%)			Tamaki et al.[79]
SPECT	4-hr RD	27	47/101 (47%)	20/31 (65%)	10/10 (100%)			Brunken et al.[136]
SPECT	24-hr RD	14	16/30 (53%)	17/31 (61%)	8/10 (80%)			Brunken et al.[141]
SPECT	Reinjection	18	27/48 (56%)		47/47 (100%)	20/20 (100%)	7/28 (25%)	Tamaki et al.[80]
SPECT	Reinjection	16	121*/166 (73%)	94†/105 (89%)	75/75 (100%)	69/78 (88%)	52/88 (59%)	Bonow et al.[145]
SPECT	Reinjection	15	135*/169 (79%)			72/77 (94%)	63/92 (68%)	Dilsizian et al.[158]
SPECT‡	Reinjection	25	135*/169 (80%)		109/112 (97%)	50/51 (98%)	86/118 (73%)	Perrone-Filardi et al.[146]

*Fixed segmental defects were subdivided into reinjection + and reinjection − defects, as listed in the last two data columns.

†The authors reported that 94 percent of partially and completely reversible ^{201}Tl defects exhibited metabolic activity on positron emission tomography but they did not provide individual data for the partially reversible and completely reversible defect categories. The 11 segments without uptake of ^{18}F-2-fluoro-2-deoxyglucose were arbitrarily assigned to the partially reversible defect category.

‡Includes data from 11 patients reported by Bonow and colleagues.[145]

RD = ^{201}Tl redistribution; Reinjection + = improvement in ^{201}Tl defect on reinjection images; Reinjection − = no improvement in ^{201}Tl defect on reinjection images; SPECT = single-photon emission computed tomography.

emission tomography. Thus, residual tissue metabolic activity was detected in 64 percent of the segments with a partially reversible ^{201}Tl defect. The four segments with completely reversible ^{201}Tl defects were normal on positron emission tomography. In addition, positron emission tomography identified seven myocardial segments with resting perfusion defects that were not detected on planar ^{201}Tl imaging. Three of these segments exhibited metabolic criteria for myocardial infarction, whereas four segments exhibited the metabolism-perfusion mismatch of myocardial ischemia. Improvement or normalization of a ^{201}Tl defect on 4-hour redistribution images was not correlated with uptake of ^{18}F-2-fluoro-2-deoxyglucose (11 of 15 versus 21 of 26, P = NS), indicating that redistribution of ^{201}Tl was not statistically associated with myocardial viability in this patient population.

In order to assess both tissue glucose metabolism and regional wall motion in myocardial segments with persistent ^{201}Tl defects, Tamaki and colleagues[135] correlated the findings on contrast left ventriculography and stress and 3-hour delayed SPECT ^{201}Tl scintigraphy with positron emission tomography in 28 patients with remote myocardial infarction. Regional function was graded on the contrast left ventriculograms according to the following scale: 2 = normal, 1 = hypokinetic, 0 = akinetic, and −1 = dyskinetic.

Positron emission tomography with ^{13}N-ammonia and ^{18}F-2-fluoro-2-deoxyglucose was performed within 2 weeks of ^{201}Tl scintigraphy. Quantitative analysis of ^{201}Tl uptake on the SPECT images and the ^{13}N-ammonia images was performed with circumferential count profile analysis techniques, whereas ^{201}Tl defects in each of five myocardial segments were visually classified as fixed (no redistribution on delayed images) or transient (partial or complete redistribution on delayed images). The ^{18}F-2-fluoro-2-deoxyglucose images were evaluated visually and compared with the ^{13}N-ammonia perfusion images. Segments with an increase in the uptake of the glucose analog were considered ischemic. In this investigation, only the segments "with ^{201}Tl fixed perfusion defects in electrocardiographically defined infarcted areas" were analyzed, whereas remote segments with perfusion defects were excluded from analysis. Thus a semiquantitative scoring system was not used to quantitate the severity of the visually defined ^{201}Tl defects, nor were all myocardial segments with ^{201}Tl perfusion defects analyzed.

All 28 patients had ^{201}Tl defects in the electrocardiographically defined infarct region. Transient ^{201}Tl defects were identified in at least one myocardial segment in 13 individuals, whereas persistent defects were identified in 15 individuals. In the 28 patients, 61 segmental ^{201}Tl defects were analyzed. Transient defects were present in 22 segments (36 percent) and persistent defects were seen in 39 segments (64 percent). On positron emission tomography, myocardial glucose metabolism was preserved in 21 of the 22 segments with transient defects (95 percent) and 15 of the 39 segments with fixed defects (38 percent, $P < .001$, see Table 71–4). This study suggested, therefore, that redistribution of ^{201}Tl in a segmental defect was more frequently associated with preservation of myocardial glucose metabolism. In agreement with the findings by Brunken and colleagues,[134] 40 percent of segments with fixed ^{201}Tl defects exhibited preserved glucose metabolism, again suggesting that analysis of relative myocardial perfusion alone underestimates the extent of tissue viability in a relatively large proportion of myocardial segments.

Brunken and coinvestigators[136] subsequently examined whether a similar discrepancy existed between ^{201}Tl SPECT and positron emission tomography. Of the 26 patients (27 studies) with angiographically confirmed coronary artery disease, 21 patients had a clinical history of 29 antecedent myocardial infarctions. The mean left ventricular ejection fraction was depressed at 32.0 ± 14 percent.

Stress ^{201}Tl scintigraphy was performed in 20 patients, rest-redistribution ^{201}Tl scintigraphy was performed in 5 patients, and dipyridamole ^{201}Tl scintigraphy was performed in 1 patient. Three observers independently assessed ^{201}Tl uptake in each of the seven myocardial segments according to the following grading scale: 0 = normal, 1 = a definite but modest defect, 2 = a severe defect, and 3 = a complete defect (equal to background).

There were 101 fixed, 31 partially reversible, and 10 completely reversible ^{201}Tl defects. Of the 101 segments with fixed defects, only 54 (53.4 percent) exhibited the concordant decreases in perfusion and glucose metabolism characteristic of completed infarction (Fig. 71–24, Table 71–4). In contrast, myocardial ischemia was observed in 24 (23.8 percent) of the segments with fixed defects, indicating residual tissue metabolic viability (Fig. 71–25). Of the 31 segments with partially reversible defects, 11 (35.5 percent) exhibited metabolic criteria for myocardial infarction, whereas myocardial ischemia was observed in 9 (29 percent) of the segments. Thus, residual tissue metabolic viability was identified in 47 (46.5 percent) of the segments with fixed ^{201}Tl defects and 20 (64.5 percent) of the segments with partially reversible ^{201}Tl defects, again indicating that ^{201}Tl scintigraphy with 4-hour redistribution images underestimates the extent of tissue viability in patients with ischemic heart disease.

Of the 10 segments with completely reversible defects, 5 (50 percent) were normal on positron emission tomography, whereas 5 (50 percent) exhibited the metabolism-perfusion mismatch. Visual improvement in a persistent ^{201}Tl defect on redistribution imaging at 4 hours was not associated with the presence of glucose metabolic activity (20 of 31 partially reversible defects versus 47 of 101

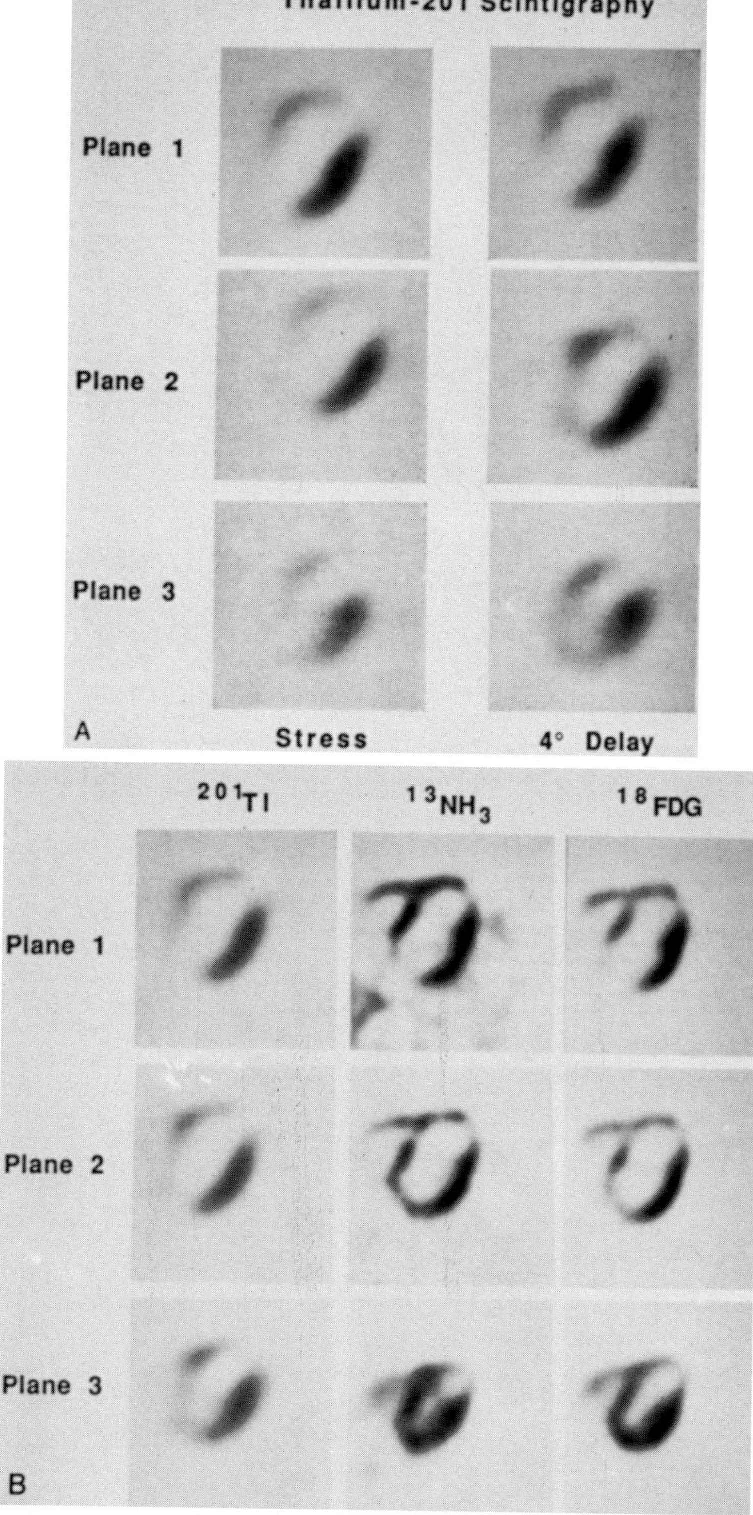

FIGURE 71–24. *Panel A,* Stress and 4-hour delayed SPECT ^{201}Tl images from the study of a 62-year-old man with a history of previous myocardial infarction and triple-vessel coronary artery disease. The ^{201}Tl images demonstrate fixed defects in the anterior and apical regions of the ventricle and partially reversible anteroseptal and inferoseptal defects. *Panel B,* The corresponding ^{13}N-ammonia (*$^{13}NH_3$*) and ^{18}F-2-fluoro-2-deoxyglucose metabolic (*^{18}FDG*) images along with the 4-hour tomographic ^{201}Tl images. Concordant reductions in myocardial perfusion and glucose metabolism are identified in the anterior, apical, and anteroseptal segments denoting completed myocardial infarction. In contrast, both perfusion and glucose metabolism are normal in the inferoseptal segment. (From Brunken, R. C., Kottou, S., Schwaiger, M., et al.: PET detection of viable tissue in myocardial segments with persistent defects at thallium-201 SPECT. Radiology 172:65, 1989, with permission.)

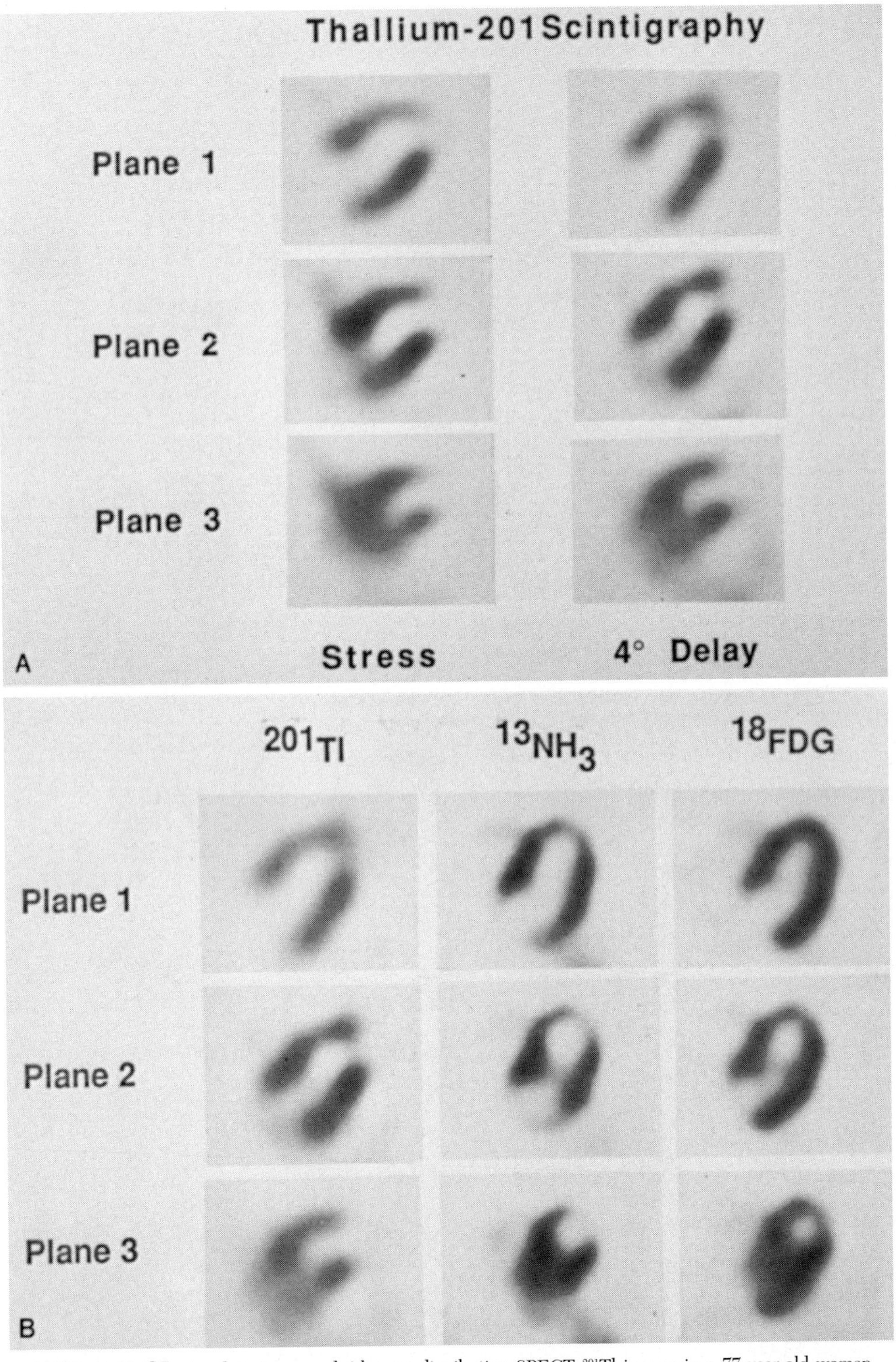

Thallium-201Scintigraphy

Plane 1

Plane 2

Plane 3

A Stress 4° Delay

^{201}Tl ^{13}NH$_3$ ^{18}FDG

Plane 1

Plane 2

Plane 3

B

FIGURE 71–25. *Panel A,* Stress and 4-hour redistribution SPECT ^{201}Tl images in a 77-year-old woman with a history of prior myocardial infarction. On the tomographic cross-sectional ^{201}Tl images there is a fixed apical defect and partially reversible septal and anterior defects. *Panel B,* Four-hour tomographic ^{201}Tl images along with the corresponding ^{13}N-ammonia perfusion (*$^{13}NH_3$*) perfusion images and ^{18}F-2-fluoro-2-deoxyglucose metabolic images (*^{18}FDG*). Although perfusion defects similar to those noted on the ^{201}Tl study are identified on the ^{13}N-ammonia perfusion images, there is preservation of glucose metabolism in the anterior and apical regions of the ventricle on the glucose metabolic images indicating myocardial viability. (From Brunken, R. C., Kottou, S., Schwaiger, M., et al.: PET detection of viable tissue in myocardial segments with persistent defects at thallium-201 SPECT. Radiology 172:65, 1989, with permission.)

fixed defects, $0.05 < P < .1$). Thus, apparent improvement in a persistent ^{201}Tl SPECT defect on redistribution images at 4 hours was not a reliable indicator of the presence or absence of tissue viability in this study population.

Delayed Thallium-201 Redistribution

Because some have proposed that 3 or 4 hours is too short a time for ^{201}Tl redistribution to occur in some individuals with tight coronary stenoses,[137] delayed ^{201}Tl redistribution imaging at 24 hours has been advocated.[138–140] For example, Kiat and coworkers[139] reported that 74 of 122 (61 percent) persistent segmental ^{201}Tl defects on 4-hour delayed images exhibited further redistribution on repeat imaging at 18 to 72 hours. Similarly, Cloninger and colleagues[138] noted that 13 of 28 (46.4 percent) patients with prior infarction and ^{201}Tl defects at 4 hours exhibit further redistribution on delayed imaging at 24 hours. Brunken and colleagues[141] compared positron emission tomography with ^{13}N-ammonia and ^{18}F-2-fluoro-2-deoxyglucose to 24-hour ^{201}Tl redistribution imaging with SPECT in 26 patients with chronic coronary artery disease, and severely impaired ventricular function (left ventricular ejection fraction = 32 ± 14 percent). On 19 stress-redistribution and 7 resting-redistribution SPECT studies, four observers visually scored ^{201}Tl activity in each of eight segments on a scale from 0 (normal) to 3 (complete defect). Using an improvement in visual score of 0.75 or greater to define redistribution, there were 100 fixed, 17 partially reversible, and 12 completely reversible defects. Glucose metabolic activity was present in 51 (51 percent) segments with fixed defects (21 ischemia, 30 normal) and 9 (53 percent) segments with partially reversible defects (five ischemia, four normal; as listed in Table 71–3 and shown in Fig. 71–26). When grouped by the 24-hour score, the proportion of fixed defects with metabolic activity varied from 84 percent (scores ≤ 1.4) to 15 percent (scores > 2.6). For partially reversible defects, only 53 percent with scores less than 2 and one of two with scores greater than or equal to 2 were considered metabolically viable on positron emission tomography. Of 12 completely reversible defects, 6 (50 percent) were

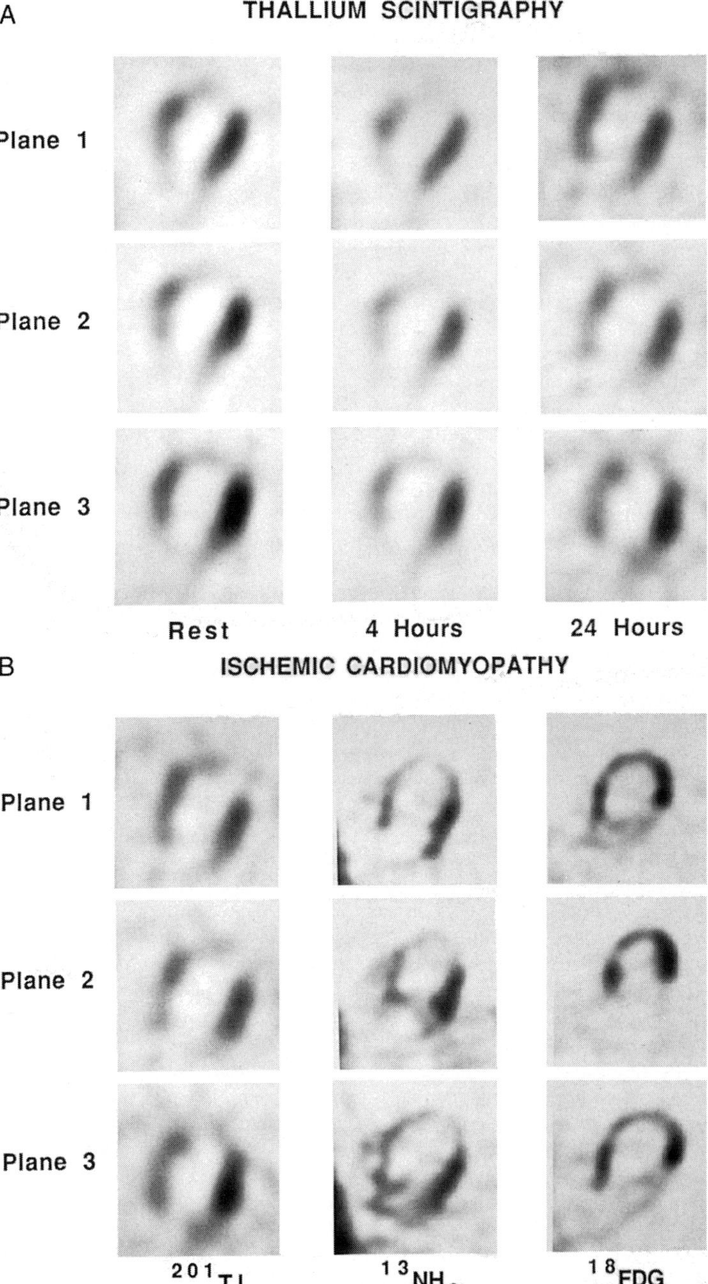

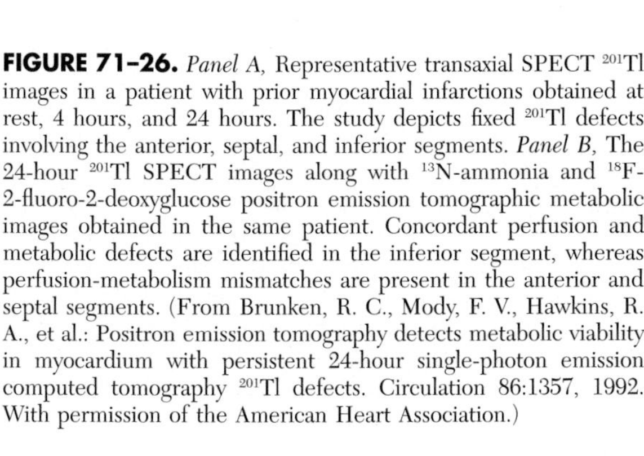

FIGURE 71–26. *Panel A,* Representative transaxial SPECT ^{201}Tl images in a patient with prior myocardial infarctions obtained at rest, 4 hours, and 24 hours. The study depicts fixed ^{201}Tl defects involving the anterior, septal, and inferior segments. *Panel B,* The 24-hour ^{201}Tl SPECT images along with ^{13}N-ammonia and ^{18}F-2-fluoro-2-deoxyglucose positron emission tomographic metabolic images obtained in the same patient. Concordant perfusion and metabolic defects are identified in the inferior segment, whereas perfusion-metabolism mismatches are present in the anterior and septal segments. (From Brunken, R. C., Mody, F. V., Hawkins, R. A., et al.: Positron emission tomography detects metabolic viability in myocardium with persistent 24-hour single-photon emission computed tomography ^{201}Tl defects. Circulation 86:1357, 1992. With permission of the American Heart Association.)

normal, 5 (42 percent) revealed persistent metabolic activity, and 1 (8 percent) had a perfusion-metabolism match. The proportion of fixed defects with metabolic activity did not depend on whether a resting or stress study was performed or on the change in visual score used to define ^{201}Tl redistribution (0.25, 0.50, 0.75, and 1.00) In a subsequent report,[142] these same investigators noted that the relative number of fixed ^{201}Tl defects on 24-hour redistribution images with metabolic viability on positron emission tomography was independent of plasma ^{201}Tl concentrations. The authors concluded that positron emission tomography identifies glucose metabolic activity in the majority of fixed 24-hour ^{201}Tl defects. However, nearly complete ^{201}Tl defects are less likely to exhibit metabolic activity than are less severe ^{201}Tl defects.

Reinjection Thallium-201 Scintigraphy

The approach of reinjection ^{201}Tl scintigraphy has been proposed to enhance the accuracy of detecting viable myocardium in patients with coronary artery disease and poor left ventricular function.[143, 144] Bonow and coworkers[145] performed stress and 4-hour redistribution ^{201}Tl SPECT imaging in 16 patients with chronic coronary artery disease and a left ventricular ejection fraction of 27±9 percent. Following redistribution imaging, an additional 1 mCi of ^{201}Tl was administered and a third set of SPECT images was obtained. The scintigraphic results were then compared with the findings on positron emission tomography with ^{15}O-water and ^{18}F-2-fluoro-2-deoxyglucose.

A ^{201}Tl defect was defined on the stress images by a relative tracer reduction to less than 85 percent of that of reference myocardium. A reversible defect was defined by an increase of 10 percent or greater in relative ^{201}Tl activity. By definition, tracer concentrations in completely reversible defects were greater than 85 percent of reference values on the redistribution or reinjection images. Defects were considered fixed if relative ^{201}Tl activity changed by less than 10 percent from the stress to redistribution or reinjection studies. Persistent defects were considered mild if relative tracer activity was between 60 and 84 percent of normal, moderate if activity was between 50 and 59 percent, and severe if activity was less than 50 percent. Any defect with a relative tracer concentration less than 50 percent of reference myocardium on the reinjection images was considered an irreversible defect. ^{18}F-2-fluoro-2-deoxyglucose counts were referenced to that in the reference region identified on the stress SPECT images. Segments with relative ^{18}F tracer concentrations less than 50 percent of reference myocardium were considered nonviable, whereas tracer concentrations 50 percent or greater were considered viable.

On the ^{201}Tl redistribution images, 166 irreversible defects were identified. On the redistribution images, metabolic activity was identified in 48 (91 percent) of 53 mild defects, 38 (84 percent) of 45 moderate defects, and 35 (51 percent) of severe defects. Of 78 defects that improved following reinjection of ^{201}Tl, 69 (88 percent) had uptake of ^{18}F-2-fluoro-2-deoxyglucose, whereas 52 (59 percent) of 88 defects without improvement on ^{201}Tl reinjection also had metabolic activity. Of the 45 segments that did not exhibit metabolic activity, 9 (20 percent) improved on the reinjection images. As the severity of the ^{201}Tl defects increased, the proportion of reinjection negative defects with metabolic activity declined from 97 percent for the mild defects to 12 percent for severe defects. The authors concluded that the reinjection of ^{201}Tl imaging enhances the ability of the imaging technique to identify viable myocardium as defined by ^{18}F-2-fluoro-2-deoxyglucose uptake.

In a subsequent study, these investigators[146] examined regional function with gated magnetic resonance imaging in 25 patients with chronic coronary artery disease and correlated these findings with relative ^{201}Tl uptake on reinjection SPECT images and with uptake of ^{18}F-2-fluoro-2-deoxyglucose on positron emission tomography. Using the methods of their prior report,[145] they identified 112 segments with improvement and 169 segments with persistent ^{201}Tl defects on 3- to 4-hour redistribution images. As anticipated, nearly all 109 (97 percent) of the 112 defects with redistribution on the 3- to 4-hour images had evidence of myocardial metabolic activity on positron emission tomography. Of the 169 defects that persisted on the redistribution images, 51 showed improvement on the reinjection images, whereas 118 did not improve. Metabolic activity was identified in 50 (98 percent) of the 51 segments with improvement and in 86 (73 percent) of the 118 segments without improvement following reinjection. As the severity of the persistent ^{201}Tl defect worsened, the relative number of defects with preserved metabolic activity also declined. Nearly all, 79 (88 percent) of 81, defects with relative ^{201}Tl activities greater than 50 percent had metabolic viability, whereas 5 (14 percent) of 35 defects with less than a 50 percent relative ^{201}Tl concentration had metabolic activity identified on positron emission tomography.

On assessment of regional anatomy and function with gated magnetic resonance imaging, the end-diastolic wall thickness in regions with perfusion defects and severely reduced ^{18}F-2-fluoro-2-deoxyglucose activity was less (8.0±3.7 mm) than in regions with matching defects and moderately reduced tracer activity (9.4±2.6 mm, $P < .01$). End-diastolic thicknesses that did not differ from normal myocardium in regions with perfusion-metabolism mismatches were significantly greater than in regions with matching perfusion and metabolic defects. Regional systolic wall thickening in the regions with the perfusion-metabolism mismatches did not differ from normal regions (2.8±2.4 versus 2.7±2.3 mm). Both were significantly greater than in segments with moderate or severe matching defects (1.7±2.7 and −0.7±2.1 mm, respectively). Systolic thickening in the regions with severe matching defects was significantly poorer than that in the regions with moderate matching defects. The large standard deviations of these values imply, however, a considerable overlap of these measurements among the various groups and suggest limitations in using such measurements to distinguish viable from nonviable myocardium.

End-diastolic wall thicknesses in regions that were normal on ^{201}Tl scintigraphy were significantly greater than in regions with reversible defects or in those with mild, moderate, or severe persistent defects. End-diastolic wall thicknesses in the latter categories did not differ from each other. Regional systolic thickening in normal regions (3.2±1.4 mm) was significantly greater than that observed in regions with reversible defects (2.0±1.4, $P < .01$) and in the regions with mild (2.0±2.4 mm), moderate (2.0±2.8 mm), and severe (0.0±2.2 mm) persistent defects. Systolic thickening in the regions with severe persistent defects on redistribution images was significantly poorer than that in the other regions. For mild and moderate persistent ^{201}Tl defects on redistribution images, systolic thickening in the reinjection positive and negative regions did not differ, whereas the regions with severe persistent defects that were reinjection-negative had significantly smaller amounts of systolic thickening. Thus, neither end-diastolic wall thicknesses nor systolic thickening reliably discriminated between myocardial regions with and those without scintigraphic criteria for myocardial viability. Furthermore, a substantial proportion (73 percent) of the myocardial regions with persistent defects on 3- to 4-hour redistribution images that did not improve following ^{201}Tl reinjection had evidence of metabolic viability on positron emission tomography with ^{18}F-2-fluoro-2-deoxyglucose.

These comparative imaging studies demonstrate that a persistent ^{201}Tl perfusion defect, whether present on 4- or 24-hour redistribution images or reinjection images does not imply the absence of tissue viability. The metabolic studies with positron emission tomography corroborate earlier findings of a postrevascularization improvement in some myocardial segments with persistent ^{201}Tl defects. In addition, the findings with positron emission tomography are in agreement with prior clinicopathologic studies indicating that some myocardial regions with extensive ^{201}Tl perfusion defects contain only small amounts of myocardial fibrosis. Thus, ^{201}Tl scintigraphy may seriously underestimate the extent of residual tissue viability in some patients with ischemic heart disease, and metabolic imaging with ^{18}F-2-fluoro-2-deoxyglucose is helpful in identifying individuals with significant amounts of viable but functionally compromised myocardium.

Reverse Thallium-201 Redistribution

Positron emission tomography has been used to explore the pathophysiologic significance of "reverse ^{201}Tl redistribution." The term reverse redistribution refers to the worsening of a stress perfusion defect or to the development of a new defect on ^{201}Tl redistribution images,[147] which may occur in patients with myocardial infarction following thrombolytic therapy or revascularization[148, 149] and in individuals with chronic coronary artery disease.[150–152] In patients with chronic coronary artery disease and prior myocardial infarction, the incidence of reverse redistribution has been reported to be as high as 18 percent.[153]

In order to better understand reverse redistribution, Ohte and coinvestigators[154] studied 16 patients 4 to 8 weeks after an acute myocardial infarction. All but three of the patients were treated with thrombolytic therapy or angioplasty at the time of infarction. Each patient underwent symptom-limited ergometer exercise, with acquisition of stress and 3- and 24-hour redistribution ^{201}Tl SPECT images. Reverse redistribution was identified in 3 of 80 regions in three patients on the 3-hour redistribution images and in 15 of 80 regions in eight patients on the 24-hour redistribution images. Each of the 15 regions had normal or only slightly reduced ^{201}Tl activity on the stress images. In two regions with reverse redistribution on the 3-hour images, defect scores worsened on the 24-hour images. Although each of the regions with reverse redistribution was supplied by patent coronary arteries, their wall motion was more impaired than in other myocardial areas with normal or mildly reduced ^{201}Tl activity. In 14 of the 15 regions with reverse redistribution, scores on the ^{18}F-2-fluoro-2-deoxyglucose images paralleled the 24-hour ^{201}Tl scores, indicating concordant perfusion and metabolic defects. In one region there was a discrepant increase in the ^{18}F-2-fluoro-2-deoxyglucose score relative to the 24-hour ^{201}Tl score, suggesting a perfusion-metabolism mismatch. The authors proposed that reverse ^{201}Tl redistribution in their patients with recent myocardial infarction was frequently indicative of a nontransmural myocardial scar, based on the concordant reductions in perfusion and metabolism scores and the presence of an associated wall motion abnormality.

In contrast to the preceding observations are the findings of Soufer and coworkers.[155] These investigators obtained planar stress and 3-hour redistribution ^{201}Tl images along with ^{13}N-ammonia and ^{18}F-2-fluoro-2-deoxyglucose images in 32 patients with chronic coronary artery disease. The findings on the imaging studies were also correlated with clinical outcomes over the ensuing 14-month period (range 9 to 19 months) of follow-up. Of the 32 subjects studied, 24 had a history of prior myocardial infarction. The other eight individuals had angiographic evidence of coronary disease or angina, or both, with a regional wall motion abnormality or ischemia on ^{201}Tl scintigraphy.

The investigators identified 50 segments with reverse redistribution in the 32 patients. In 44 of the segments with reverse redistribution, the initial ^{201}Tl distribution was normal on the stress images and abnormal on the redistribution images. Reverse redistribution was considered mild in 5 segments, moderate in 28 segments, and severe in 17 segments. In the five segments with mild reverse redistribution, four were normal on positron emission tomography, and one segment demonstrated a myocardial scar. Seventeen (61 percent) of the segments with moderate reverse redistribution were viable on positron emission tomography (9 normal, 8 perfusion-metabolism mismatches), whereas 11 (39 percent) exhibited a completed infarction. Of the 17 segments with severe reverse redistribution, 15 (88 percent) were viable (6 normal, 9 perfusion-metabolism mismatches), and only 2 (12 percent) exhibited myocardial scar. Thus, 36 (72 percent) of the 50 segments with reverse redistribution were considered viable on perfusion metabolism imaging.

In contrast to the study of Ohte and coworkers,[154] a coronary stenosis of 70 percent or greater was identified in the vessel supplying the myocardial segment with reverse redistribution in 10 of the 11 patients who underwent coronary angiography. Thus, reverse redistribution was associated with a significant coronary stenosis in nearly all the individuals who had coronary angiography. Segmental wall motion data were available for 35 of the segments with reverse redistribution, and 18 had an associated wall motion abnormality. Seven of the segments with wall motion abnormalities were viable, and 16 of the 17 segments with normal wall motion were metabolically viable. Thus, a segment with reverse redistribution and normal function was likely to be viable on metabolic imaging with ^{18}F-2-fluoro-2-deoxyglucose, but the presence or absence of viability could not be predicted in segments with reverse redistribution and abnormal wall motion.

Over the 14-month period of follow-up, 10 (31 percent) of the 32 patients had a cardiac event. Nine individuals were hospitalized for unstable angina, and one patient sustained a myocardial infarction. Five (50 percent) of the individuals with cardiac events had severe reverse redistribution and evidence of metabolic viability on positron emission tomography. In contrast, only two (9 percent) of the individuals without cardiac events exhibited these findings (P = .001). A perfusion-metabolism mismatch was three times more frequent in patients with reverse redistribution sustaining cardiac events than in the individuals with reverse redistribution who did not have events (P = .01). The authors concluded that positron emission tomography with ^{18}F-2-fluoro-2-deoxyglucose reveals preserved tissue viability in the majority of segments with reverse ^{201}Tl redistribution and provides additional important prognostic information in individuals who exhibit this scintigraphic finding on ^{201}Tl scintigraphy.

The discrepancies between these two studies likely reflect the differences in study populations as well as the period employed for redistribution imaging. In the Ohte and colleagues study, most of the patients with acute infarction were treated with either thrombolytic therapy or angioplasty, thereby successfully restoring blood flow to the infarct region. Because the coronary vessels supplying the regions with reverse redistribution were patent, it is not surprising that the findings on positron emission tomography were consistent with completed nontransmural myocardial infarction. The mechanism of reverse redistribution in these individuals likely differs from those enrolled in the Soufer and coworkers investigation, which included individuals with chronic coronary artery disease. In the latter study, the constellation of clinical symptoms and signs suggested that the myocardial regions with reverse redistribution were supplied by vessels with flow-limiting stenoses, meaning that there was a greater likelihood that the authors would identify the perfusion-metabolism mismatch characteristic of myocardial hibernation on positron emission tomography. The relatively high cardiac event rate in the patients with reverse redistribution and preserved metabolic viability is consistent with the higher cardiac event rates reported by other medical centers in medically treated patients with perfusion-metabolism mismatches (see the section on myocardial metabolic imaging for prognosis in chronic coronary artery disease).

Perfusion Defect Severity

The coronary circulation carries energy-rich substrates and molecular oxygen to the myocardium and removes the inhibitory byproducts of cellular metabolism. Blood flow is thus crucial for the maintenance of cellular life. Myocardial regions without blood flow cannot harbor viable tissue. However, the clinical observation that some hypoperfused dysfunctional myocardial regions (hibernating myocardium) improve wall motion following coronary revascularization indicates that tissue viability may be sustained in some situations in which resting blood flow is reduced but not completely absent. If a critical level of blood flow for the maintenance of tissue viability could be identified, the severity of a relative or absolute perfusion deficit might provide a means for identifying reversibly dysfunctional myocardium. If so, metabolic imaging would be unlikely to provide incremental information on tissue viability in hypoperfused ventricular regions.

Several studies have suggested that the relative severity of a perfusion defect might indeed be used for detecting clinically important viability in dysfunctional myocardium. Mori and colleagues[156] studied 17 patients with prior infarction using resting and 4-hour redistribution planar ^{201}Tl imaging. They related changes in regional wall motion following coronary revascularization to the severity of persistent defects on preoperative planar ^{201}Tl scintigrams. In 14 regions with persistent perfusion defects and improved function following revascularization, relative ^{201}Tl tracer concentrations averaged 82.3 ± 7.1 percent on 3- to 4-hour redistribution images, significantly higher than the 71.2 ± 7.0 percent noted in 23 regions with persistent perfusion defects without functional recovery. In a separate study of 37 patients undergoing coronary artery bypass surgery, Zimmermann and coworkers[157] used light microscopic morphometry to measure the percentage of interstitial fibrosis present in myocardial biopsy specimens obtained at the time of surgery. Relative ^{201}Tl concentrations in myocardium with persistent defects on preoperative reinjection planar images were correlated inversely ($r = -.85$, $P < .001$) with the percentage of interstitial fibrosis in the biopsy specimens. The planar imaging technique employed in both of these investigations compresses three-dimensional ^{201}Tl count data into two-dimensional images, and the superimposition of activity makes it difficult to accurately measure regional myocardial tracer concentrations. However, these studies do lend support to the concept that measurements of relative myocardial perfusion might aid in identifying clinically important tissue viability in dysfunctional myocardial areas.

To further explore this possibility, Dilsizian and coworkers[158] correlated the findings on stress, 4-hour redistribution, and reinjection SPECT ^{201}Tl perfusion images with the results of positron emission tomographic imaging with ^{15}O-water and ^{18}F-2-fluoro-2-deoxyglucose in 15 patients with chronic coronary artery disease. Persistent defects on the redistribution images were considered mild to moderate if relative tracer activity was 51 to 85 percent of peak activity and severe if less than or equal to 50 percent of peak activity. In addition, changes in ^{201}Tl counts from the redistribution to reinjection images in areas with persistent perfusion defects were expressed as a percent of the change in absolute ^{201}Tl counts in normal myocardial areas. This latter value, representing the incremental increase in defect ^{201}Tl counts relative to the increase in ^{201}Tl counts in normal myocardium, was termed the differential uptake.

In the 15 patients, there were 169 segments with persistent ^{201}Tl defects on the redistribution images. Of these segmental defects, 123 were mild to moderate defects and 46 were severe defects. ^{18}F-2-fluoro-2-deoxyglucose uptake was noted in 112 (91 percent) of the segments with mild to moderate reductions in ^{201}Tl activity and in 23 (50 percent) of the segments with severe (≥50 percent) reductions in ^{201}Tl activity. Thus, despite the presence of a perfusion defect on the redistribution images, half of the severely hypoperfused myocardial segments exhibited evidence of residual metabolic viability. Following ^{201}Tl reinjection, improvement was noted in 22 of the 46 segments with severe perfusion defects on the redistribution images. Of these 22 segments, preserved tissue metabolism was noted on metabolic imaging in 17 (77 percent). Relative ^{201}Tl tracer concentrations in the defects on the reinjection images were not reported.

In 24 segments, there was no significant change in relative ^{201}Tl activity between the 4-hour redistribution and reinjection images. Preserved metabolic activity was noted in six (25 percent) of these segments on imaging with ^{18}F-2-fluoro-2-deoxyglucose, meaning that tissue viability would be underestimated in about one in four segments with severe (≥50 percent reduction) perfusion defects on ^{201}Tl reinjection images. Using a differential uptake of greater than or equal to 50 percent of normal myocardium as an indicator of viability, 14 (70 percent) of the 20 segments viable by these criteria exhibited metabolic viability. In contrast, the authors reported that 9 (35 percent) of the 26 segments with differential uptakes of less than 50 percent were metabolically viable.

In this limited number of patients, therefore, metabolic viability was nearly always present in myocardial segments with mild to moderate perfusion defects on 4-hour redistribution images. However, the presence of a severe perfusion defect on either 4-hour redistribution or reinjection images did not preclude the possibility of residual tissue metabolic viability on positron emission tomography. Residual metabolic viability was present in 50 percent of severe defects on redistribution images and 25 percent of severe defects on reinjection images. In addition, about one third of the defects with small relative increases in ^{201}Tl counts from redistribution to reinjection images had residual tissue viability identified on positron emission tomography. Thus, an only slight improvement in visual defect severity from redistribution to reinjection images does not exclude the presence of residual tissue viability as identified by metabolic imaging. Therefore, this study would indicate that metabolic imaging with ^{18}F-2-fluoro-2-deoxyglucose does provide incremental information, beyond that provided by assessment of perfusion defect severity alone, about clinically important tissue viability in severely hypoperfused myocardial areas in patients with chronic coronary artery disease.

In a subsequent report from the same laboratory involving 25 patients with chronic coronary artery disease,[159] same-day resting and stress ^{99m}Tc-sestamibi SPECT perfusion images were compared with stress, 4-hour redistribution, and reinjection ^{201}Tl SPECT images and ^{15}O-water and ^{18}F-2-fluoro-2-deoxyglucose positron emission tomographic images. On the SPECT images, defects were considered mild to moderate if they had a relative tracer concentration between 51 and 85 percent of peak normal activity and were considered severe if the relative tracer concentration was less than or equal to 50 percent of peak activity.

In the 25 patients, there were 46 reversible and 27 persistent segmental defects on the ^{201}Tl SPECT studies. Twenty-eight (61 percent) of the 46 segments with reversible ^{201}Tl defects also had reversible defects on the ^{99m}Tc-sestamibi images, and nearly all of these segments—26 of 28 (93 percent)—had evidence of metabolic viability on positron emission tomographic imaging. Persistent ^{99m}Tc-sestamibi defects were identified in 18 (39 percent) segments with reversible ^{201}Tl defects, and 17 (94 percent) of these segments had metabolic viability on positron emission tomography. Four (15 percent) of the 27 segments with persistent ^{201}Tl defects had reversible defects on the ^{99m}Tc-sestamibi images and were considered nonviable on positron emission tomographic imaging with ^{18}F-2-fluoro-2-deoxyglucose. In the 23 segments in which persistent defects were noted on both ^{201}Tl and ^{99m}Tc-sestamibi images, positron emission tomography identified residual metabolic viability in 9 (39 percent) of the segments.

Of the 23 segments that had both irreversible ^{201}Tl and resting ^{99m}Tc-sestamibi defects, 6 (26 percent) had a mild to moderate reduction in ^{99m}Tc-sestamibi counts (average = 68 ± 10 percent). Five of these segments had a mild to moderate reduction in ^{201}Tl activity (mean = 63 ± 10 percent), and all five of these segments exhibited metabolic viability on positron emission tomography. Relative ^{201}Tl activity in the remaining segment was not reported, but the segment apparently was considered metabolically nonviable. In the 17 segments with severe ^{99m}Tc-sestamibi defects, ^{99m}Tc-sestamibi activity was 31 ± 13 percent of peak activity, whereas relative ^{201}Tl activity averaged 35 ± 7 percent of peak activity. Four (23 percent) of these segments with severe persistent defects exhibited residual metabolic viability on metabolic imaging with ^{18}F-2-fluoro-2-deoxyglucose. Thus, the data suggest that about one in four segments with severe perfusion defects (averaging about one third of peak myocardial activity) would be expected to exhibit evidence of residual tissue viability on metabolic imaging with ^{18}F-2-fluoro-2-deoxyglucose.

Sawada and colleagues[160] correlated the severity of resting ^{99m}Tc-sestamibi perfusion defects with the findings on positron emission tomography with ^{13}N-ammonia and ^{18}F-2-fluoro-2-deoxyglucose in 20 patients with previous myocardial infarction. Fifteen of the patients had Q waves on the electrocardiogram, whereas five had non–Q wave infarctions. Relative ^{99m}Tc-sestamibi perfusion defect activity was compared with corresponding ^{13}N-ammonia and ^{18}F-2-fluoro-2-deoxyglucose activities using a polar mapping technique.

On the ^{99m}Tc-sestamibi images, a perfusion defect was defined by relative tracer concentration less than 60 percent of peak activity. A moderate reduction in ^{99m}Tc-sestamibi activity was defined by a relative tracer concentration of 50 to 59 percent of peak myocardial activity, whereas a severe reduction was defined by relative tracer concentration of less than 50 percent of peak activity. On the ^{18}F-2-fluoro-2-deoxyglucose images, myocardial viability was defined by a relative tracer concentration greater than or equal to 60 percent of peak myocardial activity.

Comparison between perfusion defect severity and extent was performed in all the patients, whereas two individuals had ^{18}F-2-fluoro-2-deoxyglucose images that were of limited quality and were uninterpretable. In 16 patients, ^{99m}Tc-sestamibi perfusion defect extent exceeded that observed on the ^{13}N-ammonia perfusion images. As a percent of the left ventricular myocardium, the ^{99m}Tc-sestamibi perfusion defect extent averaged 28.2 ± 15 percent, whereas the mean perfusion defect extent on the ^{13}N-ammonia perfusion images was 14.6 ± 11 percent ($P < .005$).

In the 18 patients with diagnostic ^{18}F-2-fluoro-2-deoxyglucose images, there were 30 moderate and 34 severe ^{99m}Tc-sestamibi perfusion defects. Sixteen (53 percent) of the moderate and 16 (47 percent) of the severe ^{99m}Tc-sestamibi perfusion defects had relative ^{18}F-2-fluoro-2-deoxyglucose concentrations greater than or equal to 60 percent and were considered viable. In nine of the metabolically nonviable and nine of the metabolically viable segments, relative ^{99m}Tc-sestamibi concentrations were less than 40 percent of peak values. The lowest relative ^{99m}Tc-sestamibi concentration associated with metabolically viable myocardium was 29 percent, whereas the lowest concentration in the nonviable segments was 26 percent. The authors thus noted that no lower limit of ^{99m}Tc-sestamibi activity effectively precluded the presence of metabolic viability on the ^{18}F-2-fluoro-2-deoxyglucose images. However, relative ^{99m}Tc-sestamibi concentrations in the myocardial areas with severe perfusion defects with preserved metabolic viability were slightly higher than in the areas without metabolic viability (46 ± 3 percent versus 40 ± 6 percent, $P < .05$). However, relative ^{13}N-ammonia concentrations were not significantly different (60 ± 3 percent versus 55 ± 7 percent, $P < .16$). Relative ^{18}F-2-fluoro-2-deoxyglucose concentrations were by definition significantly higher in the myocardial areas with severe ^{99m}Tc-sestamibi perfusion defects and viability than in the areas without viability (67 ± 5 percent versus 50 ± 6 percent, $P = .0001$). The authors concluded that metabolic viability could frequently be identified with positron emission tomography and ^{18}F-2-fluoro-2-deoxyglucose in myocardial areas with moderate or severe resting ^{99m}Tc-sestamibi perfusion defects and that ^{99m}Tc-sestamibi perfusion defects frequently were more extensive than those identified on ^{13}N-ammonia perfusion images.

In a larger comparative study, Altehoefer and colleagues[161] correlated the severity of resting SPECT ^{99m}Tc-sestamibi perfusion defects with the results of ^{18}F-2-fluoro-2-deoxyglucose on positron emission tomography in 111 patients with chronic coronary artery disease and resting wall motion abnormalities. Ninety-four of the patients studied had a history of prior myocardial infarction. The mean left ventricular ejection fraction was 47 ± 11 percent. On both the SPECT and positron emission tomographic images, relative tracer activities were examined in 13 myocardial segments. For the resting ^{99m}Tc-sestamibi images, defect counts were normalized to counts in the region of interest with the highest counts. A perfusion defect was defined by a relative reduction in ^{99m}Tc counts to less than 70 percent of peak normal counts. On the positron emission tomographic metabolic images, counts were referenced to ^{18}F-2-fluoro-2-deoxyglucose counts in the region with the highest ^{99m}Tc-sestamibi counts on the perfusion images. Segments with ^{18}F-2-fluoro-2-deoxyglucose counts greater than 70 percent of normal were considered viable, whereas segments with ^{18}F-2-fluoro-2-deoxyglucose counts less than 50 percent of normal were considered nonviable. If the relative ^{18}F-2-fluoro-2-deoxyglucose counts were between these two groups, the segment was said to have "intermediate" uptake of the metabolic tracer.

The authors evaluated 1443 segments on the SPECT and positron emission tomographic images, of which 713 segments exhibited resting perfusion defects. On the metabolic images, ^{18}F-2-fluoro-2-deoxyglucose uptake exceeded 70 percent and therefore was considered indicative of viable tissue in 5 percent of defects with less than or equal to 20 percent relative ^{99m}Tc-sestamibi uptake (Fig. 71–27). For less severe perfusion defects, the relative number of segments with ^{18}F-2-fluoro-2-deoxyglucose activity in the "viable" category increased as the perfusion defect became less pronounced, with the highest proportion of metabolically viable segments, 61 percent, noted in perfusion defects with 61 to 70 percent of peak ^{99m}Tc-sestamibi uptake. The relative number of segments with intermediate uptake of ^{18}F-2-fluoro-2-deoxyglucose ranged from 5 percent for defects with 21 to 30 percent of peak ^{99m}Tc-sestamibi uptake to 37 percent for defects with 41 to 50 percent of peak perfusion tracer activity. Thus, the number of segments considered metabolically viable decreased as the severity of the perfusion defect increased.

The preceding studies suggest that myocardial areas with mild or moderate defects on SPECT perfusion images are likely to retain significant tissue viability as identified by positron emission tomography with ^{18}F-2-fluoro-2-deoxyglucose. Although myocardial areas with severe SPECT perfusion defects appear less likely to have perfusion-metabolism mismatches, positron emission tomography will identify residual myocardial metabolic viability in about one in every four of these areas.

These discrepancies may be explained in part by the technical difficulties inherent in measuring perfusion defect severity with the SPECT imaging technique. For example, the spatial resolution of current gamma cameras is about 15 to 20 mm. Defect counts will therefore include some "spillover" of activity from adjacent normal myocardium, especially at the borders of the defect. The anatomical extent of a defect thus influences observed defect severity, for activity in the center of large defects is less affected by spillover of counts from adjacent normal tissue than that in smaller defects. For any given tissue tracer concentration in a hypoperfused ventricular area, observed perfusion defect severity will be less pronounced for anatomically small defects than for anatomically large defects.

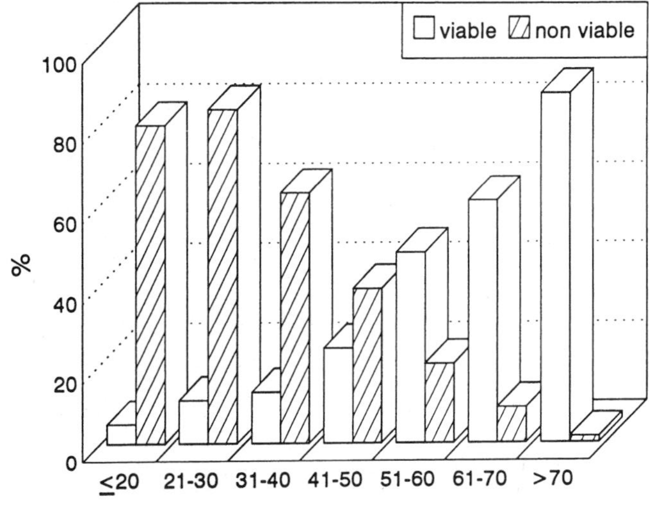

FIGURE 71–27. The relative number of hypoperfused myocardial segments with metabolic viability on positron emission tomographic imaging with ^{18}F-2-fluoro-2-deoxyglucose, according to the relative severity of the ^{99m}Tc-sestamibi perfusion defect. As the severity of the perfusion defect worsens, the likelihood of metabolic viability declines. (From Altehoefer, C., vom Dahl, J., Biedermann, M., et al.: Significance of defect severity in technetium-99m-MIBI SPECT at rest to assess myocardial viability: Comparison with F-18 2-fluoro 2-deoxyglucose PET. J. Nucl. Med. 35:571, 1994.)

In addition, both large and small perfusion defects are subject to spillover of counts from extracardiac background activity, which originates primarily from tracer within the gastrointestinal tract and lungs and can vary substantially from patient to patient and from stress to redistribution to reinjection images. Differences in background activity will have the most influence on the counts in the myocardial areas with the most pronounced reductions in blood flow. In these areas, background counts may comprise a relatively large proportion of observed defect counts because of the low number of counts present within the myocardium itself. Measured defect counts will therefore change appreciably if background activity differs between images in the same patient or between individual patients.

Measurements of SPECT perfusion defect severity are also adversely influenced by attenuation of myocardial activity. Attenuation refers to the fact that some of the photons emitted by a radioactive tracer within the heart interact with noncardiac tissues in the line of flight and are not recorded by the gamma camera. Observed SPECT image counts are therefore always less than the actual activity within the myocardium. Attenuation of cardiac activity is more problematic for some myocardial regions than for others. In particular, attenuation of anteroseptal activity by breast tissue and of inferoposterior activity by the abdominal wall are well-described problems for the relatively low-energy photons of ^{201}Tl and ^{99m}Tc and were clearly present in the study of Sawada and coworkers. Thus, differences in photon attenuation from patient to patient and from myocardial region to myocardial region make it difficult to accurately measure relative tissue tracer concentrations using current SPECT imaging techniques. Although it may eventually be possible to use simultaneously acquired transmission images to help correct for photon attenuation,[162] further studies will be needed to determine if corrected SPECT emission images accurately depict true tissue perfusion tracer concentrations.

In myocardial areas that are thinned because of prior infarction or in areas with impaired systolic thickening, the partial volume effect will also cause an underestimation of true tissue tracer concentrations.[163] For currently available gamma cameras, the smallest resolvable image volume is larger than the time-averaged wall thickness of the left ventricle. Observed myocardial counts therefore appear to originate from the entire minimal resolvable volume of the camera. The number of counts recorded by the camera relative to actual object counts (the recovery coefficient) varies nonlinearly as a function of the size of the object being imaged, and counts within larger objects are more efficiently imaged than are those in smaller objects. Myocardial regions that are thinned and do not thicken will be imaged less efficiently than will normally contracting areas. Even if a myocardial area has a normal diastolic thickness, the counts observed with the SPECT camera will be substantially less than actual tissue counts if it does not thicken during systole. This is because the "time-averaged" myocardial thickness is small and the camera is inefficient at recovering myocardial counts.

For the reasons enumerated, Go and colleagues[164] reasoned that positron emission tomography provides more accurate estimates of the relative severity of a myocardial perfusion defect. Employing ^{82}Rb, resting and dipyridamole stress perfusion imaging along with ^{18}F-2-fluoro-2-deoxyglucose imaging was performed in 145 patients with chronic myocardial infarction. Based on measurements obtained in normal individuals, a myocardial segment was considered normal if relative ^{82}Rb concentrations were equal to or exceeded 80 percent of peak activity. Persistent defects were defined by a change in relative ^{82}Rb activity of less than 15 percent between the rest and dipyridamole stress perfusion images.

Persistent ^{82}Rb perfusion defects were identified in 1252 segments in the 145 patients. Preserved glucose metabolic activity was identified in 381 (30 percent) of the segments, whereas concordant reductions in metabolic activity were noted in the remaining 871 segments. The metabolic findings in the myocardial segments with persistent ^{82}Rb perfusion defects were then correlated with relative perfusion defect severity (Fig. 71–28). When perfusion defects with relative ^{82}Rb concentrations of 70 percent or less were examined according to each 5 percent decrement in normalized tissue activity, the relative number of myocardial perfusion defects with preserved metabolic activity was remarkably constant, ranging from 23 percent for ^{82}Rb concentrations of 30 to 35 percent of peak activity to 35 percent for ^{82}Rb concentrations of 40 to 45 percent of peak activity. Thus, in this patient population, the persistence of metabolic activity and, thus, viability was independent of the severity of a persistent myocardial perfusion defect.

Tamaki and colleagues[88] also reasoned that positron emission tomography afforded a more accurate assessment of the relative severity of a myocardial perfusion defect. They studied 43 patients with chronic myocardial infarction (mean left ventricular ejection fraction = 41 percent) prior to coronary revascularization. Patients underwent both resting and stress ^{13}N-ammonia perfusion imaging along with metabolic imaging with ^{18}F-2-fluoro-2-deoxyglucose in the fasting state. Regional wall abnormalities were assessed visually on preoperative and postoperative biplanar ventriculograms, using a five-point scoring system. Function was considered to have improved if regional scores improved by one or more grades.

In the 43 patients, there were 130 asynergic segments identified on the preoperative ventriculograms. Function improved in 51 of the segments following revascularization, whereas no change in function was noted in 79 segments. In the asynergic regions, relative ^{13}N concentrations on the resting perfusion images were greater than 80 percent in 1 region, between 70 and 80 percent in 21 regions, between 60 and 70 percent in 38 regions, between 50 and 60 percent in 38 regions, between 40 and 50 percent in 21 regions, and less than 40 percent in 11 regions. As relative ^{13}N activity in the asynergic segments on the resting perfusion images

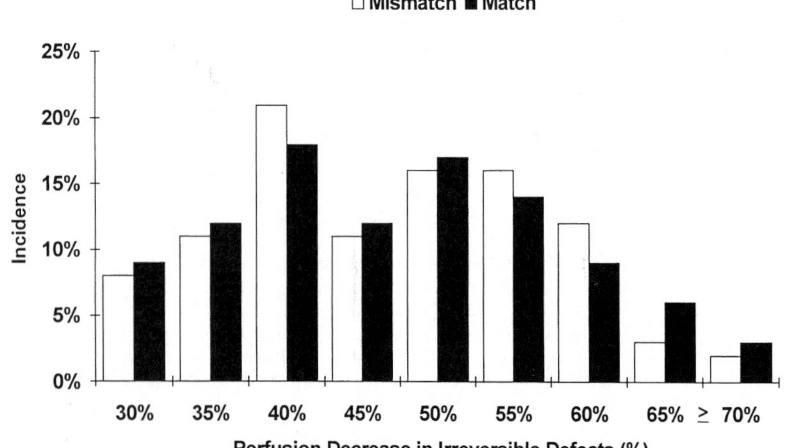

FIGURE 71–28. The relative incidence of metabolic viability in hypoperfused myocardial segments relative to the severity of the ^{82}Rb perfusion defect. The relative number of viable segments is depicted by the white bars, whereas the relative number of nonviable segments is displayed with the black bars. The relative proportion of viable segments was independent of the severity of the associated perfusion defect. (From Go, R. T., MacIntyre, W. J., Saha, G. B., et al.: Hibernating myocardium versus scar: Severity of irreversible decreased myocardial perfusion in prediction of tissue viability. Radiology 194:154, 1995.)

decreased, the proportion of regions with functional improvement after revascularization declined (Fig. 71–29). The region with a resting relative ^{13}N concentration greater than 80 percent of peak normal had improved function following revascularization, and about half of the regions with relative ^{13}N counts between 60 and 80 percent of normal had improved function. Fifteen of 38 (39 percent) regions with relative tracer concentrations between 50 and 60 percent improved following revascularization, as did 4 of 21 (19 percent) regions with ^{13}N tracer concentrations between 40 and 50 percent. None of the asynergic regions with relative ^{13}N concentrations less than 40 percent of normal had postoperative improvement in regional wall motion. The positive predictive value for a relative ^{13}N concentration greater than 50 percent for predicting improvement in function following revascularization was only 48 percent, whereas the negative predictive value for a tracer concentration less than 50 percent was 87.5 percent.

Stress-induced perfusion defects were identified in 68 of the 130 asynergic regions yet the authors provided no information regarding the relationship between stress and resting perfusion defect severity. In addition, no data were provided regarding the relationships between the severity of resting wall motion abnormalities and either the stress or resting perfusion defect severity. Of the 68 regions with reversible defects, 43 (63 percent) exhibited improved function following revascularization, whereas only 8 (13 percent) of the 62 regions without reversible defects had improved wall motion. Assessment of defect reversibility thus increased the positive predictive accuracy from 48 to 63 percent while maintaining a negative predictive accuracy of 87 percent.

On positron emission tomography with ^{18}F-2-fluoro-2-deoxyglucose, preserved glucose metabolism was identified in 59 of the 130 asynergic regions. Forty-five (76 percent) of the regions exhibited improved function following revascularization, whereas only 6 (8 percent) of the 71 regions without metabolic activity had improved wall motion. Metabolic imaging thus had a higher overall accuracy (85 percent, 110 of 130 regions) for predicting functional improvement than either the resting perfusion studies (75 of 130 regions, 58 percent) or the resting stress studies (97 of 130 regions, 75 percent, $P < .05$ versus resting or metabolic imaging). Thus, assessment of regional myocardial glucose metabolism with positron emission tomography incrementally improved the ability to discriminate between asynergic myocardial regions with and those without benefit from revascularization.

Takahashi and coworkers[165] explored the relationships between relative myocardial ^{13}N concentrations and rates of myocardial glucose consumption in 26 patients with chronic coronary artery disease. They studied 10 patients following oral glucose loading and 16 patients in the fasting state. Twenty-two of the patients had a history of remote myocardial infarction. After acquisition of a resting ^{13}N-ammonia perfusion study, dynamic positron emission tomographic imaging with ^{18}F-2-fluoro-2-deoxyglucose was performed.

The authors reported that a relative ^{13}N activity of less than 45 percent of peak activity was consistently associated with rates of glucose use of less than 0.3 $\mu mol \cdot g^{-1} \cdot min^{-1}$, for both the fasting and glucose-loaded states. Manipulation of the patient's dietary status thus had little effect on the relatively low glucose metabolic rates observed in the ventricular regions with low blood flows. In contrast, myocardial regions with relative ^{13}N concentrations greater than 45 percent of peak normal had significantly higher rates of glucose use in the glucose-loaded state than the areas with corresponding perfusion deficits in the fasting state. Rates of glucose use in the myocardial areas with relative ^{13}N concentrations less than 45 percent of peak normal were significantly lower in the glucose-loaded studies than in those in the myocardial areas with relative ^{13}N concentrations greater than 45 percent. The authors concluded that a minimal threshold of perfusion, greater than 45 percent of peak normal perfusion, exists for glucose metabolism. Unfortunately, neither absolute nor relative glucose metabolic rates were normalized to myocardial perfusion measurements, and it is not possible to ascertain if the reported metabolic rates were observed in myocardial areas with perfusion-metabolism mismatches or in areas with either incomplete or complete matching defects. Thus, it is difficult to infer from this study that myocardial viability can be reliably ascertained by either relative perfusion measurements or quantitative measurements of myocardial glucose consumption.

To determine if absolute measurements of myocardial blood flow might distinguish between viable and nonviable myocardium, Gewirtz and coworkers[166] quantitated regional myocardial blood flows in 26 chronic myocardial infarct patients with ^{13}N-ammonia. Metabolic imaging was performed with ^{18}F-2-fluoro-2-deoxyglucose. Absolute blood flows were related to relative ^{18}F-2-fluoro-2-deoxyglucose concentrations and to regional wall motion as indices of myocardial viability. Segments with greater than or equal to 75 percent of peak myocardial blood flows were considered normal, whereas infarct zones were defined by blood flows less than 50 percent of maximum. Border zones were defined by blood flow measurements between 50 and 175 percent of maximal values. Eighteen of the patients had anterior infarction and 8 had inferior infarctions. The mean time interval from the clinical infarction to positron emission tomography was 44 ± 65 months (range of 2 to 192 months). Eleven of the patients had revascularization of the clinical infarct zone prior to enrollment in the study.

In 40 normal areas, regional myocardial blood flows averaged

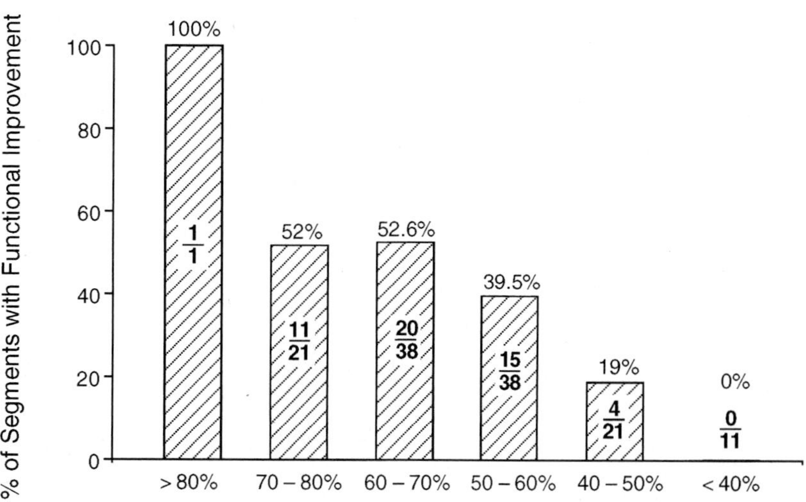

FIGURE 71–29. The relative number of hypoperfused myocardial segments with improved wall motion following coronary revascularization, according to the severity of the ^{13}N-ammonia perfusion defect on the preoperative positron emission tomographic imaging. As the severity of the resting perfusion defect decreases, the probability of functional improvement declines. (Data from Tamaki, N., Kawamoto, M., Tadamura, E., et al.: Prediction of reversible ischemia after revascularization. Perfusion and metabolic studies with positron emission tomography. Circulation 91:1699, 1995. Copyright 1995, American Heart Association.)

0.81 ± 0.32 mL · g^{-1} · min^{-1}. In 22 infarct regions, the mean myocardial blood flow was 0.27 ± 0.17 mL · g^{-1} · min^{-1}, significantly lower than that in normal areas or the mean value of 0.59 ± 0.29 mL · g^{-1} · min^{-1} observed in 16 border zones. The authors did not report the number of regional perfusion-metabolism mismatches according to each classification but did note that no mismatches were identified in any areas with less than 0.24 mL · g^{-1} · min^{-1} blood flow, a value that corresponded to 35 percent of peak counts on the perfusion images. Enhanced ^{18}F-2-fluoro-2-deoxyglucose activity relative to blood flow was noted most frequently in areas with blood flows between 40 and 70 percent of peak normal. However, enhanced uptake of ^{18}F-2-fluoro-2-deoxyglucose was also observed in areas with blood flows as great as 90 percent of normal, indicating a regional abnormality in myocardial metabolism despite relatively well-preserved resting perfusion.

On comparison with regional wall motion, each of the five segments with dyskinesis on contrast ventriculography had myocardial blood flows less than 0.25 mL · g^{-1} · min^{-1} and none of these areas exhibited enhanced uptake of ^{18}F-2-fluoro-2-deoxyglucose. Six of the 28 segments with severe hypokinesis or akinesis had blood flows less than 0.25 mL · g^{-1} · min^{-1}, and the mean blood flow for all severely hypokinetic-akinetic regions was 0.42 ± 0.21 mL · g^{-1} · min^{-1}. Four of these segments (three with akinesia, one with severe hypokinesia) had enhanced uptake of ^{18}F-2-fluoro-2-deoxyglucose. Most, that is 43 of 45 (94 percent), of the regions with normal wall motion or mild hypokinesia had resting myocardial blood flows greater than or equal to 0.39 mL · g^{-1} · min^{-1}. Enhanced uptake of ^{18}F-2-fluoro-2-deoxyglucose relative to blood flow was noted in five of these regions. Thus, although more severe myocardial blood flow reductions tended to be associated with pronounced regional dysfunction, considerable variation in absolute flows was observed when stratified by the severity of the associated wall motion abnormality. Furthermore, relatively preserved perfusion did not preclude the possibility of enhanced glucose consumption relative to substrate delivery (blood flow) on metabolic imaging, implying that myocardial metabolism may sometimes be altered in regions that are almost normal on resting perfusion imaging. The authors concluded that myocardial viability was unlikely when resting regional myocardial blood flow was less than 0.25 mL · g^{-1} · min^{-1}. However, since blood flow measurements were not correlated with changes in wall motion following revascularization, it is not possible to infer that all myocardial areas with blood flows greater than 0.25 mL · g^{-1} · min^{-1} had clinically important viability, as determined by functional improvement after restoration of blood flow.

In patients with coronary heart disease, the concept that the severity of a perfusion defect can be used to identify clinically important tissue viability has an underlying assumption. It is assumed that observed reductions in blood flow, in general, parallel the losses of viable myocytes in dysfunctional myocardial regions. For example, if activity in a perfusion defect is 65 percent of peak normal activity, the assumption would be that about 35 percent of viable tissue had been replaced by fibrous tissue. A histopathologic study by Parodi and coworkers,[167] however, challenges such an assumption. These investigators studied four patients with ischemic cardiomyopathy who were undergoing heart transplantation. ^{99m}Tc-labeled human albumin microspheres were injected into the left atrium prior to aortic cross-clamping while arterial blood was simultaneously withdrawn at a constant rate. Using the microsphere principle, the authors were able to correlate absolute myocardial blood flow measurements with gamma camera images of slices of the excised hearts and also with histologic and biochemical determinations of the percentage of fibrosis in tissue specimens.

In the patients with ischemic cardiomyopathy, mean transmural myocardial blood flows averaged 0.38 ± 0.15 mL · g^{-1} · min^{-1} and the mean percentage of fibrosis was 25 ± 28 percent. These investigators found no correlation whatsoever between myocardial blood flow and the extent of fibrosis as determined either by histologic or histochemical measurements of the excised tissue. In addition, when the relative tracer concentrations on the gamma camera images were correlated with the amount of fibrosis determined by histologic measurements, no relationship could be demonstrated. The authors concluded that the amount of myocardial fibrosis is not a primary determinant of blood flow in patients with end-stage ventricular dysfunction. Thus, inferences regarding the amount of residual tissue viability based on the severity of a perfusion abnormality would appear to be unreliable, at least in individuals with pronounced ventricular dysfunction in the setting of coronary artery disease.

Yamamoto and colleagues[168] reasoned that measurements of myocardial blood flow referenced to the amount of viable tissue within a myocardial region might prove more fruitful for examining the relationship between perfusion and myocardial viability. They proposed and employed the "perfusable tissue index," as described in Chapter 69, in 8 normal volunteers, 15 patients with chronic myocardial infarction (time to imaging = 5 to 12 months), and 11 patients with acute myocardial infarction (time to imaging = 2 ± 1 day) with successful thrombolysis of the infarct vessel. In the patients with acute infarction, echocardiographic assessment of regional wall thickening was also performed within 2 to 4 days of the infarction and 4 months later. Four regions of interest (inferior, lateral, anterior, and septal) were examined on the transaxial images. To identify myocardial areas of perfusion-metabolism matches and mismatches, uptake of ^{18}F-2-fluoro-2-deoxyglucose in asynergic zones was normalized to peak ^{18}F counts and divided by blood flow measurements normalized to peak blood flow determinations. Perfusion-metabolism mismatches were defined by a metabolic-to-perfusion ratio greater than or equal to 1.2.

In the normal volunteers, myocardial blood flows averaged 1.03 ± 0.18 mL · g^{-1} · min^{-1} of total anatomical tissue and 0.95 mL · g^{-1} · min^{-1} of water-perfusable tissue. As anticipated, the water-perfusable index was near unity in the healthy hearts—1.08 ± 0.07 g of perfusable tissue per gram of total anatomical tissue. Six patients with chronic Q-wave myocardial infarction had matching perfusion and metabolic defects, or completed infarctions, in the clinical infarct zone (average metabolism-to-flow ratio = $.79 \pm 0.29$). Blood flow in these regions averaged 0.33 ± 0.11 mL · g^{-1} · min^{-1} of anatomical tissue and 0.64 ± 0.23 mL · g^{-1} · min^{-1} of water-perfusable tissue, whereas the corresponding values for remote normal myocardium were 0.98 ± 0.25 mL · g^{-1} · min^{-1} anatomical tissue and 0.97 ± 0.25 mL · g^{-1} · min^{-1} of water-perfusable tissue, respectively. In nine patients with chronic myocardial infarction (7 Q wave, 2 non–Q wave), perfusion-metabolism mismatches were identified (mean metabolism-to-flow ratio = 1.85 ± 0.62). Blood flows in infarct zones with mismatches averaged 0.40 ± 0.17 mL · g^{-1} · min^{-1} of anatomical tissue and 0.51 mL · g^{-1} · min^{-1} of water-perfusable tissue, respectively, whereas the values for remote normal myocardium were 1.10 ± 0.23 mL · g^{-1} · min^{-1} of anatomical tissue and 1.09 ± 0.23 mL · g^{-1} · min^{-1} of water-perfusable tissue, respectively. Neither blood flow per gram of total anatomical tissue nor blood flow per gram of water-perfusable tissue reliably distinguished between myocardial infarct zones with and those without metabolic viability on imaging with ^{18}F-2-fluoro-2-deoxyglucose. However, the mean perfusable tissue index was significantly higher in the infarct areas with preserved tissue metabolism (0.75 ± 0.14 versus 0.53 ± 12; $P < .01$), suggesting that the mass of viable tissue in the perfusion-metabolism mismatch areas was greater than that in the areas with completed infarction.

In the 11 patients with acute myocardial infarction, these investigators identified 12 regions with severely impaired systolic wall thickening following thrombolytic therapy. On follow-up echocardiography at 4 months, seven regions had improved systolic wall thickening, whereas five had no functional recovery. Blood flows in regions with improved function averaged 0.61 ± 0.33 mL · g^{-1} · min^{-1} of anatomical tissue and 0.68 ± 0.32 mL · g^{-1} · min^{-1} of water-perfusable tissue and did not differ statistically from the 0.33 ± 0.15 mL · g^{-1} · min^{-1} of anatomical tissue and 0.60 ± 0.18 mL · g^{-1} · min^{-1} of water-perfusable tissue noted in the regions without recovery. Thus, measurements of absolute blood flow, whether normalized to total anatomical tissue or to the amount of water-perfusable tissue, did not reliably discriminate between regions with and those without functional recovery. However, the water-perfusable tissue index was significantly higher in the regions with functional improvement (0.88 ± 0.10 versus 0.53 ± 0.11; $P < .02$). In this small number of acute infarct patients, only those with a water-perfusable index greater than 0.7 exhibited functional improvement.

In a subsequent study from the same laboratory, de Silva and coworkers[169] examined the utility of the water-perfusable tissue index for predicting improvement in segmental function following elective coronary revascularization in 12 patients with chronic myocardial infarction. In addition, eight patients were studied with ^{18}F-2-fluoro-2-deoxyglucose. Changes in segmental function were assessed on paired echocardiographic studies performed before and 3 to 5 months after elective coronary revascularization. Preoperative echocardiograms identified 33 dysfunctional segments and 26 normally functioning control segments. Twenty-six of the 33 segments with resting wall motion abnormalities exhibited improved function following revascularization, whereas 7 segments showed no improvement. Seven akinetic and 15 hypokinetic segments had normal wall motion following revascularization, whereas four akinetic segments became hypokinetic after surgery.

Myocardial blood flows in the seven segments without functional recovery averaged 0.45 ± 0.11 mL · g^{-1} · min^{-1} perfusable tissue and were significantly lower than those in the segments with improved wall motion—0.73 ± 0.18 mL · g^{-1} · min^{-1} perfusable tissue ($P < .02$). However, there was considerable overlap in the measured blood flows for the two groups. Blood flows in the 26 control segments averaged 0.97 ± 0.22 mL · g^{-1} · min^{-1} perfusable tissue and were significantly higher than blood flows in either group of asynergic segments ($P < .001$ for both). In 13 asynergic segments with functional recovery in which comparison with metabolic images could be performed, relative ^{18}F-2-fluoro-2-deoxyglucose concentrations averaged 92 ± 17 percent of that in the control areas. Ratios of ^{18}F-2-fluoro-2-deoxyglucose concentrations relative to absolute or normalized blood flow measurements were not provided, but the mean values reported would suggest that most of the segments with functional recovery appeared to have enhanced glucose metabolism relative to blood flow or perfusion-metabolism mismatches. In the one segment without functional recovery in which correlation with the ^{18}F-2-fluoro-2-deoxyglucose images was performed, relative ^{18}F counts were 54 percent of those in control myocardium, suggesting concordant reductions in blood flow and metabolism.

In the seven segments without functional improvement, the water-perfusable tissue index averaged 0.62 ± 0.06 and was consistently less than 0.7. The mean water-perfusable tissue index in the 26 segments with improved wall motion was significantly greater—0.99 ± 0.15 ($P < .02$). Each segment with functional improvement had a water-perfusable tissue index greater than or equal to 0.70. Furthermore, the water-perfusable tissue index appeared to differentiate more clearly between hypoperfused segments with and those without functional recovery than the measurements of absolute blood flow.

For both studies, the authors concluded that 70 percent or more of the tissue mass in a dysfunctional myocardial segment must be viable if contractile function is to improve following revascularization. Thus, the water-perfusable tissue index might prove useful for identifying reversibly dysfunctional myocardium. However, the approach does not address the transmural distribution of viable myocytes and whether differences in the subendocardial and subepicardial location of viable tissue might affect ultimate recovery of function following restoration of blood flow. From a practical point of view, calculation of the water-perfusable tissue index is both technically demanding and time-consuming, rendering it less than optimal for routine clinical use.

Synopsis

Although myocardial segments with a complete absence of blood flow are unlikely to harbor viable tissue, the issue of tissue viability is more complex in situations in which resting perfusion is diminished but not totally absent. The concept of hibernating myocardium was formulated based on the clinical observation that some chronically hypoperfused myocardial regions with resting dysfunction exhibit normal or improved function following restoration of blood flow. Although several clinical studies suggest that the severity of a perfusion defect might be used to identify dysfunctional myocardial regions that would benefit from coronary revascularization, there are technical difficulties inherent in accurately measuring the severity of a perfusion defect with the SPECT imaging technique. These include differences in photon attenuation between patients and in myocardial regions, interpatient variations in background activity and in stress to redistribution reinjection images, and a nonlinear reduction in measured counts because of the partial volume effect. The severity of perfusion defect serves as an incomplete guide to the assessment of myocardial viability. Comparisons of SPECT perfusion defects with ^{18}F-2-fluoro-2-deoxyglucose uptake on positron emission tomography indicate that myocardial areas with modest (greater than 50 percent of peak normal) reductions in relative tracer activity are likely to exhibit residual tissue metabolic viability. Yet, about one in four to one in two myocardial regions with severe (activity less than 50 percent of peak normal) perfusion defects will exhibit preserved metabolic activity on ^{18}F-2-fluoro-2-deoxyglucose imaging. Thus, metabolic imaging provides incremental, clinically important information about tissue viability in myocardial areas with SPECT perfusion defects that are of moderate or more pronounced severity.

Although measurements of perfusion defect severity are more accurately made with positron emission tomography, described observations support the concept that the severity of a perfusion defect is not a reliable indicator of clinically important tissue viability in dysfunctional myocardial regions. For example, reduction in resting flow may correlate inversely in "match" regions, whereas no such correlation was found in "mismatch segments." Thus, reliance on the severity of a perfusion defect alone for the determination of the presence or absence of clinically important tissue viability would not appear to be prudent. In patients with fixed perfusion defects, noninvasive metabolic imaging with ^{18}F-2-fluoro-2-deoxyglucose and positron emission tomography offers valuable information on tissue viability and thus assists in identifying individuals who will benefit from revascularization.

Measurements of perfusion suggest that human myocardium is unlikely to be viable if transmural blood flows are less than 0.25 mL · g^{-1} · min^{-1}. However, flows greater than 0.25 mL · g^{-1} · min^{-1} cannot be assumed to denote the presence of clinically important viability. It is likely that some myocardial areas with blood flows greater than 0.25 mL · g^{-1} · min^{-1} may derive little functional benefit from revascularization. Lastly, the water-perfusable tissue index might offer information on reversibly dysfunctional myocardium. Yet, it does not discriminate between viable, although compromised, and normal myocardium.

Inotropic Stimulation

As noted in the section on regional myocardial wall motion and thickening, neither the severity of a resting wall motion abnormality nor the presence or absence of systolic thickening under basal conditions distinguishes reliably between asynergic ventricular regions with and those without metabolic viability. However, both experimental and clinical studies,[170] have suggested that inotropic stimulation of dysfunctional myocardium with sympathetic catecholamines might distinguish between reversible and irreversible tissue injury. Furthermore, the inotropic contractile reserve has been reported to be correlated to the severity of ^{201}Tl defects in patients with chronic coronary artery disease.[171] Thus, assessment of regional wall motion and systolic thickening during low-dose dobutamine stimulation might provide evidence of clinically important myocardial viability.

In order to examine the clinical utility of dobutamine stimulation relative to positron emission tomographic metabolic imaging for identifying viable myocardium, Pierard and colleagues[172] studied 17 patients with anterior myocardial infarction (13 Q wave, 4 non-Q wave) treated with thrombolytic therapy within the first 3 hours. Dobutamine echocardiography (5 and then 10 $\mu g \cdot kg^{-1} \cdot min^{-1}$) was performed at the bedside 7±4 days after thrombolytic therapy, whereas positron emission tomography was performed at 9±5 days with potassium-38 or ^{13}N-ammonia as a perfusion tracer and ^{18}F-2-fluoro-2-deoxyglucose. Follow-up resting echocardiograms and positron emission tomography were obtained at 9±7 months. A patient was considered to have myocardial viability when dobutamine infusion resulted in improved function in two or more ventricular segments, or when at least two segments in the angiographically defined risk area had normal systolic function under basal conditions or during dobutamine stress. Segments that remained akinetic or dyskinetic during dobutamine stimulation were considered nonviable.

Results correlated between the two imaging techniques in 78 segments. Of 47 segments viable on early positron emission tomography, 38 (81 percent) were considered viable on dobutamine echocardiography, whereas 24 of 31 (77 percent) nonviable segments on positron emission tomography were also considered nonviable on dobutamine echocardiography. Twenty-nine of the 31 segments with normal perfusion on the initial positron emission tomographic studies had normal perfusion and metabolism on the late positron emission tomographic studies, whereas two segments had matching perfusion and metabolic defects. In contrast, 15 of 21 (71 percent) segments with perfusion-metabolism mismatches on the early positron emission tomographic studies demonstrated matching perfusion and metabolic defects on the late positron emission tomographic studies, indicating an interval loss of viability. Of the six remaining segments, three were normal at the time of follow-up and three demonstrated persistent perfusion-metabolism mismatches.

Comparison between echocardiography and positron emission tomography was made in 82 segments on the follow-up studies. Of the 42 segments viable on positron emission tomography, only 29 (69 percent) were considered viable on echocardiography. Of the 13 segments nonviable on echocardiography, 7 had normal perfusion on positron emission tomography, whereas 6 had persistent perfusion-metabolism mismatches. Of the 40 segments nonviable on positron emission tomography, 36 (90 percent) were also nonviable on echocardiography. The authors concluded that dobutamine echocardiography might prove useful for unmasking myocardial viability in patients with acute myocardial infarction and noted that normalization of perfusion in the clinical infarct zone following thrombolysis presaged late recovery of function. In contrast, a perfusion-metabolism mismatch identified jeopardized myocardium that often progressed to completed infarction.

Using a different echocardiographic technique, Baer and colleagues[173] studied 40 patients with chronic myocardial infarction (30 with Q-wave infarction, 10 with non-Q wave infarction) using dobutamine transesophageal echocardiography and ^{18}F-2-fluoro-2-deoxyglucose and positron emission tomography. Each patient had experienced a clinical infarction 4 months or more (average = 36±47 months, range of 4 to 180 months) prior to enrollment in the study and exhibited regional akinesia or dyskinesia on contrast left ventriculography. Transesophageal stress echocardiography was performed during the intravenous infusion of 5, 10 and, in some patients, 20 $\mu g \cdot kg^{-1} \cdot min^{-1}$. Segmental function was assessed visually in 26 myocardial segments per patient on the resting and dobutamine echocardiograms. On positron emission tomography with ^{18}F-2-fluoro-2-deoxyglucose, myocardial segments were considered viable if mean segmental ^{18}F counts were equal to or greater than 50 percent of maximal activity. Regional myocardial perfusion was not assessed in the study.

Segmental function improved in response to dobutamine stress in at least one segment in 21 (53 percent) of the patients. Patients with and those without improvement in segmental function were similar with regard to age, site of clinical infarction, number of stenosed coronary vessels, or relative number of individuals with occluded vessels. Seventeen of the 29 (73 percent) patients with Q-wave infarctions did not demonstrate an improvement in function with dobutamine, whereas only 1 of 11 (9 percent) of the patients with non-Q wave infarctions failed to demonstrate an inotropic reserve. Positron emission tomography identified residual myocardial viability in the infarct zone in 25 (63 percent) of the patients, including 15 (52 percent) with Q-wave infarctions. In these 25 patients, residual inotropic reserve was noted on dobutamine echocardiography in 21 individuals (84 percent) in one or more myocardial segments. None of the 15 patients with metabolic defects revealed an inotropic response to dobutamine. Lastly, none of the patients with an inotropic reserve had a complete scar on positron emission tomography.

Of the 109 akinetic or dyskinetic segments considered viable on positron emission tomography, 88 (81 percent) were considered viable on dobutamine echocardiography. Of the 126 segments considered nonviable on positron emission tomography, 122 (97 percent) were also classified nonviable by dobutamine echocardiography. Thus, nearly all (96 percent) of the segments with akinesis or dyskinesis that improved with dobutamine stimulation were viable as defined by metabolic imaging, whereas about one in five segments (and patients) with viability on positron emission tomography did not exhibit an inotropic response to dobutamine stimulation.

In a separate report from the same institution,[174] these authors correlated the findings on imaging with ^{18}F-2-fluoro-2-deoxyglucose with low-dose (10 $\mu g \cdot kg^{-1} \cdot min^{-1}$) dobutamine gradient-echo MRI in 35 patients with chronic myocardial infarction. Each of the patients had a history of a remote myocardial infarction and exhibited regional akinesia or dyskinesia on contrast left ventriculography. The average time interval from clinical infarction to study enrollment was 18±16 months (range of 5 to 72 months). Seven of the patients had non-Q wave infarction and 28 patients had Q-wave infarction. The mean left ventricular ejection fraction of the study population was 42±16 percent. No patient with unstable angina, congestive heart failure, atrial fibrillation, a history of sustained ventricular tachycardia, or diabetes was studied.

On MRI, segments were considered viable if they showed systolic wall thickening (≥1 mm) at rest or during dobutamine infusion or if the mean end-diastolic wall thickness was 5.5 mm or greater. Positron emission tomography with ^{18}F-2-fluoro-2-deoxyglucose was performed in the glucose-loaded state. Segments were considered viable if mean segmental ^{18}F activity was greater than or equal to 50 percent of the activity in a myocardial region with normal wall motion. Myocardial perfusion imaging was not performed.

Seventeen patients (48 percent) had end-diastolic wall thicknesses greater than or equal to 5.5 mm and were considered to have viable myocardium by MRI. Each of these patients (100 percent) had residual metabolic viability on positron emission tomography, whereas 16 (94 percent) had improved systolic function during dobutamine stimulation. The other 18 individuals had end-diastolic wall thicknesses less than 5.5 mm and were considered to have completed infarction. During dobutamine infusion, three (17 percent) of these individuals had improved systolic function, and each exhibited metabolic viability. Three (20 percent) of the 15 patients without improved function during dobutamine stimulation had preserved metabolic viability on positron emission tomographic imaging. None of the patients with completed infarction on positron emission tomographic metabolic imaging had improved function during dobutamine stimulation.

If myocardial viability on MRI was defined by the presence of either an end-diastolic wall thickness greater than or equal to 5.5 mm or a positive inotropic contractile response to dobutamine infusion, or both, dobutamine gradient-echo MRI identified 263 of 299 (88 percent) of the segments that were viable on positron emission tomographic metabolic imaging. Of the 195 segments considered nonviable on MRI, residual metabolic viability was identified in 36 (18 percent). Of the 287 segments viable on MRI, scar was identified by metabolic imaging in 24 (8 percent). The authors concluded that viable myocardium is characterized on gated MRI imaging by preserved end-diastolic wall thickness and an inotropic contractile reserve. They noted that both parameters needed to be considered to maximize the utility of gated MRI imaging for identifying viable myocardium as defined by metabolic imaging with ^{18}F-2-fluoro-2-deoxyglucose.

Both investigations are limited because myocardial perfusion studies were not performed. As noted, myocardial segments that exhibit enhanced glucose use relative to blood flow are more likely to exhibit improved ventricular function following revascularization than are segments with "incomplete" (less severe) matching perfusion and metabolic defects. Thus, it is uncertain whether observed deficits in relative ^{18}F-2-fluoro-2-deoxyglucose concentrations represent perfusion-metabolism mismatches, "incomplete matches," or full matches (scar). Each of these entities has differing clinical implications regarding the degree of tissue viability remaining in the infarct region and whether revascularization might be indicated. As such, further comparative clinical studies appear to be warranted.

In summary, in clinical studies in limited numbers of patients with coronary artery disease and regional wall motion abnormalities, demonstration of a retained contractile reserve by low-dose dobutamine stimulation increases the likelihood that residual tissue metabolic viability will be identified in dysfunctional myocardium by positron emission tomography with ^{18}F-2-fluoro-2-deoxyglucose. The absence of an inotropic response to dobutamine stimulation does not preclude the presence of residual tissue metabolic activity, and about 20 percent of patients or segments that fail to demonstrate improved systolic function with dobutamine stimulation will exhibit myocardial metabolic viability on positron emission tomography. Left ventricular function appears to have been relatively well preserved in the patients in whom the initial comparative studies were performed, and it is uncertain if functional imaging with dobutamine stress testing will provide comparable results for individuals who have more pronounced degrees of left ventricular dysfunction.

Radioiodine-Labeled Fatty Acids

As described in Chapter 66, radioiodinated fatty acid analogs trace specific portions of the myocardial fatty acid metabolism. To compare ^{18}F-2-fluoro-2-deoxyglucose on positron emission tomography with iodine-123 ortho-iodophenylpentadecanoic acid (IPPA), Henrich and colleagues[175] studied 32 patients with myocardial infarction 4 weeks prior to the scintigraphic studies. The authors sought specifically to compare the uptake of these two metabolic tracers in myocardial segments with persistent defects on stress and 3- to 4-hour redistribution SPECT ^{201}Tl images. Positron emission tomography was performed with ^{18}F-2-fluoro-2-deoxyglucose 2 hours following the redistribution thallium images. Fatty acid tomography was performed following an overnight fast 4 days after the ^{201}Tl and the ^{18}F-2-fluoro-2-deoxyglucose studies.

The positron emission tomographic and SPECT images were analyzed using six contiguous short-axis slices. Normalized count data were compared with normal values derived from the study of normal subjects. Myocardial segments with a relative uptake of thallium less than the mean value -2 SD on the redistribution SPECT images were further classified with regard to the uptake of IPPA and ^{18}F-2-fluoro-2-deoxyglucose. For either of these tracers, uptake in myocardial segments less than 2 SD below the normal mean values was considered low. Of 1153 segments analyzed quantitatively, 408 segments (34.4 percent) exhibited a persistent ^{201}Tl defect. Of the myocardial segments with decreased thallium uptake, 206 (50.5 percent) had concordant reductions in both IPPA and ^{18}F-2-fluoro-2-deoxyglucose. In contrast, uptake of both IPPA and ^{18}F-2-fluoro-2-deoxyglucose appeared normal in 89 (21.8 percent) segments. Seventy-one (17.4 percent) of the segments had normal uptake of ^{18}F-2-fluoro-2-deoxyglucose with decreased IPPA uptake, whereas 42 (10.3 percent) segments had normal IPPA uptake with decreased ^{18}F-2-fluoro-2-deoxyglucose uptake. Therefore, the sensitivity of IPPA for the detection of normal ^{18}F-2-fluoro-2-deoxyglucose uptake in persistent thallium defects was 56 percent and its specificity was 83 percent. The positive and negative predictive values were 68 percent and 74 percent, respectively. The authors concluded that the sensitivity for the detection of viable myocardium using IPPA with SPECT imaging appeared to be lower than that of ^{18}F-2-fluoro-2-deoxyglucose on positron emission tomography in myocardial segments with persistent thallium defects.

Synopsis

Identification of tissue glucose metabolism in hypoperfused ventricular regions with positron emission tomography and ^{18}F-2-fluoro-2-deoxyglucose indicates the presence of viable but jeopardized tissue in patients with coronary artery disease. The presence of glucose use in hypoperfused areas reliably predicts improvement in segmental function following revascularization and frequently identifies residual tissue viability when the electrocardiogram, assessment of wall motion, and ^{201}Tl scintigraphy indicate irreversible injury. The severity of a perfusion defect is not a reliable indicator of the presence or absence of preserved metabolic viability within a myocardial segment, but the likelihood of metabolic viability appears to decline as the perfusion defect becomes more severe. Improvement in segmental wall motion during inotropic stimulation with dobutamine may also identify reversibly dysfunctional tissue, but further studies in patients with more profound degrees of left ventricular dysfunction are warranted. Thus positron emission tomography with ^{18}F-2-fluoro-2-deoxyglucose provides unique information about tissue viability that cannot be obtained by the use of routinely employed clinical tests.

MYOCARDIAL METABOLIC IMAGING FOR PROGNOSIS IN CHRONIC CORONARY ARTERY DISEASE

Although the demonstration of preserved glucose metabolism in hypoperfused myocardial regions indicates clinically important tissue viability in patients with coronary artery disease, little is known regarding the natural history of myocardium exhibiting this metabolic pattern. Glucose consumption is increased relative to substrate delivery or blood flow. Such enhanced glucose consumption presumably reflects an adaptive cellular response to an unfavorable pathophysiologic state. If the disturbances in glucose metabolism observed on positron emission tomography do indicate "distressed myocardium," the observed scintigraphic abnormalities may represent a "snapshot in time" of an unstable situation. Conceivably, progression of the disease process could exceed the adaptive capacity of the tissue and thus result in cell death and myocardial fibrosis.

The concept that perfusion-metabolism mismatches may progress to scar and eventually demonstrate matching perfusion and metabolic defects on positron emission tomography is consistent with data reported by Fragasso and coworkers.[176] In this retrospective study, the authors correlated the time interval from clinical Q-wave myocardial infarction with the results of positron emission tomography with ^{18}F-2-fluoro-2-deoxyglucose. Of 65 patients with Q-wave infarctions who were studied, 26 patients had matching perfusion and metabolic defects, whereas 39 patients had preserved metabolic activity in the clinical infarct region. On angiography, coronary artery disease severity and the relative number of patients with significant collateral vessels were similar in individuals with and those without perfusion-metabolism mismatches. In addition, the number of hypokinetic myocardial segments or the mean wall motion scores were similar for the patient groups. However, the mean time interval from clinical infarction was significantly greater in the patients with matching defects than in the patients with perfusion-metabolism mismatches (1860 ± 1333 versus 92 ± 115 days, $P < .0001$). All of the 28 patients undergoing positron emission tomography within 6 months of clinical infarction had residual

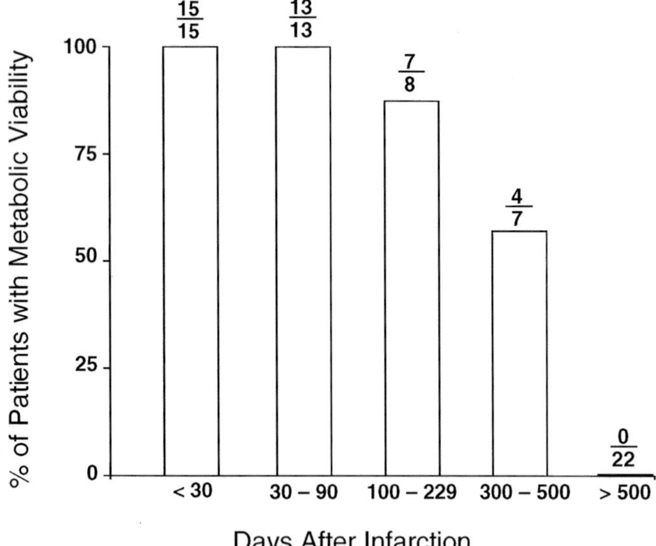

FIGURE 71–30. Relative number of patients with evidence of glucose metabolic viability on positron emission tomography with ^{18}F-2-fluoro-2-deoxyglucose in the zone of clinical infarction as a function of the time interval from the acute episode. The likelihood of preserved metabolic viability within the infarct zone declines as time progresses. (Data from Fragasso, G., Chierchia, S. L., Lucignani, G., et al: Time dependence of residual tissue viability after myocardial infarction assessed by [^{18}F]fluorodeoxyglucose and positron emission tomography. Am. J. Cardiol. 72:131G, 1993.)

tissue metabolic activity, whereas none of the patients imaged more than 500 days after infarction had evidence of metabolic viability in the zone of clinical infarction (Fig. 71–30). Thus, the likelihood that metabolic imaging would identify viable tissue in a zone of clinical infarction declined with time, consistent with the idea that some perfusion-metabolism mismatches might progress to necrosis and thus to matching defects.

If perfusion-metabolism mismatches do represent an unstable situation, patients with this finding would be at risk for clinical ischemic events as the disease progresses. Conversely, individuals who undergo successful coronary revascularization should be less likely to experience an adverse outcome. In a retrospective study, Tamaki and colleagues[177] sought to compare the prognostic value of ^{18}F-2-fluoro-2-deoxyglucose metabolic positron emission tomographic imaging with stress and 3-hour redistribution ^{201}Tl scintigraphy in medically treated patients with chronic myocardial infarction. Of an initial study population of 158 individuals, follow-up data were obtained by medical record review or telephone interview in 84 patients at a mean interval of 23.0 ± 12.7 months (Table 71–5). During the follow-up period, 17 cardiac events were observed, including 3 cardiac related deaths, 3 nonfatal myocardial infarctions, the onset of unstable angina in seven patients, and the clinical need for late coronary revascularization in four patients.

Adverse events were observed more frequently in the patients with histories of multiple prior infarctions than in those with a single infarction (5 of 17 versus 6 of 67, $P < .03$). Individuals with adverse cardiac events had a significantly greater number of diseased coronary arteries, lower left ventricular ejection fractions, a higher likelihood of ^{201}Tl redistribution, a greater number of myocardial segments with ^{201}Tl redistribution, a greater probability of having increased lung ^{201}Tl uptake, and a greater likelihood of a segmental increase in ^{18}F-2-fluoro-2-deoxyglucose uptake. On stepwise multivariate logistic regression analysis, the presence of increased uptake of ^{18}F-2-fluoro-2-deoxyglucose was the most significant predictor of a cardiac event (chi-square = 13.53), followed by the number of stenosed coronary arteries (chi-square = 7.67). The authors reported that none of the ^{201}Tl scintigraphic variables examined contributed additional prognostic value to the multivariate analysis model.

Yoshida and Gould[178] correlated ^{82}Rb washout studies and left ventricular ejection fraction with mortality at 3 years in 35 patients with coronary artery disease. Although glucose metabolic imaging with ^{18}F-2-fluoro-2-deoxyglucose was also performed, the authors relied primarily on ratios of late (120 to 360 seconds after injection) to early (15 to 110 seconds) ^{82}Rb activity on the images to define myocardial viability.[179] The mean left ventricular ejection fraction of the study population was 44 ± 12 percent (range of 19 to 60 percent) and 19 patients had sustained an acute myocardial infarction within 30 days of the imaging study.

In 14 patients with myocardial scar involving at least 23 percent of the left ventricle, the 3-year mortality rate was 43 percent, whereas the mortality rate was only 5 percent in the patients with smaller scars ($P < .02$). Similarly, the 3-year mortality rate in the 16 patients with left ventricular ejection fractions less than or equal to 43 percent was higher than that in the patients with relatively well-preserved ventricular function, 38 percent versus 6 percent ($P < .03$). As might be anticipated, the extent of the myocardial scar observed on the ^{82}Rb images was compared with the left ventricular ejection fraction by

$$\text{percent LV scar} = 130 - 3.9 \cdot \text{EF} + 0.032 \cdot (\text{EF})^2$$

where LV is left ventricular and EF is ejection fraction.

Twenty-five of the 35 patients were considered to have viable but jeopardized myocardium in the distribution of an infarct-related artery, whereas 10 patients had myocardial scar by positron emission tomographic criteria (see Table 71–5). Of the patients with viable myocardium, 5 were treated medically, whereas 20 were treated surgically. Patients were considered to have undergone revascularization if the procedure was performed anytime during the 3-year period. Thus, some with viable myocardium may have been treated medically initially and offered surgery at a later time, clouding the effects, if any, of revascularization on prognosis in these individuals. None of the five medically treated patients with viable myocardium on positron emission tomography died. Two of the 20 individuals with viable myocardium who were treated surgically died. Of the 10 patients with myocardial scar on positron emission tomography, 6 were treated medically and 4 were treated

TABLE 71–5. PATIENTS WITH ADVERSE CARDIAC EVENTS

			Viable on Positron Emission Tomography		Nonviable on Positron Emission Tomography		
Number of Patients	Left Ventricular Ejection Fraction	Follow-Up Period (months)	*Medical Treatment*	*Surgical Treatment*	*Medical Treatment*	*Surgical Treatment*	Reference
82	34 ± 13%	12	9/18 (50%)	3/26 (12%)	3/24 (13%)	1/14 (14%)	Eitzman et al.[181]
35	44 ± 12%	36	0/5 (0%)	2/20 (10%)	3/6 (50%)	2/4 (50%)	Yoshida and Gould[178]
84	≈48%	23	16/48 (33%)	—	1/36 (3%)	—	Tamaki et al.[177]
93	25 ± 6%	14	7/17 (41%)	3/26 (12%)	3/33 (9%)	1/17 (6%)	Di Carli et al.[182]
129	38 ± 16%	17	13/21 (62%)	8/49 (16%)	7/40 (18%)	2/19 (11%)	Lee et al.[180]
Totals 423	37%	18	45/109 (41%)	16/121 (13%)	17/139 (12%)	6/54 (11%)	

surgically. The 3-year mortality rate was 50 percent for each of these groups, perhaps reflecting the relatively small number of patients in each group as well as the criteria used to select the individuals for medical or surgical treatment.

Lee and coinvestigators[180] performed resting and dipyridamole ^{82}Rb perfusion imaging and ^{18}F-2-fluoro-2-deoxyglucose metabolic imaging in 129 patients with prior myocardial infarction and left ventricular dysfunction (left ventricular ejection fraction = 38 ± 16 percent). Based on clinical, angiographic, and imaging data, 61 patients were treated medically, whereas 68 were referred for coronary revascularization (50 had coronary artery bypass grafts, 16 had percutaneous transluminal coronary angioplasty and 2 had coronary atherectomy). Periodic follow-up was accomplished by clinic visit or by telephone interview for 17 ± 9 months. Three end points were examined: cardiac death, recurrent myocardial infarction, and unstable angina requiring hospitalization or urgent revascularization.

During the period of follow-up, there were 17 nonfatal cardiac events in 16 patients. All 16 patients presented with unstable angina, and 1 individual subsequently sustained a myocardial infarction. The patients with nonfatal cardiac events did not differ from the others with respect to age, presence of multivessel disease, left ventricular ejection fraction, incidence of reversible ^{82}Rb perfusion defects, or severity of anginal or heart failure symptoms. The relative number of patients with coronary revascularization tended to be higher in those without events (63 of 113, 56 percent) than in those with events (5 of 16, 31 percent) but this did not achieve statistical significance (P = .06). In contrast, 14 of the 16 (88 percent) patients with adverse ischemic events had segmentally enhanced uptake of ^{18}F-2-fluoro-2-deoxyglucose, whereas this finding was observed in 56 of the 113 (50 percent, P = .003) patients without events.

The incidence of nonfatal ischemic events in the 21 medically treated patients with enhanced uptake of ^{18}F-2-fluoro-2-deoxyglucose was 48 percent, significantly higher than the 8 percent incidence observed in the 49 surgically treated patients with enhanced uptake of ^{18}F-2-fluoro-2-deoxyglucose (P < .001), or the 5 percent incidence observed in either the medically (n = 40) or surgically treated patients (n = 19) with matching perfusion and metabolic defects (P < .001 and P < .01, respectively). Using a Cox proportional hazards model, these investigators found that the only statistically significant predictors of ischemic events were segmentally enhanced uptake of ^{18}F-2-fluoro-2-deoxyglucose (odds ratio 12.9, P < .001) and the absence of revascularization (odds ratio 5.8, P < .002). The authors also performed a Kaplan-Meier analysis that indicated that the patients with perfusion-metabolism mismatches who were treated medically sustained ischemic events more rapidly than either those treated surgically or those with matches who were treated either medically or surgically (P = .008).

Thirteen patients in the study population sustained cardiac deaths. Those who died had significantly lower ejection fractions (22 ± 13 percent) than those with nonfatal events (39 ± 14 percent) or those without events (39 ± 16 percent). In addition, those with fatal events were significantly older than those without events (69 ± 7 versus 61 ± 11 years, P = .01). In these individuals, the presence of multivessel disease, the presence of reversible ^{82}Rb perfusion defects, and the severity of angina and heart failure symptoms were not predictive of death. The incidence of cardiac death was 14 percent in the medically treated patients with mismatches, 8 percent in the surgically treated patients with mismatches, 13 percent in the medically treated patients with matching defects, and 5 percent in the surgically treated patients with matching defects. On multivariate analysis, only age (odds ratio 2.4 per 10 years of advanced age, P = .02) and left ventricular ejection fraction (odds ratio, 2.7 per 10 percent decrease in ejection fraction, P = .001) independently predicted cardiac death.

In a retrospective study, Eitzman and colleagues[181] examined the clinical status of 82 patients with advanced coronary artery disease (left ventricular ejection fraction = 34 ± 13 percent) who underwent positron emission tomography with ^{13}N-ammonia and ^{18}F-2-fluoro-2-deoxyglucose at the University of Michigan (see Table 71–5). Of 44 patients with perfusion-metabolism mismatches, 18 were treated medically and 26 underwent coronary revascularization. In the 38 patients with matching perfusion and metabolic defects, coronary revascularization was performed in 14, whereas medical therapy was provided to the other 24 patients. The positron emission tomographic findings and the type of treatment provided thus defined four patient groups: those with perfusion-metabolism mismatches treated medically, those with mismatches treated surgically, those with matching defects on positron emission tomography treated medically, and those with matching defects treated surgically. The four patient groups did not differ with respect to age, left ventricular ejection fraction, number of stenosed vessels, number of cardiac risk factors or New York Heart Association heart failure class. Patients with mismatches who underwent coronary revascularization had a slightly higher mean Canadian Cardiovascular Society anginal class than the patients in the other groups.

Telephone interviews were performed 12 months following the initial positron emission tomographic study to ascertain New York Heart Association and Canadian Cardiovascular Society classifications for heart failure and anginal symptoms and to determine the number of patients who sustained cardiac events. Such events were defined as death, nonfatal myocardial infarction, cardiac arrest, the need for coronary revascularization due to worsening symptoms, or a combination. Sixteen (19.5 percent) of the 82 patients had cardiac events during the 1-year follow-up period. There were nine deaths, three myocardial infarctions, one cardiac arrest, and three late coronary revascularizations. The individuals who sustained cardiac events did not differ from those without events with respect to age, left ventricular ejection fraction, number of stenosed vessels, number of cardiac risk factors, heart failure class, or anginal class.

The 18 patients with perfusion-metabolism mismatches who were treated medically had a cardiac event rate of 50 percent (see Table 71–5). Six of these patients died, and there were three nonfatal myocardial infarctions. In striking contrast, the cardiac event rate was only 12 percent (one death, one cardiac arrest, one late revascularization, P < .01) in the 26 patients with perfusion-metabolism mismatches who underwent revascularization. Interestingly, patients with matching perfusion and metabolic defects on the initial positron emission tomographic study had similar cardiac event rates regardless of whether medical or surgical treatment was provided. The cardiac event rate was 13 percent (two deaths, one late revascularization) in the 24 patients with matching defects treated medically and 7 percent (one late revascularization) in the 14 patients with matching defects treated surgically, similar to the cardiac event rate for the patients with mismatches treated surgically. Event rates in both patient groups with matching defects were significantly less than the rates in the medically treated patient group with perfusion-metabolism mismatches (P < .01 for both).

These investigators also determined the functional status of the patients who did not sustain cardiac events. None of the medically treated patients had an improvement in anginal class, whereas 19 of 23 (83 percent) patients with perfusion-metabolism mismatches treated surgically and 7 of 13 (54 percent) patients with matching defects treated surgically improved by one or more anginal classes. In contrast, none of the medically treated patients with perfusion-metabolism mismatches and only three (14 percent) of the medically treated patients with matching defects had an improvement in heart failure class. Eight (35 percent) patients with perfusion-metabolism mismatches treated surgically and four (31 percent) patients with matching defects treated surgically had an improvement of one or more grades in heart failure class. The authors concluded that the presence of perfusion-metabolism mismatches in patients with advanced ischemic heart disease identifies individuals at risk for adverse cardiac events and that those thus identified appear to have the most symptomatic and prognostic benefit from a revascularization procedure.

In a subsequent study, Di Carli and coinvestigators[182] retrospectively examined the clinical status of 93 patients with more pronounced ischemic left ventricular dysfunction (left ventricular ejection fraction = 25±6 percent) referred to the University of California at Los Angeles for positron emission tomography as candidates for myocardial revascularization. Of 107 consecutive patients, 13 were excluded because they were referred for heart transplantation and one was excluded because angiography demonstrated normal coronary arteries. Fifty of the remaining 93 patients were treated medically, whereas 43 underwent coronary revascularization. The medically treated and surgically treated patient groups were similar with regard to gender composition; age; number of prior clinical infarctions; individuals with New York Heart Association class III or IV heart failure symptoms; relative number of individuals with angina, diabetes, hypertension, and pulmonary disease; left ventricular ejection fraction; number of stenosed coronary arteries; and proportion of individuals with perfusion-metabolism mismatches on positron emission tomography with ^{13}N-ammonia and ^{18}F-2-fluoro-2-deoxyglucose. Telephone interviews and medical record reviews were performed by an investigator who was unaware of the imaging results. The average period of follow-up was 13.6 months.

Fourteen patients died of cardiac causes during the follow-up period. The data were analyzed using a univariate regression model incorporating sex, age, prior myocardial infarction, the presence of Q waves on the resting electrocardiogram, diabetes, hypertension, presence of angina, left ventricular ejection fraction, extent of matching and perfusion-metabolism mismatches, revascularization, heart failure class, and presence or absence of chronic obstructive pulmonary disease as variables. The only variable that was a significant predictor of survival was the extent of the perfusion-metabolism mismatch on positron emission tomographic imaging (P = .02). Chronic obstructive pulmonary disease (P = .07) and heart failure class (P = .06) were marginally significant predictors of survival. The investigators then used a stepwise Cox model analysis to ascertain the prognostic contribution of the extent of the perfusion-metabolism mismatch when the covariates with borderline significance in the univariate model were included. On this analysis, the extent of perfusion-metabolism mismatch (P = .02) and revascularization (P = .04) were the only significant predictors of survival. The relative risk of death increased by 3.5 percent for each percent increase in the percent extent of the perfusion-metabolism mismatch so that the individuals with the largest mismatches had the greatest risk of cardiac death. Conversely, revascularization decreased the risk of cardiac death by 28 percent.

In the 50 patients who were treated medically, the prevalence of angina and the severity of heart failure symptoms did not change during the period of follow-up. To determine the effect of perfusion-metabolism mismatches on survival, medically treated patients were divided into two groups based on the presence (n = 17) or absence (n = 33) of perfusion-metabolism mismatches involving 5 percent or more of the left ventricle. The cumulative annual survival in the patients with perfusion-metabolism mismatches was significantly lower than in the patients with matching defects (50 percent versus 82 percent, P = .007) (Fig. 71–31).

Of the 43 patients treated surgically, 26 had perfusion-metabolism mismatches, whereas 17 had matching defects. Following revascularization, the number of individuals with angina decreased from 19 to 3 (P < .001). Heart failure symptoms improved significantly only in the patients with mismatches preoperatively (21 of 26 in class III or IV preoperatively versus 6 of 26 postoperatively, P < .001). The patients with mismatches who had revascularization had a significantly higher annual survival probability than those treated medically (88 percent versus 50 percent, P = .03). In contrast, the survival probability for patients with matching defects treated surgically did not differ from those treated medically (94 percent versus 82 percent, P = NS). This study thus indicates that patients with coronary artery disease and pronounced left ventricular dysfunction have a significantly higher risk of cardiac death if positron emission tomographic imaging identifies a perfusion-metabolism mismatch than do individuals with comparable degrees of left ventricular dysfunction who exhibit matching perfusion and metabolic defects. The authors concluded that revascularization in patients with perfusion-metabolism mismatches benefits both survival and heart failure symptoms.

Of the five investigations in which prognosis has been correlated with the findings on positron emission tomographic imaging, only the reports of Eitzman and colleagues[181] and Di Carli and associates[182] have provided information regarding the nature of the car-

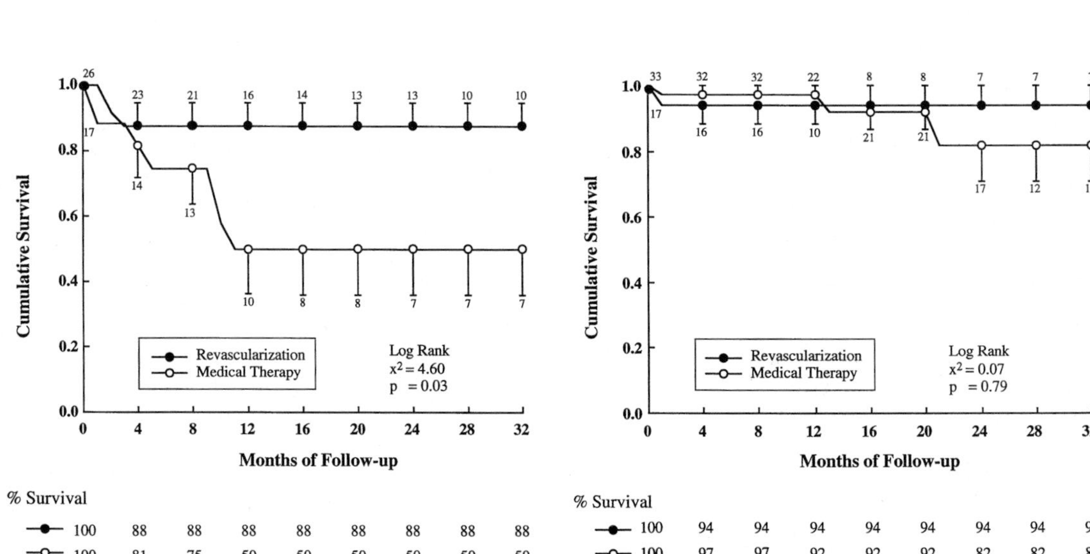

FIGURE 71–31. Cumulative annual survival of patients with ischemic cardiomyopathy according to the presence (*A*) or absence (*B*) of a perfusion-metabolism mismatch on positron emission tomography with ^{13}N-ammonia and ^{18}F-2-fluoro-2-deoxyglucose. Medically treated patients with perfusion-metabolism mismatches have a cumulative annual survival of only 50 percent, significantly lower than patients with perfusion-metabolism mismatches treated surgically or patients with matching perfusion and metabolic defects treated either medically or surgically. (From Di Carli, M. F., Davidson, M., Little, R., et al.: Value of metabolic imaging with positron emission tomography for evaluating prognosis in patients with coronary artery disease and left ventricular dysfunction. Am. J. Cardiol. 73:531, 1994, with permission.)

diac deaths sustained by their patients. In the former study, death resulted from congestive heart failure in one patient with a mismatch who was revascularized and in one patient with matching perfusion and metabolic defects who was treated medically. No deaths were observed in the patients with matching defects who were treated surgically. In contrast, death was paroxysmal in five of the six medically treated patients with mismatches: one death was sudden and four deaths were related to acute myocardial infarction. Similar findings were reported by Di Carli and coinvestigators.[182] Congestive heart failure caused two of the three deaths in the patients with matching defects treated medically and the single death in the group with matching defects treated surgically. Of the three deaths in the surgically treated patients with mismatches, two were due to congestive heart failure and one was due to postoperative sepsis. In contrast, death was sudden in five of the seven individuals with mismatches who were treated medically. The remaining two deaths in that group were due to congestive heart failure. Thus, the limited data that are available suggest that the type of cardiac death sustained by medically treated patients with perfusion-metabolism mismatches is likely to be sudden and unpredictable by conventional clinical criteria, as opposed to insidiously progressive congestive heart failure.

Synopsis

As indicated in Table 71–5, positron emission tomography frequently identifies viable tissue in hypoperfused myocardium in coronary heart disease patients with impaired left ventricular function. Tissue viability was identified in 230 (54 percent) of the 423 patients in which clinical outcomes have been correlated with the findings on initial perfusion and metabolic images. The data in Table 71–5 represent the aggregate experience for all adverse cardiac events in patients reported from five different medical centers (mean left ventricular ejection fraction = 37 percent) for an average follow-up period of 18 months after positron emission tomography. Table 71–6 presents the corresponding data for cardiac deaths only. As can be inferred from this summary, the presence of perfusion-metabolism mismatches on positron emission tomographic imaging has profound prognostic and therapeutic implications for patients with ischemic left ventricular dysfunction. Importantly, the studies of Tamaki and Lee and their associates[177, 180] further indicate that stress perfusion imaging provides little additional prognostic information beyond that afforded by a resting perfusion and ^{18}F-2-fluoro-2-deoxyglucose metabolic study alone.

Medically treated patients with perfusion-metabolism mismatches have a significant (41 percent) threefold higher risk for all adverse cardiac events (see Table 71–5) than individuals with comparable degrees of left ventricular dysfunction who do not exhibit this scintigraphic finding. The incidence of cardiac death in medically treated patients with mismatches is about twice as high as in patients with mismatches who undergo revascularization (16.5 percent versus 8.3 percent, see Table 71–6). Patients with the largest perfusion-metabolism mismatches on positron emission tomography appear to have the highest risk for adverse cardiac events. In the analysis performed by Di Carli and coinvestigators,[182] the relative risk of death increased by 3.5 percent for each 1 percent increase in the extent of the left ventricle with a perfusion-metabolism mismatch. In contrast, coronary revascularization was associated with a 28 percent reduction in cardiac mortality risk in that study. Patients with mismatches who undergo successful revascularization have adverse cardiac event rates that are similar to those of individuals with matching defects treated either medically or surgically, suggesting that restoration of blood flow favorably benefits both ventricular function and prognosis in individuals with this scintigraphic pattern.

MYOCARDIAL METABOLIC IMAGING IN CLINICAL PRACTICE

Although assessment of myocardial metabolism with positron emission tomography provides clinically useful information about the state of the myocardium in patients with ischemic heart disease, it is important to define the role of this imaging technique in the practice of clinical cardiology. Although not all patients will benefit from metabolic imaging, in well-selected individuals, the information derived from positron emission tomography will have a major impact on the patient's medical care. In this section, we identify the patients for whom metabolic imaging with positron emission tomography provides useful clinical information and discuss selected aspects of the care of the cardiac patient during myocardial metabolic imaging. Finally, we discuss how the information derived by positron emission tomography is incorporated into the clinical decision-making process for individual patient case management decisions.

Indications for Metabolic Imaging

In patients with ischemic heart disease, there are several clinical indications for myocardial glucose metabolic imaging.

1. *Detection and localization of stress-induced myocardial ischemia in patients with chest pain in whom other physiologic stress tests are inconclusive, either for establishing the diagnosis or for localizing the ischemic region or regions.*
2. *Assessment of the physiologic significance and metabolic consequence of anatomically defined stenoses in patients with known coronary artery disease by imaging with a perfusion tracer and* ^{18}*F-2-fluoro-2-deoxyglucose.* In this way, both the blood flow reserve and the metabolic reserve of the vascular territory in question can be determined. In addition, it is possible to assess the myocardial response to interventions designed to augment blood flow to ischemic myocardial regions, such as coronary artery bypass surgery or coronary angioplasty.
3. *Distinguishing myocardial regions with completed infarction from viable but ischemically compromised tissue in patients with coronary artery disease and left ventricular dysfunction.* This enables the clinician to more accurately determine the risk-to-benefit ratio of subjecting the patient to revascularization. Metabolic im-

TABLE 71–6. PATIENTS WITH CARDIAC DEATHS

Number of Patients	Viable on Positron Emission Tomography: Medical Treatment	Viable on Positron Emission Tomography: Surgical Treatment	Nonviable on Positron Emission Tomography: Medical Treatment	Nonviable on Positron Emission Tomography: Surgical Treatment	Reference
82	6/18 (33%)	1/26 (4%)	2/24 (8%)	0/14 (0%)	Eitzman et al.[181]
35	0/5 (0%)	2/20 (10%)	3/6 (50%)	2/4 (50%)	Yoshida and Gould[178]
84	3/48 (6%)	—	0/36 (0%)	—	Tamaki et al.[177]
93	7/17 (41%)	3/26 (12%)	3/33 (9%)	1/17 (6%)	Di Carli et al.[182]
129	3/21 (14%)	4/49 (8%)	5/40 (13%)	1/19 (5%)	Lee et al.[180]
Totals 423	18/109 (16.5%)	10/121 (8.3%)	14/139 (9%)	4/54 (7%)	

aging is particularly helpful in patients in whom the electrocardiogram, assessment of regional wall motion, or ^{201}Tl scintigraphy would suggest completed infarction. As noted, these routine tests frequently underestimate the extent of salvageable tissue as compared with the tissue characterization afforded by metabolic imaging. Thus, some patients with the diagnosis of completed infarction on these routine tests might actually have significant amounts of viable tissue detected on metabolic imaging with ^{18}F-2-fluoro-2-deoxyglucose and therefore be reasonable candidates for coronary revascularization. Conversely, positron emission tomography may confirm the presence of extensive infarction in some patients and may therefore influence the clinician to recommend medical therapy or cardiac transplantation rather than interventional revascularization.

4. *Discrimination of ischemic from nonischemic forms of dilated cardiomyopathies in patients with congestive heart failure of undetermined cause.* Although assessment of myocardial perfusion with ^{201}Tl might also distinguish between these two patient types, the advantage of simultaneous blood flow and glucose metabolic imaging is that it allows an independent, concurrent assessment of myocardial viability that may prove helpful in determining the need for invasive procedures such as coronary angiography.

5. *Identification of residual myocardial viability and its extent in patients with acute ischemic injury.* Blood flow and glucose metabolic imaging in these patients provide the clinician with an estimate of the amount of viable but compromised tissue in the clinical infarct zone, which will provide a rationale for instituting appropriate interventions designed to salvage endangered myocardium. In addition, positron emission tomography allows characterization of the state of function of the myocardium remote from the zone of infarction. This is likely to be most helpful in the patient presenting with an acute ischemic injury who has a history of one or more previous infarctions, enabling the clinician to ascertain the extent of jeopardized tissue throughout the left ventricle.

6. *Risk stratification in individuals with ischemic cardiomyopathy.* As noted, patients with perfusion-metabolism mismatches who are treated medically have a significantly higher risk for adverse cardiac events than do those treated surgically. As the aggregate clinical experience from five medical centers indicates, early revascularization can have a beneficial effect on prognosis and heart failure symptoms.

7. *Identification of heart transplant candidates who might benefit from surgical revascularization.* Metabolic imaging with positron emission tomography can identify patients with end-stage ischemic heart disease who have large perfusion-metabolism mismatches and therefore are likely to benefit from surgical revascularization.

As our understanding of the basic biochemistry of normal and ischemic myocardium in humans continues to grow and becomes more sophisticated, the list of clinical indications for positron emission tomography is likely to expand. For example, it may be possible to use quantitative maps of blood flow and glucose use rates obtained with dynamic positron emission tomography to predict both the extent and time course of recovery of regional and global left ventricular function in patients with ischemic left ventricular dysfunction following restoration of blood flow by coronary artery bypass surgery or by angioplasty. Thus, it is possible that metabolic imaging might prove useful in determining quantitatively the risk-to-benefit ratio of invasive interventions in individual patients with left ventricular dysfunction prior to intervention. In patients with chronic coronary artery disease, assessment of both oxidative and glycolytic metabolism as well as quantitative regional measurements of blood flow might prove more accurate for characterizing myocardial tissue, thereby improving on the prognostic utility of myocardial perfusion imaging.

Patient Care During Metabolic Imaging

By the very nature of the disease processes affecting the individual who is most likely to benefit from metabolic imaging, the patient with ischemic heart disease should be considered at risk for the development of complications during metabolic imaging. Although the information derived from metabolic imaging can significantly contribute to clinical decision-making, the clinician should be aware that it may take 1 to 2 hours for a complete perfusion and metabolic study to be performed. In some patients, therefore, it may be desirable to provide sedation prior to the positron emission tomographic study. During the imaging period it is important that a physician knowledgeable in the care of patients with ischemic heart disease be present to assist in the monitoring of unstable patients and to promptly treat any complications occurring during imaging.

Stress or dipyridamole perfusion imaging to detect coronary artery disease may provoke acute myocardial ischemia. Myocardial ischemia is capable of precipitating life-threatening arrhythmias and cardiovascular collapse. In addition, dipyridamole may provoke acute respiratory failure in patients with bronchospastic pulmonary disease. In the patient with marked left ventricular failure, care must be taken to ensure that exacerbation of cardiac dysfunction does not occur during imaging and that potentially lethal ventricular arrhythmias are adequately controlled. In addition, administration of intravenous fluids must be carefully regulated to avoid fluid overload and precipitation of acute pulmonary edema.

Because positron emission tomography is noninvasive, assessment of myocardial perfusion and metabolism in patients with acute myocardial infarction poses little additional risk to the individual beyond that engendered by the infarction itself. Whether in the intensive care unit or in the imaging suite, the key to the care of the patient with an acute infarction is careful monitoring by qualified personnel who are experienced and capable of handling the life-threatening sequelae of an acute ischemic injury. In some institutions, facilities for positron emission tomography are located next to the intensive care unit, thereby reducing the risks associated with transportation of the patient to an imaging facility. For patients undergoing positron emission tomography early in the course of an acute infarction, full electrocardiographic and hemodynamic monitoring capabilities should be available in the imaging suite. As in the intensive care unit, a crash cart with defibrillator and the drugs used to treat cardiac arrest should be readily available in case they are needed.

As with any procedure in medicine, the risks of performing the procedure must be balanced with the benefits derived. In our experience, almost any patient with a stable blood pressure and cardiac rhythm who is carefully monitored by a knowledgeable physician can derive the benefits of myocardial metabolic imaging.

Standardization of Study Conditions

Standardization of the patient's dietary state and monitoring of plasma substrate levels are important for performing metabolic imaging and, especially, for image interpretation. Plasma substrate and insulin levels markedly influence myocardial substrate metabolism and selection of the primary fuel substrate. For example, the low insulin and glucose levels and the high free fatty acid levels in plasma that are characteristically present after periods of fasting result in preferential oxidation of free fatty acids by the myocardium and reduce exogenous glucose use. Thus, myocardial time-activity curves derived from serial ^{11}C-palmitate images typically exhibit a large relative size of the rapid clearance curve component and short clearance half-times. Conversely, glucose use is often low in the fasting state, resulting in nonvisualization of normal myocardium on the ^{18}F-2-fluoro-2-deoxyglucose studies. In contrast, in the postprandial state with higher insulin and glucose levels and lower free fatty acid plasma levels, the relative size of the rapid clearance curve component on the ^{11}C-palmitate time-activity curve declines, whereas ^{18}F-2-fluoro-2-deoxyglucose accumulation in normal myocardium markedly increases. Thus, the information contained on the metabolic images in normal myocardium depends on the dietary state in a given patient.

In contrast, ischemically injured but viable myocardium appears to participate only incompletely in these metabolic responses to changes in plasma substrate levels. Use of exogenous glucose in postischemic myocardium changes with plasma glucose levels. However, these changes are markedly attenuated. Glucose use and, thus, ^{18}F-2-fluoro-2-deoxyglucose uptake in postischemic myocardium is lower than that in control myocardium during states of hyperglycemia but higher than that in control myocardium during euglycemic and low insulin states. Thus, compared with normal myocardium in humans, ischemically injured but viable myocardium characteristically will exhibit elevated ^{18}F-2-fluoro-2-deoxyglucose uptake in the fasted state and normal or slightly reduced tracer uptake in the postprandial state. Importantly, however, ^{18}F-2-fluoro-2-deoxyglucose uptake is increased relative to segmental blood flow, forming the rationale for its utility in identifying myocardial viability.

Although the effects of dietary conditions and the influence of substrate levels on the myocardial metabolic images are the subject of active investigation, patients in our laboratory are typically studied after an overnight fast and a standard oral glucose load (50 g) 1 hour prior to intravenous injection of ^{18}F-2-fluoro-2-deoxyglucose. This approach stimulates insulin secretion, lowers plasma free fatty acid levels, and characteristically results in good visualization of normal and ischemic myocardium. Circumferential profile analysis techniques are then applied to the cross-sectional perfusion and metabolic images and compared with a normal database to define abnormalities of blood flow and exogenous glucose use.

Glucose metabolic studies in the fasted state characteristically result in "hot spot" images of ischemic tissue, in which only the regions with ischemic but viable myocardium are visualized as a focal area of increased ^{18}F-activity. As quantitative analytical techniques have thus far not been developed for these images, tissue metabolic activity is assessed visually. This approach appears to be highly sensitive for the detection of ischemic but viable myocardium. It is, however, relatively nonspecific for determining whether the amount of residual tissue viability will be sufficient for an improvement of contractile function if blood flow is restored by angioplasty or bypass surgery.

Standardization of study conditions may not always be possible. This is especially true for patients studied early after an acute myocardial infarction or those admitted with acute chest pain syndromes. In these situations, the myocardial blood flow images serve as a guide to lesion identification and characterization. Myocardial areas with normal perfusion but absent or low ^{18}F-2-fluoro-2-deoxyglucose uptake are considered normal. In contrast, abnormal myocardial areas are identified by segmental decreases in blood flow. Absence of ^{18}F-2-fluoro-2-deoxyglucose uptake in these hypoperfused segments is considered indicative of completed infarction, whereas increased uptake of ^{18}F-2-fluoro-2-deoxyglucose is considered indicative of ischemic but viable tissue.

Patients with coronary artery disease and diabetes mellitus pose a particular problem. ^{18}F-2-fluoro-2-deoxyglucose uptake may be poor in nonischemic myocardium in the diabetic patient. Because of slow tracer clearance from blood, ^{18}F-2-fluoro-2-deoxyglucose images often exhibit high blood pool activity. Delayed imaging or the administration of insulin[183] may result in diagnostically acceptable myocardial images. Interestingly, ischemic but viable myocardium in the diabetic patient appears to use glucose and thus accumulates ^{18}F-2-fluoro-2-deoxyglucose. As a result, hypoperfused myocardial segments frequently exhibit increased ^{18}F-2-fluoro-2-deoxyglucose uptake that is much greater than blood pool activity. Because diabetes mellitus is frequently undiagnosed in coronary artery disease patients, we routinely determine plasma glucose levels in all patients prior to positron emission tomography. If plasma glucose levels exceed 150 mg/dL after an overnight fast, patients are not given an oral glucose load and intravenous insulin is administered if necessary. Alternatively, some institutions employ the hyperinsulinemic euglycemic clamp with excellent imaging results in patients with diabetes mellitus.[184]

Clinical Decision-Making With Metabolic Imaging

In patients with ischemic heart disease, clinical decisions are frequently based on the cardiologist's estimate of the amount of viable but jeopardized tissue that could be salvaged by interventions designed to restore myocardial blood flow. In patients with coronary heart disease and symptoms predominantly of left ventricular dysfunction rather than angina, it may be especially difficult for the clinician to identify the individuals likely to benefit from coronary revascularization. Although individuals with depressed left ventricular function have the highest risk for both coronary bypass grafting[185–187] and coronary angioplasty, the patient with the largest amount of viable but dysfunctional myocardium is the one who will benefit most symptomatically and prognostically from coronary revascularization.[188–190] Thus, distinguishing the individual with large amounts of viable tissue from the individual with extensive myocardial fibrosis is of paramount important in the management of patients with ischemic heart disease and impaired left ventricular function. The individual with large amounts of hibernating myocardium might be a candidate for coronary revascularization, whereas the individual with extensive myocardial scar formation would be a candidate for medical therapy or, in selected cases, heart transplantation.

Identification of exogenous myocardial glucose use in hypoperfused ventricular regions accurately identifies viable tissue that will benefit functionally from restoration of myocardial blood flow. As such, positron emission tomography with ^{18}F-2-fluoro-2-deoxyglucose offers a unique means of assessing myocardial viability when routine clinical tests indicate completed infarction. From the comparative studies performed both in our laboratory and at other institutions, it is clear that the extent of residual myocardial viability is seriously underestimated by conventional diagnostic tests in some patients with ischemic heart disease. It is in these individuals that metabolic imaging with positron emission tomography is likely to have the largest clinical impact, reliably identifying viable myocardium when routine tests indicate completed infarction.

In the patient with acute ischemic injury, metabolic imaging with positron emission tomography identifies residual tissue viability in the clinical infarct zone, enabling the clinician to intervene, if deemed appropriate clinically, to restore blood flow to the zone of ischemic injury. Thus, a more conservative approach might be taken in patients with acute myocardial infarction with matching perfusion and glucose metabolic defects on positron emission tomography. In contrast, individuals with large metabolism-perfusion mismatches in the clinical infarct zone might be considered candidates for coronary angiography and perhaps angioplasty of the culprit lesion earlier rather than later in the course of the infarction in an attempt to salvage viable but endangered tissue. As such, perfusion and metabolic imaging can also be used to assess the efficacy of interventions designed to restore blood flow or to reduce oxygen demand in the clinical infarct zone.

In the patient with congestive heart failure and dilated cardiomyopathy of undetermined cause, positron emission tomography with a flow tracer and ^{18}F-2-fluoro-2-deoxyglucose might be considered prior to invasive diagnostic procedures. If a relatively homogeneous perfusion and glucose metabolic pattern is observed, it is more likely that the cause of the left ventricular dysfunction is nonischemic,[191] and consideration might also be given to myocardial biopsy in addition to coronary angiography as a means of establishing the diagnosis. Conversely, if large metabolism-perfusion mismatches are identified to indicate chronic left ventricular ischemia, coronary angiography would appear warranted in most individuals to determine the suitability of coronary revascularization. Conversely, if positron emission tomography identifies only large confluent areas of completed infarction, revascularization would not likely be of clinical benefit, and medical management without coronary angiography might be proposed.

As positron emission tomography emerges into the clinical practice of cardiology, the role that metabolic imaging will assume in the decision-making process for patients with ischemic heart disease will continue to be defined and refined. A better understanding of the basic biochemical processes regulating myocardial energy production in both normal and ischemic tissue provides new and unique information that should ultimately enhance our care of the patient with ischemic heart disease and further reduce cardiac morbidity and mortality.

SUMMARY AND CONCLUSIONS

Observations made in animal experiments and in clinical studies using positron emission tomography and radioactive tracers of perfusion and substrate metabolism have provided new and unique insights into the pathophysiologic effects of acute and chronic ischemia on the human heart. This noninvasive imaging technique has helped increase our understanding of the means by which ischemic human myocardium attempts to compensate for a reduction in oxygen supply and further has provided a practical clinical method for identifying myocardium and patients at risk for future adverse ischemic events. This has decisively and directly contributed to patient care, providing the clinician information that will assist in assessing the risks and benefits of interventions directed at restoring blood flow to dysfunctional myocardial regions.

Many of the early advances in this area were initially based on semiquantitative analyses of normal and abnormal myocardial flow and metabolic function. Use of quantitative analytical techniques for measurement of blood flow rates and substrate use have further enhanced the characterization of the abnormal tissue metabolic processes resulting from myocardial ischemia. Further refinements, together with new insights that are both pathophysiologically and clinically important, are likely to be achieved as new tracers emerge and are applied to the study of human ischemic heart disease. Our challenge is to employ this newly derived knowledge in the most efficient manner to improve the detection of coronary artery disease and to reduce its human morbidity and mortality.

Acknowledgments

The authors wish to thank Diane Martin for preparing the illustrations. Further, they are grateful to Eileen Rosenfeld for her assistance in preparing this manuscript. Without her help this manuscript would not have reached the publisher.

References

1. Taegtmeyer, H.: Energy metabolism of the heart: From basic concepts to clinical applications. Curr. Probl. Cardiol. 19:57, 1994.
2. Braunwald, E., and Kloner, R. A.: The stunned myocardium: Prolonged, postischemic ventricular dysfunction. Circulation 66:1146, 1982.
3. Kloner, R., Przyklenk, K., and Patel, B.: Altered myocardial states: The stunned and hibernating myocardium. Am. J. Med. 86(Suppl. 1A):14, 1989.
4. Rahimtoola, S.: A perspective on the three large multicenter randomized clinical trials of coronary bypass surgery for chronic stable angina. Circulation 72:V-123, 1985.
5. Braunwald, E., and Rutherford, J. D.: Reversible ischemic left ventricular dysfunction: Evidence for "hibernating myocardium." J. Am. Coll. Cardiol. 8:1467, 1986.
6. Rahimtoola, S. H.: The hibernating myocardium. Am. Heart J. 117:211, 1989.
7. Bax, J., Visser, F., van Lingen, A. et al.: Feasibility of assessing regional myocardial uptake of ^{18}F-fluorodeoxyglucose using single photon emission computed tomography. Eur. Heart J. 14:1675, 1993.
8. Burt, R., Perkins, O., Oppenheim, B., et al.: Direct comparison of fluorine-18-FDG SPECT, fluorine-18-FDG PET and rest thallium-201 SPECT for detection of myocardial viability. J. Nucl. Med. 36:176, 1995.
9. Reimer, K., and Jennings, R.: Myocardial ischemia, hypoxia, and infarction: Cellular consequences of severe myocardial ischemia. *In* Fozzard, H., Haber, E., Jennings, R. (eds): The Heart and Cardiovascular System. Scientific Foundations. New York, Raven Press, 1992, pp. 1875–1973.
10. Arai, A., Grauer, S., Anselone, C., et al.: Metabolic adaptation to a gradual reduction in myocardial blood flow. Circulation 92:244, 1995.
11. Opie, L.: Fuels: Carbohydrates and lipids. *In* The Heart. Physiology and Metabolism, 2nd ed. New York, Raven Press, 1991, pp. 208–246.
12. Liedtke, A. J.: Alterations of carbohydrate and lipid metabolism in the acutely ischemic heart. Progr. Cardiovasc. Dis. 23:321, 1981.
13. Opie, L. H., Owen, P., and Riemersma, R. A.: Relative rates of oxidation of glucose and free fatty acids by ischemic and non-ischemic myocardium after coronary artery ligation in the dog. Eur. J. Clin. Invest. 3:419, 1973.
14. Heyndrickx, G., Wijns, W., Vogelaers, D., et al.: Recovery of regional contractile function and oxidative metabolism in stunned myocardium induced by 1-hour circumflex coronary artery stenosis in chronically instrumented dogs. Circ. Res. 72:901, 1993.
15. Neely, J., Whitmer, J., and Rovetto M.: Effect of coronary blood flow on glycolytic flux and intracellular pH in isolated rat hearts. Circ. Res. 37:733, 1975.
16. Most, A., Gorlin, R., and Soeldner J.: Glucose extraction by the human myocardium during pacing stress. Circulation 45:92, 1972.
17. Thomassen, A., Nielsen, T., Bagger, J., and Henningsen P.: Antianginal and cardiac metabolic effects of low-dose glucose infusion during pacing in patients with and without coronary artery disease. Am. Heart J. 118:25, 1989.
18. Lerch, R. A., Ambos, H. D., Bergmann, S. R., et al.: Localization of viable, ischemic myocardium by positron-emission tomography with ^{11}C-palmitate. Circulation 64:689, 1981.
19. Schön, H. R., Schelbert, H. R., Najafi, A., et al.: C-11 labeled palmitic acid for the noninvasive evaluation of regional myocardial fatty acid metabolism with positron computed tomography. II. Kinetics of C-11 palmitic acid in acutely ischemic myocardium. Am. Heart J. 103:548, 1982.
20. Schelbert, H. R., Henze, E., Schön, H. R., et al.: C-11 palmitic acid for the noninvasive evaluation of regional myocardial fatty acid metabolism with positron computed tomography. IV. In vivo demonstration of impaired fatty acid oxidation in acute myocardial ischemia. Am. Heart J. 106:736, 1983.
21. Rosamond, T. L., Abendschein, D. R., Sobel, B. E., et al.: Metabolic fate of radiolabeled palmitate in ischemic canine myocardium: Implications for positron emission tomography. J. Nucl. Med. 28:1322, 1987.
22. Schwaiger, M., Fishbein, M., Block, M., et al.: Metabolic and ultrastructural abnormalities during ischemia in canine myocardium: Noninvasive assessment by positron emission tomography. J. Mol. Cell. Cardiol. 19:259, 1987.
23. Fox, K. A. A., Abendschein, D. R., Ambos, H. D., et al.: Efflux of metabolized and nonmetabolized fatty acid from canine myocardium. Implications for quantifying myocardial metabolism tomographically. Circ. Res. 57:232, 1985.
24. Grover-McKay, M., Schelbert, H. R., Schwaiger, M., et al.: Identification of impaired metabolic reserve by atrial pacing in patients with significant coronary artery stenosis. Circulation 74:281, 1986.
25. Schön, H. R., Schelbert, H. R., Najafi, A., et al.: C-11 labeled palmitic acid for the noninvasive evaluation of regional myocardial fatty acid metabolism with positron computed tomography. I. Kinetics of C-11 palmitic acid in normal myocardium. Am. Heart J. 103:532, 1982.
26. Brown, M. A., Myears, D. W., and Bergmann S. R.: Noninvasive assessment of canine myocardial oxidative metabolism with ^{11}C-acetate and positron emission tomography. J. Am. Coll. Cardiol. 12:1054, 1988.
27. Buxton, D. B., Nienaber, C. A., Luxen, A., et al.: Noninvasive quantitation of regional myocardial oxygen consumption in vivo with [1-^{11}C] acetate and dynamic positron emission tomography. Circulation 79:134, 1989.
28. Brown, M. A., Myears, D. W., and Bergmann, S. R.: Validity of estimates of myocardial oxidative metabolism with carbon-11 acetate and positron emission tomography despite altered patterns of substrate utilization. J. Nucl. Med. 30:187, 1989.
29. Buxton, D. B., Schwaiger, M., Nguyen, A., et al.: Radiolabeled acetate as a tracer of myocardial tricarboxylic acid cycle flux. Circ. Res. 63:628, 1988.
30. Armbrecht, J. J., Buxton, D. B., and Schelbert, H. R.: Validation of [1-^{11}C] acetate as a tracer for noninvasive assessment of oxidative metabolism with positron emission tomography in normal, ischemic, post-ischemic and hyperemic canine myocardium. Circulation 81:1594, 1991.
31. Selwyn, A. P., Allan, R. M., Pike, V., et al.: Positive labeling of ischemic myocardium: A new approach to patients with coronary disease. Am. J. Cardiol. 47:81, 1981.
32. Allan, R., Pike, V., Maseri, A., et al.: Myocardial metabolism of ^{11}C-acetate: Experimental and patient studies. Circulation 64:IV-75, 1981.
33. Schelbert, H. R., Phelps, M. E., Selin, C., et al.: Regional Myocardial Ischemia Assessed by ^{18}Fluoro-2-Deoxyglucose and Positron Emission Computed Tomography. New York, H. W. Heiss, I, Gehard Witzstrock, 1980, pp. 437–447.
34. Camici, P., Araujo, L. I., Spinks, T., et al.: Increased uptake of ^{18}F-fluorodeoxyglucose in postischemic myocardium of patients with exercise-induced angina. Circulation 74:81, 1986.
35. Yonekura, Y., Tamaki, N., Kambara, H., et al.: Detection of metabolic alterations in ischemic myocardium by F-18 fluorodeoxyglucose uptake with positron emission tomography. Am. J. Cardiac Imaging 2:122, 1988.
36. Shen, Y., and Vatner, S.: Mechanism of impaired myocardial function during progressive coronary stenosis in conscious pigs. Hibernation versus stunning? Circ. Res. 76:479, 1995.
37. Fudo, T., Kambara, H., Hashimoto, T., et al.: F-18 deoxyglucose and stress N-13 ammonia positron emission tomography in anterior wall healed myocardial infarction. Am. J. Cardiol. 61:1191, 1988.
38. Araujo, L. I., Camici, P., Spinks, T., et al.: Abnormalities in myocardial metabolism in patients with unstable angina as assessed by positron emission tomography. Cardiovas. Drugs Ther. 2:41, 1988.
39. Patlak, C. S., Blasberg, R. G., and Fenstermacher J. D.: Graphical evaluation of blood-to-brain transfer constants from multiple-time uptake data. J. Cereb. Blood Flow Metab. 3:1, 1983.
40. Reimer, K. A., Lowe, J. E., Rasmussen, M. M., et al.: The wavefront phenomenon of ischemic cell death. I. Myocardial infarct size vs duration of coronary occlusion in dogs. Circulation 56:786, 1977.
41. Reimer, K., and Jennings R.: The "wavefront phenomenon" of myocardial ischemic cell death. II. Transmural progression of necrosis within the framework of ischemic bed size (myocardium at risk) and collateral flow. Lab. Invest. 40:633, 1979.
42. Jeremy, R., Hackworthy, R., Bautovich, G., et al.: Infarct artery perfusion and changes in left ventricular volume in the month after myocardial infarction. J. Am. Coll. Cardiol. 9:989, 1987.
43. DeWood, M., Spores, J., Notske, R., et al.: Prevalence of total coronary occlusion

during the early hours of transmural myocardial infarction. N. Engl. J. Med. 303:897, 1980.
44. Rentrop, K.: Restoration of anterograde flow in acute myocardial infarction: The first 15 years. J. Am. Coll. Cardiol. 25:1S, 1995.
45. Weaver, W.: Time to thrombolytic treatment: Factors affecting delay and their influence on outcome. J. Am. Coll. Cardiol. 25:3S, 1995.
46. Ridker, P., Marder, V., and Hennekens, C.: Large scale trials of thrombolytic therapy for acute myocardial infarction GISSI-2, ISIS-3, and GUSTO-1. Ann. Intern. Med. 120:876, 1994.
47. Grines, C., Browne, K., Marco, J., et al.: A comparison of immediate angioplasty with thrombolytic therapy for acute myocardial infarction. N. Engl. J. Med. 328:673, 1993.
48. Bergmann, S. R., Lerch, R. A., Fox, K. A. A., et al.: Temporal dependence of beneficial effects of coronary thrombolysis characterized by positron emission tomography. Am. J. Med. 73:573, 1982.
49. Knabb, R. M., Bergmann, S. R., Fox, K. A. A., et al.: The temporal pattern of recovery of myocardial perfusion and metabolism delineated by positron emission tomography after coronary thrombolysis. J. Nucl. Med. 28:1563, 1987.
50. Schwaiger, M., Schelbert, H. R., Ellison, D., et al.: Sustained regional abnormalities in cardiac metabolism after transient ischemia in the chronic dog model. J. Am. Coll. Cardiol. 6:336, 1985.
51. Schwaiger, M., Schelbert, H. R., Keen, R., et al.: Retention and clearance of C-11 palmitic acid in ischemic and reperfused canine myocardium. J. Am. Coll. Cardiol. 6:311, 1985.
52. Buxton, D., Schwaiger, M., Vaghaiwalla Mody, F., et al.: Regional abnormality of oxygen consumption in reperfused myocardium assessed with [1-^{11}C] acetate and positron emission tomography. Am. J. Cardiol. Imaging 3:276, 1989.
53. Hashimoto, T., Buxton, D., Krivokapich, J., et al.: Responses of blood flow, oxygen consumption, and contractile function to inotropic stimulation in stunned canine myocardium. Am. Heart J. 127:1250, 1994.
54. Schwaiger, M., Neese, R. A., Araujo, L., et al.: Sustained nonoxidative glucose utilization and depletion of glycogen in reperfused canine myocardium. J. Am. Coll. Cardiol. 13:745, 1989.
55. Buxton, D., and Schelbert, H.: Measurement of regional glucose metabolic rates in reperfused myocardium. Am. J. Physiol. 261:H2058, 1991.
56. Sochor, H., Schwaiger, M., Schelbert, H. R., et al.: Relationship between Tl-201, Tc-99m (Sn) pyrophosphate and F-18 2-deoxyglucose uptake in ischemically injured dog myocardium. Am. Heart J. 114:1066, 1987.
57. Melin, J. A., Wijns, W., Keyeux, A., et al.: Assessment of thallium-201 redistribution versus glucose uptake as predictors of viability after coronary occlusion and reperfusion. Circulation 77:927, 1988.
58. Marshall, R. C., Tillisch, J. H., Phelps, M. E., et al.: Identification and differentiation of resting myocardial ischemia and infarction in man with positron computed tomography ^{18}F-labeled fluorodeoxyglucose and N-13 ammonia. Circulation 67:766, 1983.
59. Schwaiger, M., Brunken, R., Grover-McKay, M., et al.: Regional myocardial metabolism in patients with acute myocardial infarction assessed by positron emission tomography. J. Am. Coll. Cardiol. 8:800, 1986.
60. Brunken, R., Schwaiger, M., and Schelbert, H.: PET detection of residual, viable tissue in acute MI. Appl. Radiol. 14:82, 1985.
61. Billadello, J., Smith, J., Ludbrook, P., et al.: Implications of "reciprocal" ST segment depression associated with acute myocardial infarction identified by positron tomography. J. Am. Coll. Cardiol. 2:616, 1983.
62. Schwaiger, M., Brunken, R., Krivokapich, J., et al.: Beneficial effect of residual antegrade flow on tissue viability as assessed by positron emission tomography in patients with myocardial infarction. Eur. Heart J. 8:981, 1987.
63. Bulkley, B., Silverman, K., Weisfeldt, M., et al.: Pathologic basis of thallium-201 scintigraphic defects in patients with fatal myocardial injury. Circulation 60:785, 1979.
64. Freifeld, A., Schuster, E., and Bulkley, B.: Nontransmural versus transmural myocardial infarction. A morphologic study. Am. J. Med. 75:423, 1983.
65. Raunio, H., Rissanen, V., Romppanen, T., et al.: Changes in the QRS complex and ST segment in transmural and subendocardial myocardial infarctions. A clinicopathologic study. Am. Heart J. 98:176, 1979.
66. Savage, R., Wagner, G., Ideker, R., et al.: Correlation of postmortem anatomic findings with electrocardiographic changes in patients with myocardial infarction. Retrospective study of patients with typical anterior and posterior infarcts. Circulation 55:279, 1977.
67. Sullivan, W., Vlodaver, Z., Tuna, N., et al.: Correlation of electrocardiographic and pathologic findings in healed myocardial infarction. Am. J. Cardiol. 43:724, 1978.
68. Brunken, R., Schelbert, H.: Acute myocardial infarction: A case for metabolic imaging. The Leading Edge: Cardiology 3:1, 1989.
69. Henes, C., Bergmann, S., Perez, J., et al.: The time course of restoration of nutritive perfusion, myocardial oxygen consumption, and regional function after coronary thrombolysis. Coronary Artery Disease 1:687, 1990.
70. Vanoverschelde, J.-L. J., Melin, J., Bol, A., et al.: Regional oxidative metabolism in patients after recovery from reperfused anterior myocardial infarction. Circulation 85:9, 1992.
71. Gropler, R., Siegel, B., Sampathkumaran, K., et al.: Dependence of recovery of contractile function on maintenance of oxidative metabolism after myocardial infarction. J. Am. Coll. Cardiol. 19:989, 1992.
72. Kalff, V., Hicks, R., Hutchins, G., et al.: Use of carbon-11 acetate and dynamic positron emission tomography to assess regional myocardial oxygen consumption in patients with acute myocardial infarction receiving thrombolysis or coronary angioplasty. Am. J. Cardiol. 71:529, 1993.
73. Chan, S., Brunken, R., Phelps, M., et al.: Use of the metabolic tracer C-11 acetate for evaluation of regional myocardial perfusion. J. Nucl. Med. 32:665, 1991.
74. Gropler, R., Siegel, B., and Geltman, E.: Myocardial uptake of carbon-11 acetate as an indirect measure of regional myocardial blood flow. J. Nucl. Med. 32:245, 1991.
75. Czernin, J., Porenta, G., Brunken, R., et al.: Regional blood flow, oxidative metabolism, and glucose utilization in patients with recent myocardial infarction. Circulation 88:884, 1993.
76. Feigl, E., Neat, G., and Huang, A.: Interrelations between coronary artery pressure, myocardial metabolism and coronary blood flow. J. Mol. Cell. Cardiol. 22:375, 1990.
77. Tillisch, J., Brunken, R., Marshall, R., et al.: Reversibility of cardiac wall motion abnormalities predicted by positron tomography. N. Engl. J. Med. 314:884, 1986.
78. Righetti, A., Crawford, M., O'Rourke, R., et al.: Interventricular septal motion and left ventricular function following coronary artery bypass surgery. Evaluation with echocardiography and radionuclide angiography. Am. J. Cardiol. 39:372, 1977.
79. Tamaki, N., Yonekura, Y., Yamashita, K., et al.: Positron emission tomography using fluorine-18 deoxyglucose in evaluation of coronary artery bypass grafting. Am. J. Cardiol. 64:860, 1989.
80. Tamaki, N., Ohtani, H., Yamashita, K., et al.: Metabolic activity in the areas of new fill-in after thallium-201 reinjection: Comparison with positron emission tomography using fluorine-18-deoxyglucose. J. Nucl. Med. 32:673, 1991.
81. Marwick, T., MacIntyre, W., Lafont, A., et al.: Metabolic responses of hibernating and infarcted myocardium to revascularization: A follow-up study of regional perfusion, function, and metabolism. Circulation 85:1347, 1992.
82. Lucignani, G., Paolini, G., Landoni, C., et al.: Presurgical identification of hibernating myocardium by combined use of technetium-99m hexakis 2-methoxyisobutylisonitrile single photon emission tomography and fluorine-18 fluoro-2-deoxy-D-glucose positron emission tomography in patients with coronary artery disease. Eur. J. Nucl. Med. 19:874, 1992.
83. Carrel, T., Jenni, R., Haubold-Reuter, S., et al.: Improvement of severely reduced left ventricular function after surgical revascularization in patients with preoperative myocardial infarction. Eur. J. Cardiothorac. Surg. 6:479, 1992.
84. Gropler, R., Geltman, E., Sampathkumaran, K., et al.: Functional recovery after coronary revascularization for chronic coronary artery disease is dependent on maintenance of oxidative metabolism. J. Am. Coll. Cardiol. 20:569, 1992.
85. Gropler, R. J., Geltman, E. M., Sampathkumaran, K., et al.: Comparison of carbon-11-acetate with fluorine-18-fluorodeoxyglucose for delineating viable myocardium by positron emission tomography. J. Am. Coll. Cardiol. 22:1587, 1993.
86. Knuuti, M., Saraste, M., Nuutila, P., et al.: Myocardial viability: Fluorine-18-deoxyglucose positron emission tomography in prediction of wall motion recovery after revascularization. Am. Heart J. 127:785, 1994.
87. vom Dahl, J., Eitzman, D., Al-Aouar, A., et al.: Relation of regional function, perfusion, and metabolism in patients with advanced coronary artery disease undergoing surgical revascularization. Circulation 90:2356, 1994.
88. Tamaki, N., Kawamoto, M., Tadamura, E., et al.: Prediction of reversible ischemia after revascularization: Perfusion and metabolic studies using positron emission tomography. Circulation 91:1697, 1995.
89. Vanoverschelde, J.-L., Wijns, W., Depre, C., et al.: Mechanisms of chronic regional postischemic dysfunction in humans: New insights from the study of noninfarcted collateral-dependent myocardium. Circulation 87:1513, 1993.
90. Maes, A., Flameng, W., Nuyts, J., et al.: Histological alterations in chronically hypoperfused myocardium: Correlation with PET findings. Circulation 90:735, 1994.
91. Depré, C., Vanoverschelde, J.-L.J., Melin, J., et al.: Structural and metabolic correlates of the reversibility of chronic left ventricular ischemic dysfunction in humans. Am. J. Physiol. 268:H1265, 1995.
92. Berry, J. J., Hoffman, J. M., Steenbergen, C., et al.: Human pathologic correlation with PET in ischemic and nonischemic cardiomyopathy. J. Nucl. Med. 34:39, 1993.
93. Delbeke, D., Lorenz, C. H., Votaw, J. R., et al.: Estimation of left ventricular mass and infarct size from nitrogen-13-ammonia PET images based on pathological examination of explanted human hearts. J. Nucl. Med. 34:826, 1993.
94. Flameng, W., Suy, R., Schwarz, F., et al.: Ultrastructural correlates of left ventricular contraction abnormalities in patients with chronic ischemic heart disease: Determinants of reversible segmental asynergy post-revascularization surgery. Am. Heart J. 102:846, 1981.
95. Weiss, J., and Hiltbrand, B.: Functional compartmentation of glycolytic vs. oxidative metabolism in isolated rabbit heart. J. Clin. Invest. 75:436, 1985.
96. Sun, D., Jguyen, N., DeGrado, T., et al.: Ischemia induces translocation of the insulin-responsive glucose transporter GLUT4 to the plasma membrane of cardiac myocytes. Circulation 89:793, 1994.
97. Chan, A., Czernin, J., Brunken, R., et al.: Effects of dietary state on the incidence of myocardial blood flow-metabolism mismatches in patients with chronic coronary artery disease. Circulation (in press).
98. Nienaber, C., Brunken, R., Sherman, C., et al.: Metabolic and functional recovery of ischemic human myocardium after coronary angioplasty. J. Am. Coll. Cardiol. 18:966, 1991.
99. Czernin, J., Porenta, G., Rosenquist, G., et al.: Loss of coronary perfusion reserve in PET ischemia. Circulation 84:II-47, 1991.
100. Sun, K., Czernin, J., Krivokapich, J., et al.: Effects of dobutamine stimulation on myocardial blood flow, glucose metabolism and wall motion in PET mismatch regions. J. Am. Coll. Cardiol. 23:117A, 1994.
101. Marwick, T., Nemec, J., Lafont, A., et al.: Prediction by postexercise fluoro-18

deoxyglucose positron emission tomography of improvement in exercise capacity after revascularization. Am. J. Cardiol. 69:854, 1992.
102. Di Carli, M., Asgarzadie, F., Schelbert, H., et al.: Quantitative relation between myocardial viability and improvement in heart failure symptoms after revascularization in patients with ischemic cardiomyopathy. Circulation (in press).
103. Goldman, L., Hashimoto, B., Cook, E. F., and Loscalzo, A.: Comparative reproducibility and validity of systems for assessing cardiovascular functional class: Advantages of a new Specific Activity Scale. Circulation 674:1227, 1981.
104. Porenta, G., Kuhle, W., Czernin, J., et al.: Semiquantitative assessment of myocardial viability and perfusion utilizing polar map displays of cardiac PET images. J. Nucl. Med. 33:1623, 1992.
105. Sun, K., De Groof, M., Yi, J., et al.: Quantification of the extent and severity of perfusion defects in canine myocardium by PET polar mapping. J. Nucl. Med. 35:2031, 1994.
106. Fedele, F. A., Gewortz, J., Capone, R. J., et al.: Metabolic response to prolonged reduction of myocardial blood flow distal to a severe coronary artery stenosis. Circulation 78:729, 1988.
107. Luu, M., Stevenson, L., Brunken, R., et al.: Delayed recovery of revascularized myocardium after referral for cardiac transplantation. Am. Heart J. 119:668, 1990.
108. Chung, E.: Myocardial Ischemia, Injury and Infarction. Baltimore, University Park Press, 1984, p. 83.
109. Durer, D., Van Lier, A., and Buller, J.: Epicardial and intramural excitation in chronic myocardial infarction. Am. Heart J. 68:765, 1964.
110. Conde, C. A., Meller, J., Espinoza, J., et al.: Disappearance of abnormal Q waves after aortocoronary bypass surgery. Am. J. Cardiol. 36:889, 1975.
111. Zeft, H. J., Friedberg, H. D., King, J. F., et al.: Reappearance of anterior QRS forces after coronary bypass surgery: An electrovectorcardiographic study. Am. J. Cardiol. 36:163, 1975.
112. Brunken, R., Tillisch, J., Schwaiger, M., et al.: Regional perfusion, glucose metabolism and wall motion in chronic electrocardiographic Q-wave infarctions. Evidence for persistence of viable tissue in some infarct regions by positron emission tomography. Circulation 73:951, 1986.
113. Horan, L., Flowers, N., and Johnson J.: Significance of the diagnostic Q wave of myocardial infarction. Circulation 43:428, 1971.
114. Hashimoto, T., Kambara, H., Fudo, T., et al.: Non-Q wave versus Q wave myocardial infarction: Regional myocardial metabolism and blood flow assessed by positron emission tomography. J. Am. Coll. Cardiol. 12:88, 1988.
115. Nakanishi, T., Takao, A., Nakazawa, M., et al.: Mucocutaneous lymph node syndrome: Clinical, hemodynamic and angiographic features of coronary obstructive disease. Am. J. Cardiol. 55:662, 1985.
116. Kato, H., Ichinose, E., and Kawasaki, T.: Myocardial infarction in Kawasaki disease: Clinical analyses in 195 cases. J. Pediatr. 108:923, 1986.
117. Yoshibayashi, M., Tamaki, N., Nishioka, K., et al.: Regional myocardial perfusion and metabolism assessed by positron emission tomography in children with Kawasaki disease and significance of abnormal Q waves and their disappearance. Am. J. Cardiol. 68:1638, 1991.
118. Bruce, R., Fisner, L., Pettinger, M., et al.: ST segment elevation with exercise: A marker for poor ventricular function and poor prognosis. Coronary Artery Surgery Study (CASS) confirmation of Seattle Heart Watch results. Circulation 77:897, 1988.
119. Chaitman B.: A Textbook of Cardiovascular Medicine. Philadelphia, W.B. Saunders, 1992, pp. 161–179.
120. Margonato, A., Chierchia, S., Xuereb, R., et al.: Specificity and sensitivity of exercise-induced ST segment elevation for detection of residual viability: Comparison with fluorodeoxyglucose and positron emission tomography. J. Am. Coll. Cardiol. 25:1032, 1995.
121. Cabin, H. S., Soni Clubbs, K., Vita, N., et al.: Regional dysfunction by equilibrium radionuclide angiography: A clinicopathologic study evaluating the relation of degree of dysfunction to the presence and extent of myocardial infarction. J. Am. Coll. Cardiol. 10:743, 1987.
122. Perone-Filardi, P., Bacharach, S., Dilsizian, V., et al.: Metabolic evidence of viable myocardium in regions with reduced wall thickness and absent wall thickening in patients with chronic ischemic left ventricular dysfunction. J. Am. Coll. Cardiol. 20:161, 1992.
123. Idecker, R., Behar, V., Wagner, G., et al.: Evaluation of asynergy as an indicator of myocardial fibrosis. Circulation 57:715, 1978.
124. Stinson, E., and Billingham, M.: Correlative study of regional left ventricular histology and contractile function. Am. J. Cardiol. 39:378, 1977.
125. Brundage, B. H., Massie, B. M., and Botvinick, E. H.: Improved regional ventricular function after successful surgical revascularization. J. Am. Coll. Cardiol. 3:902, 1984.
126. Chatterjee, K., Swan, H., and Parmley W., et al.: Influence of direct revascularization on left ventricular asynergy and function in patients with coronary heart disease. Circulation 47:276, 1973.
127. Shearn, D., and Brent, B.: Coronary artery bypass surgery in patients with left ventricular dysfunction. Am. J. Med. 80:405, 1986.
128. Cohen, M., Charney, R., Hershman, R., et al.: Reversal of chronic ischemic myocardial dysfunction after transluminal angioplasty. J. Am. Coll. Cardiol. 12:1193, 1988.
129. Melchior, J., Doriot, P., Meier, B., et al.: Improvement of left ventricular contraction and relaxation synchronism after recanalization of chronic total coronary occlusion by angioplasty. J. Am. Coll. Cardiol. 9:763, 1987.
130. Dilsizian, V., and Bonow, R. O.: Current diagnostic techniques of assessing myocardial viability in patients with hibernating and stunned myocardium. Circulation 87:1, 1993.
131. Rozanski, A., Berman, D., Gray, R., et al.: Use of thallium-201 redistribution scintigraphy in the preoperative differentiation of reversible and nonreversible myocardial asynergy. Circulation 64:936, 1981.
132. Liu, P., Kiess, M. C., Okada, R. D., et al.: The persistent defect on exercise thallium imaging and its fate after myocardial revascularization: Does it represent scar or ischemia? Am. Heart J. 110:996, 1985.
133. Gibson, R. S., Watson, D. D., Taylor, G. J., et al.: Prospective assessment of regional myocardial perfusion before and after coronary revascularization surgery by quantitative thallium-201 scintigraphy. J. Am. Coll. Cardiol. 1:804, 1983.
134. Brunken, R., Schwaiger, M., Grover-McKay, M., et al.: Positron emission tomography detects tissue metabolic activity in myocardial segments with persistent thallium perfusion defects. J. Am. Coll. Cardiol. 10:557, 1987.
135. Tamaki, N., Yonekura, Y., Yamashita, K., et al.: Relation to left ventricular perfusion and wall motion with metabolic activity in persistent defects on thallium-201 tomography in healed myocardial infarction. Am. J. Cardiol. 62:202, 1988.
136. Brunken, R. C., Kottou, S., Nienaber, C. A., et al.: PET detection of viable tissue in myocardial segments with persistent defects at Tl-201 SPECT. Radiology 172:65, 1989.
137. Gutman, J., Berman, D., Freeman, M., et al.: Time to completed redistribution of thallium-201 in exercise myocardial scintigraphy: Relation to the degree of coronary artery stenosis. Am. Heart J. 106:989, 1983.
138. Cloninger, K., DePuey, G., Garcia, E., et al.: Incomplete redistribution in delay thallium-201 single photon emission computed (SPECT) images. An overestimation of myocardial scarring. J. Am. Coll. Cardiol. 12:955, 1988.
139. Kiat, H., Berman, D. S., Maddahi, J., et al.: Late reversibility of tomographic myocardial thallium-201 defects: An accurate marker of myocardial viability. J. Am. Coll. Cardiol. 12:1456, 1988.
140. Yang, L., Berman, D., Kiat, H., et al.: The frequency of late reversibility in SPECT thallium-201 stress-redistribution studies. J. Am. Coll. Cardiol. 15:334, 1989.
141. Brunken, R., Mody, F., Hawkins, R., et al.: Positron emission tomography detects metabolic viability in myocardium with persistent 24-hour single-photon emission computed tomography ^{201}Tl defects. Circulation 86:1357, 1992.
142. Brunken, R., Mody, F., Hawkins, R., et al.: Persistent twenty-four thallium-201 concentrations and PET metabolic viability. Herz 19:28, 1994.
143. Dilsizian, V., Rocco, T., Freedman, N., et al.: Enhanced detection of ischemic but viable myocardium by the reinjection of thallium after stress-redistribution imaging. N. Engl. J. Med. 323:141, 1990.
144. Ohtani, H., Tamaki, N., Yonekura, Y., et al.: Value of thallium-201 reinjection after delayed SPECT imaging for predicting reversible ischemia after coronary artery bypass grafting. Am. J. Cardiol. 66:394, 1990.
145. Bonow, R., Dilsizian, V., Cuocolo, A., et al.: Identification of viable myocardium in patients with chronic coronary artery disease and left ventricular dysfunction: Comparison of thallium scintigraphy with reinjection and PET imaging with F-18-fluorodeoxyglucose. Circulation 83:26, 1991.
146. Perrone-Filardi, P., Bacharach, S. L., Dilsizian, V., et al.: Regional left ventricular wall thickening. Relation to regional uptake of ^{18}fluorodeoxyglucose and ^{201}Tl in patients with chronic coronary artery disease and left ventricular dysfunction. Circulation 86:1125, 1992.
147. Hecht, H., Hopkins, J., Rose, J., et al.: Reverse redistribution: Worsening of thallium-201 myocardial images from exercise to redistribution. Radiology 140:177, 1981.
148. Weiss, A., Maddahi, J., Lew, A., et al.: Reverse redistribution of thallium-201: A sign of nontransmural myocardial infarction with patency of the infarct-related coronary artery. J. Am. Coll. Cardiol. 7:61, 1986.
149. Leppo, J.: Thallium washout analysis: Fact or fiction? J. Nucl. Med. 28:1058, 1987.
150. Silberstein, E., and DeVries, D.: Reverse redistribution phenomenon in thallium-201 stress tests: Angiographic correlation and clinical significance. J. Nucl. Med. 26:707, 1985.
151. Popoma, J., Smitherman, T., Walker, B., et al.: Reverse redistribution of thallium-201 detected by SPECT imaging after dipyridamole in angina pectoris. Am. J. Cardiol. 55:1176, 1990.
152. Marin-Neto, J., Dilsizian, V., Arrighi, J., et al.: Thallium reinjection demonstrates viable myocardium in regions with reverse redistribution. Circulation 88:1736, 1993.
153. Brown, K., Benoit, L., Clements, J., et al.: Fast washout of thallium-201 from area of myocardial infarction: Possible artifact of background subtraction. J. Nucl. Med. 28:945, 1987.
154. Ohte, N., Hashimoto, T., Banno, T., et al.: Clinical significance of reserve redistribution on 24 hour delayed imaging of exercise thallium-201 myocardial SPECT: Comparison with myocardial fluorine-18-FDG-PET imaging and left ventricular wall motion. J. Nucl. Med. 36:86, 1995.
155. Soufer, R., Dey, H., Lawson, A., et al.: Relationship between reverse redistribution planar thallium scintigraphy and regional myocardial viability: A correlative PET study. J. Nucl. Med. 36:180, 1995.
156. Mori, T., Minamiji, K., Kurogane, H., et al.: Rest-injected thallium-201 imaging for assessing viability of severe asynergic regions. J. Nucl. Med. 32:1718, 1991.
157. Zimmermann, R., Mall, G., Rauch, B., et al.: Residual ^{201}Tl activity in irreversible defects as a marker of myocardial viability. Clinicopathological study. Circulation 91:1016, 1995.
158. Dilsizian, V., Freedman, N., Bacharach, S., et al.: Regional thallium uptake in irreversible defects. Magnitude of change in thallium activity after reinjection distinguishes viable from nonviable myocardium. Circulation 85:627, 1992.
159. Dilsizian, V., Arrighi, J., Diodati, J., et al: Myocardial viability in patients with chronic coronary artery disease. Comparison of ^{99m}Tc-sestamibi with thallium reinjection and [^{18}F]fluorodeoxyglucose. Circulation 89:578, 1994.

160. Sawada, S., Allman, K., Muzik, O., et al.: Positron emission tomography detects evidence of viability in rest technetium-99m sestamibi defects. J. Am. Coll. Cardiol. 23:92, 1994.
161. Altehoefer, C., vom Dahl, J., Biedermann, M., et al.: Significance of defect severity in technetium-99m-MIBI SPECT at rest to assess myocardial viability: Comparison with fluorine-18-FDG PET. J. Nucl. Med. 35:569, 1994.
162. Ficaro, E., Fessler, J., Ackermann, R., et al.: Simultaneous transmission-emission thallium-201 cardiac SPECT: Effect of attenuation correction on myocardial tracer distribution. J. Nucl. Med. 36:921, 1995.
163. Parodi, P., Schelbert, H. R., Schwaiger, M., et al.: Cardiac emission computed tomography: Underestimation of regional tracer concentrations due to wall motion abnormalities. J. Comp. Assisted Tomogr. 8:1083, 1984.
164. Go, R., MacIntyre, W., Saha, G., et al.: Hibernating myocardium versus scar: Severity of irreversible decreased myocardial perfusion in prediction of tissue viability. Radiology 194:151, 1995.
165. Takahashi, N., Tamaki, N., Kawamoto, M., et al.: Glucose metabolism in relation to perfusion in patients with ischaemic heart disease. Eur. J. Nucl. Med. 21:292, 1994.
166. Gewirtz, H., Fischman, A., Abraham, S., et al.: Positron emission tomographic measurements of absolute regional myocardial blood flow permits identification of nonviable myocardium in patients with chronic myocardial infarction. J. Am. Coll. Cardiol. 23:851, 1994.
167. Parodi, O., De Maria, R., Oltroa, L., et al.: Myocardial blood flow distribution in patients with ischemic heart disease or dilated cardiomyopathy undergoing heart transplantation. Circulation 88:509, 1993.
168. Yamamoto, Y., De Silva, R., Rhodes, C., et al.: A new strategy for the assessment of viable myocardium and regional myocardial blood flow using ^{15}O-water and dynamic positron emission tomography. Circulation 86:167, 1992.
169. de Silva, R., Yamamoto, Y., Rhodes, C. G., et al.: Preoperative prediction of the outcome of coronary revascularization using positron emission tomography. Circulation 86:1738, 1992.
170. Schulz, R., Guth, B., Pieper, K., et al.: Recruitment of inotropic reserve in moderately ischemic myocardium at the expense of metabolic recovery: A model of short-term hibernation. Circ. Res. 70:1282, 1992.
171. Panza, J., Dilsizian, V., Laurienzo, J., et al.: Relation between thallium uptake and contractile response to dobutamine. Implications regarding myocardial viability in patients with chronic coronary artery disease. Circulation 91:990, 1995.
172. Pierard, L., De Landsheere, C., Berthe, C., et al.: Identification of viable myocardium by echocardiography during dobutamine infusion in patients with myocardial infarction after thrombolytic therapy: Comparison with positron emission tomography. J. Am. Coll. Cardiol. 15:1021, 1990.
173. Baer, F., Voth, E., Deutsch, H., et al.: Assessment of viable myocardium by dobutamine transesophageal echocardiography and comparison with fluorine-18 fluorodeoxyglucose positron emission tomography. J. Am. Coll. Cardiol. 24:343, 1994.
174. Baer, F., Voth, E., Schneider, C., et al.: Comparison of low-dose dobutamine-gradient-echo magnetic resonance imaging and positron emission tomography with [^{18}F]fluorodeoxyglucose in patients with chronic coronary artery disease. A functional and morphological approach to the detection of residual myocardial viability. Circulation 91:1006, 1995.
175. Henrich, M., Vester, E., von der Lohe, E., et al.: The comparison of 2-^{18}F-2-deoxyglucose and 15-(ortho-^{123}I-phenyl)-pentadecanoic acid uptake in persisting defects on thallium-201 tomography in myocardial infarction. J. Nucl. Med. 32:1353, 1991.
176. Fragasso, G., Chierchia, S., Lucignani, G., et al.: Time dependence of residual tissue viability after myocardial infarction assessed by [^{18}F]fluorodeoxyglucose and positron emission tomography. J. Am. Coll. Cardiol. 72:131G, 1993.
177. Tamaki, N., Kawamoto, M., Takahashi, N., et al.: Prognostic value of an increase in fluorine-18 deoxyglucose uptake in patients with myocardial infarction: Comparison with stress thallium imaging. J. Am. Coll. Cardiol. 22:1621, 1993.
178. Yoshida, K., and Gould, K.: Quantitative relation of myocardial infarct size and myocardial viability by positron emission tomography to left ventricular ejection fraction and 3-year mortality with and without revascularization. J. Am. Coll. Cardiol. 22:984, 1993.
179. Gould, L., Yoshida, K., Hess, M., et al.: Myocardial metabolism of fluorodeoxyglucose compared to cell membrane integrity for the potassium analogue rubidium-82 for assessing infarct size in many by PET. J. Nucl. Med. 32:1, 1991.
180. Lee, K., Marwick, T., Cook, S., et al.: Prognosis of patients with left ventricular dysfunction, with and without viable myocardium after myocardial infarction. Circulation 90:2687, 1994.
181. Eitzman, D., Al-Aouar, Z., Kanter, H., et al.: Clinical outcome of patients with advanced coronary artery disease after viability studies with positron emission tomography. J. Am. Coll. Cardiol. 20:559, 1992.
182. Di Carli, M., Davidson, M., Little, R., et al.: Value of metabolic imaging with positron emission tomography for evaluating prognosis in patients with coronary artery disease and left ventricular dysfunction. Am. J. Cardiol. 73:527, 1994.
183. Ohtake, T., Yokoyama, I., Watanabe, T., et al.: Myocardial glucose metabolism in noninsulin-dependent diabetes mellitus patients evaluated by FDG-PET. J. Nucl. Med. 36:456, 1995.
184. Knuuti, M., Nuutila, P., Ruotsalainen, U., et al.: Euglycemic hyperinsulinemic clamp and oral glucose load in stimulating myocardial glucose utilization during positron emission tomography. J. Nucl. Med. 33:1255, 1992.
185. Alderman, E. L., Fisher, L. D., Litwin, P., et al.: Results of coronary artery surgery in patients with poor left ventricular function (CASS). Circulation 68:785, 1983.
186. Kennedy, J., Kaiser, G., Fisher, L., et al.: Clinical and angiographic predictors of operative mortality from the collaborative study in coronary artery surgery (CASS). Circulation 63:793, 1981.
187. Zubiate, P., Kay, J., and Dunne, E.: Myocardial revascularization for patients with an ejection fraction of 0.2 or less—12 years' results. West. J. Med. 140:745, 1984.
188. Bounous, E., Mark, D., Pollock, B., et al.: Surgical survival benefits for coronary disease patients with left ventricular dysfunction. Circulation 78:I-151, 1988.
189. Passamani, E., Davis, K. B., Gillespie, M. J., et al.: A randomized trial of coronary artery bypass surgery. Survival of patients with low ejection fraction. N. Engl. J. Med. 312:1665, 1985.
190. Pigott, J. D., Kouchoukos, N. T., Oberman, A., et al.: Late results of surgical and medical therapy for patients with coronary artery disease and depressed left ventricular function. J. Am. Coll. Cardiol. 5:1036, 1985.
191. Mody, F., Brunken, R., Stevenson, L., et al.: Differentiating cardiomyopathy of coronary artery disease from nonischemic dilated cardiomyopathy utilizing positron emission tomography. J. Am. Coll. Cardiol. 17:373, 1991.

CHAPTER 72 Assessment of Myocardial Perfusion and Metabolism in the Cardiomyopathies

Edward M. Geltman, M.D.

The cardiomyopathies are a diverse group of syndromes characterized by primary or secondary abnormalities of the myocardium. In general, the diagnosis of cardiomyopathy is made after excluding congenital, valvular, and pericardial disease. Some investigators would also exclude patients with ischemic and hypertensive disease, although such patients are sometimes included in separate diagnostic categories, for example, ischemic cardiomyopathy or hypertensive heart disease. The latter approach is employed in the discussion that follows.

The cardiomyopathies may be classified in either functional or etiologic terms. The functional classification separates patients into groups with dilated, restrictive, and hypertrophic physiologies. An etiologic classification is indicated in Table 72–1. The diversity of causes is great, and although the pathologic and physiologic features of many cardiomyopathies have been well described, detailed metabolic studies are often lacking.

BIOCHEMISTRY OF MYOCARDIAL ENERGETICS

The myocardium has the ability to use multiple substrates to meet its metabolic needs (Fig. 72–1). Myocardial metabolism of fatty acids and carbohydrates has been well characterized in both experimental animals and humans, using invasive assessment of substrate and metabolite levels in samples of arterial and coronary sinus blood, as well as by direct analysis of tissue. A more detailed discussion is included in Chapters 4 and 54. A few critical aspects of fatty acid and carbohydrate metabolism are discussed here. Under most physiologic conditions, the myocardium uses free fatty acids preferentially.[1] After transport across the sarcolemma by transport proteins (a reversible process, allowing back diffusion),[2] free fatty acids are activated to acetylcoenzyme A (acetyl-CoA) compounds and shuttled into the mitochondria for β-oxidation or are incorporated into triglycerides or phospholipids. Retention of free fatty acid is decreased in myocardium during oxygen supply-demand imbalance resulting from epicardial coronary disease, microvascular disease, poor substrate diffusion (due to deposition in the interstitium of collagen, amyloid, mucopolysaccharide, or other substances), or to increased metabolic demand induced by increased wall stress caused by ventricular dilatation and increased preload and afterload.[3–5]

The mitochondrial membrane is not freely permeable to high-energy intermediates. Therefore, the carnitine shuttle mechanism is employed to transport free fatty acids into the mitochondria for β-oxidation.[6, 7] Some of the cardiac metabolic effects of several diseases (including diabetes) may be mediated through alterations in levels of acyl carnitine and cytosolic free carnitine.[8] In contrast, in ischemia, glycolysis leads to lactate production with decreased availability of pyruvate and decreased citric acid cycle flux. Subsequent decreases in free acetyl-CoA and decreased activity of thiokinase (due to increased lactate levels) lead to further decreases in citric acid cycle flux and decreased intracellular trapping of free fatty acids. Increased glycolytic flux increases cytosolic levels of α-glyceryl phosphate, facilitating the storage of free fatty acids.[4] Although these abnormalities have been generally described in animal models of global or regional ischemia, they may well apply to many patients with dilated and hypertrophic cardiomyopathy. Patients with these syndromes may present with relative ischemia, either globally or of the subendocardium, caused by poor myocardial perfusion secondary to increased wall stress, compressive forces, interstitial fibrosis, or microvascular disease.[9–14] Similarly, they may experience increased metabolic demands resulting from increased circulating catecholamines and increased wall stress (both systolic and diastolic) owing to altered geometry and increased systemic vascular resistance secondary to neurohormonal activation.[11, 15, 16]

TABLE 72–1. SELECTED CAUSES OF CARDIOMYOPATHY

Inflammatory Causes	**Fibroplastic Causes**
Infective	Endomyocardial fibrosis
Viral	Endocardial fibroelastosis
Rickettsial	Loffler fibroplastic endocarditis
Bacterial	Becker disease
Mycobacterial	Carcinoid
Spirochetal	
Fungal	**Hematologic Causes**
Parasitic	Sickle cell anemia
Noninfective	Polycythemia vera
Collagen diseases	Leukemia
Granulomatosis	
Cardiac transplant rejection	**Hypersensitivity**
	Methyldopa
	Penicillin
Metabolic Causes	Sulfonamides
Nutritional	Tetracycline
Thiamine deficiency	Giant cell myocarditis
Kwashiorkor	
Pellagra	**Genetic Causes**
Endocrine	Hypertrophic cardiomyopathy
Acromegaly	With gradient
Thyrotoxicosis	Without gradient
Myxedema	Neuromuscular
Cushing disease	Duchenne muscular dystrophy
Pheochromocytoma	Fascioscapulohumeral muscular dystrophy
Diabetes mellitus	
Altered metabolism	Limb-girdle dystrophy of Erb
Gout	Myotonia dystrophica
Oxalosis	Friedreich ataxia
Porphyria	Metabolic
Electrolyte imbalance	Short-chain acyl-CoA dehydrogenase deficiency
Toxic Causes	Medium-chain acyl-CoA dehydrogenase deficiency
Alcohol	
Bleomycin	Long-chain acyl-CoA dehydrogenase deficiency
Doxorubicin	
Lead	
Cyclophosphamide	**Miscellaneous Acquired Causes**
Corticosteroids	Postpartum cardiomyopathy
Cocaine	Obesity
Infiltrative Causes	**Idiopathic Causes**
Amyloidosis	Idiopathic dilated cardiomyopathy
Hemochromatosis	Idiopathic restrictive cardiomyopathy
Neoplastic	Idiopathic hypertrophic cardiomyopathy
Glycogen storage disorders	
Sarcoidosis	**Physical Agents**
Mucopolysaccharidosis	Heat stroke
Gaucher disease	Hypothermia
Sphingolipidoses	Radiation

Adapted from Wynne, J., and Braunwald, E.: The cardiomyopathies and myocarditides. *In* Braunwald, E. (ed.): Heart Disease. A Textbook of Cardiovascular Medicine. 3rd ed. Philadelphia, W.B. Saunders, 1988, p. 1411, with permission.

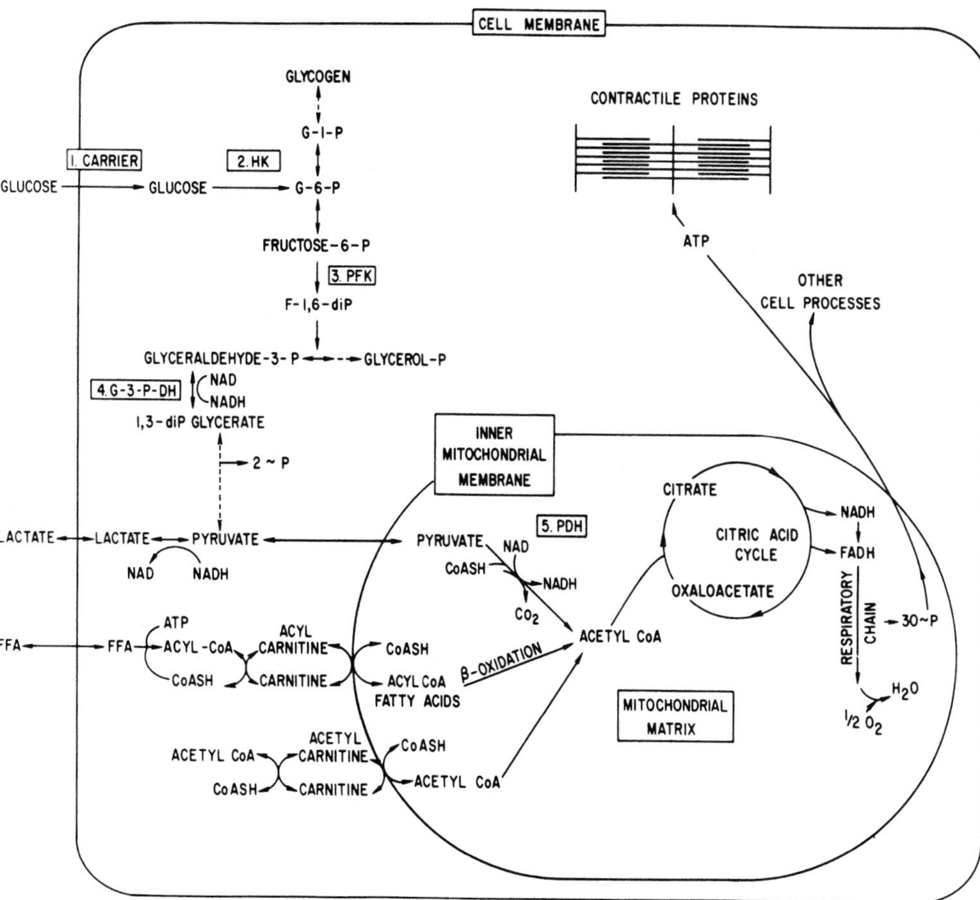

FIGURE 72–1. A schematic representation of the major pathways of metabolism of glucose, lactate, and free fatty acids, including glycolysis, the citric acid cycle, β-oxidation, and mitochondrial processes. (From Braunwald, E., Ross., J., and Sonnenblick, E.H. [eds.]: Mechanisms of Contraction of the Normal and Failing Heart. 2nd ed. Boston, Little, Brown, 1976, p. 190, with permission.)

Uptake of glucose into myocytes is carrier-mediated and not energy-dependent.[1] This process is augmented in the presence of insulin.[17] The degree to which insulin facilitates glucose uptake directly, compared with indirect effects mediated by suppressed circulating free fatty acid levels, is controversial.[1, 4] Whether accomplished directly or indirectly in intact animals and humans, increased levels of plasma glucose lead to augmented myocardial uptake and metabolism of glucose and decreased utilization of free fatty acids. In experimental animals, the rate of glycolysis increases acutely and markedly within 30 seconds after the induction of ischemia.[1] The pyruvate generated by glycolysis is converted to lactate in ischemia, and its accumulation decreases pH, eventually slowing glycolysis if ischemia is profound and prolonged.[1, 4, 18]

Defects in energy metabolism and transduction of metabolic events into myocardial contraction were thought to explain the basis of the mechanical defects observed in chronic congestive heart failure. The metabolic derangements observed in acute ischemia have been well described and delineated in Chapter 4. However, the processes involved in the slowly progressive syndrome of chronic congestive heart failure and the cardiomyopathies are less clearly defined. Although in some patients with symptoms of congestive heart failure, diastolic dysfunction predominates, in most of these patients, cardiac systolic mechanical reserve is diminished and there is a relative or absolute decrease in external cardiac work. In general, in the absence of acute ischemia due to obstructive coronary artery disease, the coronary circulation is exquisitely autoregulated. Even in patients or experimental animals with low-output congestive heart failure, total coronary blood flow and extraction of substrates (carbohydrates and free fatty acids) and oxygen (corrected for cardiac mass) remain within the normal range. There is close tracking among ventricular work, substrate use, and coronary perfusion.[19, 20]

Defects in intermediary metabolism and respiration have been sought extensively in congestive heart failure. Clearly, adenosine triphosphate (ATP) production is limited in acute severe ischemia, but in nonischemic, chronic animal models of congestive heart failure, and also in humans, it is not clear whether there is a primary defect in mitochondrial function. Some investigators have shown defects in mitochondrial energy production in animal models of heart failure and in mitochondria obtained from hearts of patients with heart failure.[21] In some animal models with hereditary cardiomyopathy (Syrian hamsters), severe depression of the ability to oxidize free fatty acids by the mitochondria has been demonstrated.[22] Yet others have found close mitochondrial coupling and respiratory mitochondrial control with essentially normal myocardial mitochondrial function in papillary muscles from cats and humans with heart failure.[23, 24] Since the mitochondrial abnormalities observed in some models of congestive heart failure are observed only late in the process, it seems likely that these abnormalities are not critical to the development of congestive heart failure in the great majority of patients. Recently, several kindreds have been described in which specific defects in fatty acid oxidation have been defined. In affected subjects with short-, medium-, and long-chain acyl coenzyme A (acyl-CoA) dehydrogenase deficiency, dilated cardiomyopathy, congestive heart failure, and sudden death can occur.[25] ATP and creatine phosphate depletion generally has not been found in experimental models of congestive heart failure or in patients, except in models with myocardial ischemia.[24, 26] In contrast, there are abundant data indicating that there are abnormalities in the contractile proteins and myofibrillar adenosine triphosphatase activity associated with congestive heart failure.[24, 27–29] Previously, such defects have been difficult to evaluate noninvasively. In vivo, nuclear magnetic resonance (NMR) spectroscopy is now feasible and as resolution improves, it may permit regional noninvasive quantitation of myocardial high-energy phosphate metabolism in patients with congestive heart failure. Magnetic resonance (MR) spectroscopy has now been performed in adults and children with dilated cardiomyopathy. Ratios of phosphocreatine

(PCr) to β-ATP generally did not separate normal subjects from patients with left ventricular hypertrophy or dilated cardiomyopathy as a group. However, patients with more advanced heart failure had lower ratios of PCr to ATP.[30] In contrast, modest separation was evident when comparing ratios of phosphodiesters to PCr, although there was substantial overlap.[31, 32] An infant with severe dilated cardiomyopathy has been studied with MR spectroscopy during dietary manipulation, with demonstration of alterations in myocardial energetics in response to substrate loading.[33] Although current spatial resolution of MR spectroscopy is low, improvements in technology are rapid, suggesting that a greater understanding of myocardial energetics in health and disease and with treatment may be forthcoming soon (see Chapter 50).

SYSTEMIC METABOLIC ABNORMALITIES IN PATIENTS WITH CARDIOMYOPATHY

With either systolic or diastolic dysfunction, there is activation of the renin-angiotensin-aldosterone system and the sympathetic nervous system.[16] These processes result in increased levels of circulating angiotensin II and aldosterone, but they also result in induction and activation of local renin-angiotensin-aldosterone systems in specific tissue beds, including the heart.[34] Similarly, systemic sympathetic activation is observed in patients with congestive heart failure with increased levels of circulating catecholamines and increased urinary excretion of catecholamine metabolites.[15, 35] The heart is richly enervated with both sympathetic and parasympathetic efferent fibers providing direct cardiac regulation, even in the absence of significant systemic sympathetic activation. In congestive heart failure, aortic coronary sinus sampling studies demonstrate excess catecholamine release into the coronary sinus during periods of myocardial stress and decompensation.[15, 35–37]

Activation of the sympathetic nervous system and the renin-angiotensin-aldosterone system can have diverse effects on cardiac metabolism, depending on their effects on the coronary circulation, loading conditions, and direct cardiac inotropic stimulation. Increases in left ventricular preload and afterload and the inotropic state induced by catecholamine stimulation in turn induce increases in myocardial oxygen consumption with acceleration of the myocardial use of acetate and fatty acids as long as regional or global myocardial ischemia is not induced.[38, 39] Conversely, high levels of exogenous catecholamines decrease myocardial glucose uptake in experimental animals.[40]

DILATED CARDIOMYOPATHY: OBSERVATIONS ON POSITRON EMISSION TOMOGRAPHY

As indicated in Table 72–1, there is a considerable variety of causative processes that may lead to the development of a cardiomyopathy. The vast majority result in a dilated cardiomyopathy, including virtually all those resulting from infectious processes, toxic agents, pregnancy and obesity, and metabolic and hematologic diseases. In most cases, there is a toxic or inflammatory process that destroys some myocytes, inducing scarring and the deposition of interstitial collagen. These processes increase the hemodynamic and metabolic burdens on the remaining viable myocytes while potentially impairing substrate delivery, particularly to the subendocardium, through fibrosis and increased left ventricular diastolic pressure with increased subendocardial wall stress. In most cases, no unique metabolic mechanism has been defined. In some dilated cardiomyopathies, the metabolic basis has been studied extensively (e.g., alcoholic cardiomyopathy[39] and hereditary carnitine deficiency)[8, 41] and specific derangements of intermediary metabolism defined, raising the hope that unique, noninvasively detectable metabolic signatures may be defined for some types of dilated cardiomyopathy.

The dilated cardiomyopathies are the most prevalent form of cardiomyopathy and, accordingly, were the first to be studied with positron emission tomography (PET).[42] Initial studies employed carbon-11-palmitate (^{11}C-palmitate) imaged in the static mode employing a multisliced PET device to define the spatial distribution of myocardial accumulation of fatty acids. Tomographic results in 17 patients with cardiomyopathies of different causes (three due to ethanol ingestion, two resulting from pregnancy and childbirth, two familial, one viral, and nine idiopathic) were compared with those of 13 normal subjects and 6 subjects with remote myocardial infarction. As expected, the tomographic images of patients with dilated cardiomyopathy demonstrated significant cardiac enlargement. Marked heterogeneity of the distribution of ^{11}C-palmitate was also observed throughout the hearts of patients with dilated cardiomyopathies (Fig. 72–2). Areas of avid accumulation of tracer were interspersed nearly randomly with zones of depressed accumulation. There was no consistent pattern to suggest a predilection for increased or decreased accumulation of ^{11}C-palmitate in any myocardial zone. Even when patients were grouped by etiologic diagnosis, no consistent patterns were detectable. Although the appearance was generally "moth-eaten," there were some small focal areas of moderately to markedly depressed accumulation of ^{11}C-palmitate.[42]

Figure 72–2. See Color Plate 35.

The patterns observed in patients with dilated cardiomyopathy were distinctly different from those of normal subjects and patients with remote myocardial infarction. In normal subjects, accumulation of ^{11}C-palmitate was homogeneous, with smooth transitions between zones of highest apparent activity and zones with lower activity. The slight variability observed in normal subjects was probably due to partial volume effects and spatial averaging in the ungated studies. Patients with remote myocardial infarction were found to have discrete zones of decreased accumulation of ^{11}C-palmitate, with homogeneous intense accumulation in remote normal zones. When analyzed quantitatively, patients with dilated cardiomyopathy demonstrated a significantly greater number of discrete zones of accumulation of ^{11}C-palmitate than did either normal subjects or patients with myocardial infarction. The distribution of tracer was also altered in patients with dilated cardiomyopathy with a flatter frequency distribution curve, a lower mean myocardial radioactivity, and a higher proportion of the myocardium demonstrating low levels of accumulation of ^{11}C-palmitate when compared with normal subjects.[42] Alterations in regional accumulation of ^{11}C-palmitate could have been caused by regional decreases in uptake resulting from decreased delivery because of microvascular disease or fibrosis, decreased extraction induced by a primary metabolic derangement, a decreased amount of myocardium in zones replaced by fibrosis, or rapid clearance of ^{11}C-palmitate due to back diffusion of unaltered ^{11}C-palmitate or rapid metabolic clearance due to β-oxidation. Alternatively, local zones with avid accumulation of ^{11}C-palmitate could have decreased clearance because of diminished β-oxidation of increased storage of the tracer as triglycerides or phospholipids.

Although the left ventricular walls of patients with cardiomyopathy tend to be thinner and demonstrate less systolic thickening than do those of normal subjects, there was no correlation between the regional wall motion abnormalities and wall thickening and zones of regionally depressed accumulation of ^{11}C-palmitate. This suggests that regional tomographic abnormalities were not attributable primarily to partial volume effects.[42]

There was also no clear association between myocardial metabolic abnormalities detected with tomography and abnormalities of myocardial perfusion detected with planar thallium-201 (^{201}Tl) scintigraphy. Among these patients, accumulation of ^{201}Tl in the myocardium was generally homogeneous except for mild apical thinning in two patients and focal defects in two additional patients, which correlated with tomographic metabolic abnormalities in only a single patient with idiopathic dilated cardiomyopathy.[42]

Subsequent studies of patients with idiopathic dilated cardiomyopathy have employed dynamic analysis of the kinetics of ^{11}C-palmitate studied in the fasting and fed states.[43, 44] In the fasting state, patients with cardiomyopathy incorporated a smaller percentage of administered ^{11}C-palmitate into the early, rapidly turning over pool (presumably that pool undergoing β-oxidation) than did normal subjects, but they did not demonstrate any alteration in the mean half-time of clearance of that early phase.[43] In normal subjects, administration of glucose decreased the fraction of radio-

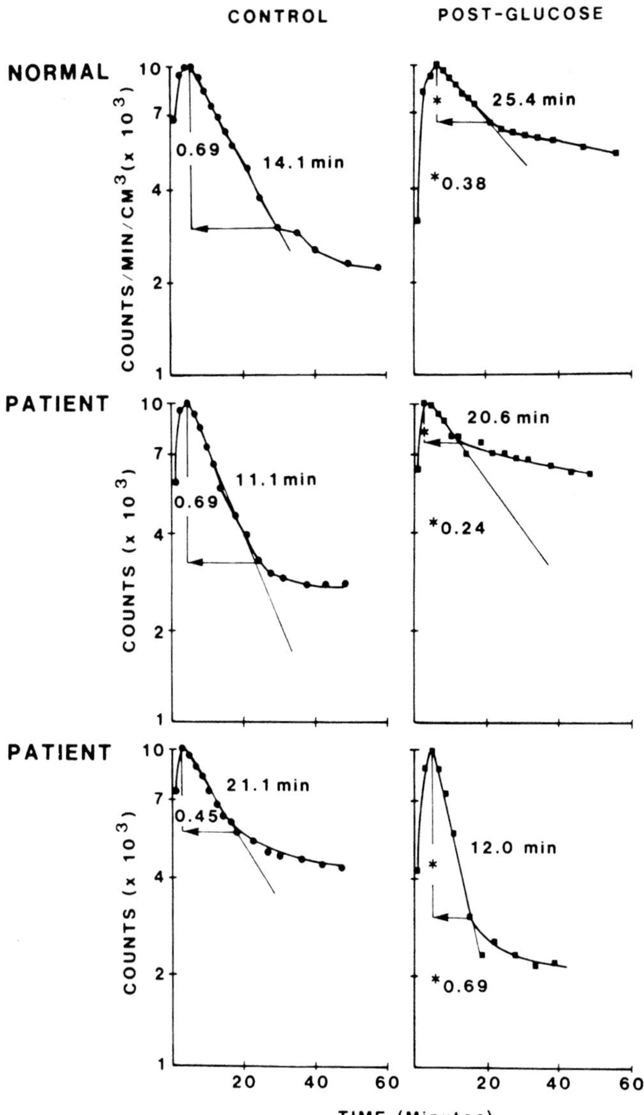

FIGURE 72–3. Myocardial time-activity curves recorded after the IV injection of ^{11}C-palmitate in a normal subject and in two patients with ventricular dysfunction. Curves recorded under fasting conditions are shown in the panels on the left, and those recorded after administration of glucose are shown in the panels on the right. In the normal subject *(top panels)*, a decreased fraction of radioactivity entered the early, rapidly turning over pool, and the rate of clearance from that pool declined after glucose. In the patient in the middle panels, the response was similar to that of the normal subject, but in the patient in the lower panels, the fraction entering the early, rapidly turning over pool increased substantially, as did the rate of clearance from that pool after administration of glucose. (From Schelbert, H.R., Henze, E., Sochor, H., et al.: Effects of substrate availability of myocardial C-11 palmitate kinetics by positron emission tomography in normal subjects and patients with ventricular dysfunction. Am. Heart J. 111:1055, 1986, with permission.)

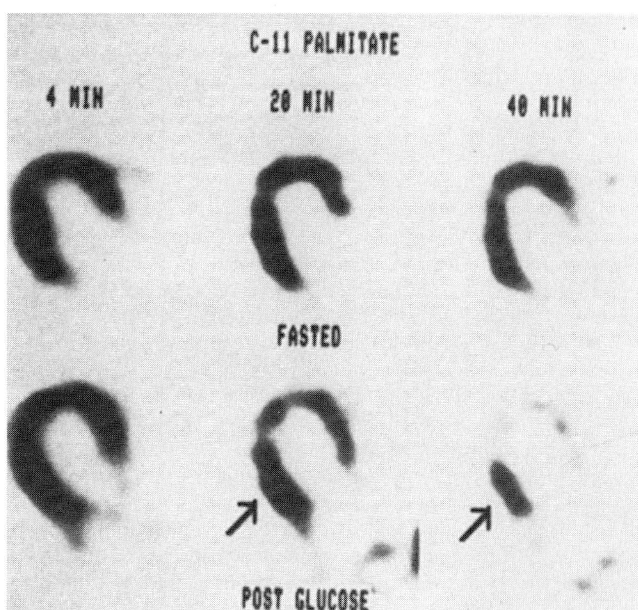

FIGURE 72–4. Serial tomographic images acquired after the IV administration of ^{11}C-palmitate in the fasting state *(top)* and after administration of glucose *(bottom)*. In these images, anterior is on the top of each image, and the right of each image represents the patient's right side. Evident in these images is substantial heterogeneity in the accumulation of tracer, which is exaggerated after glucose administration. The clearance of radioactivity is rapid from the anterior and septal walls and markedly delayed in the posterolateral wall *(arrows)*. (From Sochor, H., Schelbert, H.R., Schwaiger, M., et al.: Studies of fatty acid metabolism with positron emission tomography in patients with cardiomyopathy. Eur. J. Nucl. Med. 12[Suppl.]:S66, 1986, with permission.)

activity entering the early, rapidly turning over pool and decreased the rate of clearance of radioactivity from this pool. In patients with cardiomyopathy, the response was variable. Slightly more than half of the patients demonstrated a normal metabolic response to glucose administration. In contrast, more than 40 percent of patients with dilated cardiomyopathy demonstrated an aberrant pattern. In these patients, administration of glucose induced an increase in the fraction of radioactivity entering the early pool and markedly increased the rate of clearance from that pool (Fig. 72–3).[43]

The spatial heterogeneity previously demonstrated with static studies was confirmed with dynamic studies as well.[44] When patients with cardiomyopathy (predominantly dilated cardiomyopathy) were studied with ^{11}C-palmitate after the administration of glucose, there was significantly greater regional variability in the clearance of ^{11}C-palmitate from myocardium than occurs in normal subjects (Fig. 72–4). Similarly, there was a greater variability in the percentage of ^{11}C-palmitate taken up into the rapidly turning over pool by patients with dilated cardiomyopathy than by normal subjects.[44] There was no clear association among the rates of clearance of ^{11}C-palmitate and the cause of the cardiomyopathy, the changes in plasma substrate levels after the administration of glucose, or the heart rate and blood pressure. There was a trend toward lower ejection fractions in patients who demonstrated an abnormal metabolic response to the administration of glucose.[43] The metabolic basis for the abnormalities observed has not yet been defined, but it has been hypothesized that the pattern observed may be due to inhibition of citric acid cycle activity in the fasting state by augmented ketone body use (previously observed in some patients with congestive heart failure) that could be ameliorated by replenishment of Krebs cycle intermediates after glucose administration.[43]

Myocardial metabolism can also be assessed by tracing the activity of the Krebs cycle by following the fate of carbon-11–labeled acetate (^{11}C-acetate). Acetate plays a key role in aerobic myocardial metabolism, since it is the entry point into the Krebs cycle for fatty acids, glucose, lactate, and some amino acids (see Figure 72–1). When traced with ^{11}C-acetate, an accurate assessment of myocardial oxygen consumption is possible.[9, 38, 45–47] When the clearance of ^{11}C-acetate from the heart, assessed with PET, was compared with direct measurement of oxygen consumption (arterial-coronary sinus determinations) a strong correlation was found (r = 0.8).[9] The levels of oxygen consumption measured at rest (8.3±3 mL · min^{-1} · 100 g^{-1}) were comparable to those reported by others. When dobutamine was administered, clearance of ^{11}C-acetate increased significantly, but myocardial efficiency increased as well because of the preload and afterload reducing properties of dobutamine. Thus, wall stress was reduced and myocardial oxygen consumption increased less than external work.[9]

Although most studies of dilated cardiomyopathies with PET have focused on myocardial metabolism, the availability of methods permitting quantification of myocardial perfusion in absolute terms has led to analysis of myocardial perfusion in this entity. Both nitrogen-13–labeled ammonia (^{13}N-ammonia) and oxygen-15–labeled water (^{15}O-water) have been employed in the study of myocardial perfusion in patients with dilated cardiomyopathy. Myocardial perfusion was relatively homogeneous at rest when studied with ^{15}O-water but myocardial perfusion reserve was reduced.[48] When patients with nonischemic dilated cardiomyopathy were studied with ^{13}N-ammonia and multiple small regions of interest, heterogeneity of the resting flow was greater than that of normal subjects.[49] When patients with dilated cardiomyopathy were challenged with dipyridamole or pacing, perfusion assessed with ^{13}N-ammonia and PET was reduced significantly compared with controls, with the greatest perfusion abnormalities observed in patients with the highest left ventricular end-diastolic pressures.[12]

DIFFERENTIATION OF ISCHEMIC FROM NONISCHEMIC DILATED CARDIOMYOPATHY

It is often difficult or impossible to determine with a high degree of certainty whether this syndrome develops in a patient with congestive heart failure and an enlarged heart because of extensive coronary artery disease or because of a nonischemic dilated cardiomyopathy. When there is objective documentation of prior myocardial infarction, the diagnosis is made easily. In many other circumstances, however, the distinction is difficult. Unfortunately, the electrocardiogram is insufficiently sensitive or specific to permit clear differentiation in many instances, since patients with myocardial infarction may not exhibit Q waves and since many patients with congestive cardiomyopathy may exhibit abnormalities on the electrocardiogram that are suggestive of prior infarction. In many other instances, conduction abnormalities, such as left bundle branch block, preclude an electrocardiographic differentiation.[50–54] Similarly, chest pain suggestive of ischemia may be encountered in several conditions in which the epicardial coronary arteries are normal. This syndrome has been observed in patients whose hearts are otherwise normal but whose microvasculature is abnormal, in patients with aortic insufficiency or stenosis, and in patients with nonischemic dilated cardiomyopathy.[13, 14, 55, 56] Patients presenting with idiopathic dilated cardiomyopathy and chest pain have been found to have normal coronary blood flow at rest but limited coronary flow reserve. When assessed after the inhalation of argon gas, coronary flow averaged 78 mL · 100 g^{-1} · min^{-1} plus or minus 17 mL · 100 g^{-1} · min^{-1} at rest and increased to only 142 mL · 100 g^{-1} · min^{-1} plus or minus 38 mL · 100 g^{-1} · min^{-1} with vasodilation.[13] In contrast, coronary flow in normal subjects increased from 78 mL · 100 g^{-1} · min^{-1} plus or minus 9 mL · 100 g^{-1} · min^{-1} to 301 mL · 100 g^{-1} · min^{-1} plus or minus 64 mL · 100 g^{-1} · min^{-1} after dipyridamole infusion. Minimal coronary resistance (calculated after dipyridamole administration) correlated significantly with left ventricular end-diastolic pressure and inversely with left ventricular ejection fraction.[11, 13] In studies performed with intracoronary Doppler flow wires, coronary flow reserve correlated directly with ejection fraction and inversely with left ventricular end-diastolic pressure, left ventricular end-diastolic wall stress, and end-diastolic volume index.[11]

Assessment of regional coronary perfusion with ^{201}Tl scintigraphy has demonstrated extensive zones of depressed uptake of thallium in patients with ischemic cardiomyopathy but only minimal apical thinning in patients with nonischemic cardiomyopathy, allowing some differentiation between patient groups.[51] To detect an ischemic cardiomyopathy with this technique, however, a defect encompassing 40 percent of the circumference of the left ventricle was required, providing a relatively specific diagnostic technique but one with only modest sensitivity. More recent studies employing ^{201}Tl scintigraphy and quantitative circumferential profiles have also demonstrated substantial overlap between patients with ischemic and those with nonischemic dilated cardiomyopathy if only a single parameter such as defect size or defect severity is evaluated. When analyzed in tandem with computerized quantitative analysis, however, a reasonable separation can be achieved between patients with ischemic and those with nonischemic dilated cardiomyopathy.[57, 58] Analysis of regional wall motion assessed echocardiographically or with radionuclide ventriculography has also been employed in an attempt to differentiate patients with ischemic dilated cardiomyopathy from those with nonischemic dilated cardiomyopathy. Unfortunately, global hypokinesis is common in patients with ischemic cardiomyopathy, and some regional variability in the severity of wall motion abnormalities is commonly encountered in patients with nonischemic dilated cardiomyopathy, making accurate differentiation between these two entities difficult using traditional techniques.[50, 52, 59]

Positron Emission Tomographic Imaging

Positron emission tomography performed after intravenous (IV) administration of ^{11}C-palmitate has been used to differentiate patients with ischemic cardiomyopathy from those with nonischemic cardiomyopathy.[50] Positron emisson tomography revealed dramatic differences in the appearance of images acquired from patients with ischemic and patients with nonischemic dilated cardiomyopathy. Large defects encompassing more than 15 percent of the cross-sectional area of the left ventricle in transverse reconstructions were observed in 80 percent of patients with ischemic dilated cardiomyopathy but not in normal subjects or in patients with nonischemic dilated cardiomyopathy. In general, patients with ischemic dilated cardiomyopathy had large zones of homogeneously depressed ^{11}C-palmitate accumulations that contrasted sharply with the diffuse heterogeneity of tracer accumulation observed in patients with idiopathic dilated cardiomyopathy (Fig. 72–5). This heterogeneity was exhibited as a greater number of discrete regions of radioactivity observed in patients with nonischemic cardiomyopathy compared with those with ischemic cardiomyopathy. Similarly, the frequency distribution of radioactivity per pixel was shifted toward lower values for patients with nonischemic dilated cardiomyopathy compared with those with ischemic disease. Among patients with ischemic dilated cardiomyopathy, those with diabetes mellitus demonstrated somewhat more tomographic heterogeneity than did those without diabetes, which is in keeping with the more diffuse and severe nature of the coronary disease typically encountered in patients with diabetes mellitus. Despite this increased heterogeneity, the tomographic patterns remained distinctly different from those of patients with nonischemic dilated cardiomyopathy.[50]

Positron emission tomography using ^{13}N-ammonia and fluorine-18–labeled 2-fluoro-2-deoxyglucose (^{18}F-2-fluoro-2-deoxyglucose) has also been performed in patients with dilated cardiomyopathy. In a series of 21 patients with dilated cardiomyopathy (11 with ischemic and 10 with nonischemic disease), PET proved both

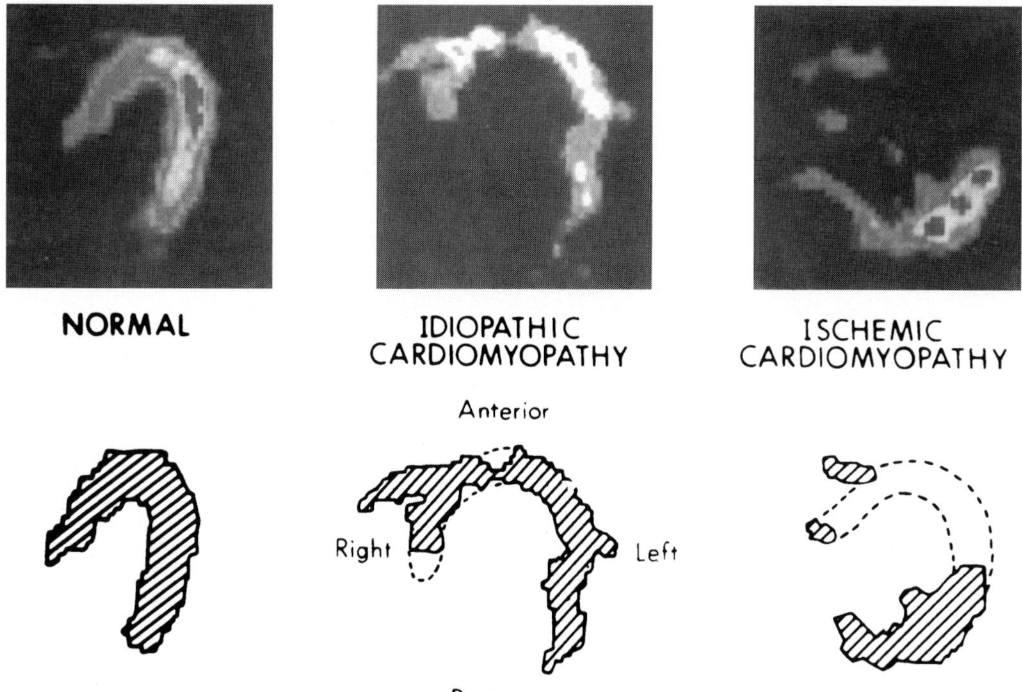

FIGURE 72–5. Representative midventricular tomograms acquired after the IV administration of ^{11}C-palmitate in a normal subject, in a patient with dilated cardiomyopathy, and in a patient with ischemic dilated cardiomyopathy. The orientation is the same as that in Figure 72–2. Schematic representations are below each image with the expected myocardial borders indicated by the interrupted lines. In patients with ischemic cardiomyopathy, large zones of homogeneously depressed accumulation of ^{11}C-palmitate are noted. In contrast, in patients with dilated nonischemic cardiomyopathy, marked spatial heterogeneity is observed without large discrete zones of decreased accumulation of tracer. (From Eisenberg, J.D., Sobel, B.E., and Geltman, E.M.: Differentiation of ischemic from nonischemic cardiomyopathy with positron emission tomography. Am. J. Cardiol. 59:1310, 1987, with permission.)

sensitive and specific for making the distinction between ischemic and nonischemic dilated cardiomyopathy.[60] Patients with ischemic cardiomyopathy had significantly more discrete perfusion defects and metabolic defects. They demonstrated patterns of infarction (reduced perfusion and glucose utilization), ischemia (reduced perfusion and preserved metabolic function), or both (Fig. 72–6). With nonischemic dilated cardiomyopathy, relatively mild defects were observed in images of perfusion and metabolism. When quantitative circumferential profiles were analyzed, the differences between groups were striking.[60]

When PET was performed with ^{13}N-ammonia and ^{18}F-2-fluoro-2-deoxyglucose in patients with ischemic and nonischemic cardiomyopathy who were to undergo heart transplantation, similar disparate patterns were observed. Patients with nonischemic cardiomyopathy demonstrated parallel patterns of perfusion and metabolism. There were only mild matched decreases in apparent uptake of ^{13}N-ammonia and ^{18}F-2-fluoro-2-deoxyglucose in the inferior wall without focal pathologic findings in this area. (Fig. 72–7). In contrast, patients with ischemic cardiomyopathy demonstrated heterogeneous, segmentally abnormal patterns of perfusion and metabolism. There was excellent correlation between zones of reduced perfusion and metabolism and areas of fibrosis identified by histologic characteristics in these hearts removed at the time of transplantation (Fig. 72–8).[53]

Comparison With Other Imaging Techniques

Many imaging techniques have been employed for the evaluation of patients with dilated cardiomyopathy. In addition to echocardiography and ^{201}Tl scintigraphy (see earlier discussion), proton magnetic resonance imaging (MRI) and single-photon scintigraphy with iodinated fatty acids have been employed for the evaluation of patients with dilated cardiomyopathy (see Chapters 49 and 65.)

Several groups have investigated global and regional mechanical function with proton MRI at rest and with pharmacologic interventions.[61, 62] Assessment of energy metabolism with phosphorus-31 (^{31}P) MR spectroscopy has also been explored.[30–33] Comparative studies of MRI and PET are few. Patients with dilated cardiomyopathy have been evaluated with proton MRI employing spin-echo techniques for comparison with PET performed after the IV administration of ^{11}C-palmitate.[63] Although cardiac structure was well delineated with high spatial resolution on MRI, the metabolic heterogeneity observed with PET was not exhibited in proton MRI studies (Fig. 72–9). Ventricular dilatation, wall thinning, and other architectural details were observed with great clarity. Within signals emanating from myocardial regions of interest, however, there were no significant differences in signal intensity between normal subjects and patients with dilated cardiomyopathy on electrocardiographic gated spin-echo images (TE = 30 msec or TE = 60 msec), in calculated T2, or in the frequency distribution of signal intensity.[63] Although some regional myocardial thinning could be observed with MRI in patients with ischemic dilated cardiomyopathy in zones of presumed infarction, the findings were often subtle and the technique did not differentiate between patients with ischemic cardiomyopathy and those with nonischemic cardiomyopathy as clearly as did PET with ^{11}C-palmitate.[63]

A number of fatty acid analogs have been synthesized and labeled with iodine-123 (^{123}I) for myocardial metabolic imaging (see Chapter 65). Several have been studied with either planar imaging or single-photon emission computed tomography in patients with dilated cardiomyopathy.[64–66] In general, the spatial heterogeneity of accumulation observed with ^{11}C-palmitate in patients with dilated

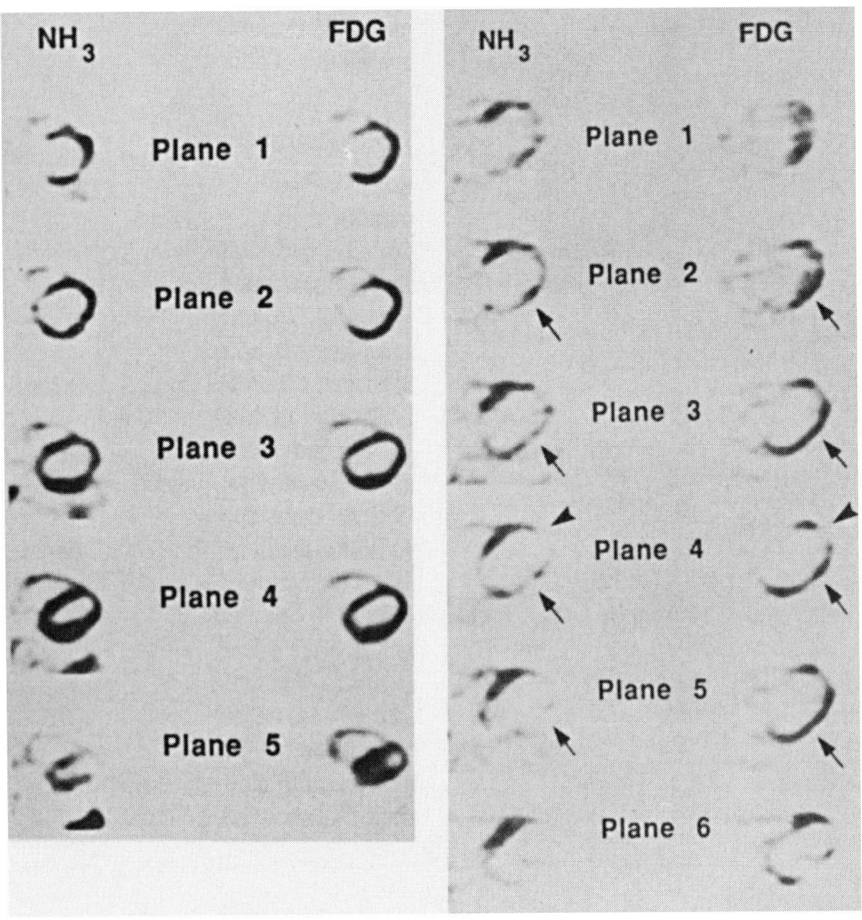

FIGURE 72–6. Left, Images of the distribution of nitrogen-13–labeled ammonia (NH_3) and fluorine-18–labeled 2-fluoro-2-deoxyglucose (FDG) in a patient with nonischemic dilated cardiomyopathy. Relative perfusion (^{13}N-ammonia) and glucose utilization (^{18}F-2-fluoro-2-deoxyglucose) are relatively homogeneous without discrete defects. *Right,* Images from a patient with ischemic cardiomyopathy. There are matched defects in both perfusion and metabolism *(arrowheads)* in the apex and inferior wall indicative of infarction. Areas of hypoperfusion with preserved ^{18}F-2-fluoro-2-deoxyglucose uptake are evident in the lateral and posterolateral wall *(arrows),* representing ischemia. Left ventricular cavity dilatation is evident in both patients. Prominent right ventricular uptake of ^{18}F-2-fluoro-2-deoxyglucose *(left)* is often associated with pulmonary hypertension. (From Vaghaiwalla Mody, F., Brunken, R.C., Warner Stevenson, L., et al.: Differentiating cardiomyopathy of coronary artery disease from nonischemic dilated cardiomyopathy utilizing positron emission tomography. J. Am. Coll. Cardiol. 17:373, 1991. Reprinted with permission from the American College of Cardiology.)

cardiomyopathy has been confirmed with the iodinated compounds. As observed with ^{11}C-palmitate, however, the spatial and kinetic abnormalities of fatty acid metabolism observed appeared relatively similar for patients with dilated cardiomyopathy of differing causes.[65, 66] Although the patterns of clearance of the single-photon emitting tracers were distinctly different from those observed with normal subjects, the pattern of altered kinetics (prolongation or acceleration) observed in patients with cardiomyopathy depended on the specific compound tested.[65, 66]

Myocardial autonomic function has also been studied with single-photon emission computed tomography and PET with iodine-123–labeled metaiodobenzylguanidine (^{123}I-metaiodobenzylguanidine) (MIBG), carbon-11–labeled hydroxyephedrine (^{11}C-hydroxyephedrine), and carbon-11–labeled CGP-12177 (^{11}C-CGP-12177), a nonselective hydrophilic β-blocker.[67–72] The distribution of sympathetic preganglionic fibers (assessed with MIBG) is homogeneous in normal myocardium but can be spatially heterogeneous in dilated cardiomyopathy, with the greatest abnormalities observed in patients with ventricular tachycardia in which regional abnormalities were detected.[68] The concentration of β-receptors in myocardium of patients with idiopathic cardiomyopathic was decreased by 53 percent compared with controls when studied with ^{11}C-GP-12177.[71] When sympathetic neuronal activity was studied with ^{11}C-hydroxyephedrine, similar reductions in tracer retention were observed. There was significant regional heterogeneity of neuronal dysfunction in some patients.[70] These findings, in concert, support the contention that there is significant sympathetic down-regulation in dilated cardiomyopathy. The ability of the myocardium to take up and retain MIBG was enhanced in patients with dilated cardiomyopathy who were treated with metoprolol, further supporting the concept that excessive norepinephrine stimulation and β-receptor occupancy may contribute to the adrenergic down-regulation in the cardiomyopathies[69] (see Chapters 67 and 72.)

HYPERTROPHIC CARDIOMYOPATHY

The hypertrophic cardiomyopathies comprise several syndromes exhibiting different pathologic findings, clinical presentations, and natural histories.[73] All demonstrate significant left ventricular hypertrophy that may be generalized throughout the heart or may predominate in the interventricular septum (particularly in the upper portion) or left ventricular apex (apical cardiomyopathy). Most are detected clinically because of abnormalities of diastolic function, characterized by pulmonary venous congestion with dyspnea. Despite signs and symptoms suggestive of left ventricular decompensation, systolic performance is generally well preserved or hyperdynamic.[73] Paradoxically, limitation of forward output can occur if ventricular performance is supernormal, hypertrophy is severe, and geometry is altered sufficiently to induce left ventricular outflow tract obstruction.

Hypertrophic cardiomyopathy may occur in either hereditary or sporadic patterns. There are numerous kindreds in which the disorder appears to be inherited as an autosomal dominant trait with variable penetrance. Up to one third of cases of hypertrophic cardiomyopathy occur in a familial pattern with equal incidence in males and females,[74] but many cases occur in a sporadic fashion. A substantial number of mutations in the β-myosin heavy-chain gene have now been mapped in patients with hypertrophic cardiomyopathy. There appears to be a significant genetic heterogeneity, even within families,[75] which may explain the apparent variable penetrance of this disease. Genetic abnormalities have also been mapped to chromosomes carrying the genes for troponin I, tropomyosin, and actin, suggesting that abnormalities of several different structural-contractile cardiac proteins can cause or predispose to the development of hypertrophic cardiomyopathy.[76] Because of the variable patterns of inheritance and the presence of significant

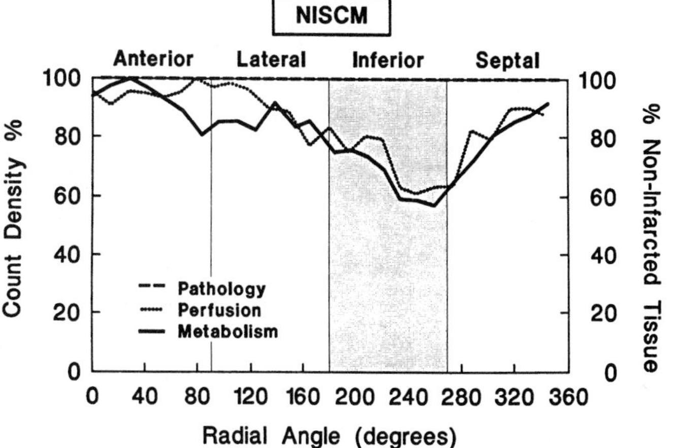

FIGURE 72–7. Correlation among perfusion, metabolism, and pathologic features in a patient with nonischemic cardiomyopathy studied with positron emission tomography (PET) and ^{13}N-ammonia and ^{18}F-2-fluoro-2-deoxyglucose and histologic appearance after explantation of the native heart at the time of orthotopic heart transplantation. The dashed line at the top indicates the lack of infarction. Metabolism and perfusion are closely matched with a mild decrease in tracer content in the inferior wall, possibly due to oblique imaging and partial volume effects. NISCM = nonischemic dilated cardiomyopathy. (From Berry, J.J., Hoffman, J.M., Steenbergen, C., et al.: Human pathologic correlation with PET in ischemic and nonischemic cardiomyopathy. J. Nucl. Med. 34:39, 1993, with permission.)

numbers of sporadic cases, it has been postulated that hereditary factors may lead to a succeptibility for the development of hypertrophic cardiomyopathy that manifests itself only if an additional stimulus, such as hypertension or hyperthyroidism, is present.[77] This concept is also supported by the observation in experimental animals of hypertrophic cardiomyopathy development in the offspring of mothers made hyperthyroid during pregnancy.[78] In many instances, hypertrophic cardiomyopathy appears only at an advanced age (about one third of patients are greater than 60 years of age at presentation) and may represent an excessive hypertrophic response to hypertension.[79, 80] Hypertrophic cardiomyopathy has also been described in patients with Friedreich ataxia, although this group makes up a small fraction of patients.[81]

Myocardial Metabolism in Hypertrophic Cardiomyopathy

Coronary blood flow in patients with hypertrophic cardiomyopathy who were assessed with arterial-coronary sinus sampling techniques was normal or increased at rest, but was reduced when corrected for left ventricular mass.[14] Myocardial oxygen consumption was normal or increased at rest and responded variably to pacing stress. Those with the highest myocardial oxygen consumption appeared to have the most extensive hypertrophy and demonstrated markedly reduced lactate extraction or lactate production with pacing, along with pacing-induced reductions in coronary blood flow or limited coronary flow reserve.[14] When analysis was localized to the anterior circulation by selective catheterization of the great cardiac vein, a similar pattern was found, with increased total regional flow at rest but reduced coronary flow reserve with pacing.[10, 82] Lactate balance was normal at rest, but lactate consumption decreased or converted to lactate production with pacing. Paradoxically, the arterial-coronary sinus oxygen difference narrowed rather than increased with pacing. Myocardial extraction of pyruvate appeared to parallel that of lactate, with decreased extraction of pyruvate demonstrated in patients who exhibited decreased extraction or production of lactate during cardiac pacing.[10] Extraction of other substrates (β-hydroxybutyrate, acetoacetate, free fatty acids, and glycerol) appeared normal at rest and with atrial pacing and did not differ in patients with hypertrophic cardiomyopathies between those who developed ischemia during atrial pacing and those who did not.[82]

Initial invasive assessments of arterial-coronary sinus plasma levels of catecholamines in small numbers of patients have demonstrated only minor alterations.[36] Recent studies have demonstrated substantial excesses of norepinephrine in great cardiac vein blood

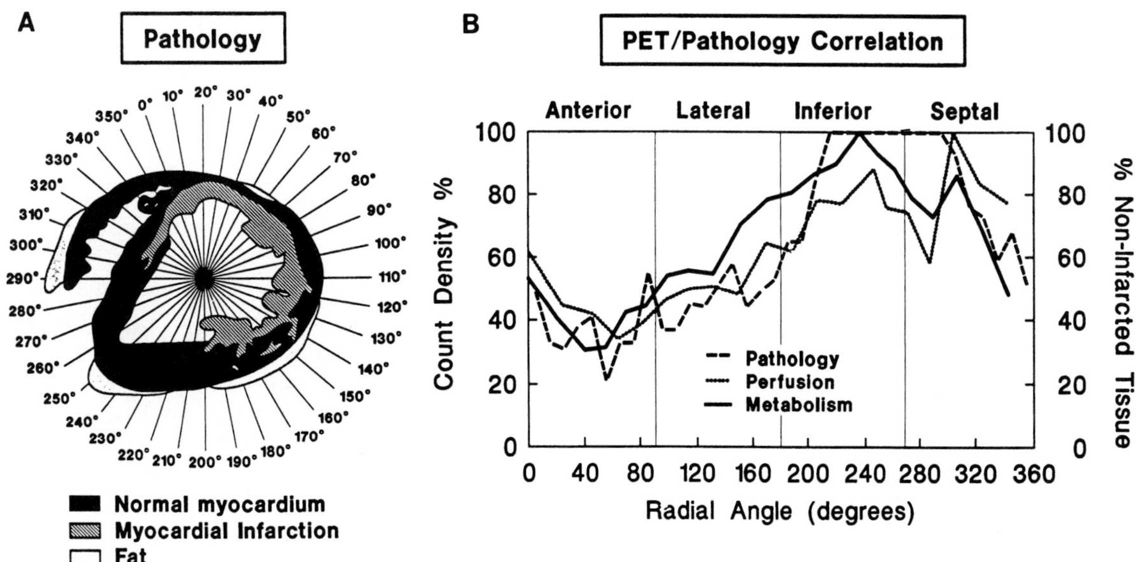

FIGURE 72–8. A schematic representation of the histologic findings in a patient with ischemic cardiomyopathy demonstrating extensive anteroseptal, anterior, and anterolateral nontransmural myocardial infarction (*A*). The regional correlations among histologic appearance, perfusion, and metabolism are displayed for the same patient (*B*). There is an excellent correlation between histologic characteristics and functional imaging. PET = positron emission tomography. (From Berry, J.J., Hoffman, J.M., Steenbergen, C., et al.: Human pathologic correlation with PET in ischemic and nonischemic cardiomyopathy. J. Nucl. Med. 34:39, 1993, with permission.)

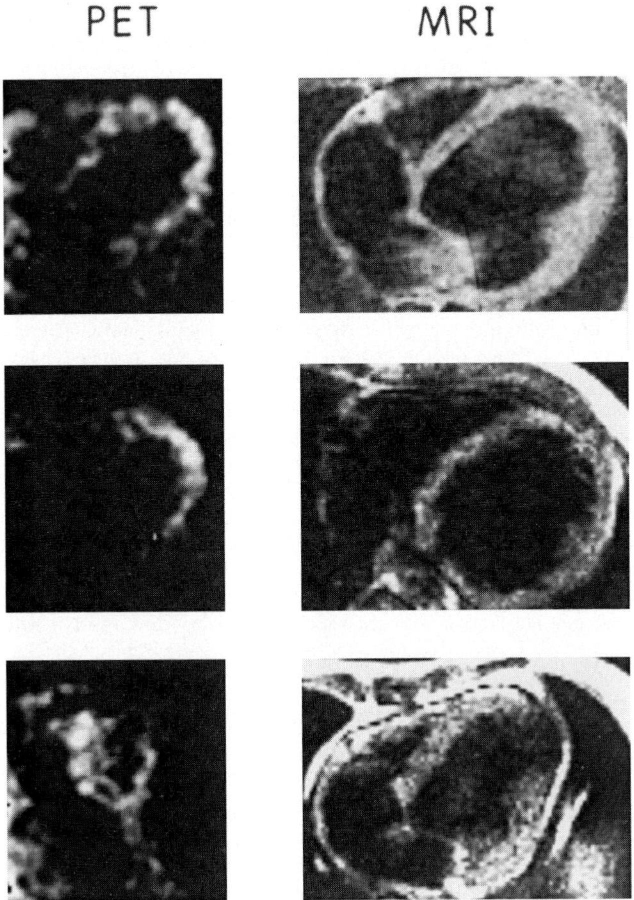

FIGURE 72–9. Transverse midventricular tomographic reconstructions acquired with PET after the IV administration of ^{11}C-palmitate *(left panels)* and, in the same patients, with proton magnetic resonance imaging (MRI) employing spin-echo technique *(right panels)*. The diagnoses were sarcoidosis *(top)*, idiopathic cardiomyopathy *(middle)*, and ischemic cardiomyopathy *(bottom)*. The two patients with nonischemic cardiomyopathy had diffuse spatial heterogeneity of metabolism reflected in the PET images. The patient with ischemic cardiomyopathy had a dense defect involving the anterior walls with an apparent transmural defect and an apparent nontransmural defect affecting the lateral wall. With MRI, the myocardial signal was essentially homogeneous for the patient in the top panel; there was fine speckling seen in the middle panel but no regional wall thinning or apparent scarring to explain the PET imaging characteristics. Conversely, this metabolic heterogeneity observed on PET was not seen with MRI. The patient with ischemic cardiomyopathy demonstrated mild apical and anterolateral thinning, but the abnormality on MRI was subtle compared with the metabolic abnormality demonstrated by PET. PET = positron emission tomography. (From Geltman, E.M., Eisenberg, J.D., Keim, S., et al.: Comparative magnetic resonance imaging and positron emission tomography in cardiomyopathy. [Abstract.] J. Am. Coll. Cardiol. 5:436, 1985. Reprinted with permission from the American College of Cardiology.)

(compared with arterial blood).[83] This appears to be due to diminished neuronal uptake of norepinephrine rather than excess release from sympathetic nerve endings. The percentage extraction of norepinephrine by patients with hypertrophic cardiomyopathy was not related to the severity of left ventricular obstruction, mean arterial pressure, coronary blood flow, or pulmonary artery occlusive pressure. In contrast, there were significant correlations among peak systolic left ventricular pressure and the arterial-coronary sinus differences in norepinephrine, arterial-coronary sinus production rate, and cardiac spillover rate of norepinephrine.[83] These findings would suggest that the myocardium of patients with hypertrophic cardiomyopathy is exposed to more norepinephrine than is that of normal subjects and that altered norepinephrine kinetics might play a role in the pathogenesis of hypertrophic cardiomyopathy.

Findings on Positron Emission Tomography

Several groups have studied patients with hypertrophic cardiomyopathy using PET and various tracers of perfusion and metabolism. The initial studies of patients with hypertrophic cardiomyopathy using PET were accomplished at rest after a brief fast using ^{18}F-2-fluoro-2-deoxyglucose, ^{11}C-palmitate, and ^{13}N-ammonia.[84] Static images of relative perfusion (^{13}N-ammonia) demonstrated apparently homogeneous flow (Fig. 72–10). When data were corrected for partial volume effects, regional perfusion in the septum was found to be mildly decreased. Initial accumulation of ^{11}C-palmitate appeared homogeneous but was also mildly reduced in the septum when corrected for partial volume effects. However, the fraction extracted into the early, rapidly turning over pool was similar in the septum and lateral walls, as was the half-time of clearance of ^{11}C-palmitate from both regions.[84] The similarity of the extraction fraction and the clearance half-time of the early rapid phase suggests that regional ischemia at rest was not the cause of any decreased extraction of ^{11}C-palmitate. The decreased extraction in the septum relative to the lateral wall may merely reflect decreased delivery of tracer, since the diminished accumula-

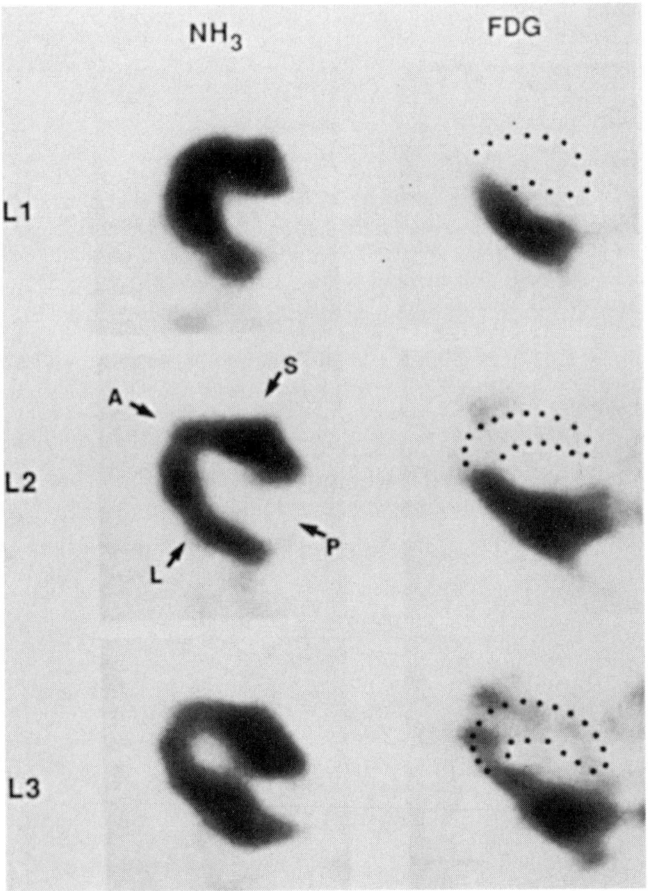

FIGURE 72–10. Transverse tomographic reconstructions acquired after the IV administration of ^{13}N-ammonia *(left)* and ^{18}F-2-fluoro-2-deoxyglucose *(right)*, acquired in the fasting state in a patient with hypertrophic cardiomyopathy. Three levels of the heart are shown: L1 is the most basal and L3 the most apical. The distribution of ^{13}N-ammonia is relatively homogeneous, but there is a markedly depressed accumulation of ^{18}F-2-fluoro-2-deoxyglucose in the interventricular septum. The location of the septum is indicated by the dotted lines. A = anterior; L = lateral; S = superior; P = posterior. (From Grover-McKay, M., Schwaiger, M., Krivokapich, J., et al.: Regional myocardial blood flow and metabolism at rest in mildly symptomatic patients with hypertrophic cardiomyopathy. J. Am. Coll. Cardiol. 13:317, 1989. Reprinted with permission from the American College of Cardiology.)

tion of ^{11}C-palmitate paralleled the reduction in accumulation of ^{13}N-ammonia.

Subsequent studies have employed modeling techniques to quantify myocardial perfusion and perfusion reserve.[85–88] Results have been variable, with either normal or reduced myocardial blood flow in the septum at rest. Endocardial to epicardial flow maldistribution has been described in patients with extreme septal hypertrophy.[89] However, there is a consistent finding of reduced myocardial perfusion reserve both in the septum and in the left ventricular free wall.[85, 88] There were also discrepancies between different groups regarding the homogeneity of resting myocardial glucose utilization. In some studies, resting glucose utilization was comparable in the septum and free wall, but in other studies, glucose utilization was higher in the free wall. When disparities were observed, they correlated with increased wall thickening in the free wall.[87] There also appears to be age-related differences, with greater disparities between glucose utilization and flow in patients in whom hypertrophic cardiomyopathy was manifested at a younger age.[86, 90] In some instances, the flow metabolism mismatches were sufficient to suggest that true ischemia can develop during stress in patients with hypertrophic cardiomyopathy (Fig. 72–11).[85, 86]

When oxygen consumption was assessed with ^{11}C-acetate and PET, the hypertrophic regions were generally found to have reduced uptake of acetate as well as reduced clearance of this tracer when compared with nonhypertrophied walls.[91, 92] These data could well be explained on the basis of increased wall motion and increased myocardial work in the thinner, more functional walls, similar to a study employing PET, ^{18}F-2-fluoro-2-deoxyglucose and ^{15}O-water.[87]

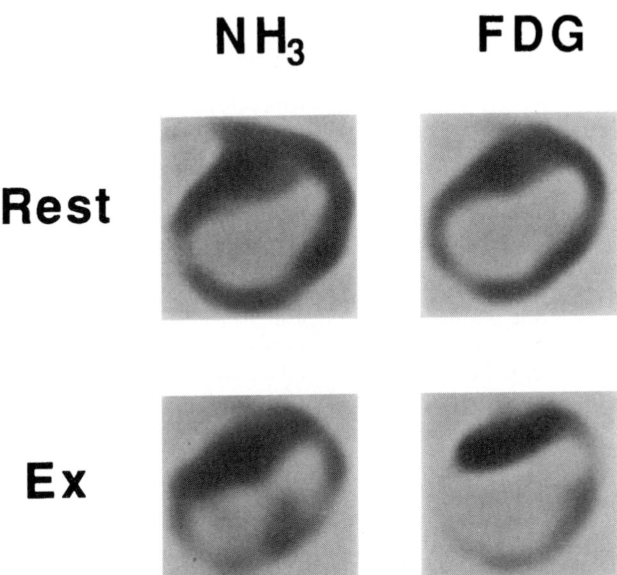

FIGURE 72–11. Tomograms of myocardial perfusion (^{13}N-ammonia, NH_3) and metabolism (^{18}F-2-fluoro-2-deoxyglucose, FDG) acquired at rest *(top)* and with exercise (Ex) *(bottom)* in a patient with hypertrophic cardiomyopathy. Calculation of myocardial blood flow and metabolic rates are performed on dynamic data. Image intensity does not necessarily match calculated flow or metabolic rates. At rest, the regional myocardial glucose utilization was 1.06 μmol · min^{-1} · g^{-1} in the septum and 1.22 μmol · min^{-1} · g^{-1} in the lateral wall; blood flow to the septum was 0.64 mL · min^{-1} · g^{-1} versus 0.94 mL · min^{-1} · g^{-1} to the lateral wall. For the exercise study, the glucose utilization was 0.72 μmol · min^{-1} · g^{-1} in the septum and 0.4 μmol · min^{-1} · g^{-1} in the lateral wall; septal blood flow fell markedly to 0.31 mL · min^{-1} · g^{-1} and remained almost unchanged in the control tissue. (From Nienaber, C.A., Gambhir, S.S., Mody, F.V., et al.: Regional myocardial blood flow and glucose utilization in symptomatic patients with hypertrophic cardiomyopathy. Circulation 87:1580, 1993, with permission. Copyright 1993, American Heart Association.)

Comparison With Other Imaging Techniques

Single-photon emission computed tomography has been performed with iodine-123–labeled betamethyl iodophenyl pentadecanoic acid (^{123}I-betamethyl iodophenyl pentadecanoic acid) (BMIPP) in patients with hypertrophic cardiomyopathy. In patients with asymmetric septal hypertrophy, there is reduced initial uptake and rapid clearance of the tracer from the septum, suggesting decreased fatty acid uptake and esterification. The metabolic heterogeneity was different from the pattern of ^{201}Tl accumulation in these same patients.[93, 94] The left ventricular cavity appeared larger on early images than on those acquired late, possibly because of delayed uptake of BMIPP in the endocardium, suggesting a metabolic abnormality of the septal endocardium. This would not be consistent with simple ischemia, since cavity size on thallium imaging was smaller than on BMIPP imaging, suggesting that subendocardial perfusion was not compromised.

NMR spectroscopy using ^{31}P has also been performed in patients with hypertrophic cardiomyopathy. Abnormalities of high-energy phosphate distribution were observed.[95] The ratio of the phosphocreatine-to-ATP peaks from the anterior heart wall was significantly reduced in patients with hypertrophic cardiomyopathy. Conversely, the ratio of phosphodiesters to PCr was higher in patients than in controls. Each of these abnormalities was most marked in patients with hypertrophic cardiomyopathy who had reduced ejection fractions (<45 percent). The abnormalities in high-energy phosphate content were not paralleled by perfusion abnormalities assessed with ^{201}Tl, indicating that the metabolic abnormalities are unlikely to be due to hypoperfusion alone.[95]

The distribution of myocardial sympathetic enervation has also been studied tomographically in patients with hypertrophic cardiomyopathy employing both single-photon and positron-emitting tracers.[69, 94, 96] MIBG is the best studied of these agents. As described in detail in Chapter 67, MIBG, a radiolabeled analog of norepinephrine, is taken up by postganglionic sympathetic nerves. Defects in accumulation of MIBG have been observed in the septum of patients with hypertrophic cardiomyopathy.[96] Focal defects have been noted in patients with hypertrophic cardiomyopathy and ventricular tachycardia as well.[68] β-Adrenergic receptors have been labeled with the nonselective hydrophilic β-blocker ^{11}C-CGP-12177.[71, 97] Patients with hypertrophic cardiomyopathy demonstrated reduced β-adrenergic density, particularly in the anterior wall. There was no correlation between receptor density and wall thickness or myocardial blood flow. Circulating catecholamine concentrations were normal at the time of study, but it was concluded that myocardial β-receptors were down-regulated, possibly resulting from high intramyocardial catecholamine levels that were not reflected by systemic plasma levels.[97]

CARDIOMYOPATHIES ASSOCIATED WITH SYSTEMIC ILLNESSES

As indicated in Table 72–1, the diversity of causes of cardiomyopathy is great. Although the molecular basis of the underlying illness is understood for some causes (e.g., nutritional deficiency, endocrine disorders, glycogen storage diseases, hypertrophic cardiomyopathy, long-chain acyl-CoA dehydrogenase deficiency),[98] and in others metabolic studies have been extensive (e.g., alcoholic heart disease, diabetes), few have been studied with PET. Duchenne muscular dystrophy is a prototype of a systemic metabolic disease that has been studied with PET.[99]

Duchenne muscular dystrophy is an X-linked recessive disorder that affects approximately 3 of every 100,000 individuals in the United States. It is caused by an abnormality in the genetic coding for dystrophin, a protein found in the sarcolemma of normal skeletal muscle but absent in patients with Duchenne dystrophy.[100] Up to one third of cases occur in a nonfamilial pattern and are believed to arise from a spontaneous mutation.[101] The disease usually becomes clinically apparent during the second year of life with a gait disturbance. Musculoskeletal abnormalities are progressive, with death, often due to pulmonary insufficiency, occurring in the second decade of life from involvement of the diaphragm and the thoracic musculature. Cardiac involvement may be discovered relatively early owing to the detection of electrocardiographic abnormalities suggesting loss of electrically active tissue in the posterobasal region of the left ventricle.[102, 103] These abnormalities correlate closely with postmortem findings in which fibrosis is found to be most extensive in the same location. Cardiac arrhythmias are prominent, including a variety of atrial arrhythmias and conduction disturbances. The illness is unique in several aspects but particularly in its predilection for involvement of a specific cardiac anatomical locus.[104]

Positron Emission Tomographic Imaging

Positron emission tomographic study of patients with Duchenne muscular dystrophy was performed in the fasting state after the IV administration of ^{13}N-ammonia for the assessment of perfusion and ^{18}F-2-fluoro-2-deoxyglucose for the evaluation of regional uptake of glucose. Regional wall motion was assessed with gated blood pool imaging, and perfusion was assessed with planar ^{201}Tl scintigraphy. Abnormal regional wall motion was detected in only 20 percent of patients in the posterobasal, lateral, or inferolateral walls, or a combination. Defects in the posterobasal or lateral walls, which were indicated by reduced accumulation of thallium, were detected in 27 percent of patients. Abnormalities were observed significantly more frequently with PET. Abnormalities in the distribution of tracers were observed in 87 percent of patients using ^{13}N-ammonia and in 92 percent of patients who had a measurable accumulation of ^{18}F-2-fluoro-2-deoxyglucose in the heart. Accumulation of ^{13}N-ammonia was decreased and accumulation of ^{18}F-2-fluoro-2-deoxyglucose was increased in the posterobasal and lateral walls of the left ventricle, which are the zones of the left ventricle known to be most affected in this illness (Fig. 72–12). In patients with wall motion abnormalities and abnormalities seen on ^{201}Tl scintigraphy, there was concordance among all techniques.[99] Necropsy of a patient studied 2 years antemortem with PET demonstrated substantial fibrosis of the posterobasal and lateral walls of the left ventricle, with normal myocardium interspersed with areas of severe fibrosis. In addition, there were foci of fibrosis in remote, relatively normal portions of the left ventricle.[99]

The biochemical explanation for the tomographic abnormalities remains speculative. The observed pattern of decreased accumulation of ^{13}N-ammonia and increased accumulation of ^{18}F-2-fluoro-2-deoxyglucose in the posterobasal wall is typical of that observed in ischemic myocardium. However, there is no other evidence of ischemia in Duchenne muscular dystrophy. Specifically, the coronary anatomy is normal in patients who were evaluated postmortem, and there are generally no electrocardiographic abnormalities or symptoms to suggest ischemia. The decreased accumulation of ^{13}N-ammonia could be due to focal fibrosis, which decreases the number of myocytes capable of accumulating ^{13}N-ammonia. Alternatively, the fibrosis could impair myocardial perfusion and diffusion, contributing to the reduced accumulation of this tracer. There could be islands of effectively ischemic cells (despite normal epicardial coronary arteries) resulting from the focal fibrosis interfering with local substrate delivery, leading to an increased accumulation of ^{18}F-2-fluoro-2-deoxyglucose in residual viable myocardium. Alternatively, phosphorylation could be augmented because of abnormal adenylate cyclase or as a compensatory mechanism due to a primary defect in free fatty acid oxidation.[99] Last, there could be a primary abnormality of membrane permeability, permitting increased diffusion of ^{18}F-2-fluoro-2-deoxyglucose into myocytes.

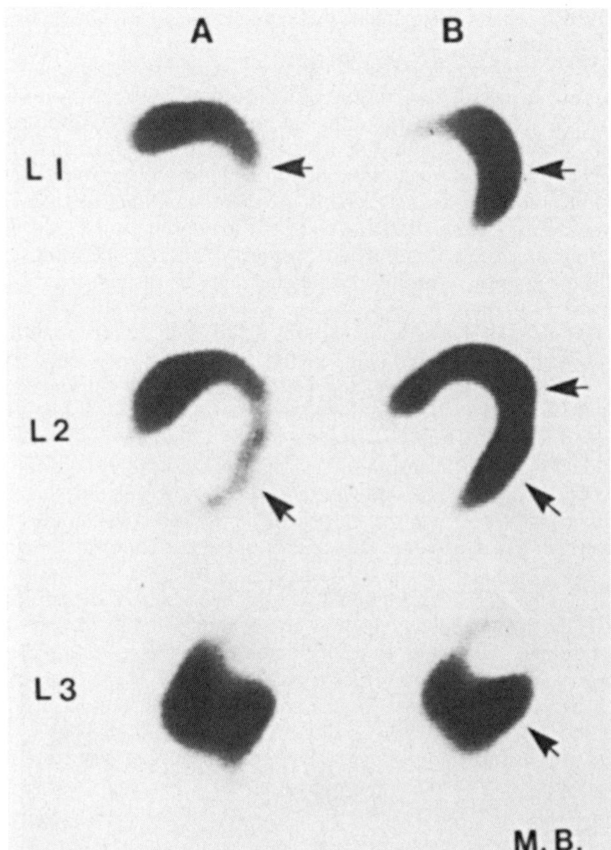

FIGURE 72–12. Regional accumulation of ^{13}N-ammonia *(A)* and ^{18}F-2-fluoro-2-deoxyglucose *(B)* in three contiguous PET transverse images of the heart in a patient with Duchenne muscular dystrophy. The images at the top are most basal and the ones at the bottom most apical. There is regionally decreased accumulation of ^{13}N-ammonia in the posterolateral region in L1 and L2 *(arrows, A)*, with relative excess accumulation of ^{18}F-2-fluoro-2-deoxyglucose in these same zones *(arrows, B)*. This patient had a moderate posterolateral thallium-201 (^{201}Tl) defect, posterolateral akinesis, and a left ventricular ejection fraction of 46 percent. (From Perloff, J.K., Henze, E., and Schelbert, H.R.: Alterations in regional myocardial metabolism, perfusion, and wall motion in Duchenne muscular dystrophy studied by radionuclide imaging. Circulation 69:33, 1984, with permission. Copyright 1984, American Heart Association)

Myotonic dystrophy is a common form of muscular dystrophy that demonstrates autosomal dominant inheritance.[106] Multiple clinical abnormalities are present in affected individuals, including frequent cardiac conduction system abnormalities and occasional abnormalities of left ventricular systolic performance in addition to the signature abnormalities of skeletal muscle.[107] Fibrosis and fatty infiltration of the myocardium and conductance system have been described.[108] Abnormalities have been mapped to chromosome 19, with alterations in the coding of the gene for a protein kinase.[109, 110]

Since myocardial involvement is common in this disorder, an abnormality of a gene coding for a protein kinase is the putative cause of the disease, and since abnormalities of glucose metabolism have been seen in brain and skeletal muscle,[111] quantitative analysis of myocardial glucose transport and utilization have been studied with dynamic PET and ^{18}F-2-fluoro-2-deoxyglucose in conjunction with the assessments of perfusion in patients with myotonic dystrophy and normal systolic function.[112] Myocardial perfusion (studied with ^{15}O-water and PET) was found to be normal in patients with myotonic dystrophy and comparable to that of control subjects. The rate constants k_1 and k_2, which describe forward and reverse transport of ^{18}F-2-fluoro-2-deoxyglucose across capillary and sarcolemmal membranes, were comparable between normal control subjects and patients with myotonic dystrophy and normal systolic performance. In contrast, k_3, which describes the rate of phosphorylation of ^{18}F-2-fluoro-2-deoxyglucose, was significantly reduced in patients when compared with controls (0.09 ± 0.07 vs 0.24 ± 0.21; $P = 0.03$). Overall glucose utilization was decreased as well (0.39 ± 0.2) compared with controls (0.64 ± 0.25, $P = 0.03$). The rate of glucose utilization and k_3 correlated inversely with the number of base pairs involved in the mutation ($r = -0.65$, $P = 0.03$; and $r = -0.85$, $P = 0.001$, respectively). Conversely, the PET-detectable metabolic abnormalities did not correlate with the electrocardiogram, echo or plasma substrate, or insulin levels. Similarly, abnormalities of myocardial glucose transport and utilization were unrelated to measured levels of myocardial perfusion. The association between the severity of abnormalities in the protein kinase gene and levels of metabolic abnormalities in the heart suggest a pathophysiologic link between the protein kinase and regulation of hexokinase in myocardium in patients with myotonic dystrophy.[112]

A number of defects in fatty acid oxidation have been recognized as causes of the metabolic derangements associated with cardiomyopathy and sudden death.[25] In a recent study of patients with long-chain acyl-CoA dehydrogenase deficiency, the myocardial metabolism of ^{11}C-palmitate and ^{11}C-acetate were evaluated in six patients and nine controls, including normal age-matched volunteers and heterozygous parents and siblings of the affected individuals. In normal subjects, the clearance kinetics of palmitate and acetate were nearly identical. In contrast, the affected individuals demonstrated reduced clearance of palmitate relative to acetate (Fig. 72–13). Accumulation and clearance of tracers was spatially uniform in the affected subjects. There was a spectrum of palmitate-to-acetate clearance ratios, with the greatest reduction of clearance of palmitate in the patients with the most severe clinical manifestation.[25] This study demonstrates that PET can provide detection of genetically determined defects in myocardial intermediary metabolism, can facilitate the understanding of the physiologic consequences of inborn errors of metabolism, and should permit the evaluation of metabolic and pharmacologic interventions in these illnesses.

Although there are a substantial number of additional systemic illnesses associated with dilated or hypertrophic cardiomyopathy, none has been studied with PET in a systematic fashion. In published studies, there are small groups with postpartum ($n = 3$) and alcoholic cardiomyopathy ($n = 4$), but in both conditions, the tomographic data acquired in the static mode after the administration of ^{11}C-palmitate were indistinguishable from the findings in other patients with dilated cardiomyopathy.[50] A single patient with sarcoidosis and dilated cardiomyopathy has been included in a previously published series.[50] In that patient, focal zones of reduced accumulation of ^{11}C-palmitate were observed in regions that were subsequently shown to represent confluent sarcoid granulomas and fibrosis when the patient was evaluated postmortem several months after tomography.

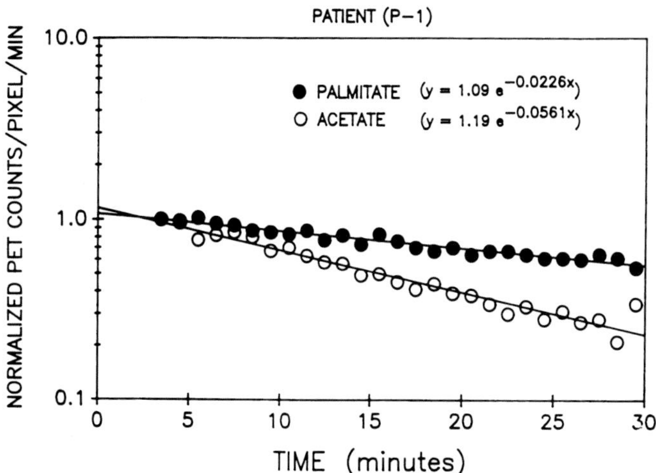

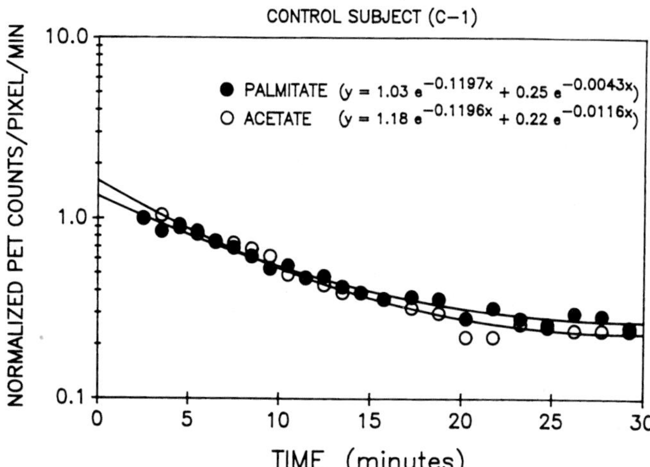

FIGURE 72–13. Representative myocardial time-activity curves from patient with long-chain acyl coenzyme A (acyl-CoA) dehydrogenase deficiency (P-1) *(top)* and from age-matched control subject (C-1) *(bottom)*. In these examples, curves are best fit by monoexponential function for patient data and by biexponential function for control subject data. Myocardial biologic half-time (after correction for isotope decay) for patient data is 12.4 minutes for acetate and 30.7 minutes for palmitate (rate of clearance [k_1] for acetate is 0.0561 min^{-1}; k_1 for palmitate is 0.0226 min^{-1}; and the k_1 ratio is 0.4). For data from the control subject, the biologic half-time for both acetate and palmitate is 5.8 minutes (k_1 for acetate is 0.1196 min^{-1}; k_1 for palmitate is 0.1197 min^{-1}; and the k_1 ratio is 1). PET = positron emission tomography. (From Kelly, D., Mendelsohn, N.J., Sobel, B.E., et al.: Detection and assessment of positron emission tomography of a genetically determined defect in myocardial fatty acid utilization [long-chain acyl-CoA dehydrogenase deficiency]. Am. J. Cardiol. 71:738, 1993, with permission.)

FUTURE DIRECTIONS

Studies of patients with dilated or hypertrophic cardiomyopathy have provided a greater understanding of some of the abnormalities of myocardial perfusion and metabolism associated with these diverse illnesses and have provided techniques for the differentiation of patients with ischemic and nonischemic dilated cardiomyopathy. Recently, several new radiopharmaceuticals have been developed that have already added substantially to our diagnostic armamentarium. ^{11}C-acetate is such a compound and is avidly extracted by myocardium and subsequently enters the citric acid cycle. In studies in experimental animals, the clearance of radioactivity from the heart after administration of ^{11}C-acetate correlated closely with ^{11}C-carbon dioxide production and myocardial oxygen consumption over a wide range of cardiac workloads.[45, 47] The correlation between ^{11}C-acetate kinetics and myocardial oxygen consumption was not affected by circulating levels of free fatty acids or glucose.[46, 47] In normal subjects, clearance of ^{11}C-acetate was homogeneous throughout the left ventricle and was augmented homogeneously by increased cardiac work induced by administration of catecholamines or dynamic exercise.[38] There was a close correlation between accelerated clearance of ^{11}C-acetate and an increased double product, an indicator of myocardial oxygen consumption.[38] The availability of this marker of oxidative metabolism is already allowing a more complete understanding of the metabolism of patients with cardiomyopathy in whom complex abnormalities of intermediary metabolism are expected. Thus, in a single patient, carbohydrate, fatty acid, and citric acid cycle flux can all be evaluated under similar conditions. As amino acids labeled with positron emitters become available, protein turnover may be evaluated as well.[105]

The addition of markers of sympathetic nervous system activity such as ^{11}C-m-hydroxyephedrine[67] and ^{11}C-CGP-12177[97] may prove of great importance in furthering the understanding of many of the cardiomyopathies, particularly hypertrophic cardiomyopathy, as they become more widely available.[69] The availability of antimyosin Fab subunits,[113] which may ultimately be labeled with positron emitters, should help in the assessment of inflammatory cardiomyopathies in which myocyte necrosis plays a significant part. Assessments of the relative roles of hypoperfusion and ischemia in the pathogenesis and clinical presentation of dilated and hypertrophic cardiomyopathies should be facilitated by the use of newly validated techniques for the assessment of myocardial perfusion with flow markers that are independent of the metabolic activity of the tissue, such as ^{15}O-water,[114–116] and the recent development of selective markers of hypoxic myocardium, such as ^{18}F-misonidazole.[117]

References

1. Neeley, J.R., Novetto, M.J., and Oram, J.F.: Myocardial utilization of carbohydrate and lipids. Prog. Cardiovasc. Dis. 15:289, 1972.
2. Fox, K.A.A., Abendschein, D.R., Ambos, D., et al.: Efflux of metabolized and nonmetabolized fatty acid from canine myocardium. Circ. Res. 57:232, 1985.
3. Rose, C.P., and Goretsky, C.A.: Constraints on the uptake of labeled palmitate by the heart. The barriers at the capillary and sarcolemmal surfaces and the control of intracellular sequestration. Circ. Res. 41:534, 1977.
4. Opie, L.H.: Metabolism of the heart in health and disease. Part I. Am. Heart J. 76:685, 1968.
5. Scheuer, J., and Brachfeld, N.: Myocardial uptake and fractional distribution of palmitate-1-C^{14} by the ischemic dog heart. Metabolism 15:945, 1966.
6. Bremer, J.: Carnitine in intermediary metabolism. The metabolism of fatty acid esters of carnitine by mitochondria. J. Biol. Cham. 237:3628, 1962.
7. Pande, S.V.: A mitochondrial carnitive acylcarnitine translocase system. Proc. Natl. Acad. Sci. U.S.A. 72:883, 1975.
8. Bremer, J., and Hokland, B.: Role of carnitine-dependent metabolic pathways in heart disease without primary ischemia. Z. Kardiol. 76(Suppl. 5):9, 1987.
9. Beanlands, R.S., Bach, D.S., Raylman, R., et al.: Acute effects of dobutamine on myocardial oxygen consumption and cardiac efficiency measured using carbon-11 acetate kinetics in patients with dilated cardiomyopathy. J. Am. Coll. Cardiol. 22:1389, 1993.
10. Cannon, R.O., III, Rosing, D.R., Maron, B.J., et al.: Myocardial ischemia in patients with hypertrophic cardiomyopathy: Contribution of inadequate vasodilator reserve and elevated left ventricular filling pressures. Circulation 71:234, 1985.
11. Inoue, T., Sakai, Y., Morooka, S., et al.: Coronary flow reserve in patients with dilated cardiomyopathy. Am. Heart J. 125:93, 1993.
12. Neglia, D., Parodi, O., Sambuceti, G., et al.: Early impairment of coronary microvascular function in dilated cardiomyopathy. J. Am. Coll. Cardiol. 160A, 1994.
13. Opherk, D., Schwarz, F., Mall, G., et al.: Coronary dilatory capacity in idiopathic dilated cardiomyopathy: Analysis of 16 patients. Am. J. Cardiol. 51:1657, 1983.
14. Pasternac, A., Noble, J., Streulens, Y., et al.: Pathophysiology of chest pain in patients with cardiomyopathies and normal coronary arteries. Circulation 65:778, 1982.
15. Levine, T.B., Francis, G.S., Goldsmith, S.R., et al.: Activity of the sympathetic nervous system and renin-angiotensin system assessed by plasma hormone levels and their relation to hemodynamic abnormalities in congestive heart failure. Am. J. Cardiol. 49:1659, 1982.
16. Packer, M.: Neurohormonal interactions and adaptations in congestive heart failure. Circulation 77:721, 1988.
17. Post, R.L., Morgan, H.E., and Park, C.R.: Regulation of glucose uptake in muscle. III. The interaction of membrane transport and phosphorylation in the control of glucose uptake. J. Biol. Chem. 236:269, 1961.
18. Opie, L.H.: Metabolism of the heart in health and disease. Part III. Am. Heart J. 767:383, 1969.
19. Bing, R.J.: Metabolic activity of intact heart. Am. J. Med. 30:679, 1961.
20. Henry, P.D., Eckberg, D., Gault, H.J., et al.: Depressed inotropic state and reduced myocardial oxygen consumption in the human heart. Am. J. Cardiol. 31:300, 1973.
21. Schwartz, A., Sordahl, L.A., Entman, M.L., et al.: Abnormal biochemistry in myocardial failure. Am. J. Cardiol. 32:407, 1973.
22. Schwartz, A., Lindenmayer, G.E., and Harigaya, S.: Respiratory control and calcium transport in heart mitochondria from the cardiomyopathic Syrian hamster. Trans. N.Y. Acad. Sci. 30(Suppl. II):951, 1968.
23. Sobel, B.E., Spann, J.R., Jr., Pool, P.E., et al.: Normal oxidative phosphorylation in mitochondria from the failing heart. Circ. Res. 21:355, 1967.
24. Chidsey, C.A., Weinbach, E.C., Pool, P.E., et al.: Biochemical studies of energy production in the failing human heart. J. Clin. Invest. 45:40, 1966.
25. Kelly, D.P., Mendelsohn, N.J., Sobel, B.E., et al.: Detection and assessment of positron emission tomography of a genetically determined defect in myocardial fatty acid utilization (long-chain acyl-CoA dehydrogenase deficiency). Am. J. Cardiol. 71:738, 1993.
26. Pool, P.E., Spann, J.R., Jr., Buiccino, R.A., et al.: Myocardial high energy phosphate stores in cardiac hypertrophy and heart failure. Circ. Res. 21:365, 1967.
27. Alpert, N.R., and Gordon, M.S.: Myofibrillar adenosine triphosphate activity in congestive failure. Am. J. Physiol. 202:940, 1962.
28. Draper, M., Taylor, N., and Alpert, N.R.: Alteration in contractile protein in hypertrophied guinea pig hearts. *In* Alpert, N. (ed.): Cardiac Hypertrophy. New York, Academic Press, 1971, pp. 313–331.
29. Luchi, R.J., Dritcher, E.M., and Thyrum, P.T.: Reduced cardiac myosin adenosine triphosphate activity in dogs with spontaneously occurring heart failure. Circ. Res. 24:5133, 1969.
30. Conway, M.A., Allis, J., Ouwerkerk, R., et al.: Detection of low phosphocreatine to ATP ratio in failing hypertrophied human myocardium by ^{31}P magnetic resonance spectroscopy. Lancet 338:973, 1991.
31. Auffermann, W., Chew, W.M., Wolfe, C.L., et al.: Normal and diffusely abnormal myocardium in humans: Functional and metabolic characterization with P-31 MR spectroscopy and cine MR imaging. Radiology 179:253, 1991.
32. Schaefer, S., Gober, J.R., Schwartz, G.G., et al.: In vivo phosphorus-31 spectroscopic imaging in patients with global myocardial disease. Am. J. Cardiol. 65:1154, 1990.
33. Whitman, G.J.R., Chance, B., Bode, H., et al.: Diagnosis and therapeutic evaluation of a pediatric case of cardiomyopathy using phosphorus-31 nuclear magnetic resonance spectroscopy. J. Am. Coll. Cardiol. 5:745, 1985.
34. Dzau, V.J., Pratt, R., and Gibbons, G.H.: Angiotensin as local modulating factor in ventricular dysfunction and failure due to coronary artery disease. Drugs 45(Suppl. 4):1, 1994.
35. Hasking, G.J., Esler, M.D., Jennings, G.L., et al.: Norepinephrine spillover to plasma in patients with congestive heart failure. Evidence of increased overall and cardiorenal sympathetic nervous activity. Circulation 73:615, 1986.
36. Haneda, T., Miura, Y., Miytazawa, K., et al.: Plasma norepinephrine concentration in the coronary sinus in cardiomyopathies. Catheter Cardiovasc. Diagn. 4:399, 1978.
37. Kawai, C., Yui, Y., Hoshino, T., et al.: Myocardial catecholamines in hypertrophic and dilated (congestive) cardiomyopathy: A biopsy study. J. Am. Coll. Cardiol. 2:834, 1983.
38. Henes, C.G., Bergmann, S.R., Walsh, M.N., et al.: Assessment of myocardial oxidative metabolic reserve with positron emission tomography and carbon-11-acetate. J. Nucl. Med. 30:1489, 1989.
39. Bing, R.J.: Cardiac metabolism: Its contribution to alcoholic heart disease and myocardial failure. Circulation 58:965, 1978.
40. Merhige, M.E., Ekas, R., Mossberg, K., et al.: Catecholamine stimulation, substrate competition, and myocardial glucose uptake in conscious dogs assessed with positron emission tomography. Circ. Res. 61(Suppl. II):II124, 1987.
41. Tripp, M.E., Katcher, M.I., Peters, H.A., et al.: Systemic carnitine deficiency presenting as familial endocardial fibroelastosis. N. Engl. J. Med. 305:385, 1981.
42. Geltman, E.M., Smith, J.L., Beecher, D., et al.: Altered regional myocardial metabolism in congestive cardiomyopathy detected by positron tomography. Am. J. Med. 74:773, 1983.
43. Schelbert, H.R., Henze, E., Sochor, H., et al.: Effects of substrate availability on myocardial C-11 palmitate kinetics by positron emission tomography in normal subjects and patients with ventricular dysfunction. Am. Heart J. 111:1055, 1986.
44. Sochor, H., Schelbert, H.R., Schwaiger, M., et al.: Studies of fatty acid metabolism with positron emission tomography in patients with cardiomyopathy. Eur. J. Nucl. Med. 12(Suppl.):s66, 1986.
45. Brown, M., Marshall, D.R., Sobel, B.E., et al.: Delineation of myocardial oxygen utilization with carbon-11-labeled acetate. Circulation 76:687, 1987.
46. Brown, M.A., Myears, D.W., and Bergmann, S.R.: Validity of estimates of myocardial oxidative metabolism with carbon-11-acetate and positron emission tomography despite altered patterns of substrate utilization. J. Nucl. Med. 30:187, 1989.
47. Buxton, D.B., Schwaiger, M., Nguyen, A., et al.: Radiolabeled acetate as a tracer of myocardial tricarboxylic acid cycle flux. Circ. Res. 63:628, 1988.
48. Merlet, P., Mazoyer, B., Hittinger, L., et al.: Assessment of coronary reserve in man: Comparison between positron emission tomography with oxygen-15–labeled water and intracoronary Doppler technique. J. Nucl. Med. 34:1899, 1993.
49. Abraham, S., Fischman, A., and Alpert, N.: Regional heterogeneity of myocardial blood flow in humans with dilated cardiomyopathy. J. Nucl. Med. 35:23P, 1994.
50. Eisenberg, J.D., Sobel, B.E., and Geltman, E.M.: Differentiation of ischemic from nonischemic cardiomyopathy with positron emission tomography. Am. J. Cardiol. 49:1310, 1987.
51. Bulkley, B.H., Hutchins, G.M., Bailey, I., et al.: Thallium-201 imaging and gated cardiac blood pool scans in patients with ischemic and idiopathic congestive cardiomyopathy. A clinical and pathologic study. Circulation 55:753, 1977.
52. Boucher, C.A., Fallon, J.T., Johnson, R.A., et al.: Cardiomyopathic syndrome caused by coronary artery disease. III. Prospective clinico-pathological study of its prevalence among patients with clinically unexplained chronic heart failure. Br. Heart J. 41:613, 1979.
53. Berry, J.J., Hoffman, J.M., Steenbergen, C., et al.: Human pathologic correlation with PET in ischemic and nonischemic cardiomyopathy. J. Nucl. Med. 34:39, 1993.
54. Schuster, E.H., and Bulkley, B.H.: Ischemic cardiomyopathy: A clinicopathologic study of fourteen patients. Am. Heart J. 100:506, 1980.
55. Cannon, R.O., III, Leon, M.B., Watson, R.M., et al.: Chest pain and "normal" coronary arteries: Role of small coronary arteries. Am. J. Cardiol. 55:50b, 1985.
56. Geltman, E.M., Henes, C.G., Senneff, M.J., et al.: Increased myocardial perfusion at rest and diminished perfusion reserve in patients with angina and angiographically normal coronary arteries. J. Am. Coll. Cardiol. 16:586, 1990.
57. Eichhorn, E.J., Kosinski, E.J., Lewis, S.M., et al.: Usefulness of dipyridamole-thallium-201 perfusion scanning for distinguishing ischemic from nonischemic cardiomyopathy. Am. J. Cardiol. 62:945, 1988.
58. Tauberg, S.G., Orie, J.E., Bartlett, B.E., et al.: Usefulness of thallium-201 for

distinction of ischemic from idiopathic dilated cardiomyopathy. Am. J. Cardiol. 71:674, 1993.

59. Glamann, D.B., Lange, R.A., Corbett, J.R., et al.: Utility of various radionuclide techniques for distinghishing ischemic from nonischemic dilated cardiomyopathy. Arch. Intern. Med. 152:769, 1992.
60. Vaghaiwalla Mody, F., Brunken, R.C., Warner Stevenson, L., et al.: Differentiating cardiomyopathy of coronary artery disease from nonischemic dilated cardiomyopathy utilizing positron emission tomography. J. Am. Coll. Cardiol. 17:373, 1991.
61. Fujita, N., Duerinekx, A.J., and Higgins, C.B.: Variation in left ventricular regional wall stress with cine magnetic resonance imaging: Normal subjects versus dilated cardiomyopathy. Am. Heart J. 125:1337, 1993.
62. Doherty, N.E., III, Seelos, K.C., Suzuki, J., et al.: Application of cine nuclear magnetic resonance imaging for sequential evaluation of response to angiotensin-converting enzyme inhibitor therapy in dilated cardiomyopathy. J. Am. Coll. Cardiol. 19:1294, 1992.
63. Geltman, E.M., Eisenberg, J.D., Keim, S., et al.: Comparative magnetic resonance imaging and positron emission tomography in cardiomyopathy. J. Am. Coll. Cardiol. 5:436, 1985.
64. Feinendegen, L.E., Vyska, K., Freundlieb, C., et al.: Noninvasive analysis of metabolic reactions in body tissues: The case of myocardial fatty acids. Eur. J. Nucl. Med. 6:191, 1981.
65. Hock, A., Freundlieb, C., Vyska, K., et al.: Myocardial imaging and metabolic studies with [17-^{123}I]iodoheptadecanoic acid in patients with idiopathic congestive cardiomyopathy. J. Nucl. Med. 24:22, 1983.
66. Ugolini, V., Hansen, C.L., Kulkarni, V., et al.: Abnormal myocardial fatty acid metabolism in dilated cardiomyopathy detected by iodine-123 phenylpentadecanoic acid and tomographic imaging. Am. J. Cardiol. 62:923, 1988.
67. Haka, M.S., Rosenspire, K.C., Gildersleeve, D.L., et al.: Synthesis of [C-11]-m-hydroxyephedrine (HED) for neuronal cardiac imaging. (Abstract.) J. Nucl. Med. 30:783, 1989.
68. Maeno, M., Ishida, Y., Hirose, Y., et al.: Characteristics of I-123 MIBG myocardial images in patients with idiopathic dilated cardiomyopathy and tachyarrhythmia. J. Nucl. Med. 35:81P, 1994.
69. Melon, P., and Schwaiger, M.: Imaging of metabolism and autonomic innervation of the heart by positron emission tomography. Eur. J. Nucl. Med. 19:453, 1992.
70. Merlet, P., Pouillart, F., Dubois-Rande, J.L., et al.: Improved adrenergic nerve function in human failing heart after beta-blocking therapy. J. Nucl. Med. 35:81P, 1994.
71. Merlet, P., Delforge, J., Synrota, A., et al.: Positron emission tomography with 11C CGP-12177 to assess beta-adrenergic receptor concentration in idiopathic dilated cardiomyopathy. Circulation 87:1169, 1993.
72. Mitrani, R.D., Klein, L.S., and Miles, W.M., et al.: Regional cardiac sympathetic denervation in patients with ventricular tachycardia in the absence of coronary artery disease. J. Am. Coll. Cardiol. 22:1344, 1993.
73. Shaver, J.A., Salerni, B., Curtiss, E.I., et al.: Clinical presentation and noninvasive evaluation of the patient with hypertrophic cardiomyopathy. Cardiovasc. Clin. 19:149, 1988.
74. Maron, B.J., and Mulvihill, J.J.: The genetics of hypertrophic cardiomyopathy. Ann. Intern. Med. 105:610, 1986.
75. Dufour, C., Causse, E., Fetler, L., et al.: Identification of a mutation near a functional site of the beta cardiac myosin heavy chain gene in a family with hypertrophic cardiomyopathy. J. Mol. Cell. Cardiol. 26:1241, 1994.
76. Watkins, H., MacRae, C., Thierfelder, L., et al.: A disease locus for familial hypertrophic cardiomyopathy maps to chromosome lq3. Nat. Genet. 3(4):333, 1993.
77. Symons, C., Olsen, E.G.J., and Hawkey, C.: Association of hyperthyroidism with hypertrophic cardiomyopathy. *In* Sekiguchi, M., and Olsen, E.G.J. (eds.): Cardiomyopathy: Clinical, Pathological and Theoretical Aspects. Tokyo, University of Tokyo Press, 1980, pp. 369–373.
78. Olsen, E.G.J., Symons, C., and Hawkey, C.M.: The effect of triac and propranolol and the developing myocardium in rats. Br. Heart J. 40:1068, 1978.
79. McKenna, W.J., and Kleinebenne, A.: Hypertrophic cardiomyopathy in the elderly. *In* Coodley, E.L. (ed.): Geriatric Heart Disease. Littleton, MA, PSG Publishing, 1985, pp. 260–268.
80. Whiting, R.B., Powell, W.J., Dinsmore, R.E., et al.: Idiopathic hypertrophic subaortic stenosis. N. Engl. J. Med. 285:196, 1971.
81. Gach, J.V., Andriange, M., and Franck, G.: Hypertrophic obstructive cardiomyopathy and Friedreich's ataxia. Am. J. Cardiol. 27:436, 1971.
82. Thompson, D.S., Naqvi, N., Juul, S.M., et al.: Effects of propranolol on myocardial oxygen consumption, substrate extraction, and haemodynamics in hypertrophic obstructive cardiomyopathy. Br. Heart J. 44:488, 1980.
83. Brush, J.E., Jr., Eisenhofer, G., Garty, M., et al.: Cardiac norepinephrine kinetics in hypertrophic cardiomyopathy. Circulation 79:836, 1989.
84. Grover-McKay, M., Schwaiger, M., Krivokapich, J., et al.: Regional myocardial blood flow and metabolism at rest in mildly symptomatic patients with hypertrophic cardiomyopathy. J. Am. Coll. Cardiol. 13:317, 1989.
85. Camici, P., Chiriatti, G., Lorenzoni, R., et al.: Coronary vasodilation is impaired in both hypertrophied and nonhypertrophied myocardium of patients with hypertrophic cardiomyopathy: A study with nitrogen-13 ammonia and positron emission tomography. J. Am. Coll. Cardiol. 17:879, 1991.
86. Nienaber, C.A., Gambhir, S.S., Vaghaiwalla, F., et al.: Regional myocardial blood flow and glucose utilization in symptomatic patients with hypertrophic cardiomyopathy. Circulation 87:1580, 1993.
87. Perroni-Filardi, P., Bacharach, S.L., and Dilsizian, V.: Regional systolic function, myocardial blood flow and glucose uptake at rest in hypertrophic cardiomyopathy. Am. J. Cardiol. 72:199, 1993.
88. Yoshida, K., Endo, M., Himi, T., et al.: Measurement of regional myocardial blood flow in hypertrophic cardiomyopathy: Application of the first-pass flow model using [^{13}N] ammonia and PET. Am. J. Physiol. Imaging 4:97, 1989.
89. Gistri, R., Cecchi, F., Choudhury, L., et al.: Effect of verapamil on absolute myocardial blood flow in hypertrophic cardiomyopathy. Am. J. Cardiol. 74:363, 1994.
90. Kagaya, Y., Ishide, N., Takeyama, D., et al.: Differences in myocardial fluoro-18 2-deoxyglucose uptake in young versus older patients with hypertrophic cardiomyopathy. Am. J. Cardiol. 69:242, 1992.
91. Maruno, H., Ishiwata, S., Senda, M., et al.: Myocardial metabolism in hypertrophic cardiomyopathy assessed by C-11 acetate, F-18 FDG and I-123 BMIPP. J. Nucl. Med. 35:110P, 1994.
92. Tadamura, E., Tamaki, N., Matsumori, A., et al.: Impaired oxidative and glucose metabolism in hypertrophic cardiomyopathy assessed by PET using C-11 acetate and FDG. J. Nucl. Med. 35:110P, 1994.
93. Takeishi, Y., Chiba, J., Abe, S., et al.: Heterogeneous myocardial distribution of iodine-123 15-(p-iodophenyl)-3-R,S-methylpentadecanoic acid (BMIPP) in patients with hypertrophic cardiomyopathy. Eur. J. Nucl. 19:775, 1992.
94. Kurata, C., Tawarahara, K., Taguchi, T., et al.: Myocardial emission computed tomography with iodine-123-labeled beta-methyl-branched fatty acid in patients with hypertrophic cardiomyopathy. J. Nucl. Med. 33:6, 1992.
95. Sakuma, H., Takeda, K., Tagami, T., et al.: ^{31}P MR spectroscopy in hypertrophic cardiomyopathy: Comparison with Tl-201 myocardial perfusion imaging.
96. Shimizu, M., Sugihara, N., Kita, Y., et al.: Long-term course and cardiac sympathetic nerve activity in patients with hypertrophic cardiomyopathy. Br. Heart J. 67:155, 1992.
97. Lefroy, D.C., de Silva, R., and Choudhury, L.: Diffuse reduction of myocardial beta-adrenoceptors in hypertrophic cardiomyopathy: A study with positron emission tomography. J. Am. Coll. Cardiol. 22:1653, 1993.
98. Schwartz, K., Carrier, L., Guicheney, P., et al.: Molecular basis of familial cardiomyopathies. Circulation 91:532, 1991.
99. Perloff, J.K., Henze, E., and Schelbert, H.R.: Alterations in regional myocardial metabolism, perfusion, and wall motion in Duchenne muscular dystrophy studied by radionuclide imaging. Circulation 69:33, 1984.
100. Ervasti, J.M., Ohlendieck, K., Kahl, S.C., et al.: Deficiency of a glycoprotein component of the dystrophin complex in dystrophic muscle. Nature 345:315, 1990.
101. Brooks, M.H.: A Clinician's View of Neuromuscular Diseases. Baltimore, Williams & Wilkins, 1979.
102. Slucka, C.: The electrocardiogram in Duchenne progressive muscular dystrophy. Circulation 38:933, 1968.
103. Perloff, J.K.: Cardiac involvement in heredofamilial neuromyopathic diseases. Cardiovasc. Clin. 4:334, 1972.
104. Perloff, J.K.: Pathogenesis of hypertrophic cardiomyopathy: Hypothesis and speculation. Am. Heart J. 14:219, 1981.
105. Henze, E., Schelbert, H.R., Barrio, J.R., et al.: Evaluation of myocardial metabolism with N-13 and C-11-labeled amino acids and positron computed tomography. J. Nucl. Med. 23:671, 1982.
106. Harper, P.: Myotonic Dystrophy: Major Problems in Neurology, Vol. 9. Philadelphia, W.B. Saunders, 1979.
107. Hawley, R.J., Milner, M.R., Gottdiener, S., et al.: Myotonic heart disease: A clinical follow-up. Neurology 41:259, 1991.
108. Nguyen, H.H., Wolfe, J.T., Holmes, D.R., et al.: Pathology of the cardiac conduction system in myotonic dystrophy: A study of 12 cases. J. Am. Coll. Cardiol. 11:662, 1988.
109. Harley, H.G., Brook, J.O., Rundle, S.A., et al.: Expansion of an unstable DNA region and phenotypic variation in myotonic dystrophy. Nature 355:545, 1992.
110. Buxton, J., Shelbourne, P., Davies, J., et al.: Detection of an unstable fragment of DNA specific to individuals with myotonic dystrophy. Nature 355:547, 1992.
111. Fiorelli, M., Duboc, O., Mazoyer, B.M., et al.: Decreased cerebral glucose utilization in myotonic dystrophy. Neurology 42:91, 1992.
112. Annane, D., Duboc, D., Mazoyer, B., et al.: Correlation between decreased myocardial glucose phosphorylation and the DNA mutation size in myotonic dystrophy. Circulation 90:2629, 1994.
113. Matsumori, A., Ohkusa, T., Matoba, Y., et al.: Myocardial uptake of antimyosin monoclonal antibody in a murine model of viral myocarditis. Circulation 79:400, 1989.
114. Bergmann, S.R., Herrero, P., Markham, J., et al.: Noninvasive quantitation of myocardial blood flow in human subjects with oxygen-15 labeled water and positron emission tomography. J. Am. Coll. Cardiol. 14:639, 1989.
115. Herrero, P., Markham, J., Myears, D.W., et al.: Measurement of myocardial blood flow with positron emission tomography: Correction for count spillover and partial volume effects. Math. Comput. Modeling 11:807, 1988.
116. Walsh, M.N., Geltman, E.M., Steele, R.L., et al.: Delineation of impaired regional perfusion by positron emission tomography with $H_2{}^{15}O$. Circulation 78:612, 1988.
117. Shelton, M.E., Dence, C.S., Hwang, D.-R., et al.: Myocardial kinetics of fluorine-18 misonidazole: A marker of hypoxic myocardium. J. Nucl. Med. 30:351, 1989.

CHAPTER

73 Positron Emission Tomography: Evaluation of Cardiac Receptors and Neuronal Function

André Syrota, M.D., Ph.D.
Pascal Merlet, M.D.

The rate and force of contraction of myocardial cells are modulated in large part by the action of autonomic neurons, which release neurotransmitters into the synaptic cleft at the neuromuscular junction. Specific molecular neurotransmitters interact with receptors on the myocardial cell surface membranes, including β- and α-adrenergic, muscarinic cholinergic, and peripheral-type benzodiazepine receptors. Receptors are membrane proteins or glycoproteins that have a high molecular affinity and selectivity for specific ligands. The binding of a neurotransmitter, or a drug, to the specific receptor site results in the opening and closing of ion channels, brought about by conformational changes of the membrane. Presynaptic neurons remove norepinephrine from the synaptic cleft and thereby terminate adrenergic action on the heart. Impairment of this process increases synaptic norepinephrine levels.[1, 2] This alteration, in association with abnormally high blood levels of norepinephrine or increased release of norepinephrine from presynaptic vesicles into the synapses of myocytes, may cause cardiac hypertrophy, myocyte calcium overload, arrhythmias, or desensitization of β-adrenergic receptors.

Normal functioning of the heart requires precise timing of atrial and ventricular contractions and a force of contraction appropriate for the energy needs of the body. Cardiac neurotransmission, especially that of the adrenergic receptor pathway, is impaired in heart disease and is the site of action of many cardiac medications. In patients with heart failure, abnormal innervation contributes to arrhythmogenesis[3, 4] and to progression of cardiac dysfunction. The prognosis of these patients depends on the degree of left ventricular dysfunction present and on the presence of ventricular arrhythmias. Sudden death from arrhythmias is still a common outcome in patients suffering from heart failure, ischemic heart disease, or primary hypertrophic cardiomyopathy; it may even reveal the presence of previously undiscovered arrhythmia. Altered adrenergic neurotransmission is also involved in the pathogenesis of arrhythmias due to idiopathic ventricular tachycardias, long-QT syndrome, or arrhythmogenic right ventricular cardiomyopathy. Therefore, the possibility of assessing the global and regional adrenergic activities of the heart is potentially of great pathophysiologic and clinical interest.

Receptor abnormalities have been documented in myocardial samples obtained by means of endomyocardial biopsy or during surgery or autopsy. Positron emission tomography (PET) now enables physicians to obtain noninvasively quantitative determination of regional receptor density and affinity in humans, as well as innervation integrity and function. These measurements are based on the synthesis of a radioligand, usually either a selective receptor antagonist or a false neurotransmitter labeled with a positron-emitting radioisotope. Mathematical compartmental models are fitted to activity-versus-time curves obtained during saturation or displacement experiments to calculate the rate constants and the receptor density in meaningful regions of interest selected in the myocardium. Several receptor classes—adrenergic, muscarinic cholinergic, and peripheral-type benzodiazepine—have thus been characterized in humans. PET has been used to evaluate changes in cardiac innervation.

ADRENERGIC NEUROTRANSMISSION OF THE HEART

Norepinephrine is synthesized in neuronal cell bodies and is transported over a period of several days through axonal microtubules to distal neuronal varicosities, where it is stored in large (75 to 95 nm) and small (45 to 55 nm) vesicles.[5] The large vesicles store norepinephrine, adenosine triphosphatase (ATPase), chromatogranin A, opioid peptides, dopamine β-hydroxylase, synapsin I, calmodulin, and neuropeptide Y. The small vesicles store norepinephrine. The amount of norepinephrine is greatest at the base of the heart and decreases progressively to the apex, corresponding to the number of adrenergic neurons.[6]

The large vesicles contain 10 times more norepinephrine than the small vesicles, and they release it during intense sympathetic activity. A single nerve impulse results in the emptying of only 30 to 40 percent of the norepinephrine content of a vesicle.[7] The prejunctional sympathetic neuronal membrane contains receptors that regulate the concentration of norepinephrine in the junctional cleft.[8, 9] Prejunctional α_2-adrenergic receptors inhibit the further release of norepinephrine when activated by norepinephrine in the junctional synaptic cleft, thereby exerting negative feedback on norepinephrine release.[9, 10] Prejunctional inhibitory muscarinic receptors (M_3 receptors), dopamine receptors, and adenosine subtype receptors (A_1-receptors), as well as histamine (H_2) and 5-hydroxytryptamine (serotonin) receptors, also inhibit norepinephrine release.[10–13] Two presynaptic receptors facilitate the release of norepinephrine: the angiotensin II receptor and the presynaptic β_2-receptor.[14, 15]

As much as 80 percent of the released norepinephrine is taken back into presynaptic nerve endings by an active transport mechanism (called uptake-1) and is returned to storage granules, from which it can be released again.[16] The uptake-1 system of adrenergic neurons is sodium- and ATP-dependent and is inhibited by cocaine, amphetamines, and some tricyclic antidepressant drugs; the uptake-2 system is far less specific and involves simple diffusion of norepinephrine.[17, 18] The neuronal norepinephrine uptake system is the principal means of terminating the action of norepinephrine. Impairment of this process results in excessive myocardial stimulation by norepinephrine, which arrives at the synapse via adrenergic nerve terminals or via coronary blood flow.

Acting through adrenergic receptors, norepinephrine increases the rate and force of contraction of the heart.[19, 20] Adrenergic receptors include the α_1- and α_2-, β_1-, β_2-, and β_3-adrenergic classes. These classes may be subdivided into subtypes, such as α_{2A} and α_{2B}, α_{1A} and α_{1B}, and others.[21–26]

The α_2-, β_1-, β_2-, and β_3-adrenergic receptors are characterized by seven helices in their structure, and in this respect they are similar to muscarinic cholinergic receptors as well as rhodopsin, the retinal color opsin; three subtypes of serotonin receptors; and substance K–receptors.[27, 28] The seven-helix receptors are attached to the cell membrane and bind ligands in the extracellular space, transducing signals through the action of one or more cytoplasmic guanosine triphosphate-binding proteins, called G proteins.

β_1-Receptors have equal affinity for both epinephrine and norepinephrine, while β_2-receptors have a higher affinity for epinephrine than for norepinephrine.[23] β_2-Receptors are involved in the control of heart rate, whereas the β_1-receptors affect both the rate and the force of cardiac contraction.[23] The widespread distribution of β-adrenergic receptors in the ventricles reflects the fact that sympathetic nerves affect all regions of the heart.[29, 30]

β_1-Adrenergic receptors are the predominant β-adrenergic receptors in the human myocardium (about 80 percent are β_1- and 20 percent are β_2-adrenergic receptors).[21, 31, 32] β_2-Receptors have also been found in the human heart, especially in the atria.[33–35] The presence of β_3-subtypes in the myocardium has been recently suggested.[36] The density of β-adrenoceptors in the heart is greater in the apex of the left ventricle than in the base[37, 38] and in the subepicardial layer than in the subendocardial layer.[39]

All subtypes of adrenergic receptors are activated during exercise.[32, 40] If β-receptors are deficient, as in heart failure, the responsiveness to catecholamine stimulation is blunted.[41]

The interaction of norepinephrine, or agonist medications, with β-receptors results in a cascade of molecular events that increase intracellular cyclic 3′,5′-adenosine monophosphate (cyclic AMP), the second messenger.[22, 42] Several proteins mediate transduction of the neurotransmitter messages. One of these proteins, called Gs, is a member of the family of guanine proteins, consisting of α-, β-, and γ-subunits. The α-subunit contains the guanine triphosphate (GTP)–binding site, possesses guanosine triphosphatase (GTPase) activity, is responsible for the specific transduction of the epinephrine signals to the effector enzyme,[42] and plays a central role in the regulation of cardiac function.[43]

The enzyme adenylyl cyclase is activated by the Gs-α-subunit when norepinephrine has been bound by its receptor. Activation of adenylyl cyclase results in the synthesis of cyclic AMP, using ATP as the substrate. Responding to hormonal or neurotransmitter stimulation, the receptors, Gs, and the enzyme adenylyl cyclase determine the level of intracellular cyclic AMP. A single neurotransmitter-receptor complex can activate many Gs-α-subunits and activate adenylyl cyclase to produce many cyclic AMP molecules. Thus, the stimulatory signal is amplified and is the mechanism by which the response to very low concentrations of extracellular agonist are maximized.

Just as there are stimulatory Gs proteins, there are three inhibitory Gi proteins.[42] The mechanism through which activation of Gi leads to inhibition of adenylyl cyclase is still incompletely understood.

α-Adrenergic receptors consist of two subtypes, α_1 and α_2.[19, 20, 23] The α_1-receptors are postsynaptic and mediate smooth muscle contraction. α_2-Receptors are found on presynaptic nerve terminals, where they mediate feedback inhibition of norepinephrine release. The α_1- and α_2-receptors can be distinguished pharmacologically by their different affinities for various agonists and antagonists. For example, yohimbine has a high selectivity for α_2-adrenergic receptors, whereas prazosin demonstrates a 1000- to 10,000-fold selectivity for α_1-adrenergic receptors. The α_1-adrenergic pathway in the human myocardium is much less developed than the β_1-adrenergic pathway, and α_1-receptor density is low.[23]

PARASYMPATHETIC INNERVATION OF THE HEART

Parasympathetic innervation of the heart is provided by efferent preganglionic parasympathetic neurons projecting to the heart from the medulla oblongata, where they synapse with postganglionic cholinergic parasympathetic neurons.[44, 45] Myocardial muscarinic receptors have been identified with autoradiography.[46] Parasympathetic innervation of the atria is well documented, but parasympathetic innervation of the ventricles is less defined. On the basis of histologic and physiologic evidence, ventricular parasympathetic innervation was thought to be lacking, but chemical and physiologic evidence indicates the existence of a direct parasympathetic innervation of the ventricles.[47] Parasympathetic ganglion cells are sparsely distributed in ventricular myocardium, if they exist at all.[29, 48] The primary vagal innervation of the canine ventricles is by way of postganglionic cholinergic axons, whose cell bodies of origin are in the atria.[45, 49] Long postganglionic axons cross the atrioventricular groove to innervate the ventricular myocardium.

Muscarinic cholinergic receptors exist in five subtypes called M_1, M_2, M_3, M_4, and M_5. The M_1-class is defined as receptors that exhibit a high affinity toward the antagonist pirenzepine, whereas the M_2-subclass is defined as receptors that exhibit a low affinity toward pirenzepine.[50, 51] The high-affinity M_1-receptor sites are primarily in the central nervous system, whereas the low-affinity M_2-receptor sites are located on peripheral effector organs. Muscarinic receptors in the heart are of the M_2-type. Development of

AF-DX 116, an M_2-antagonist, has led to the suggestion that M_2-receptors may be subdivided further into two subtypes, one with high affinity for AF-DX 116 and one with low affinity.[52, 53] Cardiac receptors have a high affinity for AF-DX 116 (M_2-subclass). The existence of the different muscarinic receptor subtypes has been confirmed by cloning and sequencing DNA genes that code the receptor proteins.[54, 55] The primary structure of a cardiac M_2-receptor from porcine atria has been determined.[28] The amino acid sequence differs in neuronal M_1-receptor from porcine brain and in cardiac M_2-receptor, each receptor being different in the 5-6 loop of the cytoplasmic region.[28, 55] The ganglia also contained smaller amounts of M_1- and M_4 mRNAs.[56]

The ventricular muscarinic receptors are localized in the sarcolemma.[57] The neurotransmitters acetylcholine and norepinephrine exert their chronotropic and inotropic effects on the heart by an opposite coupling of the cholinergic and β-adrenergic receptors to adenylate cyclase; β-adrenoreceptors activate adenylate cyclase, whereas muscarinic cholinergic receptors inhibit it.[58, 59] The cardiac conduction system and cardiac muscle have M_2-receptors[56] that mediate bradycardia and decrease cardiac contractility.

It is important to distinguish muscarinic acetylcholine receptors located on blood vessels from those on myocytes. Porcine arteries contain both M_1- and M_2-subtypes,[60] as does the coronary vasculature of the dog.[61] Relaxation of endothelial musculature in response to cholinergic agonists is mediated by the action of acetylcholine, causing the endothelium to release a vasodilating substance, endothelium-derived relaxing factor, a nitroxide.[62] The endothelial M_1-muscarinic receptor system is responsible for the redistribution of blood flow to the subendocardium during coronary vasodilation, whereas both M_1- and M_2-receptors are involved in increasing myocardial perfusion.[61] The endothelial muscarinic receptors have low affinity for the M_1-antagonist, pirenzepine,[63] as well as for the cardioselective antagonist AF-DX 116. Other vessels respond to cholinergic agonists with a contractile response mediated by muscarinic receptors.[64] Bovine coronary arteries manifest both the endothelial relaxation response and the endothelial-independent contractile response involving vascular smooth muscle. The receptors that mediate these effects have identical properties: they show low affinity for pirenzepine and AF-DX 116, and the putative M_1-selective agonist McN-A-343 produces no effect in either tissue.[65] Thus, pharmacologic studies indicate that vascular endothelium has receptors that cause them to relax. On the other hand, autoradiographic studies with ^{3}H-QNB and ^{125}I-QNB fail to reveal binding sites on endothelial cells, but reveal them only on the smooth muscle cells.[66] Furthermore, cultured endothelial cells do not have muscarinic binding sites.[67] Therefore, one can conclude that muscarinic receptors are present at least on the smooth muscles of coronary arteries and can be detected with imaging techniques, in addition to myocardial receptors.

The physiologic response after ligand binding to muscarinic receptors is mediated by the G proteins Gp, Gi, and Gk, which bind guanine nucleotides and transduce signals across the cell membrane.[42] The muscarinic M_1, M_3, and M_5 ligand-receptor complex couples with Gp, and the M_2 and M_5 complexes couple with Gi and Gk.[68–70] Stimulation of phosphatidylinositol turnover by a G protein subtype (Gp) affects the intracellular levels of cyclic AMP.[71] Cardiac sinoventricular and atrioventricular nodes and cardiac muscle have M_2-receptors.[56, 72] Their stimulation with nanomolar concentrations of acetylcholine decreases the heart rate by inhibiting the hyperpolarization-activated current involved in stimulating the rate of cardiac contraction.[73] Intermediate concentrations of acetylcholine decrease the strength and rate of contraction of cardiac muscle.[74] Both Gi and Gk protein subtypes inhibit cardiac contraction. Activation of Gi causes a decrease in levels of cyclic AMP, which reduces the activity of cyclic AMP–dependent kinases, the phosphorylation of calcium channels, and the calcium levels inside the cell. The activation of Gk increases potassium levels, causing hyperpolarization and inhibition of myocyte contractions. The α-subunit of Gk increases the conductance of potassium by coupling directly with the potassium channel,[69] whereas the β-γ-subunit of Gk stimulates phospholipase,[75] which increases potassium conductance.[76] The stimulation of muscarinic receptors with larger doses of carbachol, an M_2 agonist, has the opposite effect, increasing the strength and rate of contraction,[74] because M_2-receptors are also coupled, albeit weakly, with Gp. The increase in phosphatidylinositol turnover as a result of Gp stimulation mobilizes calcium and depolarizes myocytes by inhibition of Na^+,K^+-ATPase or by an influx of sodium through channels controlled by muscarinic receptors.[74]

Parasympathetic neurotransmission plays a lesser role than that of sympathetic neurotransmission in the diseased myocardium, but muscarinic cholinergic agonists counteract the stimulating effect of adrenergic overactivity in the heart.[77–79] In experimental cardiac failure, changes occur in cardiac muscarinic receptors,[79, 80] but no significant abnormalities have been found by in vitro binding techniques in the myocardium of patients with end-stage heart failure.[81] However, atrial myocytes isolated from failing human explanted hearts exhibited a lower resting membrane potential and reduced sensitivity to acetylcholine compared with those of control (donor) atria.[82] Whole-cell and single-channel measurements suggest that these alterations are caused by reduced muscarinic gated K^+ channel density sensitivity to M_2-cholinergic receptor–linked G protein Gi–mediated channel activation.

PRINCIPLES OF CARDIAC IMAGING OF NEUROTRANSMISSION WITH POSITRON EMISSION TOMOGRAPHY

With the advent of positron emission tomography (PET), it is now possible to obtain noninvasively quantitative determination of regional biochemical processes in the heart.[83] The procedure involves several steps. The first one is the synthesis of radioligands labeled at sufficiently high specific activities with a positron-emitting isotope, giving an externally detectable signal. The second step is the use of an imaging system that provides quantitative images of transverse sections of an organ with high sensitivity, good spatial resolution, and great accuracy. The third step is the development of mathematical models that translate radioactive concentration values into physiologic binding parameters such as receptor density and equilibrium dissociation constant. This methodology is now applied clinically for studying the perfusion and the metabolism of the human heart in vivo under normal physiologic conditions and in disease states.[84, 85] Because PET is an imaging technique that combines the advantages of quantitative autoradiography and of tomographic imaging by external detection, it has made possible both imaging and quantitative investigation of cardiac receptors. The feasibility of characterizing muscarinic acetylcholine receptors, β-adrenergic receptors, and α_1-adrenergic receptors has been shown in animals and in humans.[86] In contrast to single-photon emission computed tomography (SPECT), PET provides the exact value of the regional radioactive concentration of a tracer. It is then possible to select meaningful areas of interest in the septum or in the free wall and to plot activity-versus-time curves. Fitting these kinetic data to a mathematical model allows calculation of receptor density or drug affinity in any region of the myocardium. Furthermore, positron-emitting isotopes of natural elements have short half-lives (20 minutes for ^{11}C) and are produced at very high specific activity (400 to 1000 Ci/mmol), resulting in three advantages. First, drugs labeled by ^{11}C keep their pharmacologic properties, contrary to analogs labeled by ^{123}I (unless they naturally contain iodine). Second, the injected amount of drug usually does not exceed 10 to 50 nmol, so receptor occupancy by the tracer remains low. In addition, drugs that could have acute or chronic effects at pharmacologic doses can be used in humans (e.g., β-blockers such as ^{11}C-practolol or ^{11}C-CGP 12177). Third, for the same reason, the radiation burden is low, although the amount of radioactivity injected is relatively high (10 to 20 mCi, 370 to 740 MBq). The reverse side of the medal is the complexity and the cost of PET imaging. It is necessary to gather in the same facility a cyclotron to produce the positron emitter, a radiochemistry laboratory to synthetize in less than 40 minutes the ^{11}C-labeled molecule, and a positron tomograph to record the data.

SPECIFICITY OF IN VIVO RECEPTOR STUDIES

In vivo studies have to deal with two kinds of problems. First, the radioactive ligand that is generally intravenously injected must reach its receptor sites within the studied organ without any modification. Second, the radioligand within the organ must interact with high affinity only with its specific receptor sites and must not bind either to other receptors or to nonspecific binding sites.

Access of Ligand to Myocardium

After intravenous injection the radiotracer can bind to proteins or penetrate red blood cells, thus reducing the amount of free ligand available for binding. Ligands such as peptides can be enzymatically degraded by circulating peptidases. Other molecules can be rapidly metabolized by the liver.

Another complication of in vivo studies is the presence of different serial barriers between the site of injection (a brachial vein in humans) and the receptor sites. These barriers include the lungs, the capillary membrane, and the tissue itself. Lipophilic molecules are completely extracted during a single passage through the lung circulation. They can be metabolized by the pulmonary endothelial or epithelial cells before reaching the cardiac receptors. After intravenous injection ^{11}C-propranolol showed a 90 to 100 percent lung uptake, and the myocardium was never visualized during the 80 minutes of observation. ^{11}C-practolol is a thousand times more hydrophilic than ^{11}C-propranolol. It is not extracted by the lungs. Therefore, the myocardium is visualized a few minutes after injection. Pulmonary accumulation of drugs in patients may depend on the functional state of pulmonary cells. The extraction by the lung of ^{11}C-labeled basic amines such as ^{11}C-propranolol is reduced in patients with chronic obstructive pulmonary disease; the tissue washout half-life is significantly greater in patients with active sarcoidosis than in normal subjects.[87] The most puzzling situation was found when the authors were studying the myocardial serotonergic receptor. Ketanserin, a potent antagonist of S_2 serotonergic receptors, was labeled with ^{11}C and intravenously injected in a group of normal volunteers. A large individual variation was observed: in some subjects the myocardial concentration of ^{11}C-ketanserin was very high with low pulmonary uptake, whereas the opposite was seen in others.[88] Tobacco consumption accounted for this difference, with the radioactive ligand concentration in the lungs of smokers linearly correlated to the amount of tobacco smoke absorption. The very high ^{11}C-ketanserin concentration seems to reflect the increasing cellularity (including alveolar macrophages that have serotonergic receptors on their membranes) induced by cigarette smoking.[88] Thus, a low ligand concentration in the myocardium may be falsely attributed to a low receptor density when it only is the consequence of restricted access to receptor sites. In animals or humans, the amount of ligand that reaches the heart thus depends on its clearance from the lungs. The cardiac receptors cannot be visualized when the radioligand concentration in the lung decreases slowly, compared with the physical half-life of the isotope. The second barrier is the capillary barrier of the target organ. The problem is less acute in the heart than in the brain, where the intercellular junctions are very tight. In contrast to the blood-brain barrier, the capillary membrane is permeable to small hydrophilic molecules. The biodistribution of the radiotracer is also important to consider; it may be extracted, trapped, or metabolized by organs other than the lungs and the heart. Many drugs are transformed into metabolites in the liver. Some of these metabolites will still be labeled by the positron-emitting isotope, but their physical and pharmacologic properties may have changed. Both the lipophilicity and the affinity of the metabolites may have been modified by several orders of magnitude. The limiting step for the exchange of tracer between blood and volume of reaction depend on several parameters, for example, the structure of the capillary membrane (continuous, fenestrated, or discontinuous), the structure of the intercellular junctions (tight, leaky), the localization of the receptors (on endothelial cells, myocytes, or neuromuscular junctions), the chemicophysical properties of the labeled ligand, and, of course, the functional integrity of the myocardium itself (e.g., normal, ischemic, denervated, cardiomyopathic).

Interaction of Ligand Within the Myocardium

Additional complexities are related to the removal process of the radioligand within the myocardium, including uptake by different cells, enzymatic or chemical degradation, and intracellular trapping. A radioligand can also bind to different receptors or different receptor subtypes. The labeled ligand should ideally bind specifically to a single receptor type and even to a single receptor subtype. Cardioselective β-blockers are generally hydrophilic, whereas nonselective β-blockers are generally lipophilic, although exceptions are found. However, the affinity of the so-called cardioselective β-blockers is generally much lower than that of noncardioselective β-blockers.[89] PET detects the total radioactivity in the heart and, unlike in in vitro studies, the distinction between specific binding and nonspecific binding is not easy. In brain studies one may subtract the radioactivity in the cerebellum from that in the striatum or in the cortex when receptors are known to be absent from the cerebellum.[90] Such a correction is impossible in heart studies. Because nonspecific binding increases linearly with plasma ligand concentration, whereas specific binding is saturable, the ratio of specific to nonspecific binding can be increased by minimizing radiotracer plasma concentrations and maximizing specific radioactivity of the radioligand to detect enough radioactivity in the tissue. As a consequence, improving the affinity of a β-blocker by increasing its lipophilicity also leads to an increase in nonspecific binding. Intricate mechanisms thus interfere. The initial uptakes of two tritated antagonists of the muscarinic cholinergic receptor were compared in an isolated perfused rat heart preparation.[91] The first, ^{3}H-QNB, a very potent antagonist, is a lipophilic molecule that is widely used in in vitro binding studies.[92] The second, ^{3}H-MQNB, the methiodide salt of QNB, is a hydrophilic molecule that maintains a high affinity for the muscarinic acetylcholine receptor.[93] After rapid injection in the perfusate, a high nonspecific uptake of ^{3}H-QNB was found contrasting with a 90 percent specific binding of ^{3}H-MQNB that could be inhibited by adding an excess of unlabeled MQNB or atropine in the perfusate.[91] This example emphasizes the necessity of the search for new radioligands carefully designed for in vivo studies. It also shows the need for preliminary in vitro studies on homogenates and on isolated organs and for pharmacokinetic studies on animals before trying to label a new ligand with positron emitters.

Choice of Ligand

When preliminary studies indicate that a ligand with high specificity and nanomolar binding affinity for receptor in vitro can reach its target (e.g., β_1-adrenergic receptors) in a few minutes in vivo without being highly extracted and metabolized by other tissues (particularly the lungs and the liver), one can try to label this ligand with ^{11}C, because it then will be possible to follow with PET the tissue kinetics of ^{11}C-labeled ligand for about 100 minutes. On the other hand, when the ligand reaches the myocardial receptors very slowly, it should be labeled with a positron-emitting isotope of longer half-life, for example, ^{18}F (T1/2 = 1.8 hours), ^{75}Br (T1/2 = 1.7 hours) or ^{76}Br (T1/2 = 16.2 hours). Because ligand molecules do not generally contain a bromine or a fluorine atom, it is necessary to carefully study their binding properties in vitro; for example, the halogenation of QNB and MQNB lowers the tissue-to-blood and the specific-to-nonspecific binding ratios.

Although the 20-minute half-life of ^{11}C is a major advantage with regard to the fact that it entails minor radiation exposure of patients and has minimal side effects, it adds to the complexity of the method because the ligand must be rapidly synthesized (in less than 40 minutes). Rapid labeling of the compound ideally can be accomplished with the use of a precursor of the ligand selected. By a single chemical reaction, the precursor may then be converted into the labeled molecule. Four labeled β-blocking agents (^{11}C-propranolol, ^{11}C-practolol, ^{11}C-pindolol, and ^{11}C-CGP 12177) and the α_1-blocking agent ^{11}C-prazosin have been obtained by using ^{11}C-phosgen as the labeled precursor.[94] The muscarinic receptor antagonist ^{11}C-MQNB and the peripheral-type benzodiazepine receptor antagonist ^{11}C-PK 11195 are obtained by reaction of ^{11}C-methyl iodide with QNB.[95] Two new ^{18}F-labeled antagonists of the serotonin receptor,[96] ^{18}F-setoperone and ^{18}F-ritanserin, have been obtained by nucleophilic substitution.[97, 98] To summarize, in vivo characterization of cardiac receptors by PET requires high-affinity ligands that display both a high specificity for a subtype of receptor and a low degree of nonspecific binding in vivo. Furthermore, the labeled ligand must reach, rapidly and unmetabolized, the receptor within the myocardium. The tissue-to-blood ratio must also be high to avoid having to correct for the circulating radioactivity. Finally, side effects at saturating doses of ligand must be tolerable. Although these requirements are difficult to fulfill, several ligands have already been evaluated. It is then necessary to demonstrate that the interaction of the ligand within the myocardium detected by PET corresponds to the interaction of a drug to a receptor and not to a specific binding site unrelated to a pharmacologic effect.

Criteria for Identification of Ligand-Receptor Interaction by PET

Receptor-mediated localization of a ligand in the myocardium must be validated in vivo by the same criteria as those used for in vitro binding studies.[99]

Main Criteria

Saturability

Saturability of the ligand-receptor complex can be demonstrated by two kinds of experiments. In the displacement experiments, an excess of cold agonist or antagonist is intravenously injected some time after injection of the labeled ligand. The radioactive concentration in myocardium then rapidly decreases with time because of the competitive inhibition between the tracer and the excess of unlabeled ligand. The receptor sites can also be blocked by an excess of unlabeled ligand injected prior to the radioligand. In this case, the tracer radioactive concentration in the tissue is lower than that measured in the absence of injection of the cold molecule. Contrary to the saturation experiments used for in vitro studies, here the total amount of radioactivity cannot be increased, but the specific activity is decreased.

Stereoselectivity

Stereoselectivity is powerful proof of receptor binding. When two stereoisomers are available, one with and the other without pharmacologic activity, the displacement must be obtained only with the active isomer. The stereospecificity of the binding of the muscarinic antagonist ^{11}C-MQNB was proved in this way: only the pharmacologically active isomer of benzetimide (dexetimide) could displace ^{11}C-MQNB; the inactive isomer (levetimide) was ineffective.[100] These studies have the advantage of minimizing the effects of large amounts of cold ligand on blood flow, transport, and metabolism. However, selective effects of the active isomer on blood flow or metabolism cannot be totally excluded.

Correlation Between Binding and a Biologic Effect

This criterion is essential for distinguishing between a displaceable binding site with no signal transmission and a receptor binding site that is related to physiologic responses. A correlation between receptor binding and biologic effect was shown with ^{11}C-pindolol, ^{11}C-CGP 12177, and ^{11}C-MQNB. The percentage of ^{11}C-MQNB or ^{11}C-CGP 12177 displaced by various amounts of unlabeled atropine or propranolol was proportional to the decrease or increase in heart rate (Fig. 73–1).[100–102] Moreover, in patients with congestive heart failure due to idiopathic dilated cardiomyopathy, decreased β-receptor concentration assessed with PET and ^{11}C-CGP 12177 correlated with the β-contractile responsiveness to intracoronary dobutamine infusion ($r = .83$, $P = .003$), indicating a direct link between changes in the receptor number and its biologic function (Fig. 73–2).

Complementary Criteria

In addition to drug displacement (with agonist, antagonist, and stereoisomers) and correlation with pharmacologic activity, which are the most important and most decisive criteria, other criteria must be fulfilled: the specific regional distribution of the receptors and the high affinity of receptor sites for the radioligand. It must be noted that the receptors involved in neurotransmission have low affinity for the endogenous neurotransmitters that, however, are released at high concentrations in the synaptic cleft.[103] On the other hand, the antagonists of endogenous neurotransmitters behave like hormones; they bind with high affinity to receptors, but their blood concentration is negligible. Therefore, better results are obtained with a labeled antagonist than with a labeled agonist, which was confirmed in vivo with PET, and all the ligands used to characterize cardiac receptors up to now have been antagonists. Once all these criteria are fulfilled, it becomes possible to develop a mathematical model that transforms values of radioactive concentrations measured in selected regions of interest of PET images into values of affinity constant and of receptor density.[104]

IN VIVO RECEPTOR BINDING MODELS

Kinetic Modeling

Quantification of ligand-receptor interactions investigated in the heart requires the use of mathematical models.[105] In these models, the free ligand is first considered as it is transported from blood to tissue and then as it binds to receptor sites. In some cases, the binding of the ligand is reversible; in others, it is not. At times, the nonspecifically bound ligand fraction may be high or it may be negligible.

Figure 73–3 shows an example of a model structure that includes

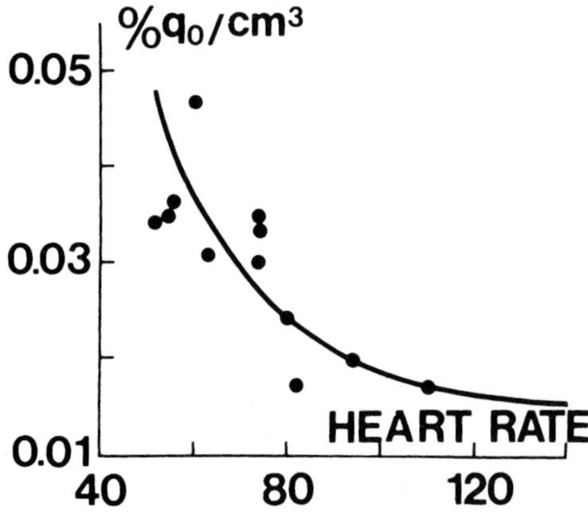

FIGURE 73–1. Dependence of ^{11}C-MQNB concentration in the ventricular septum on heart rate. In 12 individuals, the percentage of the injected dose present in 1 cm^3 of septum is plotted as a function of heart rate (expressed in beats per minute) recorded at the time of ^{11}C-MQNB injection. The uptake of ^{11}C-MQNB is higher in subjects with lower heart rate at the time of injection.

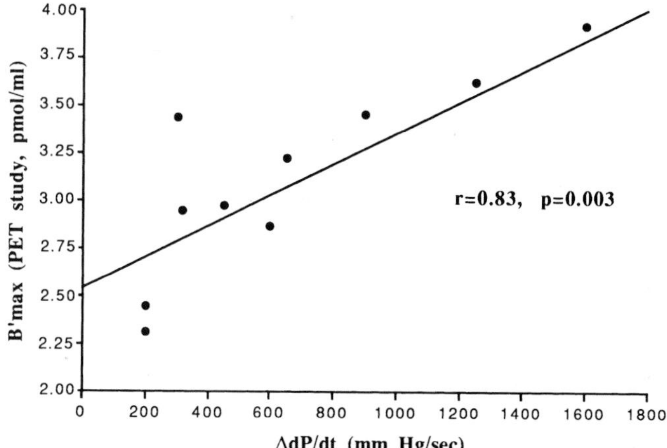

FIGURE 73–2. Correlation between the concentration of β-receptors (B'_{max}) assessed by PET and the myocardial β-contractile responsiveness to intracoronary dobutamine infusion, estimated as the net increase in left ventricular peak positive dP/dt (ΔdP/dt). Dobutamine was consecutively administered for 5-minute periods at incremental infusion rates of 25, 50, 100, 200, and 400 μg per minute using an infusion pump. The increment of infusion rate was stopped when the heart rate increased by more than 10 percent. The maximal response was taken as the maximal increase in peak positive LV dP/dt with no change in heart rate of more than 10 percent. The net increase in peak positive LV dP/dt (ΔdP/dt) was calculated as the difference between peak positive LV dP/dt at maximal intracoronary dobutamine infusion and at baseline.

nonspecific binding. The flux of free ligand that crosses the capillary membrane is equal to $p \cdot V_R \cdot C°_a(t)$, where $C°_a(t)$ is the plasma radioactive concentration at time t, p is the rate constant characterizing the transfer of ligand from blood to tissue, V_R is defined as the fraction of the region of interest delineated by PET in which the ligand can react with the receptors, and pV_R is the clearance. With a hydrophilic ligand, V_R should correspond to the fraction of extracellular fluid. The free radioactive ligand $M°_f(t)$ can either bind directly to a free receptor site or to a nonspecific site (parameter k_{+ns}) or escape with rate constant k. The binding probability depends on the rate constant (k_{+1}/V_R) and on the local concentration of available free receptors, which is equal to $[B'_{max} - M°_b(t)]$, where B'_{max} is the unknown concentration of available receptor sites, and $M°_b(t)$ the bound radioactive ligand concentration.[106] The rate constant for the dissociation of bound ligand is denoted by k_{-1}, and that for the nonspecifically bound ligand by k_{-na}.

In in vitro binding studies, the free and bound ligand concentrations are measured separately in a counter, and the nonspecific binding fraction can be evaluated after incubation of the preparation with an excess of cold ligand. The PET experimental data correspond to the sum of the concentration of labeled ligand (free, specifically or nonspecifically bound) in extravascular compartment and of a fraction of the blood concentration, F_V, which represents not only the fraction of blood present in the tissue volume but also the effect of spillover from the ventricular cavity to the myocardium.

When the experimental protocol includes injections of unlabeled ligand, it is necessary to simulate the kinetics of this unlabeled ligand, because it affects the local concentration of free receptors. Thus, the model shown in Figure 73–3 includes two parts corresponding to the labeled and unlabeled ligand kinetics, with each having the same structure and the same parameters.

Identification of model parameters requires the use of the arterial input function $C°_a(t)$, which corresponds to the nonmetabolized labeled ligand concentration in the plasma. The unlabeled arterial ligand concentration $C_a(t)$ is simulated from $C°_a(t)$ by assuming that the unlabeled ligand kinetics are similar to those of the labeled ligand. The input function is usually obtained from arterial blood samples, but it can be estimated from PET images with the use of a region of interest in the left ventricular cavity when the molecule is not metabolized and when the plasma-to-blood ratio remains constant during the entire experiment.

Such a model contains eight parameters, which have to be identified from PET data. When the number of parameter values is very large in comparison to the experimental data, the uncertainties in the parameters may be so large that the identified values are meaningless. In such a case, two solutions may be possible: the model can be simplified by a reduction of the number of parameters, or the experimental protocol can be modified to obtain more experimental data.[107]

Simplification of the model facilitates estimation of the parameters. For example, PET data are not sufficient to detect rapid nonspecific binding reaction with association-dissociation kinetic rate constants much larger than the other compartmental rate constants. If the tracer occupies a negligible fraction of the available receptors,[90, 108–110] the model becomes linear, but neither the receptor density (B'_{max}) nor the equilibrium dissociation constant K_d can be separately identified. The rate constant k_3 is equal to the

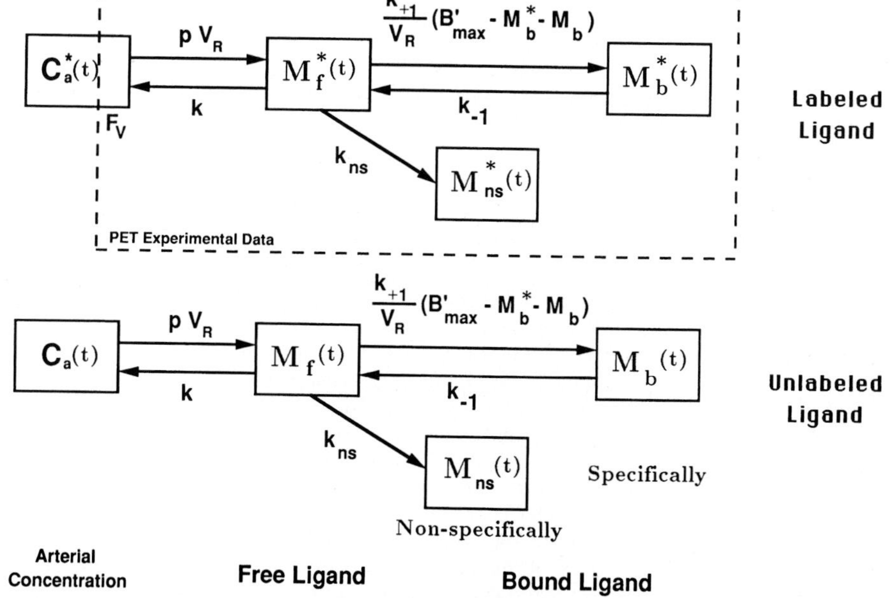

FIGURE 73–3. Compartmental model used in kinetic analysis of ligand binding to cardiac receptors. C°a is the tracer concentration (corrected for metabolites) in arterial blood. M°f, M°b, and M°T represent free, specifically bound, and total amount of tracer, respectively. The constants *P* and k are the transfer coefficients between blood and tissue; k_{+1} and k_{-1} are the association and dissociation rate constants, respectively (see the text for comments).

product (k_{+1}/V_R) · B′max) and gives an indication of the "binding potential" that reflects the capacity of a given tissue to bind a labeled molecule.[108, 110]

The equations can be further simplified when it is assumed that a steady-state condition between the blood and free ligand compartment exists and when the ligand binds irreversibly to receptor sites, that is, when $k_{-1} = 0$. When both assumptions make sense, a graphic method can then be used.[90, 111] This can be very useful because it provides a way of estimating the receptor concentration without mathematical calculations. However, validation of the graphic method is often difficult, which can lead to doubtful results. In particular, it has been shown that with ^{11}C-MQNB, the slope of the Patlak plot is not related to the binding of free ligand (parameter k_3) but corresponds to the transfer of the ligand from blood to free ligand compartment.[112] In this case, the graphic method did not provide any information on the receptor density.

The Multi-Injection Approach

The estimation of receptor concentration implies the use of an experimental protocol, including at least two injections, one of which results in a significant percentage of receptor occupancy.[106] The most general method of estimating the receptor concentration consists of the identification of all the model parameters, and it may require multiple injections.

The first example of this multi-injection approach was the study of the binding of the ^{11}C-MQNB to muscarinic receptors in dog heart.[112] The attempts to identify the model parameters from data obtained with a single tracer injection led to disappointing numerical results because most of the parameters had to be considered as unidentifiable. The possibility of improving parameter estimation with the use of a new experimental design consisting of a first tracer injection, followed 30 minutes later by an injection of the cold ligand (displacement experiment), was then investigated. However, this second protocol led to two different solutions. A biologically valid solution was obtained by using a third protocol, including both a displacement and a coinjection. A fourth injection (an injection of a large mass of unlabeled ligand) allowed the estimation of irreversible and nonspecific binding.

Such complex protocols may be unsuitable for clinical studies. Therefore, one uses results from animal experiments to set up simplified protocols applicable to the study of human beings, or to validate the assumptions made in simplified models. In the case of the investigation of muscarinic receptors, the best protocol regarding clinical feasibility consisted of a tracer injection, followed 30 minutes later by a coinjection of labeled and unlabeled ligand, to occupy about half of the receptor sites.[112]

IN VIVO CHARACTERIZATION OF CARDIAC RECEPTORS

β-Adrenergic Receptors

Four antagonists, propranolol, practolol, pindolol, and CGP 12177, have been labeled with ^{11}C for PET.[113–117] They differ in affinity, liposolubility, and subtype selectivity. ^{11}C-propranolol, a lipophilic nonselective antagonist, cannot be used for studying the β-adrenergic receptors with PET because of its high accumulation in the lungs. ^{11}C-practolol is a hydrophilic molecule that binds to the β_1 receptors. A few minutes after intravenous injection in humans, the heart is well visualized, but the tracer concentration decreases rapidly with time, even when it is injected at very high specific activity.[101] The percentage of bound tracer that can be displaced by an excess of unlabeled antagonist (practolol, propranolol, atenolol, or pindolol) 20 minutes later is also low. The results can be explained by the relatively low affinity of practolol. ^{11}C-pindolol and ^{11}C-CGP 12177 have high affinity and low lipophilicity. ^{11}C-CGP 12177 is a very potent hydrophilic β-blocker. It is usually considered to have no β-adrenoreceptor subtype selectivity, although a low β_1 selectivity has been demonstrated with rat ventricular microsomes.[118] The equilibrium dissociation constant, K_d, was 0.33 nmol/L for β_1-adrenoreceptors and 0.90 nmol/L for β_2-adrenoreceptors, suggesting a two- to threefold β_1 selectivity of ^{3}H-CGP 12177.

CGP 12177 has low nonspecific binding on membranes and low intracellular uptake.[119, 120] In addition, it does not bind to receptors that are removed from the plasma membrane and internalized during short-term desensitization.[121] Therefore, ^{3}H-CGP 12177 was used to demonstrate short-term homologous desensitization of β-adrenergic receptors in C6-glioma intact cells. Incubation of C6-cells with the agonist isoprenaline at 37° C for 15 to 20 minutes resulted in a 50 percent decrease in the number of binding sites of ^{3}H-CGP 12177, which paralleled the decrease in hormone-stimulated adenylate cyclase activity.[121] This ligand is therefore an ideal probe for specifically measuring the cell surface receptors in vivo, that is, the "functionally active" β-receptors.

A high myocardial uptake was measured after ^{11}C-CGP 12177 injection and a displacement of bound tracer was obtained after injection of an excess of cold ligand. (Figs. 73–4 and 73–5). Saturation of the β-adrenergic receptor was demonstrated by preinjection of an unlabeled β-blocker a few minutes before the injection of ^{11}C-CGP. A correlation was observed between the tracer displacement and the decrease in heart rate induced by the displacing agent (Fig. 73–6), which is a strong indication that receptor sites, and not only binding sites, are visualized.

Myocardial β-adrenergic receptor density has been found to differ among species: B_{max} = 152, 150, and 311 fmol/mg protein in rat, rabbit, and dog, respectively, using ^{3}H-dihydroalprenolol as a ligand.[122] β-Adrenoreceptor density has also been measured in biopsies of human left ventricle and found to vary between 30 and 79 fmol/mg, using ^{125}I-cyanoiodopindolol.[21, 31, 33] β-Adrenergic receptor density has been measured in the dog ventricular myocardium by PET.[123] In the left ventricular myocardium of dogs, with the use of PET with a graphic model based on a multi-injection protocol, the dissociation rate constant k_{-1} was found to be $.014 \pm .002$ min^{-1} and concentration of available binding sites B'_{max} was 31 ± 4 pmol/mL tissue.[123]

The use of PET studies with ^{11}C-CGP 12177 for clinical investigation has been validated.[124] The ability of PET used with ^{11}C-CGP 12177 to determine myocardial β-receptor changes was evaluated in patients with idiopathic dilated cardiomyopathy and in healthy persons (see Fig. 73–4). The β-receptor density obtained from PET was compared to the β-receptor density determined with endomyocardial biopsy samples by an in vitro binding technique, using ^{3}H-CGP 12177. Results obtained with the two techniques were correlated ($r = .79$, $P = .019$).

α-Adrenergic Receptors

Prazosin, a selective α_1-adrenergic blocker, was labeled with ^{11}C and injected into dogs.[125] PET scans showed a high and homogeneous myocardial uptake and a much lower pulmonary uptake. However, the criteria needed for the characterization of receptors could not be fulfilled, probably because of high nonspecific binding.

Muscarinic Acetylcholine Receptors

The radiolabeled muscarinic antagonists ^{3}H-QNB (quinuclidinyl benzylate) and ^{3}H-NMS (*N*-methylscopolamine) have widely been used in in vitro studies. QNB binds to both M_1- and M_2-receptor subtypes. When ^{3}H-QNB was used to label intact cells instead of membrane preparations, there was some trapping of the ligand within the cells, presumably by the lysosomes. The same phenomenon occurred with ^{3}H-dexetimide.[126] ^{3}H-QNB labels more sites than ^{3}H-NMS or ^{3}H-MQNB (*N*-methyl QNB), a quaternary derivative of ^{3}H-QNB.[127] It is likely that the subset of receptors detected only by ^{3}H-QNB does not participate in physiologic responses,

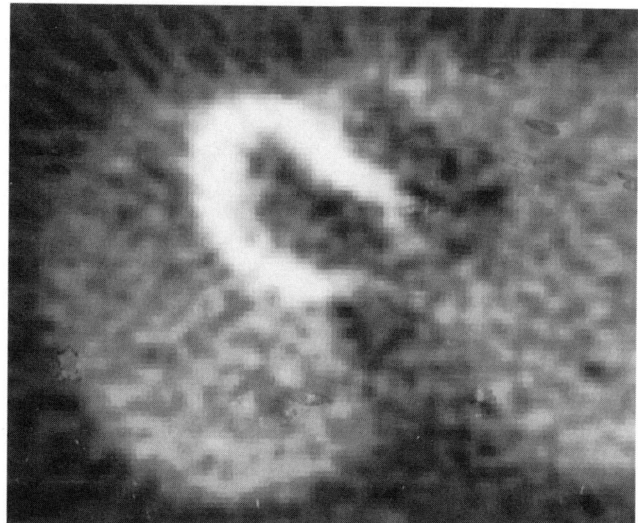

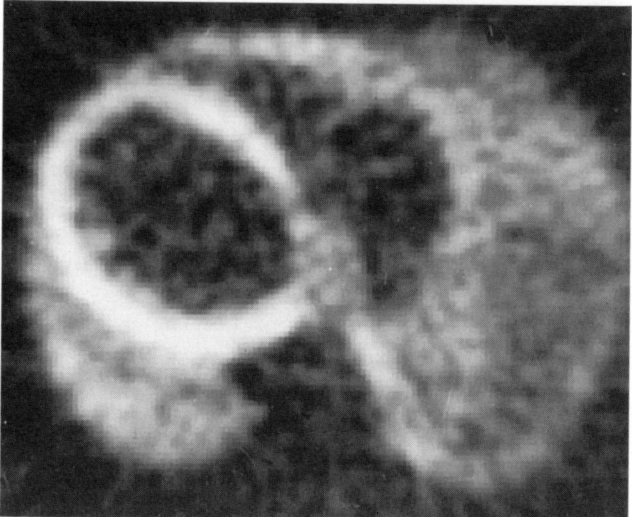

FIGURE 73–4. Myocardial distribution of ^{11}C-CGP obtained by PET (20-minute static image) in a normal subject *(top)* and in a patient with severe myocardial dysfunction related to an idiopathic dilated cardiomyopathy *(bottom)*. The left ventricle is to the left. The lateral left ventricular wall is to the left, the septum to the right, and the anterior wall is uppermost. In the patient, the myocardial uptake of labeled CGP seems to be high, contrasting with decreased concentration of available receptor sites (B'_{max}) found when using mathematical analysis, because the images are normalized.

possibly because they are sequestered in a hydrophobic compartment within the cell membrane.[127]

Therefore, the hydrophilic ligand MQNB (instead of QNB) was labeled with ^{11}C to study the muscarinic acetylcholine receptors in vivo by PET.[100] MQNB is a potent antagonist that is not extracted by the lungs and displays high affinity for the cholinergic receptors in rat heart homogenates: K_d = 0.32 nmol/L, B'_{max} = 228 fmol/mg of protein.[128] Analysis of the in vitro kinetics of ^{3}H-MQNB binding gave a k_{-1} value of 2.73 nanomolar^{-1} · min^{-1} and a dissociation rate constant k_{-1} of 0.81 min^{-1}. All the criteria needed to characterize the muscarinic receptor were validated in baboons and humans with ^{11}C-MQNB.[106]

Displacement studies have been performed in dogs with PET, using various amounts of unlabeled pirenzepine and AF-DX 116. No displacement of bound ^{11}C-MQNB was observed after injection of pirenzepine (1 mg), whereas 25 percent of the radioactivity was displaced after injection of the same dose of AF-DX 116 (unpublished personal data). These in vivo results with PET suggest that M_1-receptors are not detectable in the adult dog heart with ^{11}C-MQNB. However, the proportion of M_1- and of M_2-receptors in the myocardium seems to differ among species.

After a bolus intravenous injection of ^{11}C-MQNB at a high specific activity, the ^{11}C-MQNB blood concentration fell very rapidly to a negligible value a few minutes after intravenous injection. In contrast, the ^{11}C-MQNB concentration increased rapidly in the myocardium to reach a maximum in 1 to 5 minutes and then remained constant for 70 minutes. Rapid intravenous injection of atropine led to a rapid decrease (lasting a few minutes) in the septal ^{11}C-MQNB concentration. The maximal percentage of ^{11}C-MQNB, which could be displaced in dogs, was 94 percent. Because atropine did not discriminate between muscarinic receptor subtypes in the heart, one could assume that less than 6 percent of ^{11}C-MQNB bound in the dog or human heart corresponds to nonspecific binding. The specific binding is stereospecific because dexetimide (the pharmacologically active isomer)—but not levetimide—can displace ^{11}C-MQNB from its binding sites.[100]

The ventricles receive primarily postganglionic cholinergic fibers from ganglion cells localized in the atria.[49] Thus, the release of acetylcholine at parasympathetic nerve endings in the ventricles would depend on the activity of atrial cells mediating both the atrial chronotropic and the ventricular inotropic effects. Reduced frequency is related to a predominant vagal influence. The greater ^{11}C-MQNB binding in the septum linked to vagal stimulation could be explained by an increase in either the number or the affinity of antagonist binding sites. In the physiologically active state, the agonist is released from the receptor in a low-affinity form, and more sites are available for ^{11}C-MQNB binding.[128] The presence of two interconvertible forms of the muscarinic cholinergic receptor respectively favored by agonists and antagonists and displaying high-agonist–low-antagonist and low-agonist–high-antagonist affinities, respectively, has been demonstrated.[129] According to this hypothesis, vagal stimulation would be characterized by a conversion to a low-agonist–high-antagonist affinity form of the muscarinic receptor. These findings suggest that PET allows identification of the physiologically active conformation of the muscarinic receptor.[128]

Rate constants and B_{max} values for ^{11}C-MQNB binding to cardiac muscarinic receptors have been calculated in dogs with the three-compartment model described previously in displacement experiments with an excess of unlabeled MQNB.[112] The association rate constant k_{+1} was .6±0.1 nanomolar^{-1} · min^{-1}. The dissociation rate constant was 0.27±0.03 min^{-1}, thus yielding a K_d value of 0.49±0.14 nmol/L. The receptor density B'_{max} was 42±11 pmol/cm^3 tissue. These values can be compared to those obtained in vitro in rat heart homogenates with ^{3}H-MQNB.[128] The k_{+1}, k_{-1} and K_d values were 2.73 nanomolar^{-1} · min^{-1} and 0.3 nmol/L, respectively. The receptor density was 105 pmol/g protein or 8.6 pmol/g tissue. The experimental protocol has been optimized to make this approach suitable for human studies (Fig. 73–7) in six normal subjects with the use of a three-injection protocol: a tracer injection, followed 30 minutes later by an injection of an excess of unlabeled MQNB (displacement) and then 30 minutes later by a simultaneous injection of unlabeled and labeled MQNB (coinjection).[130] A simplified two-injection protocol (tracer injection and coinjection) was evaluated in five other normal subjects, and the results were compared to those obtained with the three-injection protocol. In the left ventricle, the mean value of the receptor concentration B′max and the equilibrium dissociation constant K_d were 26±7 and 2.0±0.5 pmol/mL tissue, respectively. The possible existence of nonspecific binding was studied in two subjects with a double-displacement protocol. The corresponding rate constant was found to be very low (0.03 min^{-1}).

Peripheral-Type Benzodiazepine Receptor

Specific high-affinity benzodiazepine binding sites have been demonstrated in several peripheral organs, including the heart.[131, 132] The ligand specificity and affinity for the peripheral-type binding site is completely different from that of the central-

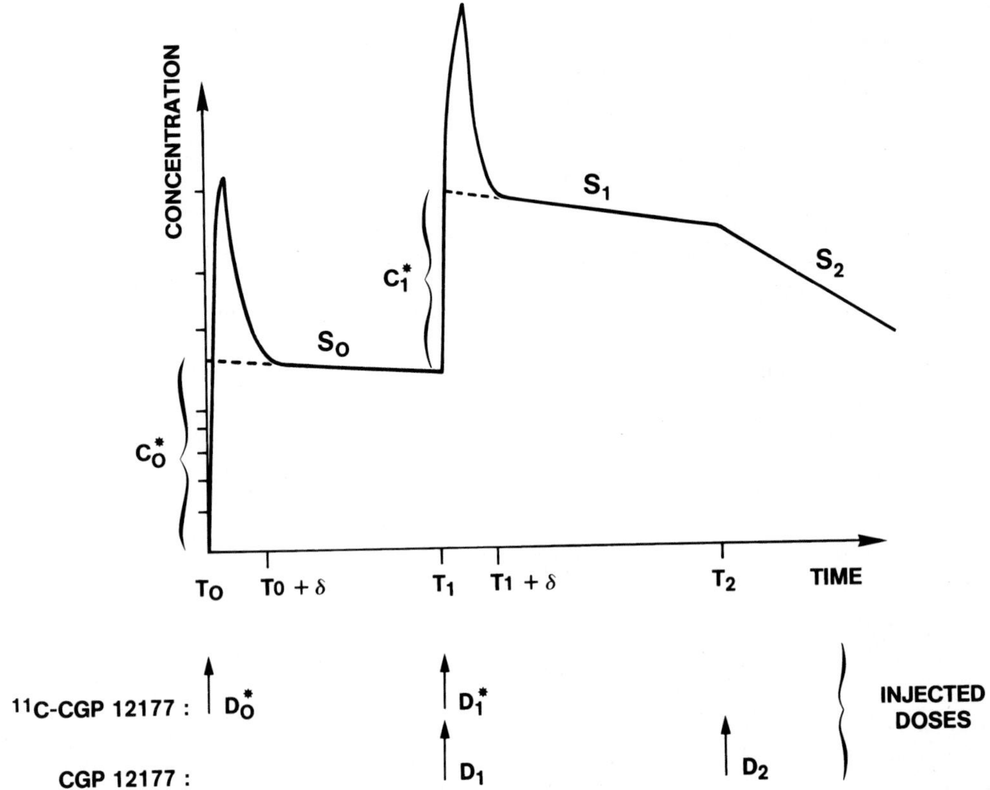

FIGURE 73–5. Schematic representation of PET curve recorded in a region of interest encompassing the left ventricular myocardium, using a coinjection protocol. The experimental protocol consists of an injection of a dose ($D_0°$) of ^{11}C-CGP at time T_0, followed 30 minutes later (T_1) by a coinjection of doses of labeled ($D_1°$) and unlabeled (D_1) CGP. Rapidly, after each ^{11}C-CGP injection, myocardial activity-concentration reaches a plateau (S_0 and S_1). From this part of the curves, the two concentrations used for the graphic method can be estimated. $C_0°$ represents the intercept on the concentration axis of the straight line corresponding to the plateau after the first injection. $C_1°$ represents the difference between the concentration at 30 minutes extrapolated from the straight line obtained after second injection and the concentration measured just before the second injection. The myocardial concentration of β-receptors is calculated from mathematical analysis, using these two values and the known injected doses of labeled and unlabeled ligand (see reference 124). The S_2 part of the curve corresponds to a displacement experiment (injection of a dose, D_2, of cold ligand).

type site.[133] The demonstration of peripheral-type benzodiazepine binding sites was first made in vitro with ^{3}H-diazepam.[131] New ligands that bind only to peripheral-type sites and do not bind to the classic central type have been synthesized. RO 5-4864 and PK 11195 are almost inactive in binding inhibition of ^{3}H-diazepam on its sites in the brain, but they have a very high affinity for peripheral sites.[134, 135] In vitro, the PK 11195 binding sites in rat cardiac membranes are specific, saturable with a K_d of 1.41 nmol/L and a B_{max} of 2250 pmol/g protein.[134, 135] PK 11195 was labeled with ^{11}C at very high specific activity[95] and injected intravenously into dogs and humans. An initial uptake of ^{11}C-PK 11195 was seen in the lung, followed by a high uptake in the heart. Benzodiazepine-binding sites were uniformly distributed.[136] The amount of PK 11195 found in the heart was proportional to the quantity injected at values below 40 nmol/kg. Above 40 nmol/kg, however, the curve showed a plateau because of saturation of the benzodiazepine-binding sites. This result agrees with the mathematical model of a ligand-receptor interaction studied in vivo.[86] A similar curve was also obtained during the study of the muscarinic acetylcholine receptor.[128] From the PK 11195 concentration values, the number of benzodiazepine binding sites in the dog ventricular myocardium (B_{max}) was found to be around 6000 pmol/cm^3 of heart tissue. Other criteria needed for identification of a ligand receptor interaction by PET were validated. Saturability was demonstrated by coinjection or displacement experiments with unlabeled PK 11195 and other ligands, which compete for peripheral-type sites, such as RO 5-4864 and diazepam. Ligands that bind only to brain-type sites, such as RO 15-1788 and clonazepam, were ineffective.[136] The physiologic function of these receptors is still largely unknown. Studies have shown that PK 11195 bind to the mitochondrial outer membrane.[75] In cardiac muscle and vascular smooth muscle, benzodiazepines have been shown to interfere with Ca^{2+} movements. PK 11195 antagonizes the effects of several calcium-channel blockers (diltiazem, nitrendipine, verapamil) and of a calcium-channel agonist (BAY K 8644) in a guinea pig papillary muscle preparation.[137] It also inhibits arrhythmias induced by ischemia and abnormalities after reperfusion in the dog heart.[137] It has been shown that the peripheral-type benzodiazepine receptor antagonists RO 5-4864 and PK 11195 increase coronary flow in isolated retrograde perfused Langendorff rat heart preparations.[138] A subpopulation of peripheral benzodiazepine receptors could also be associated with catecholaminergic neurons.[139] Chemical sympathectomy increases B_{max} in left ventricle (34 percent) 1 week after administration of 6-hydroxydopamine or reserpine. A PET study of these receptors in humans could thus be interesting in clinical situations.

IN VIVO CHARACTERIZATION OF PRESYNAPTIC NEUROTRANSMISSION

Adrenergic Neurons

Radiotracers for PET studies of cardiac nerve integrity and function have been developed only during the last few years. 6-

^{18}F-fluorometaraminol[140, 141] was the first false neurotransmitter to be used as a ligand for PET studies. Metaraminol is a high-affinity substrate for the amine pump.[142] In addition, its quantitation in tissue or perfused organ preparations is not complicated by metabolism, because of the presence of the α-methyl group, which effectively blocks the action of monoamine oxidase (MAO), and the absence of a catechol group, which confers resistance to catechol-*O*-methyltransferase. Once in the cytoplasm, metaraminol is cosequestered with norepinephrine in the synaptic vesicles. On nerve impulse, both norepinephrine and metaraminol are released by exocytosis.[143] It has been found that in vivo at least, metaraminol in tracer amounts accumulates in the storage vesicle via the energy-requiring and reserpine-sensitive vesicular transport carrier, the same carrier that transports norepinephrine into the vesicles.[144] Studies with ^{3}H-metaraminol confirmed that this false transmitter is a highly selective in vivo marker for the adrenergic nerves of the heart.[141] Studies were performed in animals to assess the tissue distribution of ^{18}F-fluorometaraminol and to validate its neuronal affinity.[141] In rats, it has been shown that ^{3}H-metaraminol and ^{18}F-fluorometaraminol had similar affinities for heart tissue and, more important, the two tracers had nearly identical heart neuronal selectivities, as determined in the 6-hydroxydopamine sympathectomized rat model. PET and ^{18}F-fluorometaraminol analyses of closed-chest dogs bearing phenol-induced, regional neuronal defects in the left ventricle clearly delineated the region of neuronal impairment.[141] Blood perfusion in the heart was normal in these dogs, as shown by $^{13}NH_3$ scans. The accumulation of ^{18}F-fluorometaraminol in these regionally denervated dog hearts correlated closely (r = .88) with endogenous norepinephrine concentrations. However, it was observed during the course of our studies with dogs that ^{18}F-fluorometaraminol sometimes produced a vasopressor response from the doses used for tomographic imaging. The mass of unlabeled and ^{18}F-fluorometaraminol in projected clinical doses was subsequently determined to be too close to pharmacologic levels to be safely used in human subjects.

The three *N*-methyl sympathomimetic amines, which could be theoretically labeled by methylation of their respective desmethyl precursors with $^{11}C\text{-}CH_3$, epinephrine, phenylephrine, and metahydroxyephedrine (HED), were tritium labeled[145] and then screened in rats. Epinephrine and HED were superior to phenylephrine in

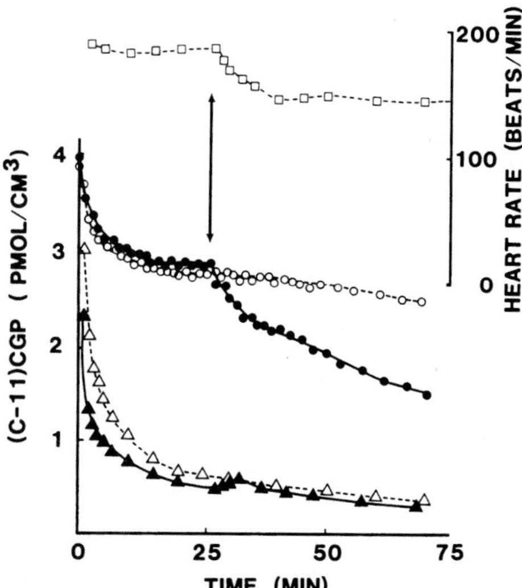

FIGURE 73–6. Control curve *(open circles)* and curve obtained after injection of an excess of unlabeled CGP 12177 (200 nmol) *(solid circles)*, 25 minutes *(arrow)* after injection of a tracer dose of ^{11}C-CGP 12177 in a dog. Measurements were made from a region of interest selected from serial PET scans in the left ventricular myocardium. Concentration values are expressed as picomoles per cubic centimeters of heart tissue. The figure also shows the correlation between the decrease in heart rate *(open squares)* and the displacement of bound ligand *(solid circles)*.

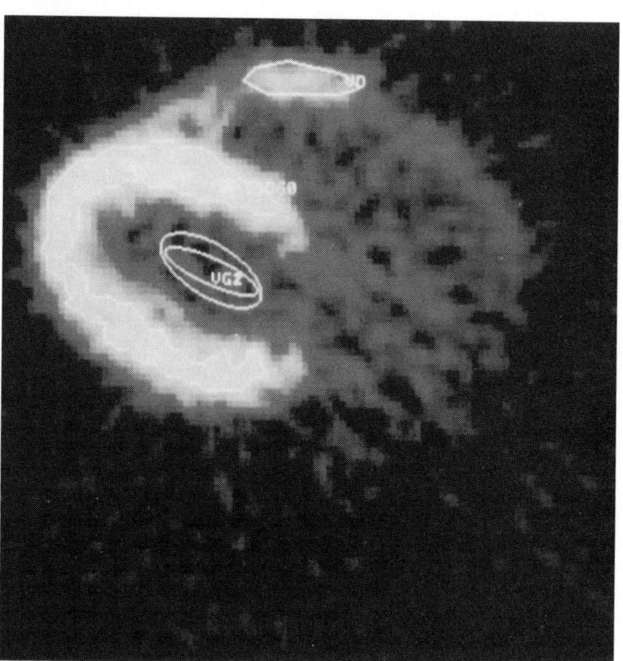

FIGURE 73–7. PET transverse section from a normal subject after intravenous injection of ^{11}C-MQNB, an antagonist of the muscarinic acetylcholine receptor. The PET is obtained 20 minutes after injection of ^{11}C-MQNB. The lateral left ventricular wall is to the left, the septum to the right, and the apex is uppermost. A high activity is seen in the myocardium. Regions of interest are positioned over the left ventricular myocardium and the left ventricular cavity area to record time-activity concentration curves. Activity in the right ventricle is lower than that in the left ventricle. Lungs and blood are not visualized.

heart neuronal imaging potential. Epinephrine, although clearly an excellent marker for cardiac nerves, would present radiolabeling difficulties because of the high in vitro chemical reactivity of its catechol group and tracer kinetic modeling problems due to its rapid in vivo metabolism. ^{3}H-HED, also an excellent neuronal marker, as shown shares the same in vivo characteristics as ^{3}H-metaraminol and ^{18}F-fluorometaraminol. ^{11}C-HED was synthesized by direct reaction of the free-base form of metaraminol with $^{11}C\text{-}CH_3I$ in DMF-DMSO (3:1) and purified by radio-HPLC.[146] Radiochemical yields approached 40 percent; specific activity ranged from 500 to 2000 Ci/mmol. In all animal models tested, ^{11}C-HED behaved identically to ^{18}F-fluorometaraminol. Metabolic studies with ^{11}C-HED in guinea pigs showed that only unchanged tracer was present in heart tissue.[146] However, ^{11}C-HED shows the presence of two metabolites in blood, α-methylepinephrine and the 3-*O*-methyl derivative of α-methylepinephrine. A rapid Sep-Pak determination of ^{11}C-HED blood levels has permitted correction of the arterial input function.[146]

The Michaelis-Menten kinetics of vesicular HED uptake have been determined with the use of bovine chromaffin-granule membranes: a K_i of 134 μmol/L was obtained for unlabeled HED inhibition of ^{3}H-norepinephrine uptake, compared with values of 23 and 27 μmol/L for metaraminol and 6-fluorometaraminol, respectively.[141] The localization of HED in the heart requires neurons that have intact plasma membranes with functioning uptake-1 carriers, requiring a constant supply of ATP. Despite the fairly high affinity of HED for the vesicular transporter, it has been found that retention of ^{11}C-HED in the neuron does not require vesicular storage. HED showed only a 50 percent decrease in heart localization in reserpine-pretreated rats, compared with that of controls 5 to 30 minutes after tracer injection, whereas desipramine-pretreated rats showed a 90 to 95 percent decrease; ^{3}H-norepinephrine in this same experiment showed an 80 to 95 percent decrease in both reserpine- and desipramine-pretreated rats.[147] Reserpine is a selective blocker of vesicular uptake; desipramine is a selective uptake-1 blocker. These findings make sense because vesicles not only store norepinephrine for subsequent quantal release but also protect norepinephrine from degradation by mitochondrial monoamine oxidase. In fact, the neuronal localization of exogenous norepinephrine is not blocked when rats are pretreated with both reserpine and a monoamine oxidase inhibitor.[148] HED is resistant to the action of monoamine oxidase because of its α-methyl group. So, when reserpine blocks entry into storage vesicles, HED can accumulate in the cytosol. Passive diffusion of HED into the synapses may occur, but uptake-1 transporter would capture most of the HED before it escaped into interstitial space. Additional evidence of this phenomenon has been brought by two facts: first, administration of desipramine after radiotracer injection markedly shortens the heart T1/2 of ^{11}C-HED but not ^{3}H-norepinephrine, suggesting that nonvesicular release of HED occurs from the neuron. Second, a stereoisomer of HED, ^{11}C-threo-(1S,2S)HED, a drug known not to displace norepinephrine from the neuron and thus not likely to be stored in the vesicles, shows initial accumulation in the dog heart nearly equal to that of ^{11}C-HED; however, in contrast with HED, the threo form rapidly effluxes from the dog heart.[147] The interaction between ^{11}C-hydroxyephedrine myocardial uptake and potential effects of elevated circulating or endogenous catecholamines has been addressed in isolated rat hearts. Increased ^{11}C-hydroxyephedrine clearance rates with increased norepinephrine concentration in perfusion have been found, suggesting that this factor should be taken into consideration in patients with high sympathetic tone.[149]

Two ^{18}F-labeled catecholamine tracers, 6-fluorodopamine and 6-fluoronorepinephrine, have been developed for heart neuronal mapping.[150–154] The use of these two PET tracers provides excellent heart images in dogs and baboons. In the baboon heart, the comparison of (+) and (−)-6-^{18}F-fluoronorepinephrine and 6-^{18}F-fluorodopamine shows striking differences in tracers' kinetics.[155] Plasma metabolization is much more important and much faster for 6-^{18}F-fluorodopamine than for 6-^{18}F-fluoronorepinephrine. The myocardial retention was greater for 6-^{18}F-fluoronorepinephrine than for 6-^{18}F-fluorodopamine. Desipramine induced a greater blocking effect for 6-^{18}F-fluoronorepinephrine than for 6-^{18}F-fluorodopamine. These findings suggest that (−)-6-^{18}F-fluoronorepinephrine is a better tracer for uptake-1 and vesicular storage assessment.[155] Racemic (+) and (−)-^{11}C-norepinephrine has been injected in monkeys, also providing good myocardial images.[156] The tracer retention was reduced by 80 percent after pretreatment with desipramine.

Another approach is the synthesis of MIBG analogs suitable for PET. Meta ^{18}F-fluorobenzylguanidine and meta ^{76}Br-bromobenzylguanidine (MBBG) have been synthesized.[157, 158] The first advantage of these tracers is that they are close to MIBG, which has proved useful for clinical studies, but they have the advantage of the absolute quantification provided by PET. Second, biodistribution and pharmacologic characteristics of these tracers in rats[157, 158] suggest that they are better norepinephrine analogs than other tracers for vesicular storage, including ^{123}I-MIBG itself. Third, the long half-life could be useful for certain applications[159] and may allow the examination of several patients for each synthesis. The pharmacologic characterization of ^{76}Br-MBBG in dogs and the first results in humans suggest a potential for the in vivo assessment of myocardial uptake-1 function similar to that reported for ^{11}C-hydroxyephedrine. This tracer also provides good myocardial images (Fig. 73–8).

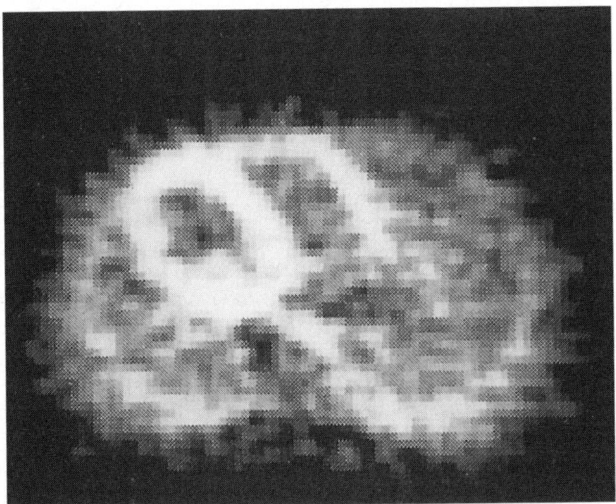

FIGURE 73–8. A 20-minute scan (transverse slice) obtained in a subject with normal cardiac function 10 minutes after injection of 1 mCi (37 MBq) of ^{76}Br-metabenzylguanidine (MBBG), an MIBG analog labeled with a PET emitter. A very high uptake is observed in the left ventricle. The right ventricle is well defined with this tracer.

Cholinergic Neurons

Radiopharmaceutical development of cholinergic nerve markers constitutes a challenge. When radiolabeled norepinephrine or analogs are injected intravenously, the majority of the dose accumulates unchanged in tissues. Conversely, intravenous acetylcholine is completely hydrolyzed almost immediately by blood and tissue cholinesterases. Another complicating factor is the low density of cholinergic neurons in the heart. Choline enters the cytosol of the nerve ending via the high-affinity choline uptake systems, is rapidly acetylated by choline-acetyltransferase, and is then shuttled into storage vesicles. The high-affinity choline uptake system is very restrictive.[160] Even close structural analogs of choline are poor substrates for the high-affinity choline uptake system; esters of choline are even poorer substrates. Although choline acetyltransferase has high specificity for choline-like analogs, the vesicular uptake system does not.[161] Thus, a cholinergic false neurotransmitter can enter the acetylcholine storage vesicle only when it satisfies the structural requirements of three systems: high-affinity choline uptake, choline acetyltransferase, and vesicular uptake. A unique binding site on the outer membrane surface of the choline acetyltransferase storage vesicle has been characterized, using vesamicol,[162–164] a compound initially synthesized as a possible analgesic.[165] Benzoderivatives of vesamicol have been found to be even more potent than vesamicol.[166, 167] Both ^{11}C- and ^{18}F-labeled benzovesamicol analogs have been synthesized.[168–172] The in vivo binding specificity and kinetic properties of ^{18}F-labeled (−)-fluoroethoxybenzovesamicol have been studied in isolated working rat hearts.[173] Data indicate that (−)-^{18}F-fluoroethoxybenzovesamicol is a moderately specific probe of vesamicol-sensitive binding in cholinergic neurons of the heart in experimental conditions that ensure adequate washout of unbound tracer. However, the utility of the radiotracer for in vivo studies with PET is likely to be limited by the low rate of specific binding in myocardium consistent with the low density of cholinergic neurons in the heart.

CLINICAL APPLICATIONS

Heart Failure

Sympathetic stimulation is one of the main compensatory mechanisms for the failing heart. As failure progresses, cardiac stores of norepinephrine are depleted,[174] but circulating norepinephrine concentration is elevated and has been directly related both to the degree of left ventricle dysfunction[175] and to the risk of death.[176] Even though the plasma levels of norepinephrine are elevated in response to heart failure, inotropic responsiveness to catecholamines is abnormal.[40, 41].

The failing heart is characterized not only by a decrease in the catecholamine content of myocytes and impairment of norepinephrine release and uptake but also by abnormalities of cardiac nerve terminals.[174, 177–180] Presynaptic uptake of norepinephrine is reduced in experimental heart failure.[177, 181] A depression of both cardiac norepinephrine release and uptake has been found in patients with mild heart failure due to volume overload caused by valvular heart disease.[179] On the other hand, patients with congestive heart failure have been observed as having a normal fractional extraction of the norepinephrine throughout the heart, which would indicate that presynaptic neuronal norepinephrine uptake is not reduced.[182] Increased release of norepinephrine in heart failure has been found by some,[182–185] but not by all researchers.[179, 180] The role of altered uptake-1 in human heart failure as a local factor for altering concentration of norepinephrine at the myocyte membranes has been demonstrated recently.[186] The effectiveness of norepinephrine in increasing the force of contraction was decreased in relation to the degree of heart failure. In contrast, the potency of norepinephrine, as expressed as the concentration producing 50 percent of the maximal effect, was increased in failing versus nonfailing hearts, whereas the potency of isoproterenol that is not a substrate of uptake-1 was reduced. Finally, this "relative supersensitivity" to extrinsic norepinephrine was related to decreased uptake-1 carrier density, measured using tritiated mazindol binding assays.[186] This alteration of uptake-1 function was demonstrated earlier, using PET with ^{11}C-hydroxyephedrine in patients suffering from heart failure, who have shown a decrease of tracer retention in comparison to control subjects.[187] However, the degree of abnormality varied regionally, indicating a heterogeneous pattern of adrenergic nerve dysfunction.

In heart failure, α-receptor density is normal or even slightly increased, suggesting that the α_1-receptor pathway has no compensatory role in supporting cardiac function.[188, 189] The uncompromised α_1-receptor pathway in the failing heart plays a role in the stimulation of cardiac hypertrophy.[190, 191] A blunted cardiac responsiveness to β-adrenergic stimulation, associated with a substantial reduction of the β-adrenergic receptor density, has been evidenced in failing human myocardium by in vitro studies.[41] Autoradiography of ^{125}I-iodocyanopindolol binding sites from failing human heart has shown that the subendocardium contained the greatest reduction in β-adrenergic receptor density.[39] Heart failure produces a loss in β_1-receptors, whereas β_2-receptor density remains constant. This relative subtype loss of β_1-receptors leads to a shift in the proportion of β_1 versus β_2-receptors from approximately 80:20 in nonfailing heart to 60:40 in failing ventricular myocardium,[192–195] and this subtype alteration is heterogeneous in transmural distribution.[196] β-Receptor density and, by inference, β_1-receptor density begin to decrease in mild heart failure and become progressively reduced as heart failure progresses.[197] A progressive 60 to 70 percent loss in β_1-receptor density leads to a marked decrease in selective β_1-agonist-stimulated adenylate cyclase activity.[198] Thus, down-regulation of β_1-receptors appears to be a main factor of the decreased β_1-agonist sensitivity of the failing heart, especially in idiopathic cardiomyopathy.[199] The β_2-receptor population, although not decreased in density, is mildly uncoupled from pharmacologic response in failing myocardium.[199] β_1-receptors appear to be uncoupled in ischemic cardiomyopathy.[199] The decreased density of β_1-adrenergic receptor density in failing human ventricular myocardium appears to be related to decreased levels of β_1-receptor mRNA.[200] Uncoupling of β_2-adrenergic receptor in idiopathic cardiomyopathy and of β_1-adrenergic receptor in ischemic cardiomyopathy is related to increased functional activity of Gi[199, 201] and receptor phosphorylation.[202]

Left ventricular concentration of β-receptors measured by PET was decreased by 53 percent in patients with idiopathic dilated cardiomyopathy, as compared to that of controls ($p < .001$), in agreement with in vitro data.[124] Moreover, decreased β-receptor concentration correlated with the contractile responsiveness to intracoronary dobutamine infusion ($r = .83$, $P = .003$), indicating a direct link between the level of down-regulation assessed by PET and the corresponding impaired biologic effect. Recently, a relationship between the decrease in β-receptor density and the neuronal norepinephrine function has been found in patients with an idiopathic dilated cardiomyopathy, using PET with ^{11}C-CGP 12177 and planar scintigraphy with ^{123}I-MIBG.[203] However, no correlation was found between plasma norepinephrine concentration and β-receptor density. This finding supports the concept of β-receptor down-regulation as a consequence of presynaptic adrenergic nerve dysfunction. This observation is also concordant with the predominance of the decrease in specific tritiated norepinephrine accumulation that paralleled a predominant β-receptor down-regulation in subendocardial regions of failing left ventricles.[204] β-Adrenergic neuroeffector abnormalities in the failing human heart are therefore likely produced by local, rather than systemic, mechanisms.[205]

Ischemic Heart Disease

Major changes in β-adrenergic receptor regulation take place in the presence of myocardial ischemia, some of which are responsible for the arrhythmias developing in the ischemic myocardium. β-Receptor density is increased in ischemic myocardium.[206–209] These results were not confirmed by others,[210] perhaps related to the duration of ischemia, reperfusion, or membrane preparations. In dog the use of ^{18}F-metaraminol as a tracer has brought evidence that short time periods of coronary occlusion affect neuronal function, indicating a high sensitivity of the sympathetic nerve terminals to ischemia.[211] Combined studies of perfusion and neuronal function, using ^{11}C-hydroxyephedrine in patients with acute myocardial infarction, have shown a neuronal dysfunction of the ischemic myocardium.[212] In patients with recent acute myocardial infarction, a decreased ^{11}C-hydroxyephedrine was found in the infarct area, and this decrease was more extensive than that of myocardial blood flow.[213] After an 8-month follow-up, no change was observed, suggesting that reinnervation does not occur, even for reversibly injured myocardium. These observations confirm and extend the results of earlier MIBG studies of patients recovering from acute myocardial infarction, which showed that the extent of the MIBG defect size was larger than that of the thallium defect size.[214–216] This reduced norepinephrine analog uptake in the ischemic myocardium is likely related to nerve energy deficiency and subsequent alteration in the uptake-1 function. Acute ischemia, as seen in myocardial areas perfused by a stenotic vessel, leads to catecholamine depletion as a first step and to decreased function of the uptake-1 system as a second step. With the prolongation of ischemia, the uptake-1 system becomes chronically impaired, and the net transport direction of the uptake-1 system is reversed. These alterations, measured by PET or single-photon emission imaging, can be of prognostic signification, as evidenced by the supersensitivity to adrenergic stimulation of denervated myocardium with absent MIBG uptake.[217]

Hypertrophy

In experimental renovascular or spontaneous hypertension, β-adrenergic receptor density is either normal[218, 219] or depressed.[220–222] With aortic banding to produce hypertension, β-adrenergic receptor number is increased[218] or unchanged.[223] In experimental left ventricular hypertrophy secondary to aortic banding, physiologic responsiveness to catecholamines is normal with increased β-adrenergic receptor density but decreased antagonist affinity.[224]

Primary hypertrophic cardiomyopathy represents a totally different clinical entity from dilated cardiomyopathy, including mainly asymmetric hypertrophy associated with hyperdynamic contractility, diastolic filling abnormalities, and propensity for arrhythmias.[225, 226] These characteristics have suggested a potential role of the altered sympathetic system in the evolution of the disease. Different clinical features may have a prognostic value, such as the importance of clinical symptoms, a family history of sudden death, the importance of hypertrophy and its mechanical consequences, and the presence of arrhythmias. However, the prognosis of this disease remains to be defined, especially in individuals.

In this disease, abnormalities include impaired catecholamine synthesis, abnormal norepinephrine neuronal release or uptake, and decreased myocardial catecholamine content.[174, 177, 227, 228] The most consistent finding is decreased presynaptic norepinephrine uptake.[229]

In vivo invasive pharmacologic methods have suggested that impaired adrenergic nerve function was involved in mechanisms of primary hypertrophic cardiomyopathy.[229] MIBG studies have reported decreased tracer uptake in patients with primary hypertrophic cardiomyopathy.[230, 231] In patients with primary hypertrophic cardiomyopathy, no change in β-adrenergic receptor density has been found, using in vitro binding studies.[33, 232, 233] However, using PET and ^{11}C-CGP 12177, a diffuse reduction in myocardial β-receptors has been evidenced in patients with primary hypertrophic cardiomyopathy without heart failure and increase in circulating norepinephrine levels.[234] This discrepancy may be attributable to patient or control subject selection, as well as to methodologic differences.

Denervation

Denervation supersensitivity occurs in patients treated with β-blockers or in naturally occurring neuronal denervation. Chronic denervation results in β-adrenergic receptor up-regulation and supersensitivity in the surgically denervated heart.[235, 236] The mechanism of supersensitivity is due to the up-regulation of β-adrenergic receptors and the lack of reuptake resulting from the absence of sympathetic nerve endings. Human studies in healthy volunteers and in heart-transplant patients demonstrated no hemodynamic effects of the compound.[237] In transplant patients, uptake was found to be reduced by 76 percent.[238] Only a small number of adrenergic neuron fibers is needed in reinnervated heart tissue to generate large functional responses.[239] If, in fact, regenerated nerves can be functional prior to the development of storage vesicles, then ^{11}C-hydroxyephedrine is likely to give a better functional map of the heart than radiolabeled norepinephrine or dopamine. Defining reinnervation in the human heart is still a controversial topic with important clinical implications.[240] Although most animal species show functional reinnervation 3 to 6 months after heart transplantation,[241, 242] a report concluded based on myocardial catecholamines levels that the transplanted human heart remains denervated for as long as 5 years after transplantation.[243] Work with ^{11}C-HED,[238] tyramine challenge studies,[244] and reports that transplant patients can experience angina pectoris[245] have demonstrated that some level of functional reinnervation is occurring.

When cardiac β-receptor sensitivity to isoprenaline in the denervated donor heart in patients with heart transplants was compared to that of the innervated recipient heart,[34] there was an increase in β-receptor density and no change in β-receptor affinity in the transplanted heart.[246, 247] However, change in β-adrenergic receptor density was found in biopsy samples from heart-transplant patients.[248] Similar results were obtained in vivo with ^{11}C-CGP.[249] These findings indicate that the observed supersensitivity of the transplanted to extrinsic catecholamines is of presynaptic origin.[249–251]

Decreased myocardial adenylate cyclase activity in response to guanine nucleotide stimulation has been recently demonstrated in denervated myocardium of transplant patients, suggesting that changes in left ventricular muscarinic receptors may occur.[250] No difference in the concentration and affinity constant of muscarinic receptors was found in transplant patients studied by means of positron emission tomography with ^{11}C-labeled MQNB compared with that of control subjects,[251] which suggests abnormalities of the signal-transduction function, such as changes in the guanine nucleotide-binding proteins.

Denervation supersensitivity is a potential mechanism of ventricular arrhythmias. Support for this concept has been provided by the reduction of ^{11}C-hydroxyephedrine retention, measured by PET in patients with a history of sustained ventricular tachycardia or sudden death, in areas showing augmented effective refactory period assessed during surgical intervention for defibrillator implantation.[252] The familial long-QT syndrome may result from congenital imbalance of sympathetic innervation of the heart caused by lower-than-normal right cardiac activity. In a small series of such patients, however no differences in ^{11}C-hydroxyephedrine retention index or ^{11}C-hydroxyephedrine uptake normalized to blood flow were evidenced, in comparison with those of control patients.[252] This discrepancy with prior MIBG studies[253] may be due to differences in tracer properties or patient selection.

In patients with diabetic neuropathy, the use of ^{11}C-hydroxyephedrine demonstrated a heterogeneous pattern of myocardial adrenergic nerve function, in comparison with that of both control subjects and diabetic patients without neuropathy. The extent of the abnormalities correlated with the severity found with conventional markers of autonomic dysfunction. Absolute myocardial tracer retention index showed a 45 percent decrease in distal, as compared to proximal, segments. This approach may represent a means for the early detection of autonomic dysfunction in diabetic patients and may help evaluate effects of therapy intervention on this complication.[254]

Cardiac toxity of cocaine, including myocardial ischemia, ventricular function alteration, and arrhythmias,[255–257] has been linked to its inhibitory effect on norepinephrine reuptake by the sympathetic nerve terminals of the heart. In dogs it has been demonstrated with ^{11}C-hydroxyephedrine and PET that cocaine induces a large and prolonged reduction in uptake-1 function, which may contribute to a large increase in norepinephrine concentration at the myocyte membrane level.

Desensitization

Desensitization is due to changes in the β-adrenergic receptor-G protein-adenylyl cyclase complex as a result of chronic exposure to high levels of β-adrenergic agonist at the receptor sites.[258–260] Homologous desensitization is characterized by a reduced responsiveness only to the specific desensitizing hormone without affecting the adenylyl cyclase enzyme's responsiveness to other hormones. Heterologous desensitization is characterized by diminished responsiveness of adenylyl cyclase to a wide spectrum of stimulators, including other hormones, fluoride, and guanine nucleotides. Human myocardium relies mainly on β-receptors to augment contractility and appears to have no or few "spare" receptors.[32, 40] A positive correlation has been found in patients with idiopathic dilated cardiomyopathy between the β-receptor concentration assessed by PET and the contractile responsiveness to intracoronary infusion of dobutamine.[124] This correlation suggests that the down-regulation of β-receptors is a main factor of the β-adrenergic desensitization, which is consistent with other findings that showed a reduced basal, Gpp(NH)p-, and isoproterenol-stimulated adenylyl cyclase activity but an unchanged forskoline-stimulated adenylyl cyclase, suggesting that reduced isoproterenol-stimulated adenylate cyclase is due to reduced β-adrenergic receptor density, rather than to increased inhibitory subunit of G protein.[261]

CONCLUSION

Researchers only recently have begun to apply PET to the study of cardiac physiology and disease. It is the only methodology able to demonstrate the physiologic regulation of receptors. Binding of neurotransmitter to receptor is an essential step in synaptic transmission. The interaction between agonist and receptor sets in motion a series of molecular events via the second messenger system, culminating in the observed response. This series of molecular interactions has been shown to be altered in several cardiac diseases. However, there is also a complex sequence of events that takes place between the nerve terminal and the postsynaptic neuron or the cardiac muscle cell. It includes synthesis and release of neurotransmitter, binding to receptor, hydrolysis of neurotransmitter in the synaptic cleft, and/or reuptake of neurotransmitter. Several pathologic and therapeutic concepts in cardiology have been based on sympathetic neuroeffector mechanisms in the heart. A limitation in evaluating these concepts has been the difficulty of measuring cardiac sympathetic function in vivo, especially the activity of the neuronal uptake process (uptake-1). It is now possible to evaluate in vivo both adrenergic innervation and adrenergic receptors noninvasively. Although the partial volume effect precludes at the present time the evaluation of the transmural distribution of the alterations of cardiac neurotransmission, one of the main advantages of PET is the possibility of studying regional abnormalities of cardiac neurotransmission, especially in arrhythmogenic cardiomyopathy. Furthermore, PET could be useful in exploring the alteration of neurotransmission in the early stages of the different diseases. As noninvasive tests, repeated PET examinations could also provide information on the effects of therapy with drugs acting on the heart and myocardial receptors.

References

1. Levy, M.N., and Blattberg, B.: The influence of cocaine and desipramine on the cardiac responses to exogenous and endogenous norepinephrine. Eur. J. Pharmacol. 48:37, 1978.
2. Masuda, Y., and Levy, M.N.: The effects of neuronal uptake blockade on the cardiac responses to sympathetic nerve stimulation and norepinephrine infusion in anesthetized dogs. J. Auton. Nerv Syst. 10:1, 1984.
3. Han, J., Garcia de Jalon, P., and Moe, G.K.: Adrenergic effects on ventricular vulnerability. Circ. Res. 14:516, 1964.
4. Inoue, H., and Zipes, D.P.: Results of sympathetic denervation in the canine heart: Supersensitivity that may be arrhythmogenic. Circulation 75:877, 1987.
5. Smith, A.D.: Summing up: Some implications of the neuron as a secreting cell. Trans. R. Soc. Lond. (Biol.) 261:423, 1971.
6. Pierpont, G.L., DeMaster, E.G., and Cohn, J.N.: Regional differences in adrenergic function within the left ventricle. Am. J. Physiol. 246:H824, 1984.
7. Dahlstom, A., Haggenda, J., and Hokfelt, T.: The noradrenaline content of the nerve terminal varicosities of the sympathetic adrenergic neurons in the rat. Acta Physiol. Scand. 67:289, 1966.
8. Langer, S.Z.: Presynaptic regulation of the release of catecholamines. Biochem. Pharmacol. 23:1793, 1974.
9. Langer, S.Z.: Presynaptic regulation of the release of catecholamines. Pharmacol. Rev. 32:337, 1981.
10. Matko, I., Feher, E., and Vizi, E.S.: Receptor mediated presynaptic modulation of the release of noradrenaline in human papillary muscle. Cardiovasc. Res. 28:700, 1994.
11. Muscholl, E., Ritzel, H., and Rossler, K.: Presynaptic muscarinic control of neuronal adrenaline release. *In* Langer, S.Z., Stark, K., Dubocovich, M.L. (eds.): Oxford, Pergamon, pp. 287–291, 1979.
12. Phillis, J.W., and Barraco, R.A.: Adenosine, adenylate cyclase and transmitter release. Adv. Cyclic Nucleotide Protein Phosphorylation Res. 19:243, 1985.
13. McGrath, M.A., and Sheperd, J.T.: Histamine and 5-hydroxytryptamine-inhibition of transmitter release mediated by H2 and 5-hydroxytryptamine receptors. Fed. Proc. 37:195, 1978.
14. Zimmerman, B.G.: Action of angiotensin on adrenergic nerve endings. Fed. Proc. 37:199, 1978.
15. Dahlof, C., Ljung, B., and Ablad, B.: Increased noradrenaline release in rat portal vein during sympathetic nerve stimulation due to activation of presynaptic β-adrenoreceptors by noradrenaline and adrenaline. Eur. J. Pharmacol. 50:75, 1978.
16. Axelrod, J.: The fate of noradrenaline in the sympathetic neuron. The Harvey Lectures, series 67. New York, Academic Press, 1972, pp. 175–197.
17. Iversen, L.L.: Inhibition of noradrenaline uptake by drugs. J. Pharm. Pharmacol. 29:62, 1965.
18. Iversen, L.L.: Role of transmitter uptake mechanisms in synaptic neurotransmission. Br. J. Pharmacol. 41:571, 1971.
19. Motulsky, H.J., and Insel, P.A.: Adrenergic receptors in man. Direct identification, physiologic regulation, and clinical alterations. N. Engl. J. Med. 307:18, 1982.
20. Stiles, G.L., Caron, M.G., and Lefkowitz, R.J.: β-Adrenergic receptors: Biochemical mechanisms of physiological regulation. Physiol. Rev. 64:661, 1984.
21. Stiles, G.L., Taylor, S., and Lefkowitz, R.J.: Human cardiac beta-adrenergic receptors: Subtype heterogeneity delineated by direct ligand binding. Life Sci. 33:467, 1983.
22. Stiles, G.L., and Lefkowitz, R.J.: Cardiac adrenergic receptors. Annu. Rev. Med. 35:149, 1984.
23. Molinoff, P.B.: Alpha- and beta-adrenergic receptor subtypes properties, distribution and regulation. Drugs 28 (Suppl. 2):1, 1984.
24. Ruffolo, R.R., Sulpizia, A.C., Nichols, A.J., et al.: Pharmacological differentiation between pre- and post-junctional alpha 2-adrenoreceptors by SKF 104078. Naunyn Schmieldebergs Arch. Pharmol. 336:415, 1987.
25. Regan, J.W., Kobilka, T.S., Yang-Feng, T.L., et al.: Cloning and expression of a human kidney cDNA for an alpha 2-adrenergic receptor subtype. Proc. Natl. Acad. Sci. U.S.A. 85:6301, 1988.
26. Emorine, L.J., Marullo, S., Briend-Sutren, M.-M., et al.: Molecular characterization of the human β_3-adrenergic receptor. Science 245:1118, 1989.
27. Bennet, J.P., Jr.: Methods in binding studies. *In* Yamamura, H.I., Enna, S.J., and Kuhar, M.J. (eds.): Neurotransmitter Receptor Binding. New York, Raven Press, 1978, pp. 57–90.
28. Peralta, E.G., Winslow, J.W., Peterson, G.L., et al.: Primary structure and biochemical properties of an M_2-muscarinic receptor. Science 236:600, 1987.
29. Tcheng, K.T.: Innervation of the dog's heart. Am. Heart J. 41:512, 1951.
30. Saito, K., Kurihara, M., Cruciani, R., et al.: Characterization of beta-1 and beta-2 adrenoreceptor subtypes in the rat atrioventricular node by quantitative autoradiography. Circ. Res. 62:173, 1988.
31. Heitz, A., Schwartz, J., and Velly, J.: Beta-adrenoceptors of the human myocardium: Determination of 1 and 2 subtypes by radioligand binding. Br. J. Pharmacol. 80:711, 1983.
32. Bristow, M.R., Kantrowitz, N.E., Ginsburg, R., et al.: Beta-adrenergic function in heart muscle disease and heart failure. J. Mol. Cell. Cardiol. S2:41, 1985.
33. Golf, S., Løfvstadt, R., and Hansson, V.: Beta-adrenoceptor density and relative number of beta-adrenoceptor subtypes in biopsies from human right atrial, left ventricular and right ventricular myocardium. Cardiovasc. Res. 19:636, 1985.
34. Hedberg, A., Kempf, F., Jr., Josephson, M.E., et al.: Coexistence of beta-1 and beta-2 adrenergic receptors in the human heart: Effects of treatment with receptor antagonists or calcium entry blockers. J. Pharmacol. Exp. Ther. 234:561, 1985.
35. Robberecht, P., Delhaye, M., Taton, G., et al.: The human heart beta-adrenergic receptors. I. Heterogeneity of the binding sites: Presence of 50% $beta_1$- and 50% $beta_2$-adrenergic receptors. Mol. Pharmacol. 24:169, 1983.
36. Kaumann, A.J.: Some aspects of heart beat adrenoreceptor function. Cardiovasc. Drugs Ther. 5:549, 1991.
37. Lathers, C.M., Levin, R.M., and Spivey, W.H.: Regional distribution of myocardial beta-adrenoceptors in the cat. Eur. J. Pharmacol. 130:111, 1986.
38. Wei, J.-W., and Sulakhe, P.V.: Regional and subcellular distribution of beta- and alpha-adrenergic receptors in the myocardium of different species. Gen. Pharmacol. 10:263, 1979.
39. Murphee, S.S., and Saffitz, J.E.: Distribution of adrenergic receptors in failing human heart: Implications for mechanisms of down regulation. Circulation 79:1214, 1989.
40. Colucci, W.S., Denniss, A.R., Leatherman, G.F., et al.: Intracoronary infusion of dobutamine to patients with and without severe congestive heart failure. J. Clin. Invest. 81:1103, 1988.
41. Bristow, M.R., Ginsburg, R., Minobe, W., et al.: Decreased catecholamine sensitivity and beta-adrenergic receptor density in failing human heart. N. Engl. J. Med. 307:205, 1982.
42. Gilman, A.G.: G proteins: Transducers of receptor-generated signals. Annu. Rev. Biochem. 56:615, 1987.
43. Robishaw, J.D., and Foster, K.A.: Role of G proteins in the regulation of the cardiovascular system. Annu. Rev. Physiol. 51:229, 1989.
44. Ardell, J.L., and Randall, W.C.: Selective vagal innervation of sinoatrial and atrioventricular nodes in canine heart. Am. J. Physiol. (Heart Circ. Physiol. 20) 251:H764, 1986.
45. Blomquist, T.M., Priola, D.V., and Romero, A.M.: Source of intrinsic innervation of canine ventricles: A functional study. Am. J. Physiol. (Heart Circ. Physiol. 21) 252:H638, 1987.
46. Hassal, C.J.S., Buckley, N.J., and Burnstok, G.: Autoradiographic localization of muscarinic receptors on guinea pig intracardiac neurons and atrial myocytes in culture. Neurosci. Lett. 74:145, 1987.
47. Levy, M.N., and Martin, P.J.: Neural regulation of the heart beat. Annu. Rev. Physiol. 43:443, 1981.
48. Napolitano, L.M., Willman, V.L., Hanlon, C.R., et al.: Intrinsic innervation of the heart. Am. J. Physiol. 208:455, 1965.
49. Takahashi, N., Barber, M.J., and Zipes, D.P.: Efferent vagal innervation of canine ventricle. Am. J. Physiol. (Heart Circ. Physiol. 17) 248:H89, 1985.
50. Hirschowitz, B.I., and Bonner, T.I. (eds.): Subtypes of muscarinic receptors. Trends Pharmacol. Sci. (Suppl):11–15, 1984.
51. Hammer, R., Berrie, C.P., Birdsall, N.J.M., et al.: Pirenzepine distinguishes between different subclasses of muscarinic receptors. Nature 283:90, 1980.
52. Giachetti, A., Micheletti, R., and Montagna, E.: Cardioselective profile of AF-DX 116: A muscarinic M2-receptor antagonist. Life Sci. 38:1663, 1986.
53. Hammer, R., Giraldo, E., Schiavi, G.B., et al.: Binding profile of a novel cardioselective muscarinic antagonist, AF-DX 116, to membranes of peripheral tissues and brain in the rat. Life Sci. 38:1653, 1986.
54. Bonner, T.I., Buckley, N.J., Young, A.C., et al.: Identification of a family of muscarinic acetylcholine receptor genes. Science 237:527, 1987.
55. Fukuda, K., Kubo, T., Akiba, I., et al.: Molecular distinction between muscarinic acetylcholine receptor subtypes. Nature 327:623, 1987.
56. Hoover, D.B., Baisden, R.H., and Ximoy, S.X.: Localization of muscarinic receptor mRNAs in rat heart and intrinsic cardiac ganglia by in situ hybridization. Circ. Res. 75:813, 1994.
57. Manalan, A.S., Werth, D.K., Jones, L.R., et al.: Enrichment, solubilization, and partial characterization of digitonin-solubilized muscarinic receptors derived from canine ventricular myocardium. Circ. Res. 52:664, 1983.
58. Nathanson, N.M.: Molecular properties of the muscarinic acetylcholine receptor. Annu. Rev. Neurosci. 10:195, 1987.
59. Bartel, S., Karczewski, P., and Krause, E.G.: Protein phosphorylation and cardiac function: Cholinergic-adrenergic interaction. Cardiovasc. Res. 27:1948, 1993.
60. Yamada, S., Yamazawa, T., Harada, Y., et al.: Muscarinic receptor subtype in porcine coronary artery. Eur. J. Pharmacol. 150:373, 1988.
61. Pelc, L.R., Gross, G.J., and Warltier, D.C.: Changes in regional myocardial perfusion by muscarinic receptor subtypes in dogs. Cardiovasc. Res. 20:482, 1986.

62. Furchgott, R.F., and Zawadzki, J.V.: The obligatory role of endothelial cells in the relaxation of arterial smooth muscle by acetylcholine. Nature 288:373, 1980.
63. Hynes, M.R., Banner, W., Jr., Yamamura, H.I., et al.: Characterization of muscarinic receptors of the rabbit ear artery smooth muscle and endothelium. J. Pharmacol. Exp. Ther. 238:100, 1986.
64. O'Rourke, S.T., and Vanhoutte, P.M.: Subtypes of muscarinic receptors on adrenergic nerves and vascular smooth muscle of the canine saphenous vein. J. Pharmacol. Exp. Ther. 241:64, 1987.
65. Duckles, S.P.: Vascular muscarinic receptors: Pharmacological characterization in the bovine coronary artery. J. Pharmacol. Exp. Ther. 246:929, 1988.
66. Stephenson, J.A., and Summers, R.J.: Autoradiographic analysis of receptors on vascular endothelium. Eur. J. Pharmacol. 134:35, 1987.
67. Peach, M.J., Singer, H.A., and Loeba, L.: Mechanisms of endothelium-dependent vascular smooth muscle relaxation. Biochem. Pharmacol. 34:1867, 1985.
68. Peralta, E.G., Ashkenazi, A., Winslow, J.W., et al.: Differential regulation of PI hydrolysis and adenylate cyclase by muscarinic receptor subtypes. Nature 334:434, 1988.
69. Yatani, A., Hamm, H., Codina, J., et al.: A monoclonal antibody to the alpha-subunit of G_k blocks muscarinic activation of atrial K^+ channels. Science 241:828, 1988.
70. Ashkenazi, A., Peralta, E.G., Winslown, J.W., et al.: Functionally distinct G proteins selectively couple different receptors to PI hydrolysis in the same cell. Cell 56:487, 1989.
71. Kikkawa, U., and Nishizuka, Y.: The role of protein kinase C in transmembrane signalling. Annu. Rev. Cell. Biol. 2:149, 1986.
72. Kubo, T., Fukuda, K., Mikami, A., et al.: Cloning, sequencing and expression of complementary DNA encoding the muscarinic acetylcholine receptor. Nature 323:411, 1986.
73. DiFrancesco, D., Ducouret, P., and Robinson, R.B.: Muscarinic modulation of cardiac rate at low acetylcholine concentrations. Science 243:699, 1989.
74. Pappano, A.J., Matsumoto, K., Tajima, T., et al.: Pertussis toxin-insensitive mechanism for carbachol-induced depolarization and positive inotropic effect in heart muscle. Trends Pharmacol. Sci. 9 (Suppl):35, 1988.
75. Anholt, R.R.H., Pedersen, P.L., De Souza, E.B., et al.: The peripheral-type benzodiazepine receptor. J. Biol. Chem. 261:576, 1986.
76. Kim, D., Lewis, D.L., Graziadei, L., et al.: G-protein beta-gamma-subunits activate the cardiac muscarinic K^+ channel via phospholipase A2. Nature 337:557, 1989.
77. Endoh, M., Yanagiasawa, T., Taira, N., et al.: Effects of new inotropic agents on cyclic nucleotide metabolism and calcium transients in canine ventricular muscle. Circulation 73 (Suppl. III):III-117, 1986.
78. Deferrari, G.M., Vanoli, E., Curcuruto, P., et al.: Prevention of life-threatening arrhythmias by pharmacologic stimulation of the muscarinic receptors with oxotremorine. Am. Heart J. 124:883, 1992.
79. Wilkinson, M., Horackova, M., and Giles, A.: Reduction of ventricular M_2-muscarinic receptors in cardiomyopathic hamster (Chf 147) at the Necrotic Stage of the Myopathy. Pflugers Arch. 426:516, 1994.
80. Vatner, D.E., Lee, D.L., Schwarz, K.R., et al.: Impaired cardiac muscarinic receptor function in dogs with heart failure. J. Clin. Invest. 81:1836, 1988.
81. Böhm, M., Gierschik, P., Jakobs, K.H., et al.: Increase of Gi alpha in human hearts with dilated but not ischemic cardiomyopathy. Circulation 82:1249, 1990.
82. Koumi, S., Arentzen, C.E., Backer, C.L., et al.: Alterations in muscarinic K^+ channel response to acetylcholine and to G protein–mediated activation in atrial myocytes isolated from failing human hearts. Circulation 90:2213, 1994.
83. Bergman, S.R., Fox, K.A.A., Geltman, E.M., et al.: Positron emission tomography of the heart. Prog. Cardiovasc. Dis. 28:165, 1985.
84. Schelbert, H.R.: Positron-emission tomography: Assessment of myocardial blood flow and metabolism. Circulation 72:IV122, 1985.
85. Sobel, B.E.: Positron tomography and myocardial metabolism: An overview. Circulation 72:IV22, 1985.
86. Syrota, A.: In vivo study of receptors for neuromediators with PET. Int. J. Nucl. Med. Biol. 13:127, 1986.
87. Pascal, O., Syrota, A., Berger, G., et al.: Lung uptake of ^{11}C-imipramine and ^{11}C-propranolol in patients with sarcoidosis evaluated by positron emission tomography. *In* Marsac, J., and Chretien, J. (eds.): Sarcoidosis and Other Granulomatous Disorders. Paris, Pergamon Press, 1981, pp. 404–408.
88. Charbonneau, P., Syrota, A., Boullais, C., et al.: Serotonin receptors and lung phagocyte recruitment induced by cigarette smoking detected in vivo by positron emission tomography. (Abstract.) J. Nucl. Med. 27:950, 1986.
89. Woods, P.B., and Robinson, M.L.: An investigation of the comparative liposolubilities of beta-adrenoceptor blocking agents. J. Pharm. Pharmacol. 33:172, 1981.
90. Wong, D.F., Gjedde, A., Wagner, H.N., Jr., et al.: Quantification of neuroreceptors in the living human brain. II. Inhibition studies of receptor density and affinity. J. Cereb. Blood Flow Metab. 6:147, 1986.
91. Chaumet-Riffaud, P., Girault, M., and Syrota, A.: Characterization of muscarinic cholinergic receptors in the isolated perfused rat heart. J. Physiol. (Lond.) 348:11P, 1984.
92. Fields, J.Z., Roeske, W.R., Morkin, E., et al.: Cardiac muscarinic cholinergic receptors. Biochemical identification and characterization. J. Biol. Chem. 253:3251, 1978.
93. Gibson, R.E., Eckelman, W.C., Vieras, F., et al.: The distribution of the muscarinic acetylcholine receptor antagonists, quinuclidinyl benzilate and quinuclidinyl benzilate methiodide (both triated) in rat, guinea pig and rabbit. J. Nucl. Med. 20:865, 1979.
94. Landais, P., and Crouzel, C.: A new synthesis of ^{11}C-labelled phosgene. Appl. Radiat. Isot. 38:297, 1987.
95. Camsonne, R., Crouzel, C., Comar, D., et al.: Synthesis of *N*-(^{11}C)methyl, *N*-(methyl-1 propyl), (chloro-2 phenyl)-1 isoquinoleine carboxamide receptors. J. Label. Compounds Radiopharmacol. 21:985, 1984.
96. Schwaiger, M., and Schelbert, H.R.: Assessment of tissue viability, in ischemic heart disease by positron emission tomography. *In* Pohost, G.M. (ed.): New Concepts in Cardiac Imaging. Chicago, Year Book, 1986, pp. 155–170.
97. Crouzel, C., Venet, M., Sanz, G., et al.: Labelling of a new serotoninergic ligand: ^{18}F-ritanserine. J. Label. Compounds Radiopharmacol. 25:827, 1988.
98. Crouzel, C., Venet, M., Irié, T., et al.: Labeling of a serotoninergic ligand with ^{18}F: ^{18}F-setoperone. J. Label. Compounds Radiopharmacol. 25:403, 1988.
99. Laduron, P.M.: Criteria for receptor sites in binding studies. Biochem. Pharmacol. 33:833, 1984.
100. Mazière, M., Comar, D., Godot, J.M., et al.: In vivo characterization of myocardium muscarinic receptors by positron emission tomography. Life Sci. 29:2391, 1981.
101. Dormont, D., Syrota, A., Berger, G., et al.: ^{11}C ligand binding to adrenergic and muscarinic receptors in the human heart studied in vivo by PET. (Abstract.) J. Nucl. Med. 24:P20, 1983.
102. Seto, M., Syrota, A., Crouzel, C., et al.: Beta adrenergic receptors in the dog heart characterized by ^{11}C-CGP 12 177 and PET. (Abstract.) J. Nucl. Med. 27:949, 1986.
103. Changeux, J.P.: The acetylcholine receptor: An "allosteric" membrane protein. Harvey Lect. 75:85, 1981.
104. Delforge, J., Syrota, A., and Mazoyer, B.M.: Identifiability analysis and parameter identification of an in vivo ligand-receptor model from pet data. I.E.E.E. Trans. Biomed. Eng. 37:653, 1990.
105. Cobelli, C., and DiStefano, J.: Parameters and structural identifiability concepts and ambiguities: A critical review and analysis. Am. J. Physiol. 239:R7, 1980.
106. Syrota, A., Paillotin, G., Davy, J.M., et al.: Kinetics of in vivo binding of antagonist to muscarinic cholinergic receptor in the human heart studied by positron emission tomography. Life Sci. 35:937, 1984.
107. Delforge, J., Syrota, A., and Mazoyer, B.: Experimental design optimization: Theory and application to estimation of receptor model parameters using dynamic positron emission tomography. Phys. Med. Biol. 34:419, 1989.
108. Mintun, M.A., Raichle, M.E., Kilbourn, M. R., et al.: A quantitative model for the in vivo assessment of drug binding sites with positron emission tomography. Ann. Neurol. 15:217, 1984.
109. Farde, L., Hall, H., Ehrin, E., et al.: Quantitative analysis of D_2-dopamine receptor binding in the living human brain by PET. Science 231:258, 1986.
110. Perlmutter, J.S., Larson, K.B., Raichle, M.E., et al.: Strategies for in vivo measurement of receptor binding using positron emission tomography. J. Cereb. Blood Flow Metab. 6:154, 1986.
111. Patlak, C.S., Blasberg, R.G., and Fenstermacher, J.D.: Graphical evaluation of blood to brain transfer constants from multiple-time uptake data. J. Cereb. Blood Flow Metab. 3:3, 1983.
112. Delforge, J., Janier, M., Syrota, A., et al.: Noninvasive quantification of muscarinic receptors in vivo with positron emission tomography in the dog heart. Circulation 82:1494, 1990.
113. Berger, G., Mazière, M., Prenant, C., et al.: Synthesis of ^{11}C-propranolol. J. Radioanal. Chem. 74:301, 1982.
114. Berger, G., Prenant, C., Sastre, J., et al.: Synthesis of a beta-blocker for heart visualization: ^{11}C-practolol. Int. J. Appl. Radiat. Isot. 34:1556, 1983.
115. Prenant, C., Sastre, J., Crouzel, C., et al.: Synthesis of ^{11}C-pindolol. J. Label. Compounds Radiopharmacol. 24:227, 1987.
116. Boullais, C., Crouzel, C., and Syrota, A.: Synthesis of 4-(3-t-butylamino-2-hydroxypropoxy)-benzimidazol-2(^{11}C)-one (CGP 12177). J. Label. Compounds Radiopharmacol. 23:565, 1986.
117. Hammadi, A., and Crouzel, C.: Asymetric synthesis of (2S) and (2R)-4-(butylamino-2-hydroxypropoxy-benzamidazol-2-^{11}C) one (S) and (R) (^{11}C CGP 12177) from optically active precursors. J. Label. Compounds Radiopharmacol. 29:681, 1991.
118. Nanoff, C., Freissmuth, M., and Schütz, W.: The role of a low beta-1 adrenoceptor selectivity of ^{3}H-CGP-12177 for resolving subtype-selectivity of competitive ligands. Naunyn Schmiedeberg's Arch. Pharmacol. 336:519, 1987.
119. Staehelin, M., and Hertel, C.: ^{3}H-CGP-12 177, a beta-adrenergic ligand suitable for measuring cell surface receptors. J. Recept. Res. 3:35, 1983.
120. Staehelin, M., Simons, P., and Jaeggik Wigger, N.: CGP-12 177. A hydrophilic beta-adrenergic receptor radioligand reveals high affinity binding of agonists to intact cells. J. Biol. Chem. 258:3496, 1983.
121. Hertel, C., Muller, P., Portenier, H., et al.: Determination of the desensitization of beta-adrenergic receptors by ^{3}H-CGP-12 177. Biochem. J. 216:669, 1983.
122. Mukherjee, A., Haghani, Z., Brady, J., et al.: Differences in myocardial alpha- and beta-adrenergic receptor numbers in different species. Am. J. Physiol. (Heart Circ. Physiol. 14) 245:H957, 1983.
123. Delforge, J., Syrota, A., Lancon, J. P., et al.: Cardiac beta-adrenergic receptor density measured in vivo using PET, CGP 12177 and a new graphical method. J. Nucl. Med. 32:739, 1991.
124. Merlet, P., Delforge, J., Syrota, A., et al.: Positron emission tomography with ^{11}C CGP-12177 to assess β-adrenergic receptor concentration in idiopathic dilated cardiomyopathy. Circulation 87:1169, 1993.
125. Ehrin, E., Luthra, S.K., Crouzel, C., et al.: Preparation of carbon 11–labelled prazosin, a potent and selective alpha-1 adrenoceptor antagonist. J. Label. Compounds. Radiopharmacol. 25:177, 1988.
126. Gossuin, A., Maloteaux, J.M., Trouet, A., et al.: Differentiation between ligand trapping into intact cells and binding on muscarinic receptors. Biochim. Biophys. Acta. 804:100, 1984.
127. Brown, J.H., and Goldstein, D.: Analysis of cardiac muscarinic receptors recog-

nized selectively by nonquaternary but not by quaternary ligands. J. Pharmacol. Exp. Ther. 238:580, 1986.

128. Syrota, A., Comar, D., Paillotin, G., et al.: Muscarinic cholinergic receptor in the human heart evidenced under physiological conditions by positron emission tomography. Proc. Natl. Acad. Sci. U.S.A. 82:584, 1985.
129. Burgisser, E., De Lean, A., and Lefkowitz, R.J.: Reciprocal modulation of agonist and antagonist binding to muscarinic cholinergic receptor by guanine nucleotide. Proc. Natl. Acad. Sci. U.S.A. 79:1732, 1985.
130. Delforge, J., Leguludee, D., Syrota, A., et al.: Quantification of myocardial muscarinic receptors with PET in humans. J. Nucl. Med. 34:981, 1993.
131. Davies, L.P., and Huston, V.: Peripheral benzodiazepine binding sites in and their interaction with dipyridamole. Eur. J. Pharmacol. 73:209, 1981.
132. Taniguchi, T., Wang, J.K.T., and Spector, S.: ^{3}H-diazepam binding sites on rat heart and kidney. Biochem. Pharmacol. 31:589, 1982.
133. Trifiletti, R.R., Lo, M.M.S., and Snyder, S.H.: Kinetic differences between type I and type II benzodiazepine receptors. Mol. Pharmacol. 26:228, 1984.
134. Le Fur, G., Perrier, M.L., Vaucher, N., et al.: Peripheral benzodiazepine binding sites: Effect of PK 11195, 1-(2-chlorophenyl)-*N*-methyl-*N*-(1-methyl-propyl)-3-isoquinoline-carboxamide. I. In vitro studies. Life Sci. 32:1839, 1983.
135. Le Fur, G., Guilloux, F., Rufat, P., et al.: Peripheral benzodiazepine binding sites: Effect of PK 11195, 1-(2-chorophenyl)-*N*-methyl-*N*-(1-methyl-propyl)-3 isoquinolinecarboxamide. II. In vivo studies. Life Sci. 32:1849, 1983.
136. Charbonneau, P., Syrota, A., Crouzel, C., et al.: Peripheral-type benzodiazepine receptors in the living heart characterized by positron emission tomography. Circulation 73:476, 1986.
137. Mestre, M., Carriot, T., Belin, C., et al.: Electrophysiological and pharmacological evidence that peripheral type benzodiazepine receptors are coupled to calcium channels in the heart. Life Sci. 36:391, 1985.
138. Grupp, I.L., French, J.F., and Matlibma, P.: Benzodiazepine RO 5-4864 coronary blood flow. Eur. J. Pharmacol. 134:143, 1987.
139. Basile, A.S., and Skolnik, P.: Tissue specific regulation of "peripheral-type" benzodiazepine receptor density after chemical sympathectomy. Life Sci. 42:273, 1988.
140. Mislankar, S.G., Gildersleeve, D.L., Wieland, D.M., et al.: 6-^{18}F fluorometaraminol: A radiotracer for in vivo mapping of adrenergic nerves of the heart. J. Med. Chem. 31:362, 1988.
141. Wieland, D.M., Rosenpire, K.C., Hutchkins, G.D., et al.: Neuronal mapping of the heart with 6-^{18}F fluorometaraminol. J. Med. Chem. 33:956, 1990.
142. Ross, S.B.: Structural requirements for uptake into catecholamine neurons. *In* Paton, D.M. (ed.): The Mechanism of Neuronal and Extraneuronal Transport of Catecholamines. New York, Raven Press, 1969, pp. 67–93.
143. Crout, J.R., Alpers, F.I.S., Tatum, E.L., et al.: Release of metaraminol (Aramine) from the heart by sympathetic nerve stimulation. Science 145:828, 1964.
144. Anton, A.H., and Berk, A.L.: Distribution of metaraminol and its relation to norepinephrine. Eur. J. Pharmacol. 44:161, 1977.
145. Van Dort, M.E., Gildersleeve, D.L., and Wieland, D.M.: Synthesis of ^{3}H-labeled sympathomimetic amines for neuronal mapping. J. Label. Compounds Radiopharmacol. 28:832, 1990.
146. Rosenpire, K., Haka, M.S., Van Dort, M.E., et al.: Synthesis and preliminary evaluation of ^{11}C-meta-hydroxyephedrine: A false transmitter agent for neuronal imaging. J. Nucl. Med. 31:1328, 1990.
147. Wieland, D.M.: Heart neuronal imaging with ^{11}C- and fluorine-18–labeled tracers. *In* van der Wall, E.E., Sochor, H., Righetti, A., et al. (eds): What's New in Cardiac Imaging? Amsterdam, Kluwer, 1992, pp. 413–426.
148. Malmfors, T.: Studies on adrenergic nerves. Acta Physiol. Scand. (Suppl. 64)248:1, 1965.
149. De Grado, T.R., Hutchins, G.D., Toorongian, S.A., et al.: Myocardial kinetics of ^{11}C-meta hydroxyephedrine: Retention mechanisms and effects of norepinephrine. J. Nucl. Med. 34:1287, 1993.
150. Eisenhofer, G.S., Hovevey-Sion, D., Kopin, I.J., et al.: Neuronal uptake and metabolism of 2- and 6-fluorodopamine: False neurotransmitters for positron emission tomographic imaging of sympathetically innervated tissues. J. Pharmacol. Exp. Ther. 248:419, 1989.
151. Goldstein, D.S., Chang, P.C., Eisenhofer, G., et al.: Positron emission tomographic imaging of cardiac sympathetic innervation and function. Circulation 81:1606, 1990.
152. Chang, P.C., Szemeredi, K., Grossman, E., et al.: Fate of tritiated 6-fluorodopamine in rats: A false neurotransmitter for positron emission tomographic imaging of sympathetic innervation and function. J. Pharmacol. Exp. Ther. 255:809, 1990.
153. Ding, Y-S., Fowler, J.S., Gatley, S.J., et al.: Synthesis of high specific activity (+)- and (−)-6-^{18}F-fluoronorepinephrine via the nucleophilic aromatic substitution reaction. J. Med. Chem. 34:767, 1991.
154. Ding, Y-S., Fowler, J.S., Gatley, S.J., et al.: Synthesis of high specific activity of 6-^{18}F-fluorodopamine for positron emission tomography studies of sympathetic nervous tissue. J. Med. Chem. 34:861, 1991.
155. Ding, Y., Fowler, J., Dewey, S., et al.: Comparison of high specific activity (−) and (+)-6-^{18}F-fluoronorepinephrine and 6-^{18}F-fluorodopamine in baboons: Heart uptake, metabolism and the effect of desipramine. J. Nucl. Med. 34:619, 1993.
156. Farde, L., Haldin, C., Nagren, K., et al.: Positron emission tomography shows high specific uptake of racemic ^{11}C-labelled norepinephrine in the primate heart. Eur. J. Nucl. Med. 21:345, 1994.
157. Vaidyanathan, G., Affeleck, D.J., and Zalutsky, M.R.: (4-^{18}F-fluoro-3-iodobenzyl) guanidine, a potential MIBG analogue for positron emission tomography. J. Med. Chem. 37:3655, 1994.
158. Loc'H, C., Mardon, K., Valette, H., et al.: Preparation and pharmacological characterization of 76-meta-bromobenzylguanidine (76-MBBG). Nucl. Med. Biol. 21:49, 1994.
159. Clerc, J., Mardon, K., Galons, J.M., et al.: Assessing intratumor distribution and uptake with MBBG versus MIBQ imaging and targeting xenografted PC-12 pheochromocytoma cell line. J. Nucl. Med. 36:851, 1995.
160. Ducis, I.: The high-affinity choline uptake system. *In* Whittaker, V.P. (ed.): The Cholinergic Synapse. New York, Springer Verlag, 1988, pp. 409–455.
161. Zimmermann, H.: Cholinergic synaptic vesicles. *In* Whittaker, V.P. (ed.): The Cholinergic Synapse. New York, Springer-Verlag, 1988, pp. 350–382.
162. Rogers, G.A., Parsons, S.M., Anderson, D.C., et al.: Synthesis, in vitro acetylcholine-storage-blocking activities, and biological properties of derivatives and analogues of trans-2-4-phenylpiperidino cyclohexanol (vesamicol). J. Med. Chem. 32:1217, 1989.
163. Marshall, I.G., and Parsons, S.M.: The vesicular acetylcholine transport system. Trends Neurosci. 10:174, 1987.
164. Kaufman, R., Rogers, G.A., Fehlmann, C., et al.: Fractional vesamicol receptor occupancy and acetylcholine active transport inhibition in synaptic vesicles. Mol. Pharmacol. 36:452, 1989.
165. Brittain, R.T., Levy, G.P., and Tyers, M.B.: The neuromuscular blocking action of 2-(4-phenylpiperidino) cyclohexanol (AH 5183). Eur. J. Pharmacol. 8:93, 1969.
166. Rogers, G.A., and Parsons, S.M.: Persistent occultation of the vesamicol receptor. Neuroreport 1:22, 1990.
167. Hicks, B.W., Rogers, G.A., and Parsons, S.M.: Purification and characterization of a nonvesicular vesamicol-binding protein from electric organ and demonstration of a related protein in mammalian brain. J. Neurochem. 57:509, 1991.
168. Kilbourn, M.R., Jung, Y.W., Haka, M.S., et al.: Mouse brain distribution of a ^{11}C-labeled vesamicol derivative: Presynaptic marker of cholinergic neurons. Life Sci. 47:1955, 1990.
169. Mulholland, G.K., Buck, F., Sherman, P.S., et al.: 4-^{18}F-fluorobenzyl-ABV: A new potential marker for central cholinergic presynaptic sites. J. Nucl. Med. 32:994, 1991.
170. Mulholland, G.K., and Jung, Y.W.: Improved synthesis of ^{11}C-methyl-aminobenzovesamicol. J. Label. Compounds Radiopharmacol. 31:253–259, 1992.
171. Mulholland, G.K., Jung, Y.W., Wieland, D.M., et al.: Synthesis of ^{18}F-fluoro-ethoxy-benzovesamicol, a radiotracer for cholinergic neurons. J. Label. Compounds Radiopharmacol. 33:583, 1993.
172. Rogers, G.A., Stoneelander, S., Ingvar, M., et al.: ^{18}F-labelled vesamicol derivatives: Syntheses and preliminary in vivo small animal positron emission tomography evaluation. Nucl. Med. Biol. 21:219, 1994.
173. Degrado, T.R., Mulholland, G.K., Wieland, D.M., et al.: Evaluation of (−)^{18}F-fluoroethoxybenzovesamicol as a new PET tracer of cholinergic neurons of the heart. Nucl. Med. Biol. 21:189, 1994.
174. Chidsey, C.A., Braunwald, E., and Morrow, A.G.: Catecholamine excretion and cardiac stores of norepinephrine in congestive heart failure. Am. J. Med. 39:442, 1965.
175. Thomas, J.A., and Marks, B.H.: Plasma norepinephrine in congestive heart failure. Am. J. Cardiol. 41:233, 1978.
176. Cohn, J.N., Levine, B.T., Olivari, M.T., et al.: Plasma norepinephrine as a guide to prognosis in patients with chronic congestive heart failure. N. Engl. J. Med. 311:819, 1984.
177. Spann, J.F., Chidsey, C.A., Pool, P.E., et al.: Mechanism of norepinephrine depletion in experimental heart failure produced by aortic constriction in the guinea pig. Circ. Res. 17:312, 1965.
178. Petch, M.C., and Nayler, W.G.: Uptake of catecholamines by human cardiac muscle in vitro. Br. Heart J. 41:336, 1979.
179. Rose, C., Burgess, J.H., and Cousineau, D.: Tracer norepinephrine kinetics in coronary circulation of patients with heart failure secondary to chronic pressure and volume overload. J. Clin. Invest. 76:740, 1985.
180. Sandoval, A.B., Gilbert, E.M., Rose, C.P., et al.: Cardiac norepinephrine uptake and release is decreased in dilated cardiomyopathy. (Abstract.) Circulation 80 (Suppl. II):393, 1989.
181. Fisher, J.E., Horst, W.D., and Kopin, I.J.: Norepinephrine metabolism in hypertrophied rat heart. Nature 207:951, 1965.
182. Hasking, G.J., Esler, M.D., Jenning, G.L., et al.: Norepinephrine spillover to plasma in patients with congestive heart failure: Evidence of increased overall and cardiorenal sympathetic nervous activity. Circulation 73:615, 1986.
183. Swedberg, K., Viquerat, C., Rouleau, J.L., et al.: Comparison of myocardial catecholamine balance in chronic congestive heart failure and in angina pectoris without failure. Am. J. Cardiol. 54:783, 1984.
184. Meredith, I.I., Broughton, A., Jennings, G.L., et al.: Evidence of a selective increase in cardiac sympathetic activity in patients with sustained ventricular arrhythmias. N. Engl. J. Med. 325:618, 1991.
185. Eisenhofer, G., Esler, M.D., Meredith, I.T., et al.: Sympathetic nervous function in human heart as assessed by cardiac spillovers of dihydroxyphenylglycol and norepinephrine. Circulation 85:1775, 1992.
186. Böhm, M., La Rosée, K., Schwinger, R.H., et al.: Evidence for reduction of norepinephrine uptake sites in the failing human heart. J. Am. Coll. Cardiol. 25:146, 1995.
187. Schwaiger, M., Hutchins, G., Rosenpire, K., et al.: Quantitative evaluation of the sympathetic nervous system in patients with cardiomyopathy. J. Nucl. Med. 31:792, 1990.
188. Vago, T., Bevilacqua, M., Norbiato, G., et al.: Identification of alpha-1 adrenergic receptor stimulation on sarcolemma from normal subjects and patients with idiopathic dilated cardiomyopathy: Characteristics and linkage to GTP-binding protein. Circ. Res. 64:474, 1989.
189. Landzberg, J.S., Parker, J.D., Gauhier, D.F., et al.: Effects of myocardial alpha-1 adrenergic receptor stimulation and blockade on contractility in humans. Circulation 84:1608, 1991.

190. Bristow, M.R., Minobe, W., Rasmussen, R., et al.: Alpha-1 adrenergic receptors in the nonfailing and failing human heart. J. Pharmacol. Exp. Ther. 247:1039, 1988.
191. Bristow, M.R., Sandoval, A.B., Gilbert, E.M., et al.: Myocardial alpha- and beta-adrenergic receptors in heart failure: Is cardiac-derived norepinephrine the regulatory signal? Eur. Heart J. 9(Suppl. H):35, 1988.
192. Bristow, M.R., Ginsburg, R., Umans, V., et al.: Beta-1 and beta-2 adrenergic receptor subpopulations in nonfailing and failing human ventricular myocardium: Coupling of both receptor subtypes to muscle contraction and selective beta-1 receptor down-regulation in heart failure. Circ. Res. 59:297, 1986.
193. Brodde, O.E., Schuler, S., Kretsch, R., et al.: Regional distribution of adrenoceptors in the human heart: Coexistence of functional beta-1 and beta-2 adrenoceptors in both atria and ventricles in severe congestive cardiomyopathy. J. Cardiovasc. Pharmacol. 8:1235, 1986.
194. Bristow, M.R., Hershberger, R.E., Port, J.D., et al.: Beta-1 and beta-2 adrenergic receptor–mediated adenylate cyclase stimulation in nonfailing and failing human ventricular myocardium. Mol. Pharmacol. 35:295, 1989.
195. Bristow, M.R., Port, J.D., and Gilbert, E.M.: The role of adrenergic receptor regulation in the treatment of heart failure. Cardiovasc. Drug. Ther. 3:971, 1989.
196. Beau, S.L., Tolley, T.K., and Saffitz, J.E.: Heterogeneous transmural distribution of beta-adrenergic receptor subtypes in failing human hearts. Circulation 88:2501, 1993.
197. Fowler, M.B., Laser, J.A., Hopkins, D.L., et al.: Assessment of the beta-adrenergic receptor pathway in the intact failing human heart: Progressive receptor down-regulation and subsensitivity to agonist response. Circulation 74:1290, 1986.
198. Vatner, D.E., Vatner, S.F., Fujii, A.M., et al.: Loss of high affinity cardiac beta adrenergic receptors in dogs with heart failure. J. Clin. Invest. 76:2259, 1985.
199. Bristow, M.R., Anderson, A.L., Port, J.D., et al.: Differences in beta-adrenergic receptor neuroeffector mechanisms in ischemic versus idiopathic dilated cardiomyopathy. Circulation 84:1024, 1991.
200. Bristow, M.R., Minobe, W.A., Raynolds, M.V., et al.: Reduced beta-1 receptor mRNA abundance in the failing human heart. J. Clin. Invest. 92:2737, 1993.
201. Neuman, J., Schmitz, W., Scholtz, H., et al.: Increase in myocardial Gi-proteins in heart failure. Lancet 22:936, 1989.
202. Ungerer, M., Böhm, M., Elce, J.S., et al: Altered expression of beta-adrenergic receptor kinase and beta-1 adrenergic receptors in the failing human heart. Circulation 87:454, 1993.
203. Merlet, P., Delforge, J., Dubois Randé, J.L., et al.: In vivo evaluation of mechanisms of down regulation in idiopathic dilated cardiomyopathy using positron emission tomography (PET) and MIBG imaging. (Abstract.) J. Nucl. Med. 33:896, 1992.
204. Beau, S.L., and Saffitz, J.E.: Transmural heterogeneity of norepinephrine in failing human hearts. J. Am. Coll. Cardiol. 23:579, 1994.
205. Bristow, M.R., Minobe, W., Rasmussen, R., et al.: β-Adrenergic neuroeffector abnormalities in the failing human heart are produced by local rather than systemic mechanisms. J. Clin. Invest. 89:803, 1992.
206. Mukherjee, A., Wong, T.M., Buja, L.M., et al.: Beta adrenergic and muscarinic cholinergic receptors in canine myocardium: Effects of ischemia. J. Clin. Invest. 64:1423, 1979.
207. Mukherjee, A., Bush, L.R., McCoy, K.E., et al.: Relationship between beta-adrenergic receptor numbers and physiological responses during experimental canine myocardial ischemia. Circ. Res. 50:735, 1982.
208. Vatner, D.E., Knight, D.R., Shen, Y.T., et al.: One hour of myocardial ischemia in conscious dogs increases beta-adrenergic receptors, but decreases adenylate cyclase activity. J. Mol. Cell. Cardiol. 20:75, 1988.
209. Maisel, A.S., Motulsky, H.J., and Insel, P.A.: Externalisation of beta-adrenergic receptors promoted by myocardial ischemia. Science 230:183, 1985.
210. Karliner, J.S., Stevens, M., Grattan, M., et al.: Beta-adrenergic receptor properties of canine myocardium: Effects of chronic myocardial infarction. J. Am. Coll. Cardiol. 8:349, 1986.
211. Schwaiger, M., Guibourg, H., Rosenpire, K., et al.: Effect of regional myocardial ischemia on sympathetic nervous systems as assessed by fluorine-18-metaraminol. J. Nucl. Med. 31:1352, 1990.
212. Allman, K., Wolfe, E., Sitomer, J., et al.: ^{11}C-hydroxyephedrine assessment of regional myocardial sympathetic neuronal function following acute myocardial infarction in man. (Abstract.) J. Nucl. Med. 32:1040, 1991.
213. Allman, K., Wieland, D., Muzik, O., et al.: ^{11}C-hydroxyephedrine with positron emission tomography for serial assessment of cardiac adrenergic neuronal function after acute myocardial infarction in human. J. Am. Coll. Cardiol. 22:368, 1993.
214. Tulli, M.M., Stanton, M.S., Mock, B.H., et al.: Comparative SPECT ^{123}I-metaiodobenzylguanidine (MIBG) and ^{201}thallium (TL) cardiac imaging following myocardial infarction. (Abstract.) J. Nucl. Med. 29:840, 1989.
215. Stanton, M.S., Tuli, M.M., Radtke, R.A., et al.: Regional sympathetic denervation after myocardial infarction in humans detected noninvasively using ^{123}I-metaiodobenzylguanidine. J. Am. Coll. Cardiol. 14:1519, 1989.
216. McGhie, I.A., Corbet, J.R., Akers, M.S., et al.: Regional cardiac adrenergic function using ^{123}I-metaiodobenzylguanidine tomographic imaging after acute myocardial infarction. Am. J. Cardiol. 67:236, 1991.
217. Minardo, J.D., Tulli, M.M., Mock, B.H., et al.: Scintigraphic and electrophysiologic evidence of canine myocardial sympathetic denervation and reinnervation produced by myocardial infarction or phenol application. Circulation 78:1008, 1988.
218. Limas, C.J.: Increased number of beta-adrenergic receptors in the hypertrophied myocardium. Biochim. Biophys. Acta 588:174, 1979.
219. Giachetti, A., Clark, T.L., and Berti, F.: Subsensitivity of cardiac beta-adrenoceptors in renal hypertensive rats. J. Cardiovasc. Pharmacol. 1:467, 1982.
220. Bobik, A., and Korner, P.: Cardiac beta adrenoceptors and adenylate cyclase in normotensive and renal hypertensive rabbits during changes in autonomic activity. Clin. Exp. Hypertens. 3:257, 1981.
221. Woodcock, E.A., and Johnson, C.I.: Changes in tissue alpha- and beta-adrenergic receptors in renal hypertension in the rat. Hypertension 2:156, 1980.
222. Ayobe, M.H., and Tarazi, R.C.: Beta-receptors and contractile reserve in left ventricular hypertrophy. Hypertension 5:192, 1983.
223. Cervoni, P., Herzlinger, H., Lai, F.M., et al.: A comparison of cardiac reactivity and beta-adrenoceptor number and affinity between aorta-coarcted hypertensive and normotensive rat. Br. J. Pharmacol. 74:517, 1981.
224. Vatner, D.E., Homcy, C.J., Sit, S.P., et al.: Effects of pressure overload left ventricular hypertrophy on β-adrenergic receptors, and responsiveness to catecholamines. J. Clin. Invest. 73:1473, 1984.
225. Wigle, E.D., Sasson, Z., Henderson, M.A., et al.: Hypertrophic cardiomyopathy: The importance of the site and the extent of hypertrophy. Prog. Cardiovasc. Dis. 28:1, 1985.
226. Maron, B.J., Bonow, R.O., Cannon, R.O., et al.: Hypertrophic cardiomyopathy. N. Engl. J. Med. 316:780, 1987.
227. Kawai, C., Yui, Y., Hishino, T., et al.: Myocardial catecholamines in hypertrophic and dilated (congestive) cardiomyopathy: A biopsy study. J. Am. Coll. Cardiol. 2:834, 1983.
228. Ganguly, P.K., Lee, S.L., Beamish, R.E., et al.: Altered sympathetic system and adrenoreceptors during the development of cardiac hypertrophy. Am. Heart J. 18:520, 1989.
229. Brush, J.E., Eisenhofer, G., Garty, M., et al.: Cardiac norepinephrine kinetics in hypertrophic cardiomyopathy. Circulation 79:836, 1989.
230. Nakajima, K., Bunko, H., Taki, J., et al.: Quantitative analysis of ^{123}I-metaiodobenzylguanidine (MIBG) uptake in hypertrophic cardiomyopathy. Am. Heart J. 119:1329, 1990.
231. Merlet, P., Dubois-Randé, J.L., Adnot, S., et al.: Myocardial β-adrenergic desensitization and neuronal norepinephrine uptake function in idiopathic dilated cardiomyopathy. J. Cardiovasc. Pharmacol. 19:10, 1992.
232. Wagner, J.A., Sax, F.L., Weisman, H.F., et al.: Calcium-antagonist receptors in the atrial tissue of patients with hypertrophic cardiomyopathy. N. Engl. J. Med. 320:755, 1989.
233. Ferry, D.R., and Kaumann, A.J.: Relationship between beta-adrenoceptors and calcium channels in human ventricular myocardium. Br. J. Pharmacol. 90:447, 1987.
234. Lefroy, D.M., De Silva, R., Choudhury, L., et al.: Diffuse reduction in myocardial beta-adrenoceptors in hypertrophic cardiomyopathy: A study with positron emission tomography. J. Am. Coll. Cardiol. 22:1653, 1993.
235. Vatner, D.E., Lavallee, M., Amano, J., et al.: Mechanisms of supersensitivity to sympathetic amines in the chronically denervated heart of the conscious dog. Circ. Res. 57:55, 1985.
236. Von Scheidt, W., Böhm, M., Schneider, B., et al.: Isolated presynaptic inotropic beta-adrenergic supersensitivity of the transplanted denervated human heart in vivo. Circulation 85:1056, 1992.
237. Schwaiger, M., Kalff, V., Rosenpire, K., et al.: Noninvasive evaluation of sympathetic nervous system in human heart by positron emission tomography. Circulation 82:457, 1990.
238. Schwaiger, M., Hutchkins, G.D., Kalff, V., et al.: Evidence for regional catecholamine uptake and storage sites in the transplanted human heart by positron emission tomography. J. Clin. Invest. 87:1681, 1991.
239. Peiss, C.N., Cooper, T., Wiliman, V.L., et al.: Circulatory response to electrical and reflex activation of the nervous system after cardiac denervation. Circ. Res. 16:153, 1966.
240. Bristow, M.R.: The surgical denervated, transplanted human heart. Circulation 82:658, 1990.
241. Willman, V.L., Cooper, T., and Hanlon, C.R.: Return of neural responses after autotransplantation of the heart. Am. J. Physiol. 207:187, 1964.
242. Kontos, H.A., Thames, M.D., and Lower, R.R.: Responses to electrical and reflex autonomic stimulation in dogs with cardiac transplantation before and after innervation. J. Thorac. Cardiovasc. Surg. 59:382, 1970.
243. Regitz, V., Bossaller, C., Strasser, R., et al.: Myocardial catecholamine content after heart transplantation. Circulation 82:620, 1990.
244. Wilson, A.A., Scheffel, U.A., Dannals, R.F., et al.: In vivo biodistribution of two ^{18}F-labelled muscarinic cholinergic receptor ligands, 2^{18}F-fluorodexetimide and 4-^{18}F-fluorodexetimide. Life Sci. 48:1385, 1991.
245. Buda, A.J., Fowles, R.A., Schroeder, J.S., et al.: Coronary artery spasm in the denervated transplanted human heart. Am. J. Med. 70:1144, 1981.
246. Lurie, K.G., Bristow, M.R., and Reitz, B.A.: Increased beta-adrenergic receptor density in an experimental model of cardiac transplantation. J. Thorac. Cardiovasc. Surg. 86:195, 1983.
247. Yusuf, S., Theodoropoulos, S., Mathias, C.J., et al.: Increased sensitivity of the denervated transplanted human heart to isoprenaline both before and after beta-adrenergic blockade. Circulation 75:696, 1987.
248. Brodde, O., Khamssi, M., and Zerbowski, A.: Beta-adrenoceptors in the transplanted human heart: Unaltered beta-adrenoceptor density, but increased proportion of beta-2 adrenoceptors with increasing post transplant time. Naunyn Schmiederbergs Arch. Pharmacol. 334:430, 1991.
249. Merlet, P., Benvenuti, C., Valette, H., et al.: Myocardial β-adrenergic receptors in heart transplanted patients: Assessment with ^{11}C-CGP 12177 and positron emission tomography. (Abstract.) Circulation 86 (Suppl. I):245, 1993.
250. Denniss, A.R., Marsh, J.D., Quigg, R.J., et al.: β-Adrenergic receptor number and adenylate function in denervated transplanted and cardiomyopathic human hearts. Circulation 79:1028, 1989.

251. Leguludec, D., Delforge, J., Syrota, A., et al.: In vivo quantification of myocardial muscarinic receptors in heart transplant patients. Circulation 90:172, 1994.
252. Calkins, H., Lehmann, M., Allman, K., et al.: Scintigraphic pattern on regional cardiac sympathetic innervation in patients with familial long QT syndrome using positron emission tomography. Circulation 87:1616, 1993.
253. Müller, K., Jakob, H., Grebe, S., et al.: ^{123}I-Metaiodobenzylguanidine scintigraphy in the detection of irregular regional sympathetic innervation in long QT syndrome. Eur. Heart J. 14:316, 1993.
254. Allman, K.C., Stevens, M.J., Wieland, D.M., et al.: Noninvasive assessment of cardiac diabetic neuropathy by ^{11}C-hydroxyephedrine and positron emission tomography. J. Am. Coll. Cardiol. 22(5):1389, 1993.
255. Lam, D., and Goldschlager, N.: Myocardial injury associated with polysubstance abuse. Am. Heart J. 115:675, 1988.
256. Zimmerman, F.H., Gustafson, G.M., and Kem, H.G.: Recurrent myocardial infarction associated with cocaine abuse in a young man with normal coronary arteries: Evidence for coronary artery spasm culminating in thrombosis. J. Am. Coll. Cardiol. 9:964, 1987.
257. Zimring, M., Fitzgerald, R.L., Engler, R.L., et al.: Intracoronary versus intravenous effects of cocaine on coronary blood flow and ventricular function. Circulation 89:1819, 1994.
258. Lefkowitz, R.J., Caron, M.G., and Sitles, G.I.: Mechanisms of receptor regulation. N. Engl. J. Med. 310:570, 1984.
259. Sibley, D.R., Daniel, K., Strader, C.E., et al.: Phosphorylation of the β-adrenergic receptor in intact cells: Relationship to heterologous and homologous mechanisms of adenylate cyclase desensitization. Arch. Biochem. Biophys. 258:24, 1987.
260. Sibley, D.R., and Lefkowitz, R.J.: Beta-adrenergic receptor-coupled adenylate cyclase. Biochemical mechanisms of regulation. Mol. Neurobiol. 1:121, 1987.
261. Feldman, A.M., Cates, A.E., Veazey, W.B., et al.: Increase of the 40,000-mol wt pertussis toxin substrate (G protein) in the failing human heart. J. Clin. Invest. 82:189, 1988.

Appendix I

Heiko Schöder, M.D.
Heinrich R. Schelbert, M.D.

RADIATION DOSIMETRY

TERMINOLOGY AND UNITS

The tables in this appendix describe estimates of the absorbed radiation doses and, whenever possible, of the effective dose equivalent. An effort has been made to compare the risk resulting from radiation with that from daily activities. The tables employ quantities in units of the Système International (SI), as established by the International Commission on Radiological Protection (ICRP) and the International Commission on Radiological Units and Measurements (ICRU).

RADIOACTIVITY. The activity of a radioactive element is a function of the rate of the disintegration of its nuclei and is defined in units of becquerel (Bq), where

$$1 \text{ becquerel (Bq)} = 1 \text{ disintegration per second (dps)} = 2.7 \times 10^{-11} \text{ Ci}$$

ABSORBED DOSE. The absorbed dose defines the amount of energy of radiation that is deposited in a unit of mass of absorbing tissue. The SI unit of absorbed dose is called gray (Gy), where

$$1 \text{ gray (Gy)} = 1 \text{ joule per kilogram of tissue} = 100 \text{ rad}$$

The amounts of absorbed doses in nuclear medicine are usually in the range of milligrays (mGy) or micrograys (μGy).

EFFECTIVE DOSE EQUIVALENT. The effective dose equivalent is a measure of the relative biologic damage resulting from radiation. For similar values of absorbed radiation, the amount of biologic damage may differ markedly between different radioactive substances because of differences in the types and energy of radiation. The degree of biologic damage depends on the density of ionization caused by a radiation particle during its transit through tissue. The density of ionization is also defined as linear energy transfer (LET) of radiation.

Calculation of the equivalent dose requires knowledge of the radiation and weighting factor (W_R), which reflects also the relative biologic effectiveness (RBE) as a function of the LET. The equivalent dose is described in units of sievert (Sv), where

$$1 \text{ sievert (Sv)} = 100 \text{ rem}$$

In medical imaging, the radiation weighting factor is 1 for most ionizing radiation. Accordingly, the equivalent dose in sieverts is numerically the same as the absorbed dose in grays. Table 1 summarizes the conversion of the various radiation measures and units.

TABLE 1. CONVERSION OF ACTIVITY AND DOSIMETRY UNITS

Radioactivity (becquerel and curie)		
1 MBq	=	2.7×10^{-8} mCi
1 mCi	=	37 MBq
Absorbed Doses (gray and rad)		
1 Gy	=	100 rad
1 rad	=	0.01 Gy = 10 mGy
Dose Equivalent (Sievert and rem)		
1 Sv	=	100 rem
1 rem	=	0.01 Sv = 10 mSv

DOSE LIMITS FOR RADIATION EXPOSURES

Dose limits as recommended by the ICRP for radiation workers and for the public differ and are listed in Table 2. Although the radiation exposures within the recommended ranges are considered relatively safe, the ICRP adopted the concept of the "dose constraint" or dose limit to which it would be feasible to adhere in the setting of clinical nuclear medicine and radiology. This dose constraint amounts to 5 mSv per year.

Exposure to ionizing radiation is unavoidable. According to Hall,[1] radiation results from several sources: (1) cosmic and terrestrial radiation; (2) radionuclides that accumulate in the body after inhalation or injection; (3) enhanced natural sources, such as exposure resulting from air travel at high altitudes, which increases cosmic ray levels, or exposure from mining or from building materials; and (4) man-made radiation (e.g., industrial, medical radiation).

The risks from radiation exposure are generally divided into *somatic* and *genetic risks.* The somatic risk for radiation exposure can be expressed by the effective (equivalent) dose. The genetic risk is expressed by the genetically significant dose, which is the effective dose for the gonads, weighted for age and gender.

MEDICAL RADIATION EXPOSURE

To estimate the risks from medical radiation exposure, effective (equivalent) doses for different diagnostic radiology and nuclear medicine procedures can be compared with data for natural background radiation. The most recent data for diagnostic medical procedures in the United States were summarized in the National Committee on Radiation Protection and Measurements (NCRP) report 100 in 1989[2] and are listed in Table 3. Data for x-ray studies from different institutions are difficult to compare. Contrary to nuclear medicine, in which the amount of injected radioactivity determines the effective dose, several technical aspects (voltage, milliamperes, filter, time of fluoroscopy, and number of films) need to be considered in radiology. Therefore, doses for the same examination may vary considerably.[3]

Averaged data, which are based on conventional x-ray imaging, are given in Table 3. Of note, radiation doses for digital imaging can be significantly lower.[4] In one recent report, for example, digital spot images or fluorographic films taken from the intensifier produced only 10 to 20 percent of the dose with a film-screen system.[5] No data on the radiation doses for a computed tomogram of the chest are available. In general, doses per computed tomogra-

TABLE 2. RADIATION DOSE LIMITS

	Dose Limit (mSv/yr)	
	Occupational	***Public***
Effective dose	20, averaged over 5 yr and not >50 mSv/yr	1, averaged over 5 years
Equivalent dose		
Lens of eye	150	15
Hands, feet	500	—
Skin (averaged over 1 cm²)	500	50

TABLE 3. ORGAN DOSES IN DIAGNOSTIC RADIOLOGY (in mSv)

Examination	Bone Marrow	Testis	Ovary	Lung	Breast	Effective Dose Equiv.
Chest x-ray, PA and LAT	0.04	0.01	0.01	0.2	0.14	0.06
CT, abdomen (based on five slices) (complete study)	4.9	0.4	0.4	—	—	1.1 7–8[15]
CT, brain						2[16]
Cerebral angiography						2.7–23.4, mean 10
IV urogram (based on five images) (complete study)	2.1	2	5.8	0.35	—	1.58 6.6[3]
Barium enema (based on four images)	3	0.6	8.0			4.06 2.8[9] 1.2–14, mean 9[3]
Lumbar spine (based on three images)	1.2	0.07	4.0	1.4	—	1.27
Thoracic spine (based on two images)	0.45	—	0.01	4.0	5.4	

Data from NCRP number 100[2] and reference 1 where not otherwise indicated.
CT = computed tomography; IV = intravenous; PA and LAT = posteroanterior and lateral views.

phy slice may vary from 5 to 15 mGy,[6] while those for a head computed tomogram have recently been reported to be higher, ranging from 20 to more than 100 mGy, with an average of 30 to 40 mGy.[7] Dose variations often result from the use of different generations of tomographs by different manufacturers and, in particular, from variable milliamperes of each product. The data on radiation doses from coronary angiography are sketchy. Averaged data for combined coronary angiography–contrast ventriculography are given in Table 4. As for all other fluoroscopy studies,[2, 5, 8–10, 14] exposure time is the most decisive factor.

Table 5 summarizes the radiation doses resulting from radiopharmaceuticals used for studies of the cardiovascular system. All the dose estimates were obtained from the U.S. Medical Internal Radiation Dose (MIRD) Committee in Oak Ridge, Tennessee, and were kindly supplied by Dr. Stubb. It should be mentioned, however, that the doses estimated by the MIRD Committee may differ from those reported by other investigators.[11, 12] These studies reported lower estimates for ^{18}F-deoxyglucose and ^{99m}Tc-sestamibi, which the table lists in parentheses.

NATURAL BACKGROUND RADIATION

Natural background exposure originates from three major sources: cosmic radiation, terrestrial radiation (radioactivity in the crust of the earth), and internal deposits of radionuclides in the human body.

TABLE 4. AVERAGE RADIATION DOSE FROM CORONARY ANGIOGRAPHY

Skin surface dose	410 mSv (40–1000)
Testis	17 mSv
Ovary	36 mSv
Bone marrow	90 mSv
Mean effective dose equivalent	5.7 mSv

Data adapted from Laubenberger and Laubenberger[6] and Coulden and Readman.[17]

Cosmic radiation results from charged particles. Because of the earth's magnetic field, these particles are generally deflected from the equator and funneled into the poles. Therefore, exposure from cosmic radiation is lowest around the equator and rises toward the poles. In addition, it rises with altitude (with rising altitude there is less atmosphere to absorb radiation). The national average for the United States (0.26 mSv per year) essentially doubles for each 2000-m rise in altitude.

Terrestrial radiation varies considerably throughout the world. For example, in the United States, radiation is highest in the Colorado plateau, where rocks and soil contain radioactive uranium and thorium.

Taken together, in Denver, Colorado, activity from cosmic rays results in about 0.5 mSv per year, and that from the earth's crust about 0.9 mSv per year. In comparison, the data for New York City are 0.25 mSv and 0.20 mSv, respectively. Because of radioactivity in rocks and soil (including building materials), inhabitants of Burgundy, a famous wine-growing district in France, receive 1.8 to 3.5 mSv per year, while individuals living in the northern Nile delta receive 3 to 4 mSv per year. The highest exposure worldwide is reported from Kerala, India (13 mSv per year).[1] Averaged data for California are 0.5 mSv per year.[13]

Radiation from *internal radioactive sources* in the body (mainly potassium-40) was estimated to be 0.39 mSv per year until recently.

The annual averaged background level for the United States is then quoted to be 1 mSv, based on averaged levels for cosmic (0.26 mSv), terrestrial (0.28 mSv), and internal radiation sources (0.39 mSv).[2]

Radiation from radioactive radon gas, which is now calculated to be as high as 2 mSv per year in the United States,[1] has been ignored until recently and is not included in these data.

ENHANCED NATURAL RADIATION

One interesting example of enhanced natural radiation is that resulting from air travel in commercial jets. As a result of cosmic radiation, a round-trip flight from Los Angeles to Paris, France, involves a dose of 48 μSv, from New York to London 29 μSv, and from Los Angeles to New York 19 μSv.[13]

TABLE 5. RADIATION DOSIMETRY FOR COMMONLY USED SINGLE-PHOTON AND POSITRON-EMITTING RADIOPHARMACEUTICALS

Organ	Thallium-201 μGy/MBq	^{99m}Tc-Sestamibi	^{99m}Tc-RBCs	^{123}I-IPPA	^{13}N-Ammonia	^{15}O-Water	^{82}Rb	^{18}F-FDG	^{11}C-Palmitate	^{11}C-Acetate
Brain	57	1.8	—	5.3	4.7	1.3	0.32	19	2.6	1.8
Thyroid	620	6.1	—	6.2	1.5	1.7	0.34	10	3.0	2.2
Liver	99	5.1	—	16.0	3.8	1.5	0.83	16	2.9	3.3
Spleen	180	5.2	12.0	11.0	1.5	1.6	0.41	37	3.1	2.7
Stomach	190	5.2	—	7.3	1.6	0.53	0.38	13	3.2	3.0
Small intestine	450	2.7	—	8.7	1.7	0.93	0.38	14	3.4	2.3
Upper large intestine	330	50	—	8.3	1.7	0.70	0.38	13	3.3	2.3
Lower large intestine	340	37	—	11.0	1.7	0.74	0.36	17	3.3	2.2
Red bone marrow	55	4.5	4.1	6.3	1.8	0.90	0.45	13	3.5	2.5
Kidneys	460	18	—	22.0	1.6	1.90	9.00	20	3.1	2.4
Urinary bladder wall	52	37	15.0	100.0	6.9	0.22	0.36	190	3.3	2.1
Ovaries	100	14	4.7	10.0	1.7	0.36	0.37	17	3.4	2.2
Testes	200	3.5	3.3	7.6	1.4	0.67	0.26	13	2.9	1.9
Effective dose Eq mSv/MBq	0.1600 (0.23)*	0.0150 (0.008)*	0.0072	.0160	0.0028 (0.002)*	0.0010 (0.00042)*	0.0012 (0.0034)*	0.0380 (0.02)*	0.0032	0.0100

*Data are taken from references 11 and 12.
IPPA = Iodophenylpentadecanoic acid; RBCs = red blood cells; ^{18}F-FDG = ^{18}F-deoxyglucose.

RISK ASSESSMENT FOR MEDICAL RADIATION EXPOSURE

The potential risks from diagnostic radiology and nuclear medicine procedures for radiation-induced cancers and heritable effects (mutations) need to be weighed against the therapeutic and prognostic benefits of these studies. Hall[1] calculates the following risks: (1) fatal cancer, 4.0 percent per Sv; (2) nonfatal cancer, 0.8 percent per Sv; and (3) heritable effects (mutations), 0.8 percent per Sv.

Medical diagnostic radiation studies represent the largest source of man-made radiation in the Developed Countries. Nevertheless, a population-based analysis shows that overall effective dose from medical radiation is less than half that from natural radiation (averaged values for United States population: 0.39 mSv per year from diagnostic x-rays, 0.14 mSv from nuclear medicine studies). The combined genetically significant dose (induction of mutations) from diagnostic x-rays (300 μGy) and nuclear medicine studies (30 μGy) is 0.33 mSv per year[1]; that is, about one third of the annual background radiation in the United States or two thirds of cosmic radiation alone in Denver, Colorado.

To perform an averaged population-based risk stratification for cancer or deaths, data for risks from medical radiation exposure should be compared to other potential risk factors (even though this may sometimes seem to be a rather rude comparison). Based on comprehensive statistics, therefore, the risk for a radiation-induced fatal cancer is 4 percent per Sv, the risk for cigarette smoking is equal to 1.37×10^{-7} per cigarette smoked (mainly due to lung cancer). The risk of highway driving is 5.6×10^{-8} deaths per mile driven.[1] From these data together, a risk assessment can be made (Table 6). Calculations for nuclear medicine studies are based on the MIRD estimates; that is, the risk for a ^{99m}Tc-sestamibi or ^{18}F-fluorodeoxyglucose study would be much lower based on other effective dose data.[11, 12]

It is not the aim of this appendix to oversimplify the potential risks resulting from medical radiation. Therefore, it should be emphasized again that each radiologic or nuclear medicine procedure should be truly indicated and that the radiation dose should be "as low as reasonably achievable" (ALARA principle). Special guidelines for the exposure of infants and pregnant women have been developed by the NCRP in the United States. Finally, guidelines for radiation exposure vary between countries; the reader is

TABLE 6. COMPARISON OF RISKS FROM MEDICAL RADIATION WITH THOSE RESULTING FROM ACTIVITIES IN DAILY LIFE

Procedure	Effective Dose (mSv)	Risk of Fatal Cancer (4% per Sv)	Equivalent to Number of Cigarettes Smoked	Equivalent to Highway Miles Driven in United States
Chest x-ray	0.06	2.4×10^{-6}	17.5	43
Bone scan	4.4	1.8×10^{-4}	1300	3200
Barium enema (four images)	4.06	1.6×10^{-4}	1160	2850
^{13}N-NH_3 PET (0.002 mSv/MBq; 555 MBq inj.)	1.11	4.4×10^{-5}	321	786
^{18}F-FDG PET (0.038 mSv/MBq; 370 MBq inj.)	14	5.6×10^{-4}	4080	10,000
^{201}Tl (0.16 mSv/MBq; 80 MBq inj.)	12.8	5.12×10^{-4}	3730	9140
^{99m}Tc-MIBI (0.015 mSv/MBq; 1000 MBq inj.)	15	6×10^{-4}	4380	10,700

PET = positron emission tomography.
Data based on effective dose equivalents given by the U.S. MIRD Committee, Oak Ridge, Tennessee, and NCRP number 100.

therefore referred to the respective national radiation protection committee for detailed information.

References

1. Hall, E.J.: Diagnostic radiology and nuclear medicine: Risk versus benefit. *In* Hall, E.J. (ed.): Radiobiology for the Radiologist. 4th ed. Philadelphia, J.B. Lippincott, 1994.
2. National Committee on Radiation Protection and Measurements (NCRP): Exposure of the U.S. population from diagnostic medical radiation: Recommendations of the National Committee on Radiation Protection and Measurements. Bethesda, MD, The Committee, 1989.
3. Calzado, A., Vano, E., Moran, P., et al.: Estimation of doses to patients from "complex" conventional X-ray examinations. Br. J. Radiol. 64:539, 1991.
4. Marshall, N.W., Faulkner, K., Busch, H.P., et al.: A comparison of radiation dose in examination of the abdomen using different radiological imaging techniques. Br. J. Radiol. 67:478, 1994.
5. Martin, C.J., and Hunter, S.: Reduction of patient doses from barium meal and barium enema examinations through changes in equipment factors. Br. J. Radiol. 67:1196, 1994.
6. Laubenberger, T., and Laubenberger, J.: Technik der medizinischen Radiologie. (Technique of Medical Radiology.) Cologne, Deutscher Aerzteverlag, 1994.
7. Conway, B.J., McCrohan, J.L., Antonsen, R.G., et al.: Average radiation dose in standard CT examinations of the head: Results of the 1990 NEXT survey. Radiology 184:135, 1992.
8. Hart, D., Haggett, P.J., Boardman, P., et al.: Patient radiation doses from enteroclysis examinations. Br. J. Radiol. 67:997, 1994.
9. Hart, D., and Wall, B.F.: Estimation of effective dose from dose-area product measurements from barium meals and barium enemas. Br. J. Radiol. 67:485, 1994.
10. Feygelman, V.M., Huda, W., and Peters, K.R.: Effective dose equivalents to patients undergoing cerebral angiography. AJNR 13:845, 1992.
11. Johannson, L., Mattson, S., Nosslin, B., et al.: Effective dose from radiopharmaceuticals. Eur. J. Nucl. Med. 19:933, 1992.
12. International Commission on Radiation Protection (ICRP): Radiation Dose to Patients from Radiopharmaceuticals. Publication N. 53. Oxford, Pergamon Press, 1988.
13. Mettler, F.: Medical Effects of Ionizing Radiation. London, Grune & Stratton, 1985.
14. Horton, D., Cook, A.M., and Taylor, A.D.: Audit in action: Significant reduction of double-contrast barium enema screening time with no loss of examination quality. Br. J. Radiol. 65:507, 1992.
15. Shrimpton, P.C., Jones, D.G., Hillier, M.C., et al.: Survey of CT Practice in the UK, Part 2: Dosimetric Aspects. NRPB-R249. London, 1991.
16. Huda, W., Sandison, G.A., and Lee, T.Y.: Patient doses from computed tomography in Manitoba from 1977–1987. Br. J. Radiol. 62:138, 1989.
17. Coulden, R.A., and Readman, L.P.: Coronary angiography: An analysis of radiographic practice in the UK. Br. J. Radiol. 66:327, 1993.

Appendix II

GLOSSARY OF NMR TERMS

Acoustic noise—vibrations of the *gradient coil* support structure create sound waves. These are caused by the interactions of the *magnetic field* created by pulses of the current through the gradient coil with the main magnetic field in a manner similar to that of a loudspeaker coil. Sound pressure is reported on a logarithmic scale called sound-pressure level expressed in *decibels (dB)* referenced to the weakest audible 1000 Hz sound pressure of 2×10^{-5} pascal. Sound level meters contain filters that simulate the ear's frequency response. The most commonly used filter provides what is called A weighting, with the letter A appended to the dB units, i.e., dBA.

Acquisition matrix—number of independent data samples in each direction: for example, in *two-dimensional Fourier transform (2DFT) imaging*, it is the number of samples in phase- and frequency-encoded directions, and in *reconstruction from projections* imaging it is the number of samples in time and angle. May be asymmetric and of a size different from the size of the reconstructed image or display matrix; for example, with *zero filling* or interpolation, or (for asymmetric sampling) by exploiting the symmetry of the data matrix. For symmetric sampling, will roughly equal the ratio of image field of view to *spatial resolution* along corresponding directions (depending on *filtering* and other processing).

Acquisition window—time in *pulse sequence* during which the magnetic resonance (MR) signal is recorded. The duration can be denoted *TAD* (for "time of *analog to digital conversion*").

Active shielding—*magnetic shielding* through the use of secondary shielding *coils* designed to produce a magnetic field that cancels the field from primary coils in regions where it is not desired. These coils may be inside the magnet *cryostat*. Can be applied to the main magnet or to the *gradient magnetic fields*.

Aliasing—consequence of *sampling* in which any components of the signal that are at a higher *frequency* than the *Nyquist limit* are "folded" in the *spectrum* so that they appear to be at a lower frequency. In *Fourier transform imaging*, this can produce an apparent wrapping around to the opposite side of the image of a portion of the object that extends beyond the edge of the reconstructed region.

Angiography—application of MRI to produce images of blood vessels; for example, with *flow effects* or *relaxation time* differences. Some common approaches use the washout of *saturated spins* from a region by blood flow to increase the relative intensity of blood vessels within images or use the variable sensitivity to motion-induced *phase* shifts provided by adjusting *gradient moments* to discriminate against the signal from stationary tissue.

Angular frequency (ω)—*frequency* of oscillation or rotation (measured, e.g., in radians per second) commonly designated by the Greek letter ω: $\omega = 2\pi f$, where f is frequency (e.g., in *hertz* [Hz]).

Angular momentum—a *vector* quantity given by the vector product of the momentum of a particle and its position vector. In the absence of external forces, the angular momentum remains constant, with the result that any rotating body tends to maintain the same axis of rotation. When a *torque* is applied to a rotating body in such a way that the direction of the rotation axis is changed, the resulting change in angular momentum results in *precession*. Atomic nuclei possess an intrinsic angular momentum referred to as *spin*, measured in multiples of Planck's constant.

Annotation—a description of the factors used in creating an image should include the types and times of the *pulse sequence*, the number of signals averaged or added *(NSA)*, the size of the reconstructed region, the size of the *acquisition matrix* in each direction, and the *slice thickness*.

Antenna—device for sending or receiving electromagnetic radiation. Electromagnetic radiation per se is not relevant to nuclear magnetic resonance (NMR), because it is the magnetic vector alone that couples the *spins* and the *coils*, and the term *coil* should be used instead.

Array coil—*RF coil* composed of multiple separate elements that can be used individually *(switchable coil)* or used simultaneously. When used simultaneously, the elements can be either (1) electrically coupled to each other *("coupled array coils")*, through common transmission lines or mutual *inductance*, or (2) electrically isolated from each other *("isolated array coils")*, with separate transmission lines and *receivers* and minimal effective mutual inductance, and with the signals from each transmission line processed independently or at different *frequencies*.

Array processor—optional component of the *computer* system specially designed to speed up numerical calculations like those needed in *magnetic resonance imaging*.

Artifacts—false features in the image produced by the imaging process. The random fluctuation of intensity due to *noise* can be considered separately from artifacts.

B_0—a conventional symbol for the constant *magnetic (induction) field* in an *NMR* system. (Although historically used, H_0 [units of *magnetic field* strength, ampere/meter] should be distinguished from the more appropriate B_0 [units of magnetic induction, *telsa*].)

B_1—a conventional symbol for the *radiofrequency magnetic* induction field used in an MR system (another symbol historically used is H_1). It is useful to consider it as composed of two oppositely rotating *vectors*, usually in a plane transverse to B_0. *At the Larmor frequency*, the vector rotating in the same direction as the *precessing spins* interacts strongly with the spins.

Bandwidth—a general term referring to a range of *frequencies* (e.g., contained in a signal or passed by a signal-processing system).

Baseline—a generally smooth background curve with respect to which either the *integrals* or the peak heights of the *resonance spectral lines* in the *spectrum* are measured.

Bloch equations—phenomenologic "classic" equations of motion for the *macroscopic magnetization vector*. They include the effects of *precession* about the *magnetic field* (static and *RF*) and the *T1* and *T2 relaxation times*.

Boltzmann distribution—if a system of particles that are able to exchange energy in collisions is in thermal equilibrium, then the relative number *(population)* of particles, N_1 and N_2, in two particular *energy levels* with corresponding energies, E_1 and E_2, is given by

$$\frac{N_1}{N_2} = \exp\,[\,-\,(E_1 - E_2)/kT\,]$$

where k is Boltzmann's constant and T is absolute temperature. For example, in *NMR* of protons at room temperature in a *magnetic field* of 0.25 *tesla*, the difference in relative numbers of spins aligned with the magnetic field and against the field is about one part in a million; the small excess of

Portions of the text were modified from Glossary of MR Terms. 3rd ed. Reston, VA, the American College of Radiology, © 1991. The pulse sequence acronyms were modified from the 1994 MResource Guide, which appeared in J. Magn. Reson. Imaging 35:25, 1993. Used with permission.

nuclei in the lower energy state is the basis of the net *magnetization* and the *resonance* phenomenon.

Chemical shift (δ)—the change in the *Larmor frequency* of a given nucleus when bound in different sites in the molecule, due to the magnetic shielding effects of the electron orbitals. Chemical shifts make possible the differentiation of different molecular compounds and different sites within the molecules in high-resolution NMR spectra. The amount of the shift is proportional to magnetic field strength and is usually specified in parts per million (ppm) of the resonance frequency relative to a standard. The actual frequency measured for a given *spectral line* may depend on environmental factors, such as effects on the local magnetic field strength due to variations of *magnetic susceptibility.*

Chemical shift imaging—a magnetic resonance imaging technique that provides mapping of the regional distribution of intensity (images) of a restricted range of *chemical shifts,* corresponding to individual *spectral lines* or groups of lines.

Chemical shift reference—a compound with respect to whose *frequency* the chemical shifts of other compounds can be compared. The standard can be either internal or external to the sample. Because of the need for possible corrections due to differential magnetic *susceptibility* between an external standard and the sample being measured, the use of an internal standard is generally preferred.

C/N—see *Contrast-to-noise ratio.*

CNR—see *Contrast-to-noise ratio.*

Coherence—maintenance of a constant *phase* relationship between rotating or oscillating waves or objects. Loss of phase coherence of the *spins* results in a decrease in the *transverse magnetization* and hence a decrease in the *MR signal.* In the quantum mechanical description of magnetic resonance, coherence refers to a transition between different states of the spin system.

Coil—single or multiple loops of wire (or other electrical conductor, such as tubing) designed either to produce a *magnetic field* from current flowing through the wire, or to detect a changing magnetic field by voltage induced in the wire.

Coil loading—in MRI, the interaction of the patient with the RF coil, which causes shifts of the *resonance frequency* and damping of the coil's resonance and hence reduction of the *quality factor* because of magnetic induction and dielectric losses in the patient.

Contrast—contrast can be defined as the relative difference of the signal intensities in two adjacent regions. In a general sense, we can consider image contrast, in which the strength of the image intensity in adjacent regions of the image is compared, or object contrast, in which the relative values of a parameter affecting the image (e.g., *spin density* or *relaxation time*) in corresponding adjacent regions of the object are compared. Relating image contrast to object contrast is more difficult in *MRI* than in conventional radiography, because there are more object parameters affecting the image, and their relative contributions are very dependent on the particular imaging technique used. As in other kinds of imaging, image contrast in NMR also depends on region size, as reflected through the modulation transfer function (MTF) characteristics. The contrast between an object (e.g., lesion) and the background also depends on the particular choice of designated background (e.g., fat, muscle).

Contrast agent—substance administered to a subject being imaged in order to alter selectively the image intensity of a particular anatomic or functional region, typically by altering the *relaxation times.*

Contrast-to-noise ratio—ratio of the absolute difference in intensities between two regions to the level of fluctuations in intensity due to *noise.*

Correlation time—the characteristic time between significant fluctuations in the local magnetic field experienced by a spin due to molecular motions. For values of the correlation time such that the magnetic field as a function of time has large *Fourier* components near the resonance frequency, the *T1 relaxation time* is shortened.

Cryogen—very low temperature liquified gas (helium or nitrogen) used to maintain superconducting magnets in a superconducting state.

Cryostat—an apparatus for maintaining a constant low temperature (as by means of liquid helium). It requires vacuum chambers to help with thermal isolation.

dB/dt—the rate of change of the *magnetic field* (induction) with time. Because changing magnetic fields can induce electrical current, this is one area of potential concern for safety limits.

Decoupling—(1) specific irradiation designed to remove the *multiplet* structure in a particular *resonance* due to *spin-spin coupling* with other nuclei; (2) techniques used to avoid interactions between *coils,* such as separate transmitting and receiving coils.

Dephasing gradient—*magnetic field gradient* pulse used to create spatial variation of phase of *transverse magnetization.* For example, it may be applied prior to signal detection in the presence of a magnetic field gradient with opposite polarity (or of the same polarity if separated by a *refocusing RF pulse*) so that the resulting *gradient echo* signal will represent a more complete sampling of the *Fourier transform* of the desired image. See also *Spoiler gradient pulse.*

Detector—portion of the *receiver* that demodulates the *RF MR signal* and converts it to a lower *frequency* signal. Most detectors now used are phase sensitive (e.g., *quadrature demodulator/detector*), and also give phase information about the RF signal.

Diamagnetic—a substance that slightly decreases a *magnetic field* when placed within it (its *magnetization* is oppositely directed to the magnetic field, i.e., with a small negative *magnetic susceptibility*).

Diffusion—the process by which molecules or other particles intermingle and migrate owing to their random thermal motion. *NMR* provides a sensitive technique for measuring diffusion of some substances.

Dipole-dipole interaction—interaction between a spin and its neighbors due to their *magnetic dipole* moments. This is an important mechanism contributing to *relaxation times.* In solids and viscous liquids, this can result in broadening of the *spectral lines.*

Dynamic range—range of signal intensities that may need to be distinguished in an image or a spectrum or that can be distinguished by the electronic components. If the signal dynamic range is too great, the need to keep the highest intensities from overloading the *digitizer* may result in the weaker features being lost in the *digitization noise.* This can be dealt with by using an *analog-to-digital converter* with a larger range of sensitivity or by using techniques to reduce the dynamic range; for example, *suppressing* the signal from water in order to detect the signal from less abundant compounds.

Echo—see *Spin echo.*

Echo offset—adjustment of *RF spin echo* and *gradient echo* to be noncoincident in time, so as to create *phase* differences between the signals from different *spectral lines.*

Echo planar imaging—a technique of *planar imaging* in which a complete planar image is obtained from one *selective excitation pulse.* The *FID* is observed while periodically switching the *y-magnetic field gradient field* in the presence of a static *x-magnetic field gradient field.* The *Fourier transform* of the resulting *spin echo* train can be used to produce an image of the excited plane.

Echo time—see *TE.*

Eddy currents—electric currents induced in a conductor by a changing magnetic field or by motion of the conductor through a *magnetic field.* It represents one of the sources of concern about potential hazard to subjects in very high magnetic fields or rapidly varying *gradient* or main magnetic fields. It can be a practical problem in the *cryostat* of *superconducting magnets.*

Energy level—in a *magnetic field,* each *spin* can exist in one of a number of distinct states having different energies; this number is determined by the *spin quantum number.*

Excitation—putting energy into the *spin* system; if a net *transverse magnetization* is produced, an *MR signal* can be observed.

Faraday shield—electrical conductor interposed between *transmitter* and/or *receiver coil* and patient to block out electric fields.

Fast Fourier transform (FFT)—an efficient computational method of performing a *Fourier transform.*

Ferromagnetic—a substance, such as iron, that has a large positive *magnetic susceptibility.*

FID—see *Free induction decay.*

Field echo—see *Gradient echo.*

Field gradient—see *Magnetic field gradient.*

Field lock—a feedback control used to maintain the static *magnetic field* at a constant strength, usually by monitoring the *resonance frequency* of a reference sample or line in the *spectrum.*

Filling factor—a measure of the geometrical relationship of the *RF coil* and the object being studied. It affects the efficiency of irradiating the object, and detecting *MR signals,* thereby affecting the *signal-to-noise ratio* and, ultimately, image quality. Achieving a high filling factor requires fitting the coil closely to the object, thus potentially decreasing patient comfort.

Flip angle—the amount of rotation of the *macroscopic magnetization vector* produced by an *RF pulse,* with respect to the direction of the static *magnetic field.*

Flow compensation—means of reducing *flow effects,* for example, *gradient moment nulling.*

Flow effects—motion of material being imaged, particularly flowing blood, can result in many possible effects in the images, including increase in the signal *("flow-related enhancement"),* decrease in the signal, or displacement of the signal (image misregistration). These effects can be understood as being caused by *time-of-flight* effects (washout or washin due to motion of nuclei between two consecutive spatially selective RF excitations, repeated in times on the order of or shorter than the relaxation times of blood) or *phase* shifts that can be acquired by excited spins moving along *magnetic field gradients.* The inconsistency of the signal resulting from pulsatile flow can lead to *artifacts* in the image; these can be reduced by *synchronization* of the imaging sequence with the heart cycle ("cardiac *gating*"), suppression of the blood signal with *saturation pulses,* or reduction of phase shifts with *gradient moment nulling.* The flow effects can also be exploited for MR *angiography* or flow measurements.

Flow-related enhancement—*the increase in intensity* that may be seen for flowing blood or other liquids with some *MR imaging* techniques, due to the washout of *saturated* spins from the imaging region.

Fourier transform (FT)—a mathematical procedure to separate out the *frequency* components of a signal from its amplitudes as a function of time, or vice versa. The Fourier transform is used to generate the *spectrum* from the FID or *spin echo* in *pulse MR* techniques and is essential to most *MRI* techniques.

Free induction decay (FID)—if *transverse magnetization* of the spins is produced (e.g., by a 90-degree pulse), a transient *MR signal* will result that decays toward zero with a characteristic time constant *T2* (or *T2**); this decaying signal is the FID. In practice, the first part of the FID is not observable because of residual effects of the powerful exciting *RF pulse* on the electronics of the *receiver,* the *receiver dead time.*

Frequency (f)—the number of repetitions of a periodic process per unit of time. For electromagnetic radiation, such as radio waves, the old unit, cycles per second (cps), has been replaced by the *SI* unit, *hertz,* abbreviated *Hz.* It is related to *angular frequency,* ω, by $f = \omega/2\pi$.

Frequency encoding—encoding the distribution of sources of *MR* signals along a direction by detecting the signal in the presence of a *magnetic field gradient* along that direction so that there is a corresponding gradient of *resonance frequencies* along that direction. In the absence of other position encoding, the Fourier transform of the resulting signal is a *projection profile* of the object.

G_x, G_y, G_z—conventional symbols for *magnetic field gradient.* Used with subscripts to denote spatial direction component of gradient, that is, direction along which the field changes.

Gadolinium—lanthanide element that is paramagnetic in its trivalent state. It has been used as the active component of some *contrast agents* in MR imaging because of its effect of strongly decreasing the *T1 relaxation times* of the tissues to which it has access. Although toxic by itself, it can be given safely in a chelated form, such as DTPA, that still retains much of its strong effect on relaxation times.

Gating—*synchronization* of imaging with a phase of the cardiac or respiratory cycles. A variety of means for detecting these cycles can be used, such as the electrocardiogram, peripheral pulse, and chest motion. The synchronization can be *prospective* or *retrospective.*

Gauss (G)—a unit of magnetic flux density in the older (CGS) system. The Earth's magnetic field is approximately one half gauss to one gauss, depending on a location. The currently preferred (SI) unit is the *tesla* (T) (1 T = 10,000 G).

Gradient—the amount and direction of the rate of change in space of some quantity, such as *magnetic field strength.* Also commonly used to refer to *magnetic field gradient.*

Gradient coils—current-carrying *coils* designed to produce a desired *magnetic field gradient* (so that the magnetic field is stronger in some locations than others). Proper design of the size and configuration of the coils is necessary to produce a controlled and uniform gradient.

Gradient echo—*spin echo* produced by reversing the direction of a *magnetic field gradient* or by applying balanced pulses of magnetic field gradient before and after a refocusing *RF pulse* so as to cancel out the position-dependent *phase* shifts that have accumulated due to the gradient. In the latter case, the gradient echo is generally adjusted to be coincident with the RF spin echo.

Gradient moment nulling—adjustment to zero at the time *TE* of the net moments of the amplitude of the waveform of the *magnetic field gradients* with time (e.g., zeroth moment is the area under the curve, first moment is the "center of gravity," etc). The aim is to minimize the *phase* shifts acquired by the *transverse magnetization* of excited nuclei moving along the gradients (including the effect of *refocusing RF pulses*), particularly for the reduction of image artifacts due to motion.

Gyromagnetic ratio (γ)—the ratio of the *magnetic moment* to the *angular momentum* of a particle. This is a constant for a given nucleus.

H_0—conventional symbol historically used for the constant *magnetic field* in an *MR system;* it is physically more correct to use B_0. A magnet provides a field strength, H; however, at a point in an object, the *spins* experience the *magnetic induction,* B.

H_1—conventional symbol historically used for the radiofrequency *magnetic field* in an *MR system;* it is physically more correct to use B_1. It is useful to consider it as composed of two oppositely rotating *vectors.* At the *Larmor frequency,* the vector rotating in the same direction as the *precessing spins* interacts strongly with the spins.

Hertz (Hz)—the standard *(SI)* unit of *frequency;* equal to the old unit cycles per second.

Homogeneity—uniformity. In *MR,* the homogeneity of the static *magnetic field* is an important criterion of the quality of the magnet. Homogeneity requirements for *MRI* are generally lower than the homogeneity requirements for NMR spectroscopy, but for most, imaging techniques must be maintained over a larger region.

I—see *Spin quantum number.*

Image acquisition time—time required to carry out an *MRI* procedure comprising only the data acquisition time. The total image acquisition time is equal to the product of the repetition time, *TR;* the number of signals averaged, *NSA;* and the number of different signals (encoded for position) to be acquired for use in image reconstruction. The additional image reconstruction time also is important in determining how quickly the image can be viewed. In comparing *sequential plane imaging* and *volume imaging* techniques, the equivalent image acquisition time per slice must be considered, as well as the actual image acquisition time.

Inductance—measure of the magnetic coupling between two current-carrying loops (mutual) reflecting their spatial relationship or of a loop (such as a *coil*) with itself (self). One of the principal determinants of the *resonance frequency* of an RF circuit.

Inhomogeneity—degree of lack of *homogeneity;* for example, the fractional deviation of the local *magnetic field* from the average value of the field.

Interpulse times—times between successive *RF pulses* used in *pulse sequences.* Particularly important are the inversion time (TI) in *inversion recovery,* and the time between the *90-degree pulse* and the subsequent *180-degree pulse* to produce a *spin echo,* which is approximately one half the *spin echo time (TE).* The time between repetitions of pulse sequences is the *repetition time (TR).*

Inversion—a nonequilibrium state in which the *macroscopic magnetization vector* is oriented opposite to the *magnetic field;* usually produced by *adiabatic fast passage* or *180-degree RF pulses.*

Inversion-recovery (IR)—*pulse NMR* technique that can be incorporated into *MR imaging,* wherein the nuclear magnetization is inverted at a time on the order of *T1* before the regular imaging pulse-gradient sequences. The resulting partial *relaxation* of the spins in the different structures being imaged can be used to produce an image that depends strongly on T1. This may bring out differences in the appearance of structures with different T1 relaxation times. Note that this does *not* directly produce an image of T1. T1 in a given region can be calculated from the change in the *NMR signal* from the region due to the inversion pulse compared with the signal with no inversion pulse or an inversion pulse with a different inversion time (TI).

Inversion-recovery-spin-echo (IRSE)—form of *inversion-recovery* imaging in which the signal is detected as a *spin echo.* For *TE* short compared to the *T2 relaxation time,* there will be only a small effect of T2 differences on image intensities; for longer TEs, the effect of T2 may be significant.

Inversion time—see *TI.*

Isotropic motion—motion that is uniform in all directions. This term is generally used in reference to molecular *diffusion* or rotation that gives rise to relaxation of the spin system through *dipole-dipole interactions.*

J-coupling—see *Spin-spin coupling.*

Kilohertz (kHz)—unit of *frequency;* equal to one thousand *hertz.*

k-space—mathematical space in which the *Fourier transform* of the image is represented. The data acquired for MR image reconstruction generally correspond to samples of k-space, that is, they represent values of the Fourier transform of the image at a particular set of locations in k-space.

Larmor equation—states that the *frequency* of precession of the nuclear *magnetic moment* is proportional to the *magnetic field.*

$$\omega = -\gamma B_0 \text{ (radians per second)}$$

or

$$f_0 = -\gamma B_0/2\pi \text{ (hertz)}$$

where ω_0 or F_0 is the frequency, γ is the *gyromagnetic ratio,* and B_0 is the magnetic induction field. The negative sign indicates the direction of the rotation.

Larmor frequency (ω_0 or f_0)—the *frequency* at which *magnetic resonance* can be excited; given by the *Larmor equation.* By varying the *magnetic* field across the body with a *magnetic field gradient,* the corresponding variation of the Larmor frequency can be used to encode position. For protons (hydrogen nuclei), the Larmor frequency is 42.58 MHz/tesla.

Lattice—by analogy to *NMR* in solids, the magnetic and thermal environment with which nuclei exchange energy in *longitudinal relaxation.*

Localization techniques—means of selecting a restricted region from which the signal is received. These can include the use of *surface coils,* with or without *magnetic field gradients.* Generally used to produce a *spectrum* from the desired region.

Longitudinal magnetization (M_z)—component of the *macroscopic magnetization vector* along the static *magnetic field.* Following excitation by *RF pulse,* M_z approaches its equilibrium value M_0, with a characteristic time constant *T1.*

Longitudinal relaxation—return of *longitudinal magnetization* to its equilibrium value after excitation; requires exchange of energy between the *nuclear spins* and the *lattice.*

Longitudinal relaxation time—see *T1.*

M—conventional symbol for *macroscopic magnetization vector.*

M_{xy}—see *Transverse magnetization.*

M_z—see *Longitudinal magnetization.*

M_0—equilibrium value of the *magnetization;* directed along the direction of the static *magnetic field.* Proportional to *spin density,* N.

Macroscopic magnetization vector—net *magnetic moment* per unit volume (a vector quantity) of a sample in a given region, considered as the integrated effect of all the individual microscopic nuclear magnetic moments. Most *MR* experiments actually deal with this.

Magnetic dipole—north and south magnetic poles separated by a finite distance. An electric current loop, including the effective current of a spinning nucleon or nucleus, can create an equivalent magnetic dipole.

Magnetic field (H)—the region surrounding a magnet (or current-carrying conductor) is endowed with certain properties. One is that a small magnet in such a region experiences a *torque* that tends to align it in a given direction. Magnetic field is a *vector* quantity; the direction of the field is defined as the direction in which the north pole of the small magnet points when in equilibrium. A magnetic field produces a magnetizing force on a body within it. Although the dangers of large magnetic fields are largely hypothetical, this is an area of potential concern for safety limits.

Formally, the forces experienced by moving charged particles, current-carrying wires, and small magnets in the vicinity of the magnet are due to *magnetic induction* (B), which includes the effect of *magnetization,* whereas the magnetic field (H) is defined so as not to include magnetization. However, both B and H are often loosely used to denote magnetic fields.

Magnetic field gradient—a *magnetic field* that changes in strength in a certain given direction. Such fields are used in *NMR imaging* with *selective excitation* to select a region for imaging and also to encode the location of *NMR signals* received from the object being imaged. Measured, for example, in *teslas* per meter.

Magnetic induction (B)—also called magnetic flux density. The net magnetic effect from an externally applied *magnetic field* and the resulting *magnetization.* B is proportional to H(B = μH), with the *SI* unit being the *tesla.*

Magnetic moment—a measure of the net magnetic properties of an object or a particle. A nucleus with an intrinsic spin has an associated *magnetic dipole* moment, so that it interacts with the *magnetic field* (as if it were a tiny bar magnet).

Magnetic resonance (MR)—*resonance* phenomenon resulting in the absorption and/or emission of electromagnetic energy by nuclei or electrons in a static *magnetic field,* after excitation by a suitable *RF* magnetic field. The peak *resonance frequency* is proportional to the magnetic field, and is given by the *Larmor equation.* Only unpaired electrons or nuclei with a nonzero *spin* exhibit magnetic resonance.

Magnetic resonance angiography (MRA)—*angiography* using MRI.

Magnetic resonance imaging (MRI)—use of MR to create images of objects such as the body. Currently, this involves primarily imaging the distribution of mobile hydrogen nuclei (protons) in the body. The image brightness depends jointly on the spin density (N(H)) and the relaxation times (T1 and T2), with their relative importance depending on the particular imaging technique and choice of interpulse times. Image brightness is also affected by any motion, such as blood flow and respiration.

Magnetic resonance spectroscopy (MRS)—use of *magnetic resonance* to study the MR *spectrum* of a sample or a tissue region. In addition to the effects of factors such as *relaxation times* that can affect the MR signal as seen in magnetic resonance imaging, effects such as *J-modulation* or the transfer of *magnetization* after selective excitation of particular *spectral lines* can affect the relative strengths of spectral lines. The *frequencies* of certain lines may also be affected by factors such as the local pH.

Magnetic shielding—means to confine the region of strong magnetic field surrounding a magnet; most commonly, the use of material with high *permeability.*

Magnetic susceptibility (χ)—measure of the ability of a substance to become magnetized.

Magnetization—(see also *Macroscopic magnetization vector*)—the magnetic polarization of a material produced by a magnetic field (magnetic moment per unit volume).

Magnetization transfer—the change in magnetization within a multicomponent spin system when one of the component peaks is selectively perturbed. This is observed as a change in relative signal intensities. One of the most common forms of perturbation in imaging is selective *saturation.* For example, this phenomenon can be exploited as part of an imaging sequence to produce image contrast based on differential amounts of magnetization transfer, *magnetization transfer contrast (MTC).*

Magnetization transfer contrast (MTC)—production of change in relative signal intensities by *magnetization transfer.* For example, *saturation* of broad *spectral lines* may produce decreases in intensity of lines not directly saturated, through exchange of magnetization between the corresponding states; more closely coupled states will show a greater resulting intensity change.

Megahertz (MHz)—unit of *frequency,* equal to one million *hertz.*

MRA—see *Magnetic resonance angiography.*

MRI—see *Magnetic resonance imaging.*

MRS—see *Magnetic resonance spectroscopy.*

MTC—see *Magnetization transfer contrast.*

Multiple echo imaging—*spin echo imaging* using spin echoes acquired as a train. Typically, a separate image is produced from each echo of the train.

Multiple slice imaging—variation of *sequential plane imaging* techniques that can be used with *selective excitation* techniques that do not affect adjacent slices. Adjacent slices are imaged while waiting for *relaxation of the first slice toward equilibrium, resulting in decreased image acquisition time* for the set of slices.

N(H)—see *Spin density.*

NEX—see *NSA.*

NMR signal—electromagnetic signal in the *radiofrequency* range produced by the *precession* of the *transverse magnetization* of the *spins.* The rotation of the transverse magnetization induces a voltage in a *coil,* which is amplified and demodulated by the *receiver;* the signal may refer only to this induced voltage.

Noise—that component of the reconstructed image (or spectrum) due to random and unpredictable processes, as opposed to the *signal* within the image itself that is due to predictable processes. Not to be confused with artifacts that are nonrandom errors in the image. Noise is commonly characterized by the standard deviation of signal intensity in the image of a uniform object (phantom) in the absence of *artifacts.* The measured noise may depend on the particular phantom used because of variable effects on the *Q* of the *receiver coil.*

NSA—number of signals averaged together to determine each distinct position-encoded signal to be used in image reconstruction.

Nuclear magnetic resonance (NMR)—the absorption or emission of electromagnetic energy by nuclei in a static *magnetic field,* after *excitation* by a suitable *RF* magnetic field. The peak *resonance frequency* is proportional to the magnetic field, and is given by the *Larmor equation.* Only nuclei with a nonzero *spin* exhibit NMR.

Nuclear spin—see also *Spin*—an intrinsic property of certain nuclei that gives them an associated characteristic *angular momentum* and *magnetic moment.*

Nuclear spin quantum number (I)—property of all nuclei related to the largest measurable component of the nuclear *angular momentum.* Nonzero values of nuclear angular momentum are quantized (fixed) as integral or half-integral multiples of ($h/2\pi$), where h is Planck's constant. The number of possible *energy levels* for a given nucleus in a fixed *magnetic field* is equal to $2I + 1$.

Nutation—a displacement of the axis of a spinning body away from the simple cone-shaped figure that would be traced by the axis during *precession.* In the *rotating frame of reference,* the nutation caused by an *RF pulse* appears as a simple precession, although the motion is more complex in the stationary frame of reference.

Nyquist limit—*frequency* of a signal beyond which *aliasing* will occur in the *sampling* process. This frequency is equal to one half the sampling rate.

Orientation—The three basic orthogonal slice orientations are transverse (T), sagittal (S), and coronal (C). The basic anatomical directions are right (R) to left (L), posterior (P) to anterior (A), and feet (F) to head (H), considered as positive directions. The location in the R/L and P/A directions can be specified relative to the axis of the magnet; the F/H location can be specified relative to a convenient patient structure.

Pacemaker effect—all implanted electronic devices are susceptible to the fields used in *MR.* The static *magnetic field* applies force to magnetic materials, and both *RF* fields and pulsed *gradients* can induce voltages in circuits. The pacemaker's susceptibility to static field and its critical role in life support have warranted special consideration. Transcutaneous control or adjustment of pacing rate is a feature of many units. Some achieve this control by using switches activated by the external application of a magnet to open or close the switch. Others use rotation of an external magnet to turn internal controls. The fringe field around an MR magnet can activate such switches or controls. Such activations are considered to be a risk. Areas with fields higher than 0.5 mT (5 G) commonly have restricted access and/or are posted as being a risk to persons with pacemakers.

Paramagnetic—a substance with a small but positive *magnetic susceptibility* (magnetizability). The addition of a small amount of paramagnetic substance may greatly reduce the *relaxation times* of water. Typical paramagnetic substances usually possess an unpaired electron and include atoms or ions of transition elements, rare earth elements, some metals, and some molecules, including molecular oxygen and free radicals. Paramagnetic substances are considered promising for use as *contrast agents* in NMR imaging.

Partial Fourier imaging—reconstruction of an image from an MR data set comprising an asymmetric sampling of *k-space.* For example, it can be used either to shorten *image acquisition time,* by reducing the number of *phase-encoding* steps required, or to shorten the *echo time, TE,* by moving the *echo* off center in the *acquisition window.* In either case, the *signal-to-noise ratio* is reduced.

Partial saturation (PS)—*excitation* technique applying repeated *RF pulses* in times on the order of or shorter than *T1.* In *NMR imaging* systems, although it results in decreased signal amplitude, there is the possibility of generating images with increased *contrast* between regions with different relaxation times. It does *not* directly produce images of T1. The change in *NMR signal* from a region resulting from a change in the *interpulse time, TR,* can be used to calculate T1 for the region. Although partial saturation is also commonly referred to as *saturation recovery,* that term should properly be reserved for the particular case of partial saturation in which recovery after each *excitation* effectively takes place from true *saturation.*

Partial saturation spin echo (PSSE)—*partial saturation* in which the signal is detected as a *spin echo.* Even though a spin echo is used, there will not necessarily be a significant contribution of the *T2 relaxation time* to image *contrast,* unless the echo time, *TE,* is on the order of or longer than T2.

Permeability (μ)—tendency of a substance to concentrate *magnetic field,* $\mu = B/H$.

Phantom—an artificial object of known dimensions and properties used to test aspects of an imaging machine.

Phase—in a periodic function (e.g., rotational or sinusoidal motion), the position relative to a particular part of the cycle.

Phase correction—(1) corrective processing of the *spectrum* so that *spectral lines* at different *frequencies* all have the *absorption-mode phase.* (2) In imaging, adjustment of the signal in different parts of the image to have a consistent phase.

Phase cycling—techniques of signal *excitation* in which the phases of the *exciting* or *refocusing* RF pulses are systematically varied, and the resulting signals are then suitably combined to reduce or eliminate certain *artifacts.*

Phase encoding—encoding the distribution of sources of *MR signals* along a direction in space with different phases by applying a pulsed *magnetic field gradient* along that direction prior to detection of the signal. In general, it is necessary to acquire a set of signals with a suitable set of different phase-encoding gradient pulses to reconstruct the distribution of the sources along the encoded direction.

Pixel—acronym for a picture element; the smallest discrete part of a digital image display. Note that the corresponding size of the pixel may be smaller than the actual spatial resolution.

Planar imaging—imaging technique in which an image of a plane is built up from signals received from the whole plane.

Precession—comparatively slow gyration of the axis of a spinning body so as to trace out a cone; caused by the application of a *torque* tending to change the direction of the rotation axis, and continuously directed at right angles to the plane of the torque. The *magnetic moment* of a nucleus with *spin* experiences such a torque when inclined at an angle to the *magnetic field,* resulting in precession at the *Larmor frequency.* A familiar example is the effect of gravity on the motion of a spinning top or gyroscope.

Probe—the portion of an *MR spectrometer* comprising the sample container and the *RF coils,* with some associated electronics. The RF coils may consist of separate *receiver* and *transmitter* coils in a *crossed-coil* configuration or, alternatively, a single coil to perform both functions.

PSSE—see *Partial saturation spin echo.*

Pulse, 90 degrees (π/2 pulse)—*RF pulse* designed to rotate the *macroscopic magnetization vector* 90 degrees in space as referred to the *rotating frame of reference,* usually about an axis at right angles to the main *magnetic field.* If the *spins* are initially aligned with the magnetic field, this pulse will produce *transverse magnetization* and an *FID.*

Pulse, 180 degrees (π pulse)—*RF pulse* designed to rotate the *macroscopic magnetization vector* 180 degrees in space as referred to the *rotating frame of reference,* usually about an axis at right angles to the main *magnetic field.* If the *spins* are initially aligned with the magnetic field, this pulse will produce inversion.

Pulse length (width)—time duration of a pulse. For an *RF pulse* near the *Larmor frequency,* the longer the pulse length, the greater the angle of rotation of the *macroscopic magnetization vector* (greater than 180 degrees can bring it back toward its original orientation). For an RF pulse of a given shape as a function of time, the longer the pulse length, the narrower the equivalent range of frequencies in the pulse.

Pulse programmer—part of the *spectrometer* or *interface* that controls the timing, duration, *phase,* and amplitude of the *pulses* (*RF* or *gradient*).

Pulse sequences—set of *RF* (and/or *gradient*) *magnetic field pulses* and time spacings between these pulses; used in conjunction with magnetic field gradients and *NMR signal* reception to produce NMR images. See also *Interpulse times.* A recommended shorthand designation of interpulse times used to generate a particular image is to list the repetition time *(TR),* the echo time *(TE),* and, if *inversion-recovery* is being used, the inversion time, *TI,* with all times given in milliseconds. For example, 2500/30/1000 would indicate an inversion-recovery pulse sequence with TR of 2500 msec, TE of 30 msec, and TI of 1000 msec. If multiple *spin echoes* are being used, as in *CPMG,* the number of the spin echo used should be stated.

Pulse sequences—acronyms

Rapid spin-echo techniques	
RARE	Rapid acquisition with relaxation enhancement
FSE	Fast spin echo
DFSE	Dual-echo, fast spin echo
MEMS	Multiecho multishot
MESS	Multiecho single shot
TSE	Turbo spin echo
Rapid gradient-echo techniques	
FFE	Fast field echo
FLASH	Fast low-angle shot
Turbo Flash	Magnetization-prepared FLASH
FISP	Fast imaging with steady-state precession
GE or GRE	Gradient-recalled echo or gradient echo
GRASS	Gradient-recalled acquisition in steady state
FGR	Fast GRASS
IRFGR	Inversion-recovery Fast GRASS
SPGR	Spoiled gradient recalled
FSPGR	Fast SPGR
SSFP	Steady-state free precession
FAST	Fourier-acquired steady-state technique
3D MP RAGE	Three-dimensional magnetization-prepared rapid gradient echo
ROAST	Resonant offset averaging in the steady state
T2-FFE	Contrast-enhanced fast field echo
Miscellaneous	
SAT	Saturation or presaturation
FATSAT	Fat saturation
RESCOMP	Respiratory compensation
GMN	Gradient moment nulling
FLOWCOMP or FC	Flow compensation

MAST	Motion-artifact suppression technique
FLAG	Flow-adjustable gradients
STEAM	Stimulated-echo acquisition model
STIR	Short-time inversion recovery
PRESS	Point-resolved spectroscopy
CHESS	Chemical shift selective
TOF	Time of flight
PC	Phase contrast

Quenching—loss of *superconductivity* of the current-carrying *coil* that may occur unexpectedly in a superconducting magnet. As the magnet becomes resistive, heat is released that can result in rapid evaporation of liquid helium in the *cryostat.* Such evaporation may present a hazard if not properly planned for.

R1—longitudinal *relaxation rate* equal to reciprocal of relaxation time (R1 = 1/T1).

R2—longitudinal *relaxation rate* equal to reciprocal of relaxation time (R2 = 1/T2).

Radian—dimensionless unit of angular measure; 360 degrees = 2π radians.

Radiofrequency (RF)—wave *frequency* intermediate between auditory and infrared. The RF used in *NMR* studies is commonly in the *megahertz* (MHz) range. The RF used in *ESR* studies is commonly in the *gigahertz* (GHz) range. The principal effect of RF *magnetic fields* on the body is power deposition in the form of heating, mainly at the surface; this is a principal area of concern for safety limits.

Ramp time—time required for a change in the *magnetic field* strength, usually measured in *tesla* per minutes depends on construction of the magnet and design of the magnet power supply.

Rapid-excitation MRI—There are several approaches to speeding up the MRI data acquisition process by repeating the *excitation* by *RF pulses* in times short compared to *T1,* typically using small *flip angles* and *gradient-echo* refocusing. When *TR* is also on the order of or shorter than *T2*, the repeated RF pulses tend to refocus transverse magnetization remaining from prior excitations, setting up a condition of *steady state free precession,* and a dependence of signal strength (and image contrast) on both T1 and T2. This dependence can be modified in various ways, particularly as follows: (1) can "spoil" the tendency to build up a steady state by reducing coherence between excitations, for example, by variation of the *phase* or timing of consecutive RF pulses or of the strength of *spoiler gradient pulses,* thus increasing the relative dependence of signal strength on T1, or (2) can acquire the signal when it is refocusing immediately prior to the next RF pulse, thus increasing the relative dependence of signal strength on T2.

Receiver—portion of the MR apparatus that detects and amplifies *RF signals* picked up by the *receiving coil.* Includes a preamplifier, amplifier, and *demodulator.*

Receiver dead time—time after exciting *RF pulse* during which *FID* is not detectable because of saturation of *receiver* electronics.

Reference compound—standard compound used as a standard reference *spectral* line for defining *chemical shifts* for a given nucleus. As recommended by the ASTM, for ^{1}H it is tetramethylsilane (TMS) and for ^{31}P it is phosphoric acid, although for practical biologic applications water and PCr have been used as secondary references for hydrogen and phosphorus spectroscopy, respectively. The reference compound can be in a capsule outside of the subject (external) or can be in the subject (internal); internal references are generally preferable when possible, as external references may be subject to different conditions.

Relaxation rates—reciprocals of the *relaxation times T1* and *T2* (*R1* = 1/T1 and *R2* = 1/T2). There is often a linear relation between the concentration of MR *contrast agents* and the resulting change in relaxation rate.

Relaxation times—after *excitation,* the *spins* tend to return to their equilibrium distribution, in which there is no *transverse magnetization* and the *longitudinal magnetization* is at its maximal value and oriented in the direction of the static *magnetic field.* It is observed that in the absence of applied *RF magnetic field,* the transverse magnetization decays toward zero with a characteristic time constant *T2*, and the longitudinal magnetization returns toward the equilibrium value M_0 with a characteristic time constant *T1.*

Repetition time—see *TR.*

Rephasing gradient—*magnetic field gradient* applied for a brief period after a *selective excitation* pulse, in the direction opposite to the *gradient* used for the selective excitation. The result of the gradient reversal is a rephasing of the *spins* (which will have become out of *phase* with each other along the direction of the selection gradient), forming a *gradient echo* and improving the sensitivity of imaging after the selective excitation process.

Resolution element—size of smallest *spatially resolved* regions in image. It may be anisotropic, for example, with an asymmetric *acquisition matrix* or *slice thickness,* and may be larger than the *pixel* or *voxel.*

Resonance—a large amplitude vibration in a mechanical or electrical system caused by a relatively small periodic stimulus with a *frequency* at or close to a natural frequency of the system; in *NMR* apparatus, resonance can refer to the NMR itself or to the tuning of the *RF* circuitry.

Resonance frequency—*frequency* at which *resonance* phenomenon occurs; given by the *Larmor equation* for *NMR;* determined by inductance and capacitance for *RF* circuits.

RF—see *Radiofrequency.*

Rotating frame of reference—a frame of reference (with corresponding coordinate systems) that is rotating about the axis of the static *magnetic field* B_0 (with respect to a stationary ["laboratory"] frame of reference) at a *frequency* equal to that of the applied *RF* magnetic field, B_1. Although B_1 is a rotating *vector,* it appears stationary in the rotating frame, leading to simpler mathematical formulations.

Safety—safety concerns in MR include *magnetic field* strength, *RF* heating *(SAR)* induced currents due to rapidly varying magnetic fields *(dB/dt),* effects on implanted devices such as *pacemakers,* magnetic *torque* effects on indwelling metal such as clips and possible "missile effect" of *magnetic forces,* and *acoustic noise.*

Sampling—conversion of the continuous (analog) signal to a series of discrete (digital) values by measurement at a set of particular times; this utilizes the *analog to digital converter.* If the rate of sampling is less than twice the highest frequency in the signal, *aliasing* will occur. The duration of sampling determines how small a difference of frequencies can be separated.

Saturation—a nonequilibrium state in *MR,* in which equal numbers of spins are aligned against and with the *magnetic field,* so that there is no net *magnetization.* Can be produced by repeatedly applying RF pulses at the *Larmor frequency* with interpulse times short compared with T1.

Saturation recovery (SR)—particular type of *partial saturation pulse sequence* in which the preceding pulses leave the *spins* in a state of *saturation,* so that recovery at the time of the next pulse has taken place from an initial condition of no *magnetization.*

Saturation transfer (or inversion transfer)—nuclei can retain their magnetic orientation through a chemical reaction. Thus, if *RF* radiation is supplied to the *spins* at a *frequency* corresponding to the *chemical shift* of the nuclei in one chemical state so as to produce *saturation* or *inversion,* and chemical reactions transform the nuclei into another chemical state with a different chemical shift in a shorter time compared with the *relaxation time,* the NMR *spectrum* may show the effects of the saturation or inversion on the corresponding, unirradiated, line in the spectrum. This technique can be used to study reaction kinetics of suitable molecules.

Scalar—a quantity having only magnitude.

SE—see *Spin echo.*

Selective excitation—controlling the *frequency spectrum* of an irradiating *RF pulse* (via *tailoring*) while imposing a *magnetic field gradient on spins,* such that only a desired region has a suitable *resonant frequency* to be excited. Originally used to excite all but a desired region, such as a plane, for excitation. Used without simultaneous *magnetic field* gradients, tailored RF pulses can be used to selectively excite a particular *spectral line* or group of lines. RF and gradient pulse combinations can be designed to select both spatial regions and spectral frequencies.

Sensitive plane—technique of selecting a plane for *sequential plane imaging* by using an oscillating magnetic field *gradient* and filtering out the corresponding time-dependent part of the *NMR signal.* The gradient used is at right angles to the desired plane, and the magnitude of the oscillating magnetic field gradient is equal to zero only in the desired plane.

Sequence time—see *TR.*

Shift reagents—*paramagnetic* compounds designed to induce a shift in the *resonance frequency* of nuclei with which they interact. For example, many rare earths have been used as shift reagents for positive metal ions, such as sodium and potassium.

Shim coils—*coils* carrying a relatively small current that are used to provide auxiliary *magnetic fields* to compensate for *inhomogeneities* in the main magnetic field of an *NMR* system.

Shimming—correction of *inhomogeneity* of the *magnetic field* produced by the main magnet of an *NMR* system due to imperfections in the magnet or to the presence of external *ferromagnetic* objects. May involve changing the configuration of the magnet or the addition of *shim coils (active shimming)* or small pieces of steel *(passive shimming).*

Signal averaging—the averaging together of signals acquired under the same or similar conditions so as to suppress the effects of random variations or random artifacts. The number of signals averaged together can be abbreviated *NSA.*

Signal-to-noise ratio (SNR or S/N)—used to describe the relative contributions to a detected signal of the true signal and random superimposed signals *("noise").* One common method for improving (increasing) the SNR is to average several measurements of the signal on the expectation that random contributions will tend to cancel out. The SNR can also be improved by sampling larger volumes (with a corresponding loss of spatial resolution) or, within limits, by increasing the strength of the magnetic field used. The SNR depends on the electrical properties of the sample or the patient being studied.

Slice—the effective physical extent of the "planar" region being imaged.

Slice thickness—the thickness of a *slice.* Because the *slice profile* may not be sharp-edged, a criterion such as the distance between the points at half the sensitivity of the maximum *(FWHM)* or the equivalent rectangular width (the width of a rectangular slice profile with the same maximal height and same area) may be useful.

S/N—see *Signal-to-noise ratio.*

SNR—see *Signal-to-noise ratio.*

Spatial resolution—the smallest distance between two points in the object that can be distinguished as separate details in the image, generally indicated as a length or a number of black and white line pairs per millimeter. The specific criterion of resolution to be used depends on the type of test used (e.g., bar pattern or contrast-detail *phantom*). As the ability to separate or detect objects depends on their *contrast* and the noise, and the different *NMR* parameters of objects affect image contrast differently for different imaging techniques, care must be taken in comparing the results of resolution phantom tests of different machines and no single simple measure of resolution can be specified. The resolution may be anisotropic. The resolution may be larger than the size corresponding to the discrete image element *(pixel),* although it cannot be smaller.

Spatially localized spectroscopy—process by which regions of tissue are selectively sampled to produce *spectra* from defined volumes in space. These methods may be employed to sample a single region in space (single voxel method) or multiple regions simultaneously (multivoxel methods). The spatial selectivity can be achieved by a variety of methods, including *surface coils,* surface coils in conjunction with *RF gradient* methods, or RF pulses in combination with switched *magnetic field* gradients, for example, *volume-selective excitation.* An indirect method of achieving spatial selectivity is the destruction of coherence of the *magnetization* in regions that lie outside the region of interest. A variety of spatial encoding schemes have been employed for multivoxel localization. See *Chemical shift imaging.*

Specific absorption rate (SAR) (W/kg)—Time varying electromagnetic fields can deposit energy in tissues. This energy is deposited mostly in the form of heat, which is considered the primary mechanism of biologic effect. The specific absorption rate (SAR) is defined as the energy dissipated in tissue (watts) per kilogram of tissue mass. Inhomogeneity of the *RF* fields leads to a local exposure where most of the power that is absorbed is applied to one body region rather than the entire person, leading to the concept of a local SAR. Averaging over the whole body leads to the global SAR.

Spectral editing—methods of selectively enhancing or suppressing the signal from a particular molecular substance by using its spin properties, typically through spin-spin coupling, e.g., *J-modulation.*

Spectral line—particular distinct *frequency* or narrow band of frequencies at which *resonance* occurs corresponding to a particular *chemical shift.*

Spectrometer—the portions of the *NMR* apparatus that actually produce the NMR phenomenon and acquire the signals, including the *magnet,* the *probe,* the *RF* circuitry, and the *gradient coils.* The spectrometer is controlled by the *computer* via the *interface* under the direction of the *software.*

Spectrum—an array of the *frequency components of the MR signal* according to frequency. Nuclei with different *resonant frequencies* show up as values at different corresponding frequencies in the spectrum. When resonances are relatively isolated, they appear as peaks or "lines" in the spectrum.

Spin—The intrinsic *angular momentum* of an elementary particle, or system of particles such as a nucleus, that is also responsible for the *magnetic moment;* or, a particle or nucleus possessing such a spin. The spins of nuclei have characteristic fixed values. Pairs of neutrons and protons align to cancel out their spins, so that nuclei with an odd number of neutrons and/or protons have a net nonzero rotational component characterized by an integer or half integer quantum *"nuclear spin number" (I).*

Spin density (N)—the density of resonating *spins* in a given region; one of the principal determinants of the strength of the *NMR signal* from the region. The *SI* units would be moles/m^3. For water, there are about 1.1×10^5 moles of hydrogen per m^3, or .11 moles of hydrogen/cm^3. True spin density is *not* imaged directly, but must be calculated from signals received with different *interpulse times.*

Spin echo—reappearance of an *NMR signal* after the *FID* has apparently died away, as a result of the effective reversal of the dephasing of the spins (refocusing) by techniques such as specific *RF pulse sequences,* e.g., *Carr-Purcell sequence (RF spin echo),* or pairs of *magnetic field gradient pulses (gradient echo),* applied in times shorter than or on the order of *T2.* Unlike RF spin echoes, gradient echoes do not refocus phase differences due to *chemical shifts* or *inhomogeneities* of the *magnetic field.*

Spin-echo imaging—any of many *MR imaging* techniques in which the *spin echo* is used rather than the *FID.* Can be used to create images that depend strongly on *T2* if TE has a value on the order of a greater than T2 of the relevant image details. Note that spin echo imaging does *not* directly produce an image of T2 distribution. The spin echoes can be produced as a train of multiple echoes, e.g., using the *CPMG pulse sequence.*

Spin-lattice relaxation time—see *T1.*

Spin number, nuclear—see *Spin quantum number.*

Spin quantum number (I)—property of all nuclei related to the largest measurable component of the nuclear *angular momentum.* Nonzero values of nuclear angular momentum are quantized (fixed) as integral or half-integral multiples of ($h/2\pi$), where h is Planck's constant. The number of possible *energy levels* for a given nucleus in a fixed *magnetic field* is equal to $2I + 1$. Similarly, an unpaired electron has a spin of 1/2 and two possible energy levels.

Spin-spin coupling—interaction between nuclei in the same molecule that results in a splitting of a single resonance line into two or more lines. For example, a ^{13}C nucleus with a directly bonded proton has two resonance frequencies corresponding to the two different orientations of the bonded proton.

Spin-spin relaxation time—see *T2.*

Spin tagging—nuclei will retain their magnetic orientation for a time on the order of *T1* even in the presence of motion. Thus, if the nuclei in a given region have their *spin* orientation changed, the altered spins will serve as a "tag" to trace the motion for a time on the order of T1 of any fluid that may have been in the tagged region.

Spin-warp imaging—a form of *Fourier transform imaging* in which phase-encoding gradient pulses are applied for a constant duration but with varying amplitude. The spin warp method, as with other Fourier imaging techniques, is relatively tolerant of nonuniformities *(inhomogeneities)* in the *magnetic fields.*

Spoiler gradient pulse—magnetic field *gradient* pulse applied to effectively remove *transverse magnetization* by producing a rapid variation of its *phase* along the direction of the gradient. For example, when used to remove the unwanted signal resulting from an imperfect 180-degree *refocusing RF pulse,* a corresponding compensating gradient pulse may be applied prior to the refocusing RF pulse in order to avoid spoiling the desired transverse magnetization resulting from the initial *excitation.* Also called homospoil pulse.

Steady-state free precession (SFP or SSFP)—method of *NMR excitation* in which strings of *RF pulses* are applied rapidly and repeatedly with interpulse intervals short compared with both *T1* and *T2.* Alternating the *phases* of the RF pulses by 180 degrees can be useful in obtaining maximal signal strength.

Stimulated echo—a form of *spin echo* produced by three-pulse *RF* sequences, consisting of two RF pulses following an initial exciting RF pulse. The stimulated echo appears at a time delay after the third pulse equal to the interval between the first two pulses. Although classically produced with 90-degree pulses, any RF pulses other than an ideal 180 degrees can produce a stimulated echo. The intensity of the echo depends in part on the *T1 relaxation time* because the excitation is "stored" as *longitudinal magnetization* between the second and the third RF pulses. For example, use of stimulated echoes with *spatially selective* excitation with orthogonal *magnetic field gradients* permits *volume-selective excitation* for spectroscopic localization.

Superconductor—a substance whose electrical resistance essentially disappears at temperatures near absolute zero. A commonly used superconductor in *NMR imaging* system magnets is niobium-titanium, embedded in a copper matrix to help protect the superconductor from *quenching.*

Suppression—one of a number of techniques designed to minimize the contribution of a particular *spectral line* to the detected *signal.* Most commonly used to suppress the strong signal from water in order to detect other components.

Surface coil—*receiver coil* that does not surround the body and is placed close to the surface of the body. Used to restrict the region of the body contributing to the detected signal.

Susceptibility—see *Magnetic susceptibility.*

T_1 or T1 ("T-one")—spin-lattice or longitudinal *relaxation time;* the characteristic time constant for *spins* to tend to align themselves with the external *magnetic field.* Starting from zero *magnetization* in the z direction, the z magnetization will grow to 63 percent of its final maximal value in a time T1.

T1-weighted (T1W)—often used to indicate an image where most of the contrast between tissues or tissue states is due to differences in tissue *T1.* This term may be misleading in that the potentially important effects of tissue density differences and the range of tissue T1 values are ignored. A T1 contrast state is approached by imaging with a TR short compared to the longest tissue T1 of interest and *TE* short compared to tissue *T2* (to reduce T2 contributions to image contrast). Because of the wide range of T1 and T2 and tissue density value that can be found in the body, an image that is T1-weighted for some tissues may not be so for others.

T_2 or T2 ("T-two")—spin-spin or transverse *relaxation time;* the *characteristic time constant for loss of phase* coherence among spins oriented at an angle to the static *magnetic field,* due to interactions between the spins, with resulting loss of *transverse magnetization* and *NMR signal.* Starting from a nonzero value of the magnetization in the xy plane, the xy magnetization will decay so that it loses 63 percent of its initial value in a time T2.

T2-weighted (T2W)—often used to indicate an image where most of the contrast between tissues or tissue states is due to differences in tissue *T2.* This term may be misleading in that the potentially important effects of tissue density differences and the range of tissue T2 values are often ignored. A T2 contrast state is approached by imaging with a *TR* long compared to tissue *T1* (to reduce T1 contribution to image contrast) and a *TE* between the longest and shortest tissue T2s of interest. A TR greater than three times the longest T1 is required for the T1 effect to be less than 5 percent. Owing to the wide range of T1 and T2 and tissue density values that can be found in the body, an image that is T2-weighted for some tissues may not be so for others.

T2* ("T-two-star")—the observed time constant of the *FID* due to loss of *phase* coherence among spins oriented at an angle to the static *magnetic field,* commonly due to a combination of magnetic field *inhomogeneities,* ΔB, and *spin-spin transverse relaxation* with resultant more rapid loss in transverse magnetization and *NMR signal.* NMR signals can usually still be recovered as a spin echo in times less than or on the order of T2. $1/T2^* \cong 1/T2 + \Delta\omega/2$; $\Delta\omega = \gamma\Delta B$.

TE—echo time. Time between middle of 90-degree *pulse* and middle of *spin echo* production. For multiple echoes, use TE1, TE2. . . .

Tesla (T)—the preferred *(SI)* unit of magnetic flux density. One tesla is equal to 10,000 *gauss,* the older (CGS) unit.

Thermal equilibrium—a state in which all parts of a system are at the same effective temperature, in particular where the relative alignment of the *spins* with the *magnetic field* is determined solely by the thermal energy of the system (in which case the relative numbers of spins with different alignments is given by the *Boltzmann distribution*).

TI—inversion time. In *inversion recovery,* time between middle of *inverting (180-degree) RF pulse* and middle of the subsequent *exciting (90-degree)* pulse to detect amount of *longitudinal magnetization.*

Time of flight—when the local magnetization of moving tissue or fluid is selectively altered in a region, e.g., by *selective excitation,* it will carry the altered magnetization with it when it moves, thus *tagging* the selected region for times on the order of the *relaxation times.* This is the source of several *flow effects.*

TR—repetition time. The period of time between the beginning of a *pulse sequence* and the beginning of the succeeding (essentially identical) pulse sequence.

Transverse magnetization (M_{xy})—component of the *macroscopic magnetization vector* at right angles to the static *magnetic field* (B_0). *Precession* of the *transverse magnetization* at the *Larmor frequency* is responsible for the detectable *NMR signal.* In the absence of externally applied *RF magnetic field,* the transverse magnetization decays to zero with a characteristic time constant of *T2* or *T2**.

Triggering—generation of an electrical pulse, on detection of a physiologic signal, that can be used to initiate a *synchronized* data-acquisition *pulse sequence.*

Tuning—process of adjusting the *resonant frequency,* e.g., of the *RF* circuit, to the desired value, e.g., the *Larmor frequency.* More generally, the process of adjusting the components of the *spectrometer* for optimal *NMR signal* strength.

Two-dimensional Fourier transform imaging (2DFT)—a form of *sequential plane imaging* using *Fourier transform imaging.*

Vector—a quantity having both magnitude and direction, frequently represented by an arrow whose length is proportional to the magnitude and with an arrowhead at one end to indicate the direction.

Volume imaging—imaging techniques in which *NMR signals* are gathered from the whole object volume to be imaged at once, with appropriate encoding *pulse RF and gradient sequences* to encode positions of the *spins.* Many *sequential plane imaging* techniques can be generalized to volume imaging, at least in principle. Advantages include potential improvement in *signal-to-noise ratio* by including signal from the whole volume at once; disadvantages include a bigger computational task for image reconstruction and longer *image acquisition times* (although the entire volume can be imaged from the one set of data). Also called simultaneous volume imaging.

Volume-selective excitation—selective excitation of spins in only a limited region of space. This can be particularly useful for spectroscopy as well as imaging, as spatial localization of the signal source may be achieved through spatially *selective excitation* and the resulting signal may be analyzed directly for the spectrum corresponding to the excited region. It is usually achieved with selective excitation. Typically, a single dimension of localization can be achieved with one selective RF excitation pulse (and a magnetic field gradient along a desired direction), while a localized volume (3-D) can be excited with a *stimulated echo* produced with three selective *RF pulses* whose selective *magnetic field gradients* are mutually orthogonal, having a common intersection in the desired region. Similar "crossed plane" excitation can be used with selective 180-degree refocussing pulses and conventional spin echoes. A degree of spatial localization of excitation can alternatively be achieved with *depth pulses,* e.g., when using surface coils for excitation as well as signal detection. An indirect application of selective excitation for volume-selected spectroscopy is to use appropriate combinations of signals acquired after selective *inversion* of different regions, in order to subtract away the signal from undesired regions.

Voxel—volume element; the element of three-dimensional space corresponding to a *pixel,* for a given slice thickness.

x—dimension in the stationary (laboratory) frame of reference in the plane orthogonal (at right angles) to the direction of the static *magnetic field* (B_0 or H_0), *z,* and orthogonal to *y,* the other dimension in this plane.

x′—dimension in the *rotating frame of reference* in the plane at right angles to the direction of the *static magnetic field* (B_0 or H_0), *z;* commonly defined to be the direction of the magnetic vector of the *exciting* RF field (B_1).

y—dimension in the stationary (laboratory) frame of reference in the plane orthogonal to the direction of the static *magnetic field* (B_0 and H_0), *z,* and orthogonal to *x,* the other dimension in this place.

y′—dimension in the *rotating frame of reference* in the plane orthogonal (at right angles) to the direction of the static *magnetic field* (B_0 *and* H_0), *z,* and orthogonal to the other dimension in the plane, *x′*.

z—dimension in the direction of the static *magnetic field* (B_0 and H_0), in both the stationary and *rotating frames of reference.*

γ—see *Gyromagnetic ratio.*

δ—see *Chemical shift.*

μ—see *Permeability.*

τ—often used to denote different time delays between RF pulses. See *Interpulse times.*

χ—see *Magnetic susceptibility.*

ω—see *Angular frequency.*

ω_0—see *Larmor frequency.*

INDEX

Note: Page numbers in *italics* refer to illustrations. Page numbers followed by t indicate tables. Plate numbers refer to color sections; Plates 1 to 21 follow page 296, and Plates 22 to 35 follow page 892.